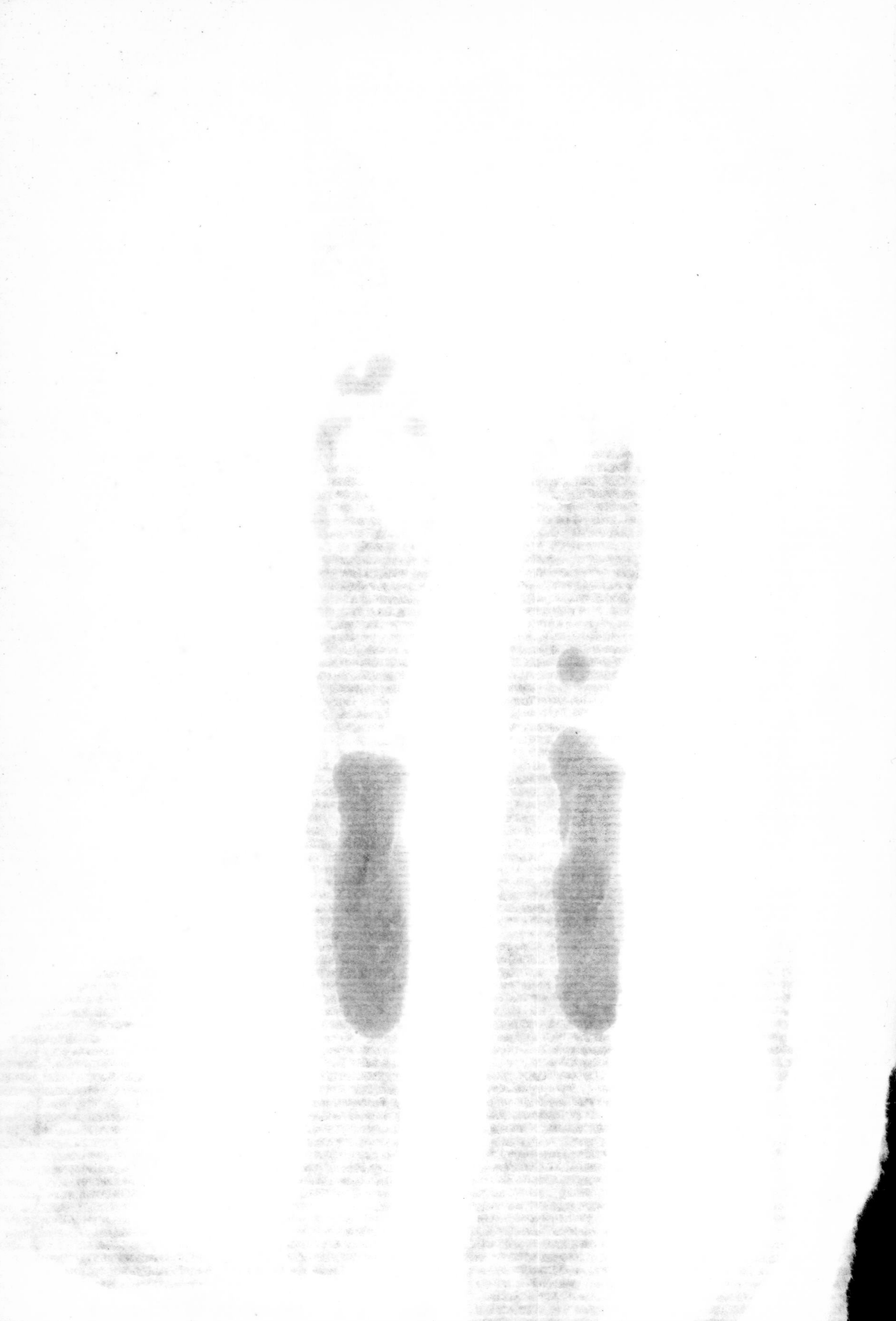

Color Atlas & Textbook of

Macropathology

by

Professor WALTER SANDRITTER

Director of the Department of Pathology,
University of Freiburg, Germany

and

Professor Dr. C. THOMAS

Department of Pathology,
University of Freiburg, Germany

Translated and edited by

W. H. KIRSTEN, M.D.

Professor of Pathology and Pediatrics
The University of Chicago

Second English Edition

With 680 Figures, of which 639 are color photographs
and 14 Tables

YEAR BOOK MEDICAL PUBLISHERS · INC.
35 East Wacker Drive · Chicago

Year Book Medical Publishers, Inc. 1976

Library of Congress Catalog Card Number: 75–34933

International Standard Book Number: 0–8151–7546–9

Dedicated to

HERWIG HAMPERL
on the occasion
of his 70th birthday

All things are one,
the eye of the senses
is the eye of the brain.

TSCHUANGTSE

Preface to the English Edition

As Doctor WARTMAN pointed out in his Preface to the *Color Atlas and Textbook of Tissue and Cellular Pathology*, the ways of writing are infinitely varied and naturally are influenced by the author's background. The translation of the German text *Makropathologie* by SANDRITTER and THOMAS was tempting for several reasons. First, there are few, if any, textbooks on Pathology that provide color photographs of high technical quality. Second, the approach used by the German authors proceeds from the gross description, that is, the observation, to the diagnosis and the scientific background of a given disease. This approach is unique and, in my experience, provides the most effective stimulus for learning. Third, it is my great appreciation of WALTER SANDRITTER as teacher and friend that has prompted me to translate this book. I have edited wherever necessary.

I am grateful to the staff of Year Book Medical Publishers for their understanding, patience and helpful advice and to Mrs. JOHNNIE BERRY for typing the manuscript.

Chicago W. H. KIRSTEN

Preface to the Third German Edition

A new edition of the *Color Atlas and Textbook of Macropathology* became necessary three years after the Second Edition. Several chapters were supplemented by new Figures, and various Figures were replaced by better ones. The text has been adapted to the most recent state of knowledge and has been expanded in part. The form and content of instruction in medicine have changed greatly as a result of the introduction of the new licensing regulations in Germany. The catalogues of teaching goals have established new standards. Formalism has won out over "free" study. Where this appeared necessary, the authors have taken the guidelines of the catalogue of teaching goals into consideration. However, anyone who wishes to *study* medicine and to *comprehend* the problems of diseases, will not be able to stick to catalogues but must concern himself intensively with the depth and breadth of pathological anatomy. In this respect, this book is not an aid for a specific section of studies but is intended to be a companion for the whole of the clinical study and for advanced medical education.

Freiburg, January 1975

W. SANDRITTER
C. THOMAS

Preface to the Second Edition

The *Color Atlas and Textbook of Macropathology* has been received unexpectedly well by students and physicians. "Anatomical thought" is evidently not yet dead. Why? The interpretation of diseases may change, but the morphological features and the related clinical aspects remain the same. Furthermore, the function of macroscopic pathology is the training for seeing, a guide to differentiation, such as the physician will constantly have to carry out in his daily practice. *Südhof's* book *Der diagnostische Blick* (The Diagnostic Glance), just like *Macropathology*, shows what is meant: Diagnosis is the comprehension of the important while recognizing the unimportant.

The First German Edition of the *Color Atlas and Textbook of Macropathology* was completely out of print after one year. The short interval did not permit the authors to carry out significant changes in the Second Edition. We hope to receive additional criticisms and suggestions, in order to improve the book for the benefit of students and physicians.

Freiburg, July 1971

W. SANDRITTER
C. THOMAS

Preface to the First German Edition

Textbooks should be enticing; this they are when the most serene and accessible aspects of knowledge and science are offered.—GOETHE

As a "bait" to learn, organ pathology is presented in this textbook in the form of a picture atlas. The accompanying text is brief and only the most basic information is given. The stimulus for learning is the photograph or schematic representation of a disease. The knowledge derived from this information should be deepened by the use of more extensive textbooks, handbooks or monographs.

Although brief accounts of histopathologic findings are presented, this *Color Atlas and Textbook of Macropathology* should be complemented by use of the third edition of the *Color Atlas and Textbook of Tissue and Cellular Pathology* by W. SANDRITTER and W. B. WARTMAN (Year Book Medical Publishers, 1969). The photographs in this textbook are presented on the left-hand pages and the corresponding text on the right-hand pages, as was done in the textbook on Tissue and Cellular Pathology. This format has resulted in presentation of the essentials in a brief, telegraphic style, to which there are advantages and disadvantages. It will be up to the reader to decide whether the "information" is still comprehensible!

The selection of photographs and the "art of omission" posed many problems. Instructive gross photographs are not obtained easily. However, the most prevalent human diseases are all included in this text. The technics used for the photographs varied somewhat. Some pictures had to be taken under water in order to reduce highlights. The color intensity is somewhat diminished under such conditions. The material was obtained from the autopsy services (approximately 16,000 autopsies) of the Departments of Pathology at the Universities of Giessen and Bonn, Germany. We should like to thank the many prosectors for their assistance. Some photographs were provided by colleagues (see below). We are grateful to Professor UEHLINGER and Doctor ADLER (Zürich) for advice and discussion on the chapter on bone diseases. Professor NOETZEL (Freiburg) assisted with the chapter on diseases of the brain, Professor OTTO (Erlangen) with the lung chapter and Professor GÖRTTLER helped write the chapter on cardiac malformations. Doctor BERTRAM has corrected the text and provided useful information. We are grateful to two medical students, Messrs. ROGG and HABERSTROH, for drawing the schemes.

The generous help and encouragement of Professor MATIS and Mr. REEG of Schattauer Verlag is greatly appreciated.

Freiburg, Summer 1970

W. SANDRITTER
C. THOMAS

Contents

Organ Systems

The following photographs were kindly provided by:

Prof. C. BECK (Freiburg): 5.4, 8
Priv.-Doz. K. Beck (Wiesbaden): 5.22, 48–50, 6.38–40
Prof. M. EDER (München): 6.23, 24
Dr. JONES-WILLIAMS (England): 5.77
Prof. W. KALKOFF: 3.31
Prof. W. W. MEYER (Mainz): 3.36
Prof. G. KERSTING (Bonn): 17.24, 26, 27
Prof. CH. MITTERMAYER (Freiburg): 5.20
Prof. H. NOETZEL (Freiburg): 17.11, 12, 37
Prof. H. OTTO (Dortmund): 4.13, 16, 19–24, 28–30
Dr. J. STAIGER (Freiburg): 2.36–39, 41, 42
Prof. R. E. TEN SELDAM (Australia): 11.1, 3
Prof. E. UEHLINGER (Zürich): 10.4–7, 13, 18, 25, 39–43, 48, 13.71

1. Introduction

General Remarks

It is the primary goal of this textbook to provide for the medical student an atlas of the most important pathologic organ changes. The material for this atlas was obtained from the morgue and from the surgical pathology service. It seems to us that most students have a thorough theoretical knowledge of organ changes in pathology but often fail to recognize or appreciate the essential gross findings in a given disease.

Aside from this practical consideration, there are other reasons that prompted us to compile a *Color Atlas and Textbook of Macropathology*. The learning process requires repeated confrontation with an "object." This is true not only for clinical diagnosis but for pathologic-anatomic descriptions as well. Organ changes in pathology usually are encountered as the final stage in the progression of a disease. The precise description of a lesion in an organ or tissue is as much a part of medical training as is the physical examination of the living patient. The student should train himself, by repeated exposure, to describe a finding without prejudging it!

The description of a lesion or an organ change eventually leads to a pathologic-anatomic diagnosis, just as various symptoms make a clinical diagnosis. In this book, we have attempted to provide a guide for this approach. Changes in organ size, form or other abnormalities are described. The diagnosis of an organ lesion is supplemented by key information concerning frequency, age, sex, differential diagnosis, pathogenesis, complications and prognosis. Remarks concerning histopathologic findings are added, although these are dealt with in the *Color Atlas and Textbook of Tissue and Cellular Pathology*. Clinical symptoms and therapeutic considerations are mentioned briefly when indicated.

Each chapter is arranged according to groups of diseases, namely:

1. Remarks on anatomy, autopsy technic and postmortem changes.
2. Malformations.
3. Changes in the size and shape of an organ.
4. Circulatory diseases.
5. Metabolic diseases.
6. Inflammations.
7. Tumors.

Definition: Most diseases are characterized at the beginning of a paragraph in order to provide the essential information necessary for the understanding of the disease.

Certain abbreviations are used throughout this book in order to accommodate maximal information:

1. *TCP* refers to the fifth edition of the *Color Atlas and Textbook of Tissue and Cellular Pathology* by W. SANDRITTER and W. B. WARTMAN (Chicago: Year Book Medical Publishers, Inc., 1976).
2. *Mi* refers to the microscopic findings.
3. The frequency *(F)*, age distribution *(A)* and sex incidence (*S*: ♂, ♀) are given.
4. *Pg* refers to the pathogenesis, which includes the development and causation of a disease.

5. Complications *(Co)* from a principal disease and the location *(Lo)* of lesions are discussed.
6. Differential diagnosis *(DD)*.
7. Clinical symptoms *(Cl)*.
8. Prognosis *(Pr)*.
9. Therapy *(Th)*.
10. $>$ = more than, $<$ = less than.

All *percentages* (%) refer to autopsy statistics unless otherwise stated.

Diagnostic Criteria

Several general problems arise in arriving at a pathologic-anatomic diagnosis. Multiple impressions of changes in organ color, shape and consistency are perceived during an autopsy. How are these impressions translated into consciousness? A large number of impressions are perceived but only some are "important." To select, retain and convert the important impressions into a diagnosis is an art that is acquired by experience only. The examiner should pay attention to every detail and be prepared to recognize the important findings from knowledge. It is a bad habit to examine organs briefly in the morgue and then speculate about these findings at length. The reverse is better!

It is the purpose of the following paragraphs to provide for the beginner certain diagnostic principles that will be helpful in recognizing the multitude of observations during an autopsy. Also included are remarks concerning the autopsy protocol, the writing of an autopsy diagnosis and principles of the autopsy technic.

Position and Shape of Organs

The autopsy technics developed by VIRCHOW or ROKITANSKY are used in most institutions. Irrespective of the technic used, the position and relationship of various organs are examined in situ instead of removing organ packages as soon as the body cavities have been opened. Positional organ changes are best diagnosed in situ. A pelvic kidney, diaphragmatic hernia (gut displaced into the thoracic cavity?), volvulus or situs inversus should be recognized immediately. Likewise, fibrous adhesions or bands are determined in relation to other organs before the organs are removed.

The shape of a diseased organ is compared with the "normal" shape or form. Deviations from the norm are common (e.g., congenital abnormal lobulation of the lung, spleen or kidney). Acquired organ deformities frequently are caused by external factors compressing an organ. For example, the finding of a saber trachea should direct the examiner's attention to the presence of a goiter. Pulmonary atelectasis points to various types of pneumothorax, etc.

Size and Weight

The size of an organ is determined by comparison with normal organ size. Although measurements of length, width and height will suffice in most cases, even these values are only approximations of the many possible shapes of diseased organs. In fact, exact measurements of organ size can be obtained only by measuring the volume of an organ, that is, the measurement of the quantity of displaced water. The density of an organ ($\frac{\text{weight}}{\text{volume}}$ = density) also can be derived from knowing its volume. A fatty liver, for example, appears larger than a normal liver of the same weight because the density of fat is less than the density of proteins. This also is true for excessive carbohydrates in an organ, e.g., glycogen storage disease of the liver. Examples of specific gravity are: granulocytes 1.070, erythrocytes 1.096, blood 1.059, blood plasma 1.027, fat 0.900.

The specific gravity of fluids is measured by the use of a urinometer. Exudates, i.e., inflammatory fluids, have a relatively high protein content; their specific gravity is 1.018 or greater. The specific gravity of transudates is 1.018 or lower.

The size of focal organ lesions should always be given in centimeters. Although it is customary to measure the size of a focal lesion on cut surface (6×4 cm.), the depth of such a lesion should be given as well (e.g., a metastasis measures 6×4×4 cm.). The size of focal lesions, stones or organs has been compared to fruits and fruit stones. A collection of various fruits and stones is given in Figure 1.1. These comparisons are inaccurate and should be avoided. The size of apples, tomatoes

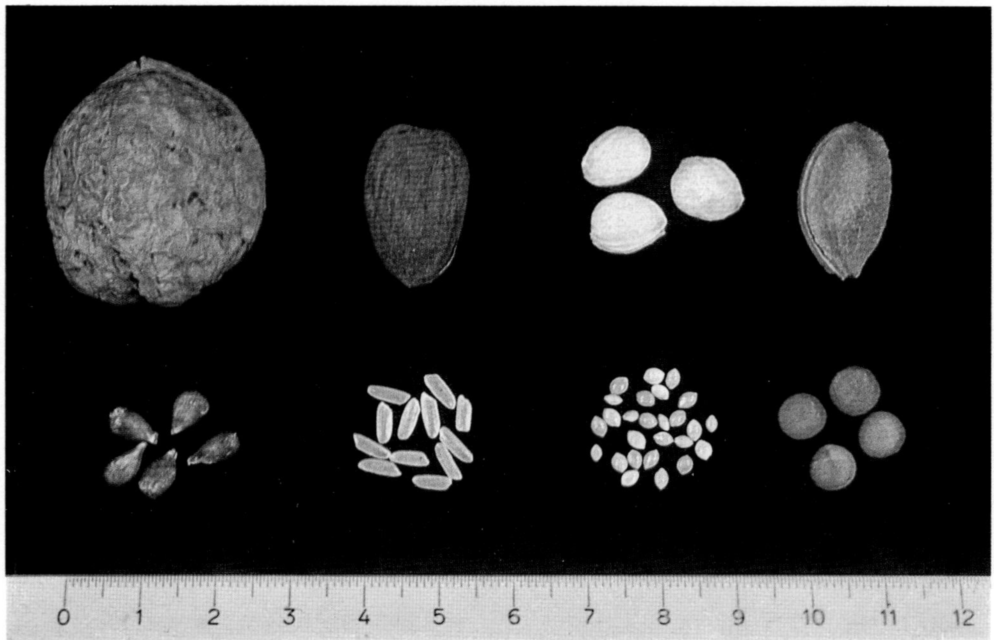

Fig. 1.1. A collection of fruits and fruit stones used in the past to describe pathologic lesions. Above: walnut, almond stone, cherry stones, plum stone. Below: apple seeds, rice corns, millet seeds, lentils.

or eggs varies considerably from season to season and from country to country. Likewise, descriptive terms such as the "size of a baby's head" or the "fist of a male" should be avoided.

The *organ size* is given in weight, which is a reliable measurement despite the above-mentioned variations due to specific gravity or density. The most important organ weights are expressed as a function of age, body weight and body height in Table 1.1. The values given in Table 1.1 are subject to variations as well. Organ weights may fluctuate by as much as 10%, especially in childhood. The organ weights of females are, in general, 20% lower than those of males. It obviously is impossible and also useless to remember all these weights. When needed, they always can be found in textbooks. However, some average weights of adults should be remembered (underlined values in Table 1.1). The following memory help has proved of some value: The heart weighs 350 Gm.; the double value of the heart weight is the weight of the lungs (700 Gm.); the half value of the heart weight is approximately the weight of the spleen (150 Gm.) or one kidney. The liver weight can be determined by multiplying the spleen weight by 10 (1,500 Gm.). The brain weighs approximately the same (minus spleen weight = 1,350 Gm.).

Organ Color

The characterization of a natural phenomenon by the eye is the single most important diagnostic aid. The eye sees more than color. *Form*, *transparency*, *luster* (dry, moist), *surface appearance* (smooth, irregular) and the *consistency* of an organ are all perceived by the eye.

Table 1.1. Size (cm.), body weight (kg.) and organ weight (Gm.) as a function of age and sex.

Age	Height		Body Weight		Heart		Lungs*)		Liver		Kidneys		Spleen		Adrenal Glands		Testes	Ovaries	Brain	
	♂	♀	♂	♀	♂	♀	♂	♀	♂	♀	♂	♀	♂	♀	♂	♀	♂	♀	♂	♀
Birth	50.6	50.2	3.4	3.3	23	21	50	47	135	134	24	23	11	10	6.2	5.2	1.1	0.25	385	365
6 mo.	66.4	65.2	7.5	7.26	28	25	60	60	160	140	31	28	14	12	3.2	2.0	1.5	0.3	300	360
1 yr.	75.2	74.2	10.0	9.7	60	55	170	170	380	330	70	60	30	25	5.6	5.4	1.9	1.0	960	960
2 yr.	87.5	86.6	12.5	12.2	65	58	190	180	420	350	77	72	35	30	6.0	5.5	2.0	1.0	970	950
5 yr.	111.3	109.7	19.4	18.7	100	90	270	266	600	450	105	105	55	52	6.6	6.0	2.8	1.8	1200	1050
10 yr.	140.3	138.6	32.6	31.8	130	120	360	310	950	800	150	125	80	70	9.0	8.0	4.0	4.0	1250	1230
15 yr.	167.8	161.1	54.8	51.4	240	200	550	500	1270	930	200	185	120	110	13.0	11.0	20.0	8.0	1340	1260
20 yr.	170.0	165.0	62.0	56.2	280	260	700	620	1560	1370	270	240	155	130	13.5	12.0	42.0	9.5	1400	1260
25 yr.	170.0	165.0	65.0	56.6	310	265	770	620	1580	1370	280	260	170	130	14.0	13.0	45.0	11.0	1400	1250
30 yr.	170.0	165.0	68.0	58.5	315	270	800	620	1580	1370	285	240	170	130	14.0	13.0	42.0	11.0	1390	1250
40 yr.	170.0	165.0	71.0	61.2	320	285	800	660	1590	1400	275	240	150	130	14.0	13.5	40.0	9.0	1380	1250
50 yr.	170.0	165.0	72.0	64.8	340	305	800	620	1600	1430	270	235	145	115	13.0	12.5	35.0	6.0	1340	1240
60 yr.	170.0	165.0	73.0	67.1	330	310	800	620	1520	1380	270	235	130	105	13.0	12.0	33.0	4.5	1300	1200
70 yr.	170.0	165.0	72.0	67.5	320	300	770	620	1400	1250	260	220	110	90	12.5	12.0	30.0	4.0	1250	1150

*) Lung weights are falsified by pulmonary edema. In cases of acute electric death (e.g., execution), the lung weight is said to be 200 Gm.

It is remarkable how little is known concerning the scientific basis of color changes in medicine. Aside from the problems of subjective color perception and the related "dualistic conflict between objectivity and subjectivity" (HEIMENDAHL, BORN), sufficiently objective color measurements are not available. We lack symbols to characterize color changes. There are many color shadings but few terms to describe them.

According to a physical definition, the color stimulus is dependent on:

1. The *hue*, i.e., the shade or tint of a color. The hue is dependent on the specific or dominant wavelength of a color (see Fig. 1.2).
2. The *saturation or chroma*, i.e., concentration or intensity of a color. The concentration of a color is dependent on the density of color particles per unit surface.
3. The *value or brightness* of a color, i.e., the gray value that is admixed to a color. The color value ranges from black to white.
4. The unsaturated color is characterized by a scale of black to white.

The role of interference colors in organ pathology is largely unknown (e.g., the colors of thin platelets).

The CIE color system (Commission Internationale de l'Éclairage; DIN 5033, WRIGHT, HASSENSTEIN) is reproduced in Figure 1.2, which represents different color qualities according to a scheme by MUNSELL. These color tables are of practical value. For example, if one wishes to determine organ colors objectively, photometric measurements by remission photometry must be

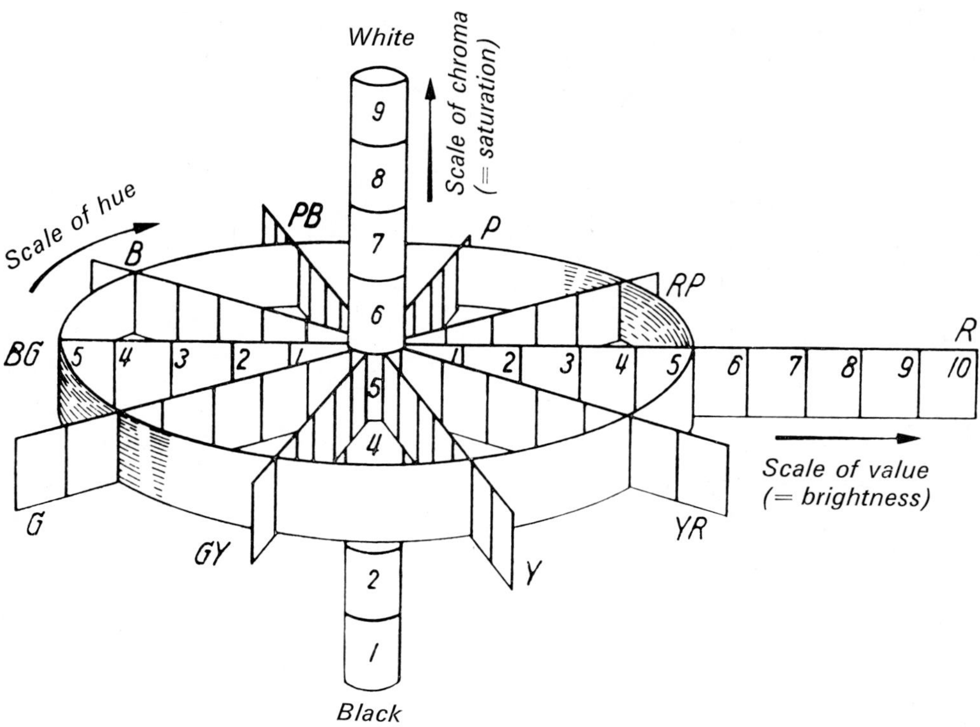

Fig. 1.2. Color circle according to MUNSELL. The equator of the color circle shows the scale of the color tone (dominant wavelength); the axis of the circle shows the scale of value or brightness from black to white; the radially arranged scales show the saturation (scale of chroma). The letters in the scale of hue are abbreviated as: R = red, YR = yellow-red, Y = yellow, GY = green-yellow, G = green, BG = blue-green, B = blue, PB = purple-blue, P = purple, RP = red-purple.

employed (see SANDRITTER and co-workers, 1964). Such color measurements show that the human eye can discriminate very accurately the hue of a color in comparison to standardized color schemes such as those shown in Figure 1.3. On the other hand, the human color discrimination deviates from a standardized color scheme when the saturation and brightness of a color are tested. The latter scales usually are overestimated. Of course, variations in daylight and background (white, black, colorful background) greatly influence such tests.

For a precise color determination in pathology, therefore, it is desirable to express organ colors in comparison to a color table. Figure 1.3 shows a collection of colors reproduced from the atlas of MUNSELL. This figure again demonstrates the scales of value (brightness) and chroma (saturation).

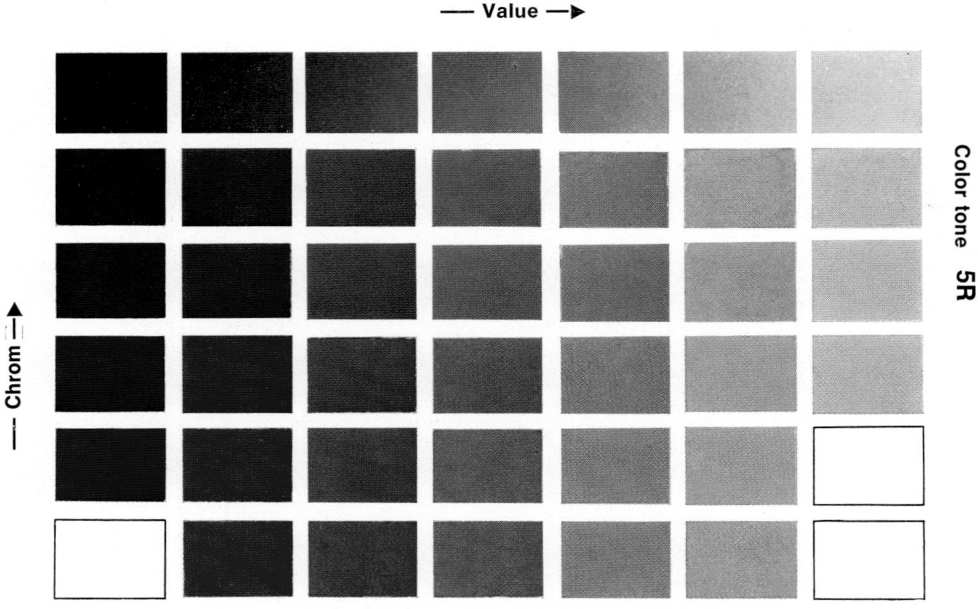

Fig. 1.3. Example of a color table (from the atlas of Munsell) for hue 5R (middle red). Various changes in the saturation (scale of chroma) are shown on the abscissa. Changes in the brightness (scale of value) are shown on the ordinate. The neutral brightness scale from black to white is seen at the top.

This method is too time-consuming for practical purposes. We must, therefore, rely on descriptions of organ colors. However, the three qualities of color, namely, *hue*, *saturation (chroma)* and *brightness (value)* should be considered when the color of a lesion or organ is described. The color *hue* is expressed by the words red, yellow-red, brown, brown-red, yellow, green-yellow, green, blue-green, blue, purple-blue, purple or red-purple. The *saturation* or *chroma* of a color is described by such terms as *dusky red*, *deep red*, *bright red*, *intensively red*, *pale red* or *weakly red*. Certain problems arise in describing the brightness or saturation of a color. For example, "bright red" can imply a minimal grayish tone or a minimal saturation. Terms like *bright red*, *dark red* or *black-red* are used to describe *color brightness*. "Dirty red" is applied when much black or brown is admixed to red (e.g., the kidney in chromoproteinuric nephrosis). The brightness of a color is enhanced by moisture or luster. Color descriptions also are compared to naturally occurring colors, although these substitutions are subject to great variation (e.g., nut brown, lemon yellow, bloody red).

Designations such as white, light gray, gray, dark gray, black or deep black are available to describe the neutral scale (see Fig. 1.3). The widely used term "pale" is not particularly accurate and should be used to modify the hue of a color (e.g., pale red) or to substitute for "light gray."

The *characterization of a color* often is critical in making a diagnosis from the descriptive part of an autopsy protocol. It is important to know which organic substances determine a given color and which substrate is responsible for color changes in pathology. Detailed information, unfortunately, is missing and only some hints can be given here.

In general, the *blood content*, that is, the red of hemoglobin, determines organ color. Oxygenated blood (e.g., active, arterial hyperemia) is responsible for a bright red organ or skin color, whereas blood poor in O_2 but rich in CO_2 imparts a dark blue-red or dusky red color to an organ. Examples are the congested kidney and the black-red, hemorrhagic lung infarction. The blood and organs are cherry red or bright red in carbon monoxide poisoning (see Fig. 17.3).

Breakdown products of hemoglobin such as *bilirubin* (red-yellow) and *biliverdin* (green-yellow) determine the discoloration of all organs in jaundice. With time, areas of hemorrhage change their color from red to red-yellow to green-yellow to yellow. These color changes reflect breakdown of hemoglobin in biliverdin.

Pigments may alter organ colors as follows:

Melanin	Black	Example: Malignant melanoma, melanuric nephrosis; black urine
Carbon	Black	Example: Anthracosis of the lungs or lymph nodes
Hemosiderin	Brown	Example: Hemosiderosis of the liver (see Fig. 6.35) or chronic congestion of the lungs (see Fig. 4.42)
Lipofuscin	Brown	Example: Brown atrophy of the heart, color of saturated fatty acids
Iron	Brown	Example: Hemosiderosis of the lungs

The *yellow color* of fat, the adrenal cortex and the corpus luteum is derived from the carotenoids (e.g., like the yellow and red feathers of birds), which cannot be synthesized by humans. They are derived only from food. Certain pathologic conditions result in a *yellow discoloration* of an organ (e.g., the fatty liver or fatty degeneration of the myocardium). Jaundice superimposed on a fatty liver results in a yellow-green hue (the so-called safran liver). Fatty degenerative changes in granulocytes also determine the *yellow color of pus*. Certain bacteria change the color of pus or granulation tissue. For example, staphylococcal pus is yellow (= fatty changes in granulocytes), streptococcal pus (phlegmon) is gray-white (determined by light scattering) and pyocyaneus pus is blue-green.

Necrotic tissues are either lighter than normal or black-red. A *fresh infarction* of the *cortex of the brain* is pale in contrast to the normal cortex, which is gray-brown from ganglion cells and their lipofuscin content. A *hemorrhagic infarction* appears black-red. The yellow to gray-yellow color of an *anemic infarction* is due to the lack of blood in the tissue and to altered light scattering (gray). Hemoglobin breakdown products from lysis of erythrocytes may determine the color of infarcted tissues as well.

Organ colors are *gray-white* after the organ is rinsed. However, extensive lipofuscin deposition imparts a brown color to an organ (liver, heart). Anemic organs likewise are gray-white.

The entire scale from *white* to *black*, mostly gray-white, is attributable to *light scattering* (Tyndall phenomenon). The degree of light scattering is dependent on particle size and the wavelength of the light. Gray to gray-white is characteristic of fresh granulocytes and all nucleated blood cells (leukemia [Greek: *leukos* white + *haima* blood], resulting in a gray-red bone marrow). Dense cell collections such as tumors with little vascular supply likewise are gray-white. When fibrin covers surfaces of organs or preformed cavities, they appear gray-white from light scattering. Clotted blood (postmortem clots) also is gray-white from light scattering; this also is characteristic of cartilage. Cartilage, however, may appear brownish in older persons because of changes in the water content, which, in turn, alters light scattering. Elastic fibers are pale yellow in contrast to connective tissue – again due to greater light scattering. In a disease called *ochronosis*, cartilage is black due to deposition of homogentisic acid. A *clean white* color is characteristic of cholesterol crystals or other crystalline deposits, e.g., cystinosis in the spleen. Thorotrast, formerly used as a contrast medium, is deposited as a white substance in the liver and spleen.

Black or green-black is the color of tissues undergoing intravital putrefaction (gangrene). Sulfur dioxide is linked to hemoglobin to produce the black sulfhemoglobin.

Surfaces and Cavities

The following criteria should be considered when the surfaces of an organ are described: markings, blood content, consistency (see below) and deposits of seemingly foreign material. The external surfaces of viscera are *smooth, glistening* and *moist* because they are covered by serosa. Visceral surfaces become dull when a fibrin exudate covers the serosa. When large fibrin masses are present, the surface may appear gray-white. Fibrin exudates usually reflect diseases of the underlying organs. For example, bronchopneumonia causes a fibrinous pleuritis, and a myocardial infarction usually is accompanied by a fibrinous pericarditis. The outer surface or cut surface of an organ may become *uneven* from fine or coarse granulations and scars (e. g., liver cirrhosis, renal infarction, renal arteriosclerosis). External and cut surfaces may appear smooth, nodular, granular, lobular or even folded (e.g., acute liver atrophy, the spleen after acute blood loss).

The cut surfaces of the liver, kidney and heart are *transparent* for a depth of approximately 0.5–1 mm. This phenomenon can be illustrated by cutting thin slices (several mm. thick), which readily transmit the background color. Normal organ slices appear darker on a black background. The tissue transparency disappears with certain retrogressive tissue changes. In *cloudy* swelling, that is, swelling of the mitochondria with strong light scattering, a tissue slice no longer is transparent. At the same time, the parenchyma projects from the cut surface so that the margins of a cut appear dull instead of sharp. The moisture of a cut surface is partly lost in cloudy swelling. Organ transparency is increased in amyloidosis, and the involved organs appear glassy. The letters of a newspaper, used as a background, can be recognized through an organ slice in amyloidosis.

Organ colors often are modified by certain surface *markings*. The best-known examples are deposition of foreign substances (anthracotic mottling of the lung). Certain pathologic conditions modify the color pattern on cut surface. The yellow-red markings of a chronically congested liver are the result of yellow, fatty streaks alternating with dark red, congested areas (nutmeg liver). The gray bands of connective tissue between brown or yellow parenchymal nodules in liver cirrhosis likewise are examples of markings on the cut surface.

The blood *content* of an organ is expressed not only by organ color but also by the quantity of blood exuding from the cut surface. The walls of blood vessels always should be examined on cut surface. Do the vessels collapse? Do they remain rigid and open (e.g., "pipestem" arteriosclerosis in the kidneys)? Hemorrhages in the brain are distinguishable from hyperemia by the fact that punctate hemorrhages cannot be wiped off the cut surface.

Deposition of foreign substances can be diagnosed best by examining the cut surface. Foreign deposits are characterized according to *size, form, color, consistency, type of delineation* (sharp or indistinct) and *type of marking* (round or streaky). Focal disease processes appear as smooth, granular, projecting or sunken lesions on the *external surface*. For example, foci of bronchopneumonia are gray-red, firm, dry, finely granular, poorly delineated and irregularly shaped.

Pathologic organ changes also can be diagnosed by the *type of material* that can be scraped off the cut surface. The knife blade normally is shiny because tissue fluid adheres to it. The knife blade is covered by fine droplets from a fatty liver and becomes dull. Foamy fluid can be expressed by the knife from an edematous lung. The fluid covering the knife blade is tenacious and gray-red as it is observed in lobar pneumonia during the stage of lysis. A stringy, elastic material adheres to the knife blade in cases of pulmonary adenomatosis or in Friedländer pneumonia.

Cystic structures or cavities in an organ should be examined according to the same principles and rules. The width of a cystic space is specified, together with the size of its opening. Moreover, the thickness and consistency of a cyst wall or cavity are recorded. The appearance of its internal surface is described. Old cavities have smooth walls, whereas fresh cavities have an irregularly frayed lining. The contents of a cyst cavity should be measured and described as liquid, doughy, clear, cloudy, floccular or stringy. The specific gravity, pH, transparency, opalescence and color of the cyst or cavity contents are determined.

Consistency

The consistency of organs or lesions is determined by touch. Although this is a relatively subjective method, the following terms can provide a fairly accurate impression: firm (e.g., the liver in cirrhosis or the lung in silicosis), hard (calcium or bone), medium-firm (certain carcinomas), doughy, soft, diffluent (septic spleen, acute liver atrophy), friable, fragile, breakable (foci of pneumonia, gangrene of the lung). A doughy consistency is characteristic of a fatty liver. A finger impression on the liver remains as it does in edema of the legs. Soft, flabby organs of diminished consistency appear collapsed and their capsule is wrinkled. Tissue slices of such organs do not "stand up" but collapse and the organ "shakes" like pudding.

The normal lung tissue is soft-elastic but firm-elastic in chronic pneumonia. An increased elasticity is characteristic of sarcomas also. The elasticity of an organ (e.g., the aorta in atherosclerosis) also can be determined by pulling.

Odor

Smelling, listening and tasting are used rarely in the diagnosis of pathologic organ changes. Nevertheless, the *odor* of an organ or the cadaver can provide important diagnostic leads. For example, patients in diabetic coma have an acetone odor resembling foul apples. Patients in hepatic coma have an odor of raw liver. Uremic patients have an ammoniacal odor (urine). Gangrenous organs have a foul, aggressive odor. When poisoning is suspected, one should remember the odor of bitter almonds in cyanide poisoning, the odor of onions in phosphorus poisoning or the odor of garlic in arsenical poisoning.

The *ear* is used to evaluate the air noise of the lung (absent or diminished in pneumonia). When organs are indurated by fibrous tissue, the noise of the cutting knife is increased (e.g., liver cirrhosis). Likewise, the noise of breaking ribs points to the presence or absence of osteoporosis. The prosector's taste buds, fortunately, are no longer needed.

Artifacts

The beginner often is misled by postmortem artifacts. Most organs are black to gray-black or green in cases of advanced postmortem putrefaction (see Fig. 6.3). Moderate degrees of a green-black discoloration are seen often on the lower liver surface near the colonic flexure (formation of sulfhemoglobin by diffusion of H_2S onto the surface of the liver). Various degrees of *postmortem oxidation* of hemoglobin can modify the color of cut surfaces. An exposed cut surface becomes bright red; a covered cut surface is dark red. *Hemoglobin* is released post mortem from erythrocytes and discolors the normally white mucosal surfaces. This common postmortem change often is mistaken as a sign of inflammation.

The gallbladder and its contents should not come into contact with other organs during an autopsy. Bile can easily impregnate various tissues, thereby mimicking jaundice.

Round or irregular impressions on organ surfaces often are artifactual. They are created by organ containers inadvertently placed on organs.

Summary

The diagnosis criteria for pathologic organ changes are summarized in Table 1.2. The criteria are organized according to principles of general pathology.

Table 1.2. Diagnostic criteria.

Position	*Cavities*	*External Surface and Cut Surface*	*Fluids*
Shape	Width	Color, markings, transparency	Quantity
Size	Wall	Lesions, deposits	Specific gravity
Weight	Content	Blood content	Color
Color		*Odor*	Transparency
Consistency			

Table 1.3. Typical gross findings arranged according to principles of general pathology.

Type of Change	Color	Shape/Weight	Consistency	Remarks
Atrophy	Mostly brown	Reduced, diminished	Firm	
Cloudy swelling	Dull	Enlarged, increased	Softer than normal (diminished)	Parenchyma protrudes from the capsule
Amyloid	Gray-red, glassy	Increased	Very firm	Transparent
Fatty degeneration	Yellow	Increased	Doughy	Knife blade "dull"
Pigments (see TCP, p. 9)				
Necrosis Anemic infarctions (heart, kidney, spleen)	Yellow		Dry, firm	Fresh: slightly protruding over cut surface; later: sunken
Hemorrhagic infarctions (lung, gut)	Dark black-red		Dry, firm	Slightly protruding over the surface
Fat necrosis	White, chalky		Firm	
Granulation tissue	Red		Soft	Granular on surfaces, sunken on cut surfaces
Scar	White, tendon-like		Firm	
Active hyperemia	Bright red	Increased	Unchanged	
Passive hyperemia (congestion)	Dark or dusky red (brown in lung, etc.)	Increased Increased	Firmer than normal, very firm	(Acute) (Chronic)
Blood aspiration Hemorrhages	Lung: bright red; hemorrhages: dark red		Normal Increased	Degradation from bilirubin to biliverdin
Inflammations Serous	Bright red	Swelling	Soft	
Purulent	Yellow pus		Soft	Phlegmonous: gray-dirty Abscess: with necrosis
Fibrinous	Gray-white		Soft	Surface dry
Chronic	Gray-red		Softer or firmer	According to age
Lobar pneumonias	Red Gray-red Yellow	Increased	Friable	Lysis: red fluid; slightly stringy; can be scraped off
Bronchopneumonias	Gray-red	Poorly demarcated foci, 3–4 cm. in diameter	Friable	Air noise missing
Gangrene	Dirty, green-black		Breaks easily, frayed	Foul odor

Type of Change	Color	Shape/Weight	Consistency	Remarks
Tuberculosis	White		Like cottage cheese	Cottage cheese
Gumma	Yellow		Gum-like	
Hodgkin's disease	Gray-white, bright yellow	Increased	Firm-elastic	Map-like, yellow areas of necrosis
Carcinomas Medullary	Gray-white	Poorly delineated nodules	Soft like the "medulla of the spinal cord"	
Solid	Gray-white	Poorly delineated		
Scirrhous	Gray-white	Diffusely infiltrative	Firm, hard	
Sarcomas	White	Large tumor nodules	Fish flesh, elastic	

Autopsy Protocol and Diagnosis

An autopsy protocol should be dictated during an autopsy or shortly thereafter. The protocol should be brief and to the point. HAMPERL has succinctly characterized the writing of an autopsy protocol as "photographing in words." The protocol should recapitulate the various sequential steps of an autopsy. The criteria listed in Table 1.2 should be applied to each organ. It is customary to arrive at a histologic diagnosis by proceeding from lower-power to higher-power magnifications. The naked-eye examination should proceed from general impressions to specific details. The knowledgeable reader should be able to make a diagnosis from the descriptive part of the protocol. Gross findings are descriptions, not interpretations. A classic protocol will be quoted as an example. The first description of liver cirrhosis by LAENNEC reads as follows:

"The liver, which was about half the size of a normal liver, was slightly warty, wrinkled and gray-yellow. The cut surfaces consisted of many round or oval nodules of the size of millet seeds or somewhat larger. Between these nodules, which were easily separated from each other, there is barely space occupied by remnants of normal liver tissue. The color of the nodules is pale brown or yellow-red and focally also greenish. The tissue is cloudy, rather moist and soft but not diffluent. When the nodules are pressed between the fingers, only parts are squeezed; the remainder resemble pieces of soft leather. The spleen was healthy."

Indeed, a plastic description of small nodular liver cirrhosis. LAENNEC called these liver changes "cirrhoses" because of their yellow color. He concluded that "cirrhosis" is a malignant neoplasm. The difference between gross descriptive findings and diagnosis can hardly be illustrated better. Diagnosis is a term for a pathologic change arrived at according to the current state of knowledge. In other words, the diagnosis may change but the description is permanent and independent of the current state of knowledge.

The order of diagnoses in an autopsy protocol varies among different institutions and hospitals. In general, the diagnoses are listed in terms of importance, ultimately leading to death. Generalized diseases are listed first; specific changes are mentioned last.

For example, in a case of death from myocardial infarction: Generalized arteriosclerosis. Hypertrophy of the left ventricle of the heart. Coronary artery sclerosis with stenosis, especially of the circumflexus branch of the right coronary artery. Fresh myocardial necrosis in the posterior walls of the left ventricle, etc.

The gross diagnosis is confirmed and modified by histologic findings.

A gross diagnosis should be understood easily by the clinician. The ultimate goals of an autopsy are to explain the cause of death, to describe pathologic changes related to clinical findings and to provide findings worthy of further investigation. *An autopsy as an exercise in itself is without value.*

The pathologist and clinician should cooperate to elucidate and understand a given disease, to explain the cause of death and to learn from these findings.

Clinicopathologic correlations are better understood, especially by the beginner, when clinical findings are contrasted with pathologic-anatomic diagnoses. In this way, the limits of both approaches are apparent, discrepancies become evident and open questions can be investigated further.

As an example, a case of intestinal lipodystrophy (Whipple's disease) is presented below (cit. Med. Welt *17* [N.F.]: 2571, 1966).

Table 1.4.

Clinical Findings	Pathologic-Anatomic Findings
I. Patient's History (Anamnesis)	
65-year-old farmer. Noticed dyspnea and palpation following physical exertion some 12 years ago	Hypertrophy and dilatation of left ventricle. Coronary artery sclerosis. Fibrous scars in the posterior wall of the left ventricle
II. Primary Disease	
Chronic cor pulmonale: dry and moist rales. X-ray: pulmonary emphysema, bilateral dilatation of the heart. ECG sinus tachycardia from cor pulmonale. Dyspnea at rest. Cyanosis of lips. Plethora. BP 150/100	Chronic bronchitis. Cylindrical bronchiectasis. Chronic, partly bullous pulmonary emphysema. Diaphragmatic grooves of the liver. Hypertrophy and dilatation of the right ventricle. Minimal arteriosclerosis of the pulmonary arteries
Fracture of right clavicle 3 months prior to death	Chronic luxation of the right acromioclavicular joint
Pain, swelling and reddening of the right leg 2 months prior to death	Old thrombosis of both femoral veins and their branches extending into the inferior vena cava
No complaints in patient's history	Intestinal lipodystrophy: marked enlargement of the mesenteric, parapancreatic and para-aortic lymph nodes. A milky, cloudy, fatty fluid exudes from the lymph nodes on cutting. Stasis of lymphatics (lacteals) of the small intestine
III. Secondary Diseases	
Right heart failure: increasing dilatation of the heart. Liver is palpable 5 cm. below the right costal margin	Dilatation of the right atrium. Congestion of the liver
Tachycardia, cyanosis of the face, profuse sweating, temperature up to 100° F.	Massive, recurrent, pulmonary emboli. Hemorrhagic infarction in the right lower lobe of the lung. Infarction-like changes in both lower lobes. Fibrinous pleuritis. Pleural hemorrhages. Acute congestion of internal organs
IV. Cause of Death	
Cardiac failure	Pulmonary emboli

General Remarks Concerning Autopsy

The physician should attempt to obtain an autopsy permit even though the cause or causes of death are readily explained by the clinical findings. An autopsy permit usually can be obtained by convincing the relatives of a deceased of the importance of and service that a postmortem examination renders to the medical profession and the welfare of other patients. The legal aspects of obtaining autopsy permits vary somewhat between states and countries. The closest relative usually is legally empowered to sign an autopsy permit. Cases of unnatural death require a postmortem examination by a Coroner's Physician or a Medical Examiner.

The autopsy should be done in a highly professional manner. Avoid mutilations, especially of the exposed parts of the body (head, face, neck, arms). Several rules should be followed when the deceased is examined:

1. Identify the body and check the body tag against the name in the medical records.
2. Age, sex, weight and length are recorded before the autopsy is started. Age and sex often point to certain diseases.
3. Determine the nutritional state, body build (muscle and bones) and hair distribution.
4. Search for external scars, evidence of trauma (especially head trauma!), needle punctures and defects (decubitus ulcer) or hemorrhages in the skin. Scars sometimes are difficult to detect after death!
5. Determine the size and equality of pupils.
6. Palpate the neck for nodules or masses (thyroid, lymph nodes!). Are the neck veins distended or collapsed (heart failure!)?
7. Examine the chest and abdomen. Is the chest symmetric? Breast masses? Look for hernias, venous distention, scars in the abdominal wall. Position of testes?
8. Measure length and circumference of extremities (thrombosis). Abnormalities of fingers and toes (clubbing)?

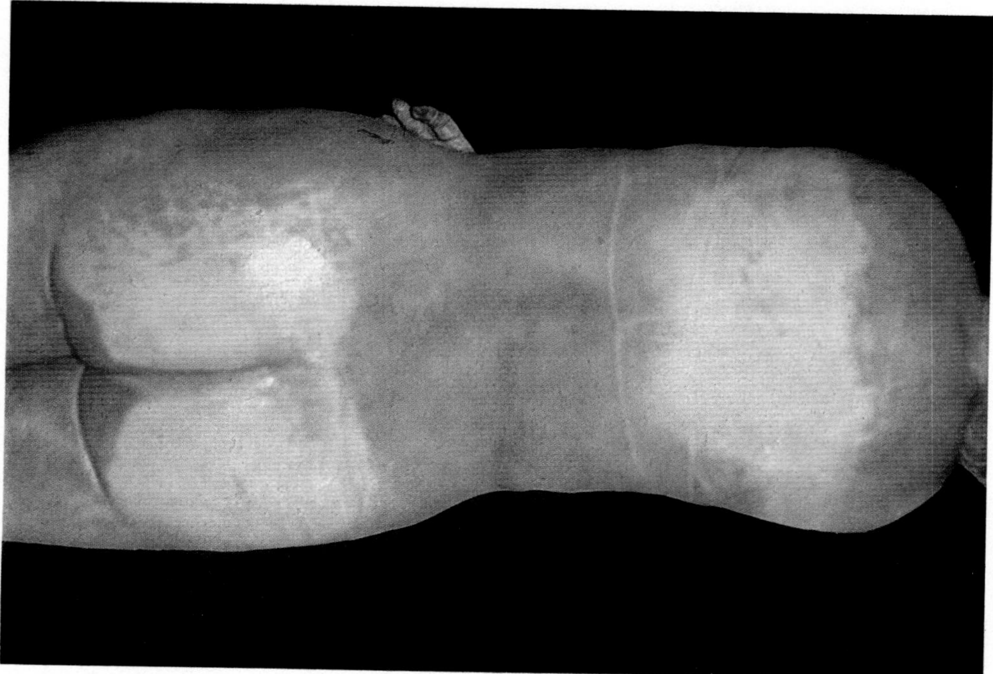

Fig. 1.4. Postmortem lividity (livores) on the back of a 45-year-old male. The livores have disappeared from pressure areas.

The following *external changes* are observed after death:

The *cornea* is cloudy and filmy because of dehydration. The tension of the *eye bulb* is reduced. *Rigor mortis* usually begins in the jaw muscles, proceeding to the neck, face, arms and lower extremities. The onset of rigor mortis usually is 2–6 hours after death and disappears 3–4 days later. *Algor mortis* (coldness of deceased). The body temperature drops hourly by 1° C. *Livor mortis* (postmortem lividity) results from the gravitational stasis of the blood in the dependent parts of the body (back). Livores are livid blue-red. After cutting, venous blood exudes from postmortem flecks. They blanch under pressure (see Fig. 1.4) and become dirty red after hemoglobin has lysed from erythrocytes.

It is important for the physician to recognize the frequency of diseases – stated in a lapidary manner: Common diseases are common – rare diseases are rare. In individual cases, however, this rule should be brought into play only in the final phase of the consideration of the diagnosis, since *statistical probabilities* are involved.

The following table (Christian, 1971) presents an abbreviated survey of the frequency of deaths in the German Federal Republic, arranged by groups of causes of death. It must be taken into consideration that, in the German Federal Republic, autopys are performed on only 10% of deceased persons and only about 1/3 of the clinically determined causes of death are in agreement with the pathological-anatomical diagnosis.

The frequency scale is clear. About 45% of the persons died of cardiac and circulatory diseases and about 20% died of malignant tumors. These values are valid for all of the world's highly civilized countries. On the other hand, infectious diseases, with a value of 1.2%, play practically no part – in contrast to the countries of the Third World.

Table 1.5. Deaths in the German Federal Republic (by Groups of Causes of Death, 1969).

Cause of Death	%
Circulatory diseases	44.2
Malignant neoplasms	18.0
Diseases of the respiratory organs	7.9
Diseases of the digestive organs	5.5
Accidents and poisoning	4.9
Symptoms and inadequately designated causes of death	4.0
Glandular disturbances with internal secretion, nutritional and metabolic diseases	2.9
Diseases of the genitourinary tract	2.4
Specific causes of perinatal mortality	1.8
Suicide and self-inflicted injuries	1.7
Mental disturbances, diseases of the nervous system and of the sense organs	1.7
Infectious and parasitic diseases	1.2
Neoplasms of the lymphatic and hematogenic organs	1.1
Congenital malformations	0.7
Complications of pregnancy, delivery, and parturition	0.1
Other Causes	1.9
	100.0

Organ Systems

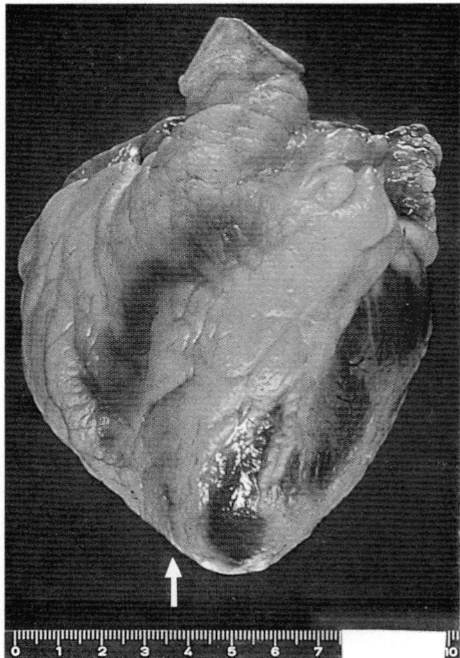

Fig. 2.1. The normal heart.

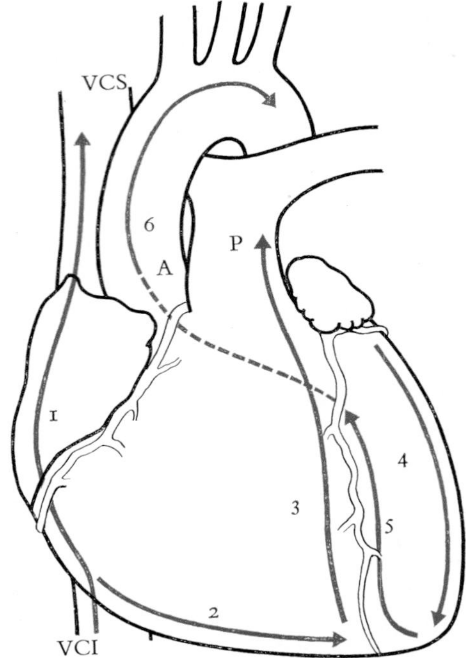

Fig. 2.2. Cut sections through the heart.
VCS = vena cava superior (cranialis)
VCI = vena cava inferior (caudalis)
A = aorta
P = pulmonary artery

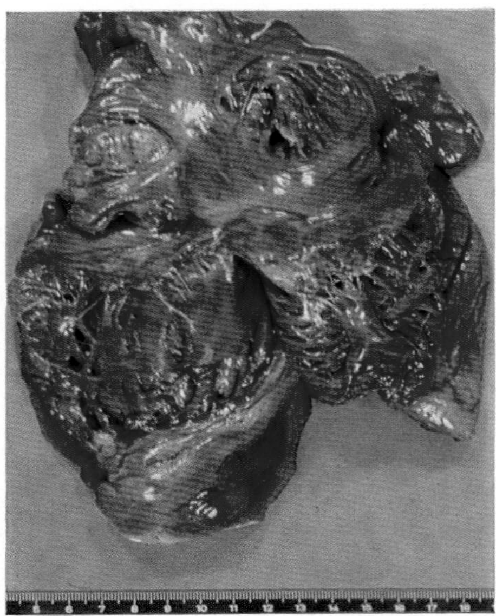

Fig. 2.3. The opened right heart (following cuts 1, 2 and 3).

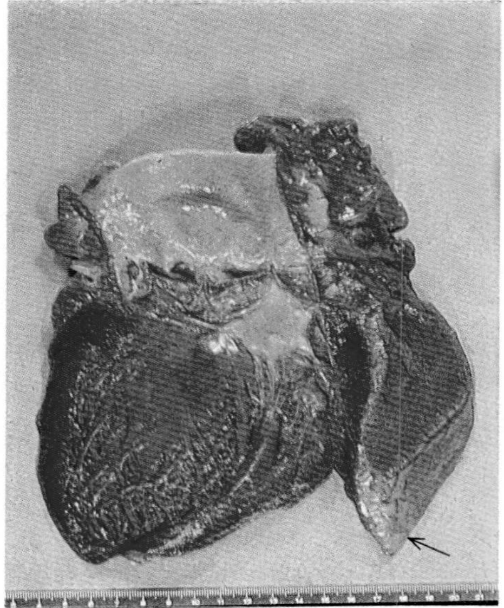

Fig. 2.4. The opened left heart (following cuts 4, 5 and 6).

2. Heart and Pericardium

Technic of Dissection

The pericardial sac is opened first by scissor cuts that correspond to an inverted Y. A distended, resilient pericardial sac suggests effusion (see Fig. 2.31). Watch for positional changes of the heart (situs inversus, dextroposition). The pericardial sac usually contains 5–10 ml. of a clear, amber fluid. As shown in Figure 2.1 *(normal heart)*, pericardium and epicardium are glistening and smooth (see highlights of photograph). The anterior wall of Figure 2.1 is found in a position usually seen at autopsy. The arrow points to the border between the left and the right ventricles. Note the abundant subepicardial fat in the area of the interventricular coronary sulcus (anterior interventricular branch of the left coronary artery). A white, tendon-like epicardial thickening often is found in the epicardium of the right ventricle (caused mechanically). The cardiac apex is formed by the left ventricle. The shape of the normal heart resembles a "gothic" arch. In contrast, the dilated heart has a rounded shape ("romanic" arch, Fig. 2.16). The size of the heart may be compared with the loosely closed fist of the patient (weight, see p. 4).

The aortic arch and ascending aorta are palpated prior to dissection of the heart. A dilated or thickened aorta is left together with the heart. The pulmonary artery is opened by a knife cut and searched for pulmonary emboli. The pulmonary artery should be opened under water when air embolism is suspected.

Cut sections through the heart are shown in Figure 2.2: The inferior and superior vena cava are connected by a cut with the enterotome (1), followed by a cut to the apex of the right ventricle (2). The cut is then extended into the pulmonary artery (3), so that a triangular, anterior right ventricular wall is prepared. The *right heart* is then inspected (Fig. 2.3).

In the right atrium, closure or slit-like or complete patency of the foramen ovale, appearance and circumference of the tricuspid valve (11 cm.), endocardium and trabeculae are examined. The thickness of the right ventricular wall (normal 3 mm.) is measured 1 cm. below the ostium of the pulmonary artery. Thickness of fat tissue, appearance of the pulmonary cusps and the circumference of the pulmonary ring (6 cm.) and pulmonary artery are determined.

The dissection of the *left heart* (Fig. 2.4) begins with a cut through the atrial wall between the pulmonary veins. The atrium and mitral valve are inspected from above. The scissors cut then extends to the left apex (4 in Fig. 2.2) without damaging or destroying lesions seen in the atrium or mitral valve. Examine the mitral valve (circumference 11 cm.). The valve is rinsed, not wiped, in order to preserve valvular deposits. The cut is continued from the apex into the aorta (5 and 6 in Fig. 2.2). The anterior left wall is thereby prepared as a sharp triangle (Fig. 2.4→). Measure the thickness of muscle 1 cm. beneath the aortic valve (1.2 cm.). Examine the endocardium for the presence of thrombi, fibrosis, fatty changes, etc. Measure the circumference of the aortic valve (7 cm.).

The left ventricular muscle can be prepared by horizontal cuts that bisect the anterior and posterior walls from the apex to the valves. Especially when subendocardial necrosis is suspected, the heart muscle may be prepared by multiple transverse cuts also.

The heart muscle usually is firm, uniformly light brown-red and transparent. A soft, dilated heart with a cloudy cut surface usually reflects postmortem changes after rigor mortis has disappeared (more than 3–4 days post mortem). Dilatation, cloudiness or a gray-red brown discoloration at an earlier time after death indicates parenchymal damage (cloudy swelling with sepsis, possibly myocarditis).

Opening of the coronary arteries. The descending branch of the left coronary is opened first with the coronary scissors. Pathologic changes, such as narrowing, usually are found 1 cm. below the coronary ostium. The circumflex branch of the left coronary is opened next, followed by the right coronary artery, which is found at the cutting margin of the right ventricle. Transverse cuts through the coronary arteries are indicated in cases of severe coronary stenosis.

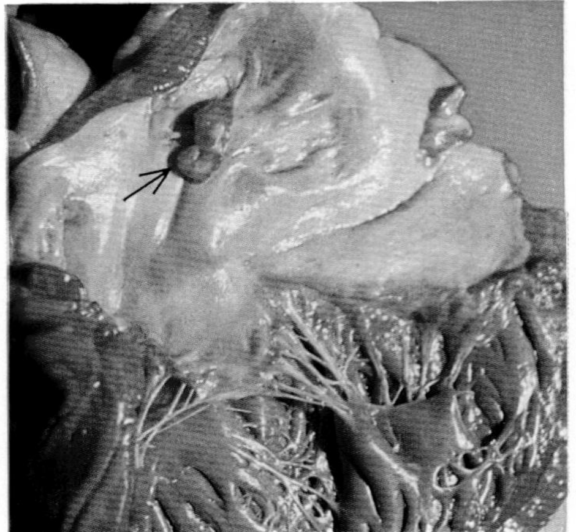

Fig. 2.5. Embolus in patent foramen ovale.

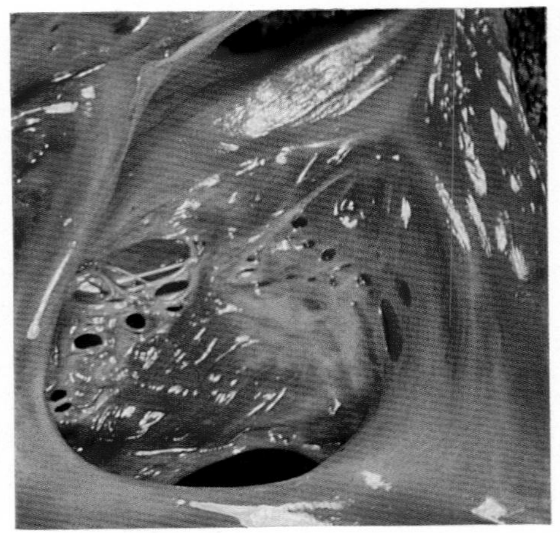

Fig. 2.6. Fenestration of the septum secundum.

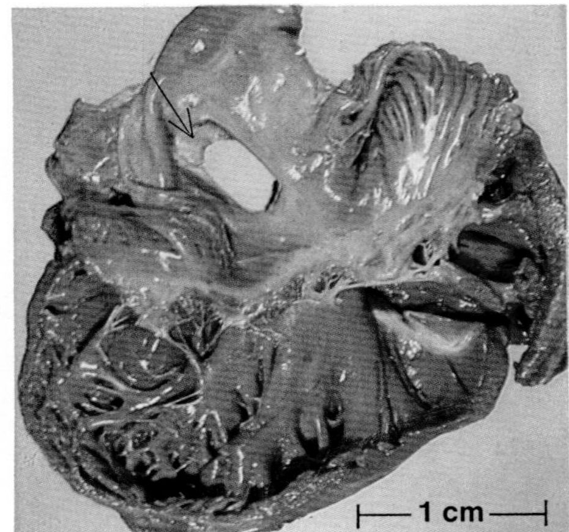

Fig. 2.7. Atrial septal defect.

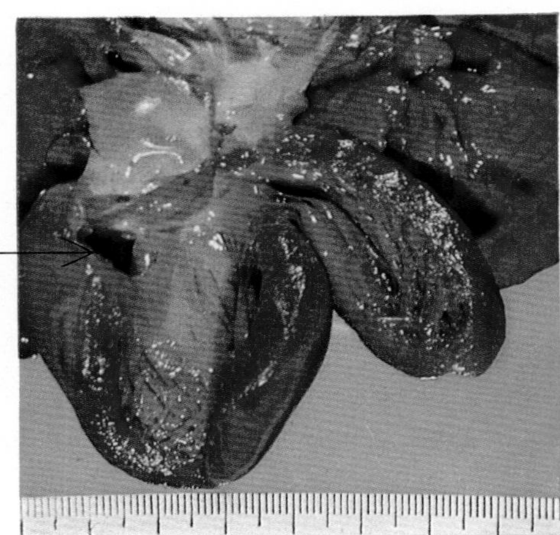

Fig. 2.8. High ventricular septal defect.

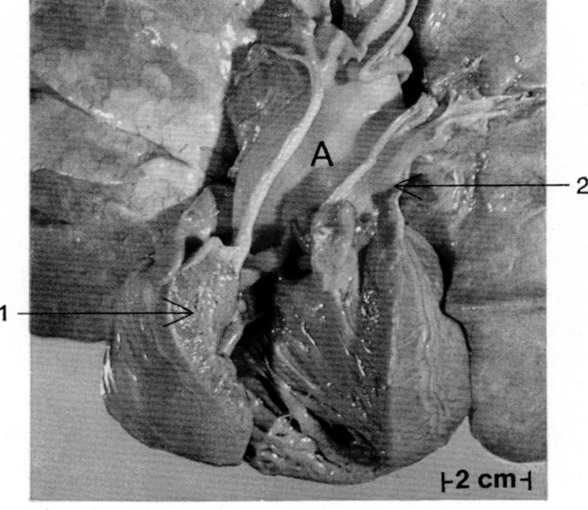

Fig. 2.9. Transposition of the aorta and pulmonary artery.

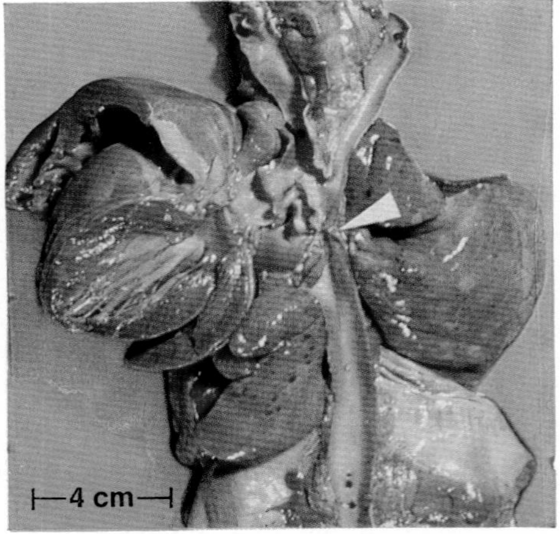

Fig. 2.10. Isthmus stenosis of the aorta.

Malformations

Cardiac malformations have attracted much attention during the past 20 years because some of these defects now can be corrected by surgery. Cardiac catheterization and angiography have considerably improved the diagnostic accuracy. In cases of cardiac congenital malformations, during autopsy, the heart, lungs and aorta should be removed in toto. The aorta, pulmonary arteries and veins should remain attached to the heart.

Congenital malformations *are structural changes in the heart that develop during the first 3 months of intrauterine life. Most cardiac malformations are either defects in the formation of the cardiac septa or rotation of the arterial heart.*

Some remarks concerning the embryogenesis of the heart are indicated for a better understanding of cardiac malformations. The paired cardiopericardial primordia, which are derived from the foregut, fuse in the midline. They form a heart tube with endocardium and a myoepicardial mantle. The heart tube grows faster than the pericardium, thereby forming an atrio-ventriculo-bulbar loop and a bayonet-like bulbotruncus. Simultaneously, the cardiac tube becomes twisted and the arterial and venous ends are twisted around each other (Fig. 2.12). The atrial and ventricular septa are formed during the rotation of the cardiac tube. The most important malformations are the result of (a) the formations of the *cardiac septa* are defective or lacking altogether (truncus arteriosus communis, atrial or ventricular septal defects), (b) the *torsion of the truncus arteriosus* is abnormal (complete or incomplete transposition with stenosis with or without deviation of the septum in the truncus arteriosus, e.g., riding aorta or pulmonary artery with stenosis), (c) the valves or blood vessels are *stenotic*, (d) the valves are *insufficient* and (e) fetal structures *persist*.

Acardia, i.e., absence of the heart, is seen only in identical twins. Vascular supply is provided by the normal twin. *Ectopia:* the heart is located in the chest wall with or without a pericardial sac. A cleft is present in the sternum.

A. **Septal defects.** *Patent foramen ovale:* This common malformation is presented in Figures 2.5–2.7. The septum primum grows from the upper dorsal atrial wall toward the ostium atrioventriculare. The septum secundum extends from the dorsocephalic atrial wall on the right atrial side of the septum primum. An opening appears in the septum primum that is covered by the septum secundum. The two septa normally suse. A slit-like, patent foramen ovale can be probed from the right atrium in 20–30% of autopsies. The feptum primum is pressed against the septum secundum because of the higher pressure in the left atrium, and hemodynamic changes usually are not observed from a patent foramen ovale. When the normal atrial pressures are reversed (lower pressure in the left than in the right atrium), the slit-like foramen ovale can be dilated and an embolus may be pushed through the foramen (Fig. 2.5). As seen from the left atrium and ventricle, a gray-red *embolus* is lodged in a slit-like *foramen ovale* (→). The other end of the embolus projects into the right atrium. This rare finding *(paradoxic embolism)* can give rise to multiple arterial emboli and infarcts in the kidney, spleen and brain or occlusion of extremity arteries.

A partial or complete developmental defect of the septum secundum likewise results in an atrial septal defect. The margins of such a defect are formed by the septum primum. Figure 2.6 shows a partially *patent foramen ovale*, viewed from the left atrium. This defect is referred to as *fenestration of the septum secundum*. A *defect of the septum secundum* is shown in Figure 2.7. The defect is viewed from the right atrium and ventricle, which are markedly dilated and hypertrophied. The upper margin of the defect shows remnants of the septum secundum (→). Hemodynamic manifestations of such a defect are apparent when the diameter of the defect exceeds 8 mm. in infants and 15 mm. in adults. Right-sided hypertrophy, dilatation of the pulmonary artery and congested lungs are symptomatic of a large atrial defect (GOERTTLER). Dominantly inherited disease, observed mostly in females. Defects of the septum secundum and persistence of foramen ovale are very commonly associated with other congenital heart diseases (70–80%).

Isolated defects of the ventricular septum (high *ventricular septal defects* without transposition, or Roger's disease) (Figs. 2.8 and 2.11.1). The isolated defect involves the area directly beneath the aortic valve between the right and the posterior cusps, the so-called pars membranacea. Septal defects sometimes are associated with malformations of the tricuspid valve or, as in our case, with marked endocardial fibrosis of the left ventricle (whitish, thickened endocardium). Septal defects account for 20–30% of all congenital malformations. A defect smaller than 5 mm. is functionally without significance; larger defects cause pulmonary hypertension. *Absence of the atrial and ventricular septum (cor biloculare) and absence of the atrial septum (cor triloculare biatrium)* frequently are associated with pulmonary artery stenosis. The *truncus arteriosus communis* (Fig. 2.11.6) consists of a single arterial trunk that divides into a pulmonary artery and aorta. The common truncus usually is combined with an atrial septal defect.

B. **Transposition complexes.** *Complete transposition of large arterial trunks with ventricular septal defect* accounts for 5–10% of all cardiac malformations (♂:♀ = 3:1) (Figs. 2.9, 2.11.7 and 2.12). The aorta and pulmonary artery emerge from the wrong ventricle: the aorta arises from a hypertrophic right ventricle and the pulmonary artery emerges from the left ventricle. *Cause:* failure of bulbus rotation. Figure 2.9 shows a markedly hypertrophic right ventricle with a thick-walled aorta emerging from it. The pulmonary artery is narrow (to the right of the aorta) and arises from the left ventricle. In partial transposition (due to incomplete bulbus rotation) and ventricular septal defect, the result is an "overriding" pulmonary

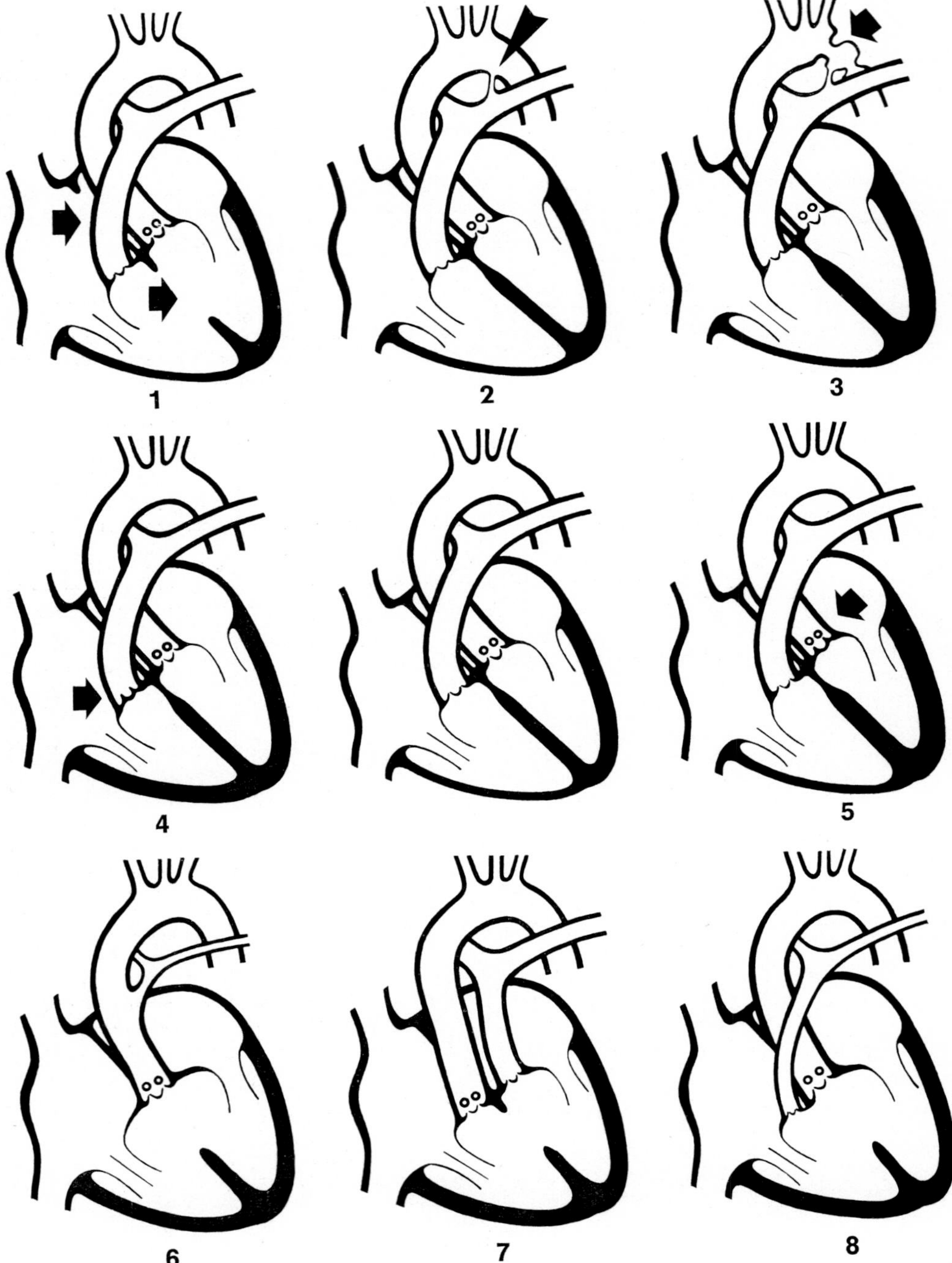

Fig. 2.11. Schematic presentation of common congenital cardiac malformations: (1) Atrial and ventricular septal defects. (2) Persistent ductus arteriosus Botalli. (3) Aortic isthmus stenosis. (4) Congenital stenosis of the pulmonary valve. (5) Congenital stenosis of the aortic valve. (6) Truncus arteriosus communis (cor triloculare). (7) Transposition of great arteries with ventricular septal defect. (8) Tetralogy of Fallot.

artery (Taussig-Bing complex; rare) or an overriding aorta with a more or less prominent dextroposition of the aorta. Complete dextroposition of the aorta refers to a malformation in which both aorta and pulmonary artery arise in the right ventricle ("double-outlet right ventricle"). The combination of right-sided hypertrophy, dextroposition of the aorta, ventricular septal defect and dilatation of the pulmonary artery formerly was called *Eisenmenger complex*. Since isolated ventricular septal defects sooner or later lead to increasing dilatation of the pulmonary artery, even without dextroposition of the aorta, the term *Eisenmenger syndrome* has gained wide acceptance. Dextroposition of the aorta with narrowing or atresia of the pulmonary artery is referred to as *tetralogy of Fallot* (1, ventricular septal defect; 2, riding aorta; 3, pulmonary artery stenosis; 4, hypertrophy of the right ventricle). *Pentalogy of Fallot* is a combination of tetralogy with atrial septal defect or patent foramen ovale. Tetralogy and pentalogy of Fallot account for 8–10% of all congenital cardiac malformations. The combination of 1, pulmonary artery stenosis, 2, right heart hypertrophy and 3, atrial septal defect is referred to as *trilogy of Fallot* (Figs. 2.11.8 and 2.12). (Tetralogy = trilogy + riding aorta.)

C. **Stenosis.** (1) *Tricuspid stenosis or atresia* occurs with right ventricular hypertrophy, with or without ventricular septal defect and anomalies of the aorta and pulmonary artery (rare malformation, approximately 3%). (2) *Stenosis of pulmonary artery* presents as either valvular or subvalvular (= muscular) stenosis. The latter also is referred to as infundibular stenosis (Fig. 2.11.4). (3) *Stenosis or atresia of the mitral valve* occurs with or without ventricular septal defect and often is associated with positional anomalies of the large arteries, including transposition. The *Lutembacher syndrome* is a congenital (occasionally also acquired) mitral stenosis and atrial septal defect. (4) *Stenosis or atresia of the aortic valve* includes valvular, subvalvular (partly pure muscular, infundibular stenosis) or supravalvular forms of stenosis. These defects frequently are accompanied by left ventricular fibroelastosis. (5) *Aortic isthmus stenosis* (10–20% of malformations, ♂>♀). (a) *Isthmus stenosis of the newborn type* (Fig. 2.11.3) is a hypoplastic stenosis of the entire isthmus, i.e., the aortic arch between the origin of the subclavian artery and the entry of the ductus arteriosus. This defect often is associated with other cardiac malformations and the prognosis is poor. (b) *Isthmus stenosis of the adult type* is shown in Figures 2.10 and 2.11.3. The stenosis is circular, often severe and limited to an area near or at the entry of the obliterated ductus arteriosus Botalli. The prognosis is better than in (a). *Pg:* heavy granulation tissue at the ostium of the ductus arteriosus, formation of scar tissue and adherence of the aorta to the pulmonary artery. *Co:* arteriosclerosis proximal to the stenotic segment (pressure!).

D. **Valvular insufficiencies.** (1) Congenital tricuspid insufficiency also is known as *Ebstein's anomaly* (less than 1% of malformations), which usually is combined with a malformation or absence of the dorsal tricuspid leaflet. (2) Congenital mitral insufficiency (rare).

E. **Persistence of fetal vessels.** (1) *Persistent ductus arteriosus Botalli* (Fig. 2.11.2) often is associated with other congenital heart malformations. The ductus normally is 4–7 mm. wide in newborns. After the first year of life, about 1% of the ducts remain open. A widely patent ductus also is observed as an isolated defect and constitutes 5–10% of all cardiac malformations. *Co:* pulmonary hypertension. (2) *Anomalies of pulmonary veins* include entry into the superior or inferior vena cava or into the coronary sinus.
The frequency of congenital malformations of the heart is 1% of autopsy cases but 5–10% of dead births. *Co:* all transpositions and larger septal defects are accompanied by cyanosis. An endocarditis may be superimposed on valvular defects, e.g., aortic valve with two cusps. *Cause:* probably genetically determined, e.g., 10% of children with Down's syndrome (autosomal trisomy of chromosome no. 21) have congenital malformations. Environmental factors are considered, e.g., chemicals (thalidomide), hypoxia, viruses (rubeola, varicella and hepatitis). Miscellaneous factors include diabetes, x-rays and hypovitaminosis.

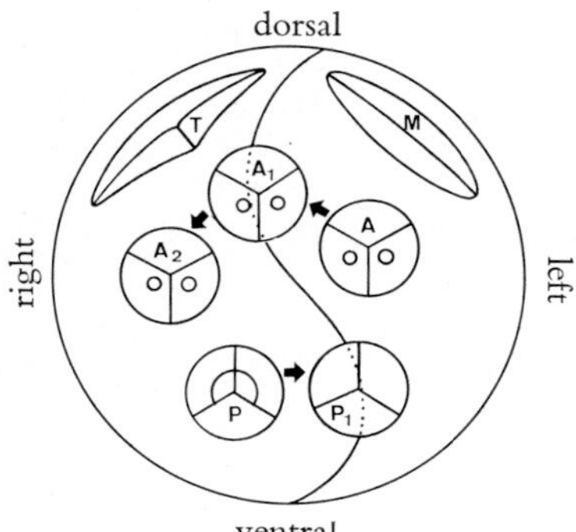

Fig. 2.12. Malformations resulting from bulbus rotation or torsion (according to GOERTTLER). Normal position of the aorta (A), pulmonary artery (P), mitral ostium (M) and tricuspid ostium (T).

A_1 = "riding aorta."
A_1 combined with pulmonary artery stenosis and right ventricular hypertrophy = tetralogy of Fallot.
A_1 combined with normal or dilated pulmonary artery = Eisenmenger complex.
A_2 Dextroposition of the aorta combined with normally positioned pulmonary artery = "double outlet right ventricle."
P (inner circle) = pulmonary artery stenosis.
P_1 = "riding pulmonary artery"; most often combined with A_2, which is then referred to as Taussig-Bing syndrome.

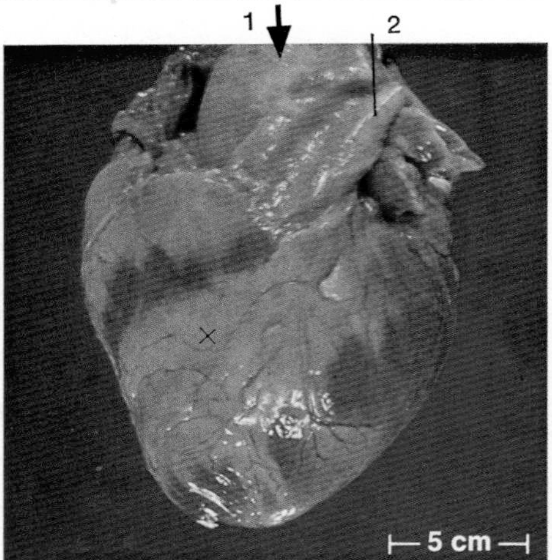

Fig. 2.13. Hypertrophy of the left ventricle.

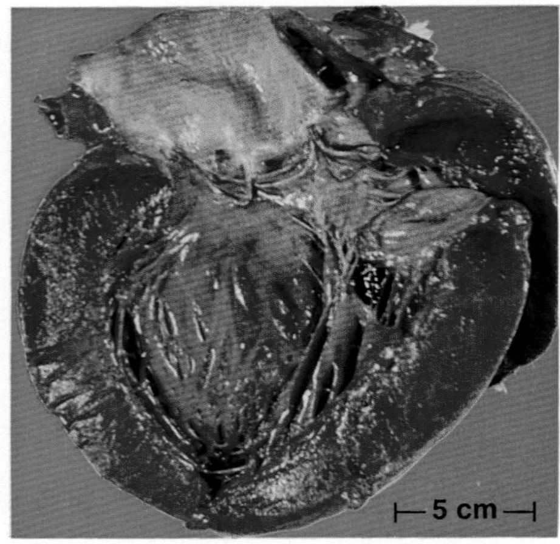

Fig. 2.14. Hypertrophy of the left ventricle.

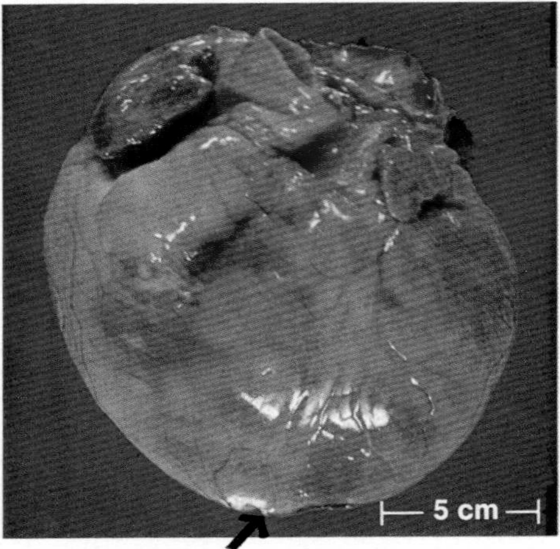

Fig. 2.15. Dilatation of the left ventricle.

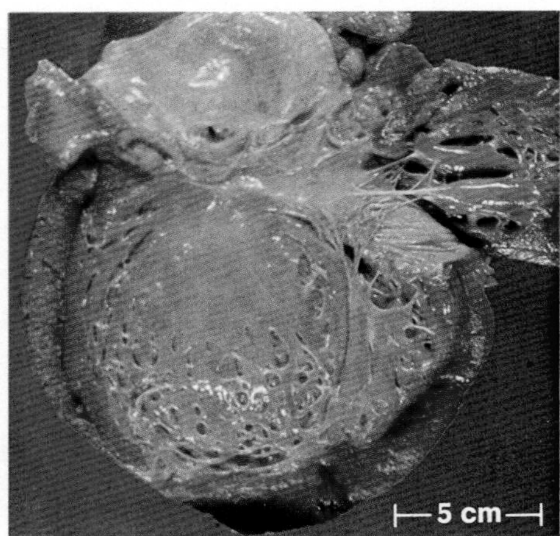

Fig. 2.16. Dilatation of the left ventricle.

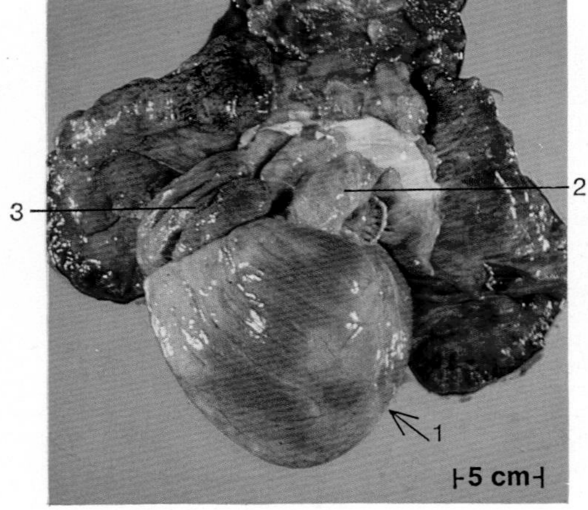

Fig. 2.17. Hypertrophy and dilatation of the right ventricle.

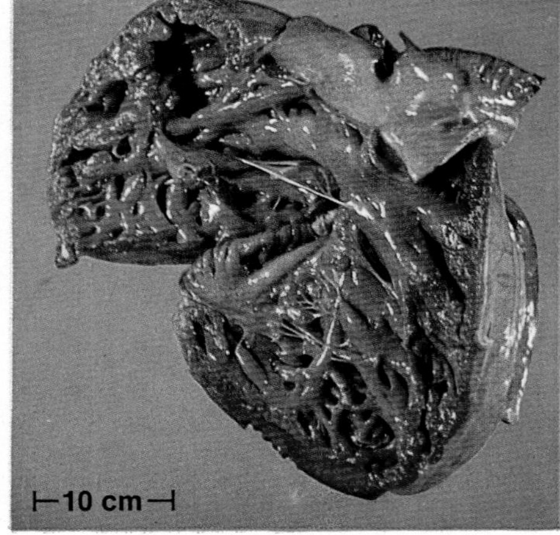

Fig. 2.18. Hypertrophy of the right ventricular wall.

Hypertrophy and Dilatation

Changes in the shape and size of the heart are reflected grossly as changes in volume and weight.

Hypertrophy of the left ventricle (Figs. 2.13, 2.14 and 2.20; TCP p. 35). *Increase in the muscle mass of the left ventricle due to increased work load (hypertension, aortic stenosis, aortic isthmus stenosis).* Also known as concentric hypertrophy because the ventricle is not dilated (clinically: no insufficiency). The heart weight is markedly increased (up to 800 Gm.). Weights above 800 Gm. usually are due to hypertrophy and dilatation. The left ventricle constitutes the major part of the heart (→1 aorta, →2 pulmonary artery, X right ventricle in Fig. 2.13). The cardiac apex is formed by the left ventricle, whereas the right ventricle is reduced to a small appendage (X in Fig. 2.13). Figure 2.14 shows the opened ventricle. The anterior wall is folded backward. The apex of the ventricle is sharply pointed, resembling a gothic arch. The left ventricular muscle is 1.8 cm. thick, brown-red and very firm. The papillary muscles project into the lumen, as in the cross section illustrated in Figure 2.20.

Hypertrophy and dilatation of the left ventricle (Figs. 2.15 and 2.21). *Eccentric hypertrophy (hypertrophy and dilatation) is defined as a decompensated, hypertrophic heart with regurgitating blood (hypertension, aortic and mitral valve defects).* The left ventricle is markedly dilated. The unopened heart is globular in shape because the right ventricle is dilated also (and sometimes hypertrophied as well) (→in Fig. 2.15 points to the border between the right and the left ventricle). The opened heart has the flattened, rounded form of a "romanic" arch. The right wall is thickened (greater than 1.1 cm.) and cross sections reveal protruding papillary muscles (Fig. 2.21). The mitral valve may become relatively insufficient due to the dilatation of the chamber and the annulus fibrosus, which, in turn, impairs blood flow.

Pg: increased work load due to changes in pressure or volume. Thickening of muscle fibers (increase in mass: a 10 μ-long strip of heart muscle weighs $200–250 \times 10^{-12}$ Gm.; the weight increases in hypertrophy to 500–600 Gm., increase in total mass up to 450×10^{-12} Gm.). The mass of a 10 μ-long fiber section does not increase beyond 600–1,000 Gm. of the total heart weight. A genuine increase in the number of heart-muscle cells in hypertrophy was demonstrated by Sandritter and Adler (1971) (normal heart-muscle count: 2×10^9; in hypertrophy: up to 4×10^9). Dilatation is caused by stretching of muscle fibers that are longer and thinner. They also are rearranged so that the number of fibers is increased per unit surface. *Causes:* essential or renal hypertension, pheochromocytoma, congenital and acquired cardiac diseases.

Dilatation of the left ventricle (Figs. 2.15 and 2.16). *Dilatation of the ventricle without hypertrophy*, which results in cardiac insufficiency with blood regurgitation. The heart is globular as in hypertrophy and dilatation, but the left ventricle is not as firm as in hypertrophy. The rounded, "romanic" arch of the left ventricle is seen again, but the muscle mass is not increased (normal weight, ventricular wall less than 1.1 cm. thick). The papillary muscles are flattened. The heart muscle is fragile, soft, gray-red or speckled (myocarditis) in acute dilatation. In chronic dilatation, multiple small fibrous-tissue scars may be seen (e.g., after healed diphtheria).

Cardiac insufficiency (hypertrophy and dilatation or dilatation alone) is due to an imbalance between work demand and work capability of the heart. The end-diastolic volume increases without a corresponding increase in the stroke volume (residual blood). Cardiac output is therefore diminished. The biochemical basis of acute insufficiency (dilatation) is damage to oxidation and phosphorylation. ATP and creatine phosphate are reduced (Type I of cardiac insufficiency). In Type II cardiac insufficiency (hypertrophy and dilatation), energy-rich phosphate is retained but not utilized because cellular permeability to calcium is impaired (electromechanical coupling is disturbed); (calcium activates ATPase! →ATP→ADP = contraction. Fleckenstein). Sudden death of heavy beer drinkers (cobalt replaces calcium!).

Hypertrophy and dilatation of the right ventricle (Figs. 2.17 and 2.18). Acute pressure and volume changes occur in the right ventricle after pulmonary embolism, shock (microthrombi in lung vessels), left ventricular failure and often without specific precipitating factors in other diseases. Hypertrophy and dilatation is the result of longstanding increases in pressure (or volume) in the pulmonary circulation (see also p. 71, cor pulmonale). Figure 2.17 shows *hypertrophy and dilatation of the right ventricle.* The rounded ventricle now forms the entire anterior heart wall

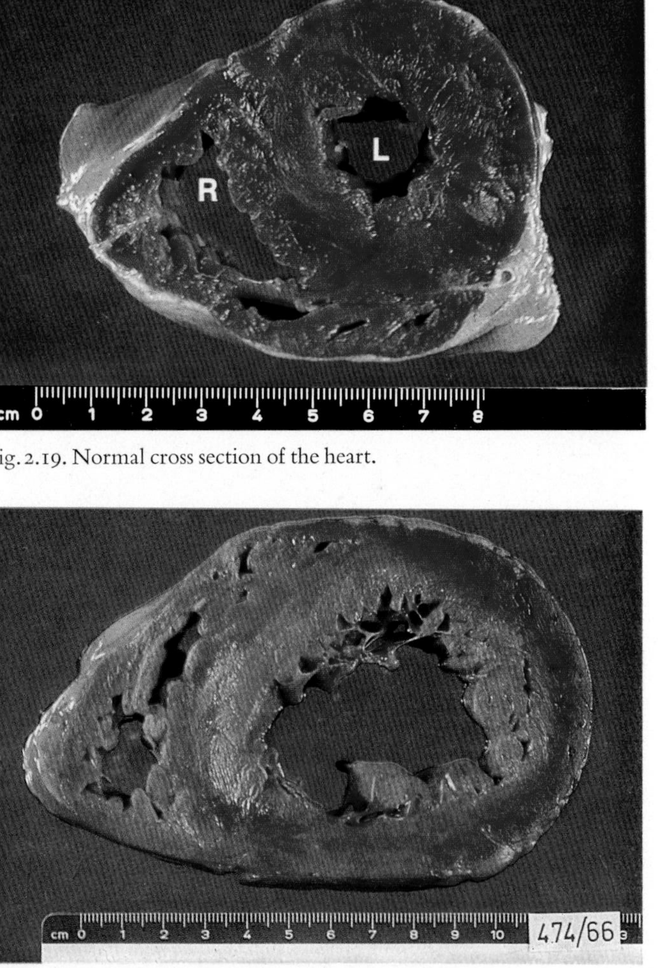

Fig. 2.19. Normal cross section of the heart.

Fig. 2.21. Eccentric hypertrophy of the left ventricle.

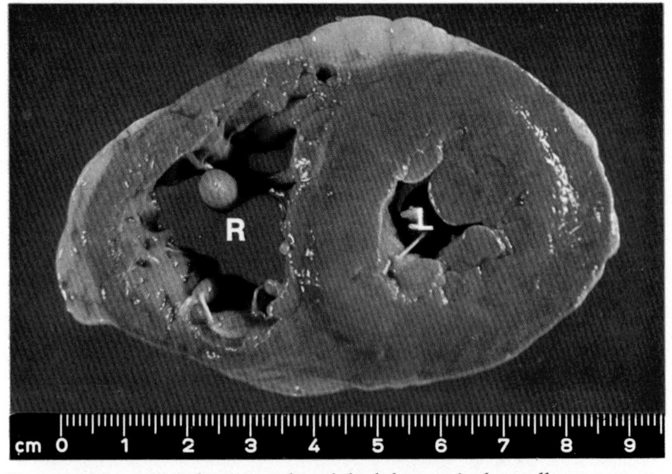

Fig. 2.20. Concentric hypertrophy of the left ventricular wall.

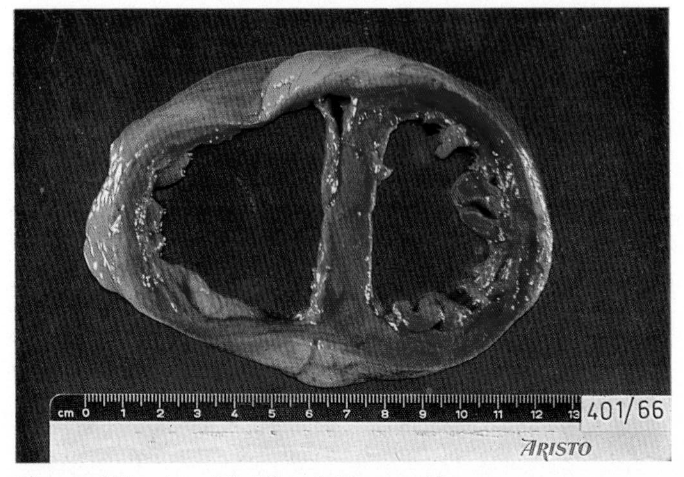

Fig. 2.22. Dilatation of the left and right ventricles.

and the cardiac apex (→1 border between left and right ventricle, →2 pulmonary artery, →3 right atrium). The right ventricle is firm to palpation but flabby with dilatation and collapses (Fig. 2.22). The *opened* heart (Fig. 2.18) shows the expanded right ventricle, especially the conus with the protruding trabeculae (musculature more than 3 mm. thick). Dilatation alone (Fig. 2.22) is seen best in cross sections. The trabeculae are flattened, and the ventricle may collapse due to reduced consistency. Acute right-sided dilatation is very common. Hypertrophy of right ventricle: 5–10% of autopsies.

Hypertension and its consequences (Fig. 2.23). Arterial hypertension (30% of persons over 60 years of age) refers to a prolonged elevation of pressure to over 160 mm Hg (systolic) and 95 mm Hg (diastolic). The most frequent form (80%) is *essential hypertension* (increased minute volume and peripheral resistance) and its cause is unknown. A steroid, "hypersterone", has recently been detected ADLERCREUTZ et al., 1973).
Renal hypertension (14% of hypertensive patients) is based on the renin-angiotensin mechanism in disturbances of renal blood supply (resistance hypertension). *Endocrine hypertensions* occur in medullo-adrenal tumors (pheochromocytoma) or cortical tumors (aldosterone: Conn's syndrome).
Pulmonary hypertension (hypertrophy of the right ventricle) particularly occurs in recurrent pulmonary embolisms, pulmonary emphysema, and pulmonary fibroses (Hamman-Rich syndrome, silicosis, etc.). Other causes are acquired or congenital heart diseases, kyphoscoliosis, polycythemia (see also cor pulmonale, page 71).

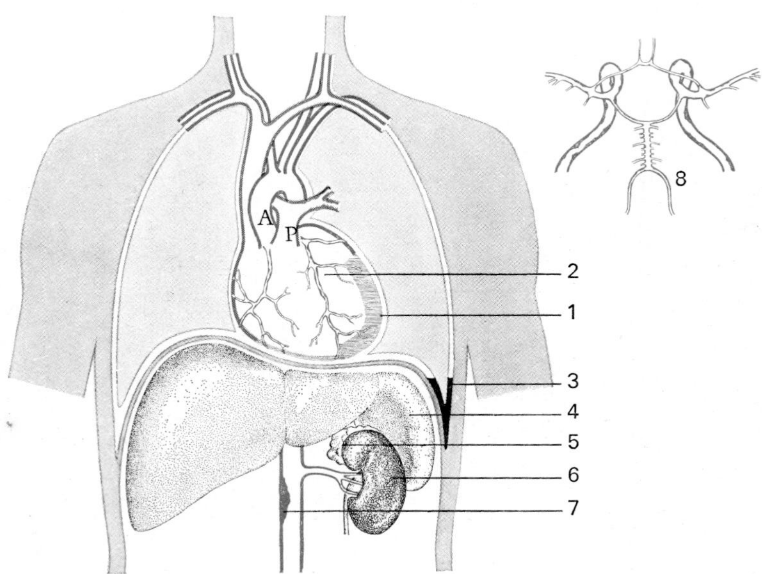

Fig. 2.23. Sequelae of arterial hypertension.
1. Hypertrophy of the left ventricular wall (60–70% of hypertensive patients).
2. Coronary sclerosis.
3. Pleural effusion.
4. Congestion of the spleen.
5. Nodular hyperplasia of the adrenal cortex.
6. Arterio-arteriolosclerosis of the kidneys.
7. Arteriosclerosis of the aorta.
8. Arteriosclerosis of basal cerebral arteries, cerebral infarctions, stroke (30–70% of hypertensive patients die from cerebral complications).
A = aorta; P = pulmonary artery.

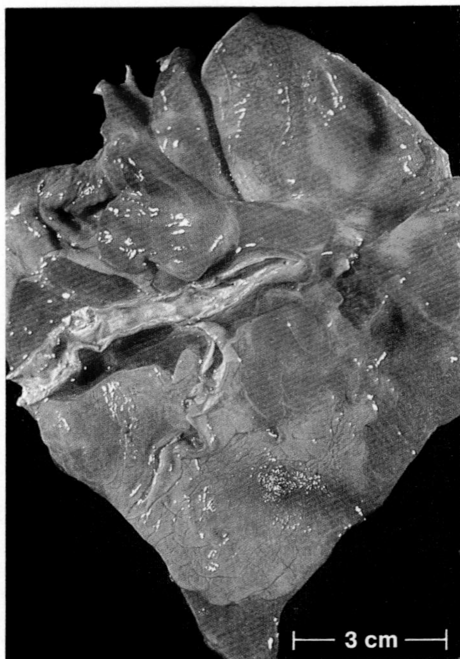

Fig. 2.24. Coronary sclerosis without narrowing of the lumen.

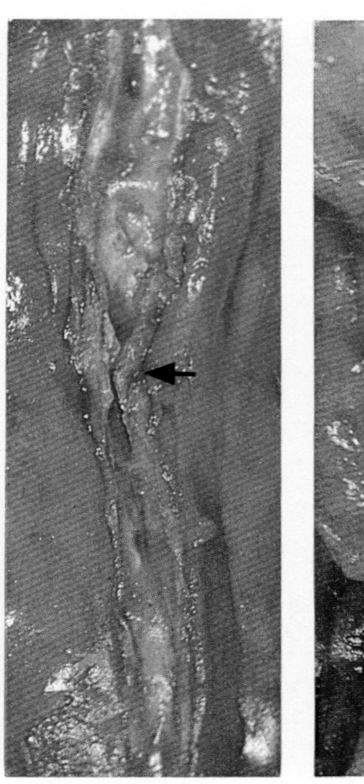

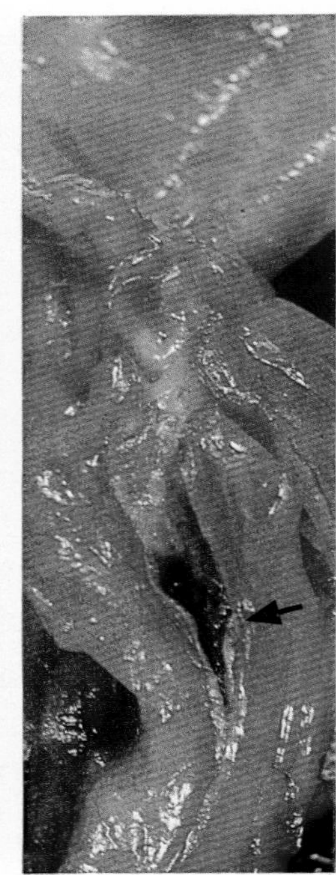

Fig. 2.25. Left: coronary sclerosis with napkin-ring narrowing of the lumen. Right: thrombosis of coronary artery.

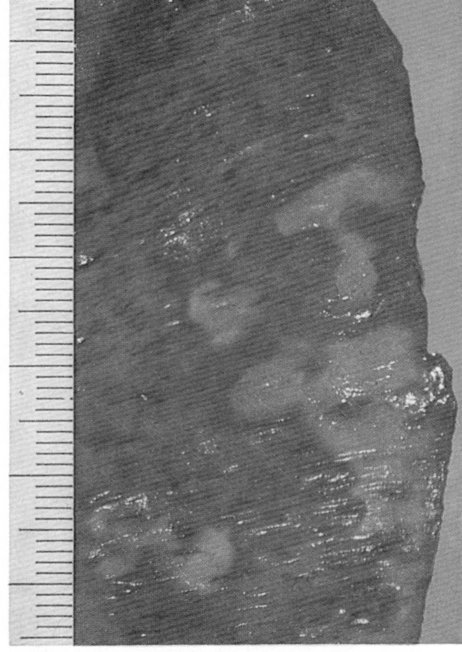

Fig. 2.26. Fresh myocardial necrosis.

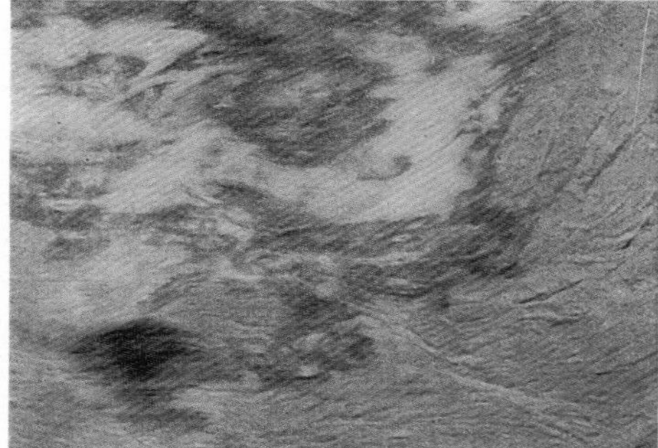

Fig. 2.27. Myocardial necrosis with granulation tissue.

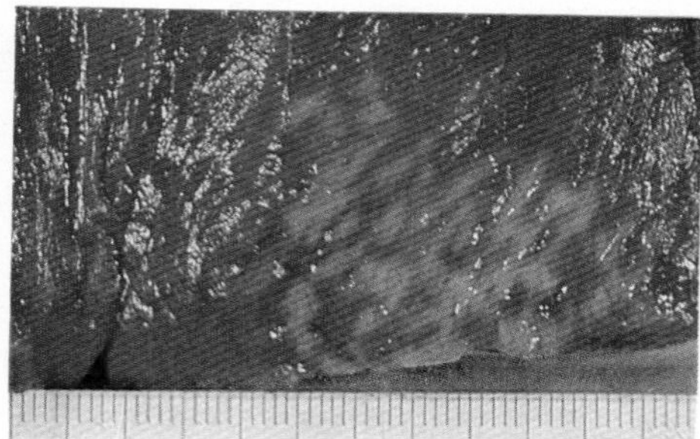

Fig. 2.28. Myocardial scars following infarction.

Myocardial Infarction

Hypoxia of large portions of the myocardium with necrosis. Most often due to coronary sclerosis or thrombosis.

Coronary sclerosis and thrombosis (Figs. 2.24 and 2.25; TCP, p. 61). Two types of coronary sclerosis may be recognized: (a) *Coronary sclerosis without narrowing of the lumen* (Fig. 2.24). The coronary artery is converted into a wide, rigid pipe with a hard wall. Our figure shows the circumflex branch and interventricular branch of the right coronary artery. Gray, splotchy epicardial changes are noted (serous atrophy of subepicardial fat). A sudden hypotensive attack can lead to a myocardial infarction (see also cerebral infarction). (b) *Constriction or stenosis* (Fig. 2.25 →left figure) is seen most commonly 1–2 cm. below the origin of the interventricular branch of the left coronary artery from the aorta. Sclerosis may be minimal in the other branches of the coronary arteries. Narrowing of the lumen in this form of sclerosis is caused by the formation of a crescent-shaped atheroma (TCP, p. 61). Sclerosis may proceed to *total luminal occlusion*. The coronary artery resembles a thin, calcium-containing pipe. The lumen cannot be opened. Coronary artery thrombosis very rarely develops in a normal or minimally sclerosed artery. An atheroma most often is the basis of coronary thrombosis. Figure 2.25 (right) shows a fresh, occlusive thrombus. It is gray-red, firm and fragile. Organization of the thrombus is seen as gray-red and firm granulation tissue. An old thrombus is white, firm and presents as white thickening of the opened wall.

Pg: coronary sclerosis usually begins as reversible foci of lipidosis, followed by sclerosis and atheromatous plaques. The lipids of the atheroma probably are derived from the blood (insudation). The role of thrombi in the development of sclerosis is emphasized by Anglo-American authors. An atheromatous plaque can be organized by connective tissue and the severity of the stenosis is thereby diminished. Sudden, total occlusion of a coronary artery lumen is precipitated by *hemorrhage* into the sclerotic plaque (intimal tears), edema with swelling or *thrombosis* (thrombosis accounts for 80–90% of cases). Thrombosis causes an infarction and is not the consequence of an infarction, as assumed previously.

Myocardial necrosis (myocardial infarction, Figs. 2.26–2.28; TCP, p. 39). Myocardial necrosis is grossly visible only after 8 hours as a yellow or clay-colored, dry, firm and slightly elevated lesion (Fig. 2.26). The size of the infarction depends on the distribution of the corresponding artery (see Fig. 2.35). The heart is dilated. Endocardial mural thrombi and fibrinous pericarditis (clinical symptomatology!) accompany myocardial infarction. A red rim of granulation tissue around the margins of the necrosis develops 1 week later. The necrotic tissue is replaced by granulation tissue, usually 4 weeks later (1 mm. necrosis is organized within 10 days). Figure 2.27 shows an extensive area of myocardial necrosis, partly replaced by granulation tissue. The latter is red (many capillaries) and sunken on cut surface (blood exudes, capillaries collapse). After 6–8 weeks, the granulation tissue becomes fibrotic (formation of collagenous fibers). The scar is white, firm and glistening like a tendon (myocardial scar, Fig. 2.28).

F: myocardial infarction: 4–6% of autopsy material. In 1924, 15% of all deaths; in 1961, 41% (!). Of 100,000 living persons 143 ♂ and 66 ♀ develop myocardial infarctions (♂:♀ = 3:1). *A:* ♂ 50–60 years. *Pg: General conditions:* 1. Size of infarction depends on *caliber* of the occluded vessel. 2. *Speed of occlusion.* 3. *Development of collaterals,* especially frequency and caliber of anastomoses (= A): Normal 9% A; cardiac hypertrophy 26% A; with stenosis 55% A; fresh occlusion 75% A; old occlusion 100% A. Diameter of A, 700–900 μ. 4. *Blood demand of heart:* with heart weights exceeding 500 Gm., the growth of the coronary arteries and their ostia does not keep pace with the weight increase of the myocardium. 5. *Heart beat and blood pressure.* 6. *Anemia and viscosity of blood.* 7. *Epinephrine:* increases oxygen demand and dilates coronary arteries.

Risk Factors

(1) *Hypertension* with increased heart weight. Hearts with infarctions weigh, on the average, 500 Gm. Sixty per cent of patients with infarctions are hypertensive. (2) *Hypercholesterolemia* (patients with more than 250 mg./100 ml. have an infarction risk of 10% within 10 years). (3) *Overweight* (is doubted by some authors). (4) *Nicotine abuse* (three times greater risk due to hypertension and increased pulse). (5) *Diabetes* (hyperlipemia, hypertension, 10% of all infarctions). (6) *Profession:* laborers have more infarctions than "chiefs." Academicians 30% fewer infarctions than nonacademicians. Also: multiple factors but not enough substantiated data are available.

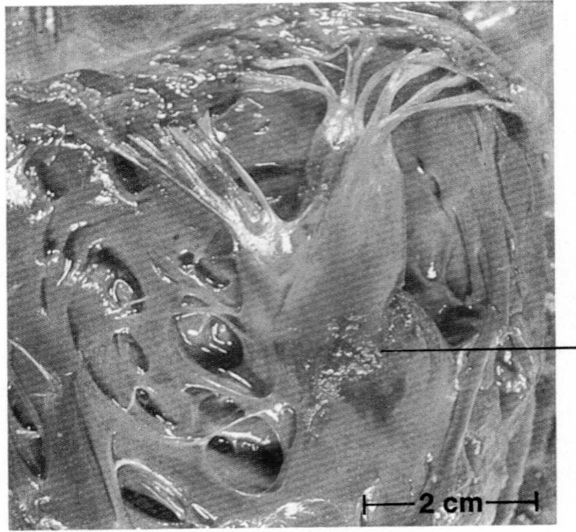

Fig. 2.29. Rupture of a papillary muscle in a myocardial infarction.

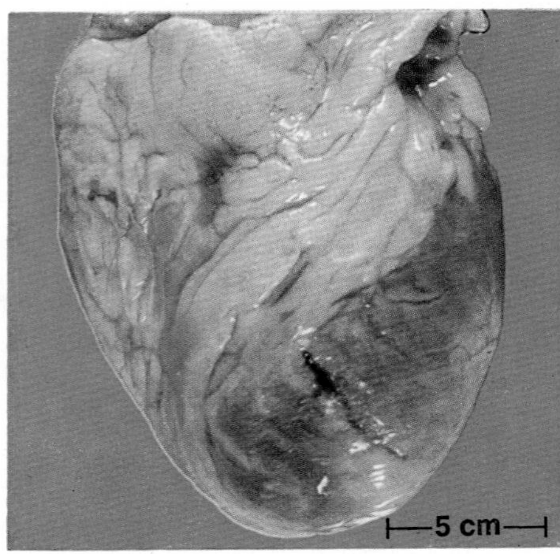

Fig. 2.30. Rupture of the heart wall.

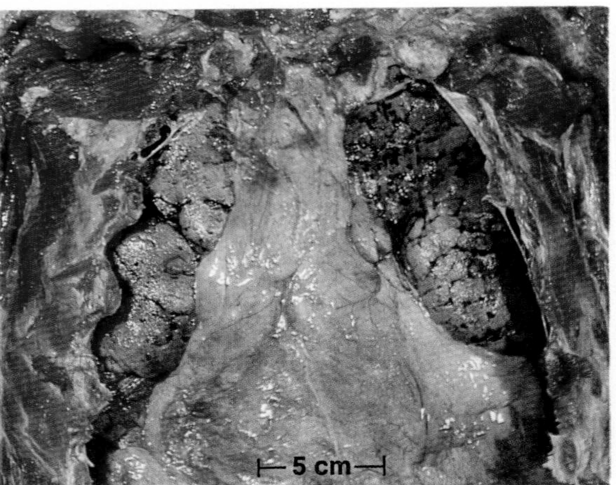

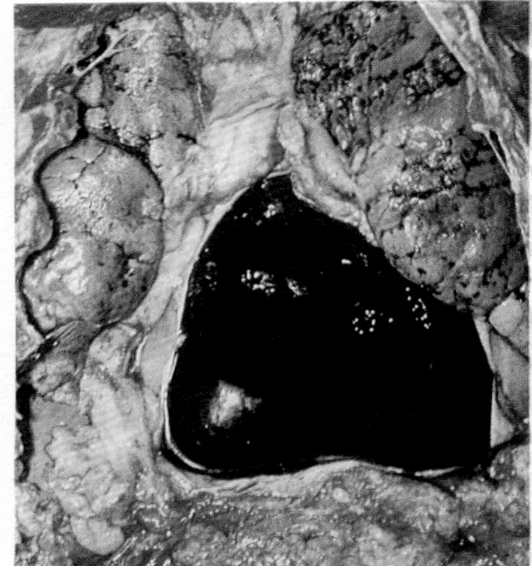

Figs. 2.31 and 2.32. Cardiac tamponade. Left: in-situ appearance. Right: opened pericardium.

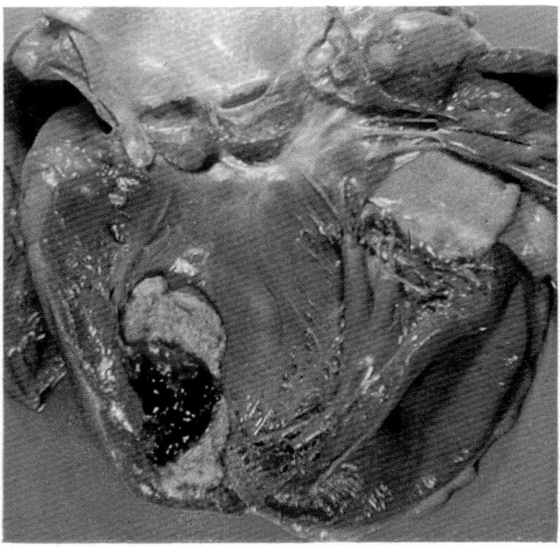

Fig. 2.33. Mural thrombi overlying the infarcted myocardium.

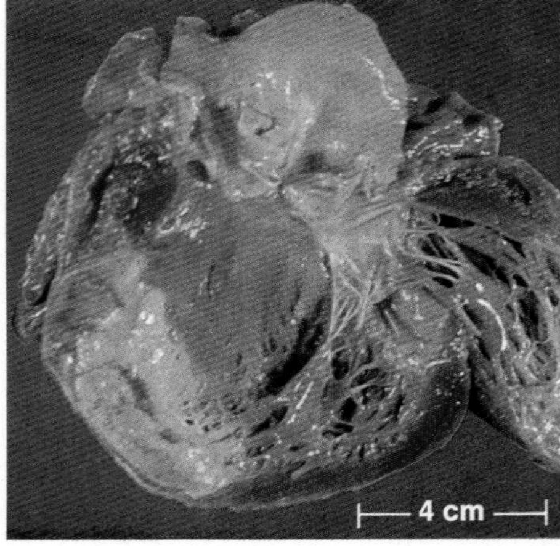

Fig. 2.34. Chronic aneurysm of the left ventricle.

Other causes of myocardial infarction are: emboli from endocarditis, very rare; *syphilis* with narrowing of the coronary artery ostia; coronary arteritis in, e.g., periarteritis nodosa; *intimal edema* in juveniles (?); traumatic factors: automobile accidents, chest wall trauma, shock, fall in blood pressure; coagulation defects, thrombus.

Co: acute cardiac insufficiency; drop in blood pressure with cardiac shock; attack of angina pectoris (5–60% are said to have no pains); atypical pain localization in upper abdomen. *DD:* perforated gastric ulcer: temperature, leukocytosis, pericardial friction rub. In 20% no EKG changes. Creatinine phosphokinase elevated in 80%. *Death* from electric heart failure (asystole, cardiac fibrillation), muscular failure, rupture, shock or secondary consequences (see Fig. 2.35).

Complications of myocardial infarction (Fig. 2.35).

Rupture of papillary muscles (Fig. 2.29). The posterior papillary muscle is ruptured in an area of yellow necrotic tissue (Fig. 2.35.1). Complete rupture leads to mitral insufficiency, thereby worsening the already damaged heart. Rupture of the myocardial wall is shown as a 2 cm.-long defect in the left ventricle (Figs. 2.30 and 2.35.2). At autopsy, the pericardial sac is distended and blue-red (Fig. 2.31). The opened pericardial sac is filled with black-red masses of clotted blood that compress the heart (*pericardial tamponade*, Fig. 2.32). Myocardial necrosis always leads to endocardial damage, which, together with hemodynamic cardiac changes (dilatation and release of tissue thrombokinase?), results in *parietal or mural thrombi* (Figs. 2.33 and 2.35.4). (Source for arterial emboli, which occurred in every other infarction prior to anticoagulation therapy, now reduced to every tenth infarction.) Red or gray-red, friable, firm thrombotic masses cover an acute aneurysm, as seen in Figure 2.33. The wall is weak and becomes dilated from the internal pressure. The *chronic aneurysm* has a thickened, fibrotic endocardial surface (the mural thrombus is organized by granulation tissue, which becomes fibrotic). The heart wall is dilated as in an aneurysm, often paper-thin and composed of scar tissue. Pericardial adhesions commonly cover the site of a previous infarction.

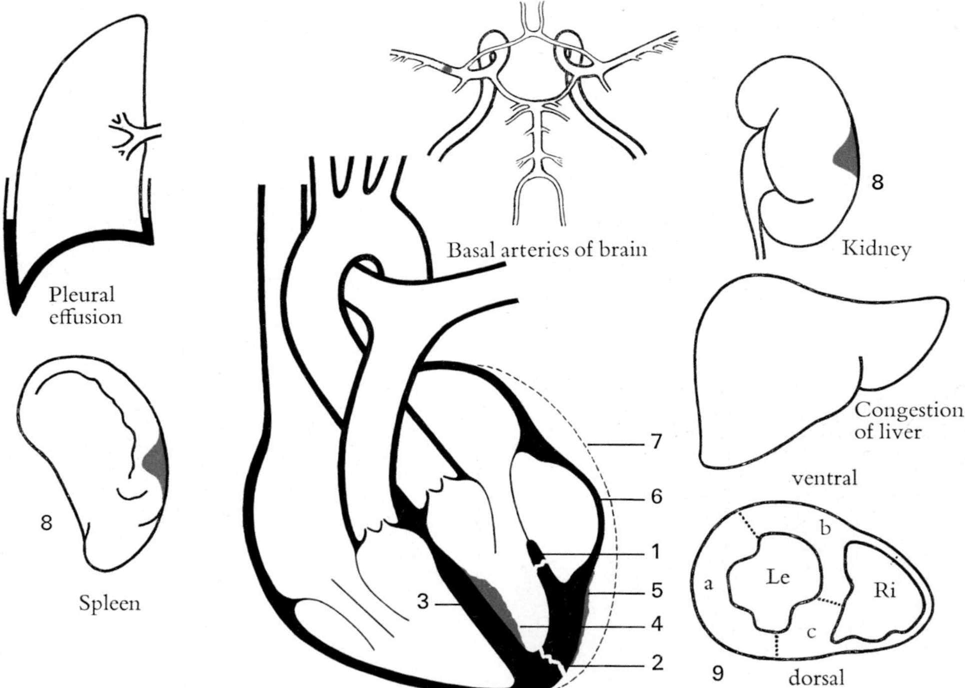

Fig. 2.35. *Complications of myocardial infarction:* (1) Rupture of papillary muscle. (2) Rupture of heart wall with tamponade (5–10% of infarctions). (3) Rupture of interventricular septum with acute cardiac failure. (4) Parietal (mural) thrombi. (5) Pericarditis. (6) Acute and chronic aneurysm. (7) Dilatation. (8) Infarctions of brain, kidneys, spleen, embolism to extremities (20%). (9) Vascular supply of heart: (a) circumflex branch of left coronary artery, (b) descending branch of left coronary artery, (c) right coronary artery.

Fig. 2.36. Coronary angiogram of a normal heart.

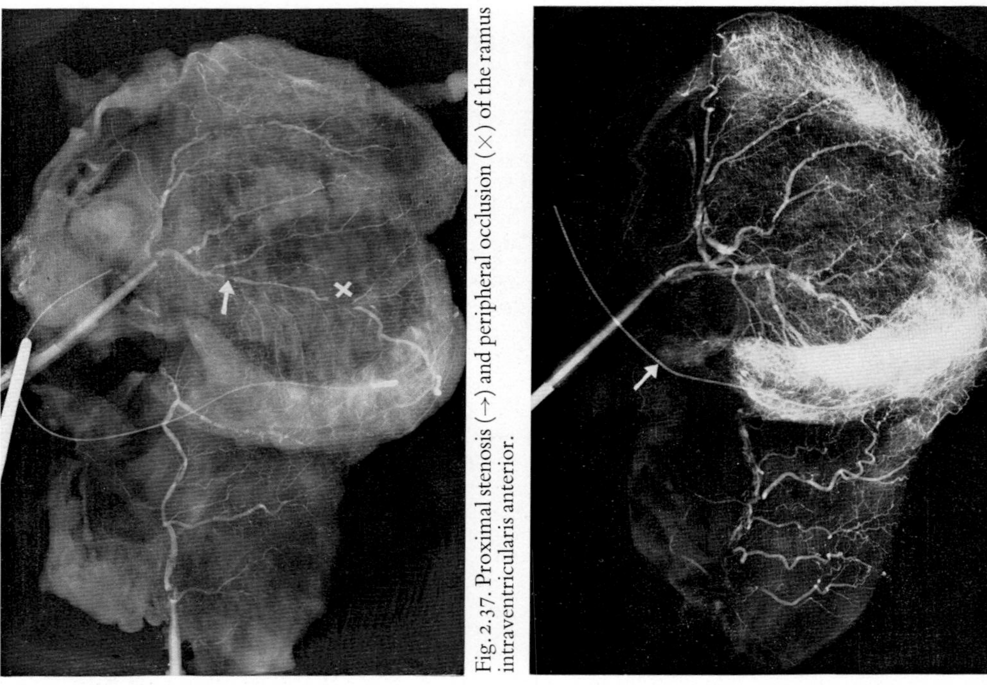

Fig. 2.37. Proximal stenosis (→) and peripheral occlusion (×) of the ramus intraventricularis anterior.

Fig. 2.38. Occlusion of the right coronary artery 5 cm after its descent from the aorta.

Fig. 2.39. Stenosing coronary sclerosis of all three large coronary artery branches.

Coronary Angiography

X-ray contrast representation of the coronary arteries presently makes possible a precise evaluation of the localization and the degree of constriction in coronary sclerosis in a patient. This technique is particularly important with respect to the possibility of operative revascularization in stenoses (so-called by-pass operation). The pathologist uses this technique post mortem, in order to be able to detect occlusions more easily.

Our figures show some examples of typical vascular occlusions which, in particular, are also intended to show the development of collaterals (up to a caliber of 50 μ in diameter). Figure 2.36 shows a normal heart (cut open; the right side of the heart is seen in the right of the photo, with a cannula at the descent of the right coronary artery from the aorta. The left side of the heart is shown on the right side of the picture). (1 = right coronary artery, 2 = ramus descendens dexter posterior, 3 = ramus interventricularis anterior, 4 = ramus circumflexus sinister). Figure 2.40 illustrates the area of spread of the left (green) and right coronary arteries of the unopened heart after filling with dyed barium sulfate (front view). A proximal stenosis (→) and a peripheral distal occlusion (×) of the ramus interventricularis anterior are shown in Figure 2.37. A detailed picture of this stenosis (constriction 70%) is shown in Figure 2.41. Occlusions of the right coronary artery are less frequent than those of the left. The consequences are largely determined by whether a so-called left supply type (21% of the hearts examined) or right supply type (9%) is present (68% normal distribution). An occlusion of the right coronary artery 5 cm (→) after its descent from the aorta (typical localization) is shown in Figure 2.38 and, in detail, in Figure 2.42. Note the numerous collaterals between left and right (×), through which a retrograde filling of the poststenotic region has taken place (→).

The worst prognosis is obtained for so-called "three-vessel diseases" (Fig. 2.39), with stenosing sclerosis of all three coronary arteries (right, left interventricular, and r. circumflexus). In this case, the anastomoses are particularly strongly developed as symptoms of the compensation in the case of severe oxygen deficiency of the myocardium. Note the pacemaker (→), the tip of whose probe is located in the right ventricle. Collaterals in the case of aortic stenosis, for example, are to be interpreted in the same way. The pressure in the aorta is greatly reduced (80–90 mm Hg), so that there is a reduced blood supply through the coronary arteries (ectatic coronary arteries, no coronary sclerosis!!). As a result of the cardiac atrophy, the vessels are dilated and the relative coronary insufficiency (O_2 deficiency) has led to the development of anastomoses.

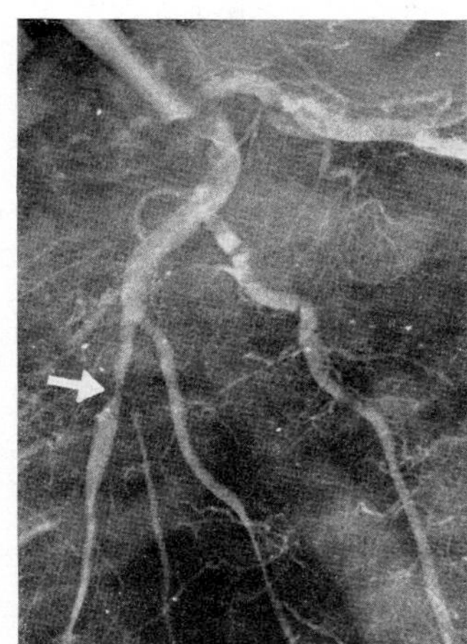

Fig. 2.41. Detail of the stenosis of Fig. 2.37.

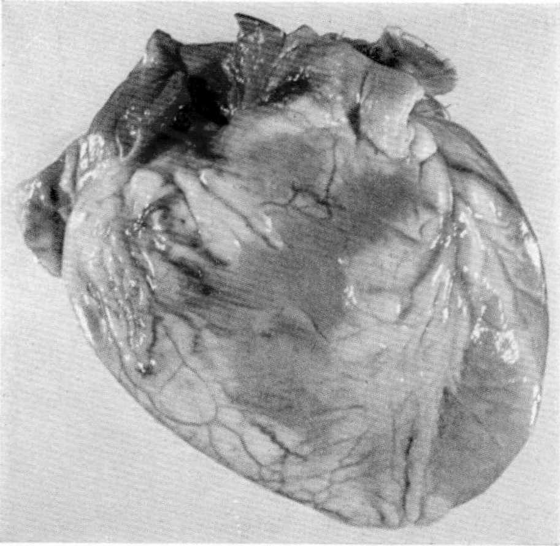

Fig. 2.40. Unopened heart. Representation of the coronary arteries with stained contrast medium: Left, green; right, red.

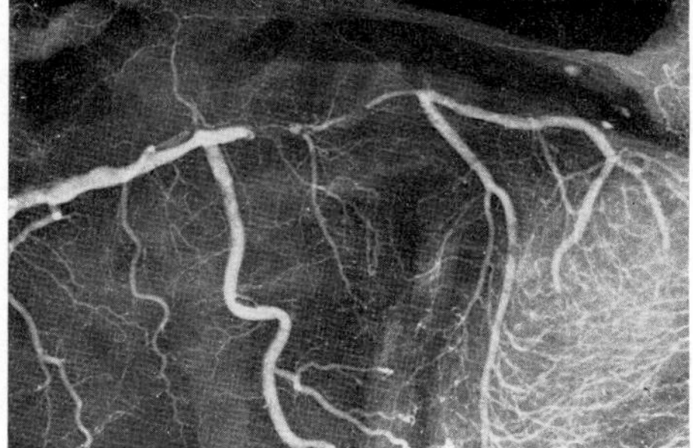

Fig. 2.42. Detail of the occlusion of Fig. 2.38.

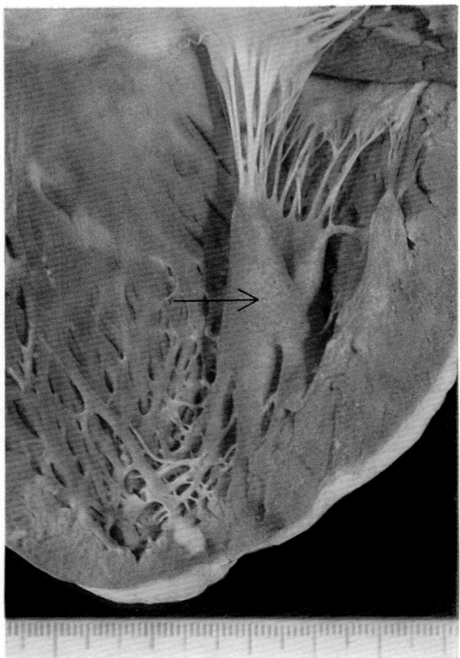

Fig. 2.43. Tigering of papillary muscles.

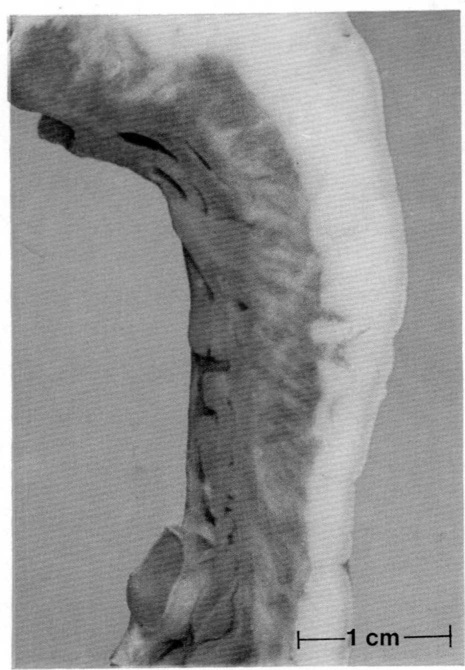

Fig. 2.44. Fatty infiltration (ingrowth).

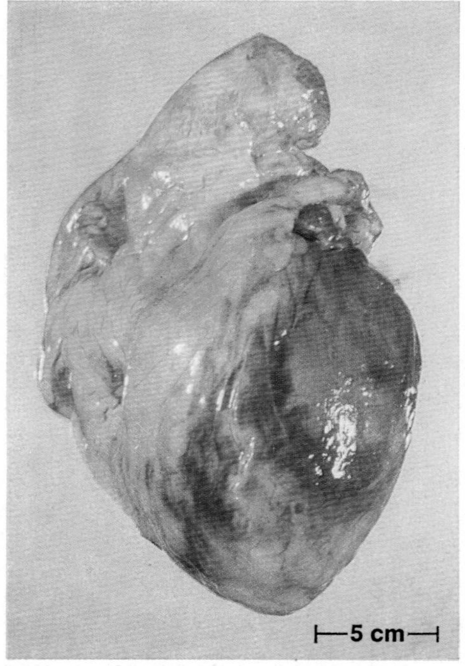

Fig. 2.45. Subepicardial hemorrhages.

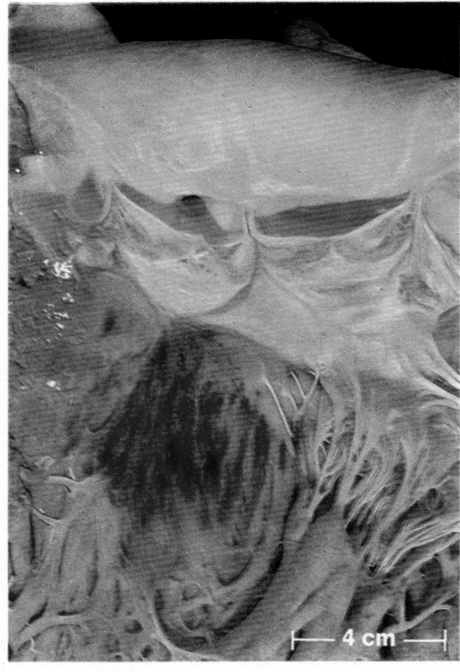

Fig. 2.46. Subendocardial hemorrhages.

Fatty degeneration of the myocardium (tigering of heart muscle, Fig. 2.43; TCP, p. 37). *Fatty metamorphosis of myocardial fibers caused by local or generalized anoxia.* Generalized hypoxia leads to tiger-skin-like markings in the myocardium, which, as seen in Figure 2.43, are especially prominent in subendocardial portions of the papillary muscles. Horizontal yellow bands anastomose with each other and alternate with brown-red muscle fibers.

Pg: the fatty areas correspond to the venous capillary loops in which O_2 content is low. Generalized hypoxia produced by high altitude, disturbances of pulmonary ventilation, anemia. *DD:* disseminated fatty degenerative foci may result from local hypoxia (spotty, yellow foci, e.g., with myocarditis) or toxic factors (diphtheria, scarlet fever, sepsis, mushroom poisoning, arsenicals, phosphorus). Phosphorus poisoning also causes fat phanerosis (release of structural fat after cytoplasmic damage → sarcolysis). Frequently, fatty degenerative changes also are seen microscopically at the margins of myocardial infarctions. *Cloudy swelling of heart muscle:* gray-red, cloudy myocardium with diminished consistency (difficult to photograph). *Hydropic degeneration:* cannot be diagnosed grossly.

Fatty infiltration of the heart (Fig. 2.44; TCP, p. 37). *Increase in the subepicardial fat tissue with infiltration of the myocardium.* A broad band of subepicardial fat tissue is seen in the dissected right ventricle near the pulmonary conus. Streaks of yellow fat extend between the muscle fibers. Subendocardial fat tissue also can occur, especially in the left ventricle.

Pg: increase in fat cells and transformation of connective tissue into adipose tissue. Therefore, no "infiltration" but rather local metaplasia. Obesity, see page 217.

Subepicardial hemorrhages occur as petechiae (small spots) or ecchymoses (larger, ill-defined foci). Figure 2.45 was obtained from a case of myeloid leukemia. Dark red, ill-defined ecchymoses partly coalesce in the subepicardial fat.

Pg: diapedesis of erythrocytes through the intact venule (bleeding per diapedesis). Bleeding per rhexis: bleeding due to rupture, e.g., apoplexy. *Causative factors:* increased pressure, slow blood flow or coagulation defects, e.g., in shock, liver cirrhosis, platelet deficiency, hypoprothrombinemia, etc. *Vascular factors:* damage of the capillary wall? Polycythemia vera rubra. Death from suffocation causes petechial hemorrhages in the heart, thymus and pleura.

Subendocardial hemorrhages (Fig. 2.43). Characteristically seen as streaky, longitudinal hemorrhages in the subaortic portions of the left ventricle. Subendocardial hemorrhages and hemorrhagic erosions in the stomach are diagnostic of increased intracranial pressure.

Cardiac atrophy (TCP, p. 35). An atrophic, a normal and a hypertrophic heart are compared in Figure 2.47. The weight of the atrophic heart is reduced (to 90 Gm.). The heart is of normal shape but the muscle mass is diminished. Note the brown color (see TCP, p. 35).

Pg: diminution in the length and width of fibers, also loss of fibers (simple and numerical atrophy). Observed in senility, malnutrition (hunger), tuberculosis, carcinomas, cachexia, physical inactivity, drop in blood pressure and Addison's disease. *DD:* the coronary arteries of a constitutionally small heart ("droplet heart") are straight but are tortuous in an atrophic heart (coronary arteries are too long). In addition, serous atrophy of the subepicardial fat, i.e., loss of fat cells and interstitial edema. A gray-dirty, soft-elastic tissue replaces the fat tissue.

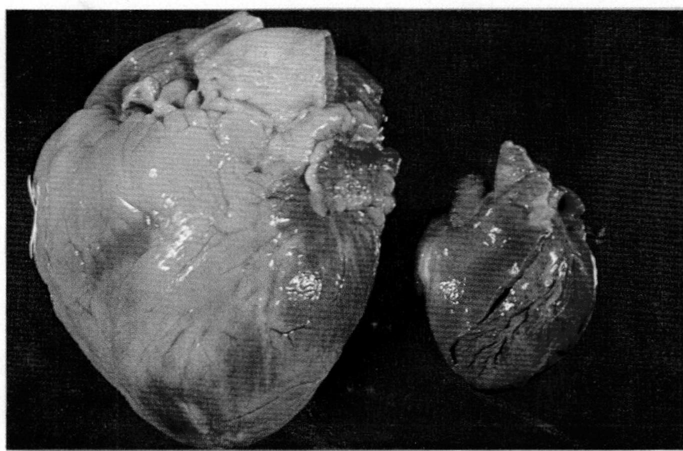

Fig. 2.47. Atrophic and hypertrophic hearts.

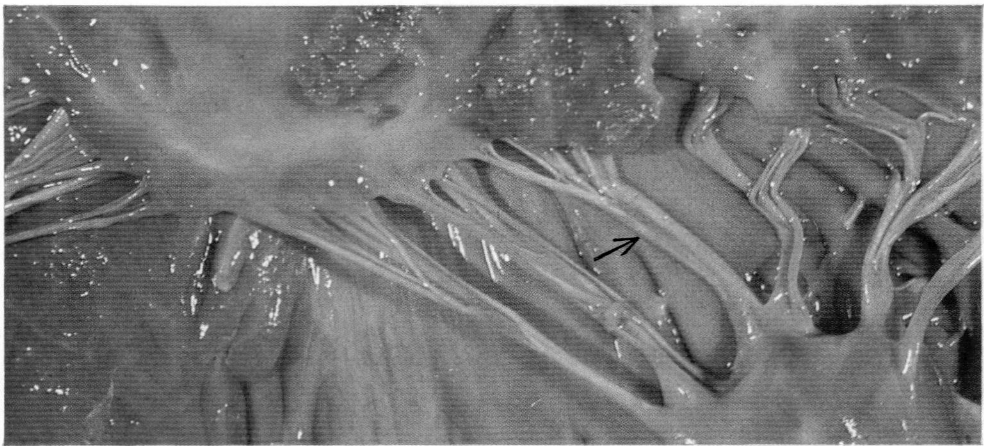

Fig. 2.48. Verrucous endocarditis of the mitral valve.

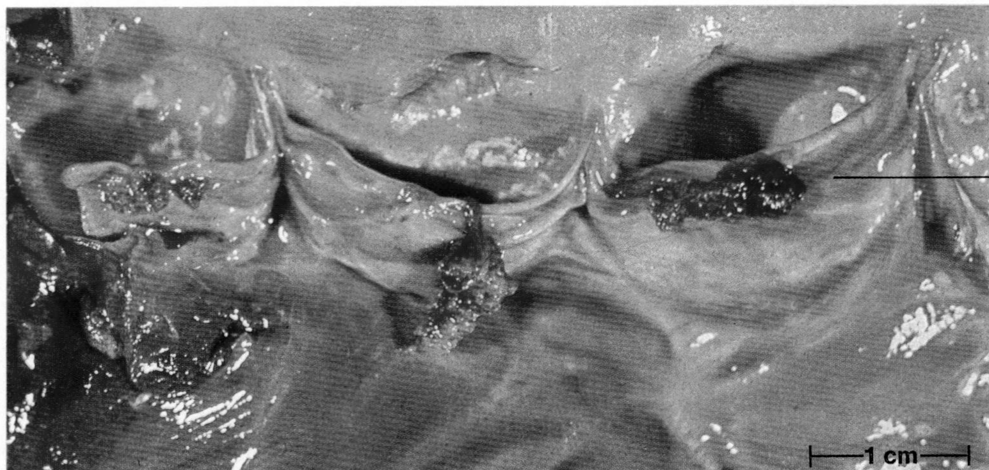

Fig. 2.49. Thrombotic-polypoid endocarditis of the aortic valve.

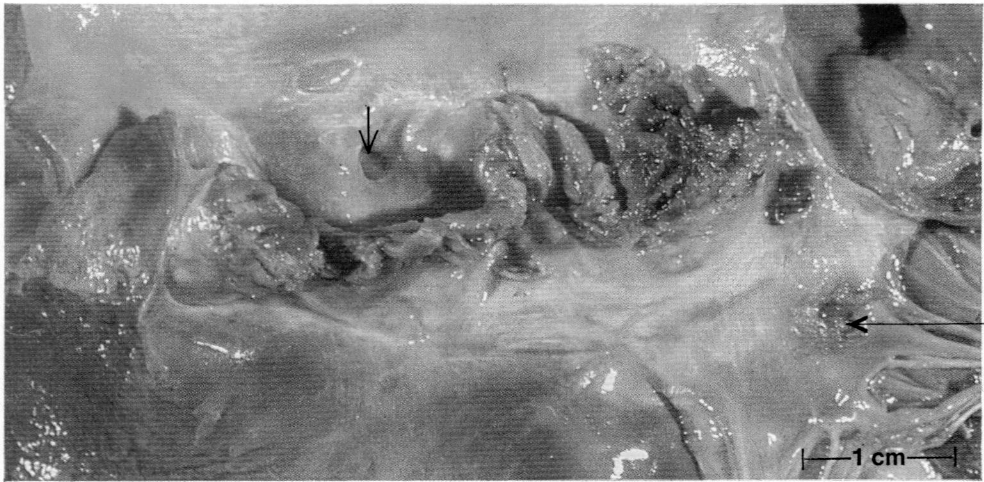

Fig. 2.50. Thrombotic, ulcerative endocarditis of the aortic valve.

Endocarditis

Nonbacterial or bacterial diseases of the cardiac valves leading to thrombotic vegetations, valve destruction or deformities.

Verrucous, marantic endocarditis (Fig. 2.48). *Nonbacterial verrucous endocarditis near or at the closing margins of the valve leaflets (mostly mitral or aortic valves, deposition of platelet thrombi).* Figure 2.48 shows gray or light gray-red, glassy vegetations at the closing margin. The verrucae are easily wiped off. The thrombi extend from the center of the valve to the chordae tendineae. The chordae are partly fused (→recurrent endocarditis).

F: rare, *A:* 60 years, *S:* ♂ = ♀, *Pg:* endothelial damage, "copying" of circulating blood platelet aggregates during valve closure. *Cf* (causative factors): found very frequently in shock or in hypercoagulability of different origins (e.g., cachexia, endocarditis marantica, in tumors: paraneoplastic "tumor endocarditis") (see Mittermayer et al., 1971; Thomas, 1974).

Thrombotic (polypoid) endocarditis (Fig. 2.49). Large, red to gray-red, polypoid, soft vegetations adhere to the aortic valve (→line of closure). *Nonbacterial: Libman-Sacks'* endocarditis of disseminated lupus erythematosus (see p. 220). A *bacterial* valvulitis develops when the causative organisms are of moderate virulence and host defense is impaired, as in our case. Transition into thrombotic-ulcerative endocarditis is possible.

Thrombotic-ulcerative endocarditis (Fig. 2.50). An *ulcerative endocarditis* is the result of a massive bacteremia [staphylococci (30% of the cases) and streptococci (50% of the cases)]. It is characterized by valvular ulcerations without formation of thrombi. *Thrombotic-ulcerative endocarditis* usually is caused by *Streptococcus viridans.* Fifty per cent of the cases are associated with a focal, embolic glomerulonephritis. Other organisms also can cause thrombotic ulcerative endocarditis. Figure 2.50 shows destruction of the aortic valve, especially of the posterior cusp, beneath the ostium of the right coronary artery (→). To the right of the coronary ostium, the cusp is ruptured and covered by thrombotic vegetations. Some thrombotic masses are dark green discolored (H_2S formation by bacteria during or after life). Note that the vegetations have extended to the posterior mitral leaflet (→in Fig. 2.50). Such a "touch infection" leads to ulceration and fibrin deposition.

Bacterial endocarditis. *F:* 3–10% of autopsies. *A:* 30–40 years. *S:* ♂ = ♀; according to some authors, 3:1. *Pg:* bacteria are implanted on the most exposed portions of the valves (closing margins). Eighty to ninety per cent of patients have experienced a previous rheumatic endocarditis. *Co:* see Figure 2.51. Mortality 20–50%. A valvular aneurysm may develop following healing of bacterial endocarditis. The clinical diagnosis is made in 45% of the cases. In 67% of the cases, only the aortic valves are affected.

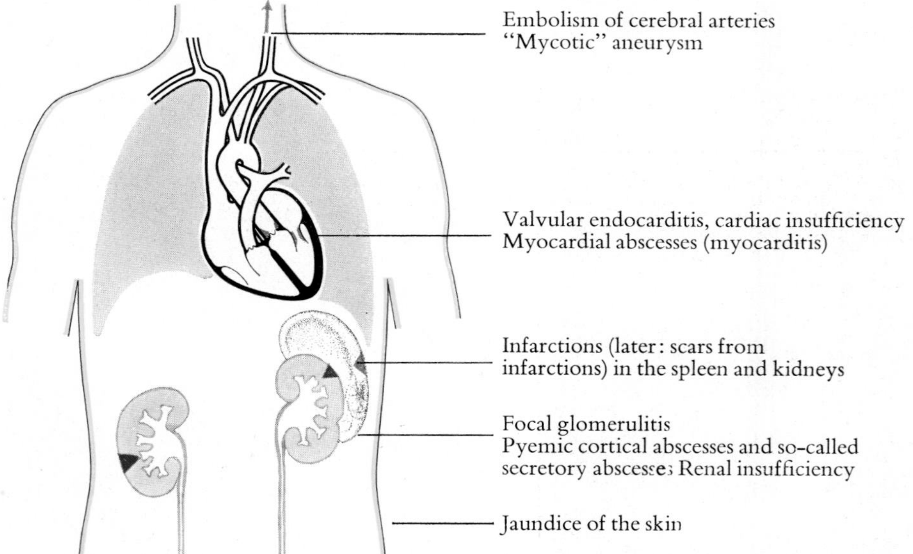

Fig. 2.51. Schematic presentation of complications arising from endocarditis.

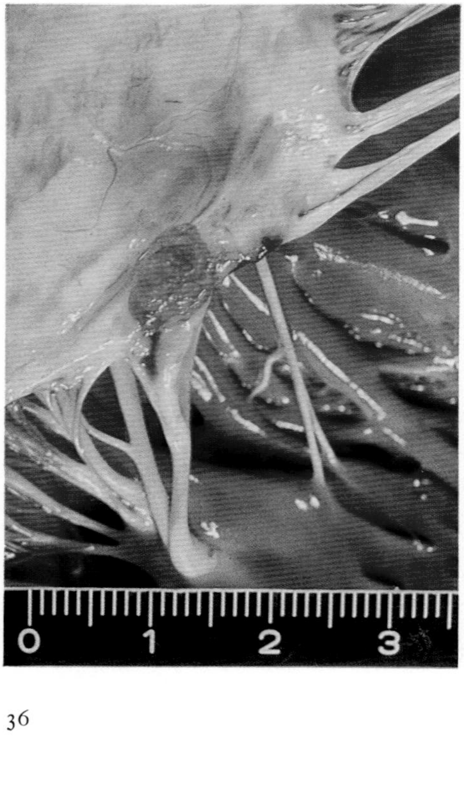

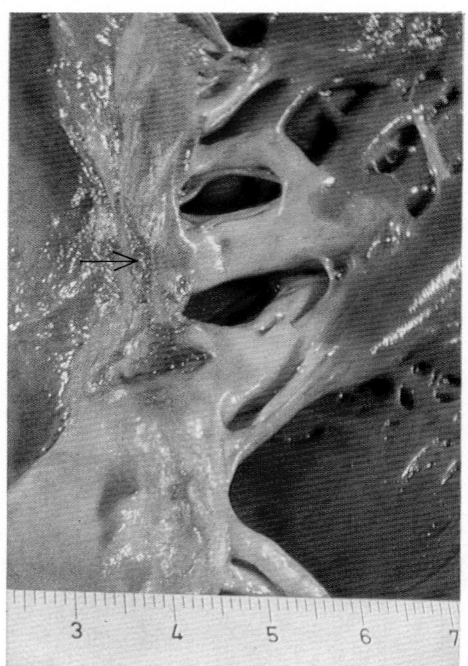

Figs. 2.52 and 2.53. Recurrent rheumatic endocarditis. Left: fresh vegetation. Right: thickened and retracted chordae tendineae.

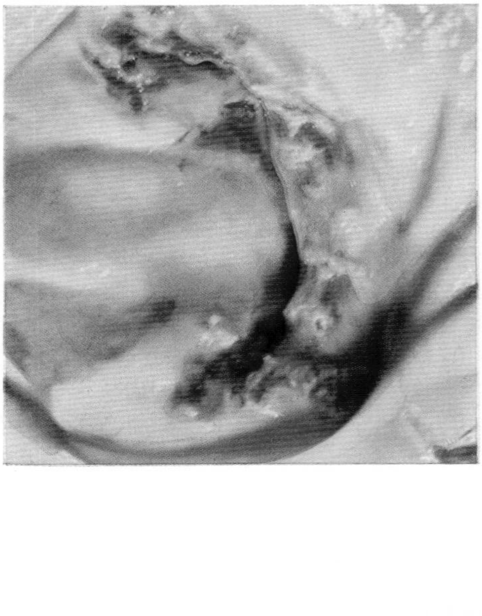

Fig. 2.54. Mitral stenosis after endocarditis.

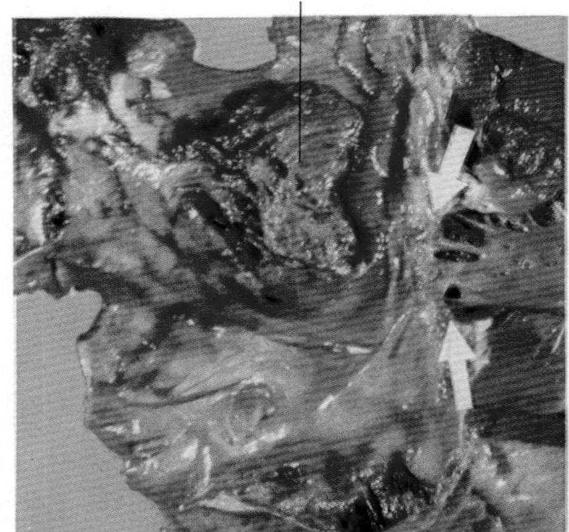

Fig. 2.55. Mitral stenosis with mural atrial thrombus.

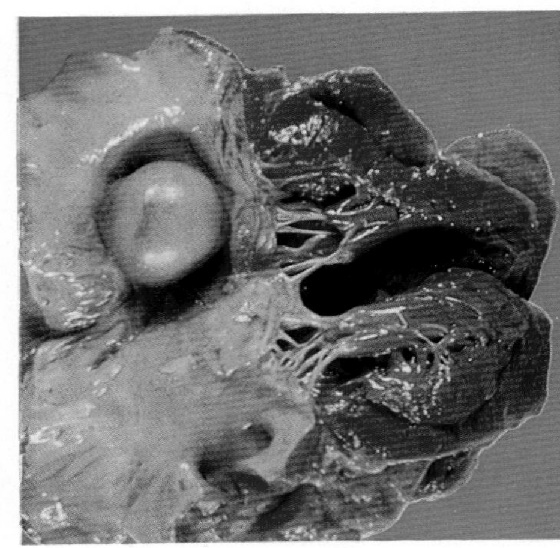

Fig. 2.56. Mitral stenosis with ball-valve thrombus.

Rheumatic Endocarditis, Valve Defects

A nonbacterial endocarditis that develops during the course of rheumatic fever and leads to valvular deformities (due to granulation tissue and scarring) (TCP, p. 49).

A fresh rheumatic endocarditis is characterized by gray-white, glassy, wart-like vegetations along the lines of closure (as in Fig. 2.48). The vegetations frequently extend to the atrial endocardium and chordae tendineae (Fig. 2.53). A recurring, verrucous rheumatic endocarditis is shown in Figure 2.52. A gray-red, tawny platelet thrombus is attached to the mitral valve. *Blood vessels* that indicate organization of platelet thrombi from an earlier endocarditis are clearly identified in the leaflet. The disease has further progressed to a recurring endocarditis, as shown in Figure 2.53. The mitral leaflets are markedly thickened, white, of firm consistency and rigid (scar tissue). Note the *pipe-like* changes in the chordae tendineae (see also Fig. 2.55). The chordae are not only thickened and rigid (due to fusion from the inflammation, which extends from the valve to the chordae) but also markedly shortened (insufficiency). The atrial endocardium is similarly thickened and white (endocardial fibrosis). A fresh, recurrent inflammatory focus with gray-red, partially organized thrombi has developed (→). In addition, a flat artifactual ulceration is seen in the center of this picture.

Mitral stenosis is the result of transverse shrinkage of the valve (or fusion of cusps) (Fig. 2.60). Figure 2.54 shows a case of mitral stenosis viewed from above. The lumen of the mitral valve resembles a small slit that permits little blood to pass through. The yellow and gray-red, irregular excrescences are caused by secondary calcium and lipid deposits in the scar tissue of the valve (superimposed arteriosclerosis). Note also the almost porcelain-white endocardial fibrosis of the atrium.

Atrial endocardial fibrosis may be confined to an area just above the mitral valve (McCallum's patch).

The sequelae of mitral stenosis are best appreciated after the heart has been opened (Fig. 2.55). The mitral valve diameter is reduced from 11 cm. to 4 cm. The white arrows point to the lateral margins of the unopened mitral valve (buttonhole or fish-mouth stenosis). The chordae are shortened and thickened. The greatly dilated atrium contains a fresh, layered mural thrombus (→). The atrial endocardium is thick and fibrotic.

Figure 2.56 demonstrates another heart with mitral stenosis. The dilated atrium contains an organized round thrombus. A valve-like occlusion of the mitral ostium (ball-valve thrombus) and sudden cardiac death are the result of a dislodged atrial thrombus. The left ventricle is atrophic because of reduced work load.

The same gross picture is observed in stenosis of the aortic valve (Figs. 2.57 and 2.58). The cusps are markedly thickened, white and project like rigid sails into the lumen. The aortic ostium is narrowed so that a triangular lumen is formed (aortic stenosis and insufficiency) (Fig. 2.57). Aortic stenosis is the result of fusion of the cusps at the closing margins and shrinkage of the fused cusps in a transverse direction (Fig. 2.60). Figure 2.58 illustrates fusion of two cusps (the two upper cusps in this picture); the lower cusp is not fused. The functional effect is stenosis. The arrow in Figure 2.58 points to a fenestrated aortic cusp above the line of closure that was without functional significance.

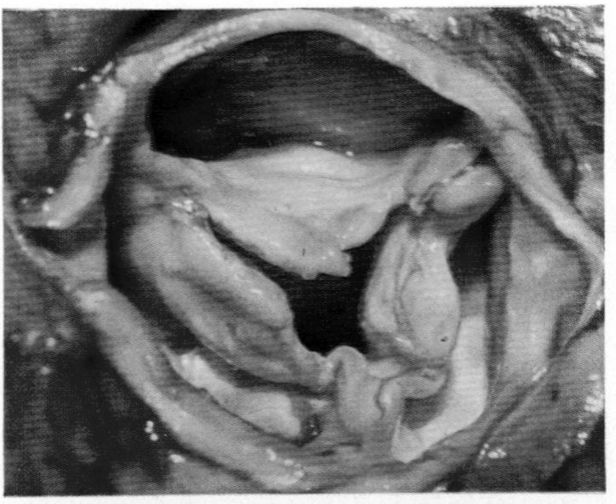

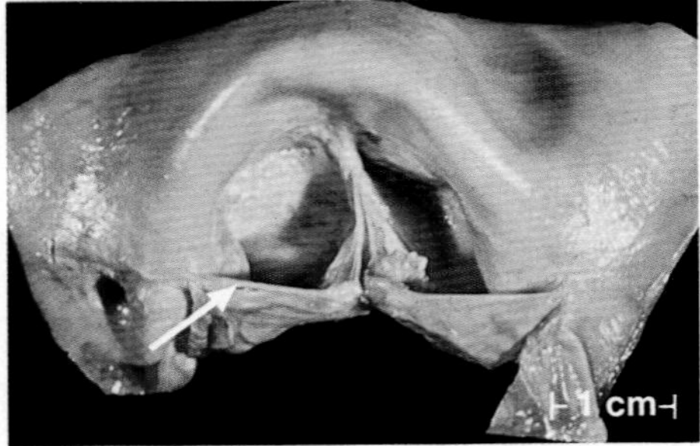

Fig. 2.57 (above) and Fig. 2.58 (below). Fusion of aortic cusps following endocarditis.

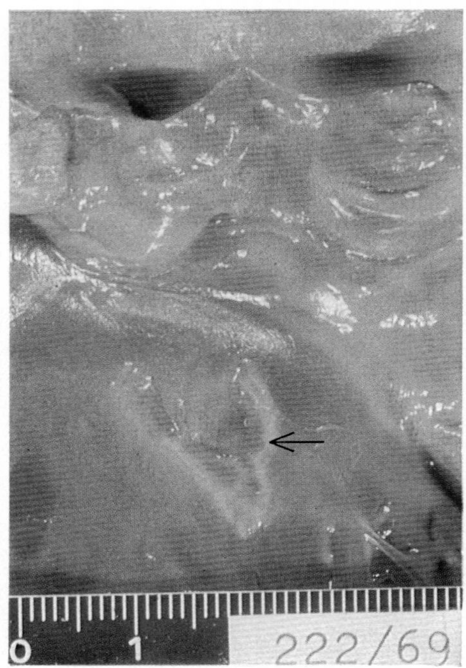

Fig. 2.59. Zahn's insufficiency sign (or pocket).

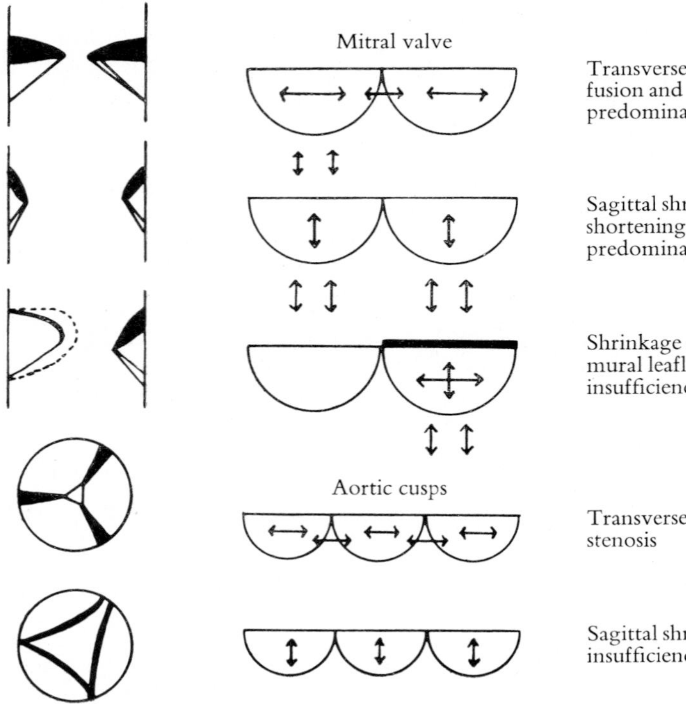

Fig. 2.60. Acquired cardiac valvular defects.

The opened heart with aortic insufficiency shows the shrinkage of the cusps, i.e., the shortening of the cusps in a sagittal direction (Fig. 2.59). Severe aortic insufficiency is diagnosed grossly by *Zahn's insufficiency sign* (Fig. 2.59): Aortic blood regurgitates during diastole, enters the left ventricle and causes focal endocardial fibrosis approximately 1 cm. beneath the aortic valve. This area of fibrosis has a semicircular shape and may transform into a pocket, as shown in Figure 2.59 (→).

Summary of acquired valve deformities (Fig. 2.60).

F: 50% of children with rheumatic fever develop valve deformities. The deformities usually become manifest between 30 and 40 years, although rheumatic endocarditis has a peak incidence between 5 and 15 years.

Mitral stenosis: transverse shrinkage and fusion of leaflets. The mitral ostium is round, rectangular, semicircular or slit-like. *Co:* dilatation and hypertrophy of the left atrium, atrophy of the left ventricle, severe chronic congestion of the lungs, dilatation and hypertrophy of the right ventricle, often relative tricuspid insufficiency. *Clinically:* relatively late complaints. *F:* 2% of autopsies.

Mitral insufficiency: sagittal shrinkage of leaflets and shortening of chordae tendineae. *Co:* blood regurgitates from the left atrium and enters the left ventricle during diastole. During systole, blood is pumped into the left atrium. The end effects are increased left ventricular volume, hypertrophy and dilatation of the left ventricle and congested peripheral organs. *Clinically:* relatively early complaints with diminished work capacity. *Variation:* occasionally, only the posterior (mural) leaflet is shrunken. This can lead to a "functional spontaneous healing" when the anterior mitral leaflet becomes dilated, thereby restoring proper closure of the mitral valve (dotted line in Fig. 2.60).

Aortic stenosis: fusion and transverse shrinkage of the cusps. *Co:* marked hypertrophy of the left ventricle (increased resistance during systole!), later dilatation and insufficiency, congestion of peripheral organs and poststenotic dilatation of the aorta. *Cl:* coronary insufficiency, since the pressure in the aorta is reduced (see Fig. 2.58).

Aortic insufficiency: shrinkage of cusps in a sagittal direction with Zahn's insufficiency sign. Severe hypertrophy and dilatation of the left ventricle, increased cardiac stroke volume (up to 200 ml.; normal 100 ml.). Increased and excessive volume of blood. *Clinically:* decompensation occurs earlier than in stenosis. Marked blood pressure amplitude.

Tricuspid stenosis or insufficiency and pulmonary stenosis are rare.

Rheumatism

Rheumatism is a generic term for various joint and muscle diseases. For a more precise definition of "rheumatism," the following classification should be kept in mind:

I. *Inflammatory rheumatic diseases* (probably immunologic in origin).
   1. *Rheumatic fever* (acute joint disease with fever and rheumatic pancarditis) (see below).
   2. *Rheumatoid arthritis* (also known as primary, chronic polyarthritis). Affects predominantly the small joints of females, 40–50 years of age (see p. 221).
   3. *Ankylosing spondylitis* (Bechterew's disease). The vertebral column of young males is affected (see p. 221).
   4. *Special forms:*
      a) *Chauffard-Still syndrome:* Atypical chronic polyarthritis in infancy (starts during the 2nd to 4th year of life) with symmetrical articular swellings (first the small, then the large joints) and hydrarthroses with granulocytes. Later ankyloses. General lymph node swellings, splenic tumor. No endocarditis. Generally streptococcal infections. Secondary amyloidosis.
      b) *Felty's syndrome:* Adult form of the Chauffard-Still syndrome.
      c) Arthritis in cases of *psoriasis, ulcerative colitis, Crohn's disease.*

II. *Degenerative rheumatism.* Primary degenerative disease of intervertebral disks and cartilage (see p. 203).

III. *So-called soft-part rheumatism.* Plays the greatest quantitative role in medical practice. Investiga tions by FASSBENDER have shown that the destruction of individual skeletal muscle fibers (myolysis) can be detected by electron microscopy, with little or no inflammatory reaction. The tendinous tissue, the synovial sheaths, bursae and articular capsules can also be affected in the form of a proliferation of fibroblasts (no inflammation).

Rheumatic fever is a systemic disease affecting the heart (pancarditis), large joints (migratory polyarthritis) and connective tissue. The disease is caused by infection with group A hemolytic streptococci (more than 50 different serotypes) and affects children or adolescents (peak incidence 8–20 years). Chief complaints are fever and migratory joint pains. Fibrinoid necrosis of collagen fibers, formation of granulomas (in the myocardium: Aschoff body) and fibrosis are morphologic manifestations of rheumatic fever. The inflammatory joint disease heals. High antistreptolysin titer. The heart is involved in 90% of the cases.

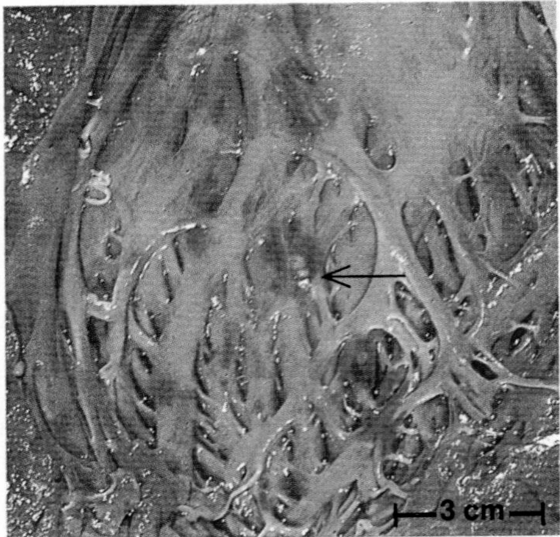

Fig. 2.61. Pyemic myocardial abscesses.

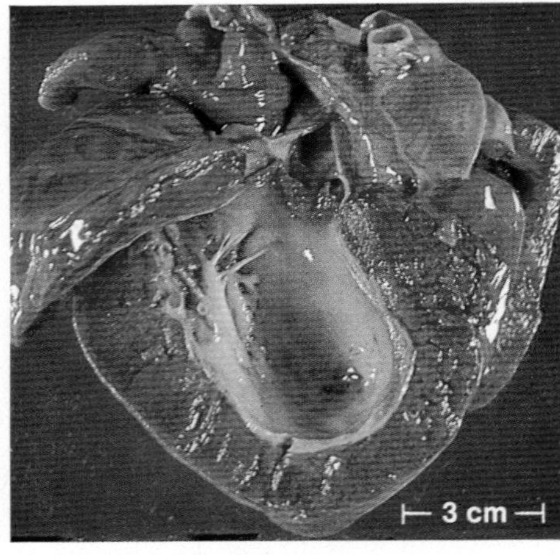

Fig. 2.62. Endocardial fibroelastosis.

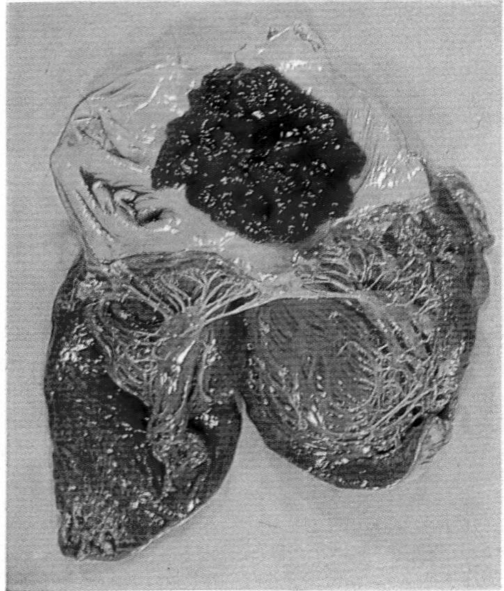

Fig. 2.63. Myxoma of the left atrium.

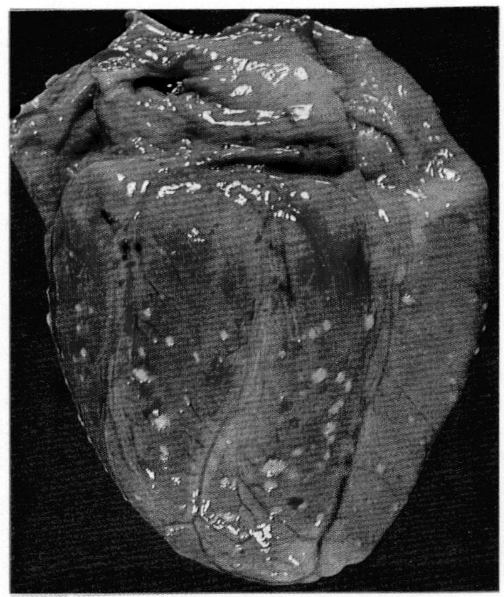

Fig. 2.64. Myocardial metastases from a bronchial carcinoma.

Myocarditis (Fig. 2.61; TCP, p. 45).

Pyemic myocardial abscesses in a case of bacterial, thrombotic-ulcerative endocarditis are shown as an example of myocarditis. The slightly elevated, yellow subendocardial foci (abscesses) measure 2–3 mm. in diameter. They are surrounded by a red zone (hemorrhagic zone of demarcation →). Yellow pus exudes from the abscess during cutting. Other forms of myocarditis are difficult to diagnose grossly. The heart usually is dilated. The myocardium is pale and contains gray to gray-yellow, indistinct foci. Tiny white scars are seen in a healed or chronic myocarditis.

F: 2–3%; others up to 10%. *A:* children predominate. Cases of myocarditis can be classified according to different points of view: (a) according to causes (frequently unknown), (b) according to the histological picture, (c) according to the manner of development: hematogenous, lymphogenous, from the environment, (d) according to the "unity of disease" (DOERR).

We prefer a subdivision according to the pathological-histological appearance:

1. *Serous myocarditis*, for example shock, burns.
2. *Purulent myocarditis* (frequently embolic).
3. *Non-purulent interstitial myocarditis:*
   a) *Toxic* (diphtheria type). Degenerative changes predominate. The right ventricular wall is predominantly affected (Fig. 2.65).
   b) *Infection-allergic myocarditis* (scarlet fever type) with lymphohistiocytic infiltration. Appears in the third week of illness after feverish infections. Most frequent form of myocarditis. The right ventricular wall is predominantly affected.
   c) *Granulomatous myocarditis: Rheumatic myocarditis* with Aschoff's nodes. The left heart is affected. *Idiopathic myocarditis* (giant-cell myocarditis, so-called Fiedler's myocarditis). Predominantly affects the left heart.
   d) *Necrotizing myocarditis, mostly viral myocarditis* (Coxsackie virus, rubella, smallpox). The left heart and ventricular septum are affected. For *Chagas' myocarditis*, see Mı.

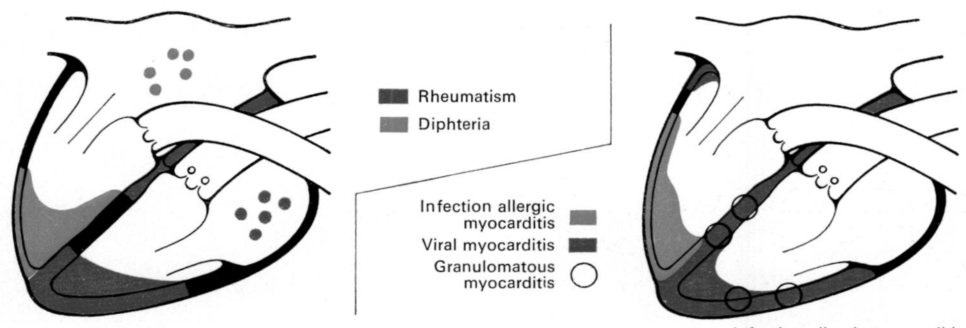

Fig. 2.65. Pattern of propagation of myocarditis (after Doerr).

Endocardial fibroelastosis is characterized by the *formation of a hyaline layer in the endocardium. This disease is of unknown etiology*. Figure 2.62 shows a white layer that covers the left ventricular endocardium, including the papillary muscles. This layer resembles a sugar coat. Although the valves are not involved in this case, they may be affected in 50% of the cases. The endocardial layer is approximately 2–3 mm. thick and sharply demarcated from the underlying muscle. The left ventricle is markedly hypertrophic (interpreted as work hypertrophy: the heart has to work against the increased resistance of the firm endocardium). Histologically, there is an increase in collagenous and elastic fibers beneath the endocardium. The collagenous tissue occasionally extends between superficial muscle fibers.

F: rare (approximately 200 cases described). *Pr:* poor. Children rarely survive beyond 1 year of age. *Pg:* suspected are malformations, hypoxia and transplacental damage. *Endocarditis parietalis fibroplastica* (Löffler) is interpreted as a healed fetal endocarditis. The endocardium is covered by granulation tissue, many eosinophilic leukocytes and thrombi. The cardiac valves usually are free. The disease heals with scarring. Seen also as secondary disease after scarlet fever, rheumatic fever and other infectious diseases. *DD:* endocardial, valvular and atrial fibrosis with the carcinoid syndrome always affects the right ventricle and tricuspid valve (serotonin effect).

Myxoma or pseudomyxoma of the left atrium is a benign "tumor" usually located in the atrial endocardium near the foramen ovale. Figure 2.63 shows a glassy, red-brown, round, pedunculated, papillary mass that measures several centimeters in diameter. Histologically, the endocardium is covered by myxomatous tissue. Elongated, star-like cells are embedded in a ground substance rich in mucopolysaccharides. Hemosiderin frequently is found in the myxomatous tissue.

F: rare. *Pg:* true myxoma (neoplasm) or myxomatous changes in an atrial thrombus ("pseudomyxoma")? *Co:* the entire tumor or parts thereof may dislodge and occlude the ostium of the mitral valve (ball-valve effect).

Myocardial metastases from bronchogenic carcinoma (Fig. 2.64). Myocardial tumor metastases are rare in contrast to metastases in the epicardium and pericardium. Several gray-white, medium-firm, irregular metastatic foci (up to 0.5 cm.) are seen in the myocardium and subepicardial tissue of Figure 2.64. The tumor was an oat-cell carcinoma of the lung.

F: 8% of all malignant tumors metastasize to the heart. *Pg:* lymphogenous or hematogenous spread from bronchogenic, mammary or thyroid carcinomas. Malignant melanomas, sarcomas and leukemias likewise.

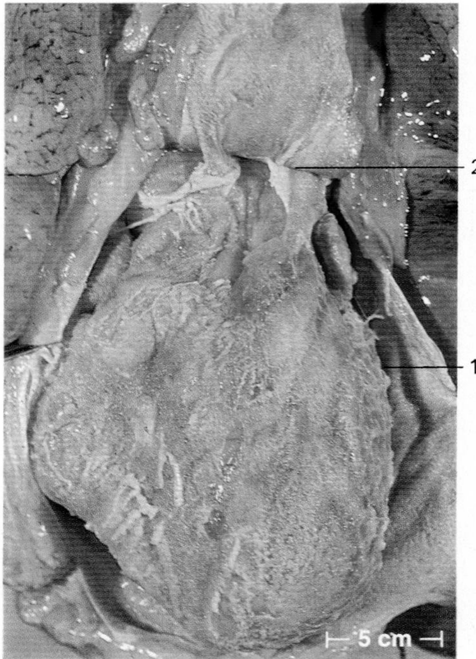

Fig. 2.66. "Bread-and-butter" pericarditis.

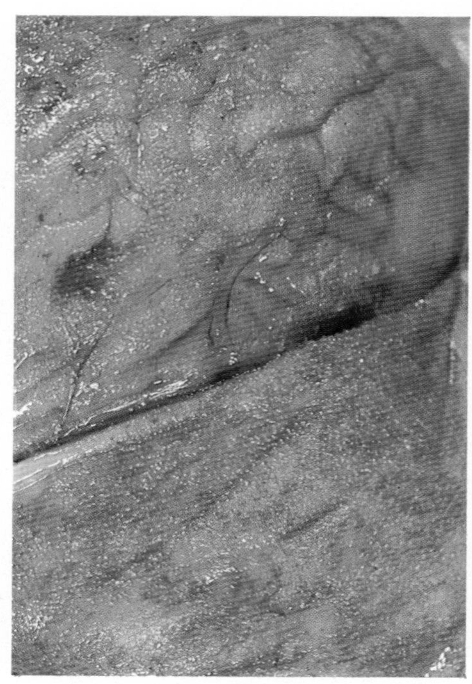

Fig. 2.67. Fibrinous pericarditis.

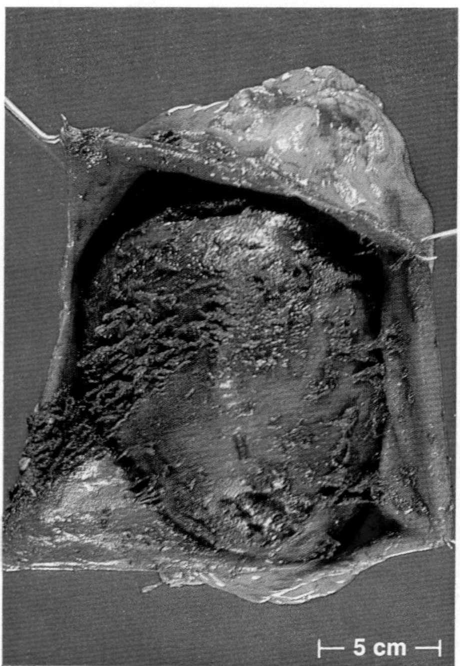

Fig. 2.68. Hemorrhagic pericarditis.

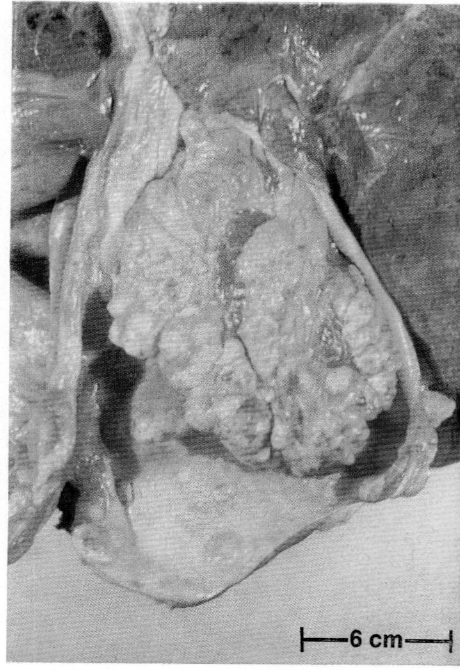

Fig. 2.69. Pericardial and epicardial metastases from a bronchogenic carcinoma.

Pericarditis

According to the type of exudate, pericardial inflammations are divided into fibrinous, serofibrinous, hemorrhagic or purulent (empyema) pericarditis (TCP, pp. 51–55). The pericardium of a fibrinous pericarditis is no longer glistening and smooth but is dull (Figs. 2.65 and 2.66). Gray-white, glassy fibrin deposits sometimes are arranged as horizontal lines (→1). Heavy fibrinous membranes can be removed easily (→2). Shaggy strands or clumps of fibrin give the appearance of "bread-and-butter" pericarditis. A layer of connective tissue is present after recurrent pericarditis as so-called concretio pericardii. In tuberculous pericarditis, calcification results in the so-called plaster mold heart. Consequence: blockage of inflow because of inhibition of the diastole.

Pg: see Figure 2.70. Inflammatory diseases from surrounding organs or myocardial diseases extend lymphogenously or hematogenously into the pericardium. *Cl:* in pericarditis sicca (without exudate), the rubbing can be heard with the stethoscope (see also pleuritis).

Hemorrhagic pericarditis (Fig. 2.68). The pericardial sac was opened. Both pericardial surfaces are covered with dark red to black fibrin. The fibrin deposits are arranged as horizontal ridges or lines that run perpendicular to the long axis of the heart. The horizontal lines form by compression of fibrin during heart contraction.

Mi: fibrin exudation and erythrocytes, often with hemorrhagic effusion. *Pg:* uremia, pericardial carcinomatosis or tuberculosis.

Pericardial carcinomatosis in a case of a bronchial oat-cell carcinoma (Fig. 2.69). Lymphogenous metastases from lung hilar lymph nodes infiltrate the pericardium. The process usually starts in the epicardium of the pulmonary artery. Very small, white subepicardial metastatic foci are seen initially. Later on, they grow into gray-white nodules that may encase the heart.

Hemopericardium (see Fig. 2.32). Occurs after myocardial rupture (infarction, trauma) and rupture of a dissecting aneurysm of the aorta.

Pneumopericardium occurs after trauma, perforated gastric ulcers, pulmonary abscesses or inflammations due to gas-forming bacteria.

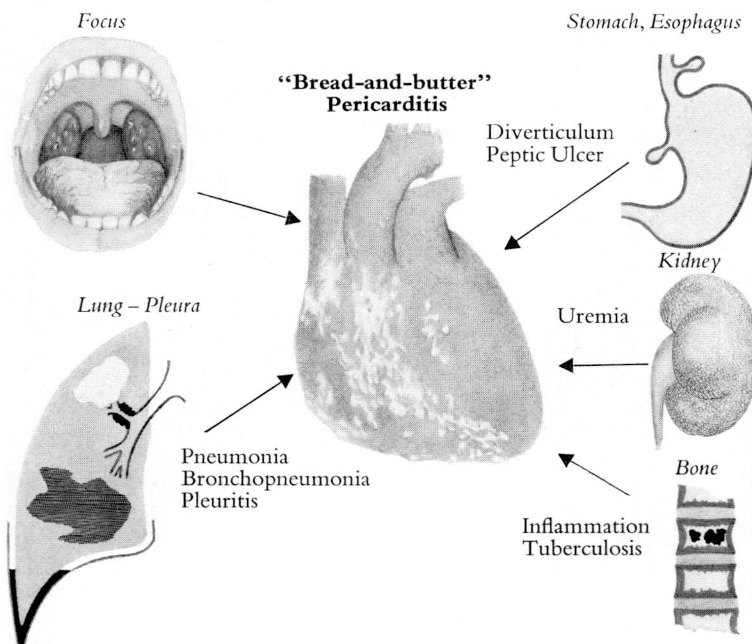

Fig. 2.70. Schematic presentation of the causes of pericarditis.

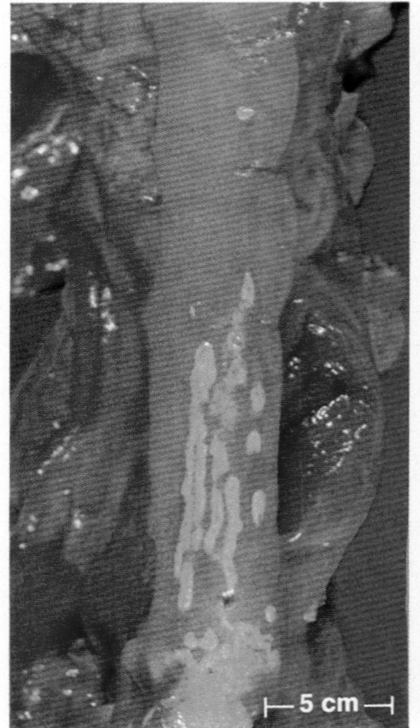

Fig. 3.1. Lipidosis of the aorta.

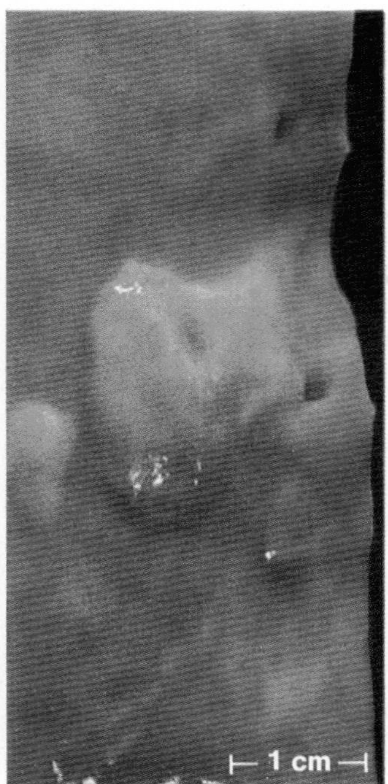

Fig. 3.2. Atheroma of the aorta.

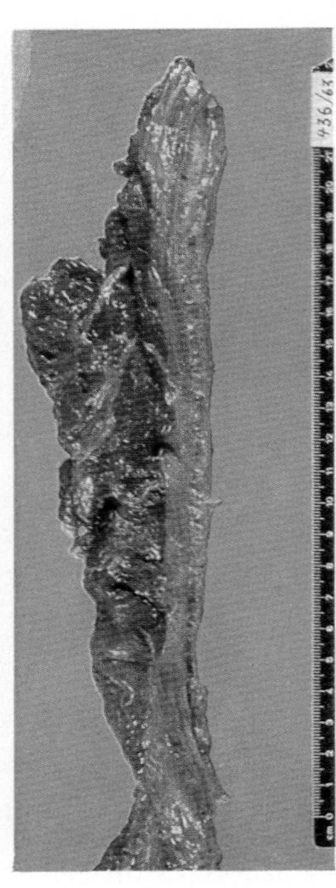

Fig. 3.3. Medial calcification.

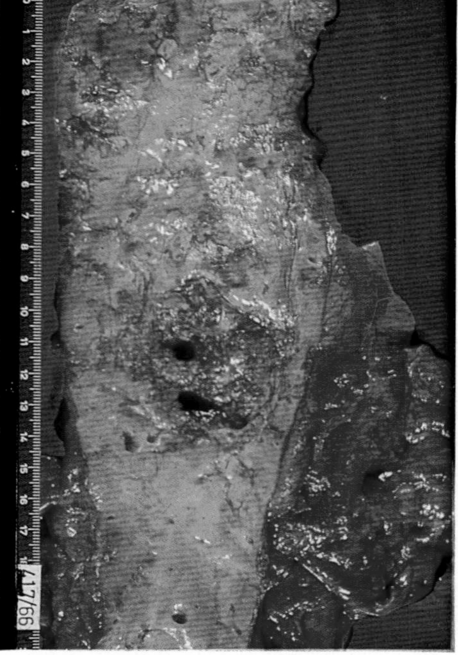

Fig. 3.4. Ulcerated atheroma of the aorta.

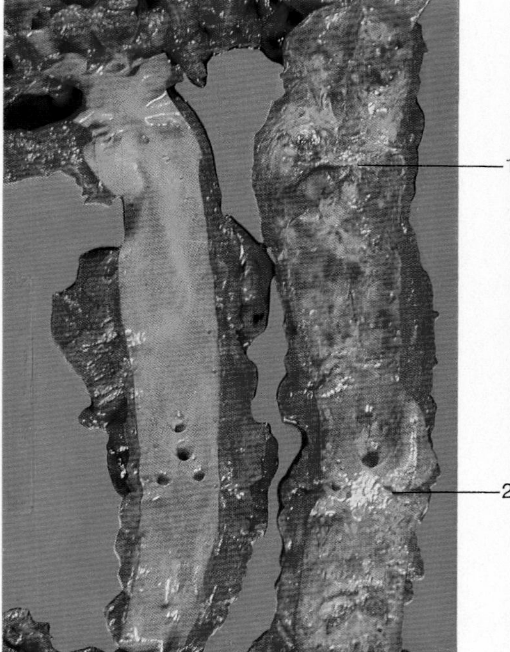

Fig. 3.5. Normal and arteriosclerotic aorta.

3. Blood Vessels

Arteriosclerosis

Diseases of the blood vessels affect the wall (degenerative changes, arteriosclerosis, inflammation) or contents (thrombosis, embolism).

Arteriosclerosis. *Collective term for chronic diseases of the vessel wall, which are characterized by deformation (stenosis, dilatation) and accompanied by metabolic changes* (LOBSTEIN, 1833). The morphologic picture depends on the type of vessel involved (TCP, p. 57). Arteries of the elastic type (aorta) show *sclerosis and atheromatosis*. Larger arteries of the muscular type (extremity arteries) develop *medial calcification*. Smaller arteries of the muscular type (coronary arteries, basal arteries of the brain, p. 313, renal arteries, p. 249) exhibit *sclerosis and elastosis*. Arterioles show *hyalinosis* (see TCP, p. 153).

Lipidosis of the aorta (Fig. 3.1; see TCP, p. 58). Reversible lipid deposition in the intima (onset of arteriosclerosis). Flat, often longitudinally arranged, yellow subintimal streaks are seen grossly in the thoracic aorta at the ostia of the intercostal arteries. Initially, the streaks are not elevated and the aorta remains elastic. With progression of lipidosis and transition into arteriosclerosis, the lipid spots enlarge, especially in the abdominal aorta. They become thickened because of continuous lipid deposition and beginning sclerosis (formation of connective tissue fibers) (*early atheroma*, Fig. 3.2). The fully developed sclerosis and atheromatosis is especially prominent in the abdominal aorta. Figure 3.4 shows an ulcerated atheromatous plaque. The plaque is flat and has irregular outlines. The thickened intima (sclerosis) is elevated (ulcerated atheroma).

A severely arteriosclerotic aorta is compared to a normal aorta in Figure 3.5. The normal aorta at the left has a smooth, yellowish red intima. The ostia of the large abdominal arteries, from top to bottom, are: celiac artery, superior mesenteric artery, renal arteries and inferior mesenteric arteries (near the lower margin of Fig. 3.5). The arteriosclerotic aorta is dilated; the transverse diameter is increased. The arteriosclerotic aorta is less elastic than the normal aorta. Slightly elevated atheromatous plaques and a white sclerotic thickening of the wall (medial calcification) are seen in the abdominal portion and extend to the thoracic aorta. The calcified wall may break during dissection. A transverse break is illustrated in Figure 3.5 (thoracic aorta →1). Extension of arteriosclerosis into the thoracic aorta is somewhat unusual. The disease usually is confined to the abdominal aorta. If the thoracic portion is affected, luetic mesaortitis or an aortitis of different etiology (e.g., rheumatic fever) with superimposed arteriosclerosis should be suspected. Our case represents arteriosclerosis only. The ostia of the renal arteries are narrowed (→2 in this picture, here opened).

Co: nephrosclerosis (Goldblatt type of hypertension).

Medial calcification of extremity arteries (Mönckeberg sclerosis). Figure 3.3 shows circular medial calcifications. They project as ridges into the lumen of the femoral artery ("gooseneck" artery on x-ray). The arterial wall is converted into an inflexible pipe. The circular calcifications can be demonstrated macroscopically in the form of black deposits by placing the arteries in a silver nitrate solution (Kossa's reaction) (MEYER). No calcifications in the vicinity of the vascular exits. Microscopically, focal calcifications of necrotic or fibrous medial tissue are seen.

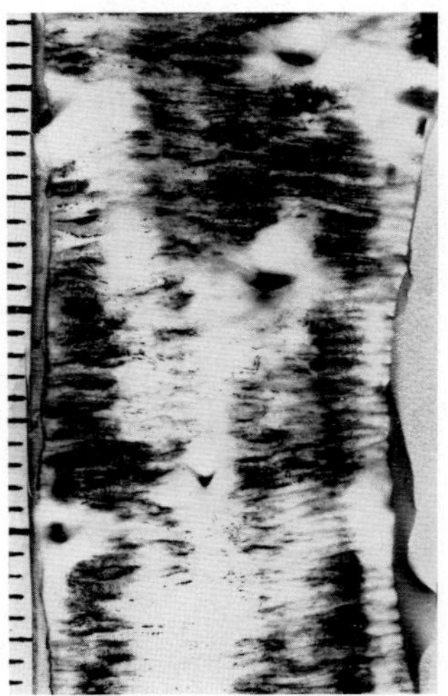

Fig. 3.6. Medial calcification of the femoral artery (after Kossa's reaction, W. W. MEYER).

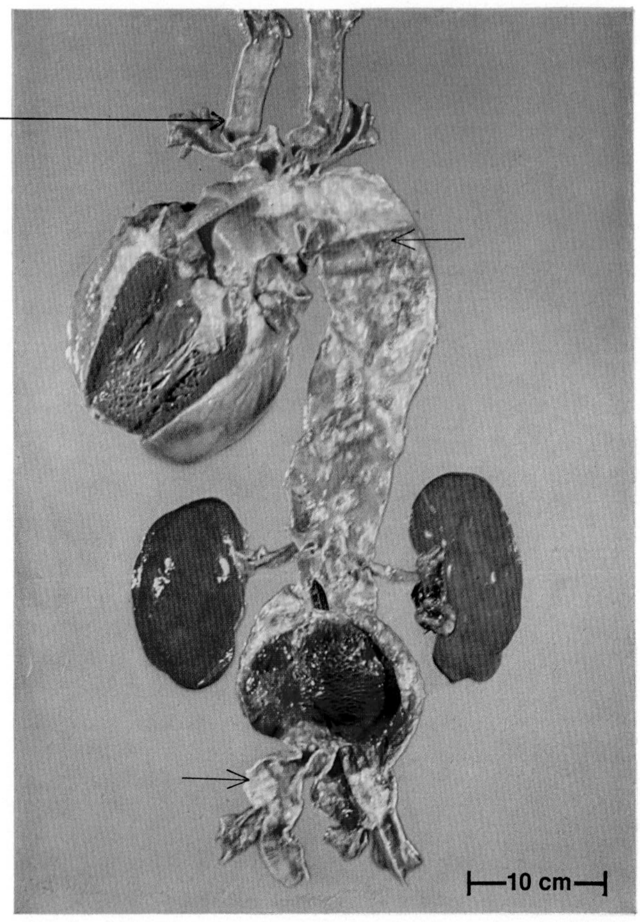

Fig. 3.7. Arteriosclerosis of the abdominal aorta with thrombosed, globular aneurysm.

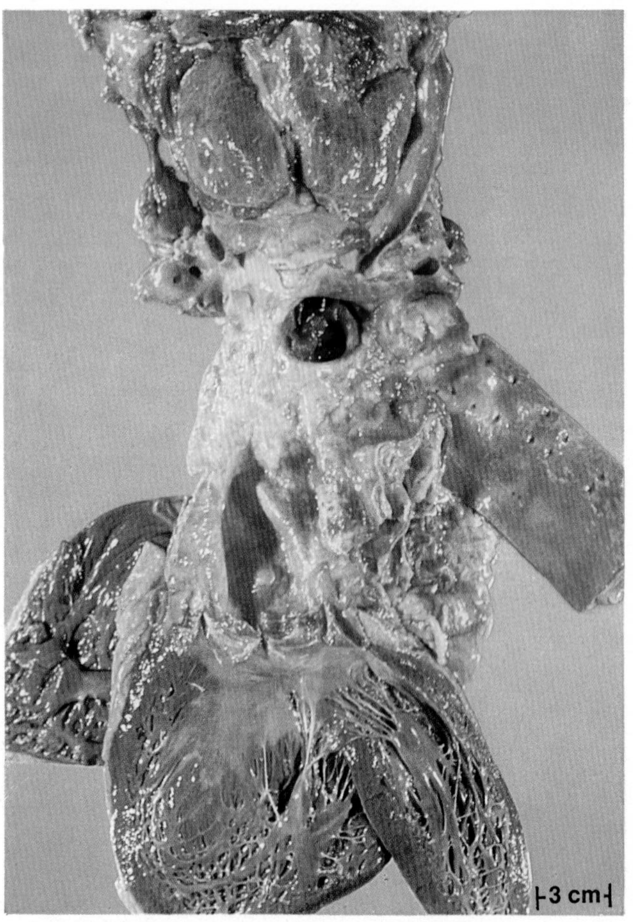

Fig. 3.8. Syphilitic mesaortitis with parietal thrombus.

Arteriosclerosis may lead to the formation of an *aneurysm* in addition to diffuse ectasia. Figure 3.7 shows the heart, aorta and kidneys. The left ventricle is hypertrophic. There is no arteriosclerosis in the ascending aorta. The origin of the major neck and arm arteries is demonstrated: the brachiocephalic truncus is at the right (left side of Fig. 3.7) and divides into the right subclavian artery and the common carotid artery (top →). At the left, the common carotid and subclavian arteries arise separately. Aortic arteriosclerosis begins near the ostia of these large arteries. Partially ulcerated atheromas (middle →) in the thoracic aorta indicate advanced arteriosclerosis. A typical complication of arteriosclerosis is found in the abdominal aorta. A saccular aneurysm with an almost occlusive mural thrombus extends from below the ostia of the renal arteries to the origin of the inferior mesenteric arteries. The local weakness of the aortic wall is a consequence of nutritional atrophy of the media, which, in turn, is caused by a thickened intima. The mural thrombus is laminated; gray platelet masses are arranged transversely across the surface. Arteriosclerotic ectasia of the iliac arteries likewise is noted (cirsoid aneurysm, bottom →).

Arteriosclerosis: *F:* cardiovascular diseases (heart, CNS) account for 30–50% of all deaths in Europe and the United States. *S:* Figure 3.9 illustrates that degenerative changes in the vessel wall begin prior to the thirtieth year of age. They increase markedly in severity with increasing age. In general, arteriosclerosis affects males more heavily than it does females, but beyond the seventieth year of age, females are affected slightly more than are males. This is true for aortic coronary arteriosclerosis. Lipidosis is always found between the tenth and thirtieth year of age in males but in only 60% of females.

Arteriosclerosis is most severe in the aorta, coronary arteries and vertebral arteries, followed by iliac, femoral and cerebral arteries. A *common combination* is arteriosclerosis of the aorta with involvement of coronary, carotid, vertebral and iliac arteries (STERNBY, 1968). *Co: rigidity of the vessel wall* results in deficient functional adaptation to fluctuations of blood pressure (cerebral and myocardial infarction). Weakness of the vessel wall leads to ectasia, aneurysm or perforation. *Narrowing of the lumen* causes myocardial and cerebral infarctions. Kidneys: scars. Mesentery arteries: Ortner's disease. Leg arteries: intermittent claudication. *Occlusive or mural thrombi* produce infarction or arterial embolism. Gangrene of leg. *Pg:* initial stage: intimal edema (?), lipidosis (lipids of blood plasma). Lipidosis of the aorta is seen in infants after a meal rich in milk, secondary sclerosis (formation of fibers), elastosis and medial calcification. Blood platelets and fibrin (thrombi) are deposited on the endothelium and become organized (DUGUID, 1946). Hypertension (either generalized or local: arteriosclerosis before aortic stenosis). *Vortex formation of the blood stream:* beginning at the ostia of the vessels. Disturbances in mucopolysaccharide metabolism (HAUSS) of the vessel wall (diminished blood supply of vessel wall. Filtration theory, ANITSCHKOV). *Disturbance in the composition of blood* (hyperlipemia as cause of arteriosclerosis. Diabetes.) *Mutation theory* (BENDITT): The smooth muscle cells of the intima of sclerotic foci belong genetically to the same cell strain and are therefore of monoclonal origin. Growth advantage of these cells? *General factors:* Higher age group. Familial disposition. Correlation to fat consumption (animal experiment!). Toxicneurogenic factors: nicotine, caffeine, epinephrine.

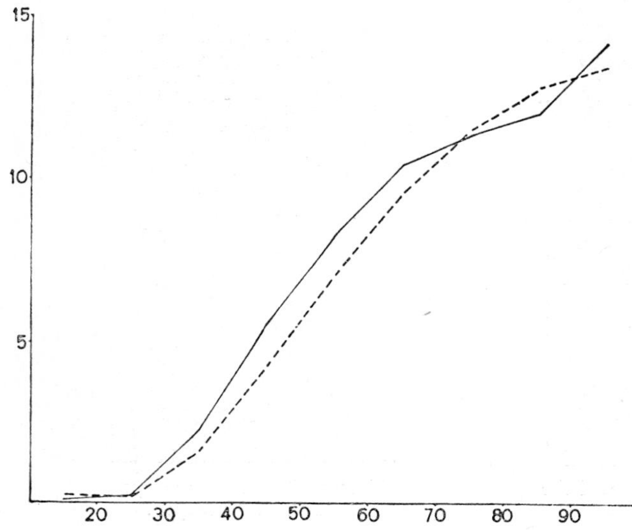

Fig. 3.9. Severity of aortic arteriosclerosis in males (solid line) and females (broken line) in Malmö (Sweden) according to STERNBY, 1968. Ordinate: severity in relative units.

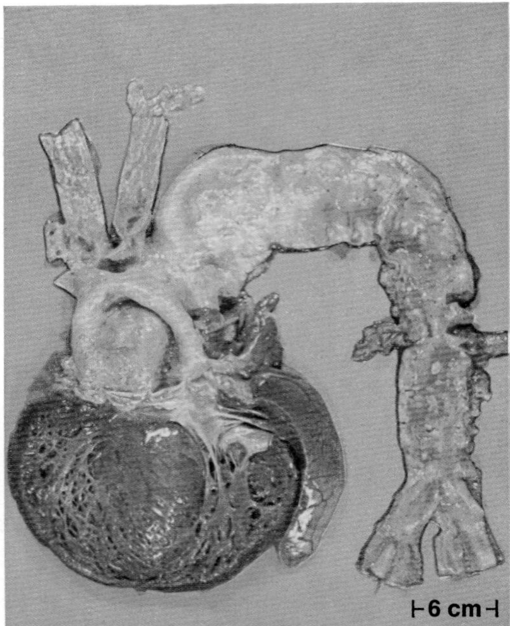

Fig. 3.10. Syphilitic aorta (mesaortitis luica).

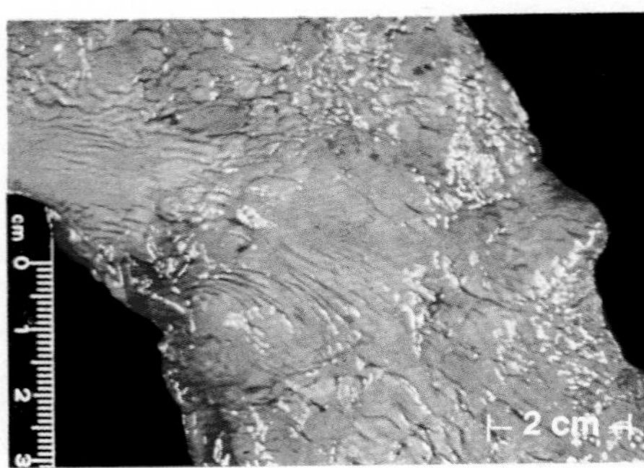

Fig. 3.11. Syphilitic mesaortitis with typical intimal tree-barking.

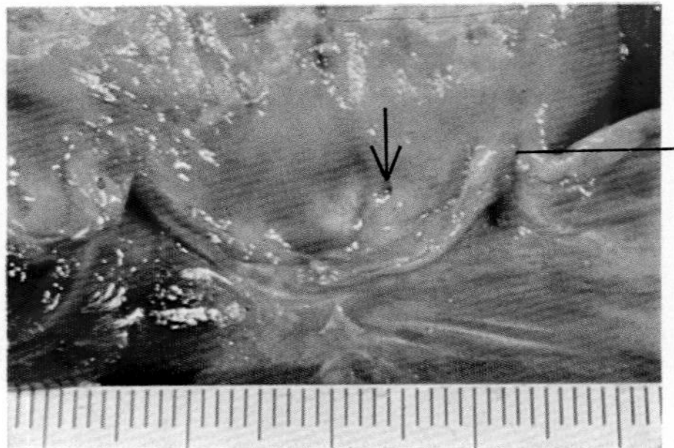

Fig. 3.12. Syphilitic mesaortitis with narrowing of the coronary ostia.

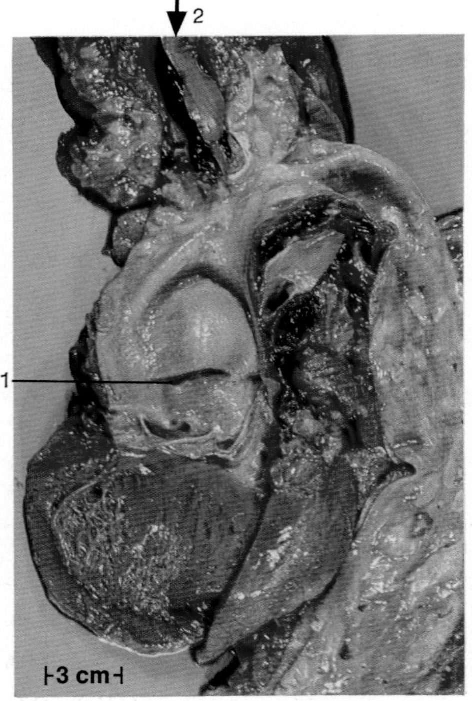

Fig. 3.13. Ruptured dissecting aneurysm of the aorta.

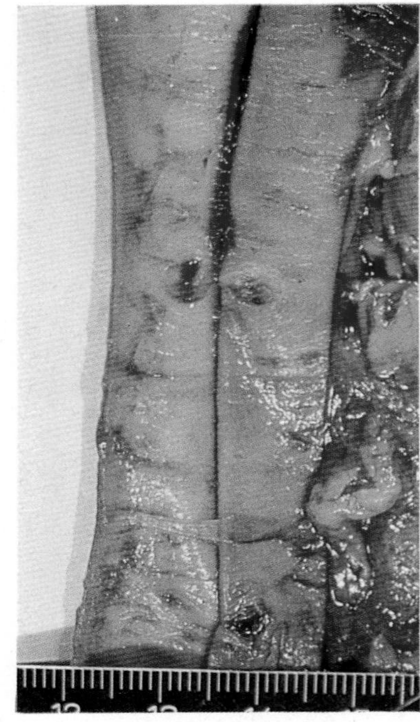

Fig. 3.14. Dissecting aneurysm. The media is folded open.

Syphilitic aortitis (Figs. 3.8 and 3.10–3.12; TCP, p. 67). *Inflammation and scar formation of the aortic media in tertiary syphilis.* The typical gross picture is characterized by diffuse aneurysmal dilatation of the ascending aorta and the aortic arch (Fig. 3.7), tree-barking and thickening of the intima (Figs. 3.10 and 3.11), narrowing of the ostia of the coronary artery and dehiscence of the cusps (grooves of Döhle, Fig. 3.12). Figure 3.8 shows aneurysmal dilatation with a mural thrombus of the ascending aorta. The process stops at the descending aorta. The intima is white and thickened. The heart is dilated and slightly hypertrophied. A close-up (Fig. 3.11) illustrates longitudinal intimal folds caused by retraction of medial scars. The fibrosis and inflammation extend into the ostia of the coronary arteries. The arteries are narrowed by contracting scar tissue, and a pinhead size opening is seen from the aorta (→ in Fig. 3.12). The cusps have been cut off in this photograph in order to demonstrate the coronary ostia. Note the dehiscence of the cusps (→ at the right): separation of the cusps by the inflammatory connective tissue (so-called Döhle's dehiscence).

F: 2%. *A:* 40–60 years. *S:* no data. *Pg:* chronic inflammation around vasa vasorum in the media with focal scar formation. Develops approximately 20 years after the primary stage. Tertiary syphilis. *Co:* perforation of aneurysm, superimposed arteriosclerosis. Myocardial infarction.

Dissecting aneurysm of the aorta with medial necrosis (Figs. 3.13 and 3.14). *Idiopathic necrosis of the aortic media, especially of the ascending aorta, with secondary rupture and formation of a dissecting aneurysm.* Figure 3.13 shows a typical case with a 6 cm.-wide, transverse tear in the intima and the inner layers of the media, approximately 5 cm. above the aortic cusp (→1). Blood has dissected the media to the iliac arteries. Often, the blood re-enters the lumen in the abdominal aorta. Figure 3.13 also illustrates that the dissection has extended into the common carotid artery, leading to a compression of the lumen (→2). Note also the ectasia of the ascending aorta (areas of wall necrosis). Figure 3.14 demonstrates the two separated walls of the dissecting aneurysm. The blood has been removed. The inner two-thirds of the media is seen at the left in this picture. At the right, the outer third of the media and the adventitia are identified. The media can be opened like the leaves of a book. It also is characteristic that during cutting, the aorta resembles blotting paper. The resistance to the dissecting scissors is markedly diminished.

A: 40–50 years. *S:* predominantly ♂. *Co:* extension of dissection into renal artery (→ compression and renal infarction), celiac or superior mesenteric arteries (→ hemorrhagic bowel infarction), carotid arteries (→ brain infarction). Perforation of blood into the pericardial sac (tamponade), lungs or peritoneal cavity. Spontaneous healing by thrombosis, granulation tissue and scar formation. *Pg:* necrosis of medial muscle and elastic fibers with an increase in acid mucopolysaccharides. (a) Circulatory disturbances of the vasa vasorum with secondary medial necrosis; for example, frequently observed after shock. (b) As part of the *Marfan syndrome:* familial disease of connective tissue with spider fingers, lens luxation, etc. Primary metabolic disease of mucopolysaccharide metabolism ("mucoid necrosis": GSELL, 1928; ERDHEIM, 1930). Experimentally produced in rats by *Lathyrus odoratus.* (c) Rarely seen with syphilitic mesaortitis.

Fig. 3.15. Types and pathogenesis of aneurysm (An.): Arteriosclerosis (1, spindle An., 2, saccular An., 3, cirsoid An.). Inflammation of vessel wall (e.g., mesaortitis: mostly diffuse aneurysmal dilatation). Erosion in tuberculosis or ulcerations (4, false An. or An. spurium). Medial necrosis (5, dissecting An.).

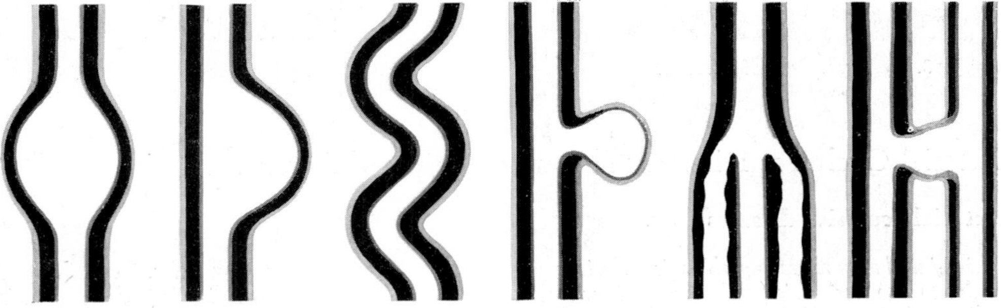

Embryonal malformation (aneurysm of the basal arteries of the brain) or embolic microaneurysms. *Co:* pressure on vertebral column and sternum, perforation, thrombosis → spontaneous healing. 6, arteriovenous An.

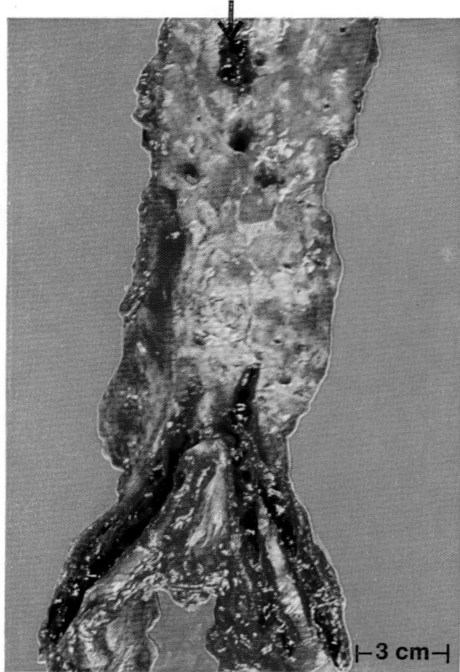

Fig. 3.16. Arteriosclerosis of the aorta with thrombosis of iliac arteries.

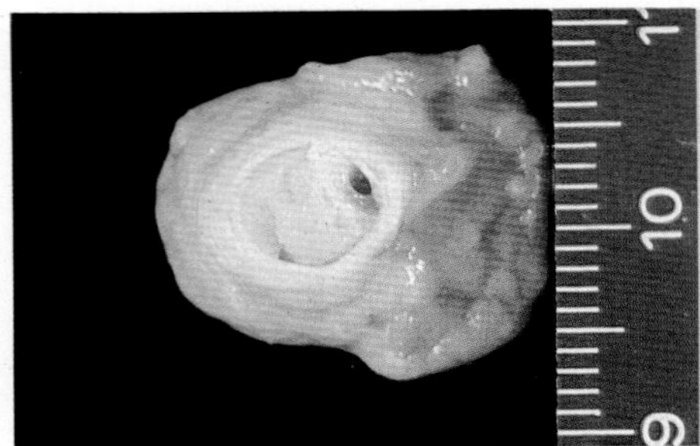

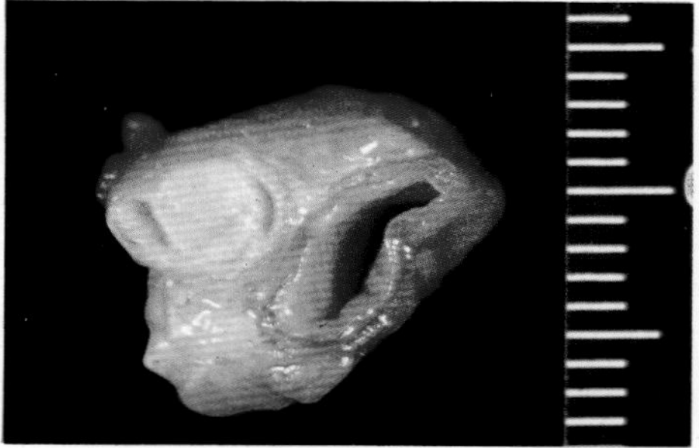

Fig. 3.17. Arterial crosssections in arteriosclerosis. Above, note the yellow atheroma. Below, thromboangiitis obliterans of te pophliteal artery.

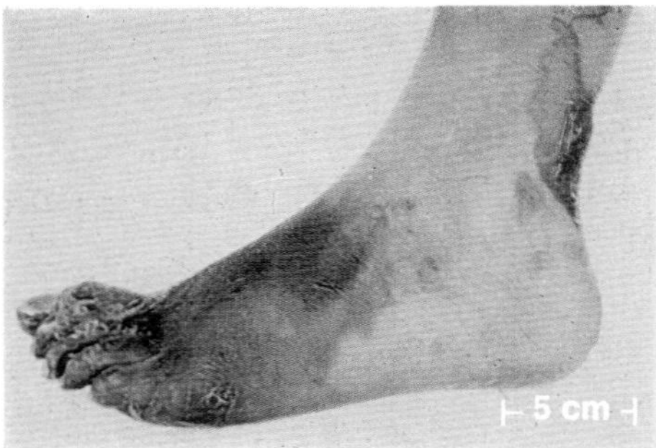

Fig. 3.18. Fresh gangrene of the foot.

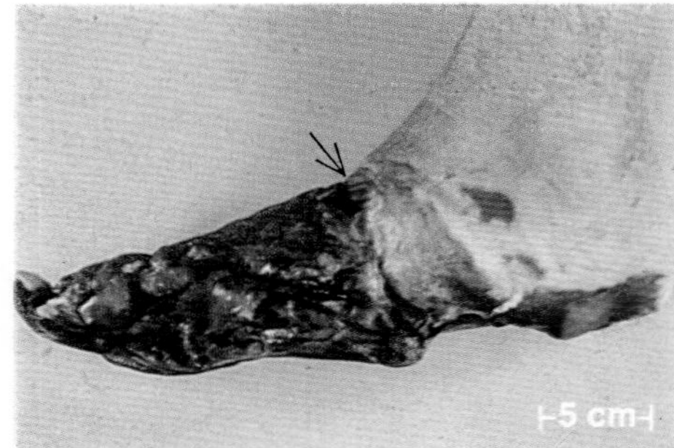

Fig. 3.19. Old, dry gangrene.

Arterial Occlusive Diseases. Thromboangiitis Obliterans. Arteritis

Arterial occlusive diseases

This clinical term refers to pathologic occlusions of arteries, mostly in the lower extremities. Occlusion may be due to arteriosclerosis (with thrombosis or embolism) or Winiwarter-Buerger's disease (thromboangiitis obliterans). Cases of arteriosclerotic occlusion are much more common than cases of thromboangiitis obliterans, both in material observed in the autopsy service and in surgical pathology. The histologic differentiation, however, sometimes is difficult.

Arteriosclerosis and embolism of the iliac artery. Figure 3.16 shows severe arteriosclerosis with multiple atheromatous plaques of the abdominal aorta. A mural thrombus (→) is attached to an atheroma above the ostia of the celiac artery. Both iliac arteries are markedly arteriosclerotic and occluded by fresh thrombi. Fresh, organizing and old thrombi also are found in the femoral arteries. The combination of fresh, organizing and old thrombotic occlusions is rather characteristic and points to recurring events. Sometimes it is impossible to decide whether the thrombi have formed locally on the basis of arteriosclerosis or whether emboli, possibly with secondary thrombi, are the cause of occlusion.

Co: gangrene of the lower legs (Figs. 3.18 and 3.19). Collateral circulation can be established when the arteriosclerotic occlusion develops slowly.

Risk factors (Fig. 3.20) for arterial occlusive disease are hypertension, cigarette smoking, hyperlipemia (see also myocardial infarction; WIDMER and co-workers).

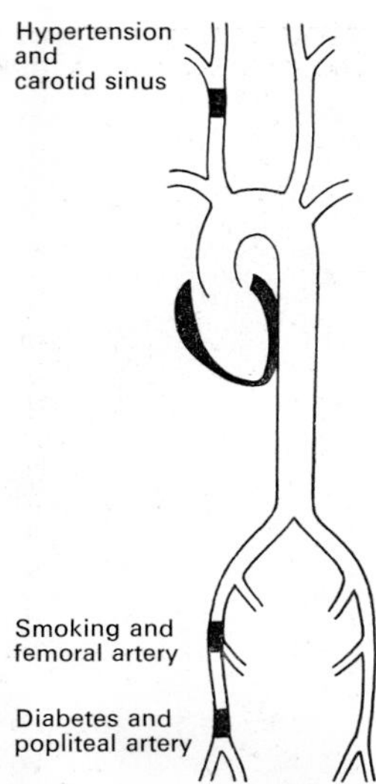

Fig. 3.20. Most common stenoses in specific vascular regions for the risk factors hypertension, smoking, and diabetes (NÜSSEL and HÖPKER).

Thromboangiitis obliterans (WINIWARTER-BUERGER) (Fig. 3.17; TCP, p. 67). *Idiopathic inflammation of myocardial, renal, mesenteric and extremity arteries)asymmetric juvenile extremity gangrene).* Figure 3.17 shows several cross sections through the popliteal artery and its branches in the lower extremity. Arteriosclerosis involves larger arteries, such as the iliac and femoral arteries.

Histologically, thromboangiitis obliterans presents as intimal fibrinoid degeneration with subsequenti inflammation and healing by scar tissue. The process is focal. Diseased portions alternate with healthy segments (segmental involvement). Veins are involved also. Arteriosclerosis affects the entire arterial wall; veins are spared.

A: 20–40 years. *S:* ♂. *Course:* 5–12 years. *Pg:* TCP, p. 67. *CP:* not known. Sixty per cent of patients are smokers. Heredity? Sometimes clinical history of cold exposure. Infectious-toxic? *Clinical:* often asymmetric; extremity without pulse. Remissions. Intermittent claudication. Also seen as isolated involvement of myocardial, renal, mesenteric and cerebral arteries. *Co:* necrosis, gangrene.

Fresh and old gangrene of the foot (Figs. 3.18 and 3.19). Gangrene is a special form of infarction with secondary bacterial infection. It is divided into:

1. **Moist gangrene** with gas-forming organisms. Grossly, a foul-smelling black-gray-green area of necrosis. The tissue is semiliquid and breaks easily (e.g., hemorrhagic lung infarction with secondary gangrene or a gangrenous appendicitis).

2. **Dry gangrene** (likewise a type of infarction). Occurs after arterial occlusions of an extremity vessel with coagulation necrosis, drying-out of the necrotic tissue and mummification (e.g., postnatal changes in the umbilical cord).

Figure 3.18 shows a fresh gangrene with a dark blue-red discoloration of the anterior foot. The tissue is friable and the skin breaks easily. Light blue areas demarcate the border to the viable tissue. Another gangrenous area is found above the heel (the yellow discoloration is due to iodine applied prior to amputation). A somewhat more advanced stage of gangrene with demarcation is shown in Figure 3.19. The anterior portion of the foot is black and the tissue is shrunken *(mummification).* The tissue is dry, firm and friable and portions of the heel have been sequestered. Demarcation of the necrosis by fresh, red granulation tissue and beginning epidermization is seen (→).

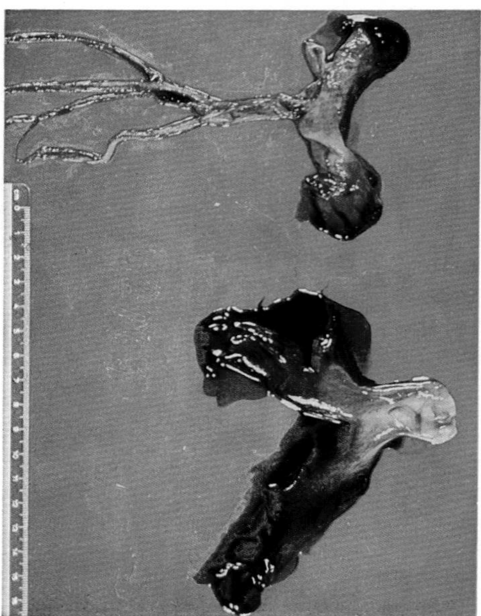

Fig. 3.21. Postmortem clots.

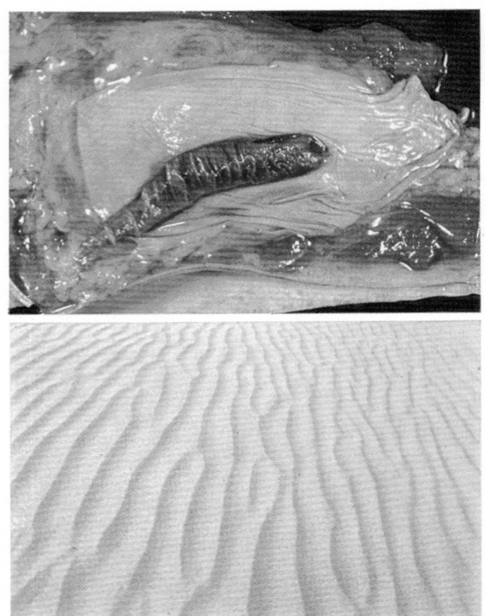

Fig. 3.22. Above, agglutination thrombus in the jugular vein. Below, sand dune (Grand Canary Island).

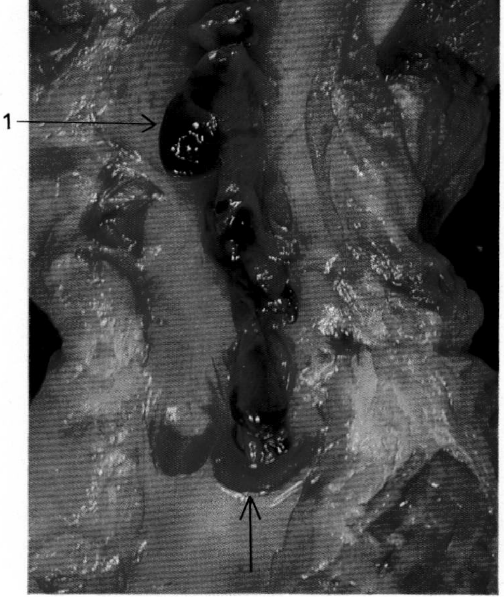

Fig. 3.23. Mixed thrombus in a femoral vein.

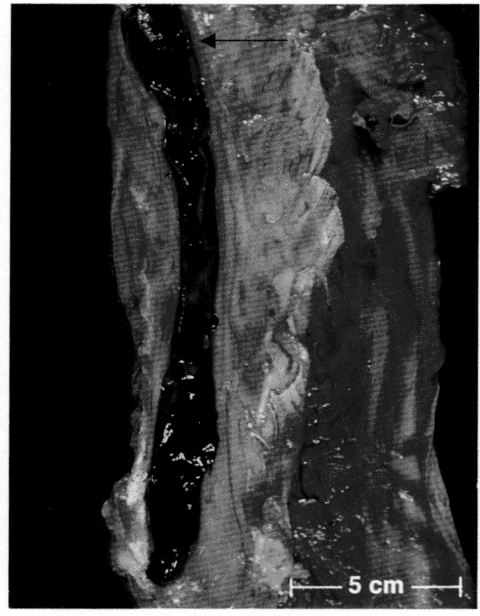

Fig. 3.24. Coagulation thrombus in a femoral vein.

Table 3.1. Summary of important inflammations of vessels.

	Periarteritis Nodosa (Panarteritis)	Wegener's Granulomatosis	Giant-cell Arteritis	Thrombo-angiitis Obliterans	Raynaud's Disease
Age (years)	20–40	30–50	50–80	20–40	20–30
Sex	♂	♂	♀	♂	♀
Involvement	Generalized	First nose, then lung, then generalized	Temporal artery	Heart, kidney, lower extremities, asymmetric	Symmetric, fingers
Localization	Focal	Arteries and veins	Media	Intima, media	Intima
Course	1 year	4 weeks – 3 years	Chronic, benign	12 years	Chronic, benign
See page	p. 251 TCP, p. 65	p. 77 –	– TCP, p. 65	p. 51 TCP, p. 67	– TCP, p. 62

Thrombosis

Chicken-fat and *currant-jelly* clots. Figure 3.21 shows a typical postmortem clot from the lung. The gray-white portions are characteristic of the chicken-fat clot, which consists almost entirely of fibrin. They typically fill the vessel, ramify and diminish in size according to the branches of the vessels. They can be removed from the vessels at autopsy. Currant-jelly clots are dark blue-red and consist of erythrocytes and little fibrin. Postmortem clots are without structure in contrast to thrombi. A typical mixed thrombus, for example, is seen in Figure 3.22. Postmortem clots are elastic in contrast to thrombi, which are firm, dry and friable. Postmortem clots do not adhere to the vessel wall. In some agonal thrombi, the distinction between postmortem clots and thrombi can be difficult.

Thrombus (TCP, pp. 68–74). *Thrombi are due to intravascular coagulation of blood during life.* Thrombi derive their structure from the blood flow. Figure 3.22 shows a typical conglutination or agglutination thrombus with a rippled surface. The white transverse bands in this picture represent gray-white rib-like projections that histologically are masses of platelets. They have been compared to the sand on a wind-swept beach or a sand dune (Aschoff). Red (in our picture black) masses of erythrocytes with little fibrin are found between the gray-red platelet scaffold. The entire thrombus is shown at the left in Figure 3.22. The lower portion consists predominantly of a coagulation thrombus. The consistency of the agglutination thrombus is firm and friable; the coagulation portion is softer but not elastic.

Figure 3.23 shows a mixed thrombus in situ in the femoral vein. The thrombus developed at a venous valve (→valve) and propagated cranially from the valve. Gray-red agglutination and red coagulation portions alternate. The upper, red, rounded coagulation portion (→1) has extended into a branch of the femoral vein. A pure coagulation thrombus of dark red color is seen in Figure 3.24. The femoral vein is totally occluded. Lines of Zahn (→) are identified in the upper portion of this thrombus; the middle portion contains gray-red platelet aggregates.

F: thrombi are found in leg veins of 30–50% of carefully examined autopsies (Cruveilhier: "La phlébite domine toute la pathologie"). Thrombi in pelvic veins are almost as common, although less significant as sources of emboli. Thrombi in cerebral sinuses occur in 10% of autopsies, especially in children; portal vein thrombosis 3–5%; renal vein thrombi are rare in children. *S:* ♀:♂ = 2:1. *Pg:* first adhesion and aggregation of platelets to the vessel wall (ADP promotes platelet aggregation; ADP sources are erythrocytes and endothelium [?]). Changes in the surface charge of endothelium and platelets (?). Platelet aggregates are surrounded by *fibrin* (activation of coagulation factors: thrombokinase converts prothrombin into thrombin, which, in turn, converts fibrinogen into fibrin). Changes in the blood flow (deceleration, vortex formation). *Predisposing factors:* Higher age group. Females predominate. Obesity. Certain weather conditions. *Co:* lung embolism (see p. 73); puriform softening (Fig. 3.28), calcification or dissolution by fibrinolysis.

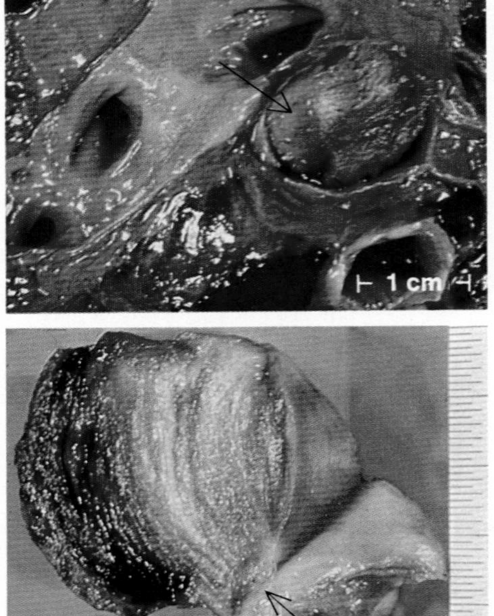

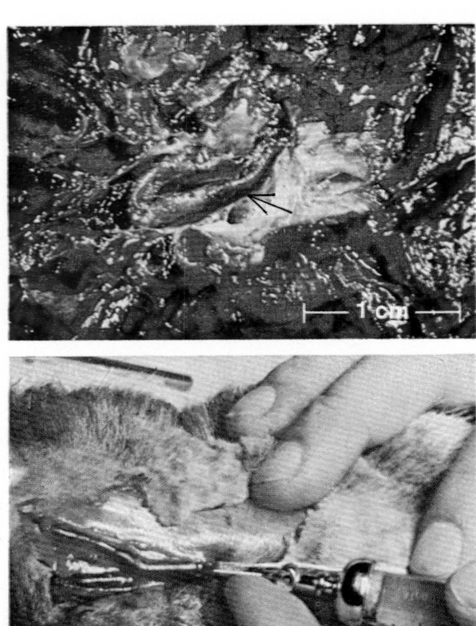

Fig. 3.25. Above, thrombus of the femoral vein, cross section.
Fig. 3.26. Below, thrombus adhering to the wall, with incipient organization (→).

Figs. 3.27 and 3.28. Thrombus (embolus) with puriform softening in a pulmonary artery. Below: experimental thrombosis.

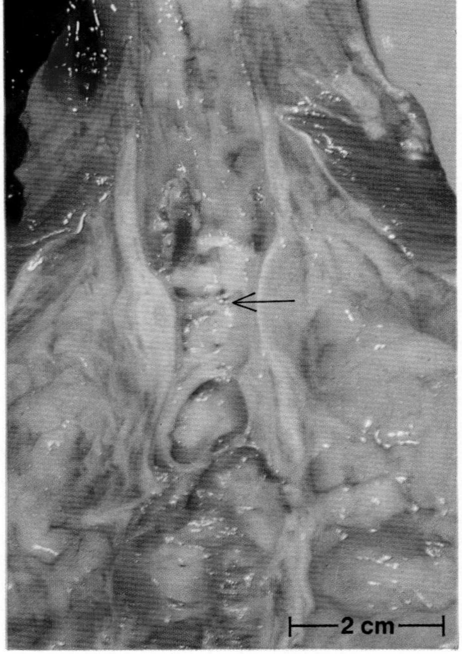

Fig. 3.29. Organized thrombosis of the femoral vein ("violin strings").

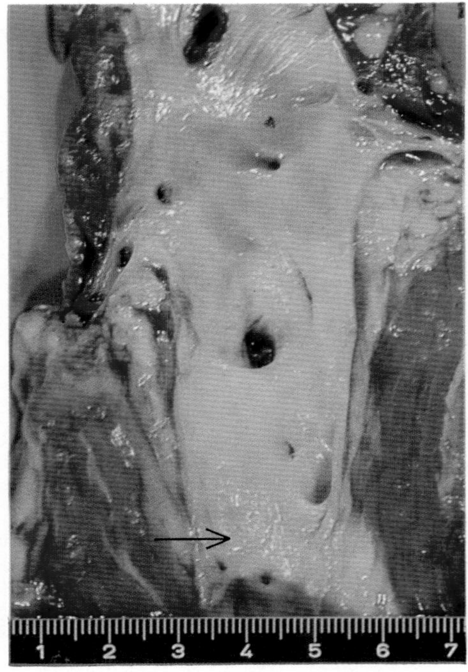

Fig. 3.30. Phlebosclerosis.

Thrombosis in the femoral vein (cross section, see Fig. 3.25): Our figure shows a photograph of a fresh, occluding agglutination thrombus (grey color). Note the coagulation thrombi in the venous side branches. There is an artery on the left side of the picture. *Wall-adhering thrombus with incipient organization* (Fig. 3.26). This is an older thrombus (or embolus) in the pulmonary artery. An attempt was made to remove the thrombus from the vessel wall. This attempt was not completely successful, since the thrombus had already firmly grown together with the wall at one point (white scar tissue →). The lamellar layering is even clearer in this picture. Puff paste-like deposits of this type are frequently seen in mural thrombi in aneurisms.

Puriform softening of a thrombus (Fig. 3.27, above). Puriform softening can result in spontaneous disappearance of thrombi. A gray-red conglutination thrombus (or pulmonary embolus) is demonstrated in Figure 3.27. Only an external, partially folded layer remains (→). The softened contents of the thrombus exudes as gray-red liquid during cutting. The softening is due to proteolytic enzymes from leukocytes.

Organized thrombus ("violin strings") (Fig. 3.29). An intimal scar is all that remains after a thrombus is organized by granulation tissue. Such a scar is shown in Figure 3.29. The wall of the vein is focally white and thickened (→). Sometimes strings or bands of connective tissue adhere to the vessel wall or project freely into the lumen *("violin strings")*. The valves of the veins usually are incorporated into the scar tissue, which is important for the function of the venous wall. Valvular insufficiency results.

Co: increased intravenous pressure with development of varices.

Post-thrombotic Syndrome (Fig. 3.31). A very frequent affliction (45% of persons between 60 and 70 years of age). The most frequent causes are recurrent thromboses with insufficiency of the venous valves or a venous-valve insufficiency of other origin (pregnancy, tumors, scars). This lengthy disease, which is resistant to therapeutic control, is accompanied by pains in the legs (80%), edemas, and varices (30–60%). A dermatitis with hyperpigmentation and depigmentation, sclerosis of the connective tissue, and ulcus cruris is also found (in 20% of the cases). It is caused by the elevated internal venous pressure as a result of a deficient fuction of the venous valves.

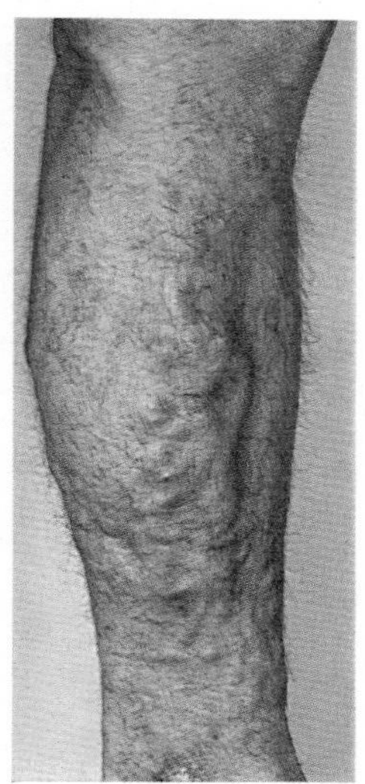

Fig. 3.31. Varicosis of the leg with ulcus cruris (lower edge of the picture).

Phlebosclerosis (Fig. 3.30). Prolonged increased intravenous pressure produces focal or diffuse white patches of intimal thickening. Histologically, there is sclerosis and elastosis of the intima. Varices are cylindrical, tortuous, diffuse or saccular dilatations of veins.

S and *A:* females predominate; 65–70 years. *Pg:* increased intravenous pressure, hereditary weakness of connective tissue.

Experimental thrombosis (Fig. 3.28). Thrombosis can be produced experimentally as follows: the jugular vein of a rabbit is prepared, ligated above the clavicle and 0.1 ml. of thrombin is injected into the engorged vein. After a short time, a coagulation thrombus forms. Its size can be manipulated experimentally (e.g., fibrinolysis). The thrombus can be seen through the venous wall. The extent of thrombus formation can be monitored by repeated blood smears (Sandritter et al.).

4. Upper Respiratory Tract, Lungs, Pleura

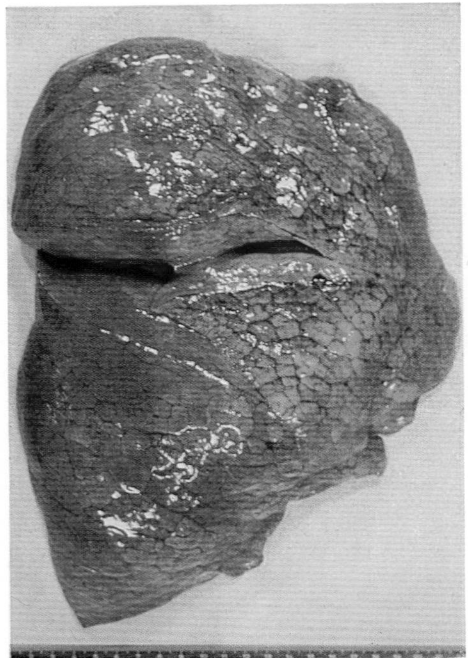

Fig. 4.1. Normal right lung.

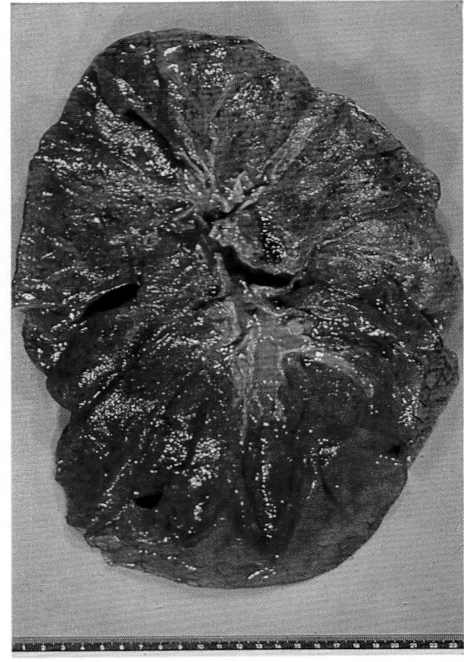

Fig. 4.2. Opened left lung.

Technic of Dissection

After removal of the sternum, the sharp mediastinal lung margins are seen to cover the lateral portions of the mediastinum. The mediastinum can be obscured by acutely hyperinflated or emphysematous lungs. The pleura is inspected (effusion, adhesion). The lungs are dissected at the hilus. The lungs are placed on the dissection board with the diaphragmatic surface facing the prosector. The hilus of the lung rests on the dissecting board (see Fig. 4.1). The sharp mediastinal margin then forms the external lung, whereas the paravertebral, rounded margin forms the internal portion of the lung. The lung hilus is palpated through the lung tissue. The lung is opened by a single longitudinal knife cut toward the hilus.

The large branches of the pulmonary artery usually are opened by this cut. An additional cut can be made to open the large bronchi (Fig. 4.2). Vessels and bronchi run parallel. The lungs are left together with the trachea when diseases of the main bronchi or hilar lung are suspected. The bronchi are then opened with scissors from the trachea.

Orientation of the dissected lung. Identify the apex and diaphragmatic surfaces with the lung resting on the hilus. In the left lung, the sharp mediastinal border is at the left and the rounded paravertebral margin at the right. The opposite is true for the right lung. Somewhat more difficult is the orientation at the hilus: *left lung:* above, pulmonary artery; middle, pulmonary vein; below, bronchus. *Right lung:* bronchus, artery and vein, from top to bottom. The pulmonary lobes (left 2, right 3) are not reliable criteria for the orientation of the lungs because variations in the numbers of lobes are common.

The lung should be dissected after formalin fixation in cases of infectious lung diseases, such as tuberculosis.

Postmortem changes in the lungs

Postmortem digestion of the stomach, diaphragm and lungs by HCl and pepsin is known as *pneumomalacia acida.* Stomach contents may enter the lungs after death via the esophagus and trachea. The lung tissue is digested and shows irregular cavities with a sour odor. The tracheal and bronchial mucosa is gray-black and dirty.

DD: gangrene: smells. Undigested food can enter the lung via the trachea and esophagus during life. Aspirated food always causes acute pulmonary emphysema.

Pneumothorax

Collection of air in the pleural cavities. Open pneumothorax: communication between pleural space and external air. *Tension pneumothorax:* partially open so that air collects in the pleural cavity during inspiration. *Closed pneumothorax:* perforation of visceral pleura. Autopsy diagnosis: a pocket is prepared from a skin flap between the intercostal muscles and the ribs. The pocket is filled with water and the intercostal space is perforated. Air bubbles escape into the water. After the thorax is opened (Fig. 4.11), the lungs are collapsed and dark blue-red. The pleural space is wider than normal.

Pg: trauma with puncture of lung or perforation from bronchoscopy.

Spontaneous pneumothorax usually is caused by tissue necrosis, e.g., perforation of a cavity or abscess, abscessive pneumonia, hemorrhagic infarctions or tumors. Pulmonary fibrosis, *emphysema* in the vicinity of scars or interstitial emphysema, malformations (congenital cystic lung or honeycomb lung, Fig. 4.19) or pleural blebs likewise may cause spontaneous pneumothorax. *Co:* acute cor pulmonale. Infection → empyema.

Dissection of neck organs

The neck organs are dissected after the heart, lungs and abdominal organs have been removed. The skin of the neck is dissected from the underlying tissues by extending the circular upper thorax incision to the inner surface of the mandible. (*Caution:* do not cut through the skin.) The floor of the mouth is dissected along the mandible; the tongue is pulled downward. Hard and soft palate are separated by knife cuts and the pharynx is prepared by a cut that runs to the vertebral column. The organs of the neck are removed by pulling the tongue forward, aided by several cuts along the vertebral column. The aorta is attached to the neck organs.

Tonsils and thyroid lobes are cut lengthwise. The trachea, aorta and esophagus are opened with the enterotome.

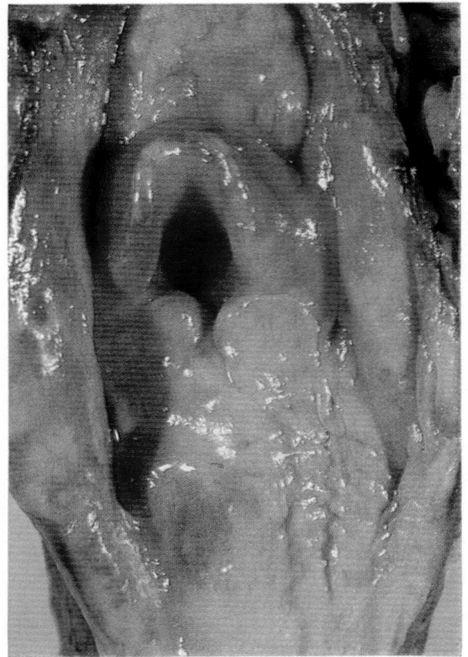

Fig. 4.3. Acute laryngeal edema.

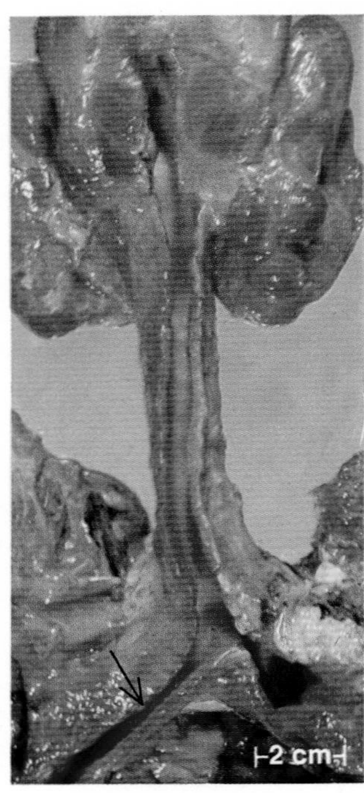

Fig. 4.4. Saber trachea.

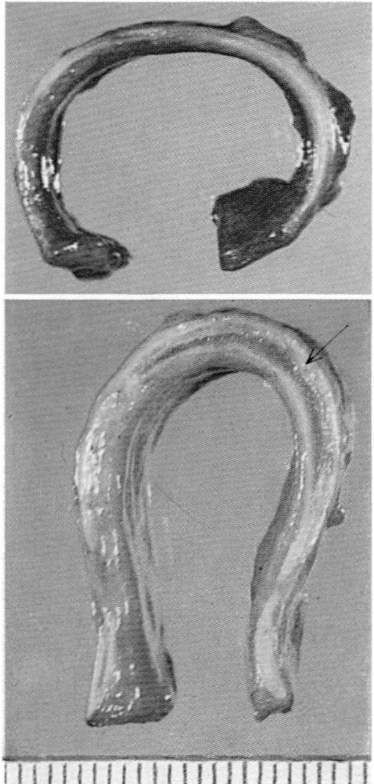

Fig. 4.5. Cross sections of the trachea. Above: normal. Below: saber trachea.

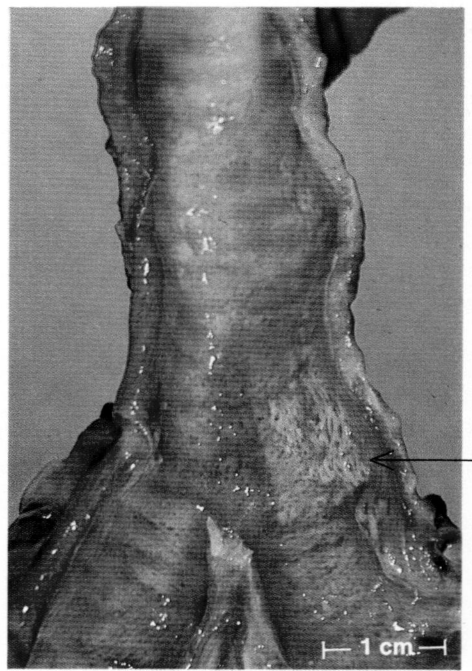

Fig. 4.6. Tracheopathia osteoplastica.

Laryngeal Edema, Diseases of the Trachea

Edema of the larynx and pharynx (Fig. 4.3). *Acute edema of the laryngeal connective tissue, especially the aryepiglottic folds.* Edema of the glottis, i.e., swelling in the immediate proximity of the vocal cords, is found only with severe degrees of edema. Figure 4.3 shows the epiglottis, hypopharynx and upper esophagus. The entire epiglottis, especially the aryepiglottic folds, are markedly swollen, slightly red and firm-elastic. A clear fluid exudes after cutting. Laryngeal edema may be difficult to demonstrate after death. The edema fluid may evaporate or collect in the dependent portions. A folded, wrinkled mucosal surface remains as the only evidence of laryngeal edema.

Pg: allergic factors (e.g., hypersensitivity to strawberries). *Angioneurotic edema* (Quincke) of unknown etiology. *Transudate* following compression of the superior vena cava. *Inflammatory edema* in diphtheria, angina. Extension of a *cellulitis* from the floor of the mouth. Laryngeal edema also may occur as so-called *laryngopathia gravidarum* together with edema of other mucosal membranes in gestational toxicosis. Acute life-threatening condition; danger of suffocation. Tracheostomy.

Acute phlegmonous inflammation of the epiglottis: The epiglottis is red and swollen. Seen in children with *Haemophilus influenzae* infection.

Saber trachea (Figs. 4.4 and 4.5). *Increase in the sagittal diameter of the trachea with corresponding decrease in the transverse diameter and marked outpouching of the membranous part* (not demonstrated in Fig. 4.4). The photograph shows a saber-like deformity of the trachea that also involves the left main bronchus (→). Cross sections of a normal trachea (upper frame) and saber trachea (lower frame) are compared in Figure 4.5. The sagittal diameter of the saber trachea is increased; the transverse diameter is reduced. The brown streak (→) near the tracheal cartilage is caused by lipid deposits and ossifications in the cartilaginous ground substance.

S: common in males past 60 years of age. *Pg:* (1) *The partial saber trachea* is due to external compression, e.g., from an enlarged thyroid (nodular colloidal goiter). (2) *The complete or total saber trachea* begins as an albuminous or cystic degeneration (e.g., arthrosis deformans) near the convexity of the tracheal cartilage. Formation of bone (osseous metaplasia) progresses from the convexity to the lateral and posterior aspects of the cartilaginous rings. Ultimately they are transformed into a rigid horseshoe-like structure – the saber trachea.

Functional aspects: The normal shape of the trachea is required in order to accommodate increased intraluminal pressure (e.g., coughing). The trachea adapts by an increase in the longitudinal and transverse diameters. The rigid saber trachea can distend in a longitudinal direction only. Pressure is exerted on the pars membranacea, which, in turn, leads to degeneration of smooth muscle bundles and elastic fibers. Consequently, the membranous part becomes dilated and overextended (Beneke).

Tracheopathia osteoplastica[1] (Fig. 4.6). Small, gray-white, firm, slightly elevated, solitary or net-like plaques are seen on gross examination in the tracheal mucosa, especially above the bifurcation (→). The tracheal lumen is somewhat dilated above the plaques (loss of elasticity proximal to a functional stenosis). Histologically, islands of bone and cartilage are found in the submucosal connective tissue above the cartilaginous rings.

F: rare. *S:* ♂=♀. *Pg:* congenital malformation. Osseous metaplasia following inflammation or hemorrhage? *DD:* ossification of the saber trachea affects the cartilage rather than the submucosa.

---

1) The first reported case came to autopsy on May 24, 1909 in the Department of Pathology, University of Freiburg, Germany (see Aschoff, 1910).

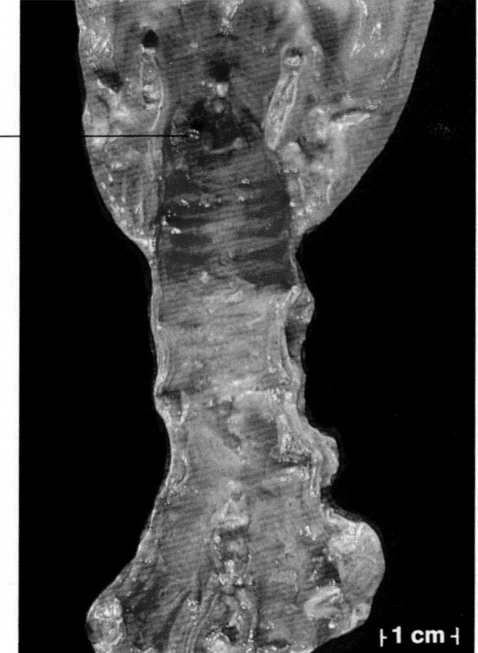

Fig. 4.7. Tracheostomy with pseudomembranous tracheitis.

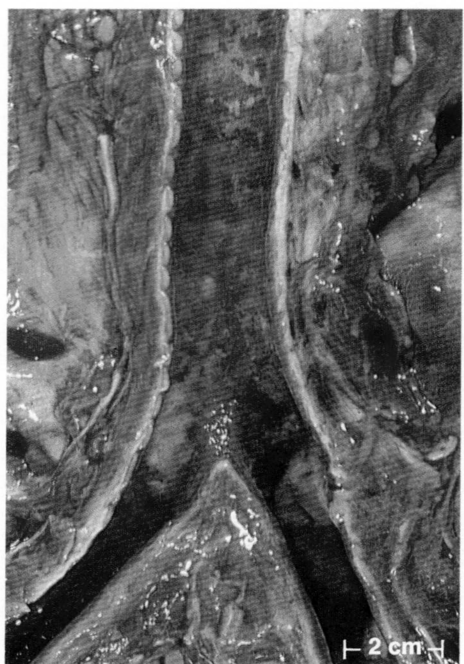

Fig. 4.8. Hemorrhagic-necrotizing tracheitis.

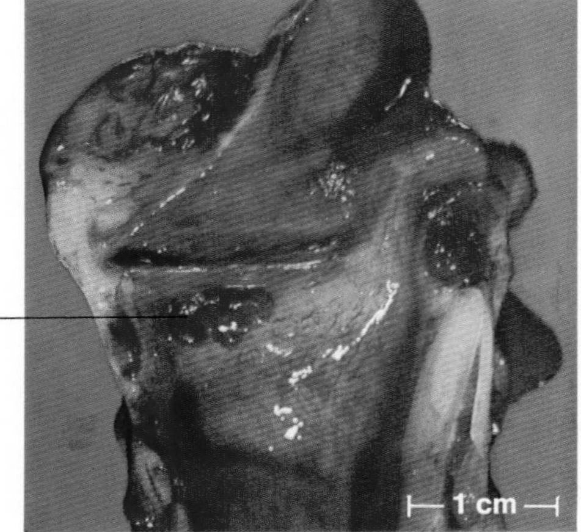

Fig. 4.9. Polyp of vocal cord (singer's node).

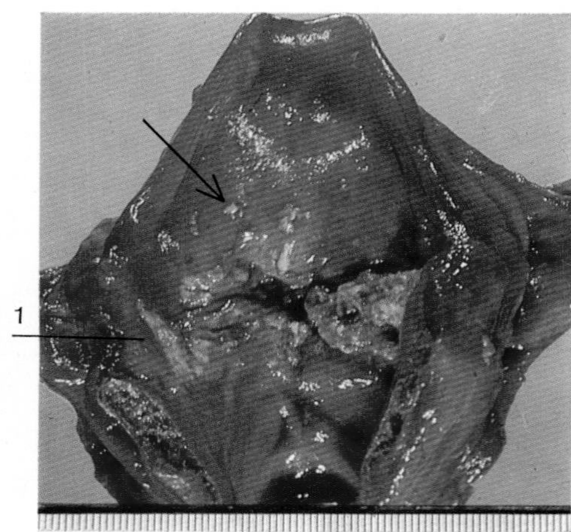

Fig. 4.10. Carcinoma of the larynx.

Tracheitis and Tumors of the Larynx

Tracheostomy with pseudomembranous tracheitis (Fig. 4.7). A tracheostomy is made in critically ill patients (poisoning, head trauma, coma) for the purpose of artificial respiration. Serious local complications may develop from the tracheostomy tube, as illustrated in Figure 4.7. A defect is seen in the wall of the upper trachea (→). Partially ossified, cartilaginous rings project over the mucosal surface (*osteochondritis dissecans:* the perichondrium is elevated by purulent exudate). Black areas of mucosal necrosis surround the defect. The upper tracheal mucosa is markedly reddened, velvety and swollen (severe inflammatory hyperemia). Yellow membranes loosely adhere to the mucosa in the lower two-thirds of the trachea. The membranes are removed easily (pseudomembranous tracheitis). Extensive ulcerations and a severe dissecting osteochondritis may occur in cases of advanced tracheitis.

Pg: secondary infection with pneumococci and streptococci through the tracheostomy tube. *Co:* tracheostomy incision rarely heals by forming cartilaginous callus. Instead, formation of connective tissue and scars eventually leads to tracheal stenosis. Other complications are: hemorrhage after trauma of larger blood vessels, mediastinal emphysema, cellulitis (phlegmon), metaplasia by squamous epithelium and tracheal fistula.

A *pseudomembranous inflammation* of the trachea can develop in diphtheria (TCP, p. 83). Rarely seen today because of vaccination!

Hemorrhagic-necrotizing influenzal tracheitis (Fig. 4.8; TCP, p. 83; see also Fig. 4.46). *Influenza is an acute infection by members of the RNA-containing influenza viruses (multiple subtypes A, B, C, etc.). Influenzal infection also may be accompanied by hemorrhagic pneumonitis.* Our picture shows a dark red and partially black-red (hyperemia and hemorrhage) tracheal mucosa. Gray-white, shiny mucosal lesions usually are the size of a pinhead but have already coalesced in our case to form larger areas of necrosis.

F: a necrotizing tracheitis is seen only in a small number of influenza cases. Hemorrhagic tracheitis is more common. *Pg:* virus replication in cells of respiratory epithelium with subsequent necrosis. Often superinfection with staphylococci. Hemorrhage is due to toxic capillary paralysis.

Polyps of the vocal cord (so-called singer's node) (Fig. 4.9). These are not true polyps but *focal, inflammatory hyperplasias* of the connective tissue in the area of the vocal cords or the ventriculus Morgagni. Our picture shows several red, glassy and round or grape-like lesions with a smooth mucosa below the free margin of the vocal cord.

S: they are more common in females than in males. *Pg:* initially gray-white areas of thickened mucosa develop (increase in connective tissue and inflammatory edema). Gray-red "polyps" with hyalinized connective tissue, chronic inflammation and thin-walled, thrombosed vessels occur at a later stage. *Pg:* misuse of voice.

Carcinoma of the larynx (Fig. 4.10). *Squamous-cell carcinomas of the anterior portion of the vocal cords (98% of all cases).* Our picture shows a gray-white, partially exophytic, irregularly nodular and superficially ulcerated tumor of soft and friable consistency (right vocal cord). The left vocal cord is ulcerated. Several mucosal metastases, measuring up to 3 mm., are seen in the vicinity of the carcinoma. These are flat to slightly elevated, gray-white lesions (→). Several white, flat areas of mucosal thickening (leukoplakia, → 1) are found near the left vocal cord.

F: 1–2% of all forms of cancer. *A:* 60–70 years. *S:* ♂ : ♀ = 10:1. *Pg:* leukoplakia → carcinoma in situ → microcarcinoma. Chronic inflammation (tuberculosis), arsenical poisoning, alcohol, tobacco. *Localization:* so-called intrinsic larynx carcinomas (60–80%) are located at or near the anterior portion of the vocal cord. Carcinomas of the epiglottis (10–15%) and carcinomas of the subglottis (5–15%) are referred to as extrinsic larynx carcinomas. *Metastases:* mucosal metastases and infiltration of the neck tissues precede regional lymph node metastases.

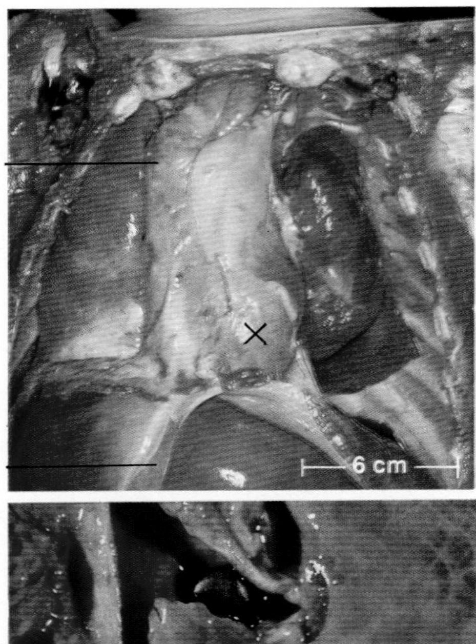

Fig. 4.11. Complete atelectasis of the left lung following occlusion of the bronchus. Below: a gravel stone is lodged in the main bronchus.

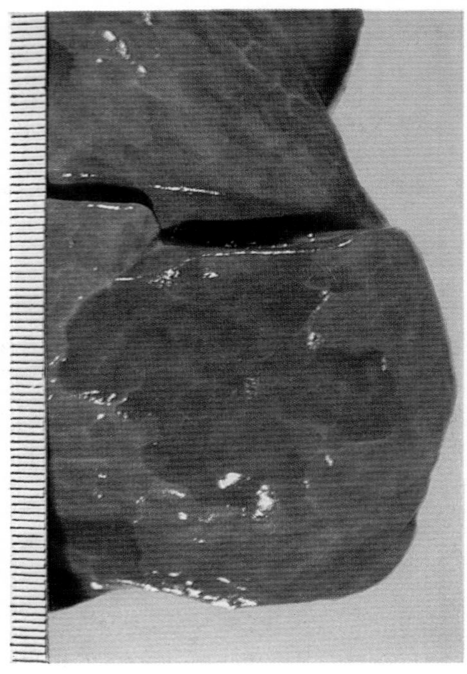

Fig. 4.12. Focal resorption atelectasis.

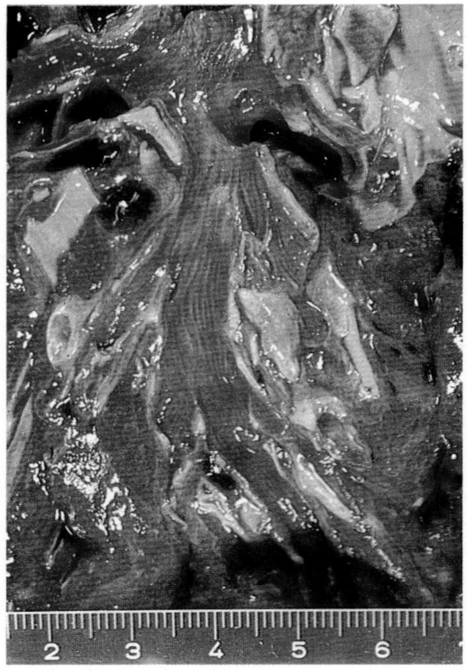

Fig. 4.14. Congestive bronchitis.

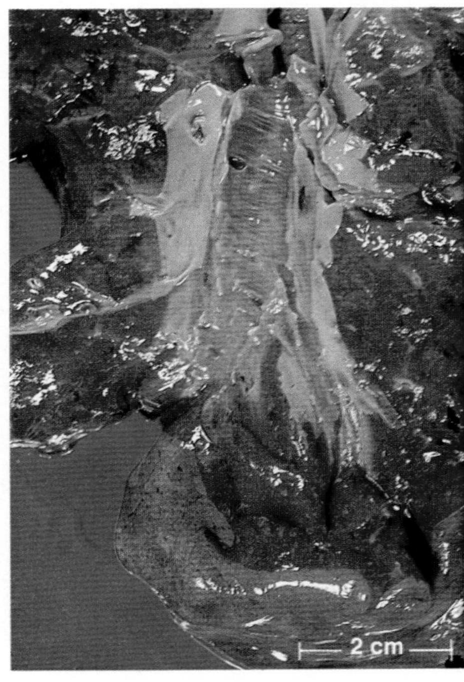

Fig. 4.15. Chronic bronchitis.

Atelectasis, Bronchitis, Bronchiectasis, Malformations

Atelectasis. *The air content of the lung is partially or completely reduced.* Figure 4.11 shows the opened thorax of a 4-year-old girl with mediastinum, thymus (upper →) and pericardial sac (X). The right heart is dilated. The right lung is somewhat hyperinflated. The lower anterior segment of the right lung is anemic. The left lung is collapsed, dark red and firm-elastic. Its cut surface likewise is dark red. The middle lobe is anemic. Air noise is absent when the knife is led over the left lung, in contrast to the normal lung. (Air noise also is missing in pneumonia.) The pleural space is widened. Note the shift of the mediastinum to the right, especially the upper mediastinum. The diaphragm is low and the liver is shifted to the left (lower →: falciform ligament of the liver). Figure 4.11, below, shows the cause of atelectasis in this case: a small gravel stone (1 cm. in diameter) was aspirated and occluded the left main bronchus. *Note:* the right main bronchus is wider than the left and originates at a shallow angle from the trachea. Foreign bodies preferentially lodge in the right bronchus. The left bronchus has a narrow, sharp angle.

A: mostly in young persons. *Pg:* prototype of resorption atelectasis: loss of air exchange → resorption of gases in the sequence of oxygen-CO_2-nitrogen despite sustained circulation. *Co:* right heart failure due to increased pulmonary resistance. Vessels constrict because of increased CO_2 tension.

Compression atelectasis is defined as diminished air content of the lung due to external pressure (tumors, cysts, pneumothorax). *Co:* cor pulmonale.

Resorption or focal atelectasis is the most common type of atelectasis (Fig. 4.12; TCP, p. 75). The blue-red, depressed areas of lung tissue correspond to the distribution of a lobulus (supplied by a bronchiolus). They are sharply demarcated from the aerated bright red lung tissue. The atelectatic areas are firm-elastic. Note the fine white markings beneath the glistening pleura (connective tissue septa, borders of lobuli). On cut surface, the atelectatic lobules are blue-red and without air noise during cutting.

Common in infants, small children and juveniles. *Types:* (1) *Fetal A.:* the lung is not aerated. Bronchi contain mucus or amniotic fluid. The surface tension lowering factor (SLF), a lipoprotein that diminishes surface tension, is missing. The alveoli become dilated. Usually newborns weighing less than 1,200 Gm. The lung sinks in water. (2) *Resorption A.:* bronchial occlusion by mucus, tumors or other factors. *Pg:* see above. *Special type: Regional A.:* develops in paravertebral lung, where agonal pressure leads to mechanical compression.

Bronchitis (Figs. 4.13–4.16). *Chronic bronchitis presents a major public health problem because of the ever-increasing air pollution in industrial regions.* According to English death statistics, 50% of the population dies from complications of chronic bronchitis (bronchiectasis, emphysema, pneumonia, cor pulmonale).

Different forms of bronchial inflammation are (TCP, p. 85): *Catarrhal-mucinous bronchitis* (Fig. 4.13). The mucosa is red (hyperemic) and covered by gray-white and partially tenacious mucus (see obstructive emphysema, p. 69). In *congestive bronchitis* (congestion of pulmonary circulation, cor pulmonale), the mucosa is somewhat more deeply red and edematous (Fig. 4.14). The mucinous-purulent bronchitis shows a marked mucosal reddening. The mucus is yellow and liquid (leukocytes). *Chronic bronchitis* (Fig. 4.15) is characterized by mucosal thickening with transverse and longitudinal mucosal folds (hypertrophic muscle bundles in the tunica propria). Figure 4.15 also shows minimal cylindrical dilatation of the bronchus. The mucosa of *atrophic bronchitis* is smooth and white. Mucosal herniations correspond to dilated excretory ducts of the mucus glands.

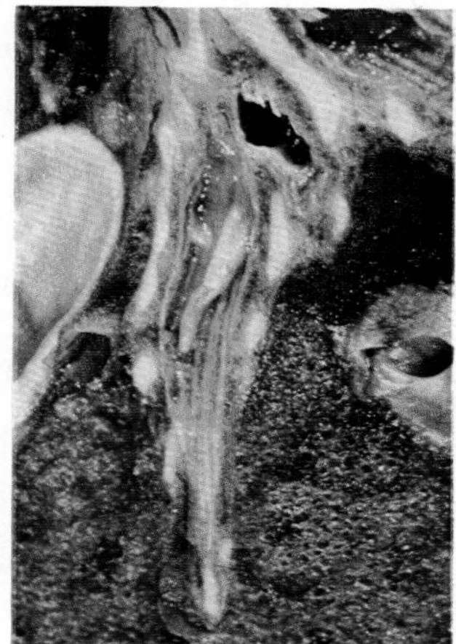

Fig. 4.13. Catarrhal-mucinous bronchitis.

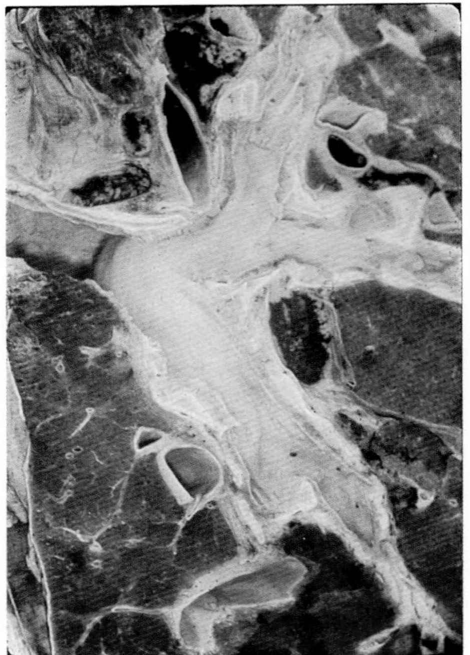

Fig. 4.16. Mucinous asthma bronchitis.

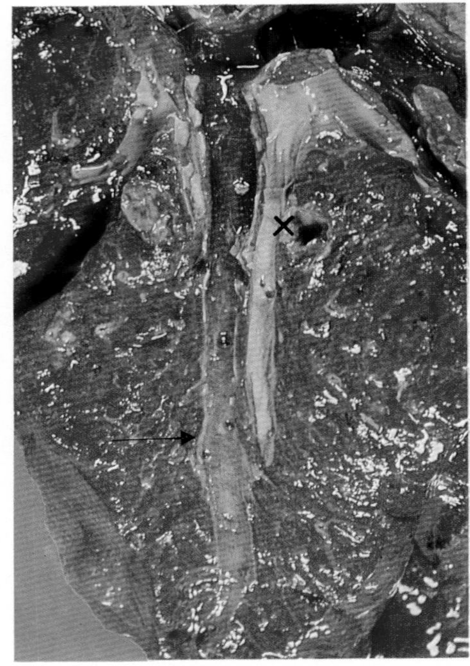

Fig. 4.17. Cylindrical bronchiectasis.

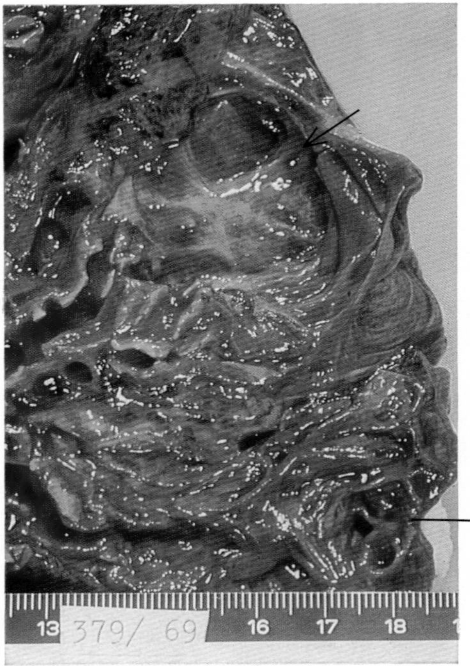

Fig. 4.18. Congenital saccular bronchiectasis.

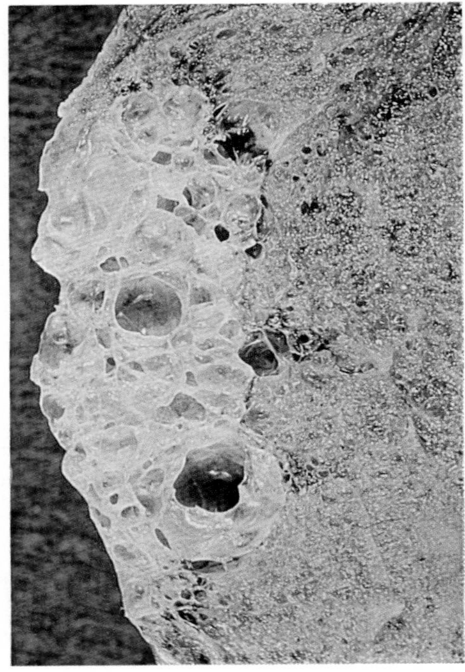

Fig. 4.19. Cystic lung.

Asthma bronchitis (Fig. 4.16). Tenacious gray-white mucus plugs can be removed from the bronchi. Smaller bronchi are filled with mucus that projects as gray-white plugs over the cut surface. Acute pulmonary emphysema usually exists (see p. 67).

S: more frequent in ♂ than in ♀. *Pg:* predisposing factors are colds, smoke, industrial gases (sulfur, ammonia). Secondary infections with *Haemophilus influenzae*, pneumococci, adenoviruses, myxoviruses. *Co:* pulmonary emphysema (see p. 67), cor pulmonale, recurrent infections and bronchiectasis.

Bronchiectases are defined as *congenital or acquired tubular, cylindrical or saccular dilatations of the bronchi.* Typical autopsy finding: the bronchi can be opened all the way to the pleura. Moreover, the bronchi are wider than pulmonary artery branches. Figure 4.17 shows a cylindrically dilated bronchus of the lower lobe. Compare its width to the adjacent small branch of the pulmonary artery. The distal portion of the bronchus (→) is almost as wide as its origin. The mucus (gray-yellow) was removed to demonstrate the mucosa, which is gray-white with minimal horizontal folding. A small pulmonary abscess (2 cm. in diameter) is seen to the right of the pulmonary artery branch (next to the X). Saccular bronchiectases (Fig. 4.18) frequently develop near pulmonary scars (e. g., tumors, see Figs. 4.70 and 4.71).

A: 40–60 years. *S:* ♂>♀. *Pg:* chronic bronchitis and inflammatory infiltrates weaken the bronchial wall. Chronic cough increases intrabronchial pressure. *Special types: Cirrhotic bronchiectases* are caused by pulmonary scars such as in tuberculosis or silicosis. *Stenotic bronchiectases* (see Fig. 4.69) occur with tumors. *Collateral bronchiectases* are seen after partial lung resection or in children with mucoviscidosis (see p. 173). *Co:* chronic, recurrent pneumonias, emphysema, brain abscess, cor pulmonale, amyloidosis. Diaphragmatic liver grooves (see p. 139).

Congenital bronchiectasis (Fig. 4.18). Malformation due to inhibition of the dichotomous division of the bronchi leads to saccular or cystic lungs. The extent of cavity formation depends on the time of inhibition. A saccular lung (early developmental stage) may affect an entire lung lobe. Smooth-walled cavities are lined by ciliated epithelium. Cartilage and muscle bundles are found in the cavity wall. Larger cystic cavities in one lobe may develop in congenital saccular bronchiectasis (congenital cystic lung). Figure 4.18 shows several large, smooth cystic spaces measuring up to 4 cm. in diameter (upper → border of the largest cystic cavity; lower → smaller cysts). The walls of the cysts, on histologic examination, contained cartilage. The congenital cystic lung often affects a small subpleural region. Figure 4.19 shows multiple small cavities.

Aspergilloma of the lung (Fig. 4.20). *Tumor form accumulations of mycelial masses of Aspergillus fumigatus in extensively epithelialized pulmonary cavities.* Aspergillomas occur, as in our figure, predominantly in the apex of the lung. The cut surface shows the grey-brown mycelial masses, which can be easily separated from the wall of the cavity (they are not adherent to the wall!). The surrounding pulmonary and pleural tissue is scarred (completed tuberculosis).

Pg: over 350 forms of Aspergillus are known, of which 13 are pathogenic to humans. Aspergillomas develop only in previously damaged tissue (in cavities found after tuberculosis, infarction, oncolysis, abscess, or in cysts). Bronchiectases are formed by the increasing internal pressure of the mycelium (not primary, since the localization is different: aspergilloma in the apex and bronchiectases in the lower lobes of the lung). Cytostatic, antibiotic, and cortisone therapy promote the development of aspergillomas. *Co:* mixed infections only after death of the fungus. No pulmonary atelectasis! *Cl:* hemoptysis.

Pulmonary aspergillosis involves a diffuse infestation of the entire lung, particularly in pre-existing cavities (pulmonary cysts and bronchiectases). Clinically, one distinguishes between allergic forms (such as bronchial asthma) and mucomembranous forms (copious expectoration).

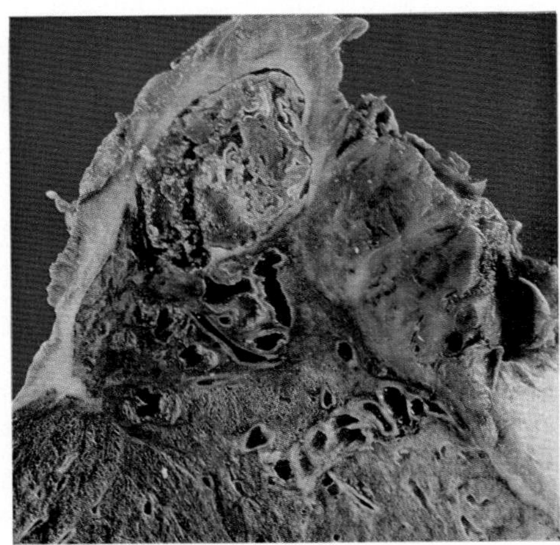

Fig. 4.20. Aspergilloma of the lung.

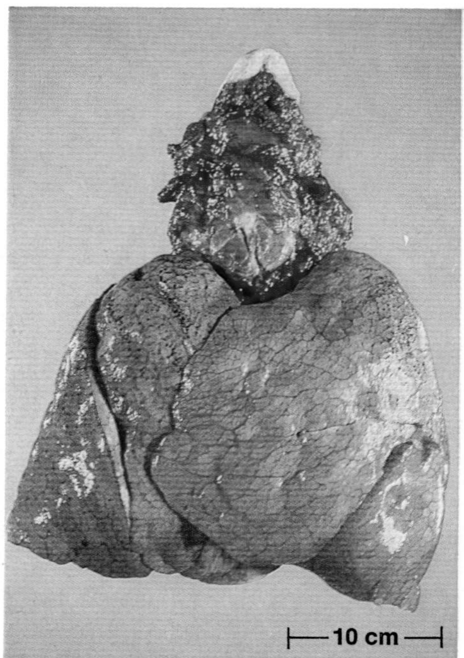

Fig. 4.21. Acute pulmonary emphysema.

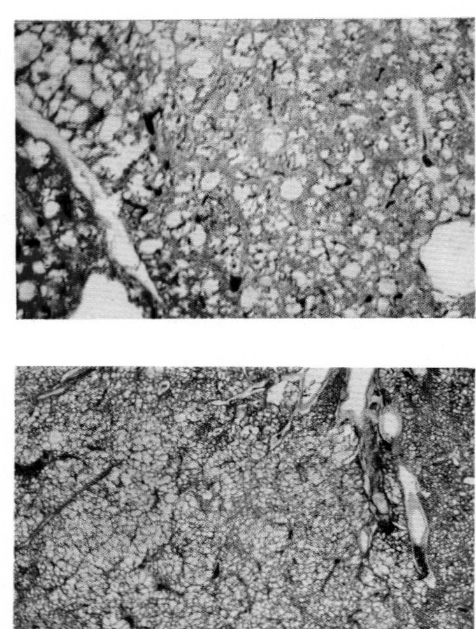

Fig. 4.22. Above: centrilobular emphysema. Below: panlobular emphysema.

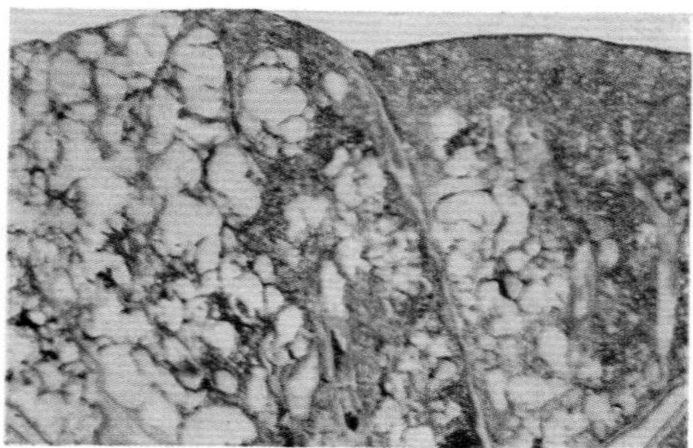

Fig. 4.23. Emphysema of an empty lobulus.

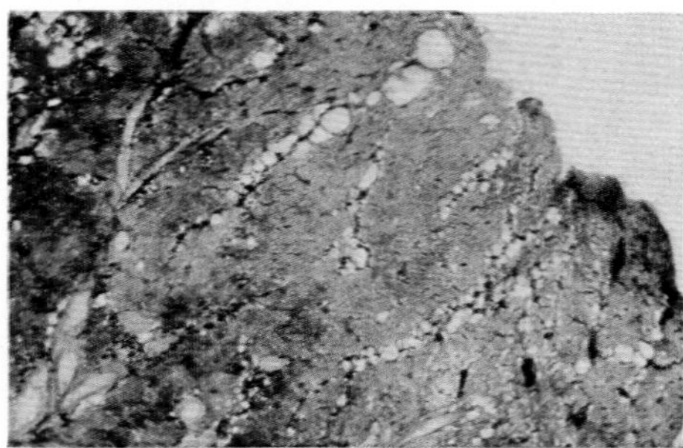

Fig. 4.24. Paraseptal emphysema.

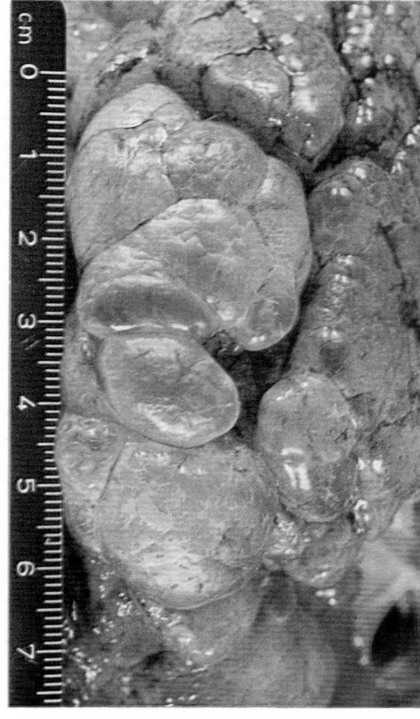

Fig. 4.25. Bullous emphysema.

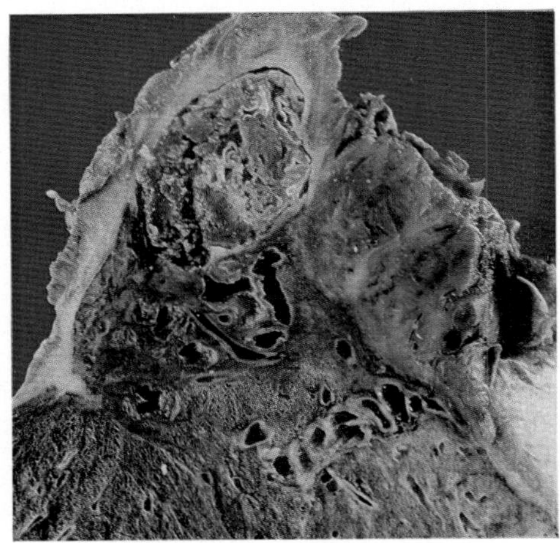

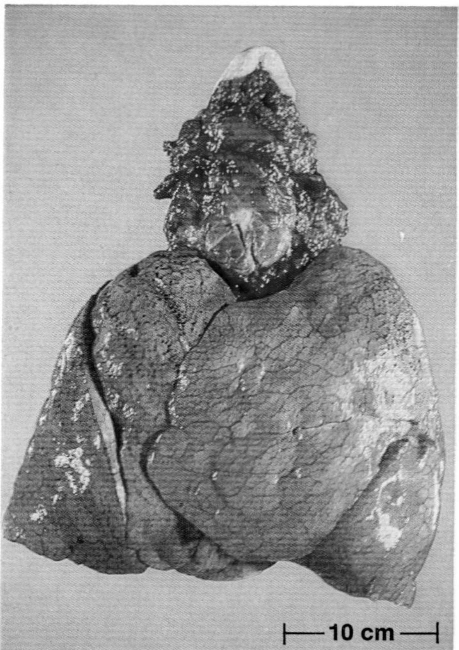

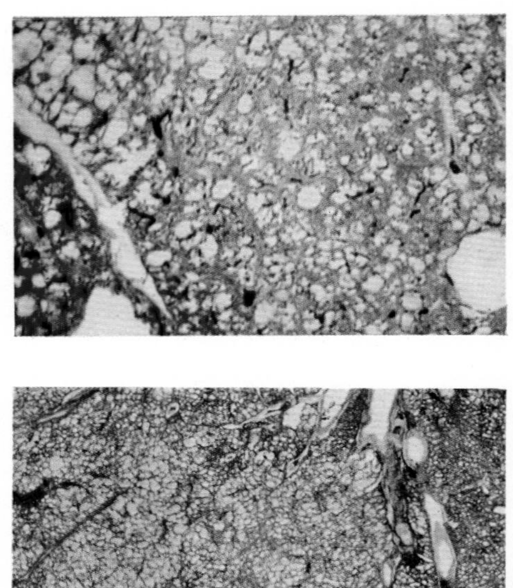

Pulmonary Emphysema

Pulmonary emphysema is defined as reversible or irreversible dilatation of air-containing spaces distal to the terminal bronchi with or without destruction of pulmonary parenchyma (TCP, p.75).

A. Acute pulmonary emphysema

Hyperinflation of the lung due to acute interference with expiration (status asthmaticus, spastic bronchitis of children, bolus death, death due to drowning). Figure 4.21 shows an acute pulmonary emphysema in a case of bronchial asthma. The lungs are light gray-red. The anterior margin is rounded (normally pointed). The lungs do not collapse after the thorax is opened and the rounded mediastinal margins touch each other. The consistency of the hyperinflated lung resembles an air-containing pillow. A finger impression remains as a small depressed focus.

B. Chronic pulmonary emphysema

Loss of pulmonary parenchyma (destructive emphysema) with reduction of the internal lung surface. Pulmonary emphysema can be classified according to morphologic or pathogenetic viewpoints. The following types can be distinguished on the basis of the *anatomic structural unit* of the lungs (lobulus or acinus[1]).

1. **Panlobular emphysema or diffuse emphysema** (Fig.4.22). The loss of parenchyma in panlobular emphysema is diffuse, even and more severe (50–80%) than in centrilobular emphysema (10–30%; Bignon).

2. **Emphysema of the empty lobulus** (Figs.4.23 and 4.29). The lobular structure has largely disappeared and, in extreme cases, the lobulus appears empty. Figure 4.29 is an enlargement (magnifying glass) of a lobulus. The alveoli are markedly dilated. Many alveolar septa have been lost, so that a large cystic space is formed. Small septa without capillaries traverse the cystic space. The almost empty lobulus is the result of functional stenosis of a lobular bronchiolus.

3. **Centrilobular emphysema** is defined as focal destruction of lung tissue in the center of a lobulus. Figure 4.21 shows a lung with "holes" of different sizes. The "holes" correspond to the central portion of the lobulus ("moth-eaten"). Several adjacent lobuli usually are affected and the end result is an empty lobulus or lobuli.

4. **Bullous emphysema** is especially seen at the margins of the lung (marginal emphysema) or near the lung apex. Bullous distention, i.e., dilatation and atrophy of lung tissue, involves one or several lobuli. Figure 4.25 shows blebs up to 1 cm. in size. The distended lung tissue is gray (anemia, pressure!). The blebs collapse after cutting. *Co:* rupture from sudden expansion of the lung and spontaneous pneumothorax.

Several morphologic forms of emphysema usually are combined in the same lung. Purely panlobular or centrilobular forms of emphysema are rare (approximately 10%). The morphologic diagnosis of emphysema can be made only on properly distended, fixed lungs, which provide information concerning the size of the blebs (vesicular, small, large or bullous) and their distribution (diffuse, panlobular, centrilobular, subpleural, focal). A morphologic classification of emphysema should be distinguished from an etiologic and pathogenetic classification.

---

[1]) A lobulus is supported by a bronchiolus that has a diameter of 1 mm. The lobulus measures approximately 2 cm. in diameter; 12–18 acini form one lobulus. The acinus is supported by a terminal bronchiolus.

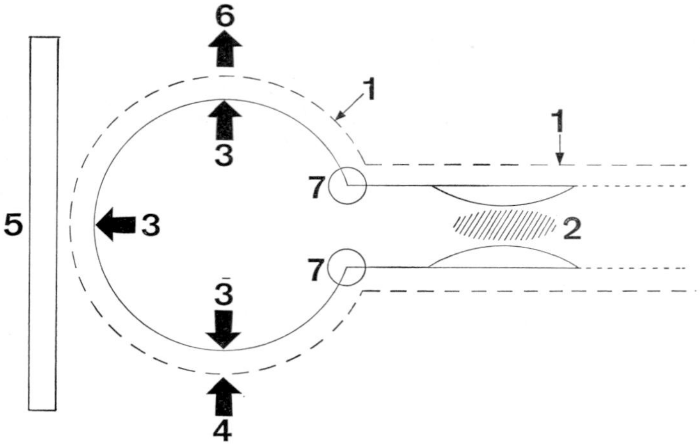

Fig. 4.26. Schematic presentation of the pathogenesis of pulmonary emphysema. (1) Hyperinflation without destruction. (2) Obstruction by mucus, spasm, bronchitis with weakening of the wall. (3) "Air-trapping." (4) Destruction (as a consequence of 2, 3 and 5). (5) Kinetic emphysema (subpleural or septal effects of adjacent tissue and organs). (6) Contraction of scars. (7) Senile emphysema (senile atrophy).

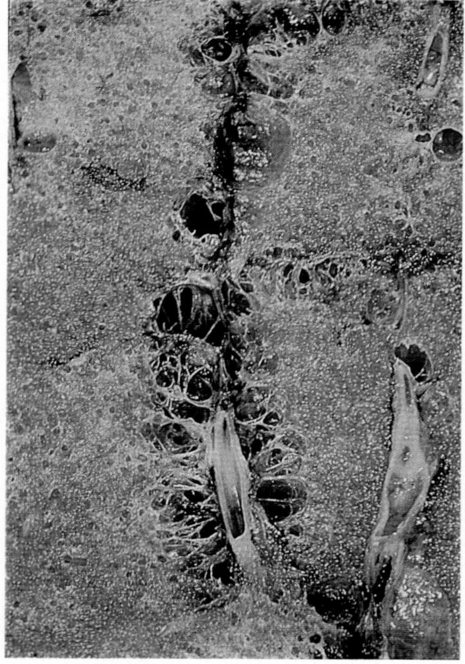

Fig. 4.28. Paraseptal emphysema.

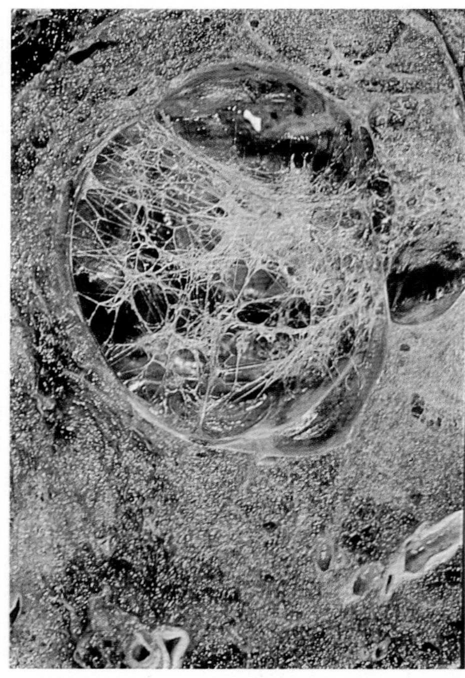

Fig. 4.29. Obstructive pulmonary emphysema.

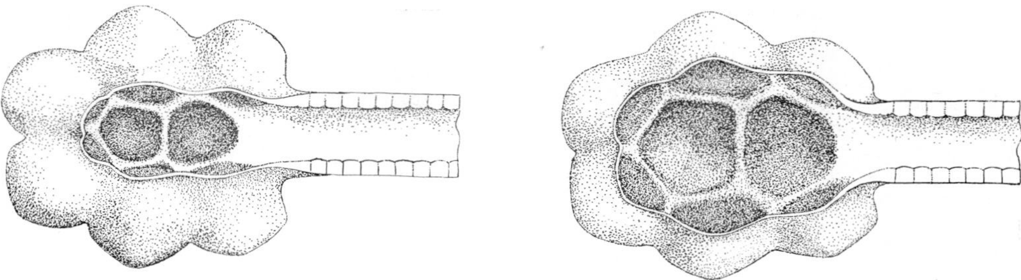

Fig. 4.27. Senile emphysema (according to OTTO). Left: normal. Right: senile emphysema.

Pathogenetic classification

Various factors leading to emphysema are summarized in Figure 4.26.

The simplest and most common form of emphysema is **senile emphysema** (atrophic senile lung or constitutional emphysema), which is the result of age-dependent atrophy of portions of alveolar septa with dilatation of alveolar ducts (Fig. 4.26.7). Senile emphysema is represented according to a model by OTTO in Figure 4.27. This process extends from the lung apex to the lower portions. The lung apex becomes rounded and the upper thorax aperture is increased (romanic dome of the senile lung in contrast to the pointed, gothic lung apex of young people). *Functional aspects:* Elastic forces of the lung are decreased and vital capacity is diminished. The lung is not "diseased," only reduced in its functional capacity. *Cor pulmonale does not develop.* Senile emphysema also can develop secondarily from bronchial obstruction.

Obstructive emphysema means *functional* and/or *organic* respiratory ventilation stenosis of bronchial lumina by *mucus* (so-called mucociliary insufficiency: overproduction of mucus from chronic irritation, diminished cleansing action by ciliated epithelium), *chronic bronchitis* (first thickening, then weakening of bronchial walls, with collapse of bronchioles during expiration: bronchial stenosis from scars of chronic bronchitis) or *congestion* (from chronic cor pulmonale). Ventilatory stenosis leads to overdistention and destruction of distal alveoli (Fig. 4.26.3). Alveoli adjacent to ventilatory stenosis likewise are compromised by overextension. As shown in Figure 4.29, individual lobules are affected; they are irregularly distributed throughout the lung. Obstructive emphysema is, at least initially, panlobular, although all other morphologic types of emphysema may develop secondarily (with the exception of emphysematous lung sclerosis or cystic lung) (see p. 67).

Obstruction can be demonstrated in approximately 80% of emphysema cases (OTTO, 1970). However, bronchial obstruction can occur without emphysema and emphysema can develop without demonstrable obstruction. Obstructive emphysema results relatively early in cor pulmonale with severe cyanosis. The widening of the thorax is a *consequence* of emphysema.

Paraseptal and subpleural emphysema (*kinetic emphysema* according to OTTO). As illustrated in Figure 4.26.5, this form of emphysema is attributed to structural changes resulting from different mechanical demands on the lung parenchyma. The lung is capable of undergoing structural changes in response to altered static or dynamic conditions (as are the bones). Alveoli disappear in order to provide increased mobility near fixed lines. Such stabile lines are the septae of the lung, as shown in Figures 4.24 and 4.28. Dilated alveoli are adjacent to septae that carry bronchioles or vessels: *paraseptal emphysema*. Another example illustrating the same pathogenetic mechanism is the *subpleural emphysema* that develops in lung segments adjacent to the thoracic wall.

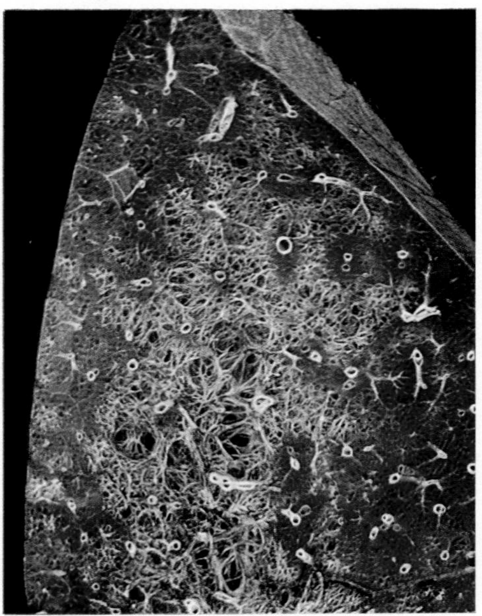

Fig. 4.30. Emphysematous pulmonary sclerosis.

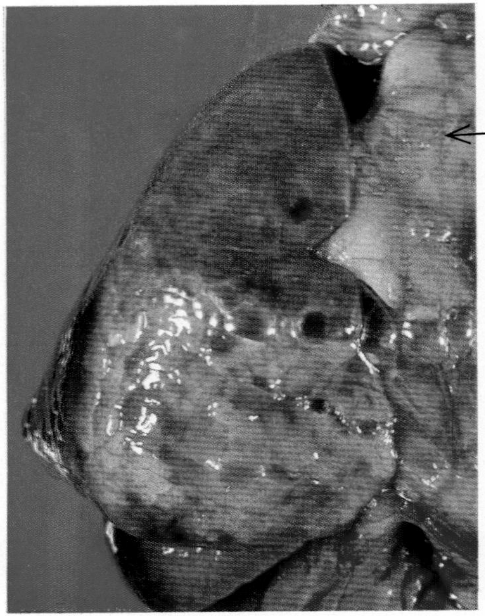

Fig. 4.31. Interstitial emphysema.

Scar emphysema. Various inflammatory processes, such as tuberculosis, silicosis, asbestosis and other pneumoconioses, produce focal pulmonary scars. The contracting scar tissue and changing dynamic conditions lead to emphysema in the vicinity of the scars (Fig. 4.30). Bands of scar tissue surround emphysematous blebs. An example is the emphysema around silicotic nodules (perinodular emphysema). *Co:* chronic bronchitis, bronchiectasis, scar carcinoma (adenocarcinoma).

Honeycomb lung (emphysematous lung sclerosis) (Figs. 4.26.6 and 4.30; TCP, p. 95). Diffuse scarring and fibrosis of the lungs is associated with interstitial fibrosis (HAMMAN-RICH syndrome), scleroderma and sarcoidosis. In addition to the structural changes (often with considerable hyperplasia of smooth muscle), the contracting scar tissue produces emphysema and dilatation of bronchioles. Grossly, the lung resembles a honeycomb.

Pulmonary emphysema. F: severe forms are encountered in 10% of autopsies. *A:* 50–60 years. *S:* ♂:♀ = 8:1. *Co:* respiratory insufficiency. Cor pulmonale in about 50% of cases because of hypoventilation, increased CO_2 in the blood and arteriolar constriction. Congestive bronchitis with right-sided cardiac failure intensifies bronchial obstruction. Recurrent pneumonias are common. Spontaneous pneumothorax.

C. Interstitial emphysema (Fig. 4.31).

Air escapes into the interstitial connective tissue following an internal lung trauma. The air bubbles resemble a string of pearls in the connective tissue septa of the lung. The air may extend into the mediastinum (→ thymus) and the subcutaneous connective tissue.

Pg: trauma (falls, concussions). Cough (during delivery, pneumonia in childhood, see Fig. 4.53). Hyperventilation under pressure. *Co:* pneumothorax, secondary infections of the opened tissue clefts (cellulitis).

Morphologic signs of pulmonary insufficiency at autopsy include: clubbed fingers, diaphragmatic grooves of the liver, cyanosis, gastric and intestinal ulcers (HARTUNG).

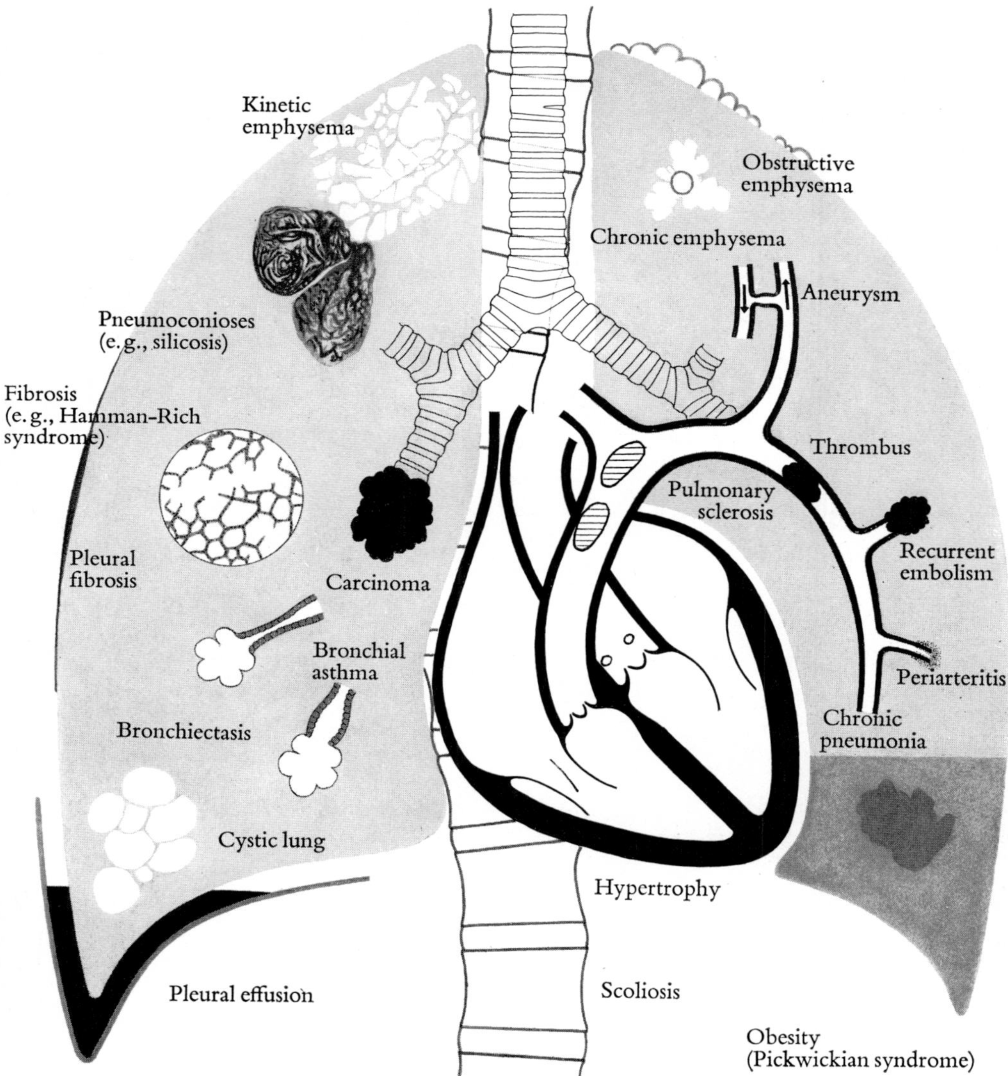

Fig. 4.32. Cor pulmonale. (1) Pulmonary causes include sclerosis of pulmonary arteries and veins (see above). (2) Extrapulmonary causes are manifold, i.e., kyphoscoliosis, obesity, Pickwickian syndrome, pleural fibrosis, pleural effusions or pleural mesotheliomas.

Cor pulmonale. Diseases of the lung that are accompanied by functional or anatomic narrowing of the pulmonary vessels produce increased pressure in the pulmonary circulation. The right ventricle first becomes dilated (acute cor pulmonale) and then hypertrophic (chronic cor pulmonale) (see also p. 23 and Figs. 2.9 and 4.22). Hypoventilation secondarily increases pulmonary resistance because of elevated CO_2 in the blood. The most important causes and consequences of cor pulmonale are summarized in Figure 4.32.

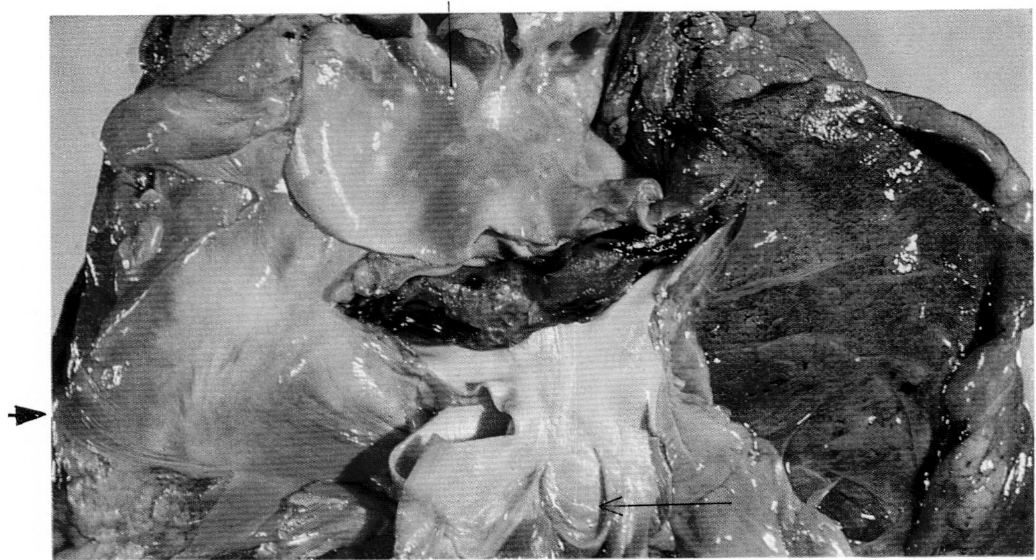

Fig. 4.33. Fatal lung embolism. Saddle embolus in the pulmonary artery.

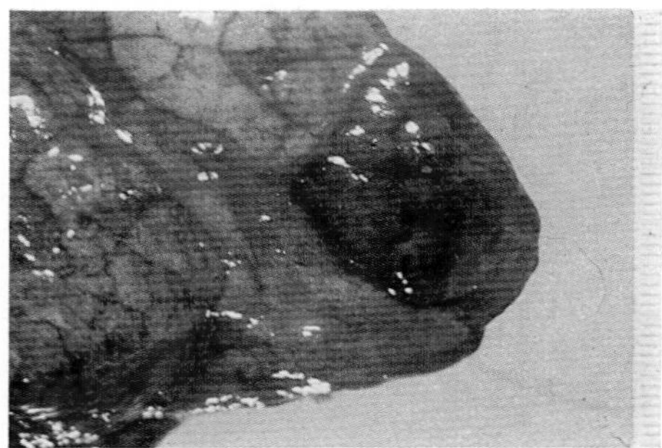

Fig. 4.34. Hemorrhagic lung infarction (external surface).

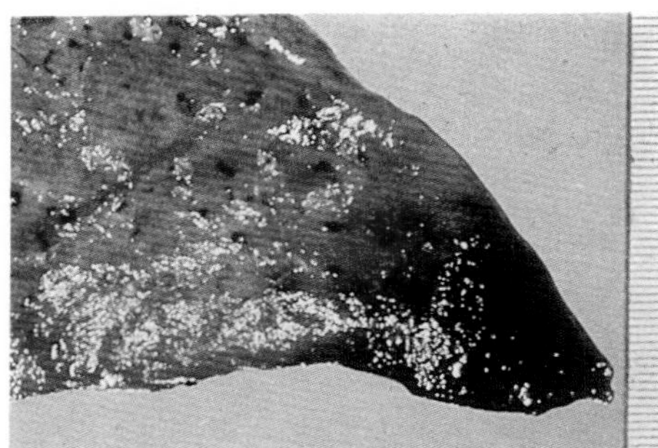

Fig. 4.35. Hemorrhagic lung infarction (cut surface).

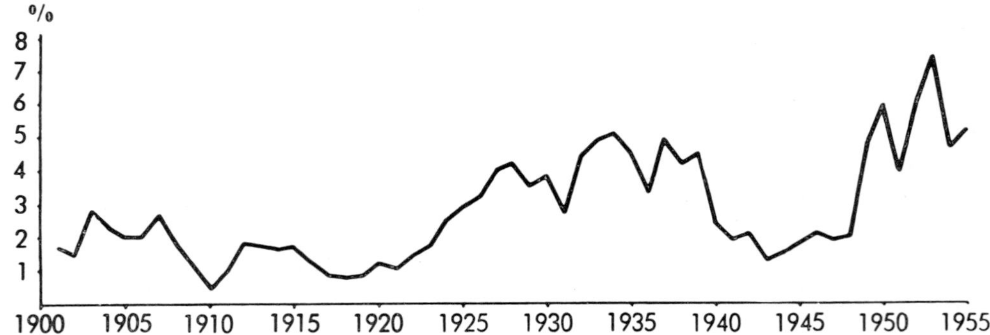

Fig. 4.36. Frequency of fatal lung embolism in Germany according to collective statistics from ten Institutes of Pathology.

Lung embolism. *Embolic occlusion of a pulmonary artery by a nonbacterial thrombus.* The fate of the patient depends on the caliber of the occluded branch of a pulmonary artery. *Fatal lung embolism* is caused by a sudden occlusion of the pulmonary artery, its main branches or several larger branches. *Nonfatal lung embolism* is caused by occlusion of one or several smaller pulmonary artery branches. Nonfatal embolism may complicate myocardial infarction or other basic diseases and thereby become fatal.

Figure 4.33 shows an occlusive embolus in the main pulmonary artery (lower →: pulmonic valve; left →: pericardial sac; upper →: aorta). The embolus is lodged at the bifurcation of the pulmonary artery and extends into its main branches. Central, gray-red portions with lines of Zahn are surrounded by red coagulation thrombosis on both ends. The embolus adheres to the wall if the patient survives for several days (organization by connective tissue).

F: between 1905 and 1955, fatal embolism accounted for 4% and nonfatal embolism for 7–8% of deaths in 51,000 autopsies. Fatal embolism accounts for less than 1% of deaths in South or Central America, Africa, Asia and Japan. Up to 2% die from fatal lung embolism in Australia, but more than 2% die from fatal embolism in Europe and the United States. In South Africa, 0.6% of Bantus but 2.8% of Europeans die from fatal embolism. Reasons for these differences: nutrition? ethnic factors? *A:* most cases of fatal lung embolism (70%) occur between 60 and 70 years of age. *S:* ♂:♀=1:2. *Pg:* see page 53. *General predisposing factors:* age, sex, nutritional state. Figure 4.36 shows the frequency of fatal lung embolism between 1900 and 1955 in Germany. At times of poor nutrition (World Wars I and II and several years thereafter), distinctly fewer fatal cases of lung embolism (2–3%) were observed than at times of good nutrition (up to 8%). Similar findings have been obtained in other European countries in contrast to the United States. Obese and well-nourished persons are affected twice as often as persons with normal weight. Figure 4.37 shows that fatal lung embolism is related to the number of thromboses, and occurs in very well-nourished persons four times more often than in malnourished persons. Obese persons have an incidence of thrombosis twice as high as persons with normal weight. Overweight must, therefore, indicate a higher tendency toward embolization from leg vein thrombosis. Cardiac and vascular diseases favor thrombosis and embolism. *Environmental factors:* certain weather conditions, such as warm and cold fronts. Leg veins are the main source of lung emboli; 25–50% of all leg vein thrombi embolize to the lung and 30% are fatal. Only one-third of all embolic events are diagnosed clinically (SANDRITTER and BENEKE)! *Co:* recurring pulmonary embolism → cor pulmonale. Hemorrhagic infarction.

Hemorrhagic lung infarction (Figs. 4.34 and 4.35; see TCP, p. 81). *Hemorrhagic necrosis of lung tissue following embolic occlusion of a pulmonary artery branch accompanied by congestion of the pulmonary circulation.* Grossly, a dark blue-red focus projects over the surface. The overlying pleura shows a fibrinous pleuritis. As seen in Figure 4.34, the adjacent lung segment above the infarction is hyperinflated. The cut surface of the infarction is of black-red color and projects above the lung surface (Fig. 4.35). Hemorrhages occur in the adjacent viable lung tissue.

Co: organization; scar; abscess; gangrene.

Anemic lung infarctions are found after occlusion of a medium-sized pulmonary artery branch, usually with lobar pneumonia.

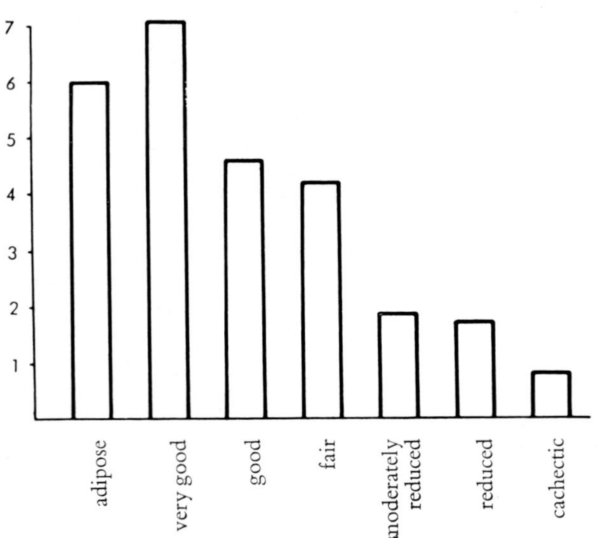

Fig. 4.37. Nutritional status and tendency of thrombi to embolize to the lungs. The data are expressed as fatal lung embolism (%) as related to the frequency of thrombosis.

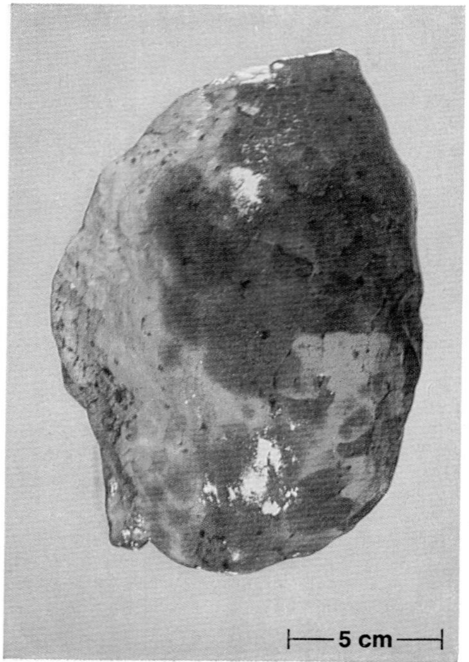

Fig.4.38. Aspiration of blood.

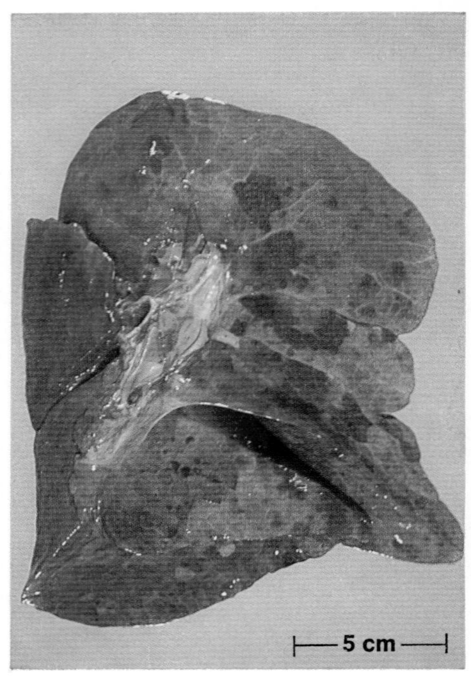

Fig.4.39. Subpleural pulmonary hemorrhages.

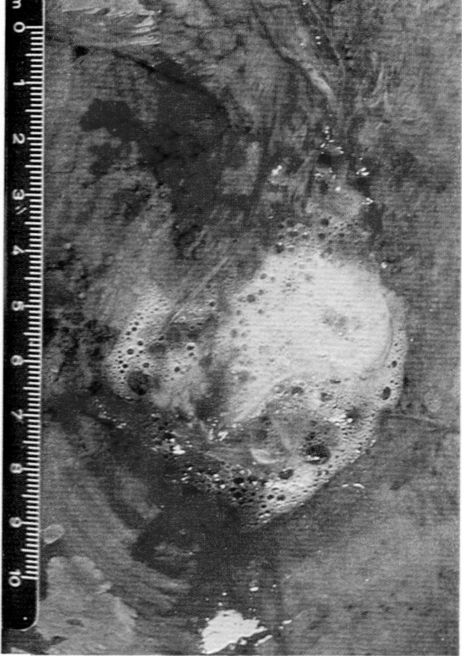

Fig.4.40. Pulmonary edema.

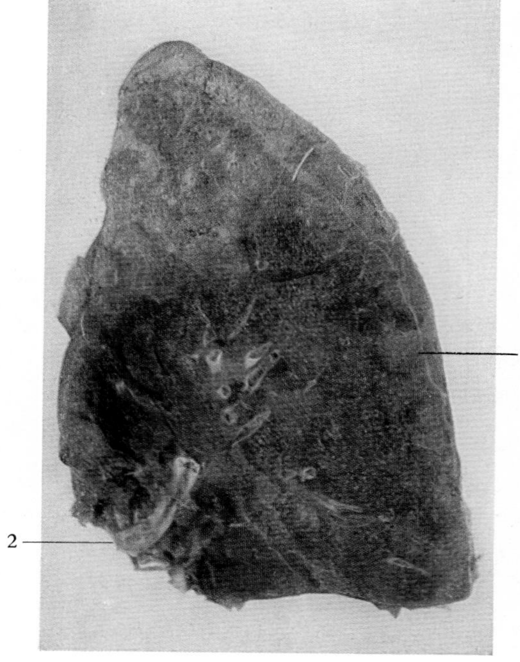

Fig.4.41. Uremic pneumonitis.

Hemorrhage, Pulmonary Edema

Aspiration of blood into the lung (Fig. 4.38). *Following hemorrhages into the upper respiratory or intestinal tract, blood is aspirated into lobar or segmental bronchi, terminal bronchioles and corresponding alveoli.*

Figure 4.38 shows the left lung with the paravertebral margin at the left. A sharply demarcated lung segment that corresponds to the distribution of a segmental bronchus is bright red. The consistency is not increased and the lung segment does not project over the surface. In contrast to a lung infarction, there is no pleuritis in the area of aspirated blood. Smaller, ill-defined foci of aspirated blood are found in the upper lobe. The cut surface of foci containing aspirated blood is soft and reddish discolored. The surrounding lung usually is hyperinflated (acute emphysema).

Pg: sources of hemorrhage are intrapulmonary and extrapulmonary. Intrapulmonary: bronchogenic carcinomas, bronchial carcinoids, tuberculosis. Extrapulmonary: after tonsillectomy, tumors, trauma of neck vessels, tracheostomy, ruptured aneurysms, esophageal varices, hemorrhages of the gastric mucosa (erosions).

Subpleural hemorrhages (Fig. 4.39). *Subpleural hemorrhages occur with hemorrhagic diathesis or suffocation. The hemorrhages are scattered throughout the lung and are not bound to anatomic lung segments.* Figure 4.39 shows extensive blue-red subpleural hemorrhages in a case of hemorrhagic diathesis from leukemia. Petechial hemorrhages are seen focally in the lower lobe. Our picture shows the hilus of the left lung; the paravertebral margin is at the left. After cutting, the blood is found in a small zone between the pleura and pulmonary tissue. No pleuritis.

Pg: the so-called suffocation hemorrhages (flecks of Tardieu) in children are small and petechial. Seen in adult patients with hemorrhagic tendencies (leukemia, aplastic anemia).

DD: a *hemorrhagic infarction* is dry, firm, dark red, triangular and causes pleuritis.

Aspirated blood is bright red, sharply demarcated, soft and involves the deeper portions of the lung.

Subpleural hemorrhages are irregularly distributed.

Traumatic intrapulmonary hemorrhages are globular and ball-type.

Hemorrhagic pneumonia (e.g., influenza) has intrapulmonary, irregular hemorrhages with bronchopneumonia.

Uremic hemorrhages are seen predominantly around the hilus and diminish in intensity toward the lung periphery.

Pulmonary edema (Fig. 4.40; see TCP, p. 75). *Exudation of serum into the lung alveoli. The most common causes are left ventricular failure or toxic substances (so-called intra-alveolar pulmonary edema).* The lung is heavier than normal (normal weight: 350 Gm. on the left, 450 Gm. on the right → up to 2,000 Gm.). A foamy, reddish fluid exudes during cutting or minor pressure (mixing of air and protein-rich fluid causes the foam. Surface tension!). Foamy edema fluid also exudes from the lumen of a main bronchus. A finger impression remains, as in edema of the lower legs.

DD: pneumonia: the lung tissue tears easily. In *chronic pulmonary edema*, the lung is firm and edema fluid can be expressed only after considerable pressure. *Mi:* conglomerated protein masses are found in lung alveoli; see TCP, pages 75 and 79. *Pg:* electron microscopic studies have revealed that edema fluid enters the lung alveoli across cell membranes. The main pathogenetic factor is increased hydrostatic pressure from left ventricular failure in the presence of a functional right ventricle. However, additional factors such as hypoxia and toxic substances also must be operative, since they are known to cause membrane damage. The most common basic disease is myocardial infarction.

Interstitial pulmonary edema occurs during shock. Dark red, hard, heavy lungs. No fluid drains off from she cut surface. Histologically, there is a broadening of she alveolar septa (see p. 15).

Hemorrhagic, fibrinous edema in uremia (so-called uremic pneumonia or pneumonitis, Fig. 4.41). *A hemorrhagic, fibrin-rich edema accumulates in the alveoli of patients with uremia.* Figure 4.41 shows a red to brown-red discoloration of the right lung. The progression of uremic pneumonitis from the hilus to the lung periphery is typical (→2, lung hilus). Note the small, unaffected subpleural zone (→1).

DD: pneumonia extends to the pleura and the involved lung is elastic or rubbery in consistency. Hemorrhagic fluid (edema and hemorrhage) exudes from the cut surface. In addition, the cut surface is granular due to alveolar fibrin plugs that project over the surface. Pleuritis may occur.

Pg: chronic uremia causes toxic endothelial damage and fibrin exudation in the pericardium, intestine and pharynx. Edema is caused by cardiac insufficiency.

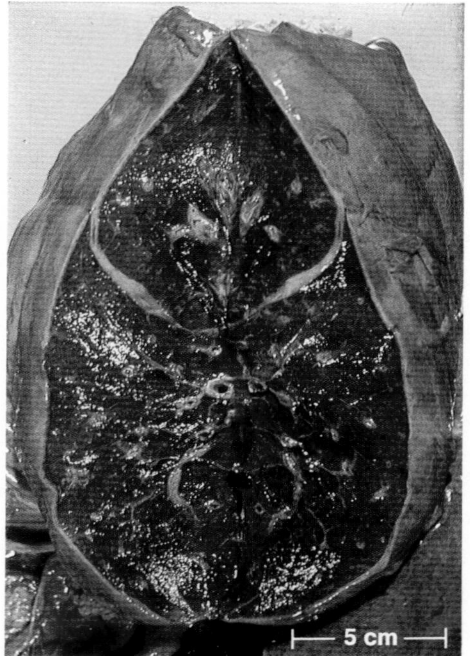

Fig. 4.42. Chronic congestion of the lungs.

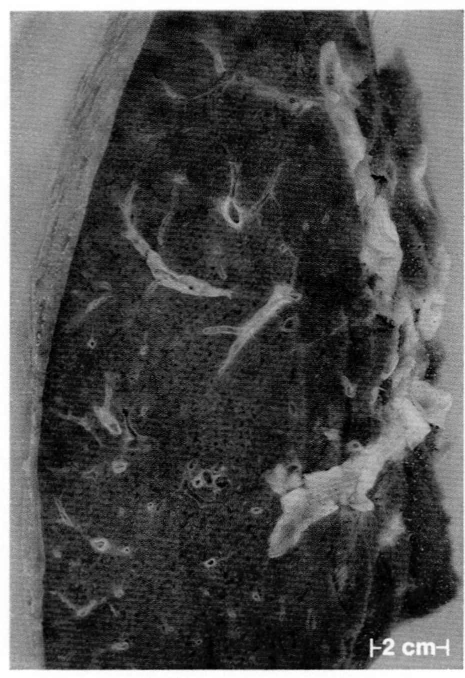

Fig. 4.43. Pulmonary hemosiderosis in a case of Goodpasture syndrome.

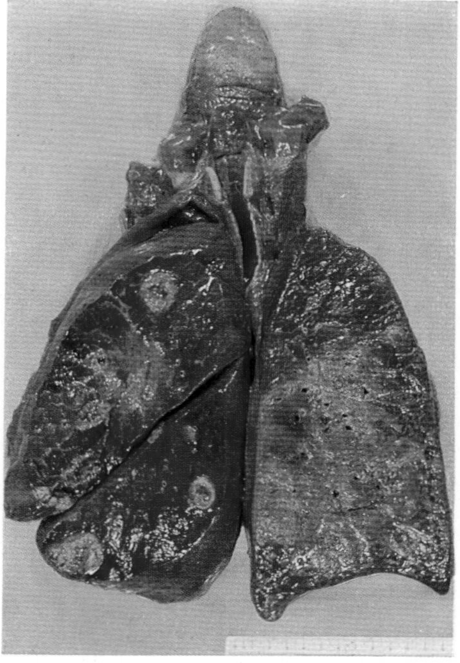

Fig. 4.44. Wegener's granulomatosis of the lungs.

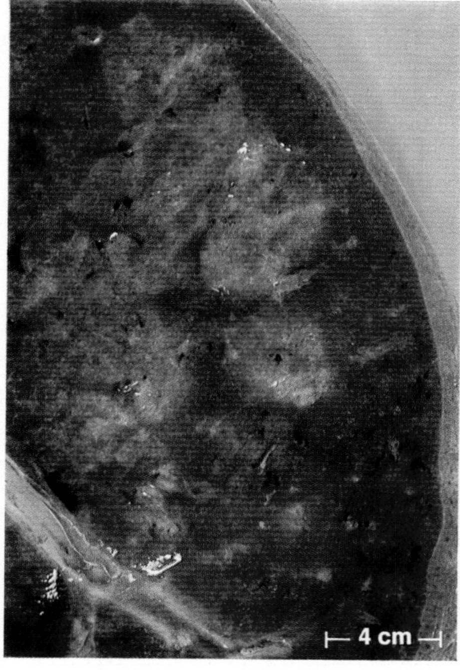

Fig. 4.45. Confluent bronchopneumonia.

Congestion of the Lung, Pneumonia

Chronic congestion of the lung (Fig. 4.42; TCP, p. 77). *Chronic, passive hyperemia due to congenital or acquired left ventricular failure.* The lungs are red or blue-red and edematous in acute congestion. They become brown with longstanding congestion. Figure 4.42 shows the homogeneous, brown cut surface of a chronically congested lung. The lung is firm; the lobes do not collapse but "stand up" (brown induration). The consistency has been compared to that of a dog's ear or the hide of a deer (ZOLLINGER). Chronic passive congestion often is accompanied by pulmonary edema. Bony-hard nodules, up to 1–2 mm. in size, can be palpated or diagnosed by x-ray in cases of severe chronic congestion, e.g., mitral stenosis (metaplastic ossification → bony lung nodules).

Pg: mitral or aortic valve defects or left ventricular failure → congestion. (Histology and consequences, see TCP, p. 77.)

Lung hemosiderosis (Fig. 4.43). *Chronic, recurring alveolar microhemorrhages with hemosiderin deposits in the alveolar epithelium, pulmonary connective tissues and elastic membranes of blood vessels. The disease occurs as primary essential lung hemosiderosis (Ceelen's disease) or is associated with glomerulonephritis (Goodpasture syndrome).* Figure 4.43 shows a uniformly brown cut surface. The lung is firm and elastic.

F: primary lung hemosiderosis (approximately 120 cases have been published): predominantly in young females. The course extends over $3^1/_2$ years. *Pg:* not known: primary, degenerative damage of elastic fibers from autoimmunity? *Secondary lung hemosiderosis (Goodpasture syndrome):* approximately 200 cases have been described. *A:* 20–30 years. *S:* ♂:♀ = 3:1. *Pg:* capillary damage → microhemorrhages, autoantibodies with glomerulonephritis.

Wegener's granulomatosis (Fig. 4.44). *Special type of a granulomatous arteritis with an unusual type of dissemination.* The disease usually begins in the nose, sinuses, pharynx, larynx or middle ear *(Stage I)*, spreads caudally (ulcerative tracheobronchitis, lung involvement) *(Stage II)* and becomes generalized (heart, liver, thyroid gland, spleen, skin) *(Stage III)*. The patient usually dies from involvement of the kidneys (→ uremia) *(Stage IV)*. Typical pulmonary manifestations are shown in Figure 4.44: several sharply delineated, yellow, firm lesions in the left lung measure up to 6 cm. in diameter. Some of these are centrally necrotic. A diffuse pneumonia of bright yellow-red color and firm-elastic consistency is found in the right lung.

Macroscopic DD: tuberculosis, Hodgkin's disease, pneumonia. The nasal, sinusoidal and pharyngeal mucosa is thickened, ulcerated and crusted. Infarctions of bright red to yellow specks as in periarteritis nodosa are found in the kidneys and spleen.

F: probably more common than the 132 cases published thus far. The disease appears to have increased in frequency during the past few years. *A:* 30–50 years. *S:* ♂:♀ = 2:1. *Pr:* 4 weeks to 3 years. *Mi: arteritis* and *phlebitis* with granuloma formation (necrosis, giant cells of foreign-body or Langhans type, epithelioid cells, fibroblasts, lymphocytes, plasma cells). *Pg:* (a) primary tuberculoid granulation tissue that secondarily extends to vessels; (b) primary arteritis with secondary granuloma formation. *Cause* is not known.

Bronchopneumonia (Fig. 4.45; TCP, pp. 87 and 89). *Multifocal pneumonia of lung lobuli without distinct anatomic boundaries.* The gross diagnosis often is difficult for the beginner. *Diagnostic criteria are:* somewhat firmer than normal, friable, poorly demarcated foci differ in size (up to 2–3 cm.). They are *slightly elevated.* The knife is led over the cut surface; irregular "elevations" are noted; a *red-cloudy liquid* adheres to the knife blade and the consolidated areas are not crepitant (no air noise). The least reliable diagnostic criterion is the *color change.* Foci of bronchopneumonia can have the same color as normal lung tissue. Sometimes they are grayish and in other cases they are gray-yellow (Fig. 4.45). The lesions in Figure 4.45 are poorly demarcated and some have fused (confluent bronchopneumonia). Lesions of various sizes and colors therefore are characteristic of fully developed bronchopneumonia because different stages of inflammation usually are encountered at autopsy. *Remember:* the initial inflammatory response is hyperemia and inflammatory edema, followed by a fibrin-rich exudate and, finally, by foci with many leukocytes. The gross picture varies accordingly. Bronchopneumonia almost always is accompanied by fibrinous pleuritis, and purulent bronchitis often coexists.

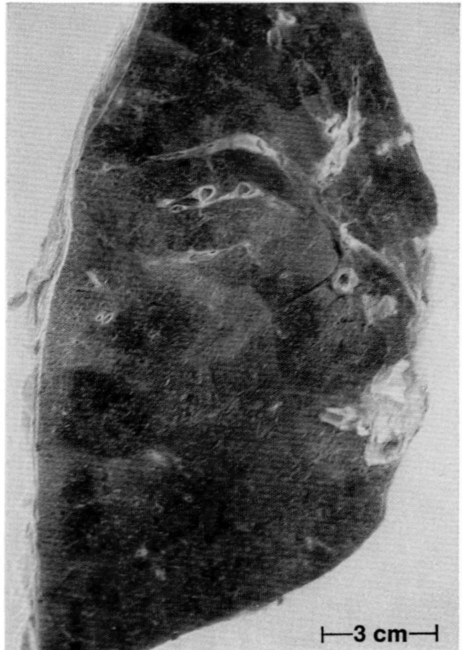

Fig. 4.46. Influenzal pneumonia.

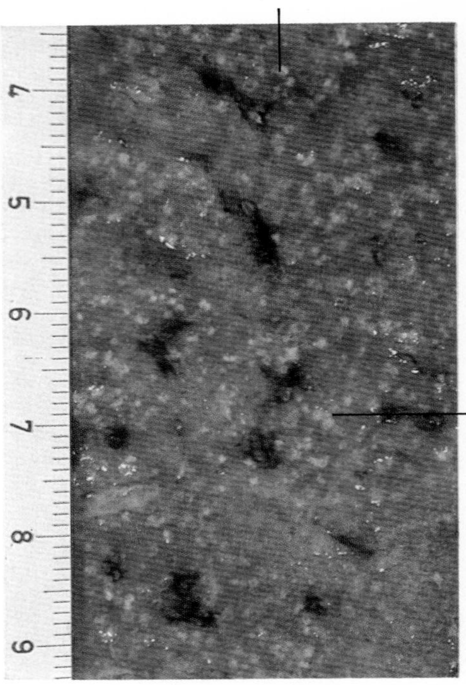

Fig. 4.47. Peribronchial focal pneumonia.

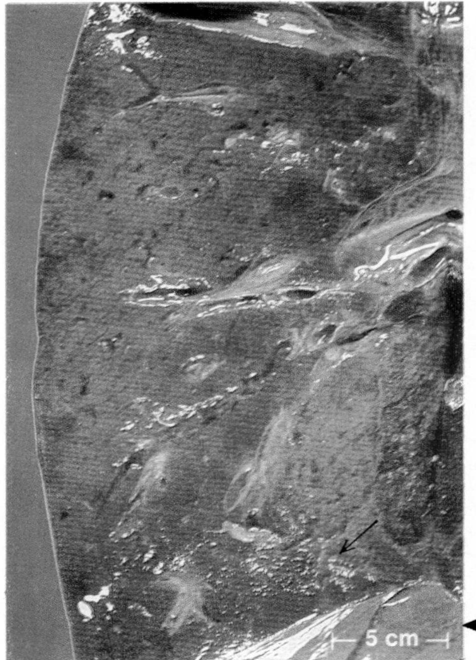

Fig. 4.48. Lobar pneumonia in the stage of gray hepatization.

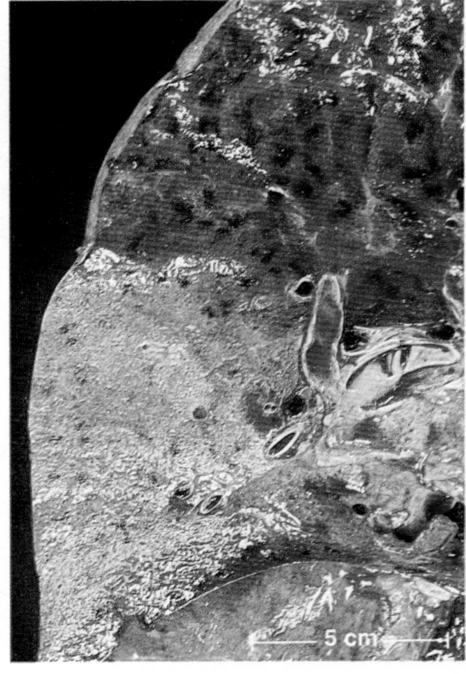

Fig. 4.49. Lobar pneumonia in the stage of yellow hepatization.

F: first peak at 2–5 years, second peak in persons past 60 years. *Pg:* bacterial infections (pneumococci, less commonly staphylococci) by diminished host resistance. Endobronchial dissemination. The so-called hypostatic pneumonia is a common form of bronchopneumonia in which red foci of consolidation are confined to the posterior, paravertebral lung (poor ventilation of lung portions that rest on the ribs → vascular disturbances → inflammation). *Co:* see lobar pneumonia.

Influenzal pneumonia (Fig. 4.46; see also p. 61; TCP, p. 89). *A special form of lobular bronchopneumonia with a marked hemorrhagic component on gross examination.* Partly confluent, red or mostly dusky red lesions occupy most of the lung, and little aerated lung remains (Fig. 4.46). Central necrosis, heavy fibrin exudates or massive infiltration with leukocytes may modify the gross picture so that the areas of consolidation are gray-yellow or red-yellow with hemorrhagic zones of demarcation. The bronchial mucosa is dusky red (trachea, see p. 61). Cases of acute, highly toxic influenzal pneumonia have been described that lack the inflammatory component and show only hemorrhages and necrosis of pulmonary parenchyma.

F: the pandemic of 1918–1919 affected all age groups, although older persons predominated. *Pg:* influenza virus with frequent secondary infection by streptococci, staphylococci or pneumococci or *Haemophilus influenzae*. The virus first causes epithelial damage, then inflammation. *Co:* abscess, empyema, chronic pneumonia, encephalitis, myocarditis. Cloudy swelling of the liver and kidney. Toxic circulatory collapse with rapid drop in blood pressure.

Peribronchial, focal pneumonia (Fig. 4.47; TCP, p. 89). *In this special type of focal pneumonia, infectious organisms penetrate the bronchial walls (rather than disseminate endobronchially) to cause peribronchial inflammation.* Accordingly, the pneumonic lesions are smaller than those of lobular bronchopneumonia and are confined to alveoli around bronchi. Figure 4.47 shows round, somewhat irregular lesions of yellow color that measure approximately 2 mm. The foci project slightly over the cut surface, as seen from the highlights at their margins. The lumen of a bronchiolus (→) may be identified as the center of consolidated foci.

DD: miliary tubercles are somewhat smaller than foci of peribronchial pneumonia, gray-white and without a central bronchiolus. *A:* mostly in children. *Pg:* measles, scarlet fever, diphtheria, influenza and whooping cough. Infection with streptococci or staphylococci.

Lobar pneumonia. *Inflammation of an entire lung lobe (or large parts thereof), with a progressive, stage-like course* (see TCP, pp. 91 and 93). Stages: *Congestion:* blood-red cut surface, foamy reddish fluid exudes (rarely seen at autopsy). *Red hepatization:* red, firm and friable cut surface.

Gray hepatization. Figure 4.48 shows the typical appearance of the lung. The cut surface of the entire left lower lobe is homogeneously gray to gray-red, dry, firm and friable (→ diaphragmatic surface of the lower lobe). The consolidated lung tissue breaks easily when finger pressure is applied. Why? Fibrin extends through the pores of Kohn into adjacent alveoli and forms a structural unit with the elastic lung tissue. The total lung elasticity is thereby reduced. (Also damage to elastic fibers?) The highlights in this picture (thin →) point to a finely granular cut surface. The granularity is due to fibrin plugs projecting from the alveoli and alveolar ducts.

Yellow hepatization. As shown in Figure 4.49, almost the entire left lower lobe is bright yellow and firm but its consistency is somewhat softer than the lung in the stage of gray hepatization (histologically: more leukocytes, beginning fibrinolysis). Thick yellow fluid can be scraped off the cut surface. Tiny plugs project from the alveoli (see highlights in this picture). Only the upper portion of the left lower lobe is aerated.

Lobar pneumonia in the stage of resolution (lysis). The lung is red and edematous. Red fluid can be scraped off the cut surface.

F: 3–6% of critically ill patients. *A:* 20–60 years. *S:* ♂:♀ = 3:1. Lethal in 10–30% but in 60–90% of patients past 60 years. *Pg:* Types I and II pneumococci in 60–80%, Type III pneumococcus mucosus in 4–6%, Type IV in 20% of lobar pneumonias. *Co:* carnification = chronic pneumonia. Anemic necrosis → sequestration; abscess, gangrene, empyema, enteritis, meningitis.

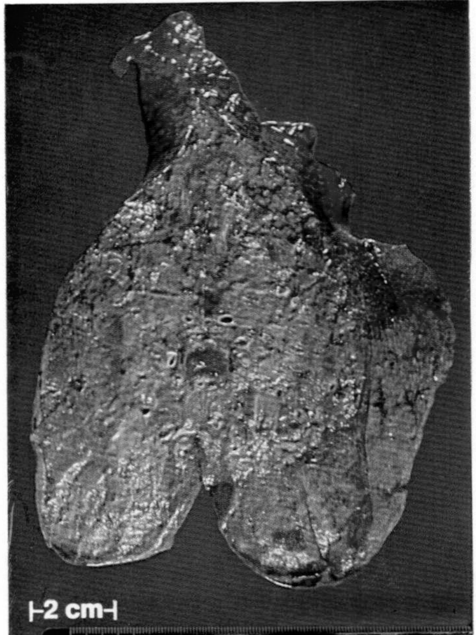

Fig. 4.50. Chronic pneumonia.

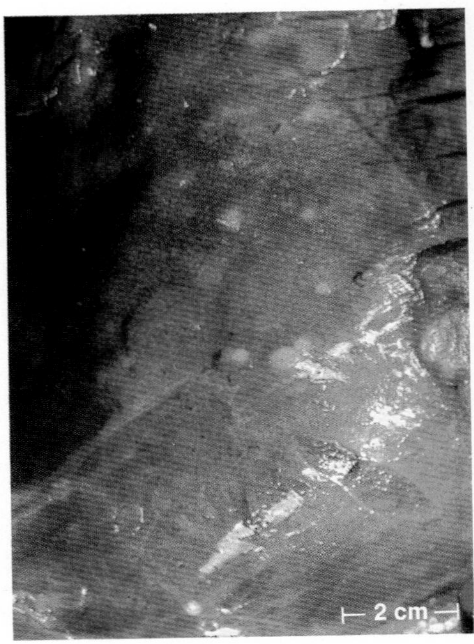

Fig. 4.51. Pyemic lung abscesses.

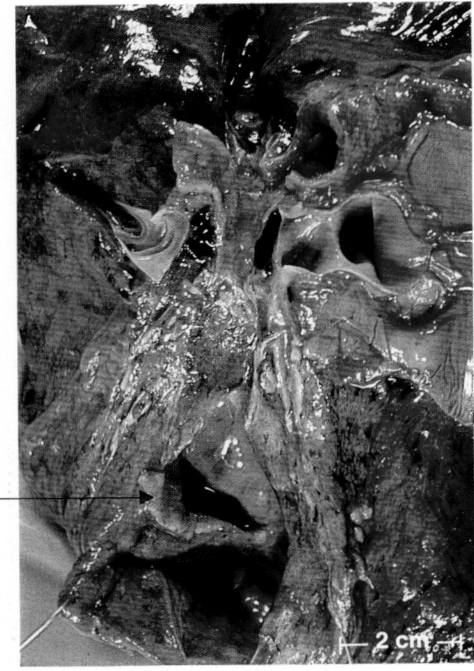

Fig. 4.52. Lung abscess.

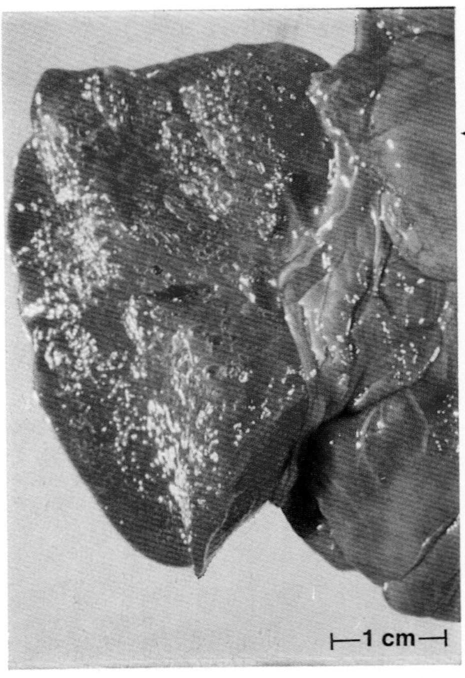

Fig. 4.53. Pneumocystis pneumonia with interstitial emphysema.

Chronic pneumonia (Fig. 4.50; TCP, p. 93). If the stage of lysis fails to develop (usually 2–3 weeks after the onset of lobar pneumonia), the fibrin exudate will be organized by granulation tissue. The result is chronic pneumonia. The gross picture is rather characteristic (Fig. 4.50). The lung is elastic, resembling fish flesh. It is focally gray-white discolored, and these foci merge with the normal surrounding lung tissue. Young granulation tissue is red in color. The relatively fresh chronic pneumonia, therefore, can be diagnosed best by palpation.

Co: cor pulmonale, pulmonary sclerosis, emphysema.

Pyemic lung abscess (Fig. 4.51; TCP, p. 81). *Occlusion of a small branch of the pulmonary artery by bacterial emboli (pyemia).* Multiple small foci from 0.5 to 1 cm. in diameter are scattered throughout the pleura. The triangular or quadrangular foci are yellow, protrude slightly and have a hemorrhagic zone of demarcation (Fig. 4.51). Yellow pus may exude after cutting. Earlier stages are yellow-gray. Pleural necrosis (white foci) frequently accompanies pyemic abscesses; fibrinous pleuritis is always present.

Source of infected (bacteria-containing) emboli: purulent thrombophlebitis, e.g., otitis media with phlebitis of cerebral sinuses, furuncle, appendicitis, diverticulitis, etc. Often accompanied by embolic glomerulonephritis (pyemic renal abscesses) (see p. 267).

Regarding terminology: bacteremia refers to infectious agents circulating in the blood stream without multiplication. Sepsis denotes a massive invasion by infectious organisms with diminished host defense. Pyemia is defined as metastatic lodging of bacteria alone or of infected emboli followed by abscess formation.

Lung abscess (Fig. 4.52). *Localized purulent necrosis of lung tissue.* Our picture shows an empty abscess, 3–4 cm. in diameter, with a gray-yellow, thin abscess membrane. The surrounding lung tissue was separated from the abscess membrane. Green-yellow pus exuded from the abscess at autopsy.

Pg: usually secondary to a pneumonia, aspiration of food, gunshot wounds or other types of trauma. Mostly caused by staphylococci or streptococci.

Interstitial pneumonia (Fig. 4.53; TCP, pp. 86 and 273). *Inflammation of interstitial lung tissue with minimal or no involvement of the alveoli.* Grossly, the lung is firmer than normal (firm-elastic) and evenly red to gray-red. A typical complication is shown in Figure 4.53: extensive interstitial emphysema with air bubbles in the interstitial tissue arranged like a string of pearls. → Thymus.

Occurs most frequently in *premature infants* (up to the ninth week of life) after infection with pneumocystis carinii. Also seen as neonatal syphilis (pneumonia alba: very rare today; gray, white-reddish, marmor-like lung cut surface). Interstitial pneumonia of *adults* is caused by viruses (influenza, psittacosis), mycoplasma or rickettsia. Measles causes interstitial pneumonia with giant cells (Warthin-Finkelday giant cells).

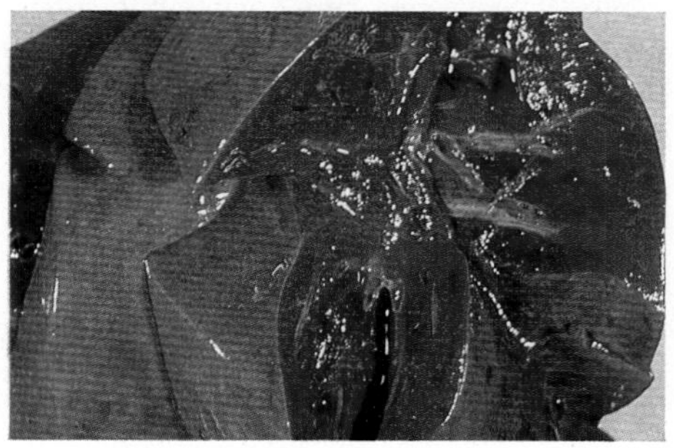

Figure 4.54. "Shock lung".

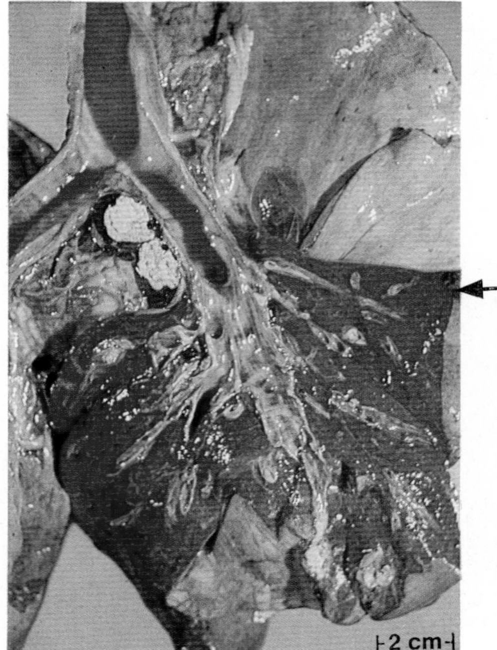

Fig. 4.55. Tuberculous primary complex.

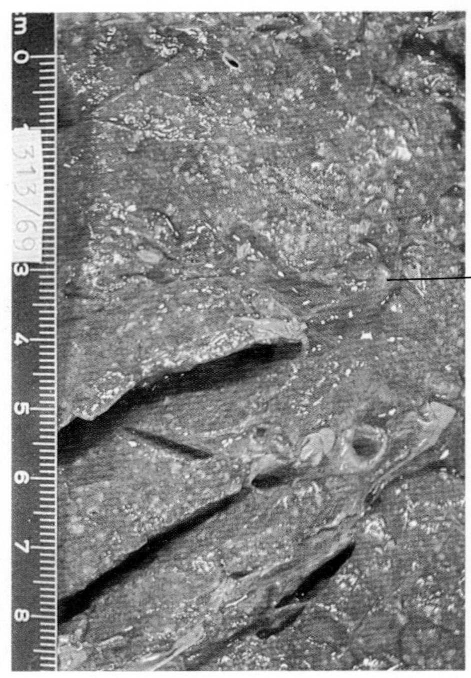

Fig. 4.56. Miliary tuberculosis.

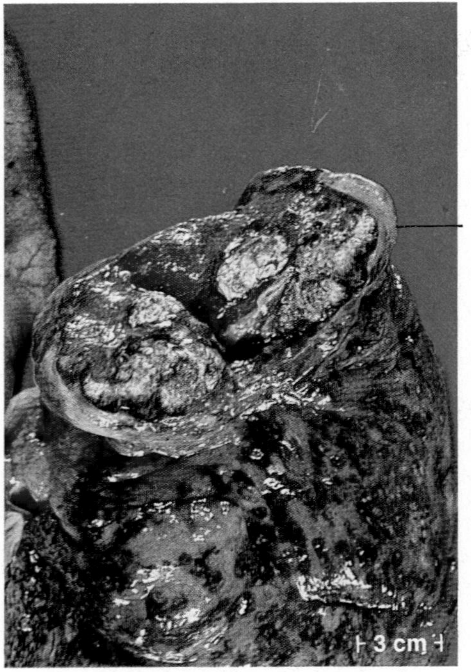

Fig. 4.57. Tuberculosis of the lung apex.

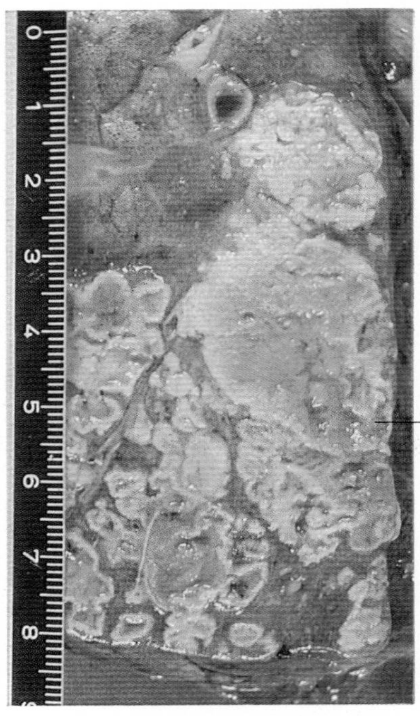

Fig. 4.58. Caseous, partially gelatinous pneumonia.

Tuberculosis of the Lung

Infectious disease due to Mycobacterium tuberculosis *with stage-like progression* (TCP, pp. 96–101). The initial aerogenous infection leads to the formation of a subpleural caseous tubercle, the so-called Ghon focus, which frequently is located in the lower portion of the right upper lobe or the upper portion of the right lower lobe. The Ghon focus soon is followed by a tuberculous lymphangitis and caseating tubercles in hilar lymph nodes *(primary complex)* (x-ray diagnosis). A primary complex is the initial response to many infections, especially tuberculosis and syphilis.

Figure 4.55 shows a tuberculous primary complex. Two hilar lymph nodes contain areas of caseation necrosis (tuberculous cheese is dry and friable, resembling cottage cheese). The primary focus in Figure 4.55 probably is represented by the gray-black subpleural lesion just below the fissure between the upper and lower lobes (→). Tiny central areas of caseation necrosis are recognized in this small (5 mm. in diameter), indurated, black scar tissue. The scar tissue is white but anthracotic pigment produces a black discoloration. Another caseous tubercle near the base of the lower lobe measures approximately 1 cm. in diameter. This focus probably developed by hematogenous spread.

Massive hematogenous dissemination and the development of miliary tuberculosis are early complications of the primary complex (see Table 4.1, p. 86). Miliary tuberculosis is observed most frequently in children but it also can occur in adults with a primary complex. Figure 4.56 illustrates a case of a 32-year-old female (see also p. 86). The entire lung is studded with gray-yellow, glassy foci measuring 1–2 mm. in diameter (→ miliary tubercle). The term "miliary" describes the size of a tubercle (milium = millet seed). Miliary tubercles may develop as single foci in other organs (liver, kidney) after hematogenous or lymphogenous spread. One has to *distinguish* between miliary tuberculosis and miliary tubercle (see Table 4.1). *The primary complex usually heals. Exogenous* or *endogenous* hematogenous reinfection most often localizes in the lung apex (apical reinfection or *Simon's apical focus*). The tuberculous apical reinfection spreads via the bronchi, and an infraclavicular infiltrate is produced *(Assmann's early infiltrate).*

Figure 4.57 shows extensive *apical tuberculosis.* Several dry, friable, white and partially chalky lesions measure up to 1 cm. in diameter. Some are surrounded by indurated scar tissue. Apical tuberculosis always involves the pleura. Such a tuberculous pleuritis heals and a gray-white pleural scar remains (→). The usual autopsy finding is an apical pleural scar and a narrow rim of indurated lung tissue beneath.

Chronic, progressive lung tuberculosis can exacerbate at any time, by either massive exogenous reinfection or diminished host resistance (war prisoners, cancer patients).

The result of exacerbation is the development of a gelatinous or caseous pneumonia. Figure 4.58 shows multiple confluent lesions, up to 10 cm. in diameter. The large central lesion (→) still has a gray-white, glassy ,gelatinous appearance (*Mi:* gelatinous areas contain cellular exudate). Other, smaller lesions (bottom of Fig. 4.58) show beginning central necrosis (*Mi:* caseation = necrosis). Cavities can arise quickly from large areas of caseation and eventually may involve an entire lung lobe (death in respiratory insufficiency or massive hemorrhage from the cavity).

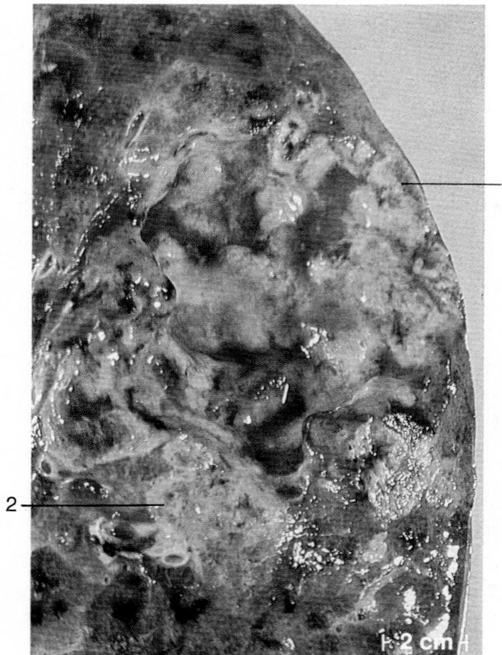

Fig. 4.59. Fresh tuberculous cavity.

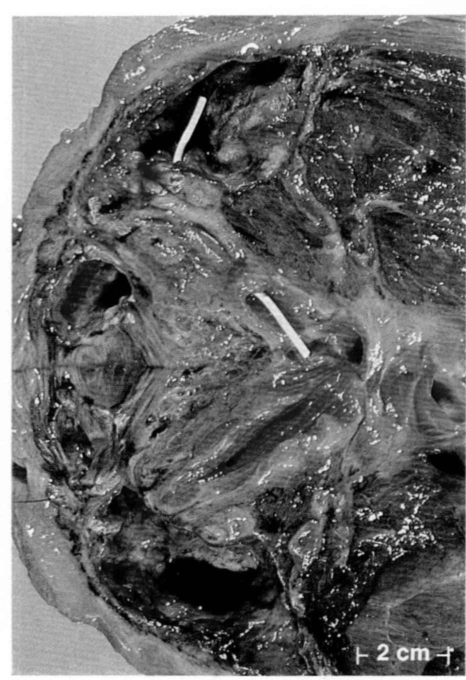

Fig. 4.60. Old, drained tuberculous cavity.

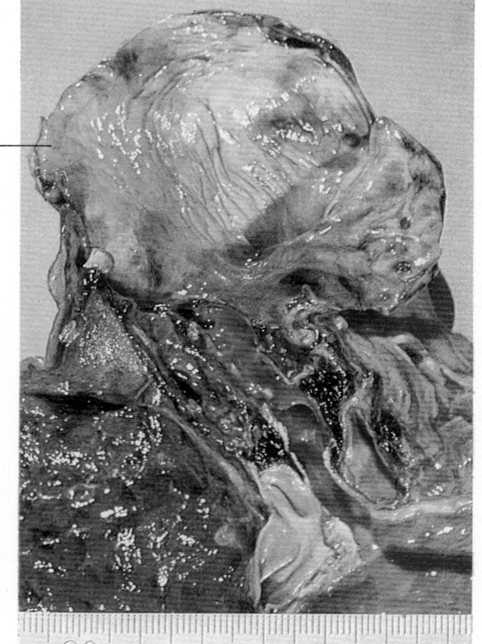

Fig. 4.61. Old tuberculous cavity with squamous metaplasia.

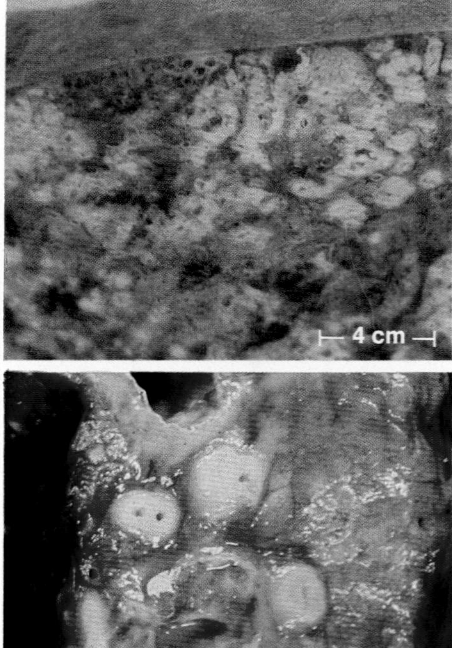

Fig. 4.62. Above: acinar-nodular tuberculosis. Below: tuberculosis of bronchial mucosa.

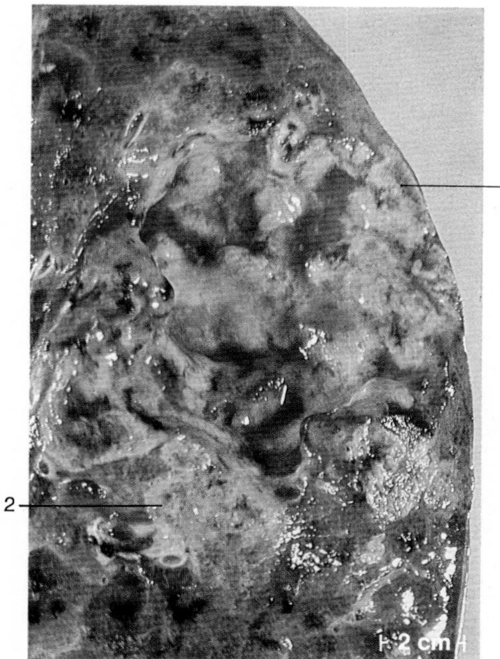

Fig. 4.59. Fresh tuberculous cavity.

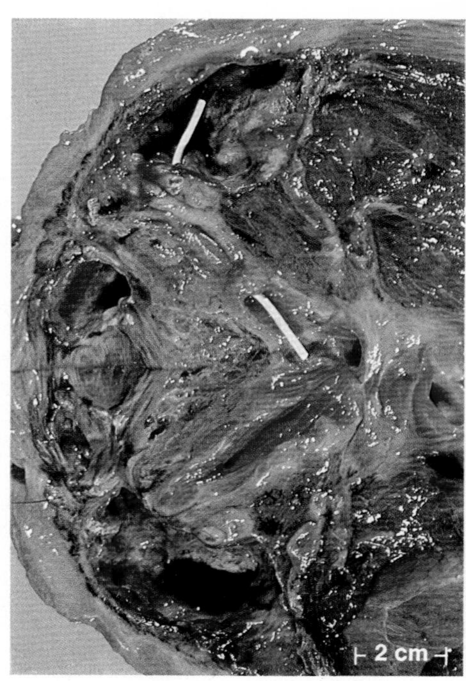

Fig. 4.60. Old, drained tuberculous cavity.

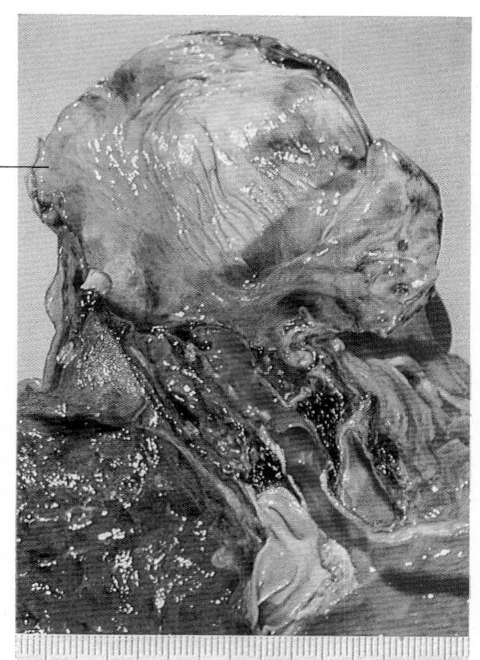

Fig. 4.61. Old tuberculous cavity with squamous metaplasia.

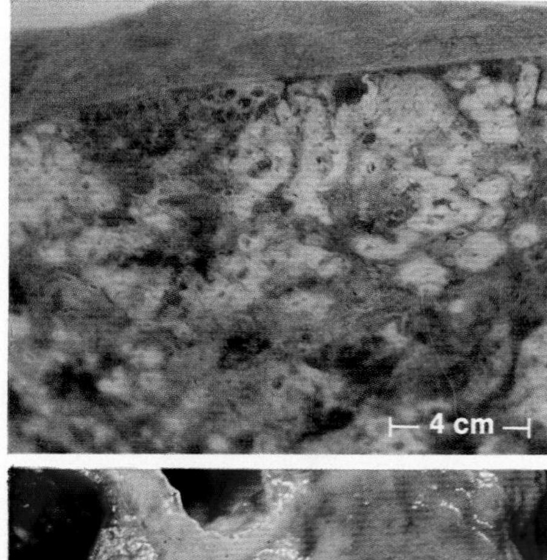

Fig. 4.62. Above: acinar-nodular tuberculosis. Below: tuberculosis of bronchial mucosa.

Tuberculosis of the Lung

Infectious disease due to Mycobacterium tuberculosis *with stage-like progression* (TCP, pp.96–101). The initial aerogenous infection leads to the formation of a subpleural caseous tubercle, the so-called Ghon focus, which frequently is located in the lower portion of the right upper lobe or the upper portion of the right lower lobe. The Ghon focus soon is followed by a tuberculous lymphangitis and caseating tubercles in hilar lymph nodes *(primary complex)* (x-ray diagnosis). A primary complex is the initial response to many infections, especially tuberculosis and syphilis.

Figure 4.55 shows a tuberculous primary complex. Two hilar lymph nodes contain areas of caseation necrosis (tuberculous cheese is dry and friable, resembling cottage cheese). The primary focus in Figure 4.55 probably is represented by the gray-black subpleural lesion just below the fissure between the upper and lower lobes (→). Tiny central areas of caseation necrosis are recognized in this small (5 mm. in diameter), indurated, black scar tissue. The scar tissue is white but anthracotic pigment produces a black discoloration. Another caseous tubercle near the base of the lower lobe measures approximately 1 cm. in diameter. This focus probably developed by hematogenous spread.

Massive hematogenous dissemination and the development of miliary tuberculosis are early complications of the primary complex (see Table 4.1, p. 86). Miliary tuberculosis is observed most frequently in children but it also can occur in adults with a primary complex. Figure 4.56 illustrates a case of a 32-year-old female (see also p. 86). The entire lung is studded with gray-yellow, glassy foci measuring 1–2 mm. in diameter (→ miliary tubercle). The term "miliary" describes the size of a tubercle (milium = millet seed). Miliary tubercles may develop as single foci in other organs (liver, kidney) after hematogenous or lymphogenous spread. One has to *distinguish* between miliary tuberculosis and miliary tubercle (see Table 4.1). *The primary complex usually heals. Exogenous* or *endogenous* hematogenous reinfection most often localizes in the lung apex (apical reinfection or *Simon's apical focus*). The tuberculous apical reinfection spreads via the bronchi, and an infraclavicular infiltrate is produced *(Assmann's early infiltrate)*.

Figure 4.57 shows extensive *apical tuberculosis*. Several dry, friable, white and partially chalky lesions measure up to 1 cm. in diameter. Some are surrounded by indurated scar tissue. Apical tuberculosis always involves the pleura. Such a tuberculous pleuritis heals and a gray-white pleural scar remains (→). The usual autopsy finding is an apical pleural scar and a narrow rim of indurated lung tissue beneath.

Chronic, progressive lung tuberculosis can exacerbate at any time, by either massive exogenous reinfection or diminished host resistance (war prisoners, cancer patients).

The result of exacerbation is the development of a gelatinous or caseous pneumonia. Figure 4.58 shows multiple confluent lesions, up to 10 cm. in diameter. The large central lesion (→) still has a gray-white, glassy ,gelatinous appearance (*Mi:* gelatinous areas contain cellular exudate). Other, smaller lesions (bottom of Fig. 4.58) show beginning central necrosis (*Mi:* caseation = necrosis). Cavities can arise quickly from large areas of caseation and eventually may involve an entire lung lobe (death in respiratory insufficiency or massive hemorrhage from the cavity).

Once a cavity has formed, pulmonary tuberculosis must be considered a chronic, progressive and recurrent disease. The primary focus rarely transforms into a cavity (early subpleural cavity). In contrast, most cavities arise from enlarging infraclavicular infiltrates either immediately or after some latent period. The upper third of the upper lobe, therefore, is the most common site of a cavity.

Figure 4.59 shows a fresh tuberculous cavity in the upper lobe. The cavity extends almost to the pleural surface. The irregularly frayed, gray-white cavity wall is 2–3 mm. thick (→1) and covered internally by gray-white caseous material. An area of recent caseation necrosis is shown (→2).

Several older tuberculous cavities are shown in Figure 4.60. A narrow zone of indurated, fibrotic lung separates the cavities from the markedly thickened pleura. Two old, round cavities with smooth walls are seen near the lung apex (at the left in this picture). They measure approximately 5 cm. in diameter. Their lumina are connected with a bronchus (white markers). The left, somewhat larger, cavity probably is of more recent origin because caseous material still adheres to its wall. The bronchial walls are thickened throughout (chronic bronchitis).

Ciliated or squamous epithelium eventually lines the internal wall if a cavity persists for a long time. The cavity then has the gray-white, smooth appearance of a drained epithelialized tuberculous cavity (Fig. 4.61). A squamous-cell carcinoma may arise later from the epithelialized cavity wall.

Bronchogenic (or intracanalicular) dissemination from a cavity leads to acinar-nodular tuberculosis. The tuberculous foci decrease in number and size from the lung apex to the base, as illustrated in Figure 4.62. Acinar-nodular tubercles are round, closely set (resembling a clover leaf) and a central bronchus can be identified in some lesions. Histologically, acinar-nodular foci represent a caseous pneumonia involving one or several acini or a peribronchial tuberculous pneumonia.

Tuberculosis also affects the bronchi that drain a cavity. The tuberculous inflammation either is confined to the mucosa or involves the entire bronchial wall. Figure 4.62 is a cross section of several white-yellowish, markedly thickened bronchi with narrow lumina. Part of a tuberculous cavity is seen at the upper margin of Figure 4.62 (below).

Bronchogenic dissemination also may take origin from a tuberculous hilar lymph node that breaks through the wall of a bronchus. A white, retracted mucosal scar is seen even years after the process has healed (Fig. 4.63 →).

Frequency of tuberculosis: 25% of persons less than 20 years of age are tuberculin-positive in Germany. A patient with open tuberculosis infects approximately 10 persons per year. Mortality: 0.14% (20 deaths daily) in Germany, Netherlands 0.03%, New York 0.56%. In some countries of Africa, the mortality is as high as 1%.

A: ♂ 50–60 years, ♀ 30–40 years; ♂:♀ = 3:2. *Therapy:* resection; 95% remain free of recurrence.

Co: tuberculous pleuritis, cor pulmonale, amyloidosis, bleeding from a cavity, late development of a carcinoma, larynx or gastrointestinal tuberculosis, pulmonary emphysema.

Nomenclature: Morbidity: percentage of diseased persons of the total population. *Mortality:* percentage of deaths of living persons. *Lethality:* percentage of deaths of diseased persons.

Lung Tuberculosis

1. **Normergic organism** (primary infection): predominantly exudative processes

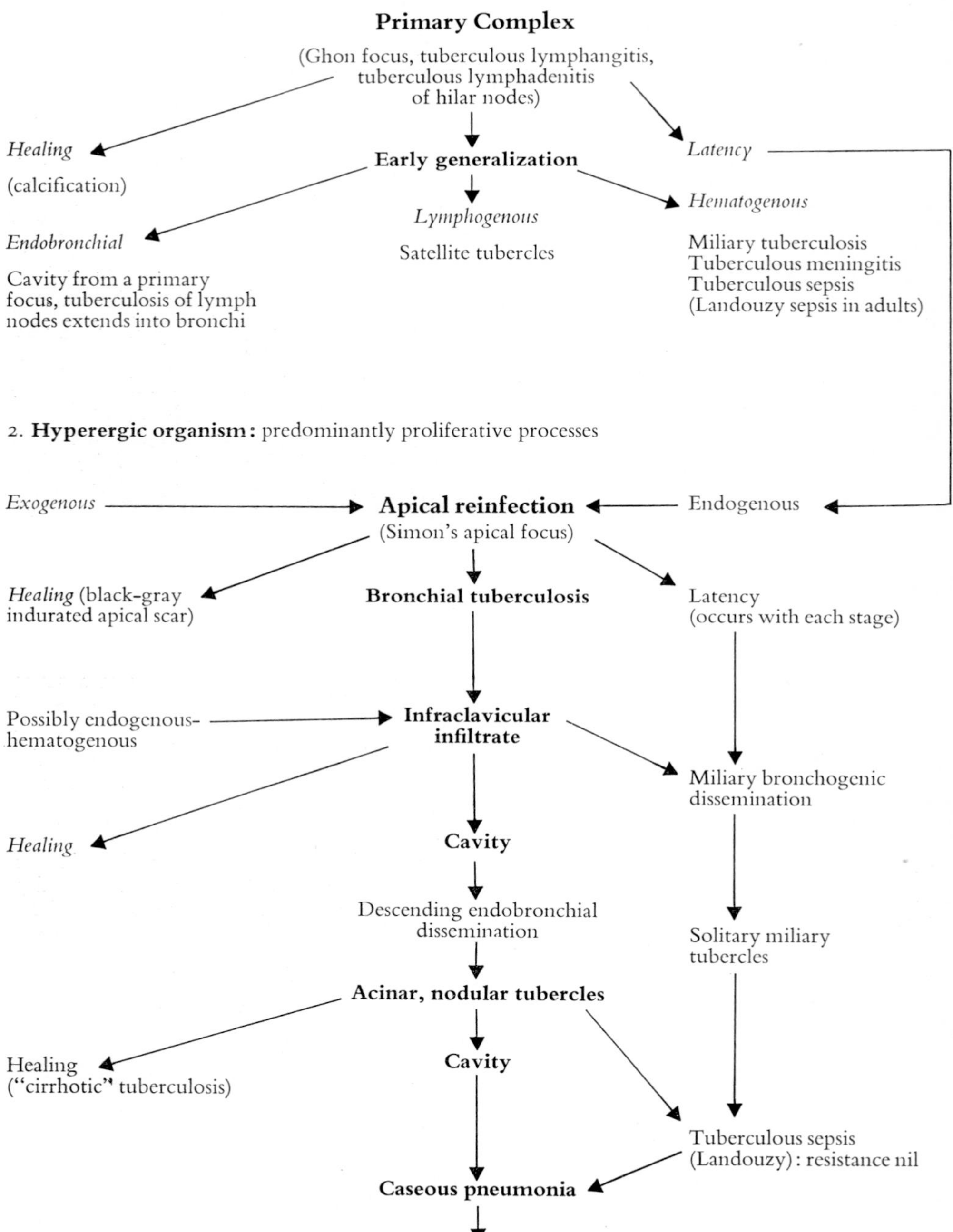

Table 4.1. Pathogenesis of tuberculosis.

Summary of pulmonary tuberculosis

Table 4.1 summarizes the evolution of pulmonary tuberculosis. The pathogenesis is easily understood provided some principles are kept in mind:

1. The primary complex is the initial response to infection with *M. tuberculosis*. A primary complex also is found in primary gastro-intestinal tuberculosis, lues and other infections. Morphologically, the primary complex consists of a primary focus, lymphangitis and regional lymphadenitis.
2. Each stage of tuberculosis either can be arrested (latency) or can heal. Healing is not necessarily permanent, since mycobacteria can be isolated from calcified tubercles. Tuberculosis can be reactivated when host resistance is impaired. Exacerbations in cancer patients (chemotherapy) are common.
3. Tuberculosis disseminates by three routes:
   a) **Lymphogenous dissemination** plays a minor role. An example is the miliary tubercle in the vicinity of a large caseous tubercle.
   b) **Hematogenous dissemination** is best exemplified by miliary tuberculosis (see p. 83) or by scattered miliary tubercles in the liver, spleen, kidneys, genital organs, bones, etc. Miliary tubercles are the source of the development of organ tuberculosis in these sites.
   c) **Bronchogenic dissemination:** tubercles enlarge and ultimately penetrate (by caseation necrosis) the walls of the bronchi. In addition, tuberculous bronchitis may develop by lymphogenous spread from distant tubercles and thereby become the source of bronchogenic dissemination. In children, extension of a caseating lymph-node tuberculosis into a main bronchus likewise leads to bronchogenic dissemination.

Pumice lung (tuff lung, Fig. 4.64). *Metastatic pulmonary calcinosis accompanying hypercalcemia.* Figure 4.64 (above) shows the fine grained, grey-white cut surface of the lung. This involves deposits of calcium salts (hydroxy-apatite), which can be histologically demonstrated with particular clarity in the region of the alveolar septa (Fig. 4.64, below, histochemical calcium detection by silvering according to Kossa).

Pg: calcifications in acid producing organs (kidneys, stomach, lungs and skin). These occur predominantly in hyperparathyroidism, paraneoplastic hypercalcemias (in renal and bronchial carcinomas), osteolytic bone metastases, and in vitamin D poisoning.

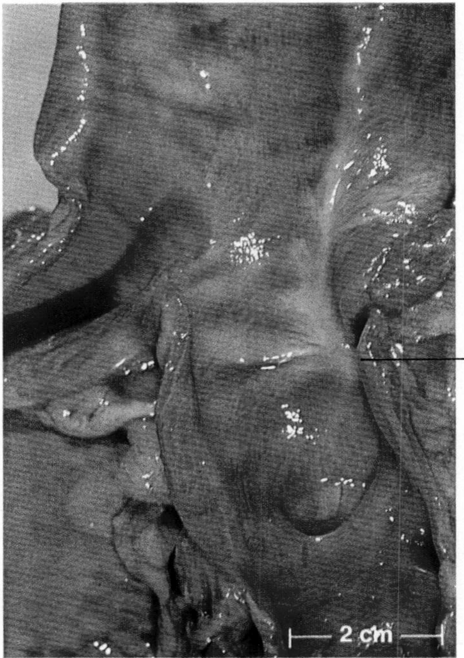

Fig. 4.63. Scar in the wall of a bronchus from extension of an adjacent lymph node with caseating tuberculosis.

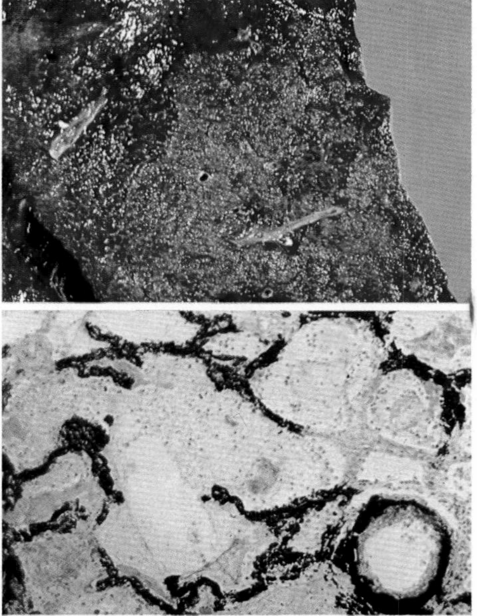

Fig. 4.64. Above, cut surface of a pumice lung. Below, calcifications of the alveolar septa (Kossa reaction).

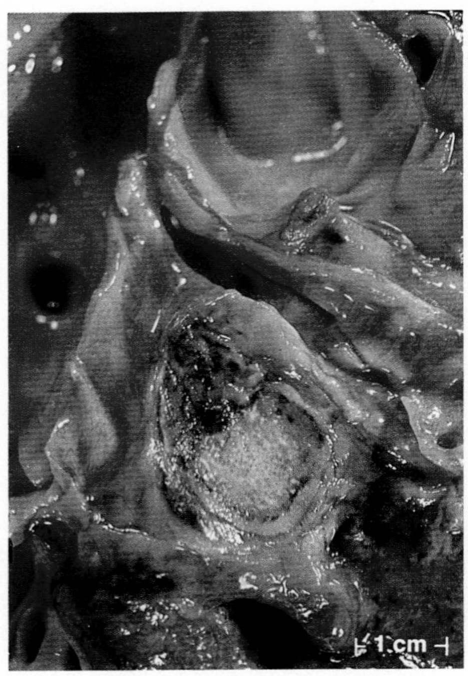

Fig. 4.65. Lymph nodes involved by sarcoidosis.

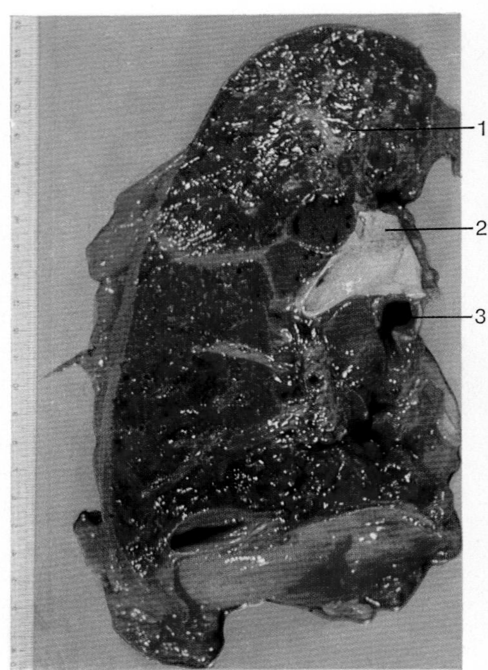

Fig. 4.66. Sarcoidosis of the lung.

Table 4.2. Frequency of organ involvement in sarcoidosis (according to WURM, SCADDING).

Mediastinal lymph nodes	100%
Tonsils	70%
Liver	65%
Lung	60%
Peripheral lymph nodes	30%
Eyes	10–30%
Heart, spleen	each 20%
Skin	10–20%
Kidney	19%
Gastrointestinal tracht	5–10%
Bone	7%
Nervous system	5%
Mucous membranes	1%
Lacrimal glands	0.5%

Summary of pulmonary tuberculosis

Table 4.1 summarizes the evolution of pulmonary tuberculosis. The pathogenesis is easily understood provided some principles are kept in mind:

1. The primary complex is the initial response to infection with *M. tuberculosis*. A primary complex also is found in primary gastrointestinal tuberculosis, lues and other infections. Morphologically, the primary complex consists of a primary focus, lymphangitis and regional lymphadenitis.
2. Each stage of tuberculosis either can be arrested (latency) or can heal. Healing is not necessarily permanent, since mycobacteria can be isolated from calcified tubercles. Tuberculosis can be reactivated when host resistance is impaired. Exacerbations in cancer patients (chemotherapy) are common.
3. Tuberculosis disseminates by three routes:
   a) **Lymphogenous dissemination** plays a minor role. An example is the miliary tubercle in the vicinity of a large caseous tubercle.
   b) **Hematogenous dissemination** is best exemplified by miliary tuberculosis (see p. 83) or by scattered miliary tubercles in the liver, spleen, kidneys, genital organs, bones, etc. Miliary tubercles are the source of the development of organ tuberculosis in these sites.
   c) **Bronchogenic dissemination:** tubercles enlarge and ultimately penetrate (by caseation necrosis) the walls of the bronchi. In addition, tuberculous bronchitis may develop by lymphogenous spread from distant tubercles and thereby become the source of bronchogenic dissemination. In children, extension of a caseating lymph-node tuberculosis into a main bronchus likewise leads to bronchogenic dissemination.

Pumice lung (tuff lung, Fig. 4.64). *Metastatic pulmonary calcinosis accompanying hypercalcemia.* Figure 4.64 (above) shows the fine grained, grey-white cut surface of the lung. This involves deposits of calcium salts (hydroxy-apatite), which can be histologically demonstrated with particular clarity in the region of the alveolar septa (Fig. 4.64, below, histochemical calcium detection by silvering according to Kossa).

Pg: calcifications in acid producing organs (kidneys, stomach, lungs and skin). These occur predominantly in hyperparathyroidism, paraneoplastic hypercalcemias (in renal and bronchial carcinomas), osteolytic bone metastases, and in vitamin D poisoning.

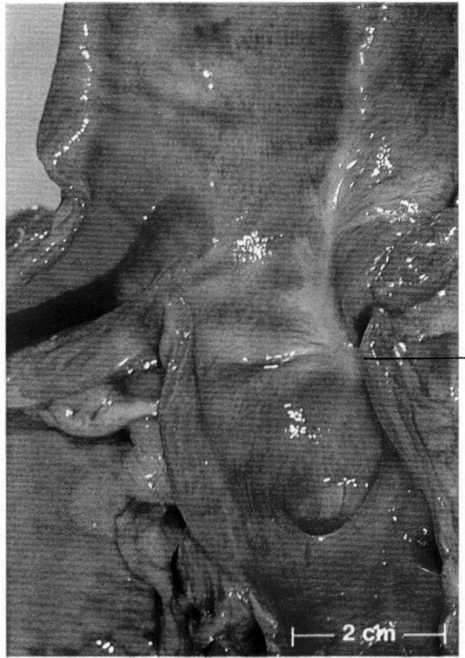

Fig. 4.63. Scar in the wall of a bronchus from extension of an adjacent lymph node with caseating tuberculosis.

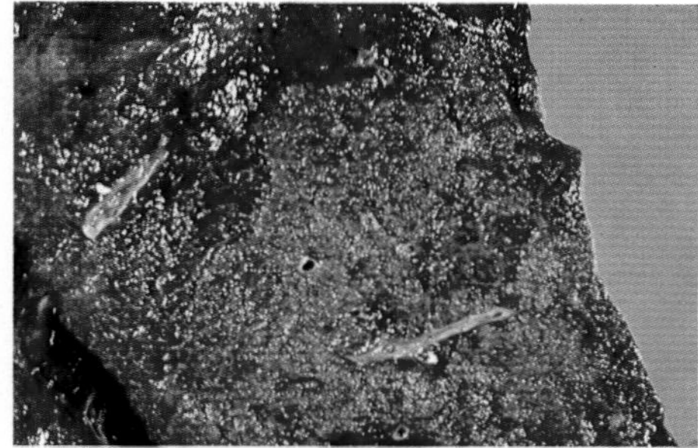

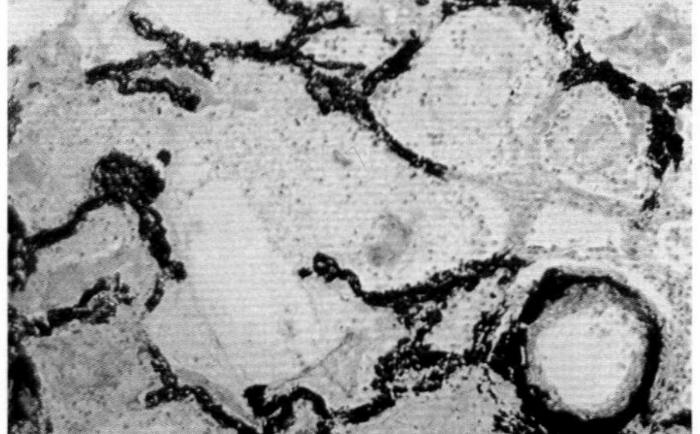

Fig. 4.64. Above, cut surface of a pumice lung. Below, calcifications of the alveolar septa (Kossa reaction).

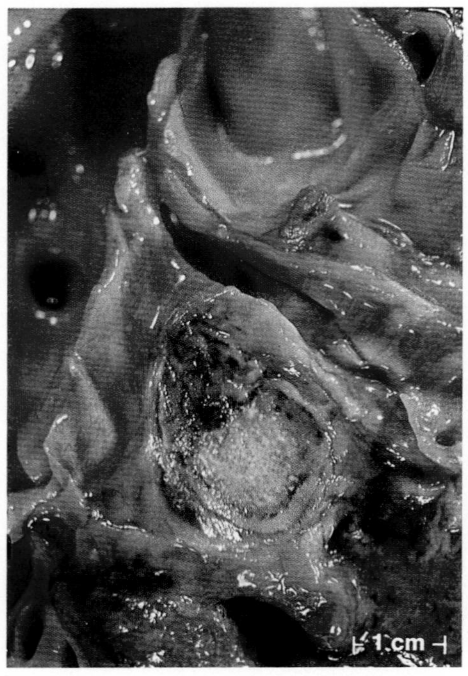

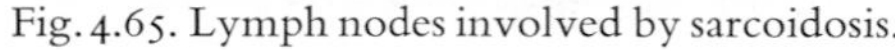
Fig. 4.65. Lymph nodes involved by sarcoidosis.

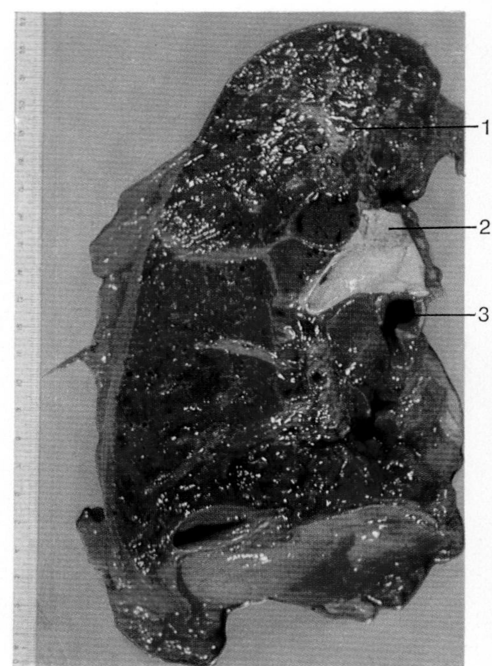

Fig. 4.66. Sarcoidosis of the lung.

Table 4.2. Frequency of organ involvement in sarcoidosis (according to Wurm, Scadding).

Mediastinal lymph nodes	100%
Tonsils	70%
Liver	65%
Lung	60%
Peripheral lymph nodes	30%
Eyes	*to*–30%
Heart, spleen	each 20%
Skin	10–20%
Kidney	19%
Gastrointestinal tracht	5–10%
Bone	7%
Nervous system	5%
Mucous membranes	1%
Lacrimal glands	0.5%

Sarcoidosis (Boeck's disease) (Figs. 4.65–4.67). *Sarcoidosis is a disease of unknown etiology. The morphologic basis is the epithelioid-cell tubercle without caseation but with scar formation.*

Sarcoidosis was recognized as a disease sui generis by BESNIER (1889), BOECK (1899) and SCHAUMANN (1914). Microscopically (TCP, Fig. 3.42, p. 98), the sarcoid granuloma is composed of epithelioid cells and giant cells of the Langhans type. The Langhans giant cell contains cytoplasmic inclusions, such as the *Schaumann body* or "conchoid bodies" (80% of the cases), asteroid bodies or centrospheres. Scar formation progresses from the periphery to the center of the granuloma and results in fibrosis. The histologic picture is not specific. The sarcoid granuloma resembles the granuloma of berylliosis and many other diseases. Mycobacteria cannot be demonstrated in sarcoid granulomas.

Practically all organs may be involved by sarcoidosis (Table 4.2). The mediastinal and lung hilar lymph nodes are affected regularly and therefore are considered the primary site of the disease. A scalene biopsy is used to establish the diagnosis. The *initial focus* (clinical Stage I) is a bilateral enlargement of the mediastinal lymph nodes (40% heal).

Figure 4.65 shows the cut surface of a hilar lymph node that is studded with soft, gray-white, glassy foci (*DD:* tuberculous lymphadenitis has a cut surface with more irregular, often larger, caseating foci).

The disease extends from the hilar lymph nodes by the lymphogenous route to the lungs (*clinical Stage II:* 40% heal, although death from dyspnea may occur). Figure 4.66 shows densely set, gray-yellow nodules measuring 3–4 mm. in diameter (usually somewhat larger lesions than the tubercles of miliary tuberculosis).

Some lesions in the upper lobe are fibrotic (→1, →2 pulmonary artery, →3 bronchus).

The sarcoid granulomas in the lung finally become scars (*clinical Stage III:* pulmonary fibrosis; 5–10% of the patients develop emphysema and cor pulmonale). Firm, gray areas of fibrosis extend along the bronchi and blood vessels, as in Figure 4.67. A similar gross picture is seen in interstitial pulmonary fibrosis (Hamman-Rich syndrome).

Hematogenous dissemination to muscles is found relatively frequently in sarcoidosis (biopsy of gastrocnemius). The liver, spleen and skin (*lupus pernio:* reddening of nose, cheeks and ears) likewise may become involved by hematogenous spread. The bronchial mucosa is involved in approximately 80% of cases (bronchial biopsy is useful for the diagnosis). *Erythema nodosum* of the lower legs is an early symptom (not a "metastasis" of the granuloma) and is associated with transient polyarthritis, colitis and uveitis. The involvement of the eyes and salivary glands (iridocyclitis and parotitis) is known as *Heerfordt syndrome.*

The short bones of hands and feet can be affected by cystic translucencies (x-ray: osteitis fibrosa cystica multiplex).

F: 1%. *A:* ♀ 35, ♂ 35–40 years (tuberculosis of lymph nodes: ♀ 35 years, ♂ 55 years). *S:* ♀:♂ = 4:1. *Pr:* cause is not known. *Hypotheses:* Tuberculosis with excellent host defense? Virus? Allergens? *Clinical diagnosis:* Kveim test: a lymph node extract with sarcoidosis is injected subcutaneously → epithelioid-cell granuloma. Tuberculin test mostly negative. *Course:* 80% survive for more than 10 years.

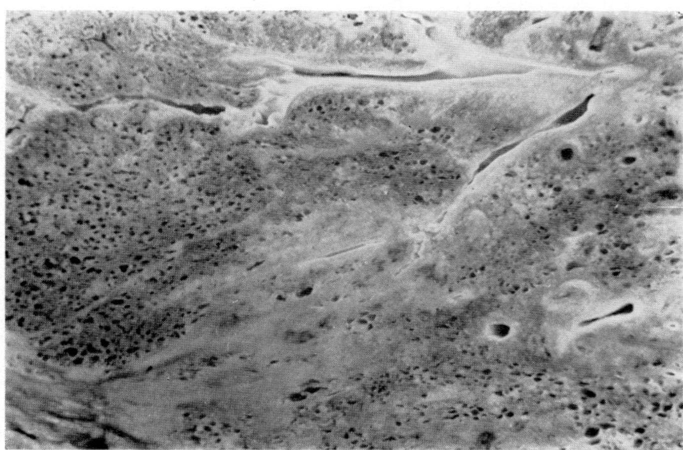

Fig. 4.67. Sarcoidosis of the lung with fibrosis.

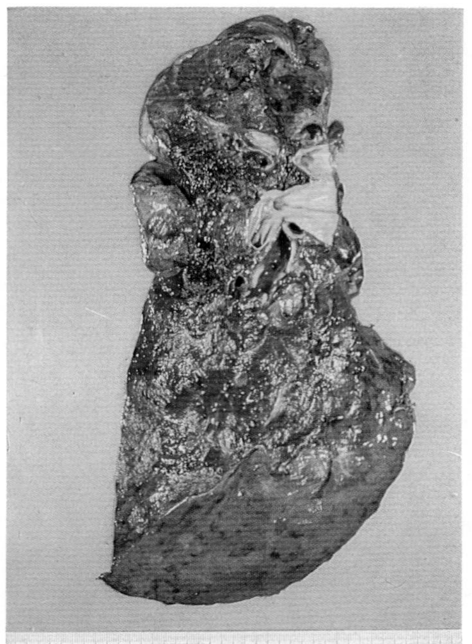

Fig. 4.68. Coarsely nodular silicosis of the lung.

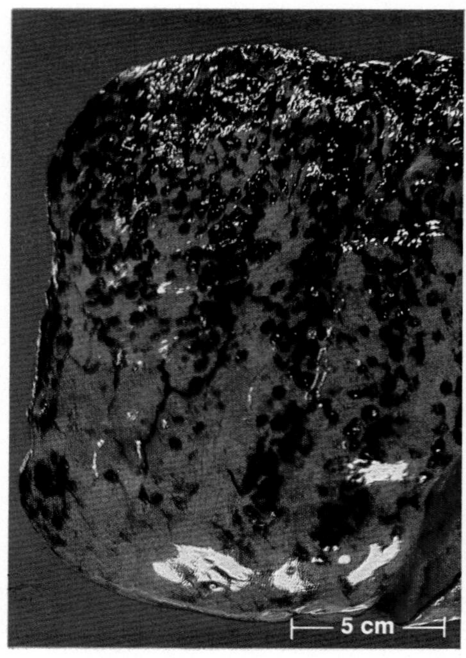

Fig. 4.69. Anthracosis of the lung.

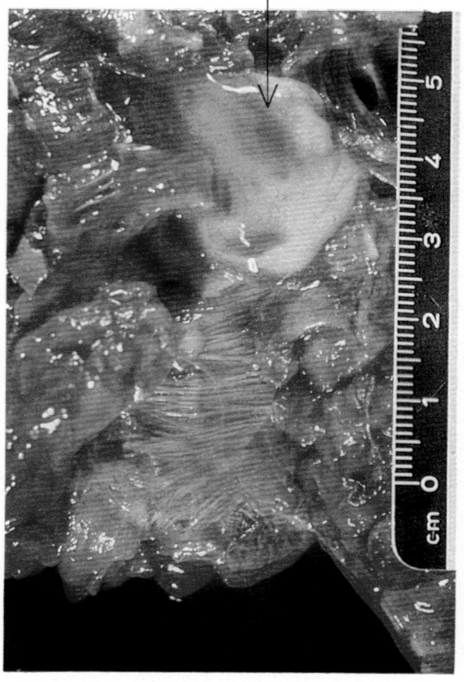

Fig. 4.70. Bronchial carcinoid with saccular bronchiectasis.

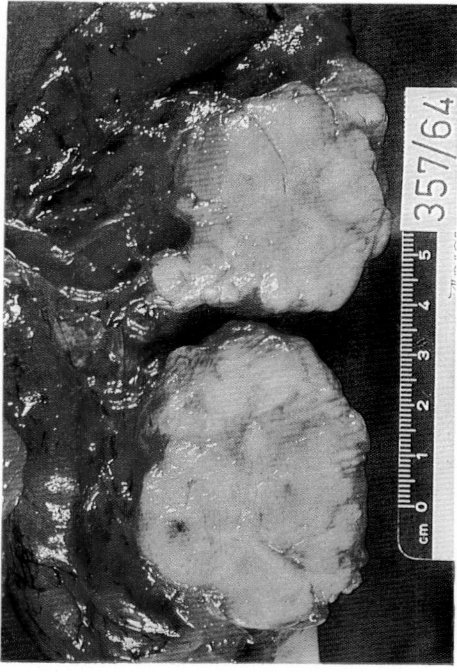

Fig. 4.71. Hamartoma (chondroma) of the lung.

Silicosis, Anthracosis, Lung Tumors

Silicosis (Fig. 4.68; TCP, p. 95). *A chronic, fibrosing pulmonary disease that results from the deposition of free (SiO_2) or bound (silicate, quartz dust) silicic acid.* Figure 4.68 shows a lung with coarse, round conglomerate nodules that measure up to 4 cm. in diameter. The involvement of the middle portions of the lung is typical. Single small nodules, 2–3 mm. in diameter, are noted in the upper and lower lobes. The silicotic small nodule can be diagnosed best by palpation rather than inspection alone. Silicotic nodules are gray, very firm, almost like calcium (scar tissue + coal pigment). The cut surface is *dry* (in anthracosis: moist). The hilar lymph nodes likewise are enlarged, firm hard, gray and dry. Silicosis often is accompanied by tuberculosis (75% of cases).

Persons afflicted are: miners, stonemasons, metal grinders, sandblasters and workers who come into contact with sandstone, quartz, ground silica, etc. Free silicic acid as quartz or talcum is particularly dangerous. *S:* almost always males. *A:* 30–50 years. *The latent period* differs: some stonemasons 5–10 years, sandblasters 3–4 years (GIESE).

Pg: silica (1–5 μ) probably does not act mechanically, but the free silicic acid presumably causes activation of fibroblasts.

Anthracosis (Fig. 4.69; TCP, p. 95). Coal pigment is found regularly in the lungs of adults. The pigment is deposited in the lymphatics and lymph nodes, but only severe anthracosis leads to minimal pulmonary fibrosis. Deposition in subpleural lymphatics results in net-like, black markings or stellate round foci (at the junction of several lymph channels). As shown in Figure 4.69, pigment-rich and pigment-free zones alternate. This distribution is explained by pressure from the ribs, which project slightly into the thoracic cavity and "milk" the coal pigment from the lymph channels. Anthracotic hilar lymph nodes are black, soft and moist. Anthracotic pigment is found occasionally in bronchi or blood vessels whereby black mucosal or intimal scars develop.

Bronchial carcinoides (Fig. 4.70). *Tumors composed of argentaffin cells (small intestine, bronchial epithelium) that may secrete serotonin, kallikrein or occasionally ACTH-like substances* (so-called paraneoplastic syndrome: Cushing's disease). Figure 4.70 shows a soft, white to gray-red tumor of the right lower lobe (→) that measures 2.5 cm. in diameter. The lumen of the bronchus is completely occluded. Note the marked dilatation of the bronchus distal to the tumor (stenotic bronchiectasis), the chronic bronchitis and the projecting transverse muscle folds of the tunica propria.

F: increase in frequency during the past few years. *A:* 30 years. *S:* ♂. Bronchial adenomas are divided on *histolic* grounds into trabecular, alveolar (cylindroma) or carcinoid types. *Pr:* Local malignancy. It is assumed that the reserve cell carcinoma represents the malignant variant of bronchial carcinoid.

Hamartoma of the lung (chondroma) (Fig. 4.71). Relatively uncommon tissue malformation. Our picture shows a firm, elastic subpleural tumor, 6 cm. in diameter. The tumor is light gray-white and sharply delineated ("coin lesion").

Remarks on nomenclature: Hamartomas are tumor-like malformations composed of tissue that is indigenous to the organ of origin (for example, cavernoma of the liver. *Choristomas* are composed of tissue foreign to the organ of origin (genuine hypernephroma of the kidney).

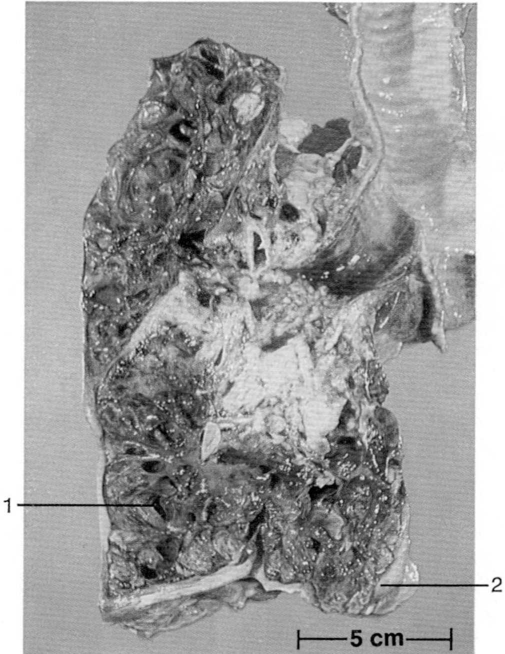

Fig. 4.72. Central bronchial carcinoma.

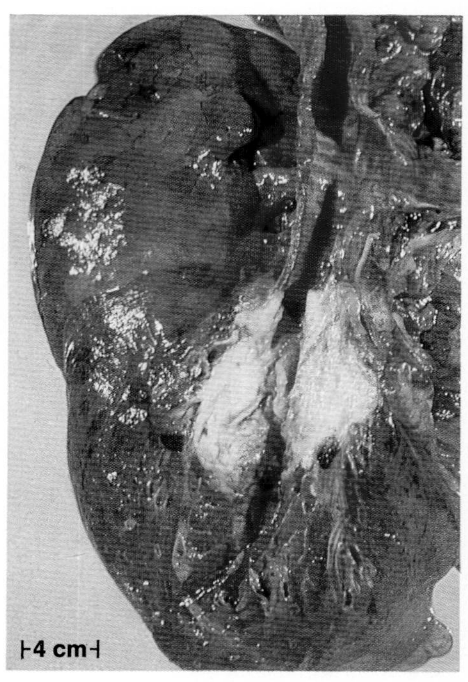

Fig. 4.73. Circular carcinoma of a lower-lobe bronchus.

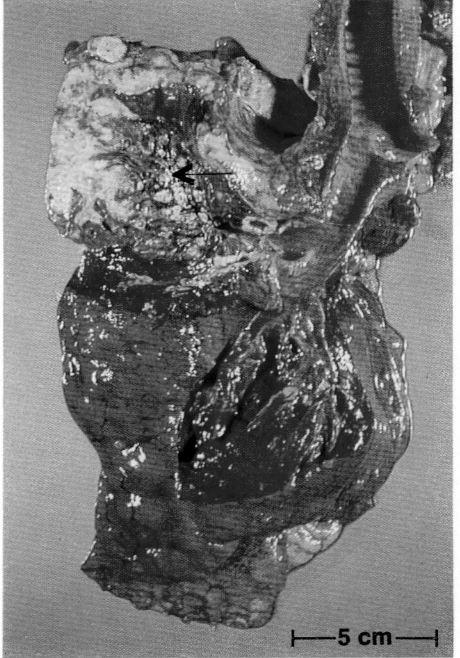

Fig. 4.74. Peripheral bronchial carcinoma (so-called Pancoast tumor).

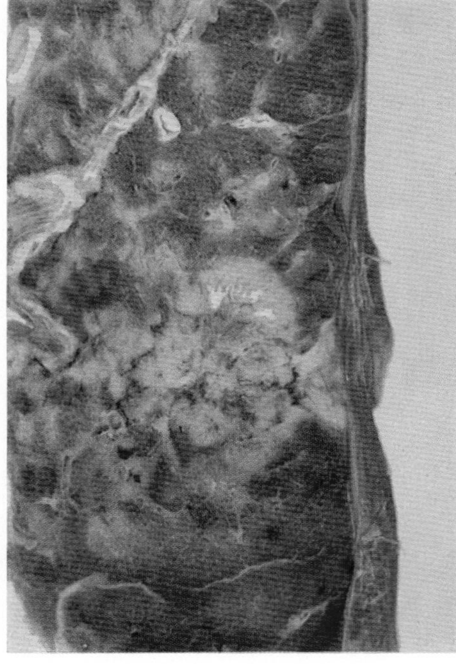

Fig. 4.75. Scar carcinoma of the lung.

Lung cancer

Bronchial or bronchogenic cancer has increased markedly in frequency during the past 40 years. It is now the most common carcinoma in males, exceeding stomach cancer.

The following gross types are distinguished according to their location: (a) *central or hilar carcinoma* (a mediastinal tumor on x-ray, but DD is difficult: Hodgkin's disease, sarcoidosis, etc.), (b) *peripheral carcinoma* (Pancoast tumor), (c) *scar carcinoma* (peripheral) and (d) *diffuse carcinoma* (grossly resembles pneumonias).

Figure 4.72 shows a *hilar bronchial carcinoma* at the bifurcation of the right lower and upper lobe bronchi. The carcinoma is centrally necrotic, white, friable and soft to firm. The microscopic diagnosis was squamous-cell carcinoma. The bronchi at the hilus are completely occluded by carcinoma. The tumor has grown along the bronchi and vessels to the periphery of the lung. Bronchial constriction or occlusion by carcinoma has led to extensive bronchiectases. Large saccular lumina in the peripheral lung are filled with mucus and pus (→1). The bronchiectatic cavities are black-green, dirty and of foul odor. Secondary infection and even gangrene of bronchiectases are not uncommon in advanced cases.

Figure 4.73 shows a *hilar carcinoma of the lung* that presented as a nodule on x-ray. At autopsy, a white tumor of firm consistency encircled and constricted the left lower lobe bronchus.

A *peripheral carcinoma of the right upper lobe* is shown in Figure 4.74. The center of the tumor (→) reveals black-gray, indurated tissue with several chalky foci. This tuberculous scar has given rise to the carcinoma, which has grown into the peripheral portions of the lung, pleura and the thoracic muscles (upper thoracic aperture). Tumor growth even extended into the clavicular fossa *(Pancoast tumor)*. Infiltration of the brachial plexus causes pains in the shoulder and arms, atrophy of the muscles of the hand and Horner's syndrome. Histologically, this tumor was a squamous-cell carcinoma. The term Pancoast tumor only implies a growth direction of a bronchogenic carcinoma.

A typical *scar cancer* is illustrated in Figure 4.75. A 3-cm. subpleural tumor is medium-firm, white and speckled black. The black indurated areas represent old tuberculous scars. Several gray-white metastases surround the main tumor mass. Scar cancers can be so small that they are not detectable by x-ray. In such instances, multiple cuts through the formalin-fixed lungs must be made at autopsy. Metastases from small scar cancers may predominate, since the size of the primary tumor does not correlate with the extent of the metastatic process. A small scar tumor may produce large metastases and a large tumor may produce few and small metastases.

F: in 1920, 5% of all carcinomas in males were lung cancers. In 1960, 12% were lung cancers. *A:* 50-60 years. *S:* ♂:♀=4:1 (but see pulmonary adenomatosis). *Localization:* the right lung is affected more often than the left.

Histologic forms: (TCP, pp. 245 and 247) 40% of all lung cancers are *squamous-cell carcinomas*. These present as round, nodular tumors. Another 40% are *oat-cell carcinomas* that tend to spread within the lung in a finger-like growth pattern. The remainder of the carcinomas are *undifferentiated* (polymorphous), *cylindrical* (6%) or *adenocarcinomas*.

Pg: sequential bronchial changes are similar to those seen in cervical carcinoma, namely metaplasia of stratified epithelium → carcinoma in situ → carcinoma. A direct malignant transformation of basal cells without precancerous changes must be considered also. Metaplasia of bronchial epithelium is associated with 40% and chronic bronchitis is evident in 50% of all bronchial carcinomas. Occupational lung cancers have been recognized in chromium workers, asbestos workers and miners working in silver mines of Schneeberg and Joachimsthal. The bronchial cancer of silver miners is attributed to the radium rays emanating from the ore. Cancer develops after a latent period of approximately 25 years. Hydrocarbons in exhaust fumes or tars likewise may act as carcinogens because bronchogenic carcinomas are much more common in urban than in rural areas. The air content of 3,4-benzpyrene is 7.7 mg./100 m^3 in cities as opposed to 0.7 mg./100 m^3 in rural areas. The content of benzpyrene in the air of a large German industrial area equals 40 cigarettes smoked daily. The increase in tobacco or cigarette consumption parallels the increase in bronchial carcinomas. Death rates from bronchial carcinomas per 100,000 males: 3.4 are nonsmokers, 11.9 are occasional smokers, 28.9 are pipe smokers and 220 are heavy cigarette smokers. Higher cancer risk in smokers and patients with tuberculosis (e.g., scar carcinoma due to cocarcinogenic actions).

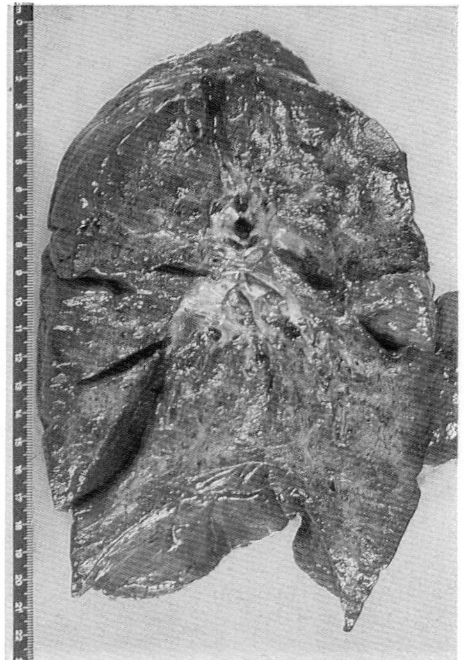

Fig. 4.76. Pulmonary adenomatosis.

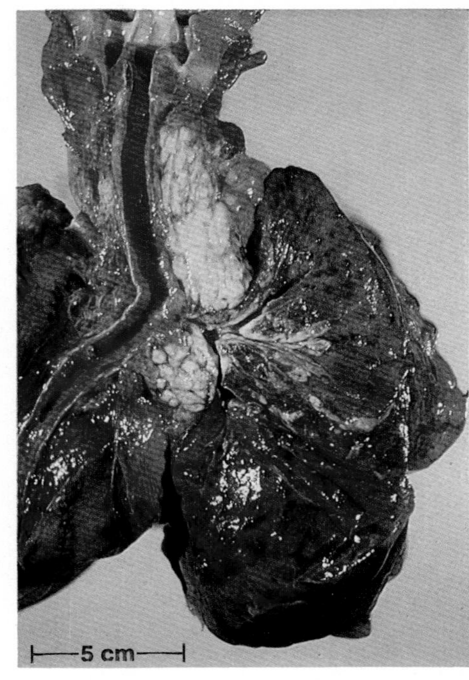

Fig. 4.77. Finger-like extension of a bronchogenic carcinoma with metatases to lymph nodes.

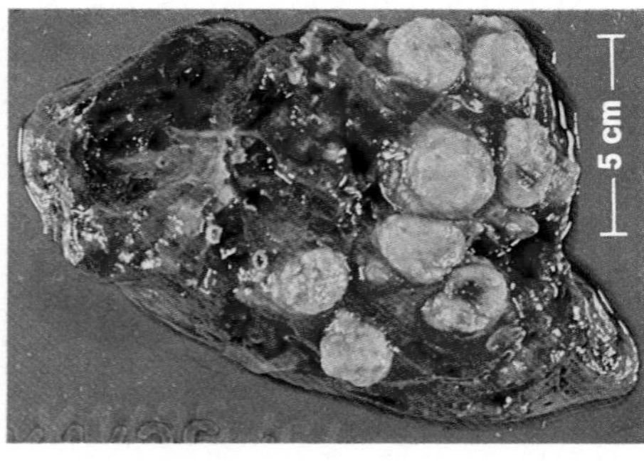

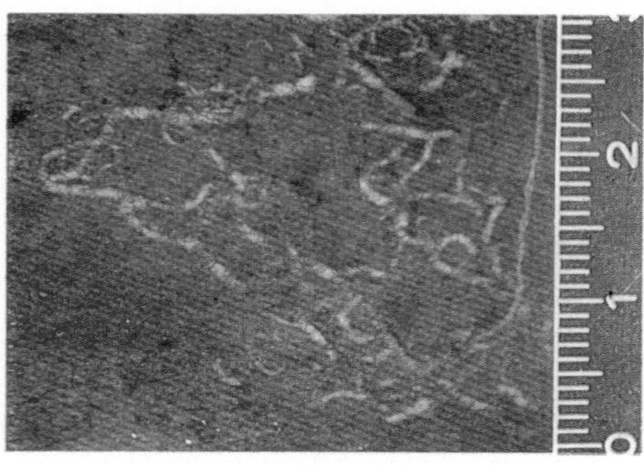

Fig. 4.78. Above: peribronchial tumor growth. Below: carcinomatous lymphangiosis.

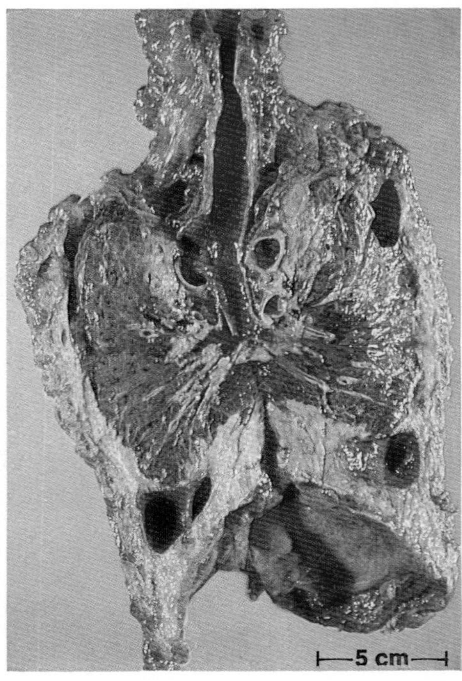

Fig. 4.79. Pleural mesothelioma.

Pulmonary adenomatosis manifests grossly and by x-ray as multifocal or even diffuse tumor growth in the lung. The distribution of the diffuse form resembles pneumonia. Figure 4.76 shows gray-white to light red, poorly demarcated, firm to elastic foci that are widely scattered throughout the lung. Fluid cannot be expressed. Other tumor infiltrates are yellow-gray amd moist, with a fibrin-like fluid on cut surface (mucus formation by tumor cells). The extent of lung involvement varies from multiple disseminated gray foci (up to 1 cm. in diameter) or smaller foci ("miliary foci") to diffuse involvement of a single lobe.

Pulmonary adenomatosis sometimes is erroneously referred to as alveolar-cell carcinoma. The alveoli are lined by cylindrical cells that are derived from the epithelium of the *respiratory bronchioli* (bronchiolar carcinoma is the correct histogenetic term). Tumor infiltration of lymph nodes and distant metastases occur relatively late ("malignant pulmonary adenomatosis"). Alveolar-cell carcinomas probably arise multicentrically, affect females, and their frequency has not increased during the past 20 years. Similarity to jaagziekte: South African driving disease of sheep (cows), which is a virus infection. *DD:* adenocarcinoma of the lung, often arises in pre-existing scars and metastasizes widely.

Bronchogenic carcinomas tend to spread within the lung by growing along *bronchi and vessels* (finger-like extension), by producing a so-called *cancerous pneumonia* (ill-defined, nodular intrapulmonary metastases) and by involving the pleural lymphatics (carcinomatous lymphangiosis).

Figure 4.77 shows a carcinoma of the left main stem bronchus that grows in a finger-like fashion in lymphatics of bronchi and vessels. Metastases are present in hilar, peribronchial and mediastinal lymph nodes (mediastinoscopy and bronchial biopsy are useful in the diagnosis).

A cross section of a lung with peribronchial tumor growth and severe narrowing of the bronchi is shown in Figure 4.78. Bronchial lumina can be identified in the centers of some tumor nodules. Figure 4.78 (below) shows a typical subpleural carcinomatous lymphangiosis (should not be called "lymphangitis" because it is not primarily an inflammation). A gray-white network extends over the pleura. The lymph channels are filled with medium-soft, white tumor emboli. Sausage-like tumor masses can be expressed after cutting.

The common metastatic sites of lung cancer are summarized in Figure 4.80. The first clinical symptoms of a bronchogenic carcinoma occasionally are attributable to metastases, e.g., brain tumor. *Co:* atelectasis, chronic pneumonia, bronchiectasis, hemorrhagic pleural effusions, tumor growth around the superior vena cava → compression and blood stasis; growth into the pericardial sac, hemoptysis.

The mean times between onset of a bronchogenic carcinoma and death are 6 months for oat-cell carcinomas and 1–2 years for squamous-cell carcinomas. *The clinical diagnosis* often is difficult. Cytology of bronchial sputum is simple and relatively accurate (92% accuracy, 3% falsely positive diagnoses; EBNER).

Pleural mesothelioma (Fig. 4.79). *Unilateral, localized or diffuse tumor of the pleura.* Figure 4.79 shows a diffuse pleural mesothelioma of the right lung. The pleural surface is approximately 4 cm. thick, firm, white and elastic. It has the appearance of fish flesh. Typical is the involvement of the costal and especially the diaphragmatic pleura. The visceral pleura of the upper lobe is not involved by the tumor. In the lower lobe, tumor growth has extended into the visceral pleura. Several encapsulated cystic spaces, filled with fibrin and fluid, lie between sheets of tumor tissue.

Diffuse pleural mesothelioma: *F:* 0.05%. *A:* 40–60 years. *S:* ♂:♀=2:1. *Pg:* a mesothelioma usually arises in the parietal and especially the diaphragmatic pleura but both pleural surfaces are involved eventually. Late metastases to liver, kidney, bones. Occupational cancer of asbestos workers, with a latent period of 20 years. Pleural mesothelioma can be induced experimentally with asbestos in animals. *Mi:* fibrous tissue with multiple epithelial tubules and trabeculae included (mesothelium). A special type is the circumscribed pleural mesothelioma: a benign, slowly growing tumor that involves the visceral pleura. Histologically, these tumors are fibromas with included epithelial structures. On occasion, pleural mesotheliomas produce hypoglycemia ("paraneoplastic syndrome").

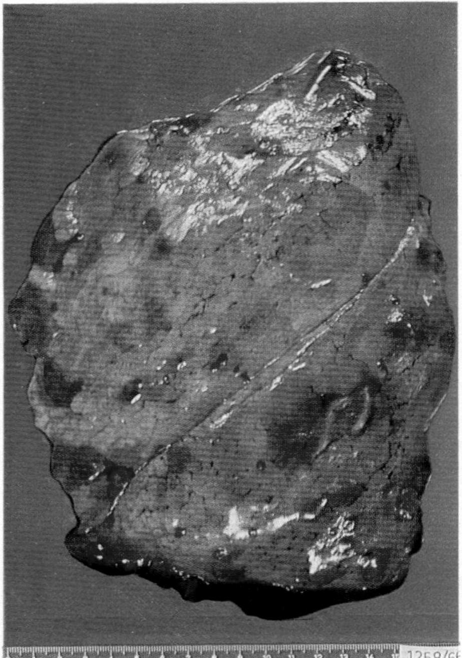

Fig. 4.81. Lung metastases from a choriocarcinoma.

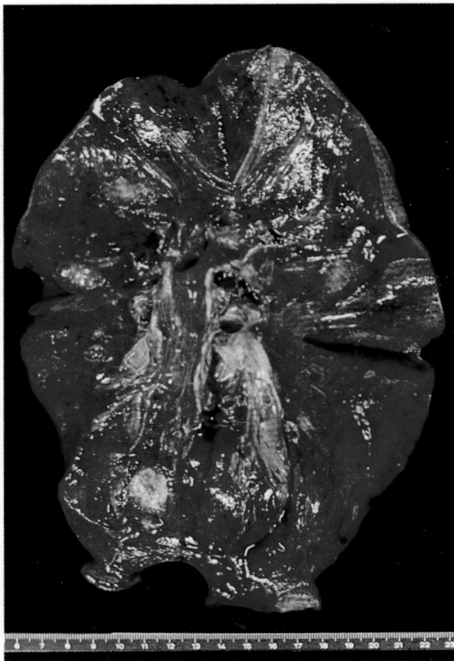

Fig. 4.82. Lung metastases from a carcinoma of the breast.

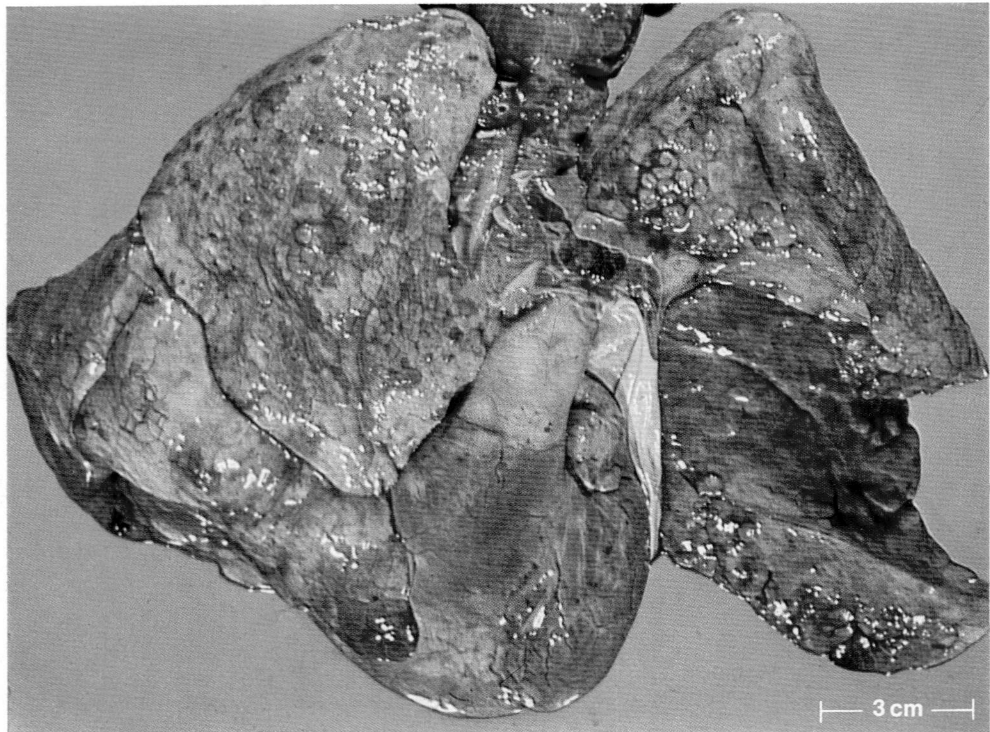

Fig. 4.83. Pleural metastases from a carcinoma of the breast.

Lung metastases (Figs. 4.81–4.83). Tumor emboli from carcinomas or sarcomas frequently reach the lungs and liver by the hematogenous route.

Figure 4.80 shows multiple, small, blood-rich metastases from a choriocarcinoma; 75% of choriocarcinomas metastasize to the lung.

Nodular, gray-white metastases from a mammary carcinoma are shown in Figure 4.82.

Several pleural metastases from a mammary carcinoma are shown in Figure 4.83. The metastases are small, flat or nodular and scattered over the lung surface. Hemorrhagic pleural effusion is a common complication from pleural or subpleural metastases.

F: Approximately 30% of all malignant tumors have metastasized to the lungs by the time of autopsy. Age and sex distribution are dependent on the primary site of the tumor. Seventy-five per cent of osteogenic sarcomas, choriocarcinomas or hypernephromas metastasize to the lungs, followed by carcinomas of the thyroid gland (65%), breast (55%) and prostate (40%). Melanoma likewise tends to metastasize to the lungs (60%). Cancers of the oral cavity or pharynx (30%), esophagus, stomach, liver or pancreas (each 20%), uterus (15%) and ovary (10%) are less likely to produce lung metastases.

Co: necrosis, hemorrhages (especially with choriocarcinoma!), cor pulmonale, secondary polycythemia, atelectasis and bronchiectasis. Unlike primary lung cancers, metastatic tumors rarely form cavities in the lung.

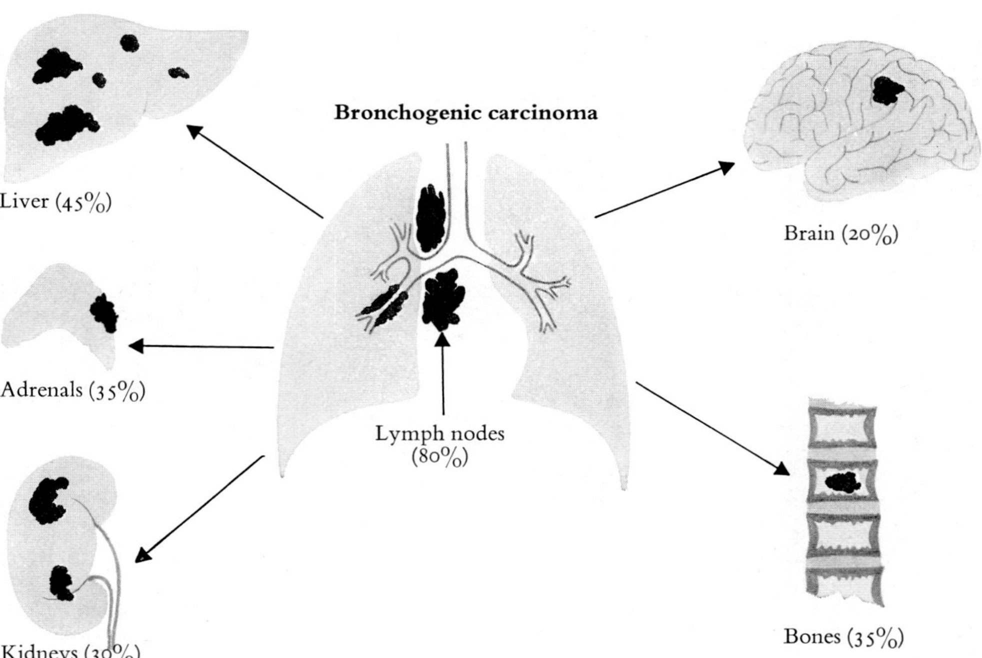

Fig. 4.80. Schematic presentation of frequency of metastases from bronchial carcinomas (according to MEHRAIN, Bonn).

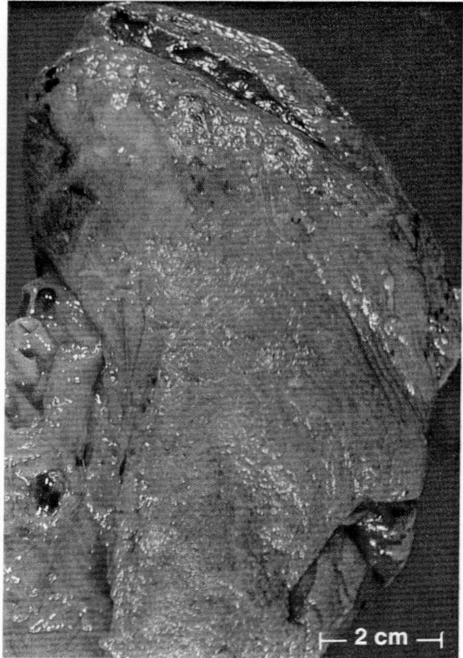

Fig. 4.84. Fibrinous pleuritis.

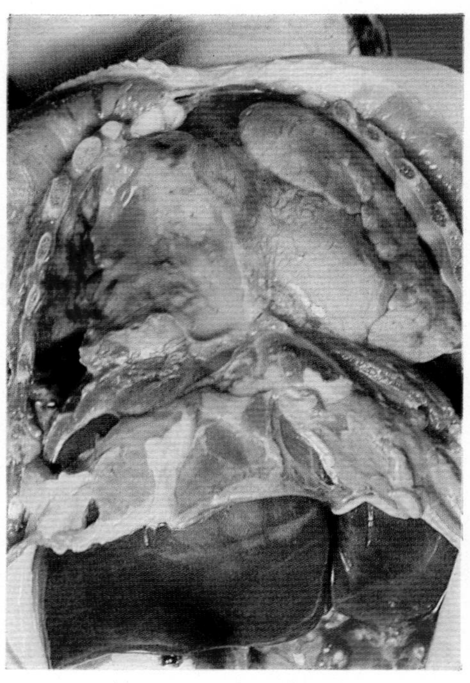

Fig. 4.85. Fibrinous-purulent pleuritis (empyema).

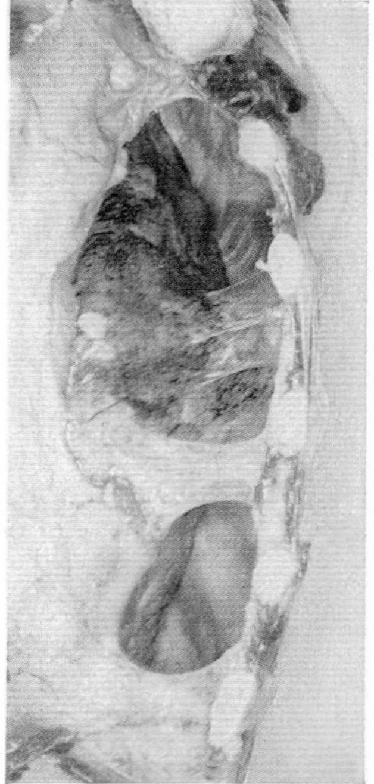

Fig. 4.86. Pleural adhesions.

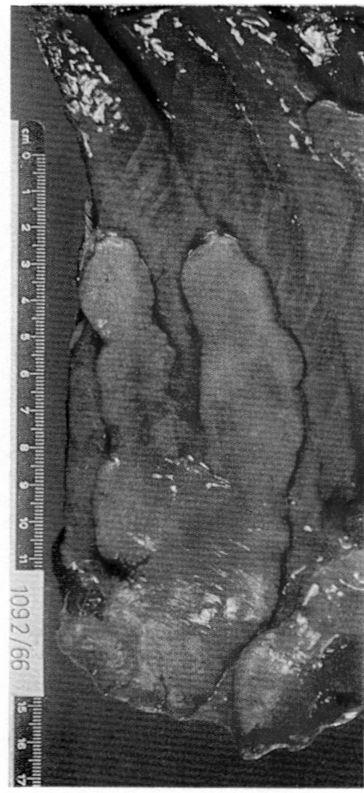

Fig. 4.87. Pleural hyalinosis.

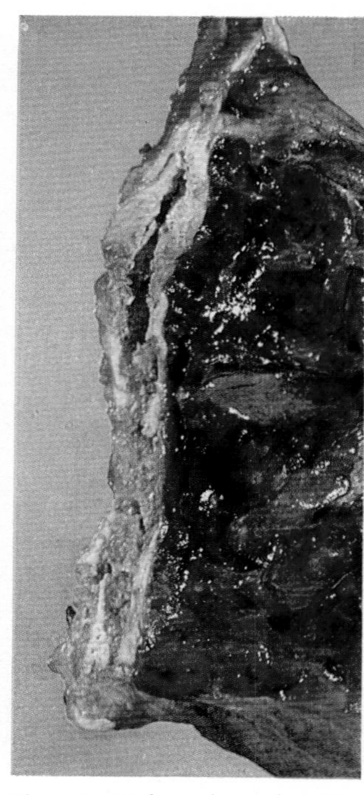

Fig. 4.88. Tuberculous pleuritis.

Pleura

Most diseases of the pleura also involve other serous membranes (pericardium, peritoneum) because of similar pathogenetic mechanisms.

Bilateral pleural effusion frequently is seen in heart diseases, especially congestive heart failure. The effusion is a transudate with a specific gravity below 1.018, and a protein content below 3%. The fluid is clear and amber (Fig. 4.89a). Bilateral pleural effusions are encountered occasionally in acute pancreatitis with pleural fat necrosis or ovarian fibromas (Meigs' syndrome: pleural effusion, ascites, ovarian fibroma).

A cloudy, gray-white effusion with flakes of fibrin is characteristic of a serofibrinous pleuritis (Fig. 4.89b). The pleura is covered by a gray-white or gray-red fibrin exudate that may resemble the "bread-and-butter" type of pericarditis. The pleura is dull, not glistening (see Fig. 4.84). Pneumonias, lung infarctions, tuberculosis and uremia are accompanied by serofibrinous pleuritis. Collection of pus in the pleural space is referred to as purulent pleuritis or empyema. Figure 4.85 shows purulent exudate in the right pleural cavity. The exudate adheres to the pleura. Note the displacement of the mediastinum and heart to the left.

Hemorrhagic effusions (Fig. 4.89c) are found in pleural carcinomatosis or tuberculosis. Band-like pleural adhesions are common sequelae of fibrinous pleuritis (Fig. 4.86). Multiple adhesions may obliterate the pleural space; commonly seen in recurrent pleuritis. The pleura is then converted into a thick plate (Fig. 4.88).

A special type of pleural scarring is pleural hyalinosis (Fig. 4.87). For practical purposes, hyalinosis affects only the parietal pleura (see also capsule hyalinosis of the spleen, p. 183). The pleura is converted into porcelain-white ("sugar-coated"), firm, flat plaques. The plaques can be diagnosed by x-ray (often with calcifications). The DD of a pleural mesothelioma must be considered. A mesothelioma usually is a nodular, diffuse growth and is thicker than the plaques of hyalinosis.

Scars in the visceral pleura present as white-gray patches of pleural thickening.

Tuberculosis of the pleura presents as miliary tubercles or as caseous necrosis of the fibrinous pleural exudate and granulation tissue (caseous pleuritis). Extensive pleural thickening with caseation and calcifications is shown in Figure 4.88. The pleural peel is white-gray; its consistency is hard like calcium or friable because of the caseous masses.

Pg: extension of infection from a tubercle near the pleura (lung, vertebrae) by lymphogenous or hematogenous spread.

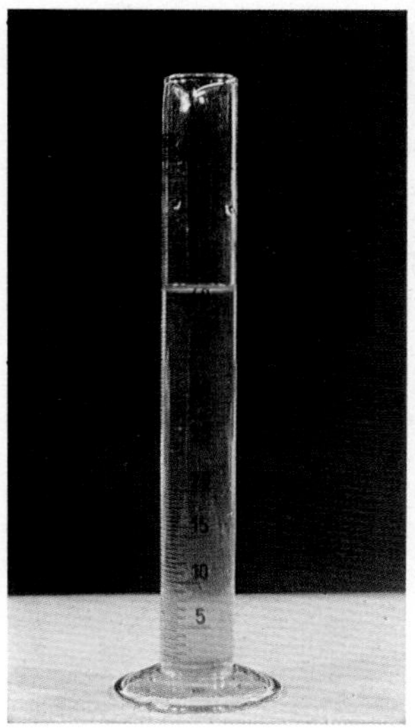

a

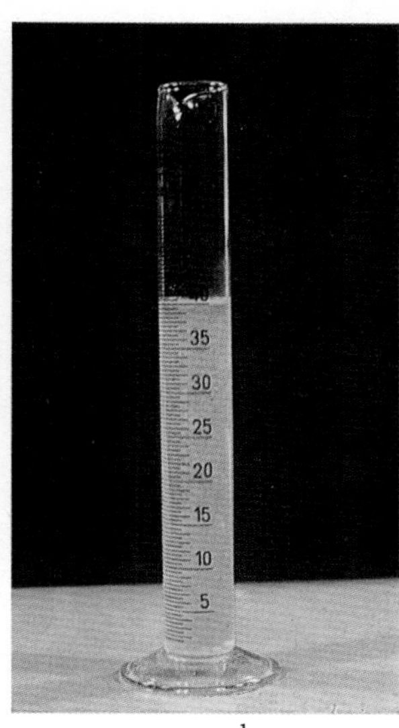

b

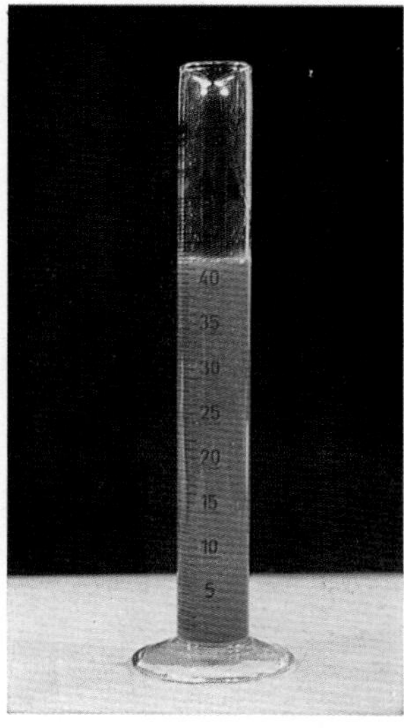

c

Fig. 4.89. Pleural effusions: (a) serous (transudate), (b) serofibrinous (exudate) and (c) hemorrhagic.

5. Gastrointestinal Tract

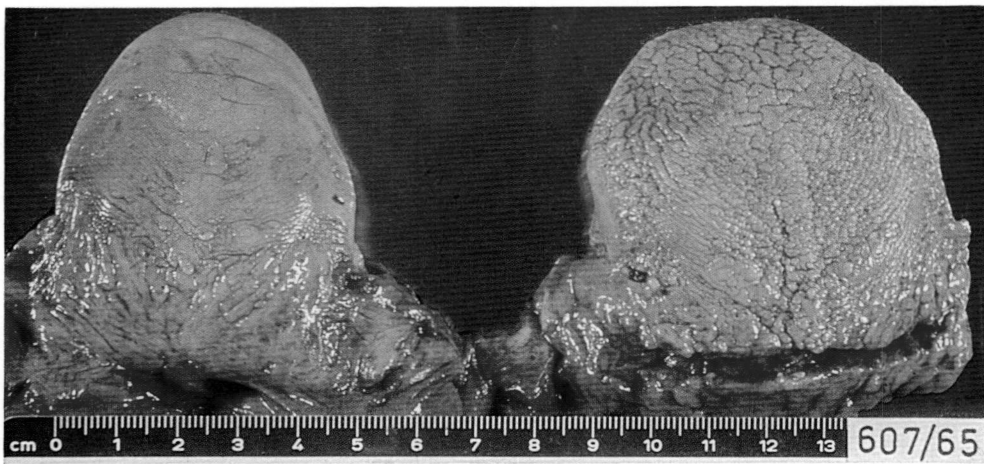

Fig. 5.1. Left: atrophy of the tongue. Right: normal tongue.

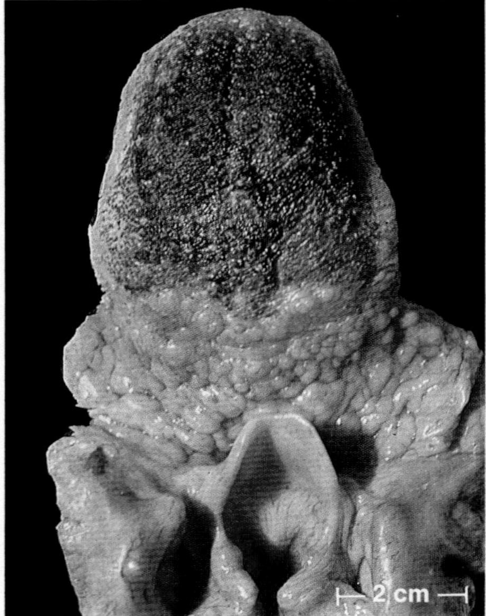

Fig. 5.2. Black hairy tongue.

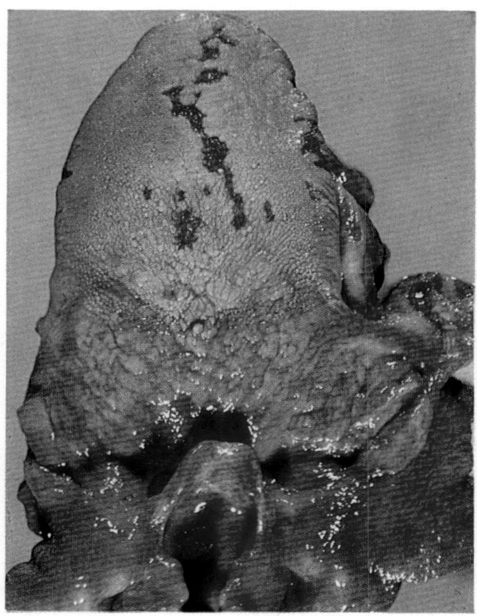

Fig. 5.3. Geographic tongue.

Technic of Dissection

The removal of the neck organs requires skill and special care. The skin should not be mutilated during the preparation of the neck organs. A circular cut is made at the level of the clavicle. The muscles of the neck are cut with a knife and dissected to the inner margin of the mandible. The tongue is freed at the inner margin of the mandible; this is followed by dissection of the soft palate at the transition to the hard palate. A knife cut is then extended to the vertebral column so that the pharynx is prepared. Tonsils are cut longitudinally. The esophagus is opened with an enterotome.

Dissection of the stomach and gut: The abdominal cavity is examined in situ (adhesions, volvulus and other changes). The colon is cut at the transition of the sigmoid to the rectum and removed in toto. The small intestine is dissected at the transition of the duodenum to the jejunum. The small intestine is opened at the root of the mesentery. The small intestine also can be prepared after the mesentery is cut off. The duodenum is opened in situ with scissors. The stomach is opened along the greater curvature. Stomach and esophagus should be left together when lesions are suspected in the fundus or esophagus (e.g., varices). The stomach content is saved until the cause of death is determined. The bile ducts are opened from the papilla of Vater after pressure is applied on the gallbladder.

Tongue

Changes in the tongue often reflect diseases of the gastrointestinal tract and blood. Figure 5.1 shows a normal tongue compared with an **atrophic tongue** mucosa (at the left in the picture). The papillae are atrophic and the mucosa is thin and bright red ("beefy tongue"). Atrophy of the tongue is symptomatic of pernicious anemia, sprue or pellagra. Atrophy of the tongue (and gastric mucosa) develops in 75% of patients with pernicious anemia (Möller-Hunter glossitis). If the atrophy involves only the margins and tip of the tongue, the condition is referred to as *Möller glossitis* (anemia in females). No blood disease was known in our case.

Black hairy tongue is a black discoloration, as shown in Figure 5.2. The condition is due to hyperplastic and hyperkeratotic filiform papillae, so that the papillae resemble small "hairs." Sulfur dioxide is produced by bacteria from remnants of food to account for the black color. (Sign of poor oral hygiene in seriously ill patients or those with hypovitaminosis.)

Lingua plicata sive scrotalis (furrowed or scrotal tongue). The tongue surface contains deep furrows that branch with a certain regularity (like the ribs of a leaf, Reichenbach). A geographic tongue is characterized by confluent, red, migratory spots and furrows (Fig. 5.3). Both types of tongues also are observed as part of the Melkersson syndrome (recurrent paresis of the facial nerve and swelling of the face).

Pg: scrotal tongue probably is a dominant, genetically determined disease. *DD:* the tongue of tertiary syphilis has deep, diffuse scars and is firm and sclerotic (lingua lobata).

Other tongue changes: Bites in the anterior portion of the tongue are seen in epileptic patients. Impressions from teeth and hemorrhages in bolus death. Dental plates may be dislodged during anesthesia, causing impressions and hemorrhages.

Tumors of the tongue. The rare granular myoblastoma (Abrisokoff) usually is a circumscribed, round tumor of the tongue or alveolar processes. The tumor consists of large lipid-laden cells. Nodular and even diffuse amyloidosis of the tongue also may resemble a tumor.

Carcinoma of the tongue usually develops at the base of the tongue. Figure 5.4 shows an exophytic carcinoma of the left lateral tongue. Carcinoma of the tongue often presents as an ulcerating lesion, as in Figure 5.4. Men between 50 and 60 years of age predominate. Metastases are to regional lymph nodes.

Carcinoma of the lips arises most often on the lower lateral lip as a small nodule with secondary ulceration (men 50–70 years of age, pipe smokers).

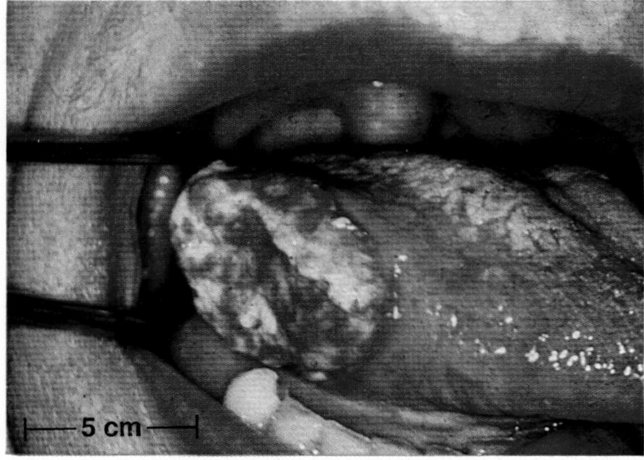

Fig. 5.4. Carcinoma of the tongue.

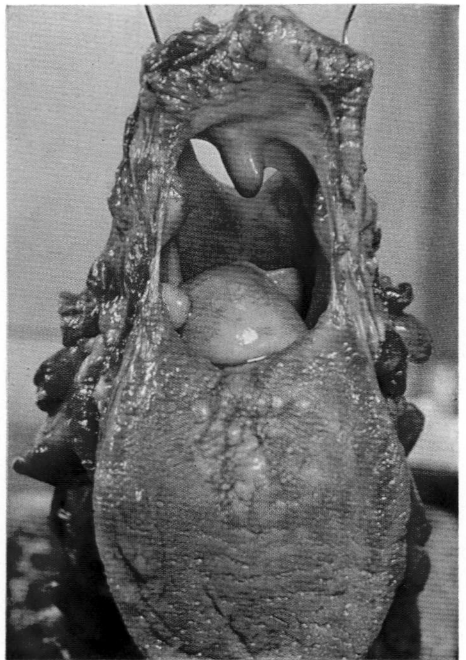

Fig. 5.5. Retention cyst at the base of the tongue.

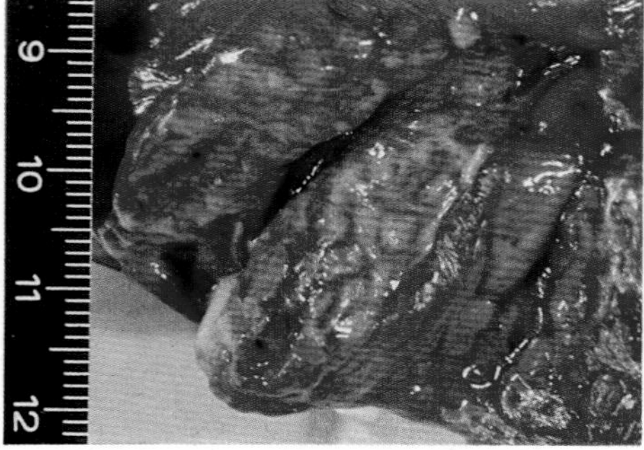

Fig. 5.6. Chronic tonsillitis.

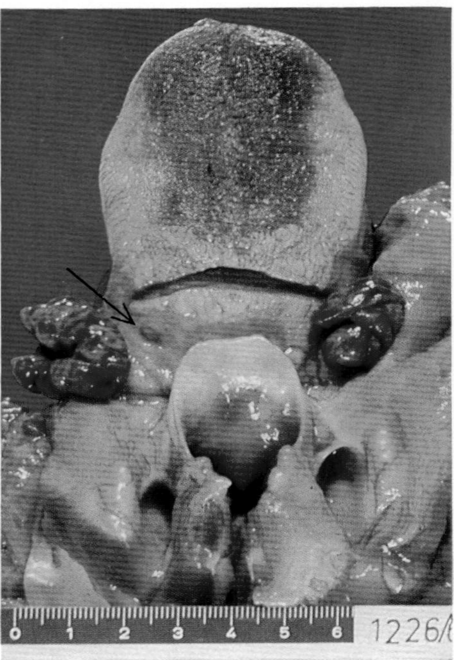

Fig. 5.7. Infiltration of the tonsils by myeloid leukemia.

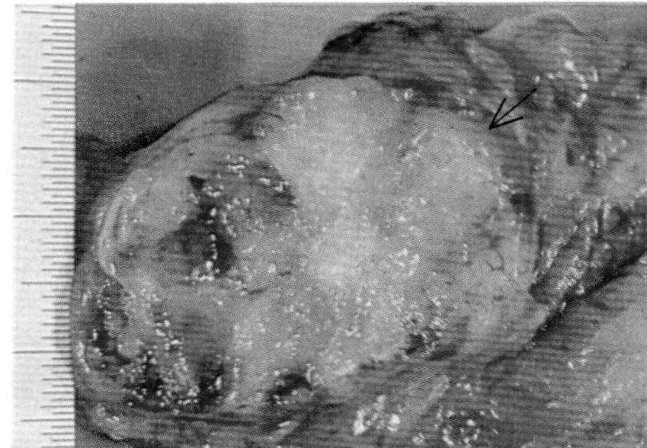

Fig. 5.8. Mixed tumor of the parotid gland.

Other tumors of the oral cavity: **Granulomatous epulis** (giant-cell reparative granuloma) is a hypertrophic inflammatory growth and not a true tumor. The epulis usually is attached to the gingiva or periosteum of the alveolar process. The central epulis (enulis) occurs in the mandible. *Mi:* a resorptive and regenerative process with many multinucleated giant cells (similar to the "brown tumors" of von Recklinghausen's disease, see p. 197). *A:* 20–40 years. *S:* ♂ : ♀ = 1 : 2.

Adamantinomas (ameloblastomas) arise from the epithelial rests of Malassez (undifferentiated epithelium of enamel organ). The tumor is anatomically benign but clinically persistent. Cubical or cylindrical cells proliferate as solid or cystic masses. Islands of squamous epithelium may be included. The primary site is the mandible, usually in the molar or premolar area. *A:* 40–60 years. *S:* ♂ : ♀ = 1 : 1.

Lingual thyroid. A developmental anomaly presenting as a round, nodular tumor near the foramen cecum at the base of the tongue. The lesion is an aberrant portion of the thyroid that may enlarge under conditions of iodine deficiency.

Retention cyst in the base of the tongue. In Figure 5.5, the tongue is pulled forward; the soft palate and uvula are retracted. The tonsils are seen at the lateral margins of the picture. A resilient, yellowish red retention cyst is found at the base of the tongue, anterior to the epiglottis. The cyst is filled with fluid secreted by mucous glands.

Tonsils, Salivary Glands

Acute inflammations of tonsils or salivary glands rarely are seen at autopsy.

Tonsillitis lacunaris. Greenish plugs of pus following streptococcal infection. A smear of the tonsil reveals granulocytes. *Co:* peritonsillar or retropharyngeal abscess, possibly mediastinitis and phlegmonous inflammation of the floor of the mouth. Sepsis → pyemia. Lacunar tonsillitis can serve as a primary focus for rheumatic fever!

Necrotizing and ulcerative tonsillitis. (a) *Plaut-Vincent angina:* painful membranous ulcerations of the tonsils caused by spirochetes and fusiform bacteria. Rare. (b) *Agranulocytosis:* extensive, dirty ulcerations. May extend from the tonsils to the gingiva or pharynx. *Mi:* areas of necrosis without cellular reaction. (c) *Diphtheria:* gray-white areas of necrosis with fibrin exudate. Extremely rare today. (d) *Scarlet fever:* Necrotizing inflammation with ulcerations caused by hemolyzing streptococci → interstitial nephritis. Glomerulonephritis.

Chronic tonsillitis. Manifested as hypertrophic tonsillitis in children. In adults, tonsillar scars after repeated bouts of tonsillitis present as white streaks on cut surface (Fig. 5.6). In addition, retention cysts in the tonsillar crypts contain white-gray plugs that can be expressed after cutting. *Mi:* the plugs are masses of cellular debris without leukocytes.

Leukemic infiltration enlarges the tonsils and the lymphatic apparatus in the oropharynx. Figure 5.7 is from a case of myeloid leukemia. The tonsils are greatly enlarged and deep red. Mucosal hemorrhages and a small necrotic area with hemorrhage (→) are seen at the base of the tongue. Leukemic infiltrates tend to become secondarily necrotic due to agranulocytosis, especially in acute undifferentiated leukemias. Chronic lymphatic leukemia also causes infiltration of tonsils and the lymphatic tissue of the oropharynx.

Mixed tumors of the parotid gland (Fig. 5.8; TCP, p. 243). Mixed tumors are pleomorphic adenomas that may arise in any of the salivary glands of the neck or oral cavity. The tumor is grossly firm-elastic, nodular, well circumscribed and surrounded by a fibrous-tissue capsule. The cut surface is white to gray-white or variable in appearance. It may contain cysts, foci of hyalinization or myxomatous and firm cartilaginous portions. The surrounding parotid gland (→) is atrophic (pressure atrophy).

F: 60% of all tumors of the parotid gland. *A:* 20–40 years. *S:* ♀>♂. Ten per cent become malignant, but more recur after excision.

Malignant mixed tumors of the parotid gland are extremely rare. Occasionally, a malignant change in a mixed tumor of the parotid is manifested as an adenocarcinoma or squamous-cell carcinoma. They can metastasize to the lung. Three times more common in females than in males.

Other types of parotid gland tumors

Mucoepidermoid carcinomas are derived from the epithelium of intercalated ducts. Histologically, the tumor is composed of epithelial and mucus-producing cells. Well-differentiated forms have a good prognosis.

S: ♀ predominate. *A:* 60–70 years.

Adenocystic carcinomas (cylindromas) are relatively benign tumors. Metastases occur relatively late. Frequently there is recurrence after excision.

Acinar cell carcinomas arise from the acini of the parotid gland, grow slowly and resemble a hypernephroma histologically.

Adenolymphoma (Warthin's tumor, cystadenoma lymphomatosum). A benign tumor composed of glands with multiple papillary proliferations from the glandular epithelium. The gland lumina contain inspissated secretion. The tumor stroma is rich in lymphocytes and lymph follicles (therefore the misnomer "lymphoma"). Warthin's tumors sometimes are mistaken for caseating lymph-node tuberculosis.

Oncocytoma (oxyphilic-cell adenoma, Hamperl). A benign tumor of the salivary glands composed of large cells with eosinophilic, finely granular cytoplasm.

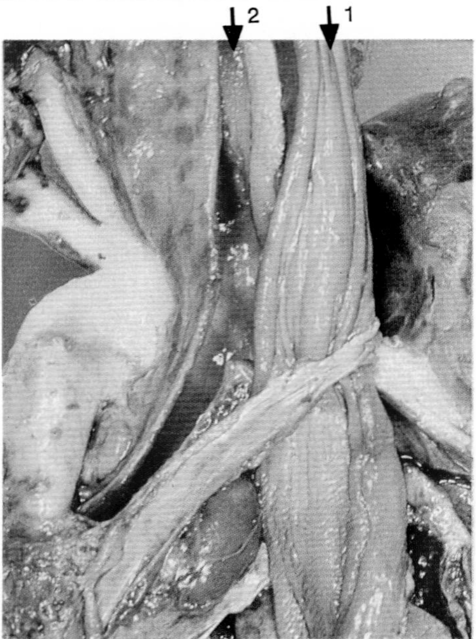

Fig. 5.9. Dysphagia lusoria.

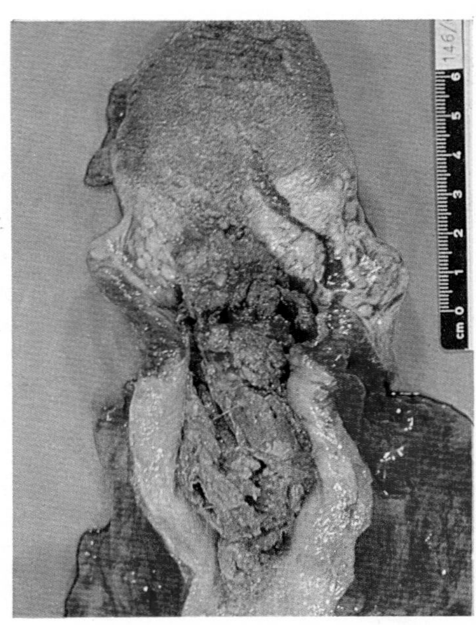

Fig. 5.10. Bolus death: occlusion of the esophagus and trachea.

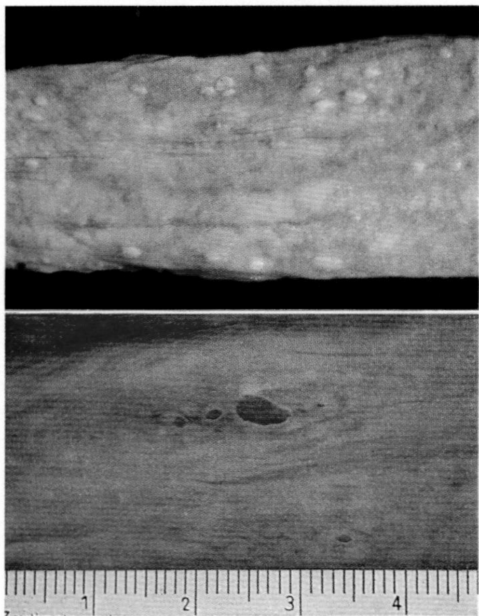

Fig. 5.11. Above: leukoplakia of the esophagus.
Fig. 5.12. Below: heterotopic gastric mucosa in the esophagus.

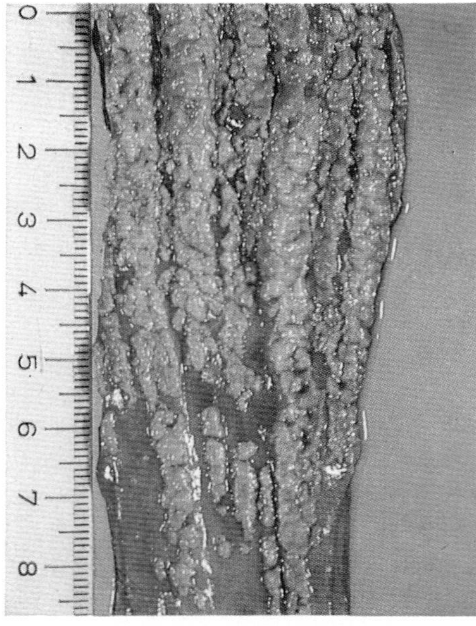

Fig. 5.13. Candidiasis (moniliasis) of the esophagus.

Esophagus

Malformations (Fig. 5.14). Despite operative corrections, malformations of the esophagus are serious and life-threatening developmental anomalies. Esophagus malformations are shown in Figure 5.14. *Agenesis:* the esophagus is not developed. *Aplasia:* only a rudimentary muscle pipe is formed. *Atresia:* partial or complete occlusion. *Stenosis:* focal narrowing. *Lower tracheo-esophageal fistula:* atresia of the upper esophagus and the lower esophagus communicates with the trachea. *Upper tracheo-esophageal fistula:* the upper esophagus communicates with the trachea (danger of aspiration!) and the lower esophagus ends blindly.
F: 1%.

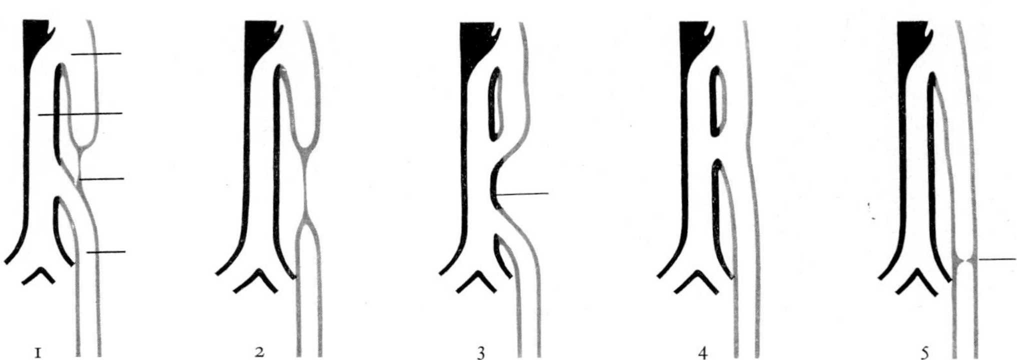

Fig. 5.14. Schematic presentation of malformations of the esophagus. Ph: pharynx; T: trachea; St: stenosis; E: esophagus; A: aplasia; F: fistula. 1. Aplasia and lower fistula, 2. aplasia, 3. upper and lower fistula, 4. simple fistula, 5. stenosis.

Dysphagia lusoria (Fig. 5.9). *Dysphagia caused by external compression of the esophagus from a deviant right subclavian artery.* Figure 5.9 shows the opened right subclavian artery, which arises as the last left arterial branch from the aortic arch. The subclavian artery runs to the right between the esophagus and the vertebral column. 1 → esophagus, 2 → trachea.

F: a rare vascular anomaly observed in approximately 0.2% of all autopsies. Much more important clinically is the arteriomesenteric ileus, likewise attributable to compression of a viscus by an artery. The horizontal portion of the duodenum is compressed or occluded by the roof of the mesentery and the superior mesenteric artery. The food-containing duodenum may add to the compression by exerting a pull on the mesenteric root. *Co:* vomitus of bile, "high" ileus and acute distention of the stomach.

Bolus death. *Sudden death from occlusion of the trachea by a foreign body.* Figure 5.10 shows the opened esophagus with a partly digested, 8 cm.-long piece of meat. The epiglottis is completely occluded by the bolus. Death also can occur from dislodged dental plates, e.g., during anesthesia. Suffocation hemorrhages (petechiae in the pericardium and pleura) and acutely emphysematous (hyperinflated) lungs are additional gross findings in bolus death.

Leukoplakia of the esophagus (Fig. 5.11). *Patchy (3–5-mm. large), white, slightly elevated areas of squamous metaplasia.* Leukoplakias also occur in the mucosa of the oral cavity, pharynx and trachea (TCP, p. 237). In contrast to leukoplakias of the tongue or gingiva, those seen in the esophagus are not considered precancerous lesions.

Heterotopic gastric mucosa in the esophagus (Fig. 5.12). *Congenital displacement of fundic mucosa into the lower third of the esophagus.* Red, circumscribed, slightly elevated islands (heterotopic fundic mucosa) (0.5 cm. long) are seen in the mucosa of the lower esophagus (Fig. 5.12). A common but mostly insignificant malformation. However, peptic ulcers (including perforation) occasionally may develop in ectopic gastric mucosa. This also is true for gastric mucosa in a Meckel's diverticulum.

Idiopathic rupture of the esophagus is seen rarely. The esophagus is ruptured longitudinally. Esophageal rupture presents a difficult clinical diagnostic problem.

Candidiasis of the esophagus (thrush or moniliasis) (Fig. 5.13; TCP, p. 273). Multiple, yellow-gray or whitish, soft and elevated patches adhere to the mucosa. The lesions consist of necrotic epithelium and hyphae of *candida albicans.* Thrush occurs in patients with weakened resistance, especially in those with cancer or leukemia during or after chemotherapy.

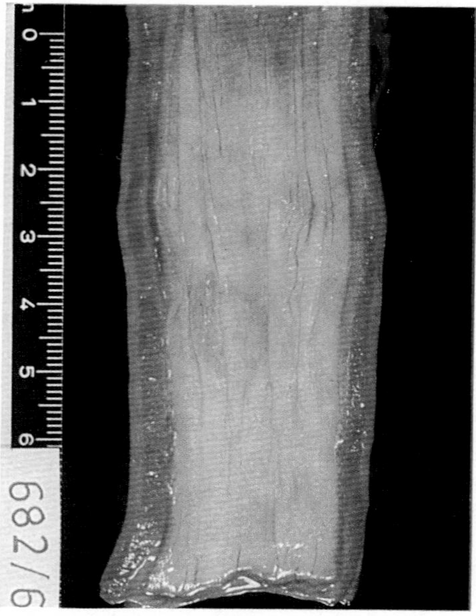

Fig. 5.15. Muscular hypertrophy of the esophagus.

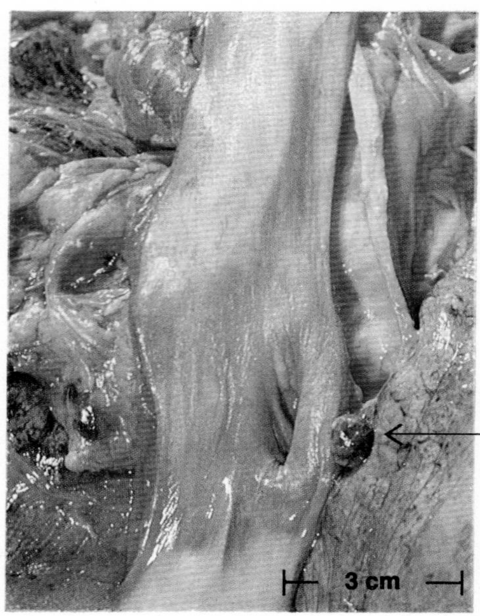

Fig. 5.16. Traction diverticulum of the esophagus.

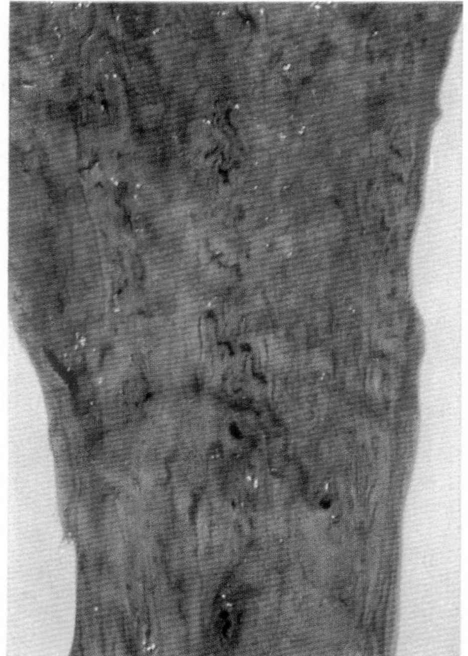

Fig. 5.17. Esophageal varices (transillumination).

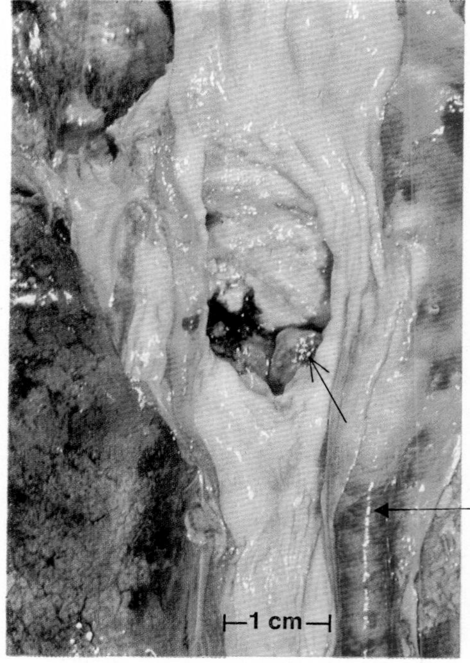

Fig. 5.18. Carcinoma of the esophagus.

Muscular hypertrophy of the esophagus. Figure 5.15 shows the wall of the esophagus, about 0.5 cm. thick, with a slightly thickened, white mucosa. Hypertrophy of the esophageal wall is observed in a congenital mega-esophagus (achalasia: wide lumen, hypertrophic wall, as in congenital megacolon) or acquired mega-esophagus (due to stenosis of the cardia or cardiospasm). The case demonstrated in Figure 5.15 was due to neither cardiospasm nor inflammation, so that a congenital malformation must be considered.
A dilation of the esophagus is found in cardiospasm (predominantly ♀) and in the *Plummer-Vinson syndrome* – esophageal membrane below the cricoid cartilage with a small opening. Atrophic gastritis. Malnutrition with hypovitaminosis.

Diverticula of the esophagus (Fig. 5.16).

A diverticulum is an outpouching of a viscus. The wall of a true diverticulum consists of mucosa, submucosa, muscularis and serosa. The false diverticulum is an outpouching or herniation of the mucosa between muscle layers. Two types are known in the esophagus:

(a) *The pulsion diverticulum* is a saccular or bottle-like, false diverticulum in the upper posterior wall at the level of the cricoid cartilage (so-called Zencker's diverticulum). Mucosa and submucosa form the wall of this developmental defect. The diverticulum becomes dilated when filled with food. *Co:* inflammation, perforation. *S:* predominantly males. *A:* 50–70 years. *Pg:* probably congenital weakness of the wall. Rarely: *epinephritic diverticula* in cardiospasm of the lower esophagus.

Co: perforation, mediastinitis, strictures, stenoses, aspiration pneumonia. *Cl:* problems in swallowing.

(b) *The traction diverticulum* results from an external adhesion and presents as a dimple or tent-like retraction of the mucosa. Figure 5.16 shows the oval stoma of a traction diverticulum. The tip of the diverticulum is attached to a hilar or paratracheal lymph node (→). Accordingly, traction diverticula occur in the middle third of the esophagus.

Pg: a nonspecific or tuberculous lymphadenitis extends into the perinodal tissue and heals by fibrosis and scarring. The scar tissue adheres to the outer wall and contracts. The traction diverticulum often has a slightly oblique position. Diverticulitis or a tracheal fistula, therefore, is a rare complication.

Esophageal varices (Fig. 5.17; see also p. 155). *Distention of venous plexus in the lower esophagus due to portal hypertension.* The esophagus was transilluminated in Figure 5.17 in order to illustrate the blue-red, blood-filled, tortuous submucosal veins. Tiny perforations or ulcerations at the apex of a tortuous vein may cause massive, sometimes fatal, hemorrhage. At autopsy, the point of perforation can be demonstrated by applying pressure to the dilated veins. The veins may collapse after a massive, fatal hemorrhage and the varices may be difficult to demonstrate.

F: in approximately 50% of patients with liver cirrhosis. *Pg:* liver cirrhosis or portal vein thrombosis causes portal hypertension, either by virtue of blood stasis (cirrhotic liver tissue) or by the presence of arteriovenous anastomoses. *Co:* caput medusae (para-umbilical veins); internal hemorrhoids. *DD:* congenital esophageal varices occur as venous tortuosities in the upper esophagus.

Carcinoma of the esophagus (Fig. 5.18). Most squamous-cell carcinomas arise in the middle third of the esophagus. Figure 5.18 shows a 5×3-cm. mucosal defect with gray-white, medium-firm tumor tissue as its base. The esophagus is perforated near the lower portion of the defect (ulcer). Gray-black hilar lymph nodes are seen at this point (→). The aorta is to the right of the esophagus. Carcinomas of the esophagus also may present as cauliflower-like, exophytic tumors that ultimately cause circular stenosis (napkin-ring stenosis). The napkin-ring, circular thickening of the wall is due to diffuse carcinomatous infiltration. Ulcerations of the mucosa frequently are found at an advanced stage of a circular carcinoma.

F: 2% of all malignant tumors. *A:* 50–60 years. *S:* ♂:♀=10:1. *Pg:* most carcinomas develop at points of physiologic narrowing: (a) entrance of the esophagus (level of the cricoid cartilage). Distance from the incisors is 16 cm, (b) intersection of the aortic arch (pulsation can be seen in the esophagoscope, 23 cm behind the incisors), (c) cardiac region (diaphragm and esophageal sphincter, 38 cm). b+c are primary sites for 60% of esophageal carcinomas. *Causative factors:* chronic, mechanical and thermal factors (e.g., carcinoma in deverticulum). Leukoplakias are not increased in frequency at points of physiologic narrowing (see above). Therefore, they are not considered precancerous changes of esophageal cancers. *Co:* 50% of the carcinomas perforate into the mediastinum, pleura or trachea; 4% infiltrate the aorta, producing fatal hemorrhage. Paralysis of recurrent laryngeal nerve. Metastases in the esophageal mucosa and to regional lymph nodes. *DD:* infiltration of the esophagus by a bronchogenic carcinoma. The DD is especially difficult when the carcinoma has been treated by x-irradiation.

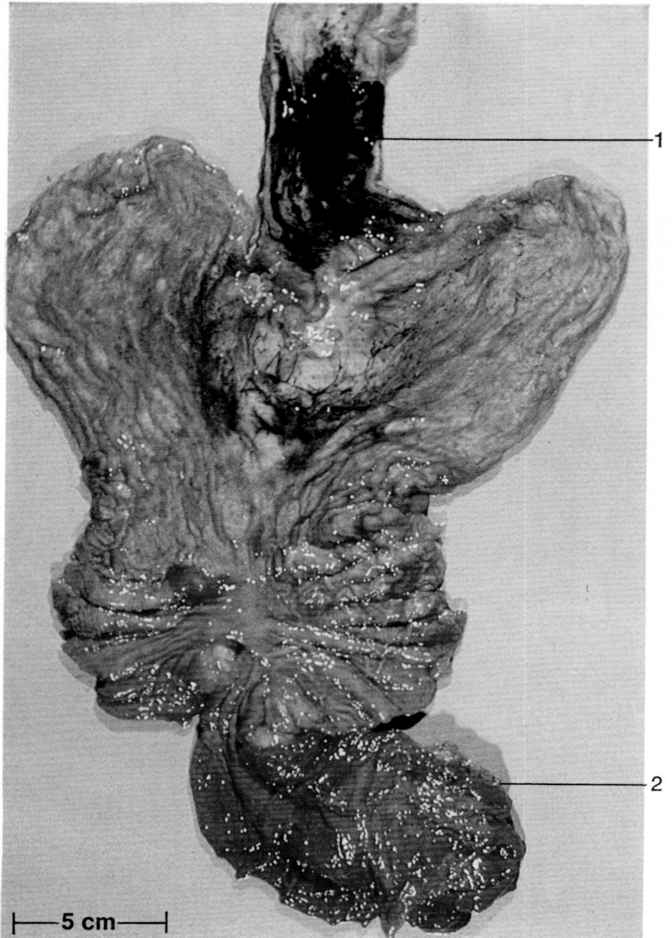

Fig. 5.19. Gastromalacia acida and reflux esophagitis.

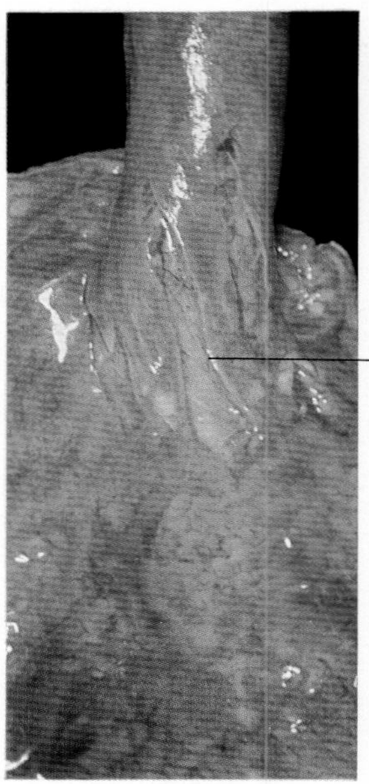

Fig. 5.20. Lacerations of the gastroesophageal mucosa and erosion in the fundus of the stomach in a case of Mallory-Weiss syndrome.

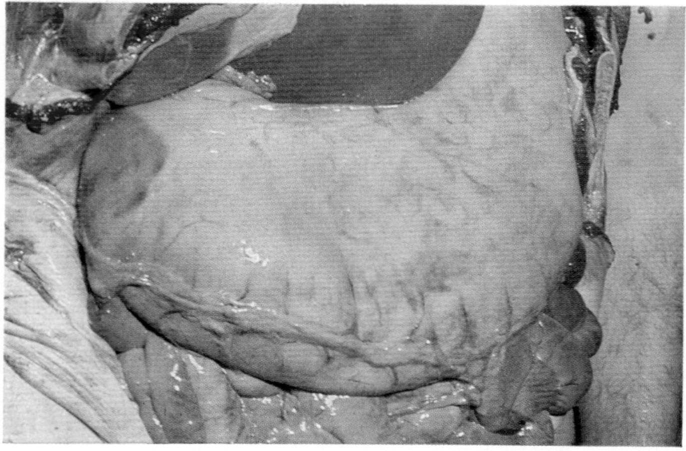

Fig. 5.21. Gastric dilatation (gastrectasia).

Stomach

Postmortem changes occur rapidly after death. Mucosal folds are no longer preserved 6–8 hours after death (probably due to the action of HCl). The mucosa is smooth and thin (misdiagnosis: atrophic gastritis). Very prominent mucosal folds suggest a hypertrophic gastritis (see Fig. 5.22). HCl and pepsin may digest not only the mucosa but also the remainder of the gastric wall (gastromalacia acida), so that the stomach perforates into the abdominal or thoracic cavity (via the diaphragm or esophagus). Dark red mucosal flecks often are seen in the stomach. They are the result of venous stasis and diffusion of hemoglobin into the gastric wall. The flecks may appear black because of formation of HCl-hemoglobin after death.

Gastromalacia acida (Fig. 5.19). The wall of the fundus is greenish black discolored and partially digested. The stomach is so thin that the blue background in this photograph can be seen through the wall. Note the black streaks in the partly digested fundus and body. The streaks are engorged veins. Hemoglobin combines with HCl to produce black HCl-hematin. The mucosa of the lower esophagus (→1) also is discolored. This is not a postmortem change but evidence of a peptic esophagitis with inflammatory hyperemia and hemorrhages (reflux esophagitis due to loss of muscle tone of the cardia). HCl-hematin has formed after death to account for the black color. →2 duodenum.

Mallory-Weiss syndrome (Fig. 5.20). *This involves longitudinal lacerations of the gastroesophageal mucosa, which occur separately or multiply (in which case they are arranged in parallel:* → in our figure) *in the lower third of the esophagus and in the gastric mucosa close to the cardia.* As a rule, the defect is confined to the internal wall layers. Perforations of the stomach or esophagus are rare (MITTERMAYER, et al., 1971).

F: about 0.2% of all autopsies. *S:* predominantly adult and in older men. *Pg:* uncoordinated vomiting (the intraesophageal pressure rises to over 150 mm Hg), alcoholism, tumor, shock with microthrombosis, radiation, may occur after cortisone therapy. Erosions of the mucosa may have a promoting effect. *Co:* severe bleeding.

Gastrectasia (Fig. 5.21) is defined as a congenital or acquired dilatation of the stomach. The condition often is combined with gastroptosis (the stomach reaches the pelvis; patients with asthenic constitution). Congenital gastrectasia is of little clinical significance. In Figure 5.21, the greater curvature of the stomach occupies the entire width of the abdominal cavity. Ribs and liver are seen at the upper margin; the colon is below. Note the large horizontal diameter of the stomach. Acute postoperative gastrectasia is attributed to a loss of gastric muscle tone (atony) and reduced gastric motility (as in paralytic ileus). An acute gastrectasia also is observed following occlusion of the mesenteric artery (see p. 105).

Congenital pyloric stenosis (Fig. 5.22). The pyloric musculature is hypertrophic, with the result of functional and anatomic stenosis. Figure 5.22 illustrates a 3 cm.-long pyloric stenosis (→). The pyloric wall is 4–6 mm. thick, gray-white and projects into the duodenum like a rigid pipe. Note the prominent longitudinal mucosal folds of the narrowed pylorus. There is marked dilatation of the stomach proximal to the stenosis. The gastric muscle layer is hypertrophic because of functional adaptation (work hypertrophy). The gastric mucosa is largely digested (postmortem change). A fresh mucosal erosion is indicated at →1. The black-brown discoloration of the erosion is caused by hematin, which forms in areas of hemorrhage by combining with HCl.

A: newborns. *S:* 80% are ♂. *Pg:* (a) congenital hyperplasia, (b) neurovegetative spasms with pyloric hypertrophy and hyperplasia. Pyloric spasms also are observed without muscle hypertrophy. *Acquired pyloric stenosis:* tumors, ulcer scars with gastrectasia.

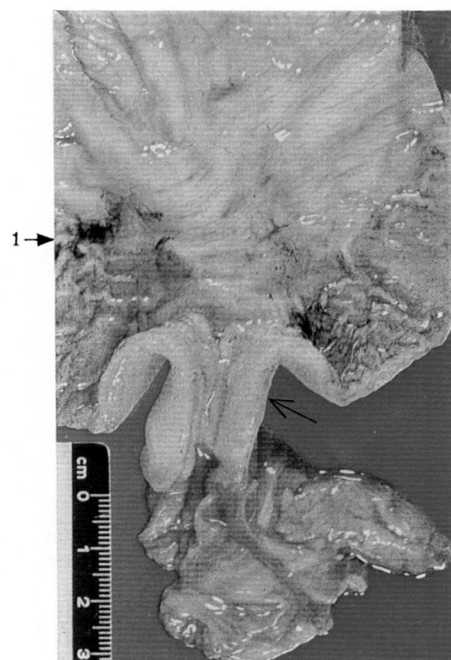

Fig. 5.22. Congenital pyloric stenosis.

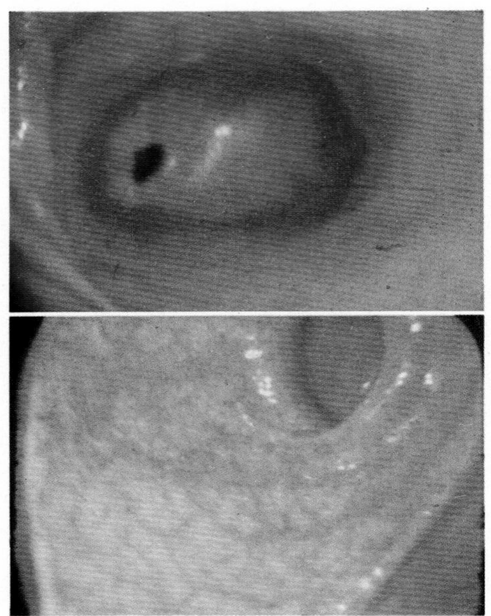

Fig. 5.23. Above: normal mucosa of the antrum. Below: chronic-atrophic gastritis. (gastroscopy).

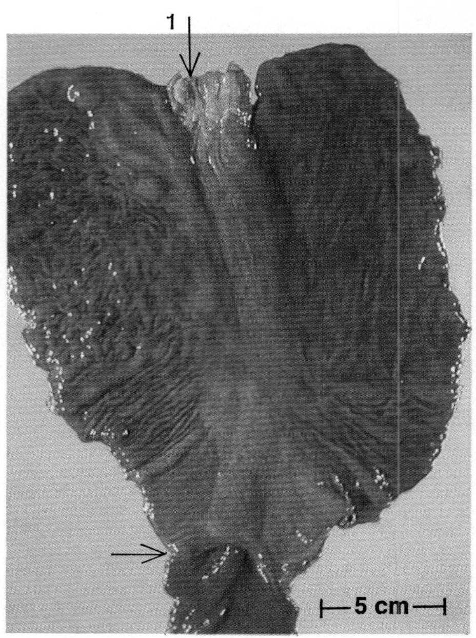

Fig. 5.24. Uremic gastritis.

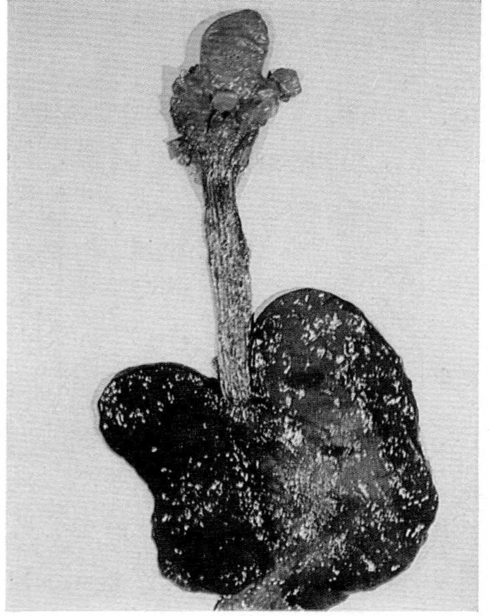

Fig. 5.25. Corrosive gastritis and esophagitis after ingestion of acetic acid.

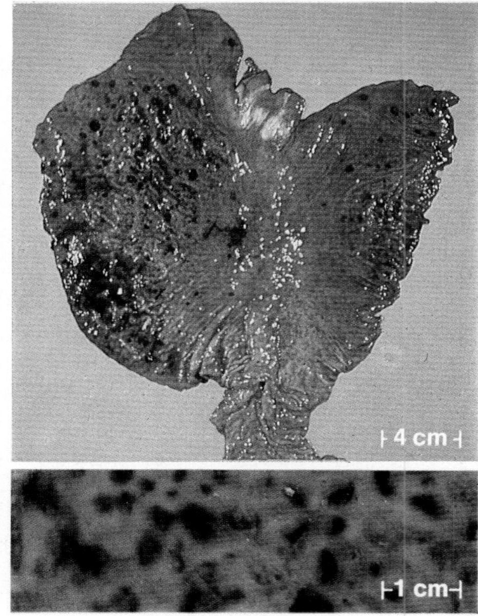

Fig. 5.26. Hemorrhagic erosions of the gastric mucosa.

Gastritis (Fig. 5.23; TCP, p. 103). Gastroscopy and gastric biopsies have contributed markedly to an understanding of gastritis. Figure 5.23 (above) shows a normal antral mucosa and pylorus. Mucosal folds are seen at the left in this illustration. The mucosa is reddened but vascular markings are inconspicuous. By comparison, Figure 5.23 (below) shows the common chronic atrophic gastritis. The mucosa is gray-white and vascular markings are conspicuous. Even small vessels are seen clearly through the thin (atrophic) mucosa.

Such subtle mucosal changes can be diagnosed by gastroscopy but rarely are preserved at autopsy (e.g., atrophic or superficial gastritis). Only advanced forms of gastritis, usually accompanied by increased mucus secretion, can be appreciated on gross examination. The mucus forms a protective layer and thereby prevents postmortem digestion. Figure 5.24 shows a uremic gastritis as an example of an acute gastritis. The gastric and duodenal mucosa is markedly reddened. The rugae are well preserved. The triangular pale zone in the photograph represents the gastric antrum; →1 points to the lower esophagus, → to the pylorus. Note the prominent longitudinal folds along the lesser curvature. The mucosa is covered by copious amounts of mucus and the gastric wall is thicker than usual (edema). A similar gross picture is observed in a chronically congested stomach (e.g., cardiac failure), the so-called congestive gastritis.

F: as judged from gastric biopsies, a normal mucosa is found in the antrum in 20%, in the cardia in 50% and in the fundus in 80% of all cases (ELSTER). In patients past 50–60 years of age, a high incidence of atrophic gastritis (50%) and of superficial gastritis (70–80%) has been reported (SIURALA). *Pg:* alcohol, dietary imbalance, autoimmunity. Uremic gastritis: excretion of urinary substances through the gastric mucosa.

Types of gastritis: (a) *simple, superficial gastritis*; (b) *chronic-atrophic gastritis*; (c) *hypertrophic gastritis* – hypertrophic gastritis, which is not generally accepted as a separate entity, probably is attributable to an increased contractility of the gastric muscle layers, thereby mimicking hypertrophic mucosal folds; (d) *glandular hyperplasia* (mucosa thicker than 1 mm. in Zollinger-Ellison syndrome; see p. 173); (e) *giant hyperplasia* with elongation of foveolar pits is characteristic of the *Ménétrier syndrome* (excessive protein loss into gastric secretions → hypoproteinemia).

Acute phlegmonous inflammation of the gastric wall is localized in the submucosa; predominantly affects males.

Corrosive gastritis and esophagitis due to ingestion of acetic acid (Fig. 5.25; TCP, p. 103). Corrosive gastritis most often affects children or persons attempting suicide. Figure 5.25 shows whitish gray, superficial areas of mucosal necrosis (coagulation necrosis) in the esophagus and black to gray-black charring of the stomach (necrosis, hemorrhage and formation of HCl-hematin). Acids and lyes continue to corrode the esophagus or stomach after death, leading to perforation.

Acids: HNO_3: bright yellow to yellow-brown scabs. H_2SO_4: charring of mucosa with black, dry scabs. *Carbolic acid:* white scabs (*Mi:* coagulation necrosis). *Sublimate:* white corrosion scabs. *Lyes: NaOH or KOH:* soft, soapy, gelatinous mucosa (liquefaction necrosis). High concentrations of ingested lyes cause scabs. *Co:* hemorrhagic-phlegmonous gastritis, perforation, ulcers, cicatricial stricture (especially esophagus). KOH corrosions are common in Egyptian children (soap is homemade).

Erosion of the gastric mucosa (Fig. 5.26; TCP, p. 105). Relatively common in autopsy material because bleeding from multiple erosions can be fatal. In severe cases, multiple, densely set, irregular, black or brown-black hemorrhages 1–5 mm. in diameter are seen (Fig. 5.26). At higher magnification, the lesions are identified as superficial mucosal defects (leopard-skin stomach). Flat, white, mucosal ulcers develop after the blood has been digested. Bloody contents in stomach and bowel.

F: 1–3%. *A:* 30–70 years. *S:* ♂=♀. *Pg:* see TCP, page 105. The necrotic material of a small mucosal hemorrhagic infarction is excavated (=erosion). Pathogenetically, hemorrhagic erosions probably precede peptic ulcers. This sequence must be rare, since erosions are much more common than ulcers. *Causes:* stress of various types: operations, shock, cerebral trauma, burns. Experimentally, erosions can be produced by histamine, hunger, gastrin (→ hyperacidity), ACTH and cortisone.

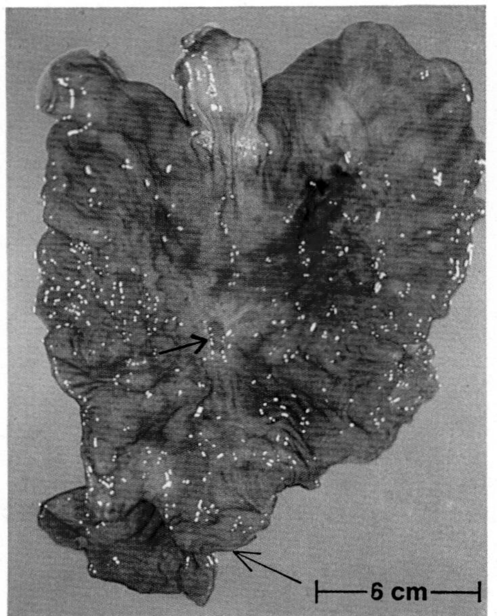

Fig. 5.27. Acute ulcer of the lesser curvature.

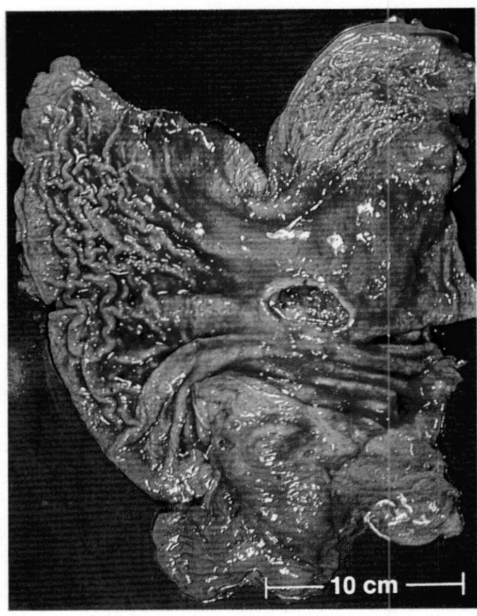

Fig. 5.28. Chronic gastric ulcer.

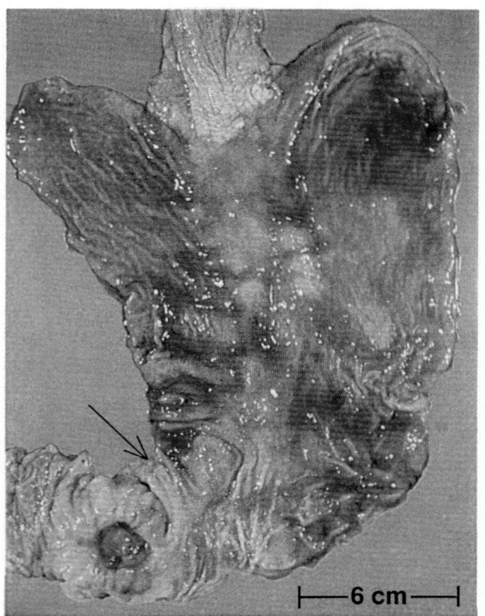

Fig. 5.29. Chronic duodenal ulcer.

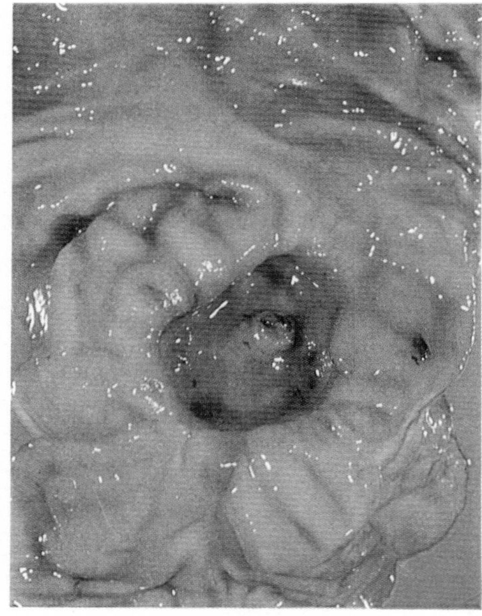

Fig. 5.30. Close-up of duodenal ulcer with an eroded vessel.

Gastric and Duodenal Ulcer

An ulcer is a defect of the gastric mucosa with involvement of the muscularis mucosae, the submucosa, and the muscularis propria. The following diagnostic criteria are important: Single or multiple ulcers (Zollinger-Ellison syndrome)? Location and size? Sharp, step-like or elevated, heaped-up, thickened margins? Consistency of ulcer margin? (*DD:* peptic ulcer – ulcerated carcinoma). Appearance of ulcer base? (Blood vessels: hemorrhage, pancreas: perforation or penetration.) The serosa of the stomach should always be examined (fibrinous exudate, penetration, perforation!). Appearance of the intact mucosa? A peptic ulcer on occasion is difficult to find in a surgically removed stomach because the ulcer may be covered by a contracted mucosa.

Acute gastric ulcer (TCP, pp. 104 and 105). Figure 5.27 includes the lower third of the esophagus at the upper margin of the photograph. The pylorus is indicated by the arrow. An oval mucosal defect with a greenish gray, smooth base is seen at the lesser curvature of the corpus. The margin of the ulcer is sharp. The entire gastric mucosa is hyperemic and reddened. The rugae are prominent and covered by mucus despite postmortem changes (seen as a glistening of the mucosa). The prominent mucosal folds are indicative of a chronic gastritis.

Chronic gastric ulcer (Fig. 5.28). Again, the ulcer is located in the middle portion (body) of the lesser curvature. The ulcer is round to oval. Its greatest diameter is perpendicular to the long axis of the stomach. The margin is firm in consistency, rounded (in contrast to a fresh ulcer), heaped up and appears whitish (scar tissue). The ulcer base is gray-red and slightly uneven (granulation tissue). In addition, small blood clots adhere to the ulcer base (hemorrhage from small vessels. *Cl:* tarry stools!). A smooth and white ulcer ground indicates that the base consists of the muscularis proper with little granulation tissue. The base of a chronic gastric ulcer also may consist of pancreas, omentum or even liver (penetrating ulcer, TCP, pp. 104 and 105). Note the chronic gastritis. The oral edge or margin of a chronic peptic ulcer can be step-like in appearance, as illustrated in Figure 5.29 (TCP, p. 104).

Chronic duodenal ulcer (Fig. 5.29). A round ulcer with rounded, slightly heaped-up margins is seen in the posterior wall of the duodenum, approximately 1 cm. below the pylorus (→). The ulcer margin and base are firm to hard in consistency, and white scar tissue is seen on the cut surface. The mucosal folds around the ulcer are gray-white, enlarged and converge in a star-like pattern toward the margin of the ulcer (compare the normal, horizontal duodenal mucosal folds on the left margin in Fig. 5.29). The ulcer base is smooth except for an occluded vessel that projects from the base. Note the reddish, well-preserved, gastric mucosal folds, which are covered by a thick layer of mucus (chronic gastritis). Most duodenal ulcers occur in the duodenal bulb.

Figure 5.30 is a higher magnification of a chronic duodenal ulcer. The step-like configuration of the oral ulcer margin contrasts with the steep margin of the aboral (distal) margin. An eroded artery projects from the base. The arterial stump is brown due to formation of hematin. An opening of a perforated artery is identified as a small, bright-red point. This patient died from massive hemorrhage.

Figure 5.31 illustrates a massive blood clot in the stomach as evidence of arterial bleeding from peptic ulcer. Blood coagulates and forms a replica of the stomach contours (→1 greater curvature, →2 pylorus). In most cases, however, an eroded artery causes massive hematemesis and/or hemorrhage into the lower gastrointestinal tract.

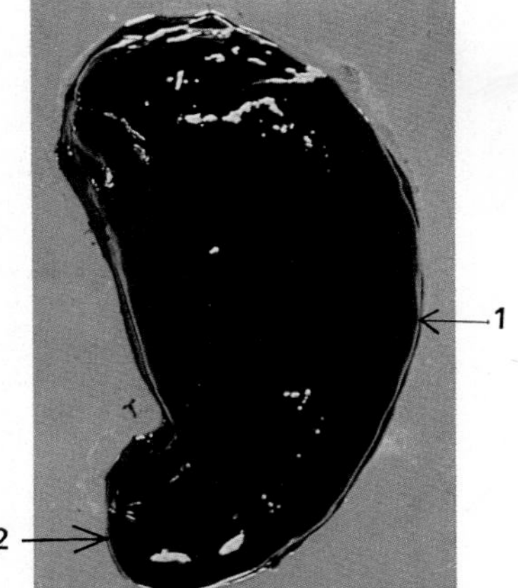

Fig. 5.31. Coagulated blood in the stomach following massive hemorrhage from a peptic ulcer.

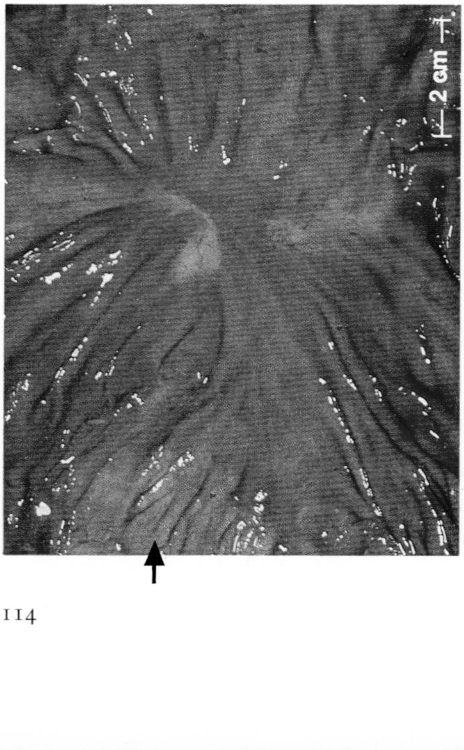

Fig. 5·32. Ulcer scar in the stomach.

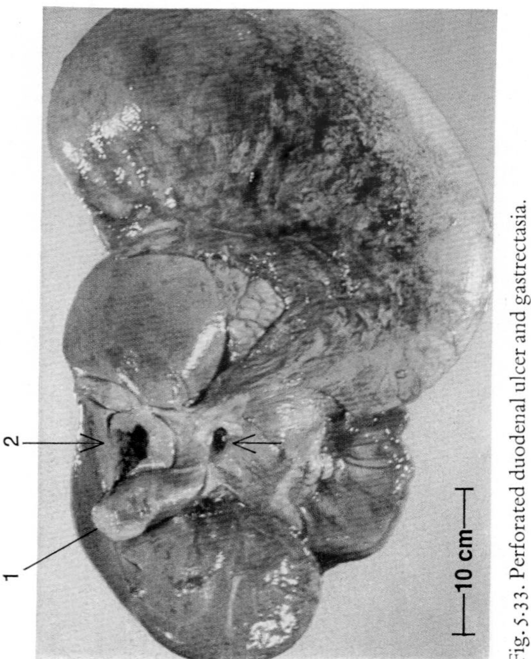

Fig. 5·33. Perforated duodenal ulcer and gastrectasia.

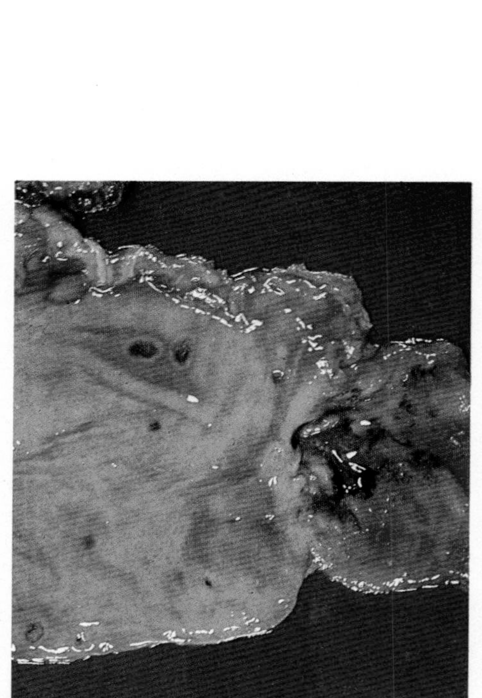

Fig. 5·34. Multiple ulcers in Zollinger–Ellison syndrome.

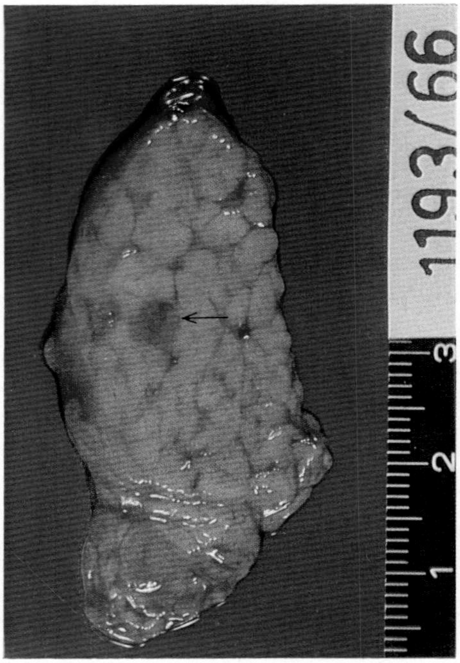

Fig. 5·35. Adenoma of pancreas in Zollinger–Ellison syndrome.

Ulcers heal by growth of granulation tissue from the base and by re-epithelialization from the margins. At this stage, the ulcer is shallow and covered by a thin, smooth, white mucosa. The end stage is an ulcer scar that presents as a small, white, sometimes retracted, sometimes star-like, area in the mucosa (Fig. 5.32). The scar is poorly vascularized and, therefore, white. The rugae converge toward the scar. Pyloric scars lead to pyloric stenosis or obstruction with dilatation of the stomach. A scar in the lesser curvature results in a foreshortened stomach (sometimes referred to as "*tobacco pouch" stomach*). Scarring and retraction of the middle portion of the body in a horizontal direction yields an "*hourglass" stomach*. In the duodenum, *pseudodiverticula* are formed by tightening of the mucosa and outpouching of adjacent wall sections.

Figure 5.33 illustrates a common complication of peptic ulcers. The unnumbered arrow in Figure 5.33 points to a perforated ulcer in the anterior duodenal wall. The stomach and duodenum are not opened, and the liver was retracted for demonstration purposes (→2, caudate lobe; →1, gallbladder). The black area of the caudate lobe covered the ulcer perforation in situ. Note the peritonitis and hemorrhages in the stomach serosa.

Zollinger-Ellison syndrome (Figs. 5.34 and 5.35). *The syndrome is characterized by single or multiple islet-cell adenomas (often associated with other endocrine tumors), hyperacidity, hypersecretion (5–6 L. gastric juice/day) and single or multiple ulcers in the stomach, duodenum or jejunum.* Figure 5.34 reveals several shallow erosions and acute ulcers in the stomach and duodenum. The ulcers are covered by clotted blood. Islet-cell adenomas (Fig. 5.35) commonly are located in the pancreatic tail and consist histologically of non-beta cells. The tumors are gray-red, medium-firm and measure 2–3 cm. in diameter. They produce gastrin, which stimulates HCl and pepsin production.

F: many cases (>100) have been published. *A:* any age group, with male predominance. *Clinical:* diarrhea. Twenty per cent of islet-cell adenomas metastasize (see p. 177).

In the Zollinger-Ellison syndrome, a *hyperplasia of the gastric mucosa* (previously designated as hypertrophic gastritis) with increased mucosal relief is found. There is a thickening of the mucosa through an increase in the number of chief cells, parietal cells, and main glands. *Other hyperplasias:* 1. *Gastropathia hypertrophica gigantea* (Ménétrier's disease). Giant folds with increase in the surface epithelium. Increased mucus production → protein loss → hypoproteinemia. 2. *Foveolar hyperplasia* in cases of chronic gastritis. Thickening of the surface epithelium.

Gastric ulcer. *F:* 10%; has increased during the past 50 years. Gastric ulcers are more common than duodenal ulcers (3:1). *S:* ♂:♀ for gastric ulcer 1:1, duodenal ulcer 9:1. *A:* ♂ 50–60 years, ♀ 30–40 and 60–70 years. *Localization:* 50% in the antral region, 25% each at the antrum-corpus boundary and pylorus, usually at the lesser curvature.

Peptic ulcers of the esophagus are located in the lower third and arise in heterotopic gastric mucosa, usually together with peptic reflux esophagitis.

Peptic ulcers of the jejunum occur postoperatively after gastroenterostomy or in a Meckel's diverticulum from heterotopic gastric mucosa.

Curling's ulcer is an acute, superficial, gastric (rarely duodenal) ulcer that may occur anywhere in the stomach. It is seen in patients with severe burns. The gastric rugal pattern is normal.

Pg: circulatory disturbances → hemorrhagic infarction of the mucosa → erosion → ulcer (this sequence is deduced from animal experiments).

Cause: imbalance between digestive (HCl, pepsin, cathepsin) and protective (mucus) factors in the presence of diminished, local resistance (circulatory disturbances, diminished epithelial regeneration).

Theories

1. Vascular theory. (a) *Embolism, arteriosclerosis:* "senile" ulcers occur without history of stomach trouble. (b) *Functional circulatory disturbances:* arteriolar constriction; spasms of the muscularis mucosae (autonomic nervous system, psychic); venous congestion; shock; head trauma. (c) *Neurogenic ulcer:* probably due to vascular constriction from brain damage (Speransky). Psychic disturbances, stimulation of vagus nerve; HCl hypersecretion; nutrition (ulcers during wartime and malnutrition). Experimentally, starved rats develop ulcers within 5–6 days.

2. Peptic theories. At the present time, it is generally assumed that *aggressive factors* predominate over the *defensive factors* in the formation of a gastric ulcer. The disturbance of the equilibrium is caused by an overproduction of HCl and pepsin, in which quantity and residence time play a part. The aggression is intensified by gastrin forming tumors, stimulation of the vagus nerve, histamine, serotonin, distention of the stomach wall, and hyperplasia of the mucosa with an increase in the number of chief and parietal cells. Pylorus spasm stenoses, scars and motility disturbances can affect the residence time of the gastric juice.

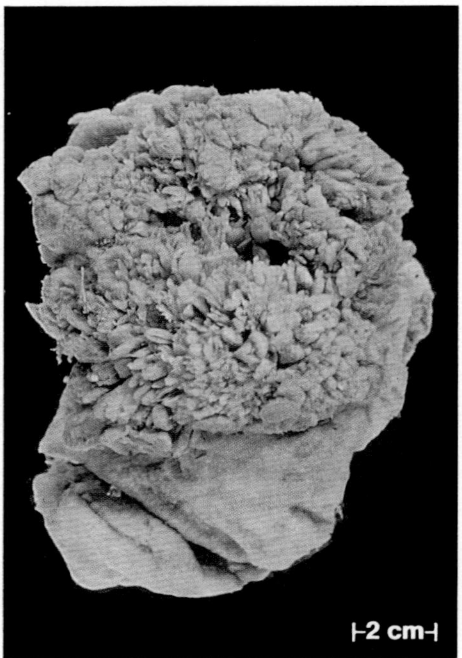

Fig. 5.36. Papillary carcinoma of the stomach.

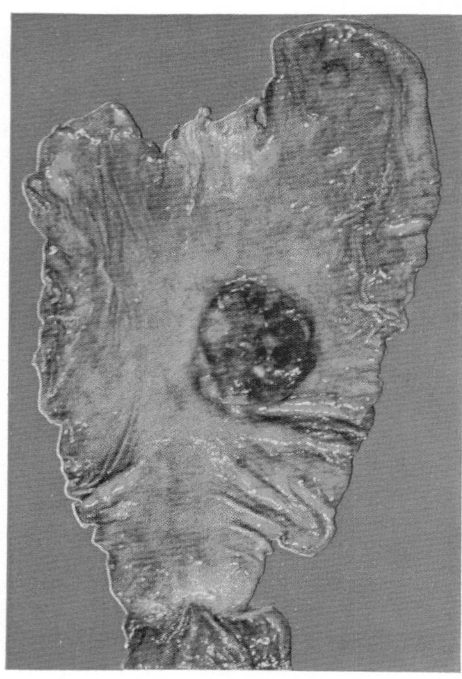

Fig. 5.37. Ulcerated carcinoma of the stomach.

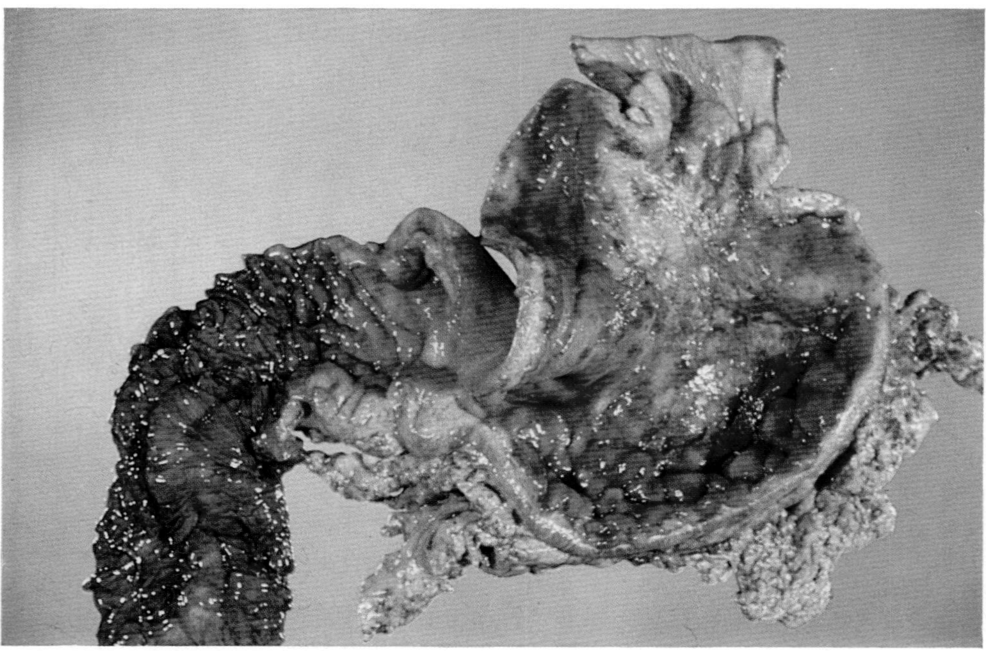

Fig. 5.38. Scirrhous carcinoma of the stomach.

Defensive factors are the *viscous surface mucus* (inhibition of mucus formation: salicylic acid derivatives, histamine, corticoids, disturbances in blood flow, HCl overproduction, mitosis inhibition), the high *regenerative power* of the surface epithelium, and the inhibition of acid formation (OEHLERT).

Other arguments in favor of the peptic theory are the fact that 50–80% of all ulcer patients show hyperacidity, 37% show normal values, and 14% show reduced acidity.

3. Inflammatory theory. Chronic gastric → ulcer. Ulcers occur in the center of small inflammatory foci in the stomach. The question is: are ulcer primary and followed by gastritis or vice versa? Eighty-six per cent of gastric ulcers and 50% of duodenal ulcers are accompanied by gastritis.

4. Hereditary faktors. Often familial incidence (30–50%); association with blood group 0.

Chronicity of peptic ulcers. The reason for the chronic course of peptic ulcers is not known. Hemorrhagic erosions normally heal rapidly. Autoimmunity or intermittent vascular changes may play a role (?). Do spasms in the gastric muscularis precipitate mechanical irritation, especially at the lesser curvature, and hyperacidity?

Co: perforation: 10% of gastrrc and 20% of duodenal ulcers (mostly those of the anterior wall) perforate Perforation of an ulcer is more common in males (12%) than in females (6%). *A perforation may be covered* by the omentum, diaphragm or liver (subphrenic empyema). Chronic peptic ulcers *penetrate* into the pancreas, liver or spleen. *Hemorrhage* from an ulcer produces hematemesis and melena (black stools in 40% of cases, more common in males than in females). Fatal hemorrhages are observed in 8% of ulcer patients but increase to 40% in senile ulcer patients. Carcinomas arise in not more than 4% of ulcers (carcinoma ex ulcero).

Tumors of the Stomach

Among the neoplasms of the stomach, carcinomas are of particular importance because of their frequency. On autopsy, gastric polyps and mesenchymal or neurogenous tumors are found less frequently.

Gastric polyps are observed *gastroscopically* more frequently during autopsy. However, in most cases, these are not genuine epithelial neoplasms but hyperplasias in cases of chronic gastritis or submucous tumors (leiomyomas, fibromas, neurinomas) which protrude into the lumen of the stomach. Genuine polyps of the gastric mucosa may occur singly or multiply and may have a villous or adenomatous histological structure. A stomach polyposis – combined with a small intestine polyposis and melanosis of the lips – can be observed in the Peutz-Jeghers syndrome.

Carcinoma of the stomach (Fig. 5.36–5.39, 5.41)

Malignant epithelial tumor originating in the gastric mucosa, and are the second most frequent malignant neoplasm in man (next to bronchial carcinoma).

The following are distinguished macroscopically:

1. The **tumorous-polypoid form** (polypoid or papillary carcinoma, Fig. 5.36). This is a broadly based tumor, with a papillary (villous) surface and a cauliflower-like shape. Figure 5.36 shows a gastric tumor of this type, which largely fills the lumen of the organ. The surface has a villous appearance, leading to the designation "*villous cancer*". This form of tumor represents about 10% of all gastric carcinomas. The light color of Figure 5.36 is to be attributed to the fact that it represents a museum specimen which has faded somewhat.

2. In the **ulcerous form** (Fig. 5.37), the gastric carcinoma shows a central involvement of the surface and a wall-like thickening of the tumor margin. The figure shows a circular carcinoma with central necrosis (ulceration) in the center of the lesser curvature of the stomach. These ulcerous tumors may represent a primary gastric carcinoma with central ulceration *(ulcerated gastric carcinoma)* or a malignantly degenerate chronic ventricular peptic ulcer *(ulcer carcinoma or degenerate ulcer)*. Gastric ulcers degenerate in about 4% of all cases. The ulcerated gastric carcinoma is seen radiologically as a niche.

3. The **infiltrative form** (gastric scirrhus, previously known as linitis plastica, Fig. 5.38) is characterized by a diffuse infiltration and thickening of the entire stomach wall. The unopened stomach resembles a leather bottle. The stomach wall has been transformed into a rigid plate and may reach a thickness of 10 mm or more. The mucosal folds are also thickened, gross, frequently nodal-humped. Macroscopically, the tumor is sharply delimited against the duodenum (at the left of the picture) and the esophagus (white mucosa, at the top of the picture). In the x-ray contrast examination, the muscular wall rigidity and the wall shrinkage are predominant.

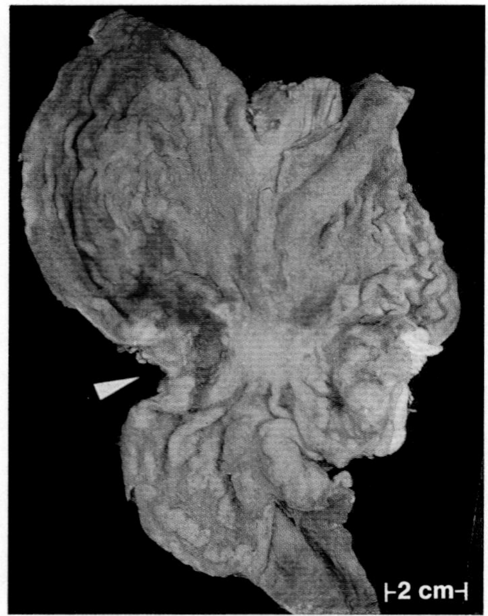

Fig. 5.39. Scirrhous carcinoma of the stomach (leather bottle stomach).

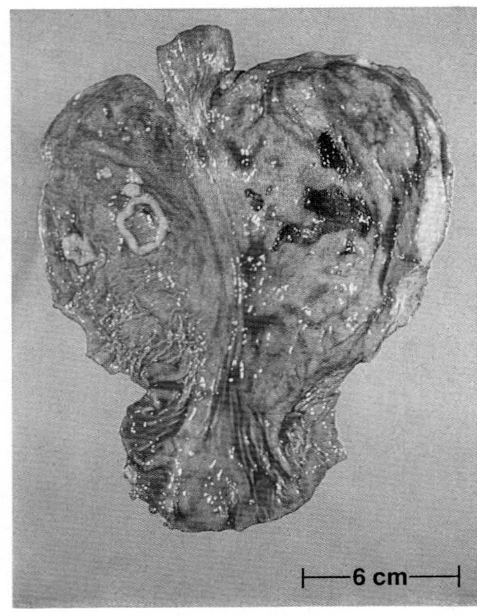

Fig. 5.40. Reticulum cell sarcoma of the stomach.

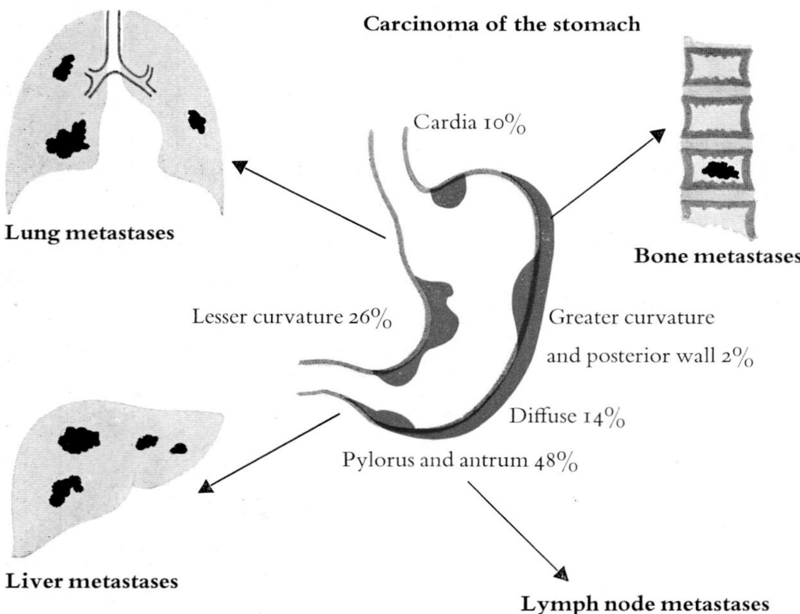

Fig. 5.41. Primary sites and metastases of gastric carcinomas.

Forms of dissemination of gastric carcinoma (Fig. 5.41)

1. **Direct growth** *(per continuitatem)* represents the most frequent form of dissemination (50% of all gastric carcinomas). The tumor can initially disseminate *in the stomach* and later spread to *adjacent organs* (liver, spleen, pancreas, esophagus, greater omentum). In the stomach, the carcinoma may show an exophytic growth or may diffusely infiltrate all layers of the wall. If the carcinoma remains confined to the corpus ventriculi, then the retraction of the connective tissue tumor components leads to a local shrinkage, so that an **hour-glass-shaped stomach** may develop (Fig. 5.39). The white arrow indicates the tumor caused retraction of the stomach. The tumor cells can disseminate in a submucous manner along the lymph vessels. In about 50% of carcinomas of the cardia, an infiltration of the esophagus is demonstrated. (Important: The infiltration of the esophagus cannot be detected macroscopically, since the mucosa is intact!) In 20–30% of pyloric and antral carcinomas, an infiltration of the duodenal wall takes place.

2. **Lymphogenous metastasis.** Dissemination of the tumors along the lymph vessels cannot be differentiated from direct growth. An involvement of the regional lymph nodes (greater and lesser curvature, less frequently parapancreatic, paraaortic or cervical lymph nodes, signal node).

3. **Hematogenous metastasis** (Fig. 5.41) occurs in 50% of all gastric carcinomas. It may take place directly through the portal vein (→ liver metastases) or through the thoracic duct into the lungs. Other preferred metastatic localizations are the bones, particularly the vertebral bodies (frequently osteoplastic).

4. **Peritoneal dissemination** (Fig. 5.42). The gastric carcinoma may permeate all layers of the wall and produce serosal metastases, which release tumor cells into the open abdominal cavity. The peritoneal infiltration may also be the result of a lymphogenous metastasis. A *hemorrhagic ascites with tumor cells* is found in the abdominal cavity. In the parietal and visceral peritoneum, numerous small tumor nodules are found (see peritoneal carcinosis), which may also spread to the ovaries *(Krukenberg's tumors)*. As a result of peritoneal carcinosis, fusions of the loops of the small intestine may take place (ileus).

F: About 30% of all carcinomas in man. 3.6% of all autopsies. Mortality rate (per 100,000 inhabitants): German Federal Republic: 30–40 per year, United States 40, Japan 70. *S:* ♂:♀ = 3:2. *Pg:* as preliminary stages or early forms: intestinal metaplasias (replacement gastritis) and foveolar hyperplasias in chronic gastritis, degeneration of chronic peptic ulcers, degeneration of polyps, early cancer (see also Lauren, Schade, Oehlert). *Cf:* exogenous carcinogenic factors play a more important role than the familial burden. Among the exogenous noxae are carcinogenic hydrocarbons (for example, in fats used for frying and in smoked meat: stomach cancer is very common in Iceland!). Contamination of rice by fungi, particularly by *Aspergillus flavus* (aflatoxin, a powerful carcinogen). High rate of stomach cancer in Japan (unhusked rice as a main component of the food!). In pernicious anemia (atrophy of the gastric mucosa with metaplasia), stomach cancer occurs 20 times as frequently as in control persons. *Lo:* the most frequent localizations of stomach cancer are summarized in Figure 5.41. *Mi:* villous adenocarcinomas, scirrhous carcinoma, dedifferentiated-medullary carcinoma, mucinous adenocarcinoma (colloid carcinoma), signet-ring cell carcinoma, squamous epithelium carcinoma (very rare). A special form of scirrhous carcinoma is carcinoma dissolutum, which consists of isolated tumor cells and an inflammatory granulation tissue (also difficult to diagnose histologically!).

Early cancer of the stomach: A carcinoma made up predominantly of signet ring cells (less frequently of glands), which permeates the mucosa and occasionally (after penetration of the muscularis mucosae) also infiltrates the submucosa, but does not spread

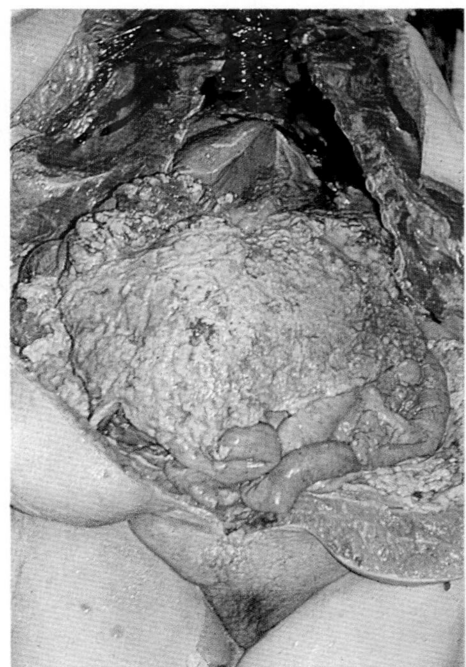

Fig. 5.42. Peritoneal carcinomatosis from a carcinoma of the stomach. Diffuse, very finely nodular tumor infiltration of the greater omentum and the parietal peritoneum.

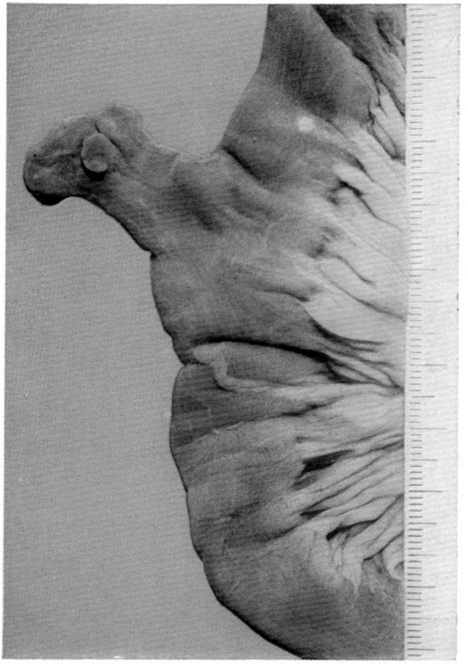

Fig. 5.43. Meckel's diverticulum.

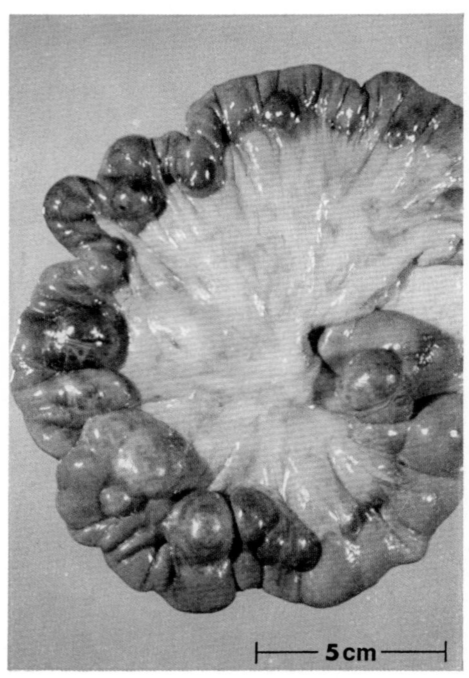

Fig. 5.44. Diverticulosis of the small intestine.

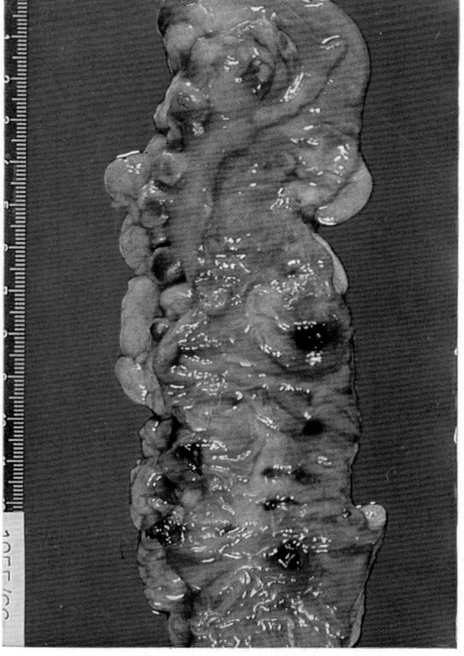

Fig. 5.45. Diverticulosis of the large intestine.

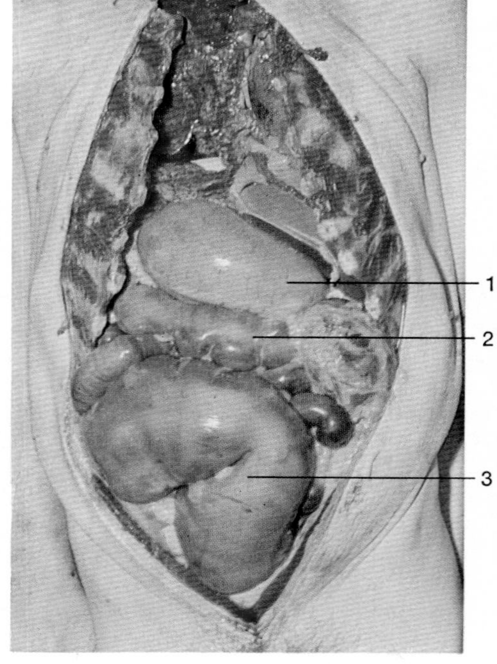

Fig. 5.46. Megacolon congenitum.

to the muscularis propria. Early cancer occurs predominantly in the antral mucosa sometimes at the margin of a chronic ulcer). Early gastroscopic diagnosis is possible; the 5-year survival rate is over 90%! *Other gastric tumors:* Benign and malignant mesenchymal and neurogenous tumors are observed, which may occur primarily or within the framework of a systemic disease (for example, Hodgkin's disease) in the stomach. Figure 5.40 shows multiple, in part central necrotic nodes of a reticulosarcoma in the region of the gastric mucosa. The differentiation between a lymphosarcoma and *pseudolymphomas* or *lymphatic hyperplasias* is of differential diagnostic importance. The latter are frequently found in women with autoaggressive diseases (OEHLERT).

Intestine

Malformations. Atresia ani (imperforate anus) develops from a persistence of the cloacal membrane. Atresia recti refers to a failure in the development of the rectum (septum urorectale misplaced). Atresia of the small intestine: with absence of mesentery.

Meckel's diverticulum is a true diverticulum (the wall consists of all layers of the intestine). A Meckel's diverticulum is located 1 meter above the ileocecal valve and can measure up to 9 cm. in length. Figure 5.43 shows a 3 cm.-long and 1 cm.-wide Meckel's diverticulum opposite the mesenteric insertion (typical). The diverticulum may contain heterotopic gastric mucosa (*Co:* ulcer formation and perforation) or pancreas.

F: in 2% of all autopsies. *Pg:* remnants of the omphaloenteric duct, which normally obliterates after birth. *When the external part of the duct is open*, the condition is known as incomplete external omphaloenteric fistula. A Meckel's diverticulum results when the *internal part* of the duct remains open. Adhesions between a Meckel's diverticulum and the gut may cause strangulation ileus.

Diverticulosis of the small intestine (Fig. 5.44). These false diverticula (i.e., prolapse of mucosa) are located at the junction of the mesentery with the intestine. The diverticula are acquired and occur in older patients. They form in a weakened area where vessels enter the bowel wall. Figure 5.44 shows multiple large outpouchings up to 1 cm. in diameter.

Diverticulosis of the large intestine (Fig. 5.45). *Multiple false diverticula of the colon, which develop with increasing age.* Figure 5.45 shows the lumen of the colon with multiple mucosal defects that are plugged by greenish black scybala (or fecaliths).

F: 5% in autopsy material of persons past 60 years of age, especially in obese patients. *S:* ♂:♀=1:1. *Pg:* herniation of the mucosa and submucosa from pressure (inspissated feces, gas). The mucosa and submucosa prolapse at both sides of the taenia near the entrance of the blood vessels. *Co:* diverticulitis, perforation (→ peritonitis, peritoneal or retroperitoneal abscesses). Thrombophlebitis → liver abscesses. Carcinomas are rare complications of colonic diverticula.

Megacolon congenitum (Hirschsprung's disease, Fig. 5.46). *A congenital dilatation and elongation of the rectosigmoid. The submucosal and myenteric ganglion cells (Auerbach and Meissner plexuses) of the distal segment are absent. The aganglionic segment is of normal width.* Figure 5.46 shows a markedly dilated sigmoid. The rectum and proximal colon were of normal width. The wall of the distended sigmoid is thickened from work hypertrophy of the muscularis. *Pg:* developmental failure in the distal, nondilated segment, usually the rectum (biopsy for diagnosis!) → stasis, dilatation and muscular hypertrophy of the proximal segment. Congenital megacolon may be associated with cryptorchidism, large viscera and spleen enlargement. In South America: Chagas' disease → acquired megacolon (KÖBERLE).

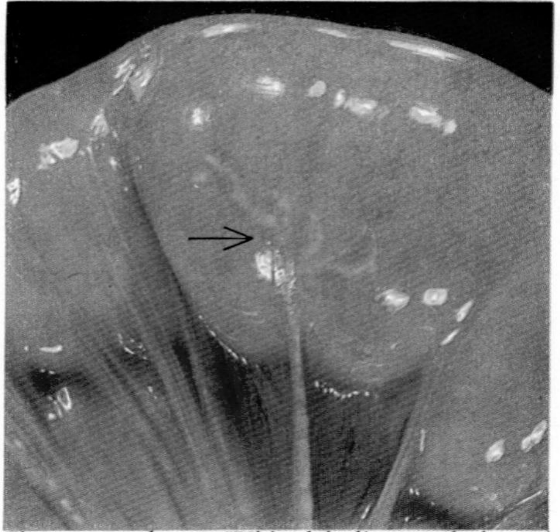

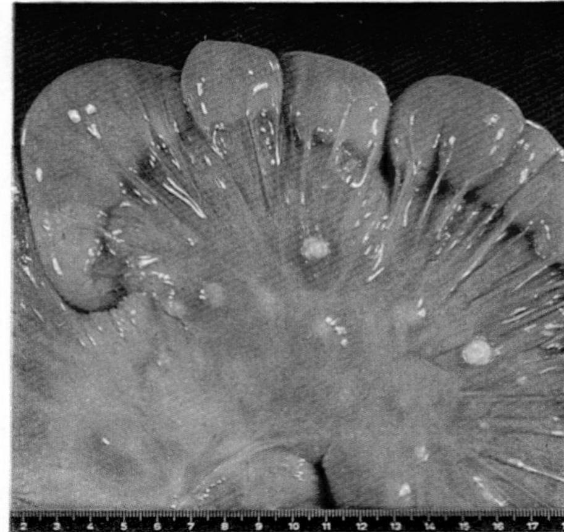

Figs. 5.47 and 5.48. Whipple's disease: chyle stasis in the small lacteals of the small intestine and mesenteric lymph nodes.

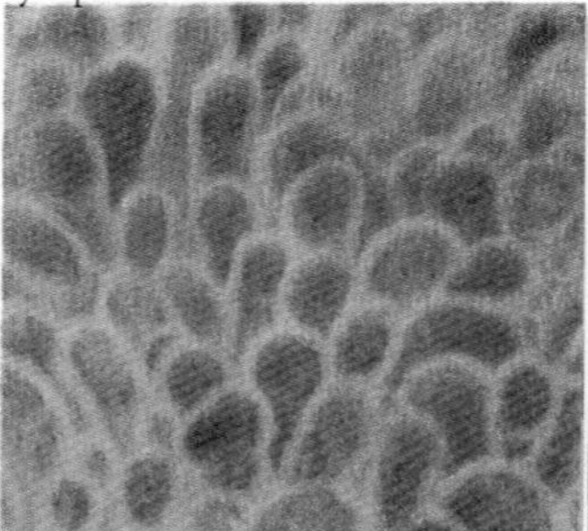

Fig. 5.49. Minimal jejunitis.

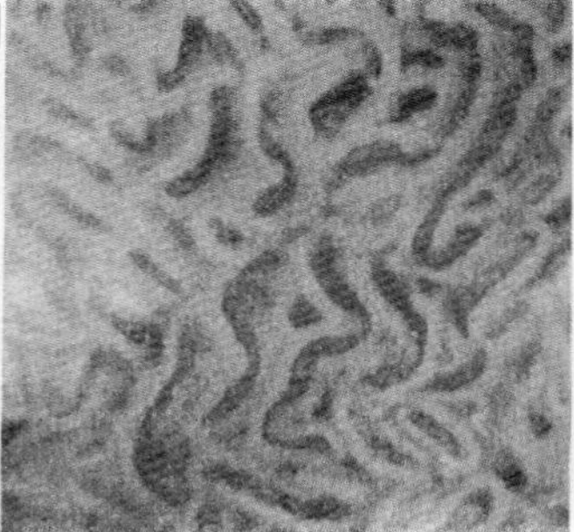

Fig. 5.50. Atrophic enteritis.

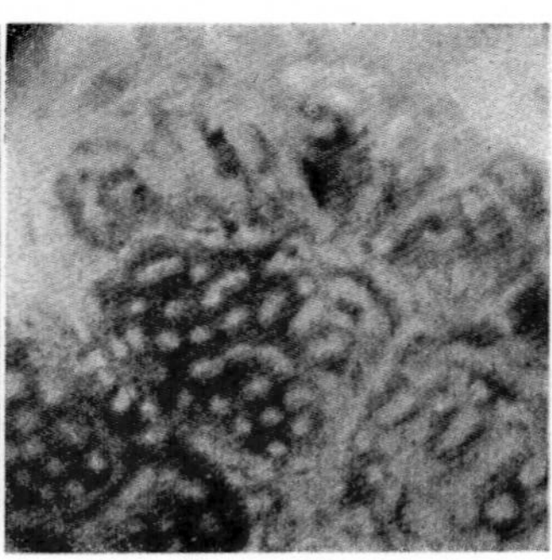

Fig. 5.51. Atrophy of villi in nontropical sprue.

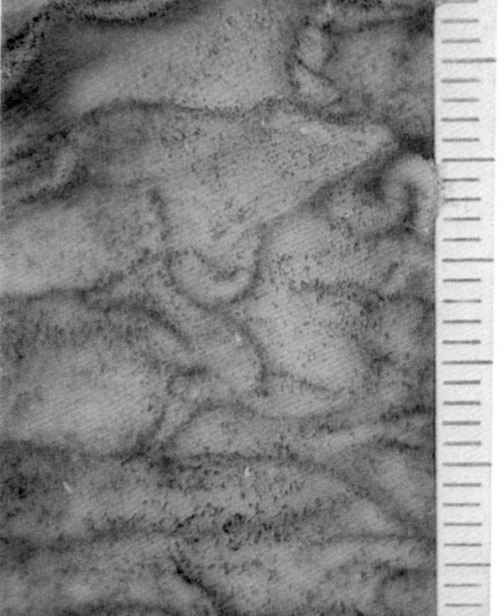

Fig. 5.52. Melanosis of small intestinal villi.

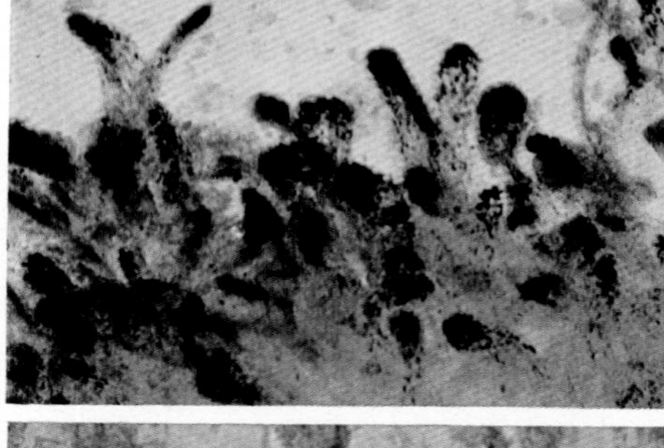

Fig. 5.53. Higher magnification (stereomicroscope) of melanosis villi. Below: melanosis after Prussian blue reaction.

Malabsorption syndrome. *Decreased absorptive ability of the small intestine due to (a) lack of digestive enzymes (diseases of the stomach or pancreas, bile production), (b) rapid food passage (enteritis) or (c) biochemical abnormalities of absorption (sprue, Whipple's disease, disaccharidase, lactase, maltase deficiencies; carrier defects for cystine, tryptophan, iron). The clinical picture is characterized by bulky, pale gray stools, steatorrhea (more than 7 Gm. fat excreted daily) and symptoms of protein, carbohydrate and vitamin deficiency.* The term *maldigestion* refers to inadequate digestion (enzymatic degradation) of the food. Absence of digestive enzymes may occur in diseases of the pancreas, gallbladder, or stomach.

Whipple's disease (Figs. 5.47 and 5.48; TCP, p. 109). *Lipodystrophia intestinalis is a granulomatous inflammation of the small intestinal mucosa and mesenteric lymph nodes. The disease probably is caused by bacteria and presents clinically as a disorder of malabsorption.* The gross findings at autopsy include yellow, chylous ascites (emulsified fat, Fig. 5.54), yellowish, net-like markings beneath the serosa (→ in Fig. 5.47) and prominent, yellow lymphatics in the mesentery of the small intestine (chyle stasis in lacteals, Fig. 5.47). The mesenteric lymph nodes are enlarged, firm, yellow and fatty fluid exudes during cutting. The cut surfaces of lymph nodes are yellow and cheesy (chyle stasis and granulomatous inflammation, Fig. 5.48). The mucosal pattern of the small intestine is coarse with villi distended in a flask-shaped manner and studded with multiple yellow flecks.

F: formerly thought to be rare, the disease appears to be increasing in frequency during the past few years. *A:* over 40 years. *S:* 80% are ♂. *Pg:* primary granulomatous inflammation of lacteals and larger lymphatics. Endothelium of lymphatic channels gives rise to granulomas with foam cells. Bacteria (coryne, hemophilus?) can be demonstrated in the cytoplasm of foam cells.

Systemic manifestations of Whipple's disease include polyarthritis and endocarditis. Symptomatic Whipple's disease refers to conditions of chyle stasis and lymphatic obstruction by tumors (e.g., bronchogenic carcinoma, Hodgkin's disease and other lymphomas) or stenosis of thoracic ductus.

Enteritis (Figs. 5.49–5.51; TCP, p. 109). *Inflammation of the small bowel due to bacterial invasion (coliform, pneumococci, dysenteric bacteria), altered flora (antibiotics) or nutritional-toxic factors (alcohol, cytostatic drugs). Enteritis is characterized morphologically by plump and shortened villi (diagnosed by stereomicroscopy).*

Figure 5.49 is a stereomicroscopic photograph of the jejunal mucosa. The villi are leaf-like, clubbed and red (normal villi are long and slender). The diagnosis is minimal enteritis. Figure 5.50 shows severe villous atrophy. The "mosaics" or "brain pattern" of the mucosa is diagnostic of chronic, atrophic enteritis.

Remember: Flattened villi impair absorption.
In children, *follicular enteritis:* edema, plump villi, and protrusion of the intestinal follicles. Found during the summer months, it is caused by bacteria or viruses. **Pseudomembranous enteritis** (rare, after antibiotics. See colon).

Sprue (Fig. 5.51). *Chronic inflammation of the small intestinal villi. The villi are shortened, plump and wider than normal.* Figure 5.51 shows flat, plump microvilli as well as loss of villi. This appearance is referred to as "sprue pattern" or "flat mucosa." This was a case of nontropical sprue, i.e., gluten-sensitive enteropathy.

Secondary sprue: Malabsorption syndrome occurs after x-ray radiation, cytostatics, amyloidosis and in scleroderma. Macroscopic description: villus atrophy.

Tropical sprue occurs in India and Central America. Due to either folic acid deficiency or abnormal bacterial flora?

F: nontropical sprue is uncommon. In childhood, the corresponding absorption defect is known as celiac disease (hereditary?). The conditions are improved or even cured by a gluten-free diet (gluten contains the polypeptide gliadin, a wheat protein).

Melanosis of villi of the small intestine (Figs. 5.52 and 5.53). *Tiny, punctate, black markings in the jejunal mucosa. Melanosis is evidence of repeated gastrointestinal hemorrhages.* Figure 5.52 shows pinhead-sized, black spots in the small intestinal mucosa. The pigmentation is confined to the tips of the villi, as seen under the dissecting microscope (Fig. 5.53, above). The tips can be stained green to blue by the Prussian blue reaction (hemosiderin) (Fig. 5.53, below). The macroscopic black color is due to H_2S.

Pg: repeated hemorrhages (e.g., peptic ulcers) → absorption of hemoglobin → hemosiderin storage in histiocytes.

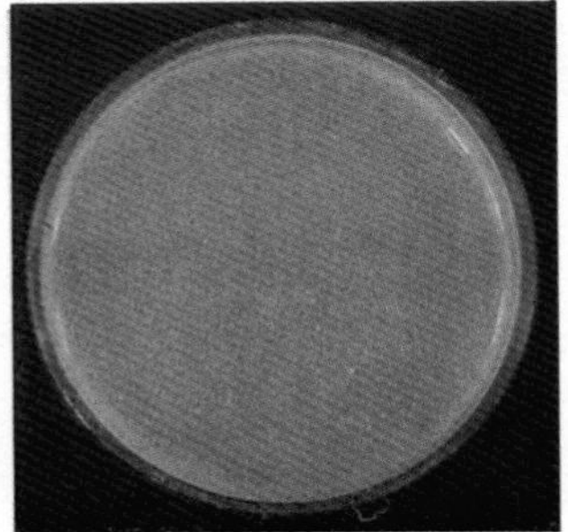

Fig. 5.54. Chylous ascites in Whipple's disease.

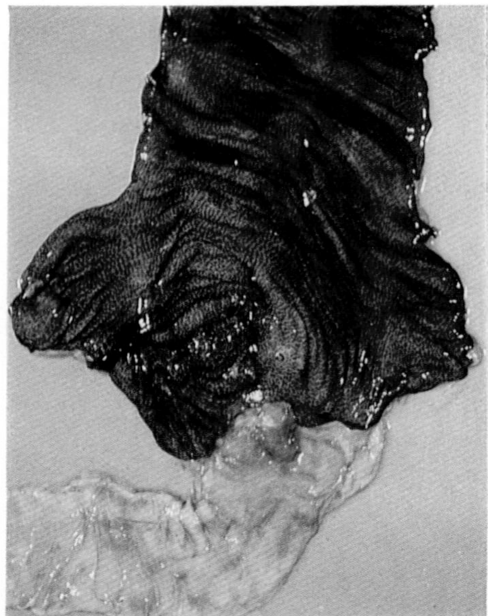

Fig. 5.55. Melanosis coli.

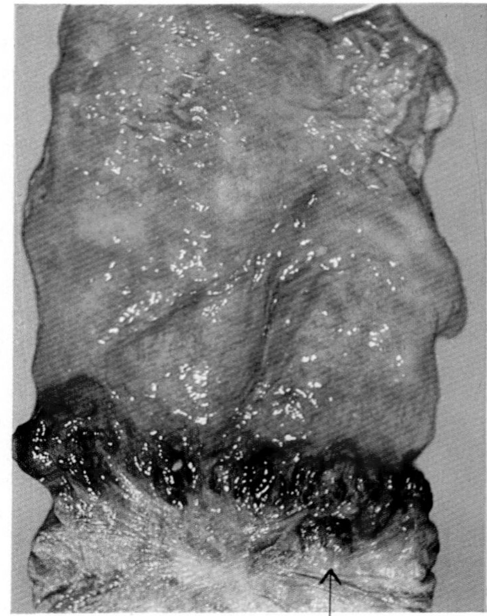

Fig. 5.56. Internal hemorrhoids.

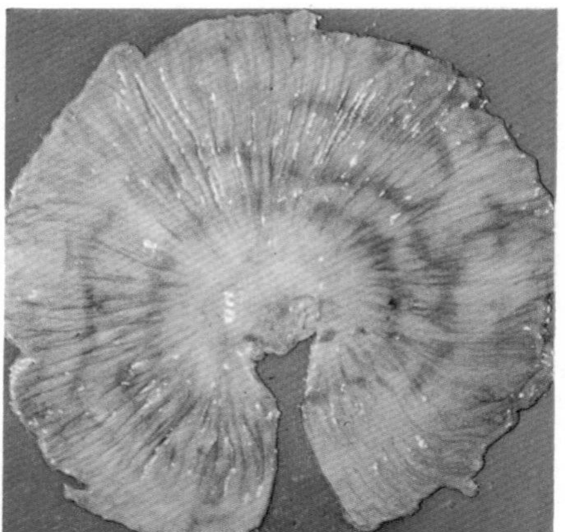

Fig. 5.57. Peritonitis manifested as red serosal streaks in the small intestine.

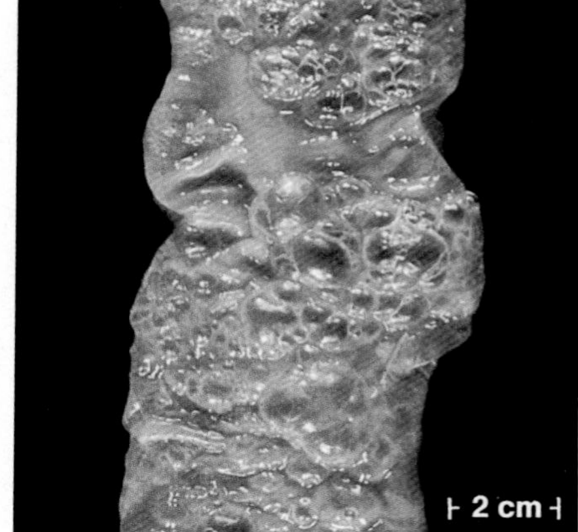

Fig. 5.58. Pneumatosis cystoides intestinalis.

Melanosis coli (so-called brown colon). Figure 5.55 (see also Fig. 5.86) shows *brown-black streaks in the mucosa against a pale brown or yellowish background (resembling tiger skin or crocodile leather)*. This change usually affects the entire colon and ends abruptly at the ileocecal junction.

Pg: not known. Observed between 30 and 50 years of age. History of constipation and abuse of laxatives. *S:* ♂ = ♀. Clinically without significance. Histologically, macrophages accumulate in the mucosa and contain a pigment resembling melanin.

Hemorrhoids (Fig. 5.56).

External hemorrhoids: Varices of the inferior hemorrhoidal vein at or below the anorectal line (blood from inferior hemorrhoidal vein is drained into the inferior vena cava). In Figure 5.56 (→), we see these external varices, which are always covered by squamous epithelium and can surround the anus in a circular pattern. These varicosities contain blue-red venous blood.

Internal hemorrhoids (Fig. 5.56) are formed proximally to the anal ring and are in the form of tightly filled protrusions of a red or blue-red color. They are arranged in a coronal pattern and are covered by mucosa. When they extend into the anal ring incompetence may occur. These are not varicosities but dilated arteriovenous anastomoses of the corpus cavernosum recti (glomera rectalia, STAUBESAND). They accordingly contain arterial blood (blood gas analyses!) and the stool shows deposits of bright red blood.

Pg: hereditary predisposition. Increased arterial blood supply? *Co:* hemorrhages, inflammations, thromboses. Their frequency of occurrence is *not* increased in cases of cirrhoses of the liver.

Ileus (Fig. 5.57). *Adynamic or paralytic ileus of the small intestine (stomach and/or large intestine), with loss of peristalsis, absorption and secretion.* The abdomen is markedly distended by gas-filled small intestinal loops. The small intestine contains gray-brown fluid and gas (x-ray: air-fluid level). Figure 5.57 shows an opened small intestinal loop. The loop is greatly dilated and 10 cm. wide instead of the normal 4 cm. The characteristic red serosal streaks (acute hyperemia) occur where two bowel loops are pressed together.

Ileus develops from

(a) Mechanical irritation: postoperatively in 0.3–5% of abdominal operations, bland or perforating abdominal trauma, mechanical bowel obstruction (strangulation ileus).

(b) Functional disturbances of peristalsis (peritonitis, pancreatitis, enteritis, vascular disturbances, infarctions).

(c) Reflex mechanisms (head, brain or spinal cord trauma; disturbances of innervation, vagotomy).

(d) Metabolic disturbances (acidosis, potassium loss, hyponatremia or hypernatremia).

Pneumatosis cystoides intestinalis (Fig. 5.58). *Development of subserosal and submucosal gas-filled blebs ("intestinal emphysema").* Figure 5.58 shows multiple, thin-walled, subserosal blebs filled with gas. The blebs measure up to 1 cm. in diameter. Seen mostly in the jejunum but also in the stomach and colon.

The condition is rare and clinically without significance. *S:* ♀. The blebs contain 80% N_2, traces of O_2 CO_2, methane and H_2. Ruptured blebs may ulcerate. *Pg:* not known. (a) *Mechanical:* small ulceration → pressure-forced entrance of gas, (b) *bacterial:* gas-forming bacteria. Gas also may enter the lymphatics.

Histologically: foreign-body giant cells often are found around the gas blebs.

DD: postmortem gas formation.

Hemorrhagic enteropathy in shock (Fig. 5.59)
Shock affects the kidneys (anuria), and later the lungs (respiratory insufficiency). However, hemorrhagic erosions of the gastric mucosa (as in the case of a hemorrhagic enteritis) are also frequently found. Figure 5.59 shows part of the small intestine with hyperemia and focal hemorrhages in the mucosa.

Histologically, a villous edema, necroses of the tips of the villi, stromal hemorrhages, and hyaline thrombi in the capillaries and venules are found (see *Mi*). These changes can be detected particularly in cases of endotoxin shock. *Cl:* bloody stools.

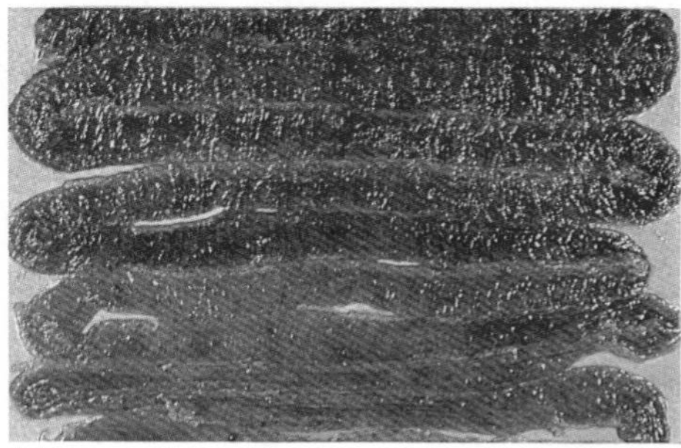

Fig. 5.59. Hemorrhagic enteropathy in shock.

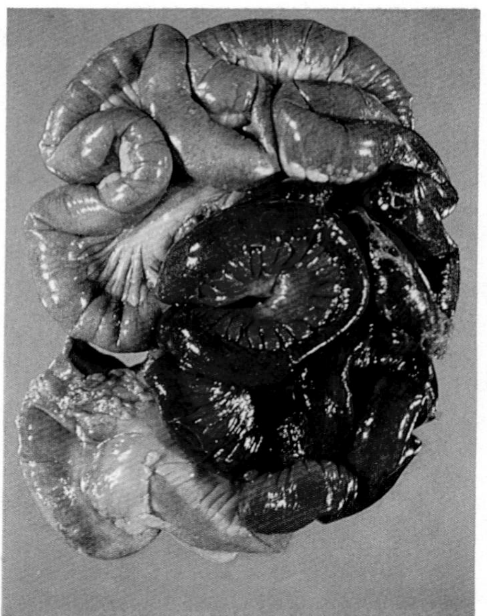

Fig. 5.61. Hemorrhagic infarction of the small intestine.

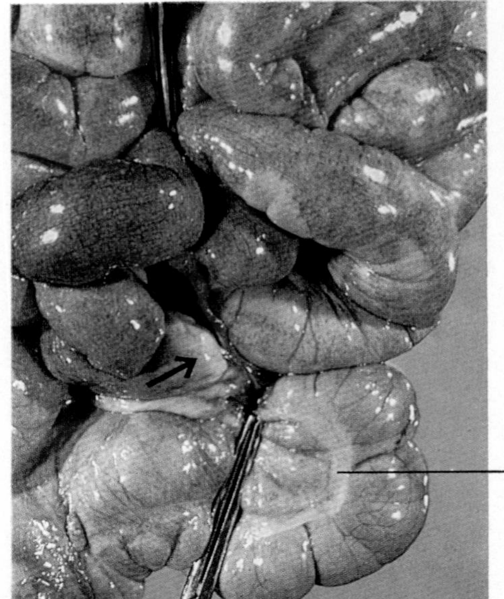

Fig. 5.62. Strangulation ileus with early infarction.

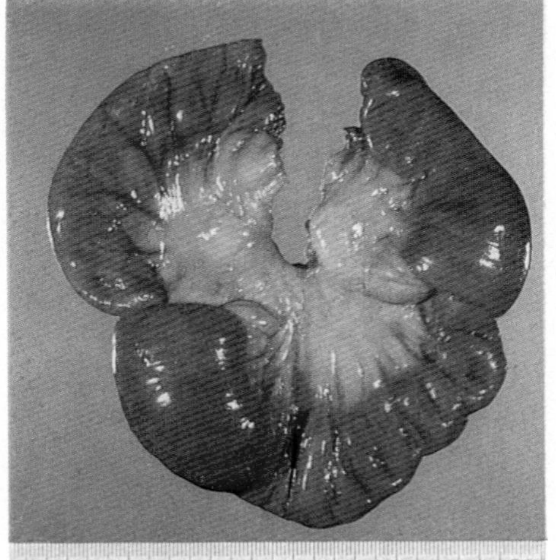

Fig. 5.63. Agonal invagination of the small intestine.

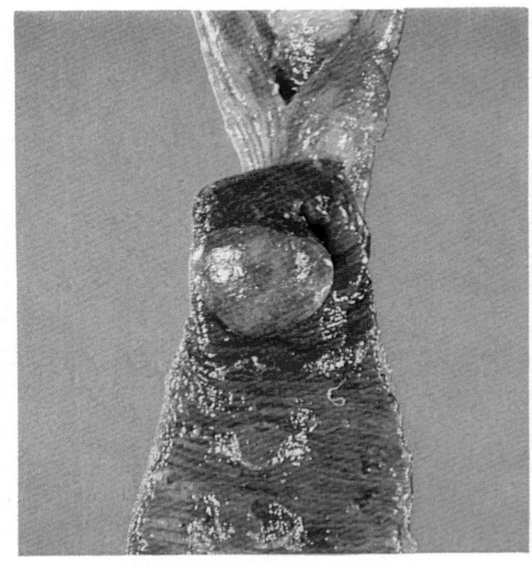

Fig. 5.64. Antemortem invagination of the small intestine by a tumor.

Hernia. *A protrusion of a viscus through the wall of a cavity into a sac covered by peritoneum.* Abdominal and especially inguinal hernias are the most common. The hernia sac contains gut or omentum. Figure 5.60 shows an indirect inguinal hernia. The major omentum has entered the hernia sac through the inguinal canal. Note the spermatic cord (→) and testis.

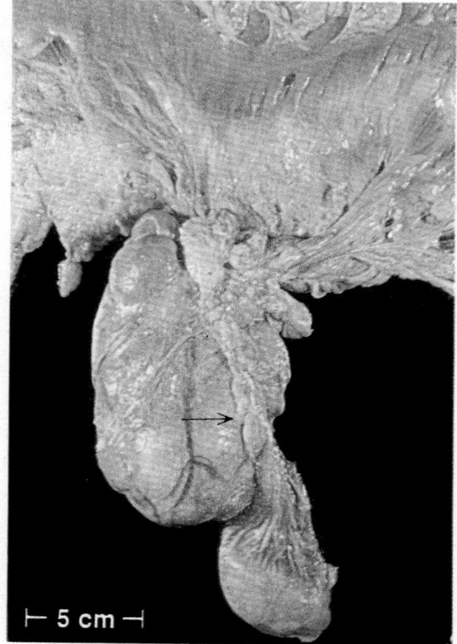

Fig. 5.60. Indirect inguinal hernia.

Direct inguinal hernia: medial to the epigastric vessels. *Femoral hernia:* protrusion through the lacuna vasorum. *Hiatus or diaphragmatic hernia:* protrusion of the stomach into the thorax through a slit in the diaphragm. *DD:* relaxatio diaphragmatica: a flabby, relaxed diaphragm causes saccular protrusion into the thorax.

Inguinal hernias: A: 50–60 years. Constitutional factors. In females after multiple deliveries.

Hemorrhagic infarction of the small intestine (Fig. 5.61). *Hemorrhagic necrosis of the small intestine due to arterial or venous occlusion.* Figure 5.61 shows several small-intestinal loops with a dark red serosa. The intestinal wall is rigid and thicker than normal. The mucosa likewise is swollen and dusky red (*Mi:* hemorrhagic necrosis). The infarcted loops contain bloody liquid chyme. Fresh thrombi are seen in veins and/or arteries. Tiny whitish fibrin deposits (fibrinous peritonitis) adhere to the serosa.

F: 0.5%. *A:* 40–60 years. *S:* ♂=♀. *Pg:* arterial embolism from mural thrombi in aorta or heart (e.g., infarction). Venous blood fills the necrotic portions to account for the hemorrhagic appearance of the infarction. Other causes are: venous thrombosis of various etiologies (e.g., descending portal vein thrombosis in liver cirrhosis, ascending thrombosis in inflammatory bowel disease or spontaneous vein thrombosis). Volvulus (torsion of mesentery → vascular occlusion), strangulation ileus (from fibrous adhesions), incarcerated hernias and intussusception also cause hemorrhagic bowel infarction.

Obstructive ileus with beginning hemorrhagic infarction (Fig. 5.62). *Several intestinal loops are obstructed or strangulated. The consequences are paralytic ileus and hemorrhagic bowel infarction.* Figure 5.62 shows a red, band-like adhesion compressing a bowel loop (in this case, remnants of the omphaloenteric duct). The occlusion apparently had existed for some time, since the serosa is whitish and thickened at the point of occlusion (→ peritoneal fibrosis). There is beginning hemorrhagic infarction of the aboral loops (distal to the obstruction) and dilatation (ileus) of loops of small intestine that are almost as wide as the colon (see free taenia: →1). Postoperative fibrous adhesions are the most common cause of obstructive ileus.

Invagination (intussusception) of the small intestine (Figs. 5.63 and 5.64). *Telescoping of a proximal portion of gut into a distal portion.* The common agonal or postmortem intussusception is caused by irregular (counter-running?) peristalsis. Figure 5.63 shows a bowel loop that is enlarged from an invaginated proximal bowel segment. There is no inflammatory reaction or hemorrhagic infarction. The invagination has, therefore, formed shortly before or after death. If an invagination occurs *during life* (Fig. 5.64), the bowel always is hemorrhagically infarcted and inflamed. Tumors of the small intestine may invaginate into the distal bowel segment during a peristaltic wave. Figure 5.64 shows a 4 cm.-large tumor at the distal end of an invaginated bowel. The tumor in this case was a solitary eosinophilic granuloma (very rare). The mucosal folds of the invaginated bowel segment are coarse. The mucosa is hemorrhagic and there are several fresh ulcers. Intussusception is common in children; the cause is not known.

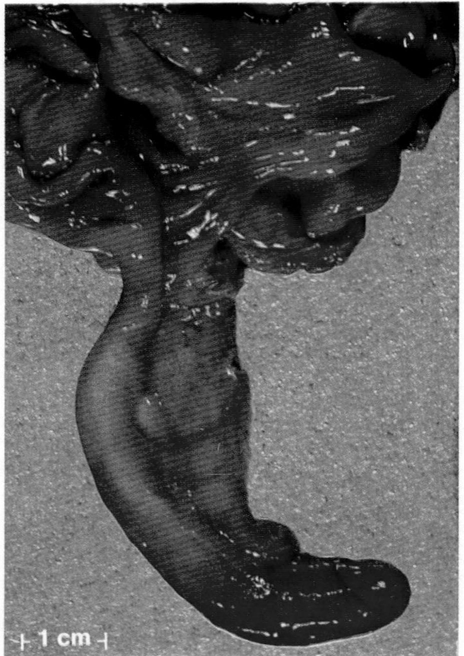

Fig. 5.65. Acute appendicitis.

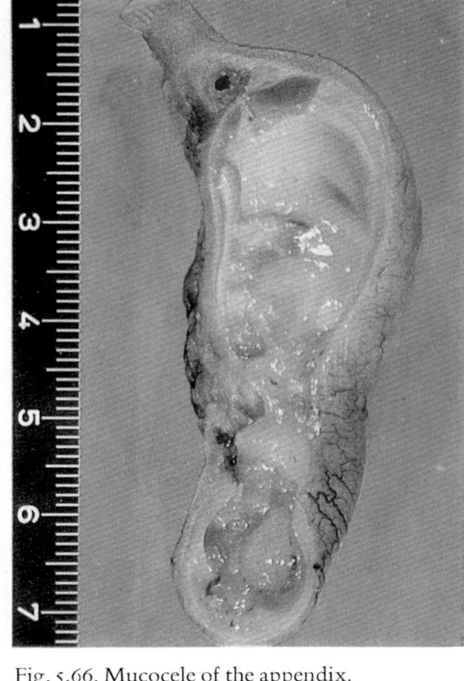

Fig. 5.66. Mucocele of the appendix.

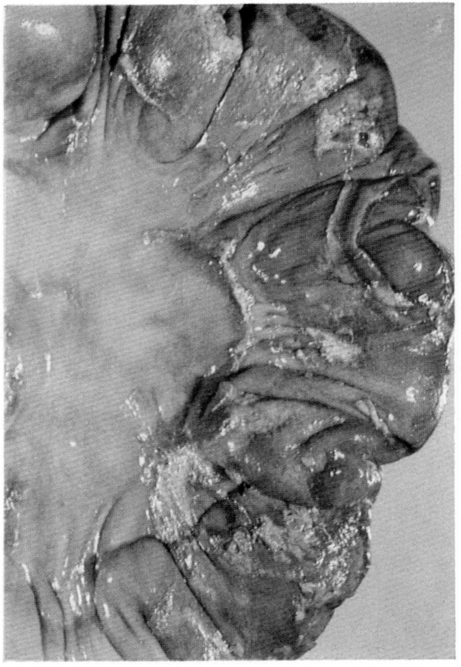

Fig. 5.67. Fresh fibrinopurulent peritonitis.

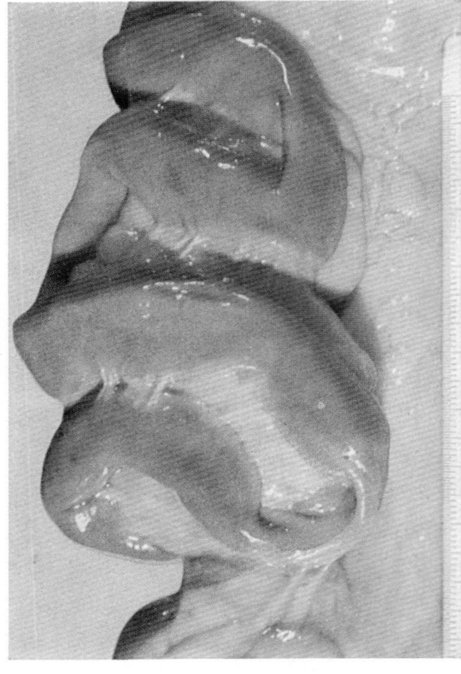

Fig. 5.68. Peritoneal adhesions following peritonitis.

Appendicitis. *Acute or chronic, recurrent inflammation of the appendix.* The most simple type is *catarrhal appendicitis.* The mucosa is edematous and infiltrated by a few leukocytes. The vascular markings of the serosa are prominent (hyperemia). *Ulcerative appendicitis* begins as single or multiple inflammatory foci in the mucosal crypts. This *primary infection* (Aschoff) is characterized by areas of epithelial necrosis, leukocytic infiltrates and fibrinous exudate. The inflammatory foci ulcerate *(ulcerative appendicitis)* or, after a brief interval, involve the entire appendix *(phlegmonous appendicitis)* (TCP, p. 113). Ulcers also can give rise to abscesses in the wall (abscessive appendicitis).

Gross diagnosis of *acute appendicitis* (Fig. 5.65): The appendix is swollen, hyperemic (red) and the serosa is covered by a fibrinous exudate. The mesenteriolum is edematous and the serosal vascular markings are prominent. The mucosa of the acutely inflamed appendix is red, swollen and ulcerated. The lumen often contains firm, dry feces or fecaliths, which cause pressure ulcers or contribute to the epithelial damage by retention of mucus, with subsequent development of an ulcerative-phlegmonous appendicitis. Microabscesses in the wall may also penetrate into the lumen of the appendix, so that ulcers are produced in this manner.

Gangrenous appendicitis: The appendix is gray-black, foul smelling and friable ("rotten") from severe inflammation and bacterial invasion.

Chronic appendicitis is a controversial problem. Lymphocytic infiltrates, scar tissue, atrophy of the lymphatic tissue and submucosal areas of adipose tissue are regular findings in the appendix of adults. The diagnosis of chronic appendicitis is justified only when heavy infiltrates of lymphocytes and plasma cells mixed with polymorphonuclear leukocytes can be demonstrated. Enlarged reactive centers in lymph follicles, especially with a starry-sky appearance, likewise are indications of a chronic appendicitis (lymphadenitis). It should be emphasized that an appendix without these strict diagnostic criteria can cause clinical symptoms (possibly by formation of scars, neuromas?). Obliteration of the lumen by fibrous tissue is the common end stage of an ulcerative appendicitis. Grossly, the appendix is firm, gray-white and its lumen is obliterated by gray-white scar tissue.

F: inflammatory changes are found in the appendix in 75–90% of adults and in 10% of persons 20–30 years of age (Aschoff). *S:* ♂ = ♀. *Pg:* the inflammation usually starts in the distal part of the appendix, which is populated by Group D streptococci and pneumococci. It is assumed that the inflammation develops through an increase in these bacteria as a result of a reduced resistance of the appendix wall. Constipation, and less frequently enterobiasis, may also play a part. In angina, a hematogenous infestation by bacteria is said to be possible. An adhesion of the small intestine and mesentery frequently occurs as a result of the local peritonitis, so that an empyema develops and the peritonitis remains localized thereby. Late sequelae: Peritoneal adhesions → adhesion ileus.

Mucocele of the appendix (Fig. 5.66). *Mucus retention due to stenosis or partial obliteration of the lumen.* In the present case, the proximal part of the appendix was obliterated by fibrous tissue. The appendix is greatly dilated (Fig. 5.66). The mucosa is white and shows prominent vascular markings. The wall is thickened, whitish and firm. The lumen contains tenacious, glassy mucus. *Hydrops* is the accumulation of predominantly serous fluid rather than thick mucus.

Rupture of a mucocele causes *localized pseudomyxoma peritonei* in the ileocecal region and lower abdominal cavity. The mucus pools are covered by loops of small bowel. A *diffuse pseudomyxoma peritonei* from an appendiceal mucocele has a poor prognosis because dislodged epithelial cells always can be demonstrated in the mucus. The mucus-producing epithelium continues to grow at sites of implantation and rarely may "metastasize" (so-called *malignant mucocele*; often misdiagnosed as mucinous adenocarcinoma!). Clinical course 5–7 years. The *pseudomyxoma of ovarian origin* (mucinous cystadenoma) always is diffuse (malignant pseudomyxoma).

Peritonitis (Figs. 5.67 and 5.68). *Fibrinous or fibrinopurulent peritoneal inflammation with or without fluid collection in the abdominal cavity. Causes:* see Ileus. Figure 5.67 shows yellow-white and gray membranes on the peritoneum, especially where loops of bowel touch each other. Peritoneal adhesions are the result of a healed fibrinous or focal purulent peritonitis (Fig. 5.68). Loops of bowel are plastered together by white, broad fibrous bands that may adhere to practically all abdominal organs.

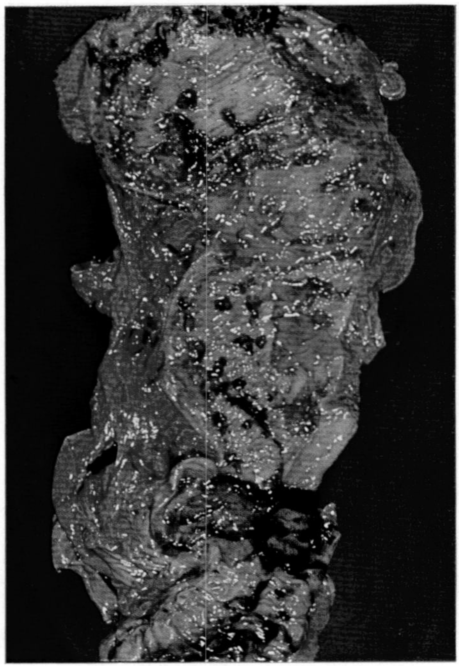

Fig. 5.69. Ulcerative colitis with fresh ulcerations.

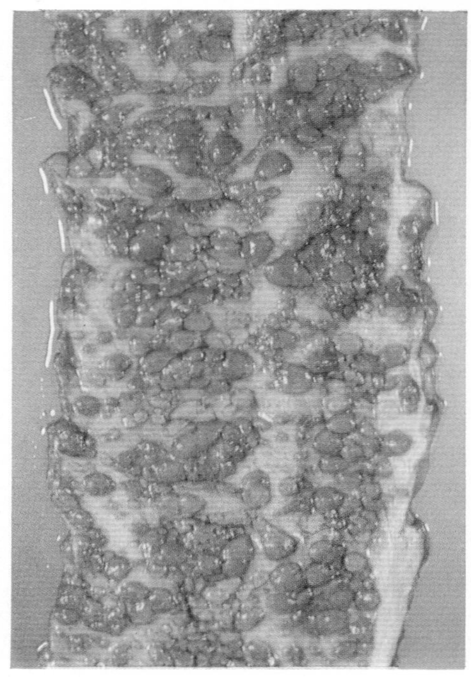

Fig. 5.70. Ulcerative colitis.

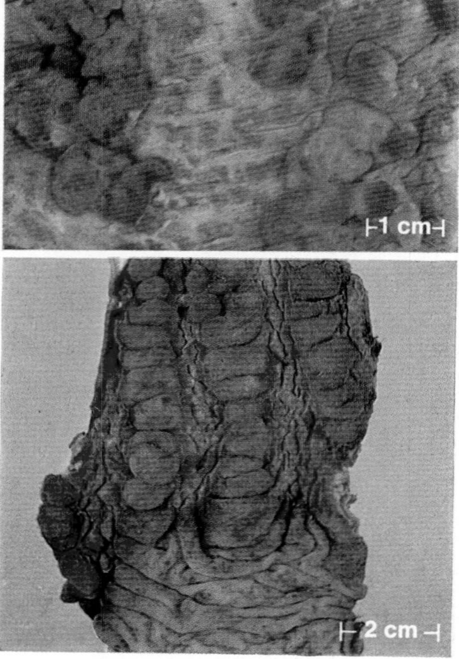

Fig. 5.71. Chronic ulcerative colitis.

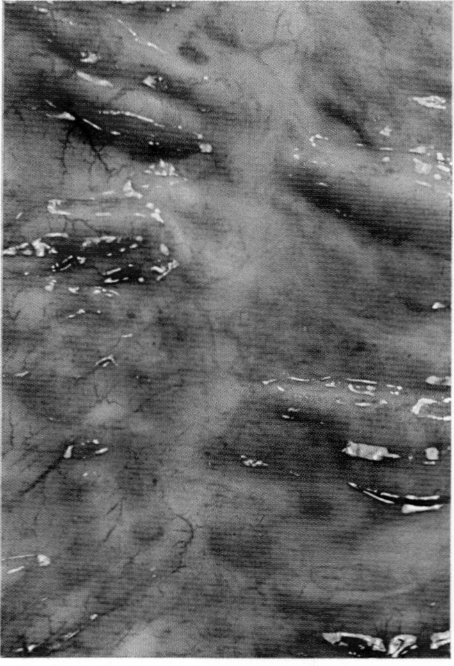

Fig. 5.72. Mucosal atrophy in ulcerative colitis.

Ulcerative Colitis

This is a chronically recurrent, noninfectious inflammation of the colon, largely confined to the mucosa, with ulcerations, formation of granulation tissue, scarring, polypoid degeneration products, and malignant degeneration. Its etiology is unknown.

Figure 5.69 shows a relatively fresh stage of an ulcerative colitis with mucosal defects in the rectum (the anal ring is at the bottom of the picture, the sigmoid colon at the top). Relatively large intact mucosal sections of a grey color, interrupted by ulcers (which appear black as a result of sulfhemoglobin formation) are seen. In addition, fresh, red-grey ulcerations are also found. The acute stage of ulcerative colitis is characterized by a mucosal edema with so-called crypt abscesses (OEHLERT) (granulocyte accumulation in the crypts with epithelial defects, Fig. 5.73). The epithelial defects lead to ulcers which expose the muscularis mucosae. A granulation tissue with telangiectatic capillaries, from which blood flows, develops at the base of the ulcer. The granulation tissue may also form pseudopolyps.

Figure 5.70 demonstrates a **chronic stage** of ulcerative colitis (pseudomembranous necrotizing colitis). Yellow, pulvinate islands of mucosa are seen, slightly projecting in a polypoid manner in part, between which there are grey sections with a smooth surface (exposed submucosa). In Figure 5.71 (below), the frequently longitudinal **ulcerations** are clearly evident. In the upper picture, the muscularis mucosae can be identified as thin horizontal muscle bundles. In the lower picture, we can also see that a segmental involvement is possible (the normal colonic mucosa is seen at the lower edge of the picture). The tumors may heal in the course of the disease; scarring leads to rigidity of the walls and intestinal shrinkage, with the **mucosa appearing completely atrophic.** Figure 5.72 shows the smooth mucosa without crypts. Vessels can be seen under the single layer epithelium.

Pg: unknown. There are many indications that an allergic process, in the sense of an autoaggressive disease, is involved. It has been demonstrated that the lymphocytes of patients with ulcerative colitis attack and destroy explanted colonic mucosa of the same patient (T lymphocytes, so-called "killer lymphocytes"). The inflammatory symptoms may perhaps be the result of a complement activation. Components intrinsic to the cell (membrane? after a virus attack?), or cross-reacting bacterial antigens are suspected as antigens in autoaggression. Another hypothesis states that a "forbidden clone" of lymphocytes is formed (BURNET), with the endogenous lymphocytes attacking the colonic mucosa (AP). Also in

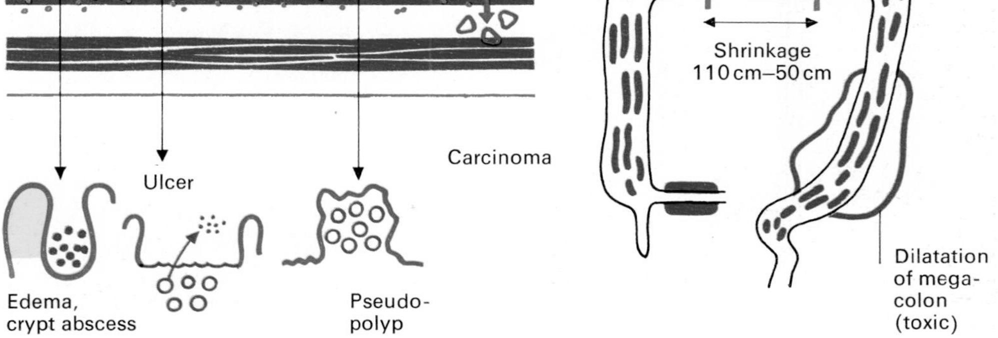

Fig. 5.73. Schematic diagram of the macroscopic and microscopic intestinal changes in ulcerative colitis.

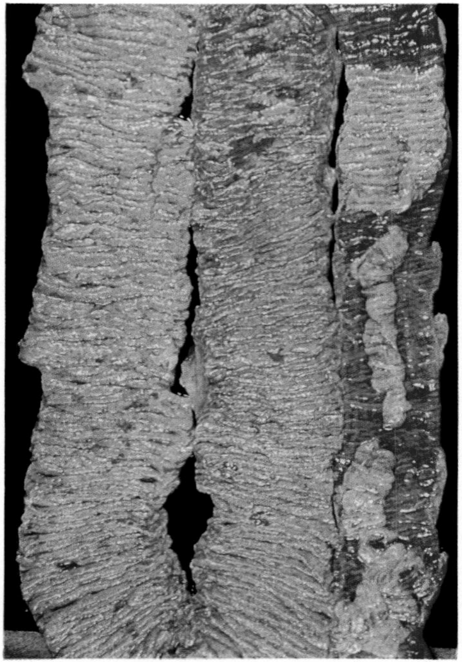

Fig. 5.75. Enterocolitis in uremia.

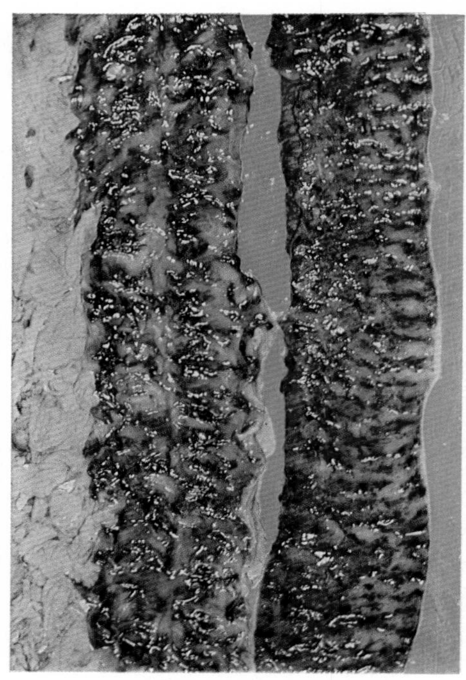

Fig. 5.76. Pseudomembranous enterocolitis.

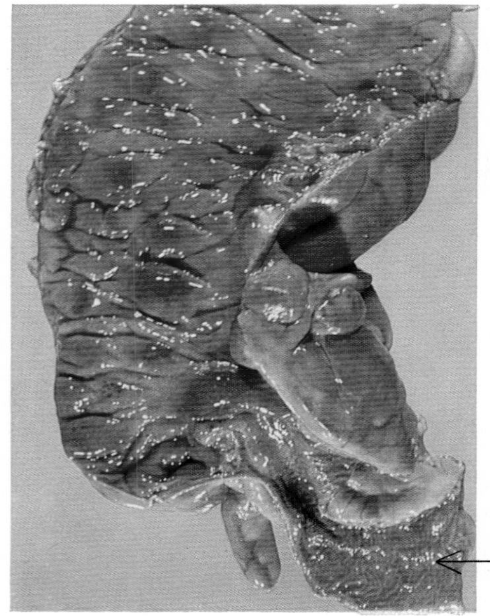

Fig. 5.77. Phlegmonous colitis.

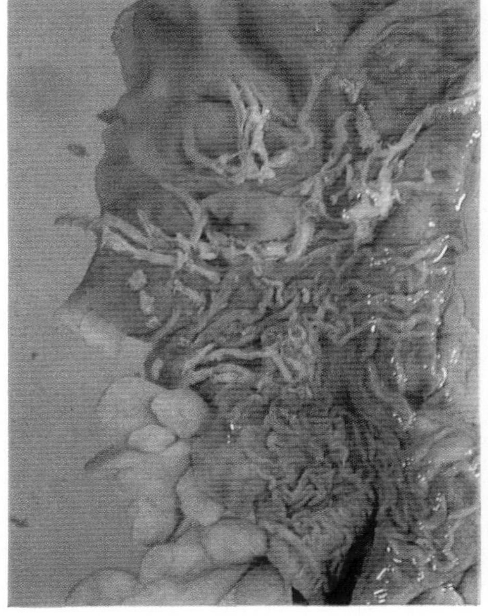

Fig. 5.78. "Colica mucosa."

Fig. 5.74. Schematic diagram of the remote actions of ulcerative colitis.

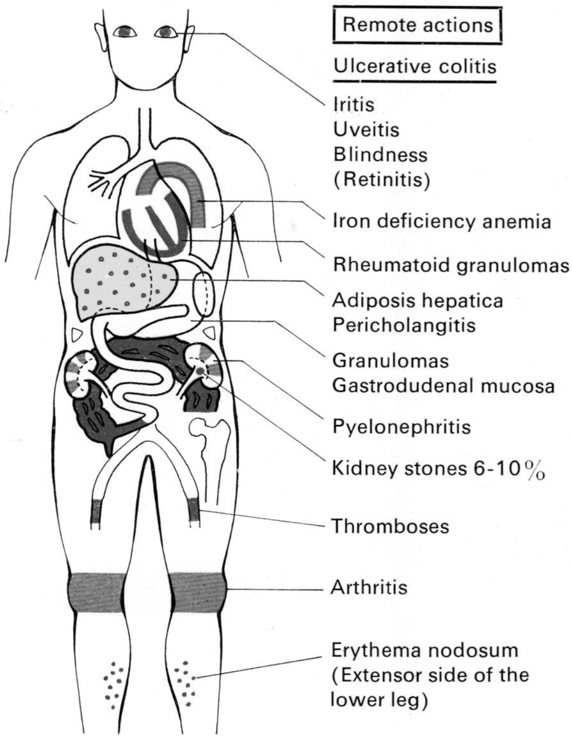

favor of an allergic genesis are the remote actions of ulcerative colitis (Fig. 5.74), with erythema nodosum (extensor side of the lower legs), rheumatoid granulomas in the heart, symptoms in the eyes and arthritides. *A:* younger, labile persons with depressions (psychotherapy!). *S:* ♂:♀ = 1:1. *Lo:* rectum and sigmoid colon alone 42% of all cases. Also spread to the lower ileum. *Co:* thromboses, pyelonephritis, kidney stones, adiposis hepatica, cholangitis, iron deficiency anemia, rheumatoid granulomas in the heart, colonic carcinomas (7% after 10 years, 40% after 25 years, "normal": 0.3%). See also Figure 5.74. *DD:* Crohn's disease.

Enterocolitis (Fig. 5.75) *can be caused by endotoxins of different pathogens, disturbances of the bacterial equilibrium in the intestines, or by toxic substances.* In the case of **bacillary dysentery,** pseudomembranous (surface fibrin exudations without major epithelial defect) or membranous inflammations primarily affecting the small intestine are seen. Figure 5.75 shows yellow pseudomembranes which can be easily removed (see the right side of the picture). The hyperemic mucosa is seen here. The *ulcerative form of dysenteric enterocolitis* is found in East Asia (Shigella dysenteriae). In this form, remote actions similar to those in ulcerative colitis are found (Fig. 5.74). Ten per cent of the cases are chronic.

Co: perforation, cicatrization.

Amebic dysentery with ulcerative colitis is caused by *Entamoeba histolytica (Mi).* Liver abscesses are formed secondarily. A hemorrhagic "enteritis" is found in shock (see page 125) and in an infarction of the small intestine, for example after thrombosis of the mesenteric veins.

Pseudomembranous enterocolitis (Fig. 5.76) is the most frequent form of enterocolitis in civilized countries. It is observed after a disturbance of the bacterial equilibrium of the intestines, for example, after antibiotic therapy. In these cases, the intestinal flora is overgrown by staphylococci. A membranous to ulcerative colitis is seen in cases of uremia and arsenic, bismuth or mercury poisoning (sublimate). Figure 5.76 shows a uremic enterocolitis with patchy, white, flat coatings (pseudomembranes and membranes) at the tip of the mucosal folds (left side of the picture). The mucosa is hyperemic and edematous. Ulcers can also be recognized in the right half of the picture.

Pg: excretion of "poisons" by the intestines.

Colonic phlegmon (Fig. 5.77). A greatly thickened wall with a paving-stone-like relief and a gelatinous grey cut surface is seen. This usually involves an inflammation spreading from the appendix and can also be observed in the small intestine (duodenum and upper jejunum).

Colica mucosa (asthma of the colon, Fig. 5.78). Allergic inflammation of the sigmoid colon and rectum characterized by increased mucus formation. Thickened masses of mucus, twisted into noodle shapes are seen accompanied by a slight reddening of the mucosa. Not universally accepted as a separate disease enfity.

Mi: infiltrates of eosinophilic granulocytes and round cells in the mucosa with a large increase in the goblet cells. *F:* young women are primarily affected.

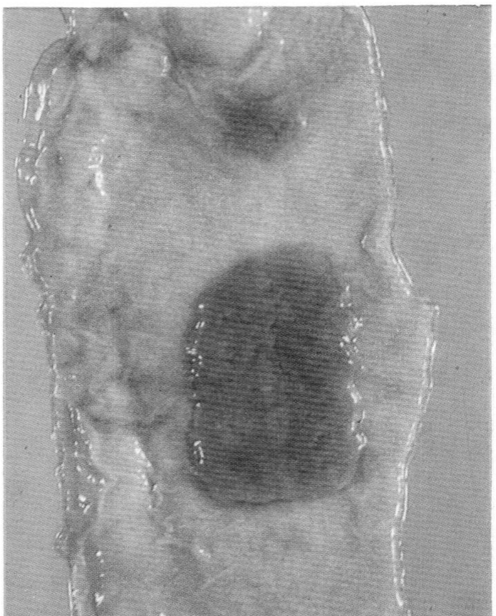

Fig. 5.79. Typhoid fever: marked inflammatory swelling.

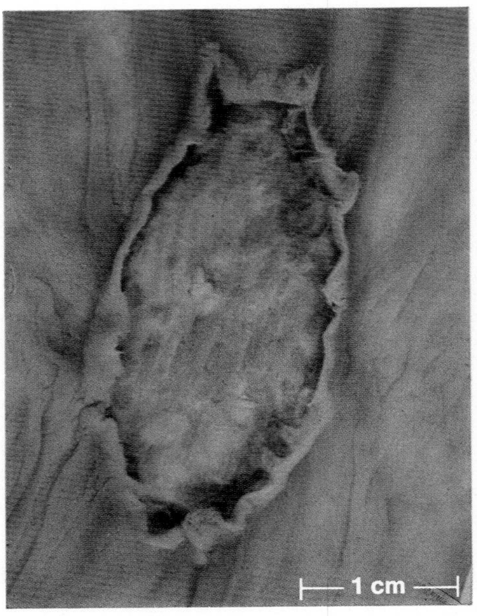

Fig. 5.80. Ulcerative intestinal tuberculosis.

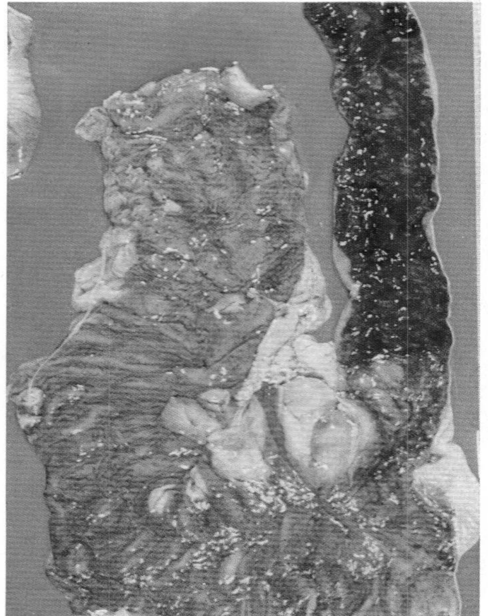

Fig. 5.81. Crohn's disease, acute inflammation.

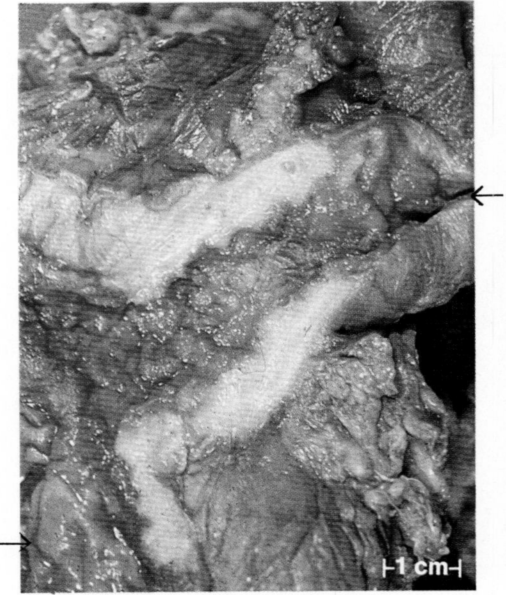

Fig. 5.82. Terminal ileitis (Crohn's disease).

Typhoid fever (Fig. 5.79; TCP, p. 111). *Infectious disease* (Salmonella typhosa), *which rarely is observed in Europe and North America. The disease affects the lower ileum and runs a limited course.* Figure 5.79 shows swelling of Peyer's patches (lymph follicles) in the lower ileum. The gray-red plaques are sharply delineated and tiny white superficial stippling suggests beginning ulceration. (*Mi:* acute lymphadenitis of lymph follicles.)

The inflammatory swelling persists for 1 week and is followed by scab formation. There is relatively little scab formation of the lesion shown in Figure 5.74. Instead, the swollen lymph follicle has ulcerated, showing typical yellow-green areas of necrosis. The third stage of typhoid fever is characterized by the formation of ulcers with the outline of Peyer's patches (TCP, p. 111). The ulcers are oval and their long axis is parallel to the long axis of the gut (*DD:* tuberculous ulcers: the largest diameter is transverse to the long axis of the gut). Typhoid ulcers have a smooth base and heal as scars. Bowel stenosis is not observed after a typhoid ulcer has healed.

Co: perforation (weeks 3–4); hemorrhages from ulcers; enlargement of the spleen. Typhoid nodules in all organs. Esophagitis, parotitis, encephalitis. Cloudy swelling of the heart, kidney and liver.

Paratyphoid fever is caused by *S. paratyphi* A, B or C. In essence, the disease clinically and pathologically is a miniature form of typhoid fever. Contaminated ice cream may be the source of infection.

Ulcerative intestinal tuberculosis (Fig. 5.80; TCP, p. 111). Intestinal tuberculosis usually is localized in the lower ileum and rarely results from a primary infection (bovine *Mycobacterium tuberculosis*). The infection most often is initiated by hematogenous spread from the lung (caseous pneumonia). Occasionally, tuberculous material is swallowed and seeded in the gastrointestinal tract. The initial response is the development of caseating tubercles in the mucosa. The mucosa soon becomes necrotic and ulcerates. The ulcer enlarges by local lymphogenous spread (tuberculous lymphangitis, see p. 83 ff.). The greatest diameter of a tuberculous ulcer is perpendicular to the long axis of the bowel, because of the circumferential distribution of the intestinal lymphatics. Figure 5.80 shows a tuberculous ulcer with shaggy, undermined margins. The ulcer base contains several small, yellowish caseous tubercles. Miliary tubercles in the serosa of the involved bowel have formed from lymphogenous extension. The serosal tubercles are not larger than 1 mm., and are white, glassy and somewhat firm (Fig. 5.80). The serosa overlying a tuberculous mucosal ulcer shows a bowl-like retraction. The mesenteric lymph nodes draining the mucosal ulcer are regularly involved by tuberculosis (primary complex).

F: see above. *Co:* stenosis, hemorrhage, tuberculous peritonitis (miliary tubercles often heal → peritoneal adhesions). *DD:* carcinomatosis of peritoneum. Foreign body granulomas caused by glove powder after operations.

Regional enteritis (terminal ileitis, Crohn's disease, Figs. 5.81–5.83, *Mi*).

Segmentally occuring, chronically recurring ulcerative and stenosing inflammation of the lower small intestine or colon with epitheoid cell granulomas and involvement of all wall layers.

Figure 5.81 shows a **regional enteritis** in the **fresh stage** with involvement of the lower ileum. The distinctly thickened and reddened mucosa, showing individual small ulcers, is seen. The cecum (at the left of the picture) is unchanged.

Figure 5.82 shows a section of intestine opened longitudinally with a whitish-coarse wall thickening (up to 2 cm thick) approximately 8 cm in length, which has led to a stenosis (lower ileum with valva ileocecalis). The mucosa shows grey-yellow ulcerations. At → 1, the muscular hypertrophy of the orally located section of intestine can be seen, a proof of stenosis. → 2: cecum.

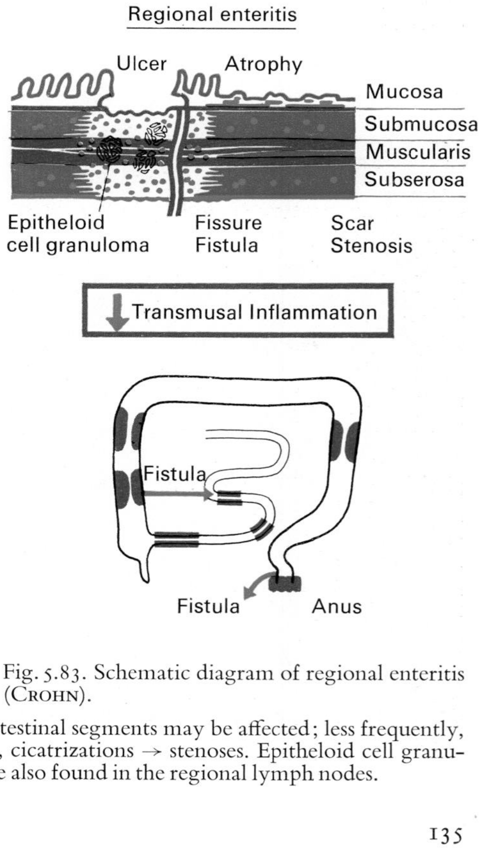

Fig. 5.83. Schematic diagram of regional enteritis (Crohn).

A: 20–40 years. *S:* more frequently in men. The most important *macroscopic and histological findings* are shown in Figure 5.83. In 20% of the cases, several intestinal segments may be affected; less frequently, also the stomach and esophagus. *Co:* fissures → fistulas, cicatrizations → stenoses. Epitheloid cell granulomas with eosinophilic granulocytes and plasma cells are also found in the regional lymph nodes.

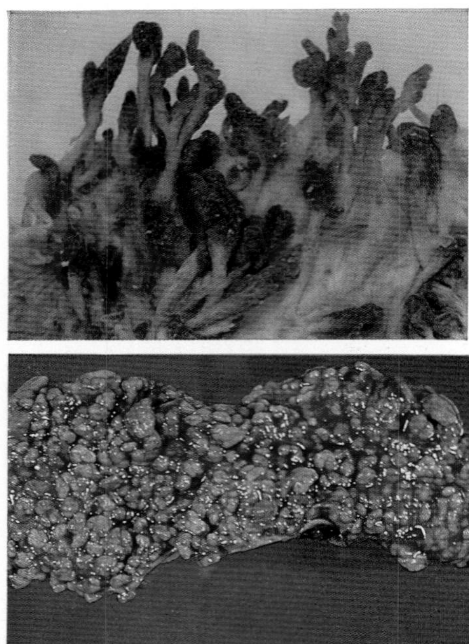

Fig. 5.84. Above: polyposis of the small intestine in Peutz-Jeghers syndrome.
Fig. 5.85. Below: polyposis of the colon.

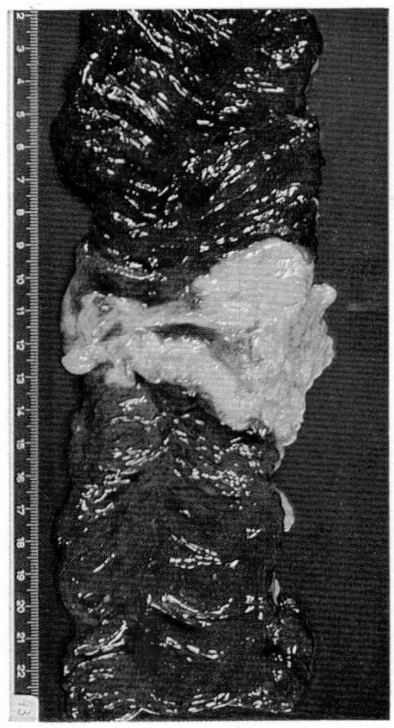

Fig. 5.86. Carcinoma of the colon. Melanosis coli.

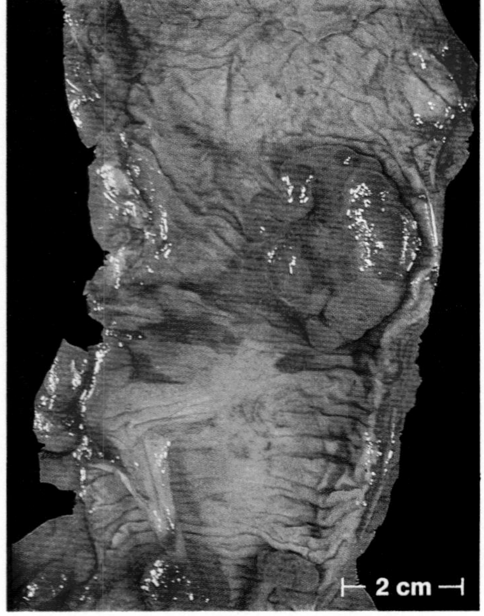

Fig. 5.87. Carcinoma of the sigmoid colon with two pedunculated polyps.

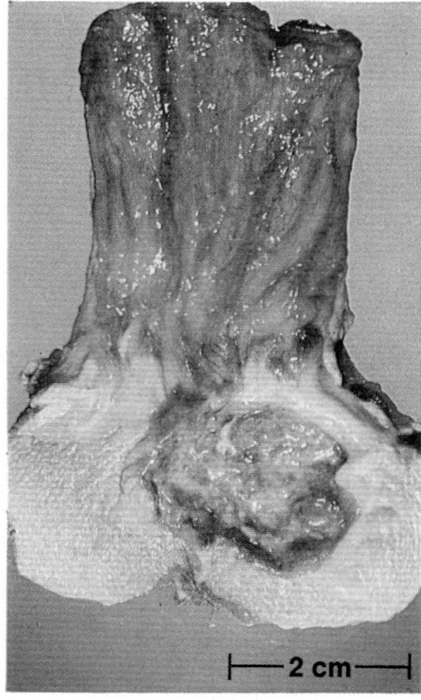

Fig. 5.88. Ulcerated carcinoma of the anus.

Intestinal Tumors

Primary, benign or malignant, epithelial, mesenchymal, and neurogenous tumors occur in the small and large intestine. Secondary tumors, that is, metastases, are extremely rare in the region of the gastro-intestinal tract (they are observed for example, in the case of metastasizing melanoma). Leiomyomas, neurinomas, lipomas (cause of invagination – ileus) and carcinoids are found in the small intestine, but carcinomas occur only in very isolated cases. In the duodenum, hyperplasias of Brunner's glands are also described (so-called Brunneriomas). Among the benign epithelial mucosal tumors are the *polyps*. The following are differentiated:

1. **Polyposis of the small intestine** (Fig. 5.84) is found in Peutz-Jeghers' syndrome – a hereditarily dominant disease with intestinal polyposis and melanosis of the lips, cheeks and fingers. Malignant changes rarely occur in the intestinal polyps. Closely adjacent, pedunculated polyps with tips distended in a flask-like manner are evident in Figure 5.84. The black discoloration of the surface of the tips is attributed to sulfhemoglobin formation.

2. Among the **colonic polyps,** the following forms can be differentiated:

a) The **juvenile colonic polyp** occurs predominantly at the age of 6 years in the region of the rectal mucosa. As a rule, it is solitary and consists of cystically broadened, mucus filled glands, which are covered by an extended mucosa. Not precancerosis, since it does not degenerate.

b) The, as a rule, solitary, pedunculated **adenomatous colonic polyp** (lower part of Fig. 5.87) shows a long, thin peduncle with a distended tip consisting of proliferated glands. Solitary polyps occur very frequently. Thirty per cent of the autopsies performed on persons 30 years of age show polyps of this type and the percentage rises to 75% in 70-year old persons. Adenomatous polyps rarely degenerate.

A special form is the **hyperplastic polyp,** which is usually observed solitarily in the rectum of sigmoid colon. It is interpreted as a transition of a hyperplasia to a polyp, since only the epithelium is proliferated and stroma formation is not yet present.

c) The **villous or papillary colonic polyp** is usually solitary and located on the mucosa with a broad base. The surface shows a friable, frond-like, velvety structure. This polyp occurs predominantly in older persons and degenerates to a carcinoma in about 30% of the cases. Polyps with a diameter of over 10 mm must be suspected of being malignant.

There are rectal polyps which cover large areas of the mucosa and, as a result of a large loss of mucus and fluid (up to 2.5 liters per day), produce electrolyte disturbances. Papillary polyps which disseminate to a large extent at the mucosal level are also interpreted as "mucosal cancers" or as carcinomas growing in situ.

d) In the case of **familial polyposis** (Fig. 5.85), multiple adenomatous polyps, up to 10 mm in diameter, which may populate the whole of the colon, are seen. These mucosal proliferations are to be differentiated from the solitary, adenomatous polyps, since they represent a dominant inherited disease. In 50% of the cases, a multicentric degeneration of these polyps takes place, as early as the age of 30–40 years. Familial polyposis may also occur in *Gardner's syndrome* (familial polyposis, fibromas and leiomyomas of the skin and the mesentery, along with osteomas and exostoses of the maxilla).

Carcinoma of the colon (Figs. 5.86 and 5.87, Mi). *Malignant epithelial tumor of the colonic mucosa.* This occurs most frequently in the rectum (61% of the cases). Other localizations are: 4% in the cecum, 5% in the ascending colon, 5.5% in the transverse colon, 3.5% in the descending colon, and 21% in the sigmoid colon. Figure 5.86 shows a circularly growing grey-red tumor, constricting the intestinal lumen, in a colonic mucosa with blackish discoloration (pseudo-melanosis coli). The tumor of Figure 5.87 is a dish-shaped rectal carcinoma with a retracted center and a periphery thickened in a wall-like manner. Two pedunculated adenomatous polyps are seen at the bottom of the picture.

F: fourth most common malignant tumor in man (in 7th place for women). 4.6% of all autopsied malignant growths. *A:* 60–70 years. *S:* ♂:♀ = 3:2. *Mi:* as a rule, this involves highly differentiated, papillary carcinomas, less frequently colloid carcinomas. *Co:* stenosis with muscular hypertrophy of the upper section of the intestine, ileus, perforation and peritonitis. In the case of colonic carcinoma of the right side, anemia is more frequent. Metastases: liver 80%, lung 15%, CNS 15%, bone marrow 5%.

Carcinoma of the anus. *This involves malignant epithelial tumors of the squamous cell carcinoma type, less frequently basal cell carcinomas.* Figure 5.88 shows an ulcerated squamous cell carcinoma 3 cm in diameter.

Benign neoplasms (anal fibromas, condylomata), precanceroses (Bowen's disease), and other malignant growths (such as melanomas) are found in the anal region. The anal fibromas or anal polyps, as a rule, are in the form of fibrosed hemorrhoidal nodes. The so-called sacral dermoid is not a genuine mixed tumor but consists of compressed hairs which lead to a chronic, granulating, and cicatrizing inflammation (the correct designation is pilonidal sinus).

Intestinal carcinoid (compare bronchial carcinoid, p. 91, Mi). *Semimalignant tumor growing in an infiltrating manner, but rarely metastasizing, derived from the argentaffin (yellow) cells of the gastro-intestinal tract.*

Carcinoid of the appendix, as a rule, is only an accidental finding during an appendextomy. In this organ, the carcinoid is always benign! Carcinoids of the ileum, on the other hand, may cause liver metastases and induce a *carcinoid syndrome:* diarrhea, flush (paroxysmal reddening of the facial skin), fibrosis of the tricuspid valves, and asthma attacks. The mesenteric arteries in the tumor region also show a pronounced proliferation of the intima with constriction of the lumen → reduced blood supply to the intestine → intestinal necroses → peritonitis. Carcinoids produce serotonin and kallikrein. There is an increase in 5-hydroxyindolacetic acid (5-HAA) in the urine. *Mi:* typical cells arranged in the form of a ball, which can be demonstrated selectively by silver staining (Bodian's reaction). *Paraneoplastic carcinoid syndromes* also occur in parvicellular bronchial carcinoma, pancreatic tumors, etc.

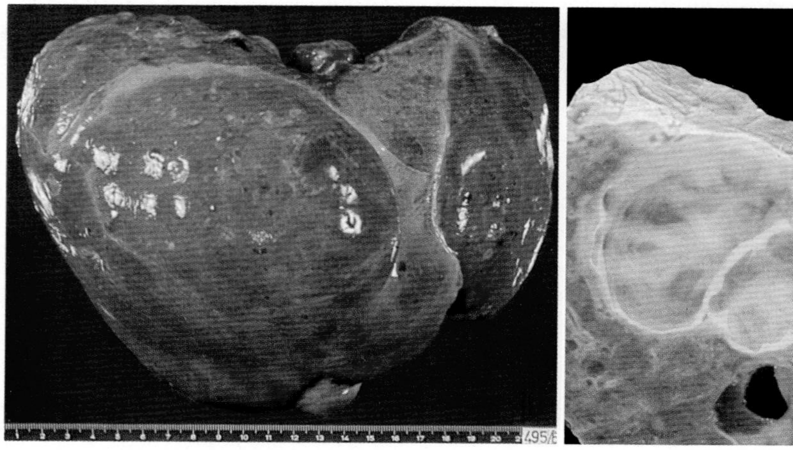

Fig. 6.1. Congenital liver cysts.

Fig. 6.2. Cut surface of liver cysts.

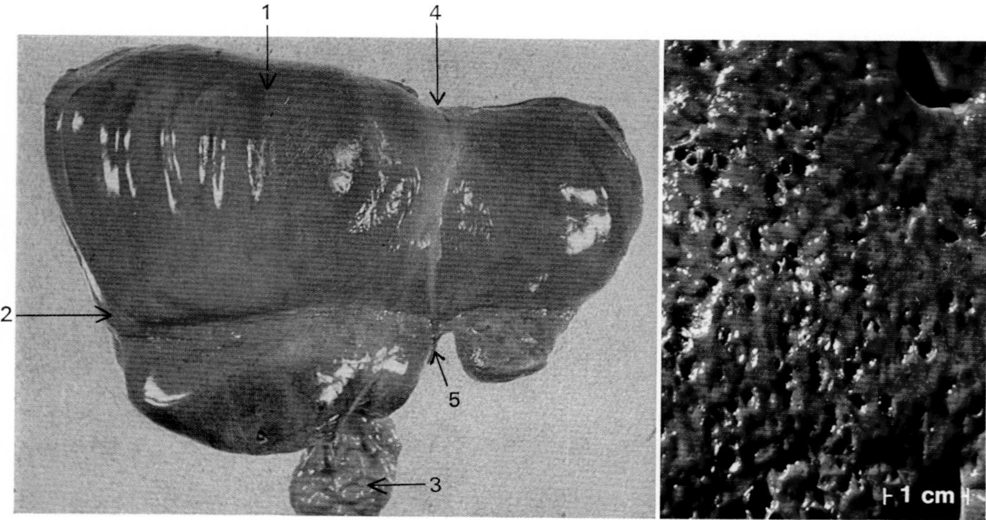

Fig. 6.3. Liver with diaphragmatic grooves, "corset" grooves and pseudomelanosis.

Fig. 6.4. Foamy liver.

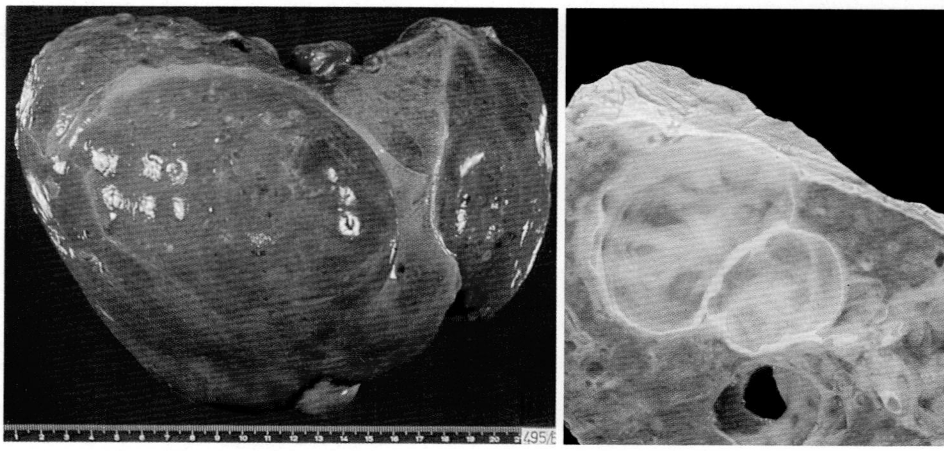

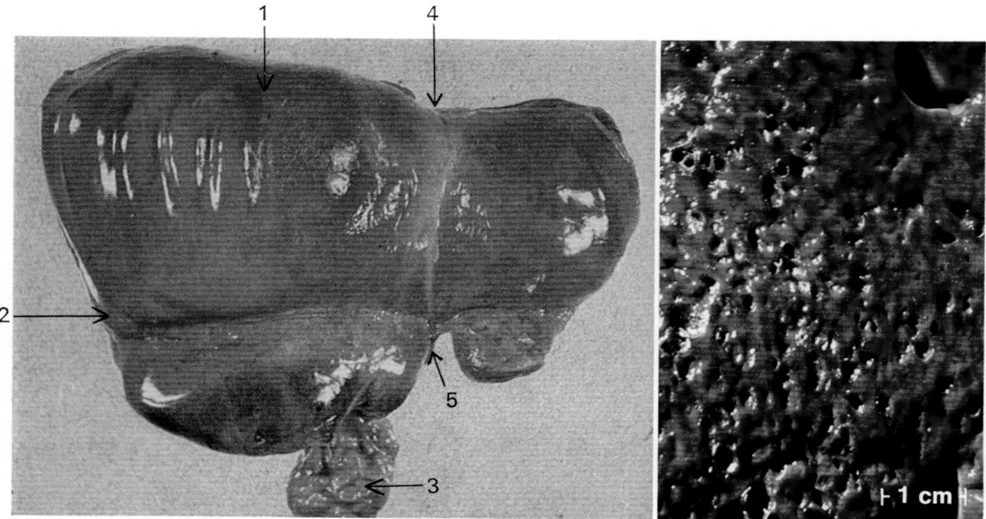

6. Liver

Dissection, Malformations, Postmortem Changes

Anatomic remarks and dissection. The liver weighs 1,500 Gm. (2% of total body weight) The falciform ligament of the anterior liver surface (→4 in Fig. 6.3) and the remnants of the umbilical vein (ligamentum teres) (→5 in Fig. 6.3) separate the right and left lobes of the liver. A line between the vena cava and the gallbladder is considered the "watershed" of the liver (separation of arterial blood supply between the two branches of the hepatic artery). This line also separates the blood flow in the portal vein. Blood does not mix in the short branch of the portal vein. The left liver lobe receives blood predominantly from the *splenic vein*, whereas the right liver lobe is supplied predominantly by the *superior and inferior mesenteric veins*. Caudate and quadrangular lobes of the liver. Pars affixa: connection of the liver with the diaphragm. The peritoneum of the liver is smooth and glistening. The consistency is firm-elastic. The cut surface of the liver is red-brown. The lobules are poorly demarcated, 1–2 mm. large. Central veins can be identified with a magnifying glass. Branches of the portal vein and hepatic artery run parallel. Hepatic veins converge toward the pars affixa, where they enter into the inferior vena cava. The hapatoduodenal ligament contains the ductus choledochus anteriorly, the hepatic artery in the middle and the portal vein in a posterior position.

The liver is dissected from the hepatoduodenal ligament and cut lengthwise by 2 or 3 knife cuts after the gallbladder is removed.

Malformations of the liver

Aplasia occurs together with other severe malformations. Hypoplasia is rare. Abnormal small lobes occur.

Liver cysts not infrequently are solitary (Figs. 6.1 and 6.2). They are located mostly near the liver surface and sometimes project over the surface. They are filled with clear fluid and appear bluish. Figures 6.1 and 6.2 show multiple cysts with a white, smooth wall on cut surface. They are lined by ciliated epithelium (derived from the gut) or cylindrical or cubical epithelium (derived from the bile ducts). Liver cysts or polycystic liver (only quantitative difference between the two) frequently are associated with polycystic kidneys or pancreas.

Commonly observed changes in the *shape of the liver:*

1. Corset liver (Fig. 6.3, → 2). A horizontal groove across the lower anterior surface that is accompanied by fibrosis of the capsule (chronic mechanical irritation). Seen in females (corset!) or in patients with ankylosing spondylitis. Due to pressure of lower thoracic aperture (ribs) on the liver surface.

2. Diaphragmatic grooves of the liver (Fig. 6.3, → 1). Vertical grooves of the right upper liver lobe caused by pressure of focally hypertrophic muscle bundles of the diaphragm in cases of chronic pulmonary diseases (frequent coughing). The diaphragm is removed and held against the light; the thick muscle bundles are clearly seen as dark bands. Note also the elongated gallbladder filled with stones in Figure 6.3 (→3).

Postmortem changes

The colon is in close proximity to the lower right liver lobe or the lower third of the anterior surface. A green-black or black discoloration of the liver surface frequently results from diffusion of gas (sulfides) (or sulfhemoglobin, in which case it is known as pseudomelanosis) (Fig. 6.3). Postmortem changes take place rapidly in the liver, depending on the body temperature. The liver becomes soft, diffluent and green-black. The cut surface becomes foamy (gas blebs from the growth of gas-forming bacteria; foamy liver). Figure 6.4 shows gas blebs in a black-purple liver. A preserved liver lobule with a central vein is seen in the upper portion of Figure 6.4.

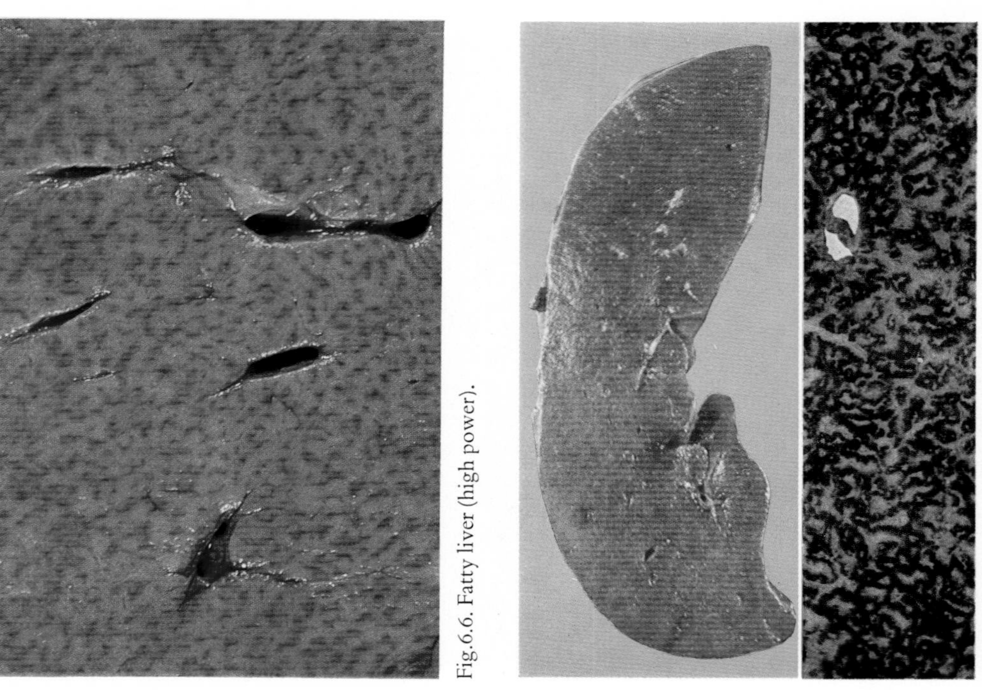

Fig.6.6. Fatty liver (high power).

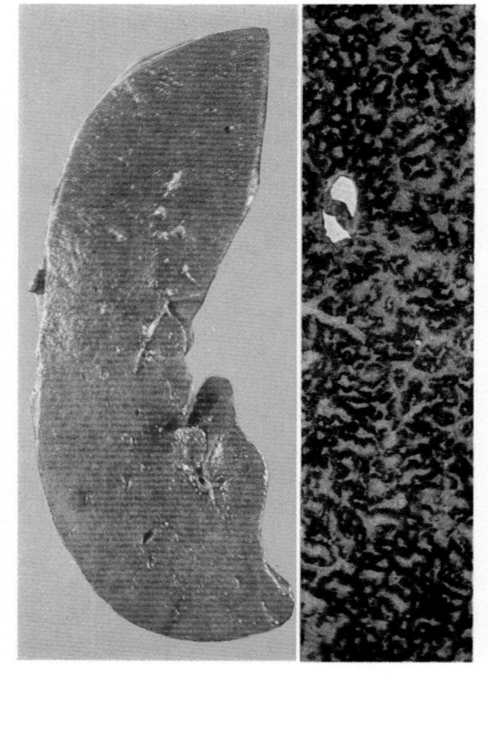

Fig. 6.8. Abve: cut surface of the liver with amyloidosis.
Fig. 6.9. Below: same after Lugol's solution was added.

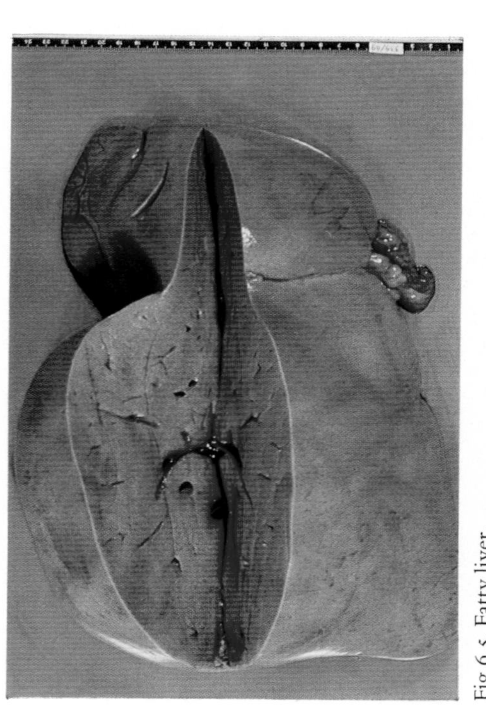

Fig.6.5. Fatty liver.

Fig. 6.7. Amyloidosis of the liver.

Metabolic Changes

Fatty liver (Figs. 6.5 and 6.6; TCP, p. 119). *Grossly visible fatty deposits in hepatocytes caused by nutritional or toxic factors (more than 50% of hepatocytes are affected).* Figure 6.5 shows an enlarged and bright yellow liver. The weight was 3,000 Gm. The margins are blunted and the consistency is doughy. A finger pressure remains and the liver tissue breaks easily. Trauma easily causes rupture. A liver slice floats on the surface of water (diminished specific weight of fat). The cutting knife meets more resistance than in a normal liver (fluid) and adheres to the cut surface. The knife blade is dull (coated with fat droplets) in contrast to the moist, glistening blade seen when cutting through normal liver. Figure 6.5 shows advanced fatty changes and, in addition, hyperemia (congestion) leading to minimal red markings. The cut surface is either diffusely yellow or, as shown in Figure 6.6, the periportal fields and the peripheral lobules are gray or gray-red (close-up) (minimal fibrosis → transition into fatty cirrhosis, Fig. 6.41). The liver becomes firmer than normal in cirrhosis.

Clinically: Zieve's syndrome: Fatty liver with mild jaundice. Alkaline phosphatase is markedly increased, SGOT only slightly elevated. Hypercholesterolemia.

Morphologic appearance of fatty liver and pathogenesis. See Figure 6.14.

Central fatty change: Yellow lobular centers with brown periphery. The cut surface is smooth in all forms of fatty degenerative changes. Depressed areas are not present as in congestion.

Causes:

(a) Damage to *energizing system* (mitochondria, ATP deficiency); seen with anoxia or toxic enzyme inhibition; e.g., arsenicals, phosphorus, mushrooms or chloroform in small doses. Severe damage – diffuse fatty changes.

(b) *Alimentary:* high dietary content of triglycerides or increased mobilization of body fats (peripheral lipolysis with alcoholism). *Morphology: peripheral large droplet fatty change:* later, also diffuse fatty changes. The role of *alcohol* has not been entirely clarified. Some authors point to the importance of choline deficiency. LIEBER and KREBS have shown experimentally a direct toxic effect of alcohol on liver metabolism (e.g., inhibition of gluconeogenesis, H. KREBS).

(c) *Substrate deficiency:* β-lipoprotein deficiency, e.g., fatty liver changes with hunger, deficiency of amino acids or choline → fatty liver in kwashiorkor (malnutrition in tropical zones). *Co:* fibrosis, fatty cirrhosis.

Amyloidosis of the liver (Figs. 6.7 and 6.8; TCP, pp. 119 and 173).

Amyloid deposition in the liver in generalized amyloidosis (spleen, kidneys, adrenals, gastrointestinal tract). The liver is wooden, nonpliable and "stands up." The cut surface is transparent, glassy and brownish tinged (Fig. 6.8). Thin liver slices are transparent (large letters of a newspaper can be identified). As first described by VIRCHOW in 1854, a brownish discoloration is elicited with the addition of Lugol's solution. The color changes to brown-black by subsequent addition of H_2SO_4 (amyloid = starch-like). VIRCHOW thought of cellulose. Pathogenesis, etc., see page 183.

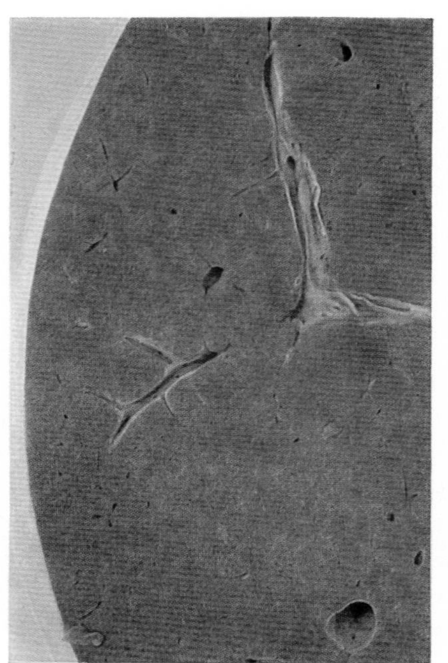

Fig. 6.10. Safran liver.

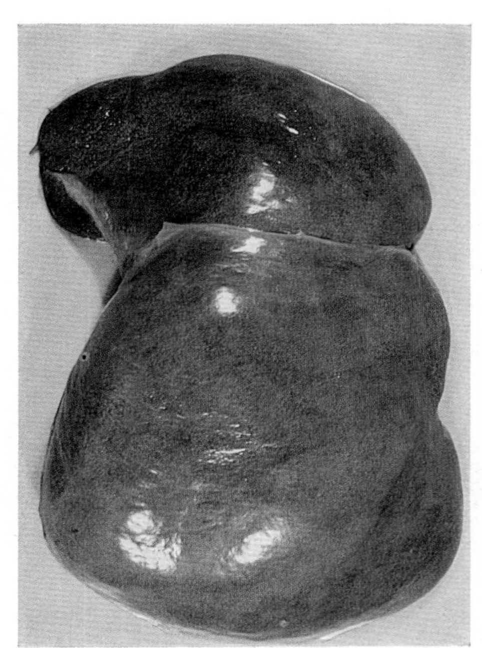

Fig. 6.11. Jaundice of the liver.

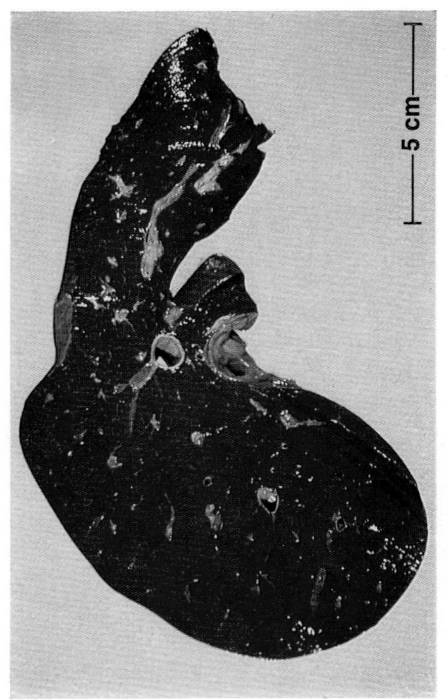

Fig. 6.12. Brown atrophy of the liver.

Fig. 6.13. Acute congestion of the liver.

Jaundice (icterus) (TCP, p. 117). *Increase in blood bilirubin concentration above 1 mg./100 ml.* Jaundice is noticed grossly when tissues are heavily impregnated with bilirubin or biliverdin. A diffuse deposition is difficult to diagnose, even microscopically. Heavy jaundice is reflected as stained protein casts in renal tubules or pigment droplets in renal tubular epithelia. Bile pigment is deposited in the liver as droplets in hepatocytes and Kupffer cells. Bile casts occur in cholangioles, bile ducts and in areas of necrosis impregnated with bile. The liver becomes greenish or golden brown. Figure 6.10 illustrates a fatty, jaundiced liver. The yellow color of fat and the green color of jaundice result in the light yellow-green of safran (so-called safran liver).

Pg: mushroom poisoning causes toxic fatty degenerative liver damage, necrosis of hepatocytes and jaundice. Stone occlusion of the ductus choledochus, as seen in Figure 6.11, produces severe obstructive jaundice. The liver is dark green.

Types of jaundice:

1. *Prehepatic (antehepatic) jaundice:* hemolytic jaundice (familial) in spherocytosis, sickle cell anemia or neonatal hemolytic disease. Toxic substances, e.g., phenylhydrazine, snake venoms. Indirect diazo reaction is positive. Bile pigment is found predominantly in the centers of the lobules on microscopic examination.

2. *Intrahepatic jaundice:* (a) hepatocellular jaundice (viral hepatitis, anoxic hepatocellular necrosis, congestion), (b) drug-induced jaundice (disturbance of conjugation with glucuronic acid), (c) intrahepatic cholestasis (congenital intrahepatic occlusion, tumors, inflammation, cirrhosis).

3. *Posthepatic jaundice:* stenosis of extrahepatic bile ducts, stones, tumors.

The diazo reaction is positive in the intrahepatic and posthepatic forms.

Brown atrophy of the liver (Fig. 6.12; TCP, p. 117). A manifestation of generalized atrophy of parenchymal organs during advanced age or malnutrition. The liver is markedly reduced in size (normal diameter of right lobe 12 cm., here 7 cm.), appears brown and firm. The reduction in size is accompanied by lipofuscin deposits (TCP, p. 117).

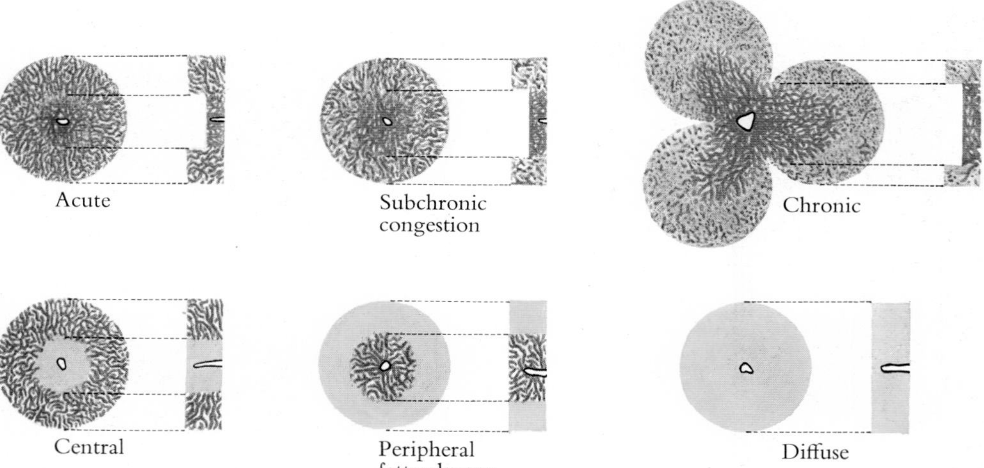

Fig. 6.14. Schematic presentation of morphologic changes in the liver occurring with congestion and fatty degenerative changes.

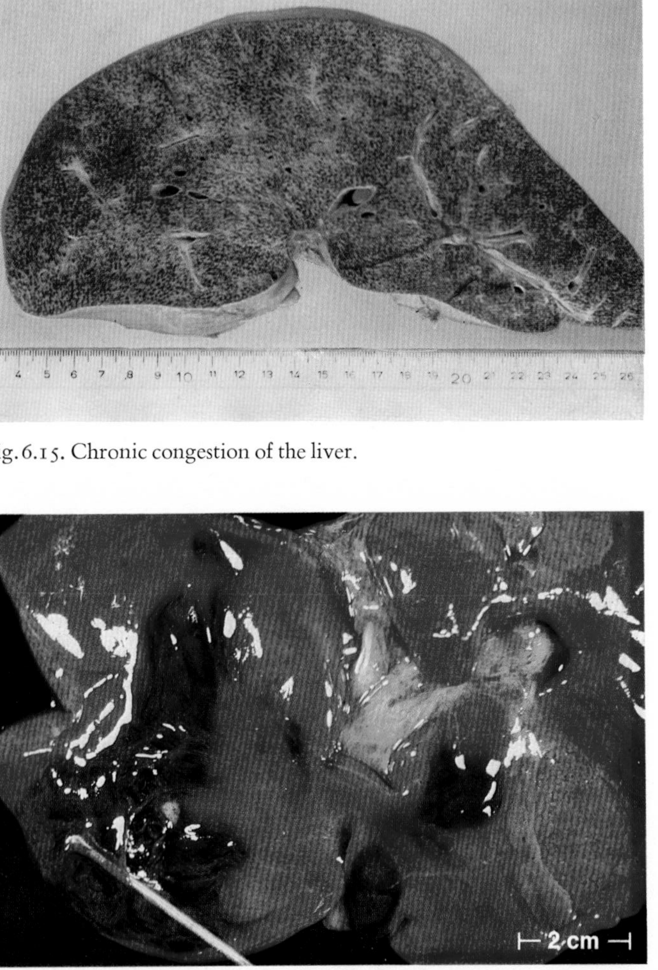

Fig. 6.15. Chronic congestion of the liver.

Fig. 6.17. Subcapsular hemorrhages in the liver.

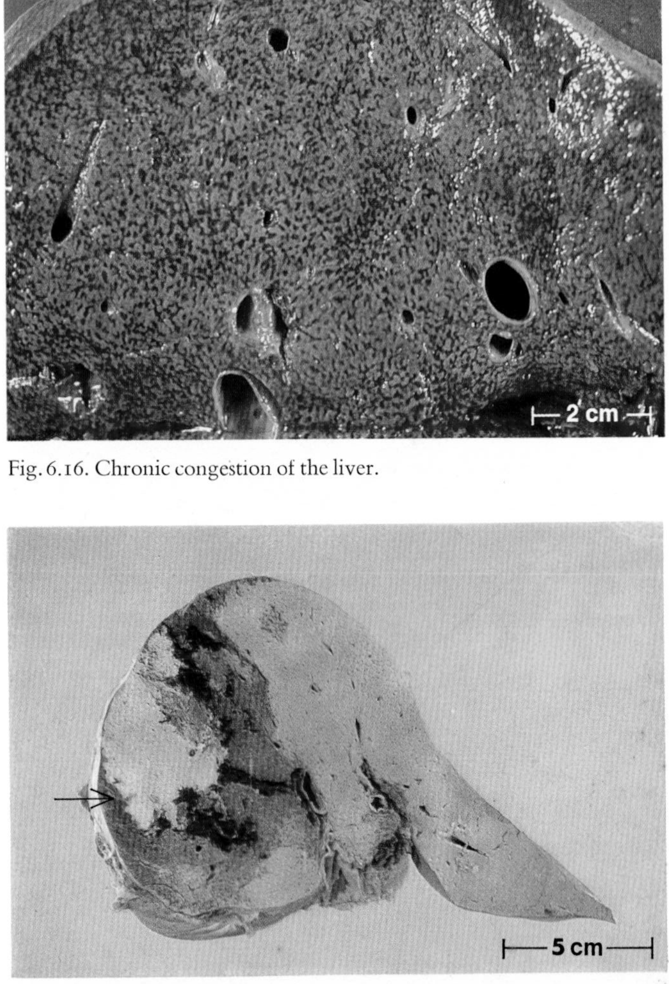

Fig. 6.16. Chronic congestion of the liver.

Fig. 6.18. Traumatic necrosis and hemorrhages of the liver.

Congestion of the liver (Figs. 6.1, 6.15 and 6.16; TCP, p. 121).

Blood stasis in hepatic sinusoids due to cardiac insufficiency.

Acute congestion is seen in the centers of the lobules. Figure 6.13 shows a close-up of the red, circular, lobular centers (extending approximately to the midzonal regions), which are surrounded by light brown, slightly yellowish peripheral zones. Note that the red portions are *sunken*, since the blood oozes from the dilated sinusoids during cutting. The hepatic cords are atrophic. The preserved, slightly fatty portions of the lobule form a slightly elevated ring around the sunken central portions. This is especially apparent on the right margin of the photograph (oblique illumination with highlights on elevated portions). The liver is enlarged, heavy, dark red and firm. The capsule is stretched.

With *prolonged congestion*, the central areas of congestion enlarge. They no longer appear round but are irregularly elongated, as already seen focally in Figure 6.13 (see also Fig. 6.14). Chronic congestion and hypoxia lead to fatty parenchymal changes, with the typical *nutmeg appearance* of the enlarged organ (Fig. 6.15). The higher magnification of Figure 6.16 reveals a network of red bridges (congestive bridges) and the remaining pale liver tissue (see also Fig. 6.14). As in liver cirrhosis, the lobular architecture is reversed: the periportal fields represent the centers of the fatty liver tissue, whereas the congestive bridges form the "periphery" of the lobule. Note that the congested portions again are sunken against the unaffected liver tissue (highlights in Fig. 6.16).

Hemorrhages in the liver are seen as subcapsular hemorrhages, especially after birth trauma. Blood collects beneath the capsule, which projects over the surface (Fig. 6.17). An intra-abdominal hematoma develops after rupture of the liver capsule (see probe in the capsule). In adults, traumatic liver rupture with massive parenchymal hemorrhages is seen after automobile accidents. Frequently, there also is rupture of the spleen.

Trauma also can lead to thrombosis or compression of branches of the hepatic artery and portal vein. Extensive liver necrosis results. Figure 6.18 shows a subcapsular, yellow, dry area of parenchymal coagulation necrosis surrounded by hemorrhages and hyperemia.

Note the yellowish white discoloration of the remaining parenchyma, which is due to anemia and fatty degenerative changes. The brown-red zone (→) between the necrotic areas and the viable liver parenchyma is a so-called *Zahn infarction*. It is caused here by portal vein thrombosis. A Zahn infarction is an area of acute hyperemia, not a true infarction with necrosis (compare with Fig. 6.19).

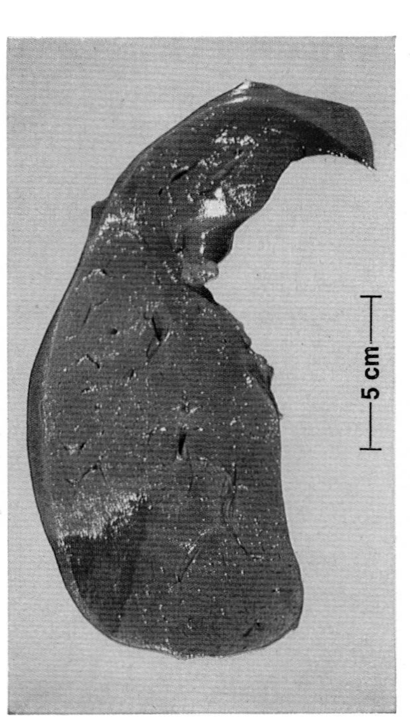

Fig. 6.19. Zahn infarction of the liver.

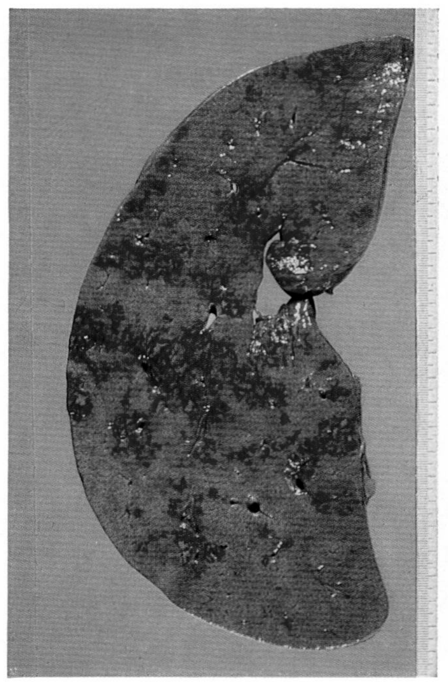

Fig. 6.20. Periarteritis nodosa of the liver.

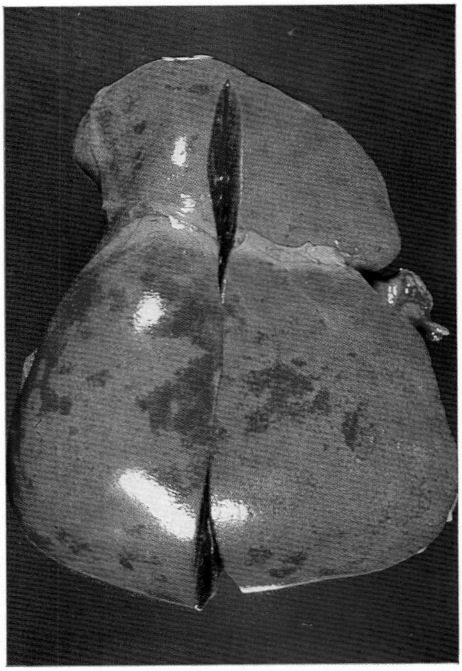

Fig. 6.21. Liver necrosis in eclampsia.

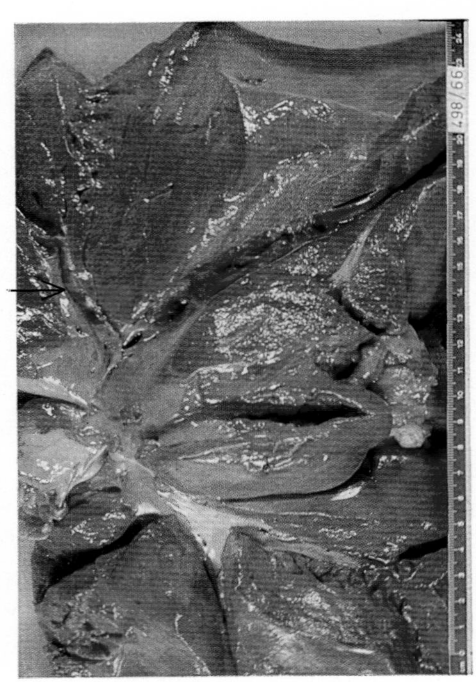

Fig. 6.22. Endophlebitis hepatica obliterans (Budd-Chiari syndrome).

Portal Vein Thrombosis, Periarteritis, Eclampsia, Endophlebitis

Thrombosis of the portal vein does not cause a sudden cessation of liver function because arterial blood is supplied by the hepatic artery. Prolonged occlusion of a main branch of the portal vein leads to *liver atrophy*, reduced bile secretion, eventually to ascites, splenomegaly and esophageal varices. Thrombosis of the portal vein is seen in liver cirrhosis and polycythemia vera rubra or after trauma. Tumor infiltration, either directly or extending through the splenic and mesenteric veins, also may result in portal vein thrombosis.

Intrahepatic portal vein thrombosis produces a so-called Zahn infarction (Fig. 6.19). The triangular, red, sunken area is not a true infarction (no necrosis) histologically but rather an area of acute hyperemia. Occlusion of the portal vein results in *atrophy* of liver parenchyma with *congestion* of the sinusoids via the hepatic veins.

Periarteritis nodosa (Fig. 6.20, see pp. 223 and 253; TCP, p. 65). Inflammation of the arterial walls (panarteritis) causes variable degrees of arterial occlusion with infarction of the liver, spleen and kidneys. In 60% of the cases, the liver contains foci of necrosis, although less frequently than the kidneys or spleen. Figure 6.20 illustrates multiple scattered areas of dry coagulation necrosis (up to 1 cm. in diameter) with hemorrhagic zones of demarcation. Liver necrosis after *occlusion of individual branches of the hepatic artery* (due to embolism or trauma) is rare because collateral circulation is abundant.

Eclampsia (Fig. 6.21; TCP, p. 121). *Toxemia of pregnancy predominantly affecting primigravidas. The disease develops during or shortly after delivery and clinically is characterized by hypertension, edema and proteinuria.* Grossly, the liver is speckled with irregular, yellow areas of anemia, necrosis and focal hemorrhages. Microscopically, fibrin thrombi are found in addition to the necrotic areas. Coagulation defects (consumption coagulopathy) are considered the cause of eclampsia.

F: 0.7% of all pregnancies, mild forms in 5–8% of all pregnancies. *A:* mostly primigravidas. *Pr:* death occurs in 4%. *Pg:* not known; coagulation defects, toxic substances of fetal origin? *Co:* shock-kidneys with interstitial edema, cerebral edema (tonicclonic convulsions). *Cl:* hepatic insufficiency with fetor hepaticus, icterus, clotting disturbances and hepatic coma. In some cases, the renal changes predominate in the clinical picture (bilateral necroses of the renal cortex).

Endophlebitis hepatica obliterans (Budd-Chiari syndrome) (Fig. 6.22). *Idiopathic thrombotic occlusion of hepatic veins of all calibers.* Figure 6.22 shows the entrance of larger hepatic vein branches into the inferior vena cava. The opened hepatic veins contain fresh thrombi (→). A thrombus projects above an opened vein. The liver is congested. When fresh or old thrombi are found in smaller veins, the gross picture is that of irregular, spotty hemorrhages on the cut surface. Congestion as a result of venous occlusion is the principal finding on microscopic examination.

Pg: not known. Recently described in Jamaica after tea consumption *(Heliotropium lasiocarbum)* (Stuart and Bros) or plants of the genus *Senecio*. Occasionally seen in polycythemia.

F: approximately 200 cases have been described. *A:* 30–40 years. *S:* ♂ = ♀.

Hepatic vein thrombosis can result *secondarily* from *tumor infiltration* (e.g., primary liver cancer or liver abscesses).

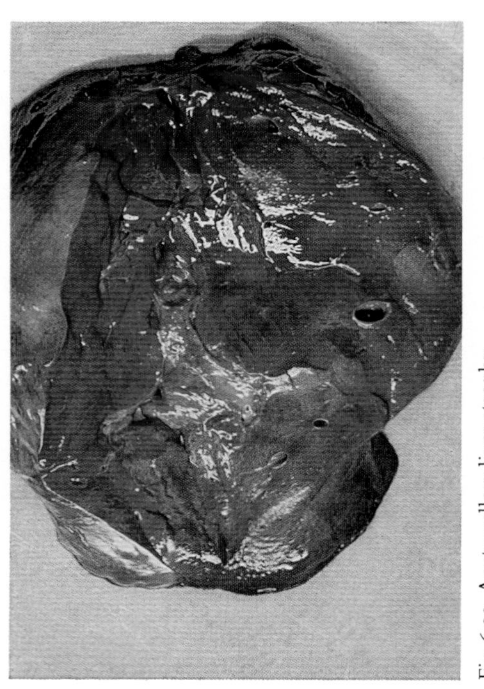

Fig. 6.23. Acute yellow liver atrophy.

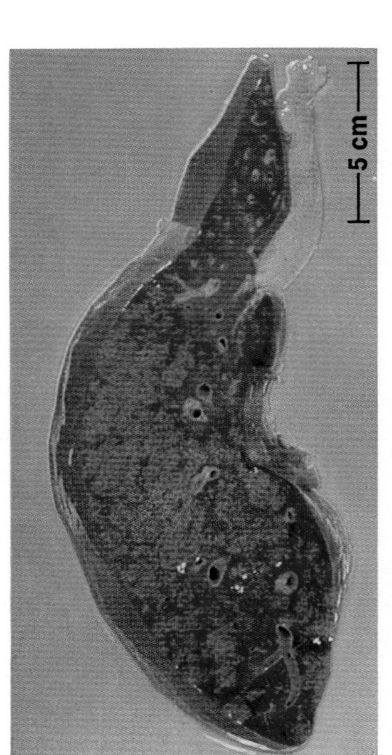

Fig. 6.24. Subacute red liver atrophy.

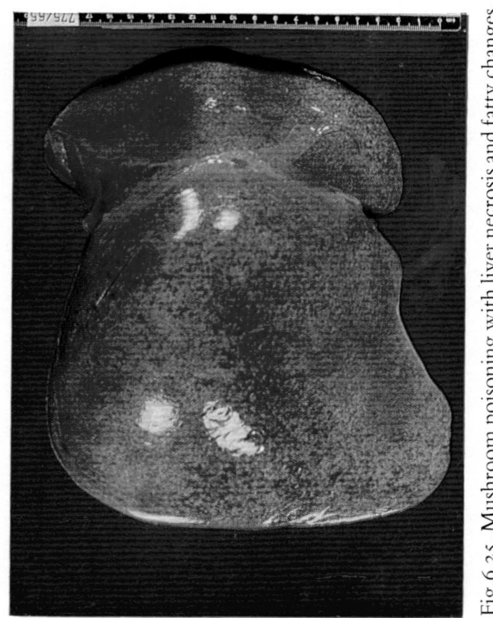

Fig. 6.25. Mushroom poisoning with liver necrosis and fatty changes.

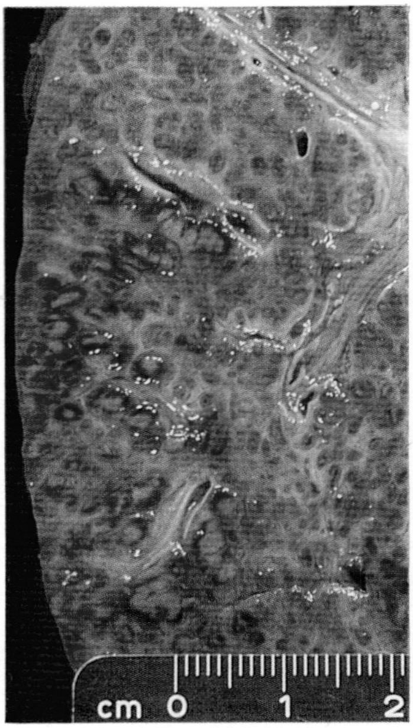

Fig. 6.26. Disseminated liver necrosis in liver cirrhosis.

Liver Atrophy and Necrosis

Acute yellow liver atrophy (Fig. 6.23; TCP, p. 129). *Acute total necrosis of the liver.* Our figure shows a very small, flabby and soft liver (weight reduced to 500 Gm.). The capsule is wrinkled because it is larger than the remaining liver tissue. The liver margins are sharp. On cut surface, the hepatic parenchyma is semiliquid, yellow to yellow-green or ocher-yellow in cases with severe fatty changes. The capsule frequently is studded with tiny white crystals (leucine or tyrosine crystals) that also may be identified post mortem on cut surface.

F: 0.05%. *A:* 30–50 years. *S:* ♂ = ♀. *Pg: toxic factors,* such as mushroom or phosphorus poisoning, arsenicals, carbon tetrachloride, formerly with salvarsan therapy. *Viral hepatitis. Nutritional-toxic factors. Clinically:* rapidly deepening jaundice, hypoglycemia, coma, hemorrhagic diathesis and death within 2–3 days.

Subacute red liver atrophy (Fig. 6.24; TCP, p. 129). *Characterized by a partial, probably slowly progressive, liver necrosis.* The liver shows red and yellow flecks on gross examination. It is smaller than normal, firm and often plate-like (weight reduced to 300 Gm.). The capsule is wrinkled. As shown in Figure 6.24, the cut surface reveals depressed *red areas* of irregular size (the necrotic liver tissue is soft in consistency and has been partially removed). The sinusoids are dilated and filled with blood: "release" hyperemia. Yellow parenchyma with fatty changes also is seen on the cut surface. The end result of the subchronic or chronic stage is liver cirrhosis (see p. 151).

Necrosis of the liver (TCP, pp. 121, 128 and 129) is divided into:

(a) *Central lobular necrosis:* (anemia, acute anoxia, congestion).

(b) "*Group*" *necrosis:* (1) irregularly distributed in eclampsia and periarteritis nodosa or as cholemic necrosis or (2) in the *midzonal* liver lobule in anoxia, diphtheria and mushroom poisoning. Necrosis of groups of liver cells can occur in acute and subacute hepatitis, predominantly in the central zones of the liver lobule.

(c) *Single-cell necrosis:* (hepatitis).

Disseminated necrosis in liver cirrhosis (Fig. 6.26).

Gray, sunken scar tissue and preserved round or oval red-yellow islands of residual parenchyma (fatty changes) are identified. Some residual liver tissue appears *bright yellow*, dry and surrounded by hemorrhagic zones of demarcation. The areas of necrosis result from contraction of the scar tissue and vascular compression, which deprives the remaining liver tissue of its blood supply. A sudden fall in the blood pressure (due to bleeding from esophageal varices) may add to hypoxia of the remaining liver tissue. An acute atrophic relapse also may occur. In this case, the entire parenchyma, which is green or yellow-green discolored, is affected.

Irregularly distributed areas of necrosis and fatty changes occur frequently in mushroom poisoning or alcoholic liver damage (chronic alcoholic hepatitis). Figure 6.25 reveals a fatty liver with focal hemorrhages and subcapsular, yellow areas of necrosis.

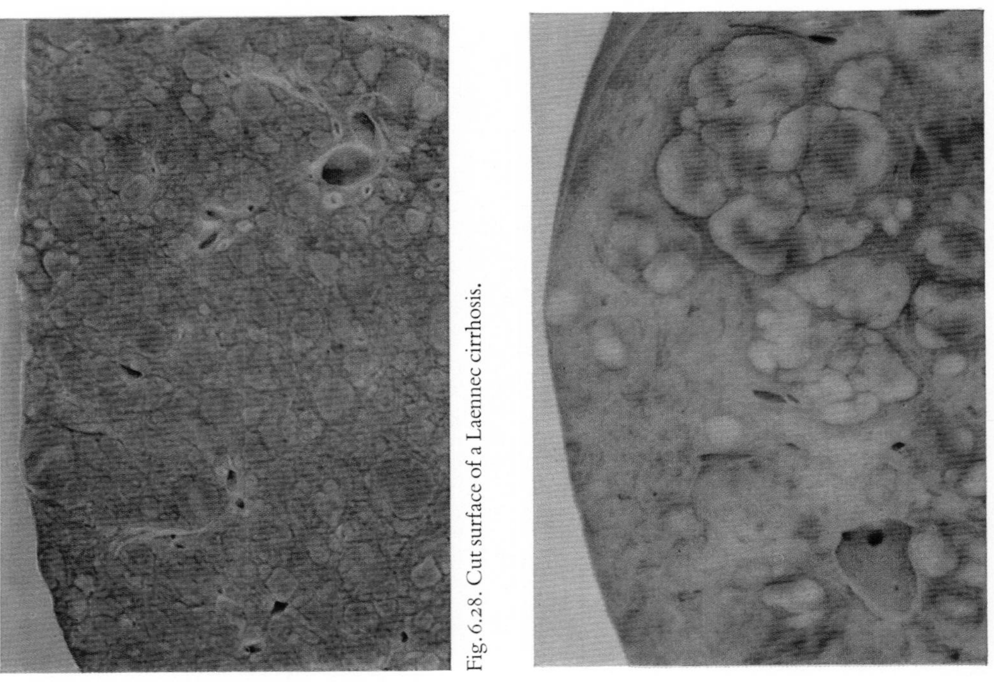

Fig. 6.27. Small nodular (Laennec) liver cirrhosis.

Fig. 6.28. Cut surface of a Laennec cirrhosis.

Fig. 6.29. Postnecrotic liver cirrhosis ("potato liver").

Fig. 6.30. Postnecrotic liver cirrhosis.

Cirrhosis of the Liver

(TCP, pp. 124, 125, 130 and 131)

Chronic progressive disease of the entire liver characterized by loss of parenchyma, lobular regeneration by connective tissue and nodular parenchymal regeneration. The disease leads to hepatic insufficiency and portal hypertension. (Definition according to Havana Conference, 1956.)

Hepatic fibrosis differs from cirrhosis: Increase in connective tissue without parenchymal loss or reconstruction. Blood flow through the liver lobule is intact, portal hypertension is absent. Hepatic fibrosis can be divided into periportal and interstitial types on histologic grounds.

Although no logical nomenclature exists to describe the various types of liver cirrhosis, pathogenetic and etiologic considerations are the basis for the existing classifications. Two main types are distinguished on the basis of *gross appearance* and *pathogenesis:*

1. **Laennec's cirrhosis:** small nudolar (so-called ordered cirrhosis of the liver) cirrhosis with parenchymal nodules ranging from 1 to 10 mm. (see also p. 11). Included in this group are septal or portal cirrhosis (fatty, biliary and pigmentary cirrhosis). A rare variant of this group is "hypertrophic cirrhosis." The liver is of normal-size or even enlarged (marked regeneration).

2. **Postnecrotic cirrhosis** (disordered cirrhosis of the liver) with parenchymal nodules 1–30 mm. in size and extended scarring areas. Postnecrotic cirrhosis must be distinguished from the *postnecrotic scar liver*, which consists of scars only, without cirrhotic reconstruction of the remaining liver tissue (e.g., only one lobe is affected, mostly the left lobe).

The *gross appearance of the cirrhotic liver basically is as follows:* The liver is smaller than usual and the lower margin is not sharp but rounded. The capsule is gray, opaque and often thickened. Nodules of various sizes and brown, yellow or green color are seen on the outer surface. The consistency is hard and leathery. The cutting knife is heard during dissection. The cut surface shows parenchymal nodules of different sizes that are delineated by connective tissue. The parenchymal nodules are brown and firm (normal liver tissue) or yellow (fatty changes) or yellow-green (fatty changes and jaundice) or green (jaundice) or yellow-green and soft (fresh necrosis) or yellow, dry and firm (fresh coagulation necrosis, see Fig. 6.25). The connective-tissue bridges are depressed below the surface of the parenchyma. The connective tissue is pink when capillaries are abundant or white-gray-silver after complete scarring (see also Fig. 6.26).

Figure 6.27 illustrates a case of Laennec's cirrhosis. Nodules of parenchymal tissue measure up to 1 cm. on the outer surface. Note the even nodularity of the surface *(hobnail liver)*. The parenchyma is yellow-brown due to minimal fatty change. Figure 6.28 shows the cut surface. The round, brown to brown-yellow nodules represent regenerative nodules. The liver cell cords or plates of the regenerative nodules are microscopically several cell layers wide and the nuclei are of irregular size. Smaller irregular islands are composed of remaining parenchyma with regular liver cell plates and small nuclei. The connective tissue bands are gray-white and depressed.

Microscopically, Laennec's cirrhosis can be subdivided into: (a) *portal, irregular* cirrhosis with broad connective-tissue bands dissecting the liver lobule ("portal" refers to regeneration arising from the periportal fields) and (b) *regular, septal* cirrhosis. The appearance resembles hog liver.

The gross appearance of postnecrotic cirrhosis varies, depending on the extent of scarring. Figure 6.29 shows a typical "potato liver." The left lobe is almost completely destroyed and converted into white scar tissue (→). In the right lobe, deeply depressed scars with funnel-like retractions and a gray-white base separate round, coarse parenchymal nodules of different sizes and yellow-brown color. Some nodules are small (in contrast to a pure *scar liver*, which has only coarse scars but no histologic evidence of a cirrhotic change). Note the flabby gallbladder, which does not contain bile. The cut surface (Fig. 6.30) illustrates the yellow parenchymal nodules of various sizes between broad, gray-red connective tissue scars.

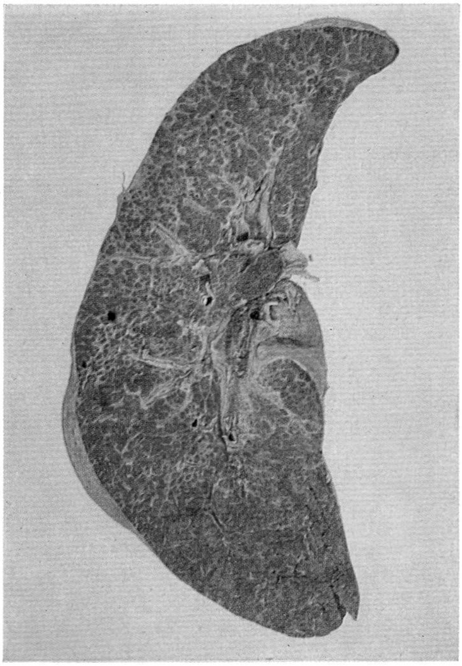

Fig. 6.33. Biliary cirrhosis of the liver.

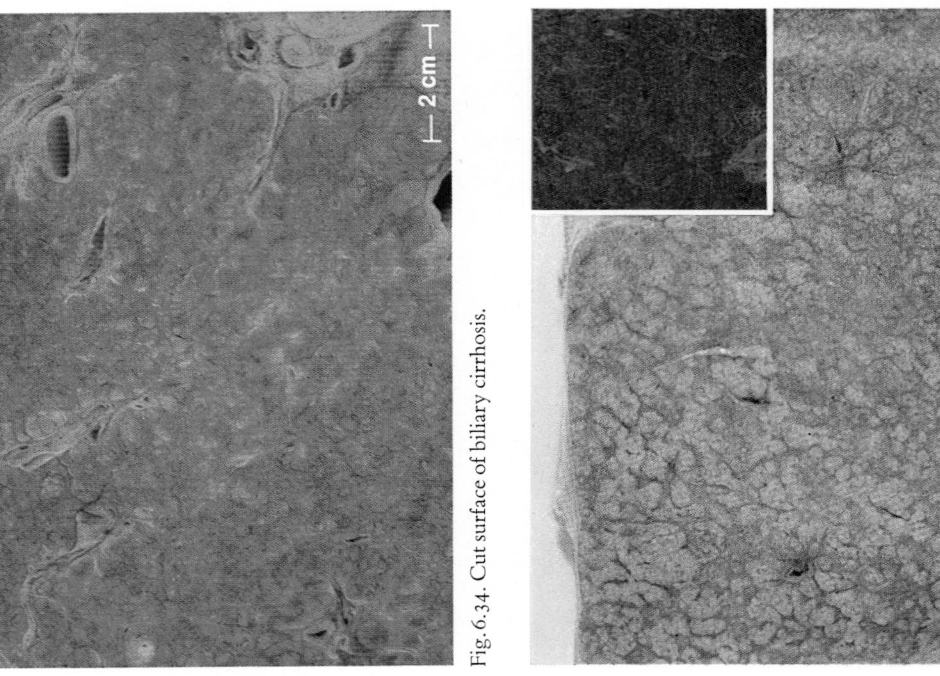

Fig. 6.34. Cut surface of biliary cirrhosis.

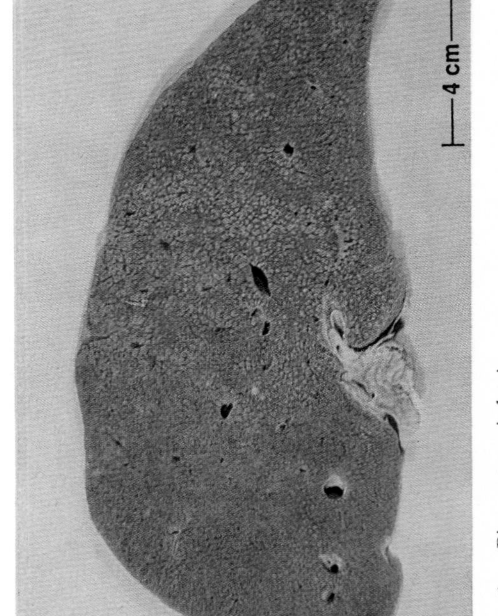

Fig. 6.35. Pigmentary cirrhosis.

Fig. 6.36. Pigmentary cirrhosis. (Inset: cut surface after Prussian blue staining.)

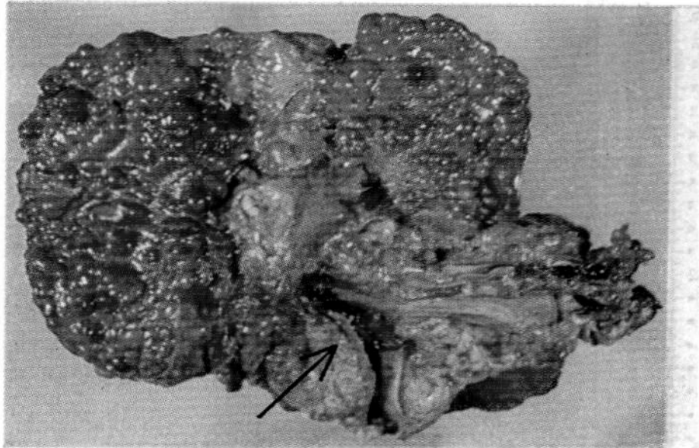

Fig. 6.31. Postnecrotic liver cirrhosis and thrombosis of the portal vein.

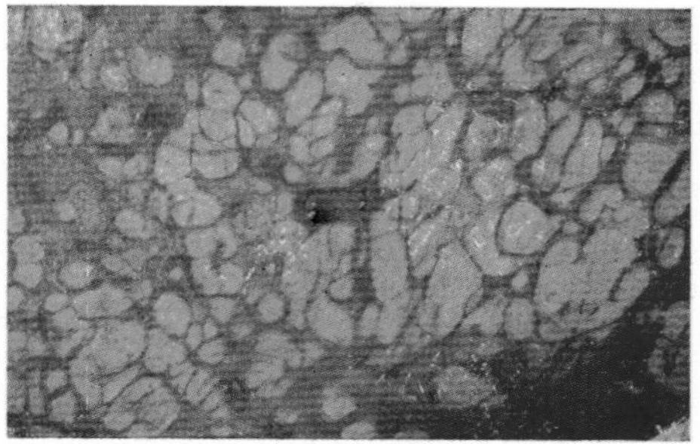

Fig. 6.32. Cut surface of a postnecrotic liver cirrhosis stained by van Gieson stain.

A different type of postnecrotic cirrhosis is illustrated in Figure 6.31. The bands of fibrous tissue are smaller than usual and irregular. The nodules differ in size and are brown. Note the fresh thrombosis of the portal vein (→), a typical complication of liver cirrhosis.

The connective-tissue strands of liver cirrhosis can be brought out in a gross specimen by the van Gieson stain, as it is used for histologic sections. The cut surface of a postnecrotic cirrhosis with bright-red bands of connective tissue and yellow islands of parenchyma is demonstrated in Figure 6.32.

F: 4–8% of all autopsy material. Portal (Laennec) cirrhosis accounts for 60% (♂:♀=4:1), postnecrotic cirrhosis for 20%, biliary cirrhosis for 13%, fatty cirrhosis for 5% and pigmentary cirrhosis for 2% of all cases of cirrhosis. *A:* 40–60 years. *S:* for all forms of cirrhosis, ♂:♀=2:1. *Pg:* see TCP, page 124. Laennec cirrhosis is caused not only by alcoholism (75%) but also by malnutrition (example: kwashiorkor, Gold Coast Bantus, especially methionine deficiency). Fatty liver → cirrhosis. *Co:* see page 155.

Biliary cirrhosis (Figs. 6.33 and 6.34). The main finding is jaundice of the liver. The surface is studded with coarse or small nodules. The cut surface reveals usually dark green parenchymal nodules surrounded by gray-white bands of connective tissue. The liver may be larger than normal in primary biliary cirrhosis.

The rare *primary biliary cirrhosis* afflicts predominantly females during the menopause. The cause is not known.

Secondary biliary cirrhosis develops as a result of chronic cholangitis and cholestasis. Occlusion of the bile ducts by stones or strictures usually is followed by an ascending infection (cholangitis and pericholangitis). On histologic examination, periportal fibrosis is prominent, but evidence of reconstruction of the lobular architecture is found only in advanced stages (TCP, p. 124).

Pigmentary cirrhosis (Figs. 6.35 and 6.36). *A consequence of a metabolic disturbance with hemosiderin deposits in the liver followed by cirrhosis.* The outer and cut surfaces resemble a Laennec cirrhosis with regard to the size and distribution of the regenerative nodules. Characteristic is the pale brown or ocher color of the parenchyma and the connective tissue. Our photographs show nodular liver parenchyma. The nodules are of even size. The brown color is due to hemosiderin storage. Hemosiderin can be stained by the Prussian blue reaction (see inset of Fig. 6.36).

A: 50–60 years. *S:* predominantly males. *Pg:* chronic hemolysis, repeated transfusions *(hemosiderotic pigmentary cirrhosis)* or a manifestation of hemochromatosis *(hemochromatotic pigmentary cirrhosis).*

Hemochromatosis is characterized by pigmentary cirrhosis of the liver and pancreas and by hemosiderosis of the pancreas, salivary glands, heart, spleen, lymph nodes and skin ("bronze diabetes").

Certain inborn errors of metabolism are accompanied by liver cirrhosis: glycogenosis (Type IV); Gaucher's disease; Wilson's disease (hepatolenticular degeneration with increased copper deposition; a deficiency of copper-binding ceruloplasmin); galactosemia; atransferrinemia; and mucoviscidosis (Thaler).

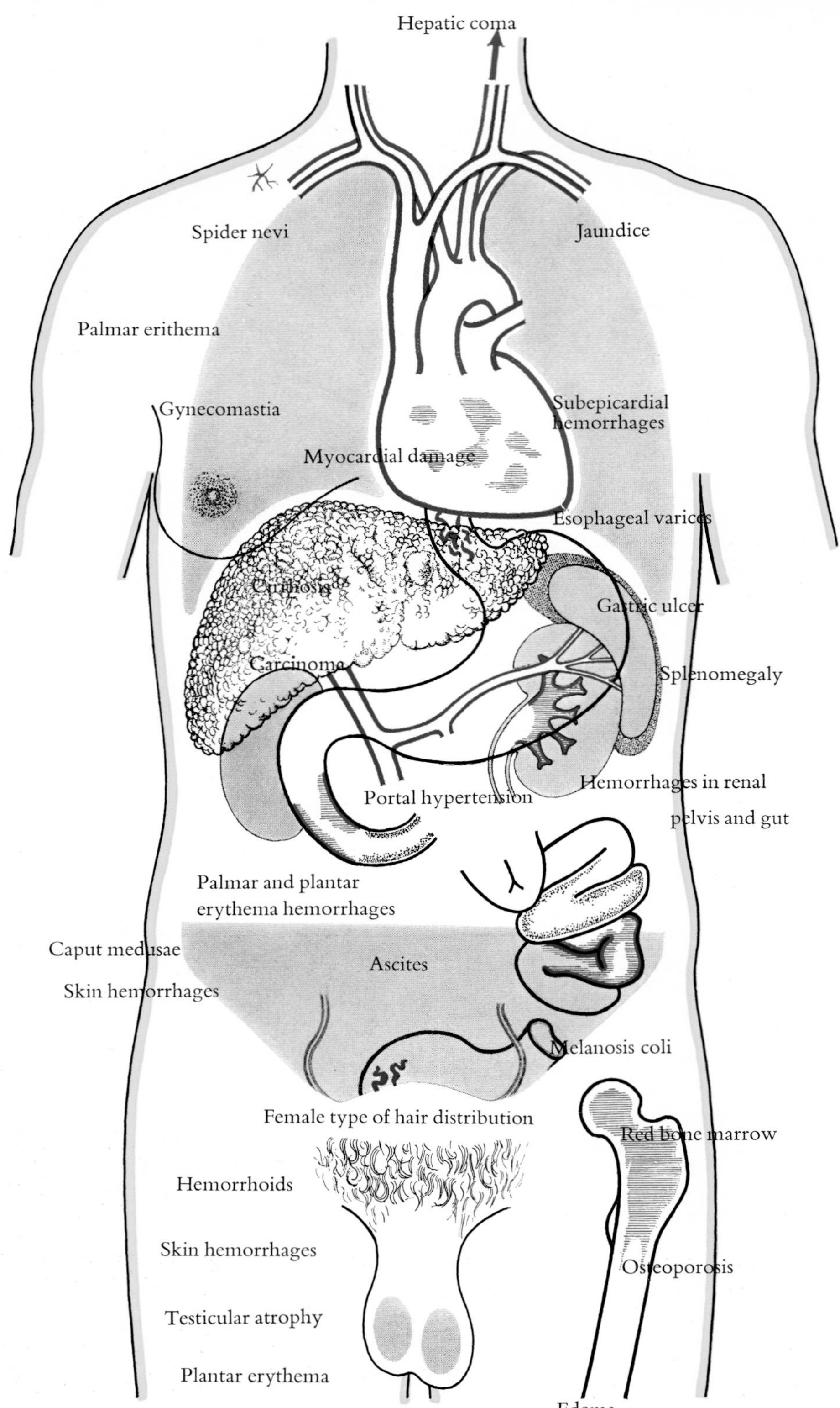

Fig. 6.37. Symptoms and complications of liver cirrhosis.

Complications of liver cirrhosis

1. **Portal hypertension** (Portal vein pressure: normal 100; 350–500 mm. H_2O in cirrhosis). *Causes:* Compression of portal vein branches by connective tissue (venous block) or intrahepatic venous anastomoses. Often secondary portal vein thrombosis due to slow blood flow. *Other causes of portal hypertension:* cardiac failure, Budd-Chiari syndrome, tumor, thrombosis.

   Co: ascites (stasis, hypoalbuminemia and loss of NaCl). *Esophageal varices* → *hemorrhage* (cause of death in 25% of cases). *Caput medusae. Congestive splenomegaly* (see p. 181). *Bone marrow inhibition* → anemia, leukocytopenia → increased incidence of infections. *Congestion* of gastrointestinal tract → *ulcerations* of the gastrointestinal tract (primary?, secondary?). Ulcers in 15% of cirrhotic patients.
2. **Hemorrhagic diathesis** (prothrombin and fibrinogen are diminished, since the total liver parenchyma is decreased). Thrombocytopenia. Hypersplenism. Latent, disseminated coagulation.
3. **Hormonal disturbances.** Estrogen is incompletely metabolized in the liver, resulting in *hyperestrogenism:* in males, testicular atrophy, female type of hair distribution, fat hips and gynecomastia. In females, menstruation ceases. Osteoporosis. Hyperaldosteronism → edema.
4. **Myocardial damage** due to hypoalbuminemia?
5. **Edema** (hypoalbuminemia, hyperaldosteronism).
6. **Icterus** (70% of cases).
7. **Hepatic coma** (cause of death in 30–60% of cases).
8. **Primary liver cell carcinoma** (3% of cases).
9. Clinical and morphologic signs of **chronic pancreatitis** (alcohol?).
10. **CNS :** so-called liver glia.

Prognosis

After a diagnosis of cirrhosis, the 5-year survival rate is 4–15%. In 50% of the cirrhoses, the diagnosis is made clinically.

Hepatitis

(TCP, p. 124–127).

Acute or chronic hepatitis rarely is seen at autopsy either because the disease heals or the patient dies later from liver cirrhosis. The liver surface can be examined directly by laparoscopy. This technic was introduced by the Dresden surgeon KELLING in 1901. A liver biopsy can be obtained simultaneously under direct visualization (in contrast to the blind biopsy introduced by IVERSEN and ROHOLM, see BECK).

Figure 6.38 shows the right liver lobe with a smooth surface. Distinct markings are seen in the area of the highlight in this picture. These correspond to liver lobules. The color is brown. The gallbladder is seen below the pointed anterior liver margin.

The liver surface is bright red in *acute viral hepatitis* (Fig. 6.39). The surface is smooth, lobular markings are distinct and the anterior margin is rounded.

Figure 6.40 illustrates a transition to *subacute hepatitis*. The liver surface is finely granular. Hyperemia, fatty changes and beginning fibrosis are evident. The white specks on the surface are interpreted as perihepatitis. In chronic hepatitis, the surface is markedly granular and brown.

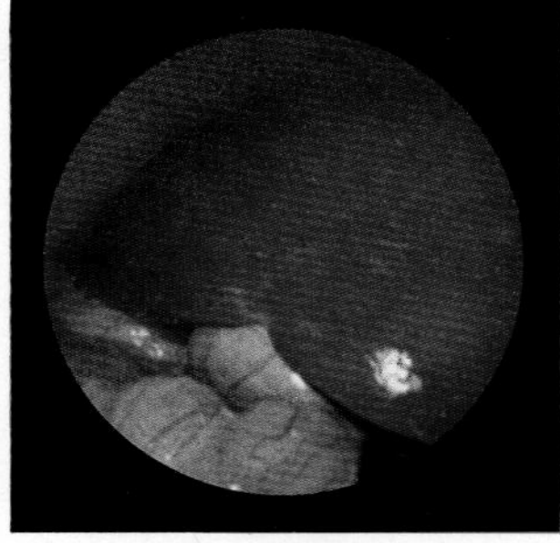

Fig. 6.38. Normal liver.

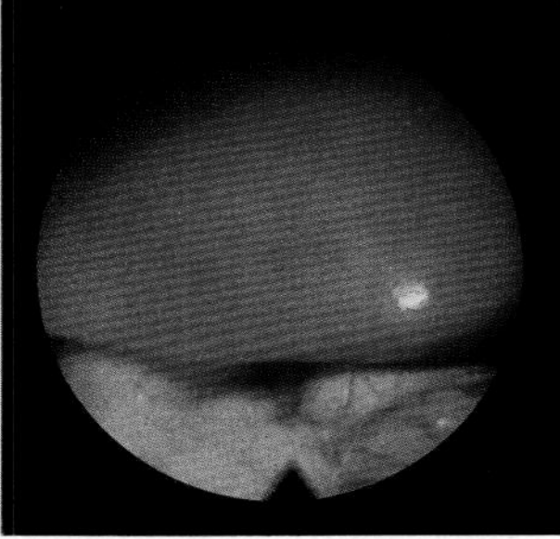

Fig. 6.39. Acute viral hepatitis.

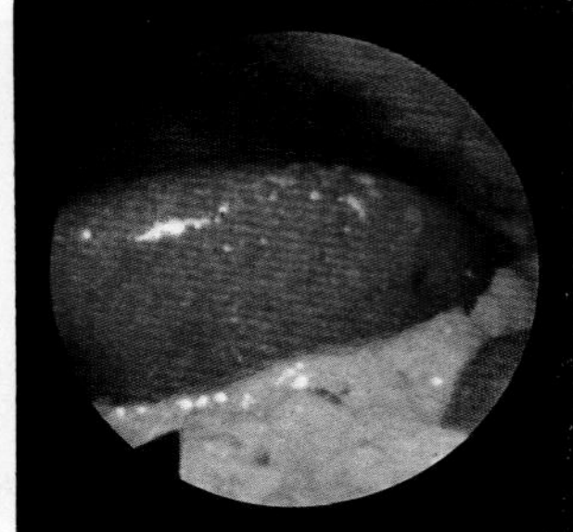

Fig. 6.40. Subacute viral hepatitis.

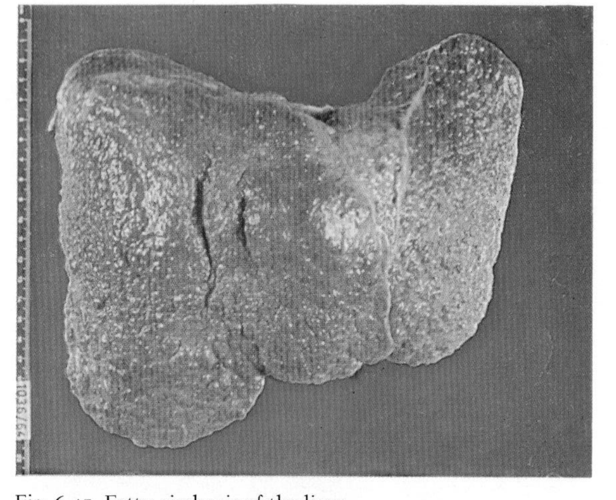

Fig. 6.41. Fatty cirrhosis of the liver.

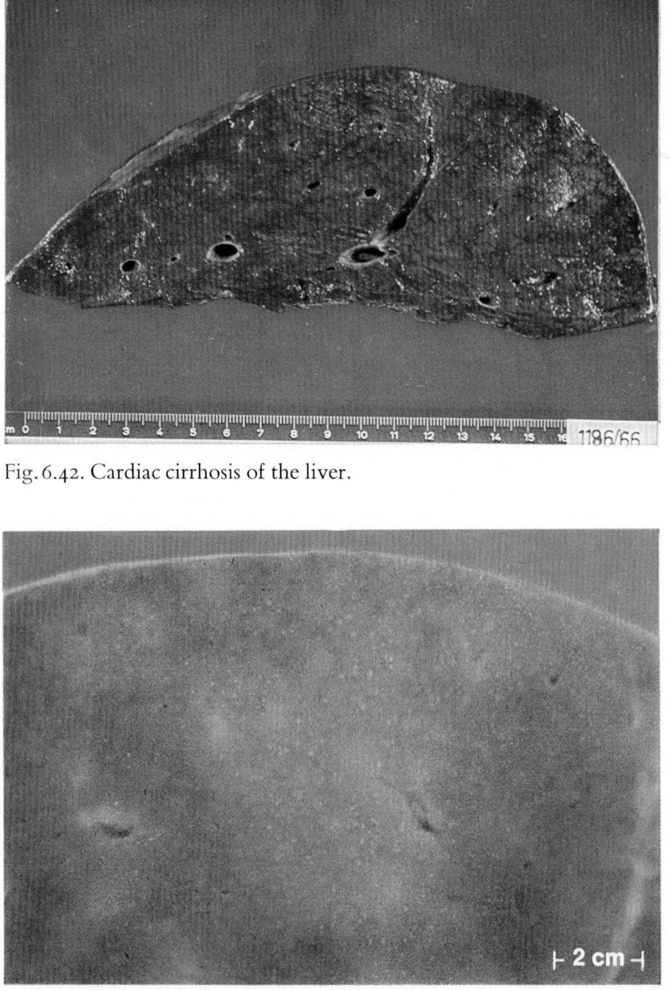

Fig. 6.42. Cardiac cirrhosis of the liver.

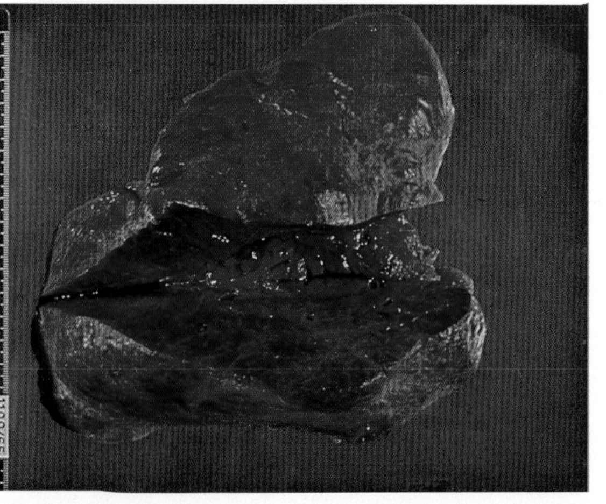

Fig. 6.43. Thorotrast liver.

Fig. 6.44. Congenital syphilis of the liver.

Course and prognosis

Approximately 10% of acute hepatitis (H.) becomes chronic. According to recent investigations, only 14% of chronic H. terminates in liver cirrhosis (effect of therapy?), previously estimated to be 30–50%. Thirty-five per cent of chronic H. heals with fibrosis, whereas a chronic, active disease process is observed for years in 51% of the cases (observation period 5 years) (VIDO and co-workers). The earlier the diagnosis is made the better the prognosis.

Chronic persistent H. has the best prognosis (lasts for up to 10 years), although transition into a chronic aggressive H. occurs in about 10% of the patients.

Chronic aggressive H. (cellular infiltrates extend into the liver parenchyma, with so-called moth-eaten necrosis) terminates as cirrhosis in only 10% of the cases, whereas 40% of chronic necrotizing H. develops into cirrhosis.

Special Types of Liver Cirrhosis and Fibroses

Fatty cirrhosis (Fig. 6.41; TCP, p. 131). Markedly enlarged liver (up to 2,500 Gm.) of firm consistency, yellow color and finely nodular surface. On cut surface, reconstruction by narrow bands of connective tissue is seen. Yellow islands of parenchyma are separated by small, gray connective-tissue bands (fibrosis without regeneration; TCP, p. 131).

F: 5% of all liver cirrhoses. *Pg:* generalized obesity. "Fatty infiltration" of the liver. In about 15% of diabetics (lipolysis). Alcoholic fatty liver ("Mallory bodies"). Malnutrition (methionine deficiency). Toxic, nutritional fatty changes in the liver represent one of the most common biopsy diagnoses.

Cardiac cirrhosis (Fig. 6.42). Chronic congestion of the liver leads to fibrosis (induration) and later to parenchymal regeneration. This is referred to as "cardiac cirrhosis." The liver is firm and dark brown-red. The capsule is thickened and the outer surface is small and nodular. The cut surface is chronically congested, the connective tissue is distinctly increased and parenchymal reconstruction is moderately severe.

F: the fully developed picture of cardiac cirrhosis is rare, since cardiac patients usually do not survive long enough. Age and sex distribution are dependent on the underlying causes (decompensated cor pulmonale, Budd-Chiari syndrome [see p. 147], constrictive pericarditis). *Pg:* replacement of areas of chronic congestion by connective tissue (TCP, p. 121).

Thorotrast liver (Fig. 6.43). *Prolonged Thorotrast storage with hepatic fibrosis* (α-emitter, 25% colloidal thorium dioxide). *Thorotrast was used in the past as an x-ray contrast medium.* Our picture shows a small liver with considerable capsular fibrosis. The parenchyma is firm and dark brown-red on cut surface. Note the white strips of connective tissue extending through the brown-red liver parenchyma.

F: Thorotrast is stored in macrophages in the RES of the liver, spleen and other organs. A progressive fibrosis develops, since Thorotrast is not metabolized or excreted and has a long half-life. *Co:* Malignant tumors (hemangioendotheliomas or carcinomas). *Mi:* Thorotrast is an α-emitter demonstrable by autoradiography. Gray, granular masses in H & E sections.

The liver in congenital syphilis (Fig. 6.44; TCP, p. 123). *Intrauterine infection with spirochetes results in diffuse hepatic fibrosis.* On gross examination, the liver is somewhat enlarged and the external surface is smooth and grayish brown. The cut surface is dirty brown and firm. Tiny, pinhead sized, grayish brown lesions are seen on cut surface at higher magnification (Fig. 6.44). These represent syphilomas (= syphilitic granulomas).

F: extremely rare in autopsy material. *Pg:* transplacental syphilitic infection.

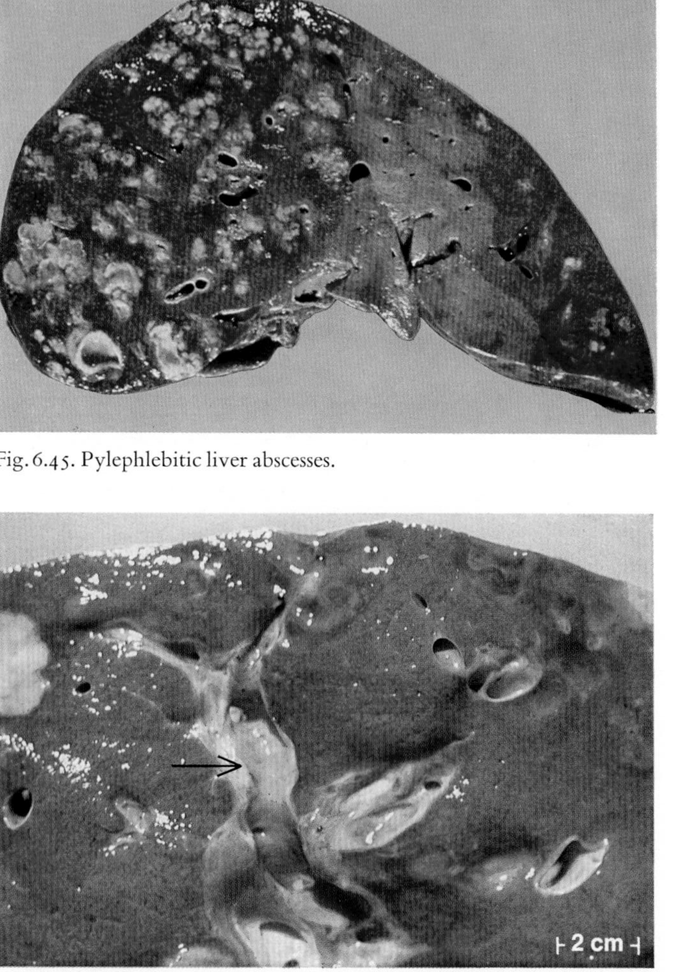

Fig. 6.45. Pylephlebitic liver abscesses.

Fig. 6.47. Cholangitic liver abscess and metastases from a carcinoma of the pancreas.

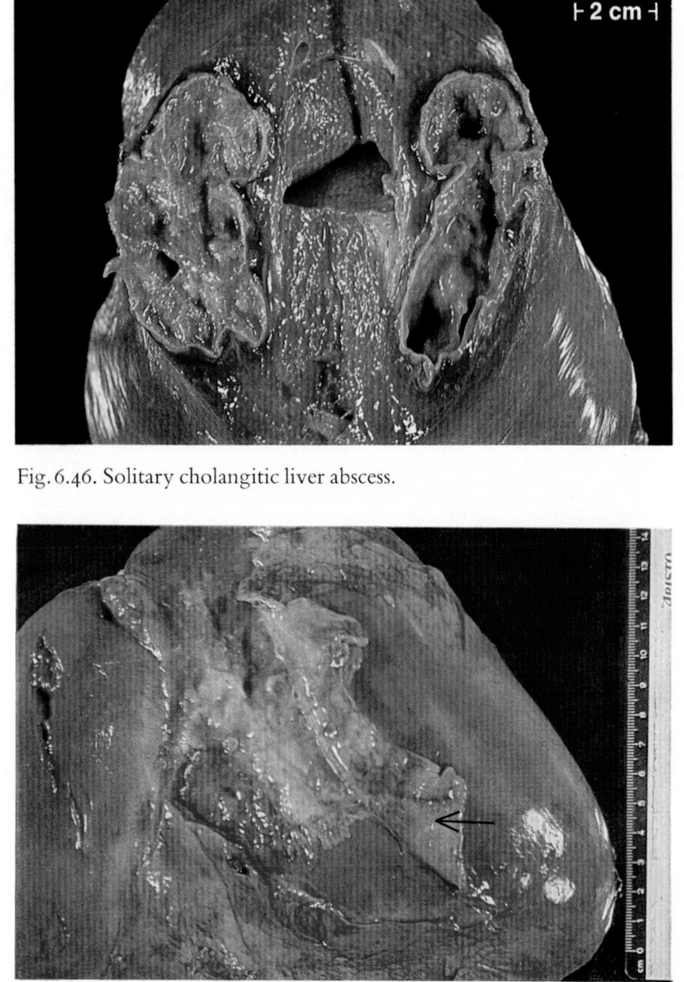

Fig. 6.46. Solitary cholangitic liver abscess.

Fig. 6.48. Subphrenic empyema.

Liver Abscesses

Pylephlebitic liver abscesses (Fig. 6.45). They are caused by purulent bacterial thrombophlebitis in the tributaries of the portal vein. Abscesses in the right liver lobe usually are due to purulent infection of the small or large intestine (appendix, diverticula). Predominant involvement of the left lobe points to the splenic vein, stomach or pancreas as the possible source of infection. Figure 6.45 shows multiple groups of necrotic foci with yellow or whitish liquid content and smooth linings. The abscess membrane is identified as a thin white membrane, which indicates an older infection (see left lower portion of Fig. 6.45). The liver tissue is dark brown-red between the abscesses (Zahn infarction).

F: rare. *Pg:* purulent bacterial thrombophlebitis in the portal vein system → septic embolism → abscess. *Causes:* in *newborns,* an infected umbilical wound (omphalitis) with inflammation of the umbilical vein (omphalophlebitis). In *adults,* most often due to a perityphlic abscess (appendicitis). Other causes are tumors of the stomach and pancreas or diverticula that become secondarily infected.
DD: (1) *cholangitic abscesses* (Fig. 6.46). Membranes and content are dark green discolored by bile, preferential subcapsular location and not confined to one liver lobe; (2) *pyemic abscess via the hepatic artery* seen especially in bacterial endocarditis. Diffuse distribution in the liver and other organs (lungs, kidneys, spleen). *Co: perforation:* subphrenic empyema, diffuse peritonitis. *Hepatic failure:* hepatic coma.

Solitary liver abscess (Fig. 6.46). This circumscribed, encapsulated, purulent process almost always is caused by a secondary infection. Figure 6.46 shows the cut surface of a liver with a solitary old abscess following *ascending cholangitis.* The peripheral folded brown band (2 mm. thick) represents the abscess wall or membrane, which is covered by chocolate-like, semiliquid material.

F: uncommon in autopsy material. *S:* ♀>♂. *Pg:* most frequently a complication of an inflamed gallbladder or bile ducts *(cholangitic solitary abscess).* In addition, a *solitary pylephlebitic abscess* may develop from an inflammatory focus in the portal vein system. In the tropics: amebic abscess!

Cholangitic liver abscesses (Fig. 6.47; TCP, p. 123). Ascending, purulent infection of intrahepatic bile ducts with severe cholestasis. Figure 6.47 shows greatly dilated and fibrosed bile ducts (→) with thick, green contents. (Most of the material was removed to demonstrate the bile ducts.) Several green cholangitic abscesses (up to 1 cm.) are seen in the subcapsular liver. In this case, the obstruction of intrahepatic bile ducts was attributed to metastatic nodules from a carcinoma of the pancreas (a metastasis is shown at the left in this picture).

Pg: common in cholelithiasis, cholecystitis or bile duct carcinomas: cholestatis with superimposed infection.

Subdiaphragmatic (subphrenic) empyema (Fig. 6.48). *Purulent inflammation in the preformed space between the upper liver surface and the diaphragm* (therefore the term empyema and not abscess!). The diaphragm is cut and folded upward (→). Yellow pus covers the liver surface. The pus has been partly removed.

Pg: subphrenic empyema usually is a complication of purulent infection in an adjacent organ, such as a perforated liver abscess, peptic ulcer or extension of pleural empyema.

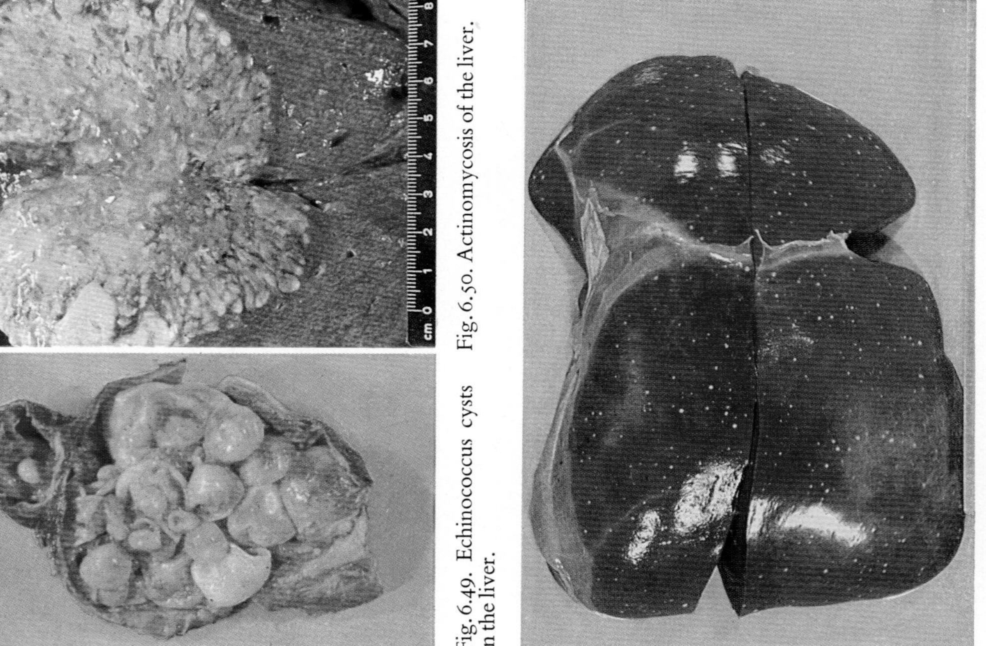

Fig. 6.49. Echinococcus cysts in the liver.

Fig. 6.50. Actinomycosis of the liver.

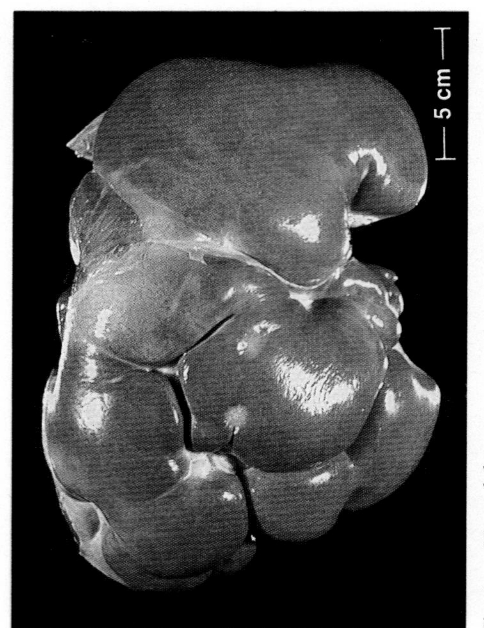

Fig. 6.51. Hepar lobatum.

Fig. 6.52. Miliary tuberculosis of the liver.

Fig. 6.53. Listeriosis of the liver.

Parasites, Specific Inflammations

Echinococcus hydatidosus *(cysticus)* of the liver (Fig. 6.49; TCP, pp. 282 and 283). *Hydatid cysts or vesicles develop in the liver of humans (intermediate host) after infection with* Taenia echinococcus *(dog tapeworm)*. Multiple daughter cysts may develop from a large unilocular cyst, as shown in this photograph of a surgical specimen. The cysts are composed of a capsule (cuticle) and contain a clear fluid, scolices (heads) or hooklets (smear!).

F: dependent on geographic factors. Example: 351 cases in Switzerland during the period 1956–1969. Infection with *Echinococcus cysticus* occurs almost exclusively in childhood. *Pg:* echinococcus eggs (oncospheres) are passed with dog's feces and swallowed by children. The eggs reach the liver from the gastrointestinal tract via the portal vein (65% of cases) or enter into the general circulation via the thoracic duct (lung, brain, bones, etc.). The hydatid vesicles may be sterile (acephalocyst) or produce daughter cysts by proliferation and secondary cystic degeneration of the scolices. *Histologically* (TCP, p. 281), cyst walls with collagenous fibrous tissue are found in these circumstances. In addition to *E. cysticus*, the liver also may be involved by *E. alveolaris*, which affects adults only. Many smaller cysts develop, together with a stroma rich in collagenous fibers. This form of echinococcus infection often is confused with a malignant tumor on gross examination.

Actinomycosis of the liver (Fig. 6.50; TCP, pp. 276 and 277). *Chronic abscessive inflammation of the liver due to hematogenous spread of* Actinomyces israeli *(bacterium, not a fungus!) from a primary infection of mucous membranes (gut) or extension from neighboring organs (pleura, lung)*. Grossly, rather large, centrally necrotic foci of gray-yellow color contain stringy pus. Actinomycosis of the liver presents as an isolated focus (as in our case) or as multiple, disseminated abscess. Larger rosette-like abscesses may form by coalescence.

F: rare. Histologically, granulation tissue with numerous foam cells in the abscess membrane is seen. In the center of the abscess, the typical fungi are shown (sulfur granules). *Co:* penetration into the peritoneum or formation of fistulous tracts through the abdominal wall. The floor of the mouth, cervical region, and lung are most frequently affected (survey by Brown, 1973).

Hepar lobatum (Fig. 6.51). The characteristic picture of a coarsely lobulated liver results from the retraction of the surface by healed syphilitic gummas (gumma = gum-like consistency). Fresh gummas are gray-yellow and soft. Later on, they become gray-white, dry and rubbery due to fibrous-tissue organization. The rubbery gumma is found at the base of the retracted surface scar.

F: very rare at autopsy (in contrast to syphilitic mesaortitis). *Pg:* tertiary lues. *DD:* postnecrotic cirrhosis of the liver; other necrotizing granulomatous inflammations (tuberculosis); tumors.

Miliary tuberculosis of the liver (Fig. 6.52). Nodular, diffuse, serosal tubercles following tuberculous dissemination. Figure 6.52 reveals gray-white foci (up to 2 mm.) that are distributed evenly throughout the outer and cut surfaces.

Miliary tuberculosis involves the liver (90%) in addition to the lung. Predominantly affected are *children* (early generalization, see p. 86) or *elderly persons* with diminished resistance (tumors). The hematogenous dissemination is initiated from exacerbated lung or lymph node lesions. A so-called *sepsis tuberculosa acutissima Landouzy* may develop in such cases. The necrotic lesions of Landouzy sepsis usually are larger than miliary tubercles. Miliary tuberculosis has to be distinguished from occasional single miliary tubercles, which occur in the liver with organ tuberculosis. *DD* for miliary tuberculosis of the liver: sarcoidosis, listeriosis, syphiloma.

Listeriosis of the liver (Fig. 6.53). *Miliary necrosis in the liver of infants. The lesions are caused by* Listeria monocytogenes *(argyrophilic, gram-positive rods)*. Grossly, diffuse, gray-yellow miliary (and smaller) lesions are found in the liver, lungs, kidneys and other organs.

F: rare granulomatous disease of newborns ("granulomatosis infantiseptica"). Histologically, the granulomas consist of histiocytes, epithelioid cells and occasional giant cells. Infections with Listeria can lead to repeated abortions.

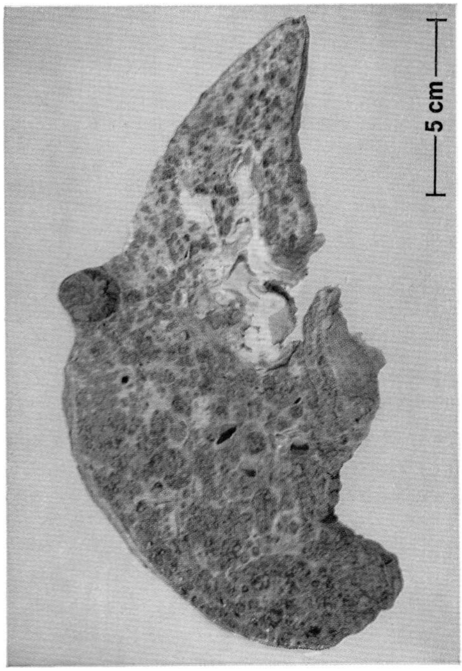

Fig. 6.54. Biliary cirrhosis and hepatocellular adenoma.

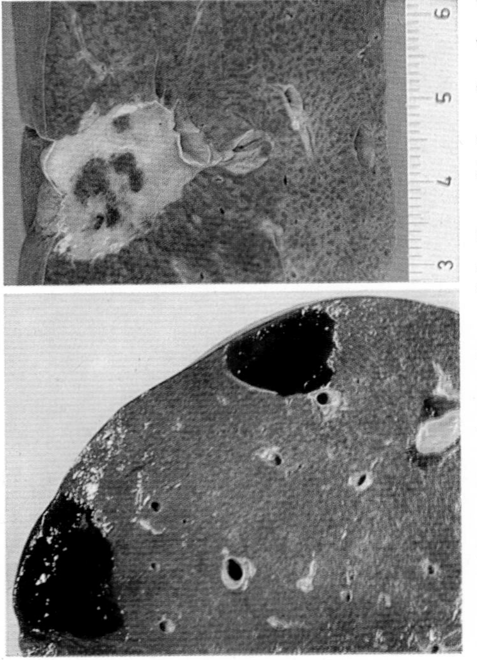

Fig. 6.55. (a) cavernous hemangioma of the liver; (b) thrombosed and organized cavernous hemangioma.

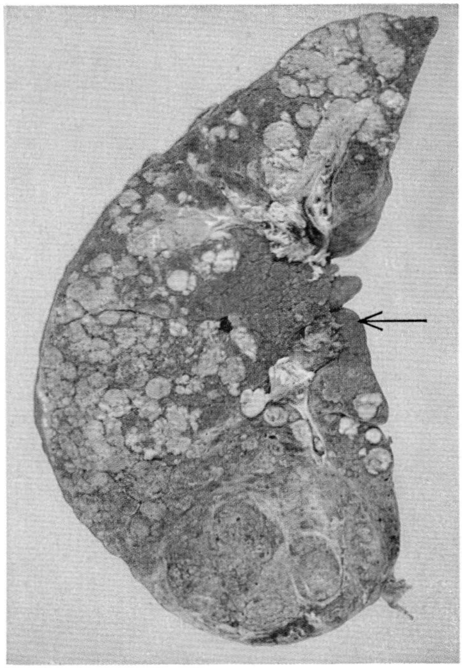

Fig. 6.56. Hepatocellular carcinoma (malignant hepatoma).

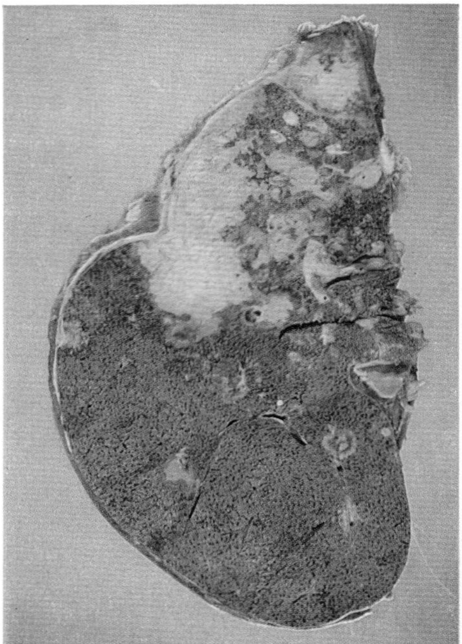

Fig. 6.57. Carcinoma of intrahepatic bile ducts (malignant cholangioma).

Tumors

Hepatocellular adenoma (benign hepatoma, Fig. 6.54; TCP, p. 241). *Circumscribed, benign tumor composed of proliferating hepatocytes.* Figure 6.54 shows a greenish discolored nodule (jaundice of adenoma) that projects over the upper surface of a liver with biliary cirrhosis. Benign hepatomas are difficult to distinguish from the nodular hyperplasia of liver cirrhosis. The adenoma grows by expansion, leading to pressure atrophy of the surrounding liver tissue.

F: rare. Histologically (TCP), an adenoma consists of liver cell plates or tubules. Fatty changes may be observed. *DD:* cholangioma (adenomas of bile duct epithelium are gray-green in color and firm in consistency); regenerating liver nodules in cirrhosis, solitary tumor metastasis, syphilitic gumma.

Cavernoma of the liver (Fig. 6.55, a and b; TCP, p. 260).

Tumor-like malformation (hamartoma) composed of cavernous capillaries. Hemangiomas usually reach the liver surface and present as dark red, sharply circumscribed foci. On cut surface, dark red venous blood exudes from a fine network after cutting.

F: not too uncommon, accidental finding, especially in older people. Histologically, blood-filled cystic spaces are lined by endothelium. *Co:* as a rule, cavernomas remain stationary for some time. Thrombi frequently develop, with subsequent organization into a fibrous mass. Such an organized cavernoma (Fig. 6.55 b) has the gray-white color of scar tissue with a central blood-containing space. A hamartoma rarely transforms into a proliferating neoplasm (hamartoblastoma), which is difficult to distinguish from a hemangioendothelioma.

Liver cell carcinoma (malignant hepatoma, hepatocellular carcinoma, Fig. 6.56).

Malignant tumor of hepatocytes, which arises in 95% of cases from a pre-existing cirrhosis. The carcinoma may consist of larger nodules or several smaller tumors (multicentric origin or intrahepatic metastases). The neoplasm is of soft consistency (scanty stroma). Hemorrhages, areas of necrosis and alternating yellow (fatty change) or green (jaundice) nodules are present. Our figure reveals multiple yellow, soft tumor nodules of various sizes, which are scattered throughout the liver. Note also the cirrhosis (→).

F: primary liver cancers are found in 0.3% of all autopsies (< 2% of malignant tumors, 3% of all seroses of the liver). *A:* 93% of patients are older than 50 years. *S:* ♂:♀ = 2:1. Liver cancer in small children (hepatoblastoma or mixed liver tumor) arises in livers without cirrhosis.

Pg: exogenous factors: arsenicals, Thorotrast. With *sufficiently long survival*, approximately 3% of all cirrhotic livers (20% of all pigmentary cirrhosis) will develop a hepatocellular carcinoma.

Metastases: intrahepatic; lymph nodes of the liver hilus and lungs. Tumor thrombosis of the portal vein. See Figure 6.58 (→1). *DD:* metastases to the liver (choriocarcinoma); hemangioendothelioma; nodular hyperplasias of liver cirrhosis.

Primary carcinoma of intrahepatic bile ducts (malignant cholangioma, cholangiocellular carcinoma; Fig. 6.57).

Glandular, stroma-rich carcinoma of larger intrahepatic bile ducts that presents as a single large tumor mass in most cases. A white, firm (connective-tissue stroma) neoplasm is found in the left liver lobe (Fig. 6.57). In our case, cirrhosis was not present and jaundice was attributed to tumor obstruction of larger bile ducts.

F: rare tumor (approximately 0.4% of all malignant tumors, five times less common than hepatocellular carcinoma). Histologically, carcinoma with small glands or alveoli, extensive stroma and mucus formation. The bile ducts of the tumor-free liver are dilated and filled with bile.

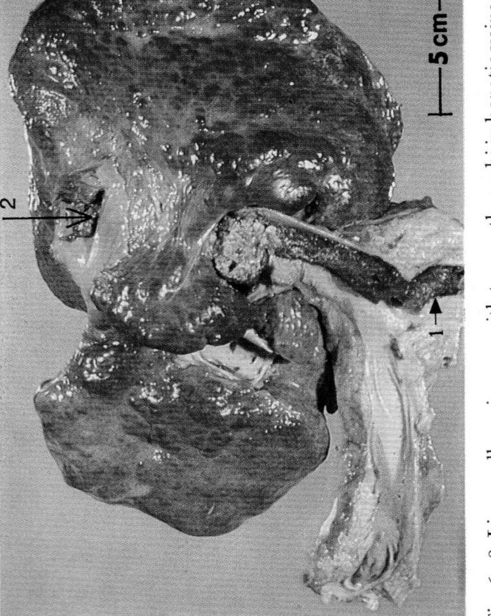

Fig. 6.58. Liver-cell carcinoma with tumor thrombi in hepatic veins.

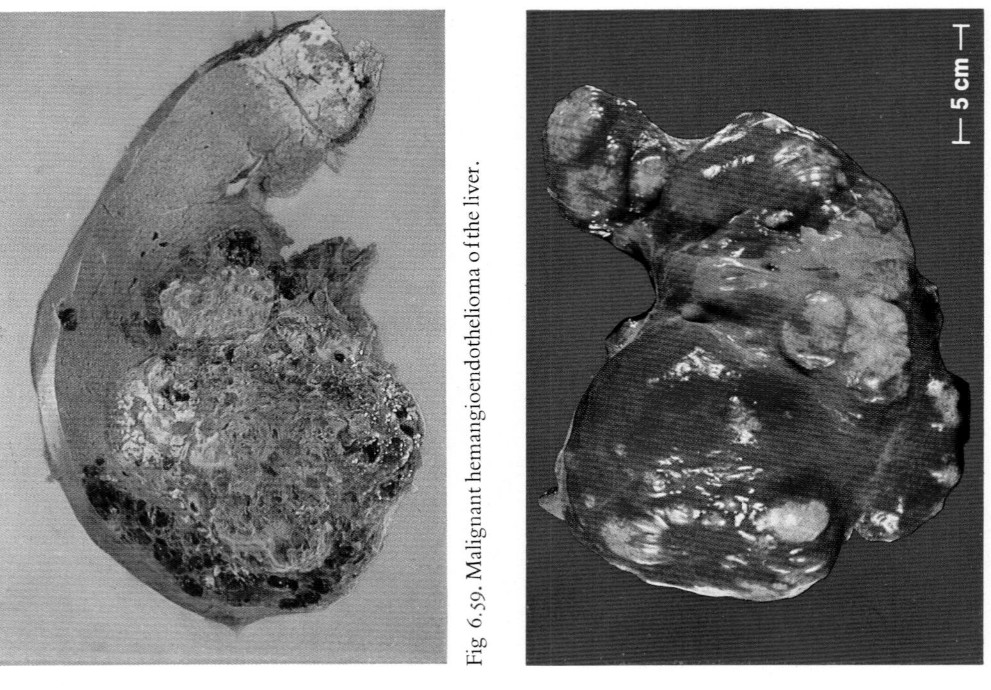

Fig 6.59. Malignant hemangioendothelioma of the liver.

Fig. 6.60. Myeloid leukemia.

Fig. 6.61. Lymphatic leukemia.

Fig. 6.62. Metastases in the liver.

Tumor thrombi in hepatic veins from a primary liver-cell carcinoma (Fig. 6.58).

Figure 6.58 shows large tumor thrombi in several lumina of the portal vein (→1) and hepatic veins (→2). The nodular, irregular lower liver margin suggests cirrhosis. The presence of tumor thrombi indicates liver-cell carcinoma. Important for DD: nodular hyperplasia, adenoma or carcinoma.

Acute portal hypertension with therapy-resistant ascites results from tumor thrombi in the portal vein.

Malignant hemangioendothelioma (Fig. 6.59).

Metastases from choriocarcinomas and primary hepatic hemangioendotheliomas give rise to blood-rich liver tumors. Figure 6.59 consists of large, hemorrhagic nodules with gray-yellow necrotic central portions. Figure 6.59 also illustrates an extensive area of parenchymal necrosis in the left lobe. Portions of the lobe were resected because the hemangioendothelioma had bled into the abdominal cavity.

F: rare tumor (approximately 0.02% of autopsies). Increased frequency with storage of Thorotrast or arsenicals. Cirrhosis coexists in 20–30% of cases. *Pg:* endothelial cells – especially Kupffer cells – are considered cells of origin. Histologically, the tumor is composed of spindle or polymorphous cells with endothelial, blood-rich clefts. *Co:* metastases to the lungs and lymph nodes; spontaneous rupture and hemorrhage in the abdominal cavity. *DD:* liver-cell carcinoma, metastasizing choriocarcinoma.

Leukemic infiltration of the liver (Figs. 6.60 and 6.61; TCP, p. 133).

The liver may be involved by such systemic diseases as leukemias, reticuloses or storage diseases. The liver becomes diffusely enlarged (up to 800 Gm.), light brown and soft.

In *myeloid leukemia* (Fig. 6.60), the lobular markings are effaced because of diffuse brown infiltrates. The lobules are better preserved in *lymphatic leukemia* (Fig. 6.61) because small, gray-white nodules are formed in the periportal fields.

F, *A* and *S:* see page 193.

Liver metastases (Fig. 6.62).

Next to the lung, the liver is the most common site of hematogenous metastases from distant primary sites. Metastases reach the liver via the portal vein (tumors of the gastrointestinal tract or pancreas, occasionally also tumors of the genital organs), hepatic artery (carcinomas of the lung, breast and thyroid) or by direct extension (the gallbladder). The tumor nodules are of various sizes and the surface is centrally retracted (cancer umbilicus = epithelial tumor. Central necrosis due to hypoxia). The tumor-free liver tissue occasionally shows a dark brown discoloration (Zahn infarction).

F: 25–36% of all malignant tumors metastasize to the liver. The frequency of liver metastases increases to 50% when primary tumors arise in organs drained by the portal vein. Liver metastases are eighteen times as common as primary liver carcinomas. The frequencies of metastases in the liver from different carcinomas are: pancreas 50%, gallbladder 40%, lung 36%, stomach and colon each 33%, breast 32%, esophagus 23%, thyroid gland 18%, uterus and ovary 12%.

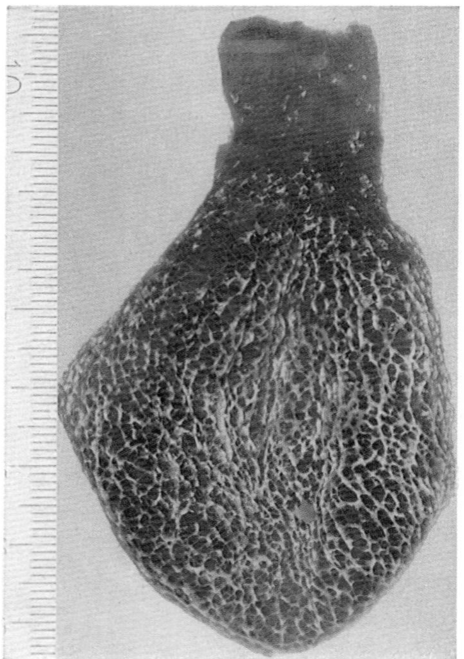

Fig. 7.1. Cholesterolosis of the gallbladder.

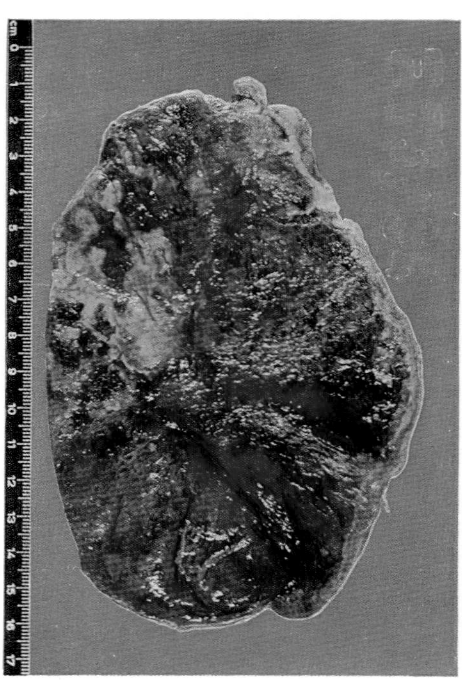

Fig. 7.2. Acute hemorrhagic necrotizing cholecystitis.

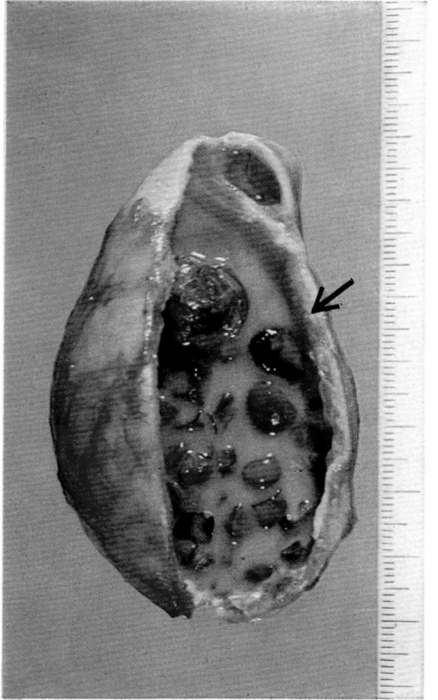

Fig. 7.3. Cholelithiasis with chronic cholecystitis and empyema.

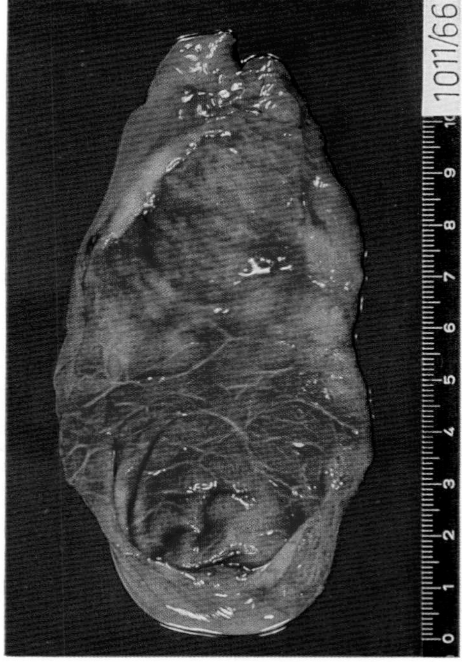

Fig. 7.4. Chronic cholecystitis (scarred gallbladder) with hydrops.

7. Gallbladder - Bile Ducts

Malformations, Cholecystitis

Malformations are rare. A *hypoplastic* gallbladder is seen occasionally (*DD:* chronic cholecystitis with shrunken gallbladder). *Cyst formation* in the ductus choledochus. Congenital *atresia* of extrahepatic bile ducts produces severe postnatal jaundice.

Cholesterolosis is a harmless change in the gallbladder without clinical significance. The wall of the gallbladder is thin (Fig. 7.1). The mucosa shows small yellow stippling or a delicate yellow network ("strawberry gallbladder"). (*Mi:* cholesterol deposits in mucosal histiocytes.)

Common in females; 40–60 years; 15% of autopsies.

Cholecystitis

Inflammation of the gallbladder frequently accompanied by cholelithiasis.

Acute hemorrhagic necrotizing cholecystitis (Fig. 7.2).

Figure 7.2 shows severe mucosal necrosis (yellow), hemorrhages (dark red) and greenish discolored areas (necrosis with bile deposits). The gallbladder is enlarged. A stone occluded the cystic duct and the gallbladder also was filled with stones. The thickened wall suggests chronic cholecystitis.

Empyema of the gallbladder (Fig. 7.3).

Empyema is the outcome of secondary infection of a chronically inflamed gallbladder that is occluded by a stone. Our figure shows a severely thickened gallbladder wall with focal calcium deposits (→). Externally, the gallbladder is porcelain-white *(porcelain gallbladder* – white hyalinized scar tissue that is similar to pleural or splenic hyalinosis). Yellow empyema fluid and cholesterol-pigment-calcium stones remain attached to the mucosa. Chronic mucosal pressure ulcers were caused by stones that had been removed in this case.

Hydrops of the gallbladder (Fig. 7.4).

Pure hydrops is due to occlusion by stones. The gallbladder contains mucus but no bile. Figure 7.4 illustrates hydrops of a dilated, thin-walled, tense-elastic gallbladder. Multiple scars are the result of a preceding ulcerating cholecystitis. Note the mucosal folding caused by scarring.

Cholecystitis: F: 15%. *A:* 40–60 years. *S:* ♂:♀=1:2. *Pg:* mostly cholelithiasis with secondary inflammation *(E. coli*, enterococci*)*. Streptococci cause phlegmon. Bacteria cannot be diagnosed in 50% of cases.

Co: (a) "Healing" = shrunken gallbladder with embedded stones.
(b) Adhesions → fistula → gallstone ileus.
(c) Ascending cholangitis (see p. 159).
(d) Perforation → peritonitis with subdiaphragmatic empyema (see also p. 159).

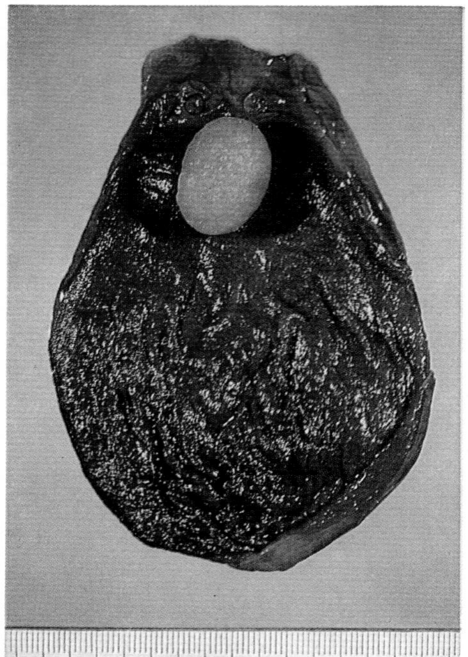

Fig. 7.5. Cholesterol stone.

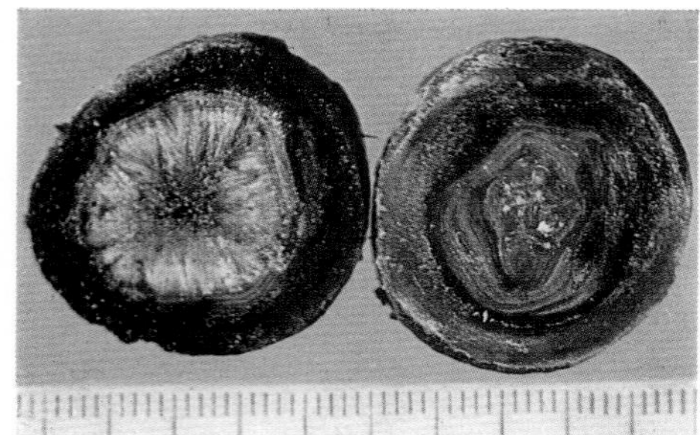

Fig. 7.6. Cholesterol-pigment-calcium stone.

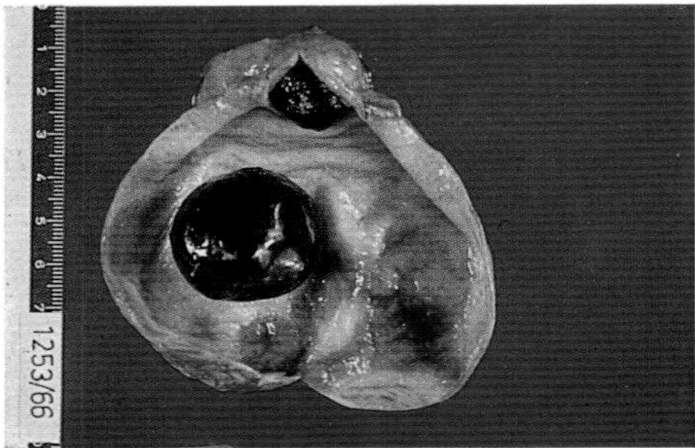

Fig. 7.7. Porcelain gallbladder with pigment stone.

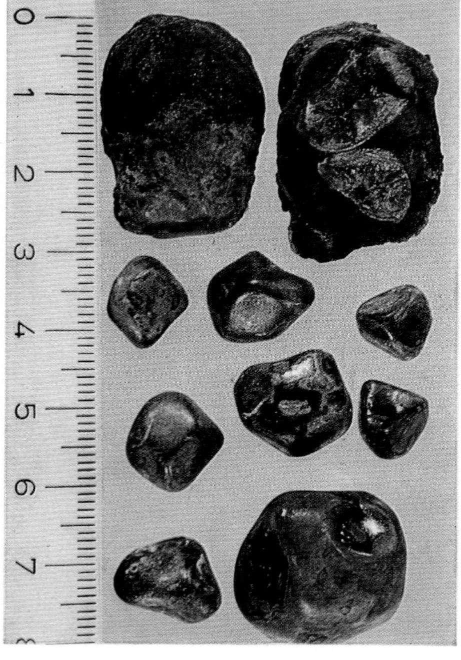

Fig. 7.8. Mixed, faceted gallbladder stones.

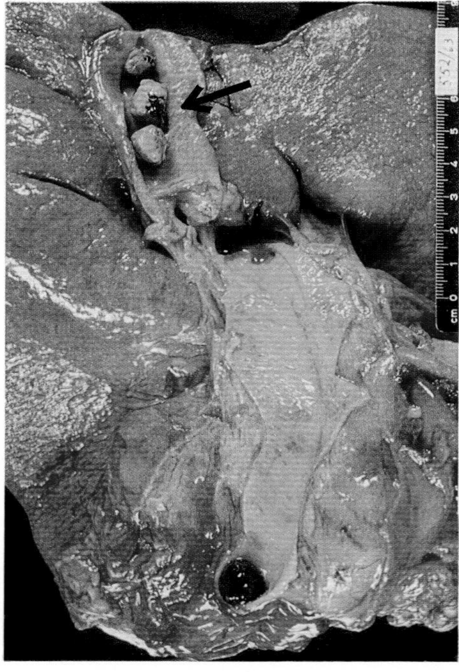

Fig. 7.9. Choledocholithiasis and shrunken gallbladder (chronic cholecystitis).

Cholelithiasis

Gallstones are common and lead to multiple complications. They are composed of cholesterol, calcium and bile (bilirubinate).

Types of stones:

(a) **Cholesterol stone** (Fig. 7.5). Spherical or ovoid, mostly solitary stone with crystalline surface and bright yellow, almost transparent, color. The cut surface is glistening and has a radiating structure that results from the light reflection of crystalline cholesterol. A "wonderful" formation of nature. A central brownish pigment nucleus may be found (pigment-calcium nucleus). As illustrated in our figure, a gallbladder containing a cholesterol stone is dilated but usually without inflammation.

(b) **Cholesterol-pigment-calcium stones** (Figs. 7.6–7.8). Eighty per cent of all gallbladder stones are mixed stones. They are composed of a small brown-black nucleus (pigment), a somewhat larger intermediate radial cholesterol portion and an external circular pigment-calcium ring (Fig. 7.6). These stones usually are round. The external pigment shell (Fig. 7.7) accounts for the black color. Figure 7.7 shows an occluding stone with hydrops of the gallbladder and a large, round, free stone.

Other stones have concentrically laminated pigment-calcium-cholesterol lamellae (Fig. 7.6). Such combinations have faceted surfaces, which may articulate with adjacent stones. They usually fill the entire gallbladder (Fig. 7.8).

(c) **Bilirubin-calcium stones.** Soft, dark green to black mulberry stones; rare; occur in large numbers.

F: 15%. *A* and *S:* 17% in males between 60 and 80 years, 40% in females of the same age.

Pg: see Urolithiasis, page 277. The cholesterol stone probably develops in the presence of sterile bile retention and/or increased cholesterol levels. Inflammation plays a primary role for all other types of stones (alkaline pH, fibrin nidus). The concentric rings suggest a chronic recurrent mode of formation.

Co: 1. *Inflammation:* acute and chronic cholecystitis; empyema; perforation, peritonitis; subphrenic empyema (abscess), porcelain or shrunken gallbladder; fistula → gallstone ileus.

2. *Carcinoma of the gallbladder.*

3. *Hemorrhagic necrosis of the pancreas* (see p. 175).

4. *Stasis* (retention): Figure 7.9 shows an occlusive stone in the ductus choledochus above the papilla with ductal dilatation, abscesses and biliary cirrhosis. Note that the liver surface is studded with small nodules.

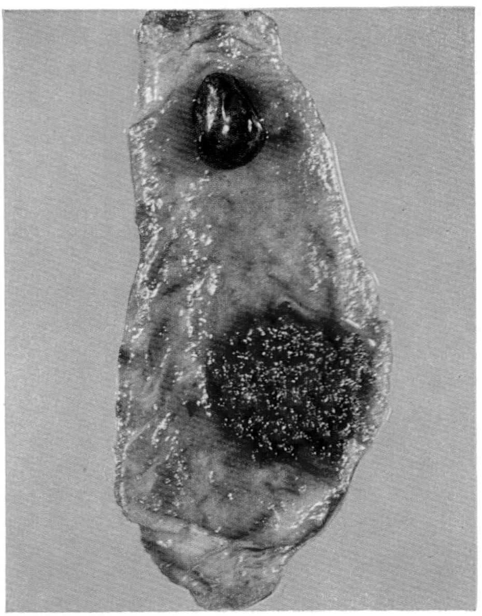

Fig. 7.10. Papilloma and stone of the gallbladder.

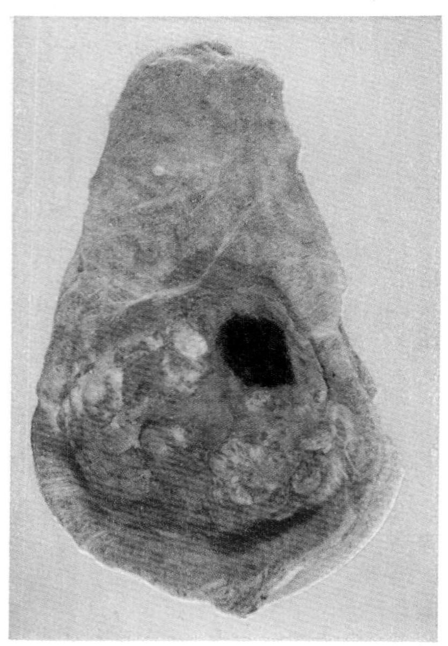

Fig. 7.11. Carcinoma of the gallbladder.

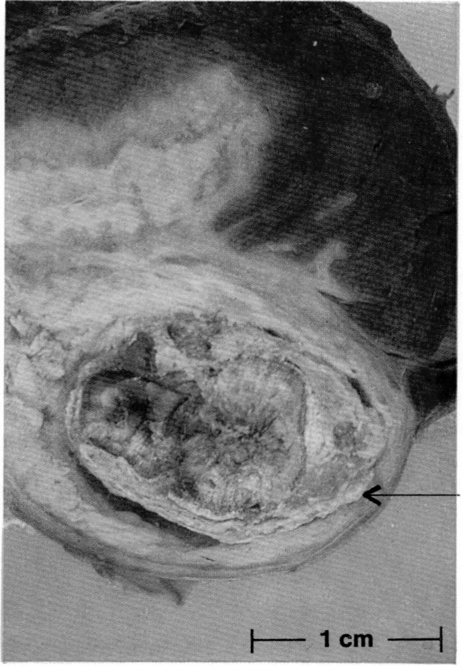

Fig. 7.12. Carcinoma of the gallbladder with chronic cholecystitis and stone.

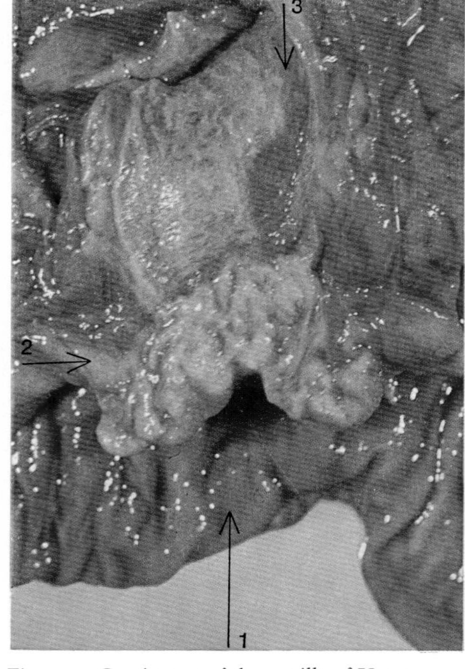

Fig. 7.13. Carcinoma of the papilla of Vater.

Tumors

Papilloma of the gallbladder (Fig. 7.10).

An uncommon benign tumor. Figure 7.10 shows a flat, red, papillary tumor measuring 3 cm. in diameter. (*Mi:* papillary proliferation.) A stone in the neck of the gallbladder caused a pressure ulcer (to the right of the stone). The gallbladder wall is slightly thickened. The bladder contains clear mucus (hydrops).

Carcinoma of the gallbladder (Figs. 7.11 and 7.12).

Usually arises in the fundus adjacent to the liver and infiltrates the liver directly.

Figure 7.11 (carcinoma of the gallbladder) shows the opened viscus with an irregular, yellow-white and red tumor that projects into the lumen. The areas of green discoloration are due to mucosal necrosis secondarily impregnated with bile. The black-dark green oval area is a pressure ulcer from a stone.

Figure 7.12 shows a gallbladder carcinoma with chronic cholecystitis and an embedded stone. Infiltration of the liver by carcinoma is shown in this cut. The gallbladder wall is markedly thickened by connective tissue (→). The cholesterol-pigment stones are firmly embedded in the wall. The posterior gallbladder wall is infiltrated by a firm, white tissue that extends into the liver. A large, compact tumor nodule is present in the liver.

DD: hepatocellular carcinoma with liver cirrhosis: multiple tumor nodules. Cholangiocellular carcinoma: infiltration of a single lobe without anatomic relationship to the gallbladder.

F: 5% of all carcinomas at autopsy. In females, 20% of all organ carcinomas. *S:* ♂:♀=1:4. *A:* 40–60 years. *Pg:* gallstones present in 90% of cases; chronic inflammation, epithelial regeneration. Specific carcinogenic substances are not known.

Metastases: lymphogenous metastases to regional lymph nodes. Peritoneal carcinomatosis. Later, hematogenous metastases to lungs and bones. *Mi:* scirrhous adenocarcinomas, rarely "medullary," mucinous or squamous-cell carcinomas.

Carcinoma of bile ducts

Circumscribed, circular and stenosing carcinoma of extrahepatic bile ducts (usually ductus choledochus) leading to retention jaundice. Males are affected more often than are females.

Carcinoma of the papilla of Vater (Fig. 7.13).

A circular, irregular, firm carcinoma at the papilla (or ampulla) causes a saccular dilatation of the choledochus duct (→1 duodenal mucosa, →2 pancreatic duct, →3 choledochus duct). *Mi:* adenocarcinomas. It often is difficult to decide whether they are derived from the epithelium of the ductus choledochus, pancreatic duct or duodenal mucosa.

DD: "benign" forms of stenosis resulting from chronic inflammation of the ampulla. Hyperplasia of ampullary folds or local glandular hyperplasia (fibroadenoma-like).

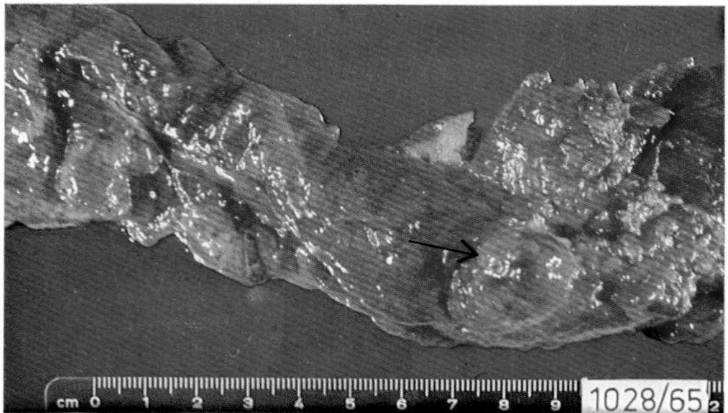

Fig. 8.1. Cystic fibrosis of the pancreas (mucoviscidosis).

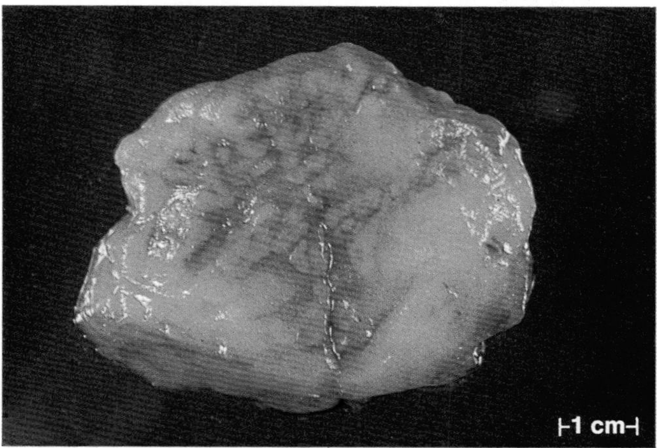

Fig. 8.2. Fatty infiltration of the pancreas.

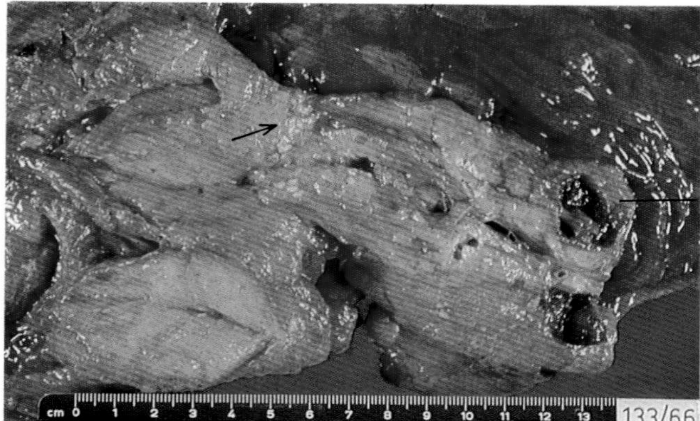

Fig. 8.3. Chronic relapsing pancreatitis.

8. Pancreas

Malformations, Fatty Infiltration, Inflammation

The pancreas is sectioned in situ by a longitudinal cut through the middle of the organ. The pancreatic duct often is opened in this way or can be prepared further by extending the longitudinal cut (width!). The duct also can be opened by transverse cuts. Pancreatic and choledochus ducts jointly enter the duodenum in the ampulla in 70% of cases. The normal pancreas is firm and lobular; softening occurs only after death.

Malformations:

Annular pancreas: the head of the pancreas encircles the descending portion of the duodenum.
Dysontogenetic cysts occur together with congenital cysts of the liver and kidneys.
Pseudocysts: brown cysts after necrosis and hemorrhage.

Cystic fibrosis of the pancreas (mucoviscidosis, Fig. 8.1; TCP, p. 115).

Autosomal, recessive disease with formation of highly viscous secretions that are deficient in enzymes but rich in NaCl, stasis of secretions and dilatation of excretory ducts with secondary inflammation. The gross findings in the pancreas and lungs are conspicuous. The pancreas of a 20-year-old male is shown in Figure 8.1. Several large (→) and multiple small cysts can be identified with the magnifying glass. In addition, the pancreas is rather firm and irregularly lobular.

F: Europe 0.1 $^0/_0$; the United States 0.2 $^0/_0$; negroes rarely are affected. No cases known in orientals. *S:* ♂ = ♀.

A: usually manifest in infants up to 6 months of age. Death from meconium ileus (thick, highly viscous meconium), sometimes perforation and peritonitis. *Infants and children:* mucus stasis in bronchi predominates, leading to *bronchiectasis*, recurring pneumonias and cor pulmonale. Fatty liver, biliary fibrosis and dilated intrahepatic biliary ducts with fibrosis are seen commonly. Some cases may even progress to focal cirrhosis. Increased mucus secretion by Brunner's glands, mucous glands of the gallbladder and salivary glands. *Cl:* deficiency of pancreatic enzymes, such as amylase, lipase and trypsin → malabsorption (celiac syndrome, see p. 123). Sweat glands are morphologically unchanged. Sweat contains increased levels of Na and Cl.

Fatty infiltration of the pancreas (lipomatosis) (Fig. 8.2). Increase in fatty tissue with increasing age or obesity accompanied by parenchymal atrophy. The islets of Langerhans remain intact. Our figure shows a piece of pancreas that resembles a piece of yellow fat. Some gray-white-yellow islands of pancreas protrude slightly over the cut surface.

Pancreatitis

Acute, serous-purulent or chronic-recurrent inflammation that accompanies infectious diseases, malnutrition and liver cirrhosis (alcohol!). Microscopically, chronic inflammation, fibrosis and loss of parenchyma are found. These changes also occur with increasing age, so that it is difficult to detect a "normal" pancreas in older patients.

The *chronic, relapsing pancreatitis* with fatty necrosis (TCP, p. 115) represents an abortive form of acute hemorrhagic pancreatitis and has a corresponding clinical symptomatology. Figure 8.3 shows multiple white areas of fat and parenchymal necrosis (→). Hemorrhagic, partly cystic areas of necrosis are found in the tail of the pancreas. The remaining tissue is firm, sclerosed and devoid of the normal lobular architecture.

Pancreatic stones (small, white, hard calcium carbonate stones) occur in ducts (head of the pancreas) as a consequence of pancreatitis. Also often seen with hypercalcemia (hyperparathyroidism).

F: 0.1% in autopsy material, probably more common because little attention is paid to the occurrence of stones.

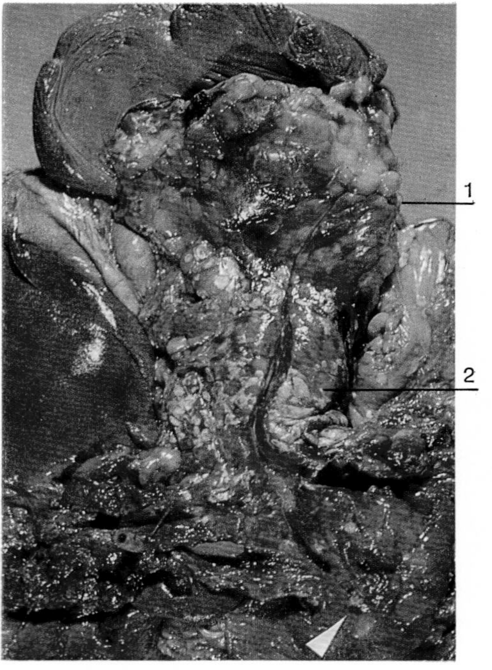

Fig. 8.4. Necrosis of the pancreas with an occlusive stone in the ampulla.

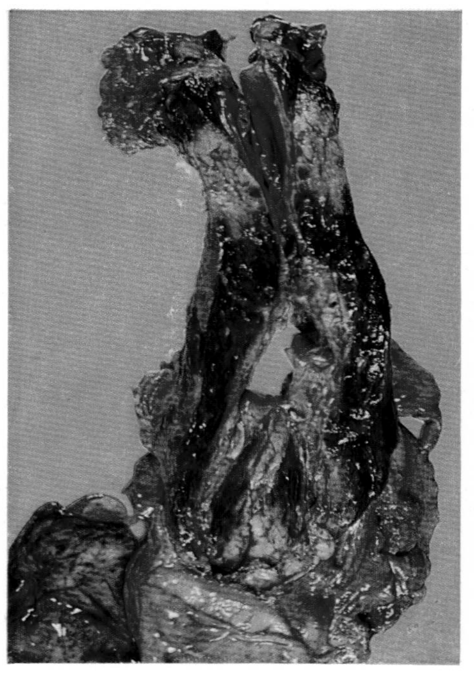

Fig. 8.5. Hemorrhagic pancreatic necrosis.

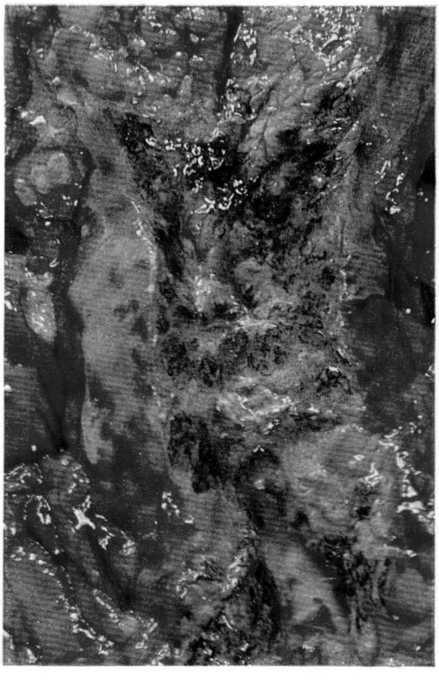

Fig. 8.6. Old hemorrhagic pancreatic necrosis.

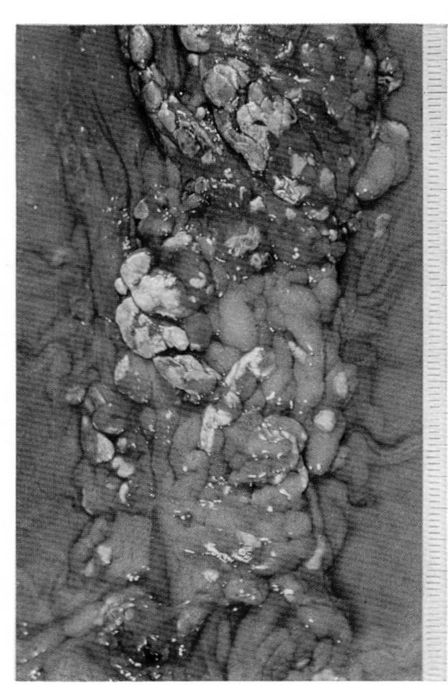

Fig. 8.7. Fat necrosis of the mesentery.

Acute hemorrhagic necrosis of the pancreas (acute pancreatitis, pancreas apoplexia) (Figs. 8.4–8.7).

Acute parenchymal necrosis of the entire pancreas with hemorrhages. Clinically manifest as "acute abdomen."

Figure 8.4 shows the entire pancreas with acute hemorrhagic necrosis. The ampulla served as a common ostium for the pancreatic duct and choledochus ducts. A gallstone is impacted in the ampulla (cholesterol-pigment-calcium stone, white arrow). The ductus choledochus was drained in this case (red drainage tube). The gray, dirty, edematous appearance of the pancreas is seen best in the tail (→1). This is typical for the early stage of pancreatic necrosis. The remaining pancreas is hemorrhagic. The body of the pancreas contains many whitish areas of fat necrosis (→ 2).

The fully developed picture of hemorrhagic pancreatic necrosis is illustrated in Figure 8.5. The pancreas is speckled black-red and gray-red (partially intact parenchyma). An unaffected portion remains in the tail, approximately 4 cm. long.

Figure 8.6 shows a somewhat older, partly hemorrhagic necrosis. Black hemorrhages, whitish necrotic parenchyma and surrounding areas of fat necrosis are seen. Intact parenchyma remains near the right margin of Figure 8.6.

Areas of fat necrosis are found in the mesentery (Fig. 8.7). These chalky white foci also may be found throughout the abdominal cavity, occasionally in the visceral pleura, bone marrow and subcutaneous fat tissues.

Brown cysts with sequestered necrotic content can be observed in patients who survive partial pancreatic necrosis.

F: 0.5%. *A:* 40–50 years. *S:* ♂:♀=1:3. Frequently obese patients. Death frequently due to shock with hyaline thrombi.

Pg: edema and circulatory disturbances are believed to develop during the initial phase (dirty, dark gray pancreas). A stage of hemorrhagic necrosis follows. Although pancreatic enzymes (trypsin, amylase, peptidase) play an important role, digestion of intact pancreatic tissue is of doubtful significance.

CP: (a) Trauma (rare).

(b) Bile stasis (occlusive stone, sclerosis of papilla).

(c) Not known.

Experimental induction: (a) Allergy: i.v. injection of egg albumin and duct ligation.

(b) Local Shwartzman-Sanarelli phenomenon: bacterial toxins in the duct; 24 hours later injected I.V. The result is hemorrhagic pancreatic necrosis.

(c) Calciphylaxis (Selye): Sensitizing agent: hypercalcemia. Challenging agent: chondroitin sulfate, Fe or other substances are administered intraperitoneally. Result: pancreatitis, calcification with hemorrhagic necrosis. Calcium enhances activation of trypsinogen to trypsin.

(d) Lysolecithin A (lecithin is present in bile), bile acid and phospholipase (abundant in bile) injected into duct → necrosis.

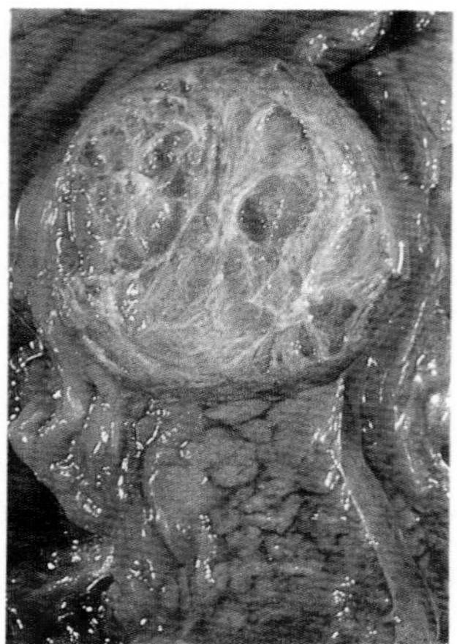

Fig. 8.8. Cystadenoma of the pancreas.

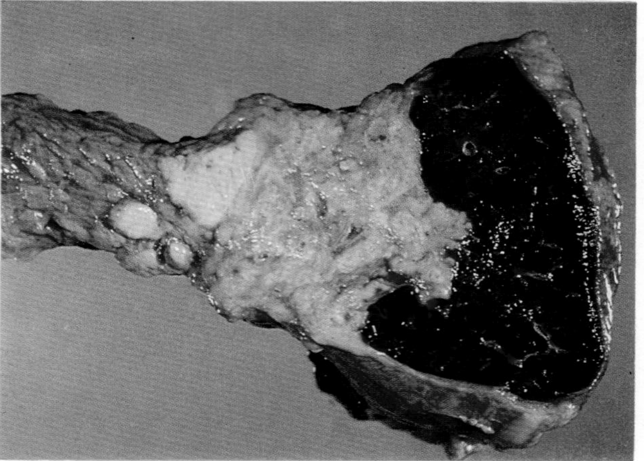

Fig. 8.9. Carcinoma of the tail of the pancreas with direct infiltration of the spleen.

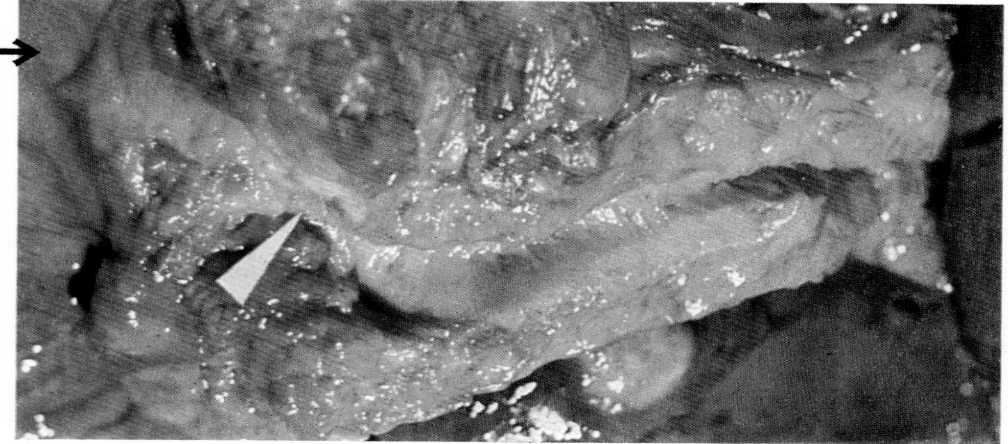

Fig. 8.10. Carcinoma of the head of the pancreas with dilatation of the pancreatic duct distal to the carcinoma.

Tumors

Cystadenoma (Fig. 8.8).

Rare tumors, derived from the duct epithelium and often located in the tail. Grossly (Fig. 8.8), the tumor is sharply delineated, firm and contains small or large cysts.

Metastases to the pancreas are rare.

Carcinoma of the pancreas (Figs. 8.9 and 8.10).

Arise most commonly in the head of the pancreas, with clinical symptoms of duct stasis (pancreatic duct and ductus choledochus). Figure 8.10 (carcinoma of the head of the pancreas) shows a gray-white, firm carcinoma, 2 cm. in diameter (white arrow). The pancreatic duct is compressed. Note the ductal dilatation distal to the stenosis; → duodenum.

Figure 8.9 shows a carcinoma of the tail of the pancreas with direct infiltration of the spleen. The gray-white, firm carcinoma and several metastases in the body of the pancreas are clearly distinguished from the normal pancreatic tissue. The tumor has invaded the hilus of the spleen. The splenic capsule is fibrotic and shows adhesions.

F: >1% in autopsy material. *A:* 60–70 years. *S:* ♂:♀=1.5:1. Fifty per cent of all carcinomas are located in the head of the pancreas. *Pg:* chronic pancreatitis is found frequently (see above). *Co:* dilatation of pancreatic duct with hemorrhagic necrosis. Compression of bile duct → retention jaundice. Infiltration of duodenum. *Metastases:* 50% to liver, 30% to lungs, 40% to regional lymph nodes; skeleton, kidneys. *Mi:* mostly adenocarcinomas. Scirrhous, cystic, papillary or mucinous variants are observed.

Tumors of the islets of Langerhans

1. Tumors derived from β cells (75%) usually are functional, i.e., they produce insulin. *Cl:* repeated hypoglycemic attacks with blood sugar levels below 30 mg./100 ml., gastrointestinal disturbances and relief from symptoms by glucose administration (Whipple's triad). Most β-cell tumors are adenomas (1–3 cm. in diameter, pink, circumscribed), rarely carcinomas.

2. Tumors derived from α cells are rare and occasionally produce excessive glucagon and diabetes mellitus.

3. The Zollinger-Ellison syndrome (see p. 115) is the clinical manifestation of islet-cell adenomas derived from non-beta or intermediate cells. The adenomas produce gastrin and stimulate the production of gastric pepsin or HCl. *Co:* intractable gastric, duodenal and/or jejunal ulcers are pathognomonic, often together with diarrhea and steatorrhea (malabsorption). Ulcers usually are missing in cases of Zollinger-Ellison syndrome with severe diarrhea. Serotonin can be extracted from the tumor tissue (histogenetic relationship to carcinoid?).

F: 0.1–1% of autopsy material; often accidental autopsy finding after careful dissection, i.e., without clinical symptoms (nonfunctioning adenoma). *A:* 40–50 years. *S:* ♂=♀. Mostly solitary tumors (85%), occasionally adenomatosis. *Lo:* 50% tail, 30% body, 20% head. Ectopic islet-cell tumors occur in the pylorus, duodenal wall or Meckel's diverticulum.

Adenomas with trabecular (winding-ribbon) or pseudotubular structure. Fifteen per cent of islet-cell adenomas metastasize early. Hyperplasias of islet cells can produce the clinical symptoms described above. Islet-cell tumors may be associated with adenomas of other endocrine organs (pituitary, adrenal, parathyroid, thyroid) in the so-called *endocrine adenomatosis*. Familial, genetically determined? Also may be acquired as the MEHA syndrome (multiple endocrine hyperplasia and adenomas).

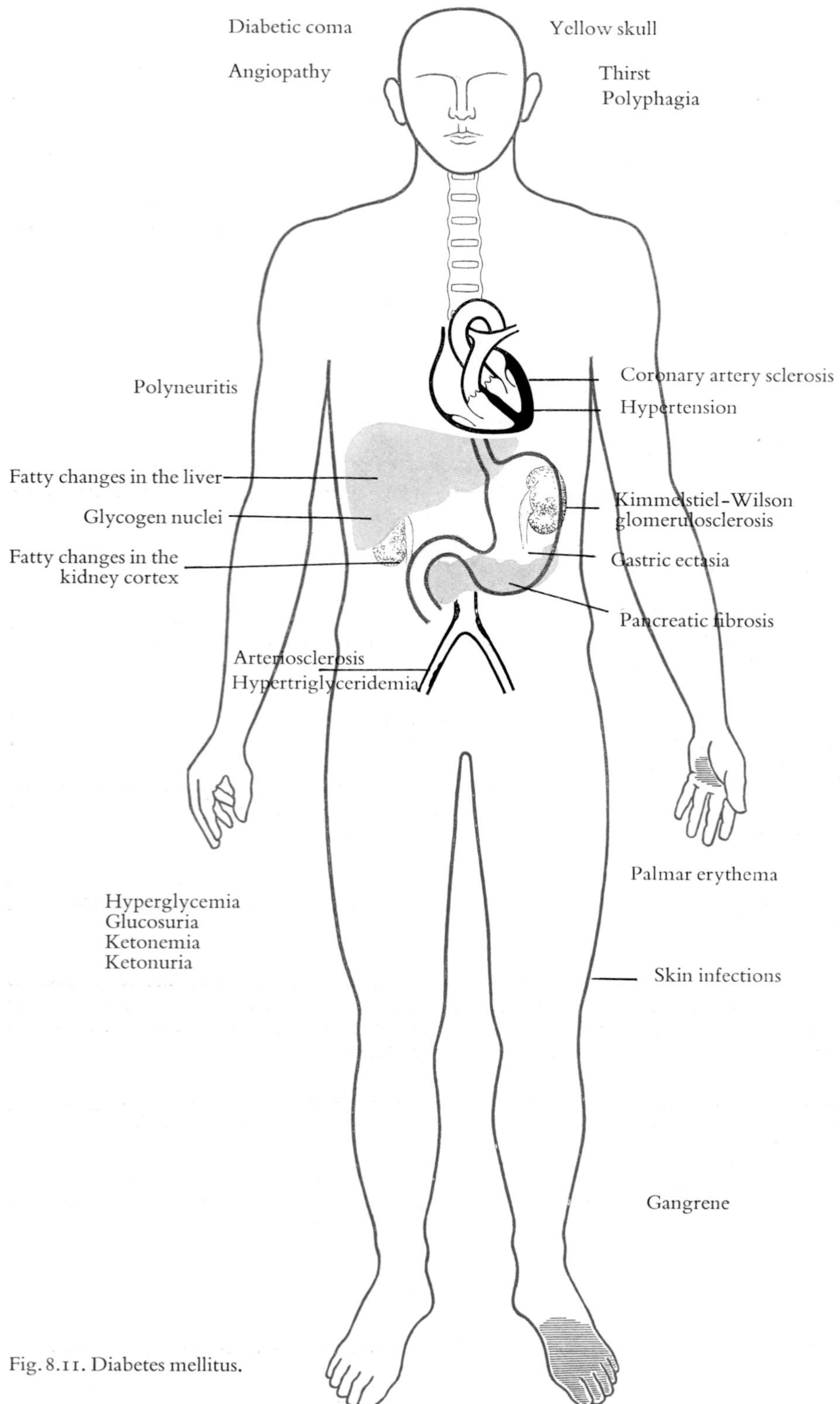

Fig. 8.11. Diabetes mellitus.

Diabetes Mellitus

Hyperglycemia and glucosuria due to absolute or relative insulin deficiency that is caused by primary or econdary insufficiency of β cells.

The most common genetic multifactorial human disease (obesity, pregnancy).

Genetics: Familial history in 30% of diabetics (anamnesis!). Diabetic disposition in 10–25% of total population. Increasing frequency during the last 10 years! Recessive inherited. Possibly dominant for juvenile diabetes.

F: 1–2% of the total population; 6–8% at 50–70 years. Ratio of diagnosed to undiagnosed cases is 1:1. Prior to World War II 0.2%; 1945–1948 1% (hunger period, e.g., occupation of Paris!).

Age, sex, forms:

1. **Infantile diabetes :** 0–10 years.

2. **Juvenile diabetes.** ♂=♀ (15 to 24 years. Infantile and juvenile are forms of insulin-deficiency diabetes). Histological: depletion of the β-cells of the islands of Langerhans.

3. **Adult and senile diabetes.** ♂:♀=1:2.

4. **Secondary diabetes** after pancreatitis, pancreatectomy, hemochromatosis (50–80% of patients develop bronze diabetes). Hypophyseal diabetes with *acromegaly:* 10% of cases; *Cushing's disease:* 15% of cases; *iatrogenic* factors (due to medication); *pheochromocytoma.*

The metabolic changes in diabetes mellitus can be summarized as follows: Relative or absolute insulin deficiency leads to glucose deficiency in muscle and fat tissues (not the liver) because glucose transport through cell membranes is diminished. Therefore diminished energy formation. Fat and protein catabolism is increased, more acetyl-coenzyme A and β-hydroxybutyric acid are produced: ketone bodies (liver) → acidosis. The basic metabolic disturbance is the result of glucose deficiency so that amino acids and fat are utilized as energy sources.

The pathologic-anatomic diagnosis of diabetes is difficult, especially death from diabetic coma (when not diagnosed clinically). According to studies by Traub, glucose and acetic acid levels are increased in the spinal fluid of the deceased.

Figure 8.11 summarizes the important *clinical symptoms* and *pathologic-anatomic findings.* Histologic changes in the pancreas usually are no longer present at autopsy (β-cell granules disappear rapidly). Amyloidosis of the islets has been described by Kief in 85% of diabetic islets (pathogenetic mechanism for senile diabetes?); formerly considered hyalinization (TCP, p. 189).

Kimmelstiel-Wilson glomerulosclerosis: 30% of longstanding diabetes causes finely granular, red, firm kidneys. Hypertension and its consequences are frequent complications of diabetes.

Pg: juvenile diabetes: accounts for 10% of diabetics. (1) Genetically determined. (2) Virus infection (mumps). *Senile diabetes:* 50–80 years; prediabetic state with hyperinsulinism and obesity → "exhaustion" of β cells, i.e., relative insulin deficiency. Questionable role of insulin antibodies or antagonists.

Th: insulin, sulfonylurea, biguanides, weight loss (diet).

Causes of death: 75% of all patients die from diabetes alone, 20% die in diabetic coma, 5% die in uremia, 10% die from infections and 40% die from consequences of arteriosclerosis.

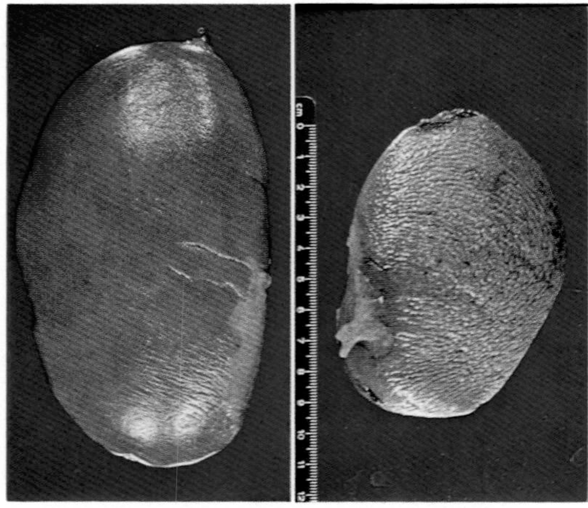

Fig. 9.1. Left: normal spleen. Right: atrophic spleen.

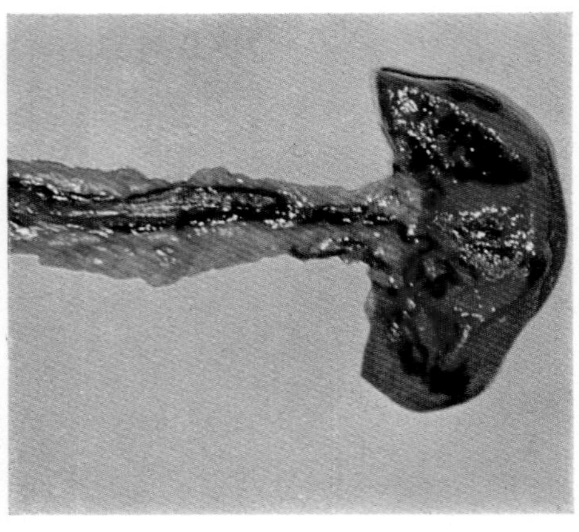

Fig. 9.2. Hemorrhagic infarctions of the spleen.

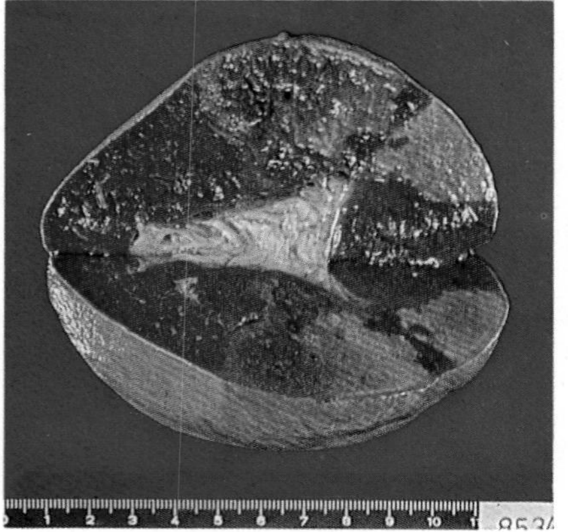

Fig. 9.3. Anemic infarctions of the spleen.

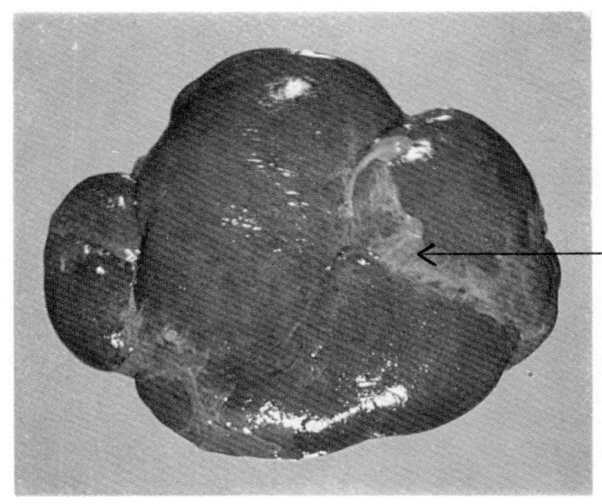

Fig. 9.4. Old splenic infarctions (scars).

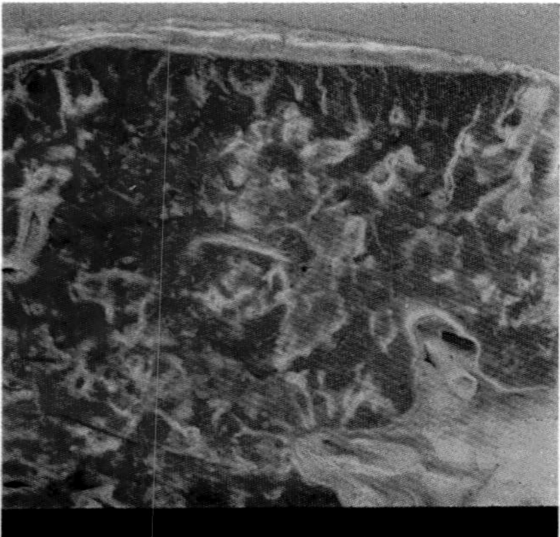

Fig. 9.5. "Fleckmilz" in periarteritis nodosa.

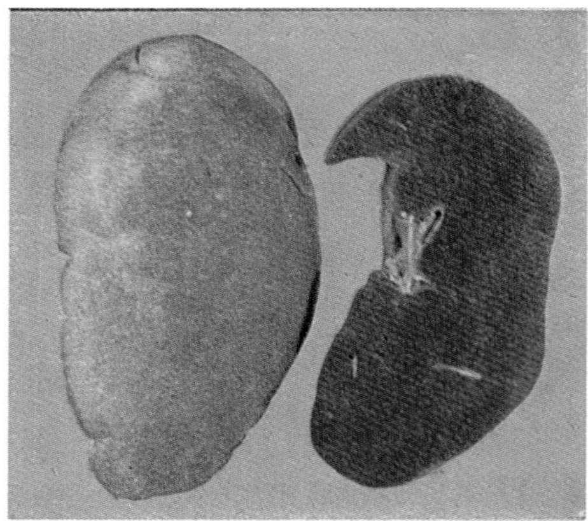

Fig. 9.6. Chronic congestion of the spleen.

9. Spleen, Lymph Nodes, Blood

The spleen (weight: 150 Gm.) is dissected by lengthwise cuts. In cases of splenomegaly, the portal veins should be opened in situ (thrombosis!). *Malformations:* Accessory spleens near the hilus are relatively common. They enlarge after splenectomy. Abnormal splenic lobes are seen occasionally. Spleen cysts (serosal, epidermoid and echinococcus cysts) are rare.

Atrophy of the spleen (Fig. 9.1). A reduction in size is observed as part of the generalized senile atrophy of internal organs. The organ is soft and elastic; the capsule is folded. On cut surface, trabecular markings are prominent, the white pulp is inconspicuous (atrophy) and the red pulp is bright red. The spleen also may become atrophic during terminal chronic heart failure ("left cardiac" spleen atrophy according to ZOLLINGER). A soft-elastic, bright red spleen with a markedly wrinkled capsule also is an indication of an acute blood loss during life, e.g., bleeding esophageal varices (emptying of blood reservoir: *collapsed spleen*).

Hemorrhagic infarction of the spleen (Fig. 9.2) occurs after splenic-vein thrombosis or arterial thrombi and emboli. Figure 9.2 shows a fresh thrombosis of the splenic vein with dark red, partly triangular, firm lesions in the spleen.

Anemic infarctions in the spleen are more common than hemorrhagic infarctions. Figure 9.3 shows typical quadrangular, yellow, dry, firm lesions that protrude slightly over the surface. Note the fibrinous perisplenitis. Depressed, retracted scars with a white base remain after an infarction is organized (Fig. 9.4). Since fibrinous perisplenitis always accompanies splenic infarctions, peritoneal adhesions point to the site of infarction (gray-white membranes, →). *Pg:* myocardial infarction with mural thrombosis is the most common cause of anemic splenic infarctions.

When multiple, smaller arteries are occluded as in periarteritis nodosa, gray-yellow infarctions localize below the capsule (so-called Fleckmilz). The cut surface in Figure 9.5 reveals several map-like infarctions, up to 2 cm. in diameter, between viable spleen tissue (see also periarteritis nodosa, p. 223).

Splenomegaly

An enlarged spleen (also called spleen "tumor") becomes clinically manifest when the spleen is heavier than 300 Gm. Splenomegaly is symptomatic of many diseases, such as:

1. **Circulatory disturbances.** (a) Chronic congestion (Fig. 9.6; TCP, p. 171). The spleen is firm and dark blue-red externally and on cut surface. The capsule is stretched. Liver cirrhosis, cardiac failure (e.g., cor pulmonale) or splenic-vein thrombosis is the main cause of circulatory splenomegaly. *Gandy-Gamna* bodies (so-called siderofibrosis) usually are present. They are grossly gray-brown and hard. Histologically, they consist of fibrous tissue, foreign-body giant cells and iron or calcium deposits. *Pg:* hemorrhages into the follicles ultimately are organized by fibrous tissue. Iron and calcium are deposited in trabeculae. (b) Splenic infarctions.

2. **Blood diseases.** (a) *Chronic myeloid leukemia* (giant spleen tumor, see p. 193). (b) *Lymphatic leukemia or lymphosarcoma.* (c) All forms of *hemolytic anemia* (small follicles). (d) *Essential thrombocytopenia* (Werlhof's disease): follicles are increased and enlarged. (e) *Extramedullary hemopoiesis* (e.g., osteomyelosclerosis, erythroblastosis, cancerous bone metastases). (f) *Panmyelophthisis* (follicles enlarged).

3. **Primary spleen tumors,** such as reticulum-cell sarcoma, lymphosarcoma or "pulpoma" (see p. 185).

4. **Metastatic diseases,** e. g., Hodgkin's disease (see p. 187) or metastases from malignant melanoma. Metastases from carcinomas are rare. Cysts, especially echinococcus cysts, also may enlarge the spleen.

5. **Storage diseases.** (a) Lipidoses: Gaucher's disease (cerebrosides), Niemann-Pick's disease (sphingomyelin), Hand-Schüller-Christian's disease (cholesterol). (b) Amyloidosis (see p. 183).

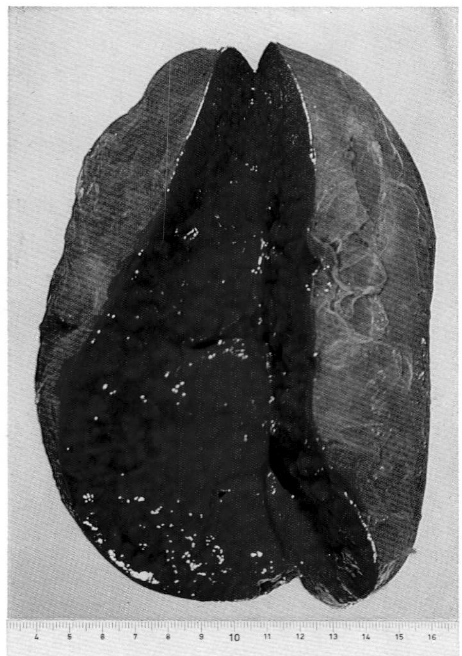

Fig. 9.7. Acute enlargement of the spleen.

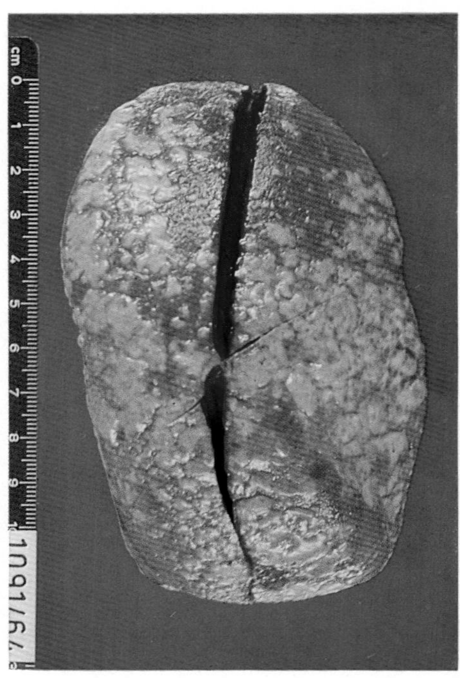

Fig. 9.8. Hyalinosis of spleen capsule ("Zuckergussmilz").

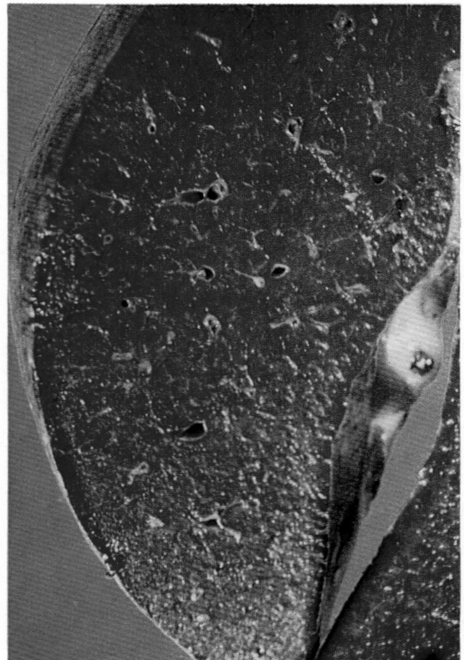

Fig. 9.9. Amyloidosis of the spleen.

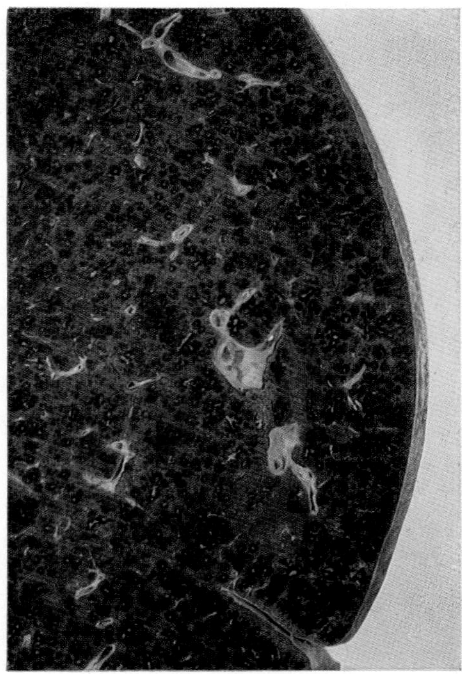

Fig. 9.10. Follicular amyloidosis ("sago spleen") after Lugol reaction.

6. **Inflammation.** (a) The most common form of splenomegaly is the inflammatory spleen enlargement ("spodogenic" spleen tumor; spodos = dust, dirt). The enlarged spleen is soft, often diffluent, fragile and gray-red (Fig. 9.7). The follicles likewise are enlarged and poorly demarcated. A turbid, gray-red juice can be scraped off the cut surface. Hyperemia of sinusoids; leukocytes and cellular debris in the red pulp; proliferation of sinus endothelium. Inflammatory spleen enlargement is a response to severe inflammations elsewhere (peritonitis, pneumonia, bacterial endocarditis, etc.) or heavy tissue destruction (malignant tumors with necrosis). The chronic inflammatory spleen "tumor" is somewhat firmer than the normal spleen. The follicles are prominent and adhesions or fibrous thickening of the capsule are found, as in our case.

The capsule of the enlarged spleen becomes edematous, covered by a fibrinous exudate and partially ruptures. Foci of fibrinous inflammation eventually are organized as hyaline scar tissue. Figure 9.8 shows white, firm and calcium-like plaques in the capsule. The condition is known as capsule hyalinosis, cartilaginous perisplenitis or Zuckergussmilz.

(b) Additional causes of *inflammatory spleen enlargement* or swelling include miliary tuberculosis (see p. 83), cavernous tuberculosis (rarely), sarcoidosis (multiple small, gray nodules), infectious mononucleosis (sometimes followed by spontaneous spleen rupture because of lymphoid hyperplasia) and malaria (a dirty-red spleen tumor). Spleen abscesses from sepsis or pyemia, rheumatoid arthritis and typhoid fever also are accompanied by splenomegaly.

Amyloidosis

(Figs. 9.9 and 9.10; TCP, p. 173)

Congenital or acquired disturbance of the immune system (immunoblasts, plasma cells of the reticuloendothelial system, connective tissue cells) with formation of light chains of antibodies which polymerize extracellularly to fibrils (70–80Å in diameter) (see Mi and AP). The following are differentiated:

1. **Typical amyloidosis** involves the kidneys, liver, stomach, adrenal glands and gastrointestinal mucosa (important: rectal biopsy for diagnosis). Diffuse amyloidosis is referred to as "bacon" or lardaceous spleen (Fig. 9.9). The spleen is enlarged, firm and rigid. The cut surface is waxy (pulp amyloidosis). In the less-common follicular form, amyloid is deposited in the follicles (*"sago spleen"*). The follicles are gray-white to red, glassy nodules and project slightly over the cut surface. Amyloid-containing follicles can be demonstrated as blue-black nodules with Lugol's solution (iodine, followed by diluted H_2SO_4) (Fig. 9.10).

2. **Atypical amyloidosis** involves the heart (endocardium, valves, myocardium), tongue, skin, brain, lungs, etc. Observed as "senile amyloidosis" in 3% of autopsies in patients past 70 years.

3. **Tumor-like amyloidosis** involves the tongue, larynx and lungs. It often is accompanied by excessive plasma cell proliferation (antibody production!).

F: 0.4%. *A:* 30–50 years. *S:* ♂>♀.

Pg: 1. **Primary inherited amyloidosis** is an inborn error of metabolism and develops without preceding disease. Chromosome aberrations are not known. Several diseases are included in hereditary amyloidosis:

(a) *Familial Mediterranean fever*, an autosomal, recessive disease accompanied by polyserositis and renal amyloidosis. A typical amyloidosis as far as organ involvement is concerned.

(b) *Amyloidosis with urticaria and deafness:* a dominantly inherited disease. Atypical amyloidosis in distribution.

(c) *Cardiac amyloidosis* involves the tongue and nerves in addition to the heart. Partly typical, partly atypical amyloidosis in distribution.

(d) *Neuropathic amyloidosis* involves the brain and nerves (atypical in distribution). Familial disease (e.g., 29% of 252 offspring of a Swiss family living in the United States were affected).

(e) In mice and golden hamsters, amyloidosis occurs *spontaneously*.

2. **Secondary or acquired amyloidosis** is always atypical amyloidosis as far as organ involvement is concerned. Preceded by chronic infections, such as tuberculosis (50% of all cases of amyloidosis) or osteomyelitis (12%), chronic pulmonary infections, especially bronchiectasis (10%) and other chronic infections (12%). Amyloidosis also develops in 20% of patients with rheumatoid arthritis.

Experimental induction of amyloidosis by repeated administration of foreign proteins. According to a suggestion by Teilum, amyloid represents atypical antibody protein that occurs spontaneously or after suppression of antibody production by cortisone, x-irradiation or nitrogen mustard treatment.

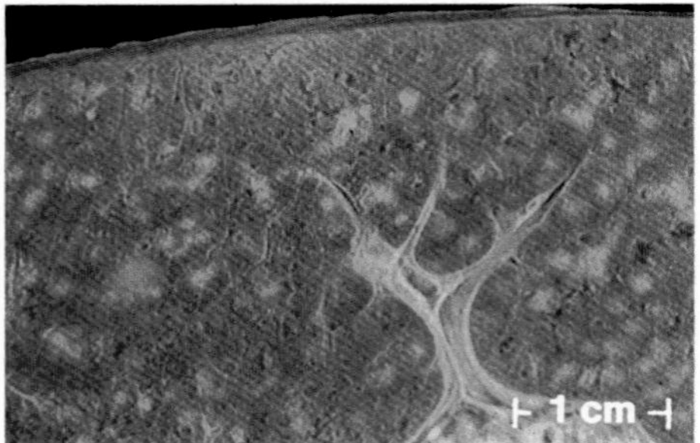

Fig. 9.11. Follicle necrosis of the spleen.

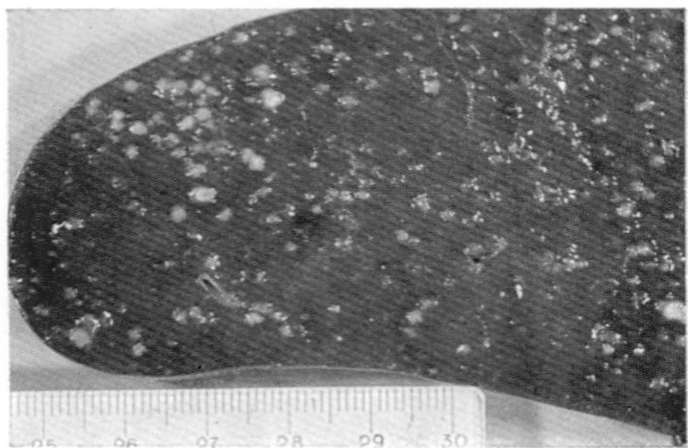

Fig. 9.12. Miliary tuberculosis of the spleen.

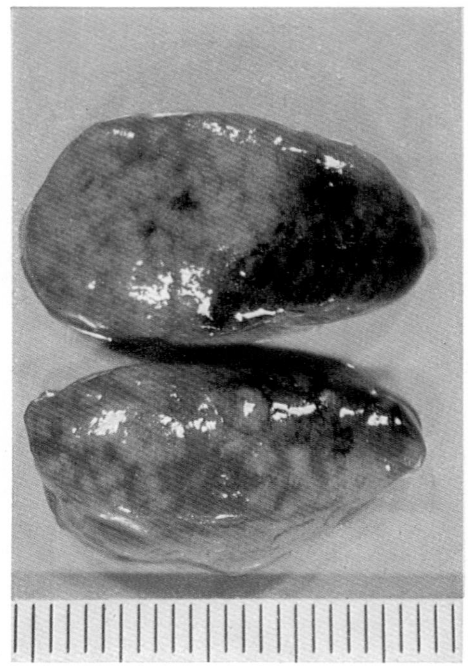

Fig. 9.13. Productive tuberculosis of lymph nodes.

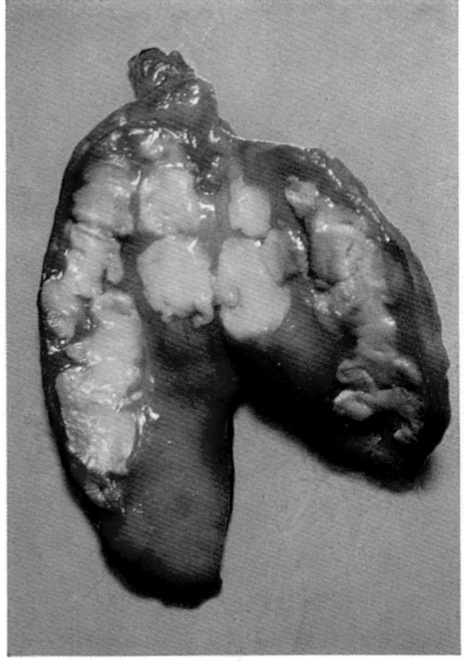

Fig. 9.14. Caseating tuberculosis of lymph nodes.

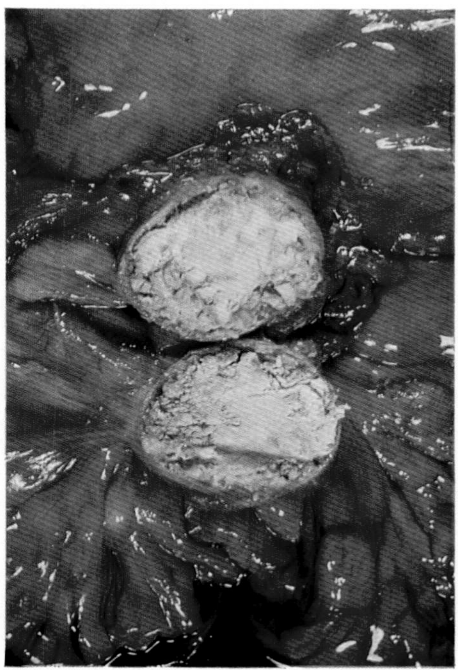

Fig. 9.15. Calcific tuberculosis of mesenteric lymph nodes.

Follicle Necrosis, Tuberculosis

Follicle necrosis of the spleen (Fig. 9.11). Multiple gray-red foci are scattered throughout the spleen. They measure up to 0.5 cm. in diameter and represent necrotic Malpighian corpuscles on histologic examination (occasionally seen in diphtheria).

The splenomegaly of the so-called Banti syndrome is now interpreted as a congestive splenomegaly caused by liver cirrhosis. The Banti syndrome often is associated with hypersplenic anemia.

Miliary tuberculosis of the spleen (Fig. 9.12). Hematogenous spread of tuberculosis almost always involves the spleen. Miliary or somewhat larger, gray-yellow nodules project slightly over the cut surface.

DD: "porphyry spleen" in Hodgkin's disease (the foci are larger than miliary tubercles and more irregular; see p. 187); so-called Landouzy sepsis of tuberculosis (distinguishable only by microscopic examination; often rather large foci); sarcoidosis (the infiltrates often coalesce); Wegener's granulomatosis (large, irregular infiltrates).

A and *Pg:* in children or adults during terminal diseases or after chemotherapy.

Tuberculosis of lymph nodes (see p. 87). *Tuberculous inflammation resulting from lymphogenous or hematogenous spread.*

Figure 9.13 shows a productive, granulomatous tuberculosis with gray-white, glassy tubercles on the cut surface. Note the anthracosis.

Mi: epithelioid-cell tubercles without caseation. They usually develop under conditions of good host defense, although caseation may occur later. A productive, granulomatous tuberculosis cannot be distinguished grossly or histologically from sarcoidosis (see p. 89). Detailed clinical data are needed for the differential diagnosis (sarcoidosis: Kveim test).

Caseating tuberculosis of lymph nodes. Figure 9.14 shows irregular, dry, yellow foci on cut surface. The foci may enlarge and thereby occupy the entire lymph node. Calcium subsequently is deposited in areas of caseation necrosis. The lymph node becomes chalky and later calcified.

Figure 9.15 shows **calcific tuberculosis of mesenteric lymph nodes** as seen frequently in intestinal tuberculosis (see p. 135). The entire lymph node is chalky-white and firm. Only a thin connective-tissue capsule remains.

Lymph node tuberculosis most often affects peribronchial lymph nodes as part of the primary complex. Epithelioid-cell tubercles with or without caseation are present; frequently they heal by fibrosis.

Tuberculosis of cervical lymph nodes (or tuberculosis of axillary lymph nodes) results from lymphogenous or hematogenous dissemination from the lungs or hilar lymph nodes. Females, 20–30 years of age, predominate.

Pg: tubercles appear first in the marginal sinus when the disease has spread lymphogenously. Hematogenous dissemination produces tubercles in the vicinity of follicles. *Co:* tuberculosis of lung hilar or mediastinal lymph nodes often is the source of hematogenous dissemination, especially with diminished host resistance (Landouzy sepsis). Liquefaction necrosis → formation of a cavity → fistula. Secondary infections.

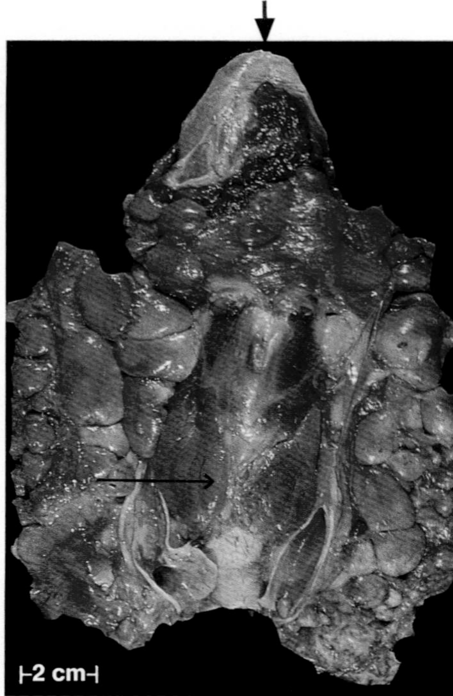

Fig. 9.16. Hodgkin's disease of cervical lymph nodes.

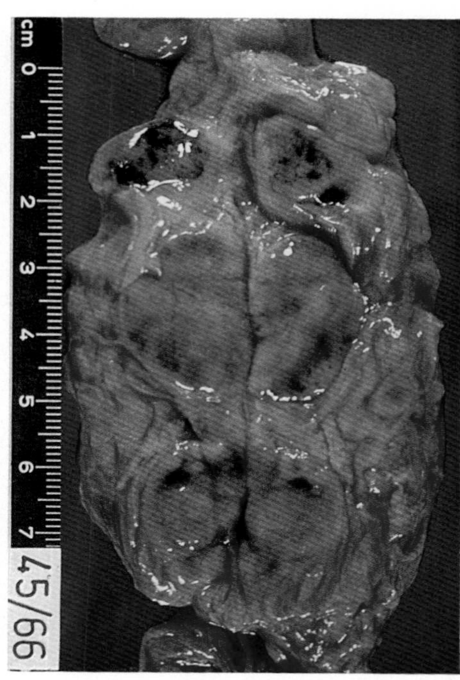

Fig. 9.17. Cut surface of lymph nodes with Hodgkin's disease.

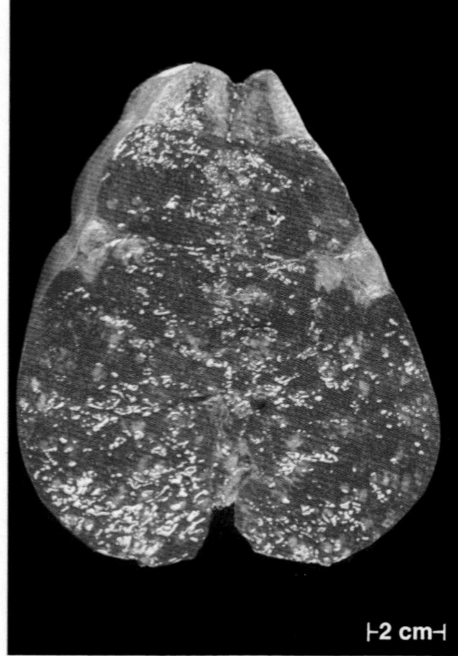

Fig. 9.18. Hodgkin's disease of the spleen ("porphyry spleen").

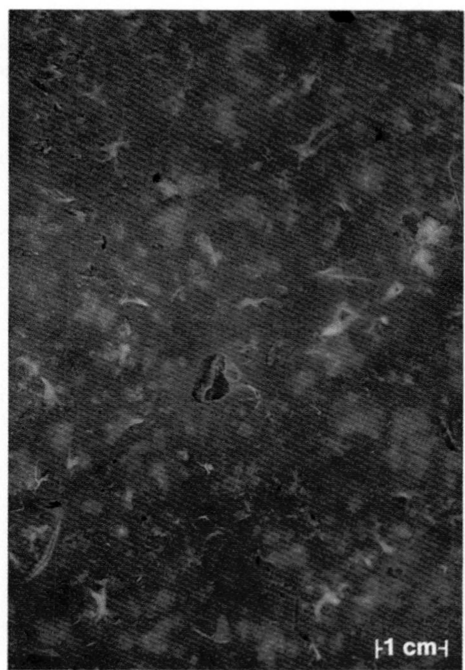

Fig. 9.19. "Porphyry spleen." Higher magnification of cut surface.

Hodgkin's Disease

(Lymphogranulomatosis) (TCP, p. 179)

Hodgkin's disease is the most common form of lymphoma (53%). The histologic pattern is characteristic. Several histologic subtypes correlate with clinical prognosis.

The lymph nodes are grossly enlarged and speckled gray-white-red. Adjacent lymph nodes are not fused during the initial course of the disease, as shown in Figure 9.16 (Hodgkin's disease of cervical lymph nodes) (→ tongue, → thyroid gland).

On cut surface (Fig. 9.17), the lymphatic tissue is replaced by a gray-white tumor tissue that is elastic to soft in consistency. Yellow, sharply demarcated areas of necrosis and/or gray-white, firm scars are seen in the later stages of the disease, especially in certain histologic forms (see below).

The spleen is involved in 75% of the cases. Figure 9.18 shows the cut surface of an enlarged "porphyry spleen." Numerous yellow and firm foci measure up to 1 cm. The larger, yellow areas are infarctions that result from vascular involvement by Hodgkin's disease. Figure 9.19 is a close-up of the cut surface (taken under water). Individual Hodgkin's disease foci are irregular, gray-brown and vary somewhat in size.

Involvement of the liver (50%), lung (20%), kidney (10%) and bone (20%) by Hodgkin's disease also is manifested by yellow, sharply circumscribed foci of relatively firm consistency.
F: 0.2% in autopsy material. *A:* 30–40 years and 50–60 years. *S:* ♂ = ♀.

Hodgkin's disease is separated into four distinct histologic subtypes, according to the recent *Rye classification* (LUKES et al.). These subtypes correlate with clinical prognosis as follows:

1. **Lymphocyte-rich forms** (LR)

(a) **Nodular lymphocyte-rich form.**
Focal involvement of the lymph nodes, predominantly lymphocytes, histiocytes, few reticular cells. Sparse Sternberg-Reed cells or Hodgkin's cells, sparse eosinophilic granulocytes.

(b) **Diffuse lymphocyte-rich form (previously called paragranulomatosis).**
Histology comparable to the nodular lymphocyte rich form, but the entire lymph node is diffusely affected. Good prognosis (Fig. 9.20). The earlier the lymphogranulomatosis is discovered, the better will be the prognosis. The nodular form may change to the diffuse form, and this, in turn, may change to the mixed form. The reticular form may then appear in the terminal stage. The lymphocyte-rich forms and the nodular sclerosis have the best prognosis (50–60% survive for over 6 years, see Fig. 9.20). In a) and b), there is usually no organ involvement. *A:* 30–40 years. *S:* ♂:♀ = 4:1. Usually appears first in the cervical lymph nodes.

Pr: involvement of one group of lymph nodes by Hodgkin's disease (e.g., cervical form) has a good prognosis (5-year survival is 60%; 35% heal). The 5-year survival is reduced to 42% when single organs are involved. Only 5% survive for 5 years when the disease has spread to multiple organs (MUSSHOFF and co-workers).

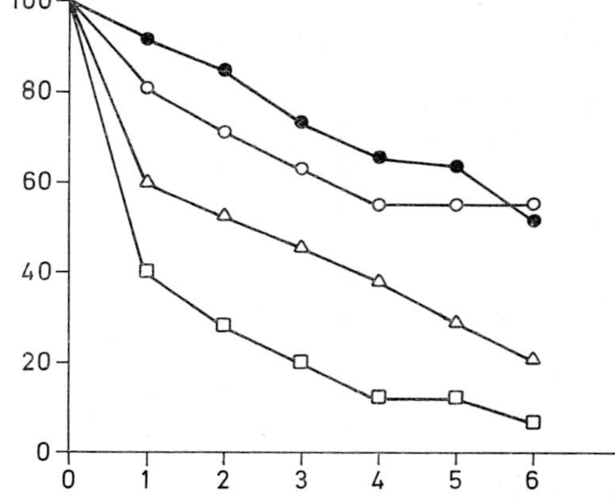

Fig. 9.20. Relationship between the survival rate and the histological type of lymphogranulomatosis (from PATCHEFSKY et al., 1973).

2. **Nodular sclerosing form** (NS).
Coarse lymph nodes rich in connective tissue. Histologically, ring-shaped bands of collagenous connective tissue (birefringent in polarized light) define granulomatous foci consisting predominantly of lymphocytes, a few reticular cells and histiocytes with light cytoplasm (so-called "lacuna cells," LUKES). **Young women are primarily affected.** A special form it does not change to any other.

3. **Mixed Form** (M). ("typical" lymphogranulomatosis) with reticular cells, lymphocytes, eosinophils, Sternberg-Reed cells, Hodgkin's cells, and areas of fibrosis and necrosis. *S:* ♂:♀ = 1:1. Survival rate: about 25% survive for more than 6 years.

4. **Lymphocyte-poor forms** (LP).

(a) **Diffuse fibrosis.** Few lymphocytes, abundant atypical reticular cells and collagenous fibrous tissue.

(b) **Reticular form** (previously called Hodgkin's sarcoma) with proliferation of highly atypical reticular cells and Sternberg-Reed cells. Sarcomatous growth with hematogenous metastases.

S: ♂:♀ = 1:1.

T: for all forms, x-ray radiation gives remarkably good results. For more meaningful therapy, the spleen is currently removed and information about the state of dissemination of the process is obtained by liver puncture and a biopsy of the iliac crest.

Cf: unknown. Virus infection? Hodgkin's disease is presently considered as a T-cell lymphoma (T = thymus dependent lymphocytes. Intracellular antibodies. Origin probably in the paracortical zone of the lymph node.

The lymphocytes cannot be stimulated with phytohemagglutinin = immunologic defect.

Tumors of Lymph Nodes (Lymphomas)

Tumors of lymph nodes present a rather uniform picture on gross examination (Hodgkin's disease, see preceding page). Only some characteristic gross findings will be discussed.

Reticulum-cell sarcoma of abdominal lymph nodes (Fig. 9.21; TCP, p. 177). The para-aortic lymph nodes are markedly enlarged and several nodes are fused together. The color is gray-white to yellow, the cut surface is rather homogeneous and the consistency is soft-elastic.

Carcinomatous metastases in lymph nodes (Fig. 9.22). In contrast to primary tumors of lymph nodes, the white tissue is somewhat more friable and dry. In addition, areas of necrosis and hemorrhage can occur.

Summary of lymphomas

F: Hodgkin's disease 53%, reticulum-cell sarcoma 12%, lymphatic leukemia 10%, lymphosarcoma 10%, giant follicular lymphoma (Brill-Symmers) 5–10%, reticuloses 0.5%.

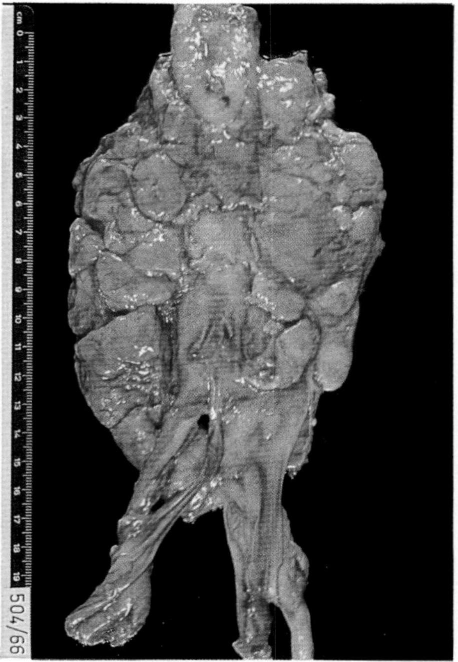

Fig. 9.21. Reticulum-cell sarcoma of abdominal lymph nodes.

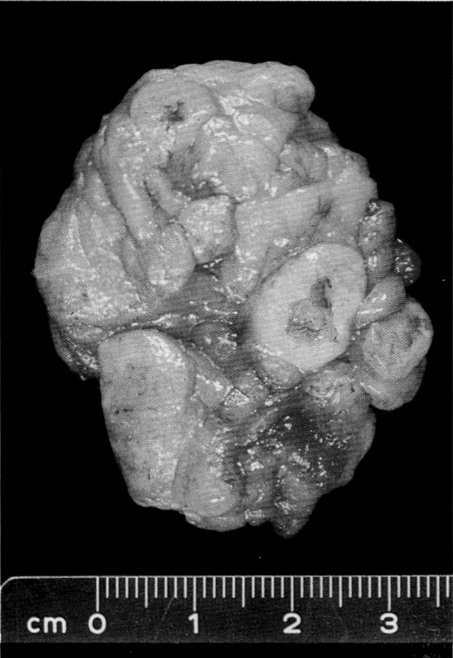

Fig. 9.22. Carcinomatous metastases in lymph nodes.

Summary of the primary lymph node tumors (lymphomas)

The malignant "non-Hodgkin lymphomas," whose classification has been greatly advanced in recent years by new methods of investigation, are differentiated from lymph-node lymphogranulomatosis. RAPPAPORT's nomenclature uses predominantly purely descriptive morphological criteria (nodular [=focal] or diffuse; histiocytic, lymphocytic; well or poorly differentiated). LUKES and LENNERT use electron microscopic and immunologic investigations (STEIN et al.) as a basis. It has been found that most lymphomas form immunoglobulins and realese these in part to the blood. Thus, certain lymphomas have been identified as descendants of B-lymphocytes. Corresponding T-cell lymphomas have also been described (T-cell lymphomas as reticulosarcomas, T-cell immunoblastic sarcoma, Hodgkin's disease). Another new feature of this classification is the recognition that there are tumors which start from the cells of the germinal centers of the lymphocytes (germinoblasts and germinocytes).

1. **Giant follicular lymphoblastoma** (BRILL-SYMMERS' disease, germinoblastoma, "follicle-center-cell tumor"). Proliferation of cells of the germinal center (predominantly germinoblasts, fewer germinocytes) which form giant follicles. Immunoglobulins can be detected in the lymph nodes and/or blood.

Ma: grey-red, relatively soft, enlarged lymph nodes. *Hi:* giant follicles (free of silver fibers) or irregular shape, no lymphocyte wall. *DD:* follicular lymphatic hyperplasia also shows giant follicles, but with many mitoses and symptoms of a nonspecific lymphadenitis. *Course:* the germinoblastoma may change to a germinoblastic sarcoma, which has the same histological appearance as a lymphoblastic sarcoma. *A:* 20–30 years and 60 years. *S:* ♂:♀ = 7:3. *Pr:* 60% survive for over 5 years, course 6–15 years.

2. **Reticulosarcoma** (reticulum cell sarcoma, immunoblastic sarcoma). Previously considered as a malignant proliferation of the reticular cells. However, RAPPAPORT assigns it to the histiocytes. Since immunoglobulins can be detected in the tumor tissue and polyribosomes are found abundantly under the electron microscope, the cells must be considered as immunoblasts (LENNERT). *Hi:* grows in a sarcomatous, destructive manner in the lymph node. The liver, spleen and bone marrow may be focally or diffusely permeated. The detection of reticular fibers is of no significance.

A: 50% of the cases are older than 50 years old. Peak incidence at 60–70 years. *S:* ♂:♀ = 3:1, other authors 1 = 1. *Pr:* course of $^1/_2$–1 year, 80% survive for less than 3 years.

3. **Lymphosarcoma.** Two types are differentiated:

a) **Lymphocytic lymphosarcoma** (germinocytoma). Diffuse proliferation of small lymphoid cells, usually generalized in all lymph nodes. IgM can frequently be detected. Frequently leukemic. Previously also designated as leukosarcomatosis. Resistant to therapy.

A: all age groups. *Course:* 6–12 months.

b) **Lymphoblastic lymphosarcoma.** This involves a diffuse proliferation of lymphoblasts. The best known representative of this group is Burkitt's lymphoma. First observed in Africa. Excessive enlargement of the cervical lymph nodes. Later generalized.

A: predominantly children. *S:* ♂:♀ = 3:1. *Cf:* Epstein-Barr virus.

4. **Lymphadenosis** (synonym: chronic lymphatic leukemia, see p. 193).

5. **Waldenström's disease** (lympho-plasmacytoid immunocytoma). Monoclonal macroglobulinemia, that is, increase in IgM immunoglobulin in the blood. In the lymph nodes, spleen and bone marrow, there is a diffuse increase of lymphoid cells, plasma cells, and their precursors. Mast cells are increased.

A: 60–70 years. *S:* ♂:♀ = 2:1. *Pr:* usually a prolonged course (30 months). Changeover to immunoblastic sarcoma. Increased susceptibility to infection. *T:* Good response to corticoids.

Table 9.1. Classification of Malignant Non-Hodgkin Lymphomas.

Old Classification	Classification According to Lennert-Lukes	Classification According to Rappaport "Malignant Lymphoma Type . . ."
Brill-Symmers disease	Nodular or diffuse germinoblastoma or "follicle-center-cell tumor"	Nodular, well differentiated, lymphocytic Nodular or diffuse, mixed Histiocytic-lymphocytic
Reticulosarcoma	Immunoblastic sarcoma	Diffuse, histiocytic
Lymphocytic lymphosarcoma	Lymphocytic sarcoma	Diffuse, poorly differentiated, lymphocytic
Lymphoblastic lymphosarcoma	Lymphoblastic lymphosarcoma, Burkitt's lymphoma	Diffuse, undifferentiated
Lymphadenosis, chronic lymphatic leukemia	Chronic lymphatic leukemia (CLL)	Diffuse, well differentiated, lymphocytic
Waldenström's disease	Lympho-plasmacytoid immunocytoma	Diffuse, well differentiated, lymphocytic

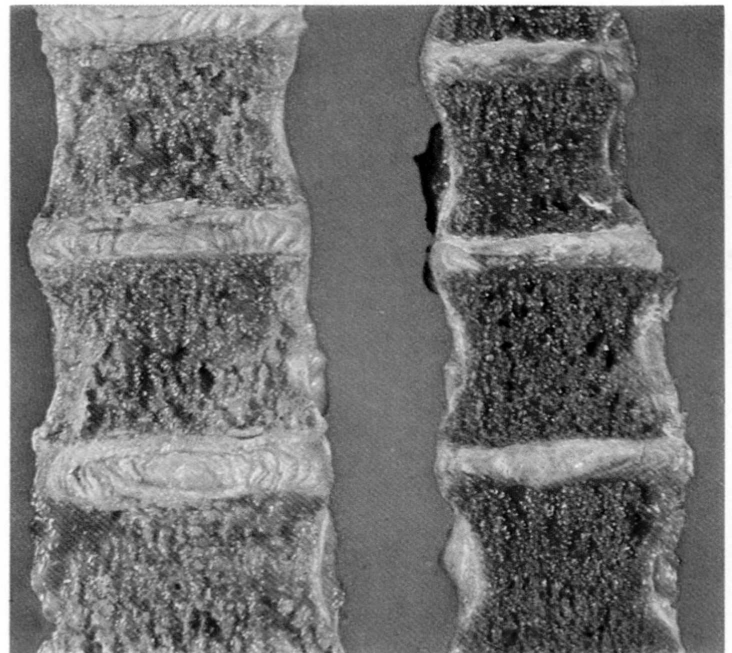

Fig. 9.23. Gray vertebral bone marrow in myeloid leukemia (normal marrow on the right).

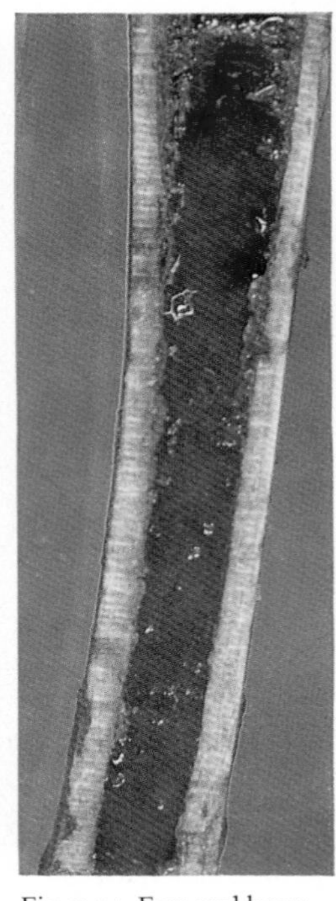

Fig. 9.24. Femoral bone marrow in myeloid leukemia.

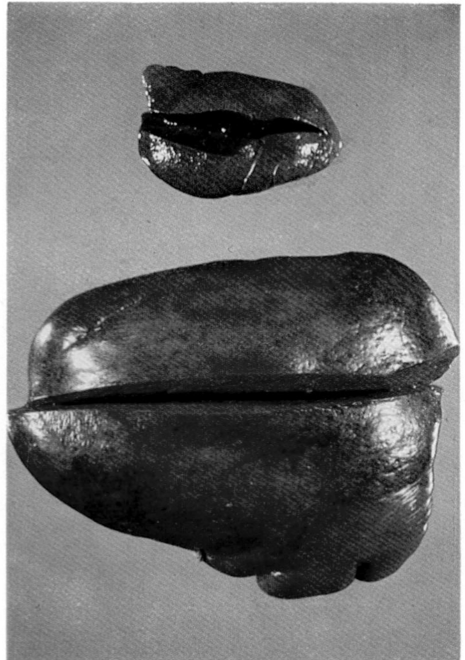

Fig. 9.25. Splenic enlargement in chronic myeloid leukemia. A normal spleen is shown above for comparison.

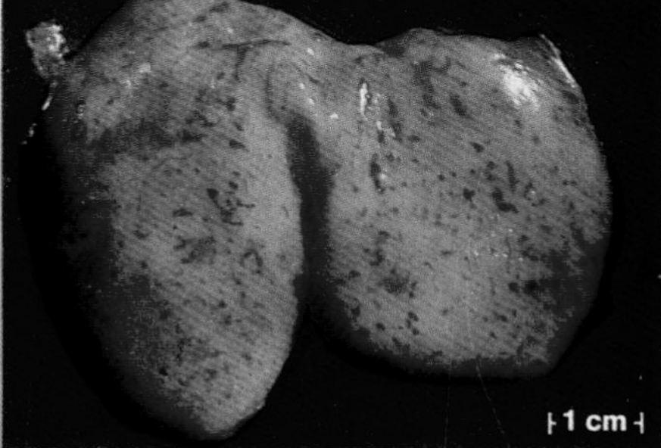

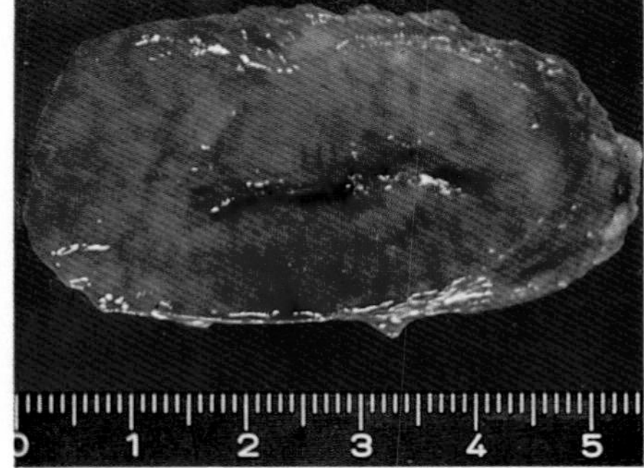

Fig. 9.26. Above: lymph nodes in chronic myeloid leukemia. Below: lymph nodes in lymphatic leukemia.

Leukemia

An increase in white blood cells in the bone marrow. The cells replace the normal cell population and disseminate into the blood (a better term is "leukosis," because leukemia is not always present). Types:

1. **Acute undifferentiated leukemias.** (a) *Blast-cell leukemias:* a differentiation is not possible on morphologic or histochemical grounds. Some of these immature forms have cells positive for peroxidase and esterase. (b) *Granulocytic types* (peroxidase type), with differentiation into paramyeloblastic, promyeloblastic or promyelocytic leukoses. The cells of these types react positively with peroxidase or naphthol-AS-D-chloracetate, which is not observed in lymphoblasts. Sometimes a so-called leukemic hiatus is found in blood smears, e.g., immature and mature cells are present without intermediate cell types. (c) *Lymphoblastic leukemias:* PAS-positive granules are present in the cytoplasm of leukemic cells. The granules do not occur in other types of leukemia. Therapy with cortisone prolongs life considerably. (d) *Monoblastic leukemias:* esterase-positive cells using α-naphthol acetate as a substrate. (e) *Monocytic leukemias* (= reticulosis with medium-large cells). Likewise esterase-positive cells. Nuclei are indented as in monocytes.

F: 45% of all leukemias. *A:* 5–10 years and 40–60 years. *S:* ♂:♀=1.5:1 (other statistics 1:1). The bone marrow is gray-red. The liver is markedly enlarged due to diffuse infiltration. The spleen and lymph nodes are minimally enlarged by infiltration with immature cells. The oral mucosa likewise may be infiltrated; frequent ulcerations. *Course:* 3–5 months. *Clinical course:* usually begins with fever (common cold; hemorrhagic diathesis and anemia. *Final course:* sepsis, fungus infections!).

2. **Chronic leukemias.** (a) *Chronic myeloid leukemia.* An increase in all cells of the granulocytic series, with predominance of immature cell types (more than 100,000/mm³). Diagnostic aberration of chromosome no. 21: Philadelphia chromosome. The spleen is greatly enlarged and may weigh up to 5 kg. The cut surface is homogeneously red to gray-red. Perisplenitis and splenic infarctions are frequent. A giant spleen is compared with a normal spleen in Figure 9.25. The marrow of the vertebral column is homogeneously gray-red (Fig. 9.23, left: leukemic marrow; right: normal vertebral marrow). The femoral marrow is gray-red to dark red (Fig. 9.24). The liver is enlarged by diffuse leukemic infiltrates (TCP, p. 133). The lymph nodes are slightly to moderately enlarged (Fig. 9.26). They are focally or diffusely gray-red in appearance.

F: 20–30% of all leukemias. *A:* 40–50 years. *S:* ♂:♀=1.5:1. *Course:* 3 years. *Cl:* splenic tumor; later, anemia and hemorrhagic diathesis. Death usually is due to cerebral hemorrhage or sepsis. *DD:* osteomyelosclerosis. Twenty per cent of the granulocytes in osteomyelosclerosis give a positive alkaline phosphatase reaction. Myeloid leukemia may develop terminally in patients with osteomyelosclerosis.

(b) *Chronic lymphatic leukemia.* (1) Mature lymphatic leukemia. Figure 9.26 shows an enlarged lymph node with a gray cut surface and several areas of hemorrhage. The spleen and liver are moderately enlarged (TCP, p. 133). Lymphoblasts and lymphocytes circulate in the *peripheral blood:* aleukemic leukemia below 3,000 cells/mm³, subleukemic below 20,000 cells/mm³, leukemic 500,000 cells/mm³. *F:* 30% of all leukemias. *A:* 60–70 years. *S:* ♂:♀ = 2:1. *Course:* 3–10 years.

(2) Immature lymphatic leukemia (leukosarcomatosis = leukemic form of lymphosarcoma); 20,000 to 40,000 lymphoblasts/mm³ in peripheral blood. Diffuse infiltration of lymph nodes, spleen and bone marrow with immature, monomorphous lymphoblasts with evidence of maturation. All age groups are affected. *Course:* 6–12 months. *DD:* lymphosarcoma: tumor *nodules* in lymph nodes and other organs.

(3) Mixed forms (tumor-forming lymphatic leukemia). Partly diffuse, partly nodular infiltration by immature lymphocytes with or without leukemic blood picture.

F: leukemias have increased in frequency during the past 50 years. Mortality in the United States: between 1921 and 1925, 2.04 ♂ and 1.54 ♀/100,000 persons; between 1951 and 1955, 7.71 ♂ and 5.32 ♀/100,000 persons. Mortality from leukemia in Germany: 6.2 ♂ and 4.8 ♀/100,000 population. *Pg:* the etiology is not known. *Virus:* RNA-tumor viruses have been demonstrated with certainty as leukemogens in animals. Similar virus-like particles also have been found in humans. *Irradiation:* increased incidence of leukemias in the population of Hiroshima and in radiologists. *Chemical substances:* e.g., leukemias after chronic exposure to benzol.

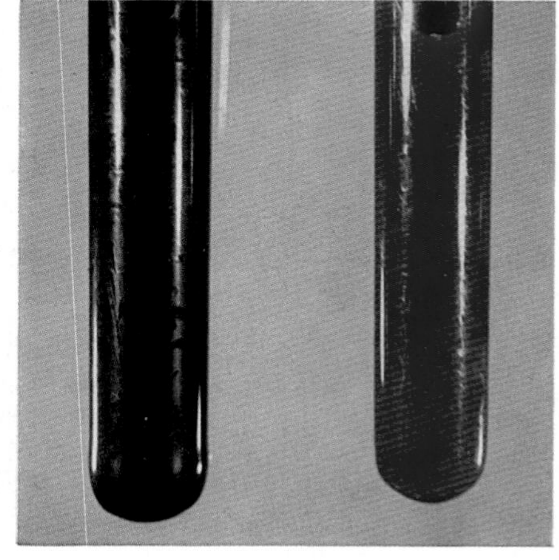

Fig. 9.27. Leukemic blood (right) and cyanotic blood (left).

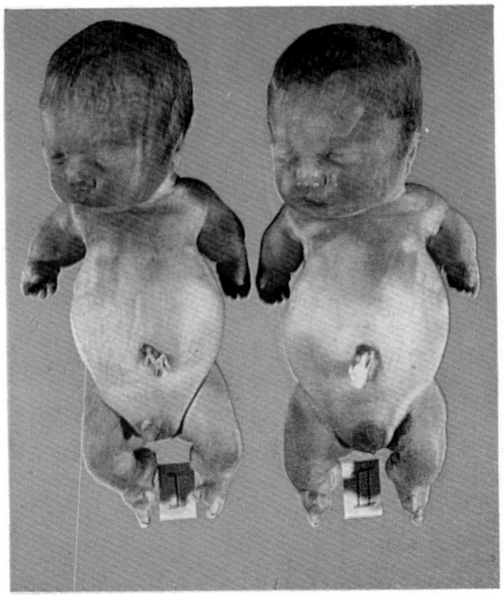

Fig. 10.1. Chondrodystrophy (achondroplasia) in twins.

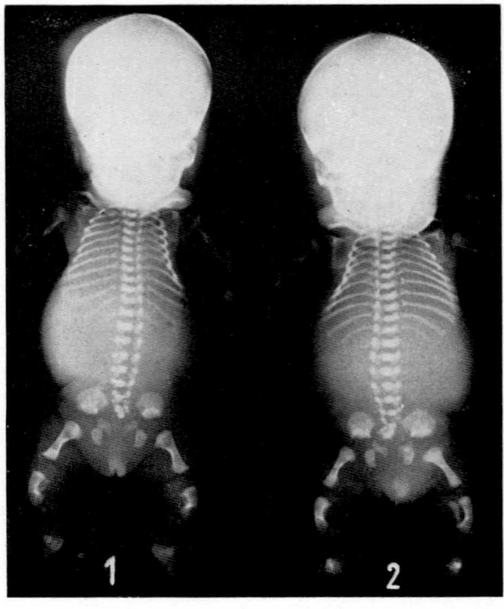

Fig. 10.2. Roentgenogram of achondroplastic twins.

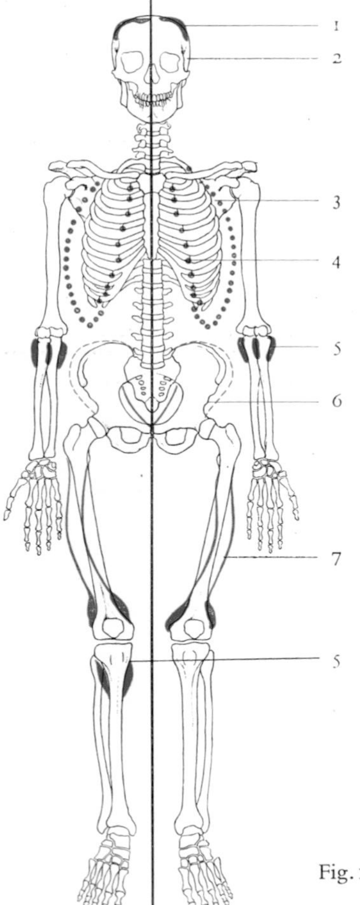

1. Caput quadratum
2. Craniotabes
3. Pigeon breast
4. Rachitic rosary
5. Trumpet-like distention of the elbow and knee joints
6. Flattened pelvis
7. Bowing of legs

Fig. 10.3. Schematic presentation of bone changes in rickets.

10. Cartilage, Bone and Soft Tissues

Chondrodystrophy, Rickets, Osteogenesis Imperfecta

Chondrodystrophy (achondroplasia, chondrodystrophia fetalis Kaufmann) (Figs. 10.1 and 10.2; TCP, p. 213). *A congenital disturbance of cartilage growth characterized by early cessation of endochondral ossification and thereby longitudinal bone growth.* Despite orderly perichondral and periosteal ossification, the typical gross appearance is that of a disproportioned dwarf (Fig. 10.1). The extremities are short and plump (micromelia), although the bones are normally formed (Fig. 10.2). The trunk is of normal configuration. The basal skull bones are somewhat smaller than normal and the forehead is prominent. Saddle nose and dorsolumbar kyphoscoliosis also are frequent manifestations of chondrodystrophy.

Pg: a dominant, genetically determined insufficiency of chondrocytes. The usual formation of the columns of cartilage is lacking (TCP, p. 213). *Co:* about 80% of those with achondroplasia are stillborn or die within the first year of life. Adult patients have normal intelligence and normal sex characteristics.

Rickets (Fig. 10.3; TCP, p. 213). *The disease is due to vitamin D insufficiency, which leads to faulty endochondral and membranous ossification of growing bones.*

Gross and histologic changes are especially noted in the zones of provisional calcification and in regions in which osteoid normally is mineralized. Metaphyseal zones of the knee and elbows are markedly enlarged. The stress of weight bearing causes anterior bowing of the tibia or a knock-knee deformity. The costochondral junctions are thickened, giving rise to the "*rachitic rosary*" of the ribs. The thorax is *bell-shaped.* The protruding sternum creates the impression of a "*pigeon breast.*" The weight-bearing pelvis is flattened. Excessive subperiosteal osteoid produces the typical "*caput quadratum.*" "*Craniotabes*" refers to thinned-out and soft occipital and parietal bones. The soft consistency of the skull bones is attributable to a lack of mineralization.

F: nowadays rickets is seen rarely at autopsy. *A:* the disease affects growing bones and, therefore, becomes manifest clinically between 6 months and 3 years of age.

Osteogenesis imperfecta (TCP, p. 213). *An inherited disorder of collagen maturation and consequently bone formation. Multiple fractures and growth retardation (short extremities, dwarfism) are the main manifestations. F:* 1 case in 2,000 births. *Pg:* recessive or dominantly inherited disorder? Two types are recognized: (1) Type *Vrolik* (lethal osteogenesis imperfecta): congenital bone fractures, blue sclerae, otosclerotic deafness, but normal lanugo hair. Life expectancy is 1 year on the average, maximally 10 years. (2) Type *Lobstein* (delayed type: osteogenesis imperfecta tarda): bone fractures develop after birth and longitudinal bone growth is retarded. Patients survive for 20 years. Brittle bones are the only manifestation of the so-called osteopsathyrosis *Ekman-Lobstein.*

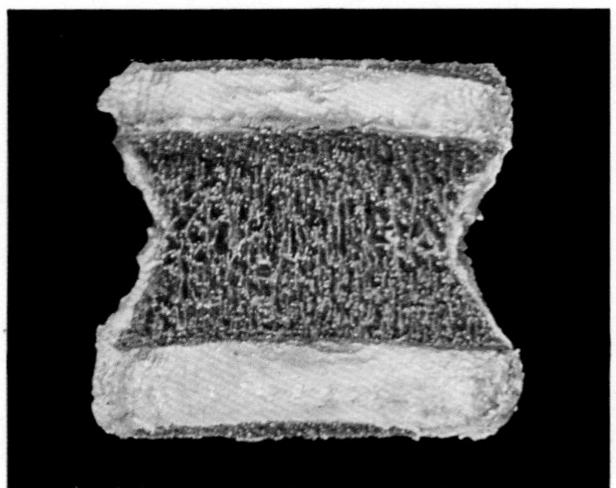

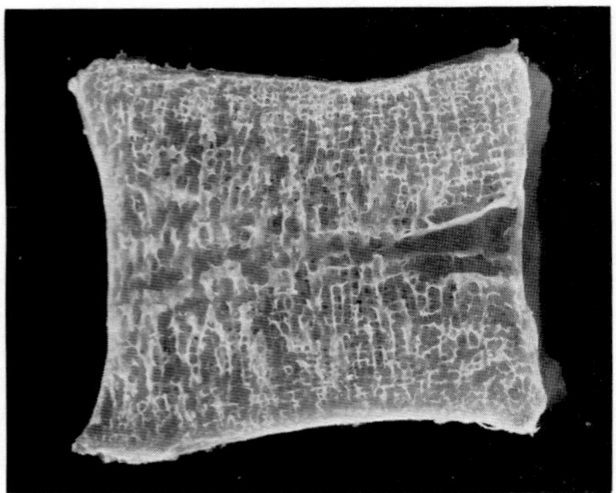

Fig. 10.4. Left: normal vertebra. Right: after decalcification.

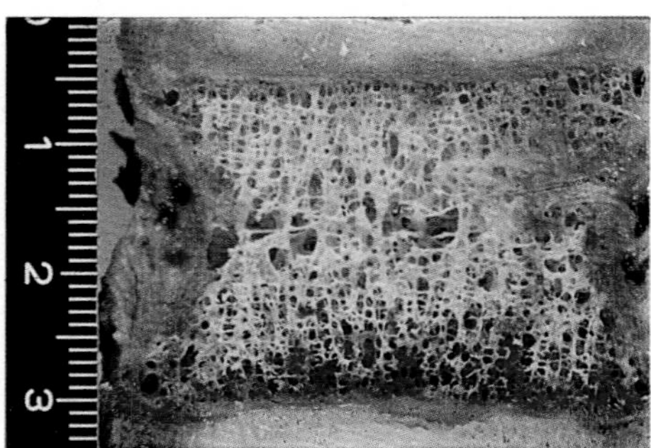

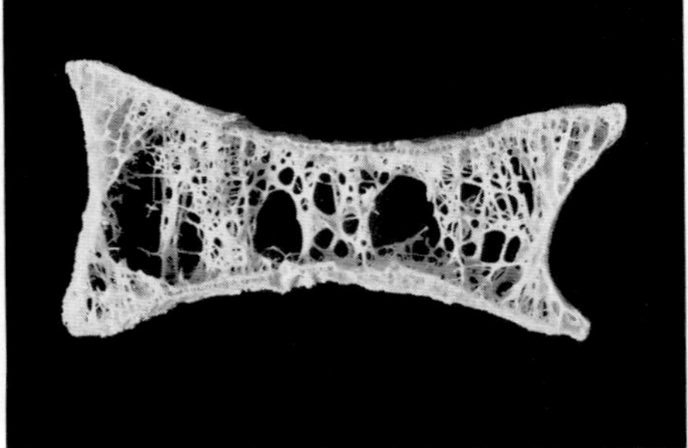

Fig. 10.5. Fresh and decalcified vertebrae from a case of osteoporosis.

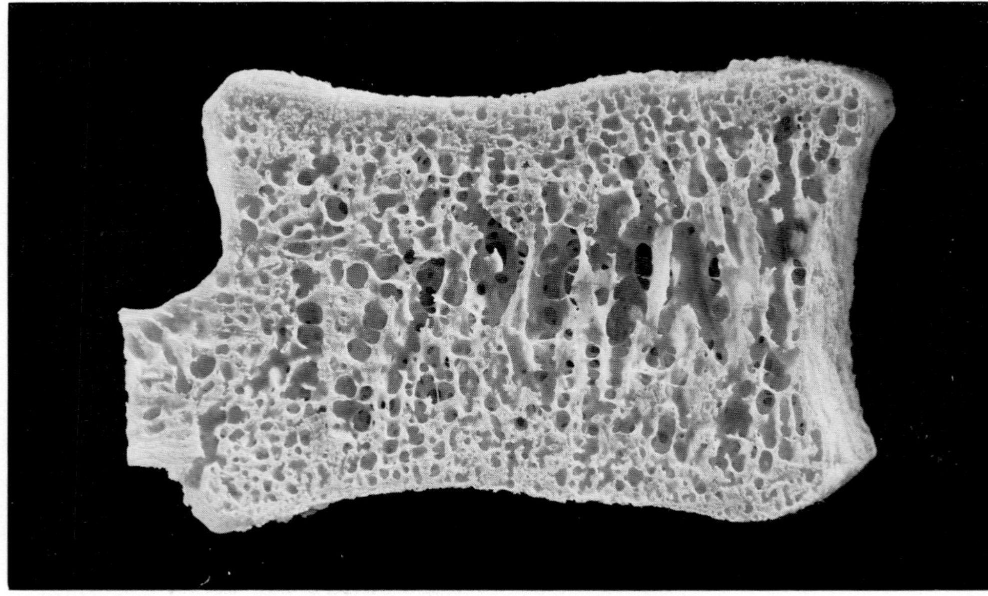

Fig. 10.7. Vertebra from a case of osteodystrophia generalisata.

Osteoporosis is a *common bone change characterized by atrophy* (Fig. 10.5; TCP, p. 215). The decrease in bone mass and corresponding increase in fatty marrow is shown in Figure 10.5. The normal vertebra has a regular, dense trabecular network (spongiosa) that encloses the hemopoietic marrow (Fig. 10.4, left). The normal, decalcified vertebra reveals axial trabeculae, which function as a carrier system, and horizontal trabeculae, which serve as a stabilization or "safety" system of the bone (Fig. 10.4, right). In osteoporosis (Fig. 10.5), the spongy trabeculae are smaller than normal and the medullary spaces become correspondingly larger. Osteoporotic atrophy first affects the horizontal trabeculae of the central areas of the vertebra. At this early stage, only excessive forces cause a compression fracture. Atrophy of the axial (i. e., longitudinal) trabeculae leads to further weakening of the carrier system and fractures are observed even after minor stress.

The neck of the femur is another common site of bone atrophy. In advanced cases, the horizontal trabeculae have almost entirely disappeared, whereas the axial trabeculae are normal or thicker than normal ("atrophic hypertrophy") (Fig. 10.6).

Pg: osteoporosis is a generic term. The pathogenesis is diverse: (1) *Senile osteoporosis:* physiologic bone atrophy after 50 years of age. (2) *Disuse or immobilization osteoporosis:* bone is resorbed when immobilized for any length of time. (3) *Endocrine osteoporosis:* examples are the *postmenopausal* osteoporosis (due to estrogen deficiency) and the *steroid osteoporosis* (e. g., Cushing's syndrome or prolonged cortisone therapy). Steroid-induced osteoporosis characteristically is confined to the vertebral column, skull and ribs. (4) *Nutritional or hunger osteoporosis:* a symptom of protein deficiency (like steroid osteoporosis). *Co:* fractures of vertebrae or femur neck with impaired healing (TCP, p. 215). Histologically, the trabeculae are thin, shortened and smooth. Osteoid seams and osteoblastic activity are missing.

Osteomalacia (adult rickets) (TCP, p. 215). *A disturbance of mineralization of the regularly formed bone matrix in adults, due to vitamin D deficiency. In severe cases, the bones are soft and flexible but not brittle.* The lack of mineralization is manifested as various deformities, such as kyphosis of the thoracic spine, a bell-shaped thorax, inward deformation of the pelvic bones, coxa vara as a result of a reduced femur angle (from 135° to 90°) or "granular" atrophy of the skull. The x-ray film shows pseudofractures (Milkman's lines).

A: predominantly senile patients are affected. Occasionally, osteomalacia is observed during the second half of pregnancy. *Pg:* faulty calcification of an otherwise normal bone matrix → unmineralized osteoid. *Cause:* vitamin D deficiency. Also observed in sprue or other malabsorption syndromes.

Osteitis fibrosa (osteodystrophia fibrosa generalisata, von Recklinghausen's disease) (Fig. 10.7; TCP, pp. 216 and 217). *A disease of increased bone formation and resorption, due to primary hyperparathyroidism.* Eighty per cent of the cases are attributable to an adenoma of the parathyroid glands. The disease clinically and pathologically is comparable to an acute osteoporosis. Figure 10.7 shows a *vertebra* with three horizontal layers. A porotic middle layer is surrounded on both ends by a dense network of spongy trabeculae, a finding typical of the disease. Small cortical cysts may develop in the *long tubular bones* due to increased focal bone resorption. Increased metaphyseal spongiosa and subsequently hyperostosis (resembling Paget's disease). The tabula externa of the skull is irregularly atrophic from bone resorption ("granular atrophy").

F, A and *S:* see hyperparathyroidism (p. 241). *Co:* pathologic fractures with hemorrhages occur throughout the skeleton in areas of bone resorption. The hemorrhages are organized by granulation tissue that contains multiple giant cells. These giant-cell granulomas often are described as "brown tumors," although they are non-neoplastic lesions. Brown tumors sometimes are mistaken for osteoclastomas!

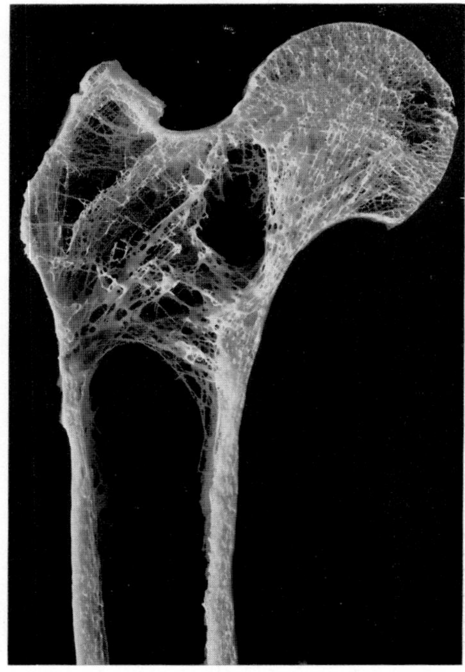

Fig. 10.6. Osteoporosis of the femur.

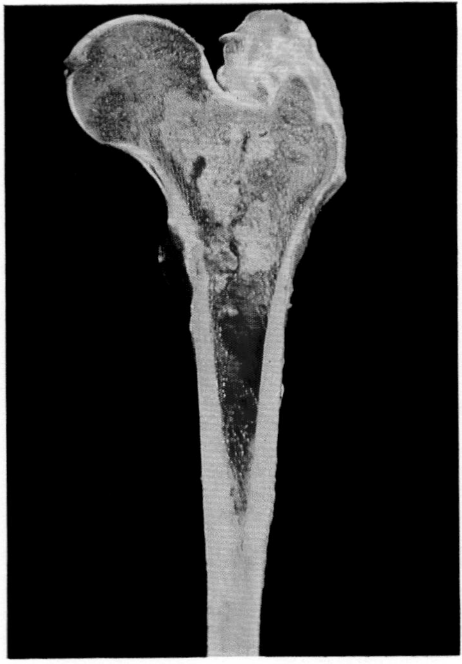

Fig. 10.8. Necrosis of the femoral marrow after prolonged cortisone therapy.

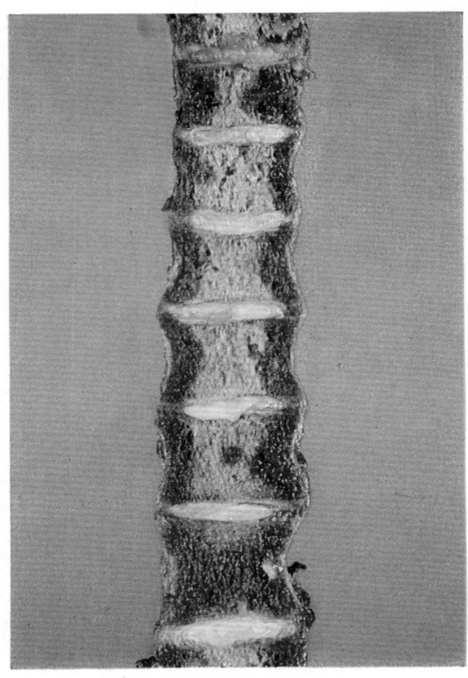

Fig. 10.9. Necrosis of vertebral marrow following x-irradiation.

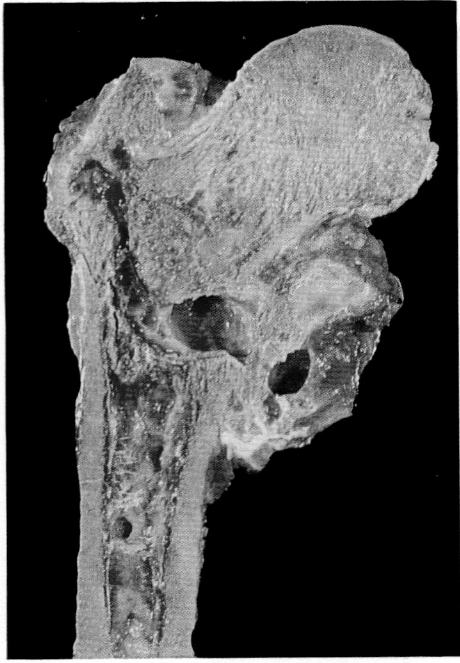

Fig. 10.10. Fracture of the neck of the femur.

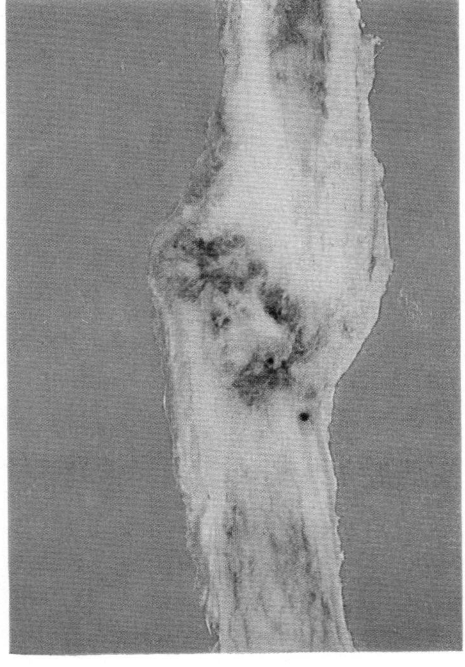

Fig. 10.11. Pseudarthrosis.

Bone Necrosis, Fracture, Pseudarthrosis

Bone necrosis (Figs. 10.8 and 10.9). Figure 10.8 shows extensive, map-like, gray-yellow areas of necrosis in the medulla of the proximal femur. The bone spicules and medullary fat are necrotic, whereas the cortex of the femur is intact. This is a case of bone necrosis from prolonged cortisone therapy.

Pg: bone necrosis and infarction are manifestations of reduced blood supply from mechanical, traumatic, thermal or other physical or chemical injury. Examples of bone necrosis are:

1. *Traumatic bone necrosis:* approximately 65% of all intracapsular fractures of the femur neck in older patients eventually develop bone necrosis from insufficient vascular supply.

2. *Bone infarctions following treatment with glucocorticoids:* the proximal femora are affected most often (♂:♀ = 2:1); less common are infarctions of the tibia, humerus and vertebrae. Seventy-five per cent of the patients are 20–50 years of age. Steroidal bone necrosis, which is independent of the dose of cortisone given, is considered the result of local ischemia (Zollinger).

3. *Caisson disease:* aseptic bone necrosis of the medullary bones of the femur, tibia, humerus and lumbar vertebrae. The ischemic necrosis is secondary to air embolism (especially nitrogen bubbles) during or after rapid decompression of atmospheric pressure (diver's disease).

4. *Thermal bone necrosis:* seen after burns or freezing of extremity bones.

5. *Chemical bone necrosis:* observed most often after phosphorus intoxication. The mandible is the site of most frequent involvement (watch-dial painters).

6. *X-ray necrosis:* Figure 10.9 shows extensive necrotic areas of the vertebral bone and marrow. Therapeutic x-irradiation was given to this patient for a carcinoma of the esophagus.

Co: infection → purulent osteomyelitis and pathologic fractures. Growth disturbances are common in children after x-irradiation.

Spontaneous, aseptic bone necrosis occurs most frequently in the epiphyses of growing bones. Aseptic emboli or local ischemia from transient arterial constriction are considered the most likely causes. The following diseases are examples of aseptic bone necrosis:

Perthes' disease (coxa plana juvenilis) is an aseptic necrosis of the femur head. The disease is detected in boys as young as 6 years of age. A flat femoral head and secondary degenerative joint changes are the late effects of Perthes' disease.

Calvé's disease (vertebrae plana osteonecrotica) refers to a collapsed necrotic vertebra with subsequent formation of angular kyphosis.

Kienböck's disease is an aseptic necrosis of the os lunatum, especially following fractures or trauma.

Köhler's disease is an aseptic necrosis of the tarsal navicular (metatarsal-phalangeal) bones.

Osgood-Schlatter's disease is an aseptic necrosis of the tibial epiphysis (tibial tubercle). The disease may occur in children and adolescents together with retarded rickets.

Bone fracture (Fig. 10.10; TCP, p. 209). Figure 10.10 shows an impacted fracture of the neck of the femur, which has been pushed into the medulla; the surrounding bone and soft parts are displaced.

Pg: most fractures are the result of trauma. Minor trauma may cause a fracture of a bone with pre-existing disease. Such *pathologic fractures* occur in bones involved with tumors, inflammations or metabolic diseases. *Co:* the normal healing of a bone fracture begins with the organization of the hematoma by a *provisional callus.* This early stage is followed by connective tissue proliferation, calcium deposition *(connective tissue callus)* and the deposition of compact spicules *(definite callus).* The healing process of a pathologic fracture is delayed or incomplete.

Pseudarthrosis (Fig. 10.11). The bony union of fractured bones is delayed or altogether missing when callus formation is defective. The result is a "false joint" or pseudarthrosis. The fractured bones are rounded and covered by firm connective tissue or a layer of cartilage. The bone remains abnormally mobile.

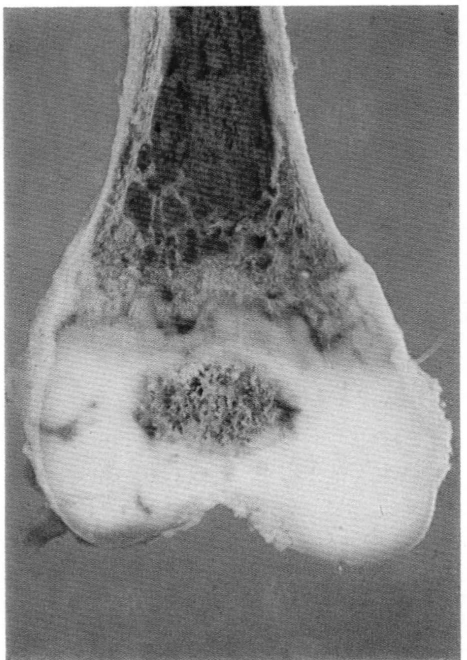

Fig. 10.12. Syphilitic osteochondritis.

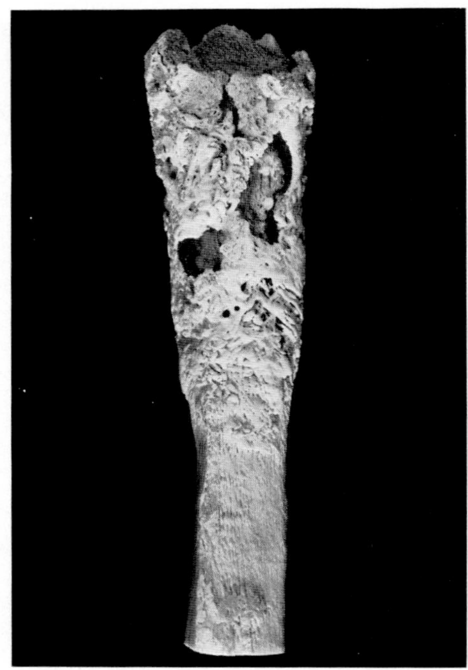

Fig. 10.13. Chronic osteomyelitis.

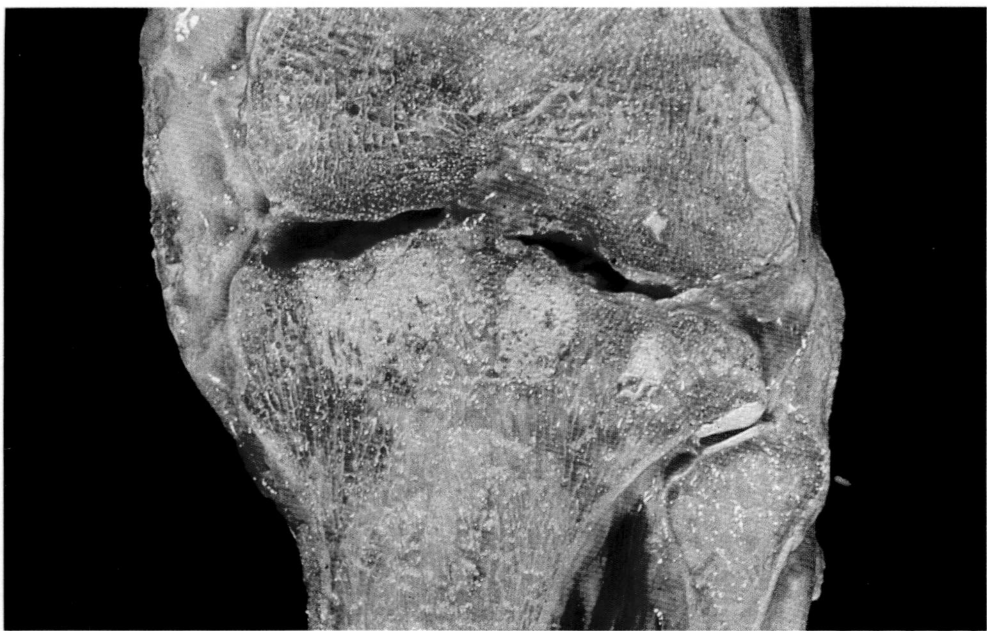

Fig. 10.14. Tuberculous osteoarthritis.

Inflammations of Bone

Syphilitic osteochondritis (osteochondritis luica; Fig. 10.12; TCP, pp. 123 and 211). *Congenital bone syphilis is a spirochetal inflammation* (Treponema pallidum) *that develops during the fifth intra-uterine month. Osteochondritis, generalized periostitis ossificans and fibrous osteomyelitis of the diaphyses of long bones may be present at birth.* Figure 10.12 shows the cut surface of the lower femur with a broad, gray-yellow, irregular (serrated) band in the provisional zone of calcification.

F: 80% of newborns with congenital syphilis develop osteochondritis. *Lo:* especially the femur, tibia and ribs. Syphilitic osteochondritis stimulates bone growth and, therefore, results in skeletal deformities. A typical example is the "saber tibia," an anterior bending and lateral flattening of the tibia.

Osteomyelitis (Fig. 10.13; TCP, p. 211). *A purulent, bacterial or fungal inflammation of the medullary bones with secondary involvement of the compact bone.* Figure 10.13 shows a decalcified tibia with considerable thickening of the proximal portion. The thickened cortical bone is due to sub-periosteal bone formation. The roughened surface is interrupted by two large defects that enter into a subcortical cavity with firm, sclerosed, bony walls. The cavity contained necrotic bone and communicated with the superficial skin by multiple sinus tracts.

F: osteomyelitis nowadays is a rare finding in autopsy material. *A:* hematogenous osteomyelitis is a disease predominantly of childhood and early adolescence; 80% of the cases occur between 2 and 16 years. *Lo:* osteomyelitis tends to localize in certain regions of the bones such as the lower end of the femur, upper and lower ends of the tibia and upper humerus. *Pg:* infection with *Staphylococcus aureus* is the most common cause of osteomyelitis. Streptococci, shigella or fungi less frequently are the cause of osteomyelitis. The inflammation eventually produces bone necrosis (bone sequestration). The necrotic bone is removed through a fistula tract or it remains enclosed and surrounded by sclerosed bone. Sequestration of the devitalized bone may last for years. *Co:* pyemia, sepsis, purulent arthritis or pathologic fractures. A squamous-cell carcinoma may develop near a fistula tract many years after the onset of osteomyelitis. Chronic osteomyelitis is one of the most common causes of secondary amyloidosis.

Special types of osteomyelitis:

1. *Brodie's abscess.* Focal osteomyelitis with abscess formation in the head of the tibia. The abscess is surrounded by a pyogenic membrane and fibrous or osseous sclerosis.
2. *Nonpurulent, sclerosing osteomyelitis Garré* is caused by microorganisms with diminished virulence. This type is seen predominantly in the jaw and is characterized by densely sclerotic, reactive new bone formation.
3. *Plasma-cell osteomyelitis* likewise is a less severe type of osteomyelitis. This type predominantly affects the jaw. A bone cavity is filled with plasma cells but reactive new bone formation is absent.
4. *Osteomyelitis of the small bones* usually presents as an osteosynovitis with early osteolysis.

Tuberculous osteoarthritis (Fig. 10.14). *Bone tuberculosis is always a manifestation of disseminated tuberculosis caused by hematogenous infection with tubercle bacilli.* Figure 10.14 shows the head of the tibia with several yellow, partly confluent lesions. They are centrally necrotic (caseation) and are referred to as *caries sicca.* The spongy bone is partly destroyed. The tuberculous process extends focally to the articular cartilage and joint space.

F: at autopsy approximately 0.4% of cases of tuberculosis have tuberculous osteoarthritis. *S:* ♂:♀ = 2:1. *A:* the disease can affect any age group, but it is more common at old age. *Lo:* vertebral column (tuberculous spondylitis), the phalanges (spina ventosa) and the shoulder joint (tuberculous omarthritis). *Co:* often healing with defects: ankylosis.

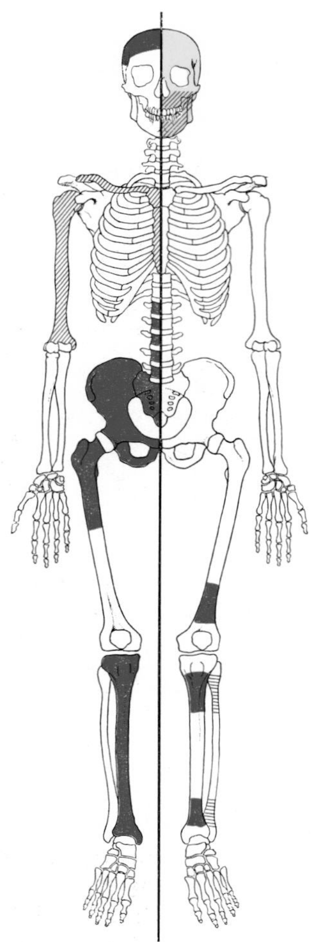

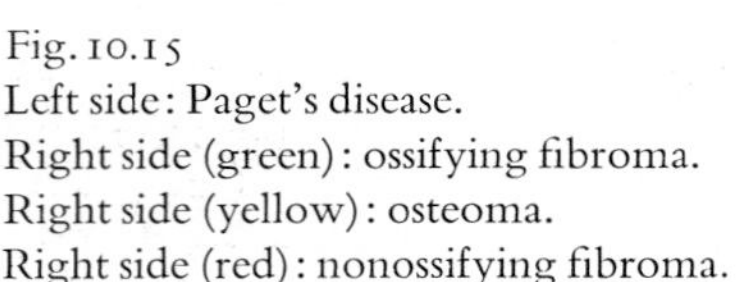

Fig. 10.15
Left side: Paget's disease.
Right side (green): ossifying fibroma.
Right side (yellow): osteoma.
Right side (red): nonossifying fibroma.

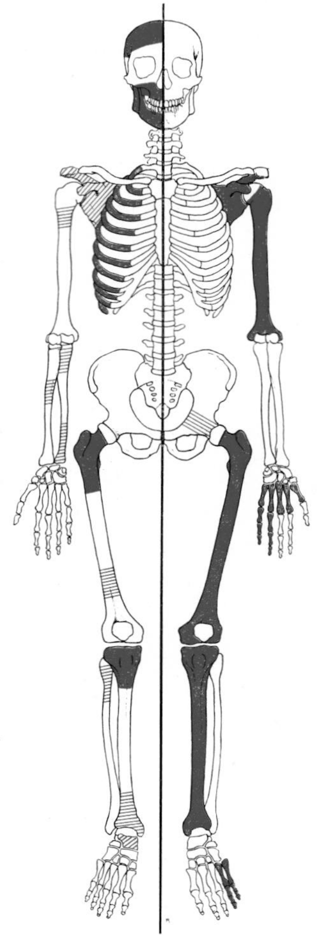

Fig. 10.16
Fibrous dysplasia.
Right side: polyostotic type.
Left side: monostotic type.

Osteitis fibrosa deformans (Paget's disease) (Figs. 10.15 and 10.17; TCP, p. 217). *A bone disease of older persons characterized by repeated waves of bone destruction and excessive bone regeneration. The disease is of unknown etiology. Skeletal deformities and irregular increases in the bony substance are the main gross manifestations.*

In Figure 10.17, the skull is increased in thickness from 0.5 to 3 cm. The tabula interna appears normal, whereas the diploë is displaced by an amorphous, spongy layer of bone. The tabula externa is irregularly roughened and sponge-like. The bones affected by Paget's disease are shown in Figure 10.15. Other bone deformities are the *saber tibia* (an anterolateral bending of the tibia), a compressed pelvis and exaggerated bowing of the vertebral column. *Monostotic Paget's disease* affects the proximal tibia or individual vertebrae.

F: next to osteoporosis and bone metastases, Paget's disease is one of the most common skeletal diseases of advanced age (approximately 3% of all autopsies on elderly patients). *S:* ♂:♀ = 4:3. *A:* usually manifest after age 50. *Co:* pathologic fractures, deformities of long extremity bones (coxa vara) and the vertebral column (kyphosis), pressure effects on nerves and blood vessels by compression of foramina. The most serious complication is the development of malignant bone tumors (malignant osteoclastoma or osteogenic sarcoma) in Paget's disease. Malignant tumors develop in 3% of severe cases of Paget's disease, with the skull and humerus especially affected. *Mi:* evidence of simultaneous osteoclastic resorption and osteoblastic regeneration. The bone trabeculae have a mosaic appearance created by the pattern of cement lines.

Fibrous dysplasia Jaffe-Lichtenstein (Figs. 10.16 and 10.18; TCP, p. 217). *A relatively common fibro-osseous disease of unknown etiology. Circumscribed areas of spongy bone are replaced by proliferating connective tissue with immature bone spicules.* Figure 10.18 shows a greatly deformed femur that resembles a "shepherd's crook." The medullary bone was occupied by a white, soft tissue that could be cut with ease. The cortex is eroded and thinned out by the proliferating medullary tissue but the periosteum is intact.

F: a disease of growing bone, common between 5 and 15 years. *S:* ♂:♀ = 1:2. *Lo:* see Figure 10.16. Fibrous dysplasia starts in the epiphysis and extends to the diaphysis. Solitary or monostotic dysplasias predominantly affect the base of the skull, the maxilla or the ribs. Fibrous dysplasia accounts for approximately 30% of benign bone diseases. *Co:* bone deformities, multiple recurrent fractures, rarely a fibrosarcoma (especially after x-irradiation). *Mi:* the spongy bone is replaced by a cellular fibrous tissue composed of delicate, horseshoe-shaped bony spicules, fibrous bone and osteoid. *Albright's syndrome* is a triad characterized by polyostotic fibrous dysplasia, patchy brown skin pigmentation (especially the skin of the trunk) and endocrine disturbances (precocious puberty, hyperthyroidism). Albright's syndrome occurs in young girls.

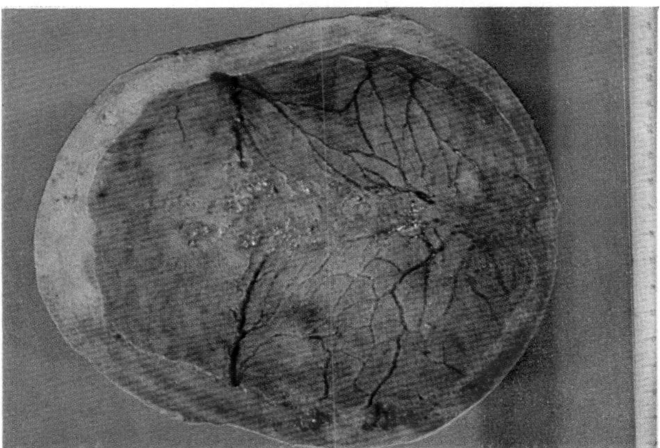

Fig. 10.17. The skull in Paget's disease.

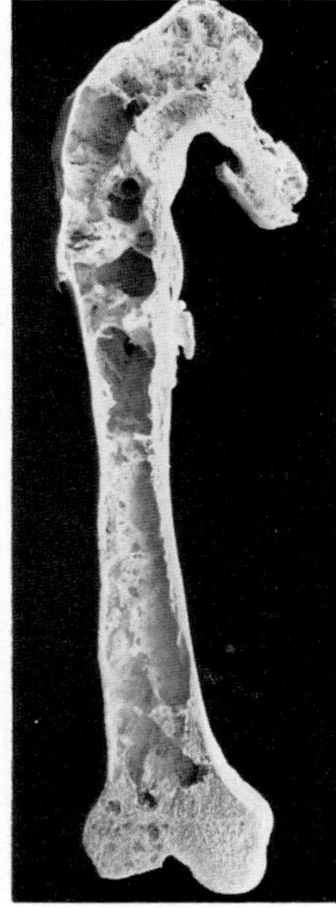

Fig. 10.18. Fibrous dysplasia of the femur.

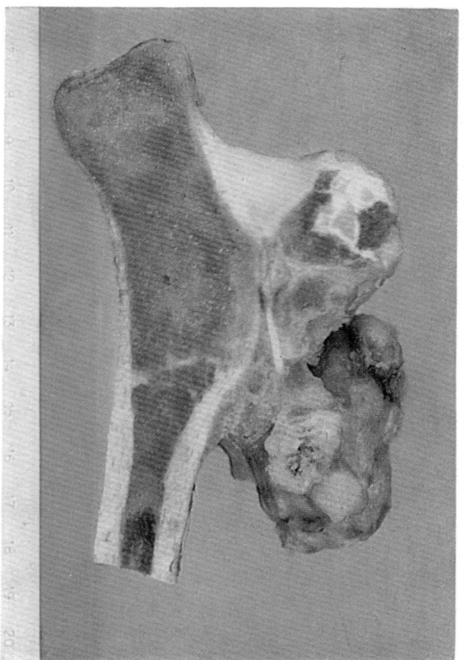

Fig. 10.19. Osteochondroma of the fibula.

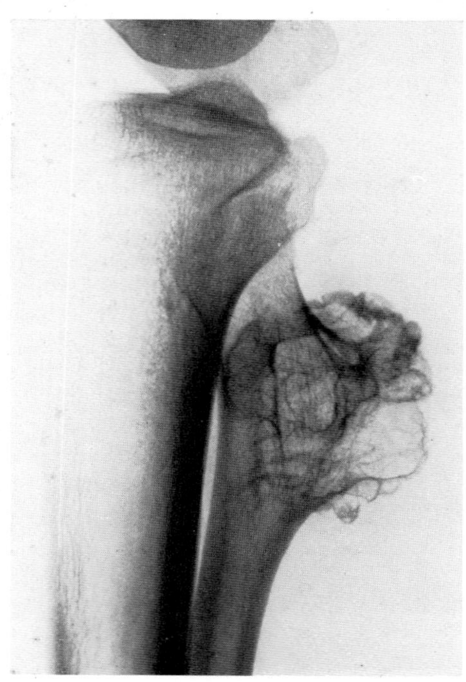

Fig. 10.20. Roentgenogram of an osteochondroma.

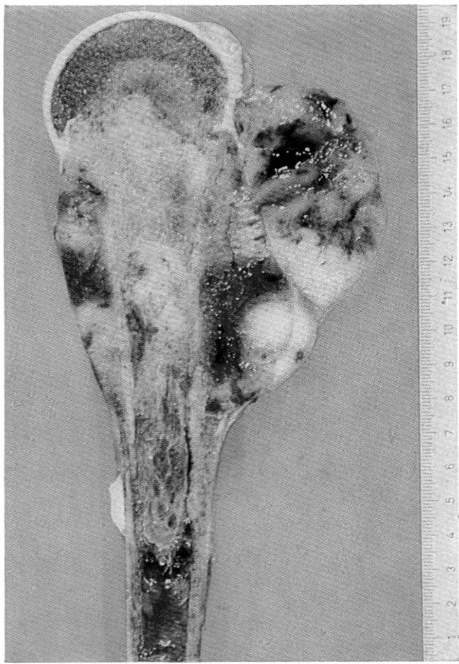

Fig. 10.21. Chondrosarcoma of the tibia.

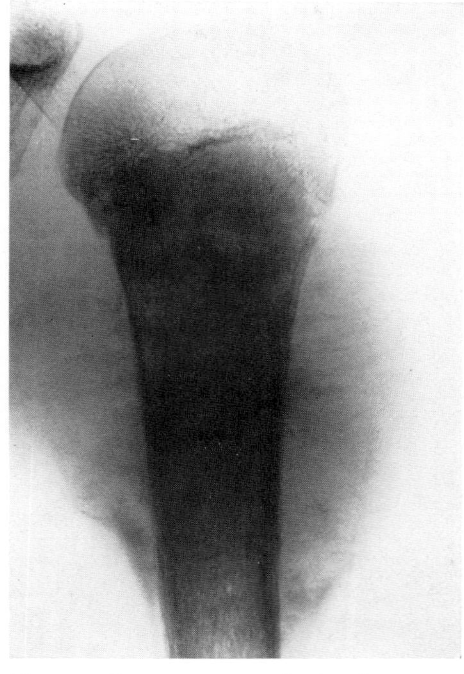

Fig. 10.22. Roentgenogram of a chondrosarcoma.

Tumors of Cartilage and Bone

Osteochondroma (ecchondroma, osteocartilaginous exostosis) (Figs. 10.19 and 10.20; TCP, p. 263). *This benign developmental malformation consists of a hyperplastic ossicle and a superficial, relatively acellular cartilaginous cap. An osteochondroma is attached to the superficial bone cortex.*

The gross picture is a bony protuberance, which may develop in all bones formed by endochondral ossification. Figure 10.19 shows the opened fibula. A sessile, cauliflower-like tumor mass is attached to the cortex. The mass is capped by a layer of cartilage approximately 2 cm. thick.

F: one of the most common tumor-like bone lesions (about 12%). *A:* mostly adolescents below 20 years of age are affected. *S:* ♂:♀ = 1:1. *Lo:* see Figure 10.34: epiphyses of long bones, scapula, pelvis, ribs and vertebrae. *Co:* malignant tumors rarely arise from an osteochondroma (less than 1%). A malignant transformation should be suspected when the cartilaginous cap of an osteochondroma is thicker than 3 cm. and when the tumor enlarges after the age of 20 years. *Mi:* the cartilaginous cap is composed of regular chondrocytes that extend as cellular columns into the underlying osseous portion. The lesion is covered by periosteum (TCP, p. 263).

Chondrosarcoma (Figs. 10.21 and 10.22; TCP, p. 265). *A malignant tumor of cartilage that continues to produce cartilage cells throughout its growth.* Figure 10.21 shows a nodular, lobulated tumor of the proximal humerus. Only a small portion of the tumor was covered by periosteum. The viable areas of the tumor are gray-white, somewhat moist and glassy in appearance (cartilage). In addition, irregular areas of partly hemorrhagic, partly gelatinous necrosis and cystic spaces (pseudocysts) are observed on cut surface. The cortex and medulla of the bone are infiltrated by white-gray, glassy tumor tissue.

F: 11% of all malignant bone tumors. *A:* primary chondrosarcomas (see below) occur after 60 years of age. Secondary chondrosarcomas are seen between 30 and 40 years. *S:* 60% ♂. *Lo:* predominantly the skeleton of the trunk (see Fig. 10.35). *Co:* recurrence after resection is frequent. A chondrosarcoma infiltrates veins and metastasizes late. Changes compatible with the diagnosis of fibrosarcoma or osteosarcoma are seen occasionally in chondrosarcomas.

Mi: tumor cells are atypical cartilage cells with plump nuclei, sometimes multinucleated. The differential diagnosis between chondroma and chondrosarcoma sometimes is difficult and always should be made on histologic grounds.

Chondrosarcomas are grouped according to their *location:* a *central* chondrosarcoma arises in the medulla of the bone, from which it infiltrates the cortex and adjacent soft parts. Areas of calcification are common in central chondrosarcomas. A *peripheral* chondrosarcoma appears first as a periosteal mass (Fig. 10.21).

According to their *mode of origin*, chondrosarcomas are divided into primary and secondary types. A secondary chondrosarcoma originates in a pre-existing benign chondroma, such as a solitary enchondroma or any of the lesions in Ollier's disease. Ten per cent of the multiple cartilaginous exostoses become malignant. The primary chondrosarcoma arises as such *ab initio*, without preceding chondroma.

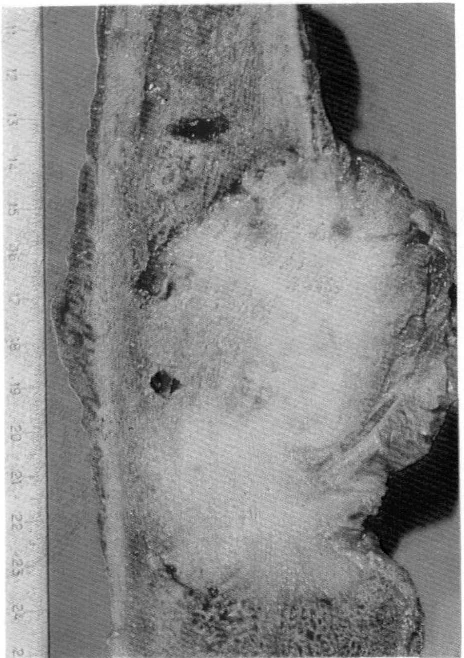

Fig. 10.23. Osteosarcoma of the tibia.

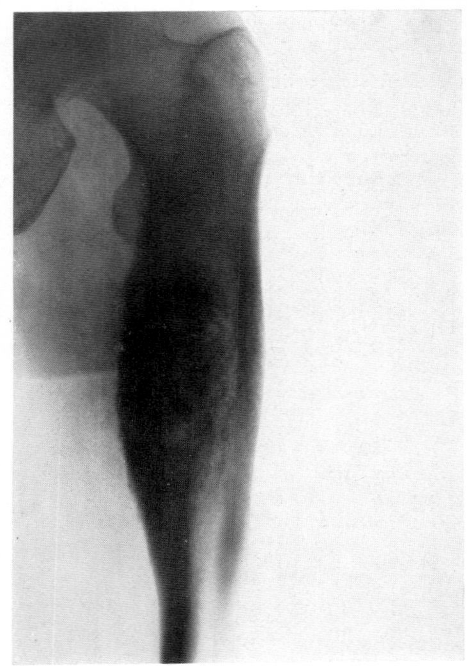

Fig. 10.24. Roentgenogram of an osteosarcoma of the femur.

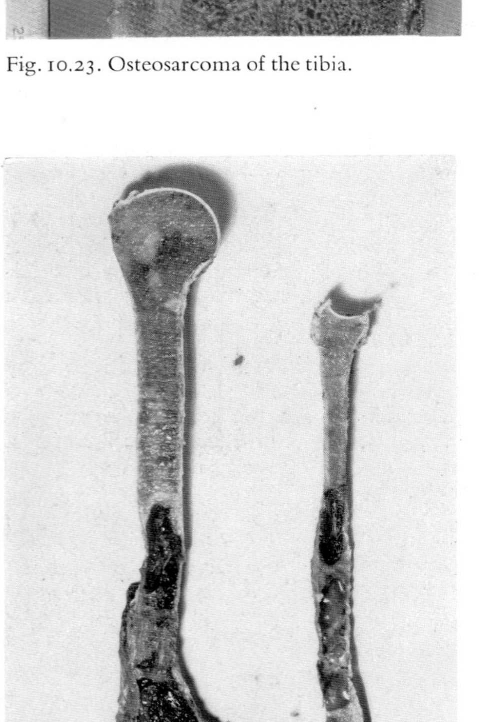

Fig. 10.25. Osteoclastoma of the humerus and ulna.

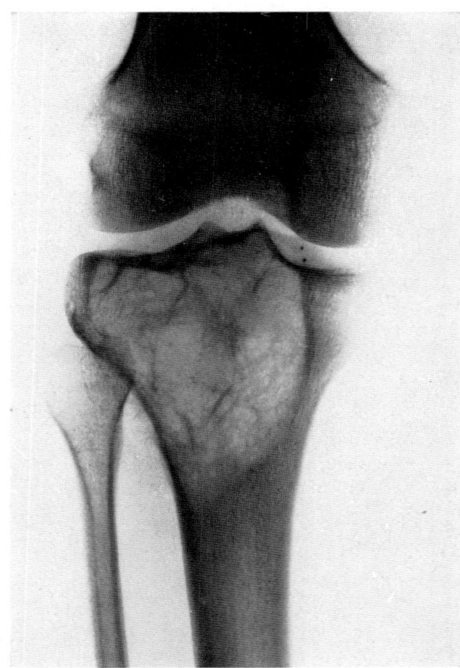

Fig. 10.26. Roentgenogram of a tibial osteoclastoma.

Osteosarcoma (osteogenic sarcoma) (Figs. 10.23, 10.24 and 10.27; TCP, p. 263). *Malignant bone tumor that forms neoplastic osteoid, cartilage and bone.*

Figure 10.23 shows the opened distal tibia. A large tumor occupies most of the medulla and destroys the cortex. The central portions of the tumor are homogeneously gray-white and bony hard, whereas the peripheral areas are softer and glassy. Cartilage and a highly cellular tumor stroma are found histologically in the periphery of the sarcoma. Reactive (non-neoplastic!) bone formation can be seen grossly and in roentgenograms as elongated bone spicules in the subperiosteal portions of the tumor. The periosteum has been elevated and separated from the bone cortex, producing the characteristic Codman's triangle. This triangle is free of neoplastic tissue and, therefore, is not suitable for diagnostic purposes (biopsy).

F: the most common malignant bone tumor (22%). *A:* 10–20 years, except for osteosarcomas arising in Paget's disease (♂ past 50 years). *S:* ♂:♀ = 6:4. *Lo:* osteosarcomas arise in actively growing bones, such as the epiphyses of the long-extremity bones (especially the knees). See Figure 10.34. *Co:* an osteosarcoma is a fast-growing tumor, usually producing a large tumor mass at the site of origin (Fig. 10.27). Hematogenous metastases to the lungs occur early. *Mi:* highly cellular tumor with evidence of differentiation into osteoid, osseous and cartilaginous tissues. Most normal bony spicules are destroyed; areas of necrosis and hemorrhage are observed frequently (see TCP, p. 263).

Osteosarcomas may present radiologically as predominantly *osteolytic* (x-ray: moth-eaten appearance) or *osteoblastic tumors*. According to their sites of origin, osteosarcomas also are divided into:

1. *Periosteal osteosarcomas* arise from the periosteum and preferentially infiltrate the surrounding soft parts. The normal bone is only superficially eroded. Periosteal osteosarcomas frequently are located in the popliteal fossa. Their x-ray appearance is that of "sunburst spicules" (due to reactive periosteal bone formation). The periosteal types have a better prognosis than the *endosteal types*.

2. *Parosteal (juxtacortical) osteosarcomas* grow slowly from the external surface of a bone and occur in an age group somewhat older than that of other osteosarcomas (76% are in females). *Lo:* posterior knee.

3. "*Paget sarcomas*" are osteogenic sarcomas that develop in bones affected by polyostotic Paget's osteitis fibrosa. Approximately 3% of Paget's disease lesions become malignant. Sites of predilection are the skull and the humerus.

Osteoclastoma (giant-cell tumor) (Figs. 10.25 and 10.26; TCP, p. 207). *A primary tumor of osseous mesenchyme with multinucleated giant cells (osteoclasts).* Osteoclastomas destroy the involved bone, frequently recur after excision and may spread to distant organs via the blood stream (approximately 7–23%). Figure 10.25 shows the humerus and the ulna with several large cystic spaces in the medulla. These pseudocysts are filled with a blood-rich, friable to soft tumor tissue. Figure 10.26 is a roentgenogram of an osteoclastoma in the proximal tibia. The translucent areas correspond to the multiloculated pseudocysts.

F: 4% of all bone tumors but 15% of all benign bone tumors. *A:* 75% of osteoclastomas occur between the ages of 20 and 40 years. An osteoclastoma should be considered malignant when the tumor occurs after the age of 40. *S:* ♂ = ♀. *Lo:* osteoclastomas arise in the epiphysis and extend to the diaphysis. Sixty-five per cent of osteoclastomas originate in the distal femur and proximal tibia. Pelvic osteoclastomas tend to become malignant. See also Figure 10.33. *DD:* "brown tumors" of von Recklinghausen's osteitis fibrosa.

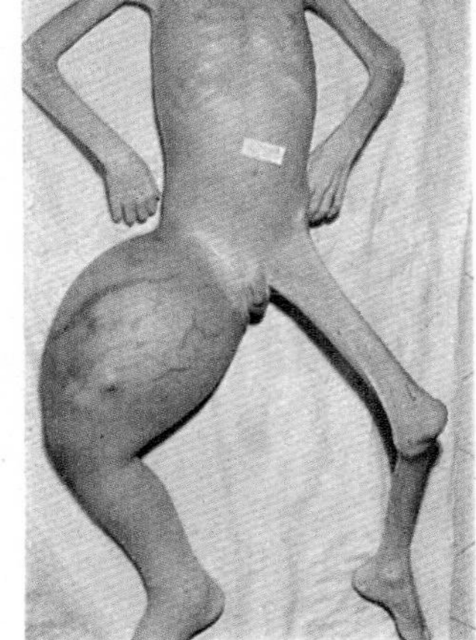

Fig. 10.27. Osteosarcoma of the femur.

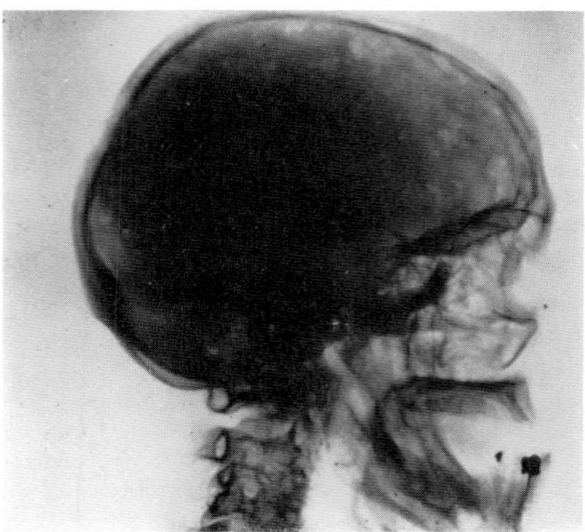

Fig. 10.28. Multiple myeloma with osteolytic lesions in the skull.

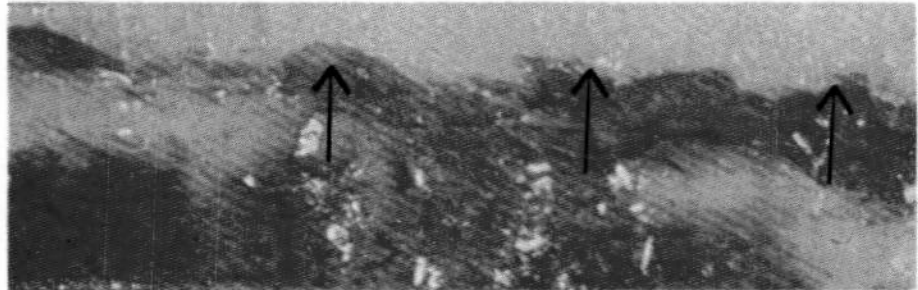

Fig. 10.29. Eroded cortex of the femur in a case of multiple myeloma.

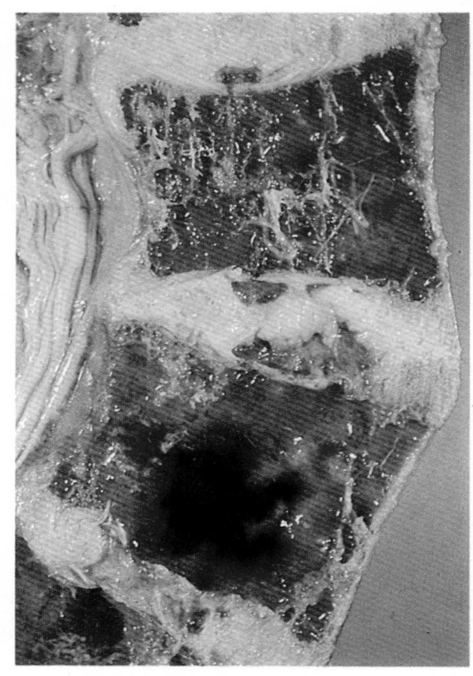

Fig. 10.30. Osteolytic foci in a vertebra in multiple myeloma.

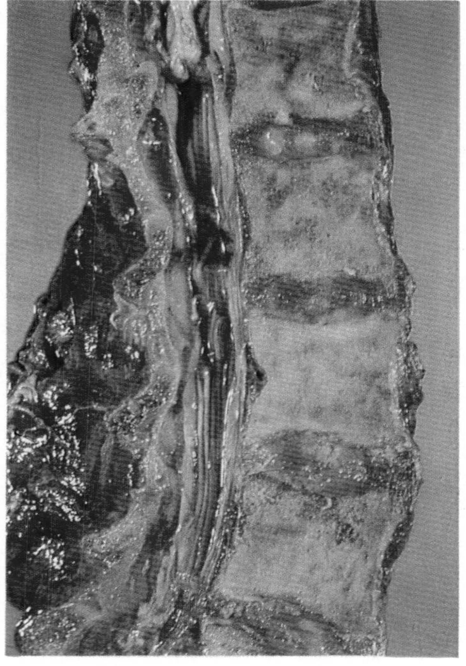

Fig. 10.31. Osteoblastic metastases in several vertebrae from a stomach carcinoma.

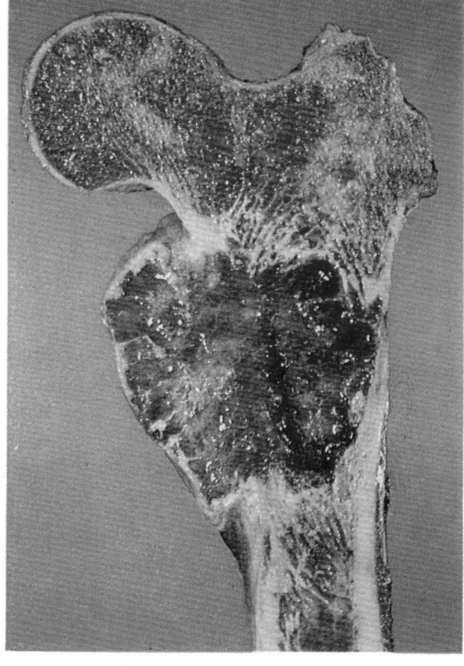

Fig. 10.32. Osteolytic metastases in the femur from a renal carcinoma.

Multiple myeloma (plasmacytoma; Figs. 10.28–10.30 and 10.36; TCP, p. 263). *A malignant tumor that arises multicentrically in the bone marrow, leading to multiple osteolytic lesions.* The gross pathologic findings are attributable to the proliferation of mature or immature plasma cells first within and later outside the bone marrow. The neoplastic plasma cells secrete abnormal proteins (myeloma proteins), which are found in the serum and multiple tissues (monoclonal gammopathy).

Figure 10.28 shows a skull roentgenogram from a patient with multiple myeloma. Multiple, punched-out areas of bone destruction are seen. Larger, red, glassy osteolytic lesions in several vertebrae are shown in Figure 10.30. A section from the femur (Fig. 10.29) reveals irregular, "moth-eaten" erosions of the cortical bone.

A: 75% of the patients with multiple myeloma are 50–70 years of age. *S:* ♂:♀ = 7:3. *Lo:* vertebrae, pelvis, sternum, ribs and skull (Fig. 10.36). *Co:* pathologic fractures (especially in the spine, with kyphosis and paralysis), anemia, multiple myeloma kidney (the result of excretion of Bence Jones protein = monoclonal light chains of antibodies), nephrocalcinosis (skeletal destruction → hypercalcemia) and uremia. Amyloidosis is observed in approximately 10% of patients with multiple myeloma.

Ewing's sarcoma. *A malignant tumor of bone probably derived from the reticular tissue and occurring in persons below the age of 25 years. The clinical course is rapidly fatal. Tumor growth sometimes is accompanied by fever and local swelling. Ewing's sarcoma metastasizes early.* The early stages of Ewing's sarcoma often are confused with an acute osteomyelitis. The diaphyses of the femur, tibia and humerus as well as the pelvic bones are affected most commonly.

Pg: the origin of Ewing's sarcoma is still controversial. It is believed to arise from the medullary tissue of bone. Some authors hold that Ewing's sarcoma represents osseous metastases of a neuroblastoma.

Reticulum-cell sarcoma. *A primary bone sarcoma derived from mesenchymal medullary tissue and occurring predominantly in males between 25 and 50 years of age.* In contrast to Ewing's sarcoma, the clinical course of a reticulum-cell sarcoma is more protracted, and a spontaneous fracture often presents as an initial symptom. Sites of predilection are similar for reticulum-cell sarcoma and Ewing's sarcoma (Fig. 10.36); therefore, reticulum-cell sarcoma was interpreted as a special form of Ewing's sarcoma. Reticulum-cell sarcomas are accompanied by zones of osteolysis and osteosclerosis, resembling Paget's disease of the bone. *Th:* Ewing's sarcoma and the osseous reticulum-cell sarcoma are radiosensitive neoplasms.

Metastases to the bone (Figs. 10.31, 10.32 and 10.37). *Most metastases in bones are due to carcinomas.* According to their growth effects and x-ray appearance, metastases may destroy bone *(osteolytic)*, elicit new bone formation *(osteoplastic)* or are indifferent (rare).

Figure 10.31 shows the opened spine. The vertebrae are uniformly gray-white, sclerosed and of hard consistency. The spongy network of the normal vertebra is missing because of multiple osteoplastic metastases from a stomach carcinoma. In contrast, Figure 10.32 shows the opened femur with a large area of cortical and medullary bone destruction by an osteolytic metastasis from a hypernephroid carcinoma of the kidney.

F, A and *S* are dependent on the primary site and type of the tumor. In order of frequency, the bones most commonly involved are the spine, sternum, ribs, femur, humerus and skull (see Fig. 10.37).

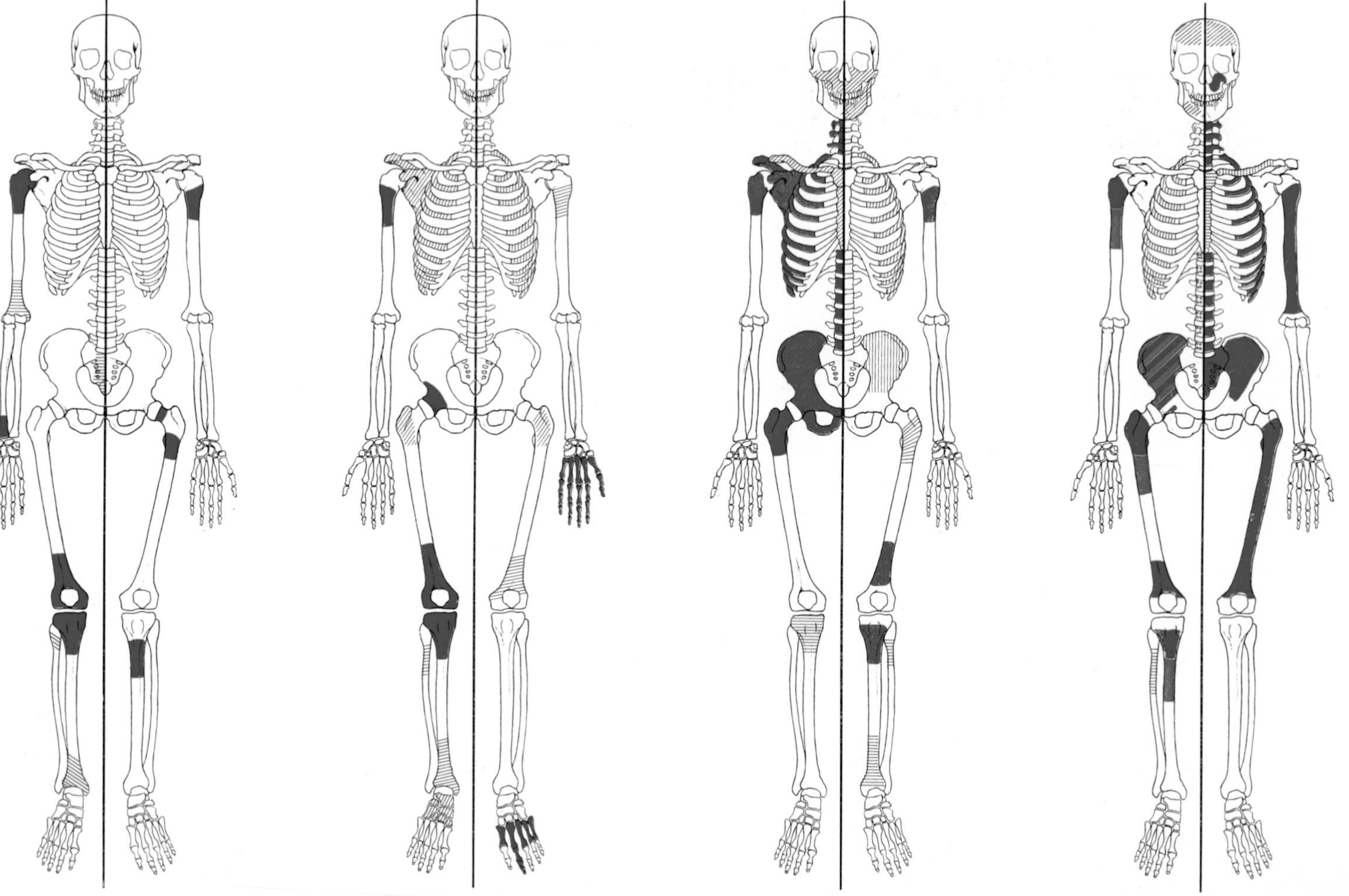

Fig. 10.33. Left: osteoclastoma. Right: juvenile bone cyst.

Fig. 10.34. Left: osteochondroma. Right: enchondroma.

Fig. 10.35. Left: chondrosarcoma. Right: osteosarcoma.

Fig. 10.36. Left (red): reticulum-cell sarcoma. Left (green): Ewing's sarcoma. Right: mul-

Bone Metastases

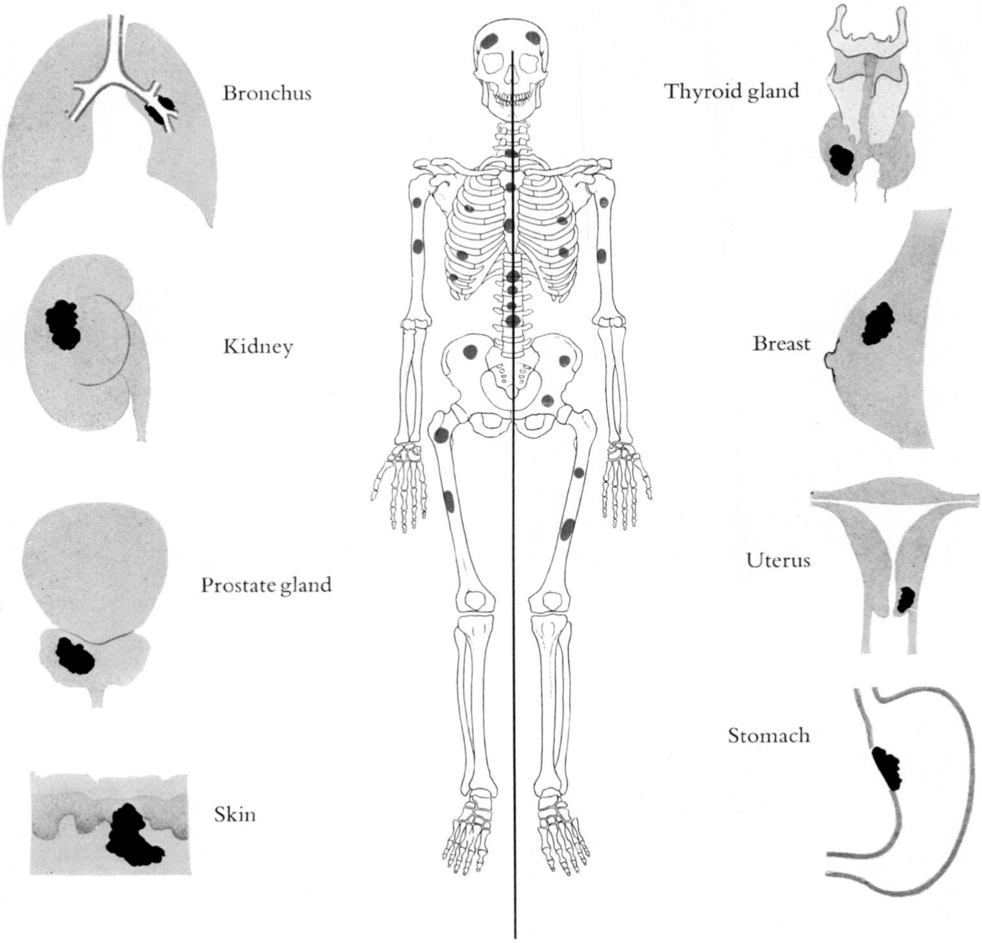

Bronchus

Thyroid gland

Kidney

Breast

Prostate gland

Uterus

Stomach

Skin

Fig. 10.37. Localization of bone metastases and primary tumor sites.

The following tumors *commonly metastasize* to the bones:

1. Breast carcinoma (approximately 47% of the carcinomas metastasize to the bones).
2. Prostate carcinoma (43%).
3. Thyroid carcinoma (31%).
4. Bronchial carcinoma (30%).
5. Hypernephroid renal carcinoma (30%).
6. Carcinoma of the skin (15%).
7. Carcinoma of the cervix (12%). See also Figure 10.37

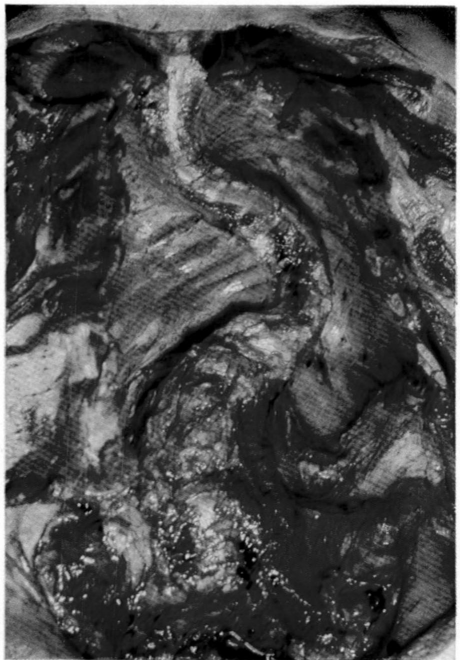

Fig. 10.38. Scoliosis of the spine.

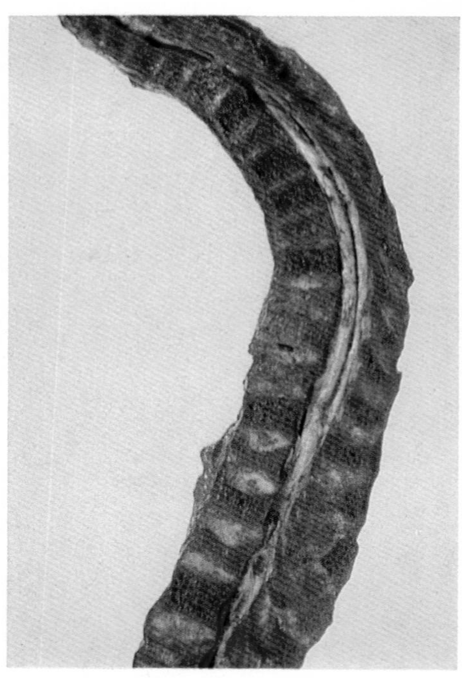

Fig. 10.39. Kyphosis of the spine in a case of osteoporosis.

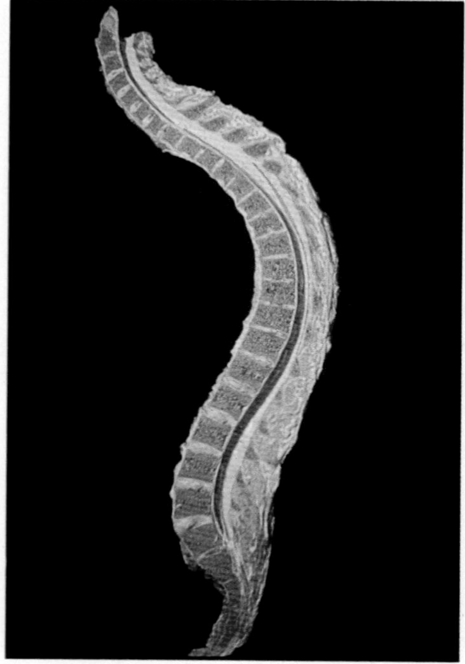

Fig. 10.40. Kyphosis of the spine in a case of deforming arthritis.

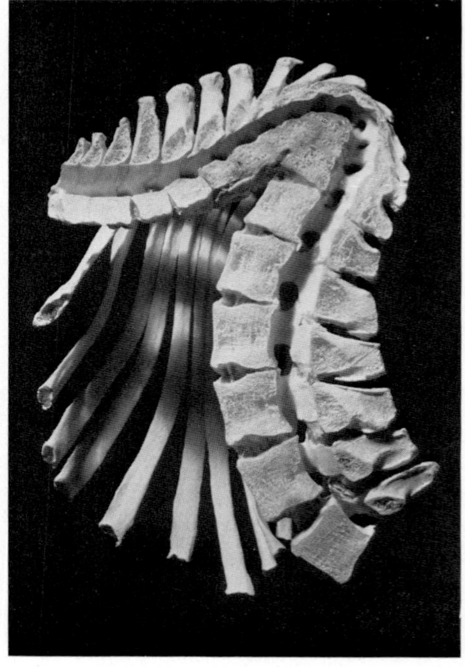

Fig. 10.41. Pott's disease of the spine (tuberculosis).

Spine

Scoliosis (Fig. 10.38). *A lateral curvature of the spine often combined with a rotation of its long axis.* On gross examination, the spine usually is curved rather than angularly bowed. *Unilateral* scoliosis refers to a single curvature. A double, S-shaped curvature is known as *bilateral* scoliosis.

F and *S:* scoliosis may be present at birth or develop during active bone growth. *Infantile scoliosis* becomes manifest during the third year, especially in boys. *Adolescent scoliosis* preferentially affects girls (10–16 years of age). *Pg:* congenital scoliosis is caused by a unilateral hemispondylus. *Idiopathic scoliosis* is of unknown etiology. *Acquired scoliosis* is the result of rickets, osteomalacia, muscular contractures or muscle paralysis (poliomyelitis). *Co:* severe deformities of the pelvis or thorax (→ cor pulmonale, see p. 71).

Kyphosis (Figs. 10.39–10.41). *A deformity of the spine characterized by an exaggerated curvature and posterior convexity.* A rounded or arch-like kyphosis is common in patients with rickets or osteomalacia (humpback) (Fig. 10.39). The more localized or *angular* kyphosis (Fig. 10.41) is the result of a collapsed vertebra (or vertebrae) from metastatic tumors, tuberculosis (Pott's disease) or metabolic diseases.

A specialform of *adolescent kyphosis* (Scheuermann's disease) is the result of a developmental anomaly. Scheuermann's disease begins in the lower thoracic spine and affects girls especially. The onset is between 7 and 12 years of age. The disease probably is the outcome of necrosis involving the vertebral epiphyses.

Lordosis. *A deformity of the spine characterized by a prominent anterior convexity, especially of the lumbar spine.* Lordosis usually is an adaptation to a thoracic kyphosis or to pelvic deformities resulting from rickets.

Degenerative disease of intervertebral disks (spondylosis deformans; Fig. 10.42; TCP, p. 221; see also p. 212). The elastic properties of the disks are reduced or lost. Consequently, pressures and vibrations are transmitted directly to the vertebral bodies and anterior longitudinal ligament. Reactive bone formation is stimulated, leading to the appearance of *osteophytes* or *lipping* of the vertebrae. The disease may progress to *intervertebral ankylosis.*

F, *A* and *S:* the most common degenerative disease of the spine. The incidence, according to some autopsy statistics, is as high as 80% in males and 60% in females past 50 years of age. In younger patients, the thoracic spine is especially involved. *Pg:* age-dependent fluid loss from intervertebral disk → loss of elasticity →buffer function of disks is reduced → vibrations and stretching act directly on the anterior ligament → formation of anterior and lateral osteophytes on vertebral bodies → fusion of osteophytes → intervertebral ankylosis. Separation or loosening of the external fibers of the vertebrae contribute to slipping of intervertebral disks. *Schmorl's nodules:* prolapse of intervertebral disks and compression by adjacent vertebrae.

Ankylosing (rheumatoid) spondylitis (Bechterew's disease, Marie-Strümpell spondylitis; TCP, p. 219; see also p. 221). Figure 10.40 shows a markedly kyphotic spine. The vertebral joints are fibrotic. Also found are cartilaginous or osseous ankylosis of the vertebral joints and ossification of the annulus fibrosis. In contrast to osteoarthritis deformans, calcification or ossification of the anterior longitudinal ligament is not observed.

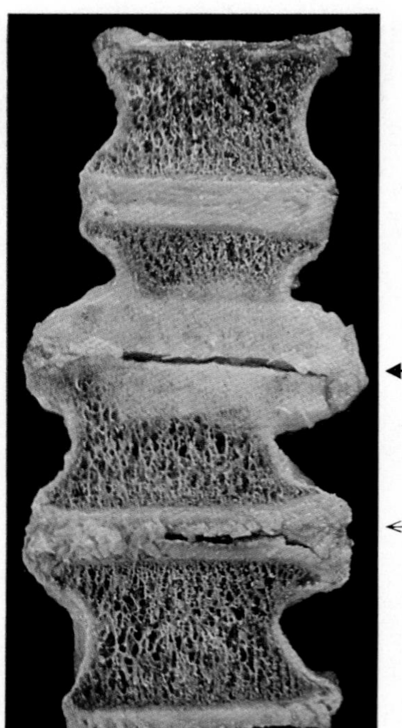

Fig. 10.42. Degenerative intervertebral disk disease.

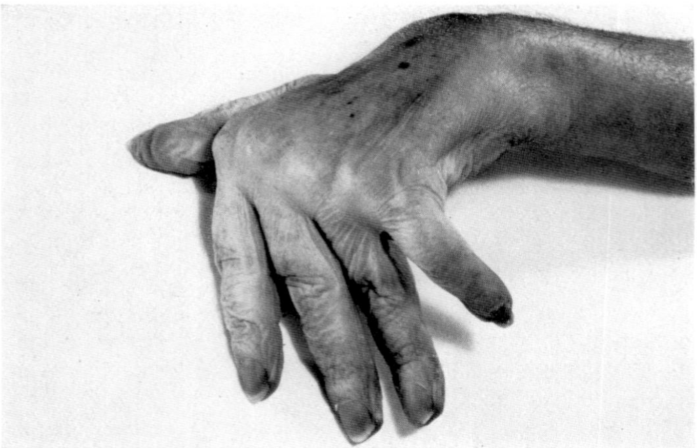

Fig. 10.43. Hand of a patient with rheumatoid arthritis.

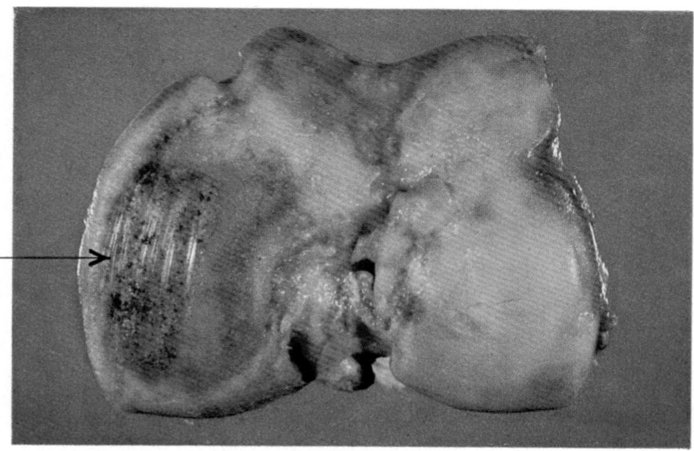

Fig. 10.44. Degenerative osteoarthritis of femur condyles.

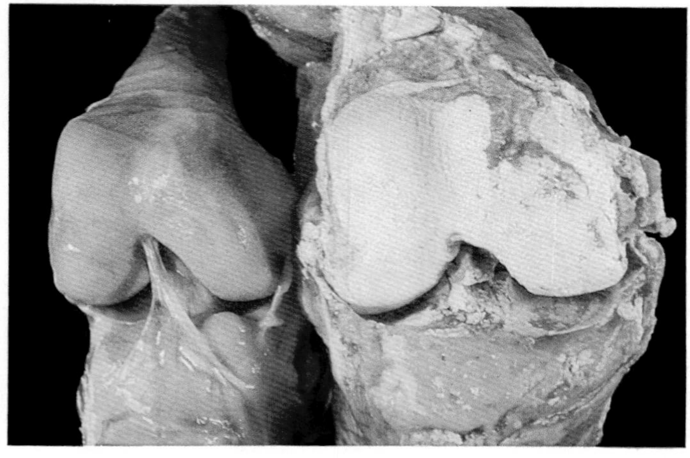

Fig. 10.45. Knee joint in gout (a normal knee joint is at the left).

Joints

Rheumatoid arthritis (Fig. 10.43). The hand of a patient with rheumatoid arthritis shows the typical ulnar abduction position of the fingers. See also p. 221. The hip, shoulder and knee joints are frequently involved.

Degenerative arthritis (osteoarthritis, Fig. 10.44; TCP, p. 221). *A primary degenerative disease of joint cartilage characterized by fibrillation and separation of small cartilage segments.* The characteristic gross findings in an advanced case are illustrated in Figure 10.44. Repeated mechanical stress produces fissuring and flattening of the central articular cartilage. The underlying bone is exposed and becomes sclerotic. The thickened bone appears smooth and brownish. Fissures (→) result from continuous movements of the articular surfaces. Bone hyperplasia at the margins of the joints gives rise to bony spurs. After the articular cartilage has been destroyed, the bone spicules are pushed into the medulla of the bone. Hemorrhages, necrosis and pseudocysts are the result.

Pg: degenerative arthritis is a common wear-and-tear phenomenon of weight-bearing articular cartilage. Occupational stress may accelerate the process. Hip and knee joints are involved. *Co:* limited joint motion.

Gouty arthritis (arthritis urica, Fig. 10.45). Chalky-white sodium or calcium urates are deposited in the articular cartilage of joints. Figure 10.45 shows a normal knee joint at the left. At the right, plaster-like urate deposits are seen. This picture was from a typical case of chronic gout.

F: approximately 2.4% of autopsies. *A:* past 40 years. *S:* ♂:♀ = 9:1. *Pg: primary gout* is a genetic (autosomal dominant), familial disease of uric acid metabolism. *Secondary* gout is observed in blood dyscrasias (increased cell turnover or cell destruction with release of nucleic acids) or renal diseases. *Lo:* metatarsal-phalangeal joints *(podagra)*, finger joints (cheiragra) and knee joints (gonagra) are affected most commonly. *Diagnosis:* elevated uric acid levels in serum (>6 mg./100 ml.). *Tophi* are uric acid deposits in soft tissues and around joints (x-ray). Tophi are common in the ear cartilage (helix and anthelix), eyelids, fingers, joint capsules and tendons. Urate deposits also are found in the kidneys and heart valves. Uric acid in tophi can be demonstrated by the murexide test: heating of tophus material with HNO_3, then addition of NH_4OH → red color.

Ankylosis (Fig. 10.46). *Severe limitation of joint mobility as a result of previous joint diseases.* The true ankylosis is the end stage of cartilage destruction and fusion of the joint space by a *fibrous* or *osseous* union. Figure 10.46 illustrates partial fusion of the knee joint following tuberculous osteoarthritis.

Limited joint motion also may be caused by a *pseudoankylosis.* There is no fibrous or osseous union. Instead, the adjacent soft parts compromise joint mobility. Examples: contracture of joint capsule *(capsular pseudoankylosis)* and muscle contractures.

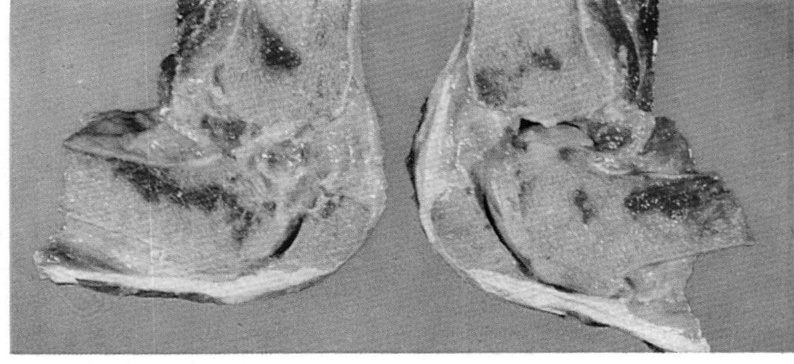

Fig. 10.46. Ankylosis of the knee joint.

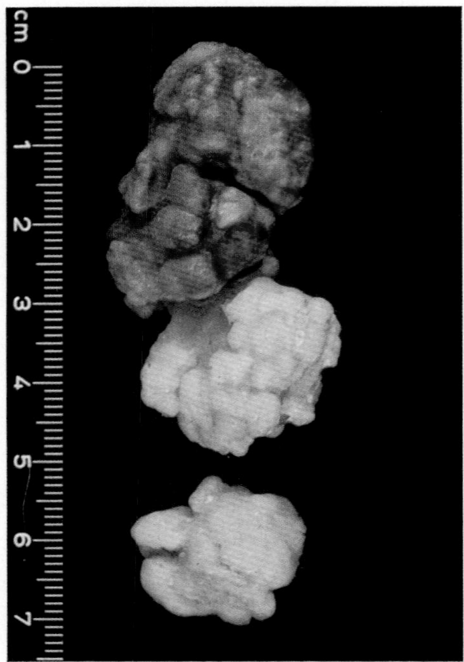

Fig. 10.47. Joint mice.

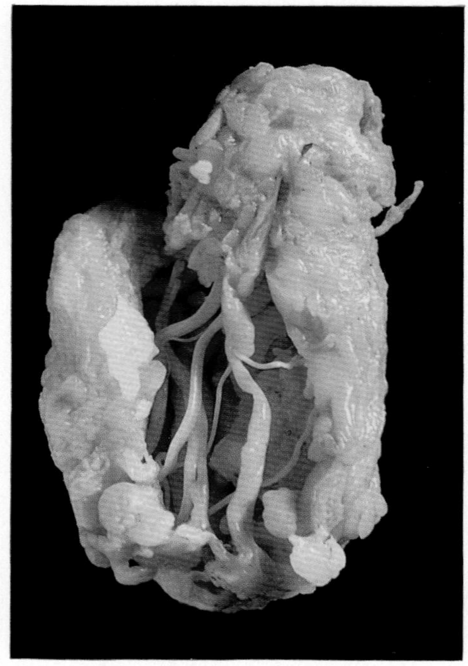

Fig. 10.48. Prepatellar bursitis.

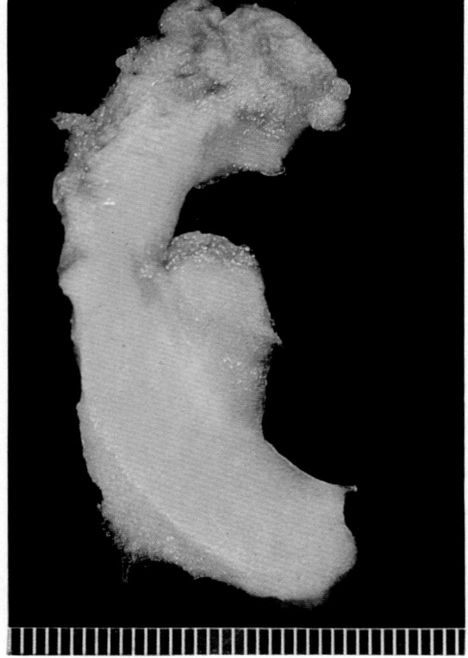

Fig. 10.49. Meniscus tear.

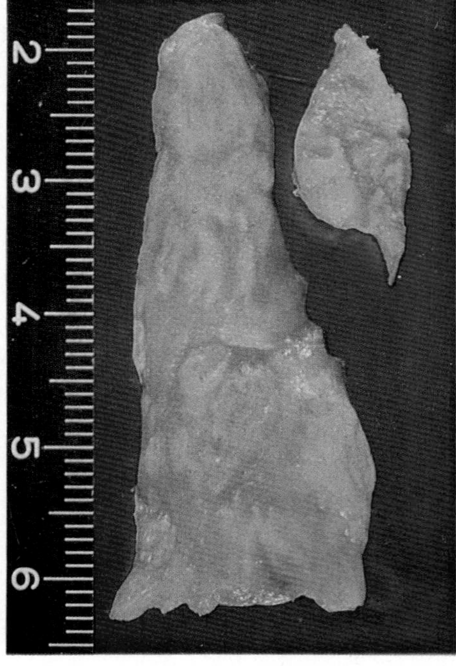

Fig. 10.50. Xanthelasma of the tendon.

Free joint mice (Fig. 10.47) are pieces of articular cartilage that become separated from the articular surface and displaced into the joint space. The articular cartilage may contain a bony nucleus.

Pg: joint mice most often are the result of traumatic separation of joint cartilage. They also occur in various forms of aseptic bone necrosis (e.g., in osteochondritis or osteoarthritis). The depression of the articular surface that remains after joint mice have been displaced is called the "mouse bed."

Co: joint mice that lodge between articular surfaces may limit joint mobility. Degenerative joint disease is a common sequela of joint mice.

Osteochondritis (or osteochondrosis) dissecans. *Aseptic bone necrosis leading to separation of cartilage and bone from the articular surfaces ("joint mice").* This disease predominantly affects the knee and elbow joints of young males (15–18 years of age).

Bursitis. Figure 10.48 shows the opened prepatellar bursa with an irregular, thickened, fibrous wall. The internal surface is warty and brownish discolored from hemosiderin deposits (old hemorrhages). The lumen of the bursa contains organized masses of fibrin (so-called *rice bodies).*

Lo: bursa of the patella (bursitis prepatellaris) and olecranon (bursitis olecrani). *DD:* ganglions are small, often cystic nodules of connective tissue with a mucoid content. They project from the joint capsule or tendon sheath, especially those of the hands and feet. A ganglion represents a traumatic myxomatous connective tissue change.

Meniscus tear (Fig. 10.49). Diseases of the meniscus are either traumatic or degenerative in nature. Any force acting on the periphery of the meniscus while the central part is fixed will tear the meniscus laterally or longitudinally (lateral tear and "bucket-handle tear," respectively). A preceding degenerative change in the ground substance of the meniscus (fatty changes or splitting of fibers) can predispose to a meniscus tear in older people. The differential diagnosis of a traumatic meniscus tear from a primarily degenerative meniscus disease can be difficult. *Lo:* tears are common in the medial as opposed to the lateral meniscus.

Xanthelasma of the tendon (Fig. 10.50). *Slowly enlarging, tumor-like nodules of tendons and tendon sheaths.* Xanthelasmas are circumscribed yellow to brownish, firm-elastic nodules or masses, as illustrated in Figure 10.50. They are located around the joints of the hands and feet. The yellowish brown discoloration is attributed to many xanthoma cells (cytoplasmic inclusions of cholesterol and neutral fats).

F: uncommon, although it may occur quite frequently in patients with familial predisposition. *A:* 20–50 years. *Pg:* not known. Tendon xanthelasmas most likely are metabolic, not neoplastic, lesions. Hypercholesterolemia, trauma and inflammation probably are of pathogenetic significance.

Tumors of tendons and tendon sheaths. The so-called xanthomatous giant-cell tumor (villonodular synovitis) is a fairly common condition of the knee joints or tendon sheaths of the fingers. Grossly, such a nodular synovial thickening consists of long, frond-like filaments that project from the synovial membrane into the joint space. The lesion is brown because of the many lipoid- or hemosiderin-laden giant cells, which resemble osteoclastic giant cells. The designation "giant-cell tumor" is inaccurate. Most observers hold that these lesions are inflammatory granulomas, possibly the result of chronic irritation and hemorrhage. They do not become malignant, rarely exceed 1–2 cm. and frequently undergo fibrous organization.

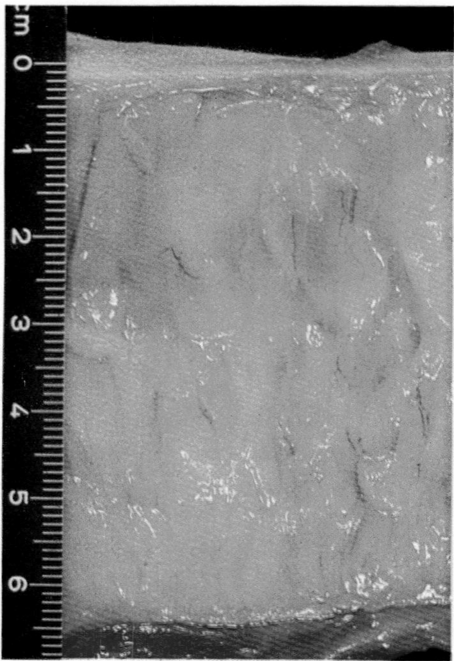

Fig. 10.51. Increased thickness of subcutaneous fat in obesity.

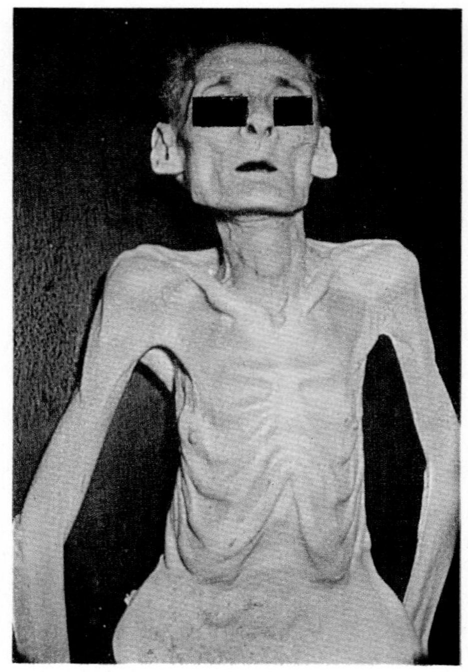

Fig. 10.52. Cachexia.

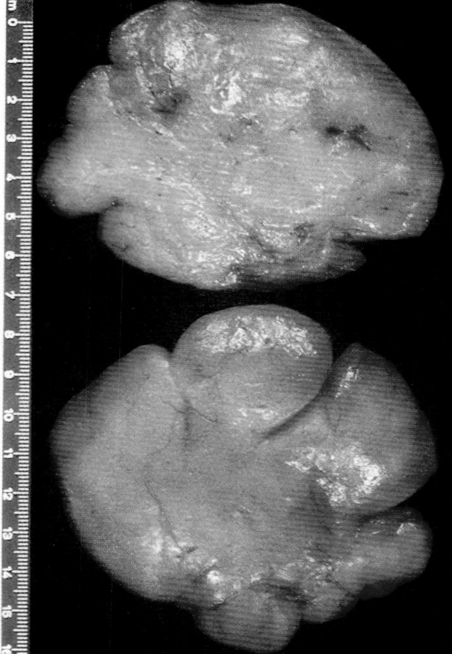

Fig. 10.53. Lipoma.

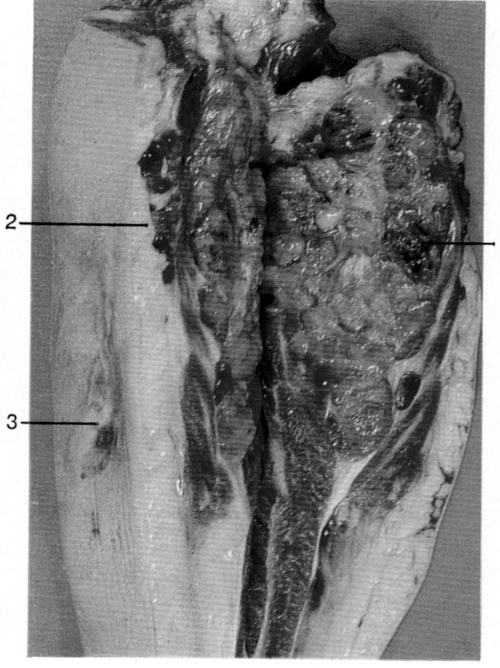

Fig. 10.54. Liposarcoma of the lower leg.

Connective and Fat Tissue

Obesity (adipositas, Fig. 10.51). *A pathologic increase in fat tissue, largely due to increased food consumption.* Obesity in *males* is most pronounced in the trunk and abdominal wall. The subcutaneous fat in these areas may increase in thickness to 6–8 cm. (Fig. 10.51). In addition to the subcutaneous fat, the adipose tissue of the mesentery, omentum, renal capsule and epicardium is abnormally large. In *females*, increased subcutaneous fat localizes in the thighs, buttocks, hips and upper arms. The predilection of adipose tissue for certain regions points to an unknown localizing factor that also can be demonstrated by skin transplantation: when a piece of abdominal skin is transplanted to the hand, a hump of fat develops in the transplanted skin with increased food consumption.
Anyone 20% or more overweight is considered as obese. About 30% of the population of the German Federal Republic is considered obese. An overweight of 10% reduces the life expectance by 18%, and an overweight of 30% reduces it by about 50%.

Pg: obesity is a numerical increase and enlargement of fat cells. The diameter of a fat cell increases from the normal value of 70–80 μ to 120 μ in obesity; in cachexia, the diameter is reduced to below 70 μ (Reh). The size of fat cells reflects the general nutritional state. Obesity is a problem of increased food consumption and diminished loss through energy dissipation. Thus far, no single metabolic cause has been detected. The regulation and psychology of "appetite" is not known. Some *genetic-constitutional* factors may play a role. *Hypothalamic lesions* (nucleus paraventricularis) may precipitate hyperphagia and subsequently obesity. *Endocrine obesity* is observed in patients with Cushing's disease and hyperinsulinism. *Co:* shortening of life span, especially with superimposed hypertension and diabetes. Other complications are myocardial infarction, fatal lung embolism and the Pickwickian syndrome (obesity, elevated diaphragm, hypoventilation, dyspnea, cyanosis, erythremia, cor pulmonale, thrombosis, embolism).

Cachexia (marasmus) *is the result of malnutrition.* An extremely cachectic patient is shown in Figure 10.52. This patient died from metastatic stomach cancer. The face is sunken, the cheekbones are prominent and the skeletal muscles are wasted. The intercostal spaces are markedly depressed. The skin is pale, dry, cold and yellowish. Atrophy of internal organs may reduce the liver weight by 30% and the heart weight by 25%. Generalized edema is due to hypoproteinemia. Basal metabolic rate and blood pressure are low. Most cachectic patients are hypoglycemic. *Mi:* hemosiderin in RES cells from muscle loss and apoferritin deficiency. Atrophy.
Tumors of soft tissues (Figs. 10.53 and 10.54; TCP p. 259). Benign and malignant soft tissue tumors are named according to the tissue of origin. The following table summarizes benign and malignant soft part tumors (with the exception of neurogenic and bone tumors).

Tissue of Origin	*Benign*	*Malignant*
Collagenous fibers	Fibroma	Fibrosarcoma
Smooth muscle	Leiomyoma	Leiomyosarcoma
Striated muscle	Rhabdomyoma	Rhabdomyosarcoma
Blood vessels	Angioma	Angiosarcoma
Fat tissue	Lipoma	Liposarcoma
Joint mesothelium	Synovioma	Malignant synovialoma

A lipoma is chosen here as an example of a benign mesenchymal tumor (Fig. 10.53). A lipoma is an encapsulated, slowly growing tumor with a glistening, moist, yellow and sometimes distinctly lobulated cut surface. Necrosis and hemorrhage are absent. Histologically, a lipoma consists of rather uniform, neoplastic fat cells with very few, if any, mitotic figures. The malignant counterpart is the liposarcoma. Figure 10.54 shows a liposarcoma arising in the lower leg. This tumor is not encapsulated and is mottled yellow-gray-brown from hemorrhages (→1). The large tumor in Figure 10.54 grows between the leg muscles and infiltrates the overlying skin (→2). The skin is dimpled from sarcoma infiltration (→3). *Criteria for the diagnosis of malignant mesenchymal tumors:* fast growth rate, absence of a capsule, evidence of infiltrative growth (vascular invasion) and retrogressive changes (necrosis and/or hemorrhages because of insufficient vascular supply). In addition, small "satellite" tumor nodules often can be observed near the primary site of a malignant mesenchymal tumor.

The frequency of benign and malignant soft tissue tumors depends on their histologic structure and site of origin. Occasionally, malignant mesenchymal neoplasms are present at birth (hepatoblastomas, Wilms' tumor).

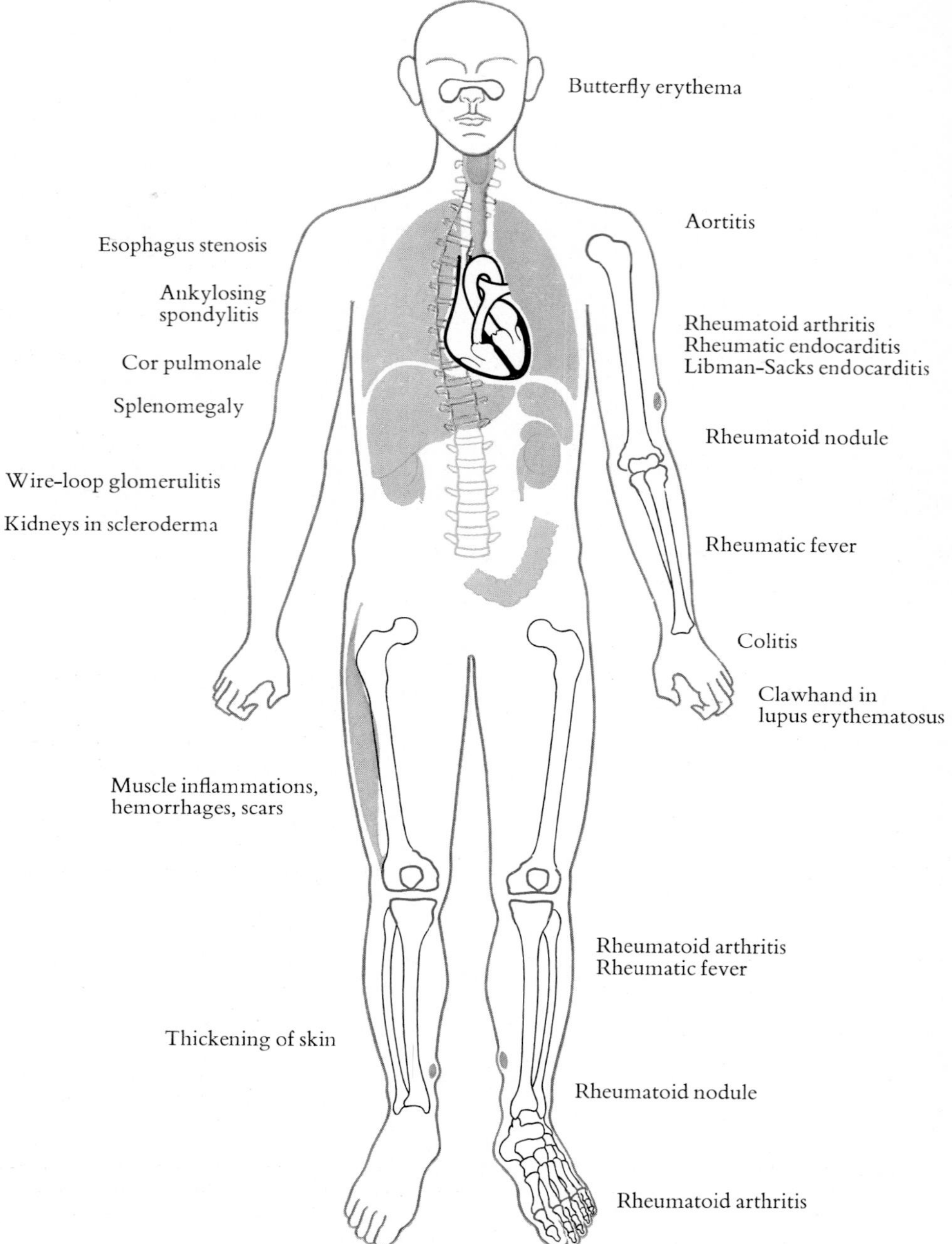

Fig. 10.55. Organ involvement in collagen diseases.

Collagen Diseases

The term collagen diseases was coined by KLEMPERER *for a group of disorders with a common morphologic and pathogenetic denominator* (Fig. 10.55). The principal pathologic findings are:

The *collagen fibers* are involved by a *stage-like inflammatory process* that begins as a degenerative fibrinoid change. The collagen fibers are swollen (as observed in the Aschoff body). Exudation of blood plasma and proteins between collagen fibers leads to the formation of so-called *precipitation hyaline* (the rheumatoid nodule is an example of precipitation hyaline). The fibrinoid changes progress to fibrinoid necrosis (as seen characteristically in periarteritis nodosa). Fibrinoid necrosis elicits a cellular reaction consisting of lymphocytes and/or histiocytic granulomas (as observed in rheumatoid arthritis). The inflammatory process is organized and heals (fibrosis and scarring).

Although the antigen(s) still are not known, some – but not all – collagen diseases are considered *immune* diseases. Autoantibodies have been shown to exist in some collagen diseases (see below).

Rheumatic fever (see p. 39; TCP, pp. 47 and 219). An exudative inflammation (with Aschoff bodies) involves the large joints of young persons (8–20 years of age) but heals without impaired joint function. A pancarditis with valve deformities develops between 30 and 40 years of age.

Rheumatoid arthritis (primary chronic or atrophic arthritis; see p. 215; TCP, p. 219). *A constitutional, chronic inflammatory disease with polyarthritis but without acute fever.* Occurs predominantly in females between 40 and 50 years of age (menopause). *S:* ♂:♀=4:1. A familial increase in frequency is observed.

As shown in the pictures in the histopathology textbook (TCP, p. 218), the small joints (fingers, toes) are inflamed initially (exudation of plasma and fibrin). This exudative inflammatory phase is followed by the development of granulation tissue *(pannus)*, which leads to bony ankylosis, loss of joint motion and joint deformities (see Fig. 10.43). The large joints may become secondarily involved. The end stage of rheumatoid arthritis is ankylosis, osteoporosis and muscular atrophy.

A nephrotic syndrome (renal amyloidosis) is observed in 30% of rheumatoid arthritis. A subcutaneous, periarticular nodule, the *rheumatoid nodule*, is found in 25% of patients. *Mi:* the rheumatoid nodule has a central zone of fibrinoid swelling or necrosis and a palisading, histiocytic demarcation (*DD:* gumma!).

The *laboratory* diagnosis of rheumatoid arthritis is based on the demonstration of the rheumatoid factor (7 S and 19 S gamma globulin complex) by the latex agglutination and bentonite agglutination tests. The morbidity is 5%. The disease starts insidiously, sometimes with subfebrile temperatures. There is morning stiffness of the finger and toe joints (symmetrical) in 80% of the cases. Transient hydrarthrosis may occur.

Pg: rheumatoid arthritis probably is an autoimmune response to connective tissue components. An experimental rheumatoid arthritis of rats can be transferred by lymphocytes from the joints to other rats. A viral infection has recently been considered as a cause.

Special types are *Still-Chauffard's disease* (rheumatoid arthritis in children, usually with prominent visceral involvement) and the *Felty syndrome* (rheumatoid arthritis in elderly females associated with skin pigmentation, splenomegaly, hypersplenic anemia and leukocytopenia). The separation of these entities from rheumatoid arthritis probably is not justified.

Ankylosing (rheumatoid) spondylitis (Bechterew's disease; see also p. 213). A type of rheumatoid arthritis with involvement of sacro-iliac and vertebral joints. The inflammatory changes of the vertebral joints and the annulus fibrosis are similar to those in rheumatoid arthritis. Progression to bony ankylosis of the intervertebral disks ultimately converts the spine into an inflexible column with kyphosis (*bamboo spine*, see Fig. 10.40). The disease usually begins in the sacro-iliac joints and extends to the spine. *S:* young males. Ankylosing spondylitis may be accompanied by aortic endocarditis, aortitis of the thoracic aorta, ulcerative colitis (30%) and uveitis (5–10%).

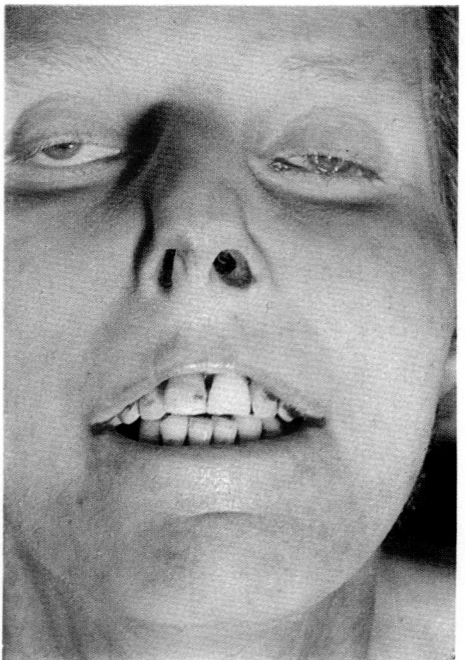

Fig. 10.56. Scleroderma.

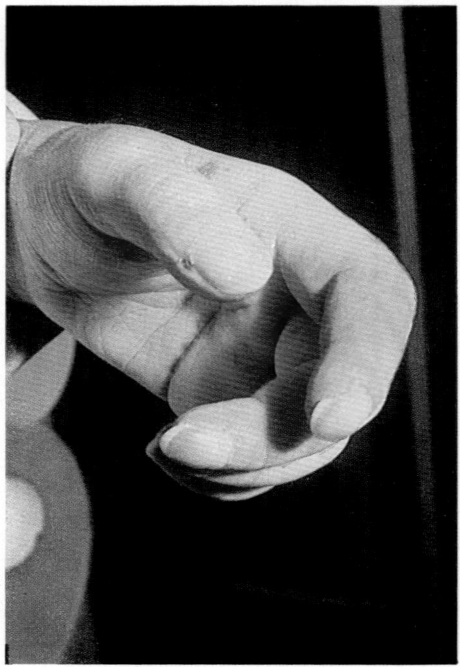

Fig. 10.57. Clawhand in scleroderma.

Lupus erythematosus. *A recurrent systemic collagen disease that predominantly affects young (20–30 years) females* (80%). *Clinically, the disease is characterized by swelling of the joints (as in rheumatoid arthritis), polyserositis and manifestations in the heart, skin and kidneys.*

F: 100,000 cases in the United States (200,000,000 inhabitants). *Course:* only 20% of the patients survive for more than 5 years. The presence of so-called LE cells in the blood, bone marrow and tissues is characteristic. LE cells are histiocytes or neutrophilic granulocytes that have engulfed pyknotic cell nuclei into the cytoplasm. The LE cell phenomenon also points to the *pathogenesis* of systemic lupus. Autoantibodies can be demonstrated against the patient's own nucleoproteins (DNA, histones). The autoantibodies are 7 S globulins, the so-called LE factor.

Organs involved in systemic lupus:

Heart: the characteristic lesions are the nonbacterial, verrucous endocarditis (Libman-Sacks endocarditis), which also involves the atrium in approximately 50%, an occasional lymphohistiocytic myocarditis and pericarditis (70%). See also page 35.

Kidney: 70% of patients with systemic lupus develop a "hyaline" thickening of the glomerular loops ("wire-loop" kidneys). Clinically, renal involvement is manifested as hypertension and death in uremia.

Vessels: arteritis with fibrinous medionecrosis and inflammatory cell infiltrates is observed in 50% of the cases. The arteritis of systemic lupus is less extensive than that in periarteritis nodosa.

Central nervous system: involved in 50% of the cases.

Serous membranes: pericarditis, pleuritis, rarely peritonitis or polyserositis.

Spleen: the spleen is enlarged in 20% of the cases. A *typical finding* is the onion-like periarterial fibrosis of the central arterioles seen in 95% of the cases.

Liver: the liver often is enlarged and contains periportal lymphohistiocytic infiltrates. This finding must be distinguished from the lupoid hepatitis in which the inflammatory cell infiltrates extend into the parenchyma ("moth-eaten"). Antinuclear antibodies also can be shown to exist in 40% of patients with viral hepatitis.

Musculature: minimal changes as in dermatomyositis.

Skin: butterfly erythema of the face and thrombocytopenic purpura.

Lung: sometimes interstitial fibrosis.

Lymph nodes: enlargement in more than half of the patients.

Panarteritis (see p. 253). The same group of forms includes **Wegener's granulomatosis** (see p. 77), **giant cell arteritis** (Mi), and **Takayasu's syndrome** (aortitis in the aortic arch with thrombosis: so-called "pulseless disease").

Dermatomyositis. *A disease that occurs predominantly in females of the middle age group. Dermatomyositis presents as fever and muscular weakness.* The skin changes are nonspecific and resemble those seen in systemic lupus erythematosus or scleroderma. Histologically, the degenerative changes in muscles include necrosis with lymphocytic and plasma-cellular infiltrates. Healing with fibrosis and scar formation. Death often is attributable to aspiration pneumonia because of muscle involvement (swallowing).

Scleroderma (Figs. 10.56 and 10.57). *A progressive, chronic sclerosis of the skin and internal organs. The disease affects predominantly females (three times more common than in males) between the ages of 30 and 50 years. The clinical course extends over a period of 5–15 years.*

The progressive skin changes pass through several stages. An initial, brawny, nonpitting edema is followed by formation of new collagen fibers. The dermis is thickened by parallel collagen fiber bundles; the dermal elastic fibers are destroyed. Ultimately, the skin becomes sclerotic, thin, smooth and fixed to the underlying muscles. Areas of brownish pigmentation alternate with patches of depigmentation. Typical is the tight, atrophic and waxy skin of the face or hands.

Figure 10.56 shows a mask-like face with a sharply pointed nose and narrowed mouth. A claw-hand (sclerodactyly) with shortened terminal phalanges and scars at the finger tips is seen in Figure 10.57.

DD: scleroderma circumscripta and sclerodactyly: benign disease without visceral involvement.

Scleroderma is a *progressive systemic sclerosis*. Systemic manifestations are *diffuse interstitial pulmonary fibrosis* (with cor pulmonale as the cause of death) and involvement of the *esophagus* (dilatation and a thickened, rigid wall) and *kidneys* (resembling malignant nephrosclerosis or systemic lupus). *Visceral scleroderma* is confined to the lungs, esophagus and kidneys. The etiology of scleroderma is not known.

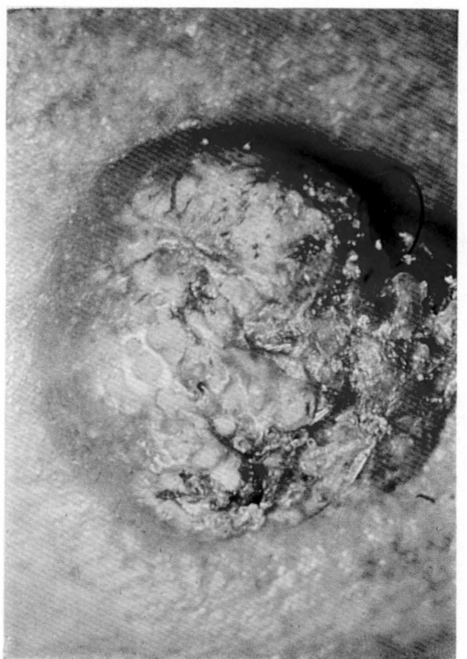

Fig. 11.1. Keratoacanthoma.

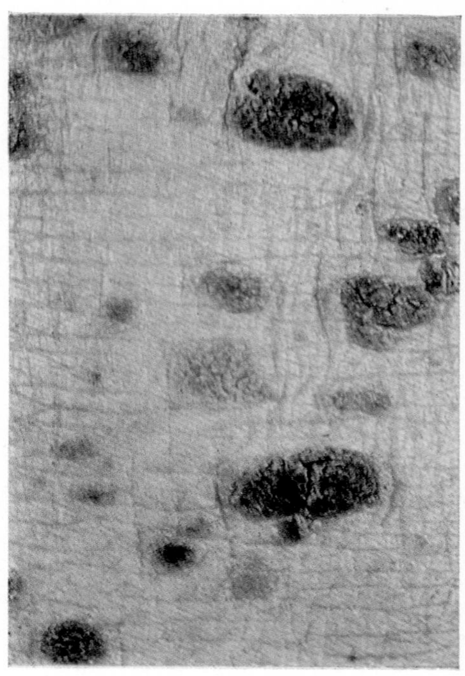

Fig. 11.2. Seborrheic keratosis.

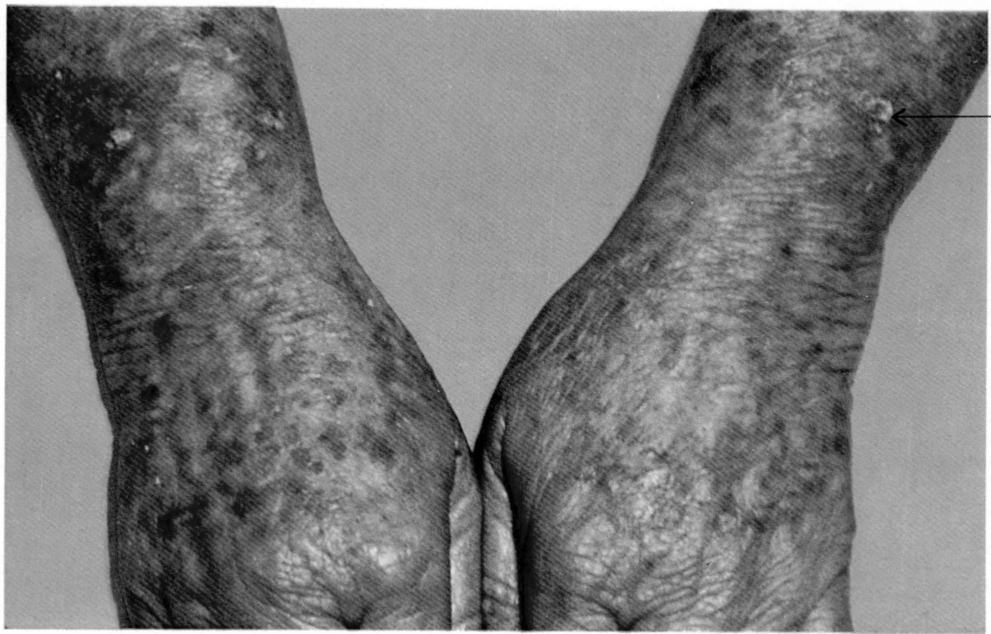

Fig. 11.3. Solar keratosis.

11. Skin and Mammary Gland

Keratoacanthoma, Seborrheic and Solar Keratoses

Remarks. Only skin lesions commonly seen in autopsy material will be discussed here. For a description of the common nonfatal skin diseases, consult any of the specialty books (see References). Some skin lesions are described in connection with systemic diseases (see postmortem spots, p. 13; scleroderma, p. 223; subcutaneous soft tissue tumors, p. 219).

Keratoacanthoma (Fig. 11.1). *A nodular, centrally keratinizing skin lesion that grows rapidly during the first 4–12 weeks but which may regress spontaneously in the following 4–6 weeks.* Figure 11.1 shows a skin nodule with a hyperkeratotic surface. The cut section reveals a keratin-covered mass filled with epithelium.

A: after 50 years. *S:* more common in males. *Lo:* keratoacanthomas are observed in sun-exposed skin, e.g., the face, ears and dorsum of the hands. *Pg:* the cause is not known (virus?). Multiple keratoacanthomas in young males probably are related to exposure to sun or tar. *Pr:* self-healing lesion; malignant changes are rare. The misdiagnosis "squamous-cell carcinoma" can be made easily when only portions of a keratoacanthoma are submitted for histologic examination.

Seborrheic keratosis (verruca senilis, Fig. 11.2). *Flat, slightly elevated, brown-to-black pigmented skin lesions measuring up to 2 cm. in diameter.* The slightly elevated seborrheic warts, as shown in Figure 11.2, have a broad base, hanging margins and a cauliflower-like surface.

F: common skin lesion, especially in males past 50 years of age. *Lo:* trunk, arms, less commonly, the face. *Pr:* benign skin lesion that should not be confused with melanoma of senile keratosis (precancerous lesion) (histologic examination!).

Mi: the epidermis is thickened due to proliferating basal cells (like basal-cell carcinoma) and circumscribed keratin pearls. However, there is no evidence of infiltrative growth.

Solar keratosis (farmer's skin). Figure 11.3 shows both forearms with melanin pigmentations of various intensities. The skin is focally thickened or atrophic. The circumscribed, yellowish areas represent hyperkeratotic epidermis (→). Solar keratosis is seen in persons who have been exposed to sunlight for a long time, especially white people living in tropical zones (South Africa, Australia).

A: older people. *Pr:* 25% of solar keratoses develop into a squamous-cell or basal-cell carcinoma. Multiple tumors often coexist on the face and arms. *Mi:* circumscribed areas of hyperkeratosis alternate with partly atrophic skin.

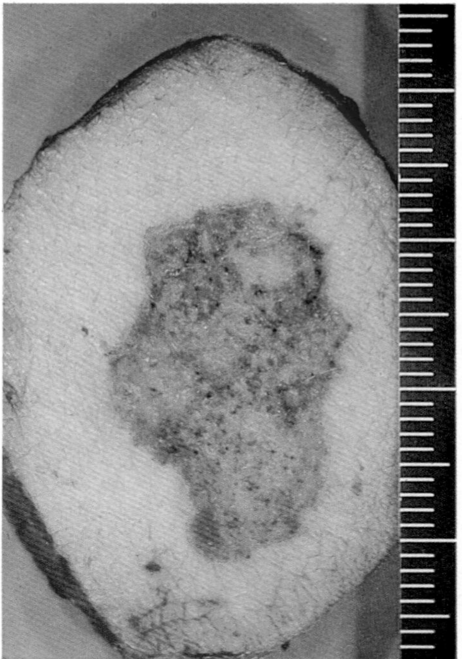

Fig. 11.4. Basal-cell carcinoma.

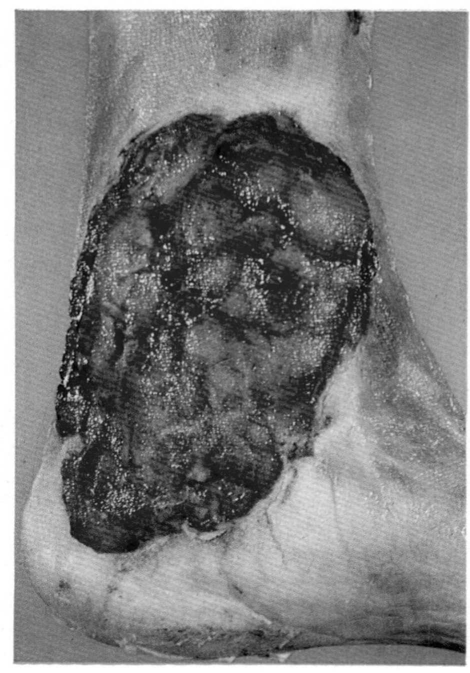

Fig. 11.5. Squamous-cell carcinoma.

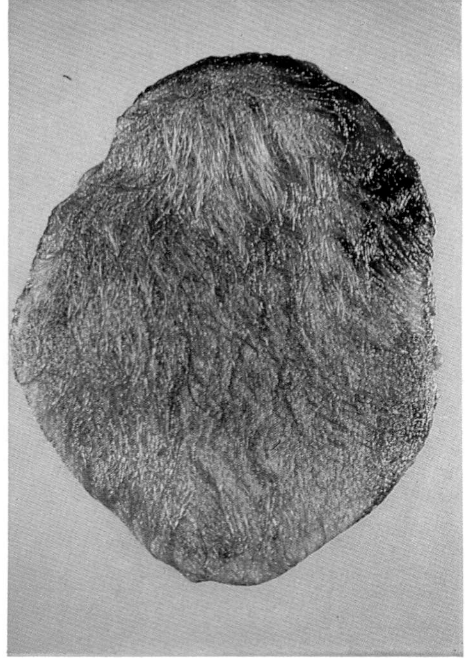

Fig. 11.6. Hairy nevus.

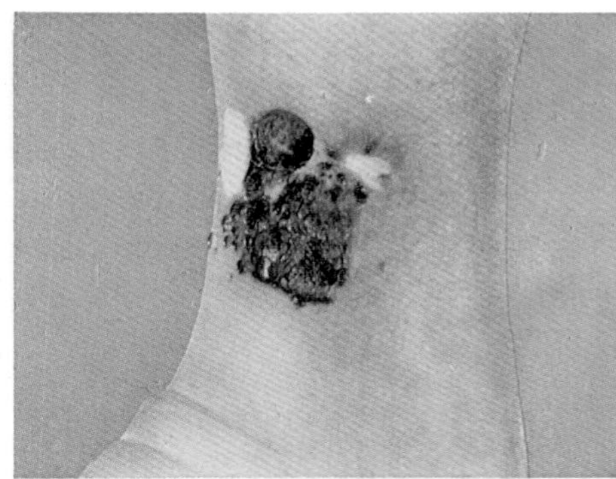

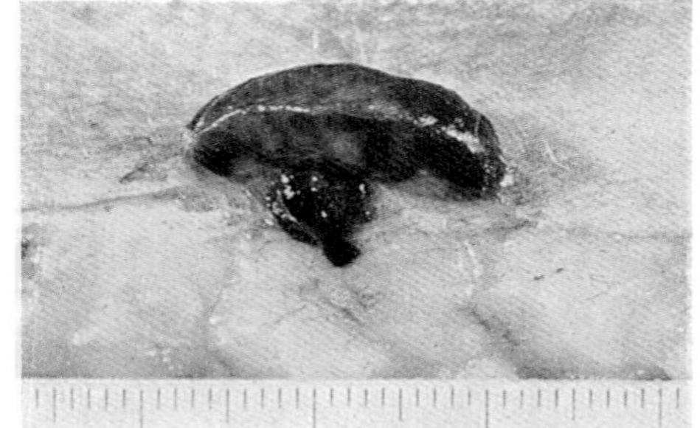

Fig. 11.7. Above: malignant melanoma above the malleolus.
Fig. 11.8. Below: cut surface of a malignant melanoma.

Skin Tumors

Basal-cell carcinoma (basaloma, Fig. 11.4; TCP, pp. 248 and 249). *An infiltrative, ulcerating epidermal tumor composed of basal cells. Distant metastases are rare.* Unprotected skin of older people is predominantly affected (face and hands). The nodular basal-cell carcinoma grows destructively into the neighboring tissues (ulcus terebrans). Figure 11.4 reveals a flat basal-cell carcinoma that does not protrude over the skin surface. The surface is reddened or discolored dark brown to black by melanin (morphea type = spot).

A: past 50 years. *S:* ♂ = ♀. White people in the tropics. *Pr:* malignant tumor that usually does not metastasize. *Mi:* solid cystic or highly differentiated (hair follicles, keratin pearls, sebaceous glands) basal-cell carcinomas.

Squamous-cell carcinoma (Fig. 11.5; TCP, pp. 246, 247, 251 and 271). *Malignant epithelial skin tumor affecting predominantly elderly males. The tumor spreads lymphogenously or hematogenously.* Figure 11.5 shows a tumor near the internal malleolus with a red tumor base.

F: approximately 1.5% of all epithelial skin tumors. *A:* elderly males; rare before 30 years of age. *Lo:* unprotected skin. *Pg:* carcinomas develop in previously damaged skin (farmer's skin, arsenical dermatosis, senile keratosis, chronic inflammation, e.g., osteomyelitis). Other precancerous lesions include old scars from burns, x-ray scars; lupus vulgaris. *Pr:* variable (self-healing squamous-cell carcinomas?). *DD:* keratoacanthoma (see above).

Nevus pigmentosus (Fig. 11.6; TCP, p. 269). Dysontogenetic malformation (hamartoma) composed of nevus cells. The lesion usually is present at birth and enlarges during puberty. Figure 11.6 shows a large hairy nevus.

Nomenclature. The term nevus refers to a malformation or hamartoma. In the narrow sense of the word, nevi are pigmented lesions. In addition, the broad definition of the term nevus includes hamartomas of the superficial skin (verrucous nevus) or skin appendages (nevi of sebaceous or sweat glands and hair follicles). *F:* pigmented nevi are found in practically all humans, with certain sites of predilection. *Pg:* they develop from melanin-producing Schwann cells (melanoblasts). *Classification: Intradermal cellular nevi* are composed of masses of nevus cells in the dermis. *Junctional nevi* show evidence of cellular proliferation and involve the basal layer of the epidermis. They can give rise to a malignant melanoma. *Compound nevi* combine features of dermal and junctional nevi.

Malignant melanoma (Figs. 11.7 and 11.8; TCP, p. 269). *Malignant tumor composed of pigmented or nonpigmented cells. Melanomas develop during or after puberty.* Figure 11.7 shows a nodular black tumor above the malleolus. The black color is due to melanin pigmentation. Only the gray-white peripheral portions of this lesion contain nonpigmented tumor cells. The cut surface clearly indicates the infiltrative growth of the melanoma (Fig. 11.8).

F: 1–2% of all malignant tumors, 20% of all malignant skin tumors. *A:* melanomas occur after puberty and increase in frequency after 40 years of age. The juvenile melanoma is biologically benign (no metastases) despite a pleomorphic histologic appearance with many mitotic figures. Fifteen per cent of juvenile melanomas occur in adults (not a malignant melanoma!). *Lo:* skin and oral cavity, mucosa of genital organs and rectum. Areas of predilection are the nail bed and foot. *Pg:* Neuroectodermal tumor derived from Schwann cells. A melanoma develops spontaneously or from a mechanically irritated pigmented nevus. Twenty-five per cent of all malignant melanomas arise from a pre-existing *melanotic precancerous dermatosis Dubreuilh. Co:* melanomas are infiltrative growths that disseminate lymphogenously and hematogenously. Metastases are widespread: one of the most malignant tumors in humans. *Mi:* carcinomatous or sarcomatous histologic pattern with many mitoses, atypical cells and evidence of infiltration into the epidermis and dermis. Proof of melanin formation by tumor cells often requires silver stains (Masson silver stain).

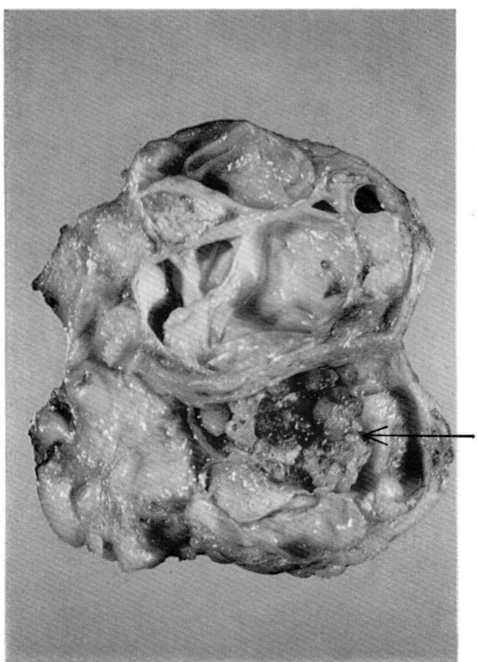

Fig. 11.9. Fibrocystic disease of the breast with intracanalicular papilloma.

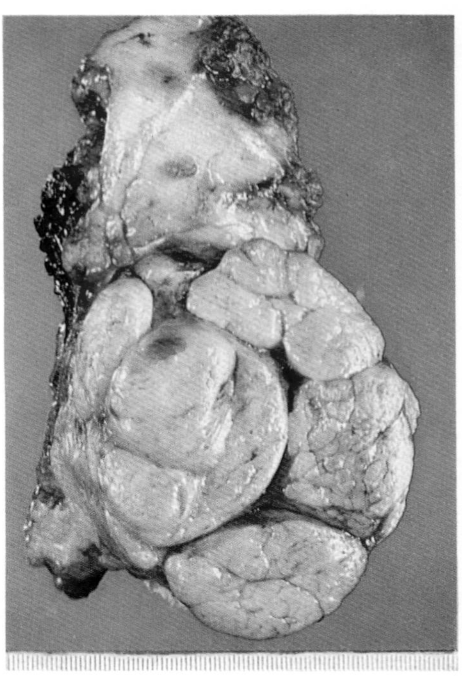

Fig. 11.10. Fibroadenoma of the breast.

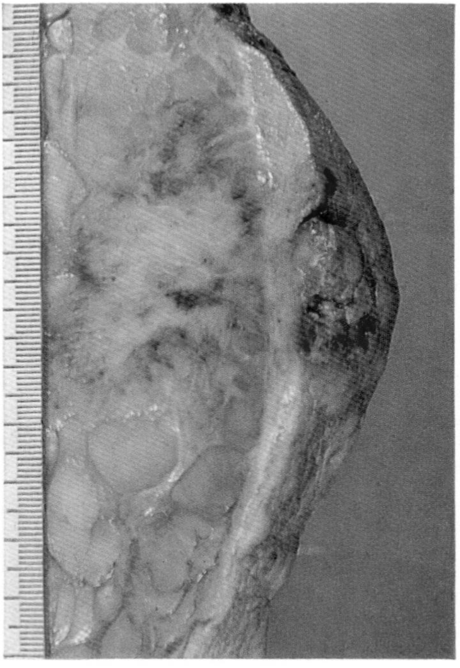

Fig. 11.11. Carcinoma of the breast.

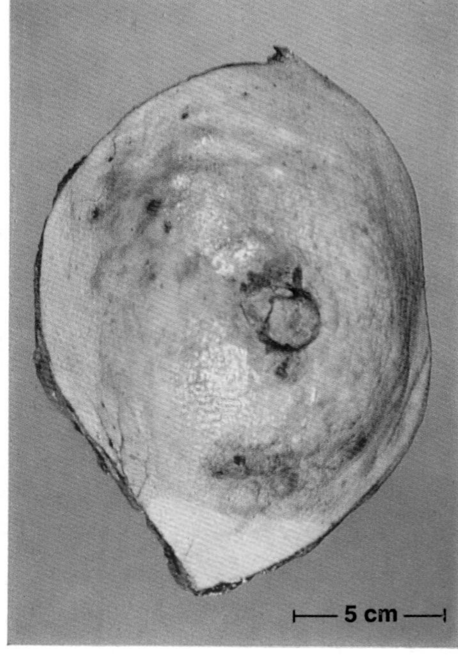

Fig. 11.12. Infiltration of the skin by a mammary carcinoma ("orange peel").

Breast

Fibrocystic disease (Fig. 11.9; TCP, p. 239). *A nodular proliferation of the breast characterized by proliferation of the stroma (fibrosclerosis) and hyperplasia of the mammary ducts (ectasia and epithelial proliferation).* A distinction sometimes is made between fibrosclerosis and adenosis, although both may occur together in the same breast. *Fibrosclerosis* refers to hyperplasia of the stromal fibrous tissue. Patients between 25 and 40 years of age are affected. *Adenosis* refers to an epithelial proliferation that forms small to medium-sized cysts lined by hyperplastic or metaplastic epithelium. The epithelium may proliferate to produce intraductal papillomas (patients 30–40 years of age; 3% of papillomas become malignant). The term *fibrocystic disease* is used when large cysts are embedded in abundant fibrous stroma (Fig. 11.9). The cysts have a smooth, glistening lining and contain a clear or slightly turbid fluid. An intraductal papilloma (→, Fig. 11.9) is present in one of them.

F: common breast lesion between 35 and 45 years of age and during early menopause (40–50 years). The clinical diagnosis of a "benign breast lesion" includes 73% fibrocystic disease and 5% fibrosclerosis. *Pg:* probably the result of estrogen.

Fibroadenoma (Fig. 11.10; TCP, p. 239). *Common benign breast tumor composed of adenomatous and fibromatous portions.* The tumor characteristically occurs in young females as a well-circumscribed, movable, nodular, firm mass. Figure 11.10 shows the coarsely nodular and gray-white cut surface of a fibroadenoma.

F: fibroadenomas account for approximately 20% of clinically benign breast lesions. *A:* a fibroadenoma develops prior to the age of 30 years and tumor growth usually ceases at this time. *Pg:* benign, hormone-dependent breast tumor. A histologically similar picture also is seen in fibrocystic disease in the form of *fibroadenomatous hyperplasia* or *microfibroadenomas. Cystosarcoma phylloides* is a giant fibroadenoma with highly cellular stroma. The tumor is rare; 5–10% metastasize.

Carcinoma of the breast (Figs. 11.11 and 11.12). *Malignant epithelial tumor of the mammary ducts or lobules occurring predominantly in females.* Figure 11.11 shows an ill-defined tumor of gray-white color and firm consistency that measures approximately 4 cm. in diameter. The surrounding breast and subcutaneous fat tissues are infiltrated by the tumor. The overlying skin is slightly protruding and wrinkled ("orange peel") from tumor infiltration (Fig. 11.12).

F: 1.6 breast cancers per 1,000 women. Mammary carcinomas account for 10% of all carcinomas and 22% of all carcinomas in females. *S:* 99% of breast cancers occur in females. In males, breast cancer is seen especially after estrogen therapy for prostate carcinoma. *A:* 40–55 years (at the beginning of the menopause). *Lo:* 50% of breast cancers arise in the upper outer quadrant. *Co:* local infiltration of the skin and pectoral muscles. Lymphogenous spread to the lymph nodes in the axilla and supraclavicular fossa. Metastases also can be observed in contralateral axillary nodes after the skin has been infiltrated. Approximately 50% of breast cancers have metastasized at the time of operation (see also p. 188). Hematogenous metastases to the pleura, lungs (see p. 97), liver and bones. Breast carcinoma not uncommonly metastasizes to the ovaries and other endocrine organs.

Histologic types. Scirrhous carcinoma (70%), *medullary carcinoma* (5–10%), *mucinous or gallert carcinoma (rare), intracanalicular carcinomas* (carcinoma cribrosum and comedo carcinoma). Carcinomas derived from the lobules are termed *lobular carcinoma;* they are confined to the lobules for some time but show signs of invasive growth in 10%. *Paget's disease of the breast* is a carcinoma of the areolar ducts with eczematous changes in the nipple due to intraepithelial growth of the carcinoma. The *Stewart-Tréves syndrome* is a lymphangiosarcoma developing from a chronic lymphedema of the upper arm following mastectomy and removal of the axillary lymph nodes.

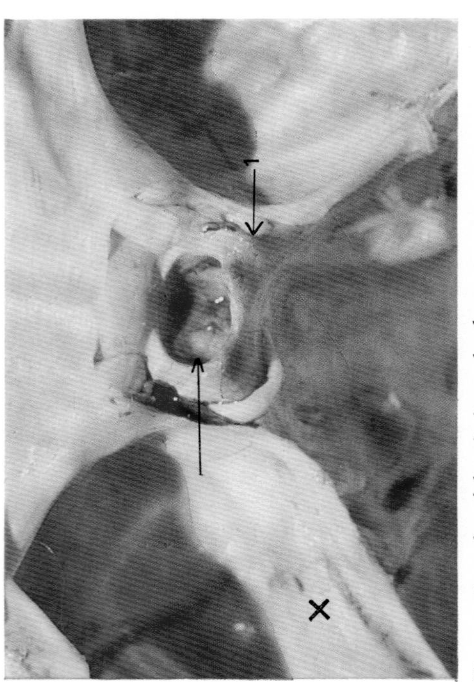

Fig. 12.1. Atrophy of the pituitary gland.

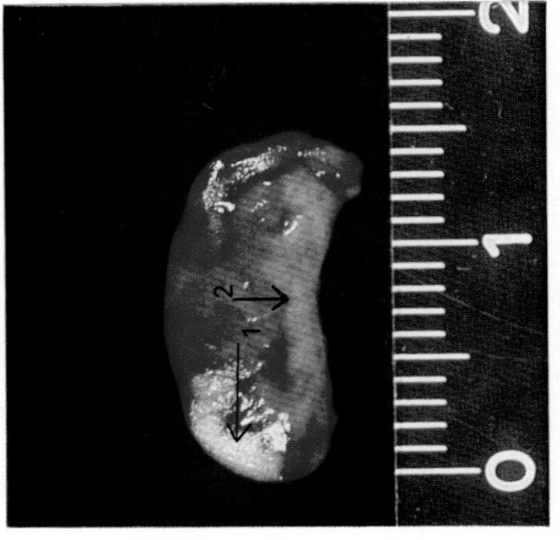

Fig. 12.2. Necrosis of the pituitary gland.

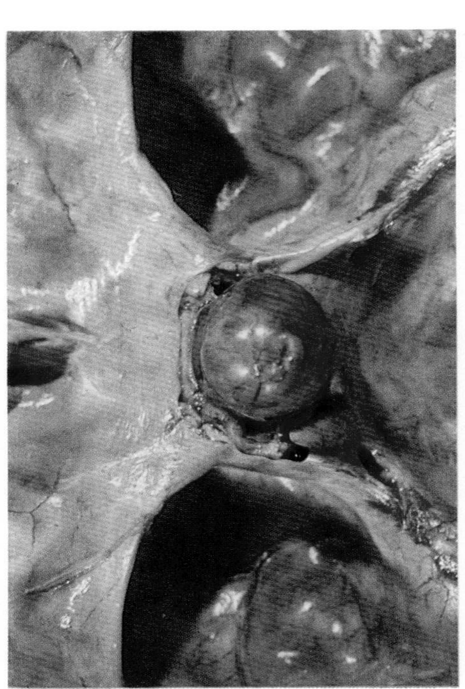

Fig. 12.3. Chromophobe pituitary adenoma.

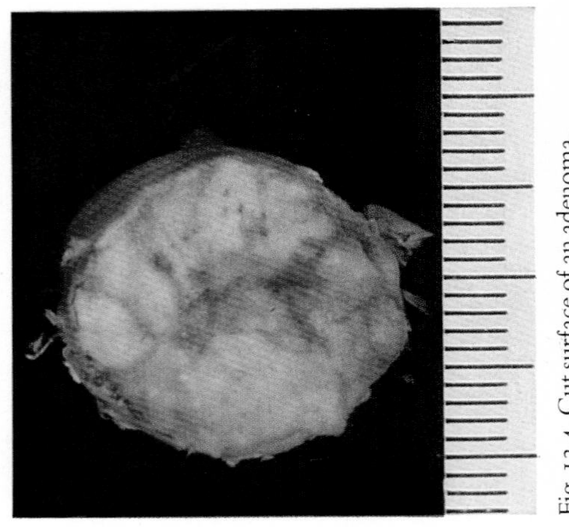

Fig. 12.4. Cut surface of an adenoma.

12. Endocrine Organs

Pituitary Gland

General remarks. The pituitary gland (hypophysis) is an oval, flat organ in the hypophyseal fossa of the sphenoid bone. The pituitary measures 11 mm. longitudinally × 16 mm. frontally × 6 mm. horizontally. The normal adult gland weighs 600–650 mg. During pregnancy, the weight may increase to 1,250 mg. The anterior lobe, or *adenohypophysis*, constitutes 75–80% of the total organ weight and develops from the roof of the ectodermal mouth (Rathke's pouch). The *neurohypophysis* includes the posterior lobe and infundibulum and accounts for 18–20% of the total organ weight. The neurohypophysis is derived from an evagination of the floor of the third ventricle. The *intermediate zone* is poorly demarcated in humans and occupies a narrow zone between the anterior and posterior lobes. Only the neurohypophysis is neurogenic in origin.

Atrophy of the pituitary gland. Figure 12.1 shows a pituitary in situ. The surface is markedly indented from pressure atrophy (bowl-like or "watch-glass" atrophy). (→ remaining pituitary, →1 optic nerve, × middle cranial fossa.) Increased intracranial pressure causes the surface indentation, since the bony sella turcica prevents the pituitary from expanding.

Pg: pressure atrophy of the pituitary is the result of pituitary tumors, cysts of the pituitary stalk, aneurysms of the carotid artery, empyema of the sphenoid bone, etc. *Small pituitary glands* also are observed after a pituitary infarction has healed or as a symptom of "exhaustion." *Co:* see page 232.

Necrosis of the pituitary gland (Fig. 12.2). Most cases are anemic infarctions of the anterior lobe following arterial occlusion. Figure 12.2 shows a dry, white area of necrosis in the anterior lobe (→1 infarction, →2 neurohypophysis).

Pg: thrombotic or embolic arterial occlusion (e.g., from thrombotic endocarditis). The *Sheehan syndrome* is defined as postpartum hypopituitarism or pituitary necrosis. *Pg* of the Sheehan syndrome: postpartum blood loss → shock with formation of thrombi → postpartum necrosis. Pituitary necrosis also is observed in young adolescent patients with diabetes mellitus; the cause is not known. *Hemorrhagic infarction of the pituitary gland* rarely is seen after local venous occlusion.

Tumors of the pituitary gland (Figs. 12.3 and 12.4). Enlargement of the pituitary may be due to hyperplasia or tumors. The anterior lobe is diffusely enlarged in hyperplasia, which can result from pregnancy (hypertrophic and hyperplastic chromophobe cells), prolonged stress or a diminished function of a peripheral endocrine organ (e.g., after castration or thyroidectomy). Tumors of the pituitary gland account for approximately 22% of all intracranial neoplasms. *Adenomas* of the anterior lobe, which may be hormonally active or inactive, are the most common pituitary neoplasms. They are divided into:

1. The *chromophobe adenoma* is the most common pituitary tumor. A chromophobe adenoma grows slowly, usually is hormonally inactive and produces symptoms of increased intracranial pressure, e.g., pressure of the optic chiasm (→ bitemporal hemianopia). Widening of the sella turcica is seen in x-ray. Figure 12.3 shows a chromophobe pituitary adenoma projecting from the sella turcica. The cut surface is gray-yellow (Fig. 12.4). The yellow portions of the adenoma are areas of necrosis.

2. *Eosinophilic adenoma:* see acromegaly and gigantism (p. 232).

3. *Basophilic adenoma:* see Cushing's disease (p. 232).

Hyperfunction of the Pituitary Gland

1. **Pituitary gigantism.** A disorder seen almost exclusively in males and defined as height exceeding 80 inches. Gigantism is the result of accelerated bone growth before the epiphyses are closed. There also is hypogonadism or late puberty.

Pg: most cases are attributable to an eosinophilic adenoma of the pituitary secreting excessive amounts of growth hormone (STH); rarely, a primary lesion of the hypothalamus is found.

2. **Acromegaly.** Excessive and prolonged STH production after epiphyseal closure (20–30 years) causes growth of flat bones (nasal bone, ribs, jaw, etc.), connective tissue and viscera *(splanchnomegaly)*. Typical gross features: a large, widened thorax, prognathism, spine abnormalities (upper spine: scoliosis; lower spine: lordosis – due to osteoporosis). Macroglossia, large hands and feet (thickening of skin and distal phalanges), large ears and nose. The expanding pituitary adenoma has other effects, e.g., visual disturbances from compression of the optic chiasm and diabetes insipidus from destruction (pressure) of the posterior lobe. In contrast to gigantism, acromegaly affects males and females equally.

3. **Cushing's disease** (see also Cushing's syndrome, p. 245). Typical manifestations are facial and truncal obesity (moon facies, buffalo hump: fat pad over upper dorsal vertebrae), plethora, osteoporosis of the spine (→ kyphosis), hypogonadism, growth of beard in females, purple-red abdominal striae, hypertension, polycythemia and hyperglycemia.

Pg: the clinicopathologic features are caused by excessive secretion of adrenocortical glucocorticoids. *Catabolic* adrenocortical functions prevail in Cushing's syndrome, in contrast to the adrenogenital syndrome. A basophilic adenoma of the pituitary is found in 30% of the patients with Cushing's disease; much more common are enlarged adrenal glands (cortical hyperplasia > adenomas or carcinomas, see p. 239). A characteristic histologic finding is the hyalinization and vacuolization of the basophilic cells in the pituitary, which have lost most cytoplasmic granules (Crooke's hyaline changes).

Hypofunction of the Pituitary Gland

1. **Hypopituitarism** results from destruction of the anterior pituitary. Endocrine function is diminished or absent.

A. During the *active growth period,* pituitary dwarfism is the main finding in hypopituitarism. The male sex is affected almost exclusively. Body growth is symmetric but diminished because epiphyseal ossification is absent. Sex organs are hypoplastic. No obesity, cachexia or psychic disturbances. *Pg:* idiopathic pituitary fibrosis, craniopharyngiomas, suprasellar cysts.

B. In the *adult,* hypopituitarism causes Simmond's disease, which is characterized by atrophy of the gonads, thyroid and adrenal cortex (cachexia, muscular atrophy, loss of hair, anorexia, hypoglycemia, low blood pressure). Postpartum necrosis or *Sheehan's syndrome:* see page 231. Hypopituitarism is clinically manifest after at least 75% of the pituitary tissue is lost.

2. In **partial hypopituitarism,** single anterior pituitary hormones are lost.

Dystrophia adiposogenitalis (Fröhlich's syndrome) is attributable to lesions of the hypothalamic-pituitary region. Gross manifestations include obesity of the trunk and thighs, hypoplasia and atrophy of the gonads, underdevelopment of secondary sex characteristics and cessation of growth (if the disease begins prior to puberty → hypophyseal dwarfism). Fröhlich's syndrome is caused by tumors (craniopharyngiomas), involvement by storage diseases, inflammations or hydrocephalus.

The **Laurence-Moon-Biedl syndrome** is a recessively inherited disease with hypogonadism, mental retardation, early obesity, retinitis pigmentosa and various malformations, such as polydactyly.

Diabetes insipidus is due to a deficiency of the antidiuretic hormone of the neurohypophysis. Tumors of the pituitary or hypothalamus and Hand-Schüller-Christian's disease account for 40% of diabetes insipidus cases. Inflammation or trauma of the hypothalamic-neurohypophyseal system also can cause diabetes insipidus.

Pg: deficiency of the neurohypophyseal antidiuretic hormone *(vasopressin)* → diminished reabsorption of water from renal tubules → loss of water; large volumes of diluted, otherwise normal, urine → compensatory polydipsia.

Pineal Gland, Thymus

Pineal gland (epiphysis cerebri). Tumors are the most common pathologic changes in the pineal gland: *pinealoblastomas* (undifferentiated, malignant, infiltratively growing), *pinealomas* or *pinealocytomas* (alveolar structure), *teratomas* and *gliomas.*

F: pineal tumors represent 5% of all intracranial neoplasms in childhood. *Co:* internal hydrocephalus due to compression of the aqueduct. Pineal tumors stimulate hypothalamic centers and thereby become endocrinologically active → pubertas praecox (in boys, premature spermatogenesis). See also adrenocortical tumors, page 241. Precocious puberty is not known to be caused by pineal tumors in females.

Thymus. The thymus is of branchiogenic origin. It diminishes in size and weight with increasing age (weight at birth: 35 Gm., reduction to 15 Gm. or less after the age of 60). Pathologic conditions include premature atrophy, inflammations (thymitis), involvement by storage diseases, hyperplasia and tumors *(thymomas).*

Hyperplasia of the thymus is observed in Graves' disease, but the reason for the enlarged thymus is not known. The term *status thymicolymphaticus* (Paltauf) frequently appeared in the old literature. This syndrome included an enlargement of lymph nodes, thymus, spleen and tonsils, together with a small heart, infantile aorta, increased subcutaneous fat and atrophic gonads. The syndrome was considered a cause of sudden death in children, but it is now held that viral infections are responsible for these findings. The formerly used term "*thymus death*" likewise is obsolete. Hyperplasia of lymphatic tissues (especially of the Waldeyer ring) is a common finding in many cases of sudden death, including traumatic death! In fact, chronic diseases cause atrophy of the lymphatic tissues, including the thymus.

Thymoma. A rare, slowly growing but often malignant, sarcomatous or carcinomatous neoplasm.

F: approximately 0.01% in autopsy material but 5% of all mediastinal tumors.

Myasthenia gravis. A chronic disease characterized by weakness of skeletal muscles, which increases with muscular fatigue. Myasthenia may affect all skeletal muscles *(generalized form),* the external ocular motor muscles only *(ophthalmologic form:* ptosis, less common diplopia) or the muscles of the face and jaw *(bulbar-paralytic form).*

F: an uncommon disease. *A:* 20–40 years. *S:* ♂:♀ = 2:2. *Pg:* > cholinesterase → hydrolysis of acetylcholine → muscular fatigability. Thymic hyperplasia is found in 50% of patients with myasthenia gravis; a thymoma is observed in another 30%. Myasthenia also is considered an autoimmune disease, since antibodies against A-bands of skeletal muscle have been demonstrated. In addition to myasthenia gravis, thymic hyperplasia and thymomas also are associated with aplastic anemias, agammaglobulinemias and Cushing's syndrome. *Co:* death from aspiration pneumonia. Muscular atrophy is seen terminally.

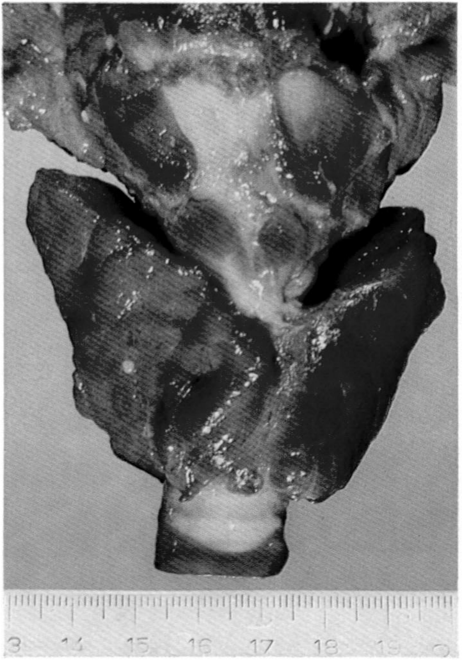

Fig. 12.5. Diffuse colloid goiter.

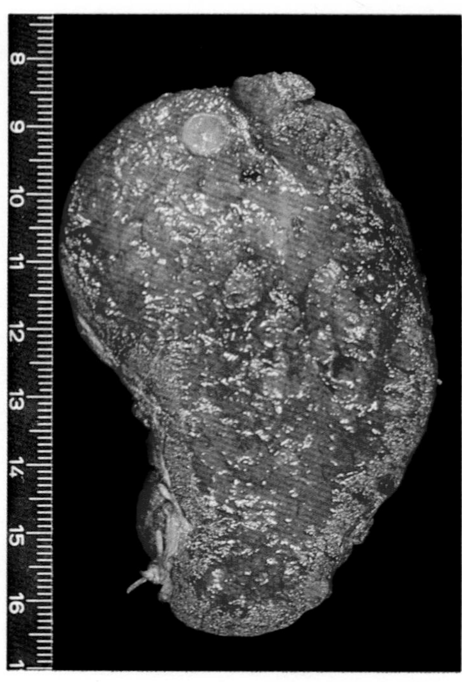

Fig. 12.6. Cut surface of a diffuse colloid goiter.

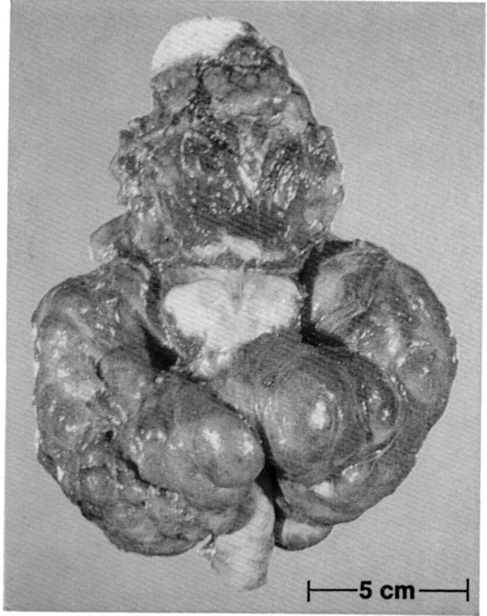

Fig. 12.7. Nodular colloid goiter.

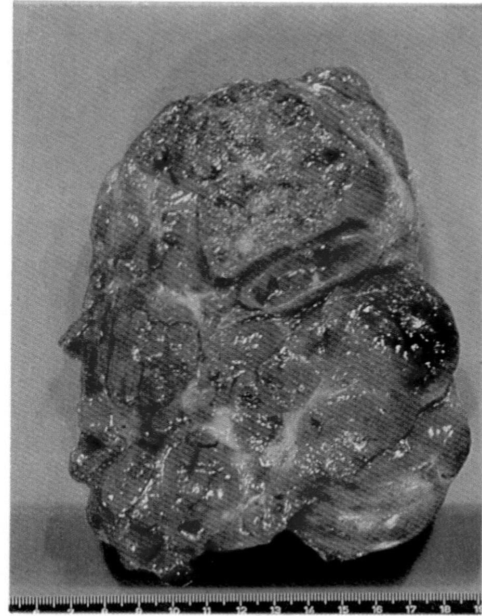

Fig. 12.8. Nodular colloid goiter with hemorrhages.

Thyroid Gland

General remarks. The thyroid gland develops from an outpouching of the floor of the mouth (ductus thyroglossus). The gland weighs 25 Gm. and consists of two lateral lobes connected by an isthmus. The cut surface is distinctly lobular and has a honey-like, glistening appearance (colloid content). Ectopic or accessory thyroid tissue is observed in the vicinity of the thyroglossal duct (base of the tongue), in cervical lymph nodes, the upper mediastinum and teratomas (so-called struma ovarii). *Function:* the endocrine function of the thyroid is regulated by the thyrotropic hormone (TSH) of the anterior pituitary gland. In the thyroid, iodide is oxidized to iodine, which is followed by iodination of tyrosine → formation of mono- and diiodotyrosine → condensation to triiodothyronine (T_3) and tetraiodothyronine or thyroxine (T_4) → T_3 or T_4 + globulin → thyroglobulin (storage form in thyroid). A proteolytic reaction releases T_3 and T_4, which binds to TBP (thyroid-binding protein. TBP regulates the transport and excretion of thyroid hormone, preventing loss by renal excretion). Thyroxine → > cell oxidation, stimulation of lymphatic tissue growth and inhibition of TSH.

Struma and **goiter** are *clinical terms for an enlarged thyroid gland.* Morphologically, the enlargement may be due to inflammation, hyperplasia or neoplasia.

Diffuse or simple goiter *is a generalized hyperplasia of the thyroid gland. The external configuration and lobular architecture of the thyroid gland are retained* (Figs. 12.5 and 12.6; TCP, p. 185). In diffuse colloid goiter (Fig. 12.5), the follicles are enlarged and rich in colloid. Lobules of various sizes can mimic a thyroid nodule *(diffuse colloid goiter with nodular hyperplasia).* Hyperplasia and hypertrophy of the follicular epithelium with diminished colloid content is the histologic basis of a *diffuse parenchymal goiter,* which occurs only in young females. The thyroid is firm, meaty and resembles the cut surface of the pancreas (Fig. 12.6). A similar appearance is characteristic of Graves' disease.

Nodular goiter (Figs. 12.7 and 12.8). The external and cut surfaces are irregularly nodular. Each nodule is surrounded by a fibrous-tissue capsule. The nodules are rich in colloid *(nodular colloid goiter)* or are more solid and cellular *(nodular, microfollicular, trabecular or tubular goiter).*

Pg: goiters occur in endemic, iodine-deficient areas or sporadically elsewhere. Endemic goiters are the result of diminished iodine uptake: iodine deficiency → diminished thyroxine production → increased TSH production → hyperplasia of the thyroid gland. Thiouracil inhibits incorporation of iodine into diiodothyroglobulin and thereby causes an enlarged thyroid. Young females often develop diffuse goiter, which may convert into a nodular colloid goiter later on. In such cases, the iodine deficiency is attributable to increased iodine demands during growth or pregnancy.

Goiter also is observed as a symptom of the following inflammatory diseases:

1. **Subacute or granulomatous thyroiditis** (De Quervain). Occurs mostly in young females. The gland is enlarged and firm. The capsule is not fixed to surrounding structures. Histologically, a granulomatous process with many giant cells (giant-cell thyroiditis). See TCP, p. 187.

Pg: not known, but autoimmunity is suspected.

2. **Chronic lymphocytic thyroiditis** (struma lymphomatosa or Hashimoto's disease; TCP, p. 187). The thyroid is symmetrically enlarged, rubbery-firm and pale yellow-gray on cut section. Females past 40 years. Histologically, there is extensive infiltration by lymphocytes (with formation of follicles) and plasma cells. Often progression to fibrosis.

Pg: probably represents an autoimmune disease, since circulating precipitins to thyroglobulin have been demonstrated in patients with Hashimoto's disease.

3. **Riedel's struma** (TCP, p. 187). This is a chronic, fibrosing thyroiditis or sclerosis of the thyroid gland. Grossly, the thyroid often is asymmetrically enlarged and "iron-hard." The capsule is fixed to adjacent organs, which are compressed.

Pg: not known. *S:* ♂:♀ = 1:3. *A:* 40–50 years.

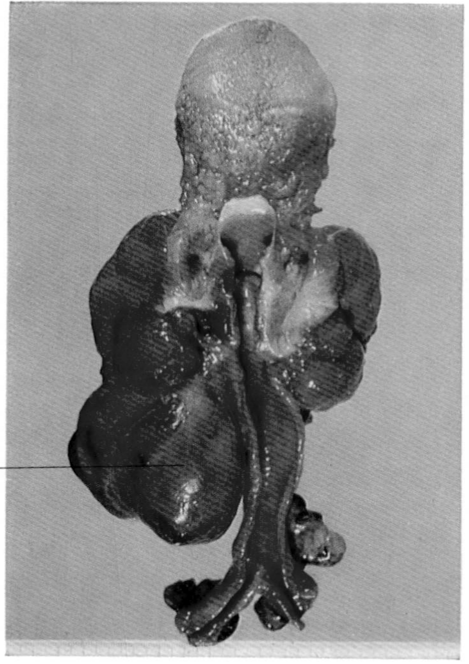

Fig. 12.9. Retrosternal goiter with compression of the trachea.

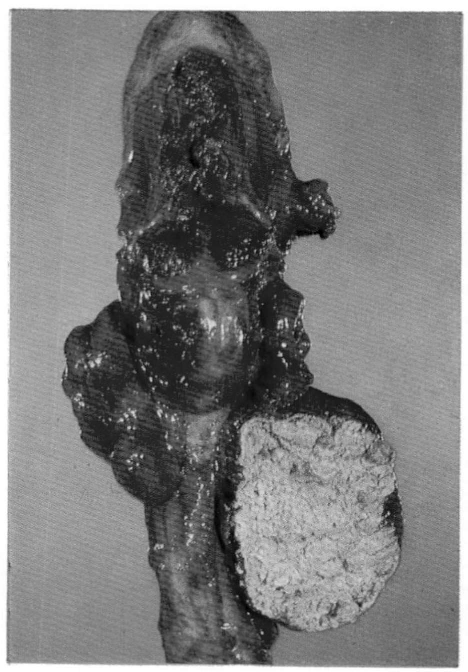

Fig. 12.10. Calcified goiter.

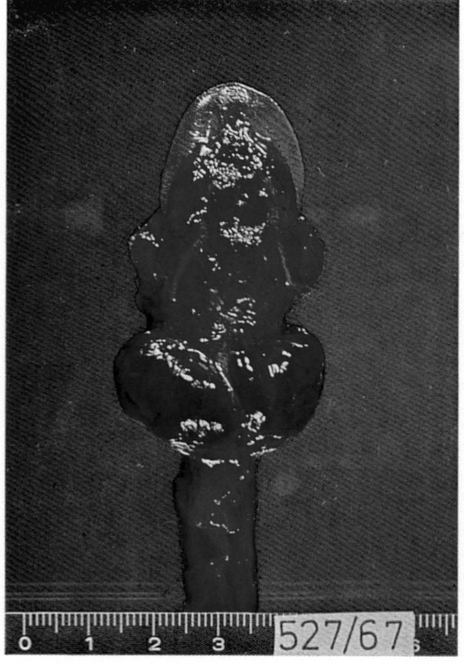

Fig. 12.11. Vascular neonatal goiter.

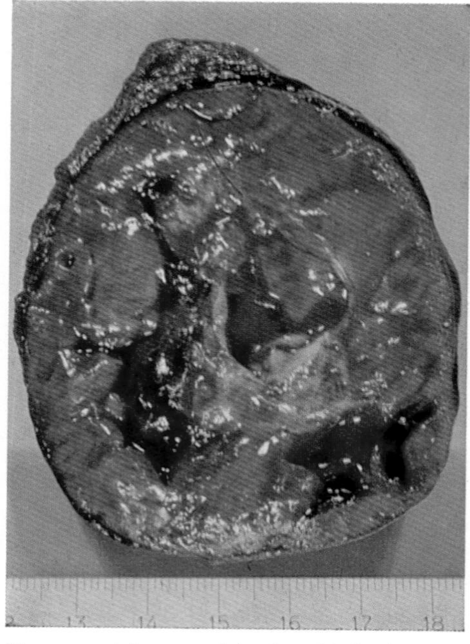

Fig. 12.12. Adenoma of the thyroid gland.

Nodular goiter with compression of the trachea. A large nodular goiter is shown in Figure 12.9. The lower goitrous nodule at the left in this figure extended behind and below the upper sternum. This is known as *substernal goiter:* a hyperplastic, accessory or ectopic thyroid gland that can reach the aortic arch. In Figure 12.9, the trachea is compressed and displaced laterally (clinically: dyspnea). Longstanding pressure from a goitrous nodule can cause necrosis of the tracheal cartilage *(tracheomalacia)*, compromise blood flow in the large neck vessels or compress the esophagus.

Retrogressive changes in a goiter (Fig. 12.10). Edema of the connective tissue, areas of parenchymal necrosis and hemorrhages are common findings in a goiter. These retrogressive changes probably are due to ischemia (see also Fig. 12.12) and can cause a sudden enlargement of a goitrous nodule. Cystic changes with fresh hemorrhages often are seen in old goitrous nodules, which also can become fibrotic, calcify or ossify.

Vascular neonatal goiter (Fig. 12.11). *A marked enlargement of the thyroid gland in newborns from severe congestion. The normal weight of the neonatal thyroid gland is 0.5 Gm. Mi:* severe hyperemia with few colloid-containing follicles. *Pg:* congestion during delivery. *DD:* true goiter from endemic cretinism should be considered.

Adenoma of the thyroid gland (Fig. 12.12). Adenomas occur as solitary or multiple nodules in an otherwise normal thyroid gland. It is not known whether the solid-cell nodules of a microfollicular nodular goiter represent areas of hyperplasia or true adenomas *(adenomatous goiter)*. The adenomatous nodules in Figure 12.12 show retrogressive changes, such as cystic softening and hemorrhages. The adenoma grew expansively, was surrounded by a capsule and compressed the adjacent thyroid.

Mi: solid, trabecular or tubular adenomas are distinguished. Adenomas are encapsulated.

The Hürthle-cell tumor is a benign adenoma composed of oncocytes.

Co: solitary thyroid adenomas sometimes are endocrinologically active. Such *toxic adenomas* present with symptoms of hyperthyroidism. Adenomas rarely become malignant, although they may resemble well-differentiated carcinomas ("metastasizing adenoma": a microfollicular, nodular goiter with hematogenous metastases).

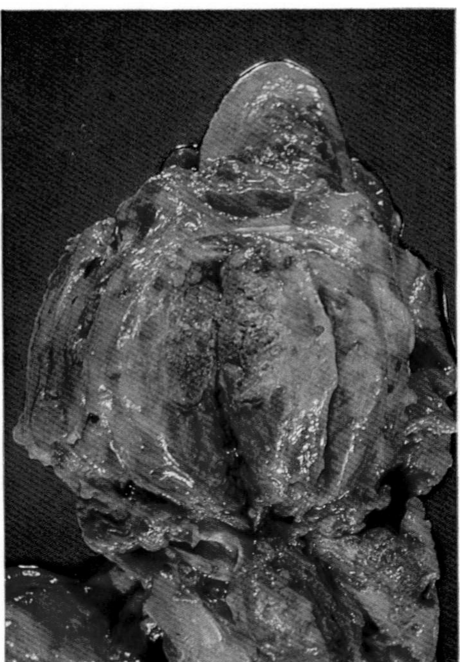
Fig. 12.13. Carcinoma of the thyroid gland.

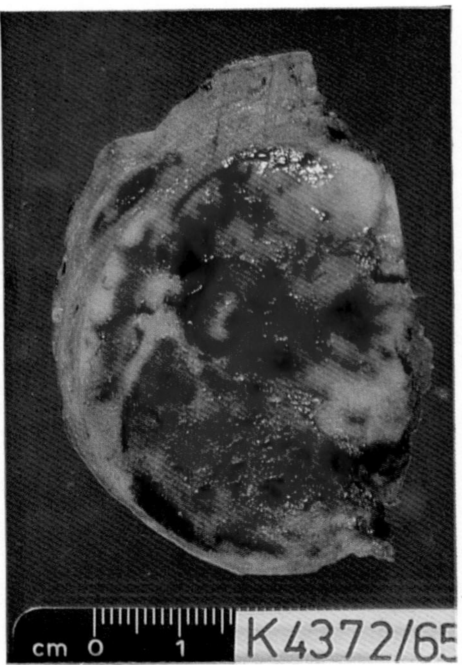

Fig. 12.14. Malignant hemangioendothelioma of the thyroid gland.

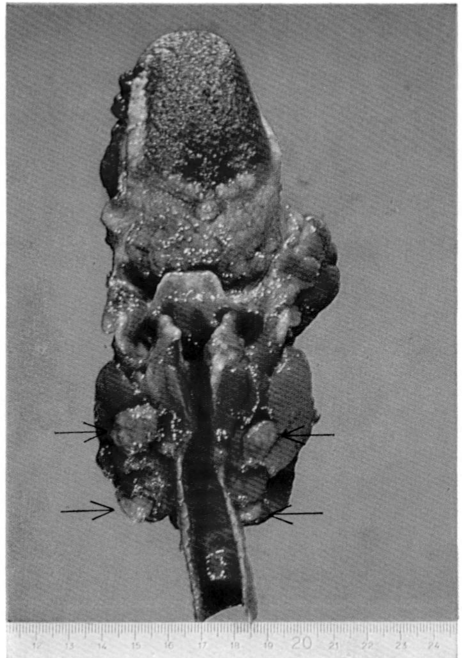
Fig. 12.15. Hyperplasia of the parathyroid glands.

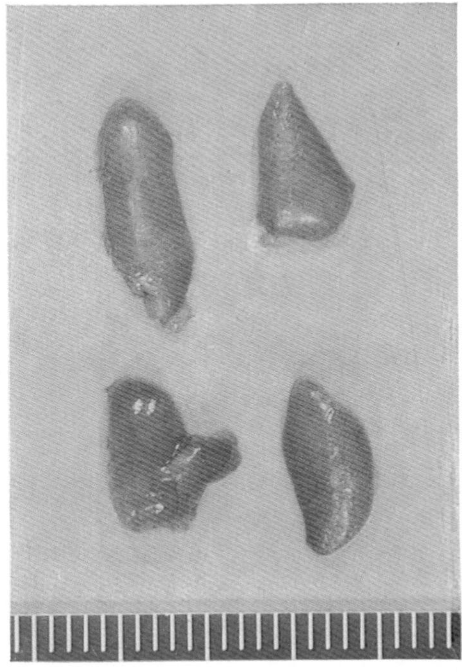
Fig. 12.16. Hyperplasia of the parathyroid glands.

Carcinoma of the thyroid (Fig. 12.13). *Thyroid carcinomas occur predominantly in elderly females.* Grossly, a thyroid carcinoma is a gray-brown, medium-firm tumor. Carcinomas may diffusely infiltrate the thyroid gland.

F: thyroid carcinomas constitute 1.6% of all malignant tumors. Approximately 12 cases are observed per 1,000,000 population per year. *A:* usually occurs after the 50th year, with the exception of papillary carcinomas, which have an earlier onset (younger females, sometimes before the age of 20 years). *S:* ♂:♀ = 1:3.

Pg: some carcinomas develop from pre-existing goiters. Approximately 2.5% of all goiters become cancerous in endemic goiter areas. The thyroid gland of children is susceptible to the carcinogenic action of x-rays. Prior to 1950, x-irradiation for thyrotoxicosis, thymic hyperplasia or lymph node tuberculosis was common practice. Thyroid carcinomas have developed in some irradiated glands after a latent period of 10–20 years.

Histologic classification of thyroid carcinomas:

1. **Papillary carcinomas** are the most common type of thyroid cancer (60%), occur predominantly in younger females and have a relatively good prognosis. Metastases in cervical lymph nodes appear after considerable time has elapsed from the onset of the cancer.

2. **Follicular carcinoma** (Langhans struma) usually is preceded by goiter and occurs in females 40–50 years of age. Follicular carcinomas account for approximately 20% of all thyroid carcinomas. These tumors are well differentiated, like the "metastasizing adenoma," although most cases are diagnosed after they have metastasized. The follicular thyroid carcinoma takes up radioactive iodine (^{131}I).

3. **Undifferentiated carcinomas** account for 18% of thyroid cancers and the peak incidence occurs in an age group older than that of papillary or medullary carcinomas. Metastases to the lungs and bones are common. Undifferentiated carcinomas are composed of small, spindle or giant cells.

A special histologic form of thyroid cancer is the **medullary carcinoma,** which is composed of cell clusters with pale cytoplasm. *Amyloid* is deposited in the tumor stroma. Medullary carcinomas arise from the so-called *parafollicular cells* (C-cells), which represent small cell clusters in the stroma of the thyroid. Parafollicular cells produce calcitonin, which decreases serum calcium and phosphate levels. Medullary carcinomas may be hormonally active.

4. **Hürthle-cell carcinomas** consist of oncocytes.

5. The rare **squamous-cell carcinoma** probably is derived from remnants of the thyroglossal duct.

Malignant hemangioendothelioma is the most common type of sarcoma of the thyroid gland (Fig. 12.14; TCP, p. 265). These highly vascular tumors contain many slit-like blood vessels. Hemangioendotheliomas probably are derived from pre-existing goiters.

S: ♀. *Co:* highly malignant tumor; hematogenous metastases to lungs, brain and other organs.

Parathyroid Glands

General remarks. Each parathyroid gland measures 3–4 mm. in length. The total weight is approximately 140 mg. They are located at or near the upper and lower posterior poles of the thyroid gland (Fig. 12.15). Occasionally, parathyroid glands are found in the thyroid, upper mediastinum and thymus.

Hyperplasia of parathyroid glands. *Parathyroid hyperplasia is a diffuse enlargement of all parathyroids, producing symptoms of hyperparathyroidism.* Figure 12.15 shows four evenly enlarged parathyroids in situ (→); the same glands are pale brown and enlarged after dissection (Fig. 12.16). Enlargement of the parathyroids may be difficult to distinguish on gross examination from lymph nodes or small thyroid adenomas. A parathyroid adenoma with hemorrhages (→) and areas of necrosis is illustrated in Figure 12.17.

Pg: see hyperparathyroidism. Adenoma and carcinoma rarely produce primary hyperparathyroidism.

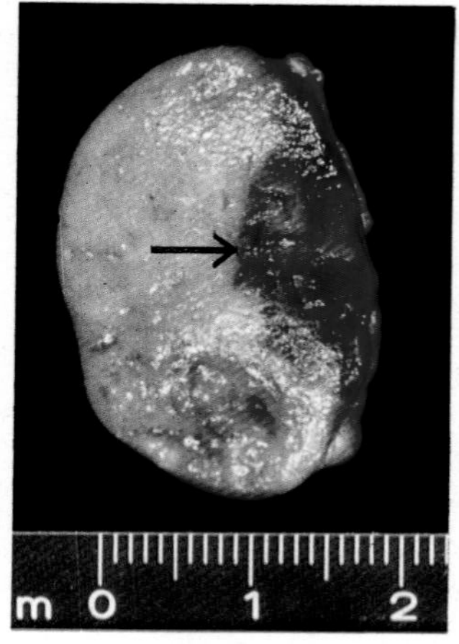

Fig. 12.17. Parathyroid adenoma.

Functional Disturbances of the Thyroid Gland

I. **Hyperfunction of the thyroid gland.** *Hyperthyroidism is defined as increased hormonal thyroid function.* The term Graves' disease includes hyperthyroidism with the triad of goiter, tachycardia and exophthalmos.

The following pathologic organ changes are observed in hyperthyroidism: *loss of weight* (elevated basal metabolic rate; normal BMR −10 to +20%), an *enlargement of the thyroid* (either diffuse or nodular enlargement from a "toxic adenoma"), *cardiac hypertrophy* (both ventricles are hypertrophied and dilated), *hyperplasia of lymphoreticular organs* (thymus, cervical lymph nodes and tonsils) and *osteoporosis* (slightly increased osteoclastic activity in vertebrae, ribs and pelvic bones). Exophthalmos is observed in 50–80% of hyperthyroid patients (considered to be due to a pituitary exophthalmos-producing substance, EPS). *Muscular atrophy* is observed in some hyperthyroid patients.

F: next to diabetes mellitus, it is one of the most common endocrinopathies. *Pg:* hyperthyroidism as a clinical disease may result from excessive pituitary or hypothalamic stimulation, a "*toxic*" *thyroid adenoma* or a euthyroid goiter that becomes secondarily hyperthyroid. The etiologic role of a long-acting thyroid stimulator (LATS) is still debated. This gamma globulin was isolated from patients with primary hyperthyroidism.

II. **Hypofunction.** *Hypothyroidism implies a diminished endocrine thyroid function manifested as myxedema or cretinism.*

1. **Myxedema.** A type of hypothyroidism characterized by an edematous swelling of the subcutaneous tissues of the face and extremities.

Pg: primary myxedema is a sequela of many thyroid diseases that extensively destroy thyroid parenchyma (inflammation, tumors, thyroidectomy). *Secondary myxedema* is caused by lesions of the hypothalamus or pituitary gland (diminished TSH secretion). *Clinical and pathologic-anatomic findings:* the basal metabolic rate is reduced (below −10%), myxedema of the skin (dry, cold, puffy, yellow), thick tongue, hypothermia, constipation, loss of hair, bradycardia and psychic changes (myxedema madness).

2. **Cretinism.** Congenital hypothyroidism occurs sporadically (congenital absence of the thyroid gland: no goiter) or endemically (with goiter in regions of iodine deficiency). The symptoms of cretinism are retarded psychic development (including total idiocy) and a typical facial expression (wrinkled skin, depressed nose, protruding jaw). Bone growth is retarded (dwarfism). The fontanelles and epiphyseal lines remain open. Hypogonadism.

Pg: sporadic cretinism is mostly a consequence of a thyroid malformation (aplasia or hypoplasia), affects children of euthyroid mothers (commonly seen as a familial disease) and is not confined to endemic areas. In contrast, endemic cretinism affects offspring of hypothyroid mothers (iodine deficiency). Overproduction of TSH activates the normal fetal thyroid gland in utero so that at the time of birth the thyroid is practically exhausted (hypothyroid).

Functional Disturbances of the Parathyroid Glands

Hyperfunction of the parathyroids

1. **Primary hyperparathyroidism** *is defined as excessive production of parathormone as a result of diffuse hyperplasia or adenomas of the parathyroid gland.*

Pg: increased osteoclastic activity → increased serum calcium levels → increased calcium excretion through the kidneys (from diminished calcium reabsorption). *Co:* the most prominent clinical manifestation is nephrolithiasis (first clinical symptom in approximately 60% of the cases). Additional manifestations are osteodystrophia fibrosa generalisata (von Recklinghausen's disease: 30% of the cases, see also p. 197), ulcers of the stomach and duodenum (in approximately 10%), increased tendency to thrombosis and pancreatitis.

2. **Secondary hyperparathyroidism** *is the result of renal acidosis and hypercalcemia.* It is considered an adaptive hyperplasia of all parathyroid glands in patients with renal insufficiency (tubular insufficiency of chronic interstitial nephritis or chronic pyelonephritis, less frequently after glomerulonephritis).

3. **Tertiary hyperparathyroidism** *is defined as secondary hyperthyroidism complicated by the formation of a parathyroid adenoma.* Seen in patients with chronic renal insufficiency and secondary hyperparathyroidism who develop a parathyroid adenoma ("autonomous secondary hyperparathyroidism"). The biochemical findings (serum, calcium and phosphorus) are similar to those of primary hyperparathyroidism.

DD: Paget's osteitis deformans, carcinomatous metastases to the bones, multiple myeloma, malabsorption syndrome, hormonal osteoporosis (Cushing's disease, hypogonadism), osteomalacia and pseudocysts of the bones.

Hypofunction of the parathyroids

1. **Hypoparathyroidism** is a syndrome of calcium deficiency (serum calcium below 9 mg./100 ml.). Clinically: tetany, but no bone changes are observed.

Pg: after operative removal of the parathyroid glands (tetany after thyroidectomy).

2. **Pseudohypoparathyroidism** *is defined as hypocalcemia independent of parathormone.* The disease is characterized by trophic changes in the skin, nails (transverse grooves), teeth (defects of dentin), eyes (cortical cataract) and manifestations of retarded bone growth (dwarfism).

Pg: the pathologic-anatomic findings in pseudohypoparathyroidism are considered the consequence of a genetically determined renal tubular disease.

3. **Pseudo-pseudohypoparathyroidism.** Dwarfism with short metacarpal bones but normal calcium and phosphorus levels in the serum.

Pg: probably inherited.

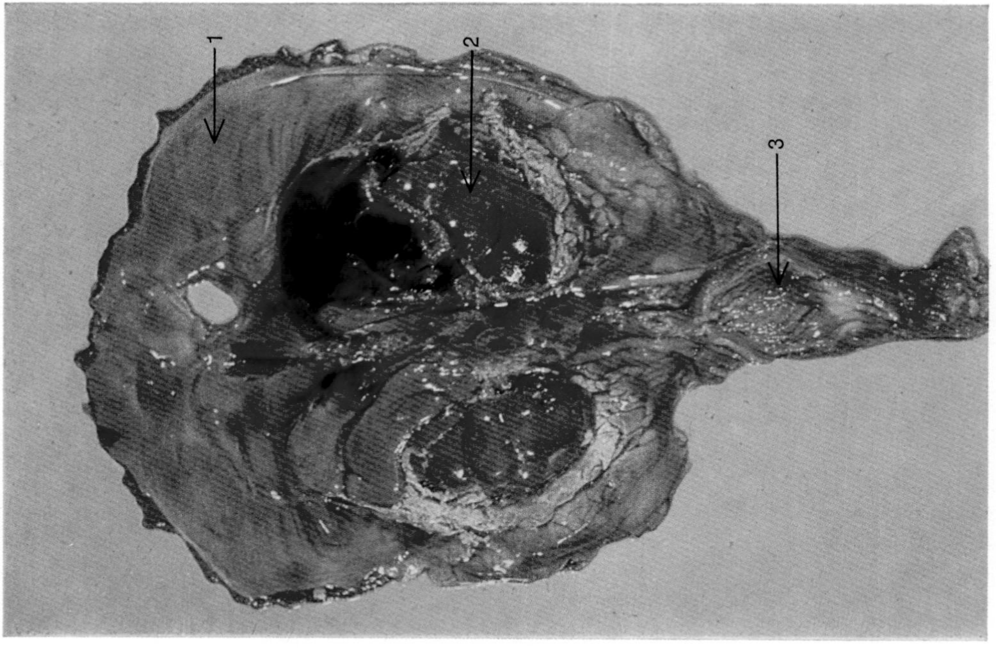

Fig. 12.19. Unilateral adrenal hemorrhages following birth trauma.

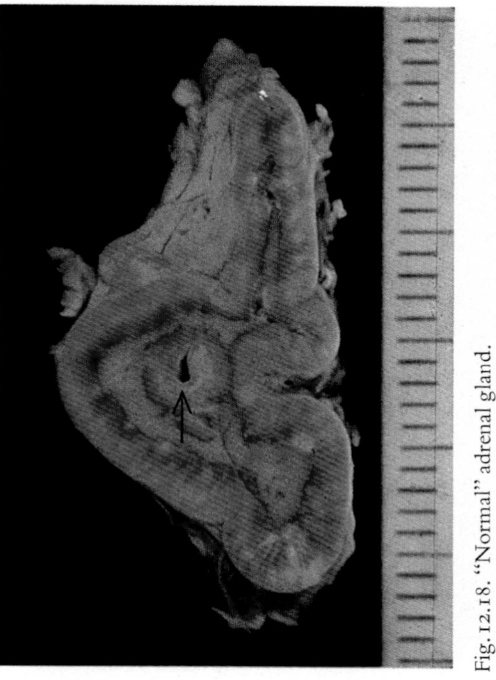

Fig. 12.18. "Normal" adrenal gland.

Fig. 12.20. Bilateral adrenal hemorrhages (Waterhouse-Friderichsen syndrome).

Adrenal Glands

General remarks. The adrenal glands are located at the upper poles of the kidneys or occasionally beneath the renal capsule. The adrenals are embedded in fat. Their total weight varies between 5 and 12 Gm. The median weight in adults is 8 Gm. (0.01% of the total body weight). The relative weights of the adrenals are considerably greater in fetuses and newborns. The adrenals weigh 0.46% of the total body weight during the fourth month of pregnancy and 0.23% of the body weight at birth.

A normal adrenal gland is shown in Figure 12.18. Four layers are identified on cut surface. A gray *medulla* is found around the central vein (→). *Three cortical zones* are recognized; these constitute approximately 75% of the adrenal weight. An external, yellowish (lipid-rich) *zona glomerulosa* and an inner, brownish (lipofuscin and iron) *zona reticularis* surround a relatively broad *zona fasciculata*. The middle layer is indistinctly delineated.

Functions of the adrenal gland. The adrenal cortex secretes steroid hormones and is regulated by the pituitary hormone ACTH. Some 40 steroids have been isolated from the adrenal cortex; these fall into five groups: *glucocorticoids, mineralocorticoids, androgens, estrogens and progestagens.* Approximately 70% of the entire adrenocortical secretion consists of *cortisol*. The most important mineralocorticoid is *aldosterone*. Diseases of overproduction of adrenocortical hormones are Cushing's disease, aldosteronism and the adrenogenital syndrome. The chromaffin adrenal medulla produces *epinephrine* (75%) and *norepinephrine* (25%). *Pheochromocytoma* is the most important disease of the adrenal medulla.

Postmortem changes. The adrenal glands undergo rapid postmortem changes. The medulla becomes soft and even liquefied, so that the brownish zona reticularis may be mistaken for medullary tissue.

Malformations. Agenesis is rare. A "unilateral adrenal agenesis" most often is the result of sloppy autopsy technic. The left adrenal gland is found near the tail of the pancreas. The right adrenal gland is positioned near or at the posterior surface of the right liver lobe. Bilateral adrenal hypoplasia is seen in anencephalic stillbirths (see p. 339).

Hemorrhages of the adrenal gland

1. **Unilateral adrenal hemorrhage** is observed frequently in premature births as a consequence of birth trauma or asphyxia. Figure 12.19 shows extensive hemorrhage in the right adrenal and the adjacent fat tissue. The diaphragm (→1), kidney (→2) and urinary bladder (→3) also are shown in Figure 12.19.

Pg: traumatic injuries in adults occasionally cause unilateral adrenal hemorrhages. Hemorrhagic infarction of the adrenal gland is observed following occlusion of adrenal veins by thrombi or tumors. *Anemic infarctions* of the adrenal gland result from occlusion of an adrenal artery by thrombi, emboli or panarteritis nodosa. *Co:* hemorrhages and/or necrosis → destruction of the adrenal cortex → acute adrenal insufficiency. Hemorrhages → resorption and organization → pseudocysts and calcifications.

2. **Bilateral toxic-bacterial adrenal hemorrhages** (Waterhouse-Friderichsen syndrome). Extensive adrenal hemorrhages are the result of severe toxic-bacterial parenchymal damage. The Waterhouse-Friderichsen syndrome presents clinically as acute adrenal failure (adrenal crisis). Figure 12.20 shows the adrenals of a child with diffuse hemorrhages and areas of necrosis.

F: the Waterhouse-Friderichsen syndrome is observed most often in small children with meningococcal sepsis. Staphylo-, strepto- or pneumococcal sepsis also can cause bilateral adrenal hemorrhages. *Pg:* toxic parenchymal damage is extensive. In addition, adrenal capillaries and veins contain hyaline thrombi that cause hemorrhagic infarction of the adrenal. Widespread purpuric skin hemorrhages develop on the same basis (consumptive coagulopathy of shock). *Co:* acute adrenal insufficiency (adrenal crisis) is a medical emergency: low blood pressure, cramping abdominal pains and high fever.

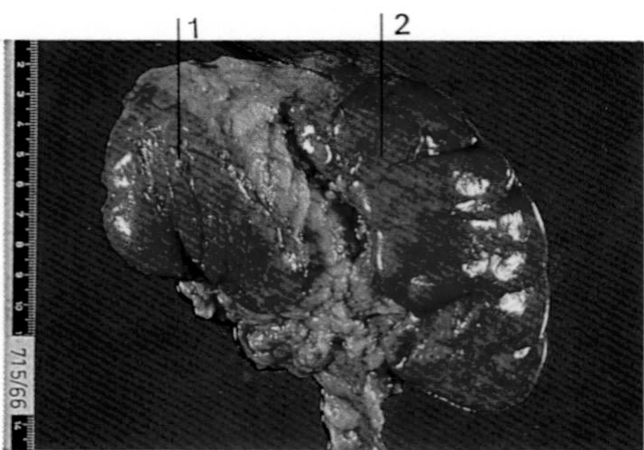

Fig. 12.21. Hyperplasia of the adrenal glands in Cushing's syndrome.

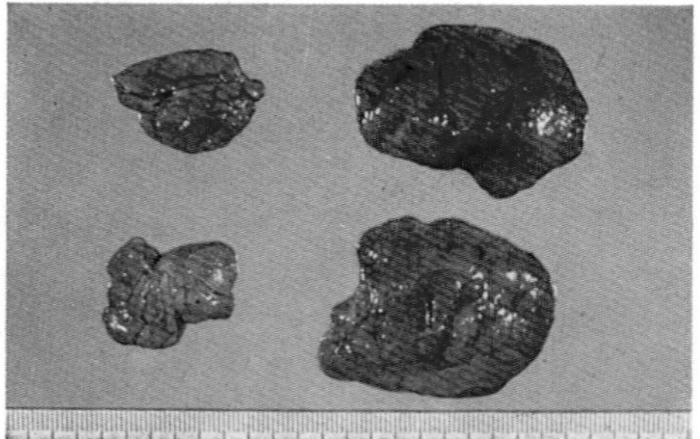

Fig. 12.22. Adrenal hyperplasia in Cushing's syndrome. The normal adrenal glands of corresponding age are shown at the left.

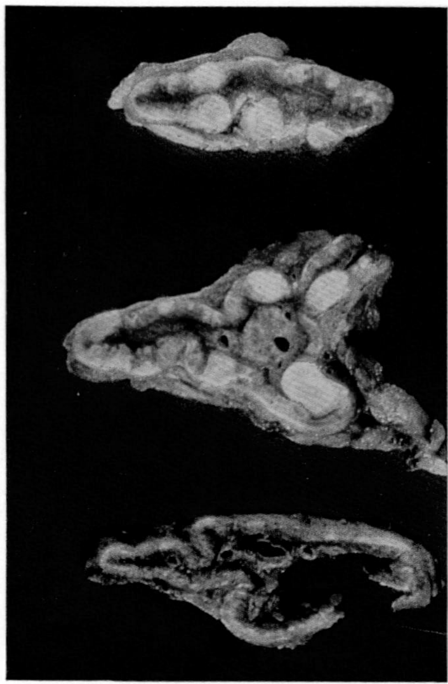

Fig. 12.23. Nodular hyperplasia of the adrenal cortex.

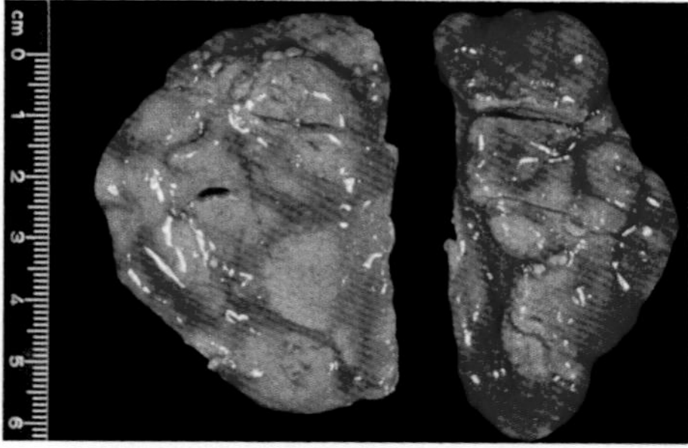

Fig. 12.24. Hyperplasia of the adrenal glands in aldosteronism.

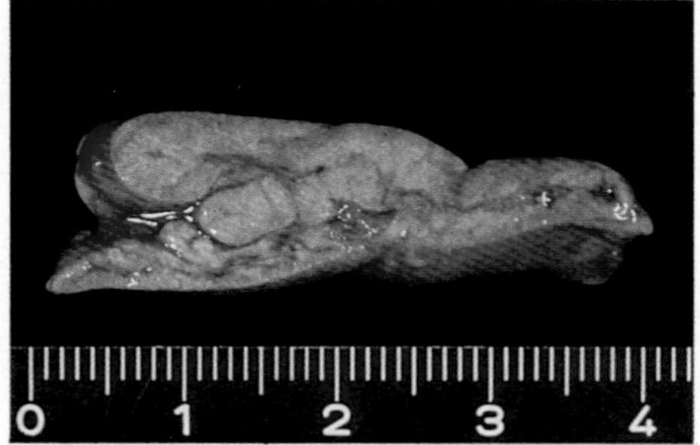

Fig. 12.25. Fatty, hyperplastic adrenal cortex in aldosteronism.

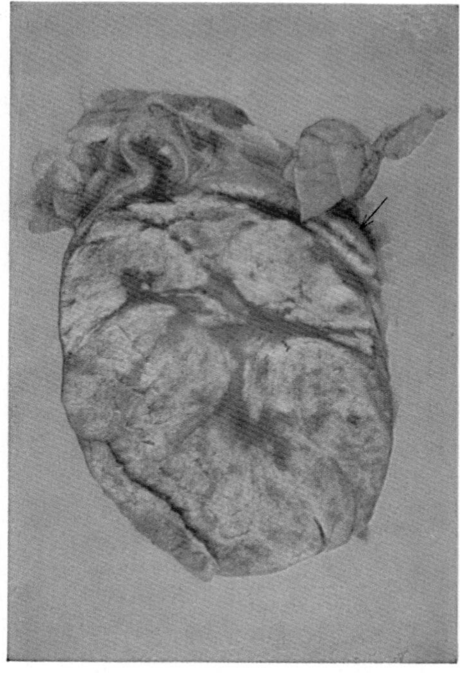

Fig. 12.26. Lipid-rich adenoma of the adrenal cortex.

Nodular hyperplasia of the adrenal cortex (Fig. 12.23). Small, circumscribed nodular proliferations of the adrenal cortex develop as an adaptation to chronic stress (especially with longstanding hypertension). Adrenocortical nodules are *not encapsulated.* They often are surrounded by atrophic cortical tissue.

In contrast, an adrenocortical adenoma is *encapsulated* (Fig. 12.26). Although most adenomas are hormonally "silent," an occasional adenoma may cause Cushing's syndrome or aldosteronism (see below). The arrow in Figure 12.26 points to the normal adrenal cortex, which is of regular thickness.

Functional Changes in the Adrenal Cortex

Chronic insufficiency of the adrenal cortex *(Addison's disease).* Adrenocortical insufficiency becomes clinically manifest after approximately 90% of the cortex is lost. The clinical symptomatology includes generalized muscle weakness, increased skin pigmentation (especially creases), frequent nausea, cachexia, low blood pressure and a small heart. The common causes are tuberculosis of the adrenal glands, rarely tumors, hemorrhages or amyloidosis. The *primary, idiopathic adrenocortical atrophy* probably is an autoimmune phenomenon. An Addisonian crisis can be precipitated by a banal infection (see also Waterhouse-Friderichsen syndrome). *Secondary adrenocortical insufficiency* is found after longstanding cortisone therapy → adrenocortical atrophy.

Cushing's syndrome is *due to overproduction of adrenocortical steroids (especially cortisone, but also mineralocorticoids, androgens and estrogens)* (Figs. 12.21 and 12.22, see also p. 232; TCP, pp. 189 and 239). In order of frequency, the clinical manifestations and gross findings are "moon face," truncal obesity, hypertension, hirsutism, purple striae, acne, hemorrhagic diathesis, osteoporosis and glucosuria.

F: Cushing's syndrome is observed predominantly in adults. *Pg:* bilateral, diffuse hyperplasia of the adrenal cortex (60% of patients with Cushing's syndrome), adrenocortical carcinomas (16%, especially in children) or adenomas (12%) and hyperplasia of aberrant adrenocortical tissue (2%). The remaining 10% present without demonstrable hyperplasia of the adrenal cortex. Half of the cases of Cushing's syndrome in childhood are attributable to adrenocortical carcinomas. A basophilic pituitary adenoma is responsible for 10–30% of Cushing's syndrome (in such instances, the term Cushing's disease is used). Cushing's syndrome also can be produced by certain nonadrenal tumors (paraneoplastic syndrome). Most clinical symptoms are attributable to cortisone excess. Fat formation causes obesity. Increased gluconeogenesis depletes muscle proteins (weakness, atrophy) and leads to osteoporosis of the spine, ribs and pelvis. Increased gluconeogenesis also causes steroid diabetes. Excessive androgen production is responsible for hirsutism and seborrhea. The pathogenesis of the arterial hypertension is still not known.

Primary aldosteronism (Conn syndrome, Figs. 12.24–12.26) *is caused by excessive secretion of mineralocorticoids, especially aldosterone independent of pituitary regulation.* Ninety per cent of the cases are caused by a unilateral, solitary adenoma of the adrenal cortex (Fig. 12.26). Multiple smaller adenomas or a diffuse hyperplasia of the adrenal cortex account for the remaining 10% of aldosteronism (Figs. 12.24 and 12.25). The typical gross finding is an enlarged, yellow adrena, cortex or an adenoma. Polyuria, polydipsia, systolic and diastolic hypertension, hypernatremial hypokalemia but absence of subcutaneous edema are the main clinical findings.

F: aldosteronism is rare. Occasionally, it is seen as a *paraneoplastic syndrome* (in cases of bronchogenic carcinoma: see Figs. 12.24 and 12.25). *S:*♂:♀ = 1:2. *A:* 30–50 years. *Pg:* aldosterone → diminished serum K and Cl levels, hypernatremia. Increased excretion of potassium but normal sodium excretion in urine. Hypertension due to Na retention → increased action of pressure substances (?). Secondary aldosteronism is characterized by excessive loss of Na and H_2O, especially from loss of plasma (burns), hypoproteinemia and renal sodium retention → edema (!).

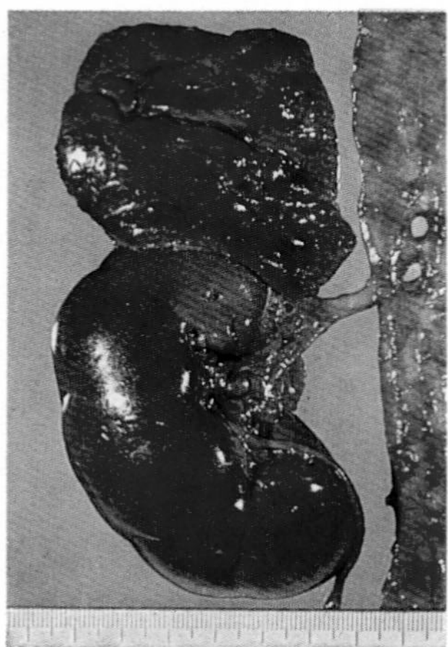

Fig. 12.27. Hyperplasia of the adrenal glands.

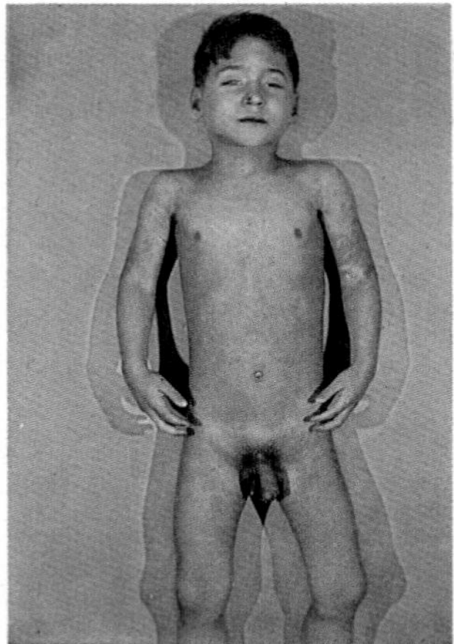

Fig. 12.28. Precocious pseudopuberty in adrenogenital syndrome.

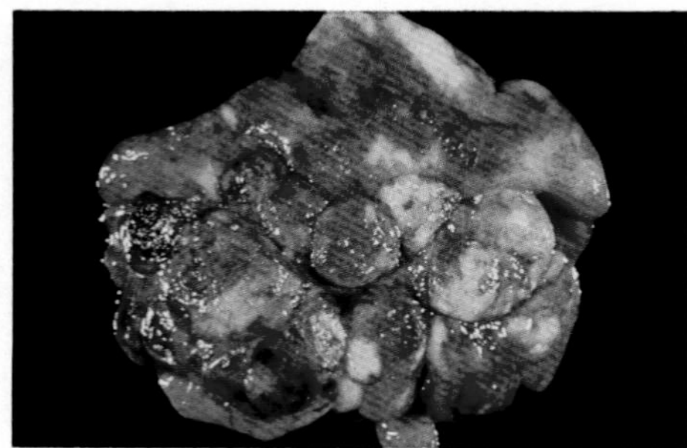

Fig. 12.30. Neuroblastoma of the adrenal glands.

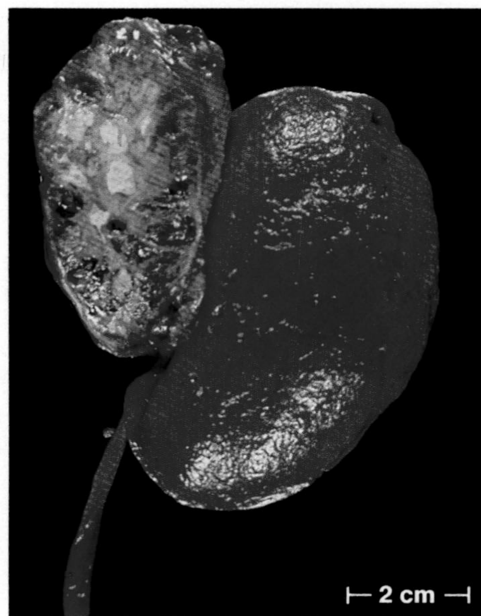

Fig. 12.31. Metastases in the adrenal gland from a bronchial carcinoma.

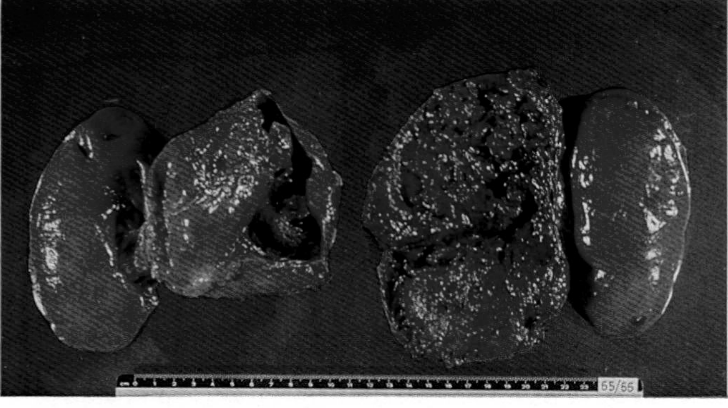

Fig. 12.29. Malignant bilateral pheochromocytoma.

Adrenogenital syndrome

1. The congenital adrenogenital syndrome (AGS) *is due to a deficiency of the enzyme 21-hydroxylase. Clinically, the disease is characterized by androgen excess* (Figs. 12.27 and 12.28).

(a) In boys, the AGS presents as precocious puberty due to the isosexual action of androgens: enlargement of the penis, small testes (dissociated virilism), growth of axillary and pubic hair prior to the fifth year and growth of a beard before the tenth year (hirsutism) (Fig. 12.28).

(b) In girls, the AGS presents as pseudohermaphroditism due to the heterosexual action of androgens: clitoris hypertrophy, premature development of pubic and axillary hair, acne and seborrhea. The uterus and ovaries are small and retarded in development. (Called pseudohermaphroditism because ovaries are present, in contrast to genetic intersexuality.)

The formation of androgens begins during the third to fifth month of pregnancy, at a time when the gonads are already differentiated but still susceptible to developmental anomalies. Androgens accelerate bone growth and closure of epiphyses. Initially, such children are somewhat taller than corresponding, age-matched children, but later a body length of 150 cm. rarely is exceeded (OVERZIER: "as children tall, as adults small"). "Hercules type" of muscle development. AGS is a familial, enzymatic defect: deficiency of 21-hydroxylase → absence of cortisol precursors → increased androgens and estrogens. This chain of events can be interrupted by giving cortisone, which normalizes ACTH secretion. Special types of the congenital AGS: (a) with hypertension, (b) with salt loss.

2. Postpubertal AGS is observed between 15 and 20 years of age. The above-mentioned effects of excessive androgen production are observed, but secretion and excretion of cortisol are normal.

3. The AGS in adults is due to adrenocortical adenomas or carcinomas causing virilization (see also Cushing's syndrome). *Feminizing adrenocortical tumors are rare.* Increased estrogen production in males causes gynecomastia.

Pheochromocytoma (Fig. 12.29; TCP, p. 189). *A chromaffin tumor that arises, in most cases, from the adrenal medulla. The peak incidence is between 20 and 40 years. Pheochromocytomas cause hypertension.* A soft, blood-rich tumor of brownish color is observed on gross examination (Fig. 12.29).

F: only 0.5% of all cases of hypertension are attributable to pheochromocytomas. *A:* 20–40 years. *Lo:* unilateral adrenal pheochromocytomas (80%), bilateral adrenal pheochromocytomas (10%) and extra-adrenal pheochromocytomas (10%) (sympathetic nerve). *S:* ♂ = ♀. *Pg:* the clinical symptomatology is dependent on hormone secretion. Hypertension is always present (epinephrine → systolic hypertension; norepinephrine → systolic and diastolic hypertension). Continued secretion → permanent hypertension; intermittent secretion → paroxysmal hypertension. *Mi:* trabecular tumor composed of polymorphous chromaffin cells. These contain catecholamines. Malignant pheochromocytomas may metastasize to the liver, lungs, lymph nodes and bones (10% of all pheochromocytomas).

Other Adrenal Tumors

Neuroblastoma (sympathicoblastoma) (Fig. 12.30). Adrenal medullary, nonchromaffin tumors are designated according to their maturity (sympathicogonioma → sympathicoblastoma → ganglioneuroma). Collectively, sympathicogoniomas and blastomas are called neuroblastomas. The ganglioneuroma is a most mature type differentiating into ganglion cells. Grossly, as shown in Figure 12.30, the tumor is gray-white, with a cut surface resembling fish flesh. Individual tumor nodules coalesce to form larger, lobulated masses.

A: especially in small children. *S:* ♂:♀ = 1:2. According to the metastatic sites: the Hutchinson type of neuroblastoma is characterized by massive hematogenous metastases in the liver and bones. The so-called Pepper type of neuroblastoma metastasizes lymphogenously; the liver is spared. *Pr:* poor.

Metastases in the adrenal glands. Hematogenous metastases from lung carcinomas (approximately 30–40%) are common (Fig. 12.31).

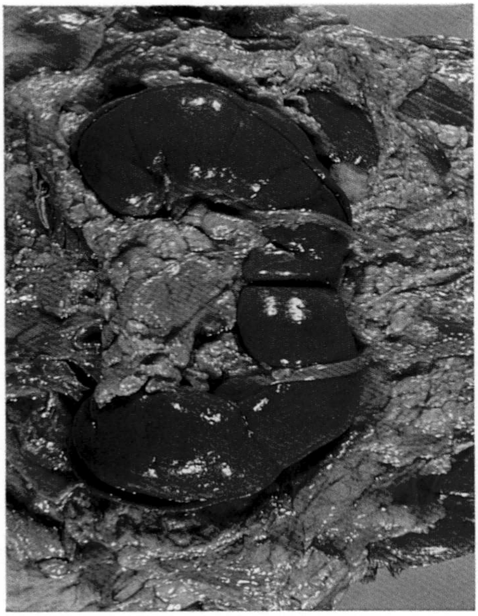

Fig. 13.1. Horseshoe kidney.

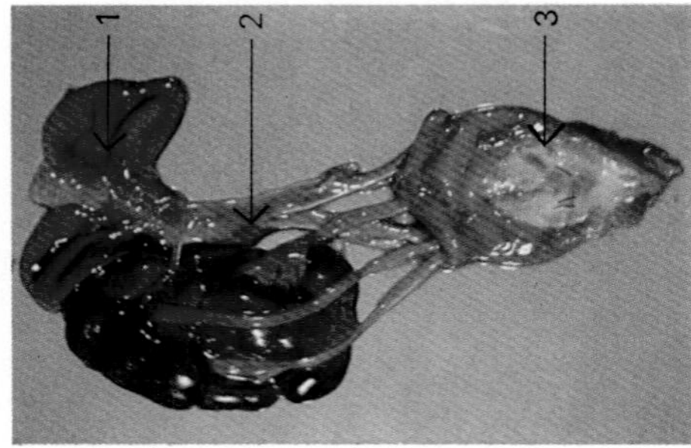

Fig. 13.2. Unilateral fusion of the kidney.

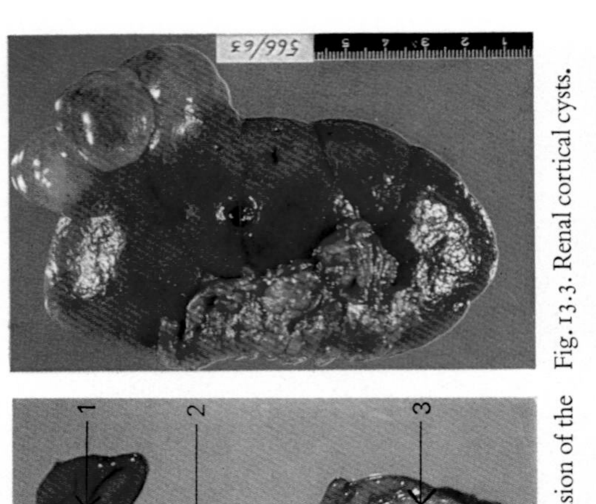

Fig. 13.3. Renal cortical cysts.

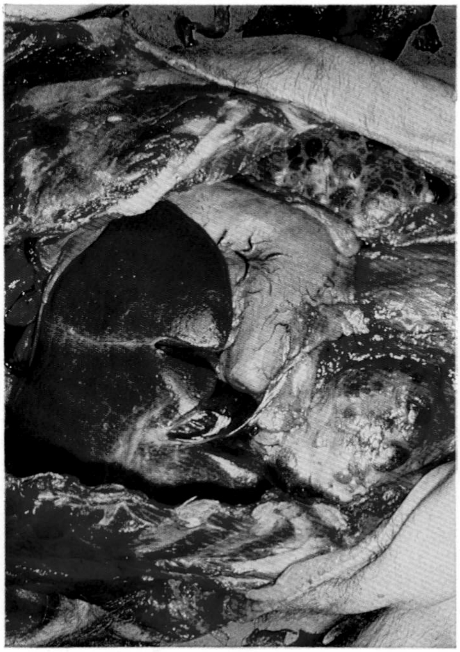

Fig. 13.4. Polycystic kidneys in situ.

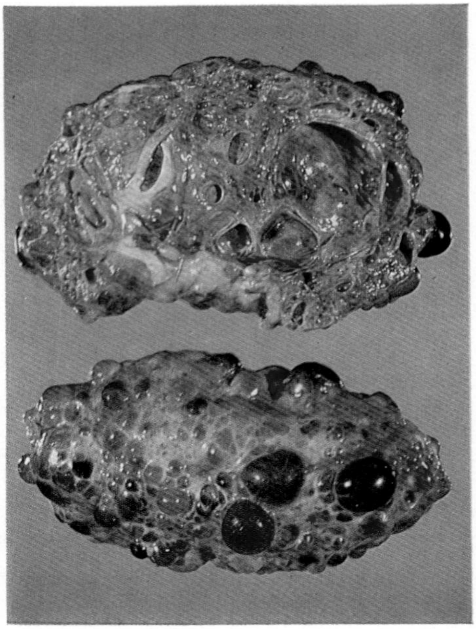

Fig. 13.5. External and cut surfaces of polycystic kidneys.

13. Kidneys and Urinary System

General remarks. The kidneys weigh between 260 and 290 Gm. (in females approximately 25 Gm. less) and measure 12×6 cm. The kidneys are visualized and inspected in situ by a cut through the peritoneum. Kidneys and ureters are not separated when the renal pelvis is dilated. When one kidney is smaller than the other, the renal arteries should be opened carefully and the kidneys should remain attached to the aorta. For orientation purposes, the left kidney is identified by a long segment of ureter, the right kidney by a short ureter. The renal capsules are stripped off. A single sagittal knife cut from the convexity toward the pelvis exposes most of the kidney cut surface. The renal pelvis is opened with scissors. The lower pole of the kidney is cut at the same time. Ureters are opened. An anterior cut from the urethra opens the urinary bladder. The ureteral ostia are located near the trigonum. The prostate gland is prepared by several longitudinal knife cuts parallel to the bladder or urethra.

Congenital Malformations

Renal malformations are found in 10% of the autopsies performed and are usually harmless in nature.

Agenesis. The renal primordium, vessels and ureters are absent. Renal agenesis is associated with flattening of the nose, recession of the chin, senile facies and low-set ears. This combination also is known as dysplasia renofacialis, a malformation with a chromosomal aberration (trisomy 18). Renal unilateral agenesis occurs also.

Aplasia. The renal primordium is present but not developed. Bilateral aplasia is incompatible with life. Unilateral aplasia is compensated for by hyperplasia and hypertrophy of the normal kidney.

Hypoplasia. The kidneys are smaller than normal and the renal arteries are narrow (*DD:* pyelonephritis hypoplasia).

Pelvic kidney. The kidneys are located in the pelvis. The renal arteries originate from the lower abdominal aorta or the iliac arteries. The ureters are short (*DD:* acquired nephroptosis).

Horseshoe kidney (Fig. 13.1). The lower kidney poles usually are fused, the upper poles rarely. The ureters pass anterior to the kidney. *Co:* Frequently pyelonephritis. Sometimes dystocia.

Pancake kidney. The kidneys likewise are fused and the hilus is displaced ventrally. Otherwise, the kidneys are smooth, as shown in Figure 13.2.

Unilateral fusion of the kidneys with three ureters and three renal pelves. The kidneys are fused caudally and the ureters arise ventrally. (Fig. 13.2: →1 adrenal glands, →2 aorta, →3 urinary bladder.)

Double ureters and double renal pelvis. This common malformation is harmless.

Mobile kidney is an acquired low (caudal) position of one or both kidneys (nephroptosis). The renal arteries arise at their usual sites. The ureters are tortuous. Hydronephrosis is a common complication.

Kidney cysts are found commonly in adult autopsies (60%). The cysts are lined by a shiny, white epithelium and filled with amber fluid (Fig. 13.3).

Polycystic kidney disease (Figs. 13.4 and 13.5). This is a hereditary familial disorder characterized by numerous renal cysts. Polycystic kidney disease may manifest after birth or in adult life.

Infantile type (Potter, Type I): Congenital polycystic kidney disease is inherited as a recessive trait. The patient usually dies during the first year of life. The kidneys are enlarged by multiple cortical and medullary cysts (predominantly, cystic dilation of the collecting tubules). Size of cysts 1–2 mm. Patients with congenital polycystic kidney disease have facial changes similar to those described for renal agenesis. The infantile type should be distinguished from small cysts in the kidneys of children who present with a nephrotic syndrome.

Adult type (Potter, Type III) (Figs. 13.4 and 13.5): Figure 13.4 shows the abdominal organs in situ. The kidneys are greatly enlarged and contain numerous cysts (up to 5 cm. in diameter). The external and cut surfaces are studded with brown-to-black cystic structures, as illustrated in Figure 13.5. The cyst content is black because of old hemorrhages. Otherwise, the cysts have smooth walls (Fig. 13.5, right). Very little normal kidney tissue remains. One-third of the patients with polycystic kidney disease have multiple cysts in the liver and pancreas (30%). Another 10–20% of these patients have berry aneurysms of the cerebral arteries. Cysts in different sections of the nephron.

A *special type* of kidney cysts is found in the sponge kidney of adults. Here, multiple cysts are confined to the medulla. The disease occurs mostly in males. *Rare forms: cystic kidneys, Type II according to* POTTER. Renal dysplasia = impairment of the complete differentiation of the renal attachment with cysts, cartilage tissue, smooth musculature, and connective tissue. No renal tissue. *Cystic kidneys, Type IV according to* POTTER: Predominantly subcapsular renal cysts with dilation of the ureter and thickening of the wall of the urinary bladder.

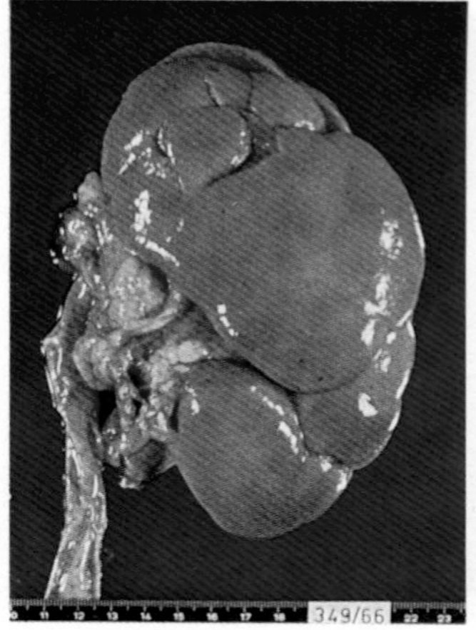

Fig. 13.6. Anemic kidney.

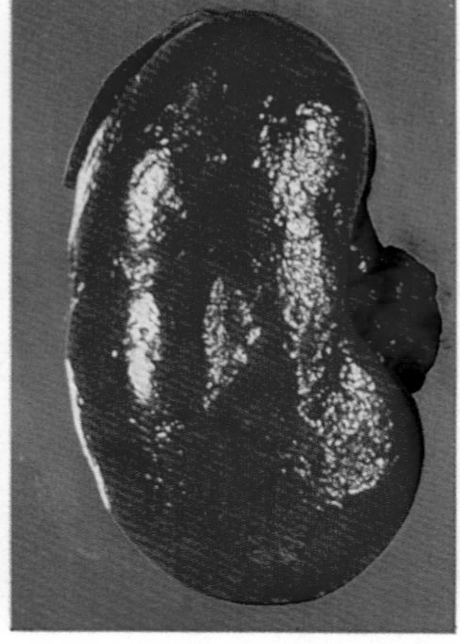

Fig. 13.7. "Normal" kidney.

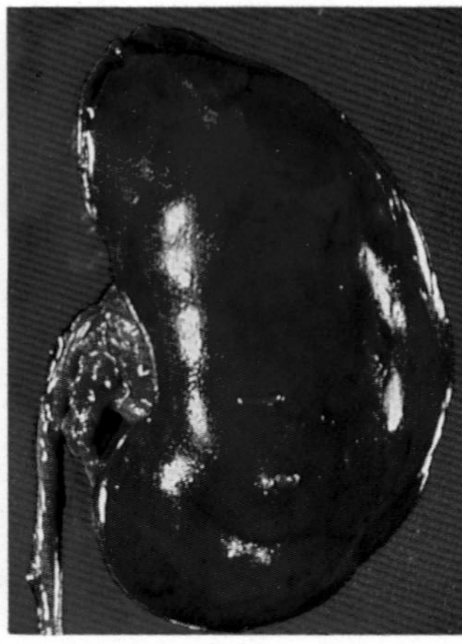

Fig. 13.8. Congested kidney.

F: polycystic kidney disease: 0.5% of autopsies; 90% are bilateral. *S:* ♂ = ♀. *A:* 40–60 years. *Pg:* the pathogenesis is still controversial. Possible mechanisms include tubular atresia, cystic dilatation as a result of focal saccular growth, persistence and cystic transformation of tubules, inhibition of dichotomous division of ureteric bud. *Co:* pyelonephritis, erythremia due to increased erythropoietin production. *Cl:* proteinuria, hypertension (60%), hematuria from ruptured cysts (30%), death in uremia.

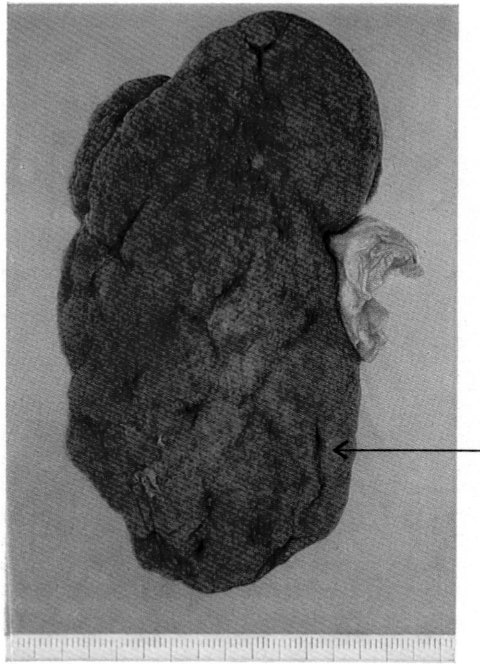

Fig. 13.9. Arteriosclerosis and arteriolosclerosis of the kidney.

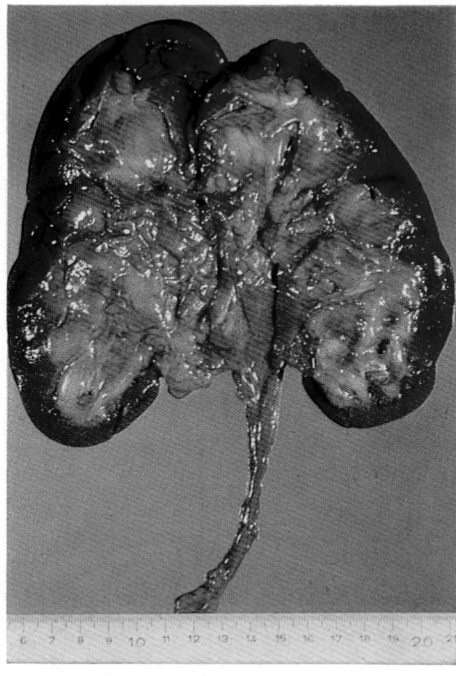

Fig. 13.10. Atrophy of the kidney with an increase in the amount of pelvic fat tissue.

Vascular Diseases of the Kidney

Vascular changes. Figure 13.7 shows a normal kidney of pale red color. The external surface is smooth and the kidney hilus contains a moderate amount of fat. The kidneys are medium-firm in consistency.

Figure 13.8 shows a kidney in acute congestion (e. g., from right cardiac insufficiency). The kidney is enlarged, dark red, moist and firm. The renal capsule is removed with ease in contrast to the normal kidney. The cut surface is dark red and the papillae are dusky red. *Mi:* Hyperemia of the capillaries and glomeruli.

In chronic congestion, the kidneys are blue-red, smaller and firmer than normal *(cyanotic induration). Mi:* glomeruli and vessels are hyperemic. The glomerular basement membranes become thicker than usual. The interstitial tissue is edematous. Protein casts and erythrocytes are found in the Bowman capsule. The tubules contain albuminous cylinders (albuminuria) and may even become atrophic.

The kidneys are pale in anemia (Fig. 13.6). The cortex is pink to pale red. The medulla is somewhat darker red. The external surface of the kidney in Figure 13.6 also shows remnants of fetal lobulations, which are always present at birth.

Arteriosclerosis and arteriolosclerosis (Figs. 13.9–13.11; TCP, p. 153. See also Figs. 13.30 and 13.61). *Kidney scars result from involvement of the renal vessels by arteriosclerosis and arteriolosclerosis. The glomeruli are hyalinized and the corresponding nephrons become atrophic.* The senile kidney is an example of minimal renal arteriosclerosis and arteriolosclerosis. The kidneys are somewhat smaller than normal and have a finely granular external surface. The cut surfaces indicate that some parenchyma has been lost and, as a consequence, the pelvic fat is more prominent than usual (Fig. 13.10). The senile kidney is part of the physiologic involution during old age (*Mi:* minimal arteriolosclerosis).

A more advanced arteriosclerosis and arteriolosclerosis is illustrated in Figure 13.9. The outer surface is uneven and finely granular from arteriosclerosis. The fine granularity is seen especially at the margins of this picture. The base of these superficial pits is dark red (dilated venules in scar tissue), whereas the granules are bright red (viable renal tissue with minimal compensatory hypertrophy) (see also Fig. 13.30, p. 260).

Figure 13.11 is a close-up of a kidney surface in arteriolosclerosis. The surface retractions are small and red, whereas the unaffected kidney tissue projects as red-gray granules. Arteriosclerotic scars are dark red and larger (2–3 mm.) and deeper than scars from arteriolosclerosis. Sclerotic vessels project from the cut surface as rigid pipes with narrow lumina ("pipestem sclerosis"). The renal capsule usually adheres to arteriosclerotic or arteriolosclerotic scars. Arteriosclerosis and arteriolosclerosis most often occur together, although separate involvement may be observed.

Renal arteriosclerosis may progress to arteriosclerotic nephrosclerosis (also known as benign nephrosclerosis). This type of nephrosclerosis always is preceded by hypertension (so-called red or genuine hypertension, see p. 25). Death from arteriosclerotic nephrosclerosis is attributable to the effects of hypertension (stroke or cardiac hypertrophy) rather than to uremia. Chronic lead poisoning also is manifested by severe renal arteriosclerosis, even in children.

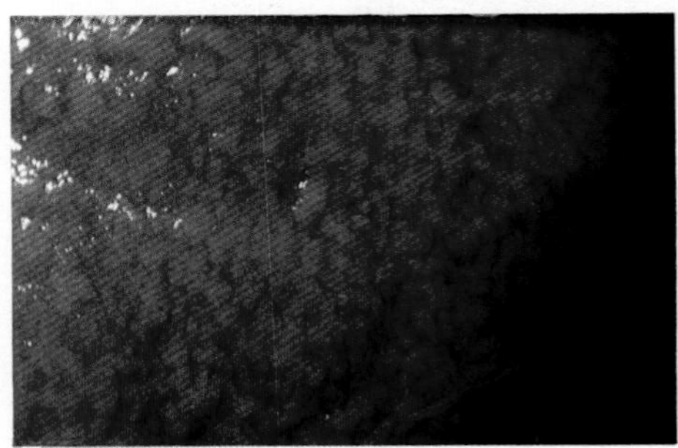

Fig. 13.11. Finely granular, arteriolosclerotic surface of the kidney.

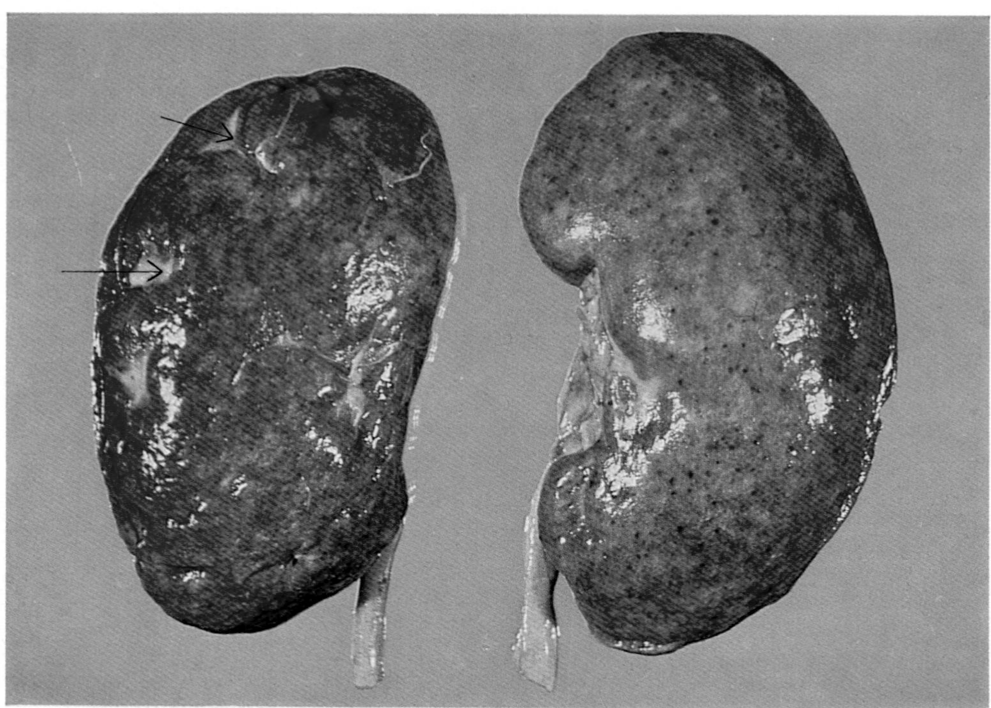

Fig. 13.12. Malignant nephrosclerosis (pinpoint petechial hemorrhages).

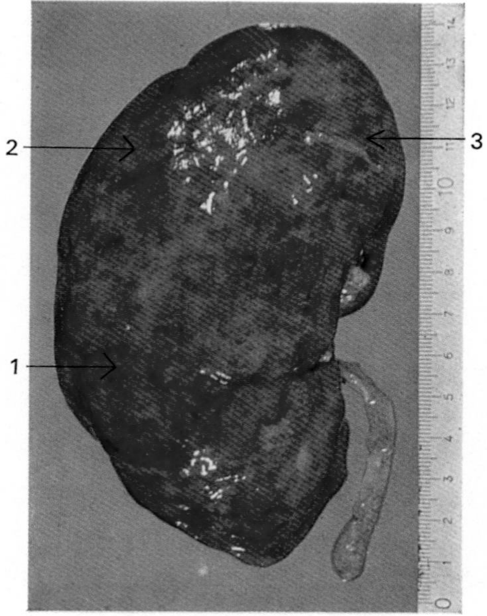

Fig. 13.13. Panarteritis nodosa of the kidney.

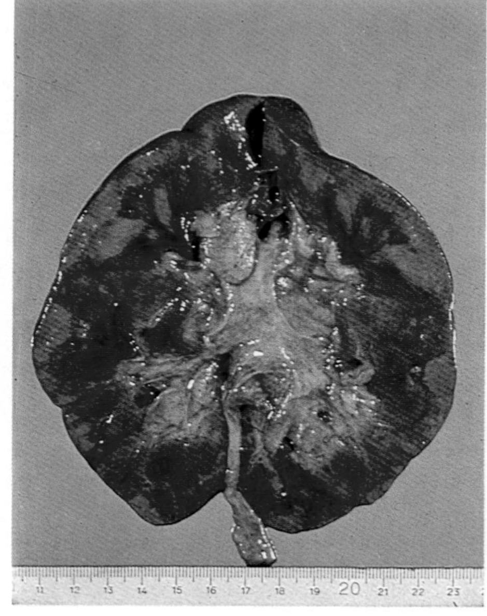

Fig. 13.14. Anemic kidney infarctions in panarteritis nodosa.

Malignant nephrosclerosis (Fig. 13.12; TCP, p. 155). *A rapidly progressive arteriolar nephropathy characterized by necrosis of arterioles and glomerular loops.* Malignant nephrosclerosis is "the malignant sister" of benign nephrosclerosis (ZOLLINGER) and causes severe hypertension.

Figure 13.12 is a typical example of malignant nephrosclerosis. The kidneys are enlarged and wet. The external surface contains *poorly delineated*, yellowish lesions, which usually do not project over the surface. These lesions correspond histologically to foci of anemia or necrosis of renal tissue. In addition, dark red punctate hemorrhages are scattered over the outer surface. The viable renal cortex is pale red. This mottled gross picture of yellow, pale red and dark red is described by the terms "speckled kidney" and "flea-bitten kidney." If malignant nephrosclerosis is superimposed on a pre-existing renal arteriolosclerosis, the kidney cortex is granular and contains the poorly delineated yellow flecks. The same yellowish flecks are seen on cut surface. Several old infarctions (→) are present in the left kidney in Figure 13.12.

F: 0.4% of all autopsies. *A:* the younger the patient (30–40 years) the more rapid the clinical course (2–3 years). Older patients (50–60 years) are prone to develop a malignant nephrosclerosis secondary to arteriolosclerosis. The clinical course then extends for 7–10 years. *S:* ♂:♀ = 3:1. *Mi:* Fibrinoid necroses of the walls of the vasa afferentia and the interlobar arteries and fibrinoid necroses of individual glomerular loops.

Pg: sudden exudation of plasma, fibrinogen and erythrocytes into the arteriolar walls and glomerular membranes → fibrinoid necrosis. It is *important* to remember that malignant nephrosclerosis is a *generalized* arteriolar disease. Arteriolar necrosis also involves the spleen (Fleckmilz), liver, adrenal glands, pancreas, heart, brain, gut, etc. There is some indication that malignant nephrosclerosis is an immune disorder. *Co:* cardiac hypertrophy, death in uremia (75%) or cerebrovascular accident.

Periarteritis (panarteritis) nodosa (Figs. 13.13 and 13.14; TCP, p. 65). *A recurrent, generalized inflammation of arterioles. Segmental involvement of the arteriolar walls leads to occlusion of arterioles and necrosis (infarctions) in multiple organs.*

The gross picture of the kidney varies with the age of the necrotic tissue. Figure 13.13 illustrates a relatively recent involvement of a kidney by periarteritis nodosa. Multiple anemic infarctions project irregularly over the renal surface (→1). The infarctions are demarcated by a hemorrhagic zone. Older infarctions are sunken and gray-yellow (→2). An accessory renal artery is indicated (→3).

On cut surface (Fig. 13.14), the cortical infarctions are seen clearly as triangular or partly rectangular, yellow lesions. Some infarctions extend into the medulla. Thickened arteriolar walls usually can be recognized on cut surface. Less severe cases of periarteritis nodosa are indistinguishable from the "speckled kidney" shown in Figure 13.12. The spleen, liver and myocardium also may contain small infarctions. Gray-white nodules may be seen around mesenteric or subepicardial arterioles as evidence of periarteritis nodosa. The nodules often are multiple and arranged like pearls on a string. They are due to adventitial involvement or small aneurysms.

F: 1%. *A:* 20–40 years with great variations. *S:* ♂:♀ = 4:1. *Pg:* sudden loss of the endothelial barrier and fibrinoid necrosis of arteriolar wall from an antigen-antibody reaction. Considered a hyperergic inflammation of arterioles because serum antibodies against vessel wall substances have been demonstrated. Experimental induction by application of foreign proteins. Secondary diseases after tonsillitis. The *clinical course* extends from 1 to 10 years, with fever, weight loss and death in uremia (80%). The clinical symptomatology may vary greatly (which is typical!).

Table 13.1. Organ involvement by periarteritis nodosa (according to pathologic studies)

Kidneys	80–100%	Pancreas	50%	Skin	30%
Heart	60–80%	Muscle	50%	Extremities	25%
Stomach, gut	50–70%	Central nervous system	40–50%	Adrenal glands	25%
Liver [1])	60%	Spleen	35%	Gallbladder	15–20%
Peripheral nervous system	60%	Testes	30%		

[1]) Especially affected are branches of the hepatic artery, less commonly the portal vein.

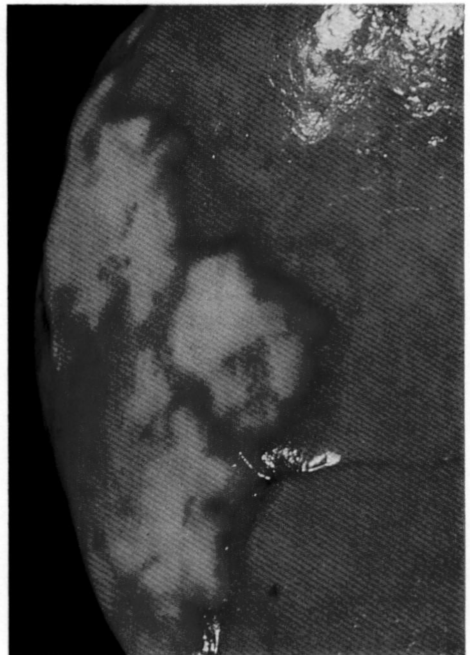

Fig. 13.15. Anemic infarction of the kidney with yellow hemorrhagic demarcation.

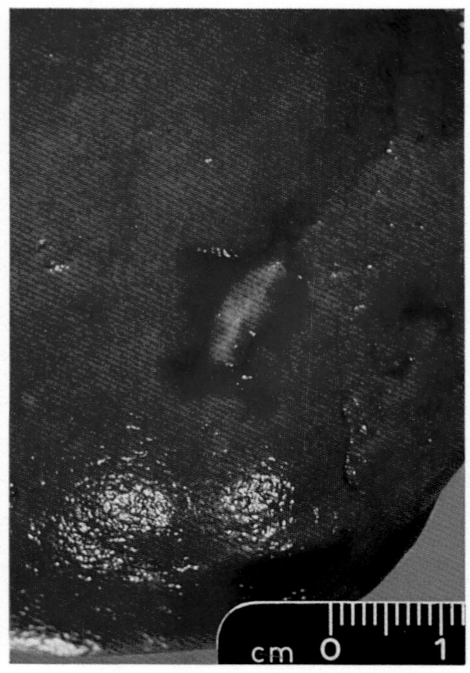

Fig. 13.16. Somewhat older, retracted infarction of the kidney with a white base.

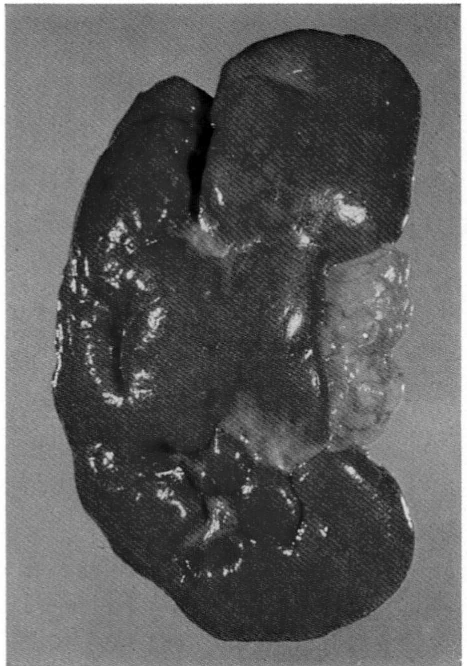

Fig. 13.17. Multiple infarction scars.

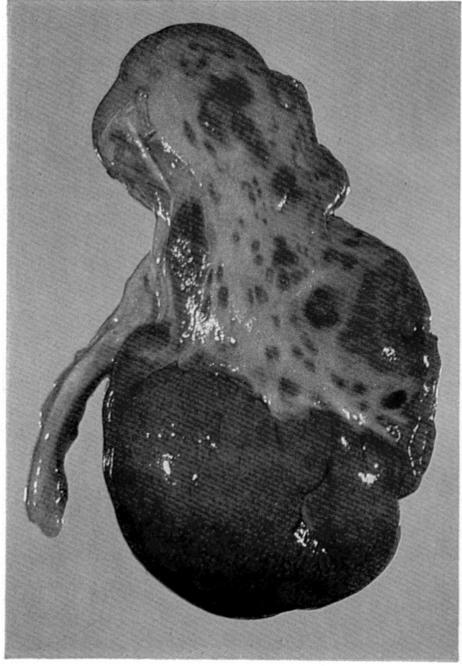

Fig. 13.18. Subtotal renal infarction.

Renal infarctions. *Areas of coagulation necrosis following sudden, complete, mostly embolic occlusion of renal artery branches. The size of the occluded artery determines the shape, position and size of a renal infarction.* Multiple renal infarctions occur in periarteritis nodosa (p. 253), shock (p. 259) and malignant nephrosclerosis (p. 253).

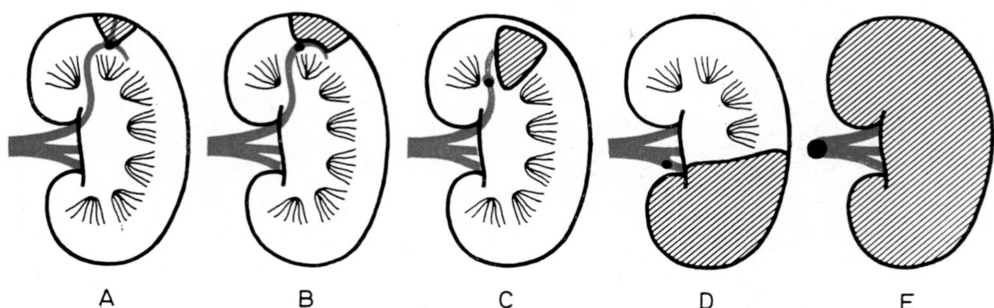

Fig. 13.19. Scheme of renal infarctions: A. *Triangular* cortical infarction (occlusion of an arteria radiata). B. *Rectangular* cortical infarction (occlusion of an arteria arcuata). C. *Triangular* corticomedullary infarction (occlusion of an arteria interlobularis). D. *Subtotal* renal infarction (occlusion of an extrarenal branch of the renal artery). E. *Total* renal infarction (sudden occlusion of the renal artery).

The gross appearance of a kidney infarction changes with time. A *fresh infarction* is slightly elevated over the outer surface, yellow and firm. The cut surface is dry, yellow and surrounded by a hemorrhagic zone. An *older infarction* (2–4 weeks after occlusion) is a depressed lesion with a yellow or gray-yellow base. An old, *organized infarction* is a deep, funnel-shaped retraction with a white base.

DD: an incomplete renal infarction from a slowly developing arterial occlusion presents as a red depression of the kidney cortex. When the main renal artery is occluded slowly, the kidney becomes small, finely granular and red (see p. 251). Old *pyelonephritic* scars are gray-white, broad indentations of the kidney surface. Fresh *pyelonephritic* scars are gray-red (see. p. 271).

Fresh anemic infarction (Fig. 13.15; TCP, p. 155). Areas of recent coagulation necrosis are yellow, sharply delineated and project slightly over the outer surface (uptake of water by necrotic tissue because of failure of sodium pump → entrance of sodium and water into cells). The fresh infarction is delineated from the normal kidney by a hemorrhagic (dark red) peripheral zone. Small hemorrhages may be seen in the infarcted tissue as well. The cut surface of a fresh infarction is similar in appearance (Fig. 13.14).

Older renal infarction. Figure 13.16 shows a deep retraction of the kidney surface with a white or gray-white base (scar). Sometimes, yellow, necrotic tissue is seen in the center of such an infarction. The more peripheral portions are deep red (granulation tissue). Multiple infarction scars in the kidney are white, firm, deep retractions, as shown in Figure 13.17. Their cut surface reveals a thin, white, firm rim of scar tissue.

Subtotal renal infarction (Fig. 13.18). An extrarenal branch of the renal artery was occluded in this case, leading to a subtotal renal infarction. Approximately two-thirds of the kidney is converted into white scar tissue. Note the whitish color of the scar tissue, which is focally reddish brown discolored (postmortem imbibition with hemoglobin). Islands of brown or red viable kidney are seen between bands of scar tissue. These islands were supplied by collateral circulation via capsular veins and did not become necrotic.

F: 4% of all autopsies. Twenty to thirty per cent of patients with myocardial infarction develop renal infarctions. *S:* ♀ > ♂. *Pg:* 90% of renal infarctions are from emboli. Common sources of emboli are mural thrombi from myocardial infarction (80%) and endocarditis (10%). In newborns, thrombosis of the ductus arteriosus is a frequent source of emboli. Arterial occlusion in small children often leads to hemorrhagic infarction of the kidney (a very broad hemorrhagic "marginal" zone of demarcation). Nephrosclerosis from emboli is extremely rare, in contrast to vascular nephrosclerosis.

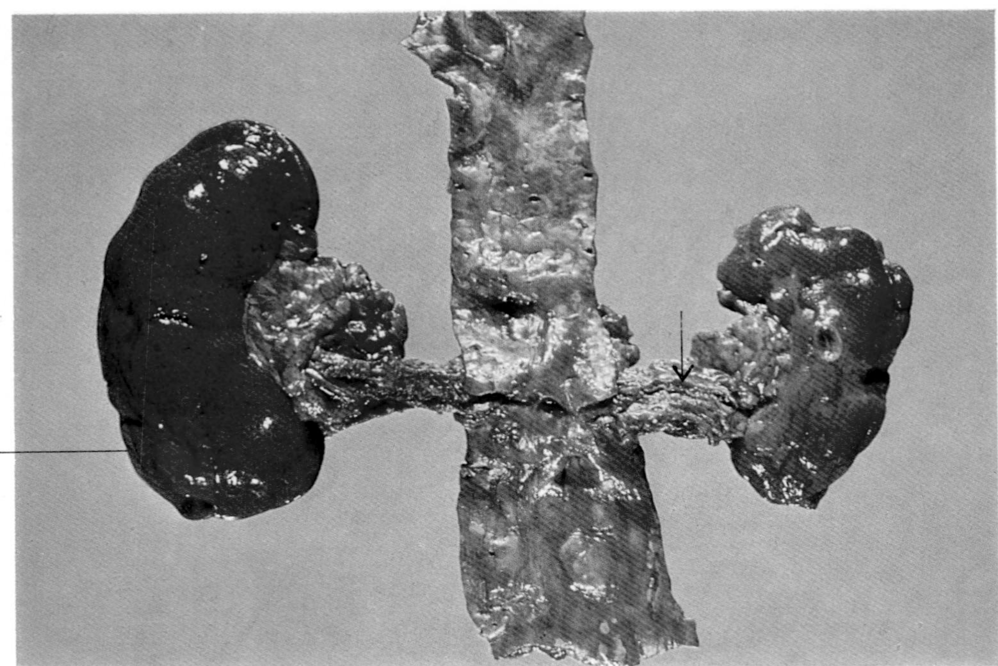

Fig. 13.20. Unilateral vascular nephrosclerosis.

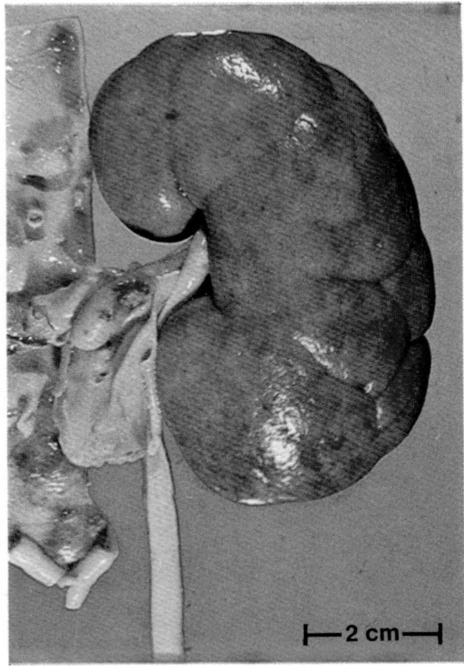

Fig. 13.21. Thrombosis of the renal vein.

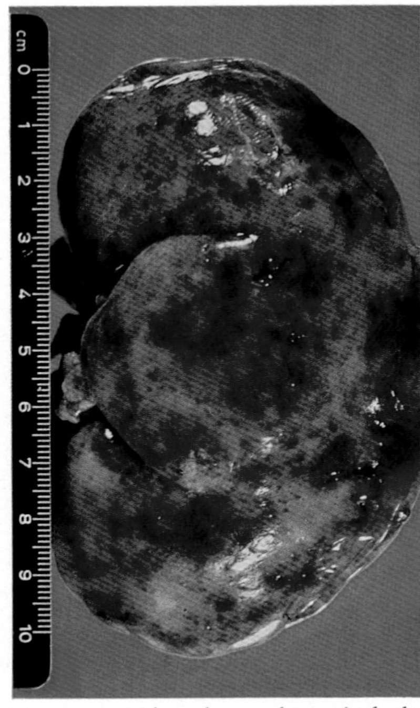

Fig. 13.22. Kidney hemorrhages in leukemia.

Unilateral vascular nephrosclerosis ("Goldblatt" kidney, Fig. 13.20). *Unilateral stenosis of the renal artery produces a gradual diminution of renal blood flow followed by nephrosclerosis (incomplete infarction) and renal hypertension (Goldblatt hypertension).*

Figure 13.20 shows the aorta and kidneys. Multiple atheromatous plaques are found in the aorta. The right kidney is much smaller than the left. There is minimal compensatory hypertrophy of the left kidney. The lumen of the entire right renal artery is markedly stenotic because of severe atherosclerosis. The arrow in Figure 13.20 points to a fibrous band that partially obstructs the arterial lumen (sclerosis and old thrombosis). Gradual arterial occlusion has resulted in an atrophic kidney (*Mi:* the glomeruli and vessels are relatively normal but the tubules are atrophic). In addition, several old infarctions are seen in the right kidney, and the lower pole of the left kidney contains a relatively fresh infarction (pale red discoloration).

F: 0.5% in autopsy material. *S:* ♂:♀ = 2:3. *Pg:* (1) narrowing of the ostium of the renal artery in cases of severe aortic atherosclerosis; (2) organized thrombosis of the renal artery. In juveniles, so-called fibromuscular dysplasia of the renal artery.

Experimental production: Hartwich and, later, Goldblatt produced unilateral or bilateral constriction of the renal artery by clamping or ligation. The result is hypertension, especially when the other kidney is removed and a salt-rich diet is given.

Therapy: Removal of the kidney after arteriographic demonstration of the stenotic artery.

The mechanism of renal hypertension can be explained as follows: Chronic obliteration of the renal vascular flow (glomerulonephritis, severe arteriosclerosis, pyelonephritis, malignant nephrosclerosis, arterial compression by tumors) enhances renin secretion from the juxtaglomerular apparatus. Tubular sodium concentration probably regulates renin secretion (Thurau) or causes change in the wall tension of the vasa afferentia. Every decrease in blood pressure in the vasa afferentia causes an increased renin secretion. Renin activates angiotensin → aldosterone (sodium retention) → hypertension. (See aldosteronism, p. 245.) Morphologically, an enlargement of the juxtaglomerular apparatus can be shown during any prolonged decrease in blood pressure.

Renal vein thrombosis with nephrotic syndrome (Fig. 13.21). A slowly progressive renal vein thrombosis in the adult interferes with glomerular permeability, which is manifested by the development of a nephrotic syndrome with proteinuria (p. 259). The histologic distinction between a nephrotic syndrome caused by renal vein thrombosis and subacute membranous glomerulonephritis may be difficult. Accordingly, some authors believe that the nephrotic syndrome is the result of a membranous glomerulonephritis whereas renal vein thrombosis is a secondary event. Figure 13.21 shows an old renal vein thrombosis. A yellow thrombus in the renal vein extends into the inferior vena cava. The kidney is enlarged and pale yellow. Renal vein thrombosis frequently is observed in cases of renal amyloidosis. Likewise, tumor thrombi in the inferior vena cava can propagate into the renal vein.

In children, renal vein thrombosis is encountered not infrequently in dehydrated patients (enteritis, infection). Hemorrhagic infarction (dark red, soft and enlarged kidneys) is diagnostic of renal vein thrombosis.

Kidney hemorrhages in leukemia. Figure 13.22 shows multiple petechial and larger, confluent hemorrhages throughout the external surface. The kidney is larger than normal and mottled gray-white from leukemic-cell infiltrates. This was a case of an undifferentiated leukemia. The bone marrow was replaced by leukemic cells, leading to thrombocytopenia and hemorrhages. The renal vessels often are infiltrated by leukemic cells that contribute to renal hemorrhages.

The kidneys in shock. *The lungs, kidneys and gut are the first target organs of shock. In addition to systemic arterial hypotension (not always present!), anuria is a reliable diagnostic sign of shock.* Morphologic manifestations of shock may be minimal in the kidneys (functional reduced blood supply to the kidneys). The kidneys usually are enlarged, soft and pale red. The cut surfaces are moist from interstitial edema. The tubules are dilated and tubular necrosis sometimes is evident histologically. Thrombi are not present. The macroscopic picture is similar to that of Figure 13.25 without the red and brown spots. Bilateral cortical necrosis and the so-called crush kidney (chromoproteinuric nephrosis) are typical findings in *severe shock*, especially *hemorrhagic shock* (exsanguination), *endotoxin shock* (abortion!) or *traumatic shock*.

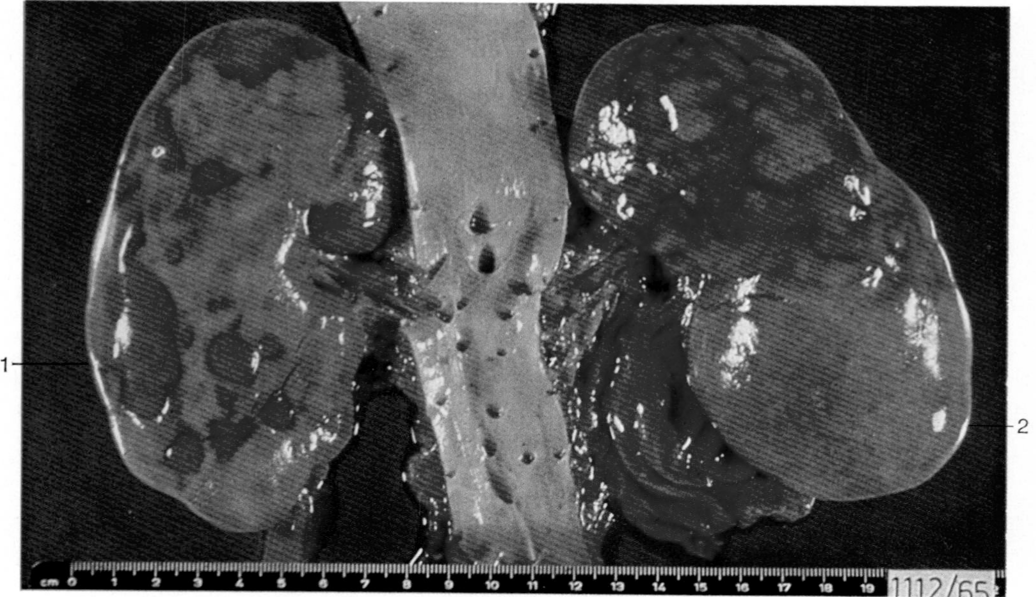

Fig. 13.23. Bilateral renal cortical necrosis in a patient with shock.

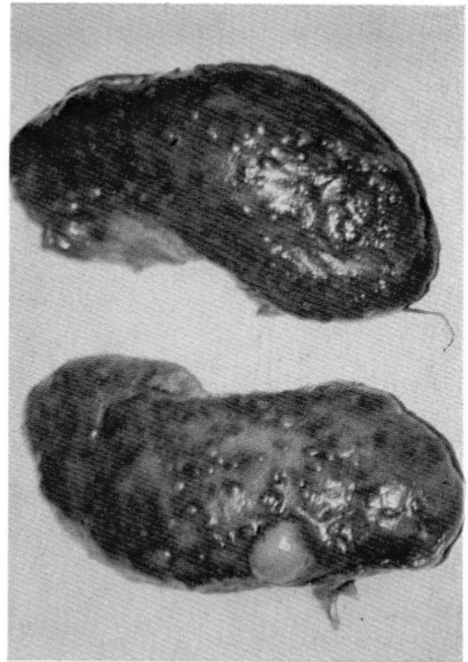

Fig. 13.24. Scars and regeneration of the kidneys following shock.

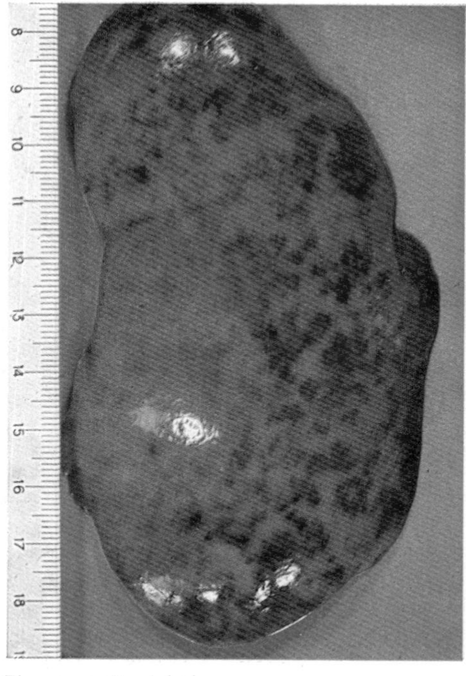

Fig. 13.25. Crush kidney.

If the initial phase of shock with kidney failure is survived, death may occur as a result of microthrombosis in the lungs (shock lung, see p. 81). A regeneration of tubular epithelia then takes place in the kidneys (clinically: polyuria).

Bilateral renal cortical necrosis from shock (Fig. 13.23). This case of hemorrhagic shock resulted from heavy blood loss. The patient was involved in an automobile accident and survived for 5 days. Almost the entire cortex of the left kidney is *necrotic* (map-like yellow areas) (Fig. 13.23). The remaining viable cortex is identified as reddish brown islands between areas of necrosis (→1). Only the upper half of the right kidney is necrotic, whereas the lower half is normal (→2). The cut surfaces of the kidneys showed extensive zones of cortical necrosis that corresponded to the yellow zones seen on the external surface. The medulla was not involved. Fibrin thrombi were found in almost all glomerular capillaries, arterioles and veins on microscopic examination. This finding explains the bilateral necrosis observed grossly.

Occasionally, a patient with bilateral renal cortical necrosis may survive for several months, especially when maintained on an artificial kidney. The kidneys of such a patient (a 20-year-old female with septic abortion) are shown in Figure 13.24. Extensive cortical scarring is evident as large, gray-white or pale brown indentations. Several white nodules are seen throughout, especially at the lower margin of Figure 13.24. They represent islands of regenerating kidney tissue. *Mi:* extensive fibrosis and regeneration of cortical parenchyma were found; only the juxtamedullary zone was intact.

Bilateral renal cortical necrosis can be induced *experimentally* in the rabbit (Fig. 13.26). Two intravenous injections of bacterial endotoxin were given within 24 hours to produce a generalized Shwartzman-Sanarelli phenomenon. The gross and histologic pictures are comparable to bilateral renal cortical necrosis in humans.

In traumatic shock, the kidneys are swollen, moist and have a dirty brown hue. Such shock kidneys are observed after extensive muscle damage, burns or chemical hemolysis (e.g., from snake venom or incompatible blood transfusions). Myoglobin or hemoglobin is released, which imparts a dirty brown hue to the kidney (Fig. 13.25, *crush kidney;* see TCP, p. 143).

Pathogenesis of shock

Shock is a manifestation of acute vascular collapse with or without loss of blood pressure. The vascular collapse is attributable to a microcirculatory failure. During the initial, *reversible phase* of shock, cardiac output and venous return to the heart are diminished. This, in turn, causes hemoconcentration and vasoconstriction (the so-called centralization of shock). Circulating platelets, various clotting factors and often fibrinogen are reduced during the early phases of shock as a result of *hypercoagulability* of the blood. Platelet aggregates and fibrin thrombi (so-called hyaline thrombi) form in the peripheral circulation (consumption coagulopathy: LASCH). Disseminated intravascular coagulation = DIC, see also AP.) Ischemia, tissue damage and necrosis are the morphologic signs of the *irreversible phase* of shock. Hemorrhages frequently accompany shock because of the consumption coagulopathy. Therapy is directed toward restoration of the blood volume and fibrinolysis (e.g., with streptokinase).

Hyaline or fibrin thrombi in the kidneys, liver, lung and pituitary gland cannot be demonstrated in all types of shock. The example of the crush kidney shows that very severe tissue damage, including necrosis, can occur even without fibrin thrombi.

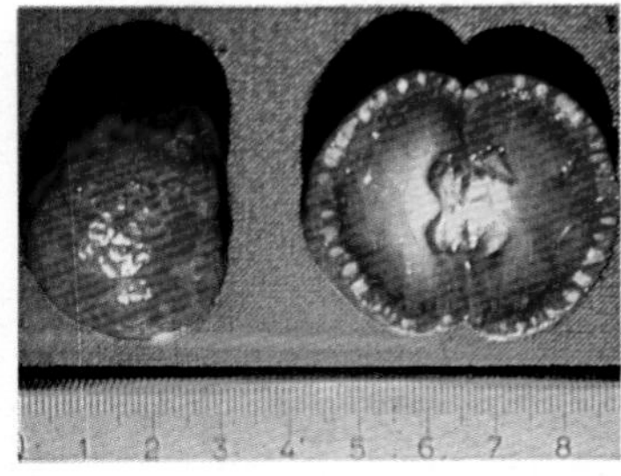

Fig. 13.26. Experimental renal cortical necrosis in the rabbit.

Noninflammatory kidney diseases (so-called nephroses)

Until recently, "degenerative" changes in the tubular system have been designated as nephroses and differentiated from inflammatory kidney diseases. This overall standpoint is no longer tenable. The following must be differentiated:

(a) Clinically: *Nephrotic syndrome:* Kidney diseases with proteinuria, hypoalbuminemia, hyperlipemia and generalized edema. Causes: Usually glomerulonephritis, amyloidosis, diabetic glomerulosclerosis, mercury and other poisonings.

(b) Pathological-anatomical: Noniflammatory kidney diseases which may or may not be accompanied by a nephrotic syndrome and in which the morbid changes are manifested in the glomerulus (glomerulonephrosis – better, glomerulopathies) or in the tubular system (tubular nephroses – better, tubulopathies).

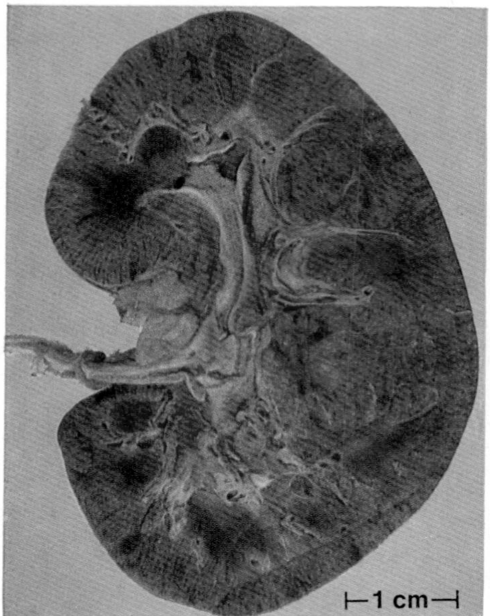

Fig. 13.27. Cholemic nephrosis.

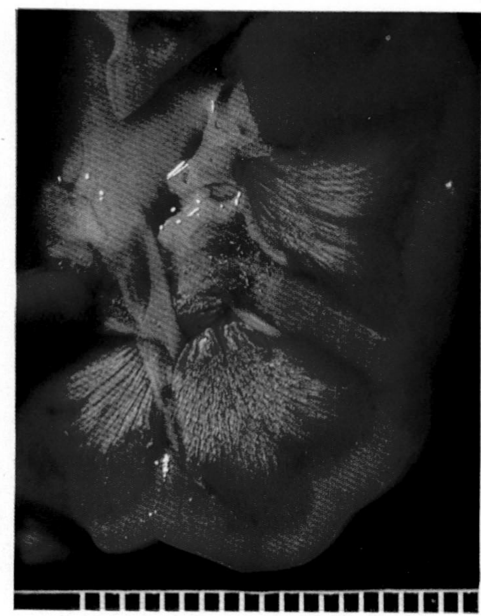

Fig. 13.28. Uric acid infarctions in the renal medulla.

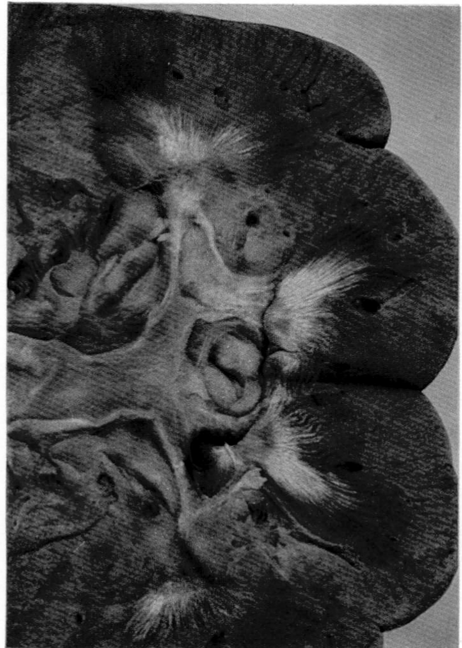

Fig. 13.29. Calcium infarctions in the renal medulla.

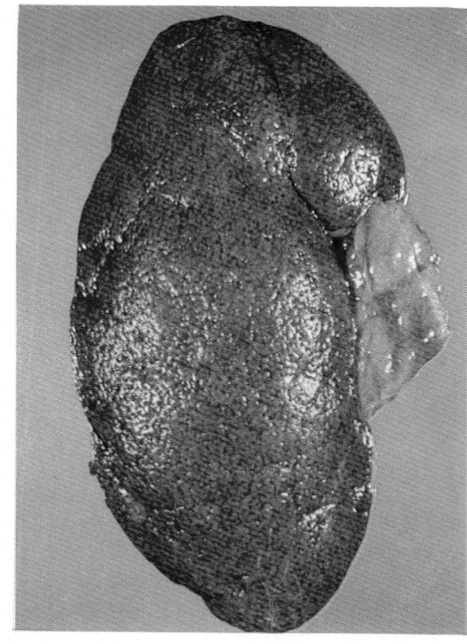

Fig. 13.30. Kimmelstiel-Wilson glomerulosclerosis.

1. Tubulopathies (tubular nephroses)

(a) **Acute tubulopathies** (acute exogenous nephrosis; TCP, pp. 143 and 145). An acute exogenous nephrosis is either due to ischemia (e.g., in patients with *shock*, burns trauma, crush kidneys, see p. 259) or attributable to the direct toxic action of poisons on the tubular system mercury chloride, sublimates, potassium chlorate, ethylene glycol, etc.). The tubular degenerative changes may progress to tubular necrosis. Grossly, the kidneys are moderately enlarged, wet, pale yellow or speckled yellow. *Clinically*, there is proteinuria or other signs of renal insufficiency but the complete nephrotic syndrome is missing.

(b) **Endogenous tubulopathies** (clinically without nephrotic syndrome). *Tubular degenerative changes result from the deposition (storage) of substances that normally are excreted.* Examples are:

Cloudy swelling is observed with certain toxic substances (see above) or renal ischemia. The kidneys are uniformly enlarged, soft and opaque (cloudy) on cut surface.

Hyaline droplet degeneration (TCP) is accompanied by severe proteinuria. Multiple causes, such as glomerulonephritis, amyloidosis or multiple myeloma (also considered a glomerular nephrosis because membrane thickening of glomeruli is present). The kidneys are enlarged, pale whitish and the tubules contain protein casts. The function of the tubules is hardly disturbed, therefore, this condition involves a secondary phenomenon in the nephrotic syndrome, indicating to us the glomerular permeability for blood proteins.

Fatty degeneration of the renal cortex with a yellow renal cortex (compare Fig. 13.38) occurs in cases of oxygen deficiency (e.g., anemia), intoxications or as a result of reabsorption of lipids in cases of severe proteinuria (lipid nephrosis).

Cholemic tubulopathy (Fig. 13.27). The kidneys are enlarged, edematous and greenish or greenish brown discolored. The discoloration is intensified in the medullary regions because of heavy bile pigmentation.

Hemosiderosis accompanies hemolysis, repeated transfusions or hemochromatosis (Prussian blue reaction of kidney slice!). The kidneys are brownish discolored and slightly enlarged.

Melanuric nephrosis. A black discolored kidney is observed in patients with metastatic melanoma.

Osmotic nephrosis is observed in patients given hypertonic solutions (sucrose). The kidneys are large and pale. *Mi:* the tubular epithelium is vacuolated. Similar changes are observed in potassium deficiency.

Hypokalemic tubulopathy. Found in cases of chronic diarrhea. *Mi:* vacuoles produced by a widening of the intercellular gaps between the tubular epithelia.

Deposition of urates: Figure 13.28 shows a so-called uric acid infarction with white to gold-yellow streaks radiating toward the tips of the papillae. (*Mi:* ammonium urate crystals in the collecting tubules.) Urate deposits are seen in newborns (decay of nucleated erythrocytes) and adults (rapid cell decay, e.g., treated leukemias). Sodium urate crystals are found in the epithelium and interstitial tissue in patients with *gout* (see p. 215). *Co:* pyelonephritis.

Calcium deposits occur secondarily following necrotizing processes (e.g., sublimate nephrosis) or metastatically in hypercalcemia (e.g., primary hyperparathyroidism, sarcoidosis, vitamin D overdose, bone metastases). Metastatic calcifications are the result of increased tubular calcium reabsorption. The gross picture is characterized by white streaks in the papillary tips (Fig. 13.29) and, on occasion, a whitish stippling of the cortex as well. Calcification of the tubular epithelium is found on microscopic examination.

Glomerular nephrosis (with nephrotic syndrome)

A primary membrane lesion of glomeruli leading to increased permeability for proteins. Glomerular nephrosis is due to either inflammatory diseases (intracapillary and membranous glomerulonephritis with secondary lipoid nephrosis) or functional membrane changes accompanying amyloidosis, renal vein thrombosis, eclampsia or Kimmelstiel-Wilson glomerulosclerosis (Fig. 13.30; TCP, p. 153). The kidneys are slightly enlarged and firm. The surface is finely granular. Renal arteriolosclerosis, which usually is present on microscopic examination, presents with a similar gross picture. However, in contrast to arteriolosclerosis, the kidneys of patients with glomerular nephrosis often are not red but vary between red and spotty yellow-red (Fig. 13.30). Kimmelstiel-Wilson glomerulosclerosis occurs in 20–30% of severe cases of diabetes mellitus. These patients usually are 60–70 years of age, with a history of diabetes of more than 10 years. *Cl:* hypertension, nephrotic syndrome, renal insufficiency.

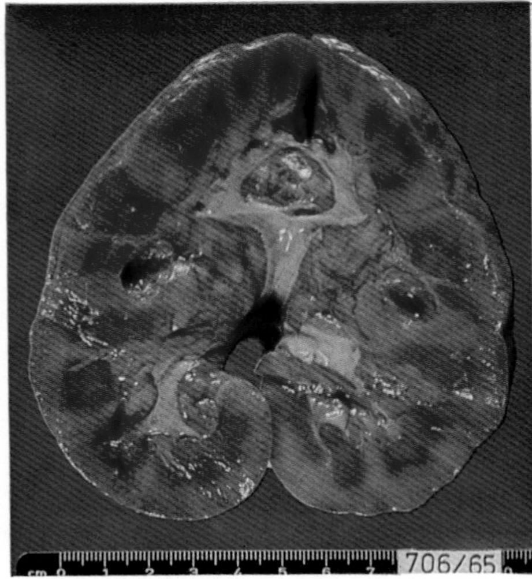

Fig. 13.31. Amyloid nephrosis.

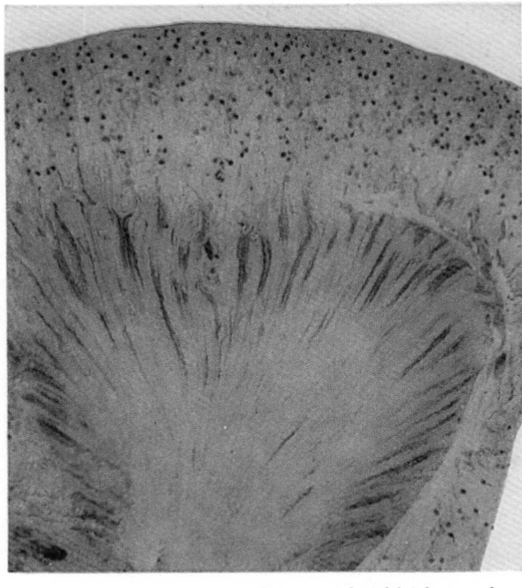

Fig. 13.32. Cut surface of an amyloid kidney after Lugol's reaction.

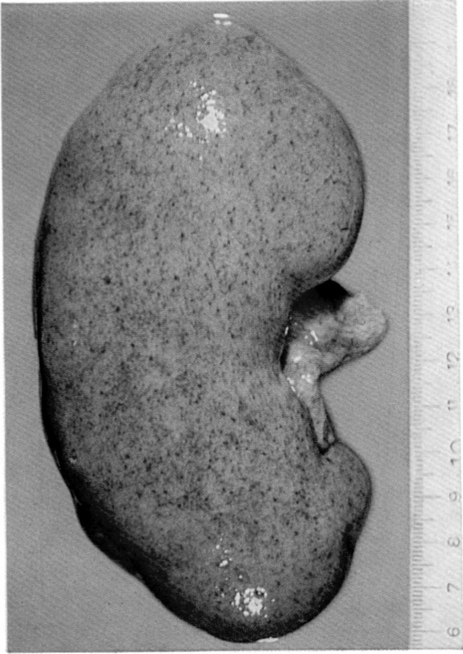

Fig. 13.33. Acute exudative (hemorrhagic) glomerulonephritis.

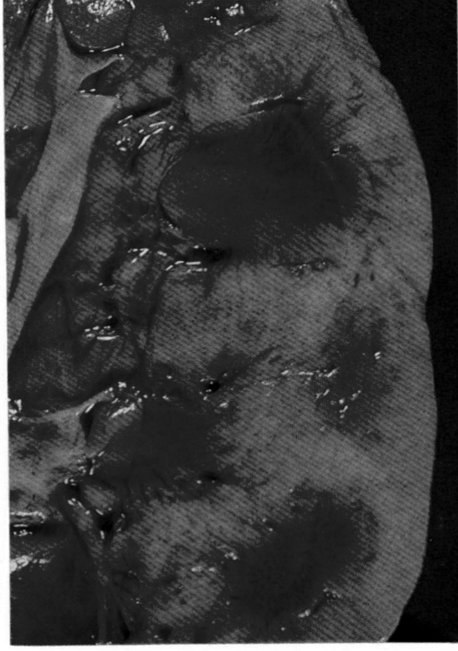

Fig. 13.34. Cut surface of a kidney in acute exudative glomerulonephritis.

Amyloidosis of the kidneys (amyloid "nephrosis," Figs. 13.31 and 13.32; TCP, p. 145). *Amyloid is deposited in the walls of the glomerular loops, arterioles and pericapillary spaces, leading to glomerular obliteration.* The classic gross picture is an enlarged, pale "white" kidney. The kidney in Figure 13.31 is pale red (almost whitish red), waxy and of wooden consistency. The cut surface is dry and transparent. The cortex is broader than usual and sharply delineated from the reddish medulla. The kidneys become small and irregularly nodular with longstanding amyloidosis. The enlarged, amyloid-containing glomeruli can be demonstrated as blue-black dots by applying Lugol's solution with subsequent H_2SO_4 treatment (Fig. 13.32). Streaks of amyloid deposits also are seen at the corticomedullary junction. *F, A, S* and *Pg:* see page 166.

Glomerulonephritis (GN)

Our knowledge of glomerulonephritis has been greatly expanded by the increasing number of kidney punctures, so that the entier area of nephritis research has been set in motion. The following table presents a survery of the present state of classification of GN, which is accepted by most authorities.

Table 17.2. Classification of glomerulonephritis (GN).

Designation	Morphology "Model"	Pathogenesis Immunology	Clinical Aspects
Exudative GN (acute exudative proliferative GN).	Granulocytes Exudation and slight mesangial and endothelial proliferation.	*Metainfective* (streptococcal infections, scarlet fever, angina). Also in serum disease. *Immune complex nephritis.* Subepithelial immune depots.	High antistreptolysin titer, RR +, albuminuria, hematuria. Frequently good prognosis, but may change to mesangial-proliferative GN.
Mesangial-proliferative GN) ("intracapillary" GN) acute → chronic.	Mesangial and endothelial proliferation.	*Metainfective* (streptococci) IgA and Ig6 *nephritis.* Immune complex nephritis. Subepithelial immune depots at the loop and/or in the mesangium.	Hematuria, proteinuria. Frequent form of GN. Steroid therapy +. Good prognosis. Occasional nephrotic course.
Intra-extracapillary proliferative GN ("extracapillary" GN) Rapid, progressive.	Proliferating parietal capsule layer "crescents". Endothelial and mesangial proliferation. Variant: necrotizing.	*Anti-basement-membrane nephritis,* e.g., in Goodpasture's syndrome. Immunoglobulins diffusely linear in the basement membrane.	*Poor prognosis.* Rapid, progressive, "subacute", RR ++.
Membranous GN (perimembranous GN)	Basement membrane greatly thickened, so-called spikes. No cell proliferation.	*Immune complex nephritis* (possibly autoantibody), subepithelial immune depots. Spikes, virus? (Aleutian minks).	*Nephrotic syndrome.* Steroid therapy + 30% healing, 50–70% persistence.
Membranoproliferative GN	Basement membrane thickened (double-contoured), mesangial proliferation.	*Hypocomplementemia,* predominantly subendothelial immune depots.	60% nephrotic syndrome. Steroid therapy +. Good healing tendency.
Minimal GN ("minimal changes")	Glomeruli normal under the optical microscope or only minimal mesangial proliferation.	?	"Genuine" lipoid nephrosis. Steroid therapy +. 60% healing.
Focal and/or segmental GN	Individual glomeruli affected and/or individual loop groups. Proliferating of sclerosing[1]).	Occurs within the scope of specific basic diseases: Schönlein-Henoch purpura, lupus erythematosus, Goodpasture's syndrome, or idiopathic.	Proliferating form: frequently favorable prognosis. Sclerosing form: frequently lipoid nephrosis.

[1]) Sclerosing = increase in the matrix of the mesangium.

According to W. Thoenes: Nieren- und Hochdruckkrankheiten **5**: (199 (1973); H. U. Zollinger: Beitr. Path. **143**: 335 (1971); P. Royer, R. Habib, H. Mathieu: Nephrologie im Kindesalter (Nephrology in Childhood). Thieme, Stuttgart 1967.

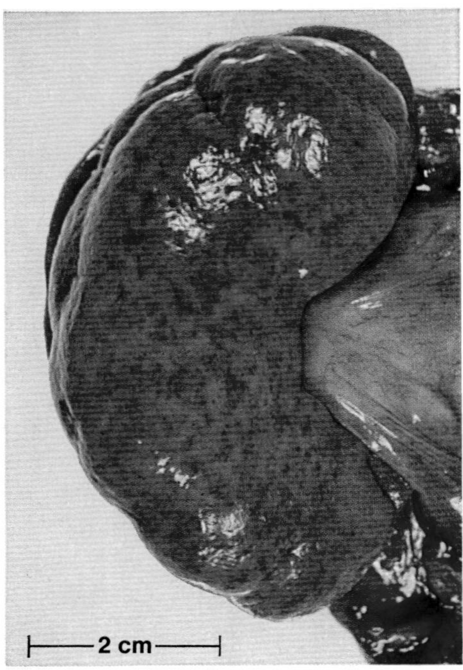

Fig. 13.35. Intra-extracapillary, proliferative glomerulonephritis.

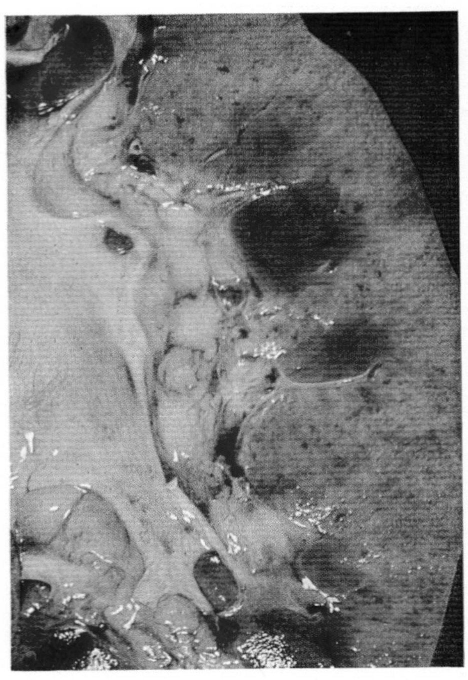

Fig. 13.36. Cut surface of a mesangial-proliferative glomerulonephritis.

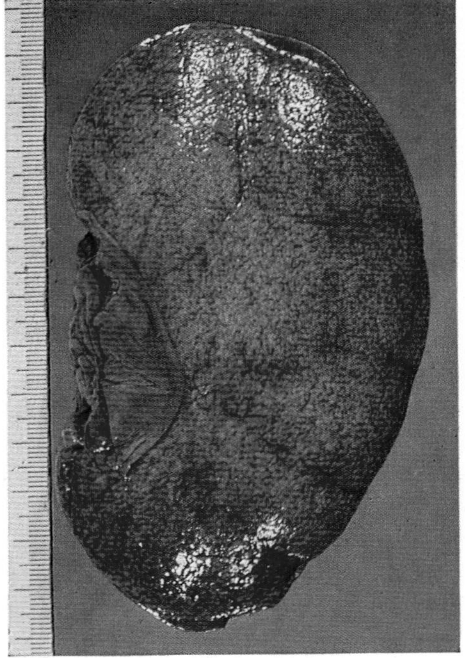

Fig. 13.37. Membranous glomerulonephritis.

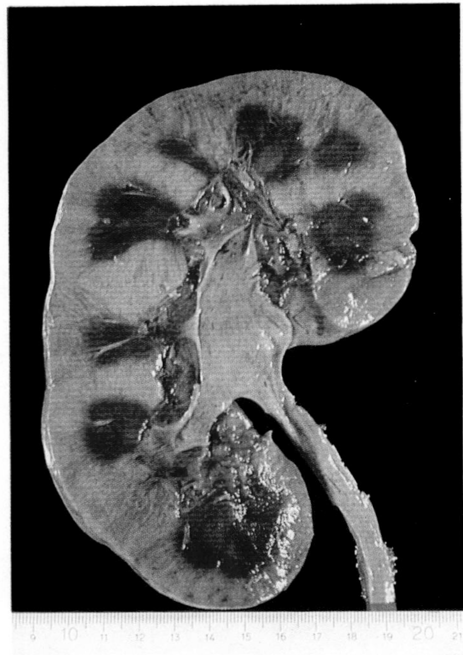

Fig. 13.38. Lipid nephrosis.

Glomerulonephritis

The classification of GN, as given in Table 17.2, is based solely on histological findings after kidney puncture. A coordination with the macroscopic picture is difficult, since, we generally see only the terminal stages of a GN in the autopsy room. Dialysis and kidney transplants have reduced the frequency of seeing earlier stages during autopsy.

Acute exudative GN (Fig. 13.33) is characterized by great enlargement of the organ. The kidneys are soft, full of fluid, and project from the capsule (relief was formerly provided by decapsulation) and are covered with flea-bite hemorrhages. The cut surface (Fig. 13.34) shows a broadened cortex, which has an edematous, yellowish appearance. At the same time, hyperemia with tiny hemorrhages is present.

DD: focal nephritis. Tiny hemorrhages, but less severe organ swelling. *Clinically:* metainfective. High antistreptolysin titer. Secondary disease after scarlet fever, angina. Immune complex nephritis. Generally favorable prognosis.

Intra-extracapillary proliferative GN (extracapillary GN according to the old nomenclature) (Fig. 13.35). This form of GN proceeds rapidly, progressively (subacute) and has a poor prognosis. The kidneys are generally enlarged, and the acute inflammatory processes cause hyperemia and small hemorrhages with diffuse yellowish spots (fatty tubular sections). Incipient cicatrizations of glomeruli can lead to fine retractions – granulation. Generally accompanied by hypertension.

Mesangial-proliferative GN (previously intracapillary GN) (Fig. 13.36). This form of GN appears acutely and may have a chronic course. Our illustration shows a subacute stage with a broadened, succulent cortex with tiny hemorrhages. As in the case of exudative GN, this involves a metainfective GN, caused by streptococci.

Membranous glomerulonephritis (Fig. 13.37). A subchronic stage with a finely granular kidney surface is shown in Figure 13.37. The kidney is hardly reduced in size and the bright yellow color of the cortex is striking. Clinically, a nephrotic syndrome is found.

Lipid nephrosis (Fig. 13.38). A magnificient golden-yellow renal cortex, which appears broadened and has a brownish marrow, is seen. The kidney surface is smooth. Histologically, lipid nephrosis can present different pictures: minimal GN, focal sclerosing GN or membranous GN. The yellow color is due to the lipids in the tubular epithelia and in the interstitium.

Chronic glomerulonephritis (Fig. 13.39). All forms of GN can enter a chronic stage, in which shrinkage of the kidney (down to 50 Gm.!) takes place with increasing hyalinization of the glomeruli. The hyalinization with obliteration of the loops by the mesangial matrix leads to a reduced blood supply to the glomeruli and thus also to the tubular system, so that this becomes atrophic. The corresponding parenchymal regions shrink and impose on the surface as retractions, whereupon intact glomeruli with compensatory hypertrophic parenchymal regions protrude as granules. If all glomeruli are in the same stage of obliteration, the result will be a shrunken kidney with a smooth surface. Figure 13–39 shows a severely shrunken kidney as compared with a normal kidney with individual cysts. Note the granular surface of the shrunken kidney, with the "granules" having a yellow appearance (fatty, compensatory hypertrophic nephrons), while the retractions between them are red (hyperemic scar tissue).

F: 1% in the autposy material. *S:* ♂:♀ = 2:1.

Causative factors:

1. *Anti-basal-membrane nephritis* (Masugi type).
Antibodies against kidney tissue (glycoproteins of the basement membrane).
Immunoglobulin diffusely linear in the basement membrane.
Antigen-antibody reaction at the basement membrane with complement activation.
Autoaggression in humans.

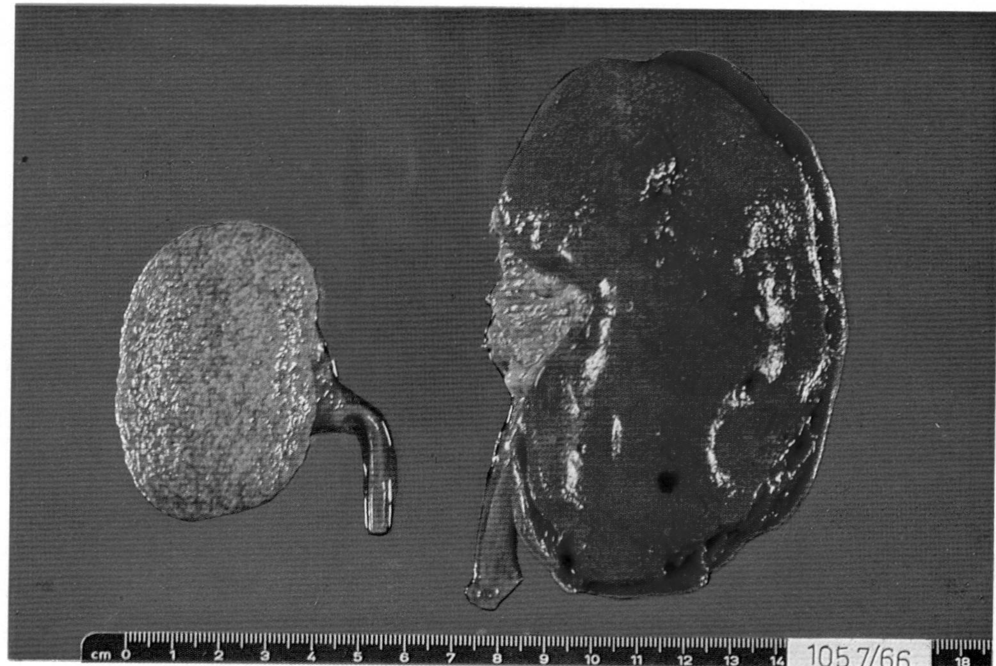

Fig. 13.39. Chronic glomerulonephritis (finely granular nephrosclerosis). A kidney of normal size for this age is shown at the right.

2. *Immune complex nephritis* (serum disease).
Antigen is a foreign protein – for slight excess of antigen.
Antigen-antibody complexes adhere to the basement membrane → complement activation
Antigen in humans consists of streptococcal components. Lupus erythematosus.
Viruses in animals. The granular immune depots are usually subepithelial.

Consequence: death from uremia (Fig. 13.40).

Uremia

The clinical syndrome of uremia results from the retention of substances that normally are excreted by the kidney. Uremia is the end stage of all progressive renal diseases. The diagnosis of uremia can be made at autopsy by the following pathologic organ changes (Fig. 13.40):

1. **Gastrointestinal tract.** *Uremic, catarrhal gastroduodenitis* (Fig. 5.23) and *pseudomembranous enterocolitis* (Fig. 5.78). These changes probably are caused by the direct action of NH_3 (from urea by urease). *Fibrinous pharyngitis.*

2. **Lung.** *Uremic pulmonary edema or pneumonitis* (Fig. 4.41). The edema is firm and rich in fibrin. Uremic edema is lysed and reabsorbed with difficulty. In addition, small parenchymal pulmonary hemorrhages are observed (see also Goodpasture syndrome). *Uremic odor* resembles the smell of NH_3.

3. **Heart.** *Fibrinous pericarditis (bread-and-butter pericarditis,* Fig. 2.66) and degenerative myocardial lesions, sometimes referred to as *myocardiosis.*

4. **Brain.** "*Firm*" *cerebral edema* (see also p. 309). Hypertensive encephalopathy from renal diseases (e.g., acute glomerulonephritis) can occur in "pseudo-uremia" without azotemia. Cerebral edema increases intracranial pressure.

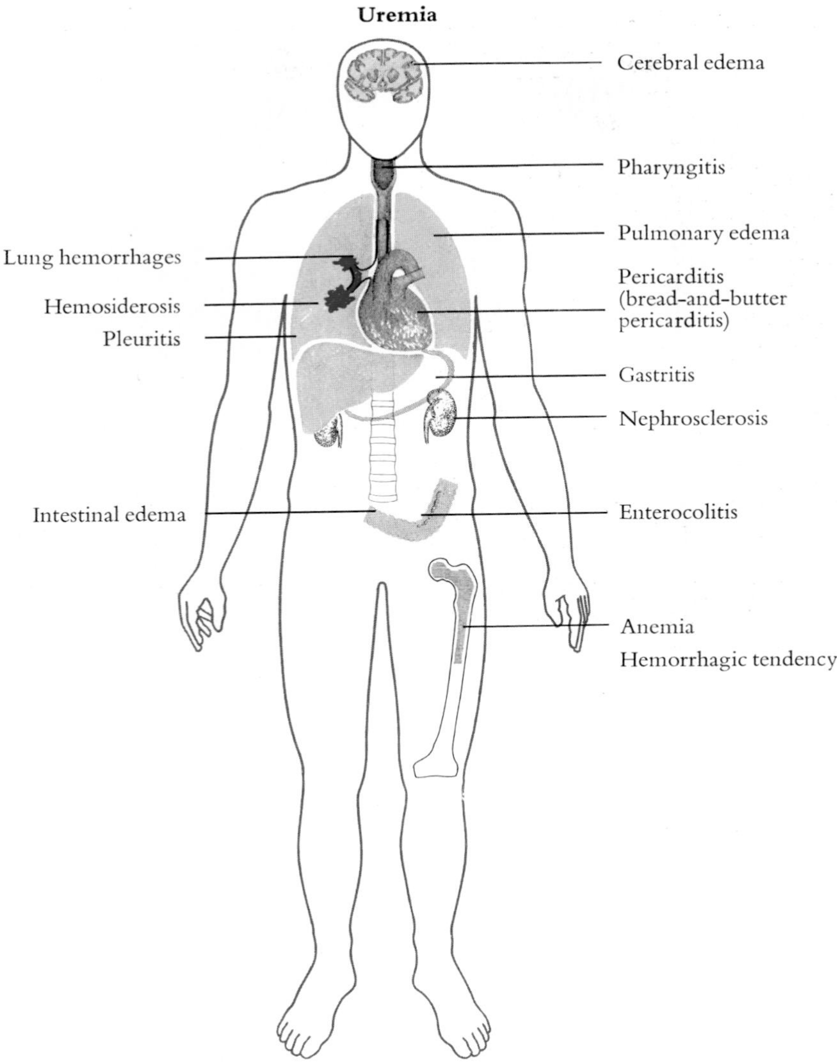

Fig. 13.40. Schematic presentation of uremia.

5. **Hemorrhagic diathesis.** Focal hemorrhages in the skin, gastrointestinal tract, renal pelvis and lung are due partly to capillary damage or abnormal clotting mechanisms.

6. **Anemia.** Probably caused by decreased erythropoietin formation.

7. **Blood of the cadaver.** Azotemia (NPN over 40 mg./100 ml., creatinine over 1.5 mg./100 ml.) still can be diagnosed from cadaver blood.

8. **Skin.** *Uremic frost* (urea crystals from sweat).

Pg: the "*poison*" of uremia still is not known; probably contained in NPN, but it is not urea. Other sources are aromatic amines (phenols). Causes of uremia: acute or chronic renal insufficiency (glomerulonephritis, pyelonephritis, renal infarctions). Extensive tissue destruction and necrosis can result in an *extrarenal uremia.*

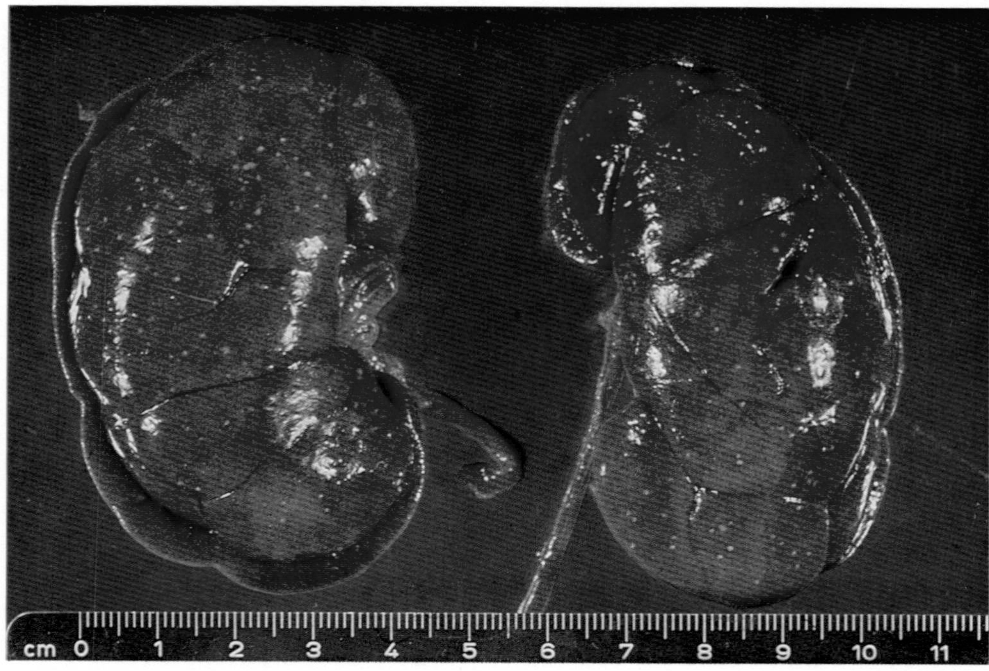

Fig. 13.41. Pyemic (embolic)abscesses of the kidneys.

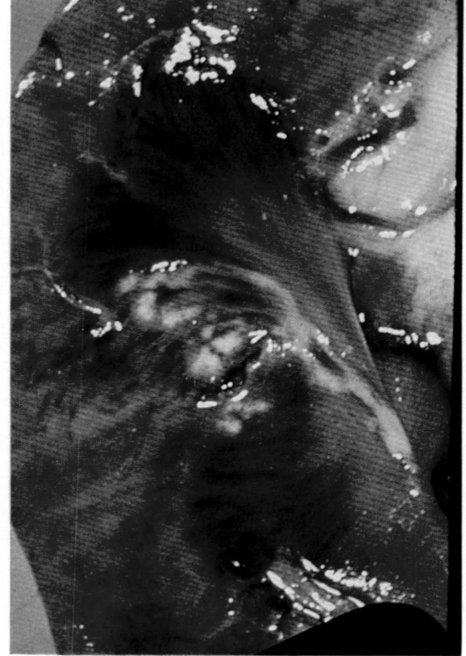

Fig. 13.42. Abscesses in the medulla of the kidney.

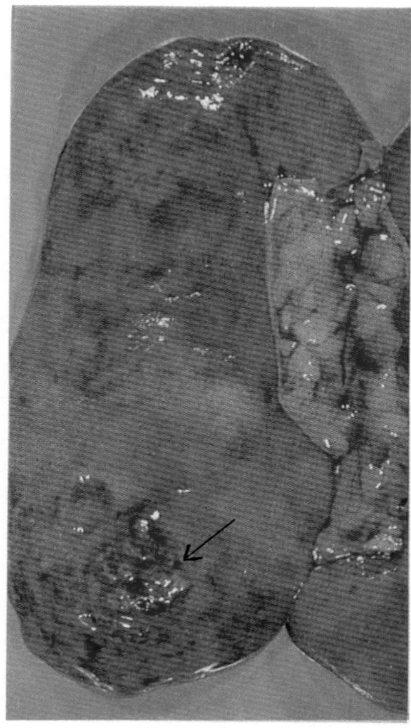

Fig. 13.43. Abscessive pyelonephritis.

Focal Glomerulonephritis

Focal glomerulonephritis implies that some glomeruli are diseased whereas others are normal. Focal glomerulonephritis affects patients *during* an infection, such as acute bacterial endocarditis (so-called Löhlein's nephritis), scarlet fever and other streptococcal infections. Also occurs in Schönlein-Henoch's purpura, lupus erythematosus, Goodpasture's syndrome and Wegener's granulomatosis. The kidneys are slightly enlarged and contain punctate hemorrhages, giving rise to the flea-bitten appearance.

Pyemic or embolic abscesses of the kidneys (Fig. 13.41; TCP p. 163). *Hematogenous, purulent focal nephritis with abscess formation in patients with sepsis or pyemia.* Figure 13.41 shows yellow, punctate (0.5–1 mm.) lesions scattered throughout the external surface of the kidneys. (*DD:* pyelonephritic abscesses are arranged in groups, as shown in Fig. 13.43.) The yellow foci are surrounded by a dark red rim and contain soft, necrotic tissue on cutting. (*Mi:* purulent, abscessive inflammation of glomeruli with bacteria in glomerular capillaries.) Superficial abscesses are torn open when the capsule is removed. Sometimes, larger single or interlinked abscesses are observed in staphylococcal sepsis (renal carbuncle).

Co: extension of the abscess to the renal capsules and fat → perinephric or paranephric abscess.

Excretion of bacteria through the glomeruli or lodging of bacterial emboli in medullary capillaries may produce yellow, streaky lesions, as shown in Figure 13.42. These converge from the cortico-medullary junctions toward the papillary tips. Central softening was noted in the medullary abscesses illustrated in Figure 13.42.

Pyelonephritis

(Figs. 13.43, 13.44 and 13.46; TCP, p. 167)

A very common, recurrent renal disease that is encountered in 10% of all autopsies. The gross findings consist of groups of renal abscesses or broad, flat kidney scars; 75% of all cases are not diagnosed clinically.

Acute pyelonephritis. Characteristically, the abscesses occur in clusters. Figure 13.43 shows a group of yellow, slightly elevated abscesses in the cortex (→). This finding is diagnostic of abscessive pyelonephritis. A somewhat more extensive involvement is illustrated in Figure 13.44, left. Multiple, densely set, yellowish white abscesses are scattered over the external surface. The cut surface (Fig. 13.44, right) reveals a gray-yellowish discoloration of individual pyramids and their corresponding cortical zones. Some lobuli are involved by abscessive pyelonephritis, others are spared. This involvement of individual renal lobuli on cut surface corresponds to the clustered abscesses seen on the external surface.

Chronic pyelonephritis results in broad, flat and irregular scars after the groups of abscesses are organized and have healed.

Figure 13.44 is an example of chronic pyelonephritis. The kidneys are markedly reduced in size (atrophy or nephrosclerosis). Flat, gray-white scars (→1) are identified on the external surface of the left kidney. The residual viable kidney tissue projects as small nodules over the external surface (→2). *Fresh* pyelonephritic scars usually are red. The cut surface (Fig. 13.44) reveals a narrow, irregularly pitted cortex. The pits correspond to cortical scars between normal parenchyma. Papillary necrosis (see p. 273), minimal hydronephrosis and hydro-ureter also are evident in this specimen from a patient with benign prostatic hyperplasia.

F: 10% of autopsy material. *S:* at an early age, predominantly ♀, later in life, predominantly ♂.

Pg: 1. *Ascending pyelonephritis* is caused by conditions that obstruct or impede urinary flow (prostatic hyperplasia or carcinoma, paralysis of the urinary bladder, neurogenic bladder, strictures, stones or diverticula). An ascending pyelonephritis occurs at an *early age* in females with a short urethra. In both instances, bacteria reach the kidney via the ureter or lymphogenously.

2. *Descending pyelonephritis:* Bacteria migrate through the mucosa of the urogenital system, enter the blood stream and produce hematogenous renal abscesses that are confined to individual lobuli (ADLER). *Proteus* and *E. coli* are the most common causative agents. *Cl:* hypertension in 40%, uremia in 30% of the

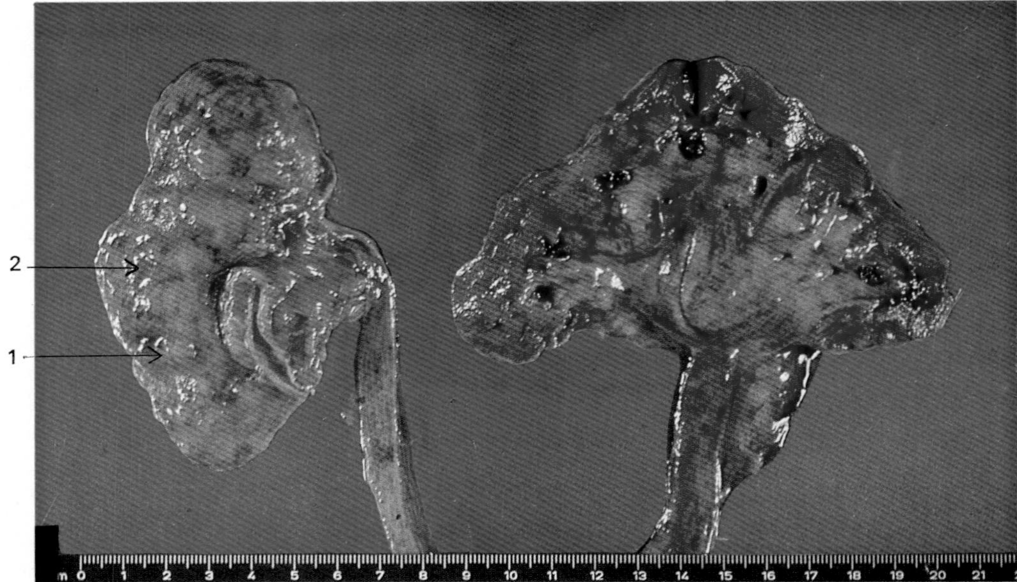

Fig. 13.44. Pyelonephritic nephrosclerosis with necrosis of the papillary tips and hydronephrosis.

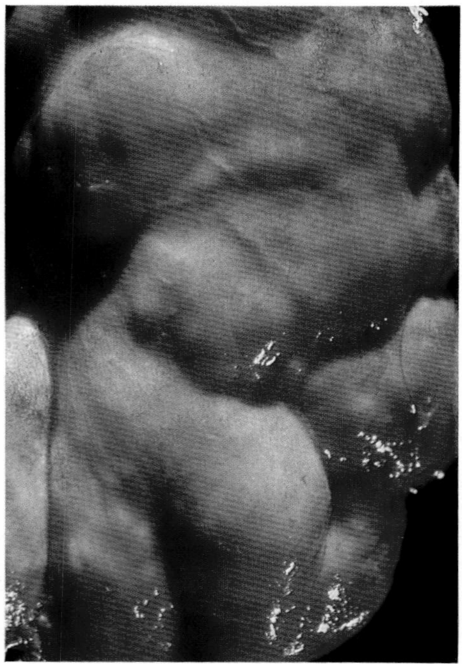

Fig. 13.45. Chronic interstitial nephritis.

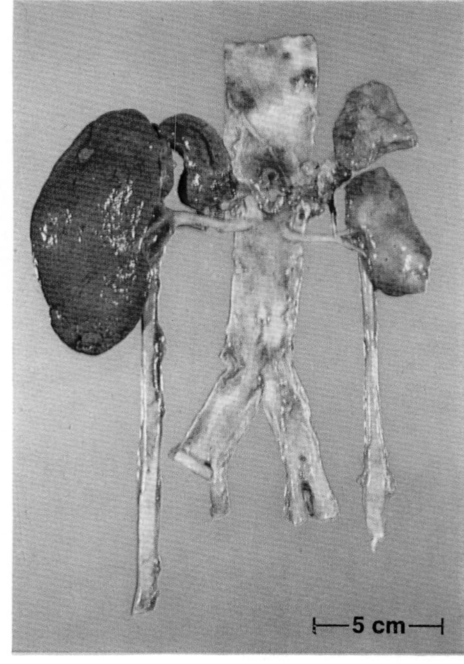

Fig. 13.46. Pyelonephritic atrophy (dwarf kidney).

cases. Pyuria, bacteria, hematuria and slight albuminuria. *Co:* Paranephritic abscess. Pyonephrosis = accumulation of pus in the renal pelvis. Pyonephroses also occur in cases of occlusion by stones, stenosis of the ureter and other diseases. In such cases, there is usually a secondary pyelonephritis. *Mi:* in the acute stage, streaky, interstitial infiltrates of granulocytes. In the chronic stage, granulomatous lympho-plasmacytic infiltrates with partial or complete atrophy of the tubuli and hyalinization of the glomeruli.

When an acute pyelonephritis is acquired during childhood, a severe pyelonephritic renal atrophy may be observed ("dwarf kidney"). Such a case is presented in Figure 13.46. Note the severe unilateral nephrosclerosis and compensatory hypertrophy of the other kidney. The small kidney si white, firm and has an irregular external surface. However, *both renal arteries are well developed and of normal width*, which excludes arterial nephrosclerosis as the cause of the unilateral renal atrophy. (See p. 257, Goldblatt kidney.) The adrenal glands near the upper kidney poles are shown for comparison with the "dwarfed" kidney.

Mi: the tubules are atrophic and contain protein casts (thyroidization). *S* and *A:* mostly females, 12–30 years of age. *Cl:* hypertension.

DD of pyelonephritic renal atrophy: (a) Congenital hypoplasia of the kidneys: the arteries also are hypoplastic (i.e., narrow); (b) Goldblatt kidney: the ostium of the renal artery is stenotic or the lumen is severely narrowed. In contrast, the renal arteries in pyelonephritic atrophy are of normal width.

Interstitial Nephritis

All kidney inflammations that do not affect the glomeruli take place in the interstitium. In this respect, pyelonephritis is also an interstitial nephritis. Of the forms of interstitial nephritis in the narrower sense, the following are differentiated:

Acute interstitial nephritis (Mi)

Acute interstitial concomitant nephritis, appearing during acute kidney failure during shock. An interstitial edema is found and, after the third day, plasmacytoid infiltrates at the cortico-medullary boundary. Clinically, a polyuria is present.

Acute interstitial nephritis, in which lympho-plasmacytoid infiltrates appear diffusely in the renal cortex. Observe on the seventh day of scarlet fever; also occurs in virus infections. *Macroscopic description:* large, grey-yellow, opaque kidneys.

Chronic interstitial nephritis (Fig. 13.45; TCP, p. 167). The characteristic gross finding is a coarse irregularity of the external surface. The gnarled surface appearance is due to flat and deep retractions representing areas of sclerosis or scarring. The viable parenchyma is "elevated" over the surface. The consistency of the kidney is firm and the color is gray-red. On cut surface, the cortex is irregularly retracted. Papillary necrosis is a common finding in chronic interstitial nephritis (see below).

F: 0.4%. *A:* 50–60 years. *Pg:* chronic interstitial nephritis and medullary (papillary) necrosis are sequelae of chronic abuse of analgesic drugs, especially phenacetin (phenacetin nephropathy). Excessive amounts of phenacetin when administered to animals do not produce the human disease. Unidentified toxic or bacterial factors probably are required to induce the disease. *Cl:* hypertension, acidosis followed by renal osteopathy, anemia and proteinuria.

Anuria

The interstitial forms of nephritis can lead to acute anuria. In cases of **anuria,** the following causes are possible by differential diagnosis:

1. **Prerenal:** *dehydration* during vomiting, diarrhea, heat stroke, salt deficiency syndrome after the administration of diuretics and *shock*.

2. **Renal:** *poisoning* (mercury, chloroform, carbon monoxide, etc.). *Glonerulonephritis. Interstitial nephritis. Pyelonephritis. Sepsis*, or septic shock. *Hepatitis, cholangitis* = hepatorenal syndrome. *Renal-artery embolism.*

3. **Postrenal:** bilateral *stone occlusion* or bilateral compression (tumors). *Adenoma of the prostate. Urethral stricture.*

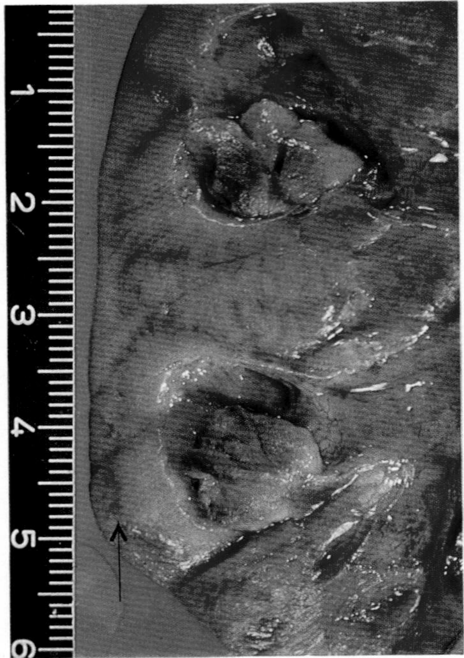

Fig. 13.47. Papillary necrosis and chronic interstitial nephritis from phenacetin abuse.

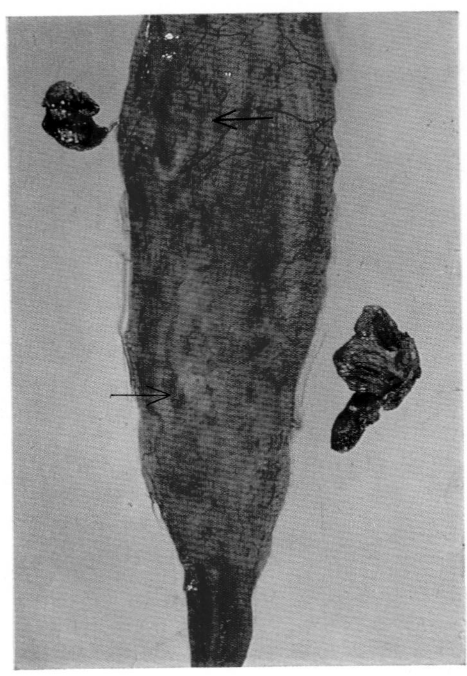

Fig. 13.48. Sequestered renal papillae in a dilated ureter (hydro-ureter).

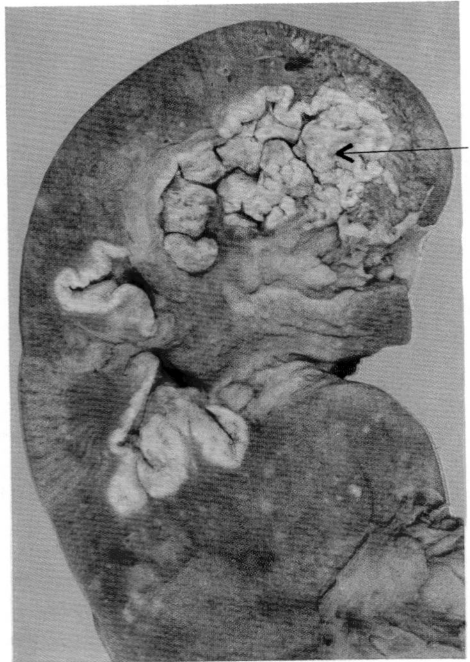

Fig. 13.49. Renal tuberculosis.

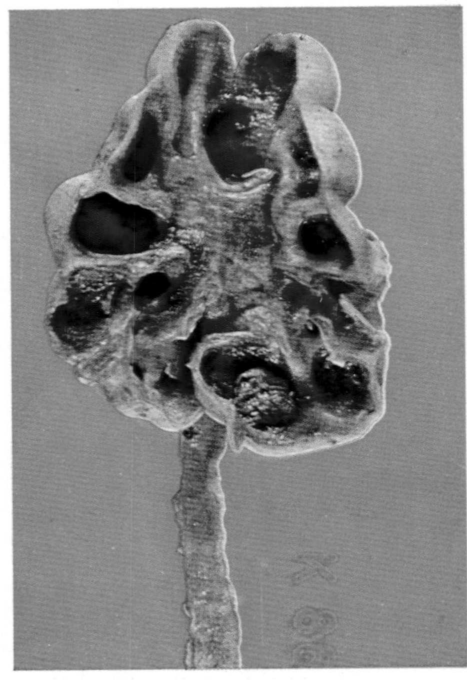

Fig. 13.50. Hydronephrosis in a case of urolithiasis.

Papillary Necrosis, Tuberculosis, Hydronephrosis

Papillary necrosis with chronic interstitial nephritis (phenacetin nephropathy; Fig. 13.47). Papillary necrosis, also known as necrotizing papillitis, may involve multiple or single pyramids or only parts thereof (tips of papillae). Our picture shows two necrotic, sequestered papillae of gray-yellow (fatty changes, necrosis) and focally black (sulfhemoglobin) color. The arrow points to the junction of cortex and medulla to demonstrate severe cortical atrophy.

Sequestered papillae may be excreted in the urine and be accompanied by colicky pain. The pain is explained by the finding illustrated in Figure 13.48. Two necrotic papillae were lodged in the ureter at points indicated by the arrows. The sequesters were removed and are shown adjacent to their original positions. The proximal ureter is dilated (hydro-ureter) and the mucosa is hyperemic. Figures 13.47 and 13.48 are from the same patient, who suffered from necrotizing papillitis and chronic interstitial nephritis following chronic phenacetin abuse.

F: necrotizing papillitis occurs commonly in patients with chronic interstitial nephritis (80%), pyelonephritis (see Fig. 13.44) and diabetes mellitus. Children with renal vein thrombosis also are prone to develop necrotizing papillitis. *Pg:* compression of vascular flow in vasa recta spuria by edema, inflammatory infiltrates and interstitial sclerosing processes.

Renal tuberculosis (Fig. 13.49). *Usually unilateral renal disease that develops after hematogenous spread of tubercle bacilli. Renal tuberculosis may manifest as late as 15–20 years after the primary complex.* Morphologic types of renal tuberculosis:

(a) Miliary tubercles are found in the cortex in 40% of all cases of *miliary tuberculosis.* Individual miliary tubercles are encountered less commonly in the kidney as a result of pulmonary tuberculosis, without otherwise generalized hematogenous spread.

(b) Single tuberculous cavities or *conglomerated tubercles* sometimes are observed in the cortex but usually they do not involve the renal pelvis.

(c) So-called *caseous* kidney: a kidney with multiple caseous lesions that may calcify.

(d) The medulla is the most common site of renal tuberculosis. Papillary tuberculosis, especially at the tips, leads to the formation of cavities. The process usually spreads to the cortex and renal pelvis **(open renal tuberculosis.)** Figure 13.49 shows a large cavity in the medulla (→). It is filled with yellow-white caseous material and communicates freely with the renal pelvis. Note the thin, folded cavity wall. Three smaller cavities also are present, in addition to miliary or somewhat larger tubercles in the cortex. Upon further progress, the tuberculosis can extend over the whole medulla and cortex and the renal pelvis, so that the kidney becomes caseous (thickened caseum = tuberculous caseous pyonephrosis). In the case of incorporation of calcium salts, one speaks of *mortar kidney*. If the tuberculosis does not penetrate into the renal pelvis, the process may be arrested by connective tissue encapsulation *(closed renal tuberculosis).*

F: 0.1%. *A:* 30–40 years. *S:* ♂ = ♀. *Co:* tuberculous pyelitis, cystitis, prostatitis or epididymitis.

Hydronephrosis (Fig. 13.50). *Retention of urine in the lower urinary tract with dilatation of the renal pelvis and calices. The kidney eventually becomes atrophic.*

The renal pelvis and calices are mildly dilated during *acute obstruction* of urinary flow. The tubules are distended and lined by a flat epithelium (eventually, tubulorrhexis).

Longstanding obstruction has different effects (Fig. 13.50). Increasing pressure atrophy involves the papillae and extends to the cortex, whereas the columns of Bertini often are unaffected. As shown in Figure 13.50, the saccular distention of the calices can even be recognized by examination of the external surface.

The kidney ultimately is transformed into a smooth bag (saccular kidney). The "capsule" is small and fibrous (severe cortical atrophy). The bag may contain 4–8 L. of fluid, which can be aspirated.

F: 4%. *S:* ♂ = ♀. *Pg:* mechanical obstruction → increased pressure in the renal pelvis above 25 mm. Hg or 10 ml. (normal capacity). Obstruction is caused by phimosis, strictures of the urethra, congenital folds in the urinary bladder, tumors of the prostate gland (see Fig. 13.53) or urinary bladder (trabeculation of urinary bladder and hydro-ureter), papillomas of the ureter (see Fig. 13.55), stones, scars, stenosis, congenital horseshoe kidney (kinking of the ureter), carcinoma of the uterine cervix (infiltration of the ureters) or a sharply angled exit of the ureter from the renal pelvis. *Co:* bilateral hydronephrosis (from low obstruction) causes uremia and pyonephrosis (secondary infection of hydronephrosis), rarely hypertension.

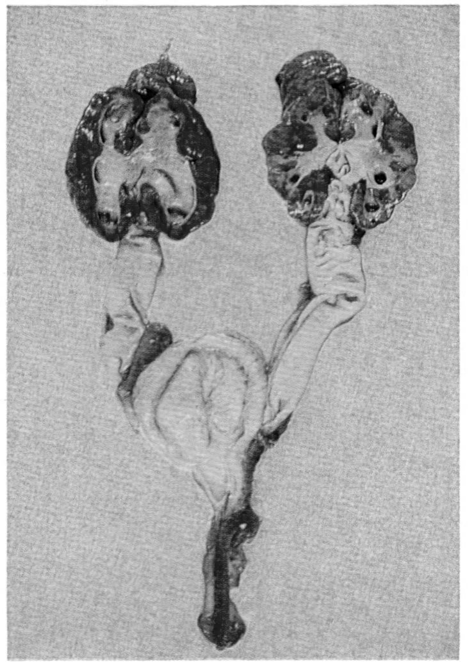

Fig. 13.51. Hydronephrosis and hydro-ureter secondary to a congenital urethral valve.

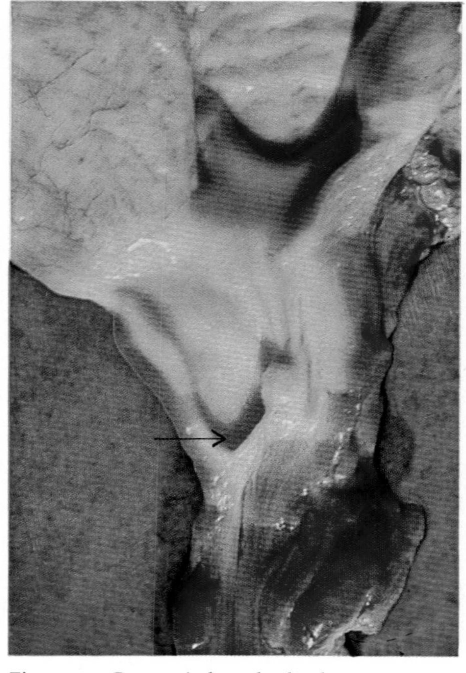

Fig. 13.52. Congenital urethral valve.

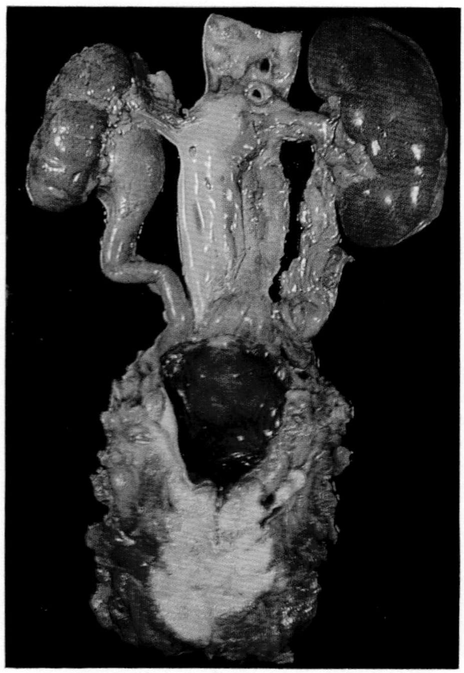

Fig. 13.53. Unilateral hydro-ureter from infiltration by a prostatic carcinoma.

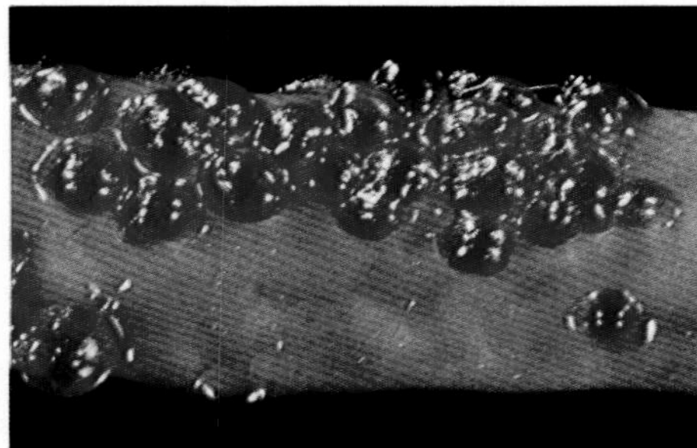

Fig. 13.54. Ureteritis cystica.

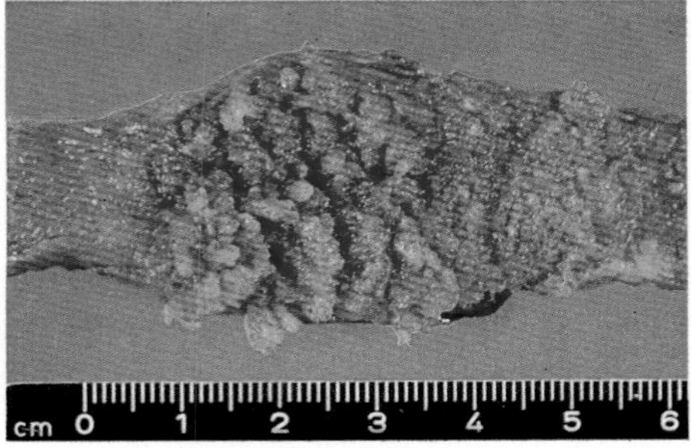

Fig. 13.55. Papilloma of the ureter.

Diseases of the Urinary Tract

Hydronephrosis and hydro-ureter with congenital urethral valve (Figs. 13.51 and 13.52). Figure 13.51 shows the kidneys with markedly dilated pelves and ureters. The urinary bladder likewise is distended and its wall is markedly hypertrophied. These findings, together with dilatation of the urethra, point to a stenosis in the lower urinary tract. Figure 13.52 is a higher magnification of the urethra. The arrow points to the level of the colliculus seminalis. When viewed from above, a transverse mucosal fold forms a pocket that also can be probed from below. Its functional effect is partial obstruction of the urinary flow (valve effect).

F: a rare congenital urethral malformation. *DD:* congenital hydronephrosis and hydro-ureters are caused more often by hypertrophy of the colliculus seminalis or by a cyst. *Co:* retention of urine → hydro-ureter → hydronephrosis → secondary inflammation and uremia.

Other malformations of the urinary system. (1) *Double renal pelvis* and *double ureter*. (2) *Hypospadia:* the urethral meatus is located at the undersurface of the penis or at the anterior wall of the vagina. (3) *Epispadia:* the urethral meatus is located at the dorsal surface of the penis or clitoris. (4) *Vesiculo-umbilical fistula:* a fistula develops between the umbilicus and the bladder from a persistence of the urachus. Incomplete obliteration of the urachus results in the formation of urachal fistula: the urachus does not obliterate and a fistulous tract connects the umbilicus and the urinary bladder. A urachal cyst may develop from incomplete obliteration of the urachus. (5) *Exstrophy or ectopia* of the urinary bladder is a congenital malformation. The pubic bones and rectus muscles are widely separated and the anterior bladder wall fails to develop. (6) *Ectopia vesicae* is associated with epispadias and other genital malformations.

Unilateral hydro-ureter from occlusion of the ureteral ostium by a prostatic carcinoma. Figure 13.53 shows a severe pyelonephritic atrophy of the right kidney (left side of the picture) together with a greatly dilated, tortuous ureter. The trigonum of the bladder and surrounding pelvic tissues are infiltrated by a yellow-white, firm tissue. The bladder mucosa is hyperemic (catarrhal cystitis). The obstruction of the ureter ostium was caused by a prostatic carcinoma.

F: unilateral or bilateral hydro-ureter is not uncommon in adults. *Pg:* multiple diseases cause partial or complete obstruction of urinary flow in the *urethra* (strictures from gonorrhea), *prostate* (benign prostatic hyperplasia: 40% cause hydronephrosis, carcinoma), *urinary bladder* (inflammations, diverticula, tumors) or *ureters* (stones; rarely tumors). Compression or infiltration of the ureters from ovarian or uterine tumors (cervical carcinoma, fibroids, pregnancy) and *neuromuscular disturbances* without mechanical obstruction (achalasia of the bladder sphincter) have similar effects.

Ureteritis cystica (Fig. 13.54) presents grossly as multiple, densely set cysts in the ureter, urinary bladder and/or renal pelvis (therefore: polyureteritis cystica). The cysts are lined by a flat epithelium and contain clear fluid. They are derived from the so-called epithelial cell nests of Brunn, which become cystically dilated.

F: single epithelial cell nests of Brunn are not uncommon in the urinary bladder (approximately 1.4% of all autopsies). A severe ureteral involvement, as shown in Figure 13.54, is relatively rare. *Pg:* pyeloureteritis cystica is the outcome of repeated nonspecific inflammations.

Papilloma of the ureter. Figure 13.55 shows a plaque-like, exophytically growing tumor that encircles the ureter. The tumor has fronds of soft, friable tissue. *Histologically*, a papilloma of transitional epithelium.

F: an isolated papilloma is rare. Papillomas usually arise multicentrically in the urinary bladder, ureter or renal pelvis. *Histology* and *Pg:* see page 283, carcinoma of the urinary bladder. *Co:* despite their relatively "benign" histologic structure, papillomas tend to recur after excision and become invasive with time.

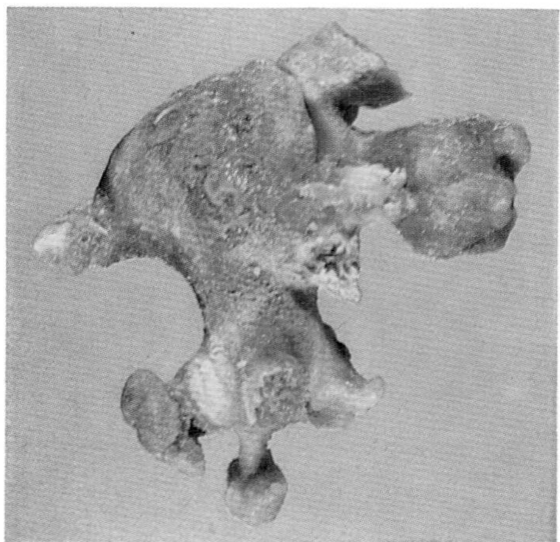

Fig. 13.56. Staghorn calculus in the renal pelvis composed of calcium phosphate.

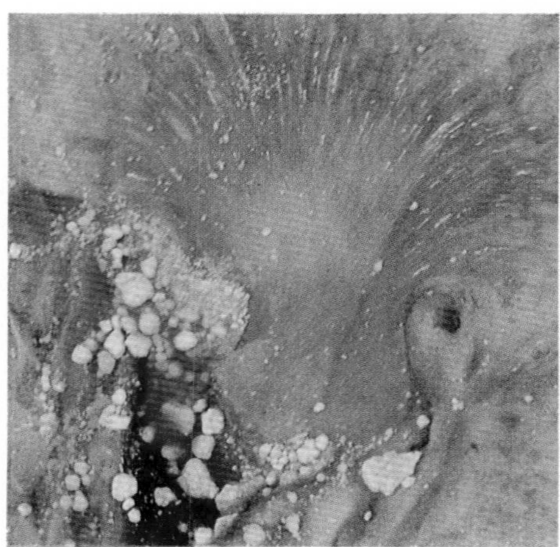

Fig. 13.57. Ammonium urate stones in leukemia.

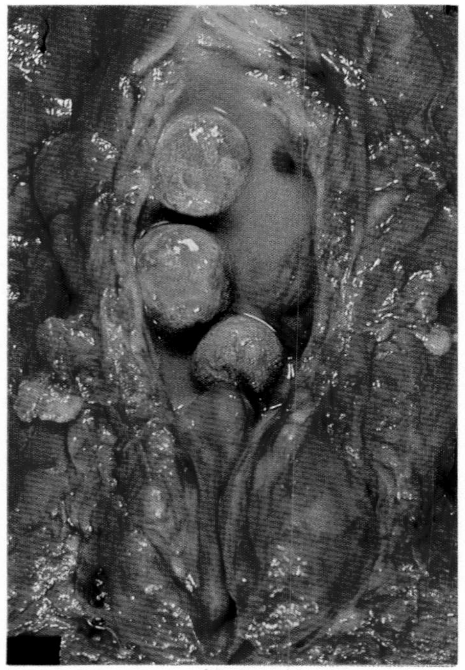

Fig. 13.58. Calcium urate stones in the urinary bladder.

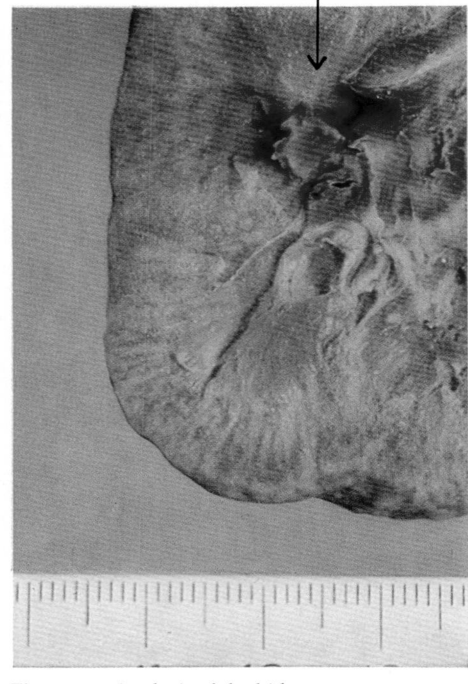

Fig. 13.59. Oxalosis of the kidney.

Urolithiasis

Calculi form by precipitation of urine in the renal pelvis, ureter or urinary bladder. These stones differ in chemical composition and appearance as follows.

Urate stones consist of Na, Mg or NH_4 urate. They are round, smooth, white (calcium) or yellowish, sometimes granular (Fig. 13.60). Uric acid stones are the most common type of urinary tract calculi. They are precipitated at an acid pH of the urine, especially in gout or leukemia.

Ammonium urate stones in leukemia. Figure 13.57 shows multiple, finely granular, yellowish calculi (up to 0.5 cm. in diameter) and granular, yellowish gravel in the renal pelvis. Note also the yellowish medullary streaks and the cortical stippling (intratubular formation of urate crystals). The urinary bladder in this case contains large (up to 1 cm. in diameter), round, smooth, whitish calcium urate stones (Fig. 13.58). Their cut surface is concentrically layered, resembling the rings of a tree (yellow-brown = predominantly urate; white = calcium) (Fig. 13.60). A slimy, cloudy residual urine was present in the urinary bladder. There also is evidence of benign prostatic hyperplasia, with formation of a prominent middle lobe.

Phosphate stones consist of Ca, NH_4 or Mg phosphates and form in an *alkaline urine*, especially after inflammations. They are whitish, brittle and chalky. Phosphate stones often surround older oxalate or urate stones like a shell. Figure 13.56 shows a large calcium phosphate stone from the renal pelvis, a so-called staghorn calculus. Its shape resembles the antler of a deer because it has formed in dilated calices. The renal pelvis in this case was slightly dilated also.

Oxalate stones consist of calcium oxalate (calcium oxalate monohydrate and calcium oxalate dihydrate) and are small, hard, mulberry-like, granular and dark brown. They form at an acid pH of the urine.

Rare stones include calcium carbonate stones (small, gray-white), cystine stones (yellow-green), xanthine stones (smooth, yellowish brown; due to xanthine-oxidase deficiency, a disease predominantly of males).

Oxalosis of the kidney is a congenital inborn error of metabolism, transmitted as an autosomal recessive trait. The disease is due to an enzyme deficiency (degradation of glycolic acid to CO_2 is lacking → formation of oxalic acid). The kidney is somewhat smaller than normal (Fig. 13.59). The surface contains multiple white stipplings as well as medullary and cortical streaks (nephrocalcinosis and nephrolithiasis). Other organs likewise are involved, such as the heart, vessels and vertebrae.

Oxalosis manifests either in childhood or past 30 years of age. The disease is complicated by a chronic interstitial nephritis. Death is from uremia.

Clinically, oxalosis is characterized by hyperoxaluria and nephrolithiasis. Most chronic renal diseases can lead to a *secondary* oxalosis. Oxalosis also is observed from *oxogenous* calcium oxalate poisoning.

Single, rosette-like calcium oxalate crystals in the kidney point to previous acidosis.

F: urolithiasis is seen in 1% of autopsies, 3–4% of the population. Stones in the urinary bladder are less common than elsewhere.

A: 30–50 years. *S:* ♂:♀ = 2:1. Urinary tract stones are unilateral in 70–90% of the cases.

Pg: (a) According to the crystallization theory, calculi are precipitated from supersaturated urine (altered pH, loss of protective colloid action). (b) The matrix theory postulates that mucopolysaccharides, urinary mucoproteins, fibrin and cellular debris bind calcium and other salts, thereby providing a nidus for a stone.

Urinary calculi are observed in *metabolic diseases*, e.g., hypercalciuria, idiopathic hypercalcemia (children with retarded growth), primary and secondary hyperparathyroidism, osteoporosis, hyperuricemia (gout, leukemias), cystinuria and oxalosis. Certain *general factors* predispose to urolithiasis: nutrition, dehydration, geographic factors (high incidence in the southern United States, North and East Africa, Persia, Thailand). Persons with little physical activity are commonly affected. (Sex: the incidence of bladder calculi in male rats is reduced after estrogen administration.) Urinary stasis. Inflammations of the urinary system. *Co:* hydro- and pyonephrosis, pyelonephritis.

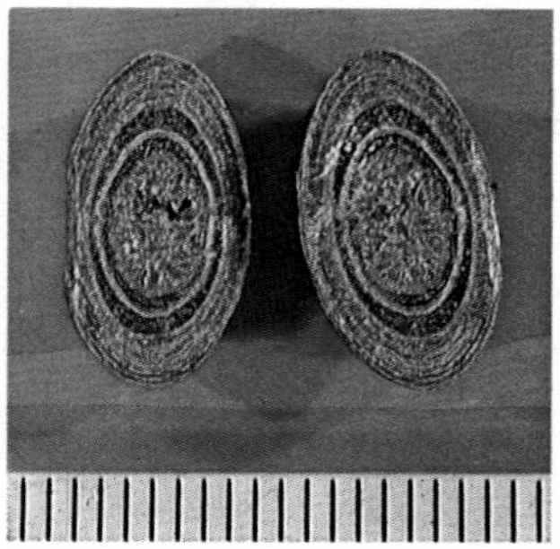

Fig. 13.60. Calcium urate stone.

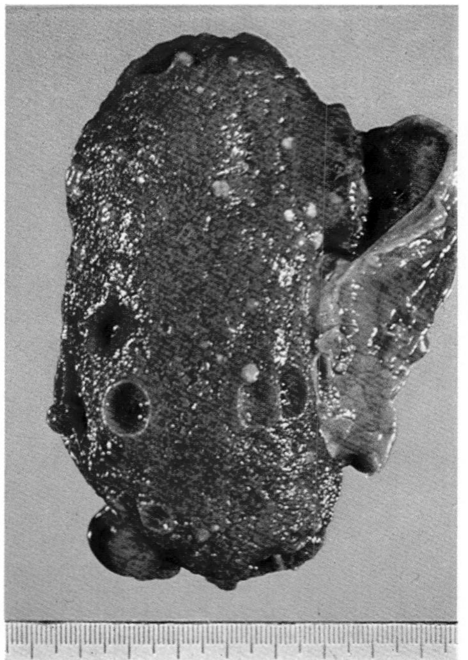

Fig. 13.61. Renal cortical adenomas and cysts.

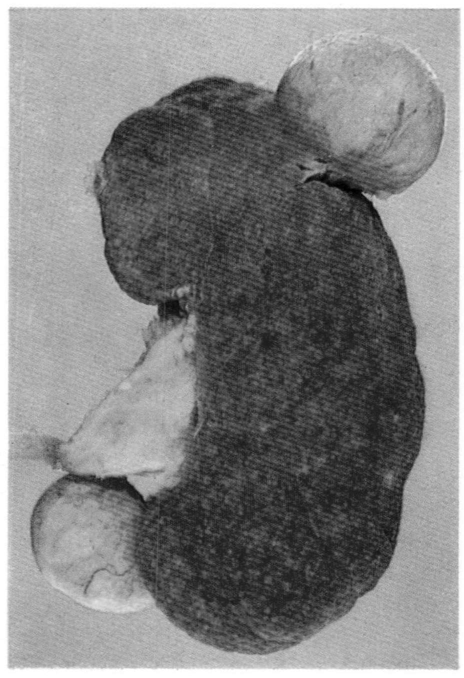

Fig. 13.62. Benign renal adenomas (hypernephroma).

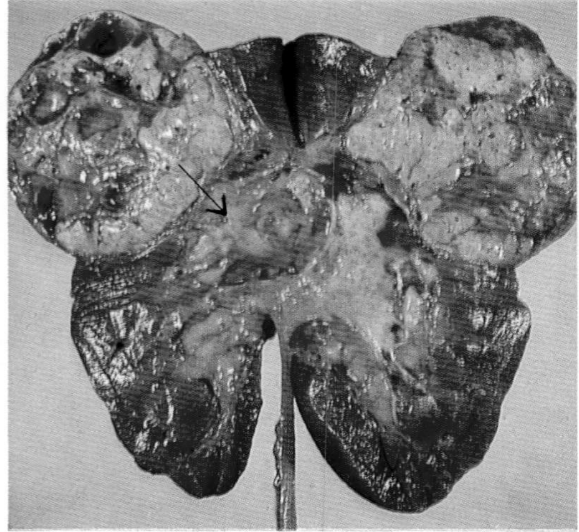

Fig. 13.63. Hypernephroid renal carcinoma with infiltration of the renal pelvis.

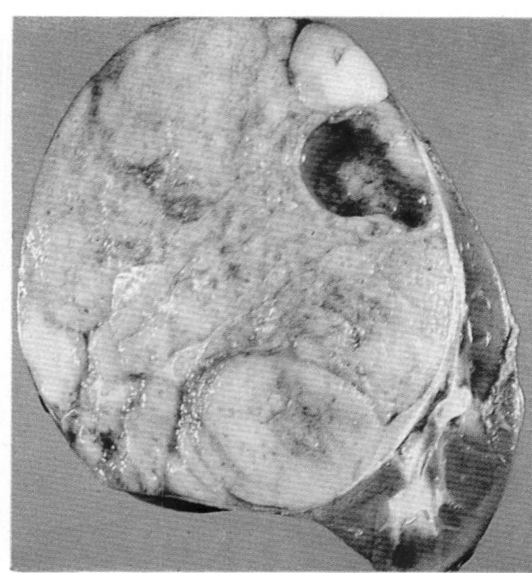

Fig. 13.64. Nephroblastoma (Wilms' tumor).

Tumors of the Kidney

Cortical adenomas (Fig. 13.61). Single or multiple cortical adenomas are found in approximately 10% of autopsies. Any type of kidney scar predisposes to the development of an adenoma (scars from arteriosclerosis, chronic glomerulonephritis or chronic pyelonephritis). A kidney with advanced arteriosclerosis is shown in Figure 13.61. The finely granular, red surface contains multiple, sharply delineated nodules of whitish or yellow color. They measure up to 2 mm. in diameter, except for a larger nodule, which projects from the left lower margin in Figure 13.61. Several cortical cysts are present also; some have ruptured during stripping of the capsule. *Mi:* the yellow nodules were tubular or papillary adenomas. *F:* the most common renal tumor. *A:* older age group. *Pg:* adenomas are considered "regenerative" tumors developing from atrophic or scarred tubules rather than hamartomas.

Displaced adrenocortical rests are golden yellow nodules in the renal cortex measuring up to 5 mm. in diameter. They resemble adrenocortical tissue on histologic examination and, therefore, are interpreted as choristomas (see p. 91).

Medullary fibromas are white, firm, circumscribed nodules in the medulla. They usually do not exceed 5 mm. in diameter. They are interpreted as hamartomas.

Angiomas also are considered hamartomatous in nature. They are red, soft and most frequently are located at or near the papillary tips.

Hypernephroma and hypernephroid renal carcinoma (Figs. 13.62 and 13.63; TCP p. 251). Tumor size is used grossly to distinguish between benign and malignant "hypernephroid" tumors. Tumors that measure less than 3 cm. in diameter are considered benign and are designated adenomas (see above) or hypernephromas, according to their histologic appearance. Tumors larger than 3 cm. in diameter are considered malignant neoplasms. They are classified as hypernephroid carcinomas or renal cell carcinomas on histologic grounds. The term "hypernephroid" was introduced by GRAWITZ, who postulated that most renal tumors are derived from displaced adrenocortical rests. Although Grawitz's theory is incorrect, the term hypernephroid is retained to describe the yellow color of such tumors on gross examination. See TCP, p. 251.

Figure 13.62 shows two (rare!) sharply circumscribed, whitish yellow tumor nodules projecting from the outer kidney surface. Each measured less than 3 cm. in diameter. A fibrous tissue capsule surrounds each tumor nodule. The cut surfaces likewise were uniformly yellow, although central white scars or hemorrhages may be seen occasionally. The gross and histologic diagnosis was hypernephroid renal adenomas.

Renal carcinomas usually measure between 5 and 15 cm. in diameter. Figure 13.63 reveals the variegated cut surface of a hypernephroid carcinoma. Areas of yellow tumor tissue alternate with white portions and hemorrhages. The carcinoma has infiltrated the renal pelvis (→). Despite the apparent sharp delineation from the normal kidney, infiltrative growth (including venous invasion) always can be demonstrated by microscopic examination.

F: 1% of all malignant tumors. *A:* 50–60 years. *S:* ♂:♀ = 1:1. *Pg:* it generally is held that renal carcinomas arise from renal adenomas, although adenomas are much more common than carcinomas.

Metastases: Renal carcinomas almost invariably infiltrate the renal pelvis (90% of cases: hematuria) or renal vein → inferior vena cava. Hematogenous metastases are common in the lungs, liver, bones and brain. The characteristically round metastases in the lung may remain stationary for years as judged from x-ray; *Th:* lobectomy. The frequency of metastases is 50% for the lungs, 30% for the liver, 20% for bones and 10% for the brain. Lymph node metastases are uncommon. *Cl:* renal mass, hematuria, hypercalcemia, low-grade fever, eventually secondary polycythemia (increased erythropoietin production).

Nephroblastoma (Wilms' tumor, embryonal adenosarcoma, Fig. 13.63). *An often congenital, metanephric neoplasm composed of epithelial and mesenchymal elements. The peak incidence is at 3 years, although nephroblastomas may occur in children up to 12 years of age.* A large, white, elastic tumor occupies most of the kidney cut surface in Figure 13.64. The tumor cut surface is composed of several nodules and some cysts. Although Wilms' tumor usually is encapsulated, infiltrative growth (including venous invasion) always can be demonstrated.

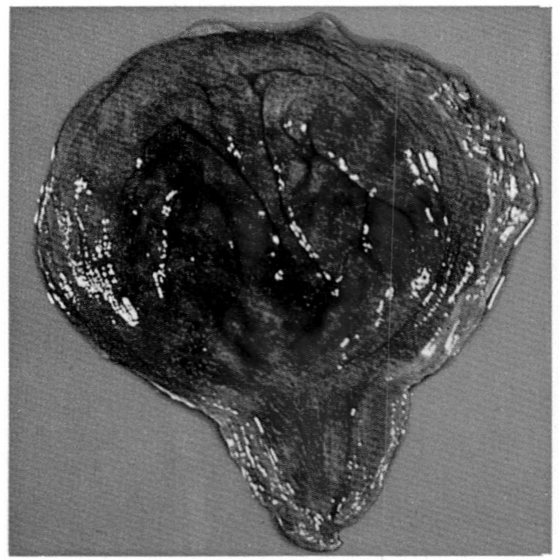

Fig. 13.65. Catarrhal and follicular cystitis.

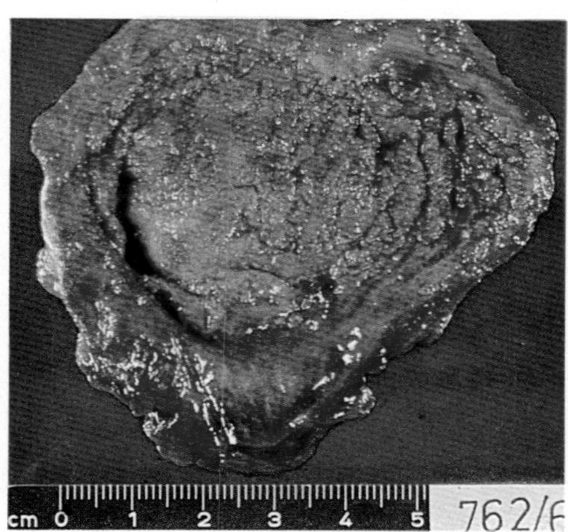

Fig. 13.66. Pseudomembranous necrotizing cystitis.

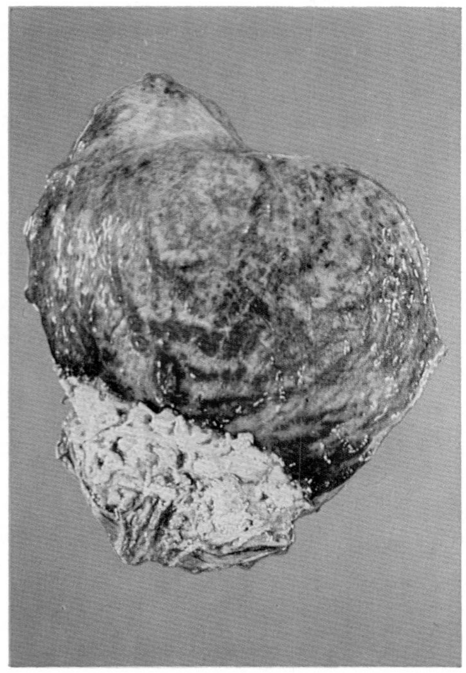

Fig. 13.67. Status after prostatectomy.

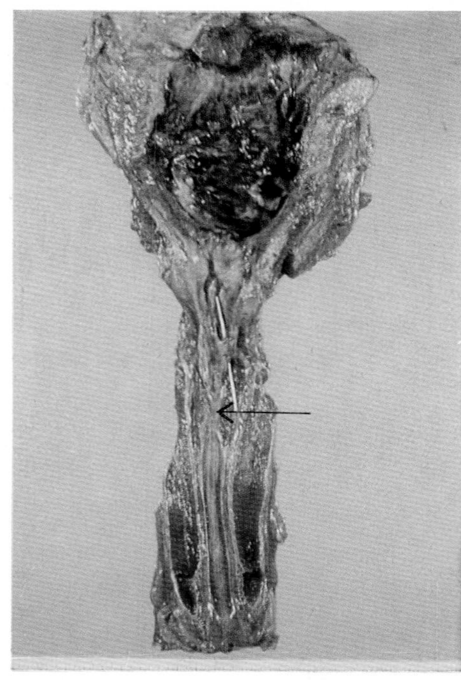

Fig. 13.68. Chronic cystitis due to urethral stricture.

Urinary Bladder

Catarrhal and follicular cystitis (Fig. 13.65). *An inflammation of the urinary bladder characterized by severe hyperemia of the mucosa and hyperplasia of the mucosal lymph follicles.* A hyperemic, edematous, nodularly thickened mucosa and tiny whitish mucosal lesions are seen in Figure 13.65. The whitish spots in the dark red mucosa represent lymph follicles (with germinal centers) in the stratum proprium of the urinary bladder. A similar gross finding, but with marked desquamation of the superficial bladder epithelium, is known as *desquamative cystitis.*

F: catarrhal, follicular or desquamative cystitis is found frequently at autopsy, especially with inflammations of the upper urinary tract. The follicular cystitis is a chronic condition that develops secondarily to chronic hydronephrosis, urolithiasis or other diseases of the urinary tract.

Pseudomembranous, necrotizing cystitis (Fig. 13.66). *An acute inflammation of the urinary bladder with the formation of membranes that adhere loosely or firmly to the mucosa.* The membranes consist of fibrin *(fibrinous cystitis)* or necrotic cell debris *(necrotizing cystitis).* Flat or deep ulcers remain after the necrotic epithelium has been desquamated *(ulcerative cystitis).* A cystitis with extensive areas of necrosis and ulceration is known as *gangrenous cystitis* (ulcers with foul odor). Figure 13.66 shows gray or brown-gray membranous material covering the mucosa of the bladder.

F and *Pg:* pseudomembranous, necrotizing cystitis is found in 4–7% of uterine or ovarian tumors that have been treated by x-ray. Severe cystitis is common in patients with diseases (tabes dorsalis) or trauma of the spinal cord (→ paralysis of the urinary bladder). *Co:* rupture, scarring or stricture of the urinary bladder.

Status after prostatectomy (Fig. 13.67). A severe fibrinous or hemorrhagic cystitis usually is observed during the first days following prostatectomy. Figure 13.67 was obtained from a 65-year-old male who presented with complaints of difficulty in urination. The prostate was enlarged and nodular. The lateral lobes were resected (*Mi:* benign prostatic hyperplasia). The patient died 2 days later from massive lung embolism. Figure 13.67 shows heavy fibrin exudates and hemorrhages in the bladder mucosa. Such areas of tissue necrosis in the operative area are common, especially after electroresection. The postoperative changes usually heal as illustrated in Figure 13.70.

Chronic cystitis and stricture of the urethra. A stricture in the middle portion of the urethra is shown in Figure 13.68. The urethral lumen is markedly narrowed at a point indicated by the arrow. A white probe is located in a defect of the urethral wall that had been perforated by a catheter. The bladder mucosa is black or blue-black focally, indicating a chronic cystitis with old hemorrhages. The lower portion of Figure 13.68 shows the opened penis with the corpus cavernosum.

F and *Pg:* urethral strictures are caused by congenital urethral valves or membranes, inflammation (such as gonorrhea) or trauma. *S:* ♂ > ♀. *Co:* retention of urine → necrotizing and even gangrenous cystitis → ascending pyelonephritis.

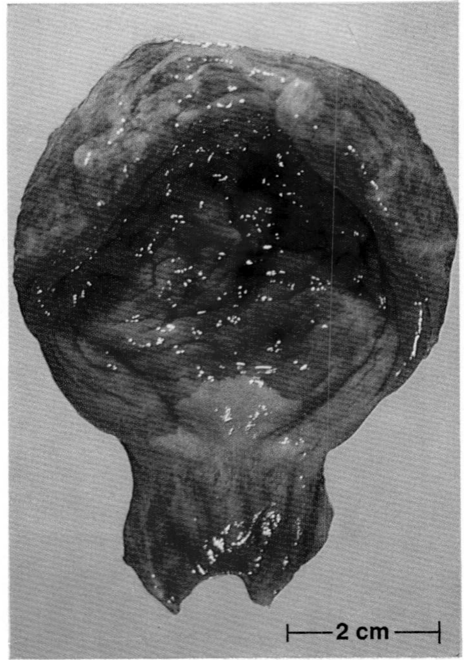

Fig. 13.69. Xerosis vesicae.

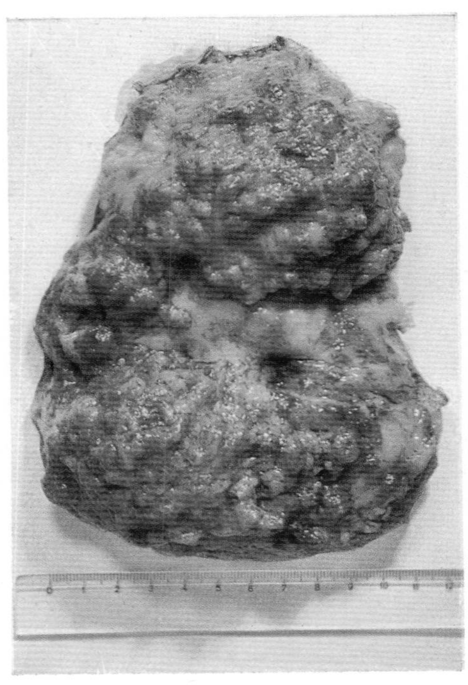

Fig. 13.71. Papilloma of the urinary bladder.

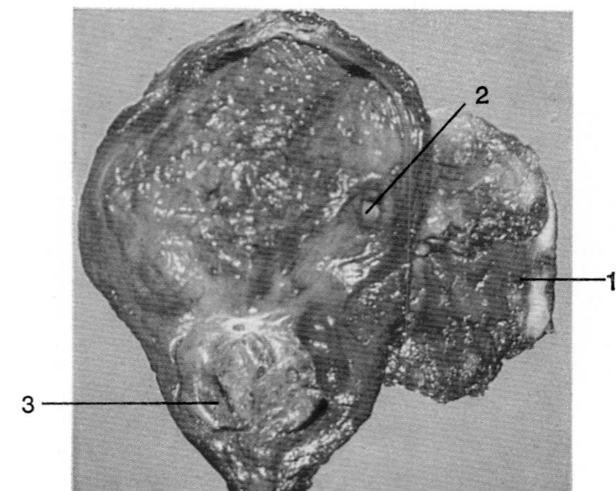

Fig. 13.70. Diverticulum of the urinary bladder. Status after prostatectomy.

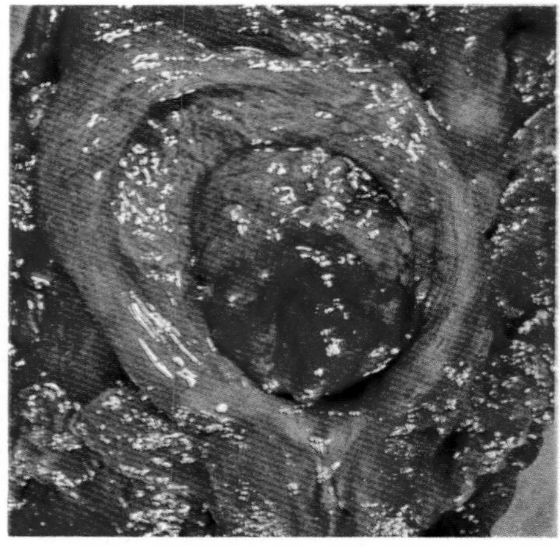

Fig. 13.72. Carcinoma of the urinary bladder.

Xerosis vesicae (leukoplakia of the urinary bladder mucosa, Fig. 13.69). *A circumscribed squamous peithelial metaplasia of the transitional epithelium of the urinary tract.* The lesions of xerosis vesicae present as slightly elevated, gray-white plaques in the mucosa. The plaques in Figure 13.69 are confined to the trigonum.

F: leukoplakias frequently are seen (60%) in the area of the trigonum. *S:* ♀ (50–60 years) are affected most commonly. *Pg:* xerosis vesicae is considered the outcome of a chronic inflammation. Histologically, the condition is due to squamous epithelial metaplasia and hyperkeratosis. *Co:* xerosis is not an obligate precancerous condition. A similar condition in the renal pelvis may present as a cholesteatoma (desquamation of horny epithelium, fatty changes).

Diverticulum of the urinary bladder and status after prostatectomy. Figure 13.70 shows a urinary bladder with moderate muscular hypertrophy (trabeculation). A large, sac-like evagination of the urinary bladder wall (diverticulum) is seen at the right in Figure 13.70. The lumen of the urinary bladder was connected with the diverticulum by a defect in the wall (stoma). The lower third of Figure 13.70 reveals focal scarring from an old, partial prostatectomy.

F and *Pg:* true diverticula are congenital in origin and consist of all layers of the urinary bladder wall. Multiple congenital diverticula are seen occasionally in the ureters as well. They are rare in contrast to the acquired pseudodiverticula (false diverticula), which represent a prolapse of the mucosa through a usually hypertrophic muscle layer. Acquired diverticula frequently are seen in a trabeculated urinary bladder (Fig. 13.70). Bladder trabeculation (submucosal cord-like ridges) is the gross manifestation of muscular hypertrophy. Benign prostatic hypertrophy, urethral strictures, stones or tumors all lead to bladder trabeculation and eventually pseudodiverticula. *Co:* cystitis from residual urine, calculus formation, ascending infections.

Papilloma of the urinary bladder (Fig. 13.71; TCP, p. 237). Papillomas are tumors of transitional epithelium (urothelium) that occur as single or multiple red, fleshy, fern-like growths. The more advanced papillomas present as sessile, friable, cauliflower-like masses (Fig. 13.71; papillomatosis of the urinary bladder).

S, A, F and *Pg:* see below. *Pr:* according to some statistics, approximately 5% of papillomas become malignant. *Mi:* a continuous morphologic spectrum is observed, ranging from simple papillomas (lined by an orderly transitional epithelium) to carcinomas in situ (thickened epithelium with atypical cells and many mitoses) to invasive carcinomas (diffuse or focal infiltration of the bladder wall).

Carcinoma of the urinary bladder. As shown in Figure 13.72, these broadly based (sessile), papillary tumors develop especially in the trigonum (near the ostia of the ureters). Bladder carcinomas also may appear as plaque-like or ulcerated or fungating, friable masses that occupy the entire bladder mucosa. Penetration of the wall usually is apparent on gross examination. The *DD* between papillomatosis and papillary carcinomas should be based on histologic examination.

F: 0.5% in autopsy material. Approximately 3% of all malignant tumors. Bladder carcinomas are rare in Japan but frequent in Egypt. *A:* 40–60 years. *S:* ♂:♀ = 3:1. *Mi:* 80% are *papillary carcinomas* (sessile, exophytic or endophytic tumors), often of multifocal origin in the urinary bladder and elsewhere in the urinary tract. The well-differentiated papillary carcinomas are of low malignancy, in contrast to *anaplastic carcinomas* (approximately 10% of bladder carcinomas) and *squamous-cell carcinomas* (2–3% of bladder carcinomas).

Pg: most carcinomas are derived from bladder papillomas. Exogenous carcinogenic agents have been identified, e.g., aromatic amines (β-naphthylamine in aniline dye workers) and *Schistosoma haematobium* (bilharziasis). These agents cause a chronic cystitis, epithelial proliferations, papillomas and carcinomas.

Staging of bladder carcinomas: Stage 1a: confined to the mucosa. Stage 1b: involvement of bladder muscle. Stage 2: extension to perivesical tissue. Stage 3: metastases to perivesical lymph nodes. Stage 4: metastases to liver, lung and bone. Fifty per cent of bladder carcinomas have metastasized at the time of autopsy, especially anaplastic carcinomas. *Pr:* 5-year survival is 25%.

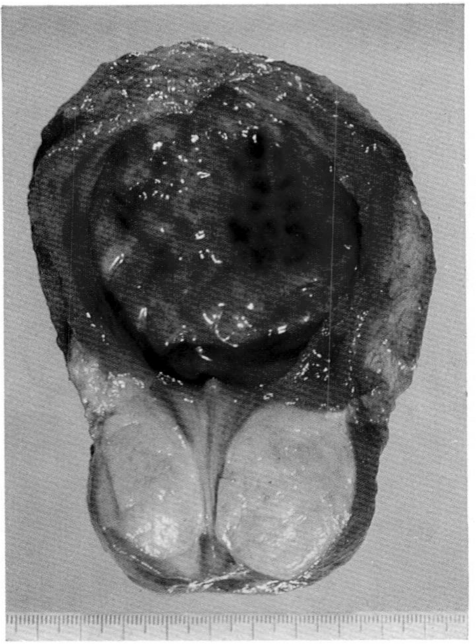

Fig. 14.1. Hyperplasia of the lateral lobes of the prostate gland with hemorrhagic cystitis.

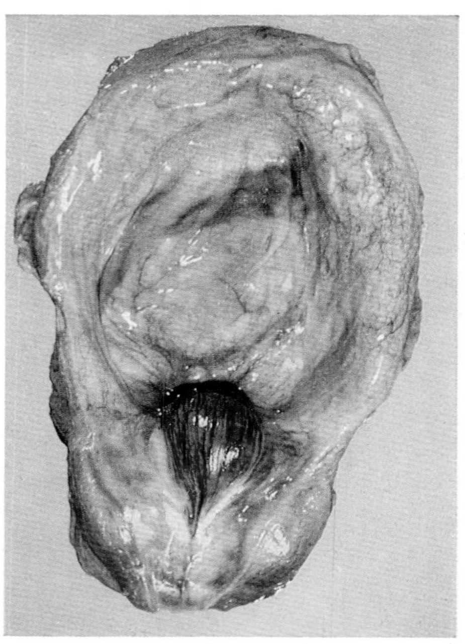

Fig. 14.2. Benign prostatic hyperplasia with formation of a median bar.

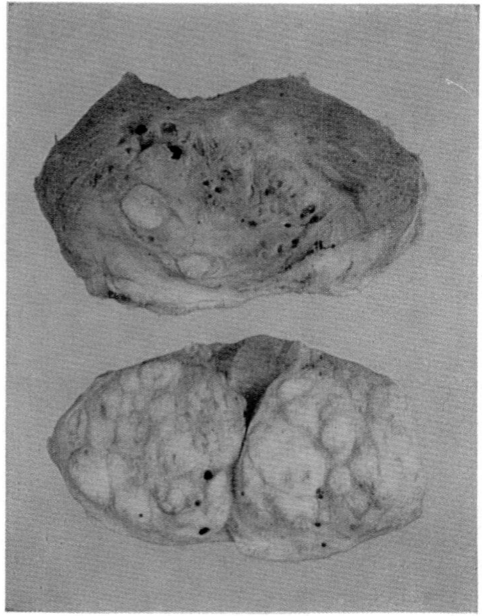

Fig. 14.3. Benign prostatic hyperplasia and prostatic concrements.

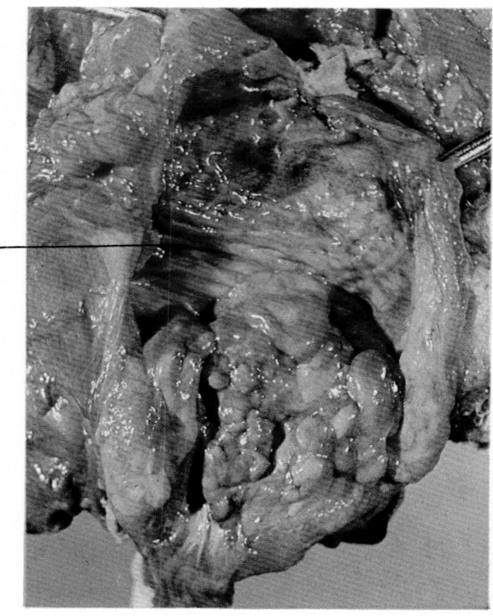

Fig. 14.4. Carcinoma of the prostate gland with infiltration of the floor of the urinary bladder.

14. Male Sex Organs

Prostate Gland

Benign prostatic hyperplasia (adenomyomatosis, nodular hyperplasia of the prostate; Figs. 14.1–14.3; TCP, p. 241). *A nodular enlargement of the prostate gland as a result of fibromuscular and glandular hyperplasia and hypertrophy.* Either the lateral lobes (Fig. 14.1), middle lobe ("median bar," Fig. 14.2) or both are enlarged. The floor of the urinary bladder becomes elevated and the internal urethral ostium is more or less narrowed. The cut surface of the prostate contains moist, gray-white, firm-elastic nodules (Fig. 14.3). The nodules are sharply delineated, bulge over the cut surface and contain tiny cysts filled with a cloudy, milky fluid.

F: progressive increase with age: 41% at 50–60 years, almost 100% past 70 years of age. *Pg:* progressive senile testicular atrophy → decreased androgen production → relative hyperestrinism → hyperplasia and hypertrophy of fibromuscular tissue and periurethral glands. *Mi:* small and large cysts, adenomatous and fibromuscular proliferation. The peripheral prostatic glands undergo pressure atrophy *(pseudocapsule or surgical prostate capsule).* A predominantly myomatous hyperplasia is observed on occasion. *Co:* the prostatic nodules encroach on the internal urethral ostium → saber-like narrowing of the prostatic urethra → retention of urine → hypertrophy and trabeculation of the bladder → hydro-ureter, hydronephrosis (see p. 283; Fig. 13.70). Incomplete emptying of bladder → residual urine → ascending ureteropyelonephritis (see p. 269).

Prostatic concrements. Figure 14.3 shows the cut surface of a prostate with nodular hyperplasia and small, brown-black prostatic concrements or corpora amylacea. They can be found prior to puberty and increase in frequency with age, especially after chronic inflammations and benign prostatic hyperplasia.

Pg: the nidus of corpora amylacea probably is formed by desquamated epithelial cells. *Mi:* corpora amylacea are homogeneous or concentrically layered, sometimes partly or completely calcified. Larger calculi (weighing >100 Gm.) are considered inspissated urinary bladder stones.

Carcinoma of the prostate gland (Fig. 14.4). *A malignant proliferation of the subcapsular prostate gland occurring predominantly past 60 years of age.* A carcinoma is recognized grossly as a homogeneous, relatively firm, often yellow lesion (*xanthomatous carcinoma:* fatty, degenerative changes in tumor cells). Prostatic carcinomas penetrate the posterior and upper prostatic capsules, infiltrate the urinary bladder floor and invade the surrounding pelvic tissues, ureters or seminal vesicles. The relatively uncommon involvement of the urethra and the rectum is remarkable. In Figure 14.4, the floor of the urinary bladder is infiltrated by a nodular prostatic carcinoma. Also note the trabeculation of the bladder wall.

F: prostatic carcinoma is rare prior to 40 years of age. In contrast, cancer is found in 30% of prostates obtained from patients past 80 years. Most of these carcinomas are discovered during routine histologic examinations. They are clinically asymptomatic, have not metastasized and are called *latent carcinomas.*

Metastases: Prostate cancers with extensive metastases (e.g., in bones → pathologic fracture) sometimes are of small size and not recognized on gross examination *(occult prostatic carcinoma).* Carcinomas of the prostate spread by *direct infiltration,* by *lymphogenous dissemination* along the perineural lymphatics to the iliac and lumbar lymph nodes and by *hematogenous dissemination,* especially to the bones *(osteoplastic bone metastases:* high acid phosphate levels).

There is no causal relationship between prostatic carcinoma and benign nodular hyperplasia. Both often coexist and a carcinoma may invade the hyperplastic fibromuscular and glandular prostate.

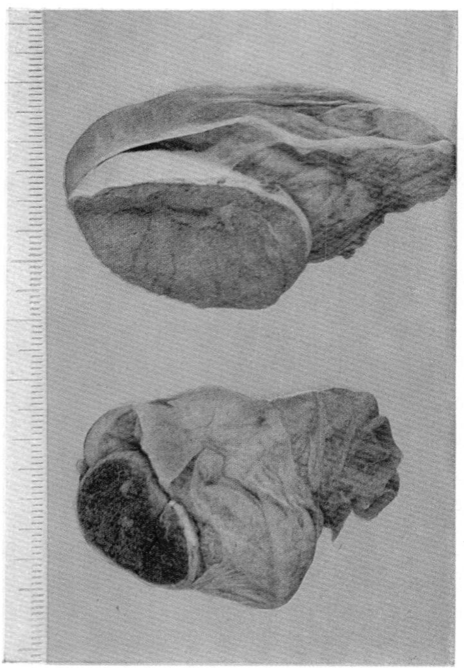

Fig. 14.5. Below: atrophy of the testis. Above: normal testis.

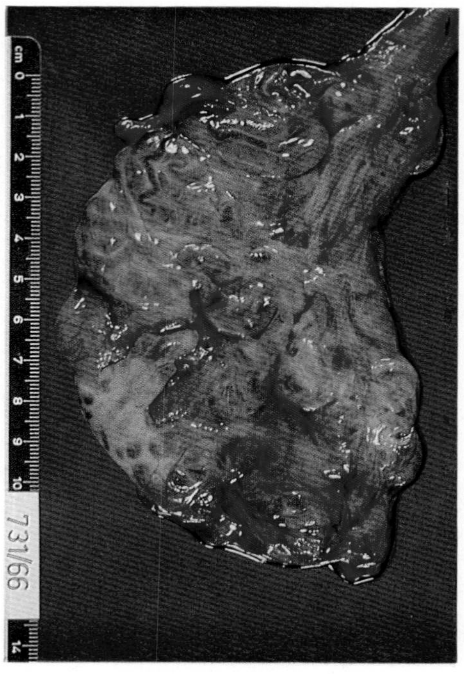

Fig. 14.6. Varicocele of the testis.

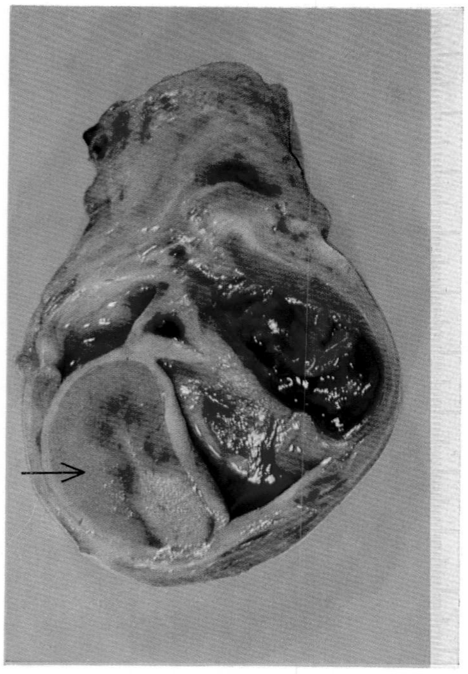

Fig. 14.7. Organized hematocele of the testis.

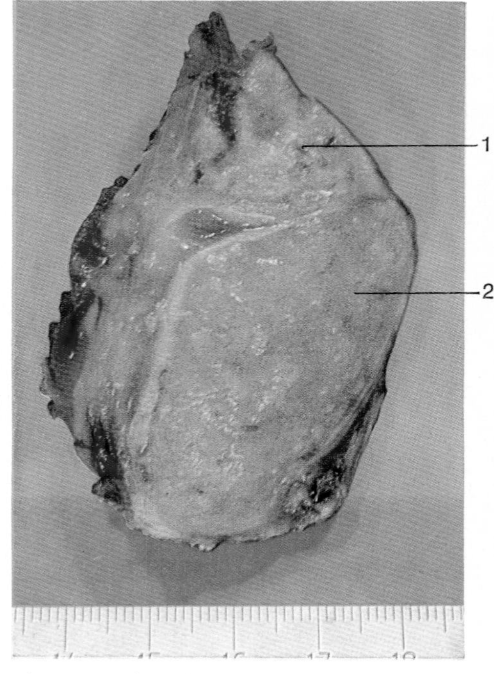

Fig. 14.8. Tuberculosis of the testis and epididymis.

Testis

Atrophy of the testis (Fig. 14.5; TCP, p. 193). *Reduction in the size of the testis due to involution and fibrosis of the seminiferous tubules.* The adult testis weighs at least 15 Gm. The atrophic testis is small, dark brown and firm instead of tan and soft on gross examination (Fig. 14.5). Seminiferous tubules cannot be plucked or strung from the cut surface.

F: very common change, especially in elderly males *(senile testicular atrophy).* Predisposing factors include arteriosclerosis, inflammations (mumps orchitis), tuberculosis, malnutrition, tumor cachexia, chemotherapeutic agents, x-rays and hormonal imbalance (hyperestrinism in liver cirrhosis). An undescended testis in the inguinal canal or abdominal cavity *(cryptorchidism)* usually is atrophic. Testicular atrophy also is found in patients with Klinefelter syndrome (see p. 332) or schizophrenia.

Varicocele of the testis (Fig. 14.6). *A varicose dilatation of the pampiniform plexus.* The veins of the tunica vaginalis and spermatic cord are dilated, elongated and tortuous. The walls of the veins are thickened.

Ninety per cent of varicoceles are left-sided (pampiniform plexus → spermatic vein → enters the left renal vein on the left side and the inferior vena cava on the right side). *Pg:* (1) idiopathic varicoceles are of unknown origin; (2) symptomatic varicoceles are due to a partial obstruction of venous flow by thrombi, tumors or hernias.

Circulatory disorders of the testis include *ischemic necrosis* (infarctions) from arterial occlusion by thrombi, emboli, periarteritis nodosa or endangiitis obliterans. Hemorrhagic infarction of the testis is, in most instances, caused by torsion of the testis (free mobility of testis → sudden twisting of the spermatic cord → strangulation of blood vessels → congestion, hemorrhage or anemic necrosis). Torsion is especially common in the cryptorchid testis.

Hematocele of the testis (Fig. 14.7). *Partly fresh, partly organized hemorrhages in the sac of the tunica vaginalis.* Hemorrhages are the result of trauma, chronic inflammations of testicular membranes (periorchitis) or hemorrhagic tendencies. The cut surface of the testis is indicated by an arrow in Figure 14.7. The wall of the tunica vaginalis is thickened. The lumen of the hematocele contains chocolate-like masses of coagulated blood, hematoidin, fibrin and cholesterol crystals. The testis may become atrophic (pressure atrophy).

Hydrocele. *A collection of serous or serofibrinous fluid in the sac of the tunica vaginalis (cavum serosum).* A hydrocele may communicate with the abdominal cavity (communicating hydrocele). The fluid of a hydrocele also may collect in a partially obliterated funicular process.

Pg: the most likely cause of a *congenital communicating hydrocele* is trauma during delivery. Acquired hydroceles, such as the *acute hydrocele,* are complications of a serofibrinous periorchitis (gonorrhea, tuberculosis), tumors or trauma. The testis usually is found in the posterior and upper portions of a hydrocele sac.

Tuberculosis of the testis and epididymis. Figure 14.8 illustrates several small and larger, discrete, centrally necrotic, yellow lesions in the epididymis (→1) and testis (→2). *Mi:* tuberculous granulomas. The epididymis is the most frequent site of genital tuberculosis. Hematogenous dissemination involves the tail of the epididymis first. The tuberculous process then extends directly or lymphogenously to the head of the epididymis and testis.

A: tuberculosis of the epididymis has a peak incidence between 20 and 40 years; testicular tuberculosis alone is a manifestation of miliary tuberculosis, usually in young children.

DD: chronic, granulomatous orchitis is characterized by a diffuse involvement. Syphilitic gummas almost exclusively are confined to the testis.

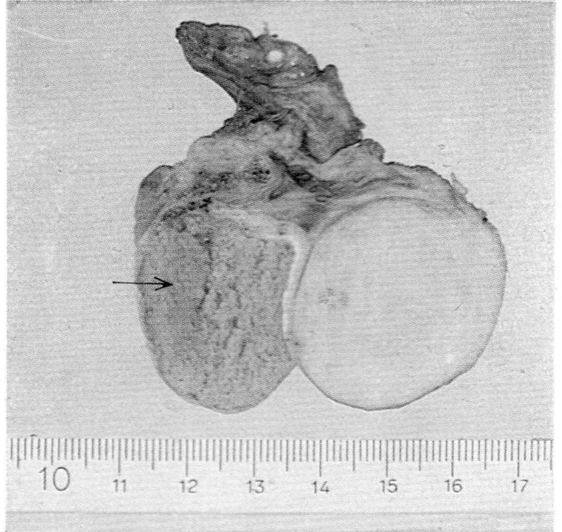

Fig. 14.9. Adenomatoid tumor of the epididymis.

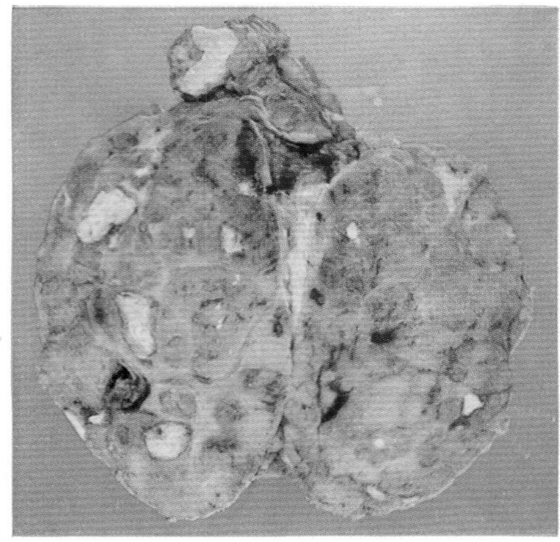

Fig. 14.10. Seminoma of the testis.

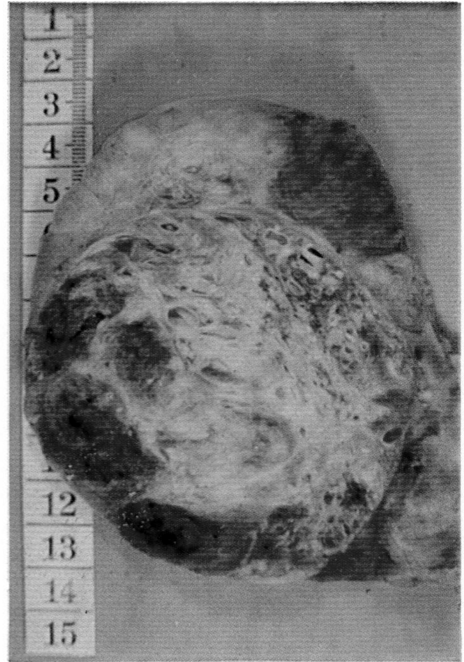

Fig. 14.11. Testicular teratoma of the trophoblastic type.

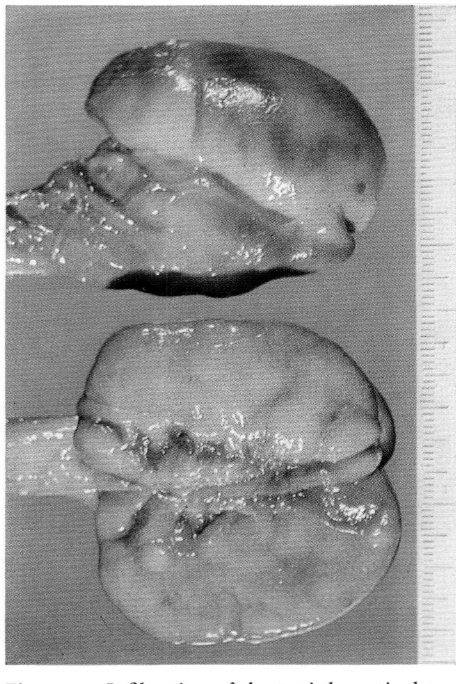

Fig. 14.12. Infiltration of the testis by reticulum-cell sarcoma.

Adenomatoid tumor of the epididymis (Fig. 14.9). This benign tumor is difficult to classify according to histogenetic principles (mesothelioma?, adenomyoma?). Figure 14.9 shows the testis (→) and a grayish white, encapsulated tumor (2.5 cm. in diameter) in the tail of the epididymis. Adenomatoid tumors grow expansively; they may occur in the spermatic cord also.

Mi: vacuolated tumor cells are arranged in cords, trabeculae or glands, separated by considerable tumor stroma with smooth muscle fibers.

Other *benign tumors and hyperplasia of the testis:* (1) *Tubular and stromal Sertoli-cell adenomas* are rare, estrogen-producing, feminizing tumors that appear as small, yellow nodules, especially in a cryptorchid testis. Sertoli-cell tumors *(androblastomas)* are the homologue to the masculinizing ovarian arrhenoblastoma. (2) Interstitial-cell tumors *(Leydig-cell tumors)* are extremely rare, yellow-tan, androgen-producing tumors. They are difficult to distinguish from nodular hyperplasia of Leydig cells. Leydig-cell tumors occur in two age groups (in boys → phallic enlargement, excessive body development; in 30–45-year-olds → no effects). Interstitial-cell tumors account for 1–2% of all testicular tumors; 5% of Leydig-cell tumors become metastatic. *Mi:* mature Leydig cells with eosinophilic, granular cytoplasm, lipid vacuoles or rod-shaped crystalloids of Reinke.

Seminoma (Fig. 14.10; TCP, p. 257). *The most common malignant tumor of the testis, composed of undifferentiated germ cells (germinoma).* Initially, a seminoma is rubbery, gray-white and fairly well demarcated from the surrounding testis. Seminomas grow rapidly and eventually may replace the entire testis. The cut surface then is gray-white or yellowish reddish, with focal hemorrhages and ischemic, map-like areas of necrosis (Fig. 14.10).

F: approximately 40–50% of all testicular tumors. *A:* 35 years and older. *Clinical course:* often early, predominantly lymphogenous metastases. *Mi:* a typical seminoma consists of large, uniform, round cells with prominent nucleoli and clear (glycogen-rich) cytoplasm. Many lymphocytes in the tumor stroma are a typical feature. The seminoma is the homologue of ovarian dysgerminomas. *Pr:* 60–80% survive for more than 5 years. Seminomas are radiosensitive.

Teratocarcinoma of the testis (Fig. 14.11; TCP, p. 253). Teratocarcinomas consist of the three germ cell layers. Figure 14.11 shows the cut surface of a teratocarcinoma; it is gray-white, cystic and mottled with dark red hemorrhages. In general, these tumors may show large areas of necrosis. Our case was a malignant teratoid tumor with areas of trophoblastic differentiation. The trophoblastic portions are represented by the blood-rich areas in Figure 14.11.

Classification of germ-cell tumors. According to normal germ cell development, germinal tumors are divided into:

1. *Seminomas* (germinomas); see above.

2. *Embryonal-cell carcinomas* are highly malignant tumors of multipotential, undifferentiated cells. They may show evidence of somatic or trophoblastic differentiation. Somatic differentiation: epithelial cell plates or layers; trophoblastic differentiation: see choriocarcinoma. *F:* embryonal-cell carcinomas account for 20% of germinal tumors.

3. *Teratoid tumors* are considered to represent parasitic malformations (see p. 335). A teratoma contains well-differentiated tissues such as thyroid, skin epithelium or neural tissues. In the adult male, teratoid tumors usually are malignant (*teratocarcinomas* 30–40% of germinal tumors). The important histologic feature is the presence of fetal or adult tissues arising from the three germ cell layers. The gross appearance almost always is cystic (resembling a honeycomb). Foci of cartilaginous tissue and calcification occasionally can be recognized grossly.

4. *Choriocarcinomas* exhibit differentiation into tissues resembling cytotrophoblastic and syncytiotrophoblastic cells. Choriocarcinomas are the most malignant but also the least common germinal tumors. They regress spontaneously on occasion despite massive metastases. *Cl:* produce gonadotropic hormones Aschheim-Zondek test).

5. *Combination types* are germinal tumors that contain areas characteristic of seminoma, embryonal-cell carcinoma, teratocarcinoma or choriocarcinoma. Figure 14.11 is an example of a teratocarcinoma with trophoblastic differentiation.

Reticulum-cell sarcoma (Fig. 14.12). Involvement of the testes by systemic malignant diseases is not uncommon (leukemias, lymphomas). Figure 14.12 shows diffuse infiltration of the testes by partly nodular, soft, yellowish brown tumor tissue. This was a case of a widely disseminated reticulum-cell sarcoma.

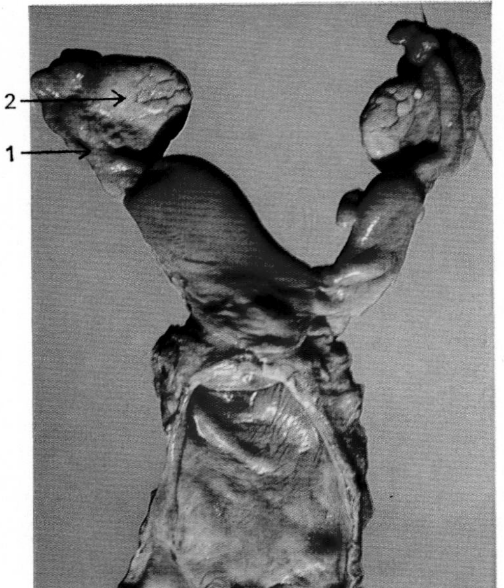

Fig. 15.1. Uterus bicornis unicollis.

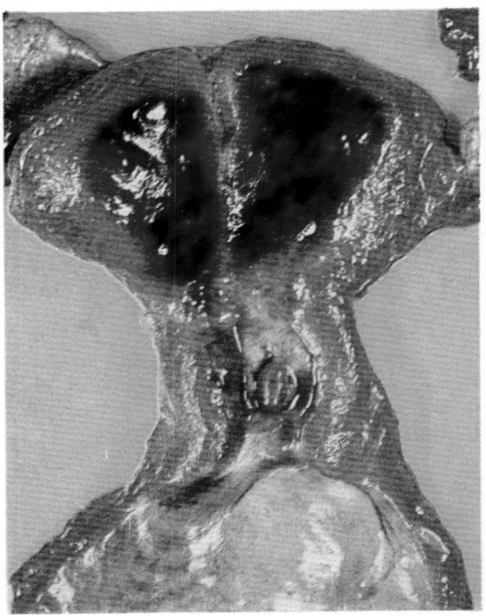

Fig. 15.2. Apoplexia of the uterus.

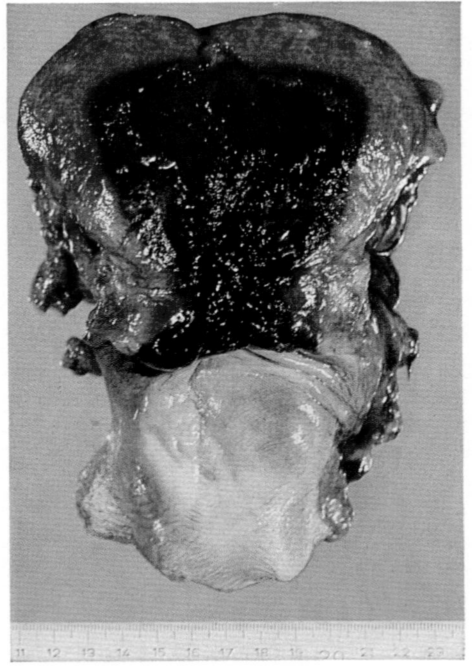

Fig. 15.3. Hemorrhagic necrotizing endometritis.

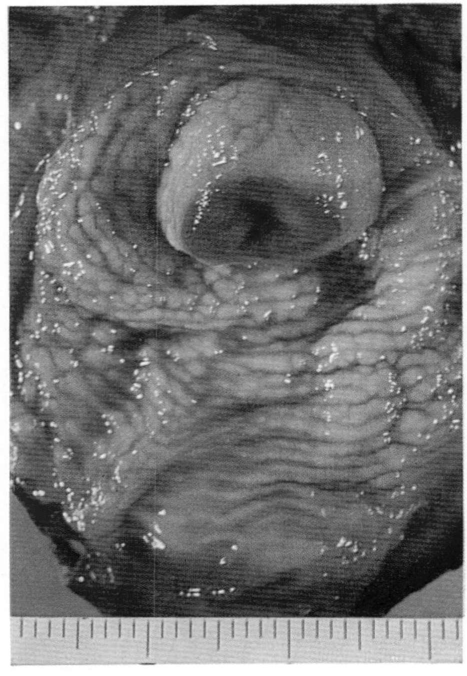

Fig. 15.4. Pseudoerosion of the cervix.

15. Female Sex Organs

Uterus

Malformations are common and often multiple in the female genital tract, especially in the uterus and the vagina. All gradations from aplasia, hypoplasia or septation to partial or complete doubling may be observed. These malformations and anomalies are readily understood from the fact that the uterus and the vagina are formed in the midline by fusion of the Müllerian ducts. *Aplasia* of the uterus is rare. *Hypoplasia* refers to a uterus that resembles the small fetal or infantile uterus (*infantilism;* see also hypogonadism in Turner's syndrome, p. 332). Malformations attributable to excess formation of certain parts of the female sex organs include complete doubling of the uterus and the vagina *(uterus didelphys or bicornis duplex separatus)* and partial doubling of the uterus (*1*, *uterus bicornis duplex* = two uteri and one septated vagina; 2, *uterus bicornis unicollis* = two uterine horns with a single cervix). The *septate uterus* has two uterine cavities but its external form is normal (no retraction).

Uterus bicornis unicollis. Figure 15.1 shows two uterine horns with a common cervix. The opened vagina is seen in the lower portion of Figure 15.1 (→1 tube, →2 ovary).

Uterine apoplexia (Fig. 15.2). *Severe, agonal congestion of the endometrium in elderly patients.* Figure 15.2 shows the opened uterus with a hemorrhagic endometrial surface. Uterine apoplexia must be distinguished from irregular menstrual bleeding.

Metrorrhagia: Acyclic uterine bleeding is observed in diseases of the uterus (polyps, tumors, cervical erosions, glandular-cystic hyperplasia or foreign bodies and systemic diseases (poisoning, hemorrhagic tendencies, typhoid fever). *Hematometra* refers to retention of blood in the uterine cavity because of congenital atresia *(gynatresia)* or acquired stenosis of the uterine outlet (senile occlusion of the internal cervical os). *Hematocolpos* refers to collection of blood in the lumen of the vagina, usually as a result of a low occlusion (e.g., *atresia of the hymen*).

Hemorrhagic necrotizing endometritis (Fig. 15.3). Inflammations of the uterus (metritis) involve the endometrium (endometritis), muscle (myometritis), serosa (perimetritis) or surrounding tissues (parametritis). Figure 15.3 shows a dilated uterine cavity lined by a blue-black mucosa. The myometrium is diffusely thickened. Such necrotizing endometritis most often is infectious in origin. Mechanical or chemical injury (e.g., abortion) also may cause an endometritis. Our case was a hemorrhagic necrotizing endometritis following abortion.

F: puerperal endometritis still is relatively common following abortion or full-term delivery. The uterus is red, soft and edematous; it may have ruptured by the time of surgery or autopsy. *Pg:* ascending endometritis from infection with streptococci, staphylococci or gonococci is more common than a descending or hematogenous endometritis. Salpingitis may involve the endometrium secondarily. Tuberculosis is an example of hematogenous endometritis.

Pseudoerosion of the cervix (Fig. 15.4). These common cervical lesions are defined as follows: an *erosion* is a chronic, inflammatory defect of the superficial cervical epithelium that extends to the underlying stroma (chronic cervicitis). Much more common is the *pseudoerosion* of the cervix, also called *ectropion or eversion.* A pseudoerosion can mimic a true erosion grossly. The swollen cervical mucosa (cylindrical epithelium) rolls out from the cervical canal covering the external os. The stroma is inflamed and, therefore, rich in blood vessels (red color!). Figure 15.4 shows the opened vagina with the typical transverse mucosal folds. The mucosa around the external os is red, whereas the remaining cervix is gray-white (lined by squamous epithelium).

F: common cervical lesion during childbearing age. *Pg:* pseudoerosions are cervical mucosal eversions following minor lacerations of the cervix. Because of chronic irritation, the everted cervical mucosa may proliferate *(glandular papillary pseudoerosion)* or may be lined by squamous epithelium. An erosion causes retention of mucus, which, in turn, produces retention cysts of the cervical glands (ovula Nabothi).

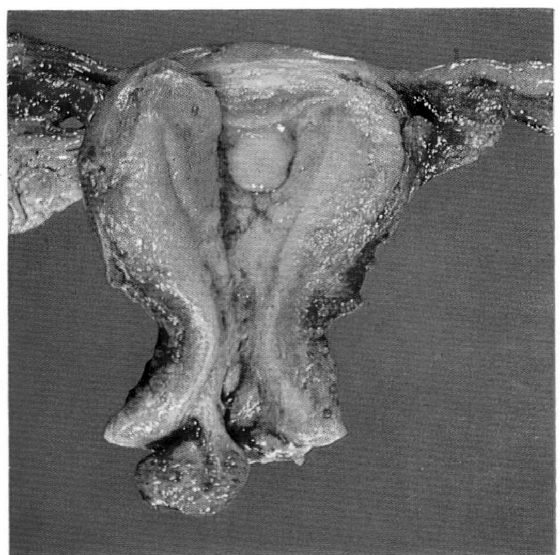

Fig. 15.5. Polyps of the endometrium and cervical mucosa.

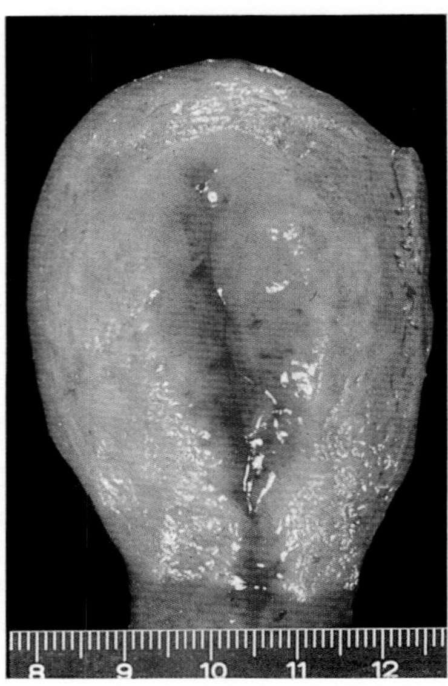

Fig. 15.6. Glandular cystic hyperplasia of the endometrium.

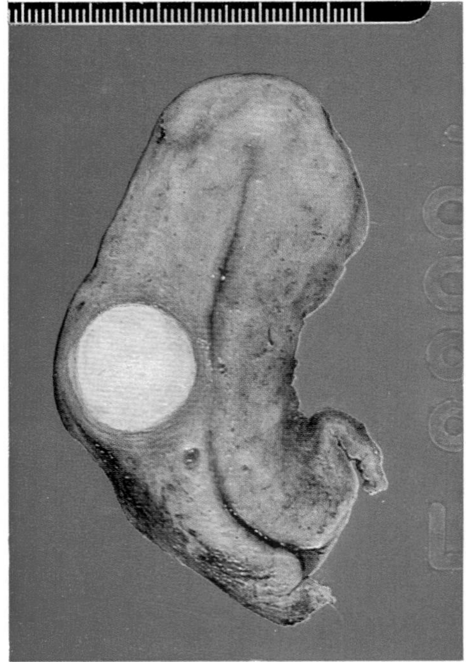

Fig. 15.7. Intramural leiomyoma of the uterus.

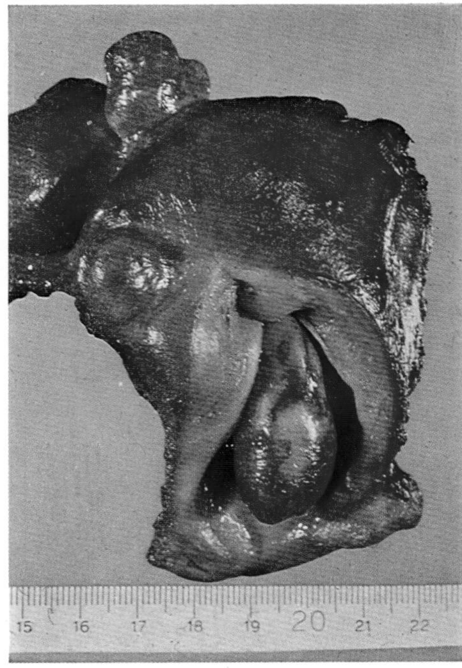

Fig. 15.8. Submucosal and subserosal leiomyomas of the uterus.

Hyperplasias of the Uterus

Polyps of the uterus (Fig. 15.5). *Circumscribed hyperplasia or neoplasia of the endometrium or cervical epithelium.* Figure 15.5 shows a broadly based or sessile polyp in the fundus and a pedunculated polyp in the cervical canal. Most endometrial polyps are composed of multiple cystically dilated endometrial glands embedded in abundant stroma. Uterine polyps may consist of functional endometrium responding to ovarian hormones. Pedunculated cervical polyps develop from ovula Nabothi.

F: a common lesion after menopause. *Co:* inflammation, superficial or total hemorrhagic infarction from pressure or torsion of the stalk. Malignant changes are rare in polyps.

Glandular cystic hyperplasia of the endometrium (metropathia hemorrhagica, Fig. 15.6; TCP, p. 191). Figure 15.6 shows a rather diffuse reddish yellow discoloration of the endometrium, which is sharply separated from the myometrium. This specimen was obtained from a case of diffuse glandular hyperplasia of the endometrium. *Mi:* typical Swiss-cheese hyperplasia.

F: common cause of abnormal bleeding (metrorrhagia). *A:* predominantly in patients prior to menopause (>40 years). *Pg:* (1) abnormal persistence of graafian follicle (or groups of follicles) → overproduction of estrogens over progesterone → glandular hyperplasia ("Swiss-cheese hyperplasia"); (2) estrogen-producing ovarian tumors (granulosa-theca cell tumors) → persistent estrogen secretion; (3) abortion or delivery → adaptive hyperplasia (is transient). *Co: adenomatous hyperplasia* (multiple, more irregular glands) is a precancerous lesion (→ endometrial carcinoma).

Leiomyomas (Figs. 15.7 and 15.8; TCP, p. 259). *Circumscribed round tumors composed of smooth muscle fibers and more or less hyalinized connective tissue.* Leiomyomas are found in the myometrium (intramural leiomyomas, Fig. 15.7), beneath the mucosa (submucosal leiomyomas) or beneath the serosa (subserosal leiomyomas, Fig. 15.8). Submucosal leiomyomas may protrude through the cervical canal into the vagina when attached to a long stalk. The cut surface of leiomyomas is gray-white or pale pink and whorled because of concentric layering of muscle bundles. Leiomyomas usually are firm-elastic, except for a young leiomyoma, which is soft and fleshy. Older leiomyomas are referred to as *fibroids.* Leiomyomas are not encapsulated but are surrounded by a pseudocapsule from which they can be shelled out.

F: very common past 50 years of age but rare before the twentieth year. *Pg:* not known but estrogenic stimulation is suspected. (Uterine leiomyomas have been compared to benign prostatic hyperplasia.) *Co:* retrogressive changes (fibrosis, myxomatous changes, telangiectasis, hemorrhages and hemorrhagic infarction from torsion of a stalk). Malignant transformation of leiomyomas is rare.

Endometriosis (Fig. 15.9). *Ectopia or heterotopia of endometrial glands or stroma or both.* The ectopic endometrial glands may be confined to the myometrium *(internal endometriosis).* The endometrial glands apparently stimulate a circumscribed hyperplasia of the smooth muscle and the uterine wall becomes thicker than 3 cm. The condition, therefore, is referred to as *adenomyosis* of the uterus. In Figure 15.9, the myometrium is of light color and contains tiny nodules (→), especially beneath the endometrium. The nodules represent hyperplastic myometrium in a case of *internal endometriosis* or adenomyosis.

External endometriosis: endometrial glands and stroma are displaced outside the uterus (ovaries, pelvic peritoneum, gut, umbilicus, appendix, laparotomy scars, even lungs). The ectopic glands respond to ovarian hormones and undergo cyclic changes (periodic pains, hemorrhages; TCP, p. 193). The ovarian "chocolate cyst" is an example of external endometriosis.

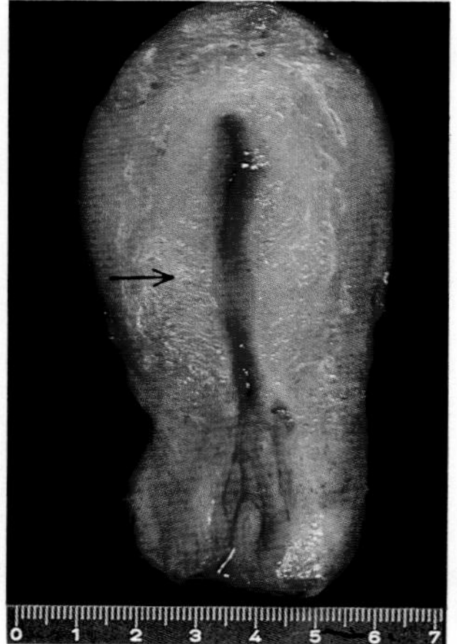

Fig. 15.9. Internal endometriosis.

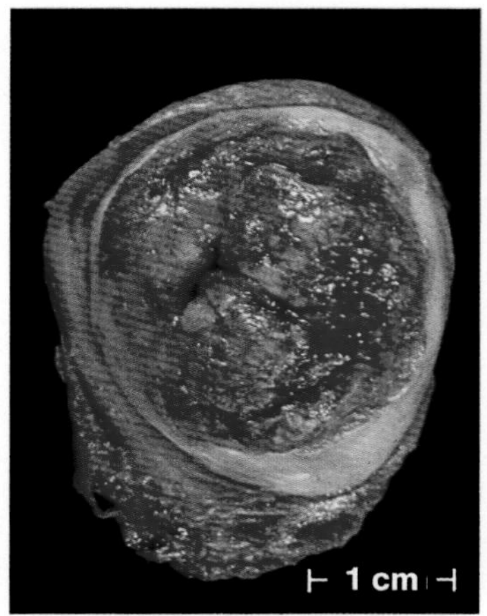

Fig. 15.10. Carcinoma of the cervix.

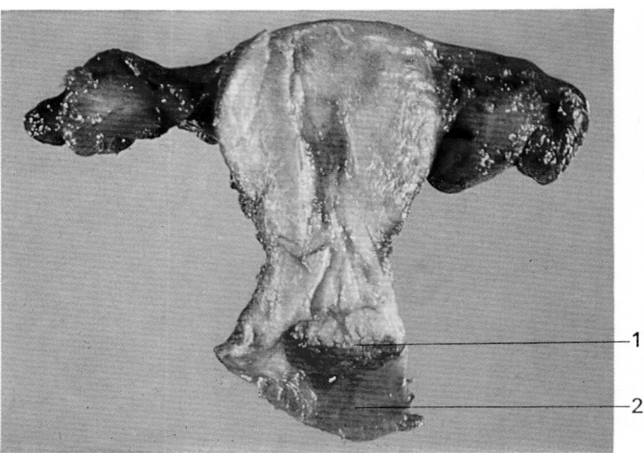

Fig. 15.11. Opened uterus with an exophytic cervical carcinoma.

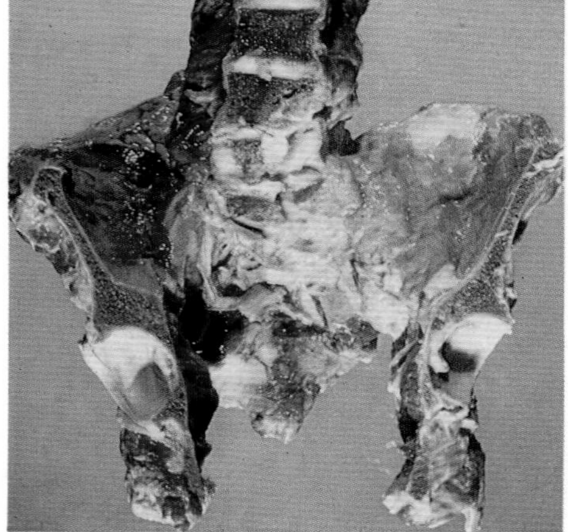

Fig. 15.12. Infiltration of the pelvis by a cervical carcinoma.

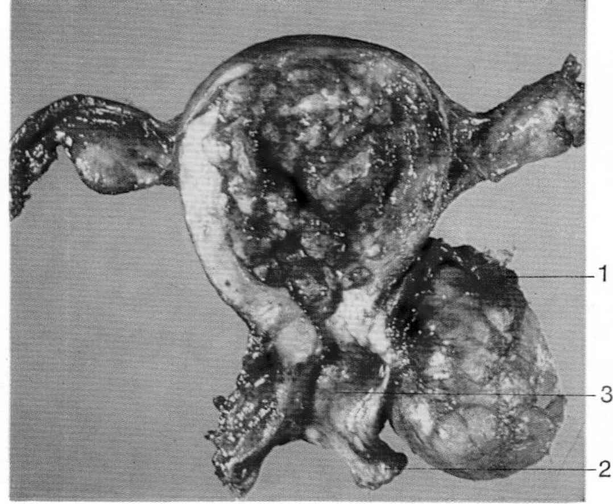

Fig. 15.13. Carcinoma of the corpus with infiltration of the parametrium.

Uterine Tumors

Carcinomas of the uterus. *Three types are distinguished according to location, histologic appearance and behavior: carcinomas of the cervix (85%), carcinomas of the endometrium (10%) and carcinomas of the exocervix (5%).*

Carcinoma of the cervix (Figs. 15.10–15.13; TCP, p. 253). *A squamous-cell or undifferentiated carcinoma developing in the area of the squamocolumnar junction of the exocervical os.* The fully developed squamous-cell carcinoma shows gross and microscopic evidence of infiltrative growth. The tumor is medium-firm and nodular or ulcerated. Cervical carcinomas sometimes are described as exophytic (everting) or endophytic (inverting) tumors. The more common *exophytic* carcinoma presents as a nodular, papillary or cauliflower-like mass growing from one lip of the cervix. The tumor bleeds freely; its superficial portions become necrotic and ulcerate. The *endophytic* carcinoma grows predominantly downward into the stroma and produces a rigid, large and sometimes nodular cervix. Figure 15.11 shows the opened uterus with a cauliflower-like cervical carcinoma (→1). The tumor was excised broadly, including the upper vagina (→2).

F: cervical carcinomas constitute approximately 16% of all malignant tumors in females. Moreover, 75% of all malignant tumors of the female genital tract occur in the area of the uterine collum.

A: the peak incidence of cervical carcinoma is around 45 years, although younger females (past 20 years of age) may develop cervical cancer. *Pg*: cervical carcinomas are uncommon in Jews and nuns but frequent in Negroes. This ethnic distribution is explained on the basis of "preventive" circumcision in males, exposure to early intercourse and the possible carcinogenic action of smegma. Genetic factors probably are operative as well.

Carcinoma in situ (preinvasive carcinoma or stage 0 carcinoma) is considered a precursor of the infiltrative cervical carcinoma (TCP, p. 253). *Spread of cervical carcinoma:* local spread to endocervical canal → uterine corpus and vagina → parametrium and later rectum, urinary bladder and pelvic bones. An example of extensive infiltration of the spine and pelvic bones by a cervical carcinoma is illustrated in Figure 15.12. Cervical carcinomas also metastasize to the iliac and para-aortic lymph nodes; hematogenous metastases to the liver or lungs are found later. Infiltration of the ureter and development of pyelonephritis are common and serious complications of cervical carcinomas.

The following stages of cervical carcinomas are distinguished:

Stage 0: so-called carcinoma in situ.

Stage I: carcinoma confined to the cervix (lymph node metastases are detectable in 2% of micro carcinomas and in 20% of small but grossly recognizable carcinomas).

Stage II: tumor has extended beyond the cervix; infiltration of the corpus and the upper two-thirds of the vagina.

Stage III: infiltration of the parametrium, pelvic wall or lower third of the vagina.

Stage IV: infiltration of the rectum and urinary bladder; metastases to distant organs.

Carcinoma of the endometrium (Fig. 15.13). *An adenocarcinoma of the uterine endometrium that grows predominantly into the uterine cavity.* Figure 15.13 shows the opened uterus, fallopian tubes and ovaries. The endometrial lining of the uterine corpus appears thickened, nodular, irregular and gray-red. The lumen of the uterine cavity was almost occluded by this tissue. Several larger tumor metastases are found in the left parametrium (→1) and fallopian tube. The cervical canal (→2) is smooth although somewhat dilated (→3).

F: carcinomas of the endometrium account for approximately 10% of all malignant epithelial uterine tumors and 5% of all malignancies in women. *A:* 50–65 years (somewhat older age group than cervical cancer!). *Co:* endometrial carcinomas remain confined to the site of origin for some time but sooner or later infiltrate the myometrium and parametrium as well as regional lymph nodes. *Mi:* 90% are well-differentiated or papillary adenocarcinomas; the remainder are *adenoacanthomas* (tumors containing nests of squamous-cell carcinoma and adenocarcinoma). *Pg:* adenomatous hyperplasia of the endometrium is observed in 80% of the patients prior to the development of a carcinoma. Excessive and prolonged ovarian estrogen stimulation of the endometrium *(hyperestrinism)*, including granulosa-theca cell tumors of the ovary → adenomatous hyperplasia → in-situ adenocarcinoma → invasive adenocarcinoma. Many patients developing endometrial carcinoma are nulliparous, obese, hypertensive and suffer from diabetes mellitus!

Adenocarcinoma of the cervix. This rare adenocarcinoma develops in the cervical canal and extends from there to the exocervix and uterine body. The advanced stage of a cervical adenocarcinoma is difficult to distinguish from cervical squamous-cell carcinoma on gross examination.

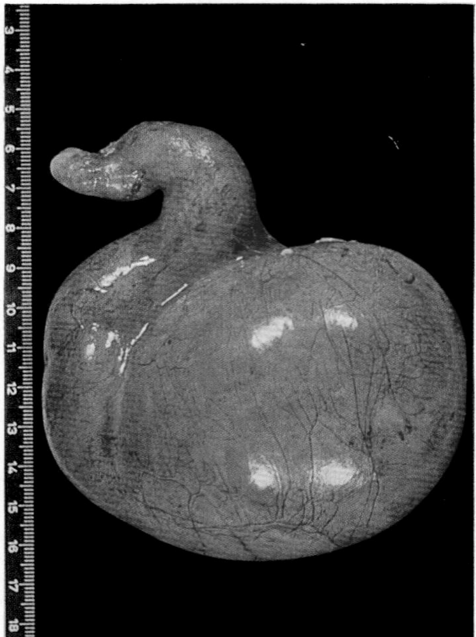

Fig. 15.14. Hydrosalpinx.

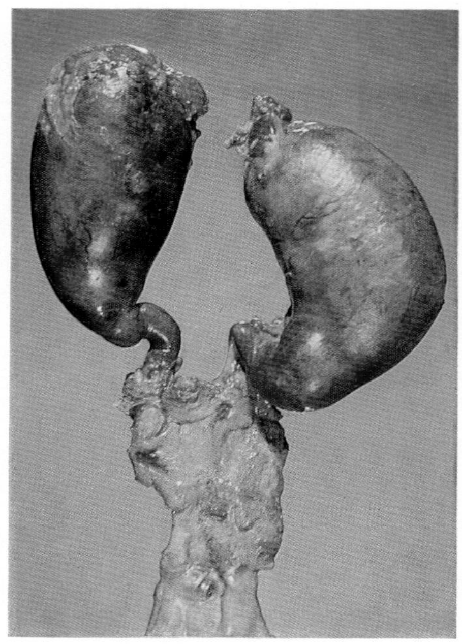

Fig. 15.15. Pyosalpinx.

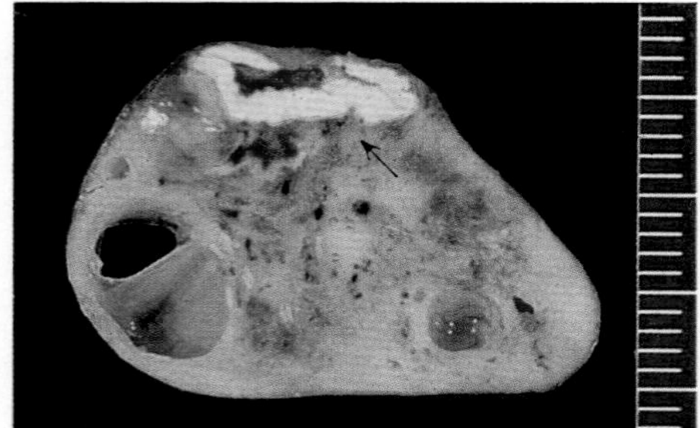

Fig. 15.16. Ovary with corpus luteum and follicle cysts.

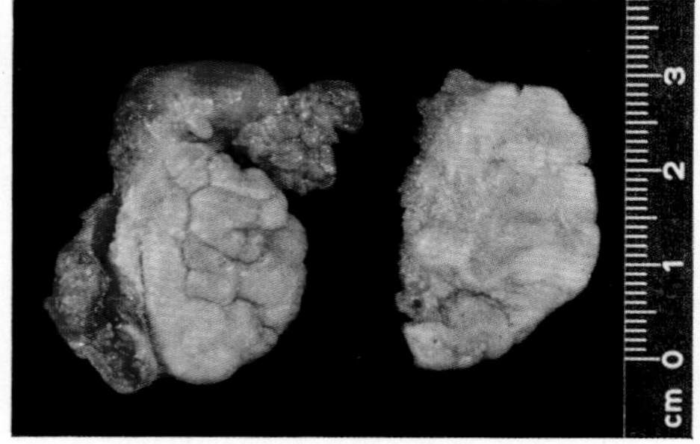

Fig. 15.17. Senile involution of the ovaries.

Tubes and Ovaries

Hydrosalpinx (Fig. 15.14). *Saccular distention of the fallopian tubes by sterile, serous fluid.* There are no signs of inflammation in the paper-thin, smooth wall (Fig. 15.14). Hydrosalpinx is a common accidental finding of unknown etiology.

Pyosalpinx. Figure 15.15 shows markedly distended, sausage-shaped tubes and the opened uterine cavity. The tubes were filled with creamy pus.

Pg: pyosalpinx most often is the result of an ascending inflammation (salpingitis); it is less commonly due to spread of pelvic or abdominal inflammations of the tubes (appendicitis or diverticulitis of the colon). Pyosalpinx is caused by staphylococci, streptococci or *E. coli*. *Hematosalpinx* is a blood-filled tube, seen in tubal pregnancy or abortion. *Tuberculous salpingitis* is the most frequent manifestation of genital tuberculosis.

Normal ovary (Fig. 15.16). The size, shape and weight of the ovaries are dependent on age. During the reproductive years, an ovary measures between 25 and 50 mm. in length. The ovaries weigh 11–15 Gm. They are attached to the anterior surface of the broad ligament by a peritoneal fold (mesovarium; see Fig. 15.21). The ovaries are glistening, convoluted and gray-white externally. Graafian follicles and yellow-orange corpora lutea may be visible through the external surface. Cut sections through the ovaries vary with age. Figure 15.16 shows a large corpus luteum (1.5 cm. in diameter) with a scalloped, bright yellow wall (→). In addition, there are present several corpora albicantia (white, fibrillar), luteinized atretic follicles (yellow-brown) and follicle cysts (left lower margin).

Menstrual corpus luteum. Following menstruation, a fresh corpus luteum with a central, dark red hematoma can be observed in most specimens. The granulosa and theca interna cells rapidly accumulate lipids after the follicle has ruptured. This corpus luteum wall is up to 3 mm. thick and consists of yellow granulosa-lutein and theca-lutein cells. The involution of the corpus luteum begins 6 days prior to the onset of menstruation. Within 6 weeks, the corpus luteum has been transformed into a *corpus albicans*. The *corpus luteum of pregnancy* is larger (>20 mm.) than the menstrual corpus luteum.

Ovarian cysts develop from a corpus luteum, graafian follicle or germinal epithelium. The *hemorrhagic corpus luteum* cyst is the result of excessive hemorrhage into a corpus luteum. Such cysts are larger than 3 cm. in diameter in contrast to the normal corpus luteum. Follicle cysts are smooth walled and rarely exceed 5 cm. in diameter. The inner wall often is lined by granulosa and/or theca cells *(granulosa-theca cysts)*. Follicle cysts sometimes are multiple, occupying most of the ovarian cortex *(polycystic ovary)*. *Germinal inclusion cysts* develop from invaginated, nipped-off ovarian surface epithelium ("germinal epithelium"). They are tiny cortical cysts of menopausal ovaries.

The *Stein-Leventhal syndrome* is characterized by oligomenorrhea or amenorrhea, mild virilism (hirsutism), sterility, a hypoplastic uterus and an enlarged clitoris. The ovaries are bilaterally enlarged, pale gray and coarsely nodular. The cut surface has a thicker than normal, sclerotic surface layer and a row of cystic follicles beneath it. The cysts are atretic graafian follicles lined by granulosa cells. The sclerotic outer cortex prevents ovulation. Therefore, corpora lutea are not formed. Wedge resection restores normal menses and fertility.

Senile involution of the ovary (atrophy, Fig. 15.17). The ovaries are small, firm, gray-white and superficially gyrated. Figure 15.17 shows the external and cut surfaces of a senile ovary. Some corpora albicantia can be identified. *Premature ovarian atrophy* may result from pressure (e.g., leiomyomas), emaciation or occasionally from surgical removal of the uterus.

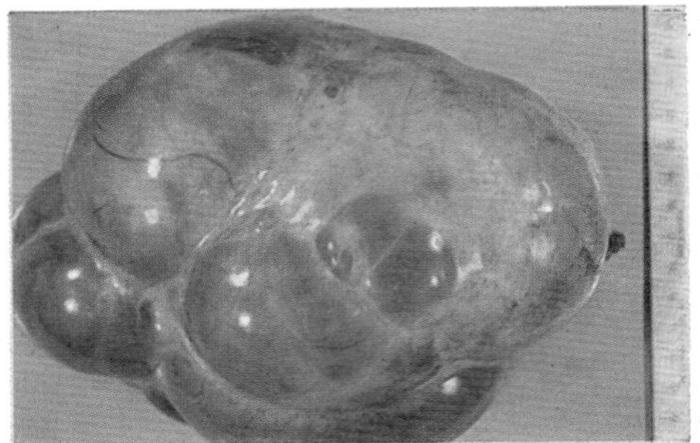
Fig. 15.18. Multilocular, serous cystadenoma of the ovary.

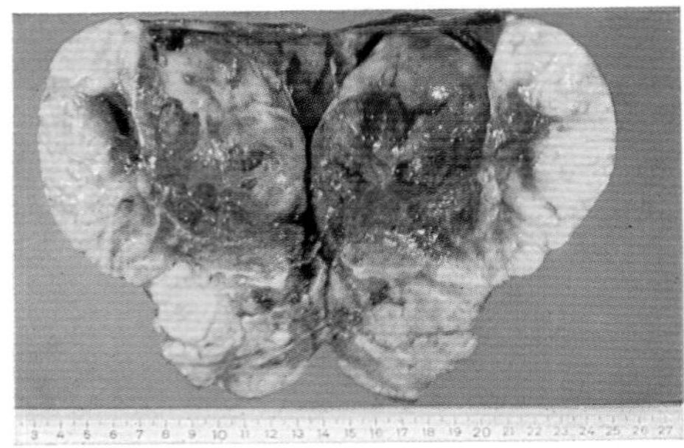
Fig. 15.19. Cystadenocarcinoma of the ovaries.

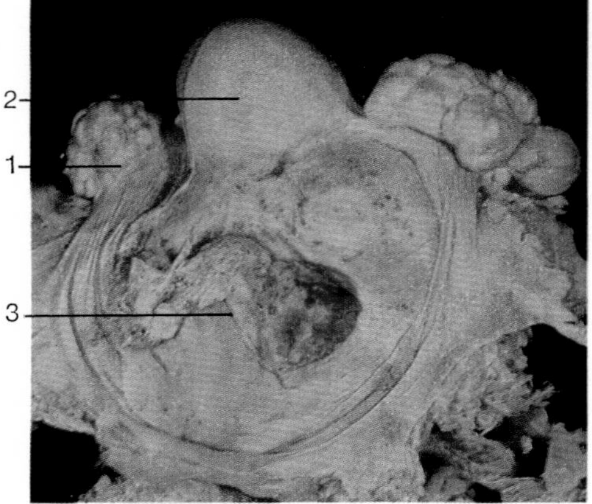

Fig. 15.20. Krukenberg tumor.

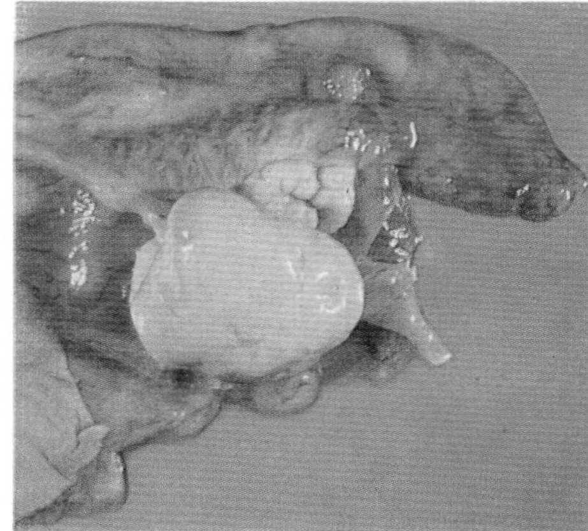
Fig. 15.21. Ovarian fibroma.

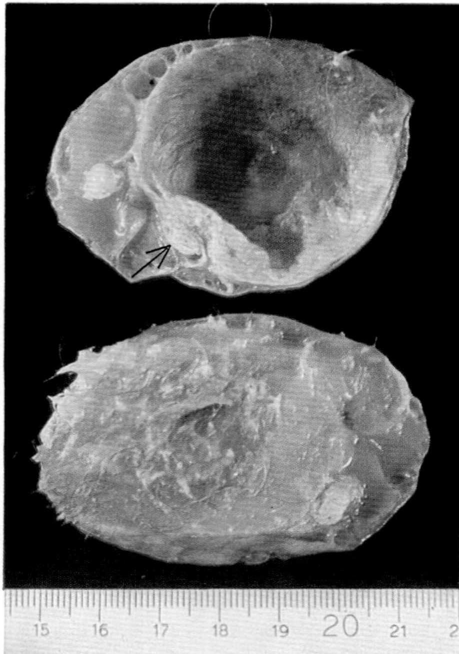
Fig. 15.22. Dermoid cysts of the ovaries.

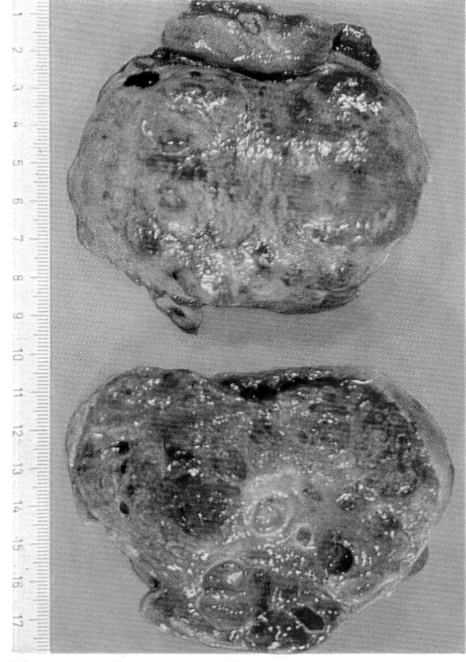
Fig. 15.23. Struma ovarii.

Ovarian Tumors

Cystadenomas of the ovary (Figs. 15.18 and 15.19; TCP, p. 243). *Unilocular or multilocular cystic tumors lined by a flat or papillary epithelium. The tumor cells elaborate pseudomucinous or serous fluid (pseudomucinous or serous cystadenomas).* A multilocular serous cystadenoma is shown in Figure 15.18. The wall is paper thin, glistening, smooth, gray-white or tinged blue. Larger blood vessels traverse the tense wall. The normal ovarian stroma is recognized as the gray-red, solid portion of the tumor.

A: the peak frequencies are 40–60 years for serous cystadenomas and 30–50 years for pseudomucinous cystadenomas. *Pg:* cystadenomas are tumors derived from the surface epithelium of the ovary. *Co:* hemorrhages into the cyst lumen; torsion and subsequent hemorrhagic infarction; rupture *(pseudomucinous cystadenoma → pseudomyxoma peritonei)*. In patients past 30 years of age, 25% of serous cystadenomas and 5% of pseudomucinous cystadenomas become malignant. Figure 15.19 is an example of a serous cystadenocarcinoma. The wall of the large cyst is irregularly thickened and contains soft, friable, partly hemorrhagic, partly gray-white tumor tissue.

Carcinoma of the ovary. Carcinomas develop either de novo or from pre-existing cystadenomas. They are divided into solid, adenomatous or papillary types according to histologic structure. Fifty per cent of ovarian carcinomas involve both ovaries (as do serous cystadenomas!). *Co:* peritoneal carcinomatosis is present at autopsy in 90% of the cases. In addition, metastases to lymph nodes, liver and lung are observed frequently.

Psammomatous carcinomas are papillary ovarian carcinomas with multiple calcifications (psammoma bodies) in the tumor tissue (TCP, p. 237).

Special types of ovarian tumors: (1) *Brenner tumors (oophoroma)* usually are benign, solid or small-cystic ovarian tumors that occur after menopause. Brenner tumors are without hormonal effects. (2) *Granulosa-cell tumors* are soft, yellowish ovarian tumors and are fairly common during the reproductive years or after menopause (approximately 10% of solid ovarian neoplasms). Metastases are observed in 20% of the cases. Granulosa-cell tumors produce estrogens (children → precocious puberty; adults → hyperplasia of endometrium). (3) *Theca-cell tumors* often are associated with granulosa-cell tumors and produce estrogens. (4) *Arrhenoblastomas* are benign, virilizing tumors of young females. (5) *Dysgerminomas* are malignant, radiosensitive "seminomas" of young girls (see p. 289).

Krukenberg tumor (Fig. 15.20). *Metastases of genital or extragenital tumors to both ovaries.* Frequent primary sites are the stomach, small or large intestine, gallbladder and breast. Figure 15.20 shows extensive metastases in the ovaries (→1), the anterior wall of the uterus (→2) and the peritoneum of the retro-uterine space (→3) from a scirrhous signet-ring-cell carcinoma of the stomach. The ovaries are enlarged by irregular metastatic tumor nodules.

Fibromas of the ovary are benign tumors that may contain doubly refractile, lipid-containing cells *(fibroma thecacellulare xanthomatodes)*. Figure 15.21 shows a firm, white, nodular fibroma.

F: mesenchymal tumors account for one-third of all ovarian neoplasms. An ovarian fibroma may cause ascites and bilateral hydrothorax *(Meigs' syndrome)*.

Teratoma (Figs. 15.22 and 15.23; TCP, p. 257). *Differentiated or undifferentiated tumors derived from the three germ cell layers.* Teratomas are divided into:

1. Cystic teratomas, which contain various organoid structures corresponding to the age of the host. Some teratomas differentiate into epidermis with appendages, gastrointestinal or respiratory epithelium, neural tissue and others. Others show only unidirectional differentiation, such as the common *dermoid cyst.* A dermoid cyst is lined by epidermis with hair follicles and sebaceous glands. Figure 15.22 shows the lumen of a dermoid cyst with sebaceous materials and hair. After removal of the cyst content, the inner surface usually reveals a slightly projecting thickening of the wall (→). This ridge often is composed of derivatives of the three germ cell layers. The *struma ovarii* likewise is a unidirectional teratoma composed only of thyroid gland. Figure 15.23 shows an ovary with large cysts containing brownish, glistening, colloid-like content. A struma ovarii can cause hyperthyroidism in rare instances.

2. Solid or *embryonal* teratomas are malignant teratomas. They are rare in the ovary (in contrast to the testes).

F: the dermoid cyst is the most common tumor of the ovary, especially during the reproductive years. *Pg:* see parasitic malformations, page 333. *Co:* primarily benign, cystic teratomas may become malignant (carcinomas or sarcomas in the thickened wall composed of the three germ cell layers).

16. Pregnancy
Fetal and Neonatal Pathology

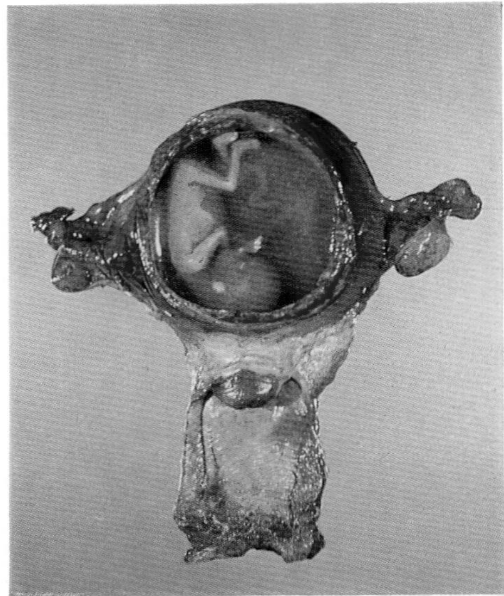

Fig. 16.1. Eutopic pregnancy.

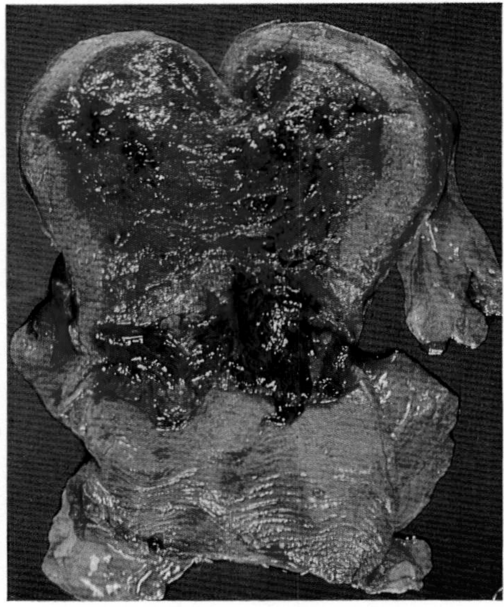

Fig. 16.2. Puerperal uterus.

Pregnancy

Normal or eutopic pregnancy. The fertilized egg normally is implanted in the anterior or posterior wall of the uterine fundus. In Figure 16.1, the anterior uterine wall has been removed to demonstrate chorion, fetus and fruit water.

The endometrium of the uterine corpus transforms into the decidua following fertilization. The decidua is poorly developed in the uterine isthmus and cervical region (present in only 25% of pregnancies). The decidua grossly is divided into the superficial *decidua capsularis*, the deep *decidua basalis* and the *decidua marginalis* (next to the implantation site). The residual decidua is referred to as the *decidua parietalis.*

Placenta. The mature human placenta is discoid, measures 16–20 cm. in diameter, 2–3 cm. in thickness and weighs approximately 500 Gm. (or $^1/_6$ of the fetal body weight). The umbilical cord roughly corresponds to the length of the fetus (50 cm.). The chorion (external covering of the egg) forms chorionic villi that are divided into an internal layer *(Langhans' layer* or *cytotrophoblast)* and an external layer *(syncytiotrophoblast)*. The lateral and uterine villi become atrophic after the sixtieth day of pregnancy *(chorion laeve)*. The *chorion frondosum* is formed by villi that are in contact with the decidua and which become large and dendritic. The decidua basalis is separated from the chorion frondosum by the *layer of Nitabuch*, an eosinophilic zone of fibrin-like material with a protective function against the histolytic action of the egg.

Diseases or abnormalities of the placenta (placentopathies) include:

1. *Infarctions*, which are found in practically all otherwise normal placentas. The "white infarction" is not a true infarction but subchorionic fibrinoid changes and fibrin deposits. Only "red infarctions" are due to thrombosis of intervillous spaces.

2. "*Polyps*," which develop following incomplete separation of the placenta. In fact, "polyps" represent remnants of the placenta in the uterine cavity covered by blood, fibrin and thrombi. *Co:* endometritis → metrorrhagia.

3. *Changes in the shape and size of the placenta* (pl.). The pl. *annulare* (ring pl.) is the result of atrophy of central villi. Pl. *accreta* and *increta* are different degrees of abnormal adherence to the myometrium. The pl. *marginalis* has a smaller fetal than maternal surface. The fetal surface is reduced to a mere central depression in the pl. *circumvallata*. The pl. *membranacea* is a very thin, flat structure. The pl. *multilobulata* is a multilobed pl.; the pl. *succenturiata* has one or more accessory lobes.

4. Ectopic location (see p. 303, extrauterine pregnancy).

5. *Inflammations* (placentitis) involve the fetal membranes *(chorioamnionitis)* and the decidua basalis. Placentitis is the result of sepsis, pyemia or specific inflammations, such as *syphilis*. The rare giant placenta of syphilis weighs more than 700 Gm.; the villi are bulbous, edematous and hyperplastic. Other specific inflammations are *tuberculosis* (especially miliary tuberculosis), *toxoplasmosis* (pale, spongy, edematous placenta), *listeriosis* (necrosis, granuloma and argyrophilic listeria organisms). *Omphalitis* refers to an umbilical inflammation; *omphalophlebitis* is an inflammation of the umbilical vein (see also p. 159).

6. In *erythroblastosis*, the placenta is pale red, greatly thickened and weighs from 1,000 to 2,000 Gm. The maternal surface has large, friable cotyledons. See Figure 16.3.

7. *Hydramnios* is an increase in the amount of amniotic fluid ($>$2,000 ml.) due to erythroblastosis, fetal cardiac malformations, congestion of the umbilical vein (from stenosis or cord nodules) or an abnormal fetal position. *Oligohydramnios:* $<$ 500 ml. of amniotic fluid.

8. *Tumors*. The *chorioangioma* is a rare, vasoformative tumor composed of multiple capillaries.

Puerperal uterus. Figure 16.2 shows an opened uterus 3 days postpartum. The endometrial surface is irregularly dark red from hemorrhages and fresh blood clots. The separation of the placenta takes place in the spongy layer of the decidua basalis. The inner surface of the uterine cavity is without epithelium for a few days. Blood lymph and leukocytes *(lochia)* are secreted during this period. The uterine cavity is completely re-epithelialized within 3 weeks.

The most important infection of the puerperal uterus is *puerperal* fever, which is manifested by:

1. *Puerperal endometritis:* (bacteria invade puerperal wound → inflammation of remnants of decidua) and

2. *Pelvic and/or femoral thrombophlebitis:* (septic thrombi → phlegmasia alba dolens or "milk leg," a thrombophlebitis of leg veins). Septic abortions → endotoxin shock (see Fig. 13.23).

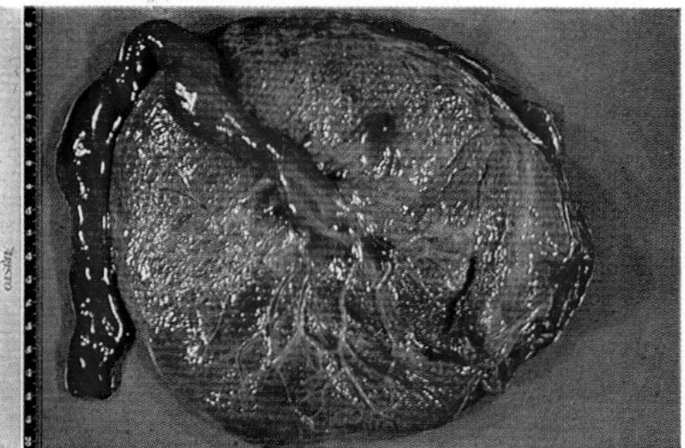

Fig. 16.3. Placenta in erythroblastosis (hemolytic disease of newborns).

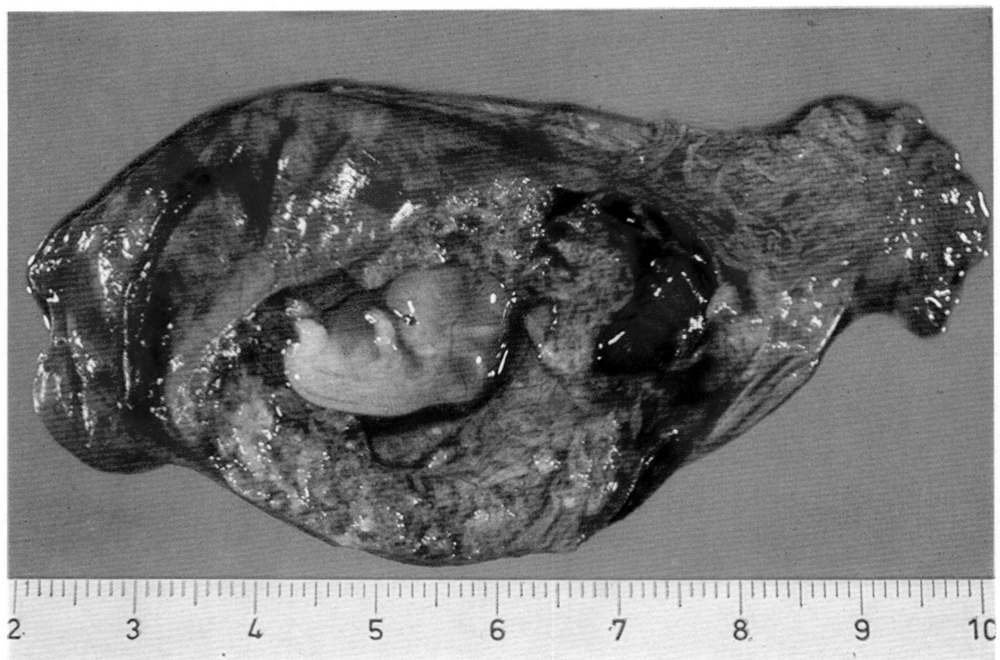

Fig. 16.4. Tubal pregnancy.

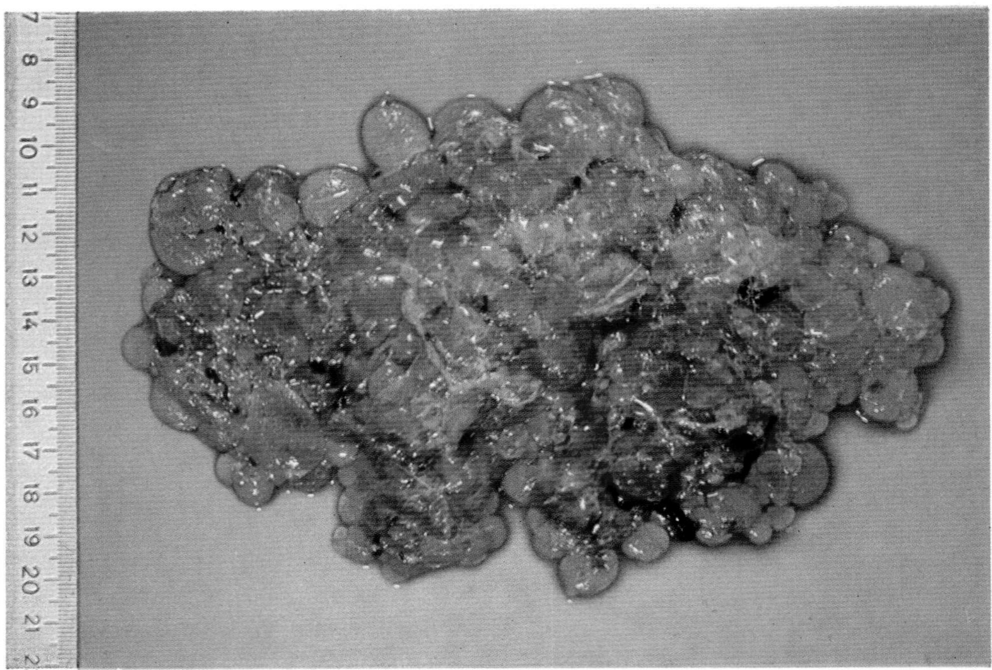

Fig. 16.5. Hydatidiform mole.

Placenta praevia refers to an atypical placentation in the uterine cavity. The placenta covers the internal os partially or completely. Delivery cannot be initiated under such circumstances. *Co:* severe hemorrhages of mother and fetus → shock → consumption coagulopathy.

Extrauterine pregnancy (Fig. 16.4). Tubal pregnancy is the most common type of extrauterine pregnancy. A markedly distended tube with a 2 cm.-long embryo is shown in Figure 16.4. Note the extensive tubal hemorrhages. Other locations of extrauterine pregnancy are the ovary and peritoneal cavity (either primary or secondary after tubal abortion). *Co:* tubal abortion and rupture → acute massive hemorrhage. As a rule, these complications occur during the first 3–4 months (especially during the 4th–8th weeks) of pregnancy.

Lithopedion is a rare outcome of an intrauterine or extrauterine pregnancy. The fetus is not expelled but becomes necrotic and mummifies. Complete "stone" formation is rare. A lithopedion usually is found in the abdominal cavity.

Hydatidiform mole (Fig. 16.5; TCP, p. 193). *A cystic, hydropic swelling of the chorionic villi and proliferation of the chorionic epithelium, especially the Langhans cells.* The uterus is markedly enlarged and contains multiple grape-like, translucent and friable clusters of chorionic villi (Fig. 16.5).

F: approximately 0.5–1% of pregnancies. *Co:* hydatidiform moles are, in most cases, spontaneously delivered between the 3d and 5th months of pregnancy. *Pg:* see TCP, page 193. *Cl:* the uterus is larger than expected for the time of pregnancy. Abnormal bleeding is common. Increased levels of chorionic gonadotropin in blood and urine. *Co:* approximately 5% of hydatidiform moles become choriocarcinomas.

Chorioadenoma destruens is a malignant variant of the hydatidiform mole. The chorionic villi infiltrate the myometrium but do not metastasize. *Co:* rupture of the uterus.

Choriocarcinoma (chorioepithelioma; TCP, p. 255). *A highly malignant, hormone-producing tumor of trophoblastic origin.* The tumor is characterized by large, friable, pale white or dark red, soft and sometimes cystic nodules in the uterine cavity, especially in the area of placentation.

Choriocarcinomas develop most often in the area of nidation either as an early or late complication of a hydatidiform mole (50–60% of choriocarcinomas) or after a full-term pregnancy. The latent period between pregnancy and the appearance of a choriocarcinoma may be as long as 10 years. Cases of choriocarcinomas have been observed to develop in patients after menopause. *Co:* direct spread to parametrial tissues. Hematogenous metastases to the liver, lung, vagina, kidneys, spleen and other organs. Some metastases, as well as the primary tumor, may regress spontaneously (immune response against foreign trophoblastic antigens?).

The *ectopic choriocarcinoma* develops in sites other than the area of nidation, usually from displaced villi of a hydatidiform mole. A common location is the vagina, rarely the ovaries, liver and gut.

F: estimates range from 1/13,000 to 1/100,000 pregnancies. More common in Asiatic females!

Fetal and Neonatal Pathology

The autopsy technic for a fetus or newborn differs only slightly from that used for adults. The body is weighed; standing and sitting heights are measured. The age of a fetus can be estimated from the body length (Haase's rule; see below). Likewise, the degree of maturity can be derived from certain external signs (see below). The skin is examined carefully for evidence of cyanosis, jaundice, macerations, injuries or skin lesions. External malformations are not uncommon and should be searched for (e.g., face: mongolism, renal agenesis?; extremities; syndactyly, etc.?; anus: perforation, exudates?). Internal organs are removed in blocks (heart-lungs-great vessels, gastrointestinal tract, kidneys-urinary tract, etc.). Umbilicus (omphalitis?), umbilical artery, umbilical vein (later: ligamentum teres), ductus omphaloentericus (Meckel's diverticulum!) and urachus are examined. Look for evidence of birth trauma during dissection of the skull and brain. The method of choice for opening the skull is to cut a large window into each parietal bone so that the falx cerebri and tentorium are preserved (lacerations, hemorrhages → birth trauma!) See Figure 16.9.

Haase has suggested that the length of the embryo (in centimeters) can be approximated during the first 5 months by squaring the number of the month of pregnancy. For example, body length at the end of the 3d month is 9 cm. (3×3). After the 5th month, body length is determined by multiplying the month by 5 (e.g., end of 9th month: $9 \times 5 = 45$ cm.) (Haase's rule).

Fetal age, organ development and organ differentiation (according to Essbach).

Age	Organ development
Embryo: up to 12 weeks of pregnancy	
Week 2	Heart, pronephros, medullary groove
Weeks 2–4	Mesonephros
Weeks 2–5	Liver
Weeks 3–4	Extremity buds
Weeks 3–5	Atrial septum
Weeks 3–8	Spleen
Weeks 5–7	Closure of diaphragm
Week 7	Closure of palate
Weeks 7–8	Testes
Week 8	Ventricular septum
Weeks 9–10	Ovaries, external genitalia
Fetus: after the 3d month of pregnancy	
Month 5	Head and lanugo hair
Month 7	Vernix caseosa
Signs of maturity after birth (after the 10th month of pregnancy)	
Body length	48–52 cm.
Body weight	3,000–3,600 Gm.
Lanugo hair	Present only around the shoulders. Hair of head approximately 12 cm. long. Eyelids and eyebrows present
Umbilicus	Between symphysis and manubrium of sternum
Nails	Reach the tips of fingers and toes
Bone	Ossification of diaphysis. Bony nuclei are present in vertebrae, epiphyseal tibia and femur (Béclard's distal femoral epiphysis is 5 mm. in diameter). Skull is hard
Bone of nose and ear cartilage	Firm
In boys	Testes descended, wrinkled scrotal skin
In girls	Clitoris and labia minora are covered by labia majora

Fetal and neonatal diseases

Most fetal and neonatal diseases are discussed in the appropriate organ chapters in this book. The following discussion is confined to definitions.

Delivery. The product of conception may be delivered viable or nonviable. Formerly, a distinction between deadbirth and stillbirth was made (absence of heartbeat, gross respiration and voluntary extremity movement). According to a recommendation by the World Health Organization, the term fetal death is substituted for stillbirth and defined as death prior to complete expulsion or extraction from the mother, irrespective of the duration of pregnancy.

Premature infants are defined as live births prior to the 37th week of pregnancy. The body weight is 2,500 Gm. or less and the crown-heel length does not exceed 47 cm. *F:* approximately 7% of all live births are premature. *Pg:* inflammations, trauma, twins, uterine myomas. The etiology remains unknown in 50% of premature infants.

Abortion is defined as expulsion of the fetus prior to the 28th week of pregnancy. According to other definitions, an abortion refers to a fetal weight of no more than 1,000 Gm. A stillbirth is defined as a nonlive birth after the 27th week of pregnancy with a maximal body length of 35 cm.

Early abortion: Gestational age less than 22 weeks; weight less than 400 Gm., length less than 28 cm.

Complete abortion: Complete delivery of all parts of the product of conception (amnion, fetus and placenta).

Incomplete abortion: Only parts expelled. Usually the placenta is retained after the 4th month of pregnancy.

Missed abortion: This term is applied when the chorionic vesicle is retained in the uterus for several weeks or months after death of the fetus. The fetus may be absorbed with very early missed abortions. At a later period of pregnancy, the fetus becomes macerated or shrinks because of water loss *(fetus papyraceus).*

Complicated abortion: An abortion complicated by inflammation of surrounding organs (myometritis, parametritis).

Pg: aside from a therapeutically induced or criminal abortion, *early abortions* are attributable to fetal malformations, disturbances of nidation or genetic factors. Repeated, *habitual abortion* after the 4th month of pregnancy may be due to syphilis, trauma, hormonal dysfunction or other factors.

The causes of intrauterine death or stillbirth may be difficult to determine at autopsy. In addition, certain morphologic findings in fetal deaths (aspiration of amniotic fluid or pulmonary hemorrhages) are not necessarily the immediate causes of death.

Common morphologic findings in fetal deaths (according to Zschoch and Mahnke)

Finding	%
Aspiration of amniotic fluid	60%
Pulmonary hemorrhages	41%
Hypoxia	33%
Trauma during delivery	33%
Malformation	20%

Causes of fetal or neonatal deaths (according to Mehlan, cited by Zschoch and Mahnke)

Cause	%
Fetal causes	42.5%
Premature birth	10.3%
Malformations	9.9%
Complications of umbilical cord	9.0%
Asphyxia	4.8%
Anomalies of the placenta	3.8%
Aspiration of amniotic fluid	2.1%
Intracranial hemorrhage and tentorium tear	1.5%
Rh incompatibility	1.1%
Maternal causes	12.7%
Abnormal delivery	10.0%
Eclampsia and toxemia	1.7%
Listeriosis, toxoplasmosis and congenital syphilis	0.5%
Chronic diseases (including diabetes)	0.5%
Diagnosis "stillbirth" without specific causes	44.8%

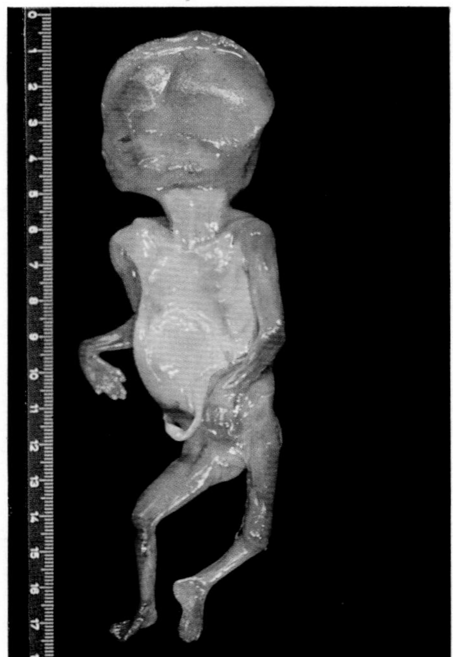

Fig. 16.6. Macerated stillbirth.

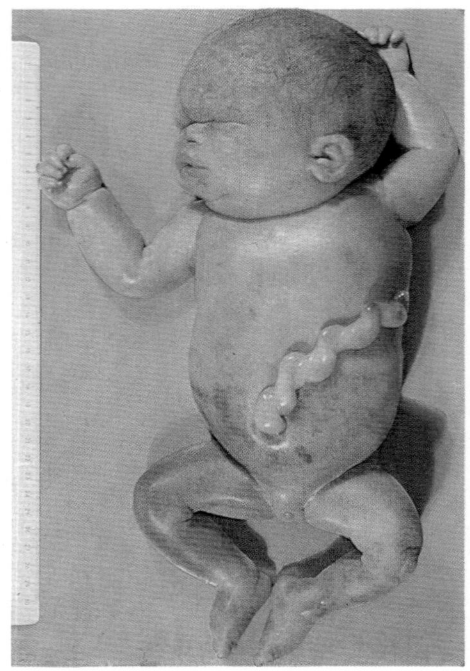

Fig. 16.7. Congenital hydrops.

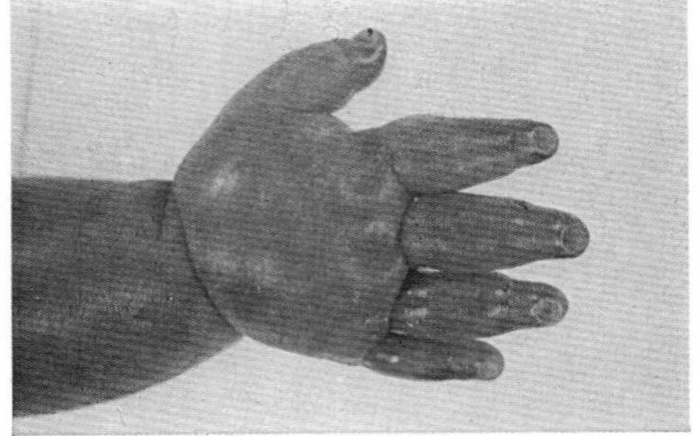

Fig. 16.8. Edema of hand in congenital hydrops.

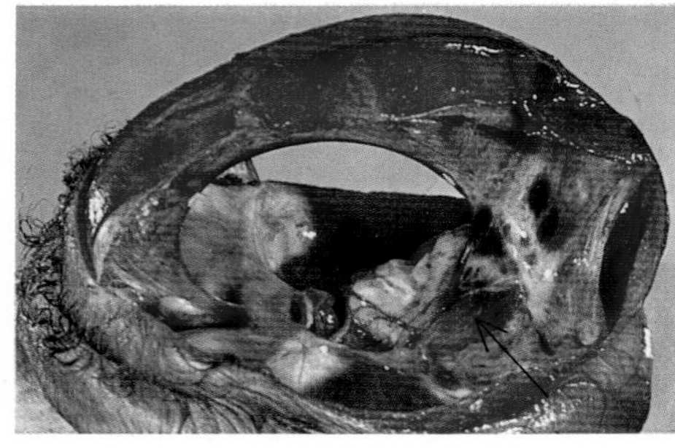

Fig. 16.9. Tear in the tentorium.

Maceration (Fig. 16.6). *Abacterial, enzymatic autolysis of intrauterine death.* Figure 16.6 shows the wrinkled skin and separated strips of epidermis.

F: see page 305. *Pg:* early after intrauterine death, the epidermis is loosened and then separated from the dermis ("skin slipping"). Fluid accumulates beneath the epidermis to produce large bullae. Finally, there is extensive autolysis of the skin and internal organs.

Congenital hydrops is a *generalized edema in the soft parts, especially the abdominal walls, dorsum of hands and feet, eyelids, scrotum or labia.* Figures 16.7 and 16.8 are representative of the edematous, resilient skin. A clear fluid exudes when the skin or soft parts are cut. A moderate amount of fluid is found in various body cavities as well. Congenital hydrops is not a disease sui generis but a manifestation of erythroblastosis, cardiac malformations and other diseases (children of diabetic mothers).

1. **Erythroblastosis or hemolytic disease of newborns.** Hemolysis is manifested in utero or shortly after birth. Erythroblastosis is due to an incompatibility between the blood groups of child and mother (incompatibility of Rh factor, rarely of AB0 blood groups).

F: 0.3–0.5% of all newborns. Erythroblastosis accounts for 1% of all perinatal mortality. *Pg:* fetal Rh factor from homozygous father → transplacental passage to Rh-negative mother → maternal antibodies → hemolysis in fetus and newborn. The morbidity regarding AB0 incompatibility is 24% of all marriages (mother has blood group 0 and child has blood group A or B). Erythroblastosis fetalis is relatively uncommon when compared to the statistically expected frequency of at least 10% of all births. This discrepancy is explained as follows: Rh-positive fetal erythrocytes are weakly antigenic, maternal antibody formation is ineffective and slow (therefore, first pregnancy without complications) or the father is heterozygous (only half of the children are Rh positive). The manifestations of erythroblastosis fetalis are:

(a) **Hemolytic anemia** (4% of autopsies) with marked pallor and hepatosplenomegaly from compensatory erythropoiesis in the spleen, liver and bone marrow.

(b) **Icterus gravis** (16% of autopsies). Increased bilirubin levels from hemolysis (up to 50 mg./100 ml.). A bright yellow discoloration (jaundice) of the basal nuclei, thalamus, cerebellum or gray matter of the brain (kernicterus). (*Note:* The yellow pigmentation of kernicterus fades within 1–2 days postmortem; section brain immediately.)

(c) **Congenital hydrops** (80% of autopsies). Most severe form of erythroblastosis due to antigen-antibody reaction in capillaries. Exudation of plasma → anasarca, often with maceration of fetus.

Erythroblastosis also may be associated with a *hemorrhagic disease of newborns.* This disease is characterized by melena and hemorrhages into the skin and mucosal surface. The hemorrhagic tendency is attributable to a prothrombin defect. The causal pathogenesis still is not known.

2. **Infants of diabetic mothers.** Newborns of diabetic or prediabetic mothers are large and heavy because of excessive fat deposits.

F: 0.32% of neonatal deaths during the first 3 months of life. *Pg:* multiple hormonal abnormalities are observed in pregnant diabetics: somatotropic hormone production is increased, insulin synthesis is diminished, chorionic gonadotropin excretion is increased whereas its production is decreased. A maturation defect of the early chorionic villi causes insufficient blood supply of the embryo and fetus → hypoxia as cause of intrauterine fetal mortality? *Co:* fetal or neonatal deaths: 25–60%. However, maternal diabetes does not appear to be a major cause of early abortion.

Laceration of the tentorium (Fig. 16.9). *A tear in the dura covering the cerebellum.* Tentorium lacerations usually are the result of birth trauma. The entire tentorium or falx is torn less commonly than the upper leaf of the tentorium. Figure 16.9 shows a skull that was opened by the bucket-handle technic. The tentorium is characteristically torn at its margin (→).

F: seen in approximately 4.5% of all perinatal deaths. Sixty per cent of cases occur in premature infants (deformity of skull!) or in babies of multiparous women (fast delivery with strong expulsive forces). *Co:* hemorrhages between the leaves of the tentorium; extension of tentorial rent into the straight sinus. Complete bilateral tentorium laceration causes increased pressure of the brain on the cerebellum → cerebellum and pons are pushed into the occipital foramen. See also hemorrhage of terminal veins, page 313.

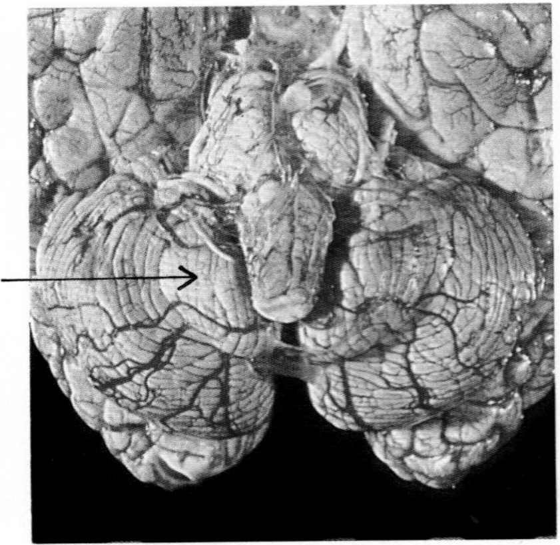

Fig. 17.1. Cerebellar pressure grooves in a case of cerebral edema.

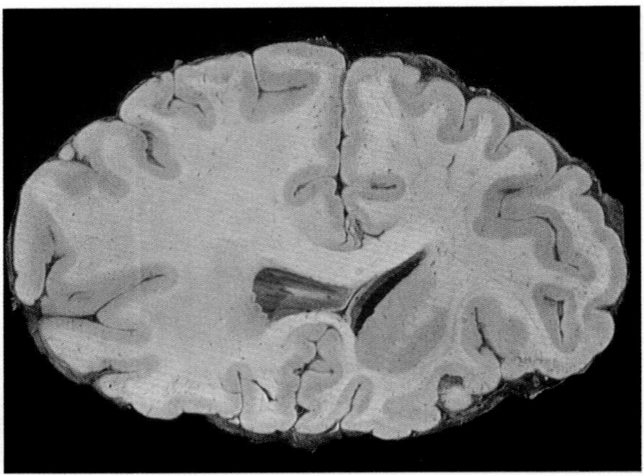

Fig. 17.2. Collateral brain edema.

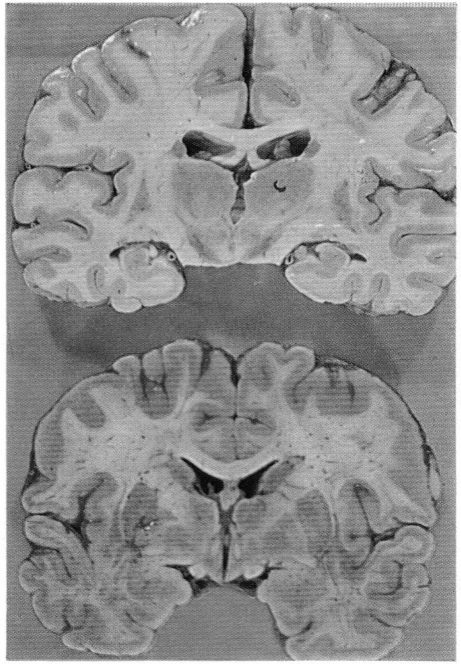

Fig. 17.3. Above: normal brain slice; below: carbon monoxide poisoning.

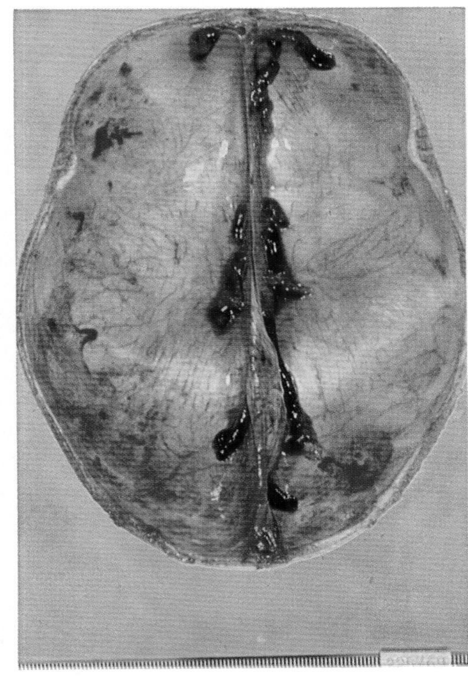

Fig. 17.4. Thrombosis of superior sagittal sinus.

17. Nervous System

Edema of the Brain, CO Poisoning, Thrombosis

Edema of the brain (Fig. 17.1). *An intracerebral collection of fluid occurring mainly in the perivascular spaces, leading to an increased total brain mass.*

The gyri are flattened and the sulci are shallow and compressed. An excessive brain volume increases intracranial pressure. Consequently, the tonsils of the cerebellum herniate into the foramen magnum and a furrow of the cerebellar tonsils is noted after the brain is removed (Fig. 17.1). The edematous brain has a moist, soft cut surface with indistinct vascular markings (increase in fluid). On occasion, an edematous brain is firm and has a dry, dull and sticky cut surface with normal vascular markings. This form of cerebral edema formerly was referred to as "brain swelling." It is observed in diabetics.

Focal or collateral brain edema is observed around tumors or abscesses. Figure 17.2 shows a unilateral brain edema caused by a solitary metastasis from a bronchogenic carcinoma (the metastasis is not shown in this picture). Characteristically, the edema is confined to one hemisphere. The ventricles are displaced laterally. The outlines of the basal nuclei are indistinct.

Pg: hemodynamic cerebral edema is due to blood stasis (e.g., right heart failure → venous congestion → transudate); *permeability edema* is caused by inflammations (increased capillary permeability in inflammatory processes: "serous" encephalitis → exudate). The *Pg* of cerebral edema associated with uremia, eclampsia or liver damage is not known. Cerebral edema also is found to accompany poisoning or cases of sudden death.

Acute carbon monoxide poisoning. Figure 17.3 compares a normal coronal brain section after formalin fixation with a coronal section following CO poisoning. Carbon monoxide poisoning causes a characteristic cherry-pink discoloration of the brain, which is retained following formalin fixation.

F: poisoning from carbon monoxide or sedatives are common causes of cerebral deaths. *Pg:* the CO concentration in illuminating gas is 8% and 4–7% in exhaust gases of internal combustion engines. CO concentrations of 0.2 vol.% in the atmospheric air are fatal. CO has a 300 times higher affinity for hemoglobin than O_2 and thereby forms a stable CO Hb. A concentration of 65% CO Hb in the blood is fatal.

Thrombosis of the superior sagittal sinus. Figure 17.4 shows the internal surface of a skull with the dura mater attached. The opened superior sagittal sinus contains multiple thrombi (predominantly coagulation thrombi). They partly occluded the lumen of the sinus. A bland sinus thrombosis must be distinguished from thrombophlebitis of the sinus. Thrombophlebitis frequently affects the sigmoid and cavernous sinuses.

Pg: bland sinus thrombi occur shortly before death (so-called marantic thrombi) or accompany infectious diseases (measles, scarlet fever and diphtheria). The sinus thrombosis of infectious diseases probably is secondary to cardiovascular failure. Thrombophlebitis of the cerebral sinuses is the result of purulent infections (purulent otitis, mastoiditis, nasal sinusitis and cellulitis of the face, mouth or nose). The infections extend to the cavernous sinus either directly or via the ophthalmic and ethmoid veins. *Co:* thrombophlebitis → purulent meningitis, brain abscess. Infarctions of the cerebral cortex (see p. 313).

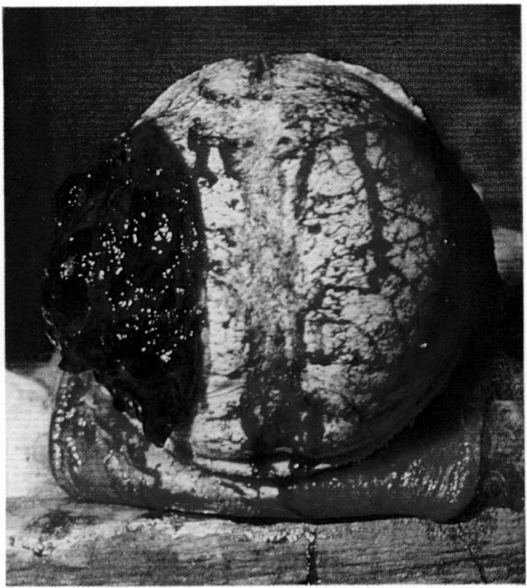

Fig. 17.5. Epidural hematoma.

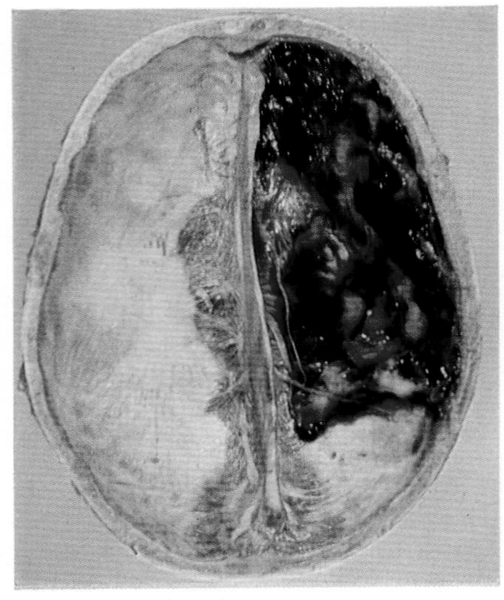

Fig. 17.6. Subdural hematoma.

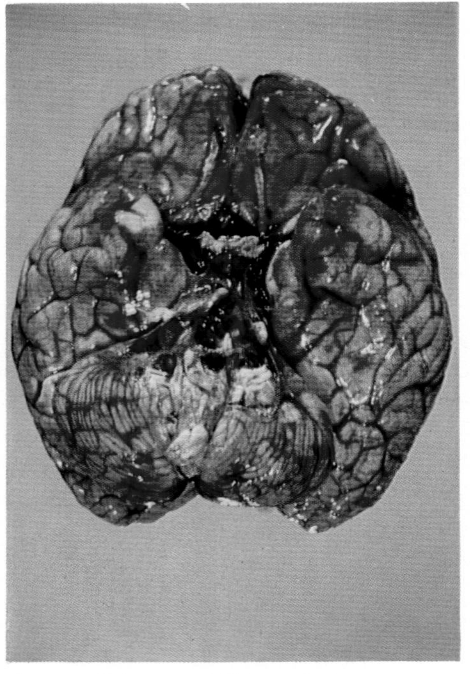

Fig. 17.7. Subarachnoid hemorrhage.

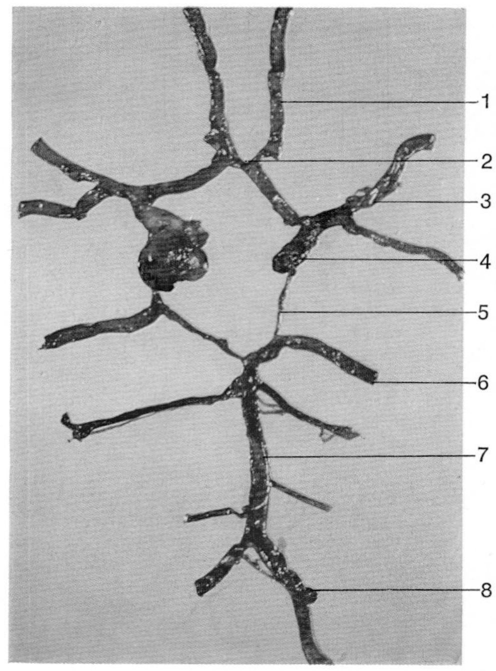

Fig. 17.8. Aneurysm of the internal carotid artery.

Hemorrhages

Epidural hematoma (Fig. 17.5). *A hemorrhage between the skull and the external surface of the dura mater. An epidural hematoma is caused by rupture of the middle meningeal artery, less commonly by lacerations of the sigmoid or transverse sinuses.* Figure 17.5 shows a massive dark red hematoma that adheres to the tense dura.

Pg: skull fracture. *Co:* a short asymptomatic interval follows the trauma until signs of increased intracranial pressure become manifest from a rapidly enlarging epidural hematoma. Death is due to respiratory arrest.

Subdural hematoma (Fig. 17.6). *A hemorrhage between the dura mater and the leptomeninges. Subdural hematomas usually are due to traumatic laceration of superficial brain veins.* Figure 17.6 shows the skull with the internal surface of the dura. An extensive hemorrhage covers the dura. The hemorrhage is unilateral, i.e., confined by the falx cerebri.

F: subdural hematomas are approximately four times more common than epidural hematomas. *Pg:* frequently severe head injuries. *Co:* signs of increased intracranial pressure and traumatic brain damage are the main clinical findings. Occasionally, acute subdural hematomas occur from a ruptured saccular aneurysm.

Subarachnoid hemorrhage (Figs. 17.7 and 17.8). *Extensive nontraumatic hemorrhages in the subarachnoid space (between the arachnoid and the pia mater). The subarachnoid hemorrhage is seen most often in the base of the brain and follows the rupture of an aneurysm of a basal artery.* Figure 17.7 shows a fresh, dark blue-red, basal hemorrhage in the vicinity of the circle of Willis. The circle of Willis was prepared as shown in Figure 17.8. A saccular aneurysm is found at the junction of the internal carotid artery and posterior communicating artery. The aneurysm had ruptured, causing the subarachnoid hemorrhage shown in Figure 17.7.

F: approximately 1% of all autopsies. *A:* rupture of an aneurysm of the basal arteries is observed most commonly between the 40th and 60th years of age (68% of all cases). *S:* ♂:♀ = 1:1.2.

The anatomy of the circle of Willis and the most frequent locations of berry aneurysms are: →1 anterior cerebral artery, →2 anterior communicating artery (45% of all aneurysms), →3 medial cerebral artery with bifurcation (15%), →4 internal carotid artery (15%), →5 posterior communicating artery (3%), →6 posterior cerebral artery (5%), →7 basilar artery (2%) and →8 vertebral artery (5%). *Congenital saccular aneurysms* (berry aneurysms) are the most common cause of subarachnoid hemorrhage. Berry aneurysms vary in size (up to 3–4 cm.) and sometimes are multiple. A coincidence of congenital aneurysms, polycystic kidneys and aortic coarctation has been noted. *Pg:* a congenital weakness of the muscle wall is suspected. Inflammatory changes in the vessel wall *(mycotic aneurysms)* are the result of infected emboli and are much less common than berry aneurysms. *Arteriosclerotic fusiform aneurysms* usually are associated with severe hypertension and sclerosis of the arteries of the circle of Willis.

Chronic subdural hematoma (pachymeningiosis hemorrhagica interna, Fig. 17.9). A highly vascular granulation tissue is present on the internal surface of the dura, especially over the convexity of both hemispheres. The lateral surfaces of the falx cerebri and the upper leaf of the tentorium are affected less commonly. Fresh hemorrhages are bright red to dark red. Older and organized hemorrhages appear brown-yellow or rusty brown from conversion of hemoglobin to hemosiderin (Fig. 17.9). They usually are encapsulated by a pseudomembrane (granulation tissue) and may contain a turbid fluid. The brain is compressed.

A: especially in small children and between 50 and 70 years. *F:* approximately 0.8% of all autopsies. *S:* 70% are ♂ among adults. *Pg:* the history of such patients often reveals minor head injuries (jars, blows), although trauma is not always elicited in the history. The chronic subdural hematoma occurs as a consequence of lacerated or torn bridging veins, with slow leakage of blood into the subdural space. Arteriosclerosis, hemorrhagic tendencies and other diseases (alcoholism) must be considered contributing factors. *Co:* a chronic, progressive disease that becomes clinically manifest by its complications (hemorrhages). *DD:* acute subdural hematoma: major trauma in history, mostly unilateral and not localized over the convexity. The chronic dural hematoma usually is bilateral and almost always affects the convexity.

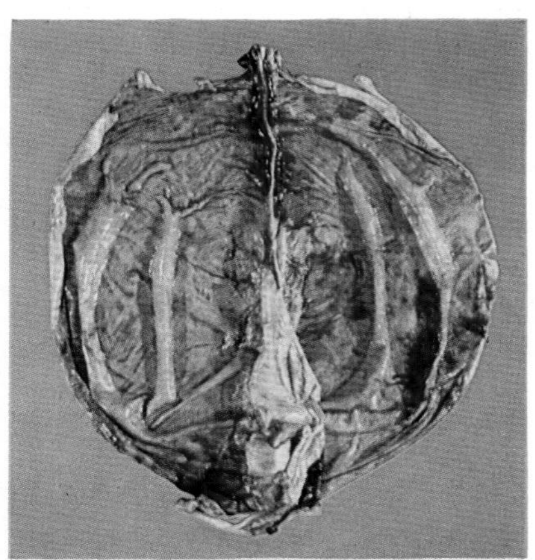

Fig. 17.9. Chronic subdural hematoma.

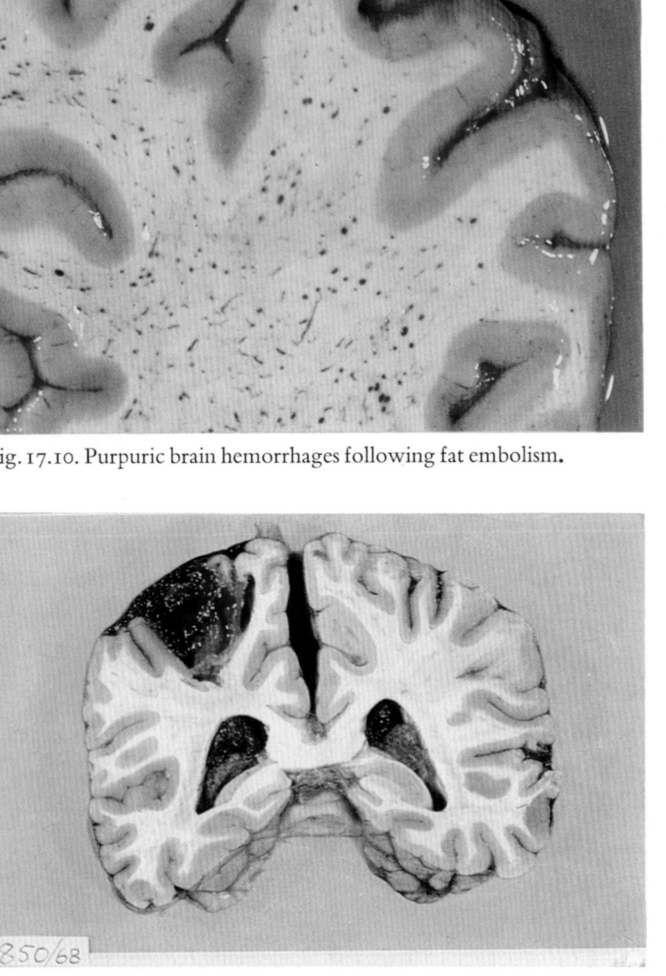

Fig. 17.10. Purpuric brain hemorrhages following fat embolism.

Fig. 17.12. Hemorrhagic brain infarction following venous thrombosis.

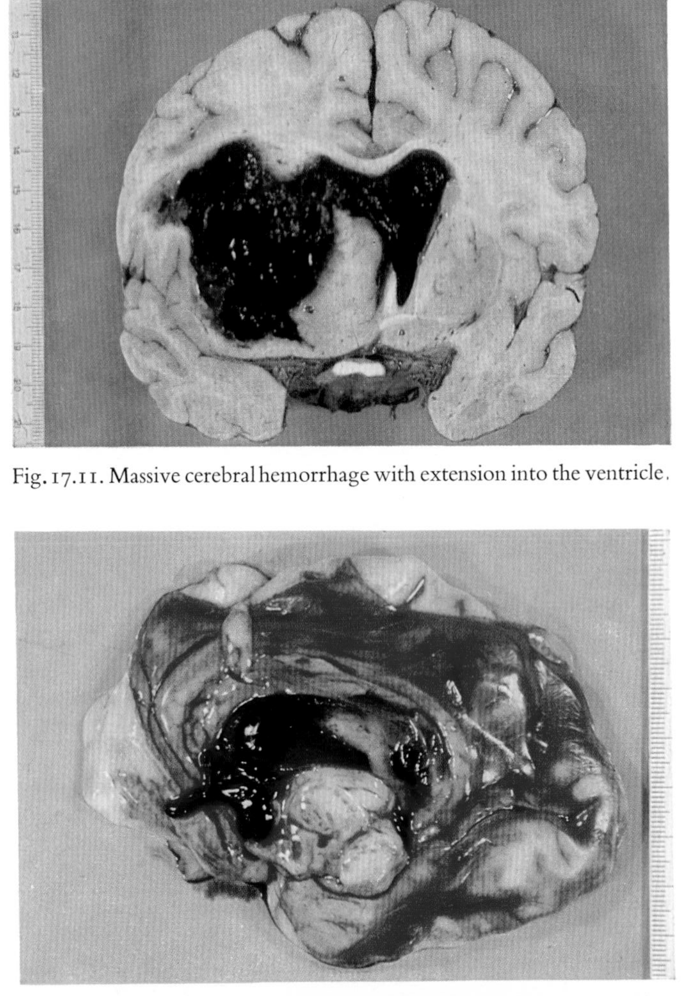

Fig. 17.11. Massive cerebral hemorrhage with extension into the ventricle.

Fig. 17.13. Internal hematocephalus after plexus hemorrhage.

Cerebral Hemorrhages

Purpuric hemorrhages following fat embolism (Fig. 17.10; TCP, p. 227). This patient sustained multiple traumatic bone fractures. Fatty bone marrow emboli occluded multiple small arterioles and capillaries. The punctate hemorrhages shown in Figure 17.10 are the gross manifestations of bone marrow embolization. The petechiae are particularly prominent in the white matter and cannot be wiped off the cut surface.

Pg: fat embolism, hyaline thrombi in shock, hemorrhagic tendencies, intoxication, allergic diseases, leukemias, infection with poxvirus, uremia, heat stroke and hemorrhagic encephalitis.

Massive cerebral hemorrhage (Fig. 17.11). *A cerebrovascular accident or "stroke" is the result of a ruptured artery, usually as a complication of longstanding hypertension.* The basal ganglia, internal capsule, cerebellum or pons is affected most commonly. Figure 17.11 shows a massive hemorrhage in the left hemisphere. The hemorrhage has ruptured into the lateral ventricle, which is filled with clotted blood: *internal hematocephalus.* The hemorrhage also may perforate into the subarachnoid space.

F and *Lo:* massive cerebral hemorrhages affect the putamen and nucleus caudatus (42%), pons (16%), thalamus (15%) and cerebellum (12%). The left and right hemispheres are affected equally. Multiple smaller hemorrhages are observed occasionally (3% of cases). *A:* 70% of cerebrovascular accidents are observed in patients between 40 and 70 years of age; 11% occur before the 40th year of age. *S:* ♂:♀ = 2:1. *Pg:* various degrees of hypertensive cerebrovascular disease (arteriosclerosis) are observed: 33% severe, 22% minimal and 25% no arteriosclerosis. The so-called *status lacunaris* is considered a precursor of hypertensive cerebral hemorrhage and often is associated with it.

DD: hemorrhages from trauma, ruptured aneurysms or angiomas. *Co:* small cerebral hemorrhages may heal by formation of a *pseudocyst.* Seventy-five per cent of massive hemorrhages rupture into the ventricular system, leading to a form of *tamponade* known as intraventricular hemorrhage or internal hematocephalus. The spinal fluid is bloody; death occurs rapidly.

Hemorrhagic cerebral infarction (Fig. 17.12). *An area of cerebral necrosis that becomes secondarily hemorrhagic from collateral congestion.* Areas of hemorrhagic necrosis are seen frequently near the origin of the dorsal superior cerebral veins. A roughly triangular, hemorrhagic cortical lesion is illustrated in Figure 17.12. Thrombosis of internal cerebral veins is less common and may cause an isolated hemorrhagic necrosis of the basal ganglia.

Co: in small children → unilateral or bilateral *porencephaly* (see p. 317).

Intraventricular hemorrhage (internal hematocephalus) after hemorrhage from the choroid plexus (Fig. 17.13). *A massive hemorrhage from the choroid plexus or the terminal vein that ruptures into the ventricles.* Figure 17.13 shows the blood-filled ventricles in a cross section of the brain. This hemorrhage from the choroid plexus characteristically occurred in a premature newborn.

F: 10% of autopsies on premature babies and 1.5% of mature newborns are due to "traumatic birth hemorrhage". *Pg:* defects in clotting mechanisms (vitamin K deficiency) or fragility of blood vessels (immaturity) → hemorrhages from the choroid plexus. A hemorrhage from the internal cerebral vein probably is the consequence of extreme stretching of the head in a sagittal direction. The rigid straight sinus or the vein of Galen becomes compressed, thereby leading to extreme venous stasis. *Co:* smaller hemorrhages usually are organized; larger hemorrhages rupture into the ventricles (→ internal hematocephalus). Anatomy of the internal cerebral or terminal vein: choroidal vein + thalamostriate vein → terminal vein → middle cerebral vein → vein of Galen → straight sinus.

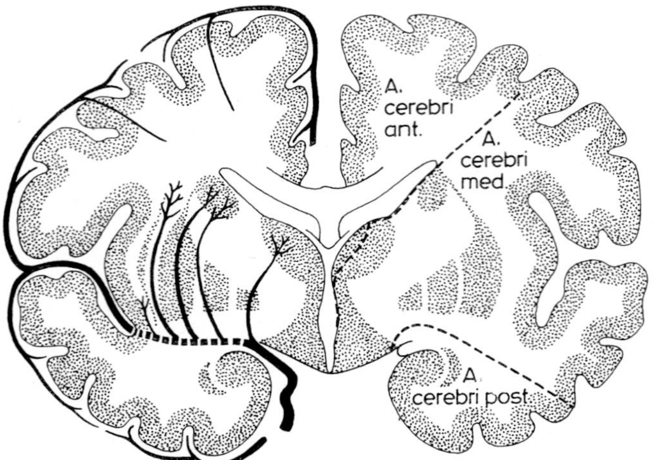

Fig. 17.14. Scheme of arterial blood supply of the brain (NOETZEL).

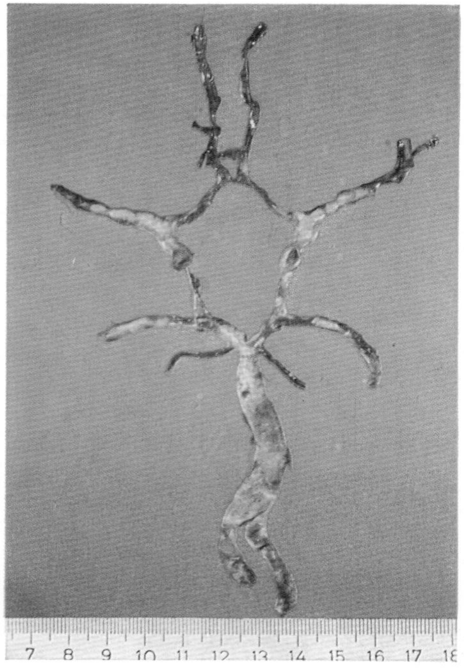

Fig. 17.15. Sclerosis of basal cerebral arteries.

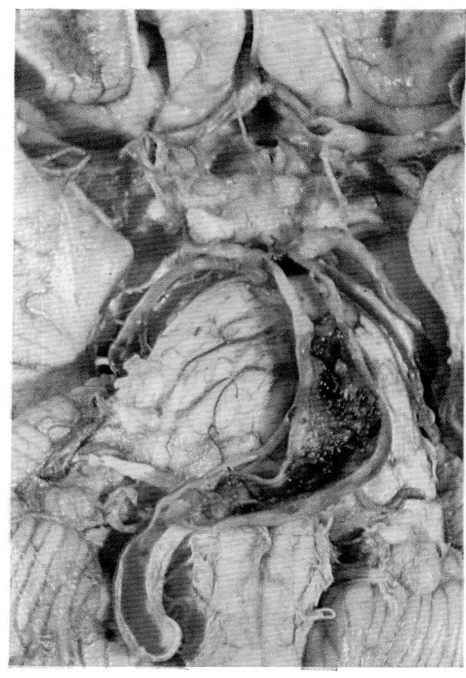

Fig. 17.16. Thrombosis of the basilar artery.

Circulatory Disorders

Normal blood supply (Fig. 17.14). The arterial blood is supplied via the carotid and vertebral arteries, which, together with the communicating branches, form the *circle of Willis* (see also p. 311). The anterior, medial and posterior cerebral arteries form the circle of Willis. The middle cerebral artery is the largest branch and supplies the major part of the cerebral surface. The anterior portions of the frontal lobes are supplied by the anterior cerebral arteries. The posterior and lower portions of the occipital lobes receive arterial blood via the posterior cerebral arteries. The basal ganglia are supplied mostly by the lenticulostriate arteries, which are branches of the middle cerebral artery.

Arteriosclerosis of basal cerebral arteries (Fig. 17.15). *Arteriosclerosis of the basal cerebral arteries is part of a generalized arteriosclerosis* (see p. 45). Basal arteriosclerosis in older persons may occur without clinical hypertension, in contrast to younger patients. Figure 17.15 shows rigid, yellowish arterial walls of the circle of Willis. The lumen of these arteries was irregularly narrowed or dilated.

Thrombosis of basal cerebral arteries (Fig. 17.16). Focal thrombosis may complicate basal cerebral arteriosclerosis. The internal carotid artery and middle cerebral artery are affected most often (75% of all cases). The remaining 25% of thromboses are distributed among the anterior and posterior cerebral arteries, basilar artery and vertebral arteries. Figure 17.16 shows multiple atheromatous plaques in a tortuous, rigid basilar artery. A circumscribed thrombus occluded the lumen.

F: 2.5% of autopsies in patients older than 20 years. *A:* 65–70 years. *S:* ♂:♀ = 2:3.6. *Pg of thrombosis:* see page 51. Arteriosclerosis and hypertension are the most common and cor pulmonale (e.g., in silicosis) the least common causes of thrombosis of the basal cerebral arteries. *DD:* the differentiation between *thrombosis* and *embolism* may be difficult. Embolism usually is observed in younger patients (around 45 years) and is characterized by occlusion of multiple smaller and larger arteries (see also p. 53). Endocarditis of mural thrombi overlying a myocardial infarction are common sources of emboli. *Co:* embolism or thrombosis → cerebral infarctions. The infarctions usually are hemorrhagic in the cortex and anemic in the white matter.

Kernicterus (bilirubin encephalopathy, Fig. 17.17). *A yellow discoloration and retrogressive changes in nerve cells, especially of the basal ganglia.* Kernicterus is the result of severe hemolytic jaundice of newborns. The globus pallidus, dentate and subthalamic nuclei, floor of the 4th ventricle, cornu Ammonis and inferior olives are affected most commonly.

F: seen in approximately 30% of severe cases of hemolytic disease of newborns (icterus gravis). *Co:* kernicterus leads to mental retardation, muscle atrophy, restricted mobility and extrapyramidal signs (tremors).

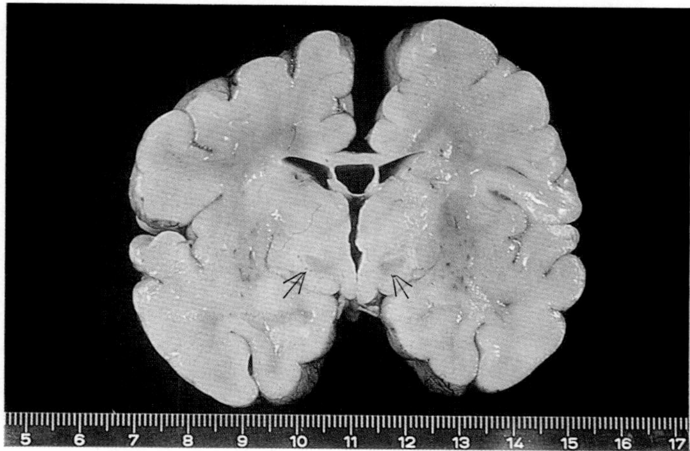

Fig. 17.17. Kernicterus.

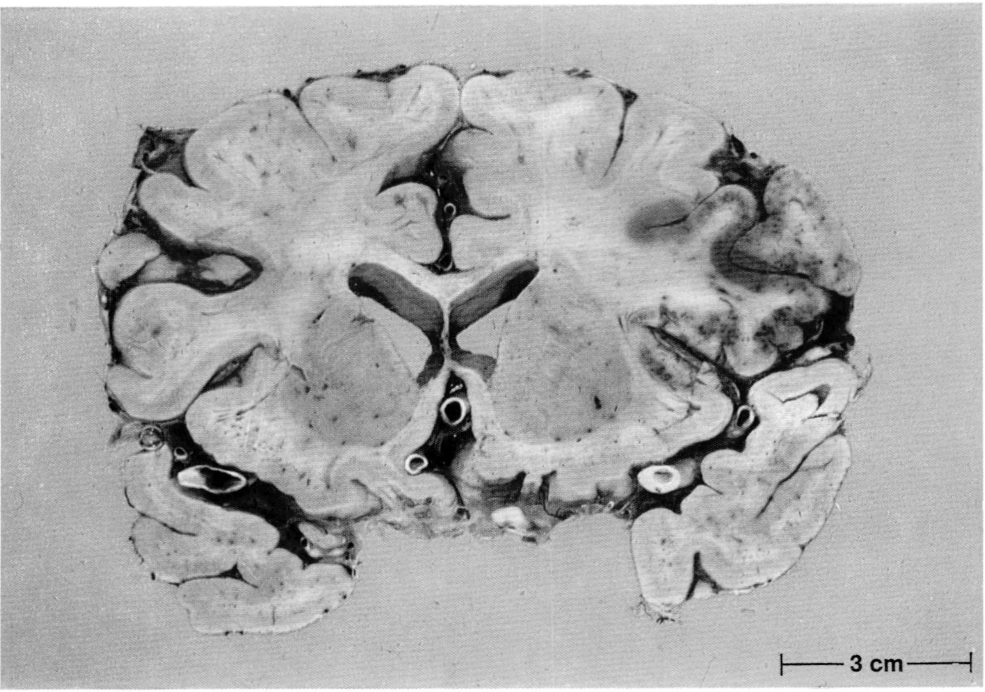

Fig. 17.18. Cortical infarctions in arteriosclerosis.

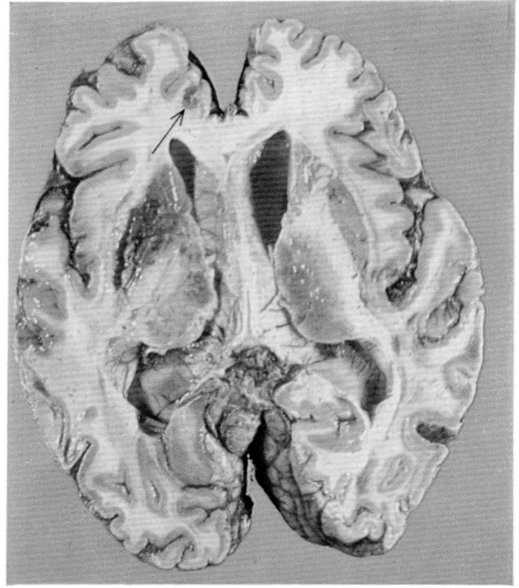

Fig. 17.19. Areas of necrosis in the cortex and basal ganglia.

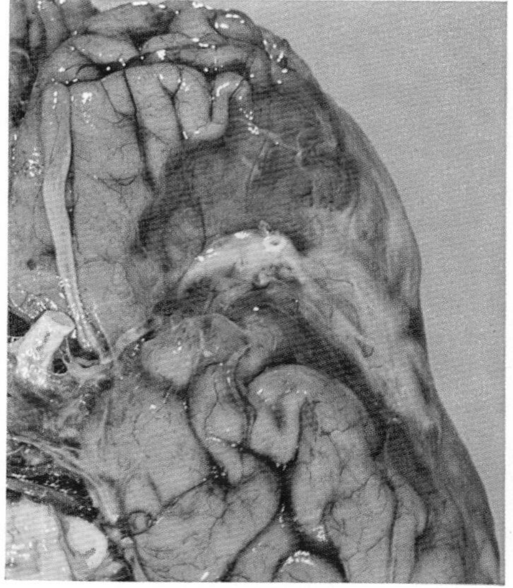

Fig. 17.20. Thickening of the leptomeninges overlying an old cerebral infarction.

Cerebral Infarctions

Cortical infarctions in advanced arteriosclerosis. Figure 17.18 shows a coronal section through the brain. The transected arteries are severely thickened due to arteriosclerosis. The arterial lumina are almost occluded in places. Fresh anemic or hemorrhagic cortical infarctions are seen in those portions of the brain supplied by the middle cerebral artery.

Pg: narrowing of the arterial lumina with or without heart failure causes hypoxia. *DD:* cortical infarctions may result from endarteritis obliterans (see p. 53), CO poisoning (see p. 309) and temporary cardiac arrest.

Cerebral infarction (white infarction, encephalomalacia, Fig. 17.19; TCP, p. 223). *A large cerebral infarction is the result of ischemic necrosis following arterial occlusion.* Figure 17.19 shows extensive areas of anemic necrosis in the cortex and basal ganglia. The necrotic areas were supplied by the middle cerebral artery and its lenticulostriate branches. A somewhat smaller infarction also was present in the frontal cortex (→), which indicates an occlusion of the anterior cerebral artery. Disseminated areas of encephalomalacia are observed commonly when the internal carotid artery is occluded.

Pg: most anemic infarctions of the brain are the result of thrombotic or embolic occlusion of a larger cerebral artery; rarely due to endarteritis obliterans. *Co:* the infarcted area is pale and indistinct 48 hours after the occlusion has occurred. This is especially well seen in the gray matter. Typical liquefaction necrosis develops 1–3 weeks later. The liquefied tissue is resorbed after 3 weeks (TCP, p. 223). *Cl:* cerebral infarctions present clinically as cerebrovascular accidents. The patients often survive, in contrast to a massive cerebral hemorrhage.

Pseudocyst after cerebral infarction (Fig. 17.20). The liquefied necrotic tissue of an anemic infarction is resorbed. The infarcted area is thereby changed into a small, sharply delineated cavity. The pseudocyst contains yellowish white fluid (resembling cerebrospinal fluid); the cyst wall is made up of gliotic tissue. The overlying meninges are thickened and gray-white (Fig. 17.20).

The location and size of pseudocysts following encephalomalacia are dependent on the size of the occluded artery. Pseudocysts in the area of the basal ganglia usually are very small (1–2 mm.) and often are surrounded by a brownish discolored brain tissue: *status lacunaris.*

Special forms in small children are:

Porencephaly. *Prenatal formation of abnormal cavities or clefts in the brain as a result of congenital malformation with arterial occlusion.* Some cases of porencephaly may present as an asymmetric absence of parts of the cerebral hemisphere. Porencephaly usually communicates with the ventricles.

Hydranencephaly. *A congenital malformation characterized by a complete or almost complete absence of cerebral hemispheres.* The normal layers of the brain (leptomeninges, cortex, medulla and ependyma) have disappeared and the space occupied by hemispheres is converted into a membranous sac filled with cerebrospinal fluid.

Pg: obstruction of blood flow in the internal carotid, anterior or middle cerebral arteries during fetal life. *Cause:* not known. *DD:* in *internal hydrocephalus*, the cerebral layers are thinner than normal but developed. Anencephaly is associated with malformations of the skull, hydranencephaly is not.

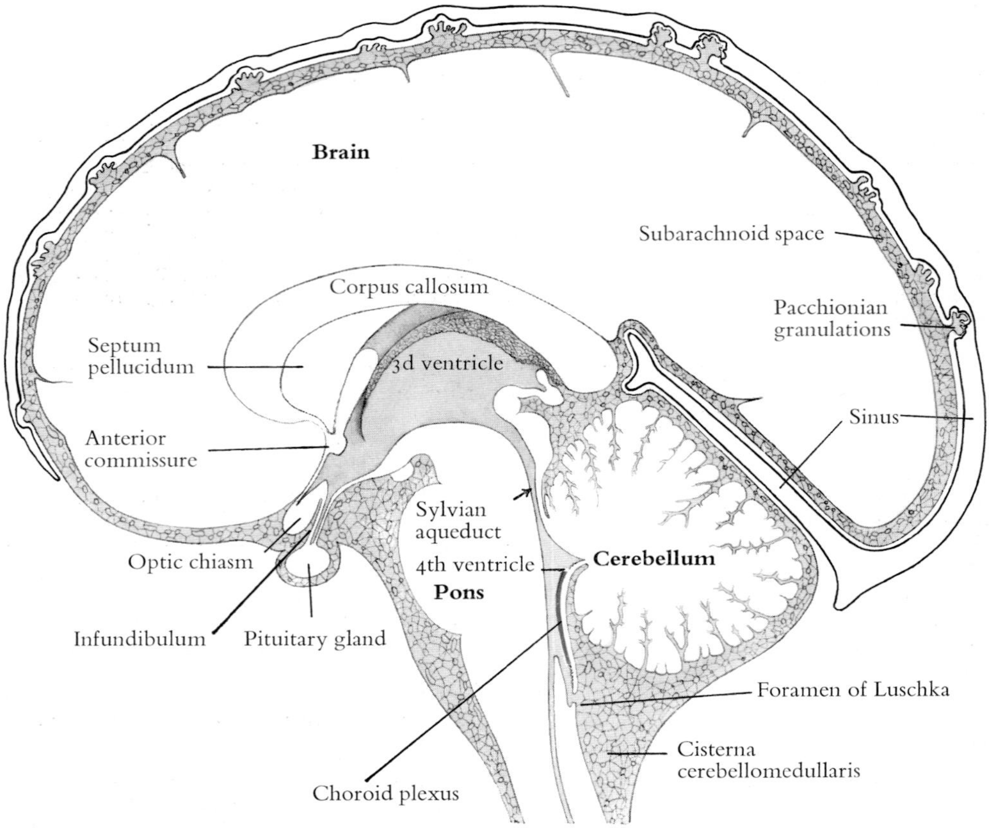

Brain
Subarachnoid space
Corpus callosum
Pacchionian granulations
Septum pellucidum
3d ventricle
Sinus
Anterior commissure
Sylvian aqueduct
Optic chiasm
4th ventricle
Cerebellum
Pons
Infundibulum
Pituitary gland
Foramen of Luschka
Cisterna cerebellomedullaris
Choroid plexus

Fig. 17.21. Schematic presentation of cerebrospinal fluid space.

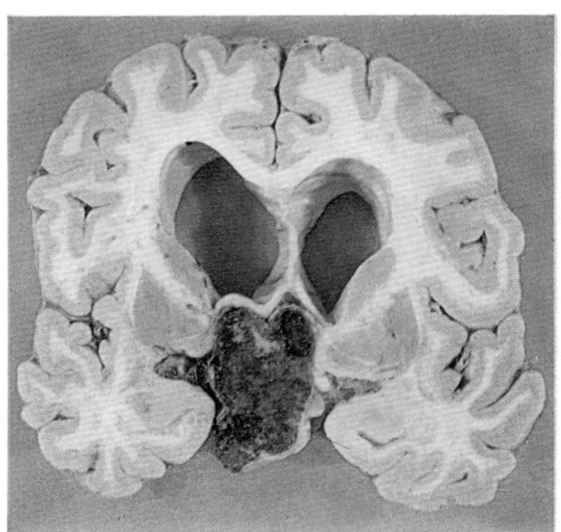

Fig. 17.22. Internal hydrocephalus in a case of craniopharyngioma.

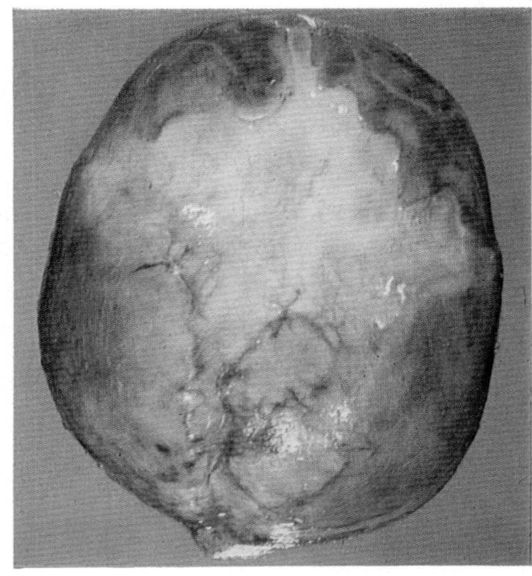

Fig. 17.23. Large anterior fontanelle in hydrocephalus.

Hydrocephalus

Hydrocephalus refers to an increase in the amount of cerebrospinal fluid.

Physiology of cerebrospinal fluid (CSF) (Fig. 17.21). CSF production and absorption are balanced under physiologic conditions. The choroid plexuses are believed to be the principal source of CSF; 95% is formed in the lateral ventricles. CSF *circulates* from the lateral ventricle through the interventricular foramen (Monro), 3d ventricle, aqueduct of Sylvius, 4th ventricle, foramen of Luschka and foramen of Magendie. This intracerebral phase is followed by *extracerebral* CSF circulation through the subarachnoid space, cisternae and surface of the brain. CSF is reabsorbed by the subarachnoid villi, especially the pacchionian granulations (large arachnoid villi in the dural venous sinuses). CSF is a clear, colorless and odorless fluid measuring 60 ml. in infants and 120–180 ml. in adults. Twenty-five per cent of CSF is found in the ventricular system and 75% in the subarachnoid space. Approximately 700 ml. of CFS is produced daily.

Internal hydrocephalus *is defined as an abnormal accumulation of CSF in the ventricular system and its connection.* Two types are distinguished: (1) *obstructive or occlusive* internal hydrocephalus, which is associated with increased intraventricular pressure, and (2) internal hydrocephalus *ex vacuo*, which is associated with normotensive intraventricular pressure.

Signs of increased CSF pressure: The meninges are tense, the convolutions are flat and the gyri are indistinct. The cut surface of the brain reveals the dilated ventricles as shown in Figure 17.22. This was a case of an internal hydrocephalus from a craniopharyngioma. Other signs of increased CSF pressure are papilledema, distention of the sella turcica (sometimes associated with atrophy of the pituitary gland), phenomenon of the "setting sun" (orbital pressure → receding eye bulbs → pupils partly covered by lower eyelids, see p. 231), projecting forehead and widening of the fontanelles (Fig. 17.23). The bones in Figure 17.23 are pale brown and consist of fibrous tissue, as does the fontanelle, which is gray-blue. The adult skull cannot adapt to increased pressure by widening of the skull. There is pressure atrophy of the brain, manifested initially by a reduction in the white matter and later in the gray matter as well. The normal layering of the brain is retained.

A: dependent on the cause of the hydrocephalus. Severe cases usually are observed in small children, less severe forms are encountered in elderly patients. *Pg:* obstruction of the intracerebral CSF flow causes an *obstructive internal hydrocephalus.* Obstructive hydrocephalus is either *symmetric* (occlusion below the aqueduct) or *asymmetric* (obstruction of a foramen of Monro). Approximately 95% of all cases of hydrocephalus are due to one of the following types of obstruction:

1. *Congenital malformations:* congenital stenosis of the aqueduct, formation of membranes or Arnold-Chiari syndrome (a tongue-like projection of the cerebellum and the dorsal medulla oblongata through the foramen magnum).

2. *Inflammations:* organized inflammatory exudates may form membranes, thereby causing an acquired stenosis or complete occlusion of the aqueduct or of the foramina of Monro, Luschka or Magendie. *Pg:* the common bacterial or nonbacterial forms of meningitis (→ ependymitis), tuberculosis (basal meningitis, p. 323) or toxoplasmosis (p. 325).

3. *Hemorrhages:* (extremely rare cause of internal hydrocephalus). Focal, organized hemorrhages of the basal cisternae or the ventricular system (aqueduct).

4. *Tumors:* ependymomas, gliomas and metastases (carcinomatous or leukemic).

The *internal or external hydrocephalus ex vacuo* is a compensatory replacement of brain substance by CSF. Progressive senile brain atrophy results in dilated ventricles and subarachnoid spaces filled with CSF. Intracranial CSF pressure is normal.

External hydrocephalus. *Diffuse or circumscribed increase in the amount of CSF in the subarachnoid space. External hydrocephalus leads to diffuse or focal atrophy of the brain.*

Pg: external hydrocephalus is the consequence of either increased CSF production (inflammations) or decreased CSF absorption (sinus thrombosis or thrombophlebitis). Late complications of recurrent subarachnoid hemorrhages or meningeal tumor infiltration rarely cause external hydrocephalus. *Co:* a *communicating* hydrocephalus may lead to an internal hydrocephalus because of retrograde CSF accumulation.

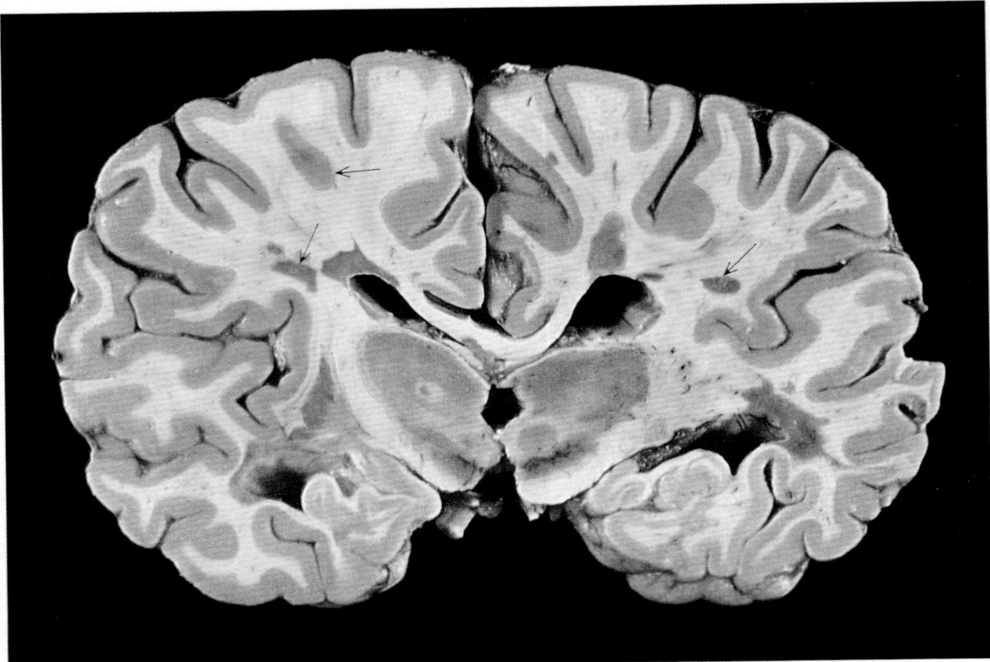

Fig. 17.24. Multiple sclerosis.

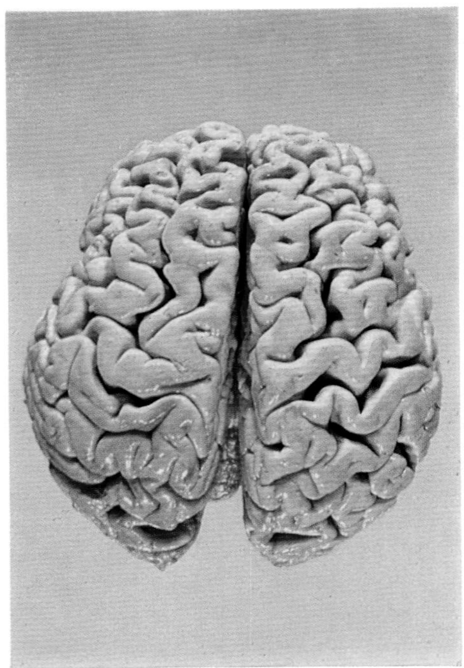

Fig. 17.25. Senile atrophy of the brain.

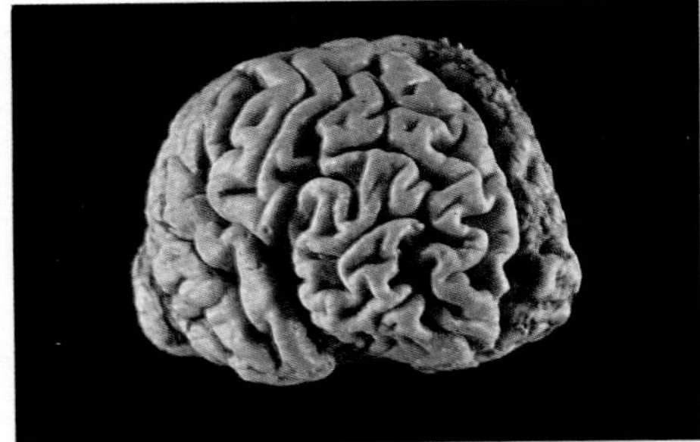

Fig. 17.26. Pick's disease.

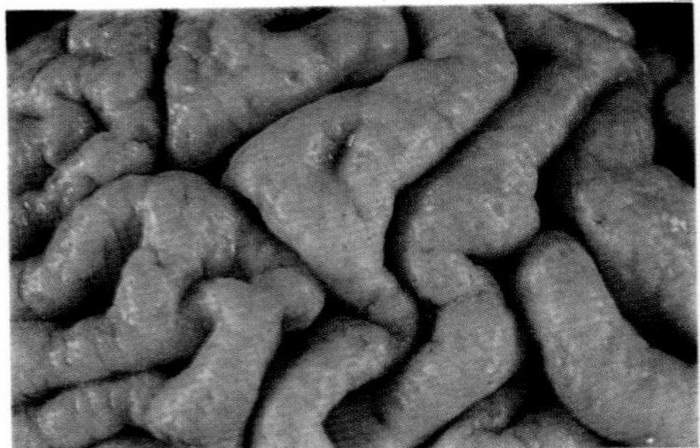

Fig. 17.27. Granular atrophy of the brain in case of endarteritis obliterans.

Demyelinating Diseases, Atrophy

Multiple sclerosis (Fig. 17.24; TCP, p. 231). *Multiple, demyelinating lesions with secondary gliosis are irregularly distributed throughout the brain and spinal cord.* Figure 17.24 shows circumscribed, gray, slightly glassy and depressed lesions (→). These must not be confused on gross examination with oblique cuts through the brain. Fresh lesions of multiple sclerosis are pink and congested rather than gray, as in Figure 17.24. The lesions affect the white matter of the optic nerve, periventricular areas, brain stem, etc.

F: 0.01% of the total population. *A:* 20–40 years. *S:* ♂:♀ = 1:2. *Pg:* the cause is still not known. Multiple sclerosis is considered an autoimmune disease by some observers; others invoke virus infections and genetic factors. *Co:* the clinical course may extend over decades, with periods of remissions and relapses alternating.

Other demyelinating diseases include:

1. *The concentric sclerosis of Baló* consists of a larger, solitary demyelinating lesion in a hemisphere. In contrast to multiple sclerosis, the concentric sclerosis of Baló is fatal within weeks or a few months.

2. *The inflammatory, diffuse sclerosis (Schilder's disease)* is a demyelinating disease of childhood that is fatal within 2 years. The white matter is extensively destroyed; the cortex is relatively spared. *Pg:* not known.

3. *Neuromyelitis optica Devic.* This demyelinating disease affects the optic nerves and spinal cord, leading to amaurosis. Transitions to multiple sclerosis have been observed.

Atrophy of the brain (Fig. 17.25). A progressive loss of brain substance occurs during old age. The atrophic brain usually weighs less than 1,200 Gm. The sulci are widened and the gyri are small. The arachnoid layer is yellowish discolored from storage of wear-and-tear pigment. Senile atrophy is most pronounced in the frontal lobes. The ventricles are somewhat dilated on cut surface (internal hydrocephalus ex vacuo).

F: usually observed past the age of 70 or 80, associated with dementia.

DD: a similar gross picture is observed in *presenile dementia (Alzheimer's disease)*, which begins between the 40th and 60th years. Atrophy is most severe in the frontal and occipital lobes. *Pick's disease or atrophy* (Fig. 17.26) is a severe atrophy of the frontal lobes. Pick's atrophy manifests clinically as personality changes between the 40th and 50th years of age. Focal atrophy of temporal lobes is observed occasionally. Pick's disease is mostly an atrophy of the cortex and is more severe than senile or presenile atrophy. The brain weighs less than 1,200 Gm.

Granular cortical atrophy in endarteritis obliterans (Winiwarter-Buerger's disease, Fig. 17.27). Obliterative endarteritis may affect the pial arteries over the convexity of the brain. The pial arteries are occluded and the brain becomes atrophic (Fig. 17.27). The granularity of the gyri reflects scarring of tiny areas of encephalomalacia.

Pg: in addition to the pial arteries, larger arteries (e.g., internal carotid arteries) may be affected also. Granular cortical atrophy also is observed in other diseases such as arteriosclerosis and CO poisoning (see p. 307).

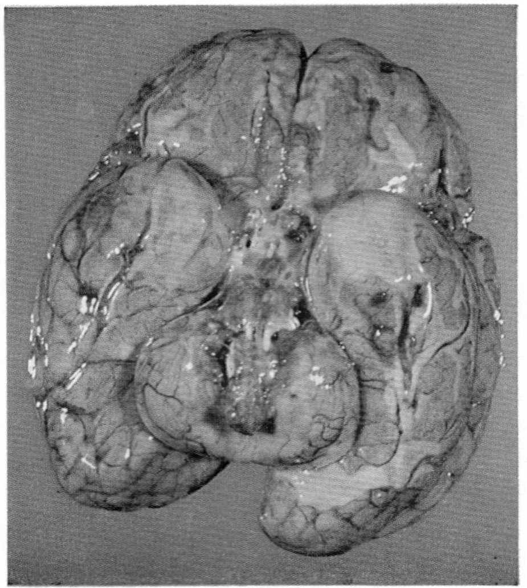

Fig. 17.28. Purulent meningitis.

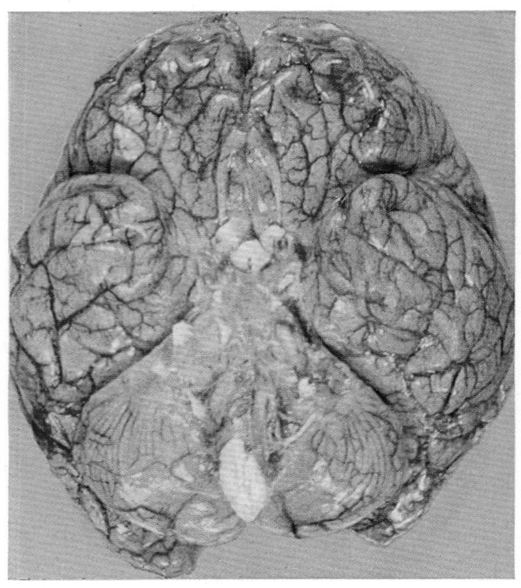

Fig. 17.29. Adhesions and fibrosis after basal tuberculous meningitis.

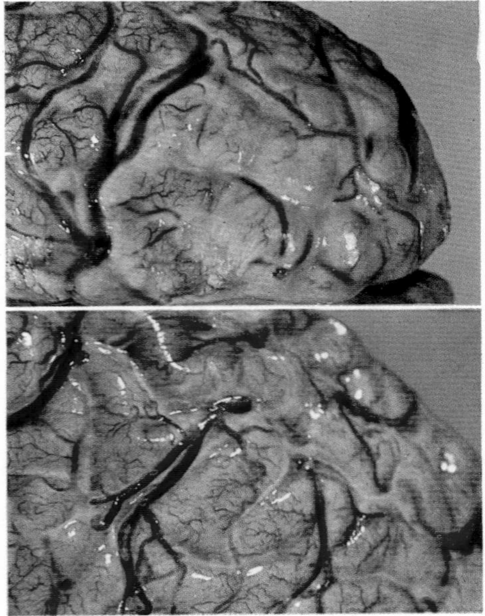

Fig. 17.30. Above: purulent meningitis.
Below: senile cloudiness of the leptomeninges.

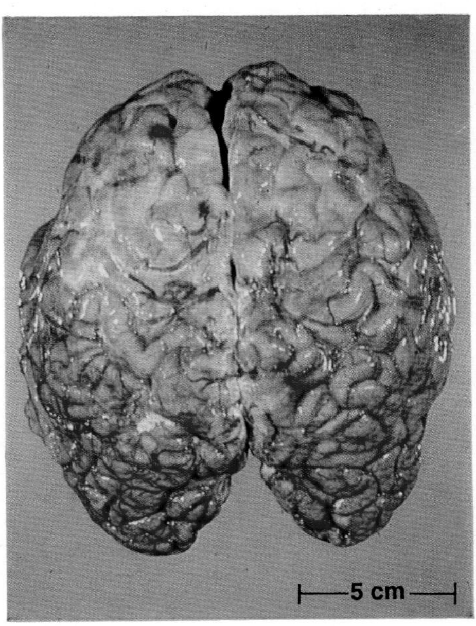

Fig. 17.31. Meningeal fibrosis in a case of progressive paralysis.

Inflammatory Diseases (TCP, p. 227)

Meningitis may present as a *bacterial* (purulent, nonpurulent or specific) or *abacterial* inflammation.

Bacterial, purulent meningitis (Figs. 17.28 and 17.30; TCP, p. 227). *Collection of pus in the subarachnoid space, especially along the blood vessels of the sulci.* The distribution of the exudate is dependent on the width of the subarachnoid space. Larger collections of pus usually accumulate over the convexity of the frontal lobes, extending to the central gyri, the temporal lobes and the base of the brain (prepontine and interpeduncular cisternae). Figures 17.28 and 17.30 are examples of purulent meningitis. Meningococci, *Haemophilus influenzae*, streptococci, staphylococci and pneumococci are the most common causes. Males are affected more often than females (70%).

1. **Meningococcal meningitis.** *A:* young children. *Pg: Neisseria meningitidis,* a gram-negative diplococcus, spreads to the brain via the lymphatics or blood stream from an infection of the nasopharynx. *Co:* fulminating clinical course, with death within 24 hours. Grossly, brain and meninges are hyperemic. Bacteria can be isolated from the cerebrospinal fluid. After 24 hours, thin, liquid pus accumulates over the base of the brain *(basal meningitis)*. The pus is poor in fibrin.

2. **Pneumococcal meningitis.** *A:* afflicted are adults; less common in infants and small children. *Diplococcus pneumoniae*, a gram-positive diplococcus, localizes in the meninges and brain following an infection of the nasopharynx or lungs. Pneumococcal meningitis is characterized by a greenish, fibrin-rich, thick pus with a tendency to localize over the frontal lobes (Fig. 17.30, above).

3. **Streptococcal and Staphylococcal meningitis.** *A:* dependent on the source of infection. Meningitis follows otitis media, sinusitis, open skull trauma or thrombophlebitis. *Co:* extension from ear or sinuses → brain abscess. Grossly, a focal collection of fibrin-poor, yellow pus.

4. **Haemophilus influenzae meningitis.** Common type of meningitis in childhood. The exudate is poor in fibrin and localizes over the convexity; often associated with venous thrombosis, hyperemia and edema during the acute phase.

Complications of meningitis: (1) *Meningoencephalitis:* secondary involvement of the superficial cortex is common in severe or extensive meningitis. (2) *Adhesive arachnoiditis:* focal adhesions between the arachnoid and the pia mater may lead to the formation of smaller and larger cysts filled with CSF *(cystic adhesive arachnoiditis)*. Such cysts are common near the cisternae cerebellomedullaris. (3) Other complications: neuritis of brain nerves (deafness, blindness), granular ependymitis, occlusive internal hydrocephalus and subdural empyema.

Tuberculous meningitis usually is confined to the basal cisternae (Fig. 17.29). The infection spreads hematogenously from a primary complex (early generalization, see p. 86) or from advanced organ tuberculosis (lung, lymph nodes, etc.). Healed cases of tuberculous meningitis are observed commonly today because of successful therapy (Fig. 17.29). Fibrous organization of the tuberculous exudate results in a fine, gray-white membrane *(pannus)*.

Co: hydrocephalus, tuberculous endarteritis of the vessels of a pannus → cerebral infarctions; neuritis.

Meningeal fibrosis in syphilitic meningoencephalitis (syphilitic progressive paralysis or general paresis; Fig. 17.31; TCP, p. 231). Progressive atrophy of the frontal lobes, fibrosis of the leptomeninges, granular ependymitis and internal hydrocephalus are manifestations of progressive paralysis. Figure 17.31 shows a typical fibrosis of the leptomeninges that is confined to the frontal lobes.

Pg: part of a neurosyphilis. *DD:* syphilitic meningoencephalitis must be distinguished from *senile meningeal thickening or cloudiness*. Senile meningeal thickening is diffuse, not localized (see Fig. 17.30, below).

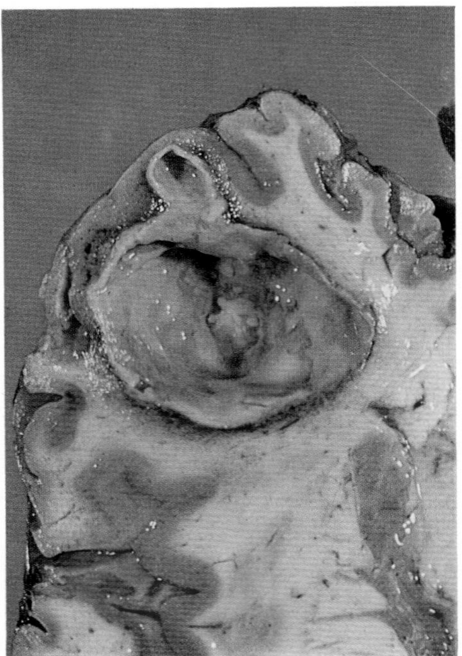

Fig. 17.32. Brain abscess.

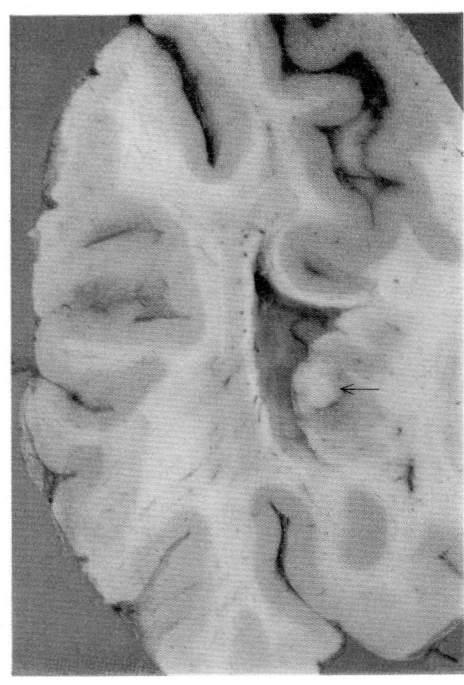

Fig. 17.33. Tuberculoma.

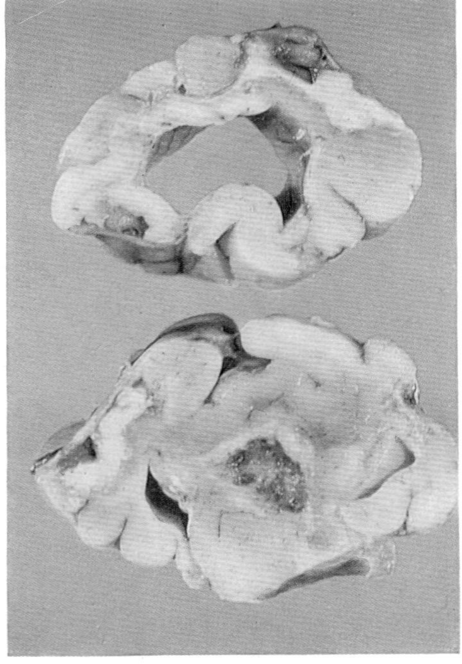

Fig. 17.34. Toxoplasmosis of the brain with necrosis and hydrocephalus.

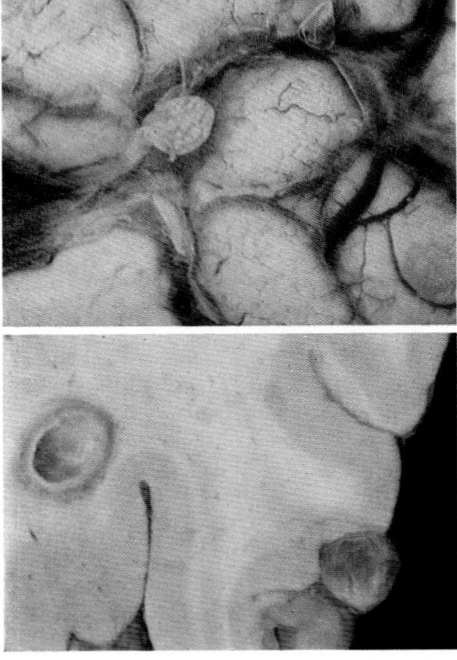

Fig. 17.35. Cysticercosis.

Brain abscess. *A circumscribed, encapsulated area of purulent necrosis in the brain.* Figure 17.32 shows a large cavity that contained pus. The cavity is lined by a gray-white wall (up to 2 mm. thick). A *fresh* brain abscess is demarcated from the surrounding brain by granulation tissue, the so-called *abscess membrane*. An *old* brain abscess is delineated by an *abscess capsule* of gray-white color. The capsule consists of connective tissue.

Pg: brain abscesses usually are the result of a hematogenous infection by strepto-, staphylo- or pneumococci. The organisms may gain access to the brain by hematogenous spread from distant sources, such as a furuncle of the face, purulent bronchiectasis, tonsillitis or endocarditis. Direct extension from otitis media, mastoiditis, sinusitis or infected head injuries is a much more common cause. "Otogenic abscesses" from otitis media often are localized in the temporal lobes or cerebellum.

Tuberculoma. Figure 17.33 shows a circumscribed, round, pale lesion with central necrosis (→). This was a conglomeration of recent tuberculous granulomas. Older tuberculomas are encapsulated, organized and may even calcify.

Pg: hematogenous conglomerate tubercles. *Lo:* cerebellum and pons are predominantly affected.

Sarcoidosis of the brain (see p. 89) is characterized by multiple small granulomas that often are arranged like rosettes around blood vessels in the so-called Virchow-Robin spaces and the basal leptomeninges.

Toxoplasmosis (Fig. 17.34; TCP, p. 229). *A granulomatous encephalitis caused by* Toxoplasma gondii *affecting mainly newborns.* Figure 17.34 shows multiple old and fresh areas of necrosis. The necrotic portions may become cystic *(porencephaly)*. The overlying leptomeninges are cloudy and thickened. The white matter and cortex are narrowed. The ventricles are dilated (internal hydrocephalus ex vacuo or by occlusion) and periventricular calcifications are common.

A and *Pg:* intrauterine infection with *toxoplasma gondii* usually results in stillbirth. Most cases of toxoplasmosis, a zoonosis, are due to transplacental infection during the first 3 months of pregnancy. Later, toxoplasma infection results in severe fetal diseases, such as chorioretinitis and microphthalmia. In adults, especially young females, toxoplasmosis usually manifests as acute lymphadenitis of cervical and axillary nodes (PIRINGER-KUCHINKA). The acute lymphadenitis usually heals, becomes chronic and the patient is without symptoms. The diagnosis is made by the Sabin-Feldman test. A titer above 1 : 50 or a rising titer is diagnostic.

Cerebral cysticercosis in man is characterized by small, solitary or racemose cysts. Racemose cysts resemble a bunch of grapes. The cysts are surrounded by a fibrous capsule that may calcify. Figure 17.35 shows the surface and cut section of the brain. A cyst is attached to the brain; another is found in the cortex. Cysts also may be found in the musculature, eyes or skin.

F: marked geographic variations; cysticercosis is common in India, Mexico and South America. In Europe, 1 : 10,000 autopsies. *A:* 20–45 years. *S:* ♂ = ♀. *Pg:* the common human tapeworm, *Taenia solium*, is transmitted from an intermediate host (pig) to humans as encysted larvae. The shells of the ova are dissolved in the stomach. The embryos penetrate the intestinal walls and are carried via the blood stream to many organs, including the central nervous system.

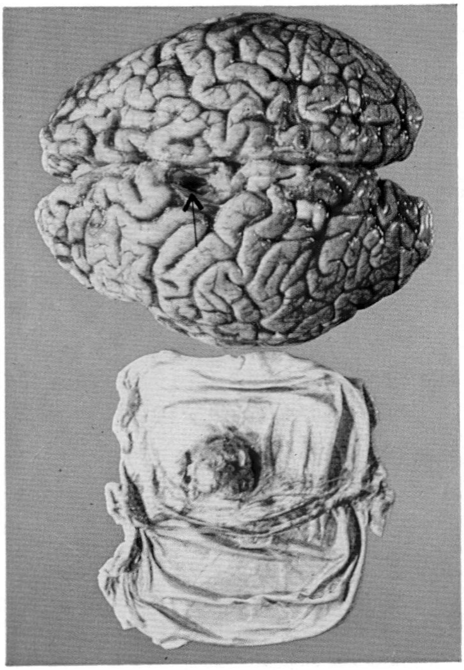

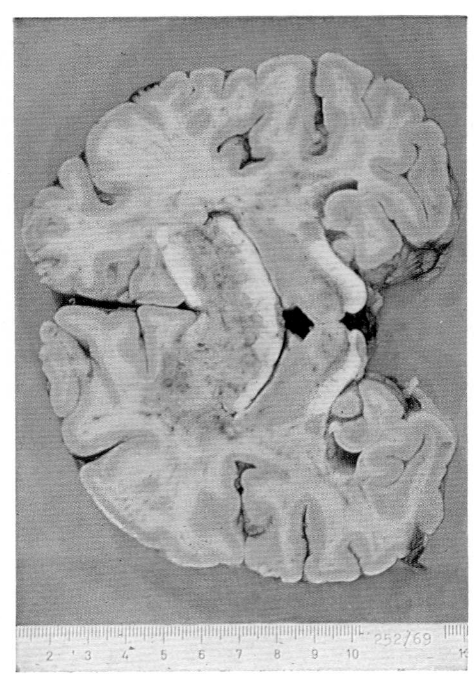

Fig. 17.37. "Butterfly" glioblastoma.

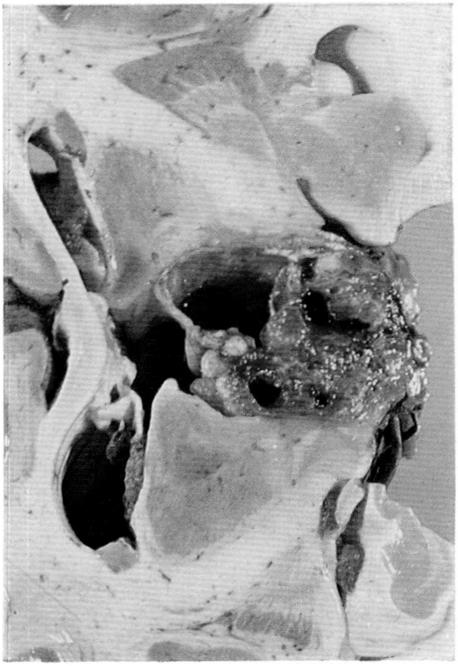

Fig. 17.39. Craniopharyngioma.

Fig. 17.36. Meningioma.

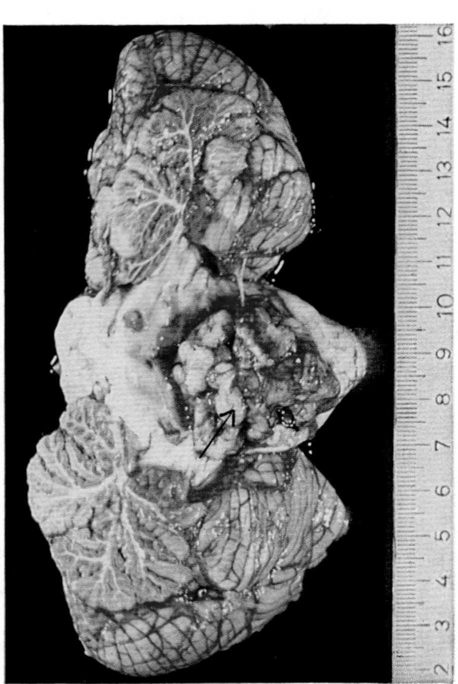

Fig. 17.38. Ependymoma.

Tumors

Meningioma (Fig. 17.36; TCP, p. 267). *A tumor that arises from arachnoidal (fibroblastic?) cells (pacchionian granulations).* A meningioma usually presents as a round, firm tumor that adheres firmly to the dura (Fig. 17.36, left). Such a slowly and expansively growing tumor eventually compresses the brain (→ in Fig. 17.36, right).

F: approximately 15–20% of all brain tumors. *A:* 40–50 years. *S:* ♂:♀ = 2:3. *Lo:* meningiomas are found most commonly next to the sagittal sinus, beneath the convexity of the skull, near the olfactory nerve or the tentorium. *Co:* the main effects are pressure symptoms. Meningiomas tend to recur after incomplete removal. Metastases are extremely rare, except for sarcomatous meningiomas. Histologically, meningiomas are divided into syncytial (meningotheliomatous), transitional (psammomatous), fibroblastic and angioblastic forms (TCP, p. 267).

Primary brain tumors have a characteristic location and age and sex distribution (Table 17.1).

Table 17.1

Tumor	F[1])	A	♂:♀	Predilection
Glioblastoma multiforme	12.3	30–60	2:1	Cerebrum
Oligodendroglioma	8.2	30–50	3:7	Cerebrum
Spongioblastoma	7.0	0–20	9:11	Cerebrum, cerebellum, pons, 4th ventricle
Astrocytoma	6.4	25–45	3:2	Cerebrum, pons
Ependymoma	4.3	0–20	6:5	Wall of ventricles
Medulloblastoma	3.8	10	5:2	Cerebellum
Papilloma of choroid plexus	0.5	all	1:1	Ventricles, cerebellopontine angle
Neurinoma	7.6	30–55	2:1	Cerebellopontine angle, spinal cord, cauda equina

[1]) % of intracranial tumors.

Figure 17.37 shows a poorly delineated glioblastoma as an example of a primary brain tumor. The tumor arose in the corpus callosum and involved both hemispheres ("butterfly glioma"). The varied cut surface is typical: areas of red hemorrhages and yellow necrosis alternate. The prognosis is poor; death usually is attributable to extensive hemorrhages (because of vascular invasion by the tumor) or massive collateral brain edema.

Ependymoma (Fig. 17.38). *A tumor derived from the lining of ventricular walls. Ependymomas arise in the cerebellum, less commonly in the cerebrum.* Figure 17.38 shows a polypoid tumor in the lumen of the 4th ventricle. The vermis of the cerebellum has been dissected.

Co: ependymomas are fast-growing tumors of poor prognosis causing occlusive hydrocephalus. *DD:* a similar gross appearance is characteristic of medulloblastomas, which almost exclusively arise in the cerebellum.

Craniopharyngioma (Fig. 17.39). *An intracranial tumor that develops from epithelial rests of Rathke's pouch (not a neurogenic tumor!).* Figure 17.39 shows a cystic tumor of brown color (old hemorrhages) at the floor of the 3rd ventricle. The ventricular system is slightly dilated, indicating incipient, occlusive hydrocephalus.

F: 2.5% of all brain tumors. *A:* 15–25 years. *S:* ♂:♀ = 2:1. *Lo:* craniopharyngiomas commonly are "suprasellar" (i.e., anterior to the pituitary stalk), rarely "intrasellar" in location. *Pg:* derived from remnants of the craniopharyngeal duct (Rathke's pouch = pituitary duct). *Co:* pressure → atrophy of the pituitary gland → infiltration of the floor of the 3rd ventricle. *Cl:* in females → amenorrhea; internal hydrocephalus. Slowly expansive growth. *Histologically*, clusters of focally squamous epithelium, cystic changes, cholesterol crystals.

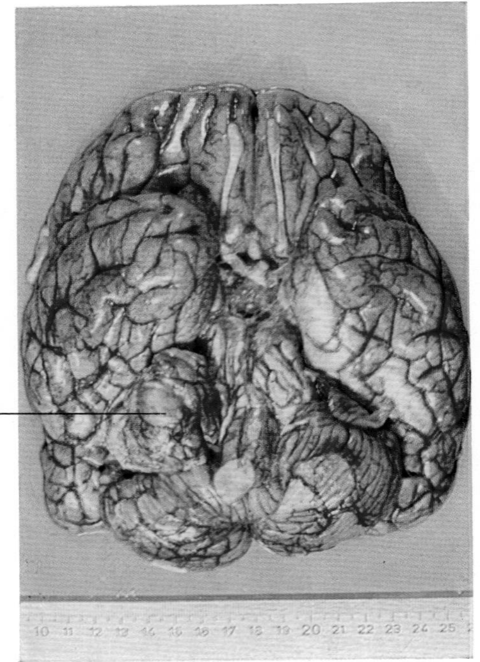

Fig. 17.40. Acoustic neurilemoma.

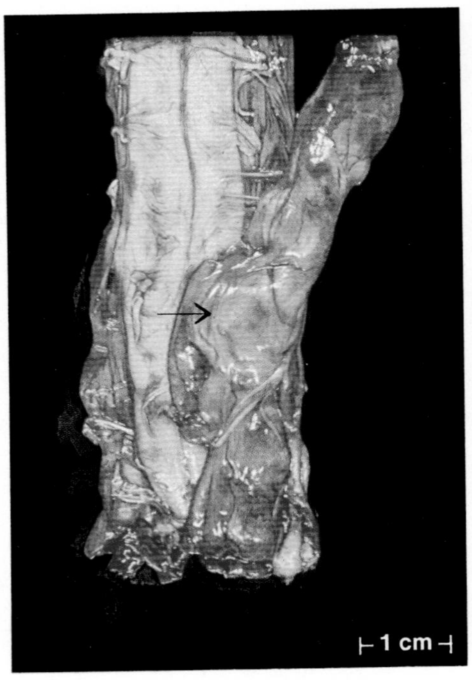

Fig. 17.41. Neurilemoma of a spinal nerve.

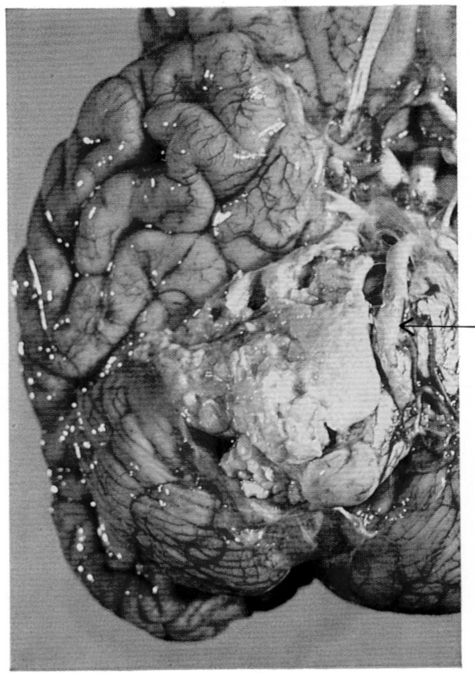

Fig. 17.42. Cholesteatoma.

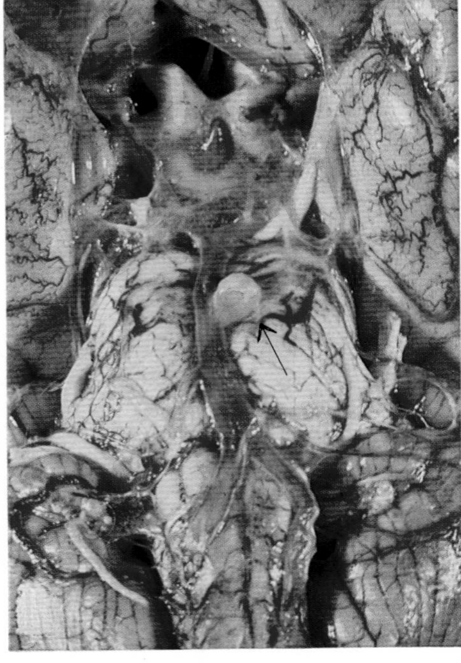

Fig. 17.43. Chordoma.

Neurilemoma (schwannoma or neurinoma; Figs. 17.40 and 17.41; TCP, p. 267). *Neurilemomas are tumors of the neuroectodermal Schwann cells. They produce little glial tissue or collagen fibers.* Neurilemomas occur intracranially or are attached to a peripheral nerve (especially cervical or brachial plexus or subcutaneous nerves). The acoustic neurilemoma is one of the most common intracranial nerve tumors. Figure 17.40 shows a tumor in the right cerebellopontine angle (→). The tumor is round, encapsulated, measuring 2×3 cm. The cut surface is fibrillar, with cystic soft areas. Histologically, this was a typical neurilemoma. Hemorrhages commonly are present on cut surface. Figure 17.41 shows a glassy, gray-white neurilemoma attached to a posterior spinal nerve (→). Neurilemomas occupy an eccentric position to the nerve of origin. They have distinct capsules composed of perineurium (in contrast to neurofibromas!).

F: see Table 17.1. *Co:* nerve pressure. Symptoms include facial paralysis, loss of hearing and compression of the medulla oblongata.

Neurofibromas consist of neoplastic Schwann cells and collagenous fibers. Neurofibromas occur as single tumors or as part of neurofibromatosis.

Phakomatoses, like hamartomas, are congenital malformations that affect the central nervous system, eyes, skin and mucous membranes. Examples are:

1. **Neurofibromatosis** (von Recklinghausen's disease). A dominantly inherited disease consisting of multiple, pedunculated tumors of the sheaths of dermal and other nerves. These skin tumors are accompanied by coffee-colored pigmentations (café au lait spots).

2. **Hippel-Lindau disease.** A phakomatosis that consists of multiple hemangiomas in the cerebellum and retina. Cysts in the pancreas, liver and kidneys also may be associated with this syndrome. *Co:* destruction of the cerebellum with corresponding symptoms; occlusion of the 4th ventricle. Degenerative pseudocysts → pressure on the medulla oblongata.

3. **Sturge-Weber-Krabbe disease.** A phakomatosis consisting of multiple hemangiomas in the skin (unilateral nevus flammeus in the area of the 1st and 2nd branches of the trigeminal nerve), the brain (tumor-like proliferation of leptomeninges and vessels with cortical calcifications → cerebral damage → epilepsy and mental retardation) and the eyes (choroidea).

4. **Tuberous sclerosis.** A phakomatosis characterized by a diffuse, tumor-like enlargement with sclerosis of the convolutions (→ mental retardation, epilepsy, paralysis), skin changes (pigmented nevi, adenoma sebaceum, subungual fibromas), renal cortical angioleiomyolipomas, rhabdomyomas of the heart and gliomas of the ventricles.

Cholesteatoma (Fig. 17.42). *Displaced, cystic epidermal rests that may occur in the leptomeninges.* Figure 17.42 shows the cerebellopontine angle with collections of horny masses resembling mother-of-pearl ("margaritomas"). The arrow points to the basilar artery.

F: rare, approximately 0.25% of all autopsies. *Pg:* not a true neoplasm but a tissue malformation (heterotopia). *Co:* pressure symptoms because of the space-occupying mass. *DD:* teratomas consist of several germ cell layers. *Cholesteatomas* of the *middle ear* may extend into the calvarium; they represent granulation tissue. *Lipomas* are yellow.

Chordoma (Fig. 17.43). *Small, shiny nodules consisting of remnants of chordal tissue. They rarely exceed 1 cm. in diameter.* Chordomas may adhere to the clivus or are attached to the arachnoid layer. Figure 17.43 shows a small chordoma (→) adjacent to the basal artery. This was not a neoplastic chordoma but remnants of chordal tissue. However, such remnants may give rise to a benign or malignant chordoma. True chordomas are observed most commonly around the sacral os and clivus. *Histologically,* a chordoma is composed of clear, glycogen-rich spindle cells. *DD:* chondroma.

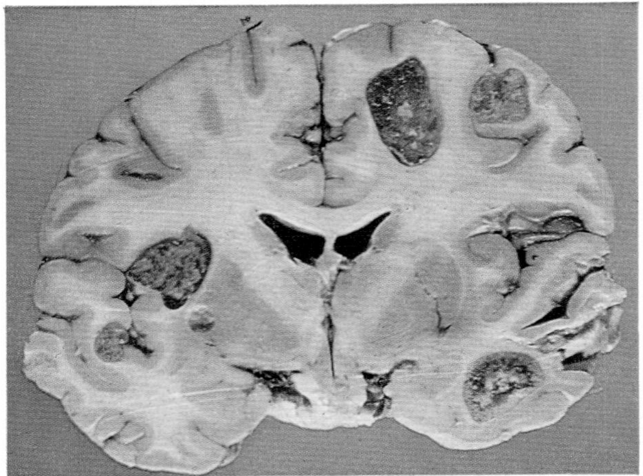

Fig. 17.44. Brain metastases from a bronchial carcinoma.

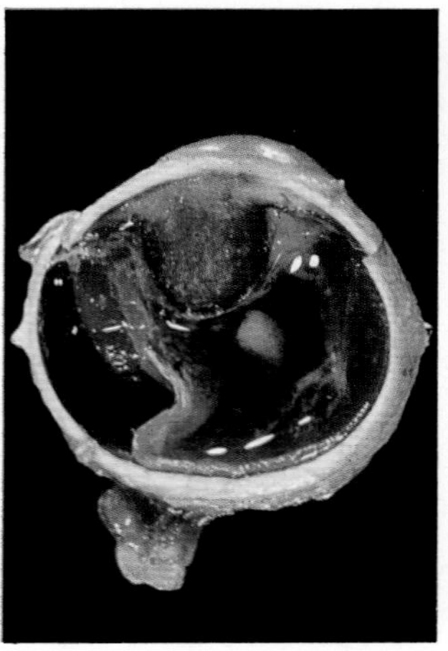

Fig. 17.46. Melanoma of the eye.

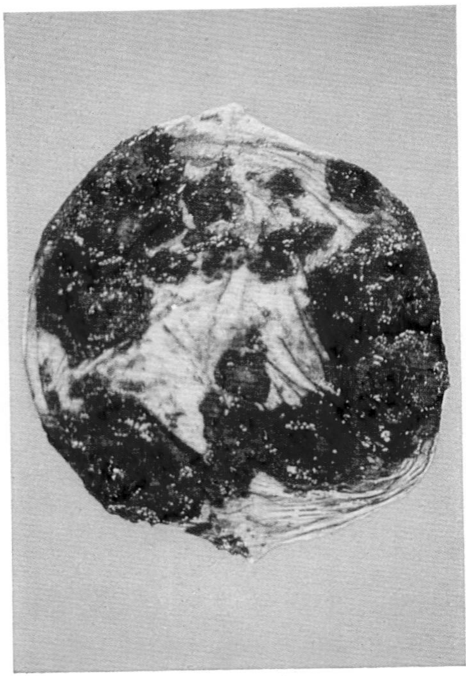

Fig. 17.45. Infiltration of the dura by a neuroblastoma.

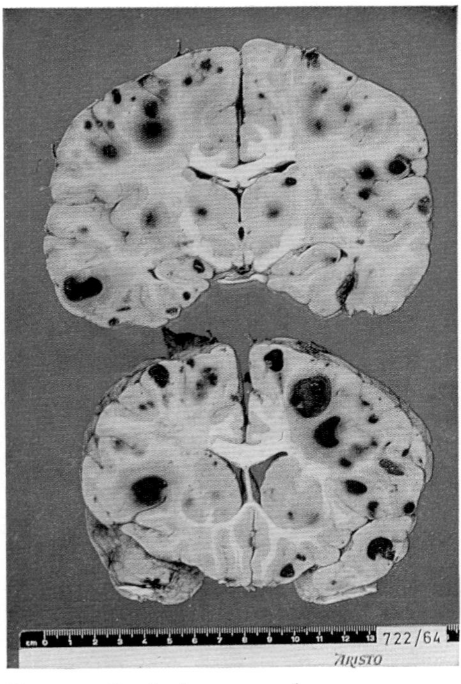

Fig. 17.47. Cerebral metastases from a malignant melanoma.

Metastases

Metastases from a bronchial carcinoma. Figure 17.44 shows a coronal section of the brain. Several gray-brownish tumor nodules of various sizes are scattered throughout. The patient died from a metastatic bronchogenic carcinoma. Relatively small cerebral metastases may be complicated by the development of extensive, unilateral brain edema (see Fig. 17.2). Metastases are grossly recognized as well-delineated nodules, frequently interspersed with areas of necrosis and hemorrhages. The metastatic tissue is yellowish or reddish discolored. The consistency of metastases varies with the primary tumor. Cystic changes frequently are observed in metastases of bronchogenic carcinomas.

F: approximately 5% of all fatal malignant neoplasms have metastasized to the brain by the time of autopsy. The most common primary tumors include bronchogenic carcinoma (brain metastases in 20–40% of the cases), breast carcinoma, renal carcinoma and melanomas. Age and sex distribution are dependent on the primary tumor. *Lo:* cerebrum, cerebellum and brain stem (in the order of frequency 4:2:1). *Co:* signs of increased cerebral pressure, collateral brain edema, growth into the ventricles and hemorrhages.

Dural metastases of a neuroblastoma. The dura and leptomeninges also may be involved in various neoplastic diseases. Figure 17.45 shows the internal surface of the dura with multiple bloody tumor nodules. The primary tumor was a neuroblastoma. Such extensive tumor infiltration of the dura and leptomeninges also is observed in metastatic stomach and breast cancers or in leukemias.

F: 60% of patients with neuroblastomas exhibit metastases in the meninges and skull. Carcinomas of the bronchus, stomach, breast, kidney and thyroid also are prone to metastasize to the dura. Age and sex distribution are dependent on the primary tumor. *Co:* hemorrhages, edema, nerve compression, hydrocephalus.

Melanoma of the eye with cerebral metastasis (Figs. 17.46 and 17.47). Melanomas commonly arise in the skin, genital region or eye. Characteristically, they metastasize widely by the hematogenous and lymphogenous routes. Figure 17.46 shows a dissected eye with a polypoid, projecting black tumor. Figure 17.47 reveals multiple black tumor nodules in the frontal lobes. The black color is due to melanin pigmentation of the tumor cells. This was a case of a melanoma of the choroid with cerebral metastases.

F: approximately 2 among 10,000 diseases of the eye. *A:* after the 60th year of age. *S:* ♂:♀ = 1:1. *Pg:* the most common primary site of intraocular melanomas is the choroidea (80%); 10% arise in the ciliary body and 6% in the iris. Some intraocular melanomas may become metastatic in the brain, liver and lungs many years after the primary tumor has been removed.

DD: (1) *Diktyoma*, a medulloepithelioma of the ciliary body or pars ciliaris of the retina, which is a tumor of small children. Histologically, diktyomas resemble adenocarcinomas. (2) *Angiomatosis* of the retina is a highly differentiated glial proliferation of the retina. (3) *Von Recklinghausen's disease* (neurofibromatosis) of the optic nerve may secondarily involve the eye. (4) *Gliomas, meningiomas*, etc.

18. Malformations

Definitions

Malformations are permanent deformities of the entire body or parts thereof. Malformations result from maldevelopment. Monsters are infants born with pronounced malformations; less severe deviations from the norm are called *anomalies.*

F: according to ZSCHOCH and MAHNKE, malformations are observed in approximately 4.6% of all newborns, account for 12% of autopsies in newborns and for 23% of all autopsies in childhood. Infants with congenital malformations have a reduced vitality, so that 40% of malformed babies die during the perinatal period. *S:* in general, ♂ = ♀, although ♀ monsters predominate. A sex predilection is known for certain malformations, e.g., 88% with a congenital dislocation of the hip are females.

Pg: normal and pathologic growth and differentiation can be separated into a period characterized by the formation and maturation of the gametes (gametogenesis), which precedes fertilization of the ovum. This period is followed by the intrauterine growth phase of the fertilized egg.

The intrauterine growth of the fertilized egg is divided into:

1. *Blastogenesis,* the period from day 1 to day 15 of pregnancy.

2. *Embryogenesis,* from the 15th day to the end of the 3rd month of pregnancy.

3. *Fetogenesis,* from the 4th month of pregnancy to the time of delivery.

Malformations may develop during each of these phases; the corresponding developmental or growth abnormalities are designated as *gameto-, blasto-, embryo- or fetopathies.*

Gametopathy. The cause of developmental abnormalities resides in the sperm or ovum, resulting in *hereditary diseases* of various types. Malformations with *dominant inheritance* include polysyndactyly and harelip. Examples of *recessively inherited malformations* are chondrodystrophy, microcephaly and spina bifida. Certain mutations likewise may cause malformations. Mutations either occur *spontaneously* (e.g., in elderly females) or are *induced* by environmental agents (e.g., x-irradiation). Some malformations are associated with distinct chromosomal changes; for example:

1. **Trisomy 21** is characteristic of *Down's syndrome (mongolism),* a relatively common disease with multiple malformations. The frequency is estimated between 1 in 6,000 and 1 in 1,000 births. ♂ are affected more commonly than ♀. *Cl:* typical mongoloid facial expression, including hypertelorism (wide eyes), epicanthus, four-finger furrow of the hand, transverse furrow of the palms, late sexual development, diminished intelligence ranging to idiocy and occasional congenital cardiac malformations or tumors (leukemia).

2. **Trisomy XXX.** Known as "superfemale," although the patients exhibit minor degrees of mental retardation.

3. **Trisomy XXY** is the most common chromosomal anomaly associated with Klinefelter's syndrome. The patients are phenotypic males, although their nuclei are chromatin positive. Klinefelter's syndrome rarely is diagnosed before puberty: *hypogonadism* with *testosterone deficiency,* eunuchoidism, infertility, gynecomastia, osteoporosis and increased gonadotropin excretion. The testes are small, atrophic and without spermatogenesis. The interstitial (Leydig) cells are hyperplastic. The hair distribution is female. *F:* approximately 0.1% of the male population. Klinefelter's syndrome is nine times more common in mentally retarded patients.

4. **Monosomy X0** is the most common chromosomal anomaly associated with Turner's syndrome. The patients are phenotypically females, although their sex chromatin usually is negative. *Cl: hypogonadism* with *estrogen deficiency.* The gonads are hypoplastic, consisting of stromal elements only. Infertility, short stature, sparse hair, hypoplastic breasts and uterus, osteoporosis, webbed neck, lymphedema of the extremities. Malformations of vessels (coarctation of the aorta), heart and kidney are not uncommon.

Embryopathies are defined as malformations that develop during the embryonal period (up to the 3rd month of pregnancy). Because of the rapid cellular growth during this period, most organ systems are susceptible to various teratogens. Malformations can be induced only prior to the end of the 3rd intra-uterine month. Teratogens include x-rays, viruses, thalidomide, hypoxia and uterine hemorrhages.

Fetopathies are defined as disturbances of growth or other diseases that develop after the 3rd month of pregnancy. In most cases, exogenous or endogenous factors result in growth disturbances or inflammatory, degenerative or neoplastic changes. Examples are the diabetic fetopathy (see p. 307; giant babies), congenital syphilis (liver damage, saddle nose, Hutchinson's triad, pneumonia alba), toxoplasmosis (internal hydrocephalus, see p. 325) or listeriosis (miliary liver granulomas, see p. 161). The persistence of certain fetal primordia also is considered a form of malformation (e.g., persistence of ductus arteriosus, Meckel's diverticulum). Amniotic bands also may cause fetopathies.

Postnatal developmental anomalies occur after birth and may become manifest as late as during puberty (e.g., local gigantism). Certain organs are not fully developed at birth and are susceptible to the development of postnatal anomalies. An example is the development of congenital pyelonephritis in an immature renal cortex. *Hamartomas* (overgrowth of tissues belonging to a particular organ) and *choristomas* (excessive growth of tissues foreign to the organ of development) are late, tumor-like malformations.

Morphologic classification of malformations (with examples)

- I. Double malformations
  - 1. Free double malformations
    - Normal: Monozygotic twins
    - Abnormal: Double malformations *(holoacardius acephalus)*
  - 2. Conjoined double malformations
    - A. Parasitic types
      - Autosite and parasite (sacral parasite)
    - B. Symmetric types
      - Incomplete *(dicephalus)*
      - Complete *(thoracopagus)*
- II. Single malformations
  - 1. Developmental failures
    - Aplasia, atresia, hypoplasia, clefts, defects, stenosis *(amelia, atresia of esophagus, stenosis of aortic isthmus, gnathopalatoschisis)*
  - 2. Excess
    - Hyperplasia, supernumerary organs, duplications *(generalized or focal gigantism, polydactyly)*
  - 3. Displacement
    - Adhesions, fusions *(amniotic adhesions, horseshoe kidney, cyclops)*
    - Duplications *(uterus bicornis)*
    - Faulty development of viscera *(cysts, diverticula)*
    - Heterotopias and ectopias *(hamartomas, pelvic kidneys, aberrant breasts)*
    - Errors of rotation, shape or position *(situs inversus, transposition of great vessels, clubfoot)*
  - 4. Persistence of fetal structures
    - *Persistence of ductus arteriosus, Meckel's diverticulum*

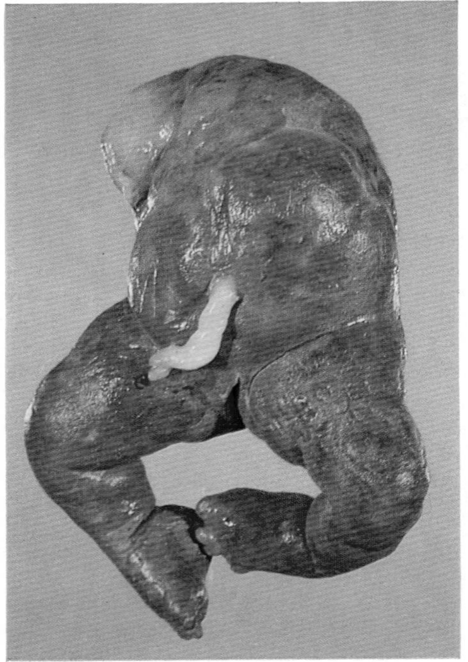

Fig. 18.1. Acardius acephalus.

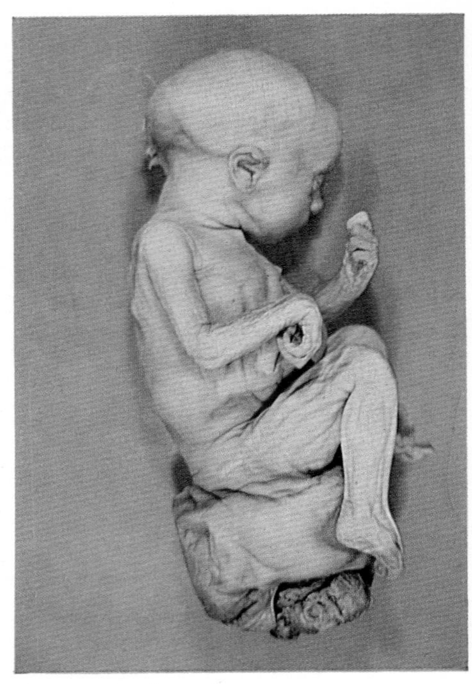

Fig. 18.2. Sacral parasite.

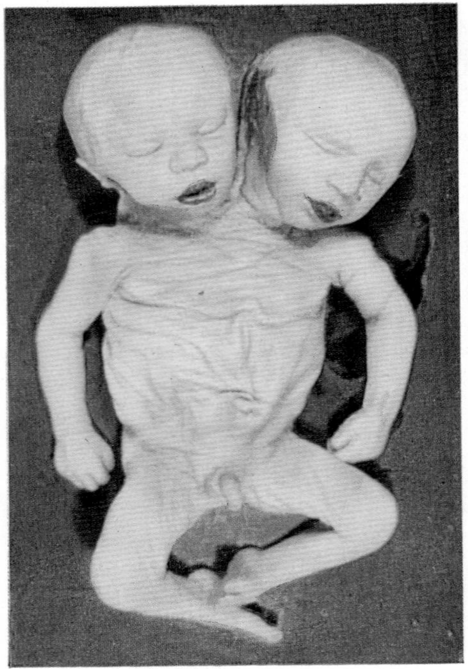

Fig. 18.3. Dicephalus.

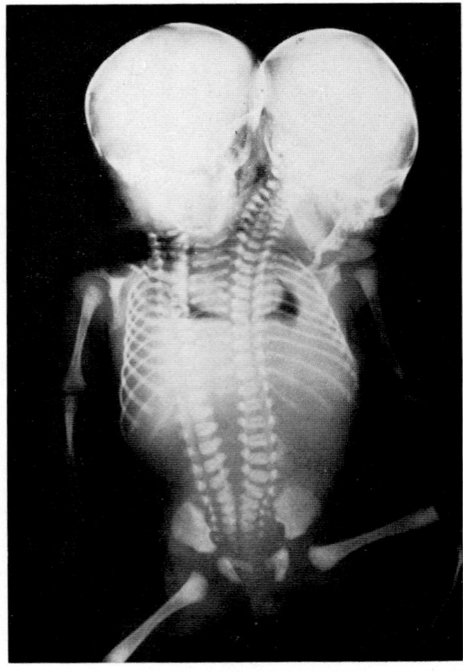

Fig. 18.4. Roentgenogram of a dicephalus.

Double Malformations

Double malformations are embryonic duplications. They may occur independently of each other (i.e., conjoined by a placenta and umbilical cord) or may be conjoined by direct junction of parts of the body. The important anatomic feature of such malformations is duplication of the body axis (head, trunk or spine). Accordingly, supernumerary fingers do not belong in the group of double malformations.

1. **Free double malformations** are termed *twins* that may be normal and fully developed (monozygotic twins) or malformed. An example of a free double malformation is the *acardius*. An acardius is observed only in monozygotic twins: the malformed twin is without a heart and the other twin has a functional heart. The *hemicardius* has a rudimentary cardiac primordium that does not function. The *acardius* may resemble a normal baby or may present as an unrecognizable mass *(A. amorphous)*. The *holoacardius* is characterized by the absence of caudal *(H. acormus)* or cranial *(H. acephalus)* portions. The head of a holoacardius occasionally may be covered in the amorphous mass and can be demonstrated only by x-ray *(H. pseudoacephalus)*.

Holoacardius acephalus. Figure 18.1 shows a malformation with recognizable trunk and lower extremities. The head is missing. This is one of the most common types of free double malformations.

2. **Joined twins** are divided into those with equal or symmetric and unequal or asymmetric organ primordia:

A. **Asymmetric, joined double malformations** also are known as parasitic double malformations. They consist of two members with unequal degrees of development. The *autosite* develops normally, whereas the *parasite* either is incomplete or presents as an amorphous mass. Autosite and parasite may be conjoined at the cranial *(epignathus)* or caudal *(sacral parasite)* portions (Fig. 18.2). A parasite also may develop within another fetus *(fetus in fetu)*. *Teratomas* likewise are considered forms of parasitic double malformation. *Mature teratomas* consist of fairly well differentiated tissues in contrast to *embryonal or immature teratomas*. Some teratomas contain only two germ cell layers (e.g., ovarian dermoid, Fig. 15.22). A teratoma may give rise to a true neoplasm by excessive growth of one or more components (e.g., choriocarcinoma in a testicular teratoma, Fig. 14.11).

B. **Symmetric double malformations** are embryonic duplications that usually are conjoined. In severe cases, partial duplication of the body axis may be observed. An example of a symmetric double malformation is the *dicephalus* (Fig. 18.3). Figure 18.4 shows the more common duplication of the spine in a dicephalus.

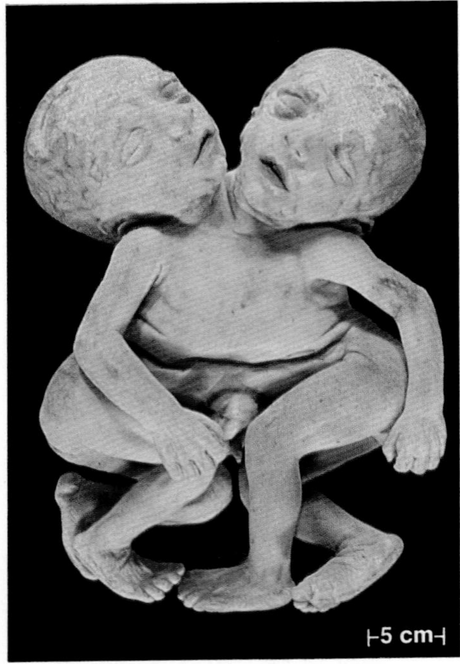

Fig. 18.5. Iliothoracopagus.

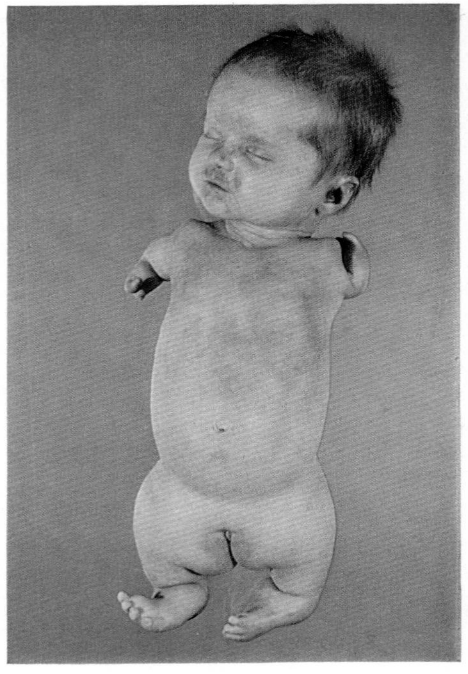

Fig. 18.6. Phocomelia.

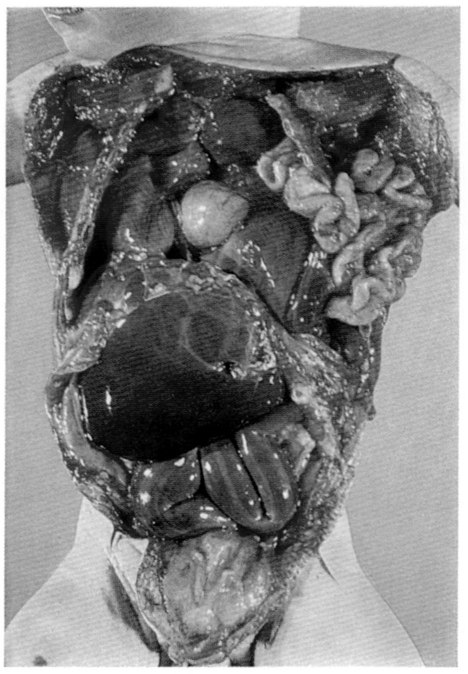

Fig. 18.7. Displacement of the abdominal organs into the left pleural cavity.

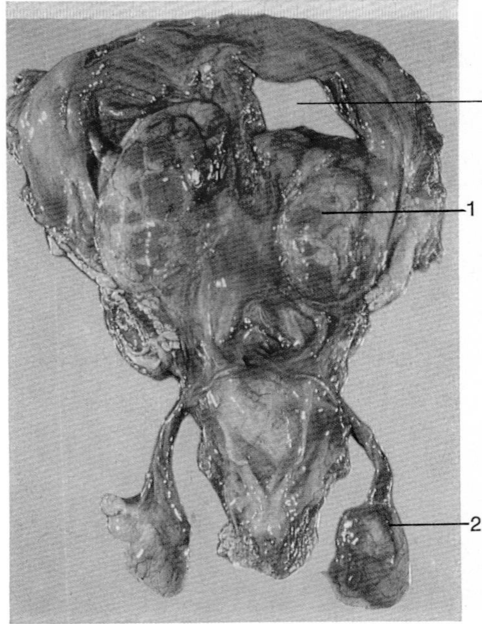

Fig. 18.8. Congenital left-sided diaphragmatic defect.

C. **Complete, symmetric double malformations** show a partial duplication between mature fetuses. The twins may be joined in the area of the head *(cephalopagus)*. An example is the mythologic Janus head, a fusion of a dorsal craniopagus with a double face (diprosopus). Twins also may be conjoined by a connection of the sternal region (*thoracopagus*, Fig. 18.5, Siamese twins) or below the umbilicus *(ilioxiphopagus)*. Extensive connections between the trunks *(ilioxiphothoracopagus)* merge morphologically with a dicephalus, especially when only two upper and two lower extremities are present (Figs. 18.3 and 18.4). *Pygopagus* refers to twins who are joined at the sacral areas. These are extremely rare but viable. *Ischiopagus* refers to a connection in the lower pelvic regions so that the heads extend in opposite directions. The lower extremities arise laterally from the trunk.

Single Malformations

Single malformations occur in single embryos (a twin must not be present), although they may be multiple. For example, Down's syndrome or the thalidomide embryopathy frequently result in multiple malformations. Multiple malformations are considered the result of *syntropy* of several developmental and growth defects. Most organ malformations are discussed in the respective organ chapters. Only some examples are listed here:

1. Developmental failures:

An organ or organ primordium may be entirely missing (aplasia or agenesis) or may be incompletely developed *(hypoplasia)*. *Dysmelias* are examples of developmental failures of the extremities. Several forms of dysmelia are recognized: *Amelia* refers to a complete absence of one or several extremities; shoulder and pelvic bones are present but often hypoplastic. *Phocomelia* (Fig. 18.6) refers to a partial defect of hands and feet that are attached to the trunk by a single, small, irregularly shaped bone. *Peromelia* is a congenital shortening of the extremities. A more common partial defect of the bony system is the *aplasia of the radius* that leads to a clubhand. Abnormally small extremities are referred to as *micromelia*. One form of micromelia is chondrodystrophy (see p. 195).

Pg: dysmelias result from damage to the embryo between the 4th and 6th weeks of pregnancy. Although known for centuries, dysmelias increased markedly in Germany between 1959 and 1962. These malformations were attributable to maternal use of thalidomide. The *dysmelia syndrome* (H. R. WIEDEMANN, 1961) includes not only developmental abnormalities of the extremities but malformations of the heart, vessels, gastrointestinal tract, urinary system and ear and nevi.

Congenital diaphragmatic hernia (Figs. 18.7 and 18.8). Most cases are not true hernias but partial defects of the diaphragm. Figure 18.8 shows such defects in the left diaphragm (→1 kidney, →2 testis). The left portion of the liver, stomach and intestinal loops are displaced into the thoracic cavity (Fig. 18.7).

F: defects of the diaphragm are observed in 4.7‰ of newborn autopsies and account for approximately 3.8% of all malformations. The left diaphragm is affected more commonly than the right (7:1) (ESSBACH). Much less common are *diaphragmatic hernias*, in which the displaced organs are surrounded by a *sac of diaphragm*.

Pg: partial agenesis of the diaphragm because of a faulty obliteration of the pleuroperitoneal duct. The duct remains open up to the 7th embryonal week.

Pr: only 15% survive the first year of life.

Other forms of atresia: *Atresias* are common in the gastrointestinal tract, e.g., atresias of the esophagus (p. 105), rectum or anus. Atresias also may manifest as congenital stenosis, e.g., in the cardiovascular system (see p. 21). Infundibular stenosis of the pulmonary artery or aortic isthmus stenosis (Fig. 2.11) are examples. *Hypoplasias of organs* include hypoplasias of the cerebellum and kidney ("dwarf kidney").

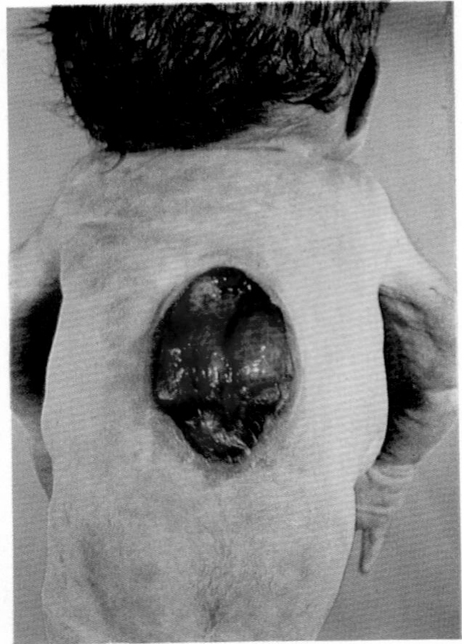

Fig. 18.9. Rachischisis.

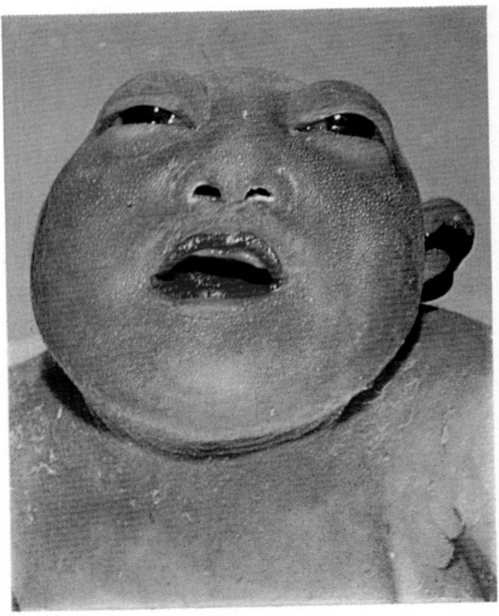

Fig. 18.10. Anencephalus.

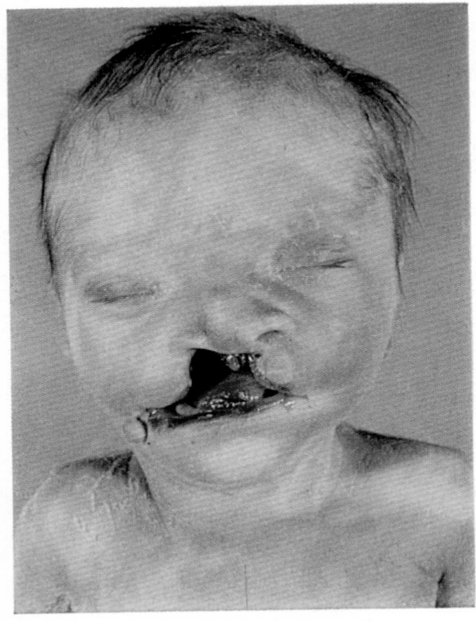

Fig. 18.11. Cheilognathopalatoschisis.

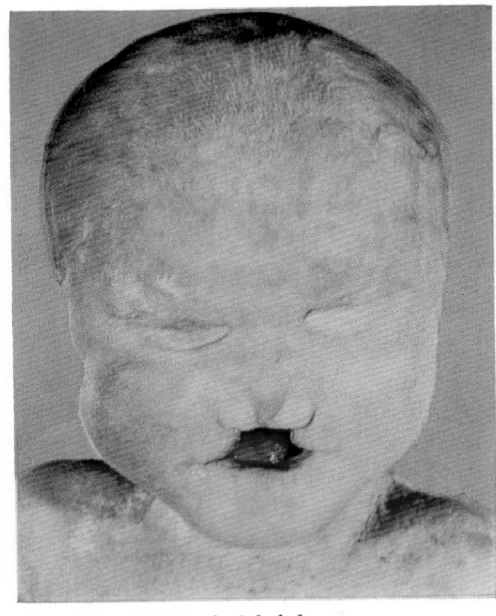

Fig. 18.12. Median facial cleft.

Common malformations are those attributable to disturbances of closure. They affect the central nervous system, usually are manifested in the dorsal median line and are most common in the lumbosacral area. *Rachischisis* refers to a congenital fissure of the spine. The gross picture is typical (Fig. 18.9): The center of the defect is oval, red, moist and spongy. This *area medullovasculosa* consists of rudimentary spinal cord tissue with many newly formed capillaries. An *area epithelo-serosa* surrounds the central portion and consists of leptomeninges that are covered by thin squamous epithelium. The most peripheral *zona dermatica* merges with the epidermis. A *myelocele* is a special form of rachischisis: a partial defect of the dorsal spinal cord is present and the central canal communicates freely with the external surface.

(a) The most simple form of rachischisis is the *occult spina bifida* – a circumscribed defect is present in the dura and the dorsal rami of one or more vertebrae. The vertebral rami fail to fuse and the spinal canal remains open (x-ray diagnosis). The area is covered by skin. *Co:* meningitis.

(b) *Meningocele* is a diverticulum-like projection of a sac that contains cerebrospinal fluid.

(c) *Meningomyelocele:* the arachnoid sac contains portions of the spinal cord, cauda equina or the area medullovasculosa (see above) and also contains cerebrospinal fluid.

(d) *Meningomyelocystocele* or *syringomyelocele:* a combination of a meningocele and *hydromyelia* (the spinal cord is ballooned because of hydropic changes in the central canal).

Anencephalus. Figure 18.10 shows the typical "frog face." The cranial vault is absent *(acrania)* and the hemispheres are either missing or markedly reduced (anencephalus). The neck is short. Anencephalus frequently is associated with other organ and skeletal malformations, especially total rachischisis (amyelia = complete aplasia of the spinal cord). The pituitary gland is missing in an anencephalus. Consequently, the adrenal glands are not stimulated and remain hypoplastic.

F: 2.1% of all autopsies in newborns and 5% of all malformations. Common cause of death of premature stillbirths or newborns. *S:* ♂ : ♀ = 1 : 3.

Clefts of the face (Figs. 18.11 and 18.12). These common malformations either occur as isolated defects or accompany other severe developmental malformations (see cyclops, p. 341). The following forms are distinguished:

(a) **Lateral clefts of the face** may occur as isolated defects or accompany other severe malformations *(cheiloschisis or harelip)* (Fig. 18.11). These clefts may extend to, and involve, the maxilla *(gnathoschisis)* or palate *(palatoschisis)*. Clefts may occur unilaterally or bilaterally (bilateral symmetric cheilognathopalato-schisis).

(b) **Median facial clefts** likewise affect lips, maxilla or palate (Fig. 18.12). The vomer is aplastic and the nose is flattened.

(c) **Oblique facial clefts** extend from the upper lip to the eyes.

F and *Pg:* simple clefts are relatively rare in autopsy material. The more complicated facial clefts represent approximately 6.3% of all malformations or 2.8% of autopsies in newborns (Zschoch and Mahnke). These malformations are inherited as a dominant trait and develop between the 8th and 10th embryonal weeks.

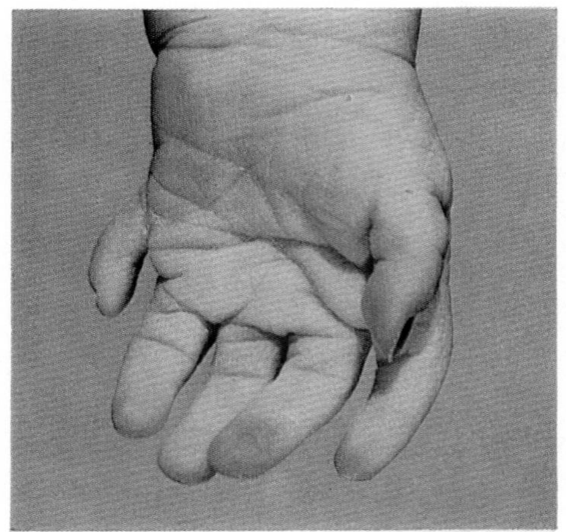

Fig. 18.13. Polydactyly.

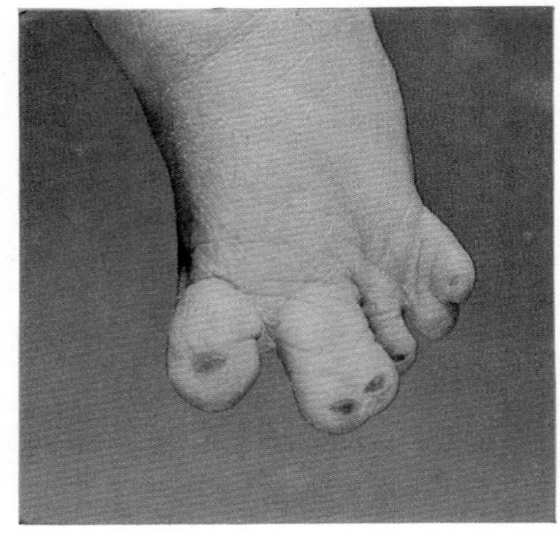

Fig. 18.14. Polysyndactyly.

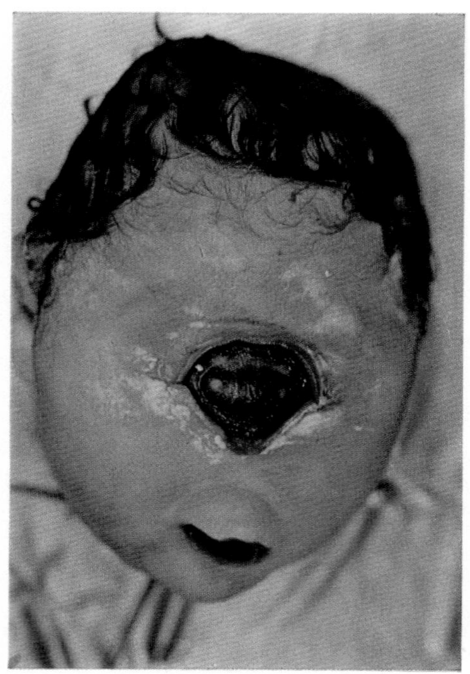

Fig. 18.15. Cyclops.

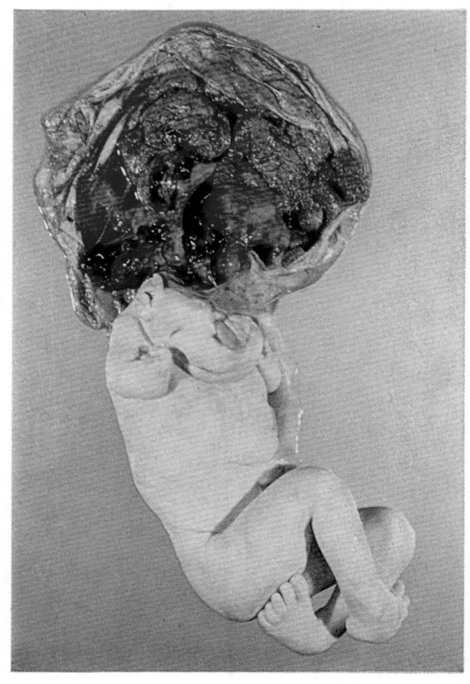

Fig. 18.16. Adhesions between the amnion, placenta and fetal head.

2. **Malformations due to excess formation of organs** include hyperplastic and supernumerary portions of the body. Excessive growth leads to hyperplasia and a generalized gigantism. The upper limit of body height is dependent on ethnic factors. Hyperplasias also can cause a local gigantism (e.g., macrodactyly or giant fingers).

Supernumerary organs are the result of duplication or partial displacement of an organ primordium. Examples are accessory spleens, unilateral double ureter and polydactyly. *Disturbances of the involution* of paired but independently developing organs (e.g., Müllerian ducts) that normally form a single organ (uterus) can lead to duplications. The uterus bicornis duplex, uterus bicornis unicollis and uterus septus are examples of organ malformations attributable to faulty involution of the Müllerian duct.

Polydactyly. Figure 18.13 shows a hand with six fingers. Polydactyly may be masked by syndactyly, i.e., fusion of several finger or toe bones (Fig. 18.14) or webbed fingers. Polydactyly is often, although not invariably, inherited as a dominant trait.

F: isolated cases of polydactyly or syndactyly are relatively uncommon (0.2%) in autopsy material of newborns.

3. **Malformations due to displacement of organs** include (1) *fusion of paired organs* (e.g.), horseshoe kidney, p. 247; cyclops, Fig. 18.15; syndactyly, Fig. 18.14), (2) *heterotopias* and *ectopias* (e.g., lung hamartomas, p. 91; liver cavernomas, p. 163; ectopias of testis or breast), (3) faulty development of viscera (e.g., congenital diverticula of the esophagus, urinary bladder, small and large intestine, p. 121), (4) formation of cysts in the lung, liver (p. 137), kidneys (p. 247) and (5) abnormal shapes and positions of feet or hands.

Cyclops is a combination of severe malformations of the eyes, nasal bones and the olfactory region. Figure 18.15 shows an orbit in the middle of the forehead. The eyelids are partially fused to form a round or ovoid organ. The eyes are partially fused *(synophthalmia)*. The nose and olfactory brain are absent *(arhinencephaly)*. Above the orbital fossa, an appendage of skin *(proboscis)* ends blindly (missing in Fig. 18.15).

F: this rare malformation is not compatible with life and accounts for 0.16% of cases of perinatal mortality (ESSBACH).

4. **Persistence of fetal primordia** involves especially organs of the gastrointestinal tract (e.g., Meckel's diverticulum) or cardiovascular system (e.g., ductus arteriosus).

Amniotic bands (Fig. 18.16). Bands of amnion adhere to the surface of the embryo, leading to severe distortions and malformations. Amniotic adhesions often are attached to the head or fingers. Fusion with the placenta is observed not uncommonly, as shown in Figure 18.16. These fibrous bands also may amputate extremities.

Selected References

1. Introduction

General

ADAMS, J. R., Jr., R. MADER: Autopsy (Chicago: Year Book Medical Publishers, Inc., 1976).
HAMPERL, H.: Leichenöffnung. Befund und Diagnose (Heidelberg: Springer-Verlag, 1962).
KOHLHAAS, M.: Deutsche med. Wchnschr. *94:* 1202 (1969).
REZEK, P. R., M. MILLARD: Autopsy Pathology (Springfield, Ill.: Charles C Thomas, Publisher, 1963).

Color

BORN, M.: Naturwissenschaften *50:* 29 (1963).
MUNSELL, A. H.: Atlas of the Munsell Color System (Malden, Mass.: Wadsworth Howland & Company, Inc., 1915).
SANDRITTER, W., W. LÜBBERS, K. NOESKE: Virchows Arch. path. Anat. *338:* 172 (1964).
WRIGHT, W. D.: The Measurement of Colour (London: Higer & Watts, 1958).

2. Heart and Pericardium

General

GOULD, S. E.: Pathology of the Heart and Blood Vessels (3rd ed.; Springfield, Ill.: Charles C Thomas, Publisher, 1968).
HUDSON, R. E.: Cardiovascular Pathology, Vol. 3 (Baltimore: The Williams & Wilkins Company, 1970).

Malformations

EDWARDS, J. E., L. S. CAREY, H. N. NEUFELD, R. LESTER: Congenital Heart Disease (Philadelphia and London: W. B. Saunders Company, 1965).
GOERTTLER, K.: In Lehrbuch der Speziellen Pathologischen Anatomie (Berlin: de Gruyter, 1968), Band I, Teil I, S. 301.
LEV, M.: Autopsy Diagnosis of Congenitally Malformed Hearts (Springfield, Ill.: Charles C Thomas, Publisher, 1953).

Hypertrophy and Dilatation

FLECKENSTEIN, A.: Verhandl. deutsch. Gesellsch. Path. *51:* 15 (1967).
SANDRITTER, W., G. SCOMMAZONI: Nature, London *202:* 100 (1964).

Infarction

FRIEDMAN, M.: Pathogenesis of Coronary Disease (New York: McGraw-Hill Book Company, Inc., 1969).
WARTMAN, W. B.: Definition of Myocardial Infarction, in James, T. N., and Keys, F. W. (eds.), The Etiology of Myocardial Infarction (Boston: Little, Brown & Company, 1961).

Atrophy

HELLERSTEIN, D., D. SANTIAGO-STEVENSON: Circulation *1:* 93 (1950).

Endocarditis

HUDSON, R. E. B.: Cardiovascular Pathology, Vol. 3 (Baltimore: The Williams & Wilkins Company, 1970).

Myocarditis

BLANKENHORN, M. A., E. A. GALL: Circulation *13:* 217 (1956).
SAPHIR, O.: Arch. path. Anat. *33:* 88 (1942).

Endocardial Fibrosis

HUDSON, R. E. B.: Cardiovascular Pathology, Vol. 3 (Baltimore: The Williams & Wilkins Company, 1970).

3. Blood Vessels

Arteriosclerosis

ANITSCHKOW, N.: Beitr. path. Anat. *56:* 379 (1913).
BÜRGER, L.: Am. J. M. Sc. *136:* 567 (1908).
DUGUID, J. B.: J. Path. & Bact. *58:* 307 (1946).
ERDHEIM, J.: Virchows Arch. path. Anat. *276:* 187 (1930).
GSELL, O.: Virchows Arch. path. Anat. *270:* 1 (1928).

LOBSTEIN, J.: Traités d'anatomie pathologique, Paris 1833.
MITCHELL, J. R. A., E. J. SCHWARTZ: Arterial Disease (Oxford: Blackwell Scientific Publications, 1965).
MÖNCKEBERG, J.: Virchows Arch. path. Anat. *171:* 141 (1903).
SCHETTLER, G.: Ergebn. inn. Med. u. Kinderh. (N. F.) *6:* 278 (1955).
SHIMAMOTO, T., F. NUMANO: Atherogenesis. Proceedings of the First International Symposium on Atherogenesis, Thrombogenesis and Pyridinolcarbamate Treatment, Tokyo (Amsterdam: Excerpta Medica Foundation, 1969).
STERNBY, N. H.: Acta path. et microbiol. scandinav. (supp.) *194:* 1 (1968).
STRANDNESS, D. E.: Peripheral Arterial Disease (Boston: Little, Brown & Company, 1969).
WEGENER, F.: Beitr. path. Anat. *102:* 36 (1939).
WINIWARTER, F. V.: Arch. klin. Chir. *23:* 202 (1879).

Circulation

HARDERS, H. (ed.): Advances in Microcirculation (Basel: Karger, 1968), Vol. 1.
HERSHEY, S. G. (ed.): Shock (Boston: Little, Brown & Company, 1964).
THAL, A. P. (ed.): Shock (Chicago: Year Book Medical Publishers, Inc., 1971).
WARTMAN, W. B.: Am. Heart J. *39:* 79 (1950).

Arteritis

LEWIS, T.: Clin. Sc. *3:* 287 (1938). (Raynaud's disease.)

Thrombosis

HARDAWAY, R. M.: Syndromes of Disseminated Intravascular Coagulation (Springfield, Ill.: Charles C Thomas, Publisher, 1966).
McKAY, D. G.: Disseminated Intravascular Coagulation (New York and London: Harper & Row, Publishers, 1965).
RODMAN, N. F., Jr., R. G. MASON, K. M. BRINKHOUS: Fed. Proc. *22:* 1356 (1963).
RODMAN, N. F., Jr., J. C. PAINTER, N. B. McDEVITT: J. Cell Biol. *16:* 225 (1963).
SANDRITTER, W., G. BENEKE: In Lehrbuch der Speziellen Pathologischen Anatomie (Berlin: de Gruyter, 1968), Band I, Teil I, S. 465.

4. Upper Respiratory Tract, Lungs, Pleura

Trachea

ASCHOFF, L.: Verhandl. deutsch. Gesellsch. Path. *14:* 125 (1910).
BENEKE, G., D. ENDERS, H. BECKER, H. NITSCHKE: Virchows Arch. path. Anat. *341:* 353 (1966).

Lungs (General)

CUMMING, G., L. B. HUNT: Form and Function in the Human Lung (Edinburgh: E. & S. Livingstone, Ltd., 1968).
LIEBOW, A. A., D. E. SMITH (eds.): The Lung (Baltimore: The Williams & Wilkins Company, 1968).
SPENCER, H.: Pathology of the Lung (London: Pergamon Press, 1968).

Emphysema, Embolism, Infarction

BIGNON, J., F. KHOURY, P. EVEN, J. ANDRE, G. BROUET: Ann. Rev. Resp. Dis. *99:* 669 (1969).
HARTUNG, W.: Ergebn. inn. Med. u. Kinderh. (N. F.) *15:* 273 (1960).
HARTUNG, W.: In Pathophysiologie und Klinik (Heidelberg: Springer-Verlag, 1964), Band XIV.
HEARD, B. E.: Pathology of Chronic Bronchitis and Emphysema (London: J. & A. Churchill, Ltd., 1969).
OTTO, H.: Handbuch der Allgemeinen Pathologie (Heidelberg: Springer-Verlag, 1970), Band III, Teil 4.
OTTO, H., R. ZEILHOFER: Respiration *26:* 226 (1969).

Lung Hemosiderosis

CEELEN, W.: In Henke, F., O. Lubarsch (eds.), Handbuch der Speziellen Pathologie (Heidelberg: Springer-Verlag, 1931), Band 3, S. 20.
GOODPASTURE, E. W.: Am. J. M. Sc. *158:* 863 (1919).
WEGENER, F.: Beitr. path. Anat. *102:* 36 (1939).

Pneumonia

HAMMAN, L., A. R. RICH: Bull. Johns Hopkins Hosp. *74:* 177 (1944).

Sarcoidosis

Proc. 3rd Internat. Congress Sarcoidosis, Acta med. scandinav., Supp. *425*, 1964.
SCADDING, J. G.: Sarcoidosis (London: Eyre & Spottiswoode, 1967).

Pulmonary Tuberculosis

Diagnostic Standards and Classification of Tuberculosis (New York: National Tuberculosis Association, 1961).

LOWELL, A. M., L. B. EDWARDS, C. E. PALMER: Tuberculosis (Cambridge, Mass.: Harvard University Press, 1969).

Bronchial Carcinoma

EBNER, H. B., B. LEDERER, W. SANDRITTER: Deutsche med. Wchnschr. *92:* 1901 (1967).

EVANS, R. W.: Histological Appearances of Tumors (2d ed.; Baltimore: The Williams & Wilkins Company, 1966).

LIEBOW, A. A.: Tumor Pathology of the Lower Respiratory Tract, Fascicle XVII, in Atlas of Tumor Pathology (Washington, D. C.: Armed Forces Institute of Pathology, 1952).

MEHRAIN, M.: Die Malignen Tumoren im Sektionsmaterial des Pathologischen Institutes der Universität Bonn von 1946 bis 1962. Bonn: Dissertation, 1966.

Pleural Mesothelioma

EVANS, R. W.: Histological Appearances of Tumors (2d ed.; Baltimore: The Williams & Wilkins Company, 1966).

5. Gastrointestinal Tract

General

BOCKUS, H. L.: Gastroenterology (3d ed.; Philadelphia: W. B. Saunders Company, 1976).

Oral Cavity

SHAFER, W. G., M. K. HINE, B. M. LEVY: A Textbook of Oral Pathology (3d ed.; Philadelphia and London: W. B. Saunders Company, 1974).

Gastritis

PALMER, E. D.: Medicine *33:* 199 (1954).

SIURALA, M., M. ISOKOSKI, K. VARIS, M. KEKKI: Scandinav. J. Gastroenterol. *3:* 211 (1968).

Gastric Carcinoma

LAUREN, P.: Acta path. et microbiol. scandinav. *64:* 31 (1965).

Small Intestine (General)

TACKRAY, A. C., F. A. JONES (eds.): The Small Intestine (Oxford: Blackwell Scientific Publications, 1965).

Malabsorption Syndrome

MCCARTHY, C. F., J. L. BORLAND, S. M. KURTZ, J. M. RUFFIN: Am. J. Path. *44:* 585 (1964).

SWANSON, V. L., R. W. THOMASSEN: Am. J. Path. *46:* 511 (1965).

TOWNLEY, R. R. W., CH. M. ANDERSON: Ergebn. inn. Med. u. Kinderh. (N. F.) *26:* 1 (1967).

Melanosis Coli

ECKER, J., D. R. DICKSON: Am. J. Gastroenterol. *39:* 363 (1963).

Carcinoma, Carcinoid

CLARK, R. L., et al.: Cancer of the Gastrointestinal Tract (Chicago: Year Book Medical Publishers, Inc., 1967).

EVANS, R. W.: Histological Appearances of Tumors (2d ed.; Baltimore: The Williams & Wilkins Company, 1966).

6. Liver

General

ELIAS, H., J. C. SHERRICK: Morphology of the Liver (New York: Academic Press, 1969).

POPPER, H., F. SCHAFFNER (eds.): Progress in Liver Disease (New York and London: Grune & Stratton, Inc., 1961).

ROULLIER, CH.: The Liver (New York: Academic Press, 1963).

VANDENBROUKE, J., J. DE GROOTE, L. O. STANDART: Advances in Hepatology (Basel: Karger, 1965).

Alcoholic and Fatty Liver
KREBS, H. A., R. A. FREDDLAND, R. HEMS, M. STUBBS: Biochem. J. *112:* 117 (1969).
LIEBER, CH. S., E. RUBIN: New England J. Med. *280:* 705 (1969).

Eclampsia
BLACK-SCHAFFER, B., D. S. JOHNSON, W. G. GOBBEL: Am. J. Path. *26:* 397 (1950).

Amyloid
VIRCHOW, R.: Arch. path. Anat. *6:* 268 (1854).

Budd-Chiari Syndrome
BUDD, G.: On Diseases of the Liver (2d ed.; London: J. & A. Churchill, Ltd., 1852).
CHIARI, H.: Beitr. path. Anat. *26:* 1 (1899).

Liver Cirrhosis
CAMERON, R., D. C. HOU: Biliary Cirrhosis (London: Oliver & Boyd, Ltd., 1962).
SHERLOCK, S.: Diseases of the Liver and Biliary System (3d ed.; Oxford: Blackwell Scientific Publications, 1963).

Hepatitis
IVERSEN, P., K. ROHOLM: Acta med. scandinav. *102:* 1 (1939).
POPPER, H., F. SCHAFFER: The Liver (New York: McGraw-Hill Book Company, Inc., 1957).
SIEDE, W., A. KLAMP: Ergebn. inn. Med. u. Kinderh. (N. F.) *18:* 283 (1962).

Tumors
STEINER, P. E., I. HIGGINSON: Acta Unio internat. contra cancrum *17:* 581 (1961).

7. Gallbladder – Bile Ducts

MOYER, C. A., J. E. RHOADS, J. C. ALLEN, H. N. HARKINS: Surgery, Principles and Practice (3d ed.; Philadelphia and Montreal: J. B. Lippincott Company, 1965).

8. Pancreas

Fibrosis, Pancreatitis and Necrosis
ANDERSON, D. H.: Ann. New York Acad. Sc. *93:* 500 (1962).
REUCH, A. V. S., M. P. CAMERON (eds.): The Exocrine Pancreas (London: J. & A. Churchill, Ltd., 1962)

Diabetes Mellitus
KIEF, H.: Zentralbl. Path. *111:* 345 (1968).
PFEIFFER, E. F.: Diabetes Mellitus (Handbuch) (München: Lehmann, 1968).
WARREN, S., P. M. LE COMPTE: The Pathology of Diabetes Mellitus (Philadelphia: Lea & Febiger, 1952).

9. Spleen, Lymph Nodes, Blood

Spleen
BLAUSTEIN, A. (ed.): The Spleen (New York: McGraw-Hill Book Company, Inc., 1963).

Lymph Nodes
LENNERT, K.: Pathologie der Halslymphknoten (Berlin: Springer-Verlag, 1964).
MARSHALL, A. H. E.: An Outline of the Cytology and Pathology of the Reticular Tissue (London: Oliver & Boyd, Ltd., 1956).

Hodgkin's Disease
LUKES, K. J., J. J. BUTLER: Cancer Res. *26:* 1063 (1966).
MUSSHOFF, K., W. OEHLERT, W. HAMANN, A. NUSS: Klin. Wchnschr. *47:* 1175 (1969).
RAPPAPORT, H.: Tumors of the Hematopoietic System (Washington, D. C.: Armed Forces Institute of Pathology, 1966).

Leukemia

AMROMIN, G. D.: Pathology of Leukemia (New York: Hoeber Medical Division, Harper & Row Publishers, 1968).

WHITBY, L. E. H., C. J. C. BRITTON: Disorders of the Blood (10th ed.; London: J. & A. Churchill, Ltd., 1969).

WINTROBE, M. M.: Clinical Hematology (7th ed.; Philadelphia: Lea & Febiger, 1974).

10. Cartilage, Bone and Soft Tissues

Bones

AERGERTER, E., J. A. KIRKPATRICK: Orthopedic Diseases (4th ed.; Philadelphia and London: W. B. Saunders Company, 1975).

HARRISON, C. V.: Diseases of Bone, in Recent Advances in Pathology (7th ed.; London: J. & A. Churchill, Ltd., 1960), Chapter IX.

Bone Tumors

ACKERMAN, L. V., J. J. SPJUT: Tumors of the Bone and Cartilage, in Atlas of Tumor Pathology (Washington, D. C.: Armed Forces Institute of Pathology, 1962), Section II, Fascicle 4.

JAFFE, H. L.: Tumors and Tumorous Conditions of the Bones and Joints (Philadelphia: Lea & Febiger, 1958).

LICHTENSTEIN, L.: Bone Tumors (St. Louis: The C. V. Mosby Company, 1959).

Joints

BENEKE, G.: Verhandl. deutsch. Gesellsch. Rheumat. *1:* 5 (1969).

Tumors of Soft Tissues

ENZINGER, F. M.: Histological Typing of Soft Tissue Tumors. International Histological Classification of Tumors (Geneva: WHO, 1969).

STOUT, A. P., R. LATTES: Tumors of Soft Tissues, in Atlas of Tumor Pathology (Washington, D. C.: Armed Forces Institute of Pathology, 1966), Second Series, Fascicle I.

Obesity

REH, H.: Virchows Arch. path. Anat. *324:* 234 (1953).

Cachexia

ASTWOOD, E. B.: Clinical Endocrinology (New York: Grune & Stratton, Inc., 1960), Vol. I.

Collagen Diseases

DORFMAN, A.: J. Chron. Dis. *10:* 365 (1959).

KLEMPERER, P.: Am. Rev. Resp. Dis. *83:* 331 (1961).

SAMTER, M., H. L. ALEXANDER (eds.): Immunological Diseases (2d ed.; Boston: Little, Brown & Company, 1971).

VASQUEZ, J. J., F. J. DIXON: Lab. Invest. *6:* 205 (1957).

11. Skin and Mammary Gland

LEVER, W. F.: Histopathology of the Skin (4th ed.; Philadelphia and Montreal: J. B. Lippincott Company, 1967).

LUND, H. Z.: Tumors of the Skin, in Atlas of Tumor Pathology (Washington, D. C.: Armed Forces Institute of Pathology, 1957), Section I, Fascicle 2.

12. Endocrine Organs

General

KUPPERMANN, H. S.: Human Endocrinology (London: Blackwell Scientific Publications, 1963).

WARNER, N. E.: Basic Endocrine Pathology (Chicago: Year Book Medical Publishers Inc., 1971).

WILLIAMS, R. H. (ed.): Textbook of Endocrinology (4th ed.; Philadelphia, London and Toronto: W. B. Saunders Company, 1968).

Pituitary Gland

BALLARD, H. S., B. FRAME, R. J. HARTSOCK: Medicine *43:* 481 (1964).

GORDON, D. A., F. M. HILL, C. EZRIN: Canad. M. A. J. *87:* 1106 (1962).

Thyroid Gland

HAZARD, J. B., D. E. SMITH (eds.): The Thyroid. International Academy of Pathology Monograph No. 5 (Baltimore: The Williams & Wilkins Company, 1964).

HEDINGER, CHR. E. (ed.): Thyroid Cancer. UICC Monograph, Vol. 12 (Berlin, Heidelberg and New York: Springer-Verlag, 1956).

HOFFMAN, W. S.: The Biochemistry of Clinical Medicine (4th ed.; Chicago: Year Book Medical Publishers, Inc., 1970).

HORN, R. C.: Cancer *7:* 234 (1954).

PIFER, J. W., L. A. HEMPERLMANN: Ann. New York Acad. Sc. *114:* 838 (1964).

RUSSEL, W. O., M. L. IBANEZ, R. L. CLARK, E. C. WHITE: Cancer *16:* 1425 (1963).

WARREN, S., M. ALVIZOURI, B. P. COLCOCK: Cancer *6:* 1139 (1953).

Hemangioendothelioma

SIMON, M. A.: Arch. Path. *27:* 571 (1939).

Parathyroid Gland

BLACK, B. K., L. V. ACKERMAN: Cancer *3:* 415 (1952).

EDER, M.: Virchows Arch. path. Anat. *334:* 301 (1961).

MARSHALL, R. B., D. K. ROBERTS, R. A. TURNER: Cancer *20:* 512 (1967).

WOOLNER, L. B., F. R. KEATING, B. M. BLACK: Cancer *5:* 1069 (1952).

Adrenal Gland

BACHMANN, K. D.: Ztschr. Kinderh. *77:* 391 (1955).

EISENSTEIN, A. B. (ed.): The Adrenal Cortex (Boston: Little, Brown & Company, 1967).

JACKSON, W. P. U., B. ZILBERG, B. LEWIS, D. MCKENZIE: Brit. M. J. *2:* 130 (1958).

Pheochromocytoma

EVANS, R. W.: Histological Appearances of Tumors (2d ed.; Baltimore: The Williams & Wilkins Company, 1966).

13. Kidneys and Urinary System

Kidney (General)

BECKER, E. L. (ed.): Structural Basis of Renal Disease (New York: Harper & Row, Publishers, 1968).

DALTON, A. J., F. HAGUENAU: Ultrastructure of the Kidney (New York and London: Academic Press, 1967).

HEPTINSTALL, R. A.: Pathology of the Kidney (Boston: Little, Brown & Company, 1966).

SANDRITTER, W., E. F. PFEIFFER: Verhandl. deutsch Gesellsch. Path. *43:* 213 (1959).

SARRE, H.: Nierenkrankheiten (Stuttgart: Georg Thieme, 1958).

ZOLLINGER, H. U.: Niere und ableitende Harnwege, in Spezielle Pathologische Anatomie (Heidelberg: Springer-Verlag, 1966).

Vascular Nephropathies

GOODPASTURE, E. W.: J. M. Sc. *158:* 863 (1919).

LASCH, H. G., D. L. HEENE, K. HUTH, W. SANDRITTER: Am. J. Cardiol. *20:* 381 (1967).

METCOFF, J. (ed.): Angiotensin Systems and Experimental Renal Diseases (Boston: Little, Brown & Company, 1963).

SANDRITTER, W., H. G. LASCH: Meth. Achiev. Exper. Path. *3:* 86 (1967).

Nephrosis, Nephritis

KASS, E. H. (ed.): Progress in Pyelonephritis (Philadelphia: F. A. Davis Company, 1965).

METCOFF, J. (ed.): Acute Glomerulonephritis (London: J. & A. Churchill, Ltd., 1967).

Kidney Tumors

KING, J. S.: Renal Neoplasia (Boston: Little, Brown & Company, 1967).

Urinary Bladder

CLEMMESEN, J. (ed.): Symposium on Cancer of the Urinary Bladder (New York: Karger, 1963).

SARMA, K. P.: Tumours of the Urinary Bladder (London: Butterworth & Co., Ltd., 1969).

14. Male Sex Organs

BALOGH, F., Z. SZENDRÖI: Cancer of the Prostate (Budapest: Akadémia i Kiadó, 1968).
COLLINS, D. H., R. C. B. PUGH: Brit. J. Urol. (supp.) *36:* 1 (1964).

15. Female Sex Organs

HAINES, M., C. W. TAYLOR: Gynecological Pathology (London: J. & A. Churchill, Ltd., 1962).
HERTIG, A. T., H. GORE: Tumors of the Genital Sex Organs, in Atlas of Tumor Pathology (Washington, D. C.: Armed Forces Institute of Pathology, 1960), Section IX, Fascicle 33.
JANOVSKI, N. A., V. DUBRAUSZLY: Atlas of Gynecologic and Obstetric Diagnostic Histopathology (New York, Toronto, Sydney and London: McGraw-Hill Book Company, Inc., 1967).
KLINEFELTER, A. F., E. C. REIFENSTEIN, F. ALBRIGHT: J. Clin. Endocrinol. *2:* 615 (1942).
MARCUSE, P. M.: Diagnostic Pathology in Gynecology and Obstetrics (New York and London: Hoeber Medical Division, Harper & Row, Publishers, 1966).
NOVAK, E. R., J. D. WOODRUFF: Gynecologic and Obstetric Pathology (7th ed.; Philadelphia: W. B. Saunders Company, 1974).

16. Pregnancy. Fetal and Neonatal Pathology

ESSBACH, H.: Paidopathologie (Leipzig: Edition, 1963).
POTTER, E. L., J. M. CRAIG: Pathology of the Fetus and Infant (3d ed.; Chicago: Year Book Medical Publishers, Inc., 1975).
ZSCHOCH, H. J., P. F. MAHNKE: Die Pathologische Anatomie des Kindesalters in der Sektionsstatistik (Jena: Gustav Fischer, 1968).

17. Nervous System

BLACKWOOD, W., W. H. MCMENEMEY, A. EYER, R. M. NORMAN, D. S. RUSSEL: In Greenfield, J. G. (ed.), Neuropathology (London: Edward Arnold & Company, 1963).
NOETZEL, H.: Med. Welt (N. F.) *20:* 1631 (1969).
NOETZEL, H.: Med. Welt (N. F.) *20:* 2605 (1969).
RUSSEL, D. S., L. J. RUBINSTEIN: Pathology of Tumours of the Nervous System (London: Edward Arnold & Company, 1963).

18. Malformations

HSIA, D. Y-Y. (ed.): Lectures in Medical Genetics (Chicago: Year Book Medical Publishers, Inc., 1966).
OVERZIER, C.: Erkrankungen der Männlichen Keimdrüse und die Intersexualität, in Klinik der Gegenwart (München and Berlin: Urban & Schwarzenberg, 1959), Band 9, S. 97.
WARKANY, J.: Congenital Malformations (Chicago: Year Book Medical Publishers, Inc., 1971).
WILLIS, R. A.: The Borderland of Embryology and Pathology (2d ed.; Washington, D. C.: Butterworth & Co., Ltd., 1962).

Index

pôr-do-sol [pordo'sɔw] *m* do-sol⟩ sunset

principiante [prĩsi'pjãtʃi] *m/f* beginner; ***curso*** *m* ***para ~s*** beginners' course

refugiado [hefu'ʒjadu] **1** *adj* refugee *atr* **2** *m*, **-a** *f* refugee

rotular [hotu'lar] ⟨1a⟩ label *tb fig* (***de*** as)

Informações gramaticais

Grammatical information

guinchar [gĩ'ʃar] ⟨1a⟩ **1** *v/t carro* tow **2** *v/i freios* screech

Entradas separadas em categorias gramaticais

Entries divided into grammatical categories

legal [le'gaw] *adj* legal; (*válido*) valid; *Bras fam* great, cool

esposa [es'poza] *f* wife, *fml* spouse

infantil [ĩfã'tʃiw] *adj* childlike; *pej* childish; MED children's *atr*

Indicadores de registro de língua

Register labels

ICM [ise'emi] *m Bras abr* (Imposto de circulação de mercadorias) sales tax, *Brit* VAT (value added tax)

Variantes britânicas

British variants

lavabo [la'vabu] *m* washbowl; *Port* **~s** *pl* rest rooms, *Brit* toilets

lacrimogêneo, *Port* **lacrimogéneo** [lakrimo'ʒeniu] *adj* ***gás*** *m* **~** tear gas

Português europeu

Continental Portuguese

ingresso [ĩ'grɛsu] *m* entry; *Bras* ticket

Português brasileiro

Brazilian Portuguese

A B C D E F G H I J K L M N O P Q R S T U V W X Z

Langenscheidt

Pocket Portuguese Dictionary

Portuguese – English
English – Portuguese

edited by the
Langenscheidt editorial staff

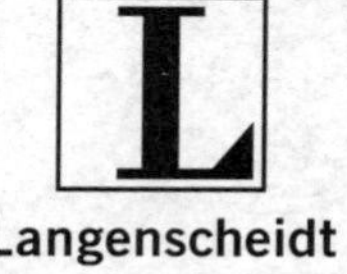

Langenscheidt

Berlin · Munich · Vienna · Zurich
London · Madrid · New York · Warsaw

Compiled by LEXUS with:

Márcia da Costa Huber · Kátia de Souza-Kirstein
Ana Maria Cortes Kollert · Barbara Epple
Sophie Cadell · Anne Heining · Peter Terrell
Cláudia Monteiro · Rafael Argenton Freire

Printed in Germany

11020 (98074)

Contents / Conteúdo

Preface

Here is a new dictionary of English and Portuguese, a tool with some 50,000 references for those who work with the English and Portuguese languages at beginner's or intermediate level.

Focusing on modern usage, the dictionary offers coverage of everyday language and this means including vocabulary from areas such as computer use and business. English is both American and British English with American being the default. Portuguese is Brazilian by default with a good coverage of Continental Portuguese.

The editors have provided a reference tool to enable the user to get straight to the translation that fits a particular context of use. Indicating words are given to identify senses. Is the *box* you use to store things in, for example, the same in Portuguese as the *box* you enter data in on a form? Is *flimsy* referring to furniture the same in Portuguese as *flimsy* referring to an excuse? This dictionary is rich in sense distinctions like this and in translation options tied to specific, identified senses.

Vocabulary needs grammar to back it up. So in this dictionary you'll find irregular verb forms, in both English and Portuguese, irregular English plural forms, guidance on Portuguese feminine endings and Portuguese plurals and on prepositional usage with verbs.

Since some vocabulary items are often only clearly understood when contextualized, a large number of idiomatic phrases are given to show how the two languages correspond in particular contexts.

All in all, this is a book full of information, which will, we hope, become a valuable part of your language toolkit.

Prefácio

Apresentamos-lhe um novo dicionário inglês-português, uma ferramenta com mais de 50.000 palavras e expressões para aqueles que utilizam a língua inglesa e a portuguesa a nível iniciante ou intermediário.

Focalizado no uso moderno, o dicionário abrange a linguagem do dia-a-dia e inclui também o vocabulário usado nas áreas da informática e de negócios.

Aqui, a língua inglesa é tanto americana quanto britânica, sendo que o padrão é o americano. O português brasileiro é o padrão para a língua portuguesa, no entanto, há também uma apresentação considerável do português europeu.

Os editores equiparam o dicionário com uma ferramenta que permite ao seu leitor chegar diretamente a uma tradução que melhor serve a certo contexto. Indicadores contextuais e semânticos são dados para a distinção entre os sentidos de uma palavra. Por exemplo, o *ponteiro* de um relógio é traduzido em inglês da mesma forma que o *ponteiro* do mouse na tela do seu computador? A tradução de *lançamento* em inglês é a mesma para o *lançamento* de um novo livro ou o *lançamento* de uma bomba? Este dicionário é rico em distinções de sentidos como estas e em outras opções de traduções vinculadas a definições mais específicas.

O vocabulário às vezes não é suficiente para a comunicação sem o apoio da gramática. Portanto, neste dicionário você encontrará verbos irregulares em inglês e em português, plurais irregulares em inglês, instruções sobre as terminações do feminino e do plural em português e, ainda, o uso das preposições com os verbos.

Uma vez que algumas palavras não podem ser muito bem compreendidas fora de contexto, o dicionário apresenta uma grande quantidade de expressões idiomáticas que ilustram como as duas línguas correspondem-se em contextos específicos.

Em resumo, esta é uma ferramenta repleta de informações que irá, esperamos, tornar-se uma parte valiosa do seu material de estudo de línguas.

How to use the dictionary

To get the most out of your dictionary you should understand how and where to find the information you need. Whether you are yourself writing text in a foreign language or wanting to understand text that has been written in a foreign language, the following pages should help.

1. How and where do I find a word?

1.1 Portuguese and English headwords. The word list for each language is arranged in alphabetical order and also gives irregular forms of verbs and nouns in their correct alphabetical order.

Sometimes you might want to look up terms made up of two separate words, for example **falling star**, or hyphenated words, for example **hands-on**. These words are treated as though they were a single word and their alphabetical ordering reflects this.

There are only two exceptions to this strict alphabetical ordering. One is made for English phrasal verbs - words like **go off**, **go out**, **go up**. These are positioned in a block directly after their main verb (in this case **go**), rather than being split up and placed apart. The other is for Portuguese feminine forms, as described in 1.2.

1.2 Portuguese feminine headwords are shown as follows:

> **acusado** [aku'zadu] *m*, **-a** *f* accused (*the feminine form is acusada*)
>
> **esquisitão** [eskizi'tãw] *m*, **-ona** *f* weirdo, oddball (*the feminine form is esquisitona*)
>
> **democrata** [demo'krata] *m/f* democrat

1.3 Running heads

If you are looking for a Portuguese or English word you can use the **running heads** printed in bold in the top corner of each page. The running head on the left tells you the *first* headword on the left-hand page and the one on the right tells you the *last* headword on the right-hand page.

1.4 How is the word spelt?

You can look up the spelling of a word in your dictionary in the same way as you would in a spelling dictionary. American English and Brazilian Portuguese are the defaults for spelling in this dictionary.

British English and Continental Portuguese variants are marked with *Brit* and *Port*.

1.5 Spelling reforms

This dictionary does not reflect spelling reforms currently (2008/9) proposed in Portugal and Brazil.

2. When an English or a Portuguese word is written with a hyphen, then this dictionary makes a distinction between a hyphen which is given just because the dictionary line ends at that point and a hyphen which is actually part of the word. If the hyphen is a real hyphen then it is repeated at the start of the following line. For example:

> **couve-flor** [kove'flor] *f* 〈*pl* couves-
> -flor〉 cauliflower

3. Swung dashes

3.1 A swung dash (~) replaces the entire headword, when the headword is repeated within an entry:

> **face** [feɪs] **1** *n* cara *f*, rosto *m*; ***~ to ~*** face a face; ***lose ~*** desonrar-se

Here ***~ to ~*** means ***face to face***.

> **ignição** [igni'sãw] *f* ignition; ***chave** f **de ~*** ignition key

Here ***chave** f **de ~*** means ***chave** f **de ignição***.

3.2 When a headword changes form in an entry, for example if it is put in the past tense or in the plural, then the past tense or plural ending is added to the swung dash - but only if the rest of the word doesn't change:

> **cobra** ['kɔbra] **1** *f* snake; ***dizer ~s e lagartos de alguém*** say bad things about s.o.

> **derive** [dɪ'raɪv] *v/t* obter; ***be ~d from*** *word* derivar de

But:

> **survive** [sər'vaɪv] **1** *v/i species, patient* sobreviver; ***how are you? – I'm surviving*** como vai? - vou levando

> **psicológico** [psiko'lɔʒiku] *adj* psychological; ***ação** f **psicológica*** psychological warfare

3.3 A swung dash after a reflexive verb which is nested in an entry replaces the reflexive form of the verb:

absorver [absoɾ'veɾ] ⟨2e⟩ *v/t* absorb; **absorver-se** *v/r* **~ *em algo*** become absorbed in sth

3.4 Double headwords are replaced by a single swung dash:

'one-track mind *hum* ***have a ~*** só ter sexo na cabeça;

4. What do the different typefaces mean?

4.1 All Portuguese and English headwords and the Arabic numerals differentiating between parts of speech appear in **bold**:

'outline 1 *n person, building etc*: perfil *m*; *plan, novel*: esboço *m* **2** *v/t plans etc* esboçar

espiar [es'pjar] ⟨1g⟩ **1** *v/t* spy on **2** *v/i* spy

4.2 *Italics* are used for :

a) abbreviated grammatical labels: *adj*, *adv*, *v/i*, *v/t* etc
b) gender labels: *m*, *f*, *mpl* etc
c) all the indicating words which are the signposts pointing to the correct translation for your needs. Here are some examples of indicating words in italics:

dead [ded] **1** *adj also fam place* morto; *battery* descarregado; *phone* cortado; *light bulb* queimado

◆ **work out 1** *v/t problem* resolver; *solution* encontrar **2** *v/i at gym* fazer ginástica; *relationship etc* ir bem

sacudir [saku'dʒiɾ] ⟨3h⟩ shake; *pó* shake off; *ombros* shrug

Synonyms or near-synonyms as indicators are given in brackets:

contract[2] [kən'trækt] **1** *v/i* (*shrink*) contrair-se **2** *v/t illness* contrair

bluff [blʌf] **1** *n* (*deception*) blefe *m* **2** *v/i* blefar

auditório [awdʒi'tɔriu] *m* (*sala*) auditorium; (*ouvintes*) audience

A colon is placed after indicators to signal a general area of usage (as opposed to identifying a typical grammatical subject or object or adjectival collocation etc):

wood [wʊd] *n* madeira *f*; *fire, stove*: lenha *f*; (*forest*) floresta *f*

corrosão [koho'zãw] *f metais*: corrosion; *fig* erosion

4.3 All phrases (examples and idioms) are given in ***bold italics***:

habit ['hæbɪt] hábito *m*; ***get into the ~ of doing sth*** criar o hábito de fazer algo

galope [ga'lɔpi] *m* gallop; ***a ~*** at a gallop; *fig* ***a todo o ~*** at full pace

gene [dʒiːn] gene *m*; ***it's in his ~s*** está em seus genes;

4.4 On the Portuguese-English side of the dictionary ***bold italics*** are also used for compounds:

mensagem [mẽ'saʒẽ] *f* message; ***~ de erro*** error message; ***~ telefônica*** telephone message; ***~ de texto*** text (message)

4.5 The normal typeface is used for the translations.

4.6 If a translation is given in italics, and not in the normal typeface, this means that the translation is more of an *explanation* in the other language and that an explanation has to be given because there just is no real equivalent:

Purple 'Heart *Am* MIL *medalha concedida a soldados americanos feridos em combate*

paio ['paiu] *m smoked pork sausage with garlic, white wine and paprika*

5. Stress

To indicate where to put the **stress** in English or Portuguese words, the stress marker ' appears before the syllable on which the main stress falls:

record[1] ['rekərd] *n* MUS disco *m*; SPORT *etc* recorde *m*;

record[2] [rɪ'kɔːrd] *v/t electronically* gravar; *in writing* registrar, *Port* registar

Panamá [pana'ma] *m* Panama; ***o canal do ~*** the Panama Canal

On the English-Portuguese side of the dictionary stress is shown either in the pronunciation or, if there is no pronunciation given, in the actual headword or compound itself:

'record holder recordista *m/f*

6. What do the various symbols and abbreviations tell you?

6.1 A solid blue diamond is used to indicate a phrasal verb:

◆ **come about** *v/i* (*happen*) acontecer

6.2 A white diamond is used to divide up longer entries into more easily digested chunks of related bits of text:

> **must** [mʌst] ◊ *necessity*: ter que; ***I ~ be on time*** tenho que ser pontual; ***I ~*** tenho
> ◊ *with negative*: ***I ~n't be late*** não posso chegar atrasado; ***you ~n't cross this line*** você não deve cruzar esta linha
> ◊ *probability*: dever; ***it ~ be about 6 o'clock*** devem ser umas seis horas; ***they ~ have arrived by now*** eles devem ter chegado agora
> ◊ ***a ~-see movie*** um filme imperdível; ***the ~-have fashion accessory*** o acessório que todos devem ter

6.3 The abbreviation *fam* tells you that the word or phrase is used colloquially rather than in formal contexts. The abbreviation *vulg* warns you that a word or phrase is vulgar or taboo. Words or phrases on the Portuguese-English side of the dictionary labeled *pop* are slang. Be careful how you use these words.

7. Does the dictionary deal with grammar too?

7.1 In general, English headwords are given a part of speech label:

> **mine**[3] [maɪn] **1** *n explosive* mina *f* **2** *v/t* minar

> **disband** [dɪs'bænd] **1** *v/t* dissolver: **2** *v/i* dissolver-se

But if a headword can only be used as a noun (in ordinary English) then no part of speech is given, since none is needed:

> **parsley** ['pɑːrslɪ] salsinha *f*

7.2 Portuguese gender markers are given for all nouns:

> **percepção** [peɾsep'sãw] *f* perception

> **perfeccionista** [peɾfeksjo'nista] *m/f* perfectionist

No part of speech is shown for Portuguese words which are only transitive verbs or only intransitive verbs or where no confusion is possible. But where confusion might exist, grammatical information is added:

> **abordar** [aboɾ'daɾ] ⟨1e⟩ **1** *v/t pessoa, problema* approach; NÁUT board **2** *v/i* NÁUT put in

> **afinar** [afi'naɾ] ⟨1a⟩ **1** *v/t* MÚS tune; TECN adjust **2** *v/i* MÚS tune up

7.3 If an English translation of a Portuguese adjective can only be used in front of a noun, and not after it or with the verb 'to be', this is marked with *atr*:

populacional [populasjo'naw] *adj* population *atr*
movimentos populacionais population movements

7.4 If an English translation of a Portuguese adjective can only be used after a noun, and not before it (or is used with the verb 'to be'), this is marked with *pred*:

aceso [a'sezu] *adj lume, luz* on *pred*, alight *pred*
a luz ficava acesa the light was on

grifado [gri'fadu] *adj* in italics *pred*, italicized
uma palavra grifada a word in italics

7.5 If the Portuguese, unlike the English, doesn't change form if used in the plural, this is marked with *inv*:

saca-rolhas [saka'hoʎas] *m* ⟨*pl inv*⟩ corkscrew

arco-íris [aɾ'kwiɾis] *mpl* ⟨*pl inv*⟩ rainbow

7.6 If the English, in spite of appearances, is not a plural form, this is marked with *nsg*:

billiards ['bɪljərdz] *nsg* bilhar *m*

measles ['miːzlz] *nsg* sarampo *m*

English translations which look like plurals but which are in fact singular nouns are given an *sg* label:

caxumba [ka'ʃũba] *f* mumps *sg*

citação [sita'sãw] *f* quotation; JUR summons *sg*

7.7 Irregular English plurals are identified and Portuguese plural forms are given in cases where there is irregularity or where there might well be uncertainty:

thesis ['θiːsɪs] ⟨*pl* theses⟩ tese *f*

thief [θiːf] ⟨*pl* thieves⟩ ladrão *m*, ladra *f*

trout [traʊt] ⟨*pl* trout⟩ truta *f*

edredom [edɾe'dõ] *m* ⟨*pl* -ns⟩ *Bras* quilt

dente-de-leão [dẽtʃidʒi'ljãw] *m* ⟨*pl* dentes-de-leão⟩ dandelion

diretor-gerente [dʒiretorʒe'rẽtʃi] *m* ⟨*pl* diretores-gerentes⟩ managing director

franco-atirador [frãkwatʃira'dor] *m* ⟨*pl* franco-atiradores⟩ sniper

Plurals of Portuguese words ending in **-ão** are only given when not formed with the regular ending **-ões**:

ganha-pão [gaɲa'pãw] *m* ⟨*pl* -pães⟩ bread-winner

7.8 Words like **physics** or **media studies** have not been given a label to say if they are singular or plural for the simple reason that they can be either, depending on how they are used.

7.9 Irregular and semi-irregular verb forms are identified:

simplify ['sɪmplɪfaɪ] *v/t* ⟨*pret & pp* ***simplified***⟩ simplificar

sing [sɪŋ] *v/t & v/i* ⟨*pret* ***sang***, *pp* ***sung***⟩ cantar

cancel ['kænsl] *v/t* ⟨*pret & pp* ***canceled***, *Brit* ***cancelled***⟩ cancelar

7.10 Portuguese verb codes are given referring to the tables of Portuguese conjugations on page 692:

simplificar [sĩplifi'kar] ⟨1n⟩ simplify

socorrer [soko'her] ⟨2d⟩ ~ ***alguém*** come to s.o.'s assistance

7.11 Grammatical information is provided on the prepositions you'll need in order to create complete sentences:

sonhar [so'ɲar] ⟨1f⟩ **1** *v/i* dream (***com*** about)

desconsideração [deskõsidʒira'sãw] *f* disregard (***de*** for)

interested ['ɪntrəstɪd] *adj* interessado; ***be ~ in sth*** estar interessado em algo

Como usar o dicionário

Para o melhor aproveitamento do seu dicionário, você deve entender como e onde encontrar a informação que precisa. Esteja você redigindo um texto em língua estrangeira ou querendo compreender um texto que foi escrito em língua estrangeira, as seguintes páginas lhe ajudarão.

1. Como e onde encontro uma palavra?

1.1 Entradas lexicais em português e em inglês. A lista de palavras para cada língua também contendo formas irregulares de verbos e substantivos está organizada em ordem alfabética.

Você pode, às vezes, querer procurar termos formados por duas palavras: **falling star**, por exemplo, ou palavras hifenizadas como **hands-on**. Estas palavras são tratadas como uma única palavra e seguem a regra da ordem alfabética.

Existem apenas duas exceções para a estrita ordem alfabética. Uma é para os phrasal verbs em inglês, termos como: **go off**, **go out**, **go up**. Estes estão posicionados num bloco diretamente depois do seu verbo principal (nesse caso, **go**) em vez de estarem separados e em posições diferentes. A outra exceção é para formas no gênero feminino em português, como descrito em 1.2.

1.2 Entradas lexicais no gênero feminino em português são exibidas como abaixo:

acusado [aku'zadu] *m*, **-a** *f* accused (*a forma feminina é acusada*)

esquisitão [eskizi'tãw] *m*, **-ona** *f* weirdo, oddball (*a forma feminina é esquisitona*)

democrata [demo'krata] *m/f* democrat

1.3 Palavras-guia

Se você estiver procurando uma palavra em português ou inglês, você pode guiar-se pelas **palavras-guia** escritas em negrito no canto superior de cada página. A palavra-guia à esquerda indica a *primeira* entrada lexical na página esquerda e a palavra-guia à direita indica a última entrada lexical na página da direita.

1.4 Qual é a ortografia de uma palavra?

Você pode procurar a ortografia de uma palavra no seu dicionário da mesma forma como num dicionário ortográfico. Inglês americano e português brasileiro são os padrões ortográficos neste dicionário. As variantes de inglês britânico e português europeu estão marcadas como *Brit* e *Port*.

1.5 Reforma ortográfica

Este dicionário não reflete as reformas ortográficas atualmente (2008/9) propostas nos países de língua portuguesa.

2. Quando uma palavra em inglês ou português é escrita com hífen, este dicionário faz uma distinção entre um hífen dado em razão do término da linha naquele ponto e um hífen que realmente faz parte da palavra. Se o hífen faz parte de uma palavra composta, ele é repetido no início da seguinte linha. Por exemplo:

> **couve-flor** [kove'flor] *f* ⟨*pl* couves-
> -flor⟩ cauliflower

3. Til

3.1 Um til (~) substitui uma entrada lexical quando repetida no verbete:

> **face** [feɪs] **1** *n* cara *f*, rosto *m*; ***~ to ~*** face a face; ***lose ~*** desonrar-se

Aqui ***~ to ~*** **significa** ***face to face.***

> **ignição** [igni'sãw] *f* ignition; ***chave** f **de ~*** ignition key

Aqui ***chave** f **de ~*** significa ***chave** f **de ignição**.*

3.2 Se uma entrada lexical muda sua forma num verbete quando, por exemplo, colocada no tempo passado ou no plural, a terminação do passado ou do plural é adicionada ao til. Isso ocorre apenas se o resto da palavra não for alterado:

> **cobra** ['kɔbra] **1** *f* snake; ***dizer ~s e lagartos de alguém*** say bad things about s.o.

> **derive** [dɪ'raɪv] *v/t* obter; ***be ~d from*** *word* derivar de

Mas:

> **survive** [sər'vaɪv] **1** *v/i species, patient* sobreviver; ***how are you? – I'm surviving*** como vai? – vou levando

psicológico [psiko'lɔʒiku] *adj* psychological; ***ação f psicológica*** psychological warfare

3.3 Um til depois de um verbo reflexivo contido num verbete substitui a forma reflexiva do verbo:

absorver [absoɾ'veɾ] ⟨2e⟩ *v/t* absorb; **absorver-se** *v/r* **~ *em algo*** become absorbed in sth

3.4 Entradas lexicais duplas são substituídas por um único til:

'one-track mind *hum* ***have a ~*** só ter sexo na cabeça;

4. O que significam diferentes fontes tipográficas?

4.1 Todas as entradas lexicais portuguesas, inglesas e numerais arábicos diferenciando partes do discurso aparecem em **negrito**:

'outline 1 *n person, building etc*: perfil *m*; *plan, novel*: esboço *m* **2** *v/t plans etc* esboçar

espiar [es'pjaɾ] ⟨1g⟩ **1** *v/t* spy on **2** *v/i* spy

4.2 *Itálico* é usado para:

a) abreviaturas de categorias gramaticais: *adj*, *adv*, *v/i*, *v/t* etc
b) gêneros: *m*, *f*, *mpl* etc
c) todos os indicadores que são sinalizadores apontando para a tradução mais adequada às suas necessidades. Abaixo, alguns exemplos de indicadores em itálico:

dead [ded] **1** *adj also fam place* morto; *battery* descarregado; *phone* cortado; *light bulb* queimado

♦ **work out 1** *v/t problem* resolver; *solution* encontrar **2** *v/i at gym* fazer ginástica; *relationship etc* ir bem

sacudir [saku'dʒiɾ] ⟨3h⟩ shake; *pó* shake off; *ombros* shrug

Sinônimos ou quase-sinônimos usados como indicadores são dados entre parênteses:

contract[2] [kən'trækt] **1** *v/i* (*shrink*) contrair-se **2** *v/t illness* contrair

bluff [blʌf] **1** *n* (*deception*) blefe *m* **2** *v/i* blefar

auditório [awdʒi'tɔriu] *m* (*sala*) auditorium; (*ouvintes*) audience

O sinal de dois pontos é colocado após indicadores para indicar uma área de uso geral (ao contrário de identificar gramaticalmente um sujeito, um objeto, ou uma colocação adjetiva etc.):

wood [wʊd] *n* madeira *f*; *fire, stove*: lenha *f*; (*forest*) floresta *f*

corrosão [koho'zãw] *f metais*: corrosion; *fig* erosion

4.3 Todas as frases (exemplos e expressões idiomáticas) são dadas em ***itálico negrito***:

habit ['hæbɪt] hábito *m*; ***get into the ~ of doing sth*** criar o hábito de fazer algo

galope [ga'lɔpi] *m* gallop; ***a ~*** at a gallop; *fig* ***a todo o ~*** at full pace

gene [dʒiːn] gene *m*; ***it's in his ~s*** está em seus genes;

4.4 No lado português-inglês do dicionário, ***itálico negrito*** também é usado para substantivos compostos:

mensagem [mẽ'saʒẽ] *f* message; ***~ de erro*** error message; ***~ telefônica*** telephone message; ***~ de texto*** text (message)

4.5 A fonte tipográfica normal é usada para as traduções.

4.6 Se uma tradução aparece em itálico e não em fonte normal, isso significa que a tradução é mais uma *explicação* do que uma tradução na outra língua. A explicação foi necessária por não haver equivalente real entre os termos:

Purple 'Heart *Am* MIL *medalha concedida a soldados americanos feridos em combate*

paio ['paiu] *m smoked pork sausage with garlic, white wine and paprika*

5. Ênfase

Para indicar onde dar-se **ênfase** em palavras em inglês ou português, o marcador de ênfase ' aparece antes da sílaba na qual a ênfase principal recai:

record[1] ['rekərd] *n* MUS disco *m*; SPORT *etc* recorde *m*;

record[2] [rɪ'kɔːrd] *v/t electronically* gravar; *in writing* registrar, *Port* registar

Panamá [pana'ma] *m* Panama; ***o canal do ~*** the Panama Canal

No lado inglês-português do dicionário, a ênfase é indicada na pronunciação ou, caso não haja pronunciação à parte, na própria entrada lexical:

'record holder recordista *m/f*

6. O que os vários símbolos e abreviaturas lhe dizem?

6.1 Um losango azul indica um phrasal verb:

♦ **come about** *v/i* (*happen*) acontecer

6.2 Um losango branco é utilizado para dividir longos verbetes em partes mais compreensíveis de textos relacionados:

must [mʌst] ◊ *necessity*: ter que; ***I ~ be on time*** tenho que ser pontual; ***I ~*** tenho

◊ *with negative*: ***I ~n't be late*** não posso chegar atrasado; ***you ~n't cross this line*** você não deve cruzar esta linha

◊ *probability*: dever; ***it ~ be about 6 o'clock*** devem ser umas seis horas; ***they ~ have arrived by now*** eles devem ter chegado agora

◊ ***a ~-see movie*** um filme imperdível; ***the ~-have fashion accessory*** o acessório que todos devem ter

6.3 A abreviatura *fam* indica que uma palavra ou frase é usada de forma coloquial em vez de formalmente.

A abreviatura *vulg* lhe adverte que uma palavra ou frase é vulgar ou tabu. Palavras ou frases no lado português-inglês do dicionário classificadas como *pop* são gírias. Cuidado ao usar estas palavras.

7. No dicionário também figuram indicações gramaticais?

7.1 Em geral são dadas as classes gramaticais das entradas lexicográficas em inglês:

mine[3] [maɪn] **1** *n explosive* mina *f* **2** *v/t* minar

disband [dɪs'bænd] **1** *v/t* dissolver: **2** *v/i* dissolver-se

Mas se uma entrada pode ser usada apenas como substantivo (em inglês comum), então, nenhuma classe gramatical é apresentada, por não haver razão para tal:

parsley ['pɑːrslɪ] salsinha *f*

7.2 Marcadores de gênero são dados pelos sustantivos portugueses:

percepção [persep'sãw] *f* perception

perfeccionista [perfeksjo'nista] *m/f* perfectionist

Nenhuma classificação gramatical é apresentada para verbos em português que podem ser apenas transitivos ou apenas intransitivos ou onde nenhuma dúvida é possível. Onde uma dúvida possa existir, a informação gramatical é apresentada:

abordar [abor'dar] ⟨1e⟩ **1** *v/t pessoa, problema* approach; NÁUT board **2** *v/i* NÁUT put in

afinar [afi'nar] ⟨1a⟩ **1** *v/t* MÚS tune; TECN adjust **2** *v/i* MÚS tune up

7.3 Se uma tradução em inglês de um adjetivo português puder ser usada apenas antes de um substantivo inglês e não após (ou com o verbo 'to be'), isso é sinalizado com *atr*:

populacional [populasjo'naw] *adj* population *atr*
movimentos populacionais population movements

7.4 Se uma tradução em inglês de um adjetivo português puder ser usada apenas depois de um substantivo inglês e não antes (ou é usada com o verbo 'to be'), esse caso é marcado com *pred*:

aceso [a'sezu] *adj lume, luz* on *pred*, alight *pred*
a luz ficava acesa the light was on

grifado [gri'fadu] *adj* in italics *pred*, italicized
uma palavra grifada a word in italics

7.5 Se uma palavra em português, diferentemente de em inglês, não alterar sua forma no plural, ela é marcada com *inv*:

saca-rolhas [saka'hoʎas] *m* ⟨*pl inv*⟩ corkscrew

arco-íris [ar'kwiris] *mpl* ⟨*pl inv*⟩ rainbow

7.6 Se a palavra em inglês, apesar das aparências, não é uma forma no plural, ela é marcada com *nsg*:

billiards ['bɪljərdz] *nsg* bilhar *m*

measles ['miːzlz] *nsg* sarampo *m*

Traduções em inglês que se parecem com plurais, mas que são de fato formas no singular, são marcadas com *sg*:

caxumba [ka'ʃũba] *f* mumps *sg*

citação [sita'sãw] *f* quotation; JUR summons *sg*

7.7 Plurais irregulares em inglês são identificados e, em português, as formas no plural são dadas em casos em que há irregularidade ou alguma incerteza:

thesis ['θiːsɪs] ⟨*pl* theses⟩ tese *f*

thief [θiːf] ⟨*pl* thieves⟩ ladrão *m*, ladra *f*

trout [traʊt] ⟨*pl* trout⟩ truta *f*

edredom [edɾe'dõ] *m* ⟨*pl* -ns⟩ *Bras* quilt

dente-de-leão [dẽʧidʒi'ljãw] *m* ⟨*pl* dentes-de-leão⟩ dandelion

diretor-gerente [dʒiretoɾʒe'ɾẽʧi] *m* ⟨*pl* diretores-gerentes⟩ managing director

franco-atirador [fɾãkwaʧiɾa'doɾ] *m* ⟨*pl* franco-atiradores⟩ sniper

O plural de palavras em português terminadas em **-ão** é dado apenas quando não formado com a terminação regular **-ões**:

ganha-pão [gaɲa'pãw] *m* ⟨*pl* -pães⟩ bread-winner

7.8 Não foram dadas classificações para palavras como **physics** ou **media studies** para dizer se são formas no plural ou no singular pela simples razão de que podem ser ambas, dependendo do seu uso.

7.9 Verbos irregulares ou semi-irregulares são identificados como em:

simplify ['sɪmplɪfaɪ] *v/t* ⟨*pret & pp* ***simplified***⟩ simplificar

sing [sɪŋ] *v/t & v/i* ⟨*pret* ***sang***, *pp* ***sung***⟩ cantar

cancel ['kænsl] *v/t* ⟨*pret & pp* ***canceled***, *Brit* ***cancelled***⟩ cancelar

7.10 Códigos de verbos portugueses são apresentados e referem-se à tabela de conjugações portuguesa na página 692:

simplificar [sĩplifi'kaɾ] ⟨1n⟩ simplify

simular [simu'laɾ] ⟨1a⟩ simulate

7.11 Alguma informação gramatical é fornecida sobre as preposições que você vai precisar para poder criar frases completas:

sonhar [so'ɲaɾ] ⟨1f⟩ **1** *v/i* dream (***com*** about)

desconsideração [deskõsidʒiɾa'sãw] *f* disregard (***de*** for)

interested ['ɪntrəstɪd] *adj* interessado; ***be ~ in sth*** estar interessado em algo

Portuguese adjectives and nouns

1 Feminine forms

In this dictionary regular adjectives are entered in their masculine form. To form the feminine change ***-o*** to ***-a***: **rico**, **rica**.

Adjectives ending in ***-or, -ol*** and ***-u*** add ***a*** to form the feminine: **conservador**, **conservadora**; **espanhol**, **espanhola**; **nu**, **nua**.

Most adjectives in ***-ês*** change ***-ês*** to **-esa**: **português**, **portuguesa**.

Most adjectives ending in ***-ão*** form their feminine by changing ***-ão*** to ***-ona*** or ***-ã***: **mandrião**, **mandriona**, **alemão**, **alemã**.

With adjectives ending in ***-e***, ***-l***, ***-m***, ***-ar*** and ***-z*** there is no difference for masculine and feminine: **breve**, **fatal**, **comum**, **solar**, **capaz**.

Important exceptions are **bom**, **boa** (*good*) *and* **mau**, **má** (*bad*).

2 Regular plural endings

Most nouns and adjectives ending in a single vowel form their plural by adding an ***-s***: **boca**, **arte, lindo**, plural **bocas, artes, lindos**.

Most nouns and adjectives ending in a consonant form their plural by adding ***-es***: **autor**, **raiz**, plural **(os) autores, (as) raízes**. Nouns ending in ***-m*** are an exception. They form their plural by changing ***-m*** to ***-ns***: **homem**, plural **(os) homens**.

Nouns ending in ***-s*** and which are not stressed on their final syllable, do not change in their plural form: **lápis**, plural **(os) lápis**.

3 Other plural endings

The plurals of nouns and adjectives ending in ***-l*** fall into two types. If the final syllable is stressed, the plural ending is ***-is***. If the final syllable is unstressed, then the plural ending is ***-eis***. Sometimes an acute accent is added to the vowel before ***i*** in the plural ending.

singular	*plural*	*examples*
-al	***-ais***	**animal** [ani'maw]; **animais** [ani'majs]
stressed ***-el***	***-éis***	**papel** [pa'pɛw]; **papéis** [pa'pejs]
unstressed ***-el***	***-eis***	**provável** [pɾo'vavew]; **prováveis** [pɾo'vavejs]
stressed ***-il***	***-is***	**barril** [ba'hiw]; **barris** [ba'his]
unstressed ***-il***	***-eis***	**fóssil** ['fɔsiw]; **fósseis** ['fɔsejs]
-ol	***-óis***	**girassol** [ʒiɾa'sɔw]; **girassóis** [ʒiɾa'sojs]
-ul	***-uis***	**azul** [a'zuw]; **azuis** [a'zuis]

Most nouns ending in ***-ão*** form their plural by changing ***-ão*** to ***-ões***: **decisão** [desi'zɐ̃w], plural **decisões** [desi'zõjs]. (The same is true for masculine forms of adjectives.) Noun plurals of this type are not given in the dictionary. However, exceptions to this rule are shown in the dictionary, for example: **mão** [mɐ̃w] *f* ⟨*pl* ~s⟩.

The pronunciation of Portuguese

The pronunciation of Portuguese given in this dictionary is Brazilian and reflects the language as it is spoken in and around São Paulo.

Consonants

b	*b*lusa	[b]	*b*ig
c	*c*olapso	[k]	*c*ollapse
ce, ci	*ce*ia, *ci*garro	[s]	*s*ystem
ç	a*ç*o	[s]	*s*illy
ch	bola*ch*a	[ʃ]	*sh*ut
d	*d*ogma	[d]	*d*og
...de (unstressed)	tar*de*	[dʒi]	*J*im
di	*di*sfarce	[dʒi]	*J*im
f	*f*icar	[f]	*f*unny
g	*g*agá	[g]	*g*aga
ge, gi	*ge*ne, *gi*z	[ʒ]	plea*sure*
h	*h*isteria		always silent
j	*J*apão	[ʒ]	plea*s*ure
k	*k*etchup	[k]	*k*etchup
l	*l*ava	[l]	*l*ava
l after a vowel	lega*l*	[w]	between an l and a diphthong
lh	agu*lh*a	[ʎ]	bi*lli*on
m	*m*agro	[m]	*m*ean
m at the end of a syllable and after a vowel makes that vowel nasal	marg*em* ['marʒẽ], pat*im* [pa'tʃĩ]		
n	*n*icotina	[n]	*n*icotine
n at the end of a syllable and after a vowel makes that vowel nasal	híf*en* ['ifẽ], bât*on* [ba'tõ]		
nh	pu*nh*o	[ɲ]	opi*ni*on, o*ni*on
p	*p*arte	[p]	*p*art
qu before a or o	ade*qu*ado, longín*quo*	[kw]	*qu*een
qu before e or i	ma*qu*eta, ma*qui*ar	[k]	*k*ing
r	a*r*ma	[ɾ]	slightly trilled
r at the beginning of a word	*r*ali	[h]	*h*appy, from the back of the throat
rr	e*rr*o	[h]	

s	*s*ussurro	[s]	*s*oft
s between two vowels	na*s*al	[z]	na*s*al
sb, sd, sg, sl, sm, sn, sr, sv	dinami*sm*o	[z]	ho*s*e
t	*t*es*t*ar	[t]	*t*est
te at the end of a word when unstressed	tes*te*	[ʧ]	*ch*eese
ti	tes*ti*ficar	[ʧ]	*ch*eese
v	*v*ídeo	[v]	*v*ideo
w	*w*indsurf	[w]	*w*hiskey
x at the start of a word or syllable	*x*á	[ʃ]	*sh*ah
x between two vowels	into*x*icado	[ks]	to*x*ic
	or		
	lagarti*x*a	[ʃ]	*sh*oe
x before ce or ci is silent	excêntrico [e'sẽtriku], excitante [esi'tãʧi]		
ex before a vowel	ine*x*ato	[z]	*z*one
z	*z*oom	[z]	*z*oom
z in final position	acide*z*	[s]	*s*it

Vowels

a, á, à	*a*cl*a*r*a*r, voc*á*bulo	[a]	f*a*ther
â	c*â*mara	[ʌ]	like the u in s*u*n
any a when followed by m or n plus consonant is nasalized	*â*mbito, ambul*â*ncia	[ã]	
ã	Ir*ã*	[ã]	as in h*ang*
e when unstressed (and not in final position)	*e*lã	[e]	as in th*ey*
e when stressed is either	*e*le	[e]	as in th*ey*
or	*é*tnico	[ɛ]	as in s*e*t
e in final position and unstressed	elefant*e*	[i]	funn*y*
é	el*é*trico	[ɛ]	as in s*e*t
ê	a-b*ê*-c*ê*	[e]	as in th*ey*
any e when followed by m or n plus consonant is nasalized	abstin*e*nte	[ẽ]	
i	*i*deal	[i]	as in s*ee*
i when followed by a is sometimes	falés*i*a	[j]	*y*es
i when followed by m or n plus consonant is nasalized	*i*mplícito, *i*nduzir	[ĩ]	

o when unstressed and not final	*o*culista	[o]	c*o*coa
final o	oc*o*	[u]	wh*o*
o when stressed is either	*o*cre	[ɔ]	h*o*t
or	*o*co	[o]	c*o*coa
ó	*ó*cio	[ɔ]	h*o*t
ô	*ô*nibus	[o]	c*o*coa
any o followed by m or n plus consonant is nasalized	p*o*mpa, L*o*ndres	[õ]	
u	t*u*ba	[u]	*too*

Diphthongs

ãe	m*ãe*	[ãj]	as in s*igh* but nasalized
ai	M*ai*o	[aj]	as in s*igh*
ao	L*ao*s	[aw]	l*ou*d
ão	mans*ão*	[ãw]	as in l*ou*d but nasalized
au	Mac*au*	[aw]	l*ou*d
ei	mant*ei*ga	[ej]	as in s*ay*
eu	m*eu*	[ew]	both e and u are pronounced
oi	n*oi*te	[oj]	as in b*oy*
ou either	t*ou*ca	[o]	as in h*o*pe
or sometimes		[ow]	o with a slight w following
õe	porta-avi*õe*s	[õj]	as in gr*oi*n but nasalized

Continental Portuguese

Some of the main differences in Continental Portuguese pronunciation are:

di	*di*sfarce	[di]	as in d*ee*d
...e (unstressed)	tard*e*, distant*e*	[ə]	as in thund*e*r without the r sound, but usually barely pronounced
r	*r*emar, e*rr*o	[ɾ]	trilled
s in final position	detrá*s*	[ʃ]	ma*sh*
s before c, f, p, qu or t	di*s*coteca, di*s*quete	[ʃ]	di*sh*
ti	diver*ti*do	[ti]	as in t*ee*nager
z in final position	lu*z*	[ʃ]	pu*sh*

Pronúncia inglesa

Vogais

[ɑː]	father	['fɑːðər]	[iː]	need	[niːd]
[æ]	man	[mæn]	[ɒː]	in-laws	['ɪnlɒːz]
[e]	get	[get]	[ɔː]	more	[mɔːr]
[ə]	about	[ə'baʊt]	[ʌ]	mother	['mʌðər]
[ɜː]	absurd	[əb'sɜːrd]	[ʊ]	book	[bʊk]
[ɪ]	stick	[stɪk]	[uː]	fruit	[fruːt]

Ditongos

[aɪ]	time	[taɪm]	[ɔɪ]	point	[pɔɪnt]
[aʊ]	cloud	[klaʊd]	[oʊ]	oath	[oʊθ]
[eɪ]	name	[neɪm]			

Consoantes

[b]	bag	[bæg]	[s]	sun	[sʌn]
[d]	dear	[dɪr]	[t]	take	[teɪk]
[f]	fall	[fɒːl]	[v]	vain	[veɪn]
[g]	give	[gɪv]	[w]	wait	[weɪt]
[h]	hole	[hoʊl]	[z]	rose	[roʊz]
[j]	yes	[jes]	[ŋ]	bring	[brɪŋ]
[k]	come	[kʌm]	[ʃ]	she	[ʃiː]
[l]	land	[lænd]	[ʧ]	chair	[ʧer]
[m]	mean	[miːn]	[dʒ]	join	[dʒɔɪn]
[n]	night	[naɪt]	[ʒ]	leisure	['liːʒər]
[p]	pot	[pɑːt]	[θ]	think	[θɪŋk]
[r]	right	[raɪt]	[ð]	the	[ðə]

['] O sinal de acento precede as sílabas acentuadas: ability [ə'bɪlətɪ]

Abbreviations / Abreviaturas

abbreviation	*abbr, abr*	abreviatura
adjective	*adj*	adjetivo
adverb	*adv*	advérbio
flying	AERO	aeronáutica
agriculture	AGR	agricultura
North American	*Am*	norte-americano
anatomy	ANAT	anatomia
architecture	ARQUIT	arquitetura
article	*art*	artigo
art	ARTE	arte
astrology	ASTROL	astrologia
attributive	*atr*	atributivo
motoring	AUTO	automobilismo
biology	BIOL	biologia
botany	BOT	botânica
Brazilian	*Bras*	brasileiro
British	*Brit*	britânico
chemistry	CHEM	química
cinema	CINE	cinema
commerce	COM	comércio
computers	COMPUT	computadores
conjunction	*conj*	conjunção
law	DIR	direito
economics	ECON	economia
education	EDUC	educação
electricity, electronics	ELEC, ELÉT	eletricidade, eletrônica
sport	ESP	esporte
especially	*esp*	especialmente
euphemism	*euph*	eufemismo
feminine	*f*	feminino
familiar, colloquial	*fam*	coloquial
railroad	FERROV	ferrovia
figurative	*fig*	figurativo
finance	FIN	finanças
physics	FÍS	física
formal	*fml*	formal
photography	FOT	fotografia
feminine plural	*fpl*	plural feminino
cooking, food	GASTR	gastronomia
geography	GEOG	geografia
geology	GEOL	geologia
grammar	GRAM	gramática
historical	*hist*	histórico
humorous	*hum*	humorístico
IT	INFORM	informática
interjection	*int*	interjeição
interrogative	*interr*	interrogativo
invariable	*inv*	invariável
ironic	*irôn*	irônico
law	LAW	direito

literature	LIT	literature
masculine	*m*	masculino
mathematics	MAT, MATH	matemática
medicine	MED	medicina
weather	METEO	meteorologia
military	MIL	militar
mining	MIN	mineração
motoring	MOT	automobilismo
masculine plural	*mpl*	plural masculino
music	MUS, MÚS	música
noun	*n*	substantivo
nautical	NAUT, NÁUT	náutica
plural noun	*npl*	substantivo plural
singular noun	*nsg*	substantivo singular
pejorative	*pej*	pejorativo
physics	PHYS	física
plural	*pl*	plural
politics	POL	política
slang	*pop*	popular, gíria
Continental Portuguese	*Port*	português europeu
past participle	*pp*	participio passado
predicative	*pred*	predicativo
preposition	*prep*	preposição
present	*pres*	presente
preterite	*pret*	pretérito
pronoun	*pron*	pronome
psychology	PSICOL, PSYCH	psicologia
chemistry	QUÍM	química
registered trademark	®	marca registrada
railroad	RAIL	ferrovia
religion	REL	religião
singular	*sg*	singular
someone	*s.o.*	alguém
something	*sth*	algo
subjunctive	*subj*	subjuntivo
also	*tb*	também
theater	TEAT	teatro
technology	TECH, TECN	técnica
telecommunications	TEL	telecomunicações
textiles	TÊX	têxteis
theater	THEA	teatro
typography, printing	TIPO	tipografia
television	TV	televisão
university	UNIV	universidade
auxiliary verb	*v/aux*	verbo auxiliar
intransitive verb	*v/i*	verbo intransitivo
reflexive verb	*v/r*	verbo reflexivo
transitive verb	*v/t*	verbo transitivo
vulgar	*vulg*	indecente
zoology	ZOOL	zoologia
and	*&*	e
see	→	veja

A

a[1] [a] **1** *art/f* the; *pl* **as** ◊ the; **com as pernas bronzeadas** with tanned legs; **ela partiu ~ perna** she broke her leg
◊ *omissão*: **~ beleza é …** beauty is … **2** *pron/f objeto*: her; *animal, coisa*: it; *Port tratamento cortês*: you

a[2] [a] *prep* ◊ *direção*: to; **vamos à minha casa** let's go to my place; **dar algo ~ alguém** give sth to s.o.
◊ *distância*: **fica ~ três quilômetros** it's 3 kilometers away, it's 3 kilometers from here; **~ poucos passos (daqui)** close by, a little way from here
◊ *temporal*: **às três** at three (o'clock); **à tarde** in the evening; **ao entrar** on entering; **ao ouvir isto** on hearing this
◊ *modo*: **~ pé / cavalo** on foot / horseback
◊ *sequência*: **passo ~ passo** step by step
◊ *meio, instrumento*: **à socapa** secretly; **à moda de** in the style of; **à brasileira** Brazilian-style
◊ *preço, números*: **~ 5 euros** at 5 euros; **aos 18 anos** at the age of 18; **~ 150 km/h** at 150 kph
◊ *comparação*: **saber / cheirar ~ vinho** taste / smell of wine
◊ **de 10 ~ 15 pessoas** from 10 to 15 people; **de segunda ~ quarta-feira** from Monday to Wednesday
◊ **aprender ~ dirigir** learn to drive

à [a] = *prep* **a** + *art f* **a**

aba ['aba] *f chapéu*: brim; *casaco*: tail; *mesa, bolso*: flap

abacate [aba'katʃi] *m* avocado

abacaxi [abaka'ʃi] *m Bras* pineapple

abade [a'badʒi] *m* abbot

abadia [aba'dʒia] *f* abbey

abafado [aba'fadu] *adj ar* stuffy; *som* muffled; *temperatura* muggy, humid

abafar [aba'faɾ] ⟨1b⟩ *grito* suppress; *som* muffle; *escândalo* hush up

abaixar [abaj'ʃaɾ] ⟨1a⟩ *v/t* lower; *cabeça* duck, bow; *som* turn down; **abaixar-se** *v/r* bend down, stoop

abaixo [a'bajʃu] **1** *adv* down, below; **as escadas ~** down the stairs; *fig* **ir(-se) ~** *pessoa* break down; *motor* stall **2** *int* **~!** get down! **3** *prep* **~ de** below, underneath; **rio ~** downstream

abaixo-assinado [abajʃwasi'nadu] *m* undersigned

abajur [aba'ʒuɾ] *m* table lamp; *Port* lampshade

abalar [aba'laɾ] ⟨1b⟩ *v/t* (*comover*) shake; (*inquietar*) worry

abalo [a'balu] *m* shock

abalroar [abaw'hwaɾ] ⟨1f⟩ hit; NÁUT ram; (*entrar em*) board

abananar [abana'naɾ] ⟨1a⟩ *fam* confuse, muddle

abanão [aba'nãw] *m* jolt, bump

abanar [aba'naɾ] ⟨1a⟩ *v/t* shake; *leque* fan; *cauda* wag; **abanar-se** *v/r* fan oneself

abandonado [abãdo'nadu] *adj* deserted; *jardim* neglected

abandonar [abãdo'naɾ] ⟨1f⟩ (*deixar*) leave, abandon; (*descuidar*) neglect; *plano* scrap, drop

abandono [abã'donu] *m* abandonment, desertion; *estado* neglect; **deixar ao ~** *jardim* neglect; *roupa etc* not look after

abarrotado [abaho'tadu] *adj* jam-packed

abarrotar [abaho'taɾ] ⟨1e⟩ *v/t* cram full; *fam* **estar a ~** be jam-packed

abastado [abas'tadu] *adj* wealthy

abastecedor [abastese'doɾ] **1** *m*, **-a** *f* supplier **2** *adj* supply *atr*

abastecer [abaste'seɾ] ⟨2g⟩ supply (**de** with); AUTO fill up

abastecimento [abastesi'mẽtu] *m* supply; *ato* supplying; *comida* provisions
abate [a'batʃi] *m* slaughter
abatedor [abate'doɾ] *m* **~ (*de gado*)** butcher
abater [aba'teɾ] ⟨2b⟩ *v/t* slaughter *tb fig*; *árvore* fell; *preço* reduce, lower; *edifício* demolish; *avião* shoot down
abatido [aba'tʃidu] *adj fisicamente* haggard; *moralmente* downcast
abatimento [abatʃi'mẽtu] *m preço*: discount; (*desânimo*) dejection; (*cansaço*) weariness; *gado*: slaughter
abaulamento [abawla'mẽtu] *m* bulge
abcesso [ab'sɛsu] *m Port* abscess
abdicação [abidʒika'sãw] *f* abdication
abdicar [abidʒi'kaɾ] ⟨1n⟩ *v/t* abdicate (***a favor de*** in favor of); **~ *de algo*** renounce sth
abdômen, *Port* **abdómen** [abi'domẽ] *m* abdomen
abdominal [abidomi'naw] *adj* abdominal; ESP ***fazer abdominais*** do situps
a-bê-cê [abe'se] *m* ABC; *fig* basics
abecedário [abese'daɾiu] *m* alphabet
abeirar-se [abej'ɾaɾsi] ⟨1a⟩ *v/r* **~ *de alguém / algo*** draw close to s.o. / sth
abelha [a'beʎa] *f* bee
abelha-rainha [abeʎaha'iɲa] *f* queen bee
abelhão [abe'ʎãw] *m* bumblebee
abelheira [abe'ʎejɾa] *f* bee hive
abelheiro [abe'ʎejɾu] *m* beekeeper
abelhudo [abe'ʎudu] *adj* nosy
abençoar [abẽ'swaɾ], **abendiçoar** [abẽdʒi'swaɾ] ⟨1f⟩ bless
aberração [abeha'sãw] *f* aberration
aberta [a'bɛɾta] *f* opening; (*clareira*) clearing; *céu*: brightening; *fig* opportunity
abertamente [abɛɾta'mẽtʃi] *adv* openly
aberto [a'bɛɾtu] *adj* open; *semáforo* green; *torneira* on; *buraco* gaping; FIN ***em ~*** outstanding
abertura [abeɾ'tuɾa] *f* opening; FOT aperture; MÚS overture; *inquérito*: launch
abeto [a'betu] *m* fir
abismo [a'bizmu] *m* abyss; *fig* gulf
abjeto, *Port* **abjecto** [abi'ʒɛtu] *adj* abject
abjurar [abʒu'ɾaɾ] ⟨1a⟩ *v/t* revoke; *crença, vício* renounce
abnegação [abnega'sãw] *f* self-denial
abnegado [abne'gadu] *adj* self-sacrificing
abóbada [a'bɔbada] *f* arch, vault
abóbora [a'bɔboɾa] *f* pumpkin, squash
abobrinha [abɔ'bɾiɲa] *f* zucchini, *Brit* courgette
abolição [aboli'sãw] *f* abolition
abolir [abo'liɾ] ⟨3f⟩ *v/t* abolish
abolorecer [abolore'seɾ] ⟨2g⟩ *v/i* go moldy, *Brit* go mouldy
abominação [abomina'sãw] *f* abomination
abominar [abomi'naɾ] ⟨1a⟩ *v/t* loathe
abominável [abomi'navew] *adj* abominable
abonado [abo'nadu] *adj* (*endinheirado*) wealthy, affluent
abonar [abo'naɾ] ⟨1f⟩ guarantee; *dinheiro* advance
abono [a'bonu] *m* guarantee; *dinheiro*: advance; **~ *de família*** child benefit; *fig* ***em ~ de*** in favor of, *Brit* in favour of
abordar [aboɾ'daɾ] ⟨1e⟩ **1** *v/t pessoa, problema* approach; NÁUT board **2** *v/i* NÁUT put in
aborígene [abo'ɾiʒeni] **1** *adj* aboriginal **2** *m* aborigine
aborrecer [abohe'seɾ] ⟨2g⟩ *v/t* bore; (*irritar*) annoy; **aborrecer-se** *v/r* get bored; **~ *com*** get annoyed about; (*estar cheio*) be fed up with
aborrecido [abohe'sidu] *adj* boring; (*irritante*) annoying
aborrecimento [abohesi'mẽtu] *m* (*transtorno*) nuisance; (*contrariedade*) annoyance; (*tédio*) boredom
abortar [aboɾ'taɾ] ⟨1e⟩ **1** *v/t* abort *tb* INFORM **2** *v/i* miscarry; *intencional* have an abortion
aborto [a'boɾtu] *m* miscarriage; **~ (*voluntário*)** abortion; ***fazer um ~*** have an abortion
abotoadura [abotwa'duɾa] *f* cuff link

abotoar [abo'twaɾ] ⟨1f⟩ button up, do up

abraçar [abɾa'saɾ] ⟨1p & 1b⟩ hug; *fig* embrace

abraço [a'bɾasu] *m* embrace, hug; ***um ~!, ~!*** best wishes; *com afeto* love; (*até logo*) bye now

abrandar [abɾã'daɾ] ⟨1a⟩ **1** *v/t* reduce; *atitude* soften **2** *v/i* calm down

abranger [abɾã'ʒeɾ] ⟨2h⟩ span, include

abrasão [abɾa'zãw] *f* abrasion

abrasileirado [abɾazilej'ɾadu] *adj* brazilianized

abrasileirar [abɾazilej'ɾaɾ] ⟨1a⟩ *v/t* brazilianize

abrasivo [abɾa'zivu] *adj* abrasive

abre-cartas [abɾi'kaɾtas] *m* ⟨*pl inv*⟩ letter opener

abre-latas [abɾi'latas] *m Port* ⟨*pl inv*⟩ can opener, *Brit* tin opener

abreviação [abɾevia'sãw] *f* abbreviation

abreviar [abɾe'vjaɾ] ⟨1g⟩ abbreviate; *texto* shorten, abridge

abreviatura [abɾevja'tuɾa] *f* abbreviation

abridor [abɾi'doɾ] *m* TECN opener; *Bras* ***~ de garrafas*** bottle-opener; ***~ de latas*** can opener, *Brit* tin opener

abrigado [abɾi'gadu] *adj* sheltered

abrigar [abɾi'gaɾ] ⟨1o⟩ *v/t* shelter; **abrigar-se** *v/r* take shelter

abrigo [a'bɾigu] *m* shelter, refuge; *fig* protection; *carro*: car port

abril [a'bɾiw] *m* April; ***em ~*** in April

abrir [a'bɾiɾ] ⟨3b; *pp* aberto⟩ **1** *v/t* open; *torneira* turn on; *apetite* whet; ***~ falência*** go bankupt; ***~ (o) caminho para*** open the way for; ***num ~ e fechar de olhos*** in the twinkling of an eye **2** *v/i* open; **abrir-se** *v/r* open; *vista*, *buraco* open up; ***~ com alguém*** open up to s.o.

ab-rogação [abhoga'sãw] *f* repeal, abolition

ab-rogar [abho'gaɾ] ⟨1o & 1e⟩ repeal, abolish

abrunheiro [abɾu'ɲejɾu] *m* plum tree

abrunho [a'bɾuɲu] *m* plum

abrupto [a'bɾuptu] *adj terreno* steep; (*repentino*) sudden; (*rude*) abrupt

abscesso [ab'sɛsu] *m* abscess

abside [ab'sidʒi] *f* ARQUIT apse

absenteísmo [absẽte'izmu] *m* absenteeism

absenteísta [absẽte'ista] *m/f* absentee

absolutamente [absoluta'mẽtʃi] *adv* absolutely; ***~ não!*** absolutely not!

absolutismo [absolu'tʃizmu] *m* absolutism

absoluto [abso'lutu] *adj* absolute; *vencedor* outright; ***não, em ~*** no, not at all

absolver [absow'veɾ] ⟨2e⟩ *v/t* acquit; REL absolve

absolvição [absowvi'sãw] *f* acquittal; REL absolution

absorção [absoɾ'sãw] *f* absorption

absorto [ab'soɾtu] *adj em pensamentos* absorbed

absorvente [absoɾ'vẽtʃi] **1** *adj* absorbent; *novela* absorbing **2** *m* ***~ higiênico*** sanitary napkin, *Brit* sanitary towel

absorver [absoɾ'veɾ] ⟨2e⟩ *v/t* absorb; **absorver-se** *v/r* ***~ em algo*** become absorbed in sth

abstêmio, *Port* **abstémio** [abs'temiu] **1** *adj* abstemious; *álcool*: teetotal **2** *m*, **-a** *f* teetotaler, *Brit* teetotaller

abstenção [abstẽ'sãw] *f* abstention

abster-se [abs'teɾsi] ⟨2xa⟩ *v/r* abstain; ***~ de*** abstain from

abstinência [abstʃi'nẽsja] *f* abstinence; ***dia*** *m* ***de ~*** day of fasting

abstinente [abstʃi'nẽtʃi] *adj álcool*: teetotal

abstração, *Port* **abstracção** [abstɾa'sãw] *f* abstraction

abstracto [abs'tɾatu] *adj Port* abstract

abstrair [abstɾa'iɾ] ⟨3l⟩ *v/t* abstract, separate

abstrato [abs'tɾatu] *adj* abstract

absurdamente [absuɾda'mẽtʃi] *adv* absurdly

absurdo [ab'suɾdu] **1** *adj* absurd **2** *m* nonsense

abundância [abũ'dãsja] *f* abundance

abundante [abũ'dãtʃi] *adj* abundant

abundar [abũ'daɾ] ⟨1a⟩ abound

abusar [abu'zaɾ] ⟨1a⟩ ***~ de alguém*** /

algo abuse s.o. / sth; ***não abuses!*** don't push it too far!
abusivo [abu'zivu] *adj* abusive
abuso [a'buzu] *m* abuse; ~ ***de drogas*** drug abuse
abutre [a'butri] *m* vulture
a/c *abr* (***ao cuidado de***) c/o (care of)
acabado [aka'badu] *adj* finished; (*exausto*) exhausted; (*gasto*) worn out
acabamento [akaba'mẽtu] *m* completion; *produto*: finish
acabar [aka'bar] ⟨1b⟩ **1** *v/t* (*terminar, aperfeiçoar*) finish **2** *v/i* finish, end; ***estar a*** ~ come to an end; *tempo, azeite* run out; ~ ***num hospital*** end up *ou* finish up in the hospital; ***acabei eu mesma fazendo isso*** I ended up *ou* finished up doing it myself; ***acabou o tempo*** time's up; ~ ***com algo*** put an end to sth; (*arruinar*) ruin sth; ~ ***com uma canção*** murder a song; ~ ***com alguém*** finish s.o. (off); *com namorado* finish with s.o.; ~ ***de fazer algo*** have just done sth; ***acabo de vê-la*** I've just seen her, I just saw her
acabrunhado [akabru'ɲadu] *adj* depressed; (*envergonhado*) embarrassed
acabrunhar [akabru'ɲar] ⟨1a⟩ *v/t* depress; (*envergonhar*) embarrass
acácia [a'kasja] *f* acacia
academia [akade'mia] *f* academy; ~ ***de ginástica*** gym; ~ ***militar*** military academy
acadêmico, *Port* **académico** [aka'dɛmiku] **1** *adj* academic **2** *m*, **-a** *f* academic
açafrão [asa'frãw] *m condimento* saffron
açafrão-da-primavera [asafrãwda-prima'vɛra] *m* crocus
acalentar [akalẽ'tar] ⟨1a⟩ *v/t* warm up; *esperança* cherish; *plano* nurture; *Bras bebê* rock to sleep
acalmar [akaw'mar] ⟨1a⟩ **1** *v/t* calm; *dor* relieve, soothe **2** *v/i vento etc* die down; **acalmar-se** *v/r* calm down
acalorado [akalo'radu] *adj* heated *tb fig*
acamado [aka'madu] *adj* bedridden
acampamento [akãpa'mẽtu] *m* camp; ~ ***de refugiados*** refugee camp
acampar [akã'par] ⟨1a⟩ *v/i* camp
acanhado [aka'ɲadu] *adj* (*tímido*) shy
acanhar-se [aka'ɲarsi] ⟨1a⟩ *v/r* go shy
acareação [akarja'sãw] *f* confrontation
acarear [aka'rjar] ⟨1l⟩ confront
acariciar [akari'sjar] ⟨1g⟩ caress
acarinhar [akari'ɲar] ⟨1a⟩ cherish; (*acariciar*) caress
ácaro ['akaru] *m* mite
acarretar [akahe'tar] ⟨1c⟩ result in, bring about
acasalar [akaza'lar] ⟨1b⟩ mate
acaso [a'kazu] *m* chance; ***ao*** ~ at random; ***por*** ~ by chance
acatar [aka'tar] ⟨1b⟩ *v/t* respect; *lei* obey; *instruções* follow
acastanhado [akasta'ɲadu] *adj* brownish
acautelado [akawte'ladu] *adj* cautious
acautelar [akawte'lar] ⟨1c⟩ *v/t* warn (***de*** of); **acautelar-se** *v/r* be careful, beware (***com*** of)
ação[1] [a'sãw] *f* action; (*ato*) act, deed; DIR ***pôr uma*** ~ bring an action, institute proceedings; ~ ***civil*** civil action; ~ ***industrial*** industrial action; ~ ***judicial*** legal action, lawsuit; ~ ***penal*** criminal action
ação[2] [a'sãw] *f* ECON share; ***cotações*** *pl* ***de ações*** share prices
acionamento [asjona'mẽtu] *m* TECN drive; ***mecanismo*** *m* ***de*** ~ gear system
acionar [asjo'nar] ⟨1f⟩ (*pôr em movimento*) set in motion; TECN operate; DIR sue
acionista [asjo'nista] *m/f* stockholder, *Brit* shareholder
acç…, acc… *Port* → ***aç…, acc…***
acedência [ase'dẽsja] *f* agreement
aceder [ase'der] ⟨2c⟩ (*alcançar*) attain; (*anuir*) agree to
aceitação [asejta'sãw] *f* acceptance; ***ter*** ~ meet with approval
aceitar [asej'tar] ⟨1a⟩ accept; *conselho* accept, take; ***você aceita um cafezinho?*** would you like a cup of coffee?

aceitável [asej'tavew] *adj* acceptable
aceleração [aselera'sãw] *f* acceleration
acelerador [aselera'doɾ] *m* AUTO gas pedal, accelerator
acelerar [asele'ɾaɾ] ⟨1c⟩ accelerate
acenar [ase'naɾ] ⟨1d⟩ wave; **~ *com a cabeça*** nod
acendedor [asẽde'doɾ] *m* lighter
acender [asẽ'deɾ] ⟨2a⟩ *lume, vela* light; *luz* switch on; *desejo* excite, inflame
aceno [a'senu] *m* gesture; *mão*: wave; *cabeça*: nod
acento [a'sẽtu] *m* accent; **~ *tônico*** stress
acentuação [asẽtwa'sãw] *f* accentuation, stress
acentuar [asẽ'twaɾ] ⟨1g⟩ accentuate, stress
acepção [ase'sãw] *f* sense, meaning
acepipe [ase'pipi] *m* delicacy; **~*s*** *pl* appetizers, hors d'œuvres
acerca [a'seɾka] *prep* **~ *de*** about, regarding
acercar(-se) [aseɾ'kaɾ(si)] ⟨1n & 1c⟩ *v/t* & *v/r* **~ *de*** approach, draw near to
acertar [aseɾ'taɾ] ⟨1c⟩ **1** *v/t alvo* hit *tb fig*; *relógio* set; **~ *contas*** settle up **2** *v/i* **~ *com algo*** (*descobrir*) hit on sth;
aceso [a'sezu] *adj lume, luz* on *pred*, alight *pred*
acessível [ase'sivew] *adj* accessible *tb fig*; *preço* reasonable, affordable; *pessoa* approachable
acesso [a'sɛsu] *m* access; MED attack, fit; ***rua*** *f* ***de* ~** access road; ***de fácil* ~** easily accessible; ***ter* ~ *a algo*** have access to sth; ***ter* ~ *à Internet*** have Internet access; **~ *de raiva*** fit of rage; **~ *remoto*** remote access
acessório [ase'sɔriu] **1** *adj* accessory; (*secundário*) minor **2** *m* TECN accessory; **~*s*** *pl* TEAT props
acetinado [asetʃi'nadu] *adj* (*liso*) smooth; (*brilhante*) gleaming; *papel* glazed
acetona [ase'tona] *f* nail polish remover; QUÍM acetone
achado [a'ʃadu] *m* (*descoberta*) find, discovery; (*idéia*) idea; ***perdidos*** *mpl* ***e* ~*s*** *pl* lost property; *oficina* lost and found, *Brit* lost property office
achar [a'ʃaɾ] ⟨1b⟩ *v/t* find; *fig* think; ***acho que não*** I guess not; ***acho que sim*** I guess so; **achar-se** *v/r* be
achatado [aʃa'tadu] *adj* flat
achatar [aʃa'taɾ] ⟨1b⟩ *v/t* flatten, squash
acidentado [asidẽ'tadu] *adj terreno* hilly, *estrada* bumpy; (*tumultuoso*) eventful, turbulent
acidental [asidẽ'taw] *adj* accidental
acidentalmente [asidẽtaw'mẽtʃi] *adv* accidentally
acidente [asi'dẽtʃi] *m* (*acaso*) chance; (*desastre*) accident; ***por* ~** by accident; **~ *de carro*** car accident; **~ *de trabalho*** industrial accident
acidez [asi'des] *f* acidity; ***grau*** *m* ***de* ~** acid content
ácido ['asidu] **1** *adj* acid **2** *m* acid; **~ *clorídrico*** hydrochloric acid
acima [a'sima] **1** *adv* above, up **2** *prep* **~ *de*** above, over; ***estar* ~ *de algo*** be above sth; ***rio* ~** upstream, upriver; **~ *de 10.000*** upwards of 10,000; **~ *de tudo*** above all
acinzentado [asĩzẽ'tadu] *adj* grayish, *Brit* greyish
aclamação [aklama'sãw] *f* acclamation
aclamar [akla'maɾ] ⟨1a⟩ cheer; (*eleger*) acclaim
aclaração [aklara'sãw] *f* METEO brightening; (*explicação*) explanation
aclarar [akla'ɾaɾ] ⟨1b⟩ light up; (*explicar*) explain, clarify; (*esclarecer*) clear up; *cor* brighten
aclimatação [aklimata'sãw] *f* acclimation, *Brit* acclimatization
aclimatar [aklima'taɾ] ⟨1b⟩ *v/t* acclimate, *Brit* acclimatize; **aclimatar-se** *v/r* become acclimated, *Brit* become acclimatized
acne ['akni] *f* MED acne
aço ['asu] *m* steel; ***nervos*** *mpl* ***de* ~** nerves of steel; **~ *inoxidável*** stainless steel
acocorar-se [akoko'ɾaɾsi] ⟨1e⟩ *v/r* squat, crouch
açoitar [asoj'taɾ] ⟨1a⟩ *v/t* whip
acolá [ako'la] *adv* over there

acolchoado [akow'ʃwadu] **1** *adj* padded, quilted **2** *m* quilt
acolchoar [akow'ʃwaɾ] ⟨1f⟩ *v/t* upholster; *vestuário* pad; *edredom* quilt
acolhedor [akoʎe'doɾ] *adj* welcoming, hospitable
acolher [ako'ʎeɾ] ⟨2d⟩ *v/t* welcome; (*receber*) receive; **acolher-se** *v/r* shelter
acolhimento [akoʎi'mẽtu] *m* (*recepção*) reception; (*refúgio*) refuge
acometer [akome'teɾ] ⟨2c⟩ (*atacar*) attack; *doença* strike
acomodação [akomoda'sãw] *f*, **acomodamento** [akomoda'mẽtu] *m* (*adaptação*) adaptation; (*alojamento*) accommodations, *Brit* accommodation
acomodar [akomo'daɾ] ⟨1e⟩ *v/t* adapt; *hóspede* accommodate
acompanhamento [akõpaɲa'mẽtu] *m* (*séquito*) accompaniment; GASTR side dish
acompanhante [akõpa'ɲãtʃi] *m/f* companion; MÚS accompanist
acompanhar [akõpa'ɲaɾ] ⟨1a⟩ **1** *v/t* accompany; *acontecimentos* follow; **~ *algo na TV*** watch sth on TV; **~ *algo pela rádio*** follow sth on the radio; **~ *alguém até a porta*** see s.o. to the door **2** *v/i* keep up
aconchegado [akõʃe'gadu] *adj* snug, cozy, *Brit* cosy
aconchegante [akõʃe'gãtʃi] *adj* cozy, *Brit* cosy
aconchegar [akõʃe'gaɾ] ⟨1a & 1o⟩ *v/t* make cozy, *Brit* make cosy; **aconchegar-se** *v/r* snuggle up, nestle
aconchego [akõ'ʃegu] *m* coziness, *Brit* cosiness
acondicionamento [akõdʒisjona'mẽtu] *m* ECON packaging
acondicionar [akõdʒisjo'naɾ] ⟨1f⟩ pack
aconselhar [akõse'ʎaɾ] ⟨1d⟩ **~ *a alguém*** advise s.o.
aconselhável [akõse'ʎavew] *adj* advisable
acontecer [akõte'seɾ] ⟨2g⟩ *v/i* (*suceder*) happen
acontecimento [akõtesi'mẽtu] *m* event, happening
acoplamento [akopla'mẽtu] *m* coupling
acoplar [ako'plaɾ] ⟨1e⟩ couple, hitch up
acordar [akoɾ'daɾ] ⟨1e⟩ **1** *v/t* wake (up); (*conceder*) grant; **~ *em fazer algo*** agree to do sth **2** *v/i* wake up
acorde [a'kɔrdʒi] *m* MÚS chord
acordeão [akoɾ'dʒiãw] *m* accordion
acordeonista [akoɾ'dʒonista] *m/f* accordionist
acordo [a'koɾdu] *m* (*conformidade*) agreement; ***de comum* ~** unanimously; ***chegar a* (*um*) ~** reach an agreement; ***de* ~** agreed; ***de* ~ *com*** in agreement with, in accordance with; ***estar de* ~ *com*** agree with
Açores [a'soris] *mpl* Azores *pl*
açoriano [aso'ɾjanu] **1** *adj* Azorean **2** *m*, **-a** *f* Azorean
acorrentar [akohẽ'taɾ] ⟨1a⟩ chain (***a*** to)
acostamento [akosta'mẽtu] *m Bras* berm, *Brit* hard shoulder
acostumado [akostu'madu] *adj* usual, customary
acostumar [akostu'maɾ] ⟨1a⟩ *v/t* accustom (***a*** to); **acostumar-se** *v/r* **~ *a*** get used to
acotovelar [akotove'laɾ] ⟨1c⟩ *v/t* nudge; **~ *alguém para fora do caminho*** elbow s.o. out of the way
açougue [a'sogi] *m Bras* butcher, *Brit* butcher's
açougueiro [aso'gejɾu] *m Bras* butcher
acre[1] ['akɾi] *adj* bitter, acrid; *fig* harsh
acre[2] ['akɾi] *m* acre
acreditado [akɾedʒi'tadu] *adj* (*reputado*) respected; (*crível*) credible; POL accredited
acreditar [akɾedʒi'taɾ] ⟨1a⟩ believe; POL accredit; **~ *em algo*** believe in sth; **~ *em alguém*** believe s.o.; *fé*: believe in s.o.
acreditável [akɾedʒi'tavew] *adj* credible, believable
acrescentar [akɾesẽ'taɾ] ⟨1a⟩ add
acréscimo [a'kɾɛsimu] *m* addition, increase
acrílico [a'kɾiliku] *adj* acrylic

acrimonioso [akrimo'njozu] *adj* acrimonious
acrobacia [akroba'sia] *f* acrobatics
acrobata [akro'bata] *m/f* acrobat
acrobático [akro'batʃiku] *adj* acrobatic
acrônimo, *Port* **acrónimo** [a'kronimu] *m* acronym
act... *Port* → ***at...***
açúcar [a'sukar] *m* sugar; ***pão*** *m* ***de ~*** sugar loaf; ***sem ~*** sugar-free; ***~ branco*** white sugar; ***~ (em) bruto*** unrefined sugar; ***~ de cana*** cane sugar; ***~ cristal*** refined sugar; ***~ mascavado*** brown sugar; ***~ em pó*** icing sugar
açucareiro [asuka'rejru] *m* sugar bowl
açude [a'sudʒi] *m* weir, dam
acudir [aku'dʒir] ⟨3h⟩ help, assist
aculturação [akultura'sãw] *f* acculturation
acumulação [akumula'sãw] *f* accumulation
acumulador [akumula'dor] *m* battery
acumular [akumu'lar] ⟨1a⟩ *v/t* accumulate, pile up; *energia* store; **acumular-se** *v/r* accumulate; *dívidas* mount up; *pessoas* gather together
acumulativo [akumula'tʃivu] *adj* cumulative
acúmulo [a'kumulu] *m* accumulation, backlog
acupuntura, *Port* **acupunctura** [akupũ'tura] *f* acupuncture
acusação [akuza'sãw] *f* accusation; DIR prosecution
acusado [aku'zadu] *m*, **-a** *f* accused
acusar [aku'zar] ⟨1a⟩ accuse; *recepção* confirm; ***~ o recebimento de*** acknowledge receipt of; ***ele me acusou de mentir*** he accused me of lying
acusatório [akuza'tɔriu] *adj* accusing
acústica [a'kustʃika] *f* acoustics
acústico [a'kustʃiku] *adj* acoustic
adaga [a'daga] *f* dagger
adaptabilidade [adaptabili'dadʒi] *f* adaptability
adaptação [adapta'sãw] *f* adaptation
adaptador [adapta'dor] *m* ELÉT adapter
adaptar [adap'tar] ⟨1a⟩ *v/t* adapt; **adaptar-se** *v/r* ***~ a algo*** adapt to sth
adaptável [adap'tavew] *adj* adaptable
adega [a'dɛga] *f* wine cellar
adentro [a'dẽtru] *adv* inside; ***correr selva ~*** run into the jungle
adepto [a'dɛptu] *m* follower, supporter
adequado [ade'kwadu] *adj* (*conforme*) suitable; (*apropriado*) appropriate
adereço [ade'resu] *m* adornment; TEAT ***~s*** *pl* props
aderência [ade'rẽsja] *f* TECN adhesion; AUTO road holding; POL supporters
aderente [ade'rẽtʃi] **1** *adj* adhesive **2** *m/f* supporter
aderir [ade'rir] ⟨3c⟩ adhere (***a*** to); POL *etc* ***~ a*** join
adesão [ade'zãw] *f* ⟨*sem pl*⟩ adhesion; ***~ a um grupo*** joining a group
adesivo [ade'zivu] **1** *adj* adhesive, sticky **2** *m* MED Band-Aid®, *Brit* sticking plaster
adestrador [adestra'dor] *m*, **-a** *f cão*: trainer
adestrar [ades'trar] ⟨1c⟩ *v/t* train
adeus [a'dews] **1** *int* ***~!*** goodbye! **2** *m* goodbye
adeusinho [adew'ziɲu] *int Port* ***~!*** bye!
adiamento [adʒia'mẽtu] *m* postponement; (*prorrogação*) adjournment
adiantado [adʒiã'tadu] *adj pagamento* advance *atr*; *tarefa* advanced; ***dinheiro*** *m* ***~*** advance; ***estar ~*** *relógio* be fast; ***chegar ~*** arrive early
adiantamento [adʒiãta'mẽtu] *m* advance
adiantar [adʒiã'tar] ⟨1a⟩ *v/t dinheiro* advance; *relógio* put forward; **adiantar-se** *v/r* advance, get ahead; *relógio* gain; ***~ a alguém*** get ahead of s.o.
adiante [a'dʒiãtʃi] **1** *int* forward **2** *adv* in front
adiar [a'dʒiar] ⟨1g⟩ postpone; (*protelar*) adjourn
adição [adʒi'sãw] *f* MAT addition
adicional [adʒisjo'naw] *adj* additional
adicionar [adʒisjo'nar] ⟨1f⟩ add
adictivo [adʒi'tʃivu] *adj Port* MED *comportamento* addictive
adido [a'dʒidu] *m* POL attaché

aditamento [adʒita'mẽtu] *m* addition; (*suplemento*) appendix; POL amendment
aditivo[1] [adʒi'tʃivu] **1** *adj* additional; ***sinal*** *m* **~** plus sign **2** *m* additive
aditivo[2] [adʒi'tʃivu] *adj Bras comportamento* addictive
adivinha [adʒi'viɲa] *f* riddle
adivinhar [adʒivi'ɲar] ⟨1a⟩ predict, foretell; *pensamento* guess; ***adivinhe!*** guess!
adivinho [adʒi'viɲu] *m*, **-a** *f* fortuneteller
adjacente [adʒa'sẽtʃi] *adj* adjacent
adjetivo [ad'ʒetʃivu] *m* adjective
adjunto [ad'ʒũtu] **1** *adj* attached; *pessoa* assistant *atr* **2** *m*, **-a** *f* assistant
administração [adʒiministra'sãw] *f* administration; **~ *de empresas*** business administration
administrador [adʒiministra'dor] *m*, **-a** *f* administrator
administrar [adʒiminis'trar] ⟨1a⟩ manage; *medicamento*, *sacramentos* administer; **~ *mal*** mismanage
administrativo [adʒiministra'tʃivu] *adj* administrative
admiração [adʒimira'sãw] *f* ⟨*sem pl*⟩ admiration; (*espanto*) wonder
admirador [adʒimira'dor] *m*, **-a** *f* admirer
admirar [adʒimi'rar] ⟨1a⟩ *v/t* admire; (*espantar*) wonder at; ***não admira*** no wonder; ***estar admirado*** be astonished; **admirar-se** *v/r* **~ *de*** be astonished at
admirável [adʒimi'ravew] *adj* admirable
admissão [adʒimi'sãw] *f* admission
admissível [adʒimi'sivew] *adj* admissible
admitir [adʒimi'tʃir] ⟨3a⟩ admit; *pessoal* take on; *ação* tolerate; ***não ~ algo*** refuse to tolerate sth
ADN [ade'ɛni] *m abr* (***ácido desoxirribonucléico***) DNA (deoxyribonucleic acid)
adoçante [ado'sãtʃi] *m* sweetener
adoção [ado'sãw] *f* adoption
adoçar [ado'sar] ⟨1p & 1e⟩ sweeten; **~ *a pílula a alguém*** sweeten the pill for s.o.
adocicado [adosi'kadu] *adj* sweetish
adoecer [adwe'ser] ⟨2g⟩ fall ill (***com*** with)
adolescência [adoles'sẽsja] *f* adolescence
adolescente [adoles'sẽtʃi] **1** *adj* adolescent; *moda* teenage *atr* **2** *m/f* teenager, adolescent
adopç…, adopt… *Port* → ***adoç…, adot…***
adorar [ado'rar] ⟨1e⟩ adore; (*respeitar*) respect; (*amar apaixonadamente*) worship
adorável [ado'ravew] *adj* adorable
adormecer [adorme'ser] ⟨2g⟩ *v/i* fall asleep, go to sleep
adormecido [adorme'sidu] *adj* asleep *pred*; *cidade* sleepy
adoptivo [ado'tʃivu] *adj* adoptive; ***pais*** *mpl* **~*s*** adoptive parents
adquirir [adki'rir] ⟨3a⟩ acquire, obtain
adrenalina [adrena'lina] *f* adrenalin
aduaneiro [adwa'nejru] **1** *adj* customs *atr* **2** *m*, **-a** *f* customs officer
adubar [adu'bar] ⟨1a⟩ manure, fertilize
adubo [a'dubu] *m* fertilizer
adulação [adula'sãw] *f* flattery
adulador [adula'dor] *m*, **-a** *f* flatterer
adular [adu'lar] ⟨1a⟩ flatter
adulterado [aduwte'radu] *adj* adulterated
adulterar [aduwte'rar] ⟨1c⟩ *v/t* falsify; *vinho etc* adulterate
adultério [aduw'tɛriu] *m* adultery; ***cometer ~*** commit adultery
adúltero [a'duwteru] **1** *adj* adulterous **2** *m*, **-a** *f* adulterer; adulteress
adulto [a'duwtu] **1** *adj* adult **2** *m*, **-a** *f* adult
advento [adʒi'vẽtu] *m* (*chegada*) advent; REL Advent
adverbial [adʒiver'bjaw] *adj* adverbial
advérbio [adʒi'vɛrbiu] *m* adverb
adversário [adʒiver'sariu] *m*, **-a** *f* adversary, opponent
adversidade [adʒiversi'dadʒi] *f* adversity
adverso [adʒi'vɛrsu] *adj* adverse; ***ser ~ a algo*** be opposed to sth

advertência [adʒiver'tẽsja] *f* warning
advertir [adʒiver'ʧir] ⟨3c⟩ *v/t* warn
advocacia [adʒivoka'sia] *f* law, legal profession
advogado [adʒivo'gadu] *m*, **-a** *f* attorney, lawyer; **~ *de defesa*** defense lawyer, *Brit* defence lawyer
advogar [adʒivo'gar] ⟨1e & 1o⟩ *v/t* advocate
aéreo [a'ɛriu] air *atr*; ***por via aréa*** by airmail
aerobarco [aɛro'barku] *m* hovercraft
aeróbica [aɛ'rɔbika] *f* aerobics
aerodinâmica [aɛrodʒi'nʌmika] *f* aerodynamics
aerodinâmico [aɛrodʒi'nʌmiku] *adj* aerodynamic
aeródromo [aɛ'rɔdrumu] *m* airfield
aeromoça [aɛro'mosa] *f Bras* flight attendant, stewardess
aeronáutica [aɛro'nawʧika] *f* aeronautics
aeronáutico [aɛro'nawʧiku] *adj* aeronautical
aeronave [aɛro'navi] *f* aircraft
aeroporto [aɛro'portu] *m* airport
aerossol [aɛro'sɔw] *m* ⟨*pl* -ssóis⟩ aerosol
aerovia [aɛro'via] *f* air route
afabilidade [afabili'dadʒi] *f* friendliness
afagar [afa'gar] ⟨1o & 1b⟩ stroke, caress
afago [a'fagu] *m* caress
afasia [afa'zia] *f* aphasia
afastado [afas'tadu] *adj* distant, remote
afastamento [afasta'mẽtu] *m* removal; (*distância*) distance; *candidato*: rejection; *fig* estrangement
afastar [afas'tar] ⟨1b⟩ *v/t* remove, take away; **afastar-se** *v/r* move away, go away; (*retirar-se*) pull away; *do caminho etc* deviate from; **~ *de um colega*** distance oneself from a colleague
afável [a'favew] *adj* friendly, affable
afazeres [afa'zeris] *mpl* (*tarefas*) business; (*deveres*) duties
afecção [afek'sãw] *f* MED illness
afect... *Port* → ***afet...***
Afeganistão [afeganis'tãw] *m* ***o*** **~** Afghanistan
afegão [afe'gãw] **1** *adj* Afghan **2** *m*, **afegã** *f* Afghan
afeição [afej'sãw] *f* affection
afeiçoado [afej'swadu] *adj* fond; (*devoto*) devoted
afeiçoar-se [afej'swarsi] ⟨1f⟩ *v/r* **~ *a alguém*** become attached to s.o.
afeminado [afemi'nadu] *adj* effeminate
afetação [afeta'sãw] *f* affectation
afetado [afe'tadu] *adj* affected, pretentious
afetar [afe'tar] ⟨1a⟩ affect; (*fingir*) feign
afetividade [afeʧivi'dadʒi] *f* affection
afetivo [afe'ʧivu] *adj* affectionate; *transtornos etc* emotional
afeto [a'fɛtu] *m* affection
afetuoso [afe'twozu] *adj* affectionate
afiado [a'fjadu] *adj* sharp
afiar [a'fjar] ⟨1g⟩ sharpen
afilado [afi'ladu] *adj* (*fino*) thin; (*bicudo*) pointed
afilhado [afi'ʎadu] *m*, **-a** *f* godchild, godson; goddaughter
afiliação [afilia'sãw] *f* membership, affiliation
afim [a'fĩ] *adj* related; (*semelhante*) similar
afinação [afina'sãw] *f* MÚS tuning
afinado [afi'nadu] *adj* MÚS in tune
afinal [afi'naw] *adv* (*finalmente*) finally, at last; **~ *de contas*** after all
afinar [afi'nar] ⟨1a⟩ **1** *v/t* MÚS tune; TECN adjust **2** *v/i* MÚS tune up
afinco [a'fĩku] *m* tenacity, persistence
afinidade [afini'dadʒi] *f* affinity
afirmação [afirma'sãw] *f* assertion; (*garantia*) assurance
afirmar [afir'mar] ⟨1a⟩ affirm, assert; **afirmar-se** *v/r* assert oneself; **~ *como*** make a name for oneself as
afirmativo [afirma'ʧivu] *adj* affirmative
afivelar [afive'lar] ⟨1c⟩ buckle
afixar [afi'ksar] ⟨1a⟩ fix; *cartaz* stick, post
aflição [afli'sãw] *f* affliction; (*ansiedade*) anxiety; ***causar aflicões a alguém*** be a source of great anxiety to s.o.

afligir [afli'ʒiɾ] ⟨3n⟩ *v/t* (*desgostar*) distress; (*preocupar*) worry
aflito [a'flitu] *adj* (*triste*) distressed; (*preocupado*) anxious
aflorar [aflo'ɾaɾ] ⟨1e⟩ *v/i* (*emergir*) emerge; *fig* (*transparecer*) appear
afluência [aflu'ẽsja] *f* flow; (*riqueza*) affluence
afluente [aflu'ẽtʃi] **1** *adj* affluent **2** *m* tributary
afluir [aflu'iɾ] ⟨3i⟩ flow; *fig* flock
afobado [afo'badu] *adj* nervous, flustered
afobar-se [afo'baɾsi] ⟨1e⟩ *v/r* get flustered
afogador [afoga'doɾ] *m* AUTO choke
afogar [afo'gaɾ] ⟨1o, *Stv* 1e⟩ *v/t* drown; **afogar-se** *v/r* drown, be drowned
afoito [a'fojtu] *adj* bold
afônico, *Port* **afónico** [a'foniku], *adj* ***estar ~*** have lost one's voice
aforrar [afo'haɾ] ⟨1e⟩ *dinheiro* save
aforro [a'fohu] *m* savings
afrescalhado [afɾeska'ʎadu] *adj fam* effeminate, camp
afresco [a'fɾesku] *m* fresco
África ['afɾika] *f* Africa
africano [afɾi'kanu] **1** *adj* African **2** *m*, **-a** *f* African
afro-brasileiro [afɾobɾazi'lejɾu] **1** *adj* Afro-Brazilian **2** *m*, **-a** *f* Afro-Brazilian
afrodisíaco [afɾodʒi'ziaku] *m* aphrodisiac
afronta [a'fɾõta] *f* affront
afrontar [afɾõ'taɾ] ⟨1a⟩ defy; (*insultar*) affront
afrouxamento [afɾoʃa'mẽtu] *m* relaxation; *aperto*: loosening; *velocidade*: deceleration
afrouxar [afɾo'ʃaɾ] ⟨1a⟩ *aperto* loosen; *tensão* relax; *dor* ease; *velocidade* slow down
afta ['afta] *f* mouth ulcer
after-shave [afteɾ'ʃejv] *m* aftershave
aftoso [af'tozu] *adj* ZOOL ***febre f aftosa*** foot-and-mouth disease
afugentar [afuʒẽ'taɾ] ⟨1a⟩ chase away
afundado [afũ'dadu] *adj* sunken *tb fig*
afundar [afũ'daɾ] ⟨1a⟩ *v/t* sink; **afundar-se** *v/r* go under, sink
agachar-se [aga'ʃaɾsi] ⟨1b⟩ *v/r* squat, crouch
agarrado [aga'hadu] *adj* (*junto*) stuck; (*forreta*) mean; (*dependente*) hooked (***a*** on)
agarrar [aga'haɾ] ⟨1b⟩ *v/t* seize, grasp; **agarrar-se** *v/r* ***~ a*** hold on to; ***~ com unhas e dentes a algo*** become set on sth
agasalhar-se [agaza'ʎaɾsi] ⟨1b⟩ *v/r* dress warmly, wrap oneself up
agasalho [aga'zaʎu] *m* (*vestuário*) warm clothing; ***~ esportivo*** sweats, *Brit* tracksuit
agência [a'ʒẽsja] *f* agency; (*escritório*) office; *banco*: branch; ***~ dos correios*** post office; ***~ de empregos*** employment agency; ***~ de notícias*** news agency; ***~ de publicidade*** advertising agency; ***~ de viagens*** travel agency
agenda [a'ʒẽda] *f* (appointments) diary; ***~ de endereços*** address book; ***~ de mesa*** desk diary
agente [a'ʒẽtʃi] **1** *m/f* agent; ***~ alfandegário*** customs officer; ***~ funerário*** *Am* mortician, undertaker; ***~ (de polícia)*** policeman; policewoman; ***~ secreto*** secret agent; ***~ de viagens*** travel agent **2** *m* QUÍM agent; ***~ tóxico*** toxic agent
ágil ['aʒiw] *adj* agile
agilidade [aʒili'dadʒi] *f* agility
agiota [a'ʒjɔta] *m/f* moneylender
agir [a'ʒiɾ] ⟨3n⟩ act, take action; ***~ como*** act as
agitação [aʒita'sãw] *f* disturbance; (*excitação*) agitation
agitado [aʒi'tadu] *adj* agitated
agitador [aʒita'doɾ] *m*, **-a** *f* agitator
agitar [aʒi'taɾ] ⟨1a⟩ agitate; (*sacudir*) shake; (*excitar*) excite; (*desinquietar*) disturb; POL stir up
aglomeração [aglomeɾa'sãw] *f* accumulation, agglomeration; *pessoas*: crowd; *carros*: mass, collection
aglomerado [aglome'ɾadu] *m* → ***aglomeração***
aglomerar [aglome'ɾaɾ] ⟨1c⟩ *v/t* heap up, pile up
agnóstico [a'gnɔstʃiku] *m/f* agnostic

agogô [ago'go] *m Afro-Brazilian musical instrument with two or three bells attached to a handle*
agonia [ago'nia] *f* agony; *fig* anguish
agoniar-se [ago'niarsi] ⟨1g⟩ *v/r* ~ ***por*** agonize over
agoniado [ago'njadu] *adj* nauseous; ***estou*** ~ I feel ill
agonizar [agoni'zar] ⟨1a⟩ *v/i* agonize; (*estar morrendo*) be dying
agora [a'gɔra] **1** *adv* now; ***de ~ em diante*** from now on; ~ ***mesmo*** right now; ~ ***não*** not now; ***por*** ~ for now; ***essa ~!*** and now this! **2** *conj* but; ~ ***que*** now that
agosto [a'gostu] *m* August; ***em*** ~ in August
agradar [agra'dar] ⟨1b⟩ **1** *v/t* please **2** *v/i* ~ ***a alguém*** please s.o.
agradável [agra'davew] *adj* pleasant, enjoyable
agradecer [agrade'ser] ⟨2g⟩ ~ ***a alguém por algo*** thank s.o. for sth
agradecidamente [agradesida'mẽtʃi] *adv* gratefully
agradecido [agrade'sidu] *adj* grateful; ***estar*** ~ be grateful
agradecimento [agradesi'mẽtu] *m* thanks; (*gratidão*) gratitude
agrado [a'gradu] *m* ***ser do ~ de alguém*** be to s.o.'s liking
agrafador [agrafa'dor] *m* stapler
agrafe [a'grafi], **agrafo** [a'grafu] *m* staple
agrafar [agra'far] ⟨1b⟩ *v/t* staple
agrário [a'grariu] **1** *adj* agrarian **2** *m*, **-a** *f* farmer
agravamento [agrava'mẽtu] *m* aggravation
agravante [agra'vãtʃi] **1** *adj circunstância* aggravating; ***testemunha*** *f* ~ witness for the prosecution **2** *f* aggravating circumstance
agravar [agra'var] ⟨1b⟩ **1** *v/t* aggravate; *estado* make worse **2** *v/i* DIR raise an objection (***de*** to); **agravar-se** *v/r* (*situação*) get worse
agravo [a'gravu] *m* DIR appeal
agredir [agre'dʒir] ⟨3d⟩ attack; (*assaltar*) assault
agressão [agre'sãw] *f* aggression; (*assalto*) assault, attack; ~ ***sexual*** sexual assault
agressivamente [agresiva'mẽtʃi] *adv* aggressively
agressividade [agresivi'dadʒi] *f* aggressiveness
agressivo [agre'sivu] *adj* aggressive
agressor [agre'sor] *m*, **-a** *f* aggressor
agreste [a'grɛstʃi] *adj* rugged, wild
agrião [agri'ãw] *m* watercress
agrícola [a'grikula] *adj* agricultural
agricultor [agrikuw'tor] *m*, **-a** *f* farmer
agricultura [agrikuw'tura] *f* agriculture, farming; ~ ***ecológica*** organic farming
agridoce [agri'dosi] *adj* GASTR sweet and sour
agronomia [agrono'mia] *f* agronomy
agrônomo, *Port* **agrónomo** [a'gronumu] *m*, **-a** *f* agronomist
agropecuária [agrope'kwarja] *f* farming and cattle raising
agro-turismo [agrotu'rizmu] *m* agritourism
agrupamento [agrupa'mẽtu] *m* grouping; (*grupo*) group
agrupar [agru'par] ⟨1a⟩ group; (*juntar*) unite; (*abranger*) cover
água ['agwa] *f* water; **~s** *pl* waters; ***isto tudo são ~s passadas*** that's all water under the bridge now; ***pescar em ~s turvas*** fish in troubled waters; ~ ***acima*** / ***abaixo*** upstream / downstream; ~ ***corrente*** running water; ~ ***engarrafada*** bottled water; ~ ***de esgoto*** sewage; ~ ***mineral*** (***com*** / ***sem gás***) (sparkling / still) mineral water; ~ ***potável*** drinking water; ~ ***salgada*** salt water; ~ ***tônica*** tonic water; **~*s da enchente*** flood waters; **~*s residuais*** sewage; **~*s territoriais*** territorial waters
aguaceiro [agwa'sejru] *m* downpour, cloudburst
água-de-colônia, *Port* **água-de-colónia** [agwadʒiko'lonja] *f* eau de Cologne
aguado [a'gwadu] *adj* watery
água-forte [agwa'fɔrtʃi] *f* ARTE etching
água-marinha [agwama'riɲa] *f* aquamarine

aguardar [agwaɾ'daɾ] ⟨1b⟩ **1** *v/t* wait for; ***aguardo notícias suas*** I look forward to hearing from you **2** *v/i* wait; ***aguarde na linha*** hold the line
aguardente [agwaɾ'dẽtʃi] *f* spirit
aguarela [agwa'rɛla] *f* watercolor, *Brit* watercolour
aguarrás [agwa'has] *f* turpentine
águas-furtadas [agwasfuɾ'tadas] *fpl* garret, attic
água-viva [agwa'viva] *f* jellyfish
aguçado [agu'sadu] *adj* sharp; (*pontiagudo*) pointed
aguçar [agu'saɾ] ⟨1p⟩ sharpen; *orelhas* prick up
agudeza [agu'deza] *f* sharpness
agudo [a'gudu] *adj* sharp; *tom* shrill, high-pitched; MED acute; ***acento*** *m* **~** acute accent
agüentar, *Port* **aguentar** [agwẽ'taɾ] ⟨1a⟩ **1** *v/t* hold up; (*tolerar*) put up with, endure **2** *v/i* last; **~ *com algo*** cope with sth; **agüentar-se** *v/r* hold out
águia ['agia] *f* eagle
agulha [a'guʎa] *f* needle; FERROV switch, *Brit* points; ***procurar ~s em palheiro*** look for a needle in a haystack; **~ *de tricô*** knitting needle
agulheiro [agu'ʎejɾu] *m* pin-cushion
ai [aj] *int* **~!** oh!; *dor*: ouch!; **~ *de mim!*** poor me!
aí [a'i] *adv* there; ***até* ~** up to there; *tempo*: up to then; ***por* ~** somewhere over there; ***espere* ~!** hang on!; ***fique por* ~** stay there; ***é por* ~** *idéia* it's going in the right direction; ***não fazem nada além de ficar por* ~** they just hang around
aidético [aj'dɛtʃiku] **1** *adj* suffering from aids **2** *m/f* aids sufferer
ainda [a'ĩda] **1** *adv* still; **~ *assim*** even so, nevertheless; **~ *bem*** just as well; **~ *bem que você ...*** it's a good job you ...; **~ *falta muito para acabar*** it's still a long way from being finished; **~ *maior*** even bigger; **~ *por cima*** on top of all that; **~ *não é a sua vez*** it's not your turn yet; **~ *não*** *enfático* still not **2** *conj* **~ *que*** even if
aipim [aj'pĩ] *m* cassava
aipo ['ajpu] *m* celery
airbag [ɛɾ'bɛg] *m* airbag; **~ *lateral*** side airbag
airbus [ɛɾ'bas] *m* airbus
airoso [aj'rozu] *adj* graceful
ajeitar [aʒej'taɾ] ⟨1a⟩ *v/t* arrange; (*alisar*) smooth out; **ajeitar-se** *v/r* **~ *a uma situação*** adapt to a situation; **~ *com algo*** be ok with sth; ***ajeita-te*** *roupa* straighten yourself out
ajoelhar [aʒoe'ʎaɾ] ⟨1a⟩ *v/i* kneel
ajuda [a'ʒuda] *f* help; (*suporte*) support; ***prestar* ~** provide help; **~ *humanitária*** humanitarian aid; **~s** *pl* ***de custo*** expenses
ajudante [aʒu'dãtʃi] *m/f* assistant, helper; MIL **~** (***-de-campo***) adjutant
ajudar [aʒu'daɾ] ⟨1a⟩ help; (*apoiar*) support
ajuizado [aʒwi'zadu] *adj* sensible, wise
ajuizar [aʒwi'zaɾ] ⟨1q⟩ *v/t* (*avaliar*) judge, assess
ajuntamento [aʒũta'mẽtu] *m* gathering
ajuntar [aʒũ'taɾ] ⟨1a⟩ → ***juntar***
ajuramentação [aʒuɾamẽta'sãw] *f* swearing in
ajuramentar [aʒuɾamẽ'taɾ] ⟨1a⟩ swear in
ajustado [aʒus'tadu] *adj* suitable
ajustagem [aʒus'taʒẽ] *f* adjustment
ajustar [aʒus'taɾ] ⟨1a⟩ adjust (***a*** to); TECN set; *roupa* take in; *preço* fix; **~ *contas*** settle *tb fig*
ajustável [aʒus'tavew] *adj* adjustable
ajuste [a'ʒustʃi] *m* adjustment; (*acordo*) agreement; **~ *de contas*** settlement of accounts; ***salário*** *m* ***por* ~** piece wages
ala ['ala] *f* wing; (*fileira*) row; MIL rank; POL **~ *direita*** right wing
alagado [ala'gadu] *adj* soaking wet
alagar [ala'gaɾ] ⟨1o & 1b⟩ flood
alameda [ala'meda] *f* avenue
álamo ['alamu] *m* poplar; **~ *branco*** white poplar
alargamento [alaɾga'mẽtu] *m* expansion
alargar [alaɾ'gaɾ] ⟨1o & 1b⟩ **1** *v/t* expand, widen; *vestuário* let out; *influência* extend **2** *v/i* broaden, extend; *tensão* relax

alarido [ala'ridu] *m* uproar, outcry
alarmante [alaɾ'mãtʃi] *adj* alarming
alarmar [alaɾ'maɾ] ⟨1b⟩ *v/t* alarm; **alarmar-se** *v/r* become alarmed
alarme [a'laɾmi] *m* alarm; (*tumulto*) tumult, panic; ***dar*** (***o sinal de***) ~ raise the alarm; ***falso*** ~ false alarm; ~ ***de incêndio*** fire alarm; ~ ***contra roubo*** burglar alarm
alarmista [a'laɾmista] *m/f* alarmist
alastrar [alas'tɾaɾ] ⟨1b⟩ **1** *v/t* spread, scatter; (*pôr peso em*) ballast **2** *v/i* encroach (***a*** on); **alastrar-se** *v/r* spread; ~ ***como fogo no palheiro*** spread like wildfire
alavanca [ala'vãka] *f* lever; AUTO ~ (***de velocidades***) gear shift, *Brit* gear lever
albanês [awba'nes] **1** *adj* Albanian **2** *m*, **albanesa** [awba'neza] *f* Albanian **3** *m lingua* Albanian
Albânia [aw'bʌnia] *f* Albania
albatroz [awba'tɾɔs] *m* albatross
albergar [awbeɾ'gaɾ] ⟨1o & 1c⟩ shelter
albergue [aw'bɛɾgi] *m* hostel; ~ ***da juventude*** youth hostel
álbum ['awbũ] *m* album; ~ ***de recortes*** scrapbook
alça ['awsa] *f* strap; *mala*: handle
alcachofra [awka'ʃɔfɾa] *f* artichoke
alçada [aw'sada] *f* (*área*) jurisdiction; (*competênica*) area of responsibility; ***não é da minha*** ~ that's outside my area of responsibility
alcagüetar [awkagwe'taɾ] ⟨1c⟩ *v/i fam* blab
alcalino [awka'linu] *adj* alkaline
alcançar [awkã'saɾ] ⟨1b⟩ reach; (*apanhar*) catch; (*obter*) obtain, get; (*perceber*) understand
alcance [aw'kãsi] *m* reach; *avião*, *arma*: range; (*compreensão*) understanding; ***ao*** ~ ***de*** within reach of; ***estar fora do*** ~ be out of reach; ***de*** (***grande***) ~ far-reaching; ***de longo*** ~ long-range
alçapão [awsa'pãw] *m* trapdoor
alcaparra [awka'paha] *f* caper
alçar [aw'saɾ] ⟨1p⟩ (*levantar*) lift up; (*erigir*) erect; put up; *voz* raise; *vela* hoist
alcateia [awka'teia] *f lobos*: pack
alcatifa [awka'tʃifa] *f Port* carpet, floor covering
alcatifado [awkatʃi'fadu] *adj Port* carpeted
alcatifar [awkatʃi'faɾ] ⟨1a⟩ *Port* carpet
alcatra [aw'katɾa] *f* rumpsteak
alcatrão [awka'tɾãw] *m* ⟨*sem pl*⟩ tar
alcatroado [awkatɾo'adu] *adj* tarred
alcatroar [awkatɾo'aɾ] ⟨1f⟩ tar; *estrada* tarmac
alce ['awsi] *m* elk
álcool ['awkɔw] *m* alcohol; ***sem*** ~ non-alcoholic
alcoólatra [aw'kɔlatɾa] *m/f* alcoholic
alcoólico [aw'kɔliku] **1** *adj* alcoholic **2** *m*, **-a** *f* alcoholic
alcoolismo [awko'lizmu] *m* alcoholism
alcoolizado [awkoli'zadu] *adj* inebriated, drunk
Alcorão [awko'ɾãw] *m* Koran
alcunha [aw'kuɲa] *f Port* nickname
aldeão [aw'deãw] *m* ⟨*mpl* -ãos, -ões⟩, **aldeã** [aw'deã] *f* villager
aldeia [aw'deja] *f* village
aleatoriamente [aliatoɾia'mẽtʃi] *adv* at random
aleatório [alia'tɔɾiu] *adj* random
alecrim [ale'kɾĩ] *m* BOT rosemary
alegação [alega'sãw] *f* allegation
alegado [ale'gadu] *adj* alleged
alegar [ale'gaɾ] ⟨1o & 1c⟩ **1** *v/t fatos* cite; *provas* claim, allege; (*afirmar*) assert **2** *v/i* (*argumentar*) argue
alegoria [alego'ɾia] *f* allegory
alegórico [ale'gɔɾiku] *adj* allegorical
alegrar [ale'gɾaɾ] ⟨1c⟩ (*causar alegria*) cheer up; *ambiente* brighten up; (*animar*) liven up
alegre [a'lɛgɾi] *adj* cheerful; (*contente*) happy; *álcool*: merry
alegremente [alɛgɾe'mẽtʃi] *adv* happily
alegria [ale'gɾia] *f* joy, happiness
aleijado [alej'ʒadu] **1** *m* cripple **2** *adj* (*deficiente*) crippled; (*magoado*) injured
aleijar [alej'ʒaɾ] ⟨1a⟩ *v/t* cripple, maim
além [a'lẽ] *adv* over there; ~ ***de*** beyond; ~ ***disso***, ~ ***de*** (*ou* ***do***) ***que***, ~

do mais in addition, besides; ***para ~ de*** on the other side of; ***o ~*** the hereafter; ***~ das possibilidades*** impossible
alemã [ale'mã] *adj/f* → ***alemão***
Alemanha [ale'maɲa] *f* ***a ~*** Germany; ***em ~, na ~*** in Germany
alemão [ale'mãw] ⟨*mpl* -ães⟩ **1** *adj* German **2** *m*, **-ã** *f* German **3** *m língua* German
além-mar [alẽ'maɾ] *adv* overseas
alento [a'lẽtu] *m* (*coragem*) courage; (*força*) strength
alergênico, *Port* **alergénico** [aleɾ'ʒɛniku] *m* allergen
alergia [aleɾ'ʒia] *f* allergy
alérgico [a'lɛɾʒiku] *adj* allergic; ***ser ~ a*** be allergic to
alerta [a'lɛɾta] **1** *adv* alert; (*na defensiva*) on the alert; ***~!*** watch out! **2** *m* alert; ***~ de tempestade*** storm warning; ***tocar ~*** sound the alert
aletria [ale'tɾia] *f* vermicelli
alfabético [awfa'bɛʧiku] *adj* alphabetical
alfabetização [awfabeʧiza'sãw] *f* ⟨*sem pl*⟩ literacy
alfabetizar [awfabeʧi'zaɾ] ⟨1a⟩ teach how to read and write
alfabetizado [awfabeʧi'zadu] *adj* literate
alfabeto [awfa'bɛtu] *m* alphabet
alface [aw'fasi] *f* lettuce
alfaiataria [awfajata'ɾia] *f* tailor's shop
alfaiate [awfa'jaʧi] *m* tailor
alfândega [aw'fʌdega] *f* customs
alfandegário [awfãde'gaɾiu] *adj* customs *atr*, ***direitos*** *mpl* ***~s*** customs duties
alfazema [awfa'zema] *f* lavender
alfinete [awfi'neʧi] *m* pin; ***~ de segurança*** safety pin
alforreca [awfo'hɛka] *f* jellyfish
algas ['awgas] *fpl* seaweed
algarismo [awga'ɾizmu] *m* numeral, digit
algazarra [awga'zaha] *f* uproar, racket
álgebra ['awʒebɾa] *f* algebra
algemas [aw'ʒemas] *fpl* handcuffs
algemar [awʒe'maɾ] ⟨1d⟩ handcuff
algibeira [awʒi'bejɾa] *f* pocket; *dinheiro*: money belt
algo ['awgu] **1** *pron* something; ***~ mais*** something else; ***~ mais?*** anything else? **2** *adv* rather, somewhat
algodão [awgo'dãw] *m* cotton; ***~ doce*** cotton candy, *Brit* candy floss; ***~ hidrófilo*** absorbent cotton, *Brit* cotton wool
algoritmo [awgo'ɾiʧimu] *m* algorithm
alguém [aw'gẽ] *pron* somebody, someone; *interrogativo*: anybody, anyone
algum [aw'gũ], **~a** [aw'guma] **1** *pron* one; *plural* some; *em frases interrogativas* one; *plural* some, any; ***você tem alguns?*** do you have any? **2** *adj* some; *em frases interrogativas*: any; ***houve ~a melhora?*** is there any improvement?; ***tem alguns copos?*** are there any glasses?; ***~a coisa*** something; ***~ dia*** one day; ***de maneira ~a, de modo ~*** in no way; ***não tenho óleo ~*** I have no oil; ***~ tempo*** for a while
algures [aw'guɾis] *adv* somewhere
alheado [a'ʎjadu] *adj* (*afastado*) distant; (*distraido*) absent-minded
alheamento [aʎja'mẽtu] *m* (*afastamento*) estrangement; (*distração*) absence
alhear-se [a'ʎjaɾsi] ⟨1l⟩ *v/r* become lost in thought; (*afastar-se*) withdraw into oneself
alheio [a'ʎeiu] *adj* foreign, alien; ***~ de*** far from; ***estar ~ a*** have nothing to do with
alheira [a'ʎejɾa] *f* spicy sausage
alho ['aʎu] *m* garlic; ***dente*** *m* ***de ~*** clove of garlic; ***cabeça*** *f* ***de ~*** garlic bulb
alho-poró [aʎo'pɔɾɔ] *m* leek
ali [a'li] *adv* there; ***por ~*** around there; that way
aliado [a'ljadu] *m*, **-a** *f* ally
aliança [a'ljãsa] *f* alliance; **~ (*de casamento*)** wedding ring; ***fazer ~ com*** form an alliance with
aliar [a'ljaɾ] ⟨1g⟩ *v/t* ally; **aliar-se** *v/r* form an alliance (***com*** with)
aliás [a'ljas] *adv* incidentally; (*a propósito*) as a matter of fact; (*de mais*

a mais) nevertheless; (*ou seja*) rather, that is
álibi ['alibi] *m* alibi
alicate [ali'katʃi] *m* pliers; **~ *de unhas*** nail clippers
alicerce [ali'sɛrsi] *m* foundations; ***lançar os ~s de*** lay the foundations for
aliciar [ali'sjar] ⟨1g⟩ entice, attract
alienação [aliena'sãw] *f* ⟨*sem pl*⟩ (*venda*) disposal, transfer; (*alheamento*) alienation; **~ *mental*** insanity
alienado [alie'nadu] *adj* alienated; (*louco*) insane
alienamento [aliena'mẽtu] *m* → ***alienação***
alienar [alie'nar] ⟨1d⟩ (*vender*) dispose of, transfer; (*alhear*) alienate
alienável [alie'navew] *adj* (*que pode ser vendido*) saleable; (*transferível*) transferable
alienígena [alie'niʒena] *m/f* alien, extraterrestrial
aligeirar [aliʒe'rar] ⟨1a⟩ lighten; (*suavizar*) relieve; *passo* speed up
alijar [a'liʒar] ⟨1a⟩ *v/t* jettison *tb fig*
alimentação [alimẽta'sãw] *f* ⟨*sem pl*⟩ food; (*sustento*) provisions; TECN supply; INFORM input
alimentar [alimẽ'tar] **1** *adj* food *atr*, eating *atr*; ***produtos*** *mpl* **~*es*** food **2** *v/t* ⟨1a⟩ feed; TECN supply; *sentimento* nurture
alimentício [alimẽ'tʃisiu] *adj* nourishing; ***gêneros*** *mpl* **~*s*** foodstuffs
alimento [ali'mẽtu] *m* food; **~ *básico*** staple
alínea [a'linja] *f* (*cláusula*) subhead
alinhamento [aliɲa'mẽtu] *m* alignment
alinhar [ali'ɲar] ⟨1a⟩ **1** *v/t* align **2** *v/i fam* join in; ***sim, alinho*** yes, I'm on
alinho [a'liɲu] *m* alignment; *fig* care
alisado [ali'zadu] *adj* smooth
alisar [ali'zar] ⟨1a⟩ smooth
alistamento [alista'mẽtu] *m* (*inscrição*) enrollment, *Brit* enrolment; MIL draft, enlistment
alistar [alis'tar] ⟨1a⟩ *v/t* (*inscrever*) enroll, *Brit* enrol; MIL draft; **alistar-se** *v/r* MIL enlist; *Brit* join up
aliviar [ali'vjar] ⟨1g⟩ alleviate; (*libertar*) liberate; (*descarregar*) lighten; *dor* relieve
alívio [a'liviu] *m* relief
alma ['awma] *f* soul; **~ *penada*** ghost; ***dia*** *m* ***das*** **~*s*** All Souls' Day; ***de ~ e coração*** with heart and soul; ***com ~*** warm, lively; ***sem ~*** heartless; **~ *de Deus!*** heavens above!
almirante [awmi'rãtʃi] *m* admiral
almoçar [awmo'sar] ⟨1p & 1e⟩ have lunch
almoço [aw'mosu] *m* lunch; **~ *de negócios*** business lunch; ***pequeno ~*** breakfast; ***tomar o pequeno ~*** have breakfast
almofada [awmo'fada] *f vestuário, sofá*: cushion; *Port cama*: pillow
almôndega [aw'mõdega] *f* meatball
alô [a'lo] *int Bras* TEL **~*?*** hello?
alocar [alo'kar] ⟨1e⟩ *v/t* allocate
alocução [aloku'sãw] *f* speech
aloirado [aloj'radu] *adj* blond
aloirar [aloj'rar] ⟨1a⟩ *v/t* GASTR brown; *cabelo* lighten
alojamento [aloʒa'mẽtu] *m* accommodations, *Brit* accommodation; TECN housing
alojar [alo'ʒar] ⟨1e⟩ *v/t pessoa* accommodate, put up
alongado [alõ'gadu] *adj* elongated
alongamento [alõga'mẽtu] *m* lengthening; (*extensão*) extension; (*dilação*) stretching
alongar [alõ'gar] ⟨1o⟩ *v/t* (*prolongar*) lengthen; (*estender*) extend; *pescoço* crane; **alongar-se** *v/r atleta etc* stretch; **~ *num assunto*** dwell on a point
alpaca [aw'paka] *f* alpaca
alpendre [aw'pẽdri] *m* porch; (*telheiro*) shed
alperce [aw'pɛrsi] *m* apricot
alperceiro [awper'sejru] *m* apricot tree
Alpes ['awpis] *mpl* ***os ~*** the Alps
alpinismo [awpi'nizmu] *m* mountaineering, climbing
alpinista [awpi'nista] *m/f* mountaineer, climber
alquimia [awki'mia] *f* alchemy
alquimista [awki'mista] *m/f* alchemist
alta ['awta] *f preços etc*: rise, increase;

ECON bull market; MED ***dar ~*** discharge; ***ter ~*** be discharged; ***alta tecnologia*** high tech, hi-tech
alta-fidelidade [awtafideli'dadʒi] *f* high-fidelity
altamente [awta'mẽtʃi] *adv* highly; ***~ confidencial*** top secret
altar [aw'taɾ] *m* altar
alta-roda [awta'hɔda] *f* high society
alteração [awteɾa'sãw] *f* alteration; (*degeneração*) falsification; (*desordem*) disturbance; (*indignação*) indignation; ***sem ~*** unaltered
alterar [awte'ɾaɾ] ⟨1c⟩ (*modificar*) alter; (*falsificar*) falsify; (*indignar*) outrage; **alterar-se** *v/r* change; (*estragar-se*) spoil; (*perturbar-se*) get angry, lose one's temper
alternadamente [awteɾnada'mẽtʃi] *adv* alternately
alternado [awteɾ'nadu] *adj* alternate; ***corrente** f **alternada*** alternating current
alternar [awteɾ'naɾ] ⟨1c⟩ **1** *v/t* (*revezar*) alternate **2** *v/i* alternate; *jogo*: take turns; **alternar-se** *v/r* alternate; *jogo*: take turns
alternativa [awteɾna'tʃiva] *f* alternative
alternativamente [awteɾnatʃiva'mẽtʃi] *adv* alternatively
alternativo [awteɾna'tʃivu] *adj* alternative
alteza [aw'teza] *f* (*altura*) height; *título* Highness
altifalante [awtʃifa'lãtʃi] *m* loudspeaker
altímetro [aw'tʃimetɾu] *m* altimeter
altitude [awtʃi'tudʒi] *f* altitude
altivez [awtʃi'ves] *f* haughtiness
altivo [aw'tʃivu] *adj* haughty
alto ['awtu] **1** *adj altura*: high; *pessoa* tall; *som* loud; ***o ~ Douro*** the upper Douro; ***~ inverno*** midwinter; ***~ verão*** midsummer; ***em voz alta*** aloud, out loud **2** *adv* high; *som*: loud; ***por ~*** superficially **3** *m* top; ***~s e baixos*** ups and downs
alto-falante [awtofa'lãtʃi] *m* loudspeaker
alto-forno [awto'foɾnu] *m* blast furnace
alto-mar [awto'maɾ] *m* open sea
altruísmo [awtɾu'izmu] *m* altruism
altruísta [awtɾu'ista] *adj* altruistic
altura [aw'tuɾa] *f* height; (*envergadura*) size; (*nível intelectual*) level; (*momento*) point, juncture; ***ter dois metros de ~*** be two meters (*ou Brit* metres) tall; ***a*** (*ou* ***em***) ***que ~?*** when?; ***nesta ~*** at this point, at this juncture; ***estar à ~ de*** be equal to, be up to; ***ficar à ~ de alguém*** *competição*: draw level with s.o.
alucinação [alusina'sãw] *f* hallucination
alucinado [alusi'nadu] *adj* hallucinating; *fam* crazy
alucinante [alusi'nãtʃi] *adj* amazing
alucinar [alusi'naɾ] ⟨1a⟩ dazzle; (*apaixonar*) bewitch
alucinogênio, *Port* **alucinogénio** [alusino'ʒeniu] **1** *adj* hallucinogenic **2** *m* hallucinogen
aludir [alu'dʒiɾ] ⟨3a⟩ ***~ a*** allude to
alugar [alu'gaɾ] ⟨1o⟩ rent; ***aluga-se*** for rent
aluguel [alu'gew] *m*, *Port* **aluguer** [alu'gɛɾ] *m* rent; *carros etc*: rental, *Brit tb* hire; ***casa** f **de ~*** rented house; ***carro** m **de ~*** rental car, *Brit tb* hire car; ***~ de carros*** car rental, *Brit tb* car hire
alumiar [alu'mjaɾ] ⟨1g⟩ ***~ alguém*** shine a light for s.o.
alumínio [alu'miniu] *m* aluminum, *Brit* aluminium
aluno [a'lunu] *m*, **-a** *f* pupil, student
alusão [alu'zãw] *f* allusion
alvejante [awve'ʒãtʃi] *m* bleach
alvejar [awve'ʒaɾ] ⟨1df⟩ *v/t* (*tomar como alvo*) aim at
alvenaria [awvena'ɾia] *f* masonry
alvitrar [awvi'tɾaɾ] ⟨1a⟩ *v/t* propose, suggest
alvitre [aw'vitɾi] *m* suggestion
alvo ['awvu] **1** *adj* white; (*limpo*) pure **2** *m* target; ***tiro** m **ao ~*** target practice; ***acertar*** (*ou* ***dar***) ***no ~*** hit the mark; ***público ~*** target audience
alvor [aw'voɾ] *m* (*brancura*) whiteness; (*brilho*) shimmer, gleam
alvorada [awvo'ɾada] *f* dawn
alvorar [awvo'ɾaɾ] ⟨1e⟩, **alvorecer**

[awvore'ser] ⟨2g⟩ dawn; ***ao ~*** at dawn
alvoroçar [awvoro'sar] ⟨1p & 1e⟩ *v/t* excite; (*sobressaltar*) startle; (*amotinar*) stir up; **alvoroçar-se** *v/r* (*insurgir-se*) get agitated; (*alegrar-se*) be pleased (***com*** about)
alvoroço [awvo'rosu] *m* commotion; (*motim*) revolt; (*sobressalto*) rush
alvura [aw'vura] *f* whiteness; (*brilho*) shine
amabilidade [amabili'dadʒi] *f* friendliness
amaciador [amasja'dor] *m* conditioner, softener
amaciante [ama'sjãtʃi] *f* fabric conditioner
amaciar [ama'sjar] ⟨1g⟩ soften
amado [a'madu] **1** *adj* dear **2** *m*, **-a** *f* loved one, sweetheart
amador [ama'dor] *m arte*: lover, collector; ESP amateur
amadorismo [amado'rizmu] *m* amateurism
amadurecer [amadure'ser] ⟨2g⟩ **1** *v/t* mature; *fruta* ripen **2** *v/i* ripen; *pessoa* mature
amadurecido [amadure'sidu] *adj* ripe, mature; *pessoa* mature
âmago ['ʌmagu] *m* BOT pith; *fig* core
amaldiçoar [amawdʒi'swar] ⟨1f⟩ curse
amálgama [a'mawgama] *f* amalgam
amamentar [amamẽ'tar] ⟨1a⟩ *v/t* breastfeed
amanhã [ama'ɲã] *adv* tomorrow; ***~ de manhã*** tomorrow morning; ***~ à noite*** tomorrow night; ***depois de ~*** the day after tomorrow
amanhecer [amaɲe'ser] ⟨2g⟩ **1** *v/i* dawn **2** *m* dawn, daybreak; ***ao ~*** at dawn
amansar [amã'sar] ⟨1a⟩ **1** *v/t* tame **2** *v/i* grow tame; **amansar-se** *v/r* grow tame; *tempestade* die down, abate
amante [a'mãtʃi] **1** *adj* loving; ***~ da paz*** peace-loving; ***ser ~ de*** like; *pessoa* love **2** *m/f* lover; ***~ de jazz*** jazz buff, jazz lover
amar [a'mar] ⟨1a⟩ love
amarelado [amare'ladu] *adj* yellowish
amarelo [ama'rɛlu] **1** *adj* yellow; (*pálido*) sallow; *sorriso* forced **2** *m* yellow
amargamente [amarga'mẽtʃi] *adv* bitterly
amargar [amar'gar] ⟨1o, *Stv* 1b⟩ **1** *v/t* make bitter, embitter **2** *v/i* taste bitter
amargo [a'margu] *adj* bitter
amargura [amar'gura] *f* bitterness
amargurado [amargu'radu] *adj* embittered
amargurar [amargu'rar] ⟨1a⟩ *v/t* embitter; (*atormentar*) torment
amarra [a'maha] *f* NÁUT anchor chain
amarrar [ama'har] ⟨1b⟩ **1** *v/t* (*fundear*) anchor; (*prender*) fasten; *cavalo* tether; *embrulho* tie up **2** *v/i barco* moor; **amarrar-se** *v/r* tie; ***~ a algo*** cling to sth
amarrotar [amaho'tar] ⟨1e⟩ *tecido, papel* crease, crumple
ama-seca [ama'seka] *f* nanny
amassar [ama'sar] ⟨1b⟩ *massa* knead; *cimento etc* mix; *tecido* crease; *papel* crumple; *carro* dent, *Brit tb* prang
amável [a'mavew] *adj* (*encantador*) kind; (*simpático*) friendly; ***pouco ~*** unfriendly
amazona [ama'zona] *f* horsewoman, rider
Amazonas [ama'zonas] *m* Amazon
amazonense [amazo'nẽŋsi] **1** *adj of the State of Amazonas* **2** *m/f person born in the State of Amazonas*
amazônico [ama'zoniku] *adj* Amazonian
âmbar ['ãbar] *m* amber
ambição [ãbi'sãw] *f* ⟨*sem pl*⟩ (*aspiração*) ambition
ambicionar [ãbisjo'nar] ⟨1f⟩ (*aspirar a*) strive for; (*cobiçar*) crave
ambicioso [ãbi'sjozu] *adj* ambitious
ambidestro [ãbi'dɛstru] *adj* ambidextrous
ambiência [ã'bjẽsja] *f* → ***ambiente***
ambiental [ãbjẽ'taw] *adj* environmental; ***impacto*** *m* ***~*** environmental impact; ***política*** *f* ***~*** environmental policy
ambientalista [ãbjẽta'lista] **1** *adj* environmental; ***associação*** *f* ***~*** envir-

onmental organization **2** *m/f* environmentalist
ambientar-se [ãbjẽ'taɾsi] ⟨1a⟩ *v/r* (*adaptar-se*) fit in, adapt
ambiente [ã'bjẽtʃi] **1** *adj* surrounding **2** *m* (*atmosfera*) atmosphere; **~ *de cortar à faca*** atmosphere you could cut with a knife; (***meio***) **~** environment; ***proteção*** *f* ***ao*** (***meio***) **~**, *Port* ***protecção*** *f* ***ao*** (***meio***) **~** environmental protection
ambigüidade, *Port* **ambiguidade** [ãbigwi'dadʒi] *f* ambiguity
ambíguo [ã'bigwu] *adj* ambiguous
âmbito ['ãbitu] *m* (*dimensão*) scope, extent; (*esfera*) range; (*enquadramento*) framework
ambivalente [ãbiva'lẽtʃi] *adj* ambivalent
ambos ['ãbus], **ambas** ['ãbas] *pron* both; **~** (***os***) ***dois*** both of them; **~ *os irmãos*** both (the) brothers
ambulância [ãbu'lãsja] *f* ambulance
ambulante [ãbu'lãtʃi] *adj* walking; (*móvel*) mobile; MED outpatient *atr*; ***vendedor*** *m* **~** commercial traveler, *Brit* commercial traveller
ameaça [a'measa] *f* threat, menace
ameaçador [ameasa'doɾ] *adj* threatening, menacing
ameaçar [amea'saɾ] ⟨1p & 1b⟩ threaten, menace
amealhar [amea'ʎaɾ] ⟨1b⟩ *v/t* save up
ameba [a'meba] *f* MED ameba, *Brit* amoeba
amedrontar [amedɾõ'taɾ] ⟨1a⟩ **1** *v/t* scare **2** *v/i* get scared; **amedrontar-se** *v/r* get frightened
ameixa [a'meʃa] *f* plum; **~ *seca*** prune
ameixoeira [ame'ʃwejɾa] *f* plum tree
amêndoa [a'mẽdwa] *f* almond; **~ *amarga*** bitter almond
amendoado [a'mẽdwadu] *adj* slanting, almond(-shaped)
amendoeira [amẽ'dwejɾa] *f* almond tree
amendoim [amẽ'dwĩ] *m* peanut
amenizar [ameni'zaɾ] ⟨1a⟩ **1** *v/t dor etc* ease; (*alegrar*) cheer up; **~ *as coisas*** smooth things over **2** *v/i* get milder, get warmer
ameno [a'menu] *adj* (*aprazível*) pleasant; (*alegre*) cheerful; (*suave*) mild
América [a'mɛɾika] *f* ***a* ~** America; ***a* ~ *Central*** Central America; ***a* ~ *Latina*** Latin America; ***a* ~ *do Norte*** North America; **~ *do Sul*** South America
americanizado [ameɾi'kanizadu] *adj* americanized
americano [ameɾi'kanu] **1** *adj* American **2** *m*, **-a** *f* American
amesquinhar [ameski'ɲaɾ] ⟨1a⟩ (*depreciar*) belittle
amestrar [ames'tɾaɾ] ⟨1c⟩ *v/t* train
ametista [ame'tʃista] *f* amethyst
amianto [a'mjãtu] *m* asbestos
amiba [a'miba] *f* ameba, *Brit* amoeba
amido [a'midu] *m* starch; **~ *de milho*** cornstarch
amiga [a'miga] *f* girlfriend
amigável [ami'gavew] *adj* amicable
amigavelmente [amigavew'mẽtʃi] *adv* amicably
amígdala [a'midala] *f* tonsil
amigdalite [amida'litʃi] *f* tonsilitis
amigo [a'migu] **1** *m* friend; **~ *de correspondência*** pen friend **2** *adj* friendly; ***ser*** (***muito***) **~ *de*** be (very good) friends with
amimar [ami'maɾ] ⟨1a⟩ *v/t* spoil
amistoso [amis'tozu] *adj* **1** *adj* friendly **2** *m* ESP friendly
amiudado [amiu'dadu] *adj* repeated
amiudar [amiu'daɾ] ⟨1q⟩ *v/t repetição*: repeat
amiúde [a'miudʒi] *adv* often, frequently
amizade [ami'zadʒi] *f* friendship; ***travar* ~ *com alguém*** make friends with s.o.
amnésia [am'nɛzja] *f* amnesia
amnistia [amnis'tʃia] *f* amnesty
amnistiar [amnis'tʃiaɾ] ⟨1g⟩ amnesty; (*perdoar*) pardon
amolar [amo'laɾ] ⟨1e⟩ *v/t* sharpen; *fam* annoy, pester
amoldar [amow'daɾ] ⟨1a⟩ *v/t* (*dar forma*) mold, *Brit* mould; **amoldar-se** *v/r* **~ *a*** *ou* ***com*** conform to
amolecer [amole'seɾ] ⟨2g⟩ **1** *v/t* soften **2** *v/i* soften; **amolecer-se** *v/r* soften; *músculo* relax
amolecimento [amolesi'mẽtu] *m fig* softening

amolgadela [amolga'dɛla] *f* → ***amolgadura***
amolgado [amow'gadu] *adj* dented
amolgadura [amolga'dura] *f* dent
amolgar [amow'gar] ⟨1o⟩ *v/t* dent; **amolgar-se** *v/r* get dented
amoníaco [amo'niaku] *m* ammonia
amontoar [amõ'twar] ⟨1f⟩ *v/t* heap up, pile up; **amontoar-se** *v/r* pile up
amor [a'mor] *m* love; (*querido*) darling; ***meu* ~** my love, darling; ***pelo*** (*ou* ***por***) **~ *de Deus*** for heaven's sake; ***fazer* ~** make love
amora [a'mɔra] *f* mulberry; **~ (*preta*)** blackberry
amoreira [amo'rejra] *f árvore* mulberry tree; *arbusto* blackberry bush
amoral [amo'raw] *adj* amoral
amordaçar [amorda'sar] ⟨1b & 1p⟩ *v/t* gag
amoroso [amo'rozu] *adj* affectionate
amor-perfeito [amorper'fejtu] *m* BOT pansy
amor-próprio [amor'prɔpriu] *m* self-esteem
amortecedor [amortese'dor] *m* shock absorber
amortecer [amorte'ser] ⟨2g⟩ **1** *v/t dor, som* deaden; *impacto* soften **2** *v/i luz, cor* fade
amortecido [amorte'sidu] *adj* deadened; (*apagado*) extinguished
amortização [amortʃiza'sãw] *f* ⟨*sem pl*⟩ (*reembolso*) repayment; COM amortization
amortizar [amortʃi'zar] ⟨1a⟩ (*pagar*) pay off
amostra [a'mɔstra] *f* sample; **~ *grátis*** free sample; **~ *aleatória*** random sample; **~ *de sangue*** blood sample
amotinação [amotʃina'sãw] *f* mutiny, rebellion
amotinar [amotʃi'nar] ⟨1a⟩ *v/i* rebel, mutiny; **amotinar-se** *v/r* mutiny
amparar [ãpa'rar] ⟨1b⟩ *v/t* (*proteger*) protect; (*auxiliar*) support; **amparar-se** *v/r* **~ *a algo*** (*apoiar-se*) lean on sth; (*seguir*) follow sth
amparo [ã'paru] *m* (*proteção*) protection; (*auxílio*) help; (*apoio*) support
ampere [ã'pɛri] *m* amp
ampliação [ãplia'sãw] *f* enlargement
ampliar [ãpli'ar] ⟨1g⟩ extend, widen; *foto* enlarge
amplificação [ãplifika'sãw] *f* enlargement; *tom*: amplification
amplificador [ãplifika'dor] *m tom*: amplifier
amplificar [ãplifi'kar] ⟨1n⟩ expand, extend; (*aumentar*) enlarge; *tom* amplify
amplitude [ãpli'tudʒi] *f* (*extensão*) extent; (*volume*) size; ELÉT amplitude
amplo ['ãplu] *adj* ample; (*espaçoso*) spacious; *conhecimentos* wide-ranging
amputação [ãputa'sãw] *f* amputation
amputar [ãpu'tar] ⟨1a⟩ amputate
amuado [a'mwadu] *adj fam* sulky
amuar [a'mwar] ⟨1g⟩ *v/i* sulk
anã [a'nã] *f* dwarf
anais [a'najs] *mpl* annals
anal [a'naw] *adj* ANAT anal
analfabetismo [anawfabe'tʃizmu] *m* illiteracy
analfabeto [anawfa'bɛtu] *m*, **-a** *f* illiterate
analgésico [anaw'ʒɛziku] **1** *adj* analgesic **2** *m* painkiller, analgesic
analisar [anali'zar] ⟨1a⟩ analyze
análise [a'nalizi] *f* analysis; ***em última* ~** in the final analysis, at the end of the day; **~*s*** *pl* ***clínicas*** laboratory tests; **~ *do mercado*** market analysis; **~ *de sangue*** blood test
analista [ana'lista] *m/f* analyst; **~ *de sistemas*** systems analyst
analítico [ana'litʃiku] *adj* analytical
analogia [analo'ʒia] *f* analogy
analógico [ana'lɔʒiku] *adj* INFORM analog, *Brit* analogue
análogo [a'nalogu] *adj* analogous
ananás [ana'nas] *m Port* pineapple
anão [a'nãw] ⟨*mpl* anões, anãos⟩ **1** *m*, **anã** *f* dwarf **2** *adj* dwarf *atr*
anarquia [anar'kia] *f* anarchy; *fig* chaos
anarquista [anar'kista] *m/f* anarchist
anatomia [anato'mia] *f* anatomy
anatômico, *Port* **anatómico** [ana'tomiku] *adj* anatomical
anca ['ãka] *f* hip
ancestral ['ãsestraw] *m/f* ancestor
anchova [ã'ʃova] *f* anchovy

ancião [ã'sjãw] ⟨*mpl* -ãos, -ães⟩ **1** *m*, **anciã** [ã'sjã] *f* old man; old woman **2** *adj* old
ancinho [ã'siɲu] *m* rake
âncora ['ãkoɾa] *f* anchor *tb* TV
ancoradouro [ãkoɾa'doɾu] *m* anchorage
ancorar [ãko'ɾaɾ] ⟨1e⟩ *v/i* anchor
andaime [ã'dajmi] *m* scaffolding
andamento [ãda'mẽtu] *m* (*continuação*) progress; (*decorrer*) course; *fig* ***dar ~ a algo*** get sth going; ***estar em ~*** be underway; ***pôr em ~*** set in motion
andar [ã'daɾ] ⟨1a⟩ **1** *v/i* go; *a pé* walk; ***~ desesperado / triste*** be desperate / sad; ***~ a fazer algo, ~ fazendo algo*** be doing sth; ***~ bem / ~ mal*** be fine / be in a bad way; ***~ mal de dinheiro*** be short of cash; ***~ bem / mal de saúde*** be well / sick; ***como anda?*** how are you?; ***vou andando*** not bad **2** *m casa*: floor; *Bras* ***~ térreo*** first floor, *Brit* ground floor
andebol [ãde'bɔw] *m Port* handball *m*
andebolista [ãdebo'lista] *m/f Port* handball player
Andes ['ãdʒis] *mpl* Andes
andino [ã'dʒinu] *adj* Andean
andorinha [ãdo'riɲa] *f* swallow
anedota [ane'dɔta] *f* anecdote
anel [a'nɛw] *m* ring; *corrente*: link; *cabelo*: curl
anemia [ane'mia] *f* anemia, *Brit* anaemia
anêmico, *Port* **anémico** [a'nemiku] *adj* anemic, *Brit* anaemic
anestesia [aneste'zia] *f* anesthetic, *Brit* anaesthetic
anestesiar [aneste'ziaɾ] ⟨1g⟩ anesthetize, *Brit* anaesthetize
anestésico [anes'tɛziku] **1** *adj* anesthetic, *Brit* anaesthetic **2** *m* anesthetic, *Brit* anaesthetic
anestesista [aneste'zista] *m/f* anesthetist, *Brit* anaesthetist
anexação [aneksa'sãw] *f* POL annexation; (*junção*) enclosure
anexar [ane'ksaɾ] ⟨1a⟩ POL annex, *Brit* annexe; (*juntar*) enclose
anexo [a'nɛksu] **1** *adj* (*junto*) attached **2** *m* enclosure; INFORM attachment; (*edifício*) annex, *Brit* annexe
anfíbio [ã'fibiu] **1** *adj* amphibious **2** *m* amphibian
anfiteatro [ãfi'tʃiatɾu] *m* amphitheater, *Brit* amphitheatre
anfitrião [ãfitɾi'ãw] *m* host
anfitriã [ãfitɾi'ã] *f* hostess
angariação [ãgaɾja'sãw] *f* (*recrutamento*) recruitment; (*fornecimento*) obtaining
angariador [ãgaɾja'doɾ] *m*, **-a** *f* agent; ***~ de seguros*** insurance agent
angariar [ãga'ɾjaɾ] ⟨1g⟩ (*recrutar*) recruit; (*arranjar*) obtain; *dinheiro tb* raise; *apoio* drum up
angina [ã'ʒina] *f* ***~ de peito*** angina pectoris
anglo-americano ['ãgloameri'kanu] *adj* Anglo-American
anglo-saxão [ãglosa'ksãw] **1** *m*, **anglo-saxã** [ãglosa'ksã] *f* Anglo-Saxon **2** *adj* Anglo-Saxon
Angola [ã'gɔla] *f* Angola
angolano [ãgo'lanu] **1** *adj* Angolan **2** *m*, **-a** *f* Angolan
angular [ãgu'laɾ] *adj* angular
ângulo ['ãgulu] *m* corner; MAT angle; *fig* point of view; ***~ agudo / obtuso / recto*** acute / obtuse / right angle
angústia [ã'gustʃia] *f* anguish, distress
angustiado [ãgus'tʃiadu] *adj* distressed
angustiante [ãgus'tʃiãtʃi] *adj* (*que causa medo*) distressing
angustiar [ãgus'tʃiaɾ] ⟨1g⟩ (*atemorizar*) distress, upset
animação [anima'sãw] *f* ⟨*sem pl*⟩ (*vida*) liveliness; (*entusiasmo*) enthusiasm; (*movimento*) bustle; INFORM animation
animado [ani'madu] *adj* lively; (*alegre*) cheerful; ***desenhos*** *mpl* ***~s*** animation
animador [anima'doɾ] **1** *adj* encouraging, promising **2** *m*, **-a** *f* host, presenter
animal [ani'maw] **1** *adj* animal; ***reino*** *m* ***~*** animal kingdom **2** *m* animal; ***~ doméstico*** domestic animal; ***~ de estimação*** pet
animar [ani'maɾ] ⟨1a⟩ *v/t* liven up;

(*consolar*) cheer up; (*encorajar*) encourage (***a*** to); **animar-se** *v/r ambiente* liven up; (*entusiasmar-se*) cheer up

ânimo ['ʌnimu] *m* spirit; (*índole*) nature; (*coragem*) courage; **(*re*)*cobrar*** (***o***) ~ pluck up courage

animosidade [animozi'dadʒi] *f* animosity

aninhar [ani'ɲaɾ] ⟨1a⟩ *v/t* nestle; **aninhar-se** *v/r* nestle

aniquilação [anikila'sãw] *f*, **aniquilamento** [anikila'mẽtu] *m* annihilation

aniquilar [aniki'laɾ] ⟨1a⟩ *v/t* annihilate

anis [a'nis] *m Port* aniseed

aniversariante [aniversa'ɾjãtʃi] *m/f* birthday boy / girl

aniversário [aniveɾ'saɾiu] *m casamento etc*: anniversary; (*dia de anos*) birthday; ***feliz ~!*** happy birthday!; ***~ de casamento*** wedding anniversary

anjo ['ãʒu] *m* angel; ***~ da guarda*** guardian angel

ano ['anu] *m* year; ***os ~s vinte / trinta*** the twenties / thirties; ***dia*** *m* ***de ~s*** birthday; ***fazer ~s*** have a birthday; ***fazer trinta ~s*** turn 30; ***ter trinta ~s*** be 30 years old; ***~ bissexto*** leap year; ***~ civil*** calendar year; ***económico*** financial year; ***~ letivo*** school year; ***Ano Novo*** New Year

anoitecer [anojte'seɾ] ⟨2g⟩ grow dark; ***ao ~*** at nightfall

ano-luz [anu'lus] *m* ⟨*pl* anos-luz⟩ light year

anomalia [anoma'lia] *f* anomaly

anômalo, *Port* **anómalo** [a'nomalu] *adj* anomalous; *comportamento* abnormal, unusual

anonimato [anoni'matu] *m* anonymity

anônimo, *Port* **anónimo** [a'nonimu] *adj* anonymous; ***sociedade*** *f* ***anônima*** stock company, *Brit* limited company

Ano-Novo [ano'novu] *m* ⟨*sem pl*⟩ New Year

anorexia [anorɛ'ksia] *f* MED anorexia

anoréxico [ano'ɾeksiku] *adj* anorexic

anormal [anoɾ'maw] *adj* abnormal

anormalidade [anoɾmali'dadʒi] *f* abnormality

anotação [anota'sãw] *f* (*observação*) annotation; (*apontamento*) note

anotar [ano'taɾ] ⟨1e⟩ annotate; (*apontar*) note

anseio [ã'seiu] *m* longing

ânsia ['ãsja] *f* ***~s*** *pl* anxiety; (*desejo*) yearning

ansiar [ã'sjaɾ] ⟨1h⟩ *v/i* ***~ por*** yearn for, long for

ansiedade [ãsie'dadʒi] *f* anxiety

ansioso [ã'sjozu] *adj* anxious; (*saudoso*) longing; (*impaciente*) eager

antagonismo [ãtago'nizmu] *m* antagonism; (*oposição*) opposition

antagonista [ãtago'nista] *m/f* antagonist; (*adversário*) opponent

antártico, *Port* **antárctico** [ã'taɾtʃiku] *adj* antarctic

Antártida, *Port* **Antárctida** [ã'taɾtʃida] *f* Antarctic

ante ['ãtʃi] *prep* before; (*em vista de*) in view of

antebraço [ãtʃi'brasu] *m* forearm

antecedência [ãtese'dẽsja] *f* ***com ~*** in advance; ***com pouca ~*** at short notice

antecedente [ãtese'dẽtʃi] **1** *adj* preceding **2** *m* antecedent **3** *m* ***~s*** *pl* ancestors; *duma pessoa* background; *duma coisa* past; ***~s*** *pl* ***penais*** criminal record; ***sem ~s*** unprecedented

anteceder [ãtese'deɾ] ⟨2c⟩ precede

antecessor [ãtese'soɾ] *m*, **-a** *f* predecessor

antecipação [ãtesipa'sãw] *f* anticipation; ECON advance (payment)

antecipado [ãtesi'padu] *adj* (*anterior*) prior; (*prematuro*) early; ***alegria*** *f* ***antecipada*** anticipation; ***pagamento*** *m* ***~*** advance payment; ***venda*** *f* ***antecipada*** advance sale

antecipar [ãtesi'paɾ] ⟨1a⟩ *v/t* anticipate; (*adiantar*) bring forward; **antecipar-se** *v/r* precede; (*adiantar-se*) anticipate; (*chegar antes*) arrive earlier (***a*** than); (*agir antes*) forestall (***a alguém*** s.o.)

antedatar [ãte'dataɾ] ⟨1b⟩ backdate

antemão [ãte'mãw] *f* ***de ~*** beforehand

antena [ã'tena] *f* aerial *tb* RÁDIO; antenna, feeler *tb* ZOOL; ***~ parabólica*** satellite dish

anteontem [ã'ʧiõtẽ] *adv* the day before yesterday
antepassado [ãtepa'sadu] *m*, **-a** *f* ancestor
anterior [ãte'rjor] *adj temporal*: previous, former; *local*: front *atr*
antes ['ãʧis] **1** *prep* **~ de** before; **~ de mais nada** above all; **~ de comer** before eating **2** *adv temporal*: before; (*de preferência, pelo contrário*) rather; **pouco ~** shortly before; **quanto ~** as soon as possible
anti... [ãʧi] *pref* anti-
antiácido [ãʧi'asidu] **1** *adj* antacid **2** *m* MED antacid
antiaderente [ãʧiade'rẽʧi] *adj* non-stick
antiaéreo [ãʧia'ɛriu] *adj* anti-aircraft
antiamericano [ãʧiameri'kanu] *adj* anti-American
antibiótico [ãʧi'bjɔʧiku] *m* antibiotic
anticiclone [ãʧisi'klɔni] *m* METEO anticyclone
anticoncepcional [ãʧikõsepsjo'naw] *adj* contraceptive
anticonstitucional [ãʧikõsʧitusiu'naw] *adj* unconstitutional
anticorpo [ãʧi'korpu] *m* antibody
antidemocrático [ãʧidemo'kraʧiku] *adj* undemocratic
antidepressivo [ãʧidepre'sivu] *adj* anti-depressant **2** *m* anti-depressant
antídoto [ã'ʧidutu] *m* antidote (**a** for)
antieconômico, *Port* **antieconómico** [ãʧieko'nomiku] *adj* uneconomic
antiespasmódico [ãʧispaʒ'mɔdʒiku] MED **1** *adj* antispasmodic **2** *m* antispasmodic
antifascista [ãʧifas'sista] **1** *adj* antifascist **2** *m/f* antifascist
antigamente [ãʧiga'mẽʧi] *adv* formerly, in the past
antigo [ã'ʧigu] *adj* old, ancient; (*anterior*) former; *móvel* antique
antigripal [ãʧigri'paw] *adj* **vacinação** *f* **~** flu vaccination
antiguidade [ãʧigwi'dadʒi] *f* antiquity; **~s** *pl* ancient monuments; (*relíquia*) antiques
anti-higiênico [ãʧii'ʒieniku] *adj* unhygienic, insanitary
anti-histamínico [ãʧiista'miniku] **1** *adj* antihistamine **2** *m* antihistamine
anti-inflamatório [ãʧiĩflama'tɔriu] *adj* anti-inflammatory
antílope [ã'ʧilopi] *m* antelope
antipatia [ãʧipa'ʧia] *f* antipathy, dislike
antipático [ãʧi'paʧiku] *adj* unfriendly
antipatizar [ãʧipaʧi'zar] ⟨1a⟩: **~ com alguém** dislike s.o.
antiquado [ãʧi'kwadu] *adj* antiquated; (*fora de moda*) old-fashioned
antiquário [ãʧi'kwariu] *m pessoa* antiques dealer; *loja de livros* secondhand bookstore, *Brit* secondhand bookshop; *loja de móveis* antique store, *Brit* antique shop
anti-rugas [ãʧi'hugas] *adj* **creme** *m* **~** anti-wrinkle cream
anti-séptico [ãʧi'sɛpʧiku] *adj* antiseptic
anti-sísmico [ãʧi'sizmiku] *adj* earthquake resistant
anti-social [ãʧiso'sjaw] *adj* antisocial
antítese [ã'ʧitezi] *f* antithesis
anti-trust [ãʧi'trast] *adj* **lei** *f* **~** anti-trust law
antitússico [ãʧi'tusiku] *m* cough medicine
antologia [ãtolo'ʒia] *f* anthology
antônimo, *Port* **antónimo** [ã'tonimu] *m* antonym
antro ['ãtru] *m* cave; *animal*: lair, den
antropófago [ãtro'pɔfagu] *m*, **-a** *f* cannibal
antropologia [ãtro'poloʒia] *f* anthropology
anual [a'nwaw] *adj* annual, yearly
anuário [a'nwariu] *m* yearbook; **~ comercial** Yellow Pages®
anuidade [anwi'dadʒi] *f* annuity
anulação [anula'sãw] *f* cancellation; (*declaração de nulidade*) annulment
anular [anu'lar] ⟨1a⟩ *v/t reserva* cancel; DIR (*declarar sem efeito*) annul; (*invalidar*) invalidate
anunciar [anũ'sjar] ⟨1g⟩ announce; (*proclamar*) herald; (*pôr anúncio*) advertise
anúncio [a'nũsiu] *m* advertisement, ad; (*proclamação*) announcement; **pôr (um) ~** advertise, place an ad-

vert; **~ classificado** classified ad; **~ luminoso** neon sign
ânus ['ʌnus] *m* anus
anzol [ã'zɔw] *m* fish-hook; *fig* **morder o ~** take the bait
ao [aw] *prep* = **a** *com art m* **o**
aonde [a'õdʒi] *interr* where; **~ quer que** wherever
aorta [a'ɔrta] *f* aorta
apagado [apa'gadu] *adj tom* muted; *pessoa* dull; *TV* off *pred*; *fogo*, *luz* out *pred*
apagar [apa'gaɾ] ⟨1o & 1b⟩ *v/t* delete, erase; *luz etc* switch off; *cigarro* stub out; *vestígio* obliterate; **apagar-se** *v/r* die down; *tom* fade away
apaixonado [apajʃo'nadu] *adj* passionate; (*enamorado*) in love (**por** with)
apaixonante [apajʃo'nãtʃi] *adj* captivating; (*excitante*) exciting
apaixonar [apajʃo'naɾ] ⟨1e⟩ *v/t* captivate; **apaixonar-se** *v/r* **~ por alguém** fall in love with s.o.; (*entusiasmar-se*) be mad about s.o.
apalpadela [apawpa'dɛla] *f* touch; *sexualmente* grope
apalpar [apaw'paɾ] ⟨1a⟩ touch, feel; *sexualmente* grope
apanhado [apa'ɲadu] **1** *adj fam* (*louco*) crazy; **bem ~** funny **2** *m* summary; **fazer um ~** summarize
apanhador [apaɲa'doɾ] *m*, **-a** *f beisebol*: catcher
apanhar [apa'ɲaɾ] ⟨1a⟩ catch; *do solo* pick up; (*agarrar*) grab; *fruta etc* pick; *febre*, *castigo* get; *Port comboio* catch; *pessoa* collect, fetch
aparador [apaɾa'doɾ] *m* hutch, *Brit* sideboard
aparafusar [apaɾafu'zaɾ] ⟨1a⟩ screw
apara-lápis [apaɾa'lapis] *m Port* ⟨*pl inv*⟩ pencil sharpener
aparar [apa'ɾaɾ] ⟨1b⟩ *golpe* parry; (*cortar*) prune, cut; *lápis* sharpen; *barba etc* trim
aparato [apa'ɾatu] *m* pomp, display; **um grande ~ policial** a big police presence
aparecer [apaɾe'seɾ] ⟨2g⟩ appear; (*vir*) turn up
aparecimento [apaɾesi'mẽtu] *m* appearance
aparelhado [apaɾe'ʎadu] *adj* ready, prepared
aparelhagem [apaɾe'ʎaʒẽ] *f* equipment, apparatus; **~ de som** stereo system
aparelhar [apaɾe'ʎaɾ] ⟨1d⟩ equip; *cavalo* harness; NÁUT rig
aparelho [apa'ɾeʎu] *m* apparatus, equipment; (*dispositivo*) device; *Bras* phone; **~ de surdez** hearing aid; **~ de televisão** television set
aparência [apa'ɾẽsja] *f* appearance, look; **salvar as ~s** save face
aparentar [apaɾẽ'taɾ] ⟨1a⟩ *v/t sinais* show
aparente [apa'ɾẽtʃi] *adj* apparent
aparição [apaɾi'sãw] *f* apparition
apartado [apaɾ'tadu] **1** *adj* (*longínquo*) remote; (*solitário*) lonely **2** *m correios*: PO box
apartamento [apaɾta'mẽtu] *m* apartment, *Brit* flat
aparte [a'paɾtʃi] *m* aside
apartidário [apaɾtʃi'daɾiu] *adj* independent
apatia [apa'tʃia] *f* apathy
apático [a'patʃiku] *adj* apathetic
apátrida [a'patɾida] **1** *adj* stateless **2** *m/f* stateless person
apavorado [apavo'ɾadu] *adj* terrified, panic-stricken
apavorar [apavo'ɾaɾ] ⟨1e⟩ terrify
apaziguador [apazigwa'doɾ] *m*, **-a** *f* peacemaker
apaziguante [apazi'gwãtʃi] *adj* peacemaking
apaziguar [apazi'gwaɾ] ⟨1m⟩ *v/t* appease
apeadeiro [apja'dejɾu] *m Port* FERROV stop
apear-se [a'pjaɾsi] ⟨1l⟩ *v/r* get off, get out
apedrejar [apedɾe'ʒaɾ] ⟨1d⟩ *v/t* stone
apegar-se [ape'gaɾsi] ⟨1c & 1o⟩ *v/r* **~ a** take a liking to; *tradição* cling to
apego [a'pegu] *m* attachment, fondness
apelação [apela'sãw] *f* DIR appeal
apelar [ape'laɾ] ⟨1c⟩ *v/i* appeal; **~ de** appeal against; **~ para** appeal to
apelidar [apeli'daɾ] ⟨1a⟩ *v/t Port* name; *Bras* nickname

apelido [ape'lidu] *m Port* surname, family name; *Bras* nickname
apelo [a'pelu] *m* appeal; ***sem ~*** irrevocable
apenas [a'penas] *adv* only, just
apêndice [a'pẽdʒisi] *m* appendix; (*aditamento*) supplement
apendicite [apẽdʒi'sitʃi] *f* appendicitis
aperceber [aperse'ber] ⟨2c⟩ *v/t* perceive; **aperceber-se** *v/r* ***~ de*** notice
aperfeiçoamento [aperfejswa'mẽtu] *m* (*acabamento*) completion; (*melhoramento*) perfection; *no trabalho* training; ***curso** m **de ~*** training course
aperfeiçoar [aperfej'swar] ⟨1f⟩ *v/t* (*melhorar*) perfect, improve; (*acabar*) complete; **aperfeiçoar-se** *v/r* improve oneself
aperitivo [aperi'tʃivu] *m* canapé; *bebida* aperitif
apertado [aper'tadu] *adj* narrow; *tempo, dinheiro* tight; (*estreito*) cramped
apertar [aper'tar] ⟨1c⟩ squeeze; (*atar*) fasten; *botão* press; *roupa* take in; *cinto, parafuso* tighten; ***~ o cinto*** fasten one's seatbelt; ***~ a mão de alguém*** shake s.o.'s hand; **apertar-se** *v/r* squeeze up
aperto [a'pertu] *m tempo etc*: pressure; *gente*: crowd; (*falta de espaço*) squeeze; (*estreitamento*) narrowing; *fig* tight spot; ***~ de mãos*** handshake
apesar [ape'zar] *conj* despite; ***~ disso*** nevertheless; ***~ de que*** in spite of the fact that, even though
apetecer [apete'ser] ⟨2g⟩ *v/t* desire; *v/i* appeal; ***não me apetece sair*** I don't feel like going out
apetecível [apete'sivew] *adj* tempting
apetite [ape'tʃitʃi] *m* appetite; (*desejo*) desire; ***falta** f **de ~*** lack of appetite; ***bom ~!*** enjoy your meal!
apetitoso [apetʃi'tozu] *adj aspecto* appetizing; (*desejável*) desirable
apetrechos [ape'treʃus] *mpl* gear
apitar [api'tar] ⟨1a⟩ **1** *v/i* whistle **2** *v/t jogo* referee
apito [a'pitu] *m* whistle; ***~ final*** final whistle
aplainar [aplaj'nar] ⟨1a⟩ *v/t* plane
aplanar [apla'nar] ⟨1a⟩ smooth *tb fig*, level; *dificuldade* smooth over
aplaudir [aplaw'dʒir] ⟨3a⟩ applaud
aplauso(s) [a'plawzu(s)] *m*(*pl*) applause
aplicação [aplika'sãw] *f* application *tb* INFORM, MED, (*zelo*) diligence; *vestido*: appliqué
aplicar [apli'kar] ⟨1n⟩ apply; *pena* sentence to; **aplicar-se** *v/r regras* apply; ***~ a*** apply oneself to
aplicável [apli'kavew] *adj* applicable
apoderar-se [apode'rarsi] ⟨1c⟩ *v/r* ***~ de algo*** seize sth
apodrecer [apodre'ser] ⟨2g⟩ *v/i* rot
apodrecimento [apodresi'mẽtu] *m* decay, rot
apogeu [apo'ʒew] *m fig* height, apogee
apoiador [apoja'dor] *adj* supportive
apoia-pés [apoja'pɛs] *m* ⟨*pl inv*⟩ footrest
apoiar [apo'jar] ⟨1l⟩ *v/t* (*auxiliar*) support; (*encostar*) lean; **apoiar-se** *v/r* ***~ em*** rest on
apoio [a'poju] *m* support; (*amparo*) backing; (*auxílio*) assistance; ***dar ~ a alguém / algo*** support s.o. / sth; ***ter o ~ de*** have the backing of
apólice [a'pɔlisi] *f* policy; ***~ de seguro*** insurance policy
apontador [aponta'dor] *m Bras* pencil sharpener
apontamento [apõta'mẽtu] *m* note; ***tomar ~s*** take notes
apontar [apõ'tar] ⟨1a⟩ *v/t* point; *arma* aim; *testemunha* name; ***~ para*** point at; *arma*: aim at
aporte [a'pɔrtʃi] *m* input
após [a'pɔs] **1** *prep* after; ***ano ~ ano*** year after year **2** *adv* afterward
aposentado [apozẽ'tadu] **1** *adj* retired **2** *m*, **-a** *f* retired person
aposentadoria [apozẽtado'ria] *f* retirement; ***plano** m **de ~*** pension plan
aposentar-se [apozẽ'tarsi] ⟨1a⟩ *v/r* retire
aposento [apo'zẽtu] *m* room
após-guerra [apɔʒ'gɛha] *m* ⟨*sem pl*⟩ post-war period
aposta [a'pɔsta] *f* bet, stake; ***fazer uma ~*** place a bet

apostar [apos'tar] ⟨1e⟩ bet (***em*** on)
apóstolo [a'pɔstulu] *m* apostle
apóstrofo [a'pɔstrufu] *m* LING apostrophe
apoteose [apote'ɔzi] *f* apotheosis *tb fig*
apreciação [apresja'sãw] *f* (*avaliação*) assessment; (*consideração*) appreciation
apreciador [apresja'dor] *m*, **-a** *f* connoisseur
apreciar [apre'sjar] ⟨1g⟩ (*estimar*) appreciate
apreciativo [apresja'tʃivu] *adj* appreciative
apreciável [apre'sjavew] *adj* appreciable
apreender [apreẽ'der] ⟨2a⟩ *pessoa* apprehend; *coisa* confiscate, seize
apreensão [apreẽ'sãw] *f* (*captura*) arrest; (*confiscação*) seizure, confiscation; (*receio*) apprehension; ***de fácil ~*** easily understood
apreensivo [apreẽ'sivu] *adj* apprehensive
aprender [aprẽ'der] ⟨2a⟩ (*estudar*) learn; (*vir a saber*) find out; ***~ a dirigir*** learn to drive; ***~ a fazer algo*** learn how to do sth
aprendiz [aprẽ'dʒis] *m* apprentice; ***~ de motorista*** student driver, *Brit* learner driver
aprendizagem [aprẽdʒi'zaʒem] *f* learning
apresentação [aprezẽta'sãw] *f* presentation; (*exibição*) performance; (*preâmbulo*) introduction; (*aparência*) appearance; ***carta** f **de ~*** letter of recommendation; ***ter boa ~*** be presentable
apresentador [aprezẽta'dor] *m*, **-a** *f* presenter
apresentar [aprezẽ'tar] ⟨1a⟩ *v/t* present; *pessoa* introduce; *pêsames* express; *projeto-lei* introduce; *queixa* lodge; *pedido* submit; MIL ***~ armas*** present arms; **apresentar-se** *v/r* introduce oneself; *repartição*: report; *eleições*: run
apressado [apre'sadu] *adj* hurried, hasty
apressar [apre'sar] ⟨1c⟩ *v/t* hurry, rush; **apressar-se** *v/r* hurry
aprofundar [aprofũ'dar] ⟨1a⟩ deepen; **aprofundar-se** *v/r* deepen
aprontar [aprõ'tar] ⟨1a⟩ *v/t* get ready, prepare; **aprontar-se** *v/r* get ready
apropriado [apropri'adu] *adj* appropriate, suitable
apropriar-se [apropri'arsi] ⟨1g⟩ *v/r* ***~ de algo*** appropriate sth
aprovação [aprova'sãw] *f* approval; (*autorização*) authorization; *exame*: passing
aprovar [apro'var] ⟨1e⟩ approve; (*autorizar*) authorize; *lei*, *exame* pass
aproveitamento [aproveta'mẽtu] *m* (*utilização*) use, utilization
aproveitar [aprovej'tar] ⟨1a⟩ **1** *v/t* (*utilizar*) use **2** *v/i* make the most of it; **aproveitar-se** *v/r* ***~ de*** take advantage of; *pej* use
aproximação [aprosima'sãw] *f* approach; (*cálculo*) approximation, rough estimate
aproximadamente [aprosimada'mẽtʃi] *adv* approximately, roughly
aproximado [aprosi'madu] *adj* approximate, rough
aproximar [aprosi'mar] ⟨1a⟩ *v/t* bring near; **aproximar-se** *v/r* get closer; ***~ de*** approach, get closer to
aproximativo [aprosima'tʃivu] *adj* approximate
aptidão [aptʃi'dãw] *f* aptitude; (*competência*) capability; ***ter aptidões para*** be skilled at
apto ['aptu] *adj* (*competente*) capable; (*apropriado*) apt
apunhalar [apuɲa'lar] ⟨1a⟩ stab
apurado [apu'radu] *adj sabor, nariz* refined
apurar [apu'rar] ⟨1a⟩ (*investigar*) investigate; *verdade* establish; (*requintar*) refine; (*aperfeiçoar*) perfect
apuro [a'puru] *m* (*perfeição*) perfection; (*delicadeza*) refinement; (*cuidado*) care; *fam* ***~s*** *pl* difficulties; ***estar em ~s*** be in a jam
aquarela [akwa'rɛla] *f* watercolor, *Brit* watercolour
aquário [a'kwariu] *m* aquarium; ASTROL ***Aquário*** Aquarius
aquático [a'kwatʃiku] *adj* aquatic

aquecedor [akese'doɾ] **1** *adj* warming **2** *m* heater
aquecer [ake'seɾ] ⟨2g & 2a⟩ **1** *v/t* warm up; *comida* heat up; *quarto* heat; **aquecer-se** *v/r tb* ESP warm up
aquecido [ake'sidu] *adj piscina* heated
aquecimento [akesi'mẽtu] *m* warming; (*calorífero*) heating; ESP warm-up; **~ *central*** central heating; **~ *a gás*** gas heating; **~ *global*** global warming
aqueduto [ake'dutu] *m* aqueduct
aquele [a'keli], **aquela** [a'kɛla] *f* **1** *adj* that; *pl* those; ***aquela casa*** that house **2** *pron* that (one); *pl* those (ones); ***quem é ~?*** who is that?
aqui [a'ki] *adv* here; ***por ~*** this way; ***ele vive por ~*** he lives around here; ***até ~*** up to here; **~ *dentro*** in here; ***está ~*** here it is; **~ *está** dando* here you are; **~ *é o João*** it's João here; ***aqui quem fala é …*** this is … speaking
aquilo [a'kilu] *pron* that
aquisição [akizi'sãw] *f* acquisition, purchase; ***Serviço** m **de Aquisição*** Procurement
ar [aɾ] *m* air; (*aragem*) breeze; (*aspecto*) look, appearance; *Port* AUTO choke; ***corrente** f **de ~*** draft, *Brit* draught; ***falta** f **de ~*** breathing difficulties; ***mudança** f **de ~es*** change of air; ***tomar ~*** get some (fresh) air; ***ao ~ livre*** in the open air; RÁDIO, TV ***no ~*** on (the) air; ***ir pelos ~es*** explode; *fig casamento etc* hit the skids; ***andar com a cabeça no ~*** go around with one's head in the clouds; ***ter** ou **dar ~es de*** look like, resemble; **~ *condicionado*** air conditioning
Arábia [a'ɾabja] *f* Arabia; **~ *Saudita*** Saudi Arabia
árabe ['aɾabi] **1** *adj* Arab; *número* Arabic **2** *m/f* Arab **3** *m lingua* Arabic
arado [a'ɾadu] *m* plow, *Brit* plough
aragem [a'ɾaʒẽ] *f* breeze
arame [a'ɾami] *m* wire; *fam* ***ir aos ~s*** freak out; **~ *farpado*** barbed wire
aranha [a'ɾaɲa] *f* spider; ***andar às ~s*** be at a loss
arar [a'ɾaɾ] ⟨1b⟩ plow, *Brit* plough
araucária [aɾaw'kaɾja] *f* BOT araucaria
arável [a'ɾavew] *adj* arable
arbitragem [aɾbi'tɾaʒẽ] *f* arbitration; ***comissão** f **de ~*** arbitration commission
arbitrar [aɾbi'tɾaɾ] ⟨1a⟩ **1** *v/t* arbitrate; *competição* judge; ESP referee; *tênis*: umpire
arbitrariedade [aɾbitɾaɾie'dadʒi] *f* arbitrariness
arbitrário [aɾbi'tɾaɾiu] *adj* arbitrary
arbítrio [aɾ'bitɾiu] *m* (*critério*) discretion; (*despotismo*) despotism; (*sentença*) (arbitral) decision; ***livre ~*** free will
árbitro ['aɾbitɾu] *m*, **-a** *f* arbitrator; *competição*: judge; ESP referee, *fam* ref; *tênis*: umpire
arborização [aɾboɾiza'sãw] *f* forestation
arborizado [aɾboɾi'zadu] *adj* wooded
arborizar [aɾboɾi'zaɾ] ⟨1a⟩ plant with trees
arbusto [aɾ'bustu] *m* shrub, bush
arca ['aɾka] *f* chest, trunk; **~ *de Noé*** Noah's Ark
arcada [aɾ'kada] *f* arcade; (*abóbada*) arch
arcaico [aɾ'kajku] *adj* archaic
arcanjo [aɾ'kãʒu] *m* archangel
arcebispo [aɾse'bispu] *m* archbishop
archote [aɾ'ʃɔtʃi] *m* torch
arco ['aɾku] *m* ARQUIT arch; MÚS bow; (*roda, anel*) hoop
arco-íris [aɾ'kwiɾis] *mpl* ⟨*pl inv*⟩ rainbow
árct… *Port* → ***árt…***
ardente [aɾ'dẽtʃi] *adj* ardent; *temperamento, sabor* fiery
arder [aɾ'deɾ] ⟨2b⟩ **1** *v/i* burn; (*abrasar*) glow; **~ *de desejo*** burn with desire; **~ *em chamas*** be ablaze **2** *v/t* burn; (*consumir*) consume
ardina [aɾ'dʒina] *m Port* paper boy
ardor [aɾ'doɾ] *m* ardor, *Brit* ardour
ardósia [aɾ'dɔzja] *f* slate
árduo ['aɾdwu] *adj* difficult, arduous
área ['aɾja] *f* area; *fig* field; **~ *editorial / bancária*** publishing / banking; ***esta não é a minha ~*** that's not my field; **~ *de acampamento*** campsite; ESP **~ *de pênalti*** penalty

area; INFORM **~ *de trabalho*** desktop; INFORM **~ *de transferência*** clipboard
areia [a'reja] *f* sand; **~ *movediça*** quicksand
arejado [are'ʒadu] *adj* airy
arejar [are'ʒar] ⟨1d⟩ **1** *v/t* air **2** *v/i* get some air
arena [a'rena] *f* arena; *circo*: ring
arenoso [are'nozu] *adj* sandy
arenque [a'rẽki] *m* herring
arfar [ar'far] ⟨1b⟩ *v/i* pant, gasp for breath
argamassa [arga'masa] *f* mortar
Argel [ar'ʒɛw] *m* Algiers
Argélia [ar'ʒɛlja] *f* Algeria
argelino [arʒe'linu] **1** *adj* Algerian **2** *m*, **-a** *f* Algerian
Argentina [arʒẽ'ʧina] *f* Argentina
argentino [arʒẽ'ʧinu] **1** *adj* Argentinian **2** *m*, **-a** *f* Argentinian
argila [ar'ʒila] *f* clay
argiloso [arʒi'lozu] *adj* clay *atr*; ***terra*** *f* ***argilosa*** clay soil
argola [ar'gɔla] *f* ring, hoop; *lata*: ring-pull; (*brinco*) hooped earring; (*batente*) door-knocker
arguido [ar'gwidu] *m*, **-a** *f Port* formal suspect
argumentação [argumẽta'sãw] *f* argumentation, line of argument
argumentar [argumẽ'tar] ⟨1a⟩ argue; **~ *contra*** argue against
argumento [argu'mẽtu] *m* argument; CINE (movie) script; **~*s*** *pl* pros and cons, arguments for and against
ária ['arja] *f* aria
aridez [ari'des] *f* dryness, aridness
árido ['aridu] *adj* arid
Áries ['aris] *m* ASTROL Aries
aristocracia [aristokra'sia] *f* aristocracy
aristocrata [aristo'krata] *m/f* aristocrat
aristocrático [aristo'kraʧiku] *adj* aristocratic
aritmética [arit'mɛʧika] *f* arithmetic
arma ['arma] *f* weapon; **~*s*** *pl* coat of arms; **~ *de fogo*** firearm; **~*s nucleares*** nuclear weapons
armação [arma'sãw] *f* frame; *óculos*: frames; ARQUIT half-timbering; *telhado*: roof truss
armada [ar'mada] *f* navy
armadilha [arma'dʒiʎa] *f* trap
armado [ar'madu] *adj* armed
armador [arma'dor] *m* NÁUT shipowner
armadura [arma'dura] *f* armor, *Brit* armour
armamento [arma'mẽtu] *m* armaments
armar [ar'mar] ⟨1b⟩ *v/t* arm; *tenda* pitch; *armadilha* set; **armar-se** *v/r* arm oneself; *fig* prepare oneself; *tempestade* be in the offing; **~ *em*** pose as, set oneself up as
armário [ar'mariu] *m* cupboard; *roupa* closet; **~ *de remédios*** medicine cabinet
armazém [arma'zẽ] *m* warehouse
armazenagem [armaze'naʒẽ] *f*, **armazenamento** [armazena'mẽtu] *m* storage; INFORM **~ *de dados*** data storage
armazenar [armaze'nar] ⟨1d⟩ *v/t* store
Armênia, *Port* **Arménia** [ar'menja] *f* Armenia
arminho [ar'miɲu] *m* ermine
armistício [armis'ʧisiu] *m* armistice
aro ['aru] *m* (*roda*) rim; (*anel*) ring
aroma [a'roma] *m* aroma; *vinho*: bouquet, nose
aromático [aro'maʧiku] *adj cheiro* aromatic; *sabor* fragrant
arpão [ar'pãw] *m* harpoon
arqueado [ar'kjadu] *adj* arched, curved; *pernas* bandy
arqueiro [ar'kejru] *m*, **-a** *f* archer; *futebol*: goalie
arquejante [arke'ʒãʧi] *adj* gasping
arquejar [arke'ʒar] ⟨1d⟩ gasp, pant
arquejo [ar'keʒu] *m* gasp
arqueologia [arkjolo'ʒia] *f* archeology, *Brit* archaeology
arqueológico [arkjo'lɔʒiku] *adj* archeological, *Brit* archaeological
arqueólogo [ar'kjɔlogu] *m*, **-a** *f* archeologist, *Brit* archaeologist
arquipélago [arki'pɛlagu] *m* archipelago
arquitect... *Port* → ***arquitet...***
arquiteto [arki'tɛtu] *m*, **-a** *f* architect;

~ de interior interior designer
arquitetônico, *Port* **arquitectónico** [aɾkite'toniku] *adj* architectural
arquitetura [aɾkite'tuɾa] *f* architecture
arquivar [aɾki'vaɾ] ⟨1a⟩ archive; INFORM store; *correspondência* file
arquivo [aɾ'kivu] *m* file; *depósito* archives; (*armário*) file cabinet, *Brit* filing cabinet; INFORM *Bras* file; ***~ somente para leitura*** read-only file
arrancada [ahã'kada] *f corrida*: spurt
arrancar [ahã'kaɾ] ⟨1n⟩ **1** *v/t* pull out; *pétala* tear off; *árvore* pull up; *dente* extract, pull out; ***~ algo a alguém*** snatch sth away from s.o.; *fig* drag sth out of s.o. **2** *v/i* set off; *motor* start
arranco [a'hãku] *m* pull, tug; (*salto*) jump
arranha-céu [ahaɲa'sɛu] *m* ⟨*pl* arranha-céus⟩ skyscraper
arranhadura [ahaɲa'duɾa] *f*, **arranhão** [aha'ɲãw] *m* scratch
arranhar [aha'ɲaɾ] ⟨1a⟩ scratch; *fam língua* have a smattering of; *guitarra* strum
arranjado [ahã'ʒadu] *adj* ***bem ~*** presentable; *irôn* ***estar bem ~*** be in a mess
arranjar [ahã'ʒaɾ] ⟨1a⟩ *v/t* repair; (*dispor*) arrange; (*arrumar*) tidy; (*procurar*) find, get; (*aprontar*) prepare, get ready; ***~ coragem*** find the courage; ***~ problemas*** get into trouble; **arranjar-se** *v/r* (*resolver-se*) sort itself out; (*ser possível*) be doable; (*vestir-se*) get dressed; ***~ com*** manage with; (*chegar a acordo*) reach an agreement with
arranjo [a'hãʒu] *m* agreement; (*disposição*) arrangement; (*conserto*) repair
arranque [a'hãki] *m* jolt; *carro, motor*: start; ESP start; ***~ final*** final spurt; AUTO ***motor*** *m* ***de ~*** starter motor; ***mecanismo*** *m* ***de ~*** automatic choke
arrasado [aha'zadu] *adj* (*destruído*) razed to the ground; (*exausto*) exhausted; (*deprimido*) devastated
arrasador [ahasa'dor] *adj notícias etc* shattering
arrasar [aha'zaɾ] ⟨1b⟩ *v/t* (*destruír*) raze to the ground, destroy; (*cansar*) exhaust; *emocionalmente* shatter
arrastado [ahas'tadu] *adj* dragging; (*lento*) slow; (*difícil*) laborious
arrastão [ahas'tãw] *m navio* trawler; *crime* hold-up
arrastar [ahas'taɾ] ⟨1b⟩ **1** *v/t* drag; ***~ a voz*** speak haltingly; ***~ os pés*** shuffle **2** *v/i* crawl; **arrastar-se** *v/r* crawl; *fig assunto* drag on; *pessoa* be worn out
arrebatado [aheba'tadu] *adj* impetuous; (*encantado*) overwhelmed
arrebatador [ahebata'doɾ] *adj* enchanting; *sentimento* overwhelming
arrebatar [aheba'taɾ] ⟨1b⟩ snatch; (*entusiasmar*) enrapture
arrebitado [ahebi'tadu] *adj fig* snooty; (*sabichão*) precocious; ***nariz*** *m* ***~*** snub nose
arrebitar [ahebi'taɾ] ⟨1a⟩ turn up; (*torcer*) twist; ***~ as orelhas*** prick up one's ears
arrecadação [ahekada'sãw] *f* storeroom; (*depósito*) storage; *impostos*: collection; (*impostos*) tax revenue
arrecadar [aheka'daɾ] ⟨1b⟩ store; (*pôr a salvo*) keep safe; *impostos* collect
arredio [ahe'dʒiu] *adj* shy
arredondado [ahedõ'dadu] *adj* rounded
arredondar [ahedõ'daɾ] ⟨1a⟩ round off; *soma* round up
arredores [ahe'dɔɾis] *mpl* environs, surrounding area; *cidade*: suburbs
arrefecer [ahefe'seɾ] ⟨2g & 2a⟩ **1** *v/t Port* cool *tb fig* **2** *v/i* cool down; *fig* cool off
arrefecimento [ahefesi'mẽtu] *m Port* cooling
arregaçar [ahega'saɾ] ⟨1p, *Stv* 1b⟩ *v/t mangas, calças* roll up
arregalado [ahega'ladu] *adj olhos* wide open
arregalar [ahega'laɾ] ⟨1a⟩ *v/t* ***~ os olhos*** stare in amazement
arreio(s) [a'heiu(s)] *m(pl) cavalo*: harness
arrelia [ahe'lia] *f Port* annoyance; ***que ~!*** how annoying!
arreliado [ahe'ljadu] *adj Port* annoying

arreliar [ahe'ljaɾ] ⟨1g⟩ *Port* annoy
arrematar [ahema'taɾ] ⟨1b⟩ (*leiloar*) auction; (*adjudicar*) award
arremessador [ahemesa'doɾ] *m*, **-a** *f* *beisebol*: pitcher; **~ de disco** discus thrower
arremessar [aheme'saɾ] ⟨1c⟩ *v/t* hurl, throw; *beisebol*: pitch; **arremessar-se** *v/r* **~ a / sobre** hurl oneself at / on
arremesso [ahe'mesu] *m* throw; ESP throw-in; **~ de dardo** javelin
arrendamento [ahẽda'mẽtu] *m Port* *ato* leasing; *quantia* lease, rent; **contrato** *m* **de ~** rental *ou* lease agreement; **tomar de ~** lease, rent
arrendar [ahẽ'daɾ] ⟨1a⟩ *Port* lease, rent; **arrenda-se** for rent
arrepender-se [ahepẽ'deɾsi] ⟨2a⟩ *v/r* **~ de algo** regret sth; **não vou me arrepender de sair daqui** I won't be sorry to leave
arrependido [ahepẽ'dʒidu] *adj* regretful, sorry; **estar ~ de algo** regret sth
arrependimento [ahepẽdʒi'mẽtu] *m* regret; REL repentance
arrepiado [ahe'pjadu] *adj* **pele** *f* **arrepiada** gooseflesh, goosebumps; **estou ~** it makes me shudder; **estou com o cabelo ~** my hair's standing on end
arrepiar [ahe'pjaɾ] ⟨1g⟩ *v/t* make shudder; (*horrorizar*) horrify; *cabelo* make stand on end; **arrepiar-se** *v/r* shudder; **arrepio-me** it gives me gooseflesh
arrepio [ahe'piu] *m* shudder; **a casa me dá ~s** the house gives me the creeps
arribação [ahiba'sãw] *f* ⟨*sem pl*⟩ migration; **ave** *f* **de ~** migratory bird
arriscado [ahis'kadu] *adj* *coisa* risky; *pessoa* daring
arriscar [ahis'kaɾ] ⟨1n⟩ *v/t* risk; **arriscar-se** *v/r* **~ a algo** risk sth; **~ a fazer algo** risk doing sth
arrivismo [ahi'vizmu] *m* pushiness
arrivista [ahi'vista] *m/f* upstart
arroba [a'hoba] *f* INFORM 'at' sign, @ sign
arrogância [aho'gãsja] *f* arrogance
arrogante [aho'gãtʃi] *adj* arrogant; **brio** *m* **~** nerve, courage
arrogar-se [aho'garsi] ⟨1o, *Stv* 1e⟩ *v/r* claim
arrojado [aho'ʒadu] *adj* bold, daring
arrombador [ahõba'doɾ] *m* burglar
arrombamento [ahõba'mẽtu] *m* DIR burglary, break-in
arrombar [ahõ'baɾ] ⟨1a⟩ (*destruir*) break down, smash; (*assaltar*) burglarize, *Brit* burgle; (*derrubar*) knock down; *cofre* crack open
arrotar [aho'taɾ] ⟨1e⟩ *v/i* burp, belch
arroto [a'hotu] *m* belch, burp
arroz [a'hos] *m* rice
arrozal [aho'zaw] *m* rice field, rice paddy
arroz-doce [ahoʒ'dosi] *m* rice pudding
arruaça [a'hwasa] *f* riot
arruaceiro [a'hwasejru] *m*, **-a** *f* rioter
arruela [a'hwɛla] *f* washer
arruinar [ahwi'naɾ] ⟨1q⟩ *v/t* ruin; *edifício* destroy; **arruinar-se** *v/r* *edifício* fall into disrepair; *pessoa* be ruined
arrumação [ahuma'sãw] *f* accommodations, *Brit* accommodation; *ato* tidying up; (*ordem*) order
arrumadeira [ahuma'deiɾa] *f* *hotel*: maid
arrumar [ahu'maɾ] ⟨1a⟩ pack; (*ordenar*) tidy up, put in order; **arrumar-se** *v/r* (*aprontar-se*) get ready; (*arranjar a roupa*) tidy oneself up; *na vida* sort oneself out
arsenal [aɾse'naw] *m* arsenal; (*apetrechos*) equipment
arsênio, *Port* **arsénio** [aɾ'seniu] *m* arsenic
arte ['aɾtʃi] *f* art; (*jeito*) skill; (*ofício*) trade; (*manha*) trick; **~ dramática** acting; **Arte Nova** Art Nouveau; **~s marciais** martial arts
artefato, *Port* **artefacto** [aɾte'fatu] *m* artifact
artéria [aɾ'tɛɾja] *f* artery
arterial [aɾte'ɾjaw] **tensão** *f* **~** blood pressure
arteriosclerose [aɾtɛɾjoskle'ɾɔzi] *f* arteriosclerosis, hardening of the arteries
artesanato [aɾteza'natu] *m* handicraft

artesão [arte'zãw] *m* ⟨*pl* -ãos⟩, **-ã** *f* artisan, craftsman; craftswoman
Ártico ['artʃiku] *m* Arctic
ártico ['artʃiku] *adj* arctic
articulação [artʃikula'sãw] *f* MED joint; TECN hinge; (*pronúncia*) articulation; ~ ***esférica*** ball-and-socket joint
articulado [artʃiku'ladu] *adj* articulated, jointed; (*dobradiço*) hinged; (*claro*) articulate
articular [artʃiku'lar] ⟨1a⟩ *v/t* join together; (*exprimir*) articulate
artífice [ar'tʃifisi] *m/f* craftsman; craftswoman; (*inventor*) inventor
artificial [artʃifi'sjaw] *adj* artificial; (*pretensioso*) affected
artifício [artʃi'fisiu] *m* (*jeito*) skill; (*truque*) trick
artigo [ar'tʃigu] *m* article; COM *tb* item; ~ ***definido*** definite article; ~ ***de fundo*** leading article, editorial; ~ ***indefinido*** indefinite article; **~*s de consumo*** consumer goods; **~*s de uso pessoal*** toiletries
artilharia [artʃiʎa'ria] *f* artillery
artilheiro [artʃi'ʎejru] *m* gunner, artilleryman; *Bras* goal scorer
artista [ar'tʃista] **1** *m/f* artist; (*artesão*) craftsman; craftswoman; ~ ***gráfico*** graphic designer **2** *adj* artistic
artístico [ar'tʃistʃiku] *adj* artistic
artrite [ar'tritʃi] *f* arthritis
árvore ['arvuri] *f* tree; *navio*: mast; TECN shaft; ~ ***de fruto*** fruit tree; ~ ***genealógica*** family tree; ~ ***de Natal*** Christmas tree
ás [as] *m naipes*: ace *tb fig*
asa ['aza] *f* wing; *chávena*: handle
asa-delta [aza'dɛlta] *f* hang glider
asbesto [az'bɛstu] *m* asbestos *sg*
ascendência [asẽ'dẽsja] *f* ascendancy; (*antepassados*) ancestry; *fig* sway, influence
ascendente [asẽ'dẽtʃi] **1** *adj* rising; (*crescente*) growing **2** *m* (*antepassado*) ancestor
ascender [asẽ'der] ⟨2a⟩ ~ ***a*** *preços*: rise to; *trono*: ascend
ascensão [asẽ'sãw] *f* ascent; *trono*: accession; REL ***Ascensão*** Ascension
ascensor [asẽ'sor] *m* elevator, *Brit* lift
asfaltado [asfaw'tadu] *adj* asphalt
asfaltar [asfaw'tar] ⟨1a⟩ asphalt
asfalto [as'fawtu] *m* asphalt
asfixia [asfi'ksia] *f* asphyxiation
asfixiado [asfi'ksjadu] *adj* asphyxiated
asfixiar [asfi'ksjar] ⟨1g⟩ *v/t* asphyxiate; **asfixiar-se** *v/r* be asphyxiated
Ásia ['azja] *f* Asia; ~ ***Menor*** Asia Minor
asiático [a'zjatʃiku] **1** *adj* Asian **2** *m*, **-a** *f* Asian
asilado [azi'ladu] *m*, **-a** *f* asylum seeker
asilo [a'zilu] *m* POL asylum; *fig* refuge; *velhos*: home; ***pedir*** ~ seek asylum; ~ ***político*** political asylum
asma ['azma] *f* asthma
asmático [az'matʃiku] **1** *adj* asthmatic **2** *m*, **-a** *f* asthmatic
asneira [az'nejɾa] *f Port* nonsense; (*estupidez*) stupidity
asno ['aznu] *m* donkey, ass *tb fig*
aspargo [as'pargu] *m Bras* asparagus
aspas ['aspas] *fpl* ***entre*** ~ in quotes
aspecto [as'pɛtu] *m* aspect; (*aparência*) appearance; (*visão*) view; (*ponto de vista*) point of view
aspereza [aspe'reza] *f* roughness; (*brusquidão*) curtness
áspero ['asperu] *adj* rough; (*brusco*) curt
aspersor [asper'sor] *m* lawn sprinkler
aspiração [aspira'sãw] *f* inhalation; TECN intake; *fig* aspiration; (*empenho*) effort
aspirador [aspira'dor] *m* vacuum cleaner; ***passar o*** ~ ***por*** vacuum
aspirante [aspi'rãtʃi] *m/f* candidate; MIL cadet
aspirar [aspi'rar] ⟨1a⟩ breathe in; TECN suck up; *carpete* vacuum; ~ ***a*** *ou* ***por*** aspire to
aspirina® [aspi'rina] *f* aspirin
asqueroso [aske'rozu] *adj* disgusting
assado [a'sadu] **1** *adj* roasted; ~ ***no forno*** roast; ~ ***na brasa*** charbroiled; ~ ***de porco*** roast pork **2** *m* roast
assalariado [asala'rjadu] **1** *m*, **-a** *f* wage-earner **2** *adj* ***trabalho*** *m* ~ salaried work

assaltante [asaw'tãtʃi] *m/f pessoa*: assailant; *na rua* mugger; *casa*, *banco*: robber, raider
assaltar [asaw'taɾ] ⟨1a⟩ *pessoa* mug; (*atacar*) attack; *banco* hold up, rob; *casa* burgle
assalto [a'sawtu] *m pessoa*: attack; *na rua* mugging; *banco*: heist, raid; *casa*: burglary, break-in; **~ *à mão armada*** armed robbery
assanhado [asa'ɲadu] *adj* (*furioso*) furious; (*vermelho*) scarlet
assar [a'saɾ] ⟨1b⟩ *frigideira*: fry; *grill*: broil, *Brit* grill; *forno*: roast
assassinar [asasi'naɾ] ⟨1a⟩ murder; POL assassinate
assassinato [asasi'natu] *m* murder; POL assassination
assassínio [asa'siniu] *m* murder; POL assassination
assassino [asa'sinu] *m*, **-a** *f* murderer; POL assassin, **~ *de aluguel*** hired killer, hitman; **~ *em série*** serial killer
asseado [a'sjadu] *adj* clean
assédio [a'sɛdʒiu] *m* **~ *moral*** bullying; **~ *sexual*** sexual harassment
assegurar [asegu'raɾ] ⟨1a⟩ assure; (*garantir*) ensure; (*pôr a salvo*) secure
asseio [a'seiu] *m* cleanliness, tidiness
assembléia [asẽ'blɛja] *f* assembly, meeting; **~ *geral anual*** annual general meeting
assemelhar [aseme'ʎaɾ] ⟨1d⟩ *v/t* liken; **assemelhar-se** *v/r* **~ *a*, ~ *com*** resemble, look like
assentar [asẽ'taɾ] ⟨1a⟩ *v/t* (*pôr em cima*) place; *fundamento* lay; *planos* fix, settle; *quantia*, *nome* enter; **assentar-se** [asẽ'taɾsi] *v/r* settle
assentimento [asẽtʃi'mẽtu] *m* agreement, assent
assento [a'sẽtu] *m* seat; **~ *na janela*** window seat; **~ *no corredor*** aisle seat
asséptico [a'sɛptʃiku] *adj* sterile
asserção [aseɾ'sãw] *f* assertion
assessor [ase'soɾ] *m*, **-a** *f* aide; adviser; **~ *de mídia*** communications officer
assíduo [a'sidwu] *adj* (*contínuo*) constant; (*aplicado*) assiduous
assim [a'sĩ] **1** *adv* like this, this way; (*portanto*) so; **~, ~** so-so; **~ *chamado*** so-called; **~ *como*** as well as; ***ainda* ~, *mesmo* ~** even so; all the same; **~ *não*** not like that; ***e* ~ *por diante*** and so forth; ***grande* / *alto* ~** that big / high; ***e* ~ *eu perdi o trem*** and so I missed the train; **~ *mesmo!*** that's it!, exactly! **2** *conj* **~ *que*** as soon as
assimetria [asime'tɾia] *f* asymmetry
assimétrico [asi'mɛtɾiku] *adj* asymmetrical
assimilação [asimila'sãw] *f* assimilation
assimilar [asimi'laɾ] ⟨1a⟩ assimilate; (*aproximar*) liken
assinalar [asina'laɾ] ⟨1b⟩ mark; (*salientar*) point out
assinante [asi'nãtʃi] *m/f revista*, *jornal*: subscriber; *contrato*: signatory
assinar [asi'naɾ] ⟨1a⟩ sign; *revista* subscribe to; (*estipular*) stipulate
assinatura [asina'tuɾa] *f* signature; (*subscrição*) subscription
assistência [asis'tẽsja] *f* (*presença*) presence; *teatro*: audience; (*apoio*) assistance; (*cuidados*) care; **~ *internacional*** foreign aid; **~ *médica*** medical care; **~ *pública*, ~ *social*** social work; **~ *técnica*** technical support
assistente [asis'tẽtʃi] *m/f* assistant; ***os* ~*s*** those present; **~ *de pesquisa*** research assistant; **~ *social*** social worker
assistir [asis'tʃiɾ] ⟨3a⟩ **1** *v/t* attend; *filme etc* watch; (*ajudar*) assist; **~ *televisão*** watch television **2** *v/i* attend; *filme etc*: watch; **~ *a um curso*** attend a course
assoalhada [aswa'ʎada] *f Port* room
assoalho [a'swaʎu] *m* floor
assoar [a'swaɾ] ⟨1f⟩ *v/t* **~ *o nariz*** blow one's nose; **assoar-se** *v/r* blow one's nose
assobiar [aso'bjaɾ] ⟨1g⟩ whistle
assobio [aso'biu] *m* whistle
associação [asosja'sãw] *f* association; **~ *comercial*** chamber of commerce; **~ *dos consumidores*** consumer association; **~ *de pais e mestres*** parent-teacher association, PTA

associado [aso'sjadu] *m*, **-a** *f* (*membro*) member; (*sócio*) partner, associate
associar [aso'sjar] ⟨1g⟩ *v/t* connect; *pensamentos* associate; (*juntar*) join; **associar-se** *v/r* associate; **~ *a*** associate with; *fig* share in
assombrado [asõ'bradu] *adj* spooky; ***este lugar é ~*** this place is haunted
assombrar [asõ'brar] ⟨1a⟩ *v/t* amaze; *lugar* haunt
assombro [a'sõbru] *m* amazement
assumir [asu'mir] ⟨3a⟩ *v/t* (*tomar sobre si*) take on, assume; (*aceitar*) accept; **~ *a responsabilidade por*** assume responsibility for
assunto [a'sũtu] *m* topic, subject; (*questão*) matter, affair
assustadiço [asusta'dʒisu] *adj* jumpy
assustado [asus'tadu] *adj* frightened, scared
assustador [asusta'dor] *adj* frightening, scary
assustar [asus'tar] ⟨1a⟩ *v/t* frighten, scare; **assustar-se** *v/r* be frightened, be scared
asterisco [aste'risku] *m* asterisk
astro ['astru] *m* star *tb fig*
astrologia [astrolo'ʒia] *f* astrology
astrólogo [as'trɔlogu] *m*, **-a** *f* astrologer
astronauta [astro'nawta] *m/f* astronaut
astronomia [astrono'mia] *f* astronomy
astronômico, *Port* **astronómico** [astro'nomiku] *adj* astronomical *tb fig*
astrônomo, *Port* **astrónomo** [as'tronumu] *m/f* astronomer
astúcia [as'tusja] *f* cunning, shrewdness
astucioso [astusi'ozu] *adj* clever
astuto [as'tutu] *adj* astute
ata ['ata] *f* minutes *pl*
atacadista [ataka'dʒista] *m/f* wholesaler
atacado [ata'kadu] *adj* ***por ~*** wholesale; ***preço*** *m* ***no ~*** wholesale price
atacador [ataka'dor] *m Port* shoelace
atacante [ata'kãtʃi] *m/f* attacker; *futebol*: forward, striker
atacar [ata'kar] ⟨1n & 1b⟩ attack; *sono* overcome
atadura [ata'dura] *f Bras* bandage
atalho [a'taʎu] *m* (*caminho mais curto*) shortcut
ataque [a'taki] *m* attack *tb* MED; **~ *de bomba*** bomb attack; **~ *cardíaco*** heart attack; **~ *epilético*** epileptic fit; **~ *de riso*** fit of laughing
atar [a'tar] ⟨1b⟩ (*amarrar*) tie; (*juntar*) fasten
atarefado [atarɛ'fadu] *adj* very busy
atarracado [ataha'kadu] *adj* stocky, thickset
atarraxar [ataha'ʃar] ⟨1b⟩ *v/t carro* clamp
até [a'tɛ] **1** *prep* up to; *lugar*: as far as; **~ *que*** until; ***podes telefonar ~ terça-feira?*** can you call by Tuesday?; **~ *que enfim!*** at last!; **~ *que foi uma surpresa!*** it was quite a surprise!; **~ *logo!*** so long!; **~ *onde posso ver*** as far as I can see; **~ *a esquina*** as far as the corner; **~ *agora tudo bem*** so far so good **2** *adv* even; **~ *mesmo*** even
atéia, *Port* **ateia** [a'teja] *f* atheist
ateísmo [ate'izmu] *m* atheism
Atenas [a'tenas] *sem art* Athens
atenção [atẽ'sãw] *f* attention; (*cortesia*) courtesy; **~, *por favor!*** your attention please!; ***prestar ~*** pay attention; ***chamar a ~ de alguém para*** call s.o.'s attention to
atenciosamente [atẽsjoza'mẽtʃi] *adv correspondência*: yours truly, *Brit* yours sincerely
atencioso [atẽ'sjozu] *adj* thoughtful, considerate
atendedor [atẽde'dor] *m Port* **~ (*de chamadas*)** answering machine
atender [atẽ'der] ⟨2a⟩ **1** *v/t cliente* serve, attend to; *doente* look after; *telefone*, *porta* answer **2** *v/i* **~ *a*** attend to; **~ *pelo nome de …*** answer to the name of …
atendimento [atẽdʒi'mẽtu] *m* ***horário de ~*** opening hours; *médico*: office hours, *Brit* surgery hours
atentado [atẽ'tadu] *m* attack; POL attempted assassination; **~ *suicida*** suicide attack; **~ *terrorista*** terrorist attack

atentar [atẽ'taɾ] ⟨1a⟩ **1** *v/t* pay attention to; (*tencionar*) plan **2** *v/i* carry out an attack (***contra*** on); **~ *contra a vida de alguém*** make an attempt on s.o.'s life
atento [a'tẽtu] *adj* attentive; **~ *à moda*** fashion-conscious
atenuante [ate'nwɐ̃tʃi] **1** *adj* extenuating **2** *f* extenuating circumstance
atenuar [ate'nwaɾ] ⟨1g⟩ (*enfraquecer*) weaken; (*suavizar*) alleviate
aterrador [ateha'doɾ] *adj* terrifying
aterragem [ate'haʒẽ] *f Port* landing
aterrar [ate'haɾ] ⟨1c⟩ **1** *v/t* ELÉT ground, *Brit* earth **2** *v/i Port avião* land
aterrissagem [atehi'saʒẽ] *f Bras* landing; **~ *forçada*** emergency landing; ***pista** f **de** ~* runway
aterrissar [atehi'saɾ] ⟨1a⟩ *v/i Bras avião* land
aterrorizar [atehori'zaɾ] ⟨1a⟩ terrify; (*perseguir*) terrorize
ater-se [a'tersi] ⟨2xa⟩ *v/r* **~ *a*** *decisão* stand by
atestado [ates'tadu] *m* certificate
atestar [ates'taɾ] ⟨1c⟩ (*testificar*) attest to; (*comprovar*) prove
ateu [a'tew] **1** *m* atheist **2** *adj* atheist
atiçar [atʃi'saɾ] ⟨1p⟩ *v/t lume* poke; *fig* incite, provoke
atingir [atʃĩ'ʒiɾ] ⟨3n⟩ reach; (*tocar*) touch; (*afetar*) affect; (*compreender*) grasp; MIL hit; *objetivo* achieve
atirador [atʃira'doɾ] *m* gunman; *polícia etc*: marksman
atirar [atʃi'raɾ] ⟨1a⟩ *v/t* throw; **~ *algo a alguém*** pelt s.o. with sth **2** *v/i* throw; *com arma* shoot; **~ *para matar*** shoot to kill; **~ *bem* / *mal*** be a good / poor shot; **atirar-se** *v/r* fling oneself
atitude [atʃi'tudʒi] *f* attitude; ***tomar uma** ~* take action
ativação [atʃiva'sɐ̃w] *f* activation
ativar [atʃi'vaɾ] ⟨1a⟩ activate
atividade [atʃivi'dadʒi] *f* activity
ativista [atʃi'vista] *m/f* activist
ativo [a'tʃivu] **1** *adj* active **2** *m* ECON **~*s*** *pl* assets
atlântico [a'tlɐ̃tʃiku] *adj* Atlantic; ***o** (**Oceano**) **Atlântico*** the Atlantic (Ocean)
atlas ['atlas] *m* atlas
atleta [a'tlɛta] *m/f* athlete
atlético [a'tlɛtʃiku] *adj Port* athletic
atletismo [atle'tʃizmu] *m* athletics; **~ *de salão*** indoor athletics
atmosfera [atʃimos'fɛra] *f* atmosphere
atmosférico [atʃimos'fɛriku] *adj* atmospheric; ***pressão** f **atmosférica*** atmospheric pressure; ***poluição** f **atmosférica*** air pollution
ato ['atu] *m* act *tb* TEAT; (*ação*) action; ***no** ~ matar* outright; *pagar* on the spot; ***ser apanhado no** ~* be caught in the act; **~ *falho*** Freudian slip
à-toa [a'toa] *adj* (*irrefletido*) rash; (*inútil*) worthless, useless
atolar-se [ato'larsi] ⟨1e⟩ *v/r* get bogged down *tb fig*
atoleiro [ato'lejru] *m* quagmire
atômico, *Port* **atómico** [a'tomiku] *adj* atomic; ***energia** f **atômica*** nuclear power
atomizador [atomiza'doɾ] *m* atomizer
átomo ['atumu] *m* atom
atônito, *Port* **atónito** [a'tonitu] *adj* astounded
ator [a'toɾ] *m* actor
atormentar [atormẽ'taɾ] ⟨1a⟩ *fig* torment
atracadouro [atraka'doru] *m* berth
atracar [atra'kaɾ] ⟨1n, *Stv* 1b⟩ *v/i* moor, tie up
atração, *Port* **atracção** [atra'sɐ̃w] *f* attraction
atract... *Port* → ***atrat***
atraente [atra'ẽtʃi] attractive
atrair [atra'iɾ] ⟨3l⟩ attract
atrapalhado [atrapa'ʎadu] *adj* (*confuso*) confused; (*desamparado*) helpless
atrapalhar [atrapa'ʎaɾ] ⟨1b⟩ (*confundir*) confuse; (*obstruir*) hamper; *tarefa* make a mess of
atrás [a'tras] **1** *adv* behind, at the back; **~ *no carro*** in the back of the car; ***dois dias** ~* two days ago **2** *prep* **~ *de*** behind; *tempo*: after
atrasado [atra'zadu] *adj* late; (*desatualizado*) overdue; *relógio* slow; ***chegar** ~* arrive late
atrasar [atra'zaɾ] ⟨1b⟩ **1** *v/t* delay; *relógio* put back; (*antedatar*) backdate

2 *v/i* be late; *relógio* be slow; **atrasar-se** *v/r* (*ficar para trás*) fall behind; *relógio* be slow; (*chegar tarde*) be late
atraso [a'trazu] *m* delay; *pagamento*: arrears; ***estar em ~*** be in arrears
atrativo [atra'tʃivu] **1** *adj* attractive **2** *m* attraction
através [atra'vɛs] *prep* ***~ de*** through; (*de um lado ao outro*) across
atravessar [atrave'sar] ⟨1c⟩ cross; (*percorrer*) pass through; *crise etc* go through
atrelado [atre'ladu] *m* AUTO trailer
atrelar [atre'lar] ⟨1c⟩ put on a leash *tb fig*; *cavalos* harness; FERROV *carruagem* couple
atrever-se [atre'versi] ⟨2c⟩ *v/r* ***~ a fazer algo*** dare to do sth
atrevido [atre'vidu] *adj* (*impertinente*) cheeky, impudent; (*audaz*) bold
atrevimento [atrevi'mẽtu] *m* (*impertinência*) cheek, insolence; (*audácia*) boldness
atribuição [atribwi'sãw] *f prémio*: awarding; *poderes*: authorization; (*distribuição*) allocation, ***atribuições*** *pl* powers
atribuir [atri'bwir] ⟨3i⟩ *cargo* confer; *poderes, direito* grant; (*distribuir*) allocate; (*imputar*) ***~ algo a*** attribute sth to
atributivo [atribu'tʃivu] *adj* GRAM attributive
atributo [atri'butu] *m* attribute
átrio ['atriu] *m* hallway
atrito [a'tritu] *m* friction *tb fig*; ***ser sem ~s*** be trouble-free
atriz [a'tris] *f* actress
atrocidade [atrosi'dadʒi] *f* atrocity
atropelamento [atropela'mẽtu] *m* collision; AUTO running over; *lei*: violation
atropelar [atrope'lar] ⟨1c⟩ *v/t peão* run over, knock down; (*menosprezar*) run down
atroz [a'trɔs] *adj* terrible, atrocious
atuação [atwa'sãw] *f* performance
atual [a'twaw] *adj* present, current
atualidade [atwali'dadʒi] *f* present; ***~s*** current affairs
atualização [atwaliza'sãw] *f* update
atualizado [atwali'zadu] *adj* up-to-date
atualizar [atwali'zar] ⟨1a⟩ *v/t* update
atualmente [atwaw'mẽtʃi] *adv* currently, at the moment
atuante [atu'ãtʃi] *adj* active
atuar [a'twar] ⟨1g⟩ **1** *v/t* set in motion **2** *v/i* act (***sobre*** on)
atum [a'tũ] *m* tuna
aturar [atu'rar] ⟨1a⟩ *v/t* endure; (*permitir*) put up with
aturdido [atur'dʒidu] *adj* dazed
audácia [aw'dasja] *f* boldness
audição [awdʒi'sãw] *f* hearing; *papel*: audition; DIR hearing
audiência [aw'djẽsja] *f* audience; DIR hearing; ***~ televisiva*** television audience
audiovisual [awdʒiovi'zwaw] *adj* audiovisual
auditor [awdʒi'tor] *m*, **-a** *f* FIN auditor
auditoria [awdʒito'ria] *f* FIN audit
auditório [awdʒi'tɔriu] *m* (*sala*) auditorium; (*ouvintes*) audience
audível [aw'dʒivew] *adj* audible
auge ['awʒi] *m* height, peak
aula ['awla] *f* lesson, class; *sala* classroom; ***~s*** *pl* tuition; ***dar ~s*** teach; ***dar ~s de inglês*** teach English; ***~ de direção*** driving lesson; ***~ noturna*** evening class
aumentar [awmẽ'tar] ⟨1a⟩ **1** *v/t quantidade* increase; *tamanho* extend, enlarge; *aquecimento* turn up **2** *v/i* increase; (*subir*) rise, go up; ***~ em valor*** increase in value
aumento [aw'mẽtu] *m* increase; (*crescimento*) growth; *preço*: rise
áureo ['awriu] *adj* golden
auriculares [awriku'laris] *mpl Port* headphones
auréola [aw'rɛula] *f* halo
aurora [aw'rɔra] *f* dawn
auscultador [awskuwta'dor] *m* TEL, ELÉT receiver; ***~es*** *pl* headphones
auscultar [awskuw'tar] ⟨1a⟩ *doente* sound; *fig* sound out
ausência [aw'zẽsja] *f* absence
ausentar-se [awzẽ'tarsi] ⟨1a⟩ *v/r* go away
ausente [aw'zẽtʃi] *adj* absent
austeridade [awsteri'dadʒi] *f* austerity

austero [aws'tɛɾu] *adj* austere; (*poupado*) thrifty
Austrália [aws'tɾalia] *f* Australia
australiano [awstɾa'ljanu] **1** *adj* Australian **2** *m*, **-a** *f* Australian
Áustria ['awstɾia] *f* Austria
austríaco [aws'tɾiaku] **1** *adj* Austrian **2** *m*, **-a** *f* Austrian
autarquia [awtaɾ'kia] *f Port* city council
autárquico [aw'taɾkiku] *adj Port* council *atr*
autenticação [awtẽtʃika'sãw] *f* authentication
autenticar [awtẽtʃi'kaɾ] ⟨1n⟩ authenticate
autenticidade [awtẽtʃisi'dadʒi] *f* authenticity
autêntico [aw'tẽtʃiku] *adj* authentic; (*fidedigno*) trustworthy
autista [aw'tʃista] *adj* autistic
auto ['awtu] *m* document; DIR *tb* record; **~s** *pl* case files
autobiografia [awtobjogɾa'fia] *f* autobiography
autocarro [awto'kahu] *m Port* bus
autocolante [awtoko'lãtʃi] *Port* **1** *adj* self-adhesive **2** *m* sticker
autoconfiante [awtoko'lãtʃi] *adj* self-confident
autocontrole [awtokõ'tɾoli] *m* self-control
autodefesa [awtode'feza] *f* self-defense, *Brit* self-defence
autodeterminação [awtodetiɾmina'sãw] *f* ⟨*sem pl*⟩ POL self-determination
autodidata, *Port* **autodidacta** [awtodʒi'data] *m/f* autodidact, self-taught person
autódromo [aw'tɔdɾumu] *m* racetrack
auto-escola [awto'skɔla] *f* driving school
auto-estima [awto'stʃima] *f* self-esteem
auto-estrada [awtos'tɾada] *f* ⟨*pl* **~** s⟩ freeway, interstate, *Brit* motorway
autografar [awtogɾa'faɾ] ⟨1b⟩ *v/t* autograph
autógrafo [aw'tɔgɾafu] *m* autograph
autolimpante [awtolĩ'pãtʃi] *adj* self-cleaning
automaticamente [awtomatʃika'mẽtʃi] *adv* automatically
automação [awtoma'sãw] *f* ⟨*sem pl*⟩ automation
automático [awto'matʃiku] *adj* automatic
automatizar [awtomatʃi'zaɾ] ⟨1a⟩ automate
automóvel [awto'mɔvew] *m* automobile, car
autonomia [awtono'mia] *f* autonomy
autônomo, *Port* **autónomo** [aw'tonumu] *adj* autonomous
autópsia [aw'tɔpsja] *f* autopsy, post-mortem
autor [aw'toɾ] *m*, **-a** *f* *texto*: author, writer; *crime*: perpetrator; ***direitos*** *mpl* ***de* ~** copyright
auto-rádio [awto'hadʒiu] *m* car radio
auto-respeito [awtohes'pejtu] *m* self-respect
auto-retrato [awtohe'tɾatu] *m* self-portrait
autoria [awto'ɾia] *f* authorship; *crime*: responsibility
autoridade [awtoɾi'dadʒi] *f* authority; (*poder*) power; ***as* ~*s*** the authorities
autoritário [awtoɾi'taɾiu] *adj* authoritarian
autorização [awtoɾiza'sãw] *f* authorization; ***~ de trabalho*** work permit
autorizar [awtoɾi'zaɾ] ⟨1a⟩ authorize
auxiliar [awsi'ljaɾ] ⟨1g⟩ **1** *v/t* (*ajudar*) help, assist **2** *adj* auxiliary **3** *m/f* assistant
auxílio [aw'siliu] *m* (*ajuda*) help, assistance
Av. *abr* (***Avenida***) Ave (Avenue)
avalanche, *Port* **avalancha** [ava'lãʃi] *f* avalanche
avaliação [avalja'sãw] *f* (*taxação*) estimate; (*classificação*) evaluation; (*juízo*) assessment
avaliar [ava'ljaɾ] ⟨1g⟩ (*taxar*) estimate (***em*** at); (*classificar*) evaluate; (*julgar*) assess
avançada [avã'sada] *f* advance
avançado [avã'sadu] **1** *adj* advanced **2** *m* ESP forward
avançado-centro [avã'sadusẽtɾu] *m* center-forward, *Brit* centre-forward

avançar [avã'saɾ] ⟨1p⟩ **1** *v/i* advance; *tempo* pass, go by **2** *v/t* advance; *relógio* put forward
avanço [a'vãsu] *m* advance; (*progresso*) progress; TECN breakthrough; **~ *rápido*** fast forward
avarento [ava'rẽtu] **1** *adj* miserly **2** *m* miser
avareza [ava'reza] *f* avarice
avaria [ava'ria] *f* damage; *carro, máquina* breakdown
avariado [ava'ɾjadu] *adj* damaged; (*estragado*) out of order
avariar [ava'ɾjaɾ] ⟨1g⟩ *v/t* damage; **avariar-se** *v/r* get damaged; *carro, máquina* break down
ave ['avi] *f* bird; **~ *marítima*** seabird; **~ *de rapina*** bird of prey
aveia [a'veja] *f* oats
avelã [ave'lã] *f* hazelnut
aveludado [avelu'dadu] *adj* velvety
avenida [ave'nida] *f* avenue
avental [avẽ'taw] *m* apron; *cirurgião*: gown
aventura [avẽ'tuɾa] *f* adventure
aventurar [avẽtu'ɾaɾ] ⟨1a⟩ *v/t* risk; *pensamentos* venture; **aventurar-se** *v/r* dare (***a*** to)
aventureiro [avẽtu'ɾejɾu] **1** *adj* adventurous **2** *m*, **-a** *f* adventurer
averiguação [averigwa'sãw] *f* (*investigação*) investigation; (*constatação*) verification
averiguar [averi'gwaɾ] ⟨1m⟩ (*certificar-se*) check; (*constatar*) verify; (*investigar*) investigate
aversão [aveɾ'sãw] *f* aversion
averso [a'vɛɾsu] *adj* averse (***a*** to)
avessas [a'vesas] ***às ~*** the wrong way around; *verticalmente* upside down; *situação* topsy-turvy
avesso [a'vesu] **1** *m* reverse; *vestuário*: back **2** *adj* ***ao ~*** *roupa* inside out
avestruz [aves'tɾus] *m* ostrich
aviação [avja'sãw] *f* ⟨*sem pl*⟩ aviation; ***campo** m **de ~*** airfield; ***~ civil*** civil aviation; ***~ militar*** air force
aviador [avja'doɾ] *m*, **-a** *f* aviator, airman; airwoman
avião [a'vjãw] *m* airplane, plane, *Brit* aeroplane; ***~ de carga*** freight plane; ***~ a jato***, *Port* ***~ a jacto*** jet; ***~ de guerra*** warplane
aviar [a'vjaɾ] ⟨1g⟩ (*despachar*) prepare for dispatch; *cliente* attend to; *receita* fill, *Brit* make up
aviário [a'vjaɾiu] **1** *m* aviary **2** *adj* bird *atr*; ***gripe** f **aviária*** bird flu
avicultor [avikuw'toɾ] *m* poultry farmer
avicultura [avikuw'tuɾa] *f* poultry farming
avidamente [avida'mẽtʃi] *adv* eagerly
avidez [avi'des] *f* eagerness; (*cobiça*) greed
ávido ['avidu] *adj* avid, eager; (*cobiçoso*) greedy
aviltante [aviw'tãtʃi] *adj* demeaning
avisado [avi'zadu] *adj* wise; ***mal ~*** unwise, misguided
avisar [avi'zaɾ] ⟨1a⟩ *v/t* notify, let know; ***~ de*** draw one's attention to; *perigo* warn of
aviso [a'vizu] *m* notice; (*ofício*) notification; (*advertência*) warning; ***sem ~*** without warning, without notice; ***~ prévio*** advance notice; ***~ de recepção*** acknowledgement of receipt
avistar [avis'taɾ] ⟨1a⟩ *v/t* catch sight of; **avistar-se** *v/r* meet
avivar [avi'vaɾ] ⟨1a⟩ *v/t* revive *tb fig*
avô [a'vo] *m* grandfather
avo ['avo] *m* MAT ***um quinze ~s*** one fifteenth
avó [a'vɔ] *f* grandmother
avós [a'vɔs] *mpl* grandparents
à-vontade [avõ'tadʒi] *m* casualness
avulso [a'vuwsu] *adj* (*solto*) loose; (*em separado*) separate, detached
avultado [avuw'tadu] *adj* bulky
axila [a'ksila] *f* armpit
axioma [a'ksjoma] *m* axiom
azar [a'zaɾ] *m* (*má sorte*) bad luck; ***jogo** m **de ~*** game of chance
azarado [aza'radu] *adj* unlucky
azedar [aze'daɾ] ⟨1c⟩ *v/i* go sour; *fig* grow embittered
azeda [a'zeda] *f* sorrel
azedar-se [aze'daɾsi] ⟨1c⟩ *v/r* turn sour; *fig* get irritated
azedo [a'zedu] *adj* sour; *fig* bad-tempered; (*irritado*) irritated, grumpy
azeite [a'zejtʃi] *m* olive oil

azeitona [azej'tona] *f* olive
azeitonado [azejto'nadu] *adj* greenish
Azerbaijão [azerbaj'ʒãw] *m* Azerbaijan
azeviche [aze'viʃi] *adj* jet-black
azevinho [aze'viɲu] *m* holly
azia [a'zia] *f* MED heartburn
azul [a'zuw] ⟨*pl* azuis⟩ **1** *adj* blue; **~ *celeste*** sky-blue **2** *m* blue
azulado [azu'ladu] *adj* bluish
azulejo [azu'leʒu] *m* (glazed) tile
azul-marinho [azuwma'riɲu] *adj* navy blue

B

baba ['baba] *f* dribble
babá [ba'ba] *f* nanny
babado [ba'badu] *m* frill
babaca [ba'baka] *m* idiot; ***seu ~!*** you idiot!
babador [baba'dor] *m* bib
babar [ba'bar] ⟨1b⟩ **1** *v/t* dribble on **2** *v/i* dribble; **babar-se** *v/r* dribble; **~ *por alguém*** drool over s.o.
babuíno [ba'bwinu] *m* baboon
bacalhau [baka'ʎaw] *m* (salt) cod; **~ *fresco*** (fresh) cod
bacalhoada [baka'ʎwada] *f* salt cod stew
bacana [ba'kana] *Bras fam* **1** *adj* great **2** *m/f* ***ele é um ~*** he's loaded
bacanal [baka'naw] *m* orgy
Bacharelado [baʃare'ladu] *m* bachelor's degree
bacia [ba'sia] *f* bowl, basin; ANAT pelvis
baço ['basu] **1** *m* ANAT spleen **2** *adj* (*sem brilho*) dull, matt
bactéria [bak'tɛrja] *f* bacterium, germ
bacteriologia [bakterilo'ʒia] *f* bacteriology
badalada [bada'lada] **1** *f sino*: stroke **2** *adj* fêted, talked about
badalar [bada'lar] ⟨1b⟩ *v/t* ring; (*dar à língua*) discuss
bafejar [bafe'ʒar] ⟨1d⟩ blow
bafo ['bafu] *m* (bad) breath; (*calor*) warmth
bagaço [ba'gasu] *m de frutos* pulp; *Port* brandy
bagageiro [baga'ʒejru] *m* luggage rack; *de teto* roof rack; *pessoa* porter
bagagem [ba'gaʒẽ] *f* luggage; **~ *de mão*** hand luggage; ***carrinho m de ~*** baggage cart, *Brit* luggage trolley; ***guiché m de ~*** baggage checkroom desk, *Brit* left luggage counter; ***seguro m de ~*** travel insurance
bagatela [baga'tɛla] *f* trinket
bago ['bagu] *m* berry; (*de chumbo*) pellet
bagunça [ba'gũsa] *f* mess; ***estar uma ~*** *quarto*, *gaveta* be a mess
bagunçado [bagũ'sadu] *adj* messy
baía [ba'ia] *f* bay
baila ['bajla] *f* ***vir à ~*** come up; *fam* ***trazer à ~*** bring up
bailado [baj'ladu] *m* ballet
bailar [baj'lar] ⟨1a⟩ *v/i* dance
bailarino [bajla'rinu] *m*, **-a** *f* dancer
baile ['bajli] *m* dance, ball
bainha [ba'iɲa] *f espada*: sheath; *saia*: hem; *calças*: cuff, *Brit* turn-up
baioneta [bejo'neta] *f* bayonet
bairro ['bajhu] *m* district, neighborhood, *Brit* neighbourhood; **~ *antigo*** old town
baixa ['bajʃa] *f preço*: reduction; *bolsa*: low; MED, MIL ***dar ~*** discharge; ***estar de ~*** to be on leave
baixa-mar [bajʃa'mar] *f Port* low tide
baixar [baj'ʃar] ⟨1a⟩ **1** *v/t* lower; (*tirar*) take down, carry down; INFORM download; *preços* drop; **~ *os faróis*** dip the headlights **2** *v/i* sink, dip; *juros*, *avião* go down; *preços etc* fall; *ter-*

reno drop; **baixar-se** *v/r* bend down; *fig* lower oneself
baixeza [baj'ʃeza] *f* meanness
baixinho [baj'ʃiɲu] **1** *adj* short **2** *adv* quietly
baixo ['bajʃu] **1** *adj* low *tb fig*; *pessoa* short; *rio* shallow; *olhar* lowered; *voz* quiet; ***baixa temporada*** low season **2** *m* MÚS bass **3** *adv* ***em ~*** low down, below; ***em (por) ~ de*** underneath; ***falar ~*** speak quietly; ***fala ~!*** keep your voice down
bajular [baʒu'laɾ] ⟨1a⟩ *v/t* suck up to
bala ['bala] *f* bullet, *Bras* boiled sweet
balada [ba'lada] *f* ballad
balança [ba'lãsa] *f* scales; ***~ comercial*** balance of trade
balançar [balã'saɾ] ⟨1p⟩ balance; (*oscilar*) shake; *em cadeira* rock; *quadris* sway, swing
balanço [ba'lãsu] *m* swing; (*oscilação*) swinging motion; ECON balance sheet; (*solavanco*) jolt; ***~ ecológico*** eco-balance; ***~ geral*** balance sheet
balão [ba'lãw] *m* balloon
balaustrada [balaws'tɾada] *f* balustrade
balbuciar [bawbu'sjaɾ] ⟨1g⟩ babble, gurgle
balbúrdia [baw'buɾdʒia] *f* hubbub
balcão [baw'kãw] *m* counter; *de informações* desk; *teatro*: circle
Balcãs [baw'kãs] *mpl* ***os ~*** the Balkans
balconista [bawko'nista] *m/f* clerk, *Brit* shop assistant
balde ['bawdʒi] *m* bucket
baldeação [bawdʒja'sãw] *f Bras* ***fazer ~*** change trains
baldio [baw'dʒiu] **1** *adj* fallow; (*vão*) pointless **2** ***terra*** *f* ***baldia*** wasteland
balé [ba'lɛ] *m* ballet
baleia [ba'leja] *f* whale
balear [ba'ljaɾ] ⟨1l⟩ *v/t* shoot
balir [ba'liɾ] ⟨3b⟩ bleat
balido [ba'lidu] *m* bleating
baliza [ba'liza] *f* (*bóia*) buoy; (*estaca*) post
balneário [baw'njaɾiu] *m* seaside resort
balofo [ba'lofu] *adj* fluffy; (*gordo*) plump
baloiçar [baloj'saɾ] ⟨1p⟩ swing
baloiço [ba'lojsu] *m Port* swing; *movimento* swinging
balsa ['bawsa] *f* raft; *barca* ferry
bálsamo ['bawsamu] *m* balm
báltico ['bawtʃiku] *adj* Baltic
baluarte [ba'lwaɾtʃi] *m* bulwark, rampart
bambo ['bãbu] *adj* slack; *pernas* limp
bambolear [bãbo'ljaɾ] ⟨1l⟩ **1** *v/t* (*oscilar*) swing; (*tremer*) shake **2** *v/i* sway; *coisa* wobble
bambu [bã'bu] *m* bamboo
banal [ba'naw] *adj* banal
banalidade [banali'dadʒi] *f* banality
banana [ba'nana] *f* banana
bananeira [bana'nejɾa] *f* banana tree
banca ['bãka] *f* bench; ***~ de jornais*** newsstand
bancada [bã'kada] *f de cozinha* counter; POL faction, *Brit* bench
bancário [bã'kaɾiu] **1** *adj* bank *atr*; ***conta*** *f* ***bancária*** bank account **2** *m*, **-a** *f* bank employee
bancarrota [bãka'hota] *f* bankruptcy; ***ir a ~*** go bankrupt
banco[1] ['bãku] *m móvel*: bench; (*escabelo*) stool; NÁUT ***~ de areia*** sandbank; ***~ dos réus*** witness stand, *Brit* witness box; AUTO ***~ traseiro*** back seat
banco[2] ['bãku] *m* FIN bank; INFORM ***~ de dados*** database; ***~ de espermas*** sperm bank; ***~ genético*** gene pool; ***Banco Mundial*** World Bank; ***~ de sangue*** blood bank
banda ['bãda] *f* band; (*faixa*) sash; *Port* ***~ desenhada*** cartoon; ***~ larga*** broadband; CINE ***~ sonora*** soundtrack
bandeira [bã'dejɾa] *f* flag, banner; *fam* ***dar ~*** give oneself away
bandeirada [bãde'ɾada] *f táxi*: taxi fare
bandeja [bã'deʒa] *f* tray
bandido [bã'dʒidu] *m* bandit, robber
bando ['bãdu] *m* group; *pássaros*: flock
bandolim [bãdo'lĩ] *m* MÚS mandolin
bangalô [bãga'lo] *m* bungalow
bangue-bangue [bãge'bãgi] *m* Western

banha ['baɲa] *f* lard, fat
banhar [ba'ɲaɾ] ⟨1a⟩ *v/t* wet; *na água* soak; **banhar-se** *v/r* to bathe
banheira [ba'ɲejɾa] *f* bathtub, *Brit* bath
banheiro [ba'ɲejɾu] *m Bras* bathroom; *Port* lifeguard; ~ ***de homens*** men's room
banhista [ba'ɲista] *m/f* bather
banho ['baɲu] *m* bath; (*chuveiro*) shower; ***tomar*** ~ take a bath / shower; ***tomar*** ~ ***de sol*** sunbathe; ~ ***de espuma*** bubble bath
banho-maria [baɲoma'ria] *m* bain-marie
banir [ba'niɾ] ⟨3a⟩ banish
banjo ['bãʒu] *m* banjo
banqueiro [bã'kejɾu] *m* banker
banqueta [bã'keta] *f* stool
banquete [bãketʃi] *m* banquet; *fig* feast
bapt... *Port* → ***bat...***
baque ['baki] *m* thud; (*contratempo*) setback; (*queda*) fall
baquear [ba'kjaɾ] ⟨1l⟩ topple over
bar [baɾ] *m* bar
barafunda [baɾa'fũda] *f* (*barulho*) racket; (*confusão*) jumble
baralhada [baɾa'ʎada] *f* jumble, confusion
baralhar [baɾa'ʎaɾ] ⟨1b⟩ *cartas* shuffle; (*confundir*) confuse
baralho [ba'ɾaʎu] *m* deck of cards; ***cortar o*** ~ cut the cards
barão [ba'ɾãw] *m* baron
barata [ba'ɾata] *f* cockroach
barato [ba'ɾatu] **1** *adj* cheap **2** *m fam* ***a festa foi um*** ~ the party was great
barba ['baɾba] *f* beard; ***fazer a*** ~ shave; ~***s do gato*** cat's whiskers; *fam* ***nas*** ~***s de*** under the nose of
barbante [baɾ'bãtʃi] *m Bras* string
barbaridade [baɾbaɾi'dadʒi] *f* cruelty; ***que*** ~***!*** that's terrible!
bárbaro ['baɾbaɾu] **1** *adj* barbaric **2** *m* barbarian
barbatana [baɾba'tana] *f* fin
barbeador [baɾbja'doɾ] *m* shaver
barbear [baɾ'bjaɾ] ⟨1l⟩ *v/t* shave; **barbear-se** *v/r* shave
barbearia [baɾbja'ɾia] *f* barber's shop
barbeiro [baɾ'bejɾu] *m* barber
barbiturato [baɾbitu'ɾatu] *m* barbiturate
barbudo [baɾ'budu] *adj* bearded
barca ['baɾka] *f* ferry; *carga*: barge
barco ['baɾku] *m* boat; ***ir de*** ~ go by boat; ~ ***a remo*** rowboat, *Brit* rowing boat; ~ ***de pesca*** fishing boat; ~ ***a vela*** sailboat, *Brit* sailing boat
barganha [baɾ'gaɲa] *f* bargain
barítono [ba'ɾitunu] *m* baritone
barlavento [baɾla'vẽtu] *m* windward
barômetro, *Port* **barómetro** [ba'ɾometɾu] *m* barometer
baronesa [baɾo'neza] *f* baroness
barqueiro [baɾ'kejɾu] *m* boatman
barra ['baha] *f ferro, ouro, sabão*: bar; *bicicleta*: crossbar; *pontuação*: slash; (*alavanca*) lever; ***segurar a*** ~ hold out; INFORM ~ ***de espaço*** space bar; ~ ***fixa*** high bar; ~***s*** *pl* ***paralelas*** parallel bars; ~ ***transversal*** crossbar
barraca [ba'haka] *f* tent; *bebidas, jornais*: kiosk, stand; (*casinha*) hut
barracão [baha'kãw] *m* shed
barragem [ba'haʒẽ] *f* (*barreira*) barrier; (*represa*) dam
barranco [ba'hãku] *m* ravine, gully
barrar [ba'haɾ] ⟨1b⟩ bar
barreira [ba'hejɾa] *f* barrier; *em corrida* hurdle; *em futebol* wall; ~ ***da língua*** language barrier; ~ ***de segurança*** security barrier
barrete [ba'hetʃi] *m* cap
barricada [bahi'kada] *f* barricade
barriga [ba'higa] *f* belly, stomach; ***fazer*** ~ bulge; ~ ***da perna*** calf
barrigudo [bahi'gudu] *adj* potbellied, paunchy
barril [ba'hiw] *m* barrel
barro ['bahu] *m* (*argila*) clay; (*lama*) mud
barroco [ba'hoku] *adj* baroque
barulhento [baɾu'ʎẽtu] *adj* noisy
barulho [ba'ɾuʎu] *m* noise; (*tumulto*) racket; ***fazer*** ~ make a racket
base ['bazi] *f* base; (*fundamento*) basis; (*alicerces*) foundation; ***na*** ~ ***de*** based on; ***com base em*** ~ on the basis of; ***sem*** ~ groundless; ~ ***aérea*** airbase; MIL ~ ***militar*** military base; ~ ***naval*** naval base; ~ ***de referência*** point of reference

B

basear [ba'zjar] ⟨1l⟩ *v/t* base; **basear-se** *v/r* ~ **em** be based on
basebol [bejze'bɔw] *m* baseball
basicamente [bazika'mẽtʃi] *adv* basically
básico ['baziku] **1** *adj* basic **2** *m* **o ~** the basics
basílica [ba'zilika] *f* basilica
basquetebol [baskɛtʃi'bɔw] *m* basketball
basta ['basta] *m* **dar um ~ em** put a stop to; **~!** that'll do!
bastante [bas'tãtʃi] **1** *adj* enough; (*muito*) quite a lot of **2** *adv* enough; *trabalhar, chover* a lot; *quente, velho* very
bastão [bas'tãw] *m* stick; **~ de beisebol** baseball bat; **~ de esqui** skipole
bastar [bas'tar] ⟨1b⟩ be enough; **basta!** that's enough!
bastardo [bas'tardu] *m/f* bastard
bastidores [bastʃi'doris] *mpl* wings; **nos ~** in the wings; **por trás dos ~** behind the scenes
basto ['bastu] *adj* (*espesso*) thick; (*denso*) dense
bata ['bata] *f* smock
batalha [ba'taʎa] *f* battle; **~ verbal** war of words; **cavalo** *m* **de ~** war horse
batalhão [bata'ʎãw] *m* battalion
batalhar [bata'ʎar] ⟨1a⟩ *v/i* battle, struggle
batata [ba'tata] *f* potato; **~ assada** jacket potato; **~ doce** sweet potato; **~s** *pl* **fritas** French fries, *Brit tb* chips; **~s** *pl* **cozidas** boiled potatoes
batatinhas fritas [batatʃiɲas'fritas] *fpl* chips, *Brit* crisps
bate-bola [batʃi'bɔla] *m* ESP practice game, knock-about
batedeira [bate'dejra] *f* whisk; **~ elétrica** mixer, blender
batedor [bate'dor] *m*, **-a** *f Bras* **~ de carteira** pickpocket
batente [ba'tẽtʃi] *m de porta* doorway; *madeira* doorpost; *fam* **no ~** at work
bate-papo [batʃi'papu] *m Bras* chat
bater [ba'ter] ⟨2b⟩ **1** *v/t* hit; *tapete etc* beat; *pé* stamp; *foto* take; *asas* flap; (*datilografar*) type; **ele batia os dentes** his teeth were chattering; **~ palmas** clap; **~ a porta** slam the door; *Bras* **~ papo** chat; **~ o pênalti** take the penalty **2** *v/i porta* slam; *coração* beat; *sol* beat down
bateria [bate'ria] *f* ELÉT battery; MÚS drums; **~ de cozinha** set of kitchenware
batida [ba'tʃida] *f à porta* knock; *coração*: beat; *polícia*: raid; *bebida cocktail made of cachaça and fruit juice*
batido [ba'tʃidu] **1** *adj caminho* beaten; *roupa* worn; *assunto* hackneyed **2** *m* **~ de leite** milkshake
batina [ba'tʃina] *f* robe
batismo [ba'tʃizmu] *m* baptism
batizado [batʃi'zadu] *m* christening
batizar [batʃi'zar] ⟨1a⟩ baptize, christen
batom [ba'tõ] *m*, **bâton** [ba'tõ] *m* lipstick
batucada [batu'kada] *f* samba percussion group
batucar [batu'kar] ⟨1n⟩ *v/i* drum in a samba rhythm
batuta [ba'tuta] *f* MÚS baton
baú [ba'u] *m* chest, trunk
baunilha [baw'niʎa] *f* vanilla
bazar [ba'zar] *m* bazaar
bazófia [ba'zɔfja] *f* bragging, boasting
beato ['bjatu] *adj* blessed; *pej* sanctimonious
bêbado ['bebadu] **1** *adj* drunk **2** *m*, **-a** *f* drunk
bebê [be'be] *m* baby; **ela vai ter um ~** she's going to have a baby
bebedeira [bebe'dejra] *f* drinking binge; (*embriaguez*) drunkenness
bêbedo ['bebedu] → **bêbado**
bebedouro [bebe'dowru] *m* drinking fountain
beber [be'ber] ⟨2c⟩ *v/t & v/i* drink; **~ em excesso** drink to excess
bebericar [beberi'kar] ⟨1n⟩ *v/t* sip
bebida [be'bida] *f* drink; **~ alcoólica / sem álcool** alcoholic / non-alcoholic drink
beco ['beku] *m* alley; **~ sem saída** dead end *tb fig*
bedelho [be'deʎu] *m* **meter o ~ em** stick one's nose into
bege ['bɛʒi] *adj* beige
beiço ['bejsu] *m* lip; **fazer ~** pout

beija-flor [bejʒa'floɾ] *m* ⟨*pl* ~ es⟩ humming bird
beijar [bej'ʒaɾ] ⟨1a⟩ *v/t* kiss; **beijar-se** *v/r* kiss
beijinho [bej'ʒiɲu] *m* peck, little kiss
beijo ['bejʒu] *m* kiss
beijoca [bejʒo'ka] *f fam* kiss
beijocar [bejʒo'kaɾ] ⟨1n, *Stv* 1e⟩ *v/t fam* kiss
beira ['bejɾa] *f* edge; *rio*: bank; ***à ~ de*** at the edge of; *fig* ***estar à ~ de*** be on the verge of
beirar [bej'ɾaɾ] ⟨1a⟩ *v/t* verge on
beira-mar [bejɾa'maɾ] *f* seaside; ***à ~*** on the beach
beisebol [bejze'bɔw] *m* baseball
belas-artes [bɛla'zaɾtʃis] *fpl* ***as ~*** fine arts; ***Academia*** *f* ***das Belas-Artes*** Academy of Fine Arts
beldade [bew'dadʒi] *f* beauty; ***ela é uma ~*** she is a beauty
beleza [be'leza] *f* beauty; ***que ~!*** this is wonderful!
belga ['bɛwga] **1** *adj* Belgian **2** *m/f* Belgian
Bélgica ['bɛwʒika] *f* Belgium
beliche [be'liʃi] *m* bunk; NÁUT berth; (*camarote*) cabin
bélico ['bɛliku] *adj atitude* bellicose, belligerent
beliscão [belis'kãw] *m* pinch
beliscar [belis'kaɾ] ⟨1n⟩ pinch; *comida* nibble
belo ['bɛlu] *adj* beautiful
bel-prazer [bɛlpɾa'zeɾ] *m* ***a seu ~*** at your convenience
bem [bẽ] **1** *adv* well; (*muito*) very; (*bastante*) quite; ***~ ..., mas*** well, ..., but; (***se***) ***~ que*** although; ***ainda ~!*** thank goodness!; ***por ~*** for the good; ***~ como*** as well as; ***estou ~*** I am well; ***está ~!*** ok!; ***~ feito!*** it serves you / him / her right!; ***gente ~*** well-to-do people; ***fica ~ ali*** it's right there; ***eu ~ que gostaria*** I'd really like to; ***~ em cima*** right at the top **2** *m* good; (*benefício*) benefit; *fig* ***meu ~*** my love; ***homem*** *m* ***de ~*** gentleman; ***querer ~ a alguém*** wish s.o. well **3** *pl* ***bens*** belongings; COM goods; (*fortuna*) assets; ***bens*** *pl* ***de consumo*** consumer goods; ***bens móveis*** real estate
bem-arrumado [bẽahu'madu] *adj* elegant
bem-comportado [bẽkõpoɾ'tadu] *adj* well-behaved
bem-conhecido [bẽkuɲe'sidu] *adj* well-known
bem-disposto [bẽdʒis'postu] *adj* on good form
bem-estar [bẽes'taɾ] *m* well-being
bem-feito [bẽ'fejtu] *adj* well-made
bemhumorado [bẽumu'ɾadu] *adj* good-tempered
bemintencionado [bẽĩtẽsjo'nadu] *adj* well-meaning
bem-passado [bẽpa'sadu] *adj* GASTR well done
bem-sucedido [bẽsuse'dʒidu] *adj* successful
bem-vindo [bẽ'vĩdu] *adj* welcome
bem-visto [bẽ'vistu] *adj* well thought of
bênção ['bẽsãw] *f* ⟨*pl* -ãos⟩ blessing
bendito [bẽ'dʒitu] *adj* blessed
bendizer [bẽ'dʒizeɾ] ⟨2t⟩ *v/t* bless
beneficência [benefi'sẽsja] *f* kindness, charity
beneficente [benefi'sẽtʃi] *adj* charitable
beneficiar [benefi'sjaɾ] ⟨1g⟩ **1** *v/t* (*favorecer*) benefit; (*melhorar*) improve; (*dar*) ***~ alguém com algo*** present sth to s.o. **2** *v/i* ***~ de*** (*ou* ***com***) benefit from; (*gozar*) enjoy
beneficiário [benefi'sjaɾiu] *m*, **-a** *f* beneficiary
benefício [bene'fisiu] *m* benefit; ***em ~ de*** in aid of
benéfico [be'nɛfiku] *adj* beneficial
benevolência [benevo'lẽsja] *f* benevolence
benevolente [benevo'lẽtʃi] *adj* benevolent
benévolo [be'nɛvulu] *adj* kind
benfeitor [bẽfej'toɾ] *m*, **-a** *f* benefactor
bengala [bẽŋ'gala] *f* walking stick
benigno [be'nignu] *adj* kind; (*suave*) gentle; MED benign
bens [bẽs] *pl* → ***bem***
bento [bẽtu] *adj* blessed, holy
benzer [bẽ'zeɾ] ⟨2a⟩ *v/t* (*consagrar*)

bless; **benzer-se** *v/r* cross oneself
berço ['bersu] *m* cradle, crib; *fig* good breeding; *fig* ***nascer em ~ de ouro*** be born with a silver spoon in one's mouth
beringela [berĩ'ʒɛla] *f* egg-plant, *Brit* aubergine
berma ['berma] *f Port* berm, *Brit* roadside
bermuda [ber'muda] *f* Bermuda shorts, Bermudas
Bermudas [ber'mudas] *fpl* ***as ~*** Bermuda
berrante [be'hãtʃi] *adj* flashy, loud
berrar [be'har] ⟨1c⟩ shout, wail; *carneiro* bleat
berro ['bɛhu] *m* shout; *carneiro*: bleating; ***~s*** *pl* (*clamor*) cries; ***aos ~s*** shouting
besouro [be'zoru] *m* beetle
besta ['besta] **1** *f* beast; *fam pessoa* fool; ***~ de carga / tiro*** beast of burden **2** *adj* stupid, silly
besteira [bes'tejra] *f fam* nonsense
bestial [bes'tʃiaw] *adj* (*animalesco*) bestial; (*bruto*) rough; *fam* cool
bestialidade [bestʃiali'dadʒi] *f* bestiality
besuntar [bezũ'tar] ⟨1a⟩ *v/t* smear
betão [be'tãw] *m* ⟨*sem pl*⟩ *m Port* concrete
beterraba [bete'haba] *f* red beet, *Brit* beetroot
betoneira [beto'nejra] *f* cement mixer
bétula ['bɛtula] *f* birch
betume [be'tumi] *m* asphalt
bexiga [be'ʃiga] *f* ANAT bladder; *de criança* balloon
bezerro [be'zehu] *m* calf
bibelô [bibe'lo] *m* ornament
biberão [bibe'rãw] *m Port* (baby's) bottle
bíblia ['biblia] *f* Bible
bíblico ['bibliku] *adj* biblical
bibliografia [bibliogra'fia] *f* bibliography
biblioteca [biblio'tɛka] *f* library
bibliotecário [bibliote'kariu] *m*, **-a** *f* librarian
bica[1] ['bika] *f* faucet, *Brit* tap; ***água f de ~*** branch water, *Brit* tap water
bica[2] ['bika] *f Port fam café*: espresso
bicada [bi'kada] *f* peck
bicentenário [bisẽte'nariu] *m* bicentennial, *Brit* bicentenary
bíceps ['biseps] *m* ⟨*pl inv*⟩ biceps
bicha ['biʃa] *f* (*parasita*) worm; *Port* line, *Brit* queue; ***fazer ~*** line up, *Brit* form a queue; ***meter-se na ~*** get in line, *Brit* queue up; *Bras fam* fairy, fag
bichinho [bi'ʃiɲu] *m* ***~ de pelúcia*** soft toy
bicho ['biʃu] *m fam* animal; *inseto* bug; ***que ~ te mordeu?*** what's gotten into you?
bicho-da-seda [biʃoda'seda] *m* silkworm
bicicleta [bisi'klɛta] *f* bicycle; ***ir (andar) de ~*** cycle, go by bike; ***~ de corridas*** racing bike; ***~ ergométrica*** exercise bike
bico ['biku] *m pássaro*: beak; (*ponta*) point; (*extremidade*) end; *bule*: spout; *caneta*: nib; *fam* ***cala o ~!*** shut your mouth!; ***~ de gás*** jet; ***~ do peito*** nipple
bicudo [bi'kudu] *adj* pointed; *fig* tricky
bidê, *Port* **bidé** [bi'de] *m* bidet
bienal [bie'naw] *adj* biennial
bife ['bifi] *m* beef; ***um ~*** a steak; ***~ bem / mal passado*** well done / rare steak; ***~ a cavalo*** *beef steak topped with fried eggs*; ***~ à milanesa*** breaded cutlet; ***~ de porco / peru*** pork / turkey steak
bifurcação [bifurka'sãw] *f* fork
bifurcar-se [bifur'karsi] ⟨1n⟩ *v/r* fork, divide
bigamia [biga'mia] *f* bigamy
bígamo ['bigamu] *adj* **1** bigamous **2** *m*, **-a** *f* bigamist
bigode [bi'gɔdʒi] *m* mustache, *Brit* moustache
bigorna [bi'gɔrna] *f* anvil
bijuteria [biʒute'ria] *f* costume jewelry, *Brit* costume jewellery
bilateral [bilate'raw] *adj* bilateral
bilhão [bi'ʎãw] *m Bras* billion
bilhar [bi'ʎar] *m* billiards *sg*
bilhete [bi'ʎetʃi] *m* ticket; (*papel*) note; ***~ eletrônico*** e-ticket
bilheteria [biʎete'ria] *f* ticket office;

TEAT box office
bilião [bi'ljãw] *m Port* billion
bilíngüe, *Port* **bilingue** [bi'lĩgi] *adj* bilingual
bilioso [bi'ljozu] *adj* bilious; *fig* bad-tempered
bílis ['bilis] *f* bile
binóculo [bi'nɔkulu] *mpl* binoculars; TEAT opera glasses
biocombustível [biokõbus'tʃivew] *m* biofuel
biodegradável [biodegra'davew] *adj* biodegradable
biodiversidade [biodʒiveɾsi'dadʒi] *f* biodiversity
biografia [bjogɾa'fia] *f* biography
biográfico [bjo'gɾafiku] *adj* biographical
biógrafo ['bjɔgɾafu] *m*, **-a** *f* biographer
biologia [bjolo'ʒia] *f* biology
biológico [bjo'lɔʒiku] *adj* biological
biólogo ['bjɔlogu] *m*, **-a** *f* biologist
biombo ['bjõbu] *m* partition, screen
biométrico [bjo'mɛtriku] *adj* biometric
biópsia ['bjɔpsja] *f* biopsy
bioquímica [bjo'kimika] *f* biochemistry
bioquímico [bjo'kimika] *m*, **-a** *f* biochemist
biotecnologia [biotɛknolo'ʒia] *f* biotechnology
bip(e) ['bip(i)] *m* TEL beep
biquíni [bi'kini] *m* bikini
Birmânia [biɾ'mʌnja] *f* Burma
birra ['biha] *f* (*teima*) obstinacy; (*aversão*) aversion; ***fazer uma ~*** have a tantrum; ***ter ~ a*** dislike
birrento [bi'hẽtu] *adj* obstinate
biruta [bi'ɾuta] *adj* crazy
bis [bis] *adv* ***~!*** encore!
bisavô [biza'vo] *m* great-grandfather
bisavó [biza'vɔ] *f* great-grandmother
bisavós [biza'vɔs] *mpl* great-grandparents
bisbilhotar [bizbiʎo'taɾ] ⟨1e⟩ *v/i* nose around, snoop
bisbilhoteiro [bizbiʎo'tejɾu] **1** *adj* nosey **2** *m*, **-a** *f* snoop
Biscaia [bis'kaja] *f* Bay of Biscay
biscoito [bis'kojtu] *m* cookie, *Brit* biscuit; (*bolacha*) cracker
bisnaga [bis'naga] *f* (*tubo*) tube; *pão*: bread roll
bisneto [bis'nɛtu] *m*, **-a** *f* great-grandchild
bispado [bis'padu] *m* bishopric
bispo ['bispu] *m* REL bishop
bissemanal [bisema'naw] *adj* twice-weekly
bissexto [bi'sestu] *adj* ***ano*** *m* ***~*** leap year
bissexual [bise'kswaw] *adj* bisexual
bisturi [bistu'ɾi] *m* scalpel
bit ['bit] *m* INFORM bit
bitola [bi'tɔla] *f* gage, *Brit* gauge
bizarro [bi'zahu] *adj* bizarre
blasfemar [blasfe'maɾ] ⟨1d⟩ *v/i* blaspheme, curse
blasfêmia, *Port* **blasfémia** [blas'femja] *f* blasphemy; (*praga*) curse
blazer ['blejzeɾ] *m* blazer
blecaute [blɛ'kawtʃi] *m Bras* power cut
blindado [blĩ'dadu] *adj* armored, *Brit* armoured
blindagem [blĩ'daʒẽ] *f* armor (-plating), *Brit* armour(-plating)
bloco ['blɔku] *m* block; POL bloc; ***voto em ~*** block vote; ***~ comercial*** office block; ***~ de notas*** notepad
blog(ue) ['blɔg(i)] *m* INTERNET blog
bloguista [blo'gista] *m/f* blogger
bloquear [blo'kjaɾ] ⟨1l⟩ *v/t* block; (*fechar*) blockade; *conta* freeze; ***~ um cheque*** stop a check
bloqueio [blo'keiu] *m* blockade; (*barricada*) barricade; MED blockage
blusa ['bluza] *f* blouse, top; ***~ de moletom*** sweatshirt
blusão [blu'zãw] *m* jacket
boa ['boa] **1** *adj/f* (→ **bom**); *int* (***essa***) ***é ~!*** *irôn* that's a good one!, yeah right! **2** *f* ZOOL boa constrictor
boas-festas [boas'fɛstas] *fpl* seasons greetings; ***votos*** *mpl* ***de ~*** happy holidays
boas-vindas [boas'vĩdas] *fpl* welcome; ***dar as ~ a alguém*** welcome s.o.
boate ['bwatʃi] *f* nightclub
boato ['bwatu] *m* rumor, *Brit* rumour
bobagem [bo'baʒẽ] *f* nonsense

B

bobina [bo'bina] *f* spool; (*cilindro*) roll
bobo ['bobu] **1** *m* fool **2** *adj* silly, foolish
boca ['boka] *f* mouth; *fogão*: ring; *túnel etc*: entrance; ***de ~ aberta*** dumbfounded, amazed; ***de dar agua na ~*** mouth-watering; ***bater ~*** argue; ***ela é boa ~*** she'll eat anything, she's a good eater; ***~ do gol*** goalmouth
bocadinho [boka'dʒiɲu] *m* little bit; *Port* ***há ~*** a little while ago
bocado [bo'kadu] *m* mouthful; *pedaço*: piece, bit; ***um ~*** quite a lot
bocal [bo'kaw] *m* (*abertura*) mouth; (*tubeira*) nozzle; MÚS mouthpiece
boçal [bo'saw] *adj* coarse, uncouth
bocejar [bose'ʒar] ⟨1d⟩ *v/i* yawn
bocejo [bo'seʒu] *m* yawn
bochecha [bo'ʃeʃa] *f* cheek
bochechar [boʃe'ʃar] ⟨1d⟩ *v/i* rinse one's mouth
bochecho [bo'ʃeʃu] *m* mouth rinse
boda(**s**) ['boda(s)] *f*(*pl*) wedding; ***~ de prata / ouro / diamante*** golden / silver / diamond wedding anniversary
bode ['bɔdʒi] *m* goat; ***~ expiatório*** scapegoat
bodega [bo'dɛga] *f* liquor store, *Brit* off-licence; (*porcaria*) piece of rubbish
body ['bɔdʒi] *m moda*: body stocking
bofetada [bofe'tada] *f*, **bofetão** [bofe'tãw] *m* punch, blow
boi [boj] *m* bullock; ***a passo de ~*** at a snail's pace
bóia ['bɔja] *f* NÁUT buoy; *crianças*: armbands; ***~ de salvação*** lifebelt
boiar [bo'jar] ⟨1k⟩ *v/i* float
boicotar [bojko'tar] ⟨1e⟩ *v/t* boycott
boicote [boj'kɔtʃi] *m* boycott
boina ['bojna] *f* beret
bola ['bɔla] *f* ball; *fam* ***ora ~s!*** oh no!; ***não dar ~ para alguém*** not care about s.o.; ***~ de beisebol*** baseball; ***~ de futebol*** football; ***~ de golfe*** golf ball; ***~ de gude*** marble; ***~ de neve*** snowball; ***~ de tênis*** tennis ball
bolacha [bo'laʃa] *f* cookie; *fig fam* wallop; ***~ de água e sal*** cracker
bolada [bo'lada] *f* jackpot; ***ganhar a ~*** hit the jackpot
bolbo ['bowbu] *m* bulb
boleia [bo'leja] *f* driver's seat; *Port* ***dar ~ a alguém*** give s.o. a ride
boletim [bole'tʃĩ] *m* report; (*informação*) bulletin; (*publicação*) newsletter; ***~ escolar*** report card; ***~ meteorológico*** weather forecast
bolha ['boʎa] *f pele*: blister; *de sabão* bubble
boliche [bo'ʎiɲa] *m* bowling
Bolívia [bo'livja] *f* Bolivia
boliviano [boli'vjanu] **1** *adj* Bolivian **2** *m*, **-a** *f* Bolivian
bolo ['bolu] *m* GASTR cake; *bacalhau etc*: pasty; ***~ de chocolate*** chocolate cake; ***~ de casamento*** wedding cake
bolor [bo'lor] *m* mold, *Brit* mould
bolorento [bolo'rẽtu] *adj* moldy, *Brit* mouldy
bolota [bo'lɔta] *f* acorn
bolsa ['bowsa] *f* (*carteira*) wallet; (*mala de mão*) purse, *Brit* handbag; UNIV ***~*** (***de estudo***) scholarship; ***~ de mercadorias*** commodities market; FIN ***~ de valores*** stock exchange; ***~ de viagem*** travel bag
bolseiro [bow'sejru] *m*, **-a** *f Port* scholarship student, scholar
bolsista [bow'sista] *m/f* scholarship holder, scholar
bolso ['bowsu] *m* pocket; ***de ~*** pocket-sized; ***~ de trás*** back pocket; ***meter a mão no ~*** put one's hand in one's pocket, give generously
bom [bõ] *adj* good; *tempo* fine; ***ficou ~*** it looks good; ***acho ~*** I think it's best; ***ele não está ~ (da cabeça)!*** he's not right in the head!; ***~ dia*** good morning; ***~, agora chega!*** ok, that's enough!
bomba ['bõba] *f* pump; MIL bomb; *fig* bombshell; ***~ de gasolina*** gas pump, *Brit* petrol pump; *Port* gas station, *Brit* petrol station; ***~ de incêndio*** fire extinguisher
bombar [bõ'bar] ⟨1a⟩ *v/i fam* ***~ em*** flunk, bomb
bombardear [bõbar'dʒiar] ⟨1l⟩ *v/t* bombard, bomb; ***~ com perguntas*** bombard with questions
bombardeio [bõbar'deiu] *m* bombardment, bombing

bombardeiro [bõbar'dejru] *m* bomber
bomba-relógio [bõbahe'lɔʒiu] *f* time-bomb
bombear [bõ'bjar] ⟨1l⟩ *v/t* pump
bombeiro [bõ'bejru] *m* fireman; ***os ~s*** the fire department, *Brit* the fire brigade
bombom [bõ'bõ] *m* chocolate
bombordo [bõ'bɔrdu] *m* NÁUT port
bonança [bo'nãsa] *f* fine weather; *fig* calm
bondade [bõ'dadʒi] *f* kindness, goodness; ***tenha a ~ de fazer ...*** be so kind as to do ...
bonde ['bõdʒi] *m Bras* cable car; *na rua* streetcar, *Brit* tram
bondoso [bõ'dozu] *adj* kind
boné [bo'nɛ] *m* cap
boneca [bo'nɛka] *f* doll
bonificação [bonifika'sãw] *f* bonus; ***~ por horas extraordinárias*** overtime
bonito [bo'nitu] *adj mulher* pretty; *homem* handsome; *dia, casa* lovely
bônus, *Port* **bónus** ['bonus] *m* ⟨*pl inv*⟩ bonus
bonzinho ['bõ'ziɲu] *adj* goody-goody
boquiaberto [bokja'bɛrtu] *adj* open-mouthed, flabbergasted
boquilha [bo'kiʎa] *f* cigarette holder
borboleta [borbo'leta] *f* butterfly
borbulha [bor'buʎa] *f* bubble; *pele*: pimple
borbulhar [borbu'ʎar] ⟨1a⟩ *v/i* (*ferver*) simmer, bubble; (*brotar*) sprout
borda ['bɔrda] *f rio*: bank; (*aresta*) edge; (*margem*) border; ***~ do passeio*** curb, *Brit* kerb
bordado [bor'dadu] *m* embroidery
bordar [bor'dar] ⟨1e⟩ *v/t* embroider; (*orlar*) border
bordel [bor'dɛw] *m* brothel
bordo ['bɔrdu] *m* NÁUT side; ***a ~*** on board
bordoada [bor'dwada] *f* ***dar uma ~ em*** hit with a stick
borla ['bɔrla] *f* tassel; ***de*** (*ou* ***à***) ***~*** tasselled
borra ['boha] *f* dregs
borracha [bo'haʃa] *f material*: rubber; *utensílio*: eraser, *Brit* rubber
borracheiro [boha'ʃejru] *m* tire fitter, *Brit* tyre fitter
borrão [bo'hãw] *m tinta*: blot; (*rascunho*) rough draft; *fig* ***é tudo um ~*** it's all a blur
borrar [bo'har] ⟨1e⟩ *v/t* smudge; *fig* blur; (*riscar*) cross out; (*sujar*) dirty
borrasca [bo'haska] *f* squall; *fig* (*tumulto*) storm
borrifar [bohi'far] ⟨1a⟩ *v/t* spray; *levemente* sprinkle; ***~ algo com algo*** spray / sprinkle sth with sth
borrifo [bo'hifu] *m agua*: spray
Bósnia ['bɔznja] *f* Bosnia
bosque ['bɔski] *m* wood
bota ['bɔta] *f* boot; *fam fig* ***bater as ~s*** kick the bucket; ***~ alta*** high-heeled boots; ***~ de borracha*** rubber boots, *Brit* Wellington boots; ***~ de esqui*** ski boots; ***~ de montar*** riding boots
bota-fora [bota'fɔra] *m* farewell party
botânica [bo'tʌnika] *f* botany
botânico [bo'tʌniku] **1** *adj* botanical **2** *m*, **-a** *f* botanist
botão [bo'tãw] *m* button; (*maçaneta*) knob; BOT bud; ***~ -de-ouro*** buttercup
botar [bo'tar] ⟨1e⟩ *v/t* put; ***~ para fora*** get off one's chest; (*vomitar*) bring up
bote ['bɔtʃi] *m* boat; ***~ salva-vidas*** lifeboat
botija [bo'tʃiʒa] *f gás*: cannister; *água quente*: pitcher, *Brit* jug
botina [bo'tʃina] *f* ankle
boutique [bu'tʃiki] *f* boutique
bovino [bo'vinu] *adj* bovine; ***gado*** *m* ***~*** cattle
boxe ['bɔksi] *m* boxing
boxeador [boksja'dor] *m* boxer
boxear [bo'ksjar] ⟨1l⟩ *v/i* box
boxes ['bɔksis] *mpl* pits
braçadeira [brasa'dejra] *f* armband; *suor*: sweatband; (*argola*) bracket
bracejar [brase'ʒar] ⟨1d⟩ wave one's arms
bracelete [brase'letʃi] *f* bracelet
braço ['brasu] *m* arm *tb da cadeira*; *fig* (*trabalhador*) hand; *fig* ***o ~ direito*** right-hand man; ***cadeira*** *f* ***de ~s*** armchair; ***de ~ dado*** arm in arm; ***enfiar o ~*** (***no ~ de***) link arms; ***receber***

de ~s abertos welcome with open arms; *fig* ***dar o ~ a torcer*** give in
bradar [bra'dar] ⟨1b⟩ *v/i* shout, yell
brado ['bradu] *m* cry; (*gritaria*) shouting
braguilha [bra'giʎa] *f* fly, flies
branco ['brãku] **1** *adj* white; (*vazio*) blank; ***pão*** *m* ***~*** white bread; ***cheque*** *m* ***em ~*** blank check, *Brit* blank cheque; ***me deu um ~*** my mind went blank; ***passar a noite em ~*** have a sleepless night **2** *m* blank; ***~ do ovo*** egg white **3** *m*, **-a** white man / woman
brancura [brã'kura] *f* whiteness
brando ['brãdu] *adj* gentle; (*suave*) soft; *tempo* mild; (*que cede*) lenient
branquear [brã'kjar] ⟨1l⟩ **1** *v/t* whiten; *roupa* bleach **2** *v/i* blanche, turn white
brasa ['braza] *f* hot coal; (*cinza*) ember; ***feito na ~*** charcoal grilled; ***estar*** (*ou* ***andar***) ***sobre ~s*** be on tenterhooks
brasão [bra'zãw] *m* coat of arms
braseiro [bra'zejru] *m* brazier
Brasil [bra'ziw] *m* Brazil; ***no ~*** in Brazil
brasileiro [brazi'lejru] **1** *adj* Brazilian **2** *m*, **-a** *f* Brazilian
Brasília [bra'zilja] *f* Brasilia
bravio [bra'viu] *adj* wild; (*fogoso*) ferocious; *clima* severe
bravo ['bravu] **1** *adj* (*corajoso*) brave; (*furioso*) angry; *animal* wild, ferocious; *clima* stormy **2** *m* brave man
bravura [bra'vura] *f* (*coragem*) courage, bravery; (*fúria*) anger; (*ferocidade*) ferocity
brecha ['brɛʃa] *f* crack, slit; *na lei* loophole; (*abertura*) gap, opening; ***abrir uma ~*** make room
brega ['brɛga] *adj fam* tacky, outdated
breu [brew] *m* tar, pitch; ***escuro como ~*** pitch black
breve ['brɛvi] **1** *adv* ***até ~*** see you soon; ***em ~*** soon, shortly **2** *adj* short, brief; ***o mais ~ possível*** as soon as possible
brevemente [brɛve'mẽtʃi] *adv* briefly
brevidade [brevi'dadʒi] *f* brevity
briefing ['brifĩ] *m* briefing
briga ['briga] *f* argument; (*pancadaria*) fight
brigada [bri'gada] *f* brigade
brigadeiro [briga'dejru] *m* MIL brigadier; (*doce*) chocolate truffle
brigão [bri'gãw], **brigona** [bri'gona] *adj* quarrelsome, pugnacious
brigar [bri'gar] ⟨1o⟩ *v/i* argue; (*lutar*) fight
brilhante [bri'ʎãtʃi] **1** *adj* shiny; *fig* brilliant **2** *m* diamond
brilhar [bri'ʎar] ⟨1a⟩ *v/i* shine *tb fig*; (*luzir*) sparkle
brilho ['briʎu] *m* shine; *estrela* brightness; *fig* splendor, *Brit* splendour
brincadeira [brĩka'dejra] *f* (*graça*) fun; *crianças*: game; ***de ~*** for fun; ***fazer uma ~*** play a trick; ***não é ~*** it's no joke
brincalhão [brĩka'ʎãw] *m*, **brincalhona** [brĩka'ʎona] *f* joker
brincar [brĩ'kar] ⟨1n⟩ *v/i* joke; *criança* play; ***estou brincando*** I'm just kidding
brinco ['brĩku] *m* earring; ***estar um ~*** be spotless
brindar [brĩ'dar] ⟨1a⟩ *v/t* toast; (*presentear*) give a gift to; ***~ alguém com algo*** give s.o. sth as a gift; ***~ à saúde de alguém*** drink to s.o.'s health
brinde ['brĩdʒi] *m* toast; (*presente*) free gift, *Brit* freebie
brinquedo [brĩ'kedu] *m* toy
brio ['briu] *m* self-respect, dignity
brioso [bri'ozu] *adj* self-respecting
brioche [bri'ɔʃi] *m* brioche
brisa ['briza] *f* breeze
britânico [bri'tʌniku] **1** *adj* British **2** *m*, **-a** *f* Briton, *fam* Brit
broca ['brɔka] *f* drill
broche ['brɔʃi] *m* brooch
brochura [bro'ʃura] *f* brochure, pamphlet
brócolos ['brɔkulus] *mpl Port* broccoli *sg*
brócolis ['brɔkulis] *mpl Bras* broccoli *sg*
bronco ['brõku] *adj* stupid
bronquite [brõ'kitʃi] *f* bronchitis
bronze ['brõzi] *m* bronze; ***de ~*** (made of) bronze

bronzeado [brõ'zjadu] bronzed; *pele* tanned, brown
bronzeador [brõzja'dor] *m* suntan lotion
bronzear [brõ'zjar] ⟨1l⟩ *v/i* tan; **bronzear-se** *v/r* get a tan
brotar [bro'tar] ⟨1e⟩ *v/i árvore* spring up; *planta* sprout; *água* flow; *fig* (*surgir*) appear
broto ['brotu] *m* bud, shoot; *pop* ***é um ~*** he / she's a real looker
browser ['brawzer] *m* INFORM browser
broxa ['brɔʃa] *f* (paint)brush
bruma ['bruma] *f* mist
brumoso [bru'mozu] *adj* misty
brusco ['brusku] *adj* brusque; (*súbito*) sudden
brutal [bru'taw] *adj* brutal
brutalidade [brutali'dadʒi] *f* brutality
brutamontes [bruta'mõtʃis] *m* thug
bruto ['brutu] **1** *adj* rough; *fig tb* coarse; ***em ~*** raw, unworked; (*diamante*) uncut; ***peso*** *m* ***~*** gross weight; ***um ~ resfriado*** a bad cold **2** *m* brute
bruxa ['bruʃa] *f* witch
bruxaria [bruʃa'ria] *f* witchcraft
Bruxelas [bru'ʃɛlas] *f* Brussels
bucha ['buʃa] *f* bung; *para fixar parafusos* rawlplug®; BOT sponge
buço ['busu] *m* down
budismo [bu'dʒizmu] *m* Buddhism
bueiro ['bwejru] *m* storm drain
búfalo ['bufalu] *m*, **-a** *f* buffalo
bufar [bu'far] ⟨1a⟩ *v/i* puff, pant; *de raiva etc* snort
bufê [bu'fe] *m* buffet
buganvília [bugã'vilja] *f* BOT bougainvillea
bugiganga [buʒi'gãga] *f* trinket
bulbo ['buwbu] *m* bulb
bule ['buli] *m* tea / coffee pot
Bulgária [buw'garja] *f* Bulgaria
búlgaro ['buwgaru] **1** *adj* Bulgarian **2** *m*, **-a** *f* Bulgarian **3** *m lingua* Bulgarian
bulha ['buʎa] *f* (*briga*) row; (*barulho*) din
bulhar [bu'ʎar] ⟨1a⟩ *v/i* row, argue
bulício [bu'lisiu] *m* (*confusão*) bustle; (*barulho*) rustling
bulimia [buli'mia] *f* MED bulimia
bulir [bu'lir] ⟨3h⟩ **1** *v/i* move, stir; ***~ em*** meddle with; ***~ com*** tease **2** *v/t* move; (*desinquietar*) disturb
bumbum [bũ'bũ] *m fam* bum, bottom
buquê [bu'ke] *m* bouquet
buraco [bu'raku] *m* hole; *agulha*: eye; ***~ da fechadura*** keyhole
burburinho [burbu'riɲu] *m* (*murmúrios*) murmur; (*barulho*) hubbub
burguês [bur'ges] *m*, **burguesa** [bur'geza] *f* middle-class, bourgeois
burguesia [burge'zia] *f* middle class, bourgeoisie
burla ['burla] *f* swindle, fraud; (*zombaria*) mockery
burlar [bur'lar] ⟨1a⟩ *v/t* cheat; (*roubar*) swindle; *lei* get around; *defesas* get past
burlão [bur'lãw] *m* swindler, fraud
burlesco [bur'lesku] *adj* burlesque
burocracia [burokra'sia] *f* bureaucracy
burocrata [buro'krata] *m/f* bureaucrat
burocrático [buro'kratʃiku] *adj* bureaucratic
burrice [bu'hisi] *f* stupidity; ***você cometeu uma ~!*** that was a stupid thing to do!
burro ['buhu] **1** *m* donkey; *fig* fool; ***~ de carga*** hard worker **2** *adj* stupid
busca ['buska] *f* search; INTERNET ***motor*** *m* ***de ~*** search engine; ***andar em ~ de*** be in search of
buscar [bus'kar] ⟨1n⟩ *v/t* seek, look for; ***ir ~, vir ~*** pick up, collect; ***mandar ~*** send for
bússola ['busula] *f* compass
busto ['bustu] *m* bust
buzina [bu'zina] *f* horn
buzinar [buzi'nar] ⟨1a⟩ *v/t* honk one's horn
búzio ['buziu] *m* seashell
byte ['bajtʃi] *m* INFORM byte

C

cá [ka] *adv* here; ***o lado de ~*** this side; ***para ~*** here, over here; ***para lá e para ~*** back and forth; ***de lá para ~*** since then
cabana [ka'bana] *f* hut, cabin
cabeça [ka'besa] **1** *f* head; (*inteligência*) brain; *lista etc*: top, head; ***~ de gado*** head of cattle; ***~ de alho*** bulb of garlic; ***quebrar a ~*** rack one's brains; ***de ~*** off the top of one's head; ***de ~ para baixo*** upside down **2** *m/f revolta*: leader; (*chefe*) head
cabeçada [kabe'sada] *f* ESP header; ***dar uma ~ a*** head-butt
cabeçalho [kabe'saʎu] *m livro*: title page; *página*: heading
cabecear [kabe'sjaɾ] ⟨1l⟩ **1** *v/i* nod **2** *v/t futebol*: head
cabeceira [kabe'sejɾa] *f* head; *mesa*: end; ***mesa** f **de ~*** bedside table
cabedal [kabe'daw] *m Port* leather
cabeleira [kabe'lejɾa] *f* head of hair; ***~ postiça*** wig
cabeleireiro [kabelej'ɾejɾu] *m*, **-a** *f* hairdresser
cabelo [ka'belu] *m* hair; ***cortar o ~*** have one's hair cut
cabeludo [kabe'ludu] *adj* hairy; (*difícil*) complicated
caber [ka'beɾ] ⟨2q⟩ *v/i* fit; (*ter cabimento*) be fitting; ***~ em alguém*** fit s.o.; ***~ a alguém fazer algo*** be up to s.o. to do sth
cabide [ka'bidʒi] *m* coathanger; (*móvel*) hat stand
cabimento [kabi'mẽtu] *m* ***não ter ~*** be out of the question
cabine [ka'bini] *f* cabin; *loja*: fitting room; *avião*: cockpit, cabin; AERO ***~ de comando*** flight deck; ***~ eleitoral*** voting booth; ***~ telefônica*** phone booth, *Brit* phone box
cabisbaixo [kabiz'bajʃu] *adj fig* dispirited; (*com a cabeça para baixo*) head down
cabo[1] ['kabu] *m* end; *vassoura*, *faca etc*: handle; ELÉT, TECN cable; ***~ de extensão*** extension cable; ***televisão** f **por ~*** cable television; *Port* ***ao ~ de*** at the end of; ***de ~ a rabo*** from beginning to end
cabo[2] ['kabu] *m* MIL corporal
Cabo-Verde [kabo'verdʒi] *m* Cape Verde
cabo-verdiano [kaboveɾ'dʒianu] **1** *adj* Cape Verdean **2** *m*, **-a** *f* Cape Verdean
cabra ['kabɾa] *f* goat
cabra-cega [kabɾa'sɛga] *f* blind man's bluff
cabrito [ka'bɾitu] *m* kid
cabular [kabu'laɾ] ⟨1a⟩ *v/i Port* skip class, *Brit* play truant
caça ['kasa] **1** *f* hunting; (*busca*) hunt; GASTR game; ***à ~ de*** in pursuit of; ***ir à ~*** go hunting; ***~ às baleias*** whaling; ***~ ao homem*** manhunt **2** *m* AERO fighter plane
caçada [ka'sada] *f* hunting trip; ***~ humana*** manhunt
caçador [kasa'doɾ] *m*, **-a** *f* hunter; ***~ clandestino, ~ furtivo*** poacher
caça-dotes [kasa'dɔtʃis] ⟨*pl* inv⟩ *m* gold-digger
caçar [ka'saɾ] ⟨1p & 1b⟩ hunt
cacarejar [kakaɾe'ʒaɾ] ⟨1d⟩ *v/i galinha* cluck
caçarola [kasa'ɾɔla] *f* (sauce)pan; GASTR casserole
caça-talentos [kasata'lẽtus] ⟨pl inv⟩ *m* talent scout
cacau [ka'kaw] *m* cocoa
cacetada [kase'tada] *f* blow with a club; ***vou dar uma ~ nele*** I'm going to give him a thrashing
cacete [ka'setʃi] *m* club; *fam* ***está quente pra ~*** it's damned hot!
cachaça [ka'ʃasa] *f Bras* sugar cane spirit
cachaçeiro [kaʃa'sejɾu] **1** *m*, **-a** *f*

drunk, drunkard **2** *adj* drunken
cachecol [kaʃe'kɔw] *m* scarf
cachimbo [ka'ʃĩbu] *m* pipe
cacho ['kaʃu] *m uvas*: bunch; *cabelo*: curl, lock
cachoeira [ka'ʃwejɾa] *f* waterfall
cachorrinho [kaʃo'hiɲu] *m* puppy
cachorro [ka'ʃohu] *m* dog
cachorro-quente [kaʃohu'kẽtʃi] *m* hot dog
cacifo [ka'sifu] *m* locker
cacique [ka'siki] *m* chief
caco ['kaku] *m* shard, fragment; (*velharia*) old crock; ***quebrar em ~s*** shatter
cacto ['kaktu] *m* cactus
caçula [ka'sula] *m/f* youngest child
cada ['kada] *adj* each; ***~ um, ~ qual*** each one, each; ***~ vez*** each time, every time; ***~ vez mais*** more and more; ***~ dois dias*** every other day, every two days
cadarço [ka'daɾsu] *m* shoelace
cadastrar [kadas'tɾaɾ] ⟨1b⟩ *v/t* register
cadastro [ka'dastɾu] *m* (*registro*) register; *ato* registration; *pessoal* file, records; *criminal* criminal record
cadáver [ka'davɛɾ] *m* corpse
cadavérico [kada'vɛɾiku] **1** *adj* cadaverous, corpse-like **2** *m* post-mortem
cadê [ka'de] *adv fam* where is / are?
cadeado [ka'dʒiadu] *m* padlock
cadeia [ka'deja] *f* (*corrente*) chain; (*prisão*) jail, prison; RÁDIO, TV network; ***~ alimentar*** food chain; ***reação** f **em ~***, *Port* ***reacção** f **em ~*** chain reaction
cadeira [ka'dejɾa] *f* chair; POL seat; (*matéria*) subject; (*função*) post; ***~ de balanço*** rocking chair; ***~ elétrica*** electric chair; ***~ de rodas*** wheelchair
cadela [ka'dɛla] *f* bitch
cadência [ka'dẽsja] *f* MÚS cadence; (*ritmo*) rhythm
caderneta [kadeɾ'neta] *f* notebook; *de professor*: register; ***~ de poupança*** savings account
caderno [ka'dɛɾnu] *m* exercise book; *de notas* notebook
cadete [ka'detʃi] *m* cadet
cadinho [ka'dʒiɲu] *m* melting pot *tb fig*
caducar [kadu'kaɾ] ⟨1n⟩ *v/i* lapse, expire; *pessoa* go senile
caduco [ka'duku] *adj* senile; *contrato* expired
caem ['kaẽ] → ***cair***
cães [kãjs] *mpl* → ***cão***
café [ka'fɛ] *m* coffee; *estabelecimento* café, coffee shop; *Bras* ***tomar ~*** have breakfast; *Port* ***~ cheio** ou **duplo*** double espresso; *Port* ***~ curto*** espresso; ***~ descafeinado*** decaffeinated coffee, *fam* decaf; ***~ com leite*** coffee with cream, *Brit* white coffee; *Bras* ***~ da manhã*** breakfast; ***~ solúvel*** instant coffee
cafeína [kafe'ina] *f* caffeine
cafetão [kafe'tãw] *m Bras* pimp
cafeteira [kafe'tejɾa] *f* coffee pot
cafezinho [kafɛ'ziɲu] *m* small black coffee, espresso
cáften ['kaftẽ] *m Port* pimp
cafundó [kafũ'dɔ] *m* ***no ~*** in the boonies, out in the sticks
cagão [ka'gãw] *m*, **cagona** [ka'gona] *f pop* ***ser ~*** be a chicken
cagar [ka'gaɾ] ⟨1o & 1b⟩ *v/i vulg* shit; **cagar-se** *v/r* shit oneself; ***~ de medo*** be shit-scared
caiar [ka'jaɾ] ⟨1b⟩ whitewash
cãibra ['kãjbɾa] *f* cramp
caída [ka'ida] *f* → ***queda***
caído [ka'idu] **1** *pp* → ***cair*** **2** *adj* fallen; *pessoa* dejected; (*pendente*) droopy; (*apaixonado*) smitten
cair [ka'iɾ] ⟨3l⟩ *v/i* fall; *dente, cabelo* fall out; *botão* fall off; *pessoa* fall down; *sol, nível* go down; ***~ no chão*** fall to the floor; ***~ bem / mal*** fit well / badly; *fig* go down well / badly; ***~ bem a alguém*** suit s.o.; ***estou caindo de sono*** I'm exhausted; ***~ em si*** come to one's senses; *fam* ***cai fora!*** clear off!
cais[1] [kajs] *m* ⟨*pl inv*⟩ NÁUT quay; *Port* FERROV platform
cais[2] [kajs] → ***cair***
caixa ['kajʃa] **1** *f* box; (*cofre*) safe; *loja*: cash desk; *cerveja*: case; ***~ acústica*** loudspeaker; ***~ do correio*** mailbox, *Brit* letterbox; INFORM mailbox;

C

INFORM ~ ***de diálogo*** dialog box; ~ ***econômica*** savings bank; *Bras* AUTO ~ ***de marchas*** gear box; *Bras* ~ ***postal*** P.O. Box; AERO ~ ***preta*** black box; *Port* AUTO ~ ***de velocidades*** gear box **2** *m/f* cashier **3** *m supermercado*: checkout; ~ ***automático*** ATM; ~ ***eletrônico*** cash dispenser

caixão [kaj'ʃãw] *m* coffin; (*caixa grande*) large box

caixeiro [kaj'ʃejɾu] *m*, **-a** *f Port* shop assistant; COM *tb Bras* ~ ***viajante*** commercial traveler, *Brit* commercial traveller

caixilho [kaj'ʃiʎu] *m* frame

caixinha [kaj'ʃiɲa] *f* small box

caixote [kaj'ʃɔtʃi] *m* crate; ~ ***do lixo*** garbage can, *Brit* dustbin

caju [ka'ʒu] *m* cashew fruit; ***castanha f de*** ~ cashew (nut)

cal [kaw] *f substância* lime

calada [ka'lada] *f* stillness; ***na*** ~ ***da noite*** in the dead of night

calado [ka'ladu] *adj* silent; (*pouco falador*) quiet; ***ficar*** ~ be quiet

calafetar [kalafe'taɾ] ⟨1c⟩ *v/t* stop up

calafrio [kala'fɾiu] *m* shudder; ***estou com*** **~*s*** I've got goosebumps

calamidade [kalami'dadʒi] *f* calamity

calamitoso [kalami'tozu] *adj* calamitous

calão [ka'lãw] *m Bras* swearword; *Port* slang; *grupo profissional*: jargon

calar [ka'laɾ] ⟨1b⟩ *v/t* be quiet; (*impor silêncio*) silence; ***cala a boca!*** shut up!; **calar-se** *v/r* go quiet; (*não dizer*) keep quiet

calça ['kawsa] *f* ~ (***s***) pants, *Brit* trousers; ~ ***do pijama*** pajama pants, *Brit* pyjama trousers

calçada [kaw'sada] *f Bras* sidewalk, *Brit* pavement

calçadeira [kawsa'dejɾa] *m* shoe-horn

calçado [kaw'sadu] *m* footwear

calção [kaw'sãw] *m* shorts; ~ ***de banho*** swimming trunks

calcanhar [kawka'ɲaɾ] *m* heel

calcar [kaw'kaɾ] ⟨1n⟩ *v/t* trample; (*pisar em*) tread on; (*comprimir*) press

calçar [kaw'saɾ] ⟨1p⟩ *v/t meias, sapatos* put on; *rua* pave

calcário [kaw'kaɾiu] **1** *adj água* hard **2** *m* limestone

calcinha(s) [kaw'siɲa(s)] *f(pl) Bras* panties, *Brit* knickers

cálcio ['kawsiu] *m* calcium

calculadora [kawkula'doɾa] *f* calculator; ~ (***de bolso***) pocket calculator

calcular [kawku'laɾ] ⟨1a⟩ *v/t* calculate; *fig* (*prever*) expect; (*imaginar*) imagine

cálculo[1] ['kawkulu] *m* calculation; MAT calculus; ~ ***mental*** mental arithmetic

cálculo[2] ['kawkulu] *m* MED stone

calculista [kawku'lista] *adj* calculating

calda ['kawda] *f* (*xarope*) syrup

caldas ['kawdas] *fpl* hot springs

caldeira [kaw'dejɾa] *f* boiler

caldeirão [kawdej'ɾãw] *m* cauldron

caldo ['kawdu] *m* broth; *fruta*: juice; ~ ***de cana*** sugar cane juice; ~ ***de galinha*** chicken stock; ~ ***verde*** potato and cabbage broth

calefação, *Port* **calefacção** [kalefa'sãw] *f* heating

calendário [kalẽ'daɾiu] *m* calendar

calha ['kaʎa] *f* (*rego*) gutter

calhar [ka'ʎaɾ] ⟨1b⟩ *v/i* ***calhou que*** it so happened that; ***a minha amiga calhou de passar*** my friend happened to pass by; ***vem mesmo a*** ~ it came at just the right time

calibrar [kali'bɾaɾ] ⟨1a⟩ *v/t* calibrate; *pneu* check the pressure of

calibre [ka'libɾi] *m* caliber, *Brit* calibre

cálice ['kalisi] *m* wine glass; REL chalice

caligrafia [kaligɾa'fia] *f* calligraphy; (*letra*) handwriting

call center [kow'sẽteɾ] *m* call-center, *Brit* call-centre

calma ['kawma] *f* calm; ***com*** ~ calmly; ***conservar a*** ~ keep calm; **~*!*** cool it!; ***tenha*** **~*!*** calm down!, cool it!

calmamente [kawma'mẽtʃi] *adv* calmly

calmante [kaw'mãtʃi] *m* MED tranquilizer, *Brit* tranquillizer

calmo ['kawmu] *adj* calm

calo ['kalu] *m* callus; *pé*: corn

calor [ka'loɾ] *m* heat; *agradável* warmth *tb fig*; ***está*** (*ou* ***faz***) ~ it's

hot; ***estar com ~*** be hot; ***~ escaldante*** extremely hot
caloria [kalo'ɾia] *f* calorie
caloroso [kalo'ɾozu] *adj* warm; *fig* enthusiastic
calota [ka'lɔta] *f* hubcap
calouro [ka'loɾu] *m*, **-a** *f* freshman, *Brit* fresher; (*novato*) novice
calúnia [ka'lunja] *f* slander
caluniar [kalu'njaɾ] ⟨1g⟩ *v/t* slander
calunioso [kalu'njozu] *adj* slanderous
calvície [kaw'visi] *f* baldness
calvo ['kawvu] *adj* bald; ***ele está ficando ~*** he's going bald; ***meio ~*** balding
cama ['kama] *f* bed; ***estar de ~*** be ill (in bed); ***ir para a ~*** go to bed; ***ir para a ~ com*** go to bed with; ***~ de campanha*** cot, *Brit* camp-bed; ***~ de casal*** double bed; ***~ de solteiro*** single bed
camada [ka'mada] *f* layer, *tinta*: coat; ***~ ~ de ouro*** gilt; ***~ de ozono*** ozone layer
camafeu [kama'few] *m* cameo
câmara ['kʌmaɾa] *f* chamber; FOT camera; ***em ~ lenta*** in slow motion; ***~ de ar*** inner tube; ***Câmara de Comércio*** Chamber of Commerce; ***Câmara dos Deputados*** House of Representatives; ***~ digital*** digital camera; ***~ escura*** dark room; ***Câmara Municipal*** town council; *Port* town hall
camarada [kama'ɾada] **1** *adj* friendly **2** *m/f* (*colega*) comrade; (*sujeito*) guy; woman
camaradagem [kamaɾa'daʒẽ] *f* comradeship, camaraderie
câmara-ardente [kʌmaɾaɾ'dẽtʃi] *f* ⟨*pl* câmaras-ardentes⟩ ***estar exposto em ~*** lie in state
camarão [kama'ɾãw] *m* shrimp; *graúdo* prawn
Camarões [kama'ɾõĩʃ] *mpl* Cameroon
camarote [kama'ɾɔtʃi] *m* NÁUT cabin; TEAT box
cambada [kã'bada] *f* horde, gang
cambalear [kãba'ljaɾ] ⟨1l⟩ *v/i* stagger, totter
cambalhota [kamba'ʎɔta] *f* somersault
câmbio ['kãbiu] *m* foreign exchange; (*preço de cambio*) rate of exchange; AUTO gearshift; ***casa** f **de ~*** bureau de change; ***~ negro*** black market; ***~ paralelo*** parallel market
cambista [kã'bista] *m/f* money changer
Camboja [kã'bɔʒa] *m* Cambodia
camélia [ka'mɛlja] *f* camelia
camelo [ka'melu] *m* camel
camelô [kame'lo] *m* street vendor
câmera ['kʌmeɾa] *f* camera
camião [kami'ãw] *m Port* truck, *Brit* lorry
caminhão [kami'ɲãw] *m Bras* truck, *Brit* lorry; ***~ de bombeiros*** fire truck. *Brit* fire engine
caminhada [kami'ɲada] *f* (*passeio*) walk; ***vou dar uma ~*** I'm going for a walk
caminhar [kami'ɲaɾ] ⟨1a⟩ *v/i* walk; *fig* progress, advance
caminho [ka'miɲu] *m* way, route; (*trilho*) path; ***indicar o ~ a alguém*** show s.o. the way; ***estar no ~*** be in the way; ***na metade do ~*** midway
caminho-de-ferro [kamiɲodʒi'fɛhu] *m* ⟨*pl* caminhos-de-ferro⟩ *Port* railroad, *Brit* railway
caminhoneiro [kamiɲo'nejɾu] *m*, **-a** *f Bras* truck driver, *Brit* lorry driver
camioneta [kamjo'neta] *f* van
camionista [kamjo'nista] *m/f Port* truck driver, *Brit* lorry driver
camisa [ka'miza] *f* shirt; *Port* ***~ de dormir, ~ de noite*** nightshirt; ***~ pólo*** polo shirt
camisa-de-forças [kamizadʒi'foɾsas] *f* ⟨*pl* camisas-de-forças⟩ straitjacket
camisa-de-Vênus, *Port* **camisa-de-Vénus** [kamizadʒi'venus] *f* ⟨*pl* camisas-de-Vénus⟩ condom
camiseta [kami'zeta] *f* T-shirt
camisinha [kami'ziɲa] *f* condom
camisola [kami'zɔla] *f Bras* nightgown; *Port* sweater; *Port* ***~ interior*** undershirt, *Brit* vest
camomila [kamo'mila] *f* camomile
campainha [kãpa'iɲa] *f* bell; ***tocar à ~*** ring the bell

C

campanha [kã'paɲa] *f* campaign; ***fazer*** ~ campaign; POL ~ ***eleitoral*** election campaign; ~ ***de marketing*** marketing campaign; ~ ***publicitária*** advertising campaign
campeão [kã'pjãw] *m*, **campeã** [kã'pjã] *f* champion
campeonato [kãpjo'natu] *m* championship; ~ ***Mundial de Futebol*** World Cup
camping ['kãpĩ] *m Bras* camping; (*lugar*) campsite
campismo [kã'pizmu] *m Port* camping; ***fazer*** ~ camp; ***parque*** *m* ***de*** ~ campsite
campista [kã'pista] *m/f* camper
campo ['kãpu] *m* field; (*oposto a cidade*) countryside; ***no*** ~ in the country; ~ ***de aviação*** airfield; ~ ***de beisebol*** ballpark; ~ ***de batalha*** battlefield; ~ ***desportivo***, *Bras* ~ ***de esportes*** playing field; ~ ***de futebol*** football pitch; ~ ***de golfe*** golf course; ~ ***petrolífero*** oilfield
camponês [kãpo'nes] *m*, **camponesa** [kãpo'neza] *f* peasant
camuflagem [kamu'flaʒẽ] *f* camouflage
camuflar [kamu'flaɾ] ⟨1a⟩ *v/t* camouflage
camundongo [kamũ'dõgu] *m Bras* mouse
camurça [ka'muɾsa] *f* suede
cana ['kana] *f* cane; ~ ***de açucar*** sugar cane
Canadá [kana'da] *m* ***o*** ~ Canada
canadense [kana'dẽsi] **1** *adj* Canadian **2** *m*, **-a** *f* Canadian
canal [ka'naw] *m* channel; *navegação*: canal; ANAT duct; ~ ***de televisão*** television channel; ***Canal da Mancha*** English Channel
canalização [kanaliza'sãw] *f* piping; *água*: plumbing
canalizador [kanaliza'doɾ] *m Port* plumber
canapé [kana'pɛ] *m Port móvel* sofa; GASTR canapé
Canárias [ka'naɾjas] *fpl* Canary Islands
canário [ka'naɾiu] *m* canary
canavial [kana'vjaw] *m* cane field
canção [kã'sãw] *f* song; ~ ***de amor*** lovesong; ~ ***infantil*** nursery rhyme
cancela [kã'sɛla] *f* (*portão*) gate
cancelamento [kãsela'mẽtu] *m* cancellation
cancelar [kãse'laɾ] ⟨1c⟩ *v/t* cancel; (*invalidar*) annul
Câncer ['kãsɛɾ] *m* ASTROL Cancer
câncer ['kãsɛɾ] *m Bras* MED cancer; ~ ***de pulmão*** lung cancer
cancerígeno [kãse'ɾiʒenu] *adj* carcinogenic
canceroso [kãse'ɾozu] **1** *adj célula* cancerous **2** *m*, **-a** *f* cancer sufferer
cancro ['kãkro] *m Port* MED cancer
candelabro [kãde'labɾu] *m* candelabra; (*lustro*) chandelier
candidatar-se [kãdʒida'taɾsi] ⟨1a⟩ *v/r* ~ ***a*** apply for; *presidência* run for, stand for
candidato [kãdʒi'datu] *m*, **-a** *f* candidate; *a cargo* applicant
candidatura [kãdʒida'tuɾa] *f a cargo* application; POL candidature
caneca [ka'nɛka] *f* mug
canela [ka'nɛla] *f* cinnamon; ANAT shin
caneta [ka'neta] *f* pen; ~ (***de tinta***) ***permanente*** permanent marker; ~ ***esferográfica*** ballpoint pen
caneta-tinteiro [kaneta'tʃĩtejru] *f* ⟨*pl* canetas-tinteiro⟩ fountain pen
canguru [kaŋgu'ɾu] *m* kangaroo
canhão [ka'ɲãw] *m* MIL cannon; GEOG canyon
canhoto [ka'ɲotu] **1** *adj* left-handed **2** *m*, **-a** *f* left-hander
canibal [kani'baw] *m/f* cannibal
canibalismo [kaniba'lizmu] *m* cannibalism
canil [ka'niw] *m* kennel, *Brit* kennels
canino [ka'ninu] **1** *adj* canine **2** *m* canine
canivete [kani'vɛtʃi] *m* pocket knife, *Brit* penknife
canja ['kãʒa] *f sopa* chicken broth; *fam* ***ser*** ~ be a piece of cake
cano ['kanu] *m* pipe; (*tubo*) tube; *bota, coluna*: top; *arma de fogo*: barrel; ~ ***de esgoto*** sewer; ~***s*** pipes, plumbing
canoa [ka'noa] *f* canoe
canoagem [ka'nwaʒẽ] *f* ESP canoeing

cansaço [kã'sasu] *m* tiredness
cansado [kã'sadu] *adj* tired; ***estar ~ de alguém / algo*** be tired of s.o. / sth; ***ficar ~*** get tired
cansar [kã'saɾ] ⟨1a⟩ **1** *v/t* tire; (*entediar*) bore **2** *v/i* tire; **cansar-se** *v/r* get tired; **~ *de*** tire of; ***ele nunca se cansa disso*** he never tires of it
cansativo [kãsa'tʃivu] *adj* tiring; (*tedioso*) tedious
cantar [kã'taɾ] ⟨1a⟩ **1** *v/t* sing; *fam* chat up **2** *v/i* sing; *galo* crow **3** *m* song
cantarolar [kãtaɾo'laɾ] ⟨1e⟩ hum
canteiro [kã'tejɾu] *m* stonemason; *flores*: flower bed; **~ *divisor*** median strip, *Brit* central reservation; **~ *de obras*** site office
cantiga [kã'tʃiga] *f* ballad; **~ *de ninar*** lullaby
cantina [kã'tʃina] *f* canteen
canto[1] ['kãtu] *m sala*, *página*: corner; (*lugar*) place; ***no ~*** in the corner
canto[2] ['kãtu] *m* song, singing
cantor [kã'toɾ] *m*, **-a** *f* singer
canudinho [kanu'dʒiɲu] *m* straw
canudo [ka'nudu] *m* straw; (*tubo*) tube
cão [kãw] *m* ⟨*pl* cães⟩ dog; **~ *de guarda*** guard dog; **~ *guia*** guide dog; **~ *pastor*** sheepdog; **~ *vadio*** stray dog
caos ['kaws] *m* ⟨*pl inv*⟩ chaos
caótico [ka'ɔtʃiku] *adj* chaotic
capa ['kapa] *f roupa* cape; (*cobertura*) cover; ***livro de ~ dura / mole*** hardback / paperback; **~ *de chuva*** raincoat
capacete [kapa'setʃi] *m* helmet
capacho [ka'paʃu] *m* doormat
capacidade [kapasi'dadʒi] *f* capacity; (*aptidão*) ability; INFORM **~ *de memória*** storage capacity; **~ *de produção*** production capacity
capar [ka'paɾ] ⟨1b⟩ *v/t animal* castrate, geld
capataz [kapa'tas] *m* foreman; *fam* slave-driver
capaz [ka'pas] *adj* capable; (*habilitado*) able; ***ser ~ de*** be capable of; ***é ~ de ser o último dia das liquidações*** it could be the last day of the sales today; ***fisicamente ~*** able-bodied
capela [ka'pɛla] *f* chapel
capelão [kape'lãw] *m* ⟨*pl* -ães⟩ chaplain
capim [ka'pĩ] *m* grass
capital [kapi'taw] **1** *adj* capital; ***pena f ~*** capital punishment **2** *f cidade* capital **3** *m* FIN capital; **~ *investido*** investment capital; **~ *imobilizado*** fixed capital
capitalismo [kapita'lizmu] *m* capitalism
capitalista [kapita'lista] *m/f* capitalist
capitalizar [kapitali'zaɾ] ⟨1a⟩ *v/t* (*tirar proveito de*) capitalize on; FIN capitalize
capitania [kapita'nia] *f* port authority
capitão [kapi'tãw] *m* ⟨*pl* -ães⟩ captain
capítulo [ka'pitulu] *m* chapter; *de novela* episode; ***transmitir em ~s*** serialize
capô [ka'po] *m* AUTO hood, *Brit* bonnet
capoeira [ka'pwejɾa] *f* (*mata*) brushwood; capoeira (*Brazilian martial art*)
capota [ka'pɔta] *f* AUTO hood, top
capotar [kapo'taɾ] ⟨1e⟩ *v/i* AUTO overturn
caprichar [kapɾi'ʃaɾ] ⟨1a⟩ *v/i* (*esforçar-se*) make an effort; **~ *em*** take trouble over
capricho [ka'pɾiʃu] *m* (*fantasia*) whim, caprice; (*obstinação*) obstinacy; (*esmero*) care
caprichoso [kapɾi'ʃozu] *adj* capricious; (*com esmero*) meticulous
Capricórnio [kapɾi'kɔɾniu] *m* ASTROL Capricorn
cápsula ['kapsula] *f* capsule; **~ *espacial*** space capsule
captar [kap'taɾ] ⟨1b⟩ *v/t* capture; *emissora* pick up; (*compreender*) catch, grasp; *águas* collect
captura [kap'tuɾa] *f* capture; **~ *de dados*** data capture
capturar [kapto'raɾ] ⟨1a⟩ *v/t* capture
capuz [ka'pus] *m* hood
cáqui ['kaki] *adj* khaki
cara ['kaɾa] *f* face; (*aspecto*) appearance; *fam homem* guy; **~ *a* ~** face to face; ***dar de ~ com*** bump into; ***de ~*** straight away; ***de ~ cheia*** drunk;

C

não ir com a ~ de alguém be ill-disposed towards s.o.; ***ser a ~ de alguém*** be the spitting image of s.o.; ***está na ~*** it's obvious; ***estar com boa ~*** look well; *comida* look good; ***~ de pau*** nerve; ***tirar ~ ou coroa*** toss a coin; ***~ ou coroa?*** heads or tails; ***~ durão*** tough guy

cara-metade [karame'tadʒi] *f fig de alguém* better half

caracol [kara'kɔw] *m* snail; (*cabelo*) curl; ***escada** f **de ~*** spiral staircase

carácter [ka'ɾateɾ] *m Port* character

característica [karakte'ɾistʃika] *f* characteristic; *cidade*: feature

característico [karakte'ɾistʃiku] *adj* characteristic

caracterização [karakteriza'sãw] *f* characterization; *ator*: make-up

caracterizar [karakteri'zaɾ] ⟨1a⟩ *v/t* characterize; TEAT make up

caramba [ka'ɾãba] *int fam **~!*** gosh! my goodness!

caramelo [kara'mɛlu] *m* caramel; *bala*: taffy, *Brit* toffee

caranga [ka'ɾãga] *f Bras* AUTO *fam* classic car

caranguejeira [karãge'ʒejɾa] *f* tarantula

caranguejo [karã'geʒu] *m* crab

carapuça [kara'pusa] *f* cap

caráter [ka'ɾateɾ] *m Bras* character; ***pessoa de ~*** person of character

caravana [kara'vana] *f* caravan

carboidrato [karboi'dratu] *m* carbohydrate

carbono [kaɾ'bonu] *m* carbon

carbonizar [karboni'zaɾ] ⟨1a⟩ *v/t* carbonize; (*queimar*) char

carburador [karbura'doɾ] *m* AUTO carbureter, *Brit* carburettor

carcaça [kaɾ'kasa] *f* (*ossada*) carcass; (*armação*) frame

cárcere ['karseri] *m* prison

cardápio [kaɾ'dapiu] *m Bras* menu

cardeal [kaɾ'dʒiaw] **1** *m* cardinal **2** *adj* cardinal

cardíaco [kaɾ'dʒiaku] **1** *adj* cardiac; ***parada** f **~*** cardiac arrest; ***ataque ~*** heart attack **2** *m*, **-a** *f* person with a heart condition

cardinal [kardʒi'naw] *adj* cardinal; ***número** m **~*** cardinal number

cardiologia [kardʒiolo'ʒia] *f* cardiology

cardiologista [kardʒiolo'ʒista] *m/f* heart specialist, cardiologist

cardiovascular [kardʒiovasku'laɾ] *adj* cardiovascular

cardume [kaɾ'dumi] *m peixes*: shoal

careca [ka'ɾɛka] **1** *adj* bald **2** *f* baldness; *cabeça* bald head; *pessoa* bald person, *fam* baldie

carecer [kare'seɾ] ⟨2g⟩ *v/i* (*precisar*) need; ***alguém carece de algo*** s.o. lacks sth

careiro [ka'ɾejɾu] *adj* expensive

carência [ka'ɾẽsja] *f* lack, shortage; (*necessidade*) need

carente [ka'ɾẽtʃi] *adj* wanting; *pessoa* needy; *carinho*: in need of affection

careta [ka'ɾeta] *f* grimace; ***fazer uma ~*** pull a face

carga ['karga] *f* (*peso*) load, burden; *navio*, *avião*: cargo; (*carregamento*) loading; ELÉT, MIL charge; ***voltar à ~*** insist; ***~ d'água*** heavy downpour; ***~ horária*** workload

cargo ['kaɾgu] *m* (*função*) post; (*encargo*) responsibility; ***ter a ~*** be in charge of; ***deixar algo a ~ de alguém*** leave s.o. in charge of sth; ***tomar ~ de*** take charge of; ***~ público*** public office

cargueiro [kaɾ'gejɾu] *m* cargo ship, freighter

cariar [kari'aɾ] ⟨1g⟩ *v/i* decay

Caribe [ka'ɾibi] *m **o ~*** the Caribbean

caricatura [karika'tuɾa] *f* caricature

caricaturar [karikato'ɾaɾ] ⟨1a⟩ *v/t* caricature

carícia [ka'ɾisja] *f* caress

caridade [kari'dadʒi] *f* charity

caridoso [kari'dozu] *adj* charitable

cárie ['kari] *f* tooth decay, caries *sg*

caril [ka'ɾiw] *m Port* curry

carimbar [karĩ'baɾ] ⟨1a⟩ *v/t* stamp; *correio*: postmark

carimbo [ka'ɾĩbu] *m* stamp; *postal* postmark

carinho [ka'ɾiɲu] *m* affection; (*carícia*) caress; ***fazer ~*** caress

carinhoso [kari'ɲozu] *adj* affectionate

carioca [ka'ɾjɔka] **1** *m/f* Rio de Janeiran **2** *adj* of Rio de Janeiro, Rio *atr*
carnal [kaɾ'naw] *adj* carnal
carnaval [kaɾna'vaw] *m* carnival; *fig* mess; ***Carnaval*** *Brazilian festival held yearly in the four days prior to Lent*
carne ['kaɾni] *f* flesh; *comida* meat; ***em ~ e osso*** in the flesh; ***ser de ~ e osso*** be human; ***~ assada*** roast beef; ***~ de boi*** beef; ***~ branca*** white meat; ***~ de novilho*** veal; ***~ picada*** ground beef, *Brit* minced meat; ***~ de porco*** pork; ***~ de vaca*** beef; ***~ de veado*** venison; ***~ vermelha*** red meat
carneiro [kaɾ'nejɾu] *m* sheep; *macho* ram; ***~ assado*** roast mutton
carnificina [kaɾnifi'sina] *f* carnage
carnívoro [kaɾ'nivuɾu] **1** *adj* carnivorous **2** *m* carnivore
carnudo [kaɾ'nudu] *adj* fleshy; *fam* beefy
caro ['karu] *adj* expensive, dear; (*estimado*) dear; ***sair ~*** work out expensive; *fig* ***pagar ~*** pay dearly
caroço [ka'rosu] *m frutos*: stone; MED lump
carona [ka'rona] *f* ride, *Brit* lift; *Bras* ***viajar de ~*** hitchhike; ***pegar uma ~*** get a ride
carpete [kaɾ'pɛtʃi] *f* carpet
carpintaria [kaɾpĩta'ria] *f* carpentry
carpinteiro [kaɾpĩ'tejɾu] *m*, **-a** *f móveis*: carpenter; TEAT stagehand
carrancudo [kahã'kudu] *adj pessoa* sullen
carrasco [ka'hasku] *m* executioner; *fig* butcher
carregado [kahe'gadu] *adj* loaded, laden *tb fig*; *céu* dark; *ambiente* charged; ***ela estava carregada de compras*** she was laden with shopping
carregador [kahega'doɾ] *m* porter; ELÉT ***~ de bateria*** battery charger
carregar [kahe'gaɾ] ⟨1o & 1c⟩ *v/t* load; *peso* carry; *pilha* charge; (*levar para longe*) carry off
carreira [ka'hejɾa] *f* (*profissão*) career; (*corrida*) running; ***às ~s*** in a hurry; ***fazer ~*** make a career
carrinho [ka'hiɲu] *m* cart, *Brit* trolley; *brinquedo* toy car; ESP sliding tackle; ***~ de bebé*** baby buggy; ***~ de mão*** wheelbarrow
carro ['kahu] *m* automobile, car; *bois etc*: cart; ***de ~*** by car; ***~ alegórico*** float; ***~ de corrida*** race car, *Brit* racing car; ***~ esporte*** sports car; ***~ de mão*** handcart, barrow; ***~ de polícia*** police car
carroça [ka'hɔsa] *f* cart
carroçeria [kaho'sejra] *f* AUTO bodywork
carrossel [kaho'sew] *m* merry-go-round, carousel
carruagem [ka'hwaʒẽ] *f* carriage, coach
carruagem-cama [kahwaʒẽ'kama] *f* ⟨*pl* carruagens-cama⟩ *Port* FERROV sleeper car
carruagem-restaurante [kahwaʒẽhestaw'ɾãtʃi] *m* ⟨*pl* carruagens-restaurante⟩ restaurant car
carta ['kaɾta] *f* letter; *de jogar* card; (*mapa*) chart; ***dar as ~s*** deal; ***~ aérea*** airmail letter; ***~ de amor*** love letter; ***~ branca*** carte blanche; *Port* ***~ de condução*** driver's license, *Brit* driving licence; ***~ de demissão*** *do emprego* notice; ***~ registrada*** registered letter; ***~ de vinhos*** winelist
cartão [kaɾ'tãw] *m* card; ***~ de crédito*** credit card; ***~ de embarque*** boarding card; ***~ de Natal*** Christmas card; *Bras* ***~ postal*** postcard; ***~ telefônico*** phone card; ***~ visita*** (calling) card
cartaz [kaɾ'tas] *m* poster; TEAT, CINE ***em ~*** on the bill; ***a peça esteve tres anos em ~*** the play had a three-year run
carteira [kaɾ'tejɾa] *f* wallet; (*cartão*) card; *móvel* (school) desk; *Port* ***~ de chá*** teabag; *Bras* ***~ de identidade*** identity card; *Bras* ***~ de motorista*** driver's license, *Brit* driving licence
carteirista [kaɾte'rista] *m/f Port* pickpocket
carteiro [kaɾ'tejɾu] *m* mailman, *Brit* postman
cartel [kaɾ'tɛw] *m* FIN cartel
cárter ['kaɾtɛɾ] *m* ***~ de óleo*** sump

cartilagem [kaɾtʃi'laʒẽ] *f* ANAT cartilage

cartógrafo [kaɾ'tɔgɾafu] *m* cartographer

cartola [kaɾ'tɔla] *f* top hat

cartolina [kaɾto'lina] *f* card

cartomante [kaɾto'mãtʃi] *m/f* tarot card reader

cartório [kaɾ'tɔriu] *m* registry office

cartucho [kaɾ'tuʃu] *m* cartridge; *dinamite*: stick; *saco*: packet

cartum [kaɾ'tũ] *m* cartoon

cartunista [kaɾtu'nista] *m/f* cartoonist

caruncho [ka'rũʃu] *m* woodworm

carvalho [kaɾ'vaʎu] *m* oak

carvão [kaɾ'vãw] *m* coal; ARTE charcoal

casa ['kaza] *f* house; (*lar*) home; COM firm; MAT decimal place; *xadrez*: square; ***em ~*** at home; ***sentir-se em ~*** feel at home; ***para ~*** home; *Port* ***~ de banho*** bathroom; *Port* ***~ de botão*** buttonhole; ***Casa Branca*** White House; ***~ de cachorro*** doghouse, *Brit* kennel ***~ de câmbio*** bureau de change; ***~ de campo*** cottage; ***~ de detenção*** detention center, *Brit* detention centre; ***~ de loucos*** madhouse; ***~ de repouso*** nursing home; ***~ de saúde*** private hospital

casaca [ka'zaka] *f* tails

casaco [ka'zaku] *m comprido*: coat; *curto*: jacket; ***~ de cabedal*** leather jacket

casado [ka'zadu] *adj* married; ***ser ~ com*** be married to

casal [ka'zaw] *m* couple

casamento [kaza'mẽtu] *m* marriage; *cerimônia* wedding; ***~ civil / religioso*** civil / church wedding; ***pedir alguém em ~*** ask for s.o's hand in marriage

casar [ka'zaɾ] ⟨1b⟩ **1** *v/t* marry; *fig* combine **2** *v/i* marry; *fig* go together; ***~ com alguém*** marry s.o.; **casar-se** *v/r* get married; *fig* combine

casarão [kaza'ɾãw] *m* mansion

casca ['kaska] *f fruta*: skin, peel; *árvore*: bark; *ovos, nozes*: shell

cascalho [kas'kaʎu] *m* gravel; *na praia* shingle

cascata [kas'kata] *f* waterfall

cascavel [kaska'vew] *m* rattlesnake

casco ['kasku] *m cavalo*: hoof; (*crânio*) skull; (*vasilha*) empty bottle; NÁUT hull; *tartaruga*: shell

caseiro [ka'zejɾu] **1** *adj* domestic; (*feito em casa*) home-made **2** *m*, **-a** *f* housekeeper

casimira [kazi'miɾa] *f* cashmere

casino [ka'sinu] *m* casino

caso ['kazu] **1** *m* case *tb* GRAM; *amoroso* affair; (*estória*) story; ***em todo ~*** in any case; ***neste ~*** in that case; ***criar ~*** cause trouble; ***não fazer ~ de alguém / algo*** take no notice of s.o. / sth; ***isso não vem ao ~*** that's beside the point **2** *conj* in case, if; ***~ contrário*** if that's not the case; ***~ necessário*** if necessary

caspa ['kaspa] *f* dandruff

casquinha [kas'kiɲa] *f de sorvete* cone

cassação [kasa'sãw] *f* withholding; *políticos*: banning

cassar [ka'saɾ] ⟨1b⟩ *v/t direitos, licença* withhold; *políticos* ban

cassete [ka'sɛtʃi] *f* cassette

casta ['kasta] *f* caste; (*estirpe*) lineage

castanha [kas'taɲa] *f* chestnut; ***~ de caju*** cashew nut

castanha-do-pará [kastaɲadopa'ɾa] *f* ⟨pl castanhas-do-para⟩ Brazil nut

castanheiro [kasta'ɲejɾu] *m* chestnut tree

castanho [kas'taɲu] *adj* brown

castelhano [kaste'ʎanu] *m língua* Spanish

castelo [kas'tɛlu] *m* castle; ***fazer*** (*ou* ***levantar***) ***~s no ar*** build castles in the air

castiçal [kastʃi'saw] *m* candlestick

castidade [kastʃi'dadʒi] *f* chastity

castigar [kastʃi'gaɾ] ⟨1o⟩ *v/t* punish

castigo [kas'tʃigu] *m* punishment; ***estar de ~*** be grounded; ***~ corporal*** corporal punishment

casto ['kastu] *adj* chaste

castor [kas'toɾ] *m* beaver

castração [kastɾa'sãw] *f* castration

castrado [kas'tɾadu] **1** *adj* castrated **2** *m* castrato

castrar [kas'tɾaɾ] ⟨1b⟩ *v/t* castrate

casual [ka'zwaw] *adj* casual; *encontro* chance *atr*

casualidade [kazwali'dadʒi] *f* chance; (*acidente*) accident
catalisador [kataliza'doɾ] **1** *m* catalyst **2** *adj* catalytic
catalogar [katalo'gaɾ] ⟨1o & 1e⟩ *v/t* catalog, *Brit* catalogue
catálogo [ka'talogu] *m* catalog, *Brit* catalogue; **~ telefônico** telephone directory
catapora [kata'pɔɾa] *f Bras* chickenpox
catapulta [kata'puwta] *f* catapult
catapultar [katapuw'taɾ] ⟨1a⟩ *v/t* catapult
catarata [kata'ɾata] *f* waterfall; MED cataract
catarro [ka'tahu] *m* catarrh
catástrofe [ka'tastɾofi] *f* catastrophe
catastrófico [katas'tɾɔfiku] *adj* catastrophic
cata-vento [kata'vẽtu] *m* ⟨*pl* ~s⟩ weathercock
catecismo [kate'sizmu] *m* catechism
cátedra ['katedɾa] *f* chair
catedral [kate'dɾaw] *f* cathedral
catedrático [kate'dɾatʃiku] *m* professor
categoria [katego'ɾia] *f* category; *hierarquia* rank; **de alta ~** first-class; **de segunda ~** second-rate
categórico [kate'gɔɾiku] *adj* categorical
cateter [kate'tɛɾ] *m* MED catheter
catinga [ka'tʃĩga] *f* stench, stink
cativante [katʃi'vãtʃi] *adj* captivating; (*encantador*) charming
cativar [katʃi'vaɾ] ⟨1a⟩ *v/t* captivate; (*escravizar*) enslave
cativeiro [katʃi'vejɾu] *m* captivity; *lugar* prison; (*servidão*) slavery
cativo [ka'tʃivu] **1** *adj* captive **2** *m*, **-a** *f* prisoner; (*escravo*) slave
catolicismo [katoli'sizmu] *m* catholicism
católico [ka'tɔliku] **1** *adj* catholic **2** *m*, **-a** *f* catholic
catorze [ka'toɾzi] *num* fourteen
caução [kaw'sãw] *f* security, guarantee; JUR bail; **sob ~** on bail
Cáucaso ['kawkazu] *m* **1** *adj* Caucasian **2** *m* **-a** *f* Caucasian
cauda ['kawda] *f* tail *tb* AERO; *vestido*: train
caudal [kaw'daw] *m água*: torrent
caudaloso [kawda'lozu] *adj* torrential
caule ['kawli] *m* stalk, stem
causa ['kawza] *f* cause; (*motivo*) motive; JUR lawsuit, case; **por ~ de** because of; **por minha ~** on my account
causador [kawza'doɾ] **1** *m* cause **2** *adj* **o elemento ~ do problema foi …** the thing that caused the problem was …
causal [kaw'zaw] *adj* causal
causar [kaw'zaɾ] ⟨1a⟩ *v/t* cause, bring about; **~ dano** cause harm; **~ agitação** cause a stir
cáustico ['kawstʃiku] *adj* caustic
cautela [kaw'tɛla] *f* caution; (*senha*) ticket; (*título*) share certificate; **com ~** cautiously
cauteloso [kawte'lozu] *adj* cautious
cauterizar [kawter'zaɾ] ⟨1a⟩ *v/t* MED cauterize
cavala [ka'vala] *f* ZOOL mackerel
cavalaria [kavala'ɾia] *f* chivalry; MIL cavalry
cavalariça [kavala'ɾisa] *f* stable
cavaleiro [kava'lejɾu] *m* rider, horseman; horsewoman; *nobreza*: knight
cavalete [kava'letʃi] *m* stand; FOT tripod; *pintor*: easel
cavalgar [kavaw'gaɾ] ⟨1o⟩ **1** *v/t* ride **2** *v/i* **~ em** ride on; **~ sobre** jump over
cavalheiro [kava'ʎejɾu] **1** *m* gentleman **2** *adj* gentlemanly, gallant
cavalo [ka'valu] *m* horse; *xadrez*: knight; **a ~** on horseback; **pode tirar o ~ da chuva!** you can forget that!; **~ de corrida** racehorse
cavalo-marinho [kavaloma'ɾiɲu] *m* seahorse
cavalo(s)-vapor [kavalu(z)va'poɾ] *m*(*pl*) horsepower
cavar [ka'vaɾ] ⟨1b⟩ dig
cave ['kavi] *f* wine-cellar
caveira [ka'vejɾa] *f* skull
caverna [ka'vɛɾna] *f* cave
caviar [ka'vjaɾ] *m* caviar
cavidade [kavi'dadʒi] *f* cavity
caxumba [ka'ʃũba] *f* mumps *sg*
CD [se'de] *m* CD
CD-Rom [sede'hɔm] *m* CD-Rom

cear [sjaɾ] ⟨1l⟩ **1** *v/t* have for supper **2** *v/i* dine
cebola [se'bola] *f* onion
cebolinha [sebo'lĩɲa] *f* chive
cecear [se'sjaɾ] ⟨1l⟩ lisp
cê-cê [se'se] *m* BO
cê-cedilha [sese'dʒiʎa] *m letra* c cedilla
cê-dê-efe [sede'ɛfi] *m/f* grind, *Brit* swot
ceder [se'deɾ] ⟨2c⟩ **1** *v/t* give up; (*dar*) hand over **2** *v/i* give in, yield; *porta, ponte* give way; **~ *a*** give in to
cedilha [se'dʒiʎa] *m* cedilla
cedo ['sedu] *adv* early; (*em breve*) soon; ***de manhã*** **~** first thing in the morning; ***mais*** **~** ***ou mais tarde*** sooner or later; ***amanhã*** **~** tomorrow morning
cedro ['sɛdɾu] *m* cedar
cédula ['sɛdula] *f* banknote; *eleitoral* ballot paper; *Bras* **~** ***de identidade*** identity card
CEE [seɛ'ɛ] *f abr* (***Comunidade Económica Europeia***) EEC (European Economic Community)
cegar [se'gaɾ] ⟨1o & 1c⟩ **1** *v/i* be dazzling **2** *v/t* blind; (*ofuscar*) dazzle
cego ['sɛgu] **1** *adj* blind; *faca* blunt **2** *m*, **-a** *f* blind man; blind woman
cegonha [se'goɲa] *f* stork
cegueira [se'gejɾa] *f* blindness
ceia ['seja] *f* supper
ceifar [sej'faɾ] ⟨1a⟩ *v/t* & *v/i* reap, harvest
cela ['sɛla] *f* cell
celebração [selebɾa'sãw] *f* celebration
celebrar [sele'bɾaɾ] ⟨1c⟩ *v/t* & *v/i* celebrate
célebre ['sɛlebɾi] *adj* famous
celebridade [selebri'dadʒi] *f* celebrity
celeiro [se'lejɾu] *m* granary; (*depósito*) barn
celeste [se'lɛstʃi], **celestial** [seles'tʃiaw] *adj* celestial, heavenly
celibatário [seliba'taɾiu] **1** *adj* unmarried, single **2** *m* bachelor; *mulher* spinster
celibato [seli'batu] *m* celibacy
celofane [selo'fani] *m* cellophane; ***papel*** **~** cling film
célula ['sɛlula] *f* cell *tb* BOT
célula-tronco [sɛlola'tɾõku] *f* ⟨pl células-tronco⟩ stem cell
celular [selu'laɾ] **1** *adj* cellular **2** *m Bras* TEL cell (phone), *Brit* mobile (phone)
celulite [selu'litʃi] *f* cellulite
celulose [selu'lɔzi] *f* cellulose
cem [sẽ] *num* one hundred; **~** ***mil*** one hundred thousand; **~** ***por cento*** one hundred per cent
cemitério [semi'tɛɾiu] *m* cemetery
cena ['sena] *f* scene; (*palco*) stage; ***em*** **~** on the stage; ***levar à*** **~** stage; ***fazer uma*** **~** make a scene
cenário [se'naɾiu] *m* scenario; TEAT scenery; (*panorama*) view; *crime*: scene
cenógrafo [se'nɔgɾafu] *m*, **-a** *f* set designer
cenoura [se'noɾa] *f* carrot
censo ['sẽsu] *m* census
censor [sẽ'soɾ] *m* censor
censura [sẽ'suɾa] *f* censorship; (*condenação*) censure
censurar [sẽsu'ɾaɾ] ⟨1a⟩ *v/t* censure; *filme, livro* censor
centavo [sẽ'tavu] *m* cent; ***estar sem um*** **~** be penniless
centeio [sẽ'teiu] *m* rye
centelha [sẽ'teʎa] *f* spark *tb fig*
centena [sẽ'tena] *f* hundred; ***às*** **~*s*** by the hundred
centenário [sẽte'naɾiu] **1** *adj* centennial, *Brit* centenary **2** *m* centennial, *Brit* centenary
centésimo [sẽ'tɛzimu] **1** *adj* hundredth **2** *m* hundredth
centímetro [sẽ'tʃimetɾu] *m* centimeter, *Brit* centimetre
cento ['sẽtu] *m* hundred; **~** ***e um*** one hundred and one; ***por*** **~** per cent
centopeia [sẽto'pɛja] *f* centipede
central [sẽ'tɾaw] **1** *adj* central **2** *f de polícia etc* headquarters; **~** ***elétrica*** power station; **~** ***nuclear*** nuclear power station; *Port* **~** ***dos telefones*** telephone exchange
centralização [sẽtɾaliza'sãw] *f* ⟨*sem pl*⟩ centralization
centralizar [sẽtɾali'zaɾ] ⟨1a⟩ *v/t* centralize

centrar [sẽ'trar] ⟨1a⟩ TECN, TIPO center, *Brit* centre
centrifugadora [sẽtrifuga'dora] *f* **~ *de roupa*** spin-dryer
centrifugar [sẽtrifu'gar] ⟨1o⟩ *v/t* spin-dry; *salada* spin
centro ['sẽtru] *m* center, *Brit* centre; *cidade* downtown, *Brit* city centre; ***no ~ de*** in the center of; ***~ comercial*** shopping center; ***~ comunitário*** community center; ***~ de convenções*** convention center; ***~ de lazer*** leisure center; ***~ de gravidade*** center of gravity
centro-avante [sẽtroa'vãtʃi] *m* ESP center-forward, *Brit* centre-forward
CEP ['sɛp] *m abr* (***código de endereçamento postal***) zip code, *Brit* post code
cepa ['sepa] *f vírus*: strain
cept... *Port* → ***cet...***
cera ['sera] *f* wax; ***fazer ~*** dawdle
cerâmica [se'rʌmika] *f* pottery, ceramics
cerâmico [se'rʌmiku] *adj* ceramic
cerca ['serka] **1** *f* fence; ***~ viva*** hedgerow; ***~ de estacas*** picket fence **2** *prep* ***~ de*** around, about
cercar [ser'kar] ⟨1n & 1c⟩ *v/t* enclose; *fig* (*por cerca em*) fence in; (*rodear*) surround; MIL besiege
cerco ['serku] *m* encirclement; MIL siege; ***pôr ~ a*** lay siege to
cereal [se'rjaw] *m* cereal; ***cereais em flocos*** breakfast cereals
cerebral [sere'braw] *adj* cerebral
cérebro ['sɛrebru] *m* brain; *fig* brains
cereja [se'reʒa] *f* cherry
cerejeira [sere'ʒejra] *f* cherry tree
cerimônia, *Port* **cerimónia** [seri'monja] *f* ceremony; ***de ~*** formal; ***sem ~*** informal; ***fazer ~*** stand on ceremony; ***~ de posse*** swearing-in ceremony
cerimonial [serimo'njaw] **1** *adj* ceremonial **2** *m* ceremonial
cerimonioso [serimo'njozu] *adj* ceremonious
cerquilha [ser'kiʎa] *f* hash sign
cerrado [se'hadu] **1** *adj* closed, shut; *punho* clenched; (*denso*) dense **2** *m* (*vegetação*) scrubland
cerrar [se'har] ⟨1c⟩ *v/t porta etc* close, shut; *passagem* block; *punho* clench; *dentes* grit; **cerrar-se** *v/r* close, shut; *noites*, *trevas* close in
certeza [ser'teza] *f* certainty; ***com ~*** certainly; ***ter ~ de*** be certain of; ***ter ~ de que*** be certain *ou* sure that; ***tem ~?*** are you sure *ou* certain?
certidão [sertʃi'dãw] *f* certificate; ***~ de nascimento*** birth certificate; ***~ de casamento*** marriage certificate
certificado [sertʃifi'kadu] *m* certificate; ***~ médico*** medical certificate; ***~ de garantia*** warranty
certificar [sertʃifi'kar] ⟨1n⟩ *v/t* certify; (*assegurar*) assure; **certificar-se** *v/r* ***~ de*** make sure of; ***~ de que algo seja feito*** make sure that sth gets done
certo ['sɛrtu] **1** *adj* (*correto*) right, correct; (*seguro*) certain, sure; ***estar ~*** *resposta*, *relógio* be right; ***um ~ Sr. Jones*** a certain Mr Jones; ***é ~ que*** it's certain that; ***tomar algo por ~*** take sth as given; ***na certa*** certainly **2** *adv* right, correctly; ***dar ~*** work out all right; ***está ~*** ok, all right
cerveja [ser'veʒa] *f* beer; ***~ lager*** lager
cervejaria [serveʒa'ria] *f* bar; *fábrica* brewery
cervical [servi'kaw] *adj* cervical
cervice [sɛr'visi] *f* cervix
cervo ['servu] *m* deer
cesariana [seza'rjana] *f* Cesarian, *Brit* Caesarian
cessão [se'sãw] *f* (*cedência*) surrender; (*transferência*) transfer
cessar [se'sar] ⟨1c⟩ *v/i & v/t* cease, stop; ***sem ~*** continually
cessar-fogo [sesar'fogu] *m* ⟨pl inv⟩ ceasefire
cesta ['sesta] *f* basket; *Bras* ***~ básica*** basket of basic food (*sold at supermarkets, sometimes included in salaries for domestic staff*); ***~ de papel*** waste basket, *Brit* waste paper basket
cesto ['sestu] *m* basket; ***~ de lixo*** litter basket
ceticismo [setʃi'sizmu] *m* skepticism, *Brit* scepticism
cético ['sɛtʃiku] **1** *adj* skeptical, *Brit* sceptical **2** *m*, **-a** *f* skeptic, *Brit* sceptic

C

cetim [se'ʧĩ] *m* TÊX satin
céu [sɛu] *m* sky; REL heaven; ***a ~ aberto*** in the open air
céu-da-boca [sɛuda'boka] *m* roof of the mouth
cevada [se'vada] *f* barley
CFC [seɛfe'se] *mpl abr* (***clorofluorcarbonos***) CFC
chá [ʃa] *m* tea; ***tomar ~ de cadeira*** *fig* be a wallflower; ***~ de bebê*** baby shower; ***~ de ervas*** herb tea; ***~ com limão*** lemon tea; ***~ de menta*** mint tea
chacal [ʃa'kaw] *m* jackal
chacina [ʃa'sina] *f* slaughter
Chade ['ʃadʒi] *m* ***o ~*** Chad
chafariz [ʃafa'ris] *m* fountain
chaga ['ʃaga] *f* MED wound; *fig fam* disease
chalé [ʃa'lɛ] *m* chalet
chaleira [ʃa'lejɾa] *f* kettle
chama ['ʃama] *f* flame; ***em ~s*** on fire, in flames
chamada [ʃa'mada] *f* call; TEL (phone)call; MIL roll call; *dos alunos* register; *no jornal* headline; ***dar uma ~ em alguém*** give s.o. a piece of one's mind; ***fazer uma ~*** make a phonecall; ***~ a cobrar*** collect call, *Brit* reverse charge call
chamar [ʃa'maɾ] ⟨1a⟩ **1** *v/t* call; (*invitar*) invite; *atenção* attract; (*dar nome*) name, call; ***mandar ~*** send for; ***nós o chamamos de Tom*** we call him Tom; ***~ alguém para jantar*** invite s.o. over to dinner **2** *v/i* call; TEL *tb* phone; **chamar-se** *v/r* be called; ***como você se chama?*** what's your name?
chamativo [ʃama'ʧivu] *adj* eye-catching; *roupa* showy
chaminé [ʃami'nɛ] *f* chimney; *navio*: funnel
champanhe [ʃã'paɲi] *m* champagne
champu ['ʃãpu] *m Port* shampoo
chamuscar [ʃamus'kaɾ] ⟨1n⟩ *v/t* scorch, singe; **chamuscar-se** *v/r* scorch oneself
chancelaria [ʃãsela'ɾia] *f* chancellery
chanceler [ʃãse'lɛɾ] *m/f* chancellor
chantagear [ʃãta'ʒjaɾ] ⟨1l⟩ *v/t* blackmail
chantagem [ʃã'taʒẽ] *f* blackmail
chantagista [ʃãta'ʒista] *m/f* blackmailer
chantilly [ʃãʧi'li] *m* whipped cream
chão [ʃãw] ⟨*pl* chãos⟩ *m* ground; (*piso*) floor
chapa ['ʃapa] **1** *f* (*placa*) plate; *metal*: sheet; *eleitoral* list; ***bife na ~*** grilled steak; ***~ ondulada*** corrugated iron **2** *m/f fam* buddy; ***oi, meu ~!*** hi, pal!
chapéu [ʃa'pɛu] *m* hat; ***~ de coco*** derby (hat), *Brit* bowler (hat); ***~ de palhinha*** straw hat; ***~ de vaqueiro*** cowboy hat
charada [ʃa'ɾada] *f* charade; (*quebra-cabeça*) puzzle
charlatão [ʃaɾla'tãw] *m* ⟨*pl* -ães⟩ charlatan
charme ['ʃaɾmi] *m* charm; ***fazer ~*** put on the charm
charmoso [ʃaɾ'mozu] *adj* charming
charneca [ʃaɾ'nɛka] *f* moor
charter ['ʃaɾtɛɾ] *m* ***vôo*** *m* ***~***, *Port* ***voo ~*** charter flight
charuto [ʃa'ɾutu] *m* cigar
chassi [ʃa'si] *m* chassis
chatear [ʃa'ʧiaɾ] ⟨1l⟩ **1** *v/t fam* upset; (*irritar*) annoy; (*entediar*) bore **2** *v/i* be upsetting; (*ser irritante*) be annoying; **chatear-se** *v/r* (*aborrecer-se*) get upset; (*zangar-se*) get annoyed
chatice [ʃa'ʧisi] *f fam* nuisance; ***que ~!*** what a nuisance!
chato ['ʃatu] **1** *adj* flat, level; (*tedioso*) boring; (*irritante*) annoying; (*grosseiro*) rude **2** *m*, **-a** *f* bore; *quem irrita* pain
chauvinista ['ʃawvinista] *adj* chauvinistic
chavão [ʃa'vãw] *m* cliché
chave ['ʃavi] *f* key; ELÉT switch; ***fechar à ~*** lock; ***guardar à ~*** lock away; ***~ de fendas*** screwdriver; ***~ inglesa*** wrench; ***~ mestra*** master key
chaveiro [ʃa'vejɾu] *m pessoa* locksmith; (*porta-chaves*) key ring
chávena ['ʃavena] *f Port* cup
checar [ʃe'kaɾ] ⟨1e⟩ check
checo ['ʃɛku] *Port* **1** *adj* Czech; ***República*** *f* ***Checa*** Czech Republic **2** *m*, **-a** *f* Czech **3** *m lingua* Czech
chefão [ʃe'fãw] *m Mafia*: godfather

C

chefe ['ʃɛfi] *m/f* head, chief; *família*: head; (*patrão*) boss; (*dirigente*) leader; **~ de estação** stationmaster; *Port* **~ de mesa** head waiter, maitre d'; **~ de polícia** police chief, *Brit* police superintendent; **~ de turma** foreman
chefia [ʃe'fia] *f* leadership; (*direção*) management; (*sede*) headquarters
chefiar [ʃe'fjar] ⟨1g⟩ *v/t* head; (*dirigir*) lead
chegada [ʃe'gada] *f* arrival; **dar uma ~** drop by
chegar [ʃe'gar] ⟨1o & 1d⟩ **1** *v/i* arrive; (*bastar*) be enough; **~ em casa** arrive home, get home; **~ a tempo** make it; **~ a uma conclusão** reach a conclusion; **chega!** that's enough!; **chega por hoje!** let's call it a day! **chega para cá!** come over here! **~ a fazer algo** manage to do sth; **~ ao fundo do poço** hit rock bottom; **estar chegando aos 40** be pushing 40; **chegar-se** *v/r* **~ a** approach
cheia ['ʃeja] *f* flood
cheio ['ʃeiu] *adj* full; (*repleto*) full up; (*gordo*) plump; *fam* fed up; **~ de si** self-important, full of oneself; *fam* **~ da nota** rich, loaded; **acertar em ~** hit the bull's eye
cheirar [ʃej'rar] ⟨1a⟩ **1** *v/t* smell **2** *v/i* smell (**a** of); **~ mal** stink
cheirinho [ʃej'riɲu] *m* whiff
cheiro ['ʃejru] *m* smell; **ter ~ de** smell of; **mau ~** stench; **sentir o ~ de algo** smell sth
cheque ['ʃɛki] *m* check, *Brit* cheque; *xadrez*: check; **~ em branco** blank check; **~ cruzado** crossed check; **~ sem fundos** bounced check; **~ de viagem** traveler's check, *Brit* traveller's cheque
chiada ['ʃjada] *f* squeak; *pneus*: screech; *vapor*: hiss
chiar [ʃjar] ⟨1g⟩ *v/i* squeak; *porta* creak; *vapor* hiss; *fritura* sizzle
chichi [ʃi'ʃi] *m Port fam* pee; **fazer ~** pee
chiclete [ʃi'klɛtʃi] *m* chewing gum
chicória [ʃi'kɔrja] *f* chicory
chicotada [ʃiko'tada] *f* lash
chicote [ʃi'kɔtʃi] *m* whip
chicotear [ʃiko'tʃiar] ⟨1l⟩ *v/t* whip
chifre ['ʃifri] *m* horn; **pôr ~ em alguém** cheat on s.o.
Chile ['ʃili] *m* Chile
chileno [ʃi'lenu] **1** *adj* Chilean **2** *m*, **-a** *f* Chilean
chilreio [ʃiw'heiu] *m* chirping
chimpanzé [ʃĩpã'zɛ] *m* chimpanzee, chimp
China ['ʃina] *f* China
chinelo [ʃi'nɛlu] *m* slipper; *praia*: sandal
chinês [ʃi'nes] **1** *adj* Chinese **2** *m*, **chinesa** [ʃi'neza] *f* Chinese person **3** *m lingua* Chinese
chip [ʃip] *m* INFORM chip
Chipre ['ʃipri] *m* Cyprus
chique ['ʃiki] *adj* chic, stylish
chiqueiro [ʃi'kejru] *m* pigsty
chocalhar [ʃoka'ʎar] ⟨1b⟩ *v/t & v/i* rattle
chocalho [ʃo'kaʎu] *m* rattle
chocante [ʃo'kãtʃi] *adj* shocking
chocar [ʃo'kar] ⟨1n & 1e⟩ **1** *v/t* shock **2** *v/i ovos* hatch; **chocar-se** *v/r* be shocked;(*colidir*) crash, collide
chocolate [ʃoko'latʃi] *m* chocolate; **barra** *f* **de ~** chocolate bar; **~ ao leite** milk chocolate; **~ meio-amargo** dark chocolate; **~ quente** hot chocolate
chocólatra [ʃo'kɔlatra] *m/f* chocaholic
chofer [ʃo'fɛr] *m/f* chauffeur
chofre ['ʃɔfri] *adv* **de ~** all of a sudden
chope ['ʃopi] *m* draft beer, *Brit* draught beer
choque ['ʃɔki] *m* shock; (*colisão*) collision; (*impacto*) impact; **estar em estado de ~** be in shock; **~ cultural** culture shock
chorão [ʃo'rãw] **1** *m* BOT weeping willow; *fam pessoa* cry-baby **2** *adj* tearful
chorar [ʃo'rar] ⟨1e⟩ *v/i & v/t* cry; **~ por alguém** grieve for s.o.
choro ['ʃoru] *m* crying; **cair no ~** burst into tears
choroso [ʃo'rozu] *adj* tearful
choupana [ʃo'pana] *f* hut
chouriço [ʃo'risu] *m* spicy sausage
chover [ʃo'ver] ⟨2d⟩ rain; *cartas* flood in; **~ a cântaros** pour down

C

chuchu [ʃu'ʃu] *m legume* chayote (*like a marrow*)
chucrute [ʃu'krutʃi] *m* sauerkraut
chulo ['ʃulu] *adj Port* vulgar
chumaço [ʃu'masu] *m* wad
chumbar [ʃũ'baɾ] ⟨1a⟩ **1** *v/t* fill with lead; *dente* fill; *fam aluno* fail **2** *no exame* fail
chumbo ['ʃũbu] *m* lead; *Port dente*: filling; ***gasolina sem ~*** unleaded
chupada [ʃu'pada] *f vulg* blowjob
chupar [ʃu'paɾ] ⟨1a⟩ *v/t* suck; (*absorver*) suck up
chupeta [ʃu'peta] *f* pacifier, *Brit* dummy
churrascaria [ʃuhaska'ɾia] *f* grill restaurant
churrasco [ʃu'hasku] *m* barbecue; *carne* grilled meat
chutar [ʃu'taɾ] ⟨1a⟩ **1** *v/t bola* kick; *fam* (*adivinhar*) guess; (*dar o fora em*) dump **2** *v/i* kick; *para o gol* shoot; *fam* (*adivinhar*) guess; ***chuta!*** guess!
chute ['ʃutʃi] *m* kick; *para o gol* shot; ***~ inicial*** kickoff; ***~ do pênalti*** penalty (kick)
chuteiro [ʃu'tejɾu] *m* football boot
chuva ['ʃuva] *f* rain; *visitantes, reclamações*: stream; *fam* ***estar na ~*** be drunk; ***~ ácida*** acid rain; ***~ de pedra*** hailstorm; ***~ radioativa*** fallout
chuveiro [ʃu'vejɾu] *m* shower
chuviscar [ʃuvis'kaɾ] ⟨1n⟩ *v/i* drizzle
chuvisco [ʃu'visku] *m* drizzle
chuvoso [ʃu'vozu] *adj* rainy
ciática ['sjatʃika] *f* sciatica; ***dor*** *f* ***~*** sciatic pains
ciático ['sjatʃiku] *adj* sciatic; ***nervo*** *m* ***~*** sciatic nerve
cibercafé [siberka'fɛ] *m* Internet café
ciberespaço [siberes'pasu] *m* cyberspace
cibernética [siber'nɛtʃika] *f* cybernetics
cicatriz [sika'tɾis] *f* scar
cicatrizar [sikatɾi'zaɾ] ⟨1a⟩ *v/i* scar; *ferida* heal
cicerone [sise'ɾoni] *m/f* tourist guide
ciciar [si'sjaɾ] ⟨1g⟩ *v/i* rustle
cicio ['sisiu] *m* rustle
cíclico ['sikliku] *adj* cyclical
ciclismo [si'klizmu] *m* cycling
ciclista [si'klista] *m/f* cyclist
ciclo ['siklu] *m* cycle
ciclone [si'kloni] *m* cyclone
ciclovia [siklo'via] *f* cycle path
cidadania [sidada'nia] *f* citizenship
cidadão [sida'dãw] ⟨*pl* -ãos⟩ *m*, **cidadã** [sida'dã] *f* citizen
cidade [si'dadʒi] *f* town; *grande* city; ***na ~*** in town; ***~ natal*** home town; ***~ fantasma*** ghost town; ***~ portuária*** port
cidade-satélite [sidadʒisa'tɛlitʃi] *f* ⟨*pl* cidades-satélites⟩ satellite (town)
ciência ['sjẽsja] *f* science; (*saber*) knowledge; ***~s*** *pl* ***sociais*** social sciences
ciente ['sjẽtʃi] *adj* aware; ***estar ~ de*** be aware of
científico [sjẽ'tʃifiku] *adj* scientific
cientista [sjẽ'tʃista] *m/f* scientist
cifra ['sifɾa] *f* figure; (*código*) cipher
cigano [si'ganu] **1** *m*, **-a** *f* gypsy **2** *adj* gypsy
cigarra [si'gaha] *f* cicada; ELÉT buzzer
cigarrilha [siga'hiʎa] *f* cigarillo
cigarro [si'gahu] *m* cigarette
cilindrada [silĩ'dɾada] *f* AUTO cubic capacity
cilíndrico [si'lĩdɾiku] *adj* cylindrical
cilindro [si'lĩdɾu] *m* cylinder; (*rolo*) roller
cílio ['siʎu] *m* eyelash
cima ['sima] *f* ***de ~*** from above; ***o / a de ~*** the top one; ***em ~*** on top; ***em ~ de*** on, on top of; ***lá em ~*** up there; ***para ~*** up; ***por ~ de*** over; ***ainda por ~*** on top of that; ***no andar de ~*** upstairs; *fam* ***dar em ~ de alguém*** hit on s.o.
cimeira [si'mejɾa] *f Port montanha, conferência*: summit
cimentar [simẽ'taɾ] ⟨1a⟩ *v/t* cement
cimento [si'mẽtu] *m* cement; *chão* concrete floor; ***~ armado*** reinforced concrete
cinco ['sĩku] *num* five
cineasta [si'njasta] *m/f* film-maker
cinema [si'nema] *m* movie theater, *Brit* cinema; *arte* cinema; ***estrela*** *f* ***de ~*** movie star; ***sessão*** *f* ***de ~*** movie showing; ***ir ao ~*** go to the movies, *Brit tb* go to the cinema

cínico ['siniku] **1** *adj* cynical **2** *m*, **-a** *f* cynic
cinqüenta, *Port* **cinquenta** [sĩŋ'kwẽta] *num* fifty
cinta ['sĩta] *f banda* sash; *de mulher* girdle
cintilar [sĩʧi'laɾ] ⟨1a⟩ *v/i* sparkle, glitter
cinto ['sĩtu] *m* belt; **~ de segurança** seatbelt; **apertar os ~s** fasten your seatbelts
cintura [sĩ'tuɾa] *f* waist; *linha* waistline
cinza ['sĩza] **1** *f* ash, ashes; **Quarta-Feira** *f* **de Cinzas** Ash Wednesday **2** *adj* gray, *Brit* grey
cinzeiro [sĩ'zejɾu] *m* ashtray
cinzel [sĩ'zɛw] *m* chisel
cinzelar [sĩze'laɾ] ⟨1c⟩ chisel
cinzento [sĩ'zẽtu] *adj* gray, *Brit* grey
cio ['siu] *m* ZOOL mating season; **estar no ~** *cadela* be on heat
cioso ['sjozu] *adj* eager
cipreste [si'pɾɛsʧi] *m* cypress (tree)
circo ['siɾku] *m* circus
circuito [siɾ'kuitu] *m* circuit; (*pista*) track; **~ fechado de televisão** closed-circuit television, CCTV
circulação [siɾkula'sãw] *f* circulation *tb* MED; *veículos etc*: traffic
circular[1] [siɾku'laɾ] **1** *adj* circular, round **2** *f* circular
circular[2] [siɾku'laɾ] ⟨1a⟩ **1** *v/t* circulate; (*estar em volta de*) encircle; (*percorrer em roda*) go around **2** *v/i* circulate; *girar, andar* go around
círculo ['siɾkulu] *m* circle; *de pessoas* ring; **fazer ~s** circle; **~ vicioso** vicious circle; **~ de amigos** circle of friends
circunferência [siɾkũfe'ɾẽsja] *f* MAT circumference
circunflexo [siɾkũ'flɛksu] *m* GRAM (**acento**) **~** circumflex (accent)
circunstância [siɾkũs'tãsja] *f* circumstance; **nestas ~s** under the circumstances; **sob ~ alguma** under no circumstances
cirrose [si'hɔzi] *f* MED cirrhosis
cirurgia [siruɾ'ʒia] *f* surgery; **~ plástica** plastic surgery; **passar por uma ~** undergo surgery
cirurgião [siruɾ'ʒjãw] *m*, **cirurgiã** [siruɾ'ʒjã] *f* surgeon; **~ plástico** plastic surgeon
cirúrgico [si'ɾuɾʒiku] *adj* surgical
cisão [si'zãw] *f* split, division; (*desacordo*) disagreement
cisma ['sizma] **1** *m* REL schism **2** *f* (*mania*) fixation; *criança*: whim; (*antipatia*) dislike; **esta ~ de que tem fantasmas aqui** this strange belief that there are ghosts here
cismar [siz'maɾ] ⟨1a⟩ **1** *v/i* **~ em** brood over; (*não gostar*) **~ com** take a dislike to **2** *v/t* **~ que** be convinced that; **~ em fazer** insist on doing
cisne ['sizni] *m* swan
cisterna [sis'tɛɾna] *f* cistern, tank
cistite [sis'ʧiʧi] *f* MED cystitis
cisto ['sistu] *m* MED cyst
citação [sita'sãw] *f* quotation; JUR summons *sg*
citadino [sita'dʒinu] *m*, **-a** *f* town-dweller
citar [si'taɾ] ⟨1a⟩ *v/t* quote; DIR summon
cítrico ['sitɾiku] *adj* citrus; **ácido** *m* **~** citric acid
ciúme ['siumi] *m* jealousy; **ter ~s de alguém** be jealous of s.o.; **um ataque de ~** a fit of jealousy
ciumento [siu'mẽtu] *adj* jealous
cívico ['siviku] *adj* civic
civil [si'viw] **1** *adj* civil; **direitos civis** civil rights; **desobediência ~** civil disobedience **2** *m* civilian
civilização [siviliza'sãw] *f* civilization
civilizado [sivili'zadu] *adj* civilized
civismo [si'vizmu] *m* public spirit
clã [klã] *m* clan
clamar [kla'maɾ] ⟨1a⟩ **1** *v/t* clamor for, *Brit* clamour for **2** *v/i* cry out
clamor [kla'moɾ] *m* outcry
clandestino [klãdes'ʧinu] *adj* clandestine
clara ['klaɾa] *f* **~** (**de ovo**) egg-white
clarabóia [klaɾa'bɔja] *f* skylight
clarão [kla'ɾãw] *m* flash
clarear [kla'ɾjaɾ] ⟨1l⟩ **1** *v/t* lighten **2** *v/i tempo* clear up
clareira [kla'ɾejɾa] *f* clearing
clareza [kla'ɾeza] *f* clarity
claridade [klaɾi'dadʒi] *f* daylight; (*luz*) brightness

C

clarinete [klaɾi'netʃi] *m* clarinet
clarividência [klaɾivi'dẽsja] *f* foresight
clarividente [klaɾivi'dẽtʃi] **1** *adj* prudent **2** *m/f* clairvoyant
claro ['klaɾu] *adj* clear; (*oposto a escuro*) bright; *cor* light; **~!** of course!; (**é**) **~** (***que sim***) sure, of course; (**é**) **~ *que não*** of course not
classe ['klasi] *f* class; **~ *alta*** upper class; **~ *baixa*** lower class; **~ *gramatical*** part of speech; **~ *média*** middle class; **~ *operária*** working class; ***de primeira* ~** first class
clássico ['klasiku] **1** *adj* classical; *muito bom, típico* classic; ***compositor*** *m* **~** classical composer **2** *m* LIT, MÚS *etc* classic
classificação [klasifika'sãw] *f* classification; ESP place, placing
classificado [klasifi'kadu] *adj* classified; *em exame* successful; *time* qualifying
classificar [klasifi'kaɾ] ⟨1n⟩ *v/t* classify; ***ficou classificada em segundo lugar*** she came second; **classificar-se** *v/r* qualify; (*chamar-se*) describe oneself
classificatório [klasifika'tɔɾiu] *adj* qualifying
claustrofobia [klawstɾofo'bia] *f* claustrophobia
cláusula ['klawzula] *f* clause
clave ['klavi] *f* MÚS key; **~ *de sol*** treble clef
clavícula [kla'vikula] *f* ANAT collar bone
clemência [kle'mẽsja] *f* clemency
clérigo ['klɛɾigu] *m* clergyman, cleric
clero ['klɛɾu] *m* clergy
clicar [kli'kaɾ] ⟨1a⟩ *v/i* INFORM **~ *em*** click on
cliché [kli'ʃe] *m* (*chavão*) cliché
cliente [kli'ẽtʃi] *m/f* client; MED patient
clientela [kliẽ'tɛla] *f* clientele; MED patients
clima ['klima] *m* climate
climático [kli'matʃiku] *adj* climatic; ***mudanças*** *fpl* ***climáticas*** climate changes
clínica ['klinika] *f* clinic; ***médico*** *m* ***de* ~ *geral*** general practitioner; **~ *ambulatorial*** outpatient clinic
clínico ['kliniku] **1** *adj* clinical **2** *m* doctor
clipe ['klipi] *m* clip; *papel*: paper clip
clique ['kliki] *m* INFORM click; ***dar um* ~ *duplo em*** double-click on
clonagem [klo'naʒẽ] *f* cloning
clonar [klo'naɾ] ⟨1f⟩ *v/t* clone
clone ['kloni] *m* clone
cloro ['klɔɾu] *m* QUÍM chlorine
clube ['klubi] *m* club; **~ *de golfe*** golf club; **~ *de jovens*** youth club
coabitar [kwabi'taɾ] ⟨1a⟩ *v/i* cohabit, live together
coação, *Port* **coacção** [kwa'sãw] *f* coercion
coador [kwa'doɾ] *m* strainer; *café*: filter bag
coagir [kwa'ʒiɾ] ⟨3n⟩ *v/t* coerce
coagular [kwago'laɾ] ⟨1a⟩ *v/i* coagulate; *sangue* clot
coágulo ['kwagulu] *m* clot
coalhada [kwa'ʎada] *f* curd
coalizão [kwali'zãw] *f* coalition
coar [kwaɾ] ⟨1f⟩ *v/t líquido* strain
co-autor [koaw'toɾ] *m*, **-a** *f* co-author; *crime*: accomplice
coaxar [kwa'ʃaɾ] ⟨1b⟩ **1** *v/i* croak **2** *m* croaking
cobaia [ko'baja] *f* guinea pig *tb fig*
cobalto [ko'bawtu] *m* cobalt
cobarde [ko'bardʒi] *Port* **1** *adj* cowardly **2** *m/f* coward
cobardia [ko'baɾdʒia] *f Port* cowardice
coberta [ko'bɛɾta] **1** *f* cover, covering; NÁUT deck **2** *adj* covered; *arena* indoor
cobertor [kobeɾ'toɾ] *m* blanket
cobertura [kobeɾ'tuɾa] *f* (*telhado*) roof; (*tampa*) covering; *apartamento* penthouse; *TV, rádio etc*: coverage; *seguros*: cover; *celular*: network coverage; **~ *da mídia*** media coverage
cobiça [ko'bisa] *f* greed
cobiçar [kobi'saɾ] ⟨1p⟩ *v/t* covet, desire
cobra ['kɔbɾa] **1** *f* snake; ***dizer* ~*s e lagartos de alguém*** say bad things about s.o. **2** *m/f fam* expert

cobrador [kobɾa'doɾ] *m dívidas, impostos*: collector; *transporte*: ticket collector
cobrança [ko'brãsa] *f* collection; (*ato de cobrar*) charging; ESP ~ ***de falta*** free kick
cobrar [ko'bɾaɾ] ⟨1e⟩ *v/t taxa* collect; *preço* charge; *pênalti* take
cobre ['kɔbɾi] *m* copper; *pop* **~s** *pl* (*moedas*) loose change
cobrir [ko'bɾiɾ] ⟨3f; *pp* coberto⟩ *v/t* cover (**de, com** with); **cobrir-se** *v/r* cover oneself; ~ ***de gelo*** freeze over
cocaína [koka'ina] *f* cocaine
coçar [ko'saɾ] ⟨1p & 1e⟩ **1** *v/t* scratch **2** *v/i* itch; **coçar-se** *v/r* scratch (oneself); ***eu não tenho tempo nem para me coçar*** I have no time to breathe
cócegas ['kɔsegas] *fpl* ***sentir*** ~ feel a tickle; ***fazer*** ~ ***a alguém*** tickle s.o.
coceira [ko'sejɾa] *f Bras* itch; *qualidade* itchiness
cochichar [koʃi'ʃaɾ] ⟨1a⟩ *v/i* whisper
cochilar [koʃi'laɾ] ⟨1a⟩ *v/i* snooze, doze
cochilo [ko'ʃilu] *m* snooze, doze
coco ['koku] *m* coconut; ***leite*** *m* ***de*** ~ coconut milk
coco, *Port* **cocó** [ko'kɔ] *m fam* poo
código ['kɔdʒigu] *m* code; ~ ***de área*** area code; ~ ***de barras*** bar code; ~ ***de ética profissional*** code of conduct; ~ ***genético*** genetic code; ~ ***postal*** zip code, *Brit* post code
codorniz [kodoɾ'nis] *f* quail
coelho ['kweʎu] *m* rabbit; ~ ***de Páscoa*** Easter bunny
coentro(s) ['kwẽtɾu(s)] *m*(*pl*) BOT coriander
coerência [kwe'ɾẽsja] *f* consistency; *fazer sentido* coherence
coerente [kwe'ɾẽtʃi] *adj* consistent; *que faz sentido* coherent
coesão [kwe'zãw] *f* cohesion
coexistência [kwizis'tẽsja] *f* coexistence
coexistir [kwizis'tʃiɾ] ⟨3a⟩ *v/i* coexist
cofre ['kɔfɾi] *m* safe *m*
cofre-forte [kɔfɾe'fɔɾtʃi] *m* strongbox
co-gestão [koʒes'tãw] *f* ⟨*sem pl*⟩ worker participation
cogumelo [kogu'mɛlu] *m* mushroom
coice ['kojsi] *m cavalo*: kick
coincidência [koĩsi'dẽsja] *f* coincidence
coincidir [koĩsi'dʒiɾ] ⟨3a⟩ *v/i* coincide; *concordar*: agree; ~ **com** coincide with
coisa ['kojza] *f* thing; ***pouca / muita*** ~ a little / a lot; ***a mesma*** ~ the same; ~ ***de*** about; *fam* ~ ***de maluco*** madness; ***uma*** ~ ***do passado*** a thing of the past; ***que*** ~**!** gosh!; ***não ser grande*** ~ be nothing special
coitado [koj'tadu] *adj* poor, ~**!** poor thing!; ~ ***do Pedro*** poor Pedro
coito ['kojtu] *m* coitus
cola ['kɔla] *f* glue; *Bras fam exame*: crib
colaboração [kolaboɾa'sãw] *f* collaboration; (*ajuda*) help; *numa atividade* partnership; ***com a*** ~ ***de*** with the help of, assisted by
colaborador [kolaboɾa'doɾ] *m*, **-a** *f* collaborator; *jornal*: contributor
colaborar [kolabo'ɾaɾ] ⟨1e⟩ *v/i* collaborate; (*ajudar*) help; (*contribuir*) contribute; ~ ***com*** work with
colapso [ko'lapsu] *m* collapse; ~ ***cardíaco*** heart failure; ~ ***nervoso*** nervous breakdown
colar[1] [ko'laɾ] *m* necklace; *animal*: collar
colar[2] [ko'laɾ] ⟨1e⟩ **1** *v/t* stick, glue; ~ ***algo em algo*** glue sth to sth **2** *v/i* stick; *Bras fam* cheat
colarinho [kola'ɾiɲu] *m* collar; *fam cerveja*: head
colarinho-branco [kulaɾiɲo'bɾãku] *m* ⟨*pl* colarinhos-brancos⟩ white-collar worker
colcha ['kowʃa] *f* bedspread
colchão [kow'ʃãw] *m* mattress
colchete [kow'ʃetʃi] *m* clasp, fastening; (*parêntese*) square bracket; ~ ***de pressão*** press stud, *Brit* popper
colchonete [kowʃo'netʃi] *m* place mat
coldre ['koldɾi] *m* holster
coleção, *Port* **colecção** [kole'sãw] *f* collection; ~ ***de selos*** stamp collection
colecionador, *Port* **coleccionador** [kolesjona'doɾ] *m*, **-a** *f* collector; ~ ***de selos*** stamp collector

C

colecionar, *Port* **coleccionar** [koles-jo'nar] ⟨1f⟩ *v/t* collect
colect... *Port* → ***colet...***
colega [ko'lɛga] *m/f* colleague; *estudos*: classmate; *time* team-mate
colégio [ko'lɛʒiu] *m* school, college; ~ ***eleitoral*** electoral college
coleira [ko'lejra] *f cão*: collar
cólera ['kɔlera] *f* wrath, rage; MED cholera
colesterol [koleste'rɔw] *m* cholesterol; ***sem*** ~ cholesterol-free
coleta [ko'lɛta] *f* levy; REL collection
coletânea [kole'tʌnja] *f* collection
coletar [kole'tar] ⟨1c⟩ *v/t* (*colher*) gather
colete [ko'letʃi] *m* vest, *Brit* waistcoat; ~ ***de salvação***, ~ ***salva-vidas*** life preserver, *Brit* life jacket
colete-de-forças [koletʃidʒi'forsas] *m* straitjacket
coletividade [koletʃivi'dadʒi] *f* totality, whole; (*sociedade*) community
coletivo [kole'tʃivu] **1** *adj* collective; ***transporte*** *m* ~ mass transit, *Brit* public transport; ***contrato*** *m* ~ pay agreement; GRAM ***nome*** *m* ~ collective noun **2** *m* collective
colheita [ko'ʎejta] *f* harvest; (*produto*) crop
colher[1] [ko'ʎer] ⟨2d⟩ *v/t* reap, harvest; INFORM *dados* gather; *fruta* pick
colher[2] [ko'ʎɛr] *f* spoon; *pedreiro*: trowel; ***me foi dado de*** ~ it was handed to me on a silver platter; ~ ***de café*** coffee spoon; ~ ***de chá*** teaspoon; ~ ***de sobremesa*** dessert spoon; ~ ***de sopa*** soup spoon
colherada [koʎɛ'rada] *f* spoonful
colibri [koli'bri] *m* hummingbird
cólica ['kɔlika] *f* colic
colidir [koli'dʒir] ⟨3a⟩ *v/i* collide; ~ ***com*** collide with, crash into
coligação [koliga'sãw] *f* coalition; ***governo*** *m* ***de*** ~ coalition government
colina [ko'lina] *f* hill
colírio [ko'liriu] *m* eye drops
colisão [koli'zãw] *f* collision; (*conflito*) conflict
coliseu [koli'zew] *m* colosseum
colite [ko'litʃi] *f* MED colitis
collants [ko'lãs] *mpl Port* pantihose, *Brit* tights
colmeia [kow'meja] *f* beehive
colo ['kɔlu] *m* neck; (*regaço*) lap; ***no*** ~ on one's lap, in one's arms
colocação [koloka'sãw] *f* placing; (*montagem*) putting up, erection; (*instalação*) installation; *corrida*: place
colocar [kolo'kar] ⟨1n & 1e⟩ *v/t* put, place; *pneus*, *tapetes* fit; (*instalar*) install; *idéia* put forward; *cartaz* put up; *maquiagem* put on; ~ ***em risco*** put at risk
Colômbia [ko'lõbja] *f* Colombia
colombiano [kolõ'bjanu] **1** *adj* Colombian **2** *m*, **-a** *f* Colombian
Colombo [ko'lõbu] *m* Columbus
colônia, *Port* **colónia** [ko'lonja] *f* colony; (*perfume*) cologne; ~ ***de férias*** summer camp
colonial [kolo'njaw] *adj* colonial
colonizar [koloni'zar] ⟨1a⟩ *v/t* colonize
colono [ko'lonu] *m* settler
coloquial [kolo'kjaw] *adj* colloquial
colorido [kolo'ridu] **1** *adj* colorful, *Brit* colourful **2** *m* (*coloração*) coloring, *Brit* colouring
colorir [kolo'rir] ⟨3f⟩ *v/t* color, *Brit* colour
colossal [kolo'saw] *adj* colossal
coluna [ko'luna] *f* column; MIL convoy ~ ***social*** gossip column; ~ ***vertebral*** spine
colunista [kolu'nista] *m/f* columnist
com [kõ] *prep* with; ***estar*** ~ ***fome*** be hungry; ~ ***cuidado*** carefully, with care; ~ ***desconfiança*** suspiciously, with suspicion; ~ ***a condição de que ...*** on condition that ...; ~ ***50 anos*** at (the age of) 50; ~ ***certeza*** certainly, surely; ***ele estava*** ~ ***ciúmes*** he was jealous
coma ['koma] *m* MED coma
comadre [ko'madri] *f* godmother of one's child; mother of one's godchild
comandante [komã'dãtʃi] *m* commander; NÁUT, AERO captain
comandante-em-chefe *m/f* commander-in-chief
comandar [komã'dar] ⟨1a⟩ *v/t* command; (*chefiar*) lead

comando [ko'mãdu] *m* command *tb* INFORM; TECN steering, navigation; **~ *à distância*** remote control
combate [kõ'batʃi] *m* combat, battle; *doença etc*: fight, battle (***a*** against); **~ *de luta livre*** wrestling match
combatente [kõba'tẽtʃi] *m/f* combatant
combater [kõba'teɾ] ⟨2b⟩ *v/t* fight, combat; (*opor-se a*) combat
combinação[1] [kõbina'sãw] *f* combination; (*acordo*) arrangement; (*plano*) scheme; QUÍM compound
combinação[2] [kõbina'sãw] *f vestuário*: slip
combinar [kõbi'naɾ] ⟨1a⟩ **1** *v/t* combine; *jantar etc* arrange; *fuga etc* plan; *fam* ***combinado!*** you're on! **2** *v/i roupas etc* go together; **~ *com*** go with, match
comboio [kõ'boju] *m* NÁUT convoy; *Port* FERROV train; **~ *expresso*** express train
combustão [kõbus'tãw] *f* combustion
combustível [kõbus'tʃivew] **1** *m* fuel; **~ *nuclear*** nuclear fuel **2** *adj* combustible
começar [kome'saɾ] ⟨1p & 1c⟩ start, begin; **~ *a fazer algo*** begin to do sth, begin doing sth; **~ *do zero*** start from scratch; ***para* ~** to begin with
começo [ko'mesu] *m* beginning, start
comédia [ko'mɛdʒia] *f* comedy
comediante [kome'dʒiãtʃi] *m/f* comedian
comemoração [komemoɾa'sãw] *f* commemoration; (*celebração*) celebration
comemorar [komemo'ɾaɾ] ⟨1e⟩ *v/t* commemorate; (*celebrar*) celebrate
comemorativo [komemoɾa'tʃivu] *adj* memorial
comensal [komẽ'saw] *m/f* diner
comentar [komẽ'taɾ] ⟨1a⟩ **1** *v/t* comment on, make comments about; ***ele comentou algo interessante*** he made an interesting comment **2** *v/i jogo etc*: commentate; **~ *no jogo*** commentate on the game
comentário [komẽ'taɾiu] *m* comment, remark; (*explicação*) commentary; ***sem* ~** no comment
comentarista [komẽta'ɾista] *m/f* commentator
comer [ko'meɾ] ⟨2d⟩ **1** *v/t* eat; *ferrugem* eat away; *xadrez*: take, capture **2** *v/i* eat; **~ *fora*** eat out
comercial [komeɾ'sjaw] **1** *adj* commercial; ***centro*** *m* **~** shopping mall **2** *m* commercial
comercializar [komeɾsjali'zaɾ] ⟨1a⟩ *v/t* commercialize; *produto, idéia* market
comerciante [komeɾ'sjãtʃi] *m/f* trader
comércio [ko'mɛɾsiu] *m* commerce; (*tráfico*) trade; (*negócio*) business; (*lojas*) stores; **~ *eletrônico*** e-commerce
comestível [komes'tʃivew] *adj* edible
cometa [ko'meta] *m* comet
cometer [kome'teɾ] ⟨2c⟩ *v/t crime, suicídio* commit; *erro* make
comichão [komi'ʃãw] *f* itch
comício [ko'misiu] *m* assembly; POL rally
cômico, *Port* **cómico** ['komiku] **1** *adj* comic(al) **2** *m*, **-a** *f* comedian
comida [ko'mida] *f* food; (*refeição*) meal; **~ *caseira*** homemade food; **~ *congelada*** frozen food
comigo [ko'migu] *pron* with me; *reflexivo* with myself; ***conta* ~** count on me
comilão [komi'lãw] **1** *adj* greedy **2** *m*, **comilona** *f* glutton
cominho(s) [ko'miɲu(s)] *m*(*pl*) cumin
comissão [komi'sãw] *f* commission; (*comitê*) committee; **~ *de vendas*** commission on sales
comissário [komi'saɾiu] *m*, **-a** *f* commissioner; **~ *de bordo*** flight attendant
comitê, *Port* **comité** [komi'te] *m* committee
comitiva [komi'tʃiva] *f* entourage
como[1] ['komu] **1** *adv* ◊ (*modo*) as; ***ela fez* ~ *eu disse*** she did as I said; **~ *se*** as if; ***seja* ~ *for*** be that as it may; ***Rodrigo Santoro* ~ *Hamlet*** Rodrigo Santoro as Hamlet
◊ (*assim como*) like; ***ela tem o cabelo escuro,* ~ *a mãe*** she has dark hair, like her mother; **~ *ela é?*** what's she like?

C

◇ *de que maneira* how; **~ *vai o trabalho?*** how's the work going?; **~ *vão as coisas?*** how are things?; ***não sei ~ fazer*** I don't know how to do it; **~?** excuse me? sorry?; **~ *assim?*** what do you mean? **2** *conj* (*porque*) as, since; **~ *estava escuro, ela acendeu a luz*** as it was dark, she turned on the light
como[2] ['komu] → ***comer***
comoção [komo'sãw] *f* (*excitação*) commotion; (*abalo*) distress, consternation
cômoda, *Port* **cómoda** ['komuda] *f* bureau, *Brit* chest of drawers
comodidade [komodʒi'dadʒi] *f* comfort; (*conveniência*) convenience
comodista [komo'dʒista] *adj* complacent
cômodo, *Port* **cómodo** ['komodu] *adj* *Bras* comfortable; (*conveniente*) convenient
comovedor [komove'doɾ], **comovente** [komo'vẽtʃi] *adj* moving
comover [komo'veɾ] ⟨2d⟩ *v/t* move; **comover-se** *v/r* be moved
comovido [komo'vidu] *adj palestra, súplica* impassioned
compactar [kõpak'taɾ] ⟨1a⟩ *v/t* INFORM compress, zip up
compacto [kõ'paktu] *adj* (*comprimido*) compact; (*denso*) solid
compadre [kõ'padri] *m fam* buddy, pal
compaixão [kõpaj'ʃãw] *f* ⟨*sem pl*⟩ compassion
companheiro [kõpa'ɲejɾu] *m*, **-a** companion; (*amigo*) friend, *fam* pal
companhia [kõpa'ɲia] *f* company, firm; MIL company; ***fazer ~ a alguém*** keep s.o. company; **~ *aérea*** airline; **~ *limitada*** limited company; **~ *de seguro*** insurance company
comparação [kõpaɾa'sãw] *f* comparison; ***em ~*** in comparison; ***não tem ~*** there's no comparison
comparar [kõpa'ɾaɾ] ⟨1b⟩ *v/t* compare (***com*** with); **comparar-se** *v/r* compare
comparativo [kõpaɾa'tʃivu] **1** *adj* comparative **2** *m* GRAM comparative
comparável [kõpa'ɾavew] *adj* comparable
comparecer [kõpaɾe'seɾ] ⟨2g⟩ *v/i* appear; **~ *a*** attend
compartilhar [kõpaɾtʃi'ʎaɾ] ⟨1a⟩ **1** *v/t* share **2** *v/i* **~ *de*** share in
compartimento [kõpaɾtʃi'mẽtu] *m* compartment; (*aposento*) room; **~ *de carga*** *avião*: hold
compasso [kõ'pasu] *m* compass; MÚS beat, time
compatibilidade [kõpatʃibili'dadʒi] *f* compatibility
compatível [kõpa'tʃivew] *adj* compatible
compatriota [kõpatɾi'ɔta] *m/f* compatriot, fellow countryman / woman
compêndio [kõ'pẽdʒiu] *m* compendium; (*livro de texto*) textbook
compensação [kõpẽsa'sãw] *f* compensation; *cheque*: clearance
compensado [kõpẽ'sadu] *m* plywood
compensar [kõpẽ'saɾ] ⟨1a⟩ *v/t* compensate for, make up for; (*equilibrar*) offset; *cheque* clear
competência [kõpe'tẽsja] *f* competence; (*responsabilidade*) responsibility; ***não é da minha ~*** that's not my responsibility
competente [kõpe'tẽtʃi] *adj* (*capaz*) competent, able; (*responsável*) responsible; (*apropriado*) appropriate
competição [kõpetʃi'sãw] *f* competition
competidor [kõpetʃi'doɾ] *m/f* competitor
competir [kõpe'tʃiɾ] ⟨3c⟩ *v/i* compete; **~ *a alguém*** be s.o.'s responsibility; (*caber*) be up to s.o.
competitividade [kõpetʃitʃivi'dadʒi] *f* competitiveness
competitivo [kõpetʃi'tʃivu] *adj* competitive
compilar [kõpi'laɾ] ⟨1a⟩ *v/t* compile
complacente [kõpla'sẽtʃi] *adj* obliging; *Port* complacent
compleição [kõplej'sãw] *f pessoa*: constitution
complementar [kõplemẽ'taɾ] **1** *v/t* ⟨1a⟩ complement **2** *adj* complementary; **complementar-se** *v/r* ***eles se complementam*** they complement

each other
complemento [kõple'mẽtu] *m* complement
completamente [kõplɛta'mẽtʃi] *adv* completely
completar [kõple'tar] ⟨1c⟩ *v/t* complete; *tanque*, *copo* top up; **~ *10 anos*** turn 10; TEL **~ *a ligação*** get through
completo [kõ'plɛtu] *adj* complete; (*cheio*) full (up); ***por* ~** completely
complexado [kõple'ksadu] *adj* with a complex, hung-up; ***estar* ~** have a complex
complexidade [kõpleksi'dadʒi] *f* complexity
complexo [kõ'plɛksu] **1** *adj* (*complicado*) complex **2** *m* PSICOL complex; **~ *de inferioridade*** inferiority complex
complicação [kõplika'sãw] *f* complication
complicado [kõpli'kadu] *adj* (*difícil*) complicated
complicar [kõpli'kar] ⟨1n⟩ *v/t* complicate
complô [kõ'plo] *m* plot, conspiracy
componente [kõpo'nẽtʃi] *m* component
compor [kõ'por] ⟨2z⟩ **1** *v/t* compose; *discurso*, *livro* write; (*arranjar*) arrange; TIPO compose, (type)set **2** *v/i* compose; **compor-se** *v/r* compose oneself; **~ *de*** consist of
comporta [kõ'pɔrta] *f* floodgate; *canal*: lock
comportamento [kõporta'mẽtu] *m* behavior, *Brit* behaviour
comportar [kõpor'tar] ⟨1e⟩ *v/t* put up with, bear; (*conter*) hold; **comportar-se** *v/r* behave; **~ *mau*** misbehave, behave badly; ***comporte-se!*** behave (yourself)!
composição [kõpozi'sãw] *f* composition; (*acordo*) compromise; TIPO composition, (type)setting
compositor [kõpozi'tor] *m*, **-a** *f* composer; TIPO compositor, typesetter
composto [kõ'postu] **1** *adj* levelheaded, composed; (*de muitos elementos*) compound, composite; **~ *de*** made up of **2** *m* compound
compota [kõ'pɔta] *f* compote; ***em* ~** *fruta* stewed
compra ['kõpra] *f* purchase; **~*s*** shopping; ***fazer* ~*s*** go shopping; **~ *online*** online shopping
comprador [kõpra'dor] *m*, **-a** *f* buyer, purchaser
comprar [kõ'prar] ⟨1a⟩ *v/t* buy, purchase; (*subornar*) bribe; **~ *a parte de*** buy out
compreender [kõpriẽ'der] ⟨2a⟩ *v/t* (*entender*) understand; (*constar de*) consist of, comprise; (*conter*) contain; (*abranger*) cover; ***chegar a* ~** realize
compreensão [kõpriẽ'sãw] *f* ⟨*sem pl*⟩ understanding; ***isso vai além da minha* ~** that's beyond me, that's beyond my comprehension
compreensível [kõpriẽ'sivew] *adj* understandable, comprehensible
compreensivo [kõpriẽ'sivu] *adj* understanding
compressa [kõ'prɛsa] *f* compress
compressão [kõpre'sãw] *f* ⟨*sem pl*⟩ compression
compressor [kõpre'sor] *m* ***rolo m* ~** steamroller
comprido [kõ'pridu] long; ***ao* ~** lengthways
comprimento [kõpri'mẽtu] *m* length; **~ *de onda*** wavelength
comprimido [kõpri'midu] **1** *adj* compressed **2** *m* pill, tablet
comprimir [kõpri'mir] ⟨3a⟩ *v/t* compress; (*apertar*) squeeze, press
comprometer-se [kõprome'tersi] ⟨2c⟩ *v/r* commit oneself; (*prejudicar-se*) compromise oneself; **~ *a*** undertake to; **~ *com alguém*** make a commitment to s.o.
compromisso [kõpro'misu] *m* commitment; (*encontro marcado*) appointment, engagement; (*acordo*) agreement; ***sem* ~** without obligation
comprovante [kõpro'vãtʃi] **1** *adj* ***o documento* ~ *de identidade*** the document giving proof of identity **2** *m* receipt
comprovar [kõpro'var] ⟨1e⟩ *v/t* prove; (*confirmar*) confirm
compulsão [kõpuw'sãw] *f* compulsion

C

compulsivo [kõpuw'sivu] *adj* compulsive
compulsório [kõpuw'sɔriu] *adj* compulsory
computador [kõputa'doɾ] *m* computer; ~ ***pessoal*** personal computer, PC; ~ ***portátil*** laptop
comum [ko'mũ] **1** *adj* common; (*não especial*) ordinary **2** *m* ***fora do ~*** out of the ordinary; ***ter bastante em ~*** have a lot in common; ***o ~ é almoçarmos no shopping*** we usually have lunch at the shopping mall
comungar [kumuɲ'gaɾ] ⟨1a & 1o⟩ *v/i* REL take communion
comunhão [komu'ɲãw] *f* communion; DIR ~ ***de bens*** joint ownership
comunicação [komunika'sãw] *f* communication; (*mensagem*) message; (*acesso*) access; ~ ***social*** media; *curso* media studies; ***meios*** *mpl* ***de ~*** means of communication
comunicado [komuni'kadu] *m* notice; POL communiqué
comunicar [komuni'kaɾ] ⟨1n⟩ **1** *v/t* communicate; (*ligar*) connect, join **2** *v/i* communicate; **comunicar-se** *v/r* communicate; ~ ***com alguém*** get in touch with s.o.
comunicativo [komunika'ʧivu] *adj* communicative
comunidade [komuni'dadʒi] *f* community; ***Comunidade*** (***Econômica***) ***Europeia*** European (Economic) Community
comunismo [komu'nizmu] *m* communism
comunista [komu'nista] **1** *m/f* communist **2** *adj* communist
comunitário [komuni'taɾiu] *adj* community *atr*; *para todos* communal
comutar [komu'taɾ] ⟨1a⟩ DIR *pena* commute
côncavo ['kõkavu] *adj* concave; (*oco*) hollow
conceber [kõse'beɾ] ⟨2c⟩ **1** *v/t* conceive; (*imaginar*) conceive of, imagine **2** *v/i* conceive, get pregnant
concebível [kõse'bivew] *adj* conceivable
conceder [kõse'deɾ] ⟨2c⟩ *v/t* (*permitir*) allow; (*outorgar*) grant; (*admitir*) concede; (*dar*) give; ~ ***em*** accede to
conceito [kõ'sejtu] *m* concept; (*opinião*) opinion; (*fama*) reputation; ***ele desceu em meu ~*** he has gone down in my estimation
conceituado [kõsej'twadu] *adj* highly regarded
concentração [kõsẽtɾa'sãw] *f* concentration; *jogadores*: training camp
concentrado [kõsẽ'tɾadu] *adj suco etc* concentrated
concentrar [kõsẽ'tɾaɾ] ⟨1a⟩ *v/t* concentrate; *num ponto* focus; (*reunir*) bring together; *molho* thicken; **concentrar-se** *v/r* concentrate; ~ ***em*** concentrate on
concepção [kõsep'sãw] *f* concept, idea; (*opinião*) opinion; BIOL conception
concertar [kõseɾ'taɾ] ⟨1c⟩ *v/t* adjust, fix; (*conciliar*) reconcile
concerto [kõ'seɾtu] *m* concert
concessão [kõse'sãw] *f* concession; (*permissão*) permission; *para TV* license, *Brit* licence
concessionária [kõsesjo'naɾja] *f* dealership
concessionário [kõsesjo'naɾiu] *m*, **-a** *f* dealer
concha ['kõʃa] *f moluscos*: shell; GASTR ladle
conciliar [kõsi'ljaɾ] ⟨1g⟩ *v/t idéias* reconcile
conciliatório [kõsilja'tɔriu] *adj* conciliatory
conciso [kõ'sizu] *adj* concise
concluir [kõklu'iɾ] ⟨3i⟩ **1** *v/t* conclude; (*acabar*) complete; ~ ***algo de algo*** conclude sth from sth **2** *v/i* conclude
conclusão [kõklu'zãw] *f* end; (*dedução*) conclusion; ***chegar a uma ~*** come to a conclusion; ***tirar conclusões precipitadas*** jump to conclusions; ***conclusões*** findings
conclusivo [kõklu'zivu] *adj* conclusive
concordância [kõkoɾ'dãsja] *f* agreement
concordar [kõkoɾ'daɾ] ⟨1e⟩ **1** *v/t* agree **2** *v/i* agree; ~ ***com*** agree with; ~ ***em fazer algo*** agree to do sth

C

concordata [kõkor'data] *f* POL concordat; FIN ***abrir ~*** go into liquidation

concorrência [kõko'hẽsja] *f* competition; *cargo*: application

concorrente [kõko'hẽtʃi] *m/f* competitor; (*candidato*) candidate

concorrer [kõko'her] ⟨2d⟩ *v/i* compete; *eleição*: run; ***~ a*** compete for, (*candidatar-se*) apply for; ***~ para*** (*contribuir*) contribute to

concorrido [kõko'hidu] *adj* popular

concretizar [kõkretʃi'zar] ⟨1a⟩ *v/t* make real; **concretizar-se** *v/r fantasías* come true; *aspirações* be realized

concreto [kõ'krɛtu] **1** *adj* concrete; (*palpável*) real **2** *m Bras* concrete; ***~ armado*** reinforced concrete

concurso [kõ'kursu] *m* contest, competition; ***~ público*** open competition

concussão [kõku'sãw] *f* MED concussion

condado [kõ'dadu] *m* county

conde ['kõdʒi] *m* count

condecoração [kõdekora'sãw] *f* decoration

condecorar [kõdeko'rar] ⟨1e⟩ *v/t soldado* decorate

condenação [kõdena'sãw] *f* condemnation; *Jur* conviction

condenado [kõde'nadu] **1** *adj* ***estar ~*** be doomed **2** *m*, **-a** *f* convicted man / woman

condenar [kõde'nar] ⟨1d⟩ *v/t* condemn; (*declarar culpado*) convict; ***~ alguém por algo*** convict s.o. of sth

condenável [kõde'navew] *adj* reprehensible

condensação [kõdẽsa'sãw] *f* condensation

condensado [kõdẽ'sadu] *adj* condensed; ***leite*** *m* ***~*** condensed milk

condensar [kõdẽ'sar] ⟨1a⟩ *v/t* (*resumir*) condense; **condensar-se** *v/r vapor* condense

condescendente [kõdesẽ'ẽtʃi] *adj* condescending

condessa [kõ'desa] *f* countess

condição [kõdʒi'sãw] *f* condition; (*social*) status; (*qualidade*) capacity; ***condições*** *dinheiro* means; ***ter ~ / condições para*** be able to; ***não me sinto em condições para isto*** I don't feel up to it; ***em boas condições*** in good condition; ***em sua ~ de líder*** in his capacity as leader; ***condições de pagamento*** terms of payment; ***condições de trabalho*** working conditions; ***com a ~ de que*** on condition that

condicionado [kõdʒisjo'nadu] *adj* ***ar*** *m* ***~*** air conditioning

condicionador [kõdʒisjona'dor] *m cabelo*: conditioner

condicional [kõdʒisjo'naw] **1** *adj* conditional **2** *m* GRAM conditional (tense)

condicionar [kõdʒisjo'nar] ⟨1f⟩ *v/t* PSICOL, TECN condition

condimento [kõdʒi'mẽtu] *m* seasoning

condoer-se [kõdo'ersi] ⟨2f⟩ *v/r* ***~ de*** sympathize with

condomínio [kõdo'miniu] *m* apartment block; ***~ fechado*** condominium

condução [kõdu'sãw] *f automóvel*: driving; (*transporte*) transport; ELÉT conduction

conduta [kõ'duta] *f* conduct, behavior, *Brit* behaviour

conduto [kõ'dutu] *m* conduit

condutor [kõdu'tor] *adj veículo*: driver; ELÉT conductor; ***fio*** *m* ***~*** wire

conduzir [kõdu'zir] ⟨3m⟩ **1** *v/t* (*levar*) lead; ELÉT conduct; *Port automóvel* drive; *negócio*, *inspeção* conduct **2** *v/i Port* drive; ***~ a*** lead to; **conduzir-se** *v/r* conduct oneself

cone ['koni] *m* cone; ***~ de sinalização*** traffic cone

conectar [konek'tar] ⟨1a⟩ *v/t* connect; **conectar-se** *v/r* INFORM log on; ***~ a*** log on to

conexão [kone'ksãw] *f* connection

confecção [kõfek'sãw] *f* (*feitura*) making; (*roupa*) off-the-peg clothing; (*loja*) clothes store, *Brit* clothes shop:

confeccionar [kõfeksjo'nar] ⟨1f⟩ *v/t* make; (*produzir*) manufacture

confederação [kõfedera'sãw] *f* confederation

conferência [kõfe'rẽsja] *f* confer-

ence; (*palestra*) lecture; ***fazer uma ~*** give a lecture; POL **~ *cimeira*** summit (conference); **~ *de imprensa*** press conference
conferencista [kõferẽ'sista] *m/f* speaker
conferir [kõfe'rir] ⟨3c⟩ **1** *v/t* (*verificar*) check; (*comparar*) compare; (*outorgar*) grant; *título* confer **2** *v/i* tally
confessar [kõfe'sar] ⟨1c⟩ *v/t & v/i* confess; **confessar-se** *v/r* REL confess
confessionário [kõfesjo'nariu] *m* REL confessional
confessor [kõfe'sor] *m* REL confessor
confiança [kõ'fjãsa] *f* confidence; (*fé*) faith (***em*** in); **~ *em si*** self-confidence; ***de ~*** trustworthy; ***dar ~ a alguém*** be on informal terms with s.o.
confiar [kõ'fjar] ⟨1g⟩ **1** *v/t* (*dar*) entrust; (*segredo*) confide; **~ *em*** rely on; **~ *a X Y*** entrust X with Y **2** *v/i* **~ *em alguém*** confide in s.o; (*ter confiança*) trust s.o
confiável [kõ'fjavew] *adj* reliable, trustworthy
confidência [kõfi'dẽsja] *f* secret; confidence; ***em ~*** in confidence
confidencial [kõfidẽ'sjaw] *adj* confidential
confinar [kõfi'nar] ⟨1a⟩ *v/t* (*enclausurar*) confine
confirmação [kõfirma'sãw] *f* confirmation
confirmar [kõfir'mar] ⟨1a⟩ *v/t* confirm
confiscar [kõfis'kar] ⟨1n⟩ *v/t* confiscate
confissão [kõfi'sãw] *f* confession *tb* REL
conflito [kõ'flitu] *m* conflict; ***entrar em ~* (*com*)** clash (with); **~ *trabalhista*** industrial dispute
conformar [kõfor'mar] ⟨1e⟩ *v/t* (*formar*) form; **conformar-se** *v/r* **~ *com*** to resign oneself to; (*acomodar-se*) conform to
conforme [kõ'fɔrmi] **1** *prep* according to; (*dependendo de*) depending on; **~ *seu costume*** as was his custom; **~ *seus caprichos*** as the fancy takes you **2** *conj* (*assim que*) as soon as; (*dependendo de*) depending on; (*à medida que*) as
conformidade [kõformi'dadʒi] *f* agreement; ***em ~ com*** in accordance with
conformista [kõfor'mista] *m/f* conformist
confortável [kõfor'tavew] *adj* comfortable
conforto [kõ'fortu] *m* comfort; ***todos os ~s da vida moderna*** all modern conveniences
confrontação [kõfrõta'sãw] *f* confrontation
confrontar [kõfrõ'tar] ⟨1a⟩ *v/t* confront; (*comparar*) compare; **confrontar-se** *v/r* face each other; **~ *com alguém / algo*** face s.o. / sth
confronto [kõ'frõtu] *m* confrontation; (*comparação*) comparison
confundir [kõfũ'dʒir] ⟨3a⟩ *v/t* confuse; **~ *X com Y*** mistake X for Y; **confundir-se** *v/r* get mixed up; *pessoa tb* get confused
confusão [kõfu'zãw] *f* confusion; (*equívoco*) mistake; (*barafunda*) chaos; (*mistura*) jumble; ***fazer ~*** (confundir-se) get confused; ***isso vai dar muita ~*** that's going to cause a lot of trouble
confuso [kõ'fuzu] *adj* confused; (*problema*) confusing; ***está tudo muito ~ aqui*** it's all very chaotic in here
congelado [kõʒe'ladu] *adj* frozen; ***comida f congelada*** frozen food
congelador [kõʒela'dor] *m* freezer, deep freeze
congelamento [kõʒela'mẽtu] *m* freezing; FIN freeze; *fig* **~ *de preços*** price freeze; **~ *do salário*** wage freeze
congelar [kõʒe'lar] ⟨1c⟩ *v/t* freeze; *motor* ice up; **congelar-se** *v/r* freeze; *motor* ice up
congênito, *Port* **congénito** [kõ'ʒenitu] *adj* congenital
congestão [kõʒes'tãw] *f* congestion
congestionado [kõʒestʃio'nadu] *adj trânsito* congested
congestionamento [kõʒestʃiona'mẽtu] *m* congestion; ***uma ~*** a traffic jam

C

conglomerado [kõglome'radu] *m* conglomerate
Congo ['kõgu] *m* ***o ~*** the Congo
congratular [kõgratu'lar] ⟨1a⟩ *v/t* congratulate; ***~ alguém por algo*** congratulate s.o. on sth
congregação [kõgrega'sãw] *f* (*reunião*) gathering; REL congregation
congregar [kõgre'gar] ⟨1c & 1o⟩ *v/t* bring together; **congregar-se** *v/r* congregate
congressista [kõgre'sista] *m/f* congressman; congresswoman
congresso [kõ'grɛsu] *m* congress; POL party conference
conhaque [ko'ɲaki] *m* cognac
conhecedor [kuɲese'dor] *m*, **-a** *f* connoisseur
conhecer [kuɲe'ser] ⟨2g⟩ **1** *v/t* know; (*travar conhecimento*) meet; (*visitar*) go to, visit; (*descobrir*) discover; ***~ de vista*** know by sight; ***passar a ~*** get to know
conhecido [kuɲe'sidu] **1** *adj* known; (*célebre*) well-known **2** *m*, **-a** acquaintance
conhecimento [kuɲesi'mẽtu] *m* knowledge; ***ter bons ~s de*** have a good knowledge of; ***sem o ~ de*** unbeknownst to; ***~ básico*** working knowledge; ***levar ao ~ de alguém*** bring to s.o.'s attention; ***tomar ~ de*** learn about
conífera [ko'nifera] *f* conifer
conjetura, *Port* **conjectura** [kõʒe'tura] *f* conjecture
conjugação [kõʒuga'sãw] *f* conjugation
conjugado [kõʒu'gadu] *adj quarto* adjoining
conjugal [kõʒu'gaw] *adj* marital, conjugal; ***cama*** *f* ***~*** double bed; ***vida ~*** married life
conjugar [kõʒu'gar] ⟨1o⟩ *v/t* (*ligar*) join; GRAM conjugate
cônjuge ['kõʒuʒi] *m* spouse
conjunção [kõʒũ'sãw] *f* (*união*) union; GRAM conjunction
conjuntivite [kõʒũʧi'viʧi] *f* MED conjunctivitis
conjuntivo [kõʒũ'ʧivu] **1** *adj* subjunctive **2** *m* subjunctive
conjunto [kõ'ʒũtu] **1** *adj* (*unido*) joint, shared **2** *m* woman's suit; (*totalidade*) whole; *músicos*: group; (*coleção*) collection; *prédios*: complex; MAT set; ***o ~*** the lot; ***em ~ com*** in conjunction with
conjuntura [kõʒũ'tura] *f* ECON state of the economy; *fig* situation, state of affairs; ***nesta ~*** at this juncture
conosco, *Port* **connosco** [ko'nosku] *pron* with us
conquista [kõ'kista] *f* conquest; *fig* achievement
conquistador [kõkista'dor] **1** *m* conqueror; (*namorador*) ladies' man **2** *adj* conquering *atr*
conquistar [kõkis'tar] ⟨1a⟩ *v/t país* conquer; *pessoa* win over; *fama etc* win, gain
consagrar [kõsa'grar] ⟨1b⟩ *v/t* REL consecrate; (*dedicar*) dedicate; *tempo* devote; *idéia*, *estilo* establish; **consagrar-se** *v/r* ***~ a*** devote oneself to
consanguíneo [kõsã'gwiniu] **1** *adj* related by blood **2** *m/f* blood relative
consciência [kõs'sjẽsja] *f* awareness, consciousness; (*moral*) conscience; (*esmero*) conscientiousness; ***perder a ~*** lose consciousness; ***está pesando na minha ~*** it's weighing on my conscience; ***~ limpa*** clear conscience; ***~ pesada*** guilty conscience
consciencioso [kõsjẽ'sjozu] *adj* conscientious
consciente [kõ'sjẽʧi] *adj* conscious
consecutivo [kõseku'ʧivu] *adj* consecutive; ***três horas consecutivas*** three hours on the trot
conseguir [kõse'gir] ⟨3o & 3c⟩ **1** *v/t* (*obter*) get, obtain; ***~ fazer algo*** manage to do sth, succeed in doing sth; ***não consegui dormir*** I couldn't get to sleep **2** *v/i* succeed; ***consegui!*** I did it!
conselheiro [kõse'ʎejru] *m*, **-a** *f* counselor, *Brit* counsellor, advisor; POL councilman, *Brit* councillor
conselho [kõ'seʎu] *m* advice; (*órgão*) council; ***um ~*** a piece of advice; ***aceitar o ~ de alguém*** take s.o.'s advice; ***Conselho de Diretoria*** board of directors; POL ***Conselho de Ministros***

Cabinet; **~ *municipal*** town council

consenso [kõ'sẽsu] *m* consensus, agreement

consentimento [kõsẽʧi'mẽtu] *m* consent

consentir [kõsẽ'ʧiɾ] ⟨3e⟩ **1** *v/t* allow, permit; (*aprovar*) agree to **2** *v/i* **~ *em*** agree to

conseqüência, *Port* **consequência** [kõse'kwẽsja] *f* consequence; ***por ~*** consequently

conseqüente, *Port* **consequente** [kõse'kwẽʧi] resultant, consequent; (*coerente*) consistent

conseqüentemente, *Port* **consequentemente** [kõsekwẽʧi'mẽʧi] *adv* consequently

consertar [kõseɾ'taɾ] ⟨1c⟩ *v/t Bras* repair, fix

conserto [kõ'seɾtu] *m Bras* repair

conserva [kõ'sɛɾva] *f vidro*: preserve; *lata*: canned food; ***em ~*** pickled

conservação [kõseɾva'sãw] *f* ⟨*sem pl*⟩ conservation; *alimentos*: preservation

conservacionista [kõseɾvasjo'nista] *m/f* conservationist

conservador [kõseɾva'doɾ] **1** *adj* conservative **2** *m*, **-a** *f* POL conservative

conservante [kõseɾ'vãʧi] *m* preservative

conservar [kõseɾ'vaɾ] ⟨1c⟩ *v/t* (*preservar*) preserve; (*guardar*) keep; (*manter*) maintain; **conservar-se** *v/r comida*: keep

conservatório [kõseɾva'tɔriu] *m* MÚS conservatory

consideração [kõsideɾa'sãw] *f* consideration; (*ponderação*) thought; (*estima*) esteem; ***levar em ~*** take into consideration; ***sem ~*** inconsiderate

considerado [kõside'ɾadu] *adj* respected

considerar [kõside'ɾaɾ] ⟨1c⟩ *v/t* consider; (*tomar em conta*) take into consideration; (*respeitar*) respect; **~ *alguém como algo*** consider s.o. to be sth; ***ser considerado responsável por*** be held accountable for

considerável [kõside'ɾavew] *adj* considerable

consignação [kõsigna'sãw] *f* consignment

consigo [kõ'sigu] *pron* with him; *f* with her; *pl* with them; (*com você*) with you

consistência [kõsis'tẽsja] *f* consistency; (*constância*) constancy

consistente [kõsis'tẽʧi] *adj* consistent; (*sólido*) solid; *mistura* thick

consistir [kõsis'ʧiɾ] ⟨3a⟩ *v/i* **~ *em*** consist of

consoante [kõ'swãʧi] **1** *prep* (*conforme*) according to **2** *conj* as; **~ *prometera*** as he had promised **3** *f* GRAM consonant

consolar [kõso'laɾ] ⟨1e⟩ *v/t* console; **consolar-se** *v/r* console oneself

consolidar [kõsoli'daɾ] ⟨1a⟩ **1** *v/t* consolidate; *vínculo* strengthen; *fratura* mend **2** *v/i* solidify; **consolidar-se** strengthen

consolo [kõ'solu] *m* consolation

consórcio [kõ'sɔɾsiu] *m* (*união*) partnership; COM consortium

conspícuo [kõs'piku] *adj* conspicuous

conspiração [kõspiɾa'sãw] *f* conspiracy

conspirador [kõspiɾa'doɾ] *m*, **-a** *f* conspirator

conspirar [kõspi'ɾaɾ] ⟨1a⟩ **1** *v/t* plot **2** *v/i* plot, conspire; **~ *contra alguém*** conspire against s.o.

constante [kõs'tãʧi] **1** *adj* steady, constant **2** *f* constant

constantemente [kõstãʧi'mẽʧi] *adv* constantly

constar [kõs'taɾ] ⟨1a⟩ *v/i* **~ *de*** consist of

constatar [kõsta'taɾ] ⟨1b⟩ *v/t* establish; (*notar*) note, notice

constelação [kõsʧila'sãw] *f* constellation; (*grupo*) cluster

consternação [kõsteɾna'sãw] *f* consternation

consternar [kõsteɾ'naɾ] ⟨1c⟩ *v/t* distress; **consternar-se** *v/r* be distressed

constipação [kõsʧipa'sãw] *f* constipation; *Port* cold

constipar-se [kõsʧi'paɾsi] ⟨1a⟩ *v/r Port* catch a cold

constitucional [kõstʃitusjo'naw] *adj* POL constitutional
constituição [kõstʃitwi'sãw] *f* POL constitution; **~ *física*** physical type
constituir [kõstʃi'twir] ⟨3i⟩ *v/t* (*representar*) constitute; (*formar*) form; (*estabelecer*) establish, set up
constranger [kõstrã'ʒer] ⟨2h⟩ *v/t* constrain; (*acanhar*) embarrass
constrangido [kõstrã'ʒidu] *adj* embarrassed
constrangimento [kõstrãʒi'mẽtu] *m* constraint; (*acanhamento*) embarrassment
construção [kõstru'sãw] *f* construction; (*terreno*) building site; (*edifício*) building; ***em*** **~** under construction
construir [kõstru'ir] ⟨3k⟩ *v/t* build, construct; ***construído numa ladeira*** built on a slope
construtivo [kõstru'tʃivu] *adj* constructive
construtor [kõstru'tor] *m*, **-a** *f*, builder
cônsul ['kõsuw] *m* ⟨*pl* cônsules⟩ consul
consulado [kõsu'ladu] *m* consulate
consular [kõsu'lar] *adj* consular
consulta [kõ'suwta] *f* consultation; MED appointment; ***horário*** *fpl* ***de*** **~** office hours, *Brit* surgery hours
consultar [kõsuw'tar] ⟨1a⟩ *v/t* consult; **~ *alguém sobre*** ask s.o's opinion about, consult s.o. about
consultor [kõsuw'tor] *m*, **-a** *f* consultant; **~ *administrativo*** management consultant
consultoria [kõsuwto'ria] *f* consultancy
consultório [kõsuw'tɔriu] *m* MED office, *Brit* surgery
consumidor [kõsumi'dor] **1** *adj* consumer *atr*; ***mercado*** *m* **~** consumer market **2** *m*, **-a** *f* consumer; **~ *final*** end-user
consumir [kõsu'mir] ⟨3h⟩ *v/t* consume; (*devorar*) eat away; (*gastar*) use up; *tempo* take up; ***melhor*** **~ *antes de*** best before; **consumir-se** *v/r* waste away
consumo [kõ'sumu] *m* consumption; ***artigos de*** **~** consumer goods; ***mercado*** *m* ***de*** **~** consumer market; **~ *de drogas*** drug abuse
conta ['kõta] *f aritmética*: count; *em restaurante* check, *Brit* bill; (*fatura*) invoice; FIN account; *vidro*: bead; (*responsabilidade*) responsibility; ***por*** **~ *própria*** of one's own accord; *trabalhar* for oneself; ***ter em*** **~** take into account; ***fazer de*** **~** pretend; ***afinal de*** **~*s*** after all is said and done; ***isso fica por sua*** **~** that's for you to deal with; ***isto é por minha*** **~** this is on me; ***dar-se*** **~ *de*** realize; ***prestar*** **~*s de*** account for; **~ *bancária*** bank account; **~ *conjunta*** joint account; **~ *corrente*** checking account, *Brit* current account; **~ *de poupança*** savings account; **~ *do telefone*** phone bill
contabilidade [kõtabili'dadʒi] *f* acountancy, book-keeping; (*departamento*) accounts department; ***fazer a*** **~** do the books
contabilista [kõtabi'lista] *m/f Port* accountant
contact... *Port* → ***contat...***
contador [kõta'dor] *m*, **-a** *f* accountant; *gás, água*: meter; **~ *de estórias*** story-teller
contagem [kõ'taʒẽ] *f* count; (*escore*) score, **~ *espermática*** sperm count; **~ *regressiva*** countdown
contagiante [kõtaʒi'ãtʃi] *adj alegría* contagious; *risada* infectious
contagiar [kõta'ʒjar] ⟨1g⟩ *v/t* infect; **contagiar-se** *v/r* become infected
contágio [kõ'taʒiu] *m* infection
contagioso [kõta'ʒjozu] *adj* contagious
conta-gotas [kõta'gotas] *m* ⟨*pl inv*⟩ dropper
container [kõ'tejnɛr] *m* container
contaminação [kõtamina'sãw] *f* contamination; *meio ambiente*: pollution; MED infection; **~ *da água*** water pollution
contaminar [kõtami'nar] ⟨1a⟩ *v/t* contaminate; *meio ambiente* pollute; MED infect
contanto [kõ'tãtu] *conj* **~ *que*** provided that, as long as
conta-quilômetros, *Port* **conta-quilómetros** [kõtaki'lometrus] *m* ⟨*pl*

inv⟩ *Port* speedometer, *fam* speedo
contar [kõ'taɾ] ⟨1a⟩ *v/t* count; (*narrar*) tell; **~ com** count on; (*esperar*) expect; **~ algo a alguém** tell s.o. sth; **ele conta que você possa ...** he expects you to be able to ...
contatar [kõtak'taɾ] ⟨1a⟩ *v/t* contact
contato [kõ'taktu] *m* contact; **entrar em ~ com** get in touch with; **manter ~ com** keep in contact with; **estar fora de ~ com** be out of touch with
contêiner [kõ'tejneɾ] *m* container
contemplação [kõtẽpla'sãw] *f* contemplation
contemplar [kõtẽ'plaɾ] ⟨1a⟩ **1** *v/t* contemplate **2** *v/i* meditate; **contemplar-se** *v/r* look at oneself
contemporâneo [kõtẽpo'ɾʌniu] **1** *adj* contemporary **2** *m*, **-a** *f* contemporary
contentamento [kõtẽta'mẽtu] *m* happiness; (*satisfação*) contentment
contentar [kõtẽ'taɾ] ⟨1a⟩ *v/t* please; (*dar satisfação*) satisfy; **contentar-se** *v/r* be satisfied; **~ com** settle for, make do with
contente [kõ'tẽʧi] *adj* happy; (*satisfeito*) pleased, content; **contentíssimo** overjoyed
conter [kõ'teɾ] ⟨2xa⟩ *v/t* contain, hold; (*reprimir*) hold back; *gastos* curb; **conter-se** *v/r* restrain oneself
conterrâneo [kõte'hʌniu] **1** *adj* fellow **2** *m*, **-a** *f* compatriot
contestação [kõtesta'sãw] *f* challenge; (*negação*) denial
contestar [kõtes'taɾ] ⟨1c⟩ *v/t* dispute, contest; (*impugnar*) challenge
conteúdo [kõte'udu] *m* **o ~** the contents; *texto*: the content
contexto [kõ'testu] *m* context; **ver algo dentro / fora do ~** look at sth in context / out of context
contigo [kõ'ʧigu] *pron* with you
continental [kõʧinẽ'taw] *adj* continental; **Europa** *f* **Continental** Continental Europe
continente [kõʧi'nẽʧi] *m* continent; **o ~** the mainland
continuação [kõʧinwa'sãw] *f* continuation; *estória*: sequel
continuar [kõʧi'nwaɾ] ⟨1g⟩ **1** *v/t* continue **2** *v/i* continue, go on; **~ fazendo algo** keep on doing sth; **ele continua teimoso como sempre** he remains as stubborn as ever; **~ com os pagamentos** keep up the payments; **continuamos em contato** we stayed in touch
continuidade [kõʧinwi'dadʒi] *f* continuity
contínuo [kõ'ʧinwu] **1** *adj* (*incessante*) continual; (*sem interrupção*) continuous **2** *m escritório*: office boy
conto ['kõtu] *m* story, tale; **~ de fadas** fairy tale
contorção [kõtoɾ'sãw] *f* contortion
contorcer [kõto'seɾ] ⟨2g & 2d⟩ *v/t* contort; **contorcer-se** *v/r* writhe
contornar [kõtoɾ'naɾ] ⟨1c⟩ *v/t* (*rodear*) go around; (*cercar*) surround; (*delinear*) outline; *problema* get around
contorno [kõ'toɾnu] *m* outline, contour
contra ['kõtɾa] **1** *prep* against; JUR versus; **ir ~** go against; **~ a lei** against the law **2** *m* **os prós e os ~s** the pros and cons
contra-atacar [kõtɾata'kaɾ] ⟨1b & 1n⟩ *v/t* counterattack
contra-ataque [kõtɾa'taki] *m* counterattack
contrabaixo [kõtɾa'bajʃu] *m* MÚS double bass
contrabalançar [kõtɾabalã'saɾ] ⟨1p⟩ *v/t* counterbalance
contrabandista [kõtɾabã'dʒista] *m/f* smuggler
contrabando [kõtɾa'bãdu] *m* smuggling; *mercadoria*: contraband
contração, *Port* **contracção** [kõtɾa'sãw] *f* contraction; (*espasmo*) spasm
contracenar [kõtɾase'naɾ] ⟨1d⟩ *v/i* **~ com** star opposite, star with
contracepção [kõtɾase'sãw] *f* ⟨*sem pl*⟩ contraception
contraceptivo [kõtɾase'ʧivu] **1** *adj* contraceptive **2** *m* contraceptive
contradição [kõtɾadʒi'sãw] *f* contradiction
contraditório [kõtɾadʒi'tɔriu] *adj* contradictory

contradizer [kõtradʒi'zer] ⟨2t⟩ *v/t* contradict; **contradizer-se** *pessoa* contradict oneself; *idéias* be contradictory
contra-espionagem [kõtraspio-'naʒẽ] *f* counterespionage
contra-indicação [kõtraĩdʒika'sãw] *f* MED contraindication
contrair [kõtra'ir] ⟨3l⟩ *v/t* contract; *hábito* pick up; *custos*, *dívidas* incur; **contrair-se** *v/r* contract, shrink
contrapartida [kõtrapar'tʃida] *f* COM counter-entry; *fig* compensation; ***em ~*** on the other hand
contrapeso [kõtra'pezu] *m* counterbalance
contrapor [kõtra'por] ⟨2z⟩ *v/t* compare; ***~ algo a algo*** set sth against sth; **contrapor-se** *v/r* ***~ a*** go against, oppose
contraproducente [kõtraprodu'sẽtʃi] *adj* counterproductive
contrariar [kõtra'rjar] ⟨1g⟩ *v/t* contradict; (*irritar*) annoy
contrariedade [kõtrarie'dadʒi] *f* annoyance
contrário [kõ'trariu] **1** *adj* opposite; *pessoa* opposed; (*adverso*) adverse **2** *m* opposite; ***ao ~*** the other way around; ***muito pelo ~*** on the contrary, quite the opposite
contra-senha [kõtra'seɲa] *f* password
contrastar [kõtras'tar] ⟨1b⟩ contrast; ***~ com*** contrast with
contraste [kõ'trastʃi] *m* contrast
contratante [kõtra'tãtʃi] **1** *adj* contracting **2** *m* contractor
contratar [kõtra'tar] ⟨1b⟩ *v/t* contract; (*empregar*) employ, take on
contratempo [kõtra'tẽpu] *m* setback; (*aborrecimento*) upset
contrato [kõ'tratu] *m* contract; ***~ de aluguel*** rental contract
contratual [kõtra'twaw] *adj* contractual
contribuição [kõtribwi'sãw] *f* contribution; (*imposto*) tax
contribuinte [kõtri'bwĩtʃi] *m/f* contributor; *impostos*: taxpayer
contribuir [kõtri'bwir] ⟨3i⟩ **1** *v/t* contribute **2** *v/i* contribute; *impostos*: pay taxes
controlador [kõtrola'dor] *m*, **-a** *f no trem* ticket collector; *pessoa neurótica* control freak; ***~ de tráfego aéreo*** air-traffic controller
controlar [kõtro'lar] ⟨1e⟩ *v/t* control; (*fiscalizar*) check; **controlar-se** *v/r* control oneself
controle [kõ'troli], *Port* **controlo** [kõ'trolu] *m* control; ***perder o ~ de*** lose control of; ***estar fora de ~*** be out of control; ***sob ~*** under control; ***~ de bagagem*** baggage check; ***~ de natalidade*** birth control; ***~ de passaportes*** passport control; ***~ de qualidade*** quality control; ***~ remoto*** remote control; ***~ de segurança*** security check
controvérsia [kõtro'vɛrsja] *f* controversy
controverso [kõtro'vɛrsu] *adj* controversial
contudo [kõ'tudu] *conj* nevertheless
contundir [kõtũ'dʒir] ⟨3a⟩ *v/t* bruise; **contundir-se** *v/r* bruise oneself
contusão [kõtu'zãw] *f* bruise
convalescença [kõvales'sẽsa] *f* convalescence
convalescer [kõvales'ser] ⟨2g⟩ *v/i* convalesce
convenção [kõvẽ'sãw] *f* convention; (*acordo*) agreement
convencer [kõvẽ'ser] ⟨2g & 2a⟩ *v/t* convince
convencido [kõvẽ'sidu] *adj* conceited, smug
convencional [kõvẽsjo'naw] *adj* conventional; ***não ~*** unconventional
conveniência [kõve'njẽsja] *f* convenience; ***com todas as ~s modernas*** with all the mod cons
conveniente [kõve'njẽtʃi] *adj* convenient; (*vantajoso*) advantageous; ***não é ~ …*** it doesn't pay to …
convênio, *Port* **convénio** [kõ'veniu] *m* convention; (*acordo*) agreement
convento [kõ'vẽtu] *m* convent
convergir [kõver'ʒir] ⟨3n & 2c⟩ *v/i* converge; ***~ para*** converge on
conversa [kõ'vɛrsa] *f* conversation; ***cair na ~ de*** be deceived by; ***ter uma ~ com alguém*** have a word

with s.o.; **~ fiada** idle talk; INFORM **~ (on line)** online chat
conversação [kõversa'sãw] *f* conversation
conversador [kõversa'dor] *adj* talkative, chatty
conversão [kõver'sãw] *f* conversion
conversar [kõver'sar] ⟨1c⟩ *v/i* talk, chat; **~ com alguém** talk to s.o.
conversível [kõver'sivew] **1** *adj* convertible **2** *m* (*auto*) convertible
converter [kõver'ter] ⟨2c⟩ *v/t* convert; **converter-se** *v/r* be converted
convés [kõ'vɛs] *m* deck
convexo [kõ'vɛksu] *adj* convex
convicção [kõvi'ksãw] *f* conviction
convicto [kõ'viktu] *adj* convinced; *criminoso* convicted; (*confirmado*) confirmed
convidado [kõvi'dadu] *m*, **-a** *f* guest
convidar [kõvi'dar] ⟨1a⟩ *v/t* invite; **~ alguém para algo** treat s.o. to sth
convincente [kõvĩ'sẽtʃi] *adj* convincing; **pouco ~** *desculpa* lame
convir [kõ'vir] ⟨3wa⟩ *v/i* agree; **~ a alguém** suit s.o.; **não convém que você ...** you shouldn't ..., it's not a good idea to ...; **quando lhe convier** when it suits you
convite [kõ'vitʃi] *m* invitation, invite
convivência [kõvi'vẽsja] *f* (*vida em comum*) cohabitation; (*familiaridade*) close contact
conviver [kõvi'ver] ⟨2a⟩ *v/i* **~ com** live with
convívio [kõ'viviu] *m* cohabitation; (*familiaridade*) familiarity
convocar [kõvo'kar] ⟨1n & 1e⟩ *v/t* summon, call upon; *reunião* call
convulsão [kõvuw'sãw] *f* MED convulsion
cooperação [koopera'sãw] *f* cooperation; **em ~ com** in collaboration with
cooperar [koope'rar] ⟨1c⟩ *v/i* cooperate
cooperativa [koopera'tʃiva] *f* COM cooperative
cooperativo [koopera'tʃivu] *adj* cooperative
coordenação [koordena'sãw] *f* coordination
coordenar [koorde'nar] ⟨1d⟩ *v/t* coordinate
copa ['kɔpa] *f* (*torneio*) cup; *aposento* breakfast room; *árvore*: top; *chapéu*: crown; **Copa do Mundo** World Cup; **~s** *pl naipes* hearts
cópia ['kɔpja] *f* copy; **tirar uma ~ de algo** make a copy of sth; **~ imprimida** printout; **~ perfeita** spitting image; **~ pirata** pirate copy
copiadora [kopja'dora] *f* (photo)copier
copiar [ko'pjar] ⟨1g⟩ *v/t* copy
co-piloto [kopi'lotu] *m* co-pilot
copo ['kɔpu] *m* glass; **um ~ de** a glass of; *fam* **ele é um bom ~** he can hold his drink; *Port* **vamos para os ~s** let's go for a drink
copo-d'água [kɔpo'dagwa] *m* ⟨*pl* copos-d'água⟩ *Port casamento*: wedding meal
coque ['kɔki] *m* (*penteado*) bun
coqueiro [ko'kejru] *m* coconut palm
coqueluche [koke'luʃi] *f* whooping cough
coquetel [koke'tew] *m* cocktail; (*festa*) cocktail party
cor[1] [kɔr] *m* **de ~** off by heart
cor[2] [kor] *f* color, *Brit* colour; **de ~** colored, *Brit* coloured
coração [kora'sãw] *m* heart; **do ~** from the heart; **de ~ partido** broken-hearted
coragem [ko'raʒẽ] *f* courage; **criar ~** take heart
corajoso [kora'ʒozu] *adj* brave, courageous
coral[1] [ko'raw] *m* coral
coral[2] [ko'raw] **1** *adj* choral **2** *m* choir
corante [ko'rãtʃi] **1** *adj* coloring *atr*, *Brit* colouring *atr* **2** *m* coloring, *Brit* colouring
corar [ko'rar] ⟨1a⟩ **1** *v/t* paint; *roupa* bleach; GASTR roast **2** *v/i* blush, color, *Brit* colour
Corão [ko'rãw] *m Port* Koran
corcunda [kor'kũda] **1** *adj* hunchbacked **2** *f* hump **3** *m/f* hunchback
corda ['kɔrda] *f* rope; *roupa*: clothes line; *relógio*: spring; MÚS string; **instrumentos** *mpl* **de ~** stringed instru-

ments; **~s** *pl* **vocais** vocal cords; **dar ~ a** *relógio* wind up; **~ fina** tightrope
corda-bamba [korda'bãba] *f* high wire
cordão[1] [kor'dãw] *m* string, twine; **~ de isolamento** cordon; **~ umbilical** umbilical cord
cordão[2] [kor'dãw] *m* Carnival group
cordeiro [kor'dejru] *m* lamb
cordel [kor'dɛw] *m Port* string; **literatura de ~** trash
cor-de-rosa [kordʒi'hɔza] *adj* pink; *situação* rosy; **revistas ~** celebrity magazines
cordial [kor'dʒiaw] **1** *adj* cordial **2** *m bebida* cordial
cordialidade [kordʒiali'dadʒi] *f* cordiality
cordilheira [kordʒi'ʎejra] *f* mountain range
coreano [ko'rjanu] **1** *adj* Korean **2** *m*, **-a** *f* Korean
Coreia [ko'reja] *f* Korea
coreografar [korjogra'far] ⟨1a⟩ *v/t* choreograph
coreografia [korjogra'fia] *f* choreography
coreógrafo [ko'rjɔgrafu] *m*, **-a** *f* choreographer
coringa [ko'rĩga] *m cartas*: joker
córnea ['kɔrnja] *f olho*: cornea
córner ['kɔrnɛr] *m* corner
corneta [kor'neta] *f* cornet; MIL bugle
coro ['koru] *m* MÚS chorus; (*cantores*) choir; **em ~** in chorus
coroa [ko'roa] *f* crown *tb dente*; *flores*: garland; *Bras fam* old codger
coroação [korwa'sãw] *f* coronation
coroar [ko'rwar] ⟨1f⟩ crown; (*premiar*) reward
coronário [koro'narjo] *adj* MED coronary
coronel [koro'nɛw] *m* colonel
coronha [ko'roɲa] *f fuzil*: butt; *revólver*: handle
corpete [kor'petʃi] *m* bodice
corpo ['korpu] *m* body; (*aparência física*) figure; *homem*: build; *vestido*: bodice; MIL corps *sg*; **ela tem um ~ bem feito** she has a good figure; **de ~ e alma** heart and soul **~ de bombeiros** fire department, *Brit* fire brigade; **~ diplomático** the diplomatic corps; **~ docente** teaching staff
corporal [korpo'raw] *adj* physical
corpulento [korpu'lẽtu] *adj* corpulent
corpúsculo [kor'puskulu] *m* corpuscle
correção, *Port* **correcção** [kohe'sãw] *f* correction; *comportamento*: correctness; **casa** *f* **de ~** reformatory; INFORM **~ ortográfica** spellcheck
correct... *Port* → **corret...**
corredor [kohe'dor] **1** *m edifício*: corridor, passageway; *avião*: aisle; *cavalo* racehorse **2** *m/f* ESP runner; **~ de barreira** hurdler
correia [ko'heja] *f* strap; *máquina*: belt; *cachorro*: leash; **~ do ventilador** fan belt
correio [ko'heiu] *m*, *tb pl* **~s** mail, post; *edifício*: post office; **por no ~** mail; **pelo ~** by mail **~ aéreo** airmail; **~ eletrônico**, *Port* **~ electrônico** e-mail; **~ terrestre** surface mail; **~ de voz** voicemail
corrente[1] [ko'hẽtʃi] *adj* (*atual*) current; *água* running; (*comum*) usual
corrente[2] [ko'hẽtʃi] *f* ELÉT, *rio*, *ar etc*: current; **~ alternada / contínua** direct / alternating current; **~ de ar** draft, *Brit* draught; **~ marítima** ocean current; **~ sangüínea** bloodstream
corrente[3] [ko'hẽtʃi] *f cadeia*, *jóia*: chain; **uma ~ de lojas** a chain of stores
correr [ko'her] ⟨2d⟩ **1** *v/i* run; *água* flow, run; *ar* flow; (*passar*) elapse; (*estar com pressa*) rush around; *em carro* speed; *boato* go around; **ela comeu correndo** she rushed through her meal; **~ pela rua** run up the street **2** *v/t risco* run
correria [kohe'ria] *f* rush; *de gente* stampede
correspondência [kohespõ'dẽsja] *f* correspondence; (*cartas no correio*) mail, *Brit* post; **~ não desejada** junk mail
correspondente [kohespõ'dẽtʃi] **1** *adj* corresponding **2** *m/f* correspondent
corresponder [kohespõ'der] ⟨2a⟩ *v/i*

correspond; *amor*: reciprocate; **~ a** correspond to; (*ser igual*) match; *expetativas* live up to; **corresponder--se** *v/r* write, correspond; **~ com** correspond with
corretagem [kohe'taʒẽ] *f* brokerage
corretamente [kohɛta'mẽtʃi] *adv* correctly; (*direito*) properly
correto [ko'hɛtu] *adj* (*certo*) correct, right; *pessoa* straight, honest; **~?** right?
corretor [kohe'toɾ] *m*, **-a** *f* broker; **~ de fundos / bolsa** stockbroker; **~ de imóveis** realtor, *Brit* estate agent; **~ ortográfico** spellchecker
corrida [ko'hida] *f* race; *ato* running; **~ de carros** motor racing; *evento* motor race; **uma ~ pelo dólar** a run on the dollar; **~ pela presidencia** race for the presidency; **~ de cavalos** horse racing; *evento* horse race; **~ de velocidade** sprint; **~ de revesamento** relay (race)
corrigir [kohi'ʒiɾ] ⟨3n⟩ *v/t* correct; *defeito*, *injustiça* put right
corrimão [kohi'mãw] *m* ⟨*pl* -ãos, -ões⟩ handrail
corriqueiro [kohi'kejɾu] *adj* common, ordinary
corroborar [kohobo'ɾaɾ] ⟨1e⟩ *v/t* corroborate
corroer [ko'hweɾ] ⟨2f⟩ *v/t metais* corrode; *fig* eat away; **corroer-se** *v/r* corrode
corromper [kohõ'peɾ] ⟨2a⟩ *v/t* corrupt; (*subornar*) bribe
corrosão [koho'zãw] *f metais*: corrosion; *fig* erosion
corrosivo [koho'zivu] **1** *adj* corrosive **2** *m* corrosive
corrupção [kohu'psãw] *f* ⟨*sem pl*⟩ corruption; (*suborno*) bribery; POL *tb* sleaze
corrupto [ko'huptu] *adj* corrupt
Córsega ['kɔrsega] *f* Corsica
cortador [korta'doɾ] *m Bras* **~ de grama**, *Port* **~ de relva** lawn mower; **~ de unha** nail clippers
cortante [koɾ'tãtʃi] *adj comentário* cutting
cortar [koɾ'taɾ] ⟨1e⟩ **1** *v/t* cut; TEL cut off; (*eliminar*) cut out; *auto* cut up; *consumo* reduce; *time*: drop; **~ o cabelo** have one's hair cut **2** *v/i* cut; (*encurtar caminho*) take a short cut; **~ em cubos** dice; **~ em fatias** slice; **cortar-se** *v/r* cut oneself
corte[1] ['kɔɾtʃi] *m* cut; (*gume*) blade; ELÉT power cut; **sem ~** *tesoura etc* blunt; **~ de cabelo** haircut; **~ representativo** cross-section
corte[2] ['koɾtʃi] *f monarca*: court; *pessoa*: retinue
cortejo [koɾ'teʒu] *m* procession; *fúnebre* cortège
cortês [koɾ'tes] *adj* polite, courteous
cortesia [koɾte'zia] *f* courtesy; **de ~** *bilhetes* complimentary
cortiça [koɾ'tʃisa] *f matéria* cork
cortiço [koɾ'tʃisu] *m* slum tenement
cortina [koɾ'tʃina] *f* drapes, *Brit* curtain; **~ de banho** shower curtain; **~ de rolo** shutters; *Brit* roller blind
cortinado [koɾtʃi'nadu] *m Port* drapes, *Brit* curtain
coruja [ko'ɾuʒa] **1** *f* owl **2** *adj pai*, *mãe* proud, doting
corvo ['koɾvu] *m* crow
cós [kɔs] *m calças*, *saia*: waistband
coser [ko'zeɾ] ⟨2d⟩ *v/t & v/i* sew
cosmético [koʒ'mɛtʃiku] **1** *adj* cosmetic **2** *m* cosmetic
cósmico ['kɔzmiku] *adj* cosmic
cosmonauta [kozmo'nawta] *m/f* cosmonaut
cosmopolita [kozmopo'lita] **1** *m/f* globetrotter **2** *adj* cosmopolitan
cosmos ['kɔzmus] *m* cosmos
costa ['kɔsta] *f* coast; **Costa do Marfim** Ivory Coast; **~ oeste** West Coast
costas ['kɔstas] *fpl* back; **de ~** on one's back; **virar as ~ para alguém** turn one's back on s.o.
costeiro [kos'tejɾu] *adj* coastal; **proteção** *f* **costeira**, *Port* **protecção** *f* **costeira** coast guard
costela [kos'tɛla] *f* ANAT rib
costeleta [koste'leta] *f* GASTR chop, cutlet; **~s** sideburns
costumar [kostu'maɾ] ⟨1a⟩ *v/t* **~ fazer algo** be in the habit of doing sth; **ele não costuma beber tanto** he doesn't normally drink so much
costume [kos'tumi] *m* custom; (*hábi-*

to) habit; ***é ~*** ... it is customary to ...; ***como de ~*** as usual; ***de ~*** usually; ***ter o ~ de fazer algo*** have a habit of doing sth

costura [kos'tuɾa] *f* sewing, needlework; (*sutura*) seam; ***sem ~*** seamless

costurar [kostu'ɾaɾ] ⟨1a⟩ *v/t & v/i* sew

costureira [kostu'ɾejɾa] *f* dressmaker; *caixa*: sewing box

cota ['kɔta] *f* (*parte*) quota, share; GEOG height

cotação [kota'sãw] *f preço* price; (*apreço*) rating

cotar [ko'taɾ] ⟨1c⟩ *v/t* rate; *ações* quote; ***~ algo em*** value sth at

cotidiano [koʧi'dʒianu] **1** *adj* daily, everyday **2** *m* ***o ~*** daily life

cotovelada [kotove'lada] *f* elbow shove; (*cutucada*) nudge; ***ele me deu uma ~ para entrar na fila*** he elbowed me out of the way to get into line

cotovelo [koto'velu] *m* elbow; (*curva*) bend; ***falar pelos ~s*** talk nineteen to the dozen

cotovia [koto'via] *f* lark

coube ['kobi], *etc* → ***caber***

couro ['koɾu] *m* leather; *animal*: hide; ***de ~*** leather; ANAT ***~ cabeludo*** scalp; ***~ envernizado*** patent leather; ***~ de porco*** pigskin

couve ['kovi] *f* kale; ***~ de Bruxelas*** Brussels sprout

couve-flor [kove'flɔɾ] *f* ⟨*pl* couves--flor⟩ cauliflower

cova ['kɔva] *f* (*buraco*) pit; (*sepultura*) grave; (*caverna*) cavern

covarde [ko'vaɾdʒi] *Bras* **1** *adj* cowardly **2** *m/f* coward

covardia [ko'vaɾdʒia] *f* cowardice

coxa ['koʃa] *f* thigh

coxia [ko'ʃia] *f* aisle, gangway

cozer [ko'zeɾ] ⟨2d⟩ *v/t & v/i* cook; *pão etc* bake

cozido [ko'zidu] **1** *pp* → ***cozer***, cooked; *ovo* hard-boiled **2** *m* stew

cozinha [ko'ziɲa] *f* kitchen; *navio*: galley; *preparação da comida* cookery; *estílo de cozinhar* cuisine

cozinhar [kozi'ɲaɾ] ⟨1a⟩ **1** *v/t* cook; ***~ demais*** overcook **2** *v/i* cook

cozinheiro [kozi'ɲejɾu] *m*, **-a** *f* cook

crachá [kɾa'ʃa] *m* badge

crânio ['kɾʌniu] *m* ANAT skull

craque ['kɾaki] *m* ace, expert; *futebol*: football star

C

cratera [kɾa'tɛɾa] *f* crater

cravar [kɾa'vaɾ] ⟨1b⟩ *v/t prego etc* drive in; *pedra* set; *com os olhos* stare at; **cravar-se** *v/r* stick

cravejar [kɾave'ʒaɾ] ⟨1d⟩ *v/t* nail; ***~ alguém de balas*** spray s.o. with bullets

cravo ['kɾavu] *m especiaria* clove; BOT carnation; *pele*: blackhead; MÚS harpsichord; (*prego*) nail

creche ['kɾɛʃi] *f* crèche

credibilidade [kɾedʒibili'dadʒi] *f* credibility

creditar [kɾedʒi'taɾ] ⟨1a⟩ *v/t* credit; ***~ um valor em uma conta*** credit an amount to an account

crédito ['kɾɛdʒitu] *m* credit; ***a ~*** on credit; ***linha** f **de ~*** line of credit; ***digno de ~*** reliable; ***dar ~ a alguém*** give s.o. credit; ***cartão** m **de ~*** credit card

credo ['kɾɛdu] **1** *m* creed **2** *int fam* ***~!*** heavens!

credor [kɾe'doɾ] *m*, **-a** *f* FIN creditor

crédulo ['kɾɛdulu] *adj* credulous, gullible

creio ['kɾeiu] *etc* → ***crer***

cremação [kɾema'sãw] *f* cremation

crematório [kɾema'tɔɾiu] *m* (***forno** m*) ***~*** crematorium

creme ['kɾemi] **1** *m cosmético, leite*: cream; ***~ Chantilly*** whipped cream; ***~ hidratante*** moisturizer; ***~ de proteção solar***, *Port* ***~ de protecção solar*** sun cream **2** *adj* cream

cremoso [kɾe'mozu] *adj* creamy

crença ['kɾẽsa] *f* belief

crente ['kɾẽʧi] **1** REL *adj* believing; ***estar ~ que*** think that **2** *m/f* believer

crepe ['kɾɛpi] *m* GASTR crepe

crepitação [kɾepita'sãw] *f lume*: crackling

crepitar [kɾepi'taɾ] ⟨1a⟩ *v/i lume* crackle; *motor* sputter

crepúsculo [kɾe'puskulu] *m* twilight, dusk

crer [kɾeɾ] ⟨2k⟩ *v/i & v/t* believe (***em*** in); (*julgar*) think; ***~ que*** think (that)

crescente [kɾes'sẽʧi] **1** *adj* growing;

C

lua crescent **2** *m* crescent
crescer [kres'ser] ⟨2g⟩ *v/i* grow; *pão etc* rise
crescimento [kresi'mẽtu] *m* growth; **~ *de capital*** capital growth; **~ *zero*** zero growth
crespo ['krespu] *adj cabelo* frizzy
cretino [kre'ʧinu] *m* cretin
cria ['kria] *f* ZOOL baby animal
criação [kria'sãw] *f* creation *tb* REL; *crianças*: upbringing; *gado*, *galinhas etc*: breeding; ***filho de ~*** adopted child
criada [kri'ada] *f* maid
criado [kri'adu] **1** *adj* ***bem ~*** well behaved; ***mal ~*** badly behaved, naughty **2** *m* (male) servant
criador [kria'dor] *m* creator *tb* REL, maker; ***~ de caso*** troublemaker; ***~ de gado*** cattle breeder
criança [kri'ãsa] **1** *f* child, *fam* kid; ***ela é muito ~ para entender*** she's too young to understand; ***~ de colo*** infant; ***não seja ~!*** grow up! **2** *adj* childish
criar [kri'ar] ⟨1g⟩ *v/t* create; *animais* rear; *criança* raise, bring up; (*amamentar*) suckle, nurse; ***~ coragem*** pluck up courage; ***~ caso*** make trouble
criativo [kria'ʧivu] *adj* creative
criatura [kria'tura] *f* creature
crime ['krimi] *m* crime; ***~ organizado*** organized crime
criminal [krimi'naw] *adj* criminal
criminalidade [kriminali'dadʒi] *f* crime
criminoso [krimi'nozu] **1** *adj* criminal **2** *m*, **-a** *f* criminal
crina ['krina] *f cavalo*: mane
cripta ['kripta] *f* crypt
crisântemo [kri'zãtemu] *m* chrysanthemum
crise ['krizi] *f* crisis; MED attack, fit; ***ter uma ~ de choro*** cry; ***ela teve uma ~ de choro assim que ...*** she burst into tears when ...; ***~ de crédito*** credit crunch
cristã [kris'tã] → ***cristão***
cristal [kris'taw] *m* crystal; (*vidro*) glass; ***de ~*** crystal
cristaleira [krista'lejra] *f* dresser
cristalizar [kristali'zar] ⟨1a⟩ *v/i* crystallize; **cristalizar-se** *v/r* crystallize
cristão [kris'tãw] ⟨*mpl* -ãos⟩ **1** *adj* Christian **2** *mpl*, **-ã** *f* Christian
cristianismo [krisʧia'nizmu] *m* Christianity
Cristo ['kristu] *m* Christ
critério [kri'tɛriu] *m* criterion; (*juízo*) discretion, judgment; ***deixo isso ao seu ~*** I'll leave that to your discretion
crítica ['kriʧika] *f* criticism; (*análise*) critique; *livro*, *filme*: review
criticar [kriʧi'kar] ⟨1n⟩ *v/t* criticize; *livro* review
crítico ['kriʧiku] **1** *adj* critical **2** *m*, **-a** *f* critic; ***~ de teatro*** theater critic, *Brit* theatre critic
crivar [kri'var] ⟨1a⟩ *v/t* (*furar*) riddle; *de perguntas* bombard
Croácia [kro'asja] *f* Croatia
croata [kro'ata] **1** *adj* Croatian **2** *m/f* Croat **3** *m lingua* Croatian
crochê, *Port* **croché** [kro'ʃe] *m* crochet; ***fazer ~*** crochet
crocodilo [kroko'dʒilu] *m* crocodile
croissant [krwa'sã] *m* croissant
cromo [kro'mu] *m* chrome
crônica, *Port* **crónica** ['kronika] *f* chronicle; *jornal*: feature
crônico, *Port* **crónico** ['kroniku] *adj* chronic
cronista [kro'nista] *m/f* chronicler; *jornal*: columnist
cronologia [kronolo'ʒia] *f* chronology
cronológico [krono'lɔʒiku] *adj* chronological
cronometrar [kronome'trar] ⟨1c⟩ *v/t* time
cronômetro, *Port* **cronómetro** [kro'nometru] *m* stopwatch; *forno etc*: timer
croquete [kro'kɛʧi] *m* croquette
crosta ['krosta] *f* crust; MED scab
cru [kru] *adj* raw; *tom*, *palavra* harsh; *linguagem* crude
crucial [kru'sjaw] *adj* crucial
crucificação [krusifika'sãw] *f* crucifixion
crucificar [krusifi'kar] ⟨1n⟩ *v/t* crucify
crucifixo [krusi'fiksu] *m* crucifix
cruel [kru'ew] *adj* cruel
crueldade [kruew'dadʒi] *f* cruelty

crustáceos [krus'tasius] *mpl* crustaceans
cruz [kɾus] *f* cross; ***fazer o sinal da ~*** do the sign of the cross, cross oneself; ***Cruz Vermelha*** Red Cross
cruzamento [kɾuza'mẽtu] *m* cross; *idéias*: crossover; *ruas*: crossroads *sg*, junction
cruzar [kɾu'zaɾ] ⟨1a⟩ **1** *v/t* cross; ***~ os braços*** fold one's arms; ***~ as pernas*** cross one's legs **2** *v/i* cruise; ***~ com alguém*** pass s.o.; **cruzar-se** *v/r* cross; *pessoas* pass each other
cruzeiro [kɾu'zejɾu] *m* NÁUT cruise; (*cruz*) cross; ***fazer um ~*** go on a cruise
cu [ku] *m vulg* ass, *Brit* arse; ***vai tomar no ~*** fuck off!
Cuba ['kuba] *f* Cuba
cubano [ku'banu] **1** *adj* Cuban **2** *m*, **-a** *f* Cuban
cubículo [ku'bikulu] *m* cubicle
cúbico ['kubiku] *adj* cubic
cubo ['kubu] *m* cube; *roda*: hub
cuca ['kuka] *f fam* head; ***use a ~!*** use your loaf!
cuco ['kuku] *m* cuckoo
cueca ['kwɛka] *f*, *Port* **cuecas** ['kwɛkas] *fpl* underpants; *mulher*: panties
cuidado [kui'dadu] **1** *adj* careful **2** *m* care; MED ***~s pl intensivos*** intensive care; ***~!*** watch out!, careful!; ***aos ~s de*** in the care of; ***com ~*** carefully; ***ter ~*** be careful, take care; ***~ com o degrau!*** mind the step!
cuidadosamente [kuidadoza'mẽtʃi] *adv* carefully
cuidadoso [kuida'dozu] *adj* careful; (*meticuloso*) thorough
cuidar [kui'daɾ] ⟨1a⟩ *v/i* ***~ de*** take care of; **cuidar-se** look after oneself; ***cuide-se!*** take care!; ***cuide de sua vida!*** mind your own business!
cujo, cuja ['kuʒu, 'kuʒa] *pron* (*de quem*) whose; (*de que*) of which
culinária [kuli'naɾja] *f* cookery
culinário [kuli'naɾiu] *adj* culinary
culminante [kuwmi'nãtʃi] *adj* ***ponto m ~*** highest point
culminar [kuwmi'naɾ] ⟨1a⟩ *v/i* culminate (***com*** in)
culpa ['kuwpa] *f* fault; JUR guilt; ***pôr a ~ em*** put the blame on; ***sentimento de ~*** guilty conscience; ***é ~ sua*** it's your fault
culpabilidade [kuwpabili'dadʒi] *f* guilt
culpado [kuw'padu] **1** *adj* guilty **2** *m*, **-a** *f* culprit
culpar [kuw'paɾ] ⟨1a⟩ *v/t* blame; (*acusar*) accuse; ***~ alguém de algo*** blame s.o. for sth
culpável [kuw'pavew] *adj* guilty
cultivar [kuwtʃi'vaɾ] ⟨1a⟩ *v/t terras* cultivate; *plantas* grow; *talento* nurture
cultivo [kuw'tʃivu] *m* AGR cultivation; *plantas*: growing
culto ['kuwtu] **1** *adj pessoa* cultured; *povo* civilized **2** *m* cult
cultura [kuw'tuɾa] *f* culture; AGR cultivation; ***~ geral*** general knowledge
cultural [kuwtu'ɾaw] *adj* cultural
cúmplice ['kũplisi] *m/f* accomplice; JUR accessory
cumprimentar [kũpɾimẽ'taɾ] ⟨1a⟩ *v/t* greet; (*elogiar*) compliment
cumprimento [kũpɾi'mẽtu] *m* (*saudação*) greeting; (*elogio*) compliment; *regra*: compliance; (*realização*) fulfilment, *Brit* fulfillment
cumprir [kũ'pɾiɾ] ⟨3a⟩ **1** *v/t* carry out; *promessa* keep; *lei* obey; *pena* serve; ***~ os seus deveres*** do one's duty; ***~ trinta anos*** turn thirty **2** *v/i* be necessary; **cumprir-se** *v/r* be fulfilled
cúmulo ['kumulu] *m* height; ***é o ~!*** that's the limit!
cunha ['kuɲa] *f* wedge
cunhada [ku'ɲada] *f* sister-in-law
cunhado [ku'ɲadu] *m* brother-in-law
cupom [ku'põ] *m* coupon
cúpula ['kupula] *f* ARQUIT dome, cupola; *abajur*: shade; POL leadership; POL ***reunião f de ~*** summit (meeting)
cura[1] ['kuɾa] *f carne*: curing; MED cure; (*tratamento*) treatment; ***ter ~*** be curable
cura[2] ['kuɾa] *m* curate, priest
curandeiro [kuɾã'dejɾu] *m* healer, medicine man
curar [ku'ɾaɾ] ⟨1a⟩ *v/t carne, doença* cure; *ferida* treat; **curar-se** *v/r* be cured, recover
curativo [kuɾa'tʃivu] *m* dressing

curiosidade [kuɾjozi'dadʒi] *f* curiosity; (*raridade*) oddity; ***por ~*** out of curiosity
curioso [ku'ɾjozu] *adj* curious; ***eu ficaria ~ em saber ...*** I would be curious to know ...
curral [ku'haw] *m* pen, enclosure
currículo [ku'hikulu] *m* curriculum; (*curriculum*) résumé, *Brit* curriculum vitae, *Brit* CV
curso ['kuɾsu] *m* course; ***~ de pós-graduação*** post-graduate degree course; ***~ de administração*** business studies; ***~ intensivo*** crash course; ***~ primário*** primary school; ***~ de revisão*** refresher course; ***~ secundário*** secondary school; ***~ superior*** degree course
cursor [kuɾ'soɾ] *m* INFORM cursor
curta-metragem [kuɾtame'tɾaʒẽ] *f* short (movie)
curtir [kuɾ'tʃiɾ] ⟨3a⟩ **1** *v/t couro* tan; *fam* enjoy **2** *v/i* enjoy oneself
curto ['kuɾtu] short; *conhecimento, inteligência* limited; (*rápido*) quick; ***~ e grosso*** terse
curto-circuito [kuɾtusiɾ'kuitu] *m* ⟨*pl* curtos-circuitos⟩ short-circuit
curva ['kuɾva] *f* curve, *Brit tb* bend; ***fazer a ~*** round the corner; ***~ fechada*** hairpin curve; ***~ cega*** blind corner
curvar [kuɾ'vaɾ] ⟨1a⟩ *v/t* bend; **curvar-se** *v/r* stoop; *dor*: double up; ***~ a*** submit to
curvatura [kuɾva'tuɾa] *f* curvature
curvo ['kuɾvu] *adj* curved; *estrada* winding
cuspe ['kuspi] *m* spit, spittle
cuspir [kus'piɾ] ⟨3h⟩ **1** *v/t* spit out **2** *v/i* spit
custa(s) ['kusta(s)] *f(pl)* ***à ~*** (*ou* ***às ~s***) ***de*** at the expense of; ***viver à ~ de alguém*** sponge off s.o.
custar [kus'taɾ] ⟨1a⟩ *v/i* cost; (*ser difícil*) be difficult; (*demorar*) take a long time; ***~ caro*** be expensive; ***custam 150 cada*** they're *ou* they cost 150 each; ***custe o que ~!*** no matter what!
custear [kus'tʃiaɾ] ⟨1l⟩ *v/t* bear the cost of
custo ['kustu] *m* cost; ***a ~*** with difficulty; ***a todo ~*** at all costs; ***~s*** *pl* ***de produção*** production costs; ***~ unitário*** unit cost; ***~ de vida*** cost of living
cutelo [ku'tɛlu] *m* cleaver
cutícula [ku'tʃikula] *f* cuticle
cútis ['kutʃis] *f* (*pele*) skin; (*tez*) complexion
cutucar [kutu'kaɾ] ⟨1n⟩ *v/t* poke, prod; ***~ o nariz*** pick one's nose

D

da [da] *prep* ***de*** + *art f* ***a***
dá [da] → ***dar***
dado[1] ['dadu] *m* die, dice; ***lançar os ~s*** throw the dice; *fig* ***os ~s estão lançados*** the die is cast
dado[2] ['dadu] **1** *m* fact, piece of information; ***~s*** *pl* data; ***banco*** *m* ***de ~s*** database; ***processamento*** *m* ***de ~s*** data processing; ***~s pessoais*** personal details **2** *adj* given; ***~ que*** given that; ***ser ~ a algo*** be prone to sth
dado[3] *pp* → ***dar***
daí [da'i] *prep* = ***de*** + *adv* ***aí***; *lugar*: from there; *momento*: from then; *fam relato*: then; *fam* ***e ~*** so what?
dali [da'li] *prep* = ***de*** + *adv* ***ali*** from there
dália ['dalia] *f* dahlia
daltônico, *Port* **daltónico** [daw'toniku] *adj* color-blind, *Brit* colour-blind
daltonismo [dawto'nizmu] *m* color-blindness, *Brit* colour blindness
dama ['dama] *f* lady; *xadrez*: queen; ***jogo*** *m* ***das ~s*** checkers *sg*, *Brit*

draughts *sg*; ~ ***de honra*** bridesmaid; POL ***primeira*** ~ First Lady

damasco [da'masku] *m* apricot; *tecido* damask

danado [da'nadu] *adj* (*furioso*) furious; (*condenado*) damned; *criança* naughty; ***estar*** ~ ***para*** be desperate to; ***uma ressaca danada*** a terrible hangover; ***estou com uma fome danada*** I'm absolutely starving; *fam* ***ele é*** ~ ***de bom*** he's damn good

dança ['dãsa] *f* dance; *atividade* dancing; ~ ***folclórica*** folk dance / dancing; ***entrar na*** ~ get involved

dançar [dã'saɾ] ⟨1p⟩ *v/i* dance; *fam* ***ele dançou*** he's out

dançarino [dãsa'ɾinu] *m*, **-a** *f* dancer

danificar [danifi'kaɾ] ⟨1n⟩ *v/t* damage

daninho [da'niɲu] *adj* harmful; ***erva*** *f* ***daninha*** weed

dano ['dãu] *m moral* harm; *a uma pessoa* injury; ***causar*** ~ harm

dantes ['dãtʃis] *adv* before, formerly

dão [dãw] → ***dar***

daquele [da'keli], **-a** *prep* ***de*** + *pron* ***aquele***, ***aquela*** from that

daqui [da'ki] *prep* ***de*** *com adv* ***aqui***; from here; *temporal* from now; ~ ***a duas horas*** in two hours from now; ~ ***para lá*** from here to there; ~ ***a pouco*** in a little while

dar [daɾ] ⟨1r⟩ **1** *v/t* give; *festa* hold; *problemas* cause; *cartas* deal; *frutas* produce; *caminhada* take; ~ ***algo a alguém*** give sth to s.o. **2** *v/i* ~ ***com*** *pessoa* meet, *coisa* find; *roupas* match, go with; ~ ***certo*** work out; ***dá para*** it is possible; ***dá para trocar dinheiro aqui?*** can I change money here?; ***dá para todo mundo*** is there enough for everyone?; *Bras* ~ ***ré*** *carro* reverse; **dar-se** *v/r* ~ ***com alguém*** get along with s.o.

dardo ['daɾdu] *m* dart; *grande* spear; ESP javelin

dás [das] → ***dar***

data ['data] *f* date; *época* time; ***de longa*** ~ of long standing; ***nós nos conhecemos de longa*** ~ we go back a long way; ~ ***de entrega*** delivery date; ~ ***de nascimento*** date of birth; ~ ***de validade*** sell-by date

datar [da'taɾ] ⟨1b⟩ **1** *v/t* date **2** *v/i* ~ ***de*** date from

datilografar [datʃilogɾa'faɾ] ⟨1a⟩ *v/t* type

datilógrafo [datʃi'lɔgɾafu] *m*, **-a** *f* typist

de [de] *prep* ◊ *proveniência*: from; ***ele é*** ~ ***Recife*** he's from Recife; ~ ***lá para cá*** from there to here

◊ *posse*: of; ***o nome da rua*** the name of the street; ***a moto do Pedro*** Pedro's bike; ***é do Pedro*** it's Pedro's, it belongs to Pedro

◊ *meio*: ~ ***ônibus*** / ***trem*** by bus / train

◊ *tempo*: ~ ***noite*** / ***dia*** by day / night; ~ ***manhã*** in the morning; ***antes das 6*** before 6

◊ *descrição*: ***um prato*** ~ ***macarrão*** a plate of pasta; ***um bilhete*** ~ ***trem*** a train ticket; ***um álbum*** ~ ***foto*** a photo album; ~ ***prata*** made of silver; ***vestir-se*** ~ ***amarelo*** dress in yellow

◊ *comparativo*: than; ***mais*** ~ ***dez*** more than ten; ***ele é mais esperto do que o seu pai*** he is cleverer than his father

◊ *razão*: ***morrer*** ~ ***algo*** die of sth, die from sth; ***gritar*** ~ ***medo*** / ***alegria*** scream with joy / fear; ***difícil*** ~ ***ouvir*** difficult to hear

dê [de] → ***dar***

debaixo [de'bajʃu] **1** *adv* below, underneath **2** *prep* ~ ***de*** under, beneath

debate [de'batʃi] *m* debate; (*disputa*) argument

debater [deba'teɾ] ⟨2b⟩ *v/i & v/t* debate, discuss

débil ['dɛbiw] **1** *adj* weak **2** *m* ~ ***mental*** mentally handicapped person; *fam* idiot

debilidade [debili'dadʒi] *f* weakness

debilitado [debili'tadu] *adj* weak, debilitated

debitar [debi'taɾ] ⟨1a⟩ **1** *v/t* debit; ~ ***a conta de alguém*** debit s.o's account **2** *v/i* ~ ***em*** charge to

débito ['dɛbitu] *m* debit; ***estar com um*** ~ ***de 800 dólares na conta*** be 800 dollars overdrawn

deboche [de'bɔʃi] *m* jibe

debruçar [debru'saɾ] ⟨1p⟩ *v/t* bend

over; **debrucar-se** *v/r* bend over; **~ *sobre algo*** lean over sth
debutante [debu'tãʧi] *f* débutante
década ['dɛkada] *f* decade; ***a ~ dos 60*** the sixties
decadência [deka'dẽsja] *f* decadence
decadente [deka'dẽʧi] *adj* decadent
decair [deka'iɾ] ⟨3l⟩ *v/i* decline; *qualidade, distrito* go downhill; *planta* wilt
decantar [dekã'taɾ] ⟨1a⟩ *v/t líquido* decant; (*purificar*) purify
decapitar [dekapi'taɾ] ⟨1a⟩ *v/t* decapitate
decência [de'sẽsja] *f* decency
decênio, *Port* **decénio** [de'seniu] *m* decade
decente [de'sẽʧi] *adj* decent
decepção [desep'sãw] *f* disappointment; ***foi uma ~*** it was a let-down
decepcionante [desepsjo'nãʧi] *adj* disappointing
decepcionar [desepsjo'naɾ] ⟨1f⟩ *v/t* disappoint, let down
decerto [de'sɛrtu] *adv* certainly
decibel [desi'bɛw] *m* decibel
decidido [desi'dʒidu] *adj pessoa* determined; *questão* settled
decidir [desi'dʒiɾ] ⟨3a⟩ *v/t* decide; (*solucionar*) resolve; **decidir-se** *v/r* make up one's mind; **~ *por*** decide on
decíduo [de'siduu] *adj* deciduous
decifrar [desi'fɾaɾ] ⟨1a⟩ *v/t* decipher; *futuro* foretell
decilitro [desi'litɾu] *m* deciliter, *Brit* decilitre
decimal [desi'maw] **1** *adj* decimal **2** *m número* decimal
décimo ['dɛsimu] **1** *adj* tenth **2** *m* tenth
decisão [desi'zãw] *f* decision; *personalidade*: decisiveness, resolution; ***tomar uma ~*** make a decision; ***chegar a uma ~*** come to a decision; ***a ~ é sua*** it's up to you; **~ *por pênalti*** penalty shoot-out
decisivo [desi'zivu] *adj* decisive; ***o jogo ~*** the decider
declamar [dekla'maɾ] ⟨1a⟩ **1** *v/t* recite **2** *v/i pej* rant
declaração [deklaɾa'sãw] *f* declaration; **~ *de amor*** declaration of love; **~ *de imposto de renda*** income tax return
declarar [dekla'ɾaɾ] ⟨1b⟩ *v/t* declare; *veredicto* bring in; **~ *alguém inocente / culpado*** find s.o. not guilty / guilty; **declarar-se** *v/r* **~ *inocente / culpado*** plead not guilty / guilty
declinação [deklina'sãw] *f* GRAM declension
declinar [dekli'naɾ] ⟨1a⟩ **1** *v/i sol* go down; *terreno* slope down; *força, coragem* ebb away **2** *v/t* GRAM decline; *convite* turn down, decline
declínio [de'kliniu] *m* decline; *economia*: downturn
declive [de'klivi] *m* (downward) slope; *na rua* dip
decodificar [dekodʒifi'kaɾ] ⟨1a & 1n⟩ *v/t* decode
decolagem [deko'laʒẽ] *f* AERO takeoff
decolar [deko'laɾ] ⟨1e⟩ *v/i* AERO take off
decompor [dekõ'poɾ] ⟨2z⟩ **1** *v/i* decompose, rot **2** *v/t* (*analisar*) break down; **decompor-se** *v/r* decompose, rot
decomposição [dekõpozi'sãw] *f* ⟨*sem pl*⟩ decomposition; (*análise*) breakdown
decoração [dekoɾa'sãw] *f* decoration; TEAT scenery; (*aprendizagem*) learning off by heart; **~ *de interiores*** interior design
decorador [dekoɾa'doɾ] *m*, **-a** *f casa*: interior designer
decorar [deko'ɾaɾ] ⟨1e⟩ *v/t* decorate; (*aprender*) learn by heart
decorativo [dekoɾa'ʧivu] *adj* decorative
decoro [de'koɾu] *m* decorum
decorrer [deko'heɾ] ⟨2d⟩ **1** *v/i tempo* pass; (*acontecer*) take place, happen; **~ *de*** result from **2** *m* ***no ~ do tempo*** over the course of time
decotado [deko'tadu] *adj roupa* low-cut
decote [de'kɔʧi] *m vestido*: low neckline; **~ *em V*** V-neck
decrépito [de'kɾɛpitu] *adj* decrepit
decrescer [dekɾes'seɾ] ⟨2g⟩ *v/i* decrease, diminish

decretação [dekɾeta'sãw] *f* announcement
decretar [dekre'taɾ] ⟨1c⟩ *v/t* decree, order; (*anunciar*) announce; (*determinar*) determine
decreto [de'krɛtu] *m* decree, order
decreto-lei [dekɾɛto'lej] *m* ⟨*pl* decretos-lei(s)⟩ act, law
decurso [de'kuɾsu] *m* (*decorrer*) course; ***no ~ de*** in the course of
dedal [de'daw] *m* thimble
dedão [de'dãw] *m* thumb; *pé*: big toe
dedicação [dedʒika'sãw] *f* dedication
dedicado [dedʒi'kadu] *adj* (*zeloso*) dedicated; (*fiel*) devoted
dedicar [dedʒi'kaɾ] ⟨1n⟩ *v/t livro etc* dedicate; *tempo* devote; **dedicar-se** *v/r* ***~ a*** dedicate oneself to
dedicatória [dedʒika'tɔɾja] *f* dedication
dedilhar [dedʒi'ʎaɾ] ⟨1a⟩ *v/t guitarra* pluck
dedinho [de'dʒiɲu] *m* little finger
dedo ['dedu] *m* finger; *pé*: toe; ***cheio de ~s*** all fingers and thumbs; ***~ indicador*** index finger; ***~ polegar*** thumb
dedo-duro [dedo'duɾu] ⟨**dedos-duros**⟩ *m* blabbermouth
dedução [dedu'sãw] *f* MATH *etc* subtraction; (*conclusão*) deduction
deduzir [dedu'ziɾ] ⟨3m⟩ *v/t* deduct; (*concluir*) deduce
defasado [defa'zadu] *adj* out of synch
defeito [de'fejtu] *m* defect; ***com ~*** damaged; COM ***produtos com ~*** rejects; ***botar ~ em*** find fault with; ***~ de fala*** speech impediment; ***~ de projeto*** design fault
defeituoso [defej'twozu] *adj* defective, faulty
defender [defẽ'deɾ] ⟨2a⟩ *v/t* defend; (*proteger*) protect (***de*** from); ESP *gol* save; *tradição* uphold; **defender-se** *v/r* defend oneself
defensiva [defẽ'siva] *f* ***na ~*** on the defensive
defensivamente [defẽsiva'mẽtʃi] *adv* defensively
defensivo [defẽ'sivu] *adj* defensive
defensor [defẽ'soɾ] *m*, **-a** *f* defender; *advogado* defense counsel, *Brit* counsel for the defence
deferência [defe'ɾẽsja] *f* deference
deferente [defe'ɾẽtʃi] *adj* deferential
deferir [defe'riɾ] ⟨3c⟩ **1** *v/t* grant; *prêmio* award **2** *v/i* ***~ a um pedido*** agree to a request; ***~ para alguém*** refer to s.o.
defesa [de'feza] **1** *f* defense, *Brit* defence; ***legítima ~*** self-defense **2** *m/f* ESP defender, back
défice ['dɛfisi] *m* deficit
deficiência [defi'sjẽsja] *f* deficiency; *pessoa*: disability; ***~ visual*** visual impairment; ***~ física*** physical handicap
deficiente [defi'sjẽtʃi] **1** *adj* defective; (*aleijado*) handicapped **2** *m/f* ***~ físico*** physically handicapped person
déficit ['dɛfisit] *m* deficit
deficitário [defisi'taɾiu] *adj* in deficit
definição [defini'sãw] *f* definition
definido [defi'nidu] *adj* definite
definir [defi'niɾ] ⟨3a⟩ *v/t* define; **definir-se** *v/r* (*decidir-se*) make a decision; (*explicar-se*) make one's position clear
definitivamente [definitva'mẽtʃi] *adv* definitively; *certeza*: definitely
definitivo [defini'tʃivu] *adj* definitive, final
deflagração [deflagɾa'sãw] *f* explosion; *guerra*: outbreak
deflagrar [defla'gɾaɾ] ⟨1b⟩ **1** *v/i* explode; *fig* break out **2** *v/t* set off, trigger
deflorar [deflo'ɾaɾ] ⟨1e⟩ *v/t* deflower
deformação [defoɾma'sãw] *f corpo*: deformation; *imagem, pensamento*: distortion
deformar [defoɾ'maɾ] ⟨1e⟩ *v/t* deform; *imagem, pensamento* distort; **deformar-se** *v/r madeira* warp
deformidade [defoɾmi'dadʒi] *f* deformity
defraudar [defɾaw'daɾ] ⟨1a⟩ *v/t* defraud; ***~ alguém de algo*** cheat s.o. out of sth
defronte [de'fɾõtʃi] **1** *adv* opposite **2** *prep* ***~*** (***de***) across from, opposite
defumado [defu'madu] *adj* smoked
defumador [defuma'doɾ] *m* REL incense burner
defumar [defu'maɾ] ⟨1a⟩ *v/t* smoke
defunto [de'fũtu] **1** *adj* dead, de-

D

ceased **2** *m*, **-a** *f* dead person, deceased
degelo [de'ʒelu] *m* thaw
degeneração [deʒenera'sãw] *f* degeneration; *moral* degeneracy
degenerar [deʒene'rar] ⟨1c⟩ *v/i* degenerate; **~ em** degenerate into
degradação [degrada'sãw] *f* degradation
degradante [degra'dãʧi] *adj* degrading
degradar [degra'dar] ⟨1b⟩ *v/t* degrade, debase; **degradar-se** *v/r* demean oneself
degradável [degra'davew] *adj* degradable
degrau [de'graw] *m* step; *escada de mão*: rung
degredar [degre'dar] ⟨1c⟩ *v/t* exile
degredo [de'gredu] *m* exile
degustação [degusta'sãw] *f vinho*: tasting
dei [dej] → ***dar***
deitada [dej'tada] *f* ***dar uma ~*** have a lie-down
deitado [dej'tadu] *adj* lying down; *na cama* in bed
deitar [dej'tar] ⟨1a⟩ *v/t* lay down; *crianças* put to bed; (*pôr*) put; *Port* (*atirar*) throw; *Port líquido* pour; ***~ a fazer algo*** start doing sth; **deitar--se** *v/r* lie down; (*ir para cama*) go to bed
deixa ['dejʃa] *f* cue
deixar [dej'ʃar] ⟨1a⟩ *v/t* ◇ leave; (*abandonar*) abandon; *passageiro* drop off; ***~ alguém em casa*** drop s.o. off at home; ***~ em paz*** leave alone; ***deixe-me fora disso*** leave me out of this; ***a professora me deixou de castigo*** the teacher kept me in; ***~ alguém esperando*** keep s.o. waiting; ***~ algo abandonado*** leave sth unattended; ***~ algo de lado*** give sth a miss
◇ (*parar*) stop; *emprego* quit; ***~ de fazer algo*** stop doing sth; (*não fazer*) omit to do sth; ***não posso ~ de perguntar*** I can't help but ask; ***deixa para lá!*** forget it!
◇ ***~ alguém louco*** drive s.o. crazy; ***~ inconsciente*** knock unconscious; ***~ alguém mais independente*** make s.o. more independent
◇ (*permitir*) let; ***~ alguém fazer algo*** let s.o. do sth; ***deixe-o entrar!*** let him in!; ***~ cair*** drop
dela ['dɛla] = *prep* **de** + *pron f* **ela**
delatar [dela'tar] ⟨1b⟩ *v/t pessoa* inform on; *abusos* reveal; *polícia*: report
delator [dela'tor] *m* informer
dele ['deli] = *prep* **de** + *pron m* **ele**
delegação [delega'sãw] *f* delegation
delegacia [delega'sia] *f* office; ***~ de homicídios*** homicide department; *Bras* ***~ de polícia*** police station
delegado [dele'gadu] *m*, **-a** *f* delegate; ***~ de polícia*** police chief
delegar [dele'gar] ⟨1o & 1c⟩ *v/t* delegate
deleitar-se [delej'tarsi] ⟨1a⟩ *v/r* ***~ com*** revel in
deleito [de'lejtu] *m* delight
deletar [dele'tar] ⟨1c⟩ *v/t* INFORM delete
delgado [dew'gadu] *adj* slim, slender
deliberação [delibera'sãw] *f* deliberation; (*decisão*) decision
deliberadamente [deliberada'mẽʧi] *adv* deliberately
deliberado [delibe'radu] *adj* deliberate
deliberar [delibe'rar] ⟨1c⟩ **1** *v/t* (*decidir*) decide **2** *v/i* ***~ sobre*** deliberate over
delicadamente [delikada'mẽʧi] *adv* delicately
delicadeza [delika'deza] *f* delicacy; (*cortesia*) politeness; (*sensibilidade*) gentleness, kindness; ***ela repondeu à sua carta com ~*** she answered his letter politely
delicado [deli'kadu] *adj* delicate; (*cortês*) polite; (*sensível*) sensitive; *corpo* slight
delícia [de'lisja] *f* delight; (*prazer*) pleasure; ***uma ~*** delicious; ***que ~*** how lovely!
delicioso [deli'sjozu] *adj* delicious; (*encantador*) lovely
delimitação [delimita'sãw] *f* delimitation
delimitar [delimi'tar] ⟨1a⟩ *v/t* delimit
delineador [delinja'dor] *m* eyeliner

delinear [deli'njar] ⟨1l⟩ *v/t* outline
delinqüência, *Port* **delinquência** [delĩ'kwẽsja] *f* delinquency; **~ *juvenil*** juvenile delinquency
delinqüente, *Port* **delinquente** [delĩ'kwẽtʃi] **1** *adj* delinquent **2** *m* delinquent, criminal; **~ *juvenil*** juvenile delinquent; **~ *primário*** first-time offender
delirante [deli'rãtʃi] *adj* MED delirious *tb fig*
delirar [deli'rar] ⟨1a⟩ *v/i com febre* be delirious, rave; *fig* go wild
delírio [de'liriu] *m* delirium
delito [de'litu] *m* offense, *Brit* offence; **~ *sexual*** sex crime
delonga [de'lõga] *f* ***sem mais*** **~** without more ado
demais [dʒi'majs] **1** *adv* too much; (*muitíssimo*) a lot; ***grande / quente*** **~** too big / hot; ***é bom*** **~** it's really good **2** *adj* ***tem arroz*** **~** there's too much rice; ***tem problemas*** **~** there are too many problems; ***já é*** **~*!*** this is too much!; *fam* ***foi*** **~*!*** it was great! **3** *pron* ***os / as*** **~** the rest (of them)
demanda [de'mãda] *f* JUR lawsuit; (*disputa*) claim; (*requisição*) request; ECON demand; ***em*** **~** ***de*** in search of
demarcação [demarka'sãw] *f* demarcation
demarcar [demar'kar] ⟨1n & 1b⟩ *v/t* demarcate
demasia [dema'zia] *f* excess; ***em*** **~** *comida etc* too much; *cartas etc* too many
demasiado [dema'zjadu] **1** *adj* too much; *plural* too many **2** *adv* too much; **~ *grande*** too big
demência [de'mẽsja] *f* insanity; MED dementia
demente [de'mẽtʃi] **1** *adj* insane, demented **2** *m/f* demented person
demissão [demi'sãw] *f* dismissal; (***pedido de***) **~** resignation; ***pedir*** **~** resign
demitir [demi'tʃir] ⟨3a⟩ *v/t* dismiss, *fam* fire; ***ser demitido*** be fired; **demitir-se** *v/r* resign
democracia [demokra'sia] *f* democracy
democrata [demo'krata] *m/f* democrat
democraticamente [demokratʃika'mẽtʃi] *adv* democratically
democrático [demo'kratʃiku] *adj* democratic
democratização [demokratʃiza'sãw] *f* ⟨*sem pl*⟩ democratization
democratizar [demokratʃi'zar] ⟨1a⟩ democratize
demográfico [demo'grafiku] *adj* demographic
demolição [demoli'sãw] *f* ⟨*sem pl*⟩ demolition
demolir [demo'lir] ⟨3f⟩ *v/t edifício* demolish; *carro* total, write off
demoníaco [demo'niaku] *adj* demonic
demônio, *Port* **demónio** [de'moniu] *m* demon; *fam criança* brat; ***o*** **~** the Devil
demonstração [demõstra'sãw] *f* demonstration
demonstrar [demõs'trar] ⟨1a⟩ *v/t* demonstrate; *emoção* show; **~ *respeito por*** show respect for
demonstrativo [demõstra'tʃivu] *adj* demonstrative *tb* GRAM
demonstrável [demõs'travew] *adj* demonstrable
demora [de'mɔra] *f* delay; ***sem*** **~** at once, without delay
demorado [demo'radu] *adj* time-consuming
demorar [demo'rar] ⟨1e⟩ **1** *v/t* delay; ***quanto tempo demora?*** how long does it take? **2** *v/i* take; (*permanecer*) stay; (*levar muito tempo*) take a long time; (*tardar a vir*) be late; ***vai*** **~** ***muito?*** will it take long?; **demorar-se** *v/r* linger, stay for a long time; ***não se demore*** don't be long
demos ['dɛmus], **dêmos** ['demus] → ***dar***
dendê [dẽ'de] *m* palm oil; BOT oil palm
denominação [denomina'sãw] *f* REL denomination
denominador [denomina'dor] *m* MAT **~ *comum*** common denominator
denominar [denomi'nar] ⟨1a⟩ *v/t* name; **denominar-se** *v/r* be called; *a si mesmo* call oneself

denotar [deno'taɾ] ⟨1e⟩ *v/t* denote
densamente [dẽsa'mẽtʃi] *adv* densely; **~ habitado** densely populated
densidade [dẽsi'dadʒi] *f* density
denso ['dẽsu] *adj* dense; (*espesso*) thick
D
dentada [dẽ'tada] *f* bite; **dar uma ~** take a bite
dentado [dẽ'tadu] *adj* serrated
dentadura [dẽta'duɾa] *f* teeth; *artificial* dentures
dental [dẽ'taw] *adj* dental
dente ['dẽtʃi] *m* tooth; *alho*: clove; **ranger os ~s** grind one's teeth; **~ de leite** milk tooth; **~ do siso** wisdom tooth
dente-de-leão [dẽtʃidʒi'ljãw] *m* ⟨pl dentes-de-leão⟩ dandelion
dentista [dẽ'tʃista] *m/f* dentist
dentro ['dẽtɾu] **1** *adv* inside; **de ~** from within; **por ~** on the inside, inwardly; **para ~** *ir* inside **2** *prep* **~ de** inside, *tempo* inside of, within; **~ das minhas possibilidades** within my power; **~ de casa** indoors; **~ do limite** within limits; **~ em breve** soon, before long; **aí ~** in there; *fam* **estar por ~** be in the know; **estar por ~ de algo** be up to date about sth
dentuço [dẽ'tusu] *adj* buck-toothed
denúncia [de'nũsja] *f* denunciation; (*acusação*) accusation; *de roubo* report
denunciante [denũ'sjãtʃi] *m/f* informant
denunciar [denũ'sjaɾ] ⟨1g⟩ *v/t* denounce; **~ alguém à polícia** report s.o. to the police
deparar-se [depa'ɾaɾsi] ⟨1b⟩ *v/r* **~ com** stumble across
departamento [depaɾta'mẽtu] *m* department; **~ de marketing** marketing department
depenar [depe'naɾ] ⟨1d⟩ *v/t* pluck
dependência [depẽ'dẽsja] *f* dependence; *colonial* dependency; (*cômodo*) room
dependente [depẽ'dẽtʃi] **1** *adj* dependant **2** *m/f* dependant
depender [depẽ'deɾ] ⟨2a⟩ *v/i* depend; **~ de** depend on; **depende!** it depends!

depilação [depila'sãw] *f* depilation
depilar [depi'laɾ] ⟨1a⟩ *v/t* remove the hair from; **~ as pernas** wax one's legs
depilatório [depila'tɔɾiu] *m* hair-remover, depilatory
deplorar [deplo'ɾaɾ] ⟨1e⟩ *v/t* deplore; (*lamentar*) regret; *morte*, *perda* lament
deplorável [deplo'ɾavew] *adj* deplorable; (*lamentável*) regrettable
depoimento [depoi'mẽtu] *m* deposition, testimony; *polícia*: statement
depois [de'pojs] **1** *adv* afterward, later **2** *prep* **~ de** after; **~ de comer** after eating; **~ de amanhã** the day after tomorrow; **~ de escurecer** after dark; **~ disso** after that
depor [de'poɾ] ⟨2z⟩ **1** *v/t armas* lay down; *rei*, *presidente* depose **2** *v/i polícia*: give a statement; DIR testify
deportação [depoɾta'sãw] *f* deportation
deportar [depoɾ'taɾ] ⟨1e⟩ *v/t* deport
deposição [depuzisãw] *f* deposition, overthrow
depositar [depozi'taɾ] ⟨1a⟩ *v/t* deposit; *confiança* place
depositário [depozi'taɾiu] *m*, **-a** trustee; *fig* confidant(e)
depósito [de'pɔzitu] *m* deposit; (*armazém*) warehouse, depot; *lixo*: dump; *gasolina*: tank; *carro*: pound; **~ a prazo fixo** fixed term deposit; **~ de bagagens** baggage checkroom, *Brit* left-luggage office
depravado [depɾa'vadu] *adj* depraved
depreciação [depɾesja'sãw] *f* depreciation; (*menosprezo*) deprecation
depreciar [depɾe'sjaɾ] ⟨1g⟩ *v/t* devalue; (*menosprezar*) belittle; **depreciar-se** *v/r* depreciate, lose value; (*menosprezar-se*) be self-deprecating
depreciativo [depɾe'sjaɾ] *adj* deregatory
depressa [de'pɾɛsa] *adv* quickly, fast; **vamos ~!** hurry!
depressão [depɾe'sãw] *f* PSICOL, ECON, GEOG depression
depressivo [depɾe'sivu] *adj* depressive
deprimente [depɾi'mẽtʃi] *adj* depres-

sing
deprimido [depri'midu] *adj* depressed
deprimir [depri'mir] ⟨3a⟩ *v/t* depress; **deprimir-se** *v/r* get depressed
depurar [depu'rar] ⟨1a⟩ *v/t água* purify
deputado [depu'tadu] *m*, **-a** *f* deputy; *Am* congressman; congresswoman, *Brit* Member of Parliament
der [dɛr], **dera** ['dɛra], *etc* → ***dar***
deriva [de'riva] *f* NÁUT ***ir à ~*** drift; ***à ~*** adrift
derivação [deriva'sãw] *f* derivation
derivado [deri'vadu] *m* derivative
derivar [deri'var] ⟨1a⟩ **1** *v/t* derive; (*desviar*) divert **2** *v/i* (*ir à deriva*) drift; **derivar-se** *v/r palavra* be derived; (*ir à deriva*) drift; ***~ de*** derive from, be derived from
dermatologia [dermatolo'ʒia] *f* dermatology
dermatologista [dermatolo'ʒista] *m/f* dermatologist
derradeiro [deha'dejru] *adj* last, final
derramamento [dehama'mẽtu] *m* spill; ***~ de sangue*** bloodshed
derramar [deha'mar] ⟨1a⟩ *v/t* spill; *sangue*, *lágrimas* shed; **derramar-se** *v/r* spill; *lágrimas* stream
derrame [de'hami] *m* hemorrhage, *Brit* haemorrhage; ***~ cerebral*** stroke
derrapagem [deha'paʒẽ] *f* skid; *ação* skidding
derrapar [deha'par] ⟨1b⟩ *v/i* skid
derreter [dehe'ter] ⟨2c⟩ *v/t & v/i* melt; **derreter-se** *v/r* melt; ***~ por alguém*** fall for s.o.
derrocada [deho'kada] *f* (*desmoronamento*) collapse; (*queda*) downfall
derrota [de'hɔta] *f* defeat
derrotar [deho'tar] ⟨1e⟩ *v/t* defeat; *time* beat; ***ser derrotado*** be defeated
derrotista [deho'ʧista] *adj* defeatist
derrubar [dehu'bar] ⟨1a⟩ *v/t* knock down; *governo* overthrow; *mesa* knock over; *árvore* chop down; *porta* break down; *avião* shoot down, bring down
dês [des] → ***dar***
desabafar [dezaba'far] ⟨1b⟩ **1** *v/t emoções* give vent to **2** *v/i* unburden oneself
desabafo [deza'bafu] *m* confession; *de sentimentos* outburst
desabamento [dezaba'mẽtu] *m* collapse; ***~ de terra*** landslide
desabar [deza'bar] ⟨1b⟩ *v/i* collapse; *chuva* pour down
desabitado [dezabi'tadu] *adj* uninhabited
desabituado [dezabi'twadu] *adj* ***estar ~ a algo*** no longer be used to sth
desabotoar [dezabo'twar] ⟨1f⟩ *v/t* unbutton
desabrido [deza'bridu] *adj* brusque, rude
desabrigado [dezabri'gadu] *adj* (*sem casa*) homeless; (*exposto*) exposed; ***os ~s*** the homeless
desabrochar [dezabro'ʃar] ⟨1e⟩ **1** *v/i* blossom, bloom **2** *m* blossoming
desacelerar [dezasele'rar] ⟨1c⟩ *v/i & v/t* slow down, decelerate
desacertado [dezarse'tadu] *adj palavras* unfortunate
desacompanhado [dezakõpa'ɲadu] *adj* unaccompanied, alone
desaconselhar [dezakõse'ʎar] ⟨1d⟩ *v/t* advise against; ***~ algo a alguém*** advise s.o. against sth
desaconselhável [dezakõse'ʎavew] *adj* inadvisable
desacordo [deza'kordu] *m* disagreement; (*desarmonia*) discord; ***estar em ~ com*** disagree with
desacostumado [dezakostu'madu] *adj* unaccustomed; ***estar ~ a*** be unaccustomed to
desacostumar [dezakostu'mar] ⟨1a⟩ *v/t* ***~ alguém de algo*** get s.o. out of the habit of sth
desacreditado [dezakredʒi'tadu] *adj* discredited
desacreditar [dezakredʒi'tar] ⟨1a⟩ *v/t* discredit
desact... *Port* → ***desat...***
desafiador [dezafja'dor] *adj* defiant; *emprego*, *projeto* challenging
desafiar [deza'fjar] ⟨1g⟩ *v/t* challenge; (*opor-se*) defy; ***~ alguém a fazer algo*** dare X to do Y
desafinado [dezafi'nadu] *adj* out of tune
desafinar [dezafi'nar] ⟨1a⟩ **1** *v/t* put

out of tune 2 *v/i* MÚS play out of tune; *cantor* sing out of tune
desafio [deza'fiu] *m* challenge; ESP match, game; ***em ~ a*** in defiance of
desafivelar [dezafive'lar] ⟨1c⟩ *v/t* unbuckle
desafogado [dezafo'gadu] *adj* (*livre*) free; (*desimpedido*) clear
desafogo [deza'fogu] *m* (*alívio*) relief; (*folga*) leisure
desaforado [dezafo'radu] *adj* insolent
desaforo [deza'foru] *m* insolence; ***um ~*** a liberty
desafortunado [dezafortu'nadu] *adj* unfortunate, unlucky
desagradar [dezagra'dar] ⟨1b⟩ **1** *v/t* displease **2** *v/i* ***~ a*** displease
desagradável [dezagra'davew] *adj* unpleasant
desagrado [deza'gradu] *m* displeasure; (*aversão*) distaste
desagravo [deza'gravu] *m* amends
desagregação [dezagrega'sãw] *f* ⟨*sem pl*⟩ separation; (*dissolução*) disintegration
desagregar [dezagre'gar] ⟨1o & 1c⟩ *v/t* (*separar*) separate; (*desunir*) break up, split; **desagregar-se** *v/r* break up, split
desaguar [deza'gwar] ⟨1m⟩ **1** *v/t* drain **2** *v/i* ***~ em*** flow into
desajeitado [dezaʒej'tadu] *adj* awkward, clumsy
desajustado [dezaʒus'tadu] *adj pessoa* maladjusted; *peças* out of adjustment
desajuste [deza'ʒustʃi] *m* maladjustment; *mecânico* malfunction
desalentar [dezalẽ'tar] ⟨1a⟩ *v/t* discourage; (*deprimir*) depress
desalento [deza'lẽtu] *m* discouragement
desalinhado [dezali'ɲadu] *adj pessoa* disheveled, *Brit* dishevelled, untidy
desalinho [deza'liɲu] *m* (*desordem*) untidiness; ***ele estava vestido com ~*** he was shabbily dressed
desalmado [dezaw'madu] *adj* inhuman, cruel
desalojar [dezalo'ʒar] ⟨1e⟩ *v/t* dislodge; (*expulsar*) oust; *inquilino* turn out
desamarrar [dezama'har] ⟨1b⟩ **1** *v/t* untie **2** *v/i* NÁUT cast off
desamparado [dezãpa'radu] *adj* abandoned; (*sem apoio*) helpless
desamparar [dezãpa'rar] ⟨1b⟩ *v/t* abandon
desamparo [dezã'paru] *m* helplessness; (*abandono*) abandonment
desanimado [dezani'madu] *adj* discouraged, dispirited; *festa* lifeless
desanimador [dezanima'dor] *adj* disheartening
desanimar [dezani'mar] ⟨1a⟩ **1** *v/t* dishearten **2** *v/i* lose heart, be discouraged; **desanimar-se** *v/r pessoa* lose heart
desânimo [de'zʌnimu] *m* discouragement
desanuviado [dezanu'vjadu] *adj* cloudless
desaparafusar [dezaparafu'zar] ⟨1a⟩ *v/t* unscrew
desaparecer [dezapare'ser] ⟨2g⟩ *v/i* disappear; *tradição, espécie tb* die out
desaparecido [dezapare'sidu] **1** *adj* missing **2** *m/f* missing person
desaparecimento [dezaparesi'mẽtu] *m* disappearance
desapercebido [dezaperse'bidu] *adj* unnoticed
desapertar [dezaper'tar] ⟨1c⟩ *v/t* loosen
desapiedado [dezapie'dadu] *adj* pitiless
desapontado [dezapõ'tadu] *adj* disappointed
desapontador [dezapota'dor] *adj* disappointing
desapontamento [dezapõta'mẽtu] *m* disappointment
desapontar [dezapõ'tar] ⟨1a⟩ *v/t* disappoint
desapossar [dezapo'sar] ⟨1e⟩ *v/t* ***~ alguém de algo*** take sth away from s.o.; **desapossar-se** *v/r* ***~ de algo*** give sth up
desaprender [dezaprẽ'der] ⟨2a⟩ *v/t* & *v/i* forget; ***~ a fazer algo*** forget how to do sth
desaprovação [dezaprova'sãw] *f* disapproval; ***com ~*** disapprovingly

desaprovar [dezapro'var] ⟨1e⟩ *v/t* disapprove of
desarmamento [dezarma'mẽtu] *m* disarmament
desarmar [dezar'mar] ⟨1b⟩ **1** *v/t* disarm *tb fig*; (*desmontar*) dismantle; *bomba* defuse; *barraca* take down; **desarmar-se** *v/r* disarm
desarmonia [dezarmo'nia] *f* discord
desarranjo [deza'hãʒu] *m* disarray; MED **~ *intestinal*** upset stomach
desarrolhar [dezaho'ʎar] ⟨1e⟩ *v/t* uncork
desarrumação [dezahuma'sãw] *f* disarray, disorder
desarrumado [dezahu'madu] *adj* untidy, messy
desarrumar [dezahu'mar] ⟨1a⟩ *v/t* mess up; *mala* unpack
desarvorado [dezarvo'radu] *adj* disoriented
desassociar [dezaso'sjar] ⟨1g⟩ *v/t* disassociate; **desassociar-se** *v/r* **~ *de algo*** disassociate oneself from sth
desassossego [dezasose'segu] *m* disquiet
desastrado [dezas'tradu] *adj* (*desajeitado*) clumsy
desastre [de'zastri] *m* disaster; (*acidente*) accident; *avião*: crash; ***~ de trânsito*** car crash
desastroso [dezas'trozu] *adj* disastrous
desatar [deza'tar] ⟨1b⟩ **1** *v/t nó* undo, untie; *cinto* unfasten **2** *v/i* ***~ a chorar*** burst out crying; ***~ a rir*** burst out laughing
desatarraxar [dezataha'ʃar] ⟨1b⟩ *v/t* unscrew
desatencioso [dezatẽ'sjozu] *adj* inattentive; (*descortês*) impolite
desatento [deza'tẽtu] *adj* inattentive; (*irrefletido*) absent-minded
desativado [dezatʃi'vadu] *adj* deactivated; (*não funcionando*) out of action
desativar [dezatʃi'var] ⟨1a⟩ *v/t* shut down; *bomba* deactivate, defuse
desatualizado [dezatwali'zadu] *adj* out of date; *pessoa* out of touch
desautorizar [dezawtori'zar] ⟨1a⟩ *v/t prática* disallow; (*deacreditar*) discredit
desavença [deza'vẽsa] *f* (*briga*) quarrel; (*discórdia*) disagreement; ***em ~*** at loggerheads
desavergonhado [dezavergo'ɲadu] *adj* shameless; (*insolente*) insolent
desbaratar [dezbara'tar] ⟨1b⟩ *v/t* ruin; *dinheiro* waste, squander; *inimigos* crush; (*pôr em desordem*) mess up
desbastar [dezbas'tar] ⟨1b⟩ *v/t cabelo*, *plantas* thin (out); *vegetação* trim
desbotado [dezbo'tadu] *adj cor* faded
desbotar [dezbo'tar] ⟨1e⟩ **1** *v/t* discolor, *Brit* discolour **2** *v/i* fade
desbravar [dezbra'var] ⟨1b⟩ *v/t terra* make arable; *caminho* clear; *fig* ***ele desbravou seu caminho*** he carved his own path
descabido [deska'bidu] *adj* improper; (*inoportuno*) inappropriate
descafeinado [deskafej'nadu] **1** *adj* decaffeinated **2** *m* decaf
descalçar [deskaw'sar] ⟨1p⟩ *v/t sapatos* take off; **descalçar-se** *v/r* take one's shoes off
descalço [des'kawsu] *adj pé* bare; ***estar ~*** be barefoot
descambar [deskã'bar] ⟨1a⟩ *v/i* ***~ de algo para algo*** denegerate from sth to sth
descampado [deskã'padu] *m* open country
descansado [deskã'sadu] *adj* relaxed; (*vagaroso*) slow; ***esteja ~!*** don't worry!; ***ele pode ficar ~ que …*** he can rest assured that …
descansar [deskã'sar] ⟨1a⟩ **1** *v/t* rest, (*apoiar*) lean **2** *v/i* rest; ***sem ~*** tirelessly
descanso [des'kãsu] *m* rest; *prato*: mat; (*pausa*) break
descaradamente [deskarada'mẽtʃi] *adv* impudently; (*na cara*) blatantly; ***ele mentiu ~*** he told a blatant lie
descarado [deska'radu] *adj* impudent, fresh
descaramento [deskara'mẽtu] *m* impudence
descarga [des'karga] *f* discharge *tb* ELÉT; COM offloading; ***dar a ~*** flush the toilet

descarnado [deskar'nadu] *adj* scrawny
descarregado [deskahe'gadu] *adj pilha* dead
descarregamento [deskahega'mẽtu] *m carga*: offloading; ELÉT discharge
descarregar [deskahe'gar] ⟨1o & 1c⟩ **1** *v/t carga* offload; ELÉT discharge; (*aliviar*) relieve; *fúria etc* vent; *arma* fire **2** *v/i pilha* run out; **~ em cima de alguém** take it out on s.o.
descarrilhamento [deskahiʎa'mẽtu] *m* derailment
descarrilhar [deskahi'ʎar] ⟨1a⟩ **1** *v/t* derail **2** *v/i* be derailed; *fig* go off the rails
descartar [deskar'tar] ⟨1a⟩ *v/t* discard; *possibilidade* exclude; (*eliminar*) eliminate
descartável [deskar'tavew] *adj* disposable
descascar [deskas'kar] ⟨1n & 1b⟩ **1** *v/t fruta etc* peel; *ervilhas* shell **2** *v/i pele* peel; **descascar-se** *v/r pele, tinta* peel
descaso [des'kazu] *m* neglect
descendência [desẽ'dẽsja] *f* descent, ancestry; **de ~ portuguesa** of Portuguese descent
descendente [desẽ'dẽtʃi] **1** *adj* (*oposto a ascendente*) going down; *ordem* descending **2** *m* descendant
descender [desẽ'der] ⟨2a⟩ *v/i* **~ de** be descended from
descentralização [desẽtraliza'sãw] *f* decentralization
descentralizar [desẽtrali'zar] ⟨1a⟩ *v/t* decentralize
descer [de'ser] ⟨2g⟩ **1** *v/t escada* go down; *bagagem* take down; *página* scroll down; *preço* bring down **2** *v/i* (*saltar*) get off; (*baixar*) go down; *preço, temperatura* drop, go down; *avião* descend; *do carro* get out; *do cavalo* dismount; *da montanha* climb down; *da escada* get down; **~ a pique** *avião* dive; *pássaro* swoop
descida [de'sida] *f* descent; (*declive*) slope; *preço, temperatura*: fall, drop
desclassificação [desklasifika'sãw] *f* disqualification
desclassificar [desklasifi'kar] ⟨1n⟩ *v/t* ESP disqualify; (*desacreditar*) discredit
descoberta [desko'bɛrta] *f* discovery; *crime, criminoso*: detection
descoberto [desko'bɛrtu] *adj* uncovered; (*nu*) naked, bare; (*desprotegido*) exposed; *piscina etc* open-air; *conta* overdrawn; **a ~** overdrawn
descobridor [deskobri'dor] *m* discoverer
descobrimento [deskobri'mẽtu] *m* discovery
descobrir [desko'brir] ⟨3f⟩ *v/t* discover; (*expor*) uncover; *panela* take the lid off; *enigma* solve
descolagem [desko'laʒẽ] *f Port* AERO take-off
descolar [desko'lar] ⟨1e⟩ **1** *v/i Port* AERO take off **2** *v/t* unstick
descoloração [deskolora'sãw] *f* ⟨*sem pl*⟩ discoloration, *Brit* discolouration
descolorir [deskolo'rir] ⟨3f⟩ **1** *v/t* discolor, *Brit* discolour; *cabelo* bleach **2** *v/i* fade
descomprimir [deskõpri'mir] ⟨3a⟩ *v/t* INFORM unzip, decompress
descomunal [deskomu'naw] *adj* (*não comum*) extraordinary; (*enorme*) huge, enormous
desconcertado [deskõser'tadu] *adj* disconcerted
desconcertante [deskõser'tãtʃi] *adj* disconcerting
desconcertar [deskõser'tar] ⟨1c⟩ *v/t* disconcert; (*atrapalhar*) puzzle; **desconcertar-se** *v/r* get upset; (*atrapalhar-se*) be thrown
desconectado [deskonek'tadu] *adv* INFORM off line
desconexo [desko'nɛksu] *adj pessoa* incoherent; *estória, filme* disjointed; *fato* unrelated
desconfiado [deskõ'fjadu] *adj* suspicious; (*que duvida*) distrustful
desconfiança [deskõ'fjãsa] *f* distrust; (*suspeita*) suspicion
desconfiar [deskõ'fjar] ⟨1g⟩ *v/i* **~ de alguém** distrust s.o., be suspicious of s.o.; **~ que** have the feeling that
desconfortável [deskõfor'tavew] *adj* uncomfortable
desconforto [deskõ'fortu] *m* discom-

fort
descongelar [deskõʒe'laɾ] ⟨1c⟩ *v/t* defrost; AERO de-ice; FIN unfreeze; **descongelar-se** *v/r freezer* defrost
descongestionar [deskõʒestʃio'naɾ] ⟨1f⟩ *v/t trânsito, cabeça* clear; MED, *estrada* decongest
desconhecer [deskuɲe'seɾ] ⟨2g⟩ *v/t* not to recognize; (*não saber*) not to know; *método etc* be unfamiliar with
desconhecido [deskuɲe'sidu] **1** *adj* unknown; *método etc* unfamiliar **2** *m/f* stranger
desconhecimento [deskuɲesi'mẽtu] *m* ignorance
desconsideração [deskõsidʒiɾa'sãw] *f* disregard (***de*** for)
desconsolado [deskõso'ladu] *adj* disconsolate
descontar [deskõ'taɾ] ⟨1a⟩ *v/t* discount; (*abater*) deduct; ***~ algo em alguém*** take sth out on s.o.
descontentamento [deskõtẽta'mẽtu] *m* discontent; (*desprazer*) displeasure
descontentar [deskõtẽ'taɾ] ⟨1a⟩ *v/t* displease
descontente [deskõ'tẽtʃi] *adj* dissatisfied; (*aborrecido*) discontented; ***estar ~ com o serviço*** be unhappy with the service
descontínuo [deskõ'tʃinwu] *adj conversa, telefonema etc* disjointed; (*quebrado*) broken
desconto [des'kõtu] *m preço:* discount; (*dedução*) deduction; ESP ***tempo de ~*** injury time; ***~ por quantidade*** volume discount; ***~ à vista*** cash discount
descontraído [deskõtɾa'idu] *adj* casual, laid-back
descontrair [deskõtɾa'iɾ] ⟨1i⟩ *v/t* relax; **descontrair-se** *v/r* relax
descontrolado [deskõtɾo'ladu] *adj* out of control; *adolescente, festa* wild
descontrole [deskõ'tɾoli] *m* lack of control
descortesia [deskoɾte'zia] *f* impoliteness
descoser [desko'zeɾ] ⟨2d⟩ *v/t* unstitch; *roupa* tear apart; **descoser-se** *v/r* ***o vestido se descoseu do lado*** the side of the dress came unstitched
descrédito [des'kɾɛdʒitu] *m* discredit
descrença [des'kɾẽsa] *f* disbelief
descrente [des'kɾẽtʃi] *adj* skeptical, *Brit* sceptical, disbelieving
descrer [des'kɾeɾ] ⟨2k⟩ *v/t* disbelieve; ***~ de*** not to believe in
descrever [deskɾe'veɾ] ⟨2c; *pp* descrito⟩ *v/t* describe
descrição [deskɾi'sãw] *f* description
descritivo, *Port* **descriptivo** [deskɾi'tʃivu] *adj* descriptive
descuidadamente [deskuidada'mẽtʃi] *adv* carelessly
descuidado [deskui'dadu] *adj* careless; *aparência* unkempt
descuidar [deskui'daɾ] ⟨1a⟩ **1** *v/t* neglect **2** *v/i* ***~ de*** neglect
descuido [des'kuidu] *m* neglect; *em trabalho, dever* carelessness; ***um ~*** an oversight; ***por ~*** inadvertently, accidentally
desculpa [des'kuwpa] *f* excuse; (*perdão*) pardon; ***pedir ~s a alguém*** apologize to s.o.
desculpar [deskuw'paɾ] ⟨1a⟩ *v/t* excuse; (*perdoar*) forgive, pardon; ***desculpe*** I'm sorry; *pedindo licença* excuse me; **desculpar-se** *v/r* apologize; ***~ por algo*** apologize for sth
desde ['dezdʒi] **1** *prep* ◊ *lugar* from; ***~ … até …*** from … to …; ***dirigimos ~ Recife até Olinda*** we drove from Recife to Olinda
◊ *tempo* since; ***~ então*** since then, from then on, ***~ já*** from now on; *logo* right away; ***o conheço ~ 1975*** I've known him since 1975 **2** *conj* ***~ que*** since; ***~ que você se foi*** since you left; ***~ que você volte na hora*** as long as you come back on time
desdém [dez'dẽ] *m* disdain; ***com ~*** disdainfully
desdenhar [dezde'ɲaɾ] ⟨1d⟩ *v/t* disdain, look down on
desdenhoso [dezde'ɲozu] *adj* disdainful
desdentado [dezdẽ'tadu] *adj* toothless
desdita [dez'dʒita] *f* misfortune
desdizer [dezdʒi'zeɾ] ⟨2t⟩ **1** *v/t* take

back, withdraw **2** *v/i* ***você vai ~?*** will you take back what you said?

desdobramento [dezdobra'mẽtu] *m* implication, ramification; *obra etc*: spin-off

D

desdobrar [dezdo'brar] ⟨1e⟩ *v/t* unfold; *dados, contas* break down; *empenhos* increase; *bandeira* unfurl; **desdobrar-se** *v/r* unfold; (*esforçar-se*) go to a lot of trouble, bend over backwards

desejar [deze'ʒar] ⟨1d⟩ *v/t* want, desire; ~ ***ardentemente*** long for; ***deixar tudo a ~*** leave a lot to be desired; ***~ tudo de bom a alguém*** wish s.o. well

desejável [deze'ʒavew] *adj* desirable; ***não ~*** undesirable

desejo [de'zeʒu] *m* wish; *forte* desire; ***~ forte*** craving

desejoso [deze'ʒosu] *adj* ***estar ~ de*** *ou* ***por*** wish for; ***~ de fazer algo*** eager to do sth

deselegante [dezele'gãtʃi] *adj* inelegant

desembalar [dezẽba'lar] ⟨1b⟩ *v/t* unwrap, unpack

desembaraçado [dezẽbara'sadu] *adj* confident, undaunted; (*desinibido*) uninhibited; *cabelo* untangled

desembaraçar [dezẽbara'sar] ⟨1p & 1b⟩ *v/t* (*livrar*) free; *cabelo* untangle; **desembaraçar-se** *v/r* lose one's inhibitions; (*tomar a iniciativa*) show initiative; ***~ de*** get rid of

desembaraço [dezẽba'rasu] *m* (*facilidade*) ease; (*segurança*) confidence

desembarcar [dezẽbar'kar] ⟨1n & 1b⟩ **1** *v/t pessoas* let off; *mercadoria* unload **2** *v/i* disembark

desembargador [dezẽbarga'dor] *m*, **-a** *f* supreme court judge

desembarque [dezẽ'barki] *m* COM *mercadoria*: unloading; AERO disembarkation; *seção no aeroporto* arrivals *sg*

desembocadura [dezẽboka'dura] *f rio*: mouth

desembocar [dezẽbo'kar] ⟨1n & 1e⟩ *v/i* ***~ em*** flow into; *rua* lead into

desembolsar [dezẽbow'sar] ⟨1a⟩ **1** *v/t dinheiro* spend **2** *v/i* ***sou o único que desembolsa*** I am the only one that ever coughs up

desembolso [dezẽ'bowsu] *m* expenditure

desembrulhar [dezẽbru'ʎar] ⟨1a⟩ *v/t* unwrap

desempacotar [dezẽpako'tar] ⟨1e⟩ *v/t* unpack

desempatar [dezẽpa'tar] ⟨1a⟩ **1** *v/t jogo* decide **2** *v/i* break the tie, decide the match

desempate [dezẽ'patʃi] *m* ESP ***jogo*** *m* ***de ~*** decider, play-off

desempenar [dezẽpe'nar] ⟨1d⟩ **1** *v/t* (*endireitar*) straighten; **desempenar-se** *v/r* stand up straight

desempenhar [dezẽpe'ɲar] ⟨1d⟩ *dever* carry out, fulfill, *Brit* fulfil; *papel* play; TEAT perform

desempenho [dezẽ'peɲu] *m* performance; *obrigações*: fulfillment, *Brit* fulfilment

desemperrar [dezẽpe'har] ⟨1c⟩ *v/i* & *v/t* loosen

desempregado [dezẽpre'gadu] *adj* unemployed

desemprego [dezẽ'pregu] *m* unemployment; ***~ em massa*** mass unemployment

desencadear [dezẽka'dʒiar] ⟨1l⟩ *v/t* set off, trigger; **desencadear-se** break loose; *tempestade* break

desencaixar [dezẽkaj'ʃar] ⟨1a⟩ *v/t* dislodge; **desencaixar-se** *v/r* become dislodged

desencaminhar [dezẽkami'ɲar] ⟨1a⟩ *v/t* lead astray; *fundos* embezzle

desencantado [dezẽkã'tadu] *adj* disenchanted

desencantar [dezẽkã'tar] ⟨1a⟩ *v/t* disenchant

desencontrar-se [dezẽkõ'trarsi] *v/r* fail to meet, miss each other

desencontro [dezẽ'kõtru] *m* ***houve um ~ entre os dois*** the two of them failed to meet

desencorajamento [dezẽkoraʒa'mẽtu] *m* discouragement

desencorajar [dezẽkora'ʒar] ⟨1b⟩ *v/t* discourage

desenferrujar [dezẽfehu'ʒar] ⟨1a⟩ *v/t* remove the rust from; *pernas* stretch;

língua brush up
desenfreado [dezẽfɾi'adu] *adj* unbridled
desenganar [dezẽga'naɾ] ⟨1a⟩ *v/t* disabuse; *doente* declare incurable; **~ alguém de algo** disabuse s.o. of sth; **desenganar-se** *v/r* (*sair de erro*) realize the truth, lose one's illusions
desenganchar [dezẽgã'ʃaɾ] ⟨1a⟩ *v/t* unhook; (*soltar*) loosen
desengatado [dezẽga'tadu] *adj motor* idling
desengatar [dezẽga'taɾ] ⟨1b⟩ *v/t* unhitch; AUTO declutch
desenhar [deze'ɲaɾ] ⟨1d⟩ *v/t* draw; TECN design
desenhista [deze'ɲista] *m/f* designer; *artista* artist, *desenho animado*: cartoonist; **~ técnico** draftsman, *Brit* draughtsman
desenho [de'zeɲu] *m* drawing; TECN design; (*esboço*) sketch; **~ animado** cartoon
desenlaçar [dezẽla'saɾ] ⟨1b⟩ *v/i estória* unfold
desenlace [dezẽ'lasi] *m* outcome
desenredar [dezẽhe'daɾ] ⟨1c⟩ *v/t* unravel
desenrolar [dezẽho'laɾ] ⟨1e⟩ *v/t* unroll; *fita* unwind; (*desenvolver*) develop; **desenrolar-se** *v/r* unfold; *fita* unwind
desentender [dezẽtẽ'deɾ] ⟨2a⟩ *v/t* misunderstand; **fazer-se desentendido** pretend not to understand; **desentender-se** *v/r* **~ com** have a disagreement with
desentendimento [dezẽtẽdʒi'mẽtu] *m* misunderstanding
desenterrar [dezẽte'haɾ] ⟨1c⟩ *v/t* unearth; (*procurar*) dig out
desentupir [dezẽtu'piɾ] ⟨3a & 3h⟩ *v/t cano*, *tubo* unblock
desenvolver [dezẽvow'veɾ] ⟨2e⟩ *v/t* develop; **desenvolver-se** *v/r* develop
desenvolvimento [dezẽvowvi'mẽtu] *m* development; **país** *m* **em ~** developing country
desequilibrado [dezikili'bradu] *adj* unbalanced
desequilibrar-se [dezikili'brarsi] ⟨1a⟩ *v/r* lose one's balance
desequilíbrio [deziki'libriu] *m* imbalance
deserção [dezeɾ'sãw] *f* MIL desertion
deserdar [dezeɾ'daɾ] ⟨1c⟩ *v/t* disinherit
desertar [dezeɾ'taɾ] ⟨1c⟩ *v/t & v/i* desert
desertificação [dezeɾtʃifika'sãw] *f* ⟨*sem pl*⟩ GEOG desertification
deserto [de'zɛrtu] **1** *adj* deserted; **ilha deserta** desert island **2** *m* desert
desertor [dezeɾ'toɾ] *m*, **-a** *f* MIL deserter
desesperado [dezespe'ɾadu] *adj* desperate; (*furioso*) furious
desesperar [dezespe'ɾaɾ] ⟨1c⟩ *v/t* drive to despair; (*enfurecer*) infuriate; **desesperar-se** *v/r* despair; (*enfurecer-se*) get infuriated
desespero [dezes'peɾu] *m* despair; (*raiva*) fury; **levar ao ~** drive to despair; **ele me deixa em ~** I despair of him
desestabilização [dezestabiliza'sãw] *f* ⟨*sem pl*⟩ destabilization
desestabilizador [dezestabiliza'doɾ] *adj* destabilizing
desestabilizar [dezestabili'zaɾ] ⟨1a⟩ *v/t* destabilize
desfalecer [desfale'seɾ] ⟨2g⟩ *v/i* faint; (*enfraquecer*) weaken
desfalecimento [desfalesi'mẽtu] *m* (*enfraquecimento*) weakening; (*desmaio*) faint
desfalque [des'fawki] *m dinheiro*: embezzlement
desfavorável [desfavo'ɾavew] *adj* unfavorable, *Brit* unfavourable
desfavorecer [desfavore'seɾ] ⟨2g⟩ *v/t* disfavor, *Brit* disfavour
desfazer [desfa'zeɾ] ⟨2v⟩ *v/t costura* undo; *dúvidas* remove; *mala* unpack; *cama* strip; *contrato* break; *mistério* clear up; *grupo* break up; **desfazer-se** *v/r* come undone; *casamento* break up; **~ em lágrimas** burst into tears; **~ de** get rid of
desfecho [des'feʃu] *m* ending, outcome
desfeita [des'fejta] *f* affront

D

desfeito [des'fejta] *adj contrato, promessa* broken; *quebra-cabeça* undone; *cama* unmade
desfiar [des'fjar] ⟨1g⟩ *v/t tecido* unravel; **desfiar-se** *v/r tecido* fray
D
desfigurar [desfigu'rar] ⟨1a⟩ *v/t* disfigure; (*deformar*) distort; (*degradar*) deface; *prosa* mutilate
desfiladeiro [desfila'dejru] *m* (*canhão*) canyon; *em montanha* pass
desfilar [desfi'lar] ⟨1a⟩ *v/i* parade; *modelo* model
desfile [des'fili] *m* procession, parade; *~ de carros* motorcade; *~ militar* military parade; *~ de modas* fashion show
desflorestamento [desfloresta'mẽtu] *m* deforestation
desflorestar [desflores'tar] ⟨1c⟩ *v/t* deforest
desforra [des'foha] *f* revenge; (*reparação*) redress; *tirar ~* take one's revenge
desfrutar [desfru'tar] ⟨1a⟩ **1** *v/t* enjoy **2** *v/i ~ de* enjoy; *desfrute!* enjoy it!, make the most of it!
desfrute [des'frutʃi] *m* (*prazer*) enjoyment
desgastado [dezgas'tadu] *adj ~ pelo clima* weather-beaten
desgastar [dezgas'tar] ⟨1b⟩ *v/t pessoa* exhaust, wear out; *objeto* wear away, erode; **desgastar-se** *v/r* be worn away; *pessoa* be worn out
desgaste [dez'gastʃi] *m equipamento etc*: wear and tear; *pessoa*: stress
desgostar [dezgos'tar] ⟨1e⟩ **1** *v/t* displease; (*afligir*) upset **2** *v/i ~ de* dislike; **desgostar-se** *v/r ~ de* go off; *~ com* be offended by
desgosto [dez'gostu] *m* displeasure; (*aflição*) unhappiness
desgostoso [dezgos'tozu] *adj* sad, upset; (*irritado*) annoyed; *ficar ~ com algo* get upset about sth
desgraça [dez'grasa] *f* disgrace; (*infortúnio*) misfortune; (*miséria*) misery; *é uma ~* it's a disgrace
desgraçado [dezgra'sadu] **1** *adj* (*infeliz*) wretched; *está fazendo um calor ~* it's damned hot **2** *m*, **-a** *f* wretch
desgraçar [dezgra'sar] ⟨1b⟩ *v/t* disgrace
desgrenhado [dezgre'ɲadu] *adj* unkempt; *cabelo* tousled
desgrudar [dezgru'dar] ⟨1a⟩ **1** *v/t* unstick; *~ uma coisa da outra* take one thing off another **2** *v/i ~ de* tear oneself away from
desidratação [dezidrata'sãw] *f* ⟨*sem pl*⟩ dehydration
desidratado [dezidra'tadu] *adj* dehydrated
desidratar [dezidra'tar] ⟨1b⟩ *v/t* dehydrate
design [de'zajn] *m* design
designação [dezigna'sãw] *f* designation; *a uma posição* appointment
designar [dezi'gnar] ⟨1a⟩ *v/t* designate; (*nomear*) appoint; *encontro* fix
desígnio [de'zigniu] *m* (*intenção*) intention; (*objetivo*) purpose
desigual [dezi'gwaw] *adj* unequal; *paisagem* uneven; *briga* one-sided; *qualidade* patchy; *tamanho* irregular
desigualdade [dezigwaw'dadʒi] *f* inequality
desiludido [dezilu'dʒidu] *adj* disillusioned; (*decepcionado*) disappointed
desiludir [dezilu'dʒir] ⟨3a⟩ *v/t* disillusion; (*decepcionar*) disappoint
desilusão [dezilu'zãw] *f* disillusionment
desimpedido [dezĩpe'dʒidu] *adj* unimpeded; *pessoa* unattached
desimpedir [dezĩpe'dʒir] ⟨3r⟩ *v/t* unblock; *congestionamento* ease
desinchar [dezĩ'ʃar] ⟨1a⟩ **1** *v/t* MED ease the swelling on **2** *v/i minha perna desinchou* the swelling in my leg went down
desinfetante, *Port* **desinfectante** [dezĩfe'tãtʃi] *m* disinfectant
desinfetar, *Port* **desinfectar** [dezĩfe'tar] ⟨1a⟩ *v/t* disinfect
desinflamar [dezĩfla'mar] ⟨1a⟩ *v/t* eliminate the infection in; **desinflamar-se** *v/r* become less inflamed
desininbido [dezini'bidu] *adj* uninhibited
desininbir [dezini'bir] ⟨3a⟩ *v/t* make less inhibited; **desininbir-se** *v/r* let go of one's inhibitions

desintegração [dezĩtegra'sãw] *f* ⟨*sem pl*⟩ disintegration
desintegrar [dezĩte'grar] ⟨1c⟩ *v/t* break up, separate; **desintegrar-se** *v/r* disintegrate
desinteressado [dezĩtere'sadu] *adj* disinterested; *atitude* off-hand
desinteressante [dezĩtere'sãʧi] *adj* uninteresting
desinteressar-se [dezĩtere'sarsi] ⟨1c⟩ *v/r* lose interest
desinteresse [dezĩte'resi] *m* disinterest
desintoxicação [dezĩtoksika'sãw] *f* drug withdrawal; (*limpeza*) detoxification
desintoxicar [dezĩtoksi'kar] ⟨1a & 1n⟩ *v/t* detoxify; **desintoxicar-se** *v/r da bebida* dry out
desistência [dezis'tẽsja] *f* giving up; *idéia*: abandonment
desistir [dezis'ʧir] ⟨3a⟩ *v/i* give up; *da escola* drop out; **~ de algo** give sth up
deslavado [dezla'vadu] *adj roupa* worn out; (*insípido*) boring; *fig* shameless; *mentira* blatant
desleal [dez'leaw] *adj* disloyal
deslealdade [dezleaw'dadʒi] *f* disloyalty
desleixado [dezlej'ʃadu] *adj* sloppy; *no vestir* scruffy
desleixo [dez'lejʃu] *m* sloppiness; *no vestir* scruffiness
desligado [dezli'gadu] *adj* disconnected; *eletricidade* off *pred*, switched off; *pessoa* vague, absent-minded
desligar [dezli'gar] ⟨1o⟩ *v/t luz, TV etc* turn off; *computador* shut down, turn off; *telefone* hang up; (*desconetar*) disconnect; *na tomada* unplug; **desligar-se** *v/r* **~ de** *família, tradição* break away from; *problema etc* turn one's back on
deslizar [dezli'zar] ⟨1a⟩ *v/i* slide; (*escorregar*) slip *tb fig*
deslize [dez'lizi] *m* (*escorregadela*) slip; *fig* slip-up
deslocamento [dezloka'mẽtu] *m* dislocation; (*movimentação*) moving; *de oficial* transfer
deslocado [dezlo'kadu] *adj* dislocated; *fig* out of place
deslocar [dezlo'kar] ⟨1n & 1e⟩ *v/t* move; *ombro etc* dislocate; *funcionário, tropas* transfer; **deslocar-se** *v/r* be dislocated; (*mover-se*) move; ***ele se dislocou até lá*** he went all the way there
deslumbrante [dezlũ'brãʧi] *adj* dazzling; (*impressionante*) striking; *lugar, festa* amazing
deslumbrar [dezlũ'brar] ⟨1a⟩ **1** *v/t* (*cegar*) dazzle, blind; (*maravilhar*) amaze; (*chamar*) engage **2** *v/i* be dazzling
desmaiar [dezma'jar] ⟨1b⟩ *v/i* faint
desmaio [dez'maiu] *m* faint; ***ter um ~*** faint
desmancha-prazeres [dezmãʃapra'zeris] *m/f* ⟨*pl inv*⟩ spoilsport, kill-joy
desmanchar [dezmã'ʃar] ⟨1a⟩ *v/t acordo* break; *costura* undo; *penteado* mess up; *sonhos* shatter; *tricô* unravel; *noivado* break off
desmantelar [dezmãte'lar] ⟨1c⟩ *v/t* (*desmontar*) dismantle, take to pieces; *edifício* demolish
desmarcar [dezmar'kar] ⟨1n & 1b⟩ *v/t encontro* cancel
desmascaramento [dezmaskara'mẽtu] *m pessoa desonesta*: exposure
desmascarar [dezmaska'rar] ⟨1n & 1b⟩ *v/t* unmask; *fig* expose
desmatamento [dezmata'mẽtu] *m* deforestation
desmatar [dezma'tar] ⟨1b⟩ *v/t* clear (of forest)
desmazelado [dezmaze'ladu] *adj* messy; (*negligente*) slovenly
desmedido [dezme'dʒidu] *adj* excessive
desmentido [dezmẽ'ʧidu] *m* denial; (*contradição*) contradiction
desmentir [dezmẽ'ʧir] ⟨3e⟩ *v/t* **~ algo** (*negar*) deny sth; (*contradizer*) **~ alguém** contradict s.o.
desmesurado [dezmezu'radu] *adj* huge, enormous
desmiolado [dezmio'ladu] *adj* (*esquecido*) forgetful, empty-headed
desmobiliado [dezmobi'ladu] *adj* unfurnished
desmontar [dezmõ'tar] ⟨1a⟩ **1** *v/t*

máquina dismantle, take to pieces; *andaime* take down **2** *v/i do cavalo* dismount
desmoralizado [dezmoɾali'zadu] *adj* demoralized
desmoralizante [dezmoɾali'zãʧi] *adj* demoralizing
desmoralizar [dezmoɾali'zaɾ] ⟨1a⟩ *v/t* demoralize
desmoronamento [dezmoɾona'mẽtu] *m terras*: landslide; (*queda*) collapse
desmoronar [dezmoro'naɾ] ⟨1f⟩ **1** *v/t edifício* knock down **2** *v/i* collapse; **desmoronar-se** *v/r* collapse
desnatar [dezna'taɾ] ⟨1b⟩ *v/t leite* skim; ***leite** m **desnatado*** skimmed milk
desnaturado [deznatu'ɾadu] **1** *adj* heartless **2** *m/f* monster
desnecessário [deznese'saɾiu] *adj* unnecessary; *comentário* uncalled-for
desnível [dez'nivew] *m* unevenness; *fig* difference
desnorteado [deznoɾ'ʧiadu] *adj* disoriented, *Brit* disorientated
desnudar [deznu'daɾ] ⟨1a⟩ *v/t* strip; (*expor*) expose; **desnudar-se** *v/r* undress, strip
desnutrição [deznutɾi'sãw] *f* ⟨*sem pl*⟩ malnutrition
desnutrido [deznu'tɾidu] *adj* malnourished
desobedecer [dezobedʒi'seɾ] ⟨2g⟩ **1** *v/t* **~ *a*** disobey **2** *v/i* disobey
desobediência [dezobe'djẽsja] *f* disobedience
desobediente [dezobe'djẽʧi] *adj* disobedient
desobrigar [dezobri'gaɾ] ⟨1o⟩ *v/t* **~** (***de***) release from; **~ *de fazer algo*** release from doing sth
desobstruir [dezobistɾu'iɾ] ⟨3k⟩ *v/t* unblock
desocupação [dezokupa'sãw] *f casa*: vacating; (*lazer*) leisure; (*desemprego*) unemployment
desocupado [dezoku'padu] *adj casa* unoccupied; (*desempregado*) unemployed; (*livre*) free
desocupar [dezoku'paɾ] ⟨1a⟩ *v/t casa* vacate; (*soltar*) free
desodorante [dezodo'ɾãʧi] *m Bras* deodorant
desodorizante [dezodoɾi'zãʧi] *m Port* deodorant
desolação [dezola'sãw] *f* desolation; (*pesar*) grief
desolado [dezo'ladu] *adj* desolate; *pessoa* inconsolable
desolar [dezo'laɾ] ⟨1e⟩ *v/t pessoa* distress; *lugar* devastate
desonestidade [dezonesʧi'dadʒi] *f* dishonesty
desonesto [dezo'nɛstu] *adj* dishonest
desonra [de'zõha] *f* dishonor, *Brit* dishonour; ***trazer* ~ *a*** bring dishonor on
desonrar [dezõ'haɾ] ⟨1a⟩ *v/t* dishonor, *Brit* dishonour, disgrace; **desonrar-se** *v/r* disgrace oneself
desonroso [dezõ'hozu] *adj* dishonorable, *Brit* dishonourable
desopilar [dezopi'laɾ] ⟨1a⟩ **1** *v/t* MED unblock; *mente* clear **2** *v/i fam* get going
desordeiro [dezoɾ'dejɾu] **1** *adj* troublemaking *atr* **2** *m/f* troublemaker
desordem [de'zɔɾdẽ] *f* disorder; (*confusão*) confusion; ***em* ~** *casa, quarto* untidy
desordenado [dezoɾdʒi'nadu] *adj* disorganized; *vida* disordered
desordenar [dezoɾdʒi'naɾ] ⟨1a⟩ *v/t* disorganize; (*desarrumar*) mess up
desorganização [dezoɾganiza'sãw] *f* ⟨*sem pl*⟩ disorganization
desorganizado [dezoɾgani'zadu] *adj* disorganized
desorganizar [dezoɾgani'zaɾ] ⟨1a⟩ *v/t* disorganize; (*separar*) break up
desorientação [dezoɾjẽta'sãw] *f* ⟨*sem pl*⟩ disorientation; (*confusão*) confusion; (*perplexidade*) bewilderment
desorientado [dezoɾjẽ'tadu] *adj* disoriented, *Brit* disorientated; (*perplexo*) bewildered; (*confuso*) confused
desorientar [dezoɾjẽ'taɾ] ⟨1a⟩ *v/t* throw off course; (*confundir*) confuse; **desorientar-se** *v/r* lose one's way; (*confundir-se*) get confused
desossar [dezo'saɾ] ⟨1e⟩ *v/t galinha* bone

despachado [despa'ʃadu] *adj* efficient
despachante [despa'ʃãtʃi] *m/f* COM shipping agent; *de documentos* agent
despachar [despa'ʃar] ⟨1b⟩ **1** *v/t* (*mandar*) dispatch, send off; (*tratar*) deal with; (*despedir*) fire **2** *v/i empregado* work
despacho [des'paʃu] *m* dispatch; *comércio*, *negócios*: handling; (*reunião*) meeting; (*decisão*) ruling; **~ alfandegário** customs clearance
desparafusar [desparafu'zar] ⟨1a⟩ *v/t* unscrew
despedaçar [despeda'sar] ⟨1p & 1b⟩ *v/t* smash; (*rasgar*) tear to pieces; **despedaçar-se** *v/r* smash, shatter
despedida [despe'dʒida] *f* farewell; (*demissão*) dismissal; **~ de solteiro** bachelor party, *Brit* stag party
despedir [despe'dʒir] ⟨3r⟩ *v/t emprego* dismiss; **despedir-se** *v/r* **~ de alguém** say goodbye to s.o., see s.o. off
despeito [des'pejtu] *m* spite; **a ~ de** in spite of, despite
despejar [despe'ʒar] ⟨1d⟩ *v/t* (*esvaziar*) empty; *líquido* pour; *inquilino* evict
despejo [des'peʒu] *m inquilino*: eviction; **ordem** *f* **de ~** eviction order
despenhadeiro [despeɲa'dejru] *m* cliff, precipice
despensa [des'pẽsa] *f* larder
despenteado [despẽ'tʃiadu] *adj cabelo* tousled, unkempt
despentear [despẽ'tʃiar] ⟨1l⟩ *v/t cabelo* let down; *de outra pessoa* ruffle
despercebido [desperse'bidu] *adj* unnoticed; **passar ~** pass unnoticed
desperdiçar [desperdʒi'sar] ⟨1p⟩ *v/t dinheiro* squander; *tempo* waste
desperdício [desper'disiu] *m* waste
despertador [desperta'dor] *m relógio* alarm clock
despertar [desper'tar] ⟨1c⟩ **1** *v/t* wake; *recordação* revive; *sentimento* arouse; *apetite* whet **2** *v/i* wake up; **despertar-se** *v/r* **~ para algo** wake up to sth
desperto [des'pɛrtu] *adj* awake
despesa [des'peza] *f* expense; **~s** *pl* expenses; **~s** *pl* **de viagem** travel expenses; COM **~s gerais** overhead, *Brit* overheads; **reduzir ~s** cut costs
despido [des'pidu] *adj* bare, stripped; (*livre*) free; **~ de** stripped of
despir [des'pir] ⟨3c⟩ *v/t pessoa* undress; *roupa* strip off; (*despojar*) strip; **despir-se** *v/r* undress
despistar [despis'tar] ⟨1a⟩ *v/t* throw off the track; **~ alguém** give s.o. the slip
despojar [despo'ʒar] ⟨1e⟩ *v/t* strip (**de** of); *pessoas* rob
despojo [des'poʒu] *m* spoils, loot; **~s mortais** mortal remains
despontar [despõ'tar] **1** ⟨1a⟩ *v/i* emerge; *sol* rise; *estrelas etc* come out **2** *m* **ao ~ do dia** at daybreak
desportista [despor'tʃista] *m/f Port* sportsman; sportswoman
desportivo [despor'tʃivu] *adj Port* sporting *atr*; **carro ~** sports car
desporto [des'portu] *m Port* sport
déspota ['dɛsputa] *m/f* despot
despótico [des'pɔtʃiku] *adj* despotic
despovoado [despo'vwadu] **1** *m* wilderness **2** *adj* uninhabited
despovoar [despo'vwar] ⟨1f⟩ *v/t* depopulate
despovoamento [despovwa'mẽtu] *m* depopulation
despregar [despre'gar] ⟨1o & 1c⟩ *v/t* remove, detach; **despregar-se** *v/r* come off
desprender [des'prẽder] ⟨2a⟩ *v/t* detach; *da parede* take down; **desprender-se** *v/r alça etc* come off; *pessoa* distance oneself
despreocupado [despreoku'padu] *adj* carefree; *sem preocupação* unconcerned
despreparado [desprepa'radu] *adj* unprepared
despretensioso [despretẽ'sjozu] *adj pessoa*, *estilo*, *hotel* unpretentious
desprevenido [despreve'nidu] *adj* (*não preparado*) unprepared; **pegar alguém ~** catch s.o. unawares
desprezar [despre'zar] ⟨1c⟩ *v/t* despise; (*ignorar*) ignore, disregard; *idéia*, *sugestão* scorn
desprezível [despre'zivew] *adj* despicable; (*vergonhoso*) shameful

desprezo [des'prezu] *m* contempt, scorn; ***com ~*** scornfully
desprivilegiado [desprivili'ʒjadu] *adj* underprivileged
despromover [despromo'ver] ⟨2d⟩ demote
D
desproporção [despropor'sãw] *f* disproportion
desproporcionado [desproporsjo'nadu] *adj* disproportionate; (*irregular*) unequal
despropositado [despropozi'tadu] *adj* preposterous, absurd
desprotegido [desprote'ʒidu] *adj* defenseless, *Brit* defenceless; (*desabrigado*) unprotected
desprovido [despro'vidu] *adj* deprived; ***~ de*** lacking
desqualificação [deskwalifika'sãw] *f* disqualification
desqualificado [deskwalifi'kadu] *adj* disqualified
desqualificar [deskwalifi'kar] ⟨1n⟩ *v/t* disqualify
desregrado [deshe'gradu] *adj* unruly; (*desorganizado*) disorderly; (*exagerado*) immoderate
desregulamentar [deshegulamẽ'tar] ⟨1a⟩ *v/t* deregulate
desrespeitar [deshespej'tar] ⟨1a⟩ *v/t* disrespect; *regras* ignore, flout
desrespeito [deshes'pejtu] *m* disrespect
desrespeitoso [deshespej'tozu] *adj* disrespectful
desse[1] ['desi], **dessa** ['dɛsa] = *prep* ***de*** + *pron* ***esse, essa*** → ***deste***
desse[2] ['dɛsi], *etc* → ***dar***
dessegregar [desegre'gar] ⟨1c & 1o⟩ *v/t* desegregate
dessemelhante [deseme'ʎãtʃi] *adj* dissimilar
destacado [desta'kadu] *adj* outstanding; (*desprendido*) detached
destacamento [destaka'mẽtu] *m* MIL detachment
destacar [desta'kar] ⟨1n & 1b⟩ **1** *v/t* detach; (*realçar*) highlight; (*enfatizar*) emphasize **2** *v/i* stand out; **destacar-se** *v/r* stand out; (*desprender-se*) come off; *pessoa* be outstanding
destacável [desta'kavew] *adj* detachable
destampar [destã'par] ⟨1a⟩ *v/t* remove the lid of
destapar [desta'par] ⟨1b⟩ *v/t* uncover
destaque [des'taki] *m* distinction, prominence; *notícias*: headline; ***pôr em ~*** highlight
deste[1] ['destʃi], **desta** ['dɛsta] *prep* ***de*** + *pron* ***este, esta***
deste[2] ['dɛstʃi] *etc* → ***dar***
destemido [deste'midu] *adj* fearless
desterrar [deste'har] ⟨1c⟩ *v/t* exile; *fig* banish
desterro [des'tehu] *m* exile
destilação [destila'sãw] *f* ⟨*sem pl*⟩ distillation
destilados [desti'ladus] *mpl* spirits
destilar [desti'lar] ⟨1a⟩ **1** *v/t* distill, *Brit* distil
destilaria [destila'ria] *f* distillery
destinação [destʃina'sãw] *f* destination
destinar [destʃi'nar] ⟨1a⟩ *v/t* destine (***para*** for); *área* designate; *carta* address (***a*** to); *dinheiro* ***~ para*** set aside for
destinatário [destʃina'tariu] *m*, **-a** *f* addressee
destino [des'tʃinu] *m* destiny; *viagem*: destination; ***com ~ a*** heading for, bound for; ***sem ~*** aimless
destituir [destʃi'twir] ⟨3i⟩ *v/t do cargo* remove; (*despedir*) dismiss; *Presidente* impeach; ***~ de*** deprive of
destrancar [destrã'kar] ⟨1n⟩ *v/t* unlock
destravar [destra'var] ⟨1b⟩ *v/t carro* take the brake off; *fechadura* unlock
destreza [des'treza] *f* dexterity, skill
destro ['dɛstru] *adj* skillful, *Brit* skilful; *na letra etc* right-handed; (*ágil*) agile
destroçar [destro'sar] ⟨1o & 1e⟩ *v/t* destroy, wreck; (*arruinar*) ruin; (*quebrar*) smash; *lugar* smash up
destroço [des'trosu] *m* ***~s*** *pl* wreckage
destruição [destrui'sãw] *f* destruction
destruido [destru'idu] *adj* destroyed
destruidor [destrui'dor] *adj* destructive

destruir [destɾu'iɾ] ⟨3k⟩ *v/t* destroy; *ilusões* shatter; (*eliminar*) wipe out; ***destruído pela guerra*** ravaged by war
destrutivo [destɾu'ʧivu] *adj* destructive
desumano [dezu'manu] *adj* inhuman; (*cruel*) cruel
desunião [dezu'njãw] *f* ⟨*sem pl*⟩ disunity; (*separação*) separation
desunir [dezu'niɾ] ⟨3a⟩ *v/t* separate; TECN disconnect; (*lançar discórdia*) cause a rift between
desuso [de'zuzu] *m* disuse; ***em ~*** outdated; ***cair em ~*** go out of date
desvairado [dezvaj'ɾadu] *adj* crazy, demented; (*confuso*) bewildered; *multidão* frenzied
desvairar [dezvaj'ɾaɾ] ⟨1a⟩ **1** *v/t* drive mad **2** *v/i* rant and rave
desvalorização [dezvaloɾiza'sãw] *f* FIN devaluation
desvalorizar [dezvaloɾi'zaɾ] ⟨1a⟩ *v/t* devalue; **desvalorizar-se** *v/r* undervalue oneself; *moeda* lose value; *máquina* depreciate
desvantagem [dezvã'taʒẽ] *f* disadvantage; (*inconveniente*) drawback; ***estar em ~*** be at a disadvantage
desvantajoso [dezvãta'ʒozu] *adj* disadvantageous
desvelar [dezve'laɾ] ⟨1c⟩ *v/t estátua* unveil; *situação* clarify; *segredo* reveal; *complô* uncover
desvendar [dezvẽ'daɾ] ⟨1a⟩ *v/t segredo* reveal; *mistério* solve; (*tirar a venda*) remove the blindfold from
desventura [dezvẽ'tuɾa] *f* misfortune; (*tristeza*) unhappiness
desviar [dez'vjaɾ] ⟨1g⟩ **1** *v/t trânsito*, *atenção* divert; *avião etc* reroute; *golpe* deflect; *olhos* avert; *dinheiro* embezzle; ***~ o olhar*** look away **2** *v/i carro*, *motorista* swerve; *da rua* turn off; **desviar-se** *v/r* deviate; *do assunto* digress; ***~ de*** avoid
desvio [dez'viu] *m trânsito*: detour, *Brit* diversion; (*curva*) curve; *fig* deviation; *mercadorias*: misappropriation; *linha ferroviária* siding; *dinheiro*: embezzlement
detalhadamente [detaʎada'mẽʧi] *adv* in detail
detalhado [deta'ʎadu] *adj* detailed
detalhar [deta'ʎaɾ] ⟨1a⟩ *v/t* describe in detail; ***~ melhor*** elaborate on
detalhe [de'taʎi] *m* detail; ***em ~*** in detail; ***~ técnico*** technicality
detectar [detek'taɾ] ⟨1a⟩ *v/t* detect
detector [detek'toɾ] *m* detector; ***~ de fumo*** smoke detector; ***~ de mentiras*** lie detector
detenção [detẽ'sãw] *f* detention; (*prisão*) imprisonment; ***casa*** *f* ***de ~*** detention center, *Brit* detention centre
detento [de'tẽtu] *m*, **-a** *f* detainee
detentor [detẽ'toɾ] *m*, **-a** *f título etc*: holder
deter [de'teɾ] ⟨2xa⟩ *v/t* (*reter*) keep; (*parar*) stop; (*prender*) detain, arrest; *riso* hold back; *poder* hold; **deter-se** *v/r* stay; (*parar*) stop; (*conter-se*) restrain oneself
detergente [deteɾ'ʒẽʧi] *m* detergent; ***~ em pó*** washing powder; ***~ líquido*** dishwashing liquid, *Brit* washing-up liquid
deterioração [deterioɾa'sãw] *f* deterioration; (*estrago*) decay
deteriorado [deterio'ɾadu] *adj* rotten, bad
deteriorar [deterio'ɾaɾ] ⟨1e⟩ *v/t* damage; **deteriorar-se** *v/r* deteriorate, get worse
determinação [deteɾmina'sãw] *f* determination; (*resolução*) resolution
determinar [deteɾmi'naɾ] ⟨1a⟩ *v/t* determine; (*decretar*) order; (*causar*) cause; (*decidir*) decide (on)
detestar [detes'taɾ] ⟨1c⟩ *v/t* detest, hate
detestável [detest'tavew] *adj* detestable
detetive, *Port* **detective** [dete'ʧivi] *m* detective
detonação [detona'sãw] *f* detonation
detonador [detona'doɾ] *m* detonator
detonar [deto'naɾ] ⟨1f⟩ **1** *v/t* detonate **2** *v/i* detonate, go off
detrás [de'tɾas] **1** *adv* behind **2** *prep* ***~ de*** behind; ***por ~ de*** from behind
detrimento [detɾi'mẽtu] *m* detriment; ***em ~ de*** to the detriment of
detrito [de'tɾitu] *m* (*lixo*) garbage, *Brit*

D

rubbish; *restos* remains; (*resíduo de líquido*) dregs
deturpar [detur'par] ⟨1a⟩ *v/t* misrepresent; (*distorcer*) distort
deu [dew] → ***dar***
deuce [dews] *m tênis*: deuce
Deus [dews] *m* God; **~ *me livre!*** God forbid!; **~ *o abençoe!*** God bless you! ***se* ~ *quiser!*** God willing; ***pelo amor de* ~!** for God's sake!
deus [dews] *m* god
deusa ['dewza] *f* goddess
devagar [deva'gar] *adv* slowly
devanear [devani'ar] ⟨1l⟩ **1** *v/i* daydream **2** *v/t* dream up
devaneio [deva'neiu] *m* daydream
devassar [deva'sar] ⟨1b⟩ *v/t* expose
devassidão [devasi'dãw] *f* debauchery
devasso [de'vasu] *adj* debauched
devastador [devasta'dor] *adj* devastating; *maioria* overwhelming
devastar [devas'tar] ⟨1b⟩ *v/t campo, cidade* devastate
devedor [deve'dor] **1** *m*, **-a** *f* debtor **2** *adj* in debt; ***saldo* ~** debit balance
dever [de'ver] ⟨2c⟩ **1** *v/t* owe; **~ *desculpas a alguém*** owe s.o. an apology
2 *v/aux* ◇ *obrigação*: should; ***deveria estar envergonhado de si mesmo*** you should be ashamed of yourself; ***você não deveria fazer isso*** you shouldn't do that; ***você não deve …*** you are not supposed *ou* allowed to …
◇ *exclamação*: ***você deveria tê-lo visto!*** you should have seen him!; ***você deve ser dotado de telepatia!*** you must be telepathic!
◇ *necessidade*: must; ***candidatos devem ter …*** applicants must have …
◇ *probabilidade, conjetura*: ***ele deve chegar daqui a pouco*** he should arrive soon; ***devemos ter passado a saída*** we must have missed the turnoff; ***deve ser longo o suficiente*** that should be long enough, that ought to be long enough
3 *m* duty; **~ *de casa*** homework
devidamente [devida'mẽtʃi] *adv* duly
devido [de'vidu] *adj* due; **~ *a*** due to
devoção [devo'sãw] *f* (*religiosidade*) worship; (*dedicação*) devotion
devolução [devolu'sãw] *f* return; *de dinheiro* refund
devolver [devow'ver] ⟨2e⟩ *v/t* give back; *favor, convite* return; *saúde* restore; **~ *algo a alguém*** give sth back to s.o.; **~ *algo à loja*** take sth back to the store
devorar [devo'rar] ⟨1e⟩ *v/t* devour; (*aniquilar*) destroy
devotado [devo'tadu] *m*, **-a** *f* devotee
devotar [devo'tar] ⟨1e⟩ *v/t* devote; **devotar-se** *v/r* **~ *a*** devote oneself to
devoto [de'vɔtu] *adj* devout
dez [dɛs] *num* ten
dezanove [deza'nɔvi] *num Port* nineteen
dezasseis [deza'sejs] *num Port* sixteen
dezassete [deza'sɛtʃi] *num Port* seventeen
dezembro [de'zẽbru] *m* December; ***em* ~** in December
dezena [de'zena] *f* ten; ***uma* ~ *de*** about ten
dezenove [deze'nɔvi] *num Bras* nineteen
dezesseis [deze'sejs] *num Bras* sixteen
dezessete [deze'sɛtʃi] *num Bras* seventeen
dezoito [de'zojtu] *num* eighteen
dia ['dʒia] *m* day; ***que* ~ *é hoje?*** what day is it today?; **~ *a* ~** day to day; **~ *após* ~** day in, day out; ***um* ~ *destes*** one of these days; ***o* ~ *todo*** all day (long); ***o outro* ~** the other day; ***de um* ~ *para o outro*** overnight; ***no* ~ *primeiro de abril*** on April 1st; ***estar em* ~** be up to date; ***pôr em* ~** update, bring up to date; **~ *do casamento*** wedding day; **~ *de eleição*** election day; **~ *de folga*** day off; ***Dia das Mães*** Mother's Day; **~ *de Natal*** Christmas Day; **~ *de pagamento*** payday; **~ *útil*** workday
diabetes [dʒia'bɛtʃis] *f* diabetes *sg*
diabético [dʒia'bɛtʃiku] **1** *adj* diabetic **2** *m*, **-a** *f* diabetic
diabinho [dʒia'biɲu] *m fam* little devil
diabo ['dʒiabu] *m* devil; *fam* ***que* ~*s***

você está fazendo? what the hell are you doing?
diabólico [dʒia'bɔliku] *adj* diabolical; (*danado*) devilish
diafragma [dʒia'fɾagma] *m* ANAT, MED diaphragm
diagnosticar [dʒiagnostʃi'kaɾ] ⟨1n⟩ *v/t* diagnose
diagnóstico [dʒia'gnɔstʃiku] *m* MED diagnosis
diagonal [dʒiago'naw] *adj* diagonal
diagonalmente [dʒiagonaw'mẽtʃi] *adv* diagonally
diagrama [dʒia'gɾama] *m* diagram
dialeto, *Port* **dialecto** [dʒia'lɛtu] *m* dialect
dialogar [dʒialo'gaɾ] ⟨1o & 1e⟩ *v/i* talk; POL hold discussions; *iniciar* enter into dialog
diálogo ['dʒialogu] *m* dialog, *Brit* dialogue
diamante [dʒia'mãtʃi] *m* diamond
diâmetro ['dʒiʌmetɾu] *m* diameter
diante ['dʒiãtʃi] **1** *adv* ***para ~*** forward; ***ir por ~*** go on, continue; ***e assim por ~*** and so on; ***de agora em ~*** from now on; ***a ~!*** let's move on! **2** *prep* ***~ de*** before; *posição* in front of; *problemas etc* in the face of; ***~ dos nossos olhos*** before our very eyes
dianteiro [dʒiã'tejɾu] *adj* front; ***o assento ~*** the front seat
diapositivo [dʒiapozi'tʃivu] *m* FOT slide
diária ['dʒiaɾja] *f* (*salário*) allowance; *hotel*: daily rate; ***~ completa*** full board
diário ['dʒiaɾiu] **1** *adj* daily **2** *m* diary; (*jornal*) (daily) newspaper; ***~ de bordo*** log book
diarista [dʒia'ɾista] *f Bras* domestic help
diarreia [dʒia'hɛja] *f* diarrhea, *Brit* diarrhoea
dica ['dʒika] *f* pointer, tip
dicção [dʒi'ksãw] *f* diction
dicionário [dʒisjo'naɾiu] *m* dictionary
dicotomia [dʒikoto'mia] *f* dichotomy
didática, *Port* **didáctica** [dʒi'datʃika] *f* education
didático, *Port* **didáctico** [dʒi'datʃiku] *adj* didactic; (*instrutivo*) educational
diesel ['dʒizew] *m* diesel
dieta ['dʒiɛta] *f* diet; ***de ~*** on a diet; ***~ básica*** staple diet; ***~ intensiva*** crash diet
difamação [dʒifama'sãw] *f* defamation
difamar [dʒifa'maɾ] ⟨1a⟩ *v/t* defame; *nome* blacken
difamatório [dʒifama'tɔɾiu] *adj* defamatory
diferença [dʒife'ɾẽsa] *f* difference; ***~ de horário*** time difference; ***não faz ~ alguma*** it doesn't make any difference; *fig* ***~s*** *pl* differences
diferencial [dʒifeɾẽ'sjaw] **1** *f* MAT, AUTO differential **2** *adj* differential
diferenciar [dʒifeɾẽ'sjaɾ] ⟨1g⟩ *v/t* differentiate
diferente [dʒife'ɾẽtʃi] *adj* different; ***~ de*** different from, unlike
diferentemente [dʒifeɾẽtʃi'mẽtʃi] *adv* differently
diferir [dʒife'ɾiɾ] ⟨3c⟩ **1** *v/i* differ **2** *v/t* (*adiar*) defer
difícil [dʒi'fisiw] *adj* difficult; (*improvável*) unlikely
dificilmente [dʒifisiw'mẽtʃi] *adv* ***ele ~ completará o curso*** he is unlikely to complete the course; ***~ acredito nele*** I find it hard to believe him
dificuldade [dʒifikuw'dadʒi] *f* difficulty; *de situação, problema* delicacy; ***com / sem ~*** with / without difficulty
dificultar [dʒifikuw'taɾ] ⟨1a⟩ *v/t* ***isso vai ~ as coisas*** that's going to make things difficult
difteria [dʒifte'ɾia] *f* diphtheria
difundido [dʒifũ'dʒidu] *adj* widespread
difundir [dʒifũ'dʒiɾ] ⟨3a⟩ *v/t* spread; *rádio*: broadcast; *luz, calor* diffuse; **difundir-se** *v/r* spread
difusão [dʒifu'zãw] *f* diffusion
difuso [dʒi'fuzu] *adj* diffuse
diga ['dʒiga], **digo** ['dʒigu] *etc* → ***dizer***
digerir [dʒiʒe'ɾiɾ] ⟨3c⟩ *v/t* digest *tb fig*
digerível [dʒiʒe'ɾivew] *adj comida* digestible
digestão [dʒiʒes'tãw] *f* ⟨*sem pl*⟩ digestion; ***fazer a ~*** digest
digestivo [dʒiʒes'tʃivu] **1** *adj* diges-

tive **2** *m* GASTR digestif
digitação [dʒiʒita'sãw] *f* keying
digitador [dʒiʒita'dor] *m*, **-a** *f* keyboarder
digital [dʒiʒi'taw] *adj* digital; ***impressões*** *fpl* ***digitais*** fingerprints

D

digitar [dʒiʒi'tar] ⟨1a⟩ *v/t dados* key in
dígito ['dʒiʒitu] *m* digit
dignar-se [dʒig'narsi] ⟨1a⟩ *v/r* ***~ a*** deign to
dignidade [dʒigni'dadʒi] *f* dignity
dignitário [dʒigna'tariu] *m*, **-a** *f* dignitary
digno ['dʒignu] *adj* worthy; (*nobre*) dignified; ***~ de*** worthy of
dilapidação [dʒilapida'sãw] *f prédio*: demolition; *dinheiro*: squandering
dilapidado [dʒilapi'dadu] *adj* dilapidated
dilapidar [dʒilapi'dar] ⟨1a⟩ *v/t dinheiro* squander; *prédio* demolish
dilatação [dʒilata'sãw] *f* ⟨*sem pl*⟩ dilation; *metal*: expansion
dilatar [dʒila'tar] ⟨1b⟩ *v/t* MED dilate; (*aumentar*) expand; *narina* flare; **dilatar-se** *v/r pupila* dilate; *metal* expand
dilema [dʒi'lema] *m* dilemma
diletante [dʒile'tãtʃi] **1** *m/f* dilettante; ESP amateur **2** *adj* dilettante
diligência [dʒili'ʒẽsja] *f* diligence; (*investigação*) inquiry; (*carruagem*) stagecoach
diligente [dʒili'ʒẽtʃi] *adj* diligent, industrious
diluir [dʒi'lwir] ⟨3i⟩ *v/t* dilute
diluvio [dʒi'luviu] *m* deluge
dimensão [dʒimẽ'sãw] *f* dimension; (*tamanho*) extent, scale
diminuir [dʒimi'nwir] ⟨3i⟩ **1** *v/t* reduce, decrease; *fumo* cut down on; *som* turn down; *interesse* lessen **2** *v/i* lessen, diminish; *preço* go down; *motorista*, *carro* slow down; *dor* wear off; *ruído* die down; ***ir diminuindo*** peter out
diminutivo [dʒiminu'tʃivu] **1** *m* diminutive **2** *adj* diminutive
diminuto [dʒimi'nutu] *adj* minute
Dinamarca [dʒina'marka] *f* Denmark
dinamarquês [dʒinamar'kes] **1** *adj* Danish **2** *m*, **dinamarquesa** [dʒinamar'keza] *f* Dane
dinâmica [dʒi'nʌmika] *f* dynamic
dinâmico [dʒi'nʌmiku] *adj* dynamic; *empresário* high-powered
dinamismo [dʒina'mizmu] *m* dynamism
dinamitar [dʒinami'tar] ⟨1a⟩ *v/t* blow up
dinamite [dʒina'mitʃi] *f* dynamite
dínamo ['dʒinamu] *m* dynamo
dinastia [dʒinas'tʃia] *f* dynasty
dinheiro [dʒi'ɲejru] *m* money; ***pagar em ~*** pay (in) cash; ***~ adiantado*** cash in advance; ***~ falso*** counterfeit money; ***~ trocado*** small change; ***~ vivo*** ready cash; ***~ para pequenas despesas*** petty cash
dinossauro [dʒino'sawru] *m* dinosaur
diploma [dʒi'ploma] *m* diploma; *universidade*: degree
diplomacia [dʒiploma'sia] *f* diplomacy
diplomar-se [dʒiplo'marsi] ⟨1a⟩ *v/r* graduate
diplomata [dʒiplo'mata] *m/f* diplomat
diplomático [dʒiplo'matʃiku] *adj* diplomatic
dique ['dʒiki] *m* dyke
dirá [dʒi'ra], **dirão** [dʒi'rãw] *etc* → ***dizer***
direção, *Port* **direcção** [dʒire'sãw] *f* (*sentido*) direction; (*gerência*) management; (*condução*) driving; (*manuseio do volante*) steering; ***em ~ a*** toward; ***em ~ leste*** eastward ***nessa ~*** that way, in that direction; ***sob sua ~*** under his direction / management; ***~ hidráulica*** power steering; ***~ à direita / esquerda*** left- / right-hand drive
direct... *Port* → ***diret...***
direi [dʒi'rej] → ***dizer***
direita [dʒi'rejta] *f* right; POL right-wing; *lado* right-hand side; ***à ~*** on the right; ***virar à ~*** turn right; ***mantenha-se à ~*** keep right
direito [dʒi'rejtu] **1** *adj* right; *lado* right, right-hand; (*honesto*) honest; (*vertical*) straight **2** *adv* right, properly; (*em linha reta*) straight; *sentar-se* straight, upright **3** *m* right; DIR law; ***ter o ~ de*** be entitled to, have

the right to; ~ ***ao voto*** right to vote; ***ser formado em*** ~ have a law degree; ~***s autorais*** copyright; ~***s civis*** civil rights; ~ ***empresarial*** corporate law; ~***s humanos*** human rights
diretiva [dʒire'tʃiva] *f* directive
direto [dʒi'rɛtu] **1** *adj* direct; *trem* non-stop, direct **2** *adv* straight, directly; ***ir*** ~ ***ao assunto*** cut to the chase, get straight to the point; ***transmissão direta*** live broadcast
diretor [dʒire'tor] **1** *m*; **-a** *f* director; *escola*: principal, *Brit* headteacher; *jornal*: editor; ~ ***assistente*** assistant director **2** *adj* directing *atr*
diretor-gerente [dʒiretorʒe'rẽtʃi] *m* ⟨*pl* diretores-gerentes⟩ managing director
diretor-presidente [dʒiretorprezi'dẽtʃi] *m* ⟨*pl* diretores-presidentes⟩ CEO, chief executive officer
diretriz [dʒire'tris] *f* directive
dirigente [dʒiri'ʒẽtʃi] **1** *adj* leading; *classe* ruling **2** *m/f* leader; (*gerente*) manager; (*diretor*) director
dirigir [dʒiri'ʒir] ⟨3n⟩ **1** *v/t* direct; *empresa* manage; *Bras carro*, *barco* drive **2** *v/i Bras* drive; ~ ***embriagado*** drink (and) drive; **dirigir-se** *v/r* ~ ***a*** speak to, address; *energias* be directed to; (*ir*) make one's way; (*consultar*) turn to; *autoridade* apply to
discar [dʒis'kar] ⟨1a & 1n⟩ *Bras* TEL dial
discernidor [dʒiserni'dor] *adj* discerning
discernir [dʒiser'nir] ⟨3c⟩ *v/t* discern; (*distinguir*) distinguish
discernível [dʒiser'nivew] *adj* discernible
disciplina [dʒisi'plina] *f* discipline
disciplinar [dʒisipli'nar] ⟨1a⟩ **1** *adj* disciplinary **2** *v/t* discipline; **disciplinar-se** *v/r* discipline oneself
discípulo [dʒis'sipulu] *m*, **-a** *f* disciple
disc-jóquei [dʒisk'ʒɔkej] *m* disc-jockey, DJ
disco ['dʒisku] *m* disc; INFORM disk; ESP discus; MÚS record; *fig* ***mudar o*** ~ change the record; ~ ***compacto*** compact disc, CD; ~ ***de demonstração*** demo disk; INFORM ~ ***flexível*** floppy disk; ~ ***rígido*** hard disk; ~ ***voador*** flying saucer
discordância [dʒiskor'dãsja] *f* disagreement; *opinião*: difference
discordar [dʒiskor'dar] ⟨1e⟩ *v/i* ~ **(*de*)** disagree (with)
discórdia [dʒis'kɔrdʒia] *f* discord, dissent
discoteca [dʒisko'tɛka] *f* discotheque, disco
discrepância [dʒiskre'pãsja] *f* discrepancy; (*desigualdade*) mismatch
discretamente [dʒiskrɛta'mẽtʃi] *adv* discreetly
discreto [dʒis'krɛtu] *adj* discreet; (*reservado*) reserved; (*modesto*) modest; *roupa* plain
discrição [dʒiskri'sãw] *f* ⟨*sem pl*⟩ discretion; (*reserva*) reserve; (*modéstia*) modesty
discriminação [dʒiskrimina'sãw] *f* discrimination; (*descrição*) description
discriminar [dʒiskrimi'nar] ⟨1a⟩ **1** *v/t* distinguish; *contas* break down, itemize **2** *v/i* ~ ***entre*** discriminate between
discriminatório [dʒiskrimina'tɔriu] *adj* discriminatory
discursar [dʒiskur'sar] ⟨1a⟩ *v/i* give a speech, speak
discurso [dʒis'kursu] *m* speech; ***fazer um*** ~ give a speech, make a speech
discussão [dʒisku'sãw] *f* discussion; (*briga*) argument; ***ter uma*** ~ have words
discutir [dʒisku'tʃir] ⟨3a⟩ **1** *v/t* discuss (***sobre algo*** sth) **2** *v/i* (*brigar*) argue (***sobre*** about)
discutível [dʒisku'tʃi] *adj* debatable
disenteria [dʒizẽte'ria] *f* MED dysentery
disfarçado [dʒisfar'sadu] *adj* disguised, in disguise; ***ele estava*** ~ ***de ...*** he was disguised as …
disfarçar [dʒisfar'sar] ⟨1p & 1b⟩ **1** *v/t* disguise **2** *v/i* pretend; **disfarçar-se** *v/r* disguise oneself
disfarce [dʒis'farsi] *m* diguise; (*máscara*) mask; *fig* masquerade
disforme [dʒis'fɔrmi] *adj* deformed; (*horrendo*) hideous

D

D

dislexia [dʒizle'ksia] *f* dyslexia
disléxico [dʒiz'lɛksiku] *adj* dyslexic
disparar [dʒispa'rar] ⟨1b⟩ **1** *v/t arma* fire **2** *v/i* fire; *arma* go off; *preços* shoot up; (*sair correndo*) shoot off
disparate [dʒispa'ratʃi] *m* nonsense; *ação* blunder
disparidade [dʒispari'dadʒi] *f* disparity
disparo [dʒis'paru] *m* shot
dispendioso [dʒispẽ'djozu] *adj* costly
dispensa [dʒis'pẽsa] *f* exemption; *de dívida*: cancellation; REL dispensation
dispensar [dʒispẽ'sar] ⟨1a⟩ *v/t* (*distribuir*) dispense; (*desobrigar*) excuse (***de*** from); (*deixar de lado*) dispense with; (*conferir*) grant
dispensável [dʒispẽ'savew] *adj* expendable
dispersar [dʒisper'sar] ⟨1c⟩ **1** *v/t* disperse; *energias* waste **2** *v/i* disperse; **dispersar-se** *v/r* disperse
disperso [dʒis'pɛrsu] *adj família, chuvas etc* scattered
disponibilidade [dʒisponibili'dadʒi] *f* availability; FIN liquid assets; ***segundo ~*** subject to availability
disponível [dʒispo'nivew] *adj* available; (*livre*) free
dispor [dʒis'por] ⟨2z⟩ **1** *v/t móveis, talheres* arrange, lay out; (*pôr em ordem*) put in order **2** *v/i **~ de*** have at one's disposal; (*ter*) have, own; ***~ sobre*** talk about; ***disponha!*** feel free!; ***disponho de tempo para ...*** I have plenty of time to ...; **dispor-se** *v/r **~ a*** be prepared to, be willing to; (*oferecer-se*) volunteer to; (*decidir*) decide to
disposição [dʒispozi'sãw] *f* (*vontade*) willingness; *espírito*: frame of mind; (*arranjo*) arrangement; ***estar** ou **ficar à ~ de alguém*** be at s.o's disposal
dispositivo [dʒispozi'tʃivu] *m* device; *lei*: provision; MED ***~ intra-uterino*** intra-uterine device, IUD; ***~ de segurança*** security operation
disposto [dʒis'postu] *adj* arranged; (*pronto*) prepared, willing; ***estar ~ a fazer algo*** be willing to do sth; ***estar bem / mal ~*** be on good / bad form
disputa [dʒis'puta] *f* dispute, argument; (*competição*) contest; ESP ***~ final*** decider
disputar [dʒispu'tar] ⟨1a⟩ **1** *v/t* dispute; (*tentar ganhar*) compete for; ***~ uma corrida*** run a race **2** *v/i* (*discutir*) argue
disquete [dʒis'kɛtʃi] *f* INFORM diskette, floppy disk
dissabor [dʒisa'bor] *m* sorrow; (*dificuldade*) trouble
disse ['dʒisi] *etc* → ***dizer***
dissecação [dʒiseka'sãw] *f* dissection
dissecar [dʒise'kar] ⟨1n & 1c⟩ *v/t* dissect
dissertação [dʒiserta'sãw] *f* (*tese*) dissertation; (*conferência*) lecture
dissertar [dʒiser'tar] ⟨1c⟩ *v/i* speak (***sobre*** about)
dissidente [dʒisi'dẽtʃi] **1** *adj* dissident **2** *m/f* dissident
dissimulação [dʒisimula'sãw] *f* ⟨*sem pl*⟩ dissimulation
dissimulado [dʒisimu'ladu] *adj* devious, sly
dissimular [dʒisimu'lar] ⟨1a⟩ **1** *v/t* hide; (*fazer de conta*) feign **2** *v/i* dissimulate
dissipar [dʒisi'par] ⟨1a⟩ **1** *v/t* disperse; (*gastar*) squander; *dúvida, suspeitas* dispel; **dissipar-se** *v/r dúvidas etc* be dispelled; *nevoeiro* clear
dissociação [dʒisosja'sãw] *f* ⟨*sem pl*⟩ dissociation
dissociar [dʒiso'sjar] ⟨1g⟩ *v/t **~ algo*** separate sth; **dissociar-se** *v/r **~ de algo*** dissociate oneself from sth
dissolução [dʒisolu'sãw] *f* dissolution; *amizade, matrimônio*: break-up
dissolver [dʒisow'ver] ⟨2e⟩ *v/t* dissolve; (*dispersar*) disperse; **dissolver-se** *v/r* dissolve; *grupo* disband
dissonância [dʒiso'nãsja] *f* dissonance
dissuadir [dʒiswa'dʒir] ⟨3b⟩ *v/t* dissuade; ***~ alguém de fazer algo*** dissuade s.o. from doing sth
distância [dʒis'tãsja] *f* distance; ***à ~*** from a distance; *longe* in the distance; ***de longa ~*** long-distance; ***a grande ~*** far away; ***qual é a ~ até***

... ? how far away is ...?; ***a três quilômetros de ~*** three kilometers away

distanciar [dʒistã'sjar] ⟨1g⟩ *v/t* distance; (*colocar espaço entre*) space out; **distanciar-se** *v/r* distance oneself; *duas pessoas, dois barcos* drift apart

distante [dʒis'tãtʃi] *adj* distant; *antepassado* remote; *fig* aloof

distender [dʒistẽ'der] ⟨2a⟩ *v/t* expand; (*inchar*) distend; (*esticar*) stretch; *músculo* pull; **distender-se** *v/r* expand

distinção [dʒistʃĩ'sãw] *f* distinction

distinguir [dʒistʃĩ'gir] ⟨3o⟩ *v/t* distinguish; (*perceber*) make out; ***~ entre*** distiguish between; **distinguir-se** *v/r* stand out

distintivo [dʒistʃĩ'tʃivu] **1** *adj* distinctive **2** *m* badge; *policial*: shield, *Brit* badge

distinto [dʒis'tʃĩtu] *adj* distinct; (*diferente*) different; *senhor* distinguished; (*fino*) refined

distorção [dʒistor'sãw] *f* distortion; MED sprain

distorcer [dʒistor'ser] ⟨2g & 2d⟩ *v/t* distort

distração, *Port* **distracção** [dʒistra'sãw] *f* distraction; (*passatempo*) diversion

distraidamente [dʒistraida'mẽtʃi] *adv* absent-mindedly

distraído [dʒistra'idu] *adj* distracted; (*não atento*) absent-minded

distrair [dʒistra'ir] ⟨3l⟩ **1** *v/t* distract; (*divertir*) amuse; **distrair-se** *v/r* get distracted; (*divertir-se*) amuse oneself

distribuição [dʒistribwi'sãw] *f* distribution

distribuidor [dʒistribwi'dor] *m* distributor

distribuir [dʒistri'bwir] ⟨3i⟩ *v/t* distribute; *tarefas* share out; *cartas* deliver; (*passar*) pass around

distrito [dʒis'tritu] *m* district; ***~ eleitoral*** constituency; ***~ federal*** federal area; ***~ policial*** *Am* station house, police station

disturbio [dʒis'turbiu] *m* MED disorder; POL ***~s*** unrest

ditado [dʒi'tadu] *m* dictation; (*provérbio*) saying

ditador [dʒita'dor] *m*, **-a** *f* dictator

ditadura [dʒita'dura] *f* dictatorship

ditar [dʒi'tar] ⟨1a⟩ *v/t* dictate

ditatorial [dʒitatori'aw] *adj* dictatorial

dito ['dʒitu] **1** *pp* → ***dizer***; ***~ e feito*** no sooner said than done **2** *m* remark

dito-cujo [dʒito'kuʒu] *m* ⟨*pl* ditos-cujos⟩ said person

ditongo [dʒi'tõgu] *m* diphthong

DIU ['dʒiu] *m abr* (***dispositivo intra-uterino***) IUD (intra-uterine device)

diurético [dʒiu'rɛtʃiku] **1** *adj* diuretic **2** *m* diuretic

diurno ['dʒiurnu] *adj* daytime *atr*

divã [dʒi'vã] *m* couch

divagação [dʒivaga'sãw] *f* digression

divergência [dʒiver'ʒẽsja] *f* divergence; (*desacordo*) disagreement; ***estar em ~ com*** be at odds with

divergir [dʒiver'ʒir] ⟨3n & 3c⟩ *v/i* diverge; (*diferir*) differ; (*discordar*) disagree; ***~ de alguém*** disagree with s.o.

diversão [dʒiver'sãw] *f* diversion; (*divertimento*) amusement; ***parque*** *m* ***de diversões*** amusement park

diversificação [dʒiversifika'sãw] *f* diversification

diversificar [dʒiversifi'kar] ⟨1n⟩ *v/i* diversify

diverso [dʒi'vɛrsu] *adj* different; ***~s*** various

divertido [dʒiver'tʃidu] *adj* (*cômico*) funny; (*que se curte*) enjoyable

divertimento [dʒivertʃi'mẽtu] *m* enjoyment, fun; ***foi um grande ~*** it was great fun

divertir [dʒiver'tʃir] ⟨3c⟩ *v/t* entertain, amuse; **divertir-se** *v/r* enjoy oneself, have fun; ***divirta-se!*** have a good time!, have fun!

dívida ['dʒivida] *f* debt; (*compromisso*) indebtedness; ***estar com ~s*** be in debt; ***~ externa*** foreign debt; ***~ incobrável*** bad debt; ***~ pública*** national debt

dividendo [dʒivi'dẽdu] *m* FIN dividend

dividir [dʒivi'dʒir] ⟨3a⟩ *v/t* divide; (*compartilhar*) share; (*separar*) sepa-

rate; ~ ***ao meio*** halve; **dividir-se** *v/r* be divided
divindade [dʒivĩ'dadʒi] *f* divinity; (*deus*) deity
divino [dʒi'vinu] *adj* divine *tb fig*
divirto [dʒi'virtu] *etc* → ***divertir***
divisão [dʒivi'zãw] *f* division; *país*: partition
divisível [dʒivi'zivew] *adj* divisible
divorciado [dʒivor'sjadu] **1** *adj* divorced **2** *m*, **-a** *f* divorcee
divorciar [dʒivor'sjar] ⟨1g⟩ *v/t* divorce; **divorciar-se** *v/r* get divorced
divórcio [dʒi'vɔrsiu] *m* divorce; ***obter um*** ~ get a divorce
divulgar [dʒivuw'gar] ⟨1o⟩ *v/t* divulge; *notícias* spread; *livro* publish; COM market
diz [dʒis] → ***dizer***
dizer [dʒi'zer] ⟨2t⟩ **1** *v/t* say; ~ ***algo a alguém*** tell s.o. sth; (*falar*) say sth to s.o.; ~ ***para alguém fazer algo*** tell s.o. to do sth; ~ ***a alguém que …*** tell s.o. that …; ***por assim*** ~ so to speak; ***querer*** ~ mean; ***quer*** ~ that is to say; **dizer-se** *v/r* claim to be; ***como se diz isso em … ?*** how do you say that in …?; ***diz-se que …*** it's said that … **2** *m* saying
dizia [dʒi'zia] → ***dizer***
dizimar [dʒizi'mar] ⟨1a⟩ *v/t* decimate
do [du] = *prep* ***de*** + *art m* ***o***
dó [dɔ] *m* pity; MÚS C; ***ter*** ~ ***de*** pity
doação [dwa'sãw] *f* donation
doador [dwa'dor] *m*, **-a** *f* donor; ~ ***de sangue / órgão*** blood / organ donor
doar [dwar] ⟨1f⟩ *v/t* donate
dobra ['dɔbra] *f* fold; *calça*; cuff, *Brit* turn-up; *saia*: pleat
dobradiça [dobra'dʒisa] *f* hinge
dobrar [do'brar] ⟨1e⟩ **1** *v/t* fold; *perna* bend; *esquina* turn; *manga* roll up; *quantia* double **2** *v/i* double; **dobrar-se** *v/r* *arame etc* bend; *pessoa* bend over
dobrável [do'brar] *adj cadeira* folding
dobro ['dobru] *m* double; ***o*** ~ twice as much
doca ['dɔka] *f* NÁUT dock
doce ['dosi] **1** *adj* sweet; (*suave*) gentle; ***água*** *f* ~ fresh water **2** *m* (*sobremesa*) dessert, sweet; (*chocolates etc*) sweet; ***ela é um*** ~ she's a sweetie; ~***s*** confectionary; ~ ***em calda*** compote; ~ ***de fruta*** caramelized fruit; ~ ***de leite*** fudge
docente [do'sẽtʃi] *adj* ***corpo*** *m* ~ teaching staff
dócil ['dɔsiw] *adj* docile
documentação [dokumẽta'sãw] *f* documentation; (*papéis*) paperwork; ~ ***do veículo*** driver's logbook
documentar [dokumẽ'tar] ⟨1a⟩ *v/t* document
documentário [dokumẽ'tariu] *m* TV documentary
documento [doku'mẽtu] *m* document; ~***s*** *pl* papers, documents; ~ ***de identidade*** identification, ID
doçura [do'sura] *f* sweetness; (*ternura*) gentleness; *pessoa* sweetie
doença ['dwẽsa] *f* disease, illness; ~ ***mental*** mental illness; ~ ***sexualmente transmissível*** sexually transmitted disease
doente ['dwẽtʃi] **1** *adj* ill, sick; ***estar*** ~ be ill; ***deixar*** ~ sicken, disgust; ***gravemente*** ~ seriously ill **2** *m/f* sick person; (*paciente*) patient; ~ ***mental*** mentally ill person; ~ ***terminal*** terminally ill person
doentio [dwẽ'tʃiu] *adj* sickly; *interesse* sick; *clima* unhealthy
doer [dwer] ⟨2f⟩ *v/i* hurt; *músculo*, *cabeça* ache
dogma ['dɔgma] *m* REL dogma
dogmático [dog'matʃiku] *adj* dogmatic
doido ['dojdu] **1** *adj* mad, crazy; ~ ***por*** obsessed by **2** *m*, **-a** *f* madman; madwoman; ~ ***varrido*** raving lunatic
doído [do'idu] → ***dolorido***
dois [dojs] *num m*, **duas** *f* ['duas] two; ***os*** ~, ***as duas*** the two (of them), both (of them); ESP ~ ***a*** ~ two all; ***conversa a*** ~ tête-à-tête; ~ ***pontos*** colon
dólar ['dɔlar] *m* dollar
doleiro [do'lejru] *m*, **-a** *f* (unofficial) dollar dealer
dolorido [dolo'ridu] *adj* sore; *fig* sorrowful
doloroso [dolo'rozu] *adj* painful; (*lastimoso*) distressing

dom [dõ] *m* gift; ***ter o ~ da palavra*** have the gift of the gab
domador [doma'doɾ] *m*, **-a** *f* tamer
domar [do'maɾ] ⟨1f⟩ *v/t* tame
doméstico [do'mɛstʃiku] *adj* domestic; ***animal*** *m* **~** pet
domiciliado [domisi'ljadu] *adj* resident
domicílio [domi'siliu] *m* domicile; ***entrega*** *f* ***ao*** **~** home delivery
dominação [domina'sãw] *f* domination; **~ *mundial*** world domination
dominador [domina'doɾ] *adj* domineering
dominante [domi'nãtʃi] *adj* dominant; (*predominante*) predominant; *partido* ruling
dominar [domi'naɾ] ⟨1a⟩ **1** *v/t* dominate; *fisicamente* overpower; *língua* have a command of **2** *v/i* dominate, prevail; **dominar-se** *v/r* control oneself
domingo [do'mĩgu] *m* Sunday; ***no*** **~** on Sunday; **~ *de ramos*** Palm Sunday
domínio [do'miniu] *m* command; (*poder*) power; (*território, esféra*) domain
donde ['dõdʒi] *prep Port* ***de*** + *pron* ***onde***: from where; **~ *você veio?*** where did you come from?
dono ['donu] *m*, **-a** *f* owner; ***mudar de*** **~** change hands; ***dona de casa*** housewife; **~ *da estrada*** road hog; ***Dona X*** Miss X
dopar [do'paɾ] ⟨1e⟩ *v/t* dope, drug; **dopar-se** *v/r atleta* take drugs
dor [doɾ] *f* pain; *menos forte* ache; **~ *de cabeça*** headache; **~ *nas costas*** backache; **~ *de estômago*** stomach-ache; **~ *de ouvido*** earache; **~*es*** *pl* (***de parto***) labor pains, *Brit* labour pains
dormente [doɾ'mẽtʃi] *adj* numb
dormida [doɾ'mida] *f estado* sleep; *lugar* place to sleep; ***dar uma*** **~** have a sleep
dorminhoco [doɾmi'ɲoku] *m*, **-a** *f* sleepyhead
dormir [doɾ'miɾ] ⟨3f⟩ *v/i* sleep; **~ *até tarde*** sleep late, *Brit* sleep in; **~ *como uma pedra*** sleep like a log; ***hora de*** **~** bedtime; ***pôr para*** **~** *criança* put to bed
dormitório [doɾmi'tɔriu] *m* bedroom; *comunitário* dormitory
dorsal [doɾ'saw] *adj* ***coluna*** *f* **~** spine
dorso ['doɾsu] *m* (*costas*) back; *livro*: spine; *nariz*: bridge
dosagem [do'zaʒẽ] *f* dosage
dosar [do'zaɾ] ⟨1e⟩ *v/t* measure out
dose ['dɔzi] *f* dose; *uísque etc*: shot, measure; *Port* GASTR portion; **~ *excessiva*** overdose
dossiê [do'sie] *m* file
dotado [do'tadu] *adj* gifted; **~ *de*** endowed with
dotar [do'taɾ] ⟨1e⟩ *v/t* **~ *alguém de algo*** endow s.o. with sth
dote ['dɔtʃi] *m* dowry; *característica física* endowment; (*dom*) gift
dou [dow] → ***dar***
dourado [dow'ɾadu] **1** *adj* golden **2** *m* gilt; *cor* golden color, *Brit* golden colour
dourar [dow'ɾaɾ] ⟨1a⟩ *v/t* gild; GASTR brown
doutor [dow'toɾ] *m*, **-a** *f* doctor; **~ *em medicina*** doctor of medecine
doutorado [dowto'ɾadu] *m* doctorate, PhD
doutrina [dow'tɾina] *f* doctrine
doutrinar [dowtɾi'naɾ] ⟨1a⟩ *v/t* indoctrinate
download [dawn'lod] *m* download; ***fazer o*** **~ *de algo*** download sth
doze ['dozi] *num* twelve
Dr *abr* (***Doutor***) Dr. (Doctor)
Dra *abr* (***Doutora***) Dr. (Doctor)
dragão [dɾa'gãw] *m* dragon
dragar [dɾa'gaɾ] ⟨1b⟩ *v/t canal* dredge
drama ['dɾama] *m* drama *tb fig*; (*peça*) play; ***ser um*** **~** be an ordeal; ***causar um*** **~** make a scene
dramático [dɾa'matʃiku] *adj* dramatic
dramatização [dɾamatʃiza'sãw] *f* dramatization
dramatizar [dɾamatʃi'zaɾ] ⟨1a⟩ *v/t estória* dramatize *tb fig*
dramaturgo [dɾama'tuɾgu] *m*, **-a** *f* dramatist
drástico ['dɾastʃiku] *adj* drastic
drenagem [dɾe'naʒẽ] *f* drainage
drenar [dɾe'naɾ] ⟨1d⟩ *v/t* drain
dreno ['dɾenu] *m* drain

driblar [dɾi'blaɾ] ⟨1a⟩ ESP dribble
drinque ['dɾĩki] *m Bras* drink
drive ['dɾajvi] *m* INFORM drive; **~ *de CD-ROM*** CD-Rom drive
droga ['dɾɔga] *f* drug; **~ *leve*** soft drug; ***viciado*** *m* ***em ~s*** drug addict; ***usar ~s*** be on drugs; ***que ~!*** damn!; ***ser uma ~*** be a drag
drogado [dɾo'gadu] **1** *adj* high on drugs, drugged-up **2** *m/f fam* junkie
drogar [dɾo'gaɾ] ⟨1e⟩ *v/t* drug; **drogar-se** *v/r* take drugs
drogaria [dɾoga'ɾia] *f* drug store, *Brit* chemist's shop
duas ['duas] *num f* two; → ***dois***
dublagem [du'blaʒẽ] *f* dubbing
dublar [du'blaɾ] ⟨1a⟩ *v/t* dub; **~ *em francês*** dub into French
ducha ['duʃa] *f Bras* shower; MED douche
duelo ['dwɛlu] *m* duel
duende ['dwẽdʒi] *m* elf
dueto [du'etu] *m* MÚS duet
dum [dũ], **duma** ['duma] = *prep* ***de*** + *art* ***um, uma***
duna ['duna] *f* dune; **~ *de areia*** sand dune
duo [duo] *m* MÚS duo
duodeno [duo'denu] *m* duodenum
duplicar [dupli'kaɾ] ⟨1n⟩ **1** *v/t* duplicate **2** *v/i (dobrar)* double
duplicata [dupli'kata] *f* duplicate; **~ *de chave*** duplicate key
duplo ['duplu] **1** *adj* double; **~ *clique*** *m* double click; ***fazer ~ clique em*** double click on; ***cama dupla*** double bed **2** *fpl tênis*: ***duplas*** doubles
duque ['duki] *m* duke
duquesa [du'keza] *f* duchess
durabilidade [duɾabili'dadʒi] *f* durability
duração [duɾa'sãw] *f* duration; **~ *do vôo*** flight time
duradouro [duɾa'doɾu] *adj* lasting
durante [du'ɾãtʃi] *prep* during; **~ *quatro anos*** for four years; **~ *o dia*** by day, in the daytime; **~ *a minha vida*** in my lifetime, throughout my life; **~ *todo*** throughout
durar [du'ɾaɾ] ⟨1a⟩ *v/i* last; **~ *mais que*** outlast
durável [du'ɾavew] *adj* durable; *relação* lasting
durex® [du'ɾɛks] *m* Scotch tape®, *Brit* sellotape®
dureza [du'ɾeza] *f* hardness; *(crueldade)* harshness
durmo ['duɾmu] *etc* → ***dormir***
duro ['duɾu] *adj* hard; *castigo* harsh; *carne, pessoa* tough; *fam* ***estar ~*** *sem dinheiro* be broke; *fam* ***dar um ~ em alguém*** come down hard on s.o.
dúvida ['duvida] *f* doubt; *(pergunta)* query; ***estar em ~*** be in doubt; ***pôr em ~*** question; ***sem ~*** undoubtedly; ***ter ~*** have doubts; ***não há ~*** there's no doubt
duvidar [duvi'daɾ] ⟨1a⟩ **1** *v/i* have one's doubts; **~ *que*** doubt that; **~ *de*** doubt **2** *v/t* doubt
duvidoso [duvi'dozu] *adj* doubtful; *(suspeito)* dubious
duzentos [du'zẽtus] *num* two hundred
dúzia ['duzja] *f* dozen; ***meia ~ (de)*** half a dozen
DVD [deve'de] *m* DVD

E

e [e] *conj* and; **~ *a minha mãe?*** what about my mother?; **~ *assim por diante*** and so on
é [ɛ] → ***ser***
ébano ['ɛbanu] *m* ebony
ébrio ['ɛbɾiu] **1** *adj* drunk **2** *m/f* drunkard
ebulição [ebuli'sãw] *f* ⟨*sem pl*⟩ *água*:

boiling; ***ponto*** *m* ***de ~*** boiling point
ebuliente [ebuli'ẽtʃi] *adj* boiling
eclesiástico [ekle'zjastʃiku] **1** *adj* ecclesiastical **2** *m* clergyman
eclético [e'klɛtʃiku] *adj* eclectic
eclipsar [ekli'psaɾ] ⟨1a⟩ *v/t* eclipse *tb fig*; **eclipsar-se** *v/r* disappear
eclipse [e'klipsi] *m* eclipse *tb fig*; ***~ da lua / do sol*** eclipse of the moon / sun
eco ['ɛku] *m* echo; ***ter ~*** have repercussions
ecoar [e'kwaɾ] ⟨1f⟩ *v/i & v/t* echo
ecografia [ɛkogɾa'fia] *f* MED ultrasound
ecologia [ekolo'ʒia] *f* ecology
ecologicamente [ekoloʒika'mẽtʃi] *adv* ecologically; ***~ correto*** ecologically friendly
ecológico [eko'lɔʒiku] *adj* ecological; (*que respeita o meio ambiente*) green; ***reserva*** *f* ***ecológica*** nature reserve; ***sistema*** *m* ***~*** ecosystem
ecologista [ekolo'ʒista] *m/f* ecologist
economia [ekono'mia] *f* economy; (*poupança*) savings; *ciência* economics *sg*; ***fazer ~s*** save; ***~ informal*** black market economy; ***~ livre de mercado*** free market economy; ***~ de mercado*** market economy; ***~ mundial*** global economy
economicamente [ekonomika'mẽtʃi] *adv* economically
econômico, *Port* **económico** [eko'nomiku] *adj* economic; (*que não gasta*) economical; *pessoa* thrifty; (*barato*) cheap; ***classe*** *f* ***econômica*** economy class; ***crescimento*** *m* ***~*** economic growth; ***ser ~ com*** be sparing with
economista [ekono'mista] *m/f* economist
economizador [ekonomiza'doɾ] *adj pessoa* economical
economizar [ekonomi'zaɾ] ⟨1a⟩ **1** *v/t* economize on, save; (*poupar*) save up; ***~ em*** economize on; ***~ para*** save up for **2** *v/i* economize; (*poupar*) save up
ecossistema [ɛkosis'tema] *m* ecosystem
ecoturismo [ɛkotu'ɾizmu] *m* ecotourism
ecrã, écran [ɛ'kɾã] *m Port* screen; ***~ táctil*** *ou* ***sensível ao toque*** touch screen
ecumênico, *Port* **ecuménico** [eku'meniku] *adj* ecumenical
eczema [ek'zema] *f* eczema; (*irritação*) rash
edição [edʒi'sãw] *f* (*publicação*) publication; (*conjunto de exemplares*) edition; TV editing; ***~ extra*** special edition; ***~ de imagem*** video editing
edicto [e'dʒitu] *m Port* edict
edificação [edʒifika'sãw] *f* ⟨*sem pl*⟩ construction; *fig moral* edification
edificar [edʒifi'kaɾ] ⟨1n⟩ **1** *v/t* construct; *fig* edify **2** *v/i* be edifying
edifício [edʒi'fisiu] *m* building
edital [edʒi'taw] *m* announcement
editar [edʒi'taɾ] ⟨1a⟩ *v/t* edit; (*publicar*) publish
edito [e'dʒitu] *m Bras* edict
editor [edʒi'toɾ] *m* publisher; (*redator*) editor; ***~ de esportes / política*** sports / political editor
editora [edʒi'toɾa] *f* (***casa*** *f*) ***~*** publishing company
editoração [edʒitoɾa'sãw] *f* ***~ eletrônica*** desktop publishing
editoria [edʒito'ɾia] *f* section; ***~ de esportes*** sports desk
editorial [edʒito'ɾjaw] **1** *adj* publishing *atr* **2** *m* editorial
edredão [edɾe'dãw] *m Port* quilt
edredom [edɾe'dõ] *m* ⟨*pl* -ns⟩ *Bras* quilt
educação [eduka'sãw] *f* education; (*criação*) upbringing; *de animais* training; (*maneiras*) manners; ***sem ~*** uneducated; (*grosseiro*) rude; ***é falta de ~ …*** it is rude to …
educadamente [edukada'mẽtʃi] *adv* politely
educado [edu'kadu] *adj* (***bem***) ***~*** polite; (*com boas maneiras*) well-mannered
educador [eduka'doɾ] *m*, **-a** *f* educator
educar [edu'kaɾ] ⟨1n⟩ *v/t* educate; (*criar*) bring up; *animal* train
educativo [eduka'tʃivu] *adj* educational

efect... *Port* → ***efet...***
efeito [e'fejtu] *m* effect; (*resultado*) result; ***fazer ~*** work, have an effect; ***com ~*** indeed ***~ colateral*** side effect; CINE ***~s*** *pl* ***especiais*** special effects; ***~ de estufa*** greenhouse effect; ***~s*** *pl* ***sonoros*** sound effects
efêmero, *Port* **efémero** [e'femeru] *adj* ephemeral
efeminado [efemi'nadu] *adj* effeminate
efervescência [eferves'sẽsja] *f* fizz; *fig* effervescence
efervescente [eferves'sẽtʃi] *adj* fizzy; *fig* effervescent
efetivar [efetʃi'var] ⟨1a⟩ *v/t* bring into effect; (*realizar*) carry out; *professor, estagiário* take on permanently
efetividade [efetʃivi'dadʒi] *f* effectiveness; (*realidade*) reality
efetivo [efe'tʃivu] **1** *adj* (*eficaz*) effective; (*real*) actual, real; (*permanente*) permanent **2** *m* FIN liquid assets
efetuar [efe'twar] ⟨1g⟩ *v/t* carry out; ***~ um ataque*** carry out an attack; **efetuar-se** *v/r* happen, take place
eficácia [efi'kasja] *f método*: effectiveness; *pessoa*: efficiency
eficaz [efi'kas] *adj pessoa* efficient; *meio, método* effective
eficiência [efi'sjẽsja] *f* → ***eficácia***
eficiente [efi'sjẽtʃi] *adj* → ***eficaz***
Egi(p)to [e'ʒitu] *m* Egypt
egípcio [e'ʒipsiu] **1** *adj* Egyptian **2** *m*, **-a** *f* Egyptian
ego ['ɛgu] *m* PSICOL ego
egocêntrico [ego'sẽtriku] *adj* egocentric
egoísmo [ego'izmu] *m* selfishness, egoism
egoísta [ego'ista] **1** *adj* selfish, egoistic **2** *m/f* egoist
égua ['ɛgwa] *f* mare
eiró [ej'rɔ] *f* → ***enguia***
eis [ejs] *pron* here is; *pl* here are
eixo ['ejʃu] *m* axle; MAT axis; *de máquina* shaft; ***entrar nos ~s*** get back on the straight and narrow; ***pôr algo nos ~s*** get sth straight; ***sair dos ~s*** step out of line
ejaculação [eʒakula'sãw] *f* ejaculation
ejacular [eʒaku'lar] ⟨1a⟩ **1** *v/t* ejaculate; *líquido* spurt **2** *v/i* ejaculate
ejetar [eʒe'tar] ⟨1c⟩ **1** *v/t* eject **2** *v/i de um avião* eject
ela ['ɛla] *pron* she; *coisa* it; *com prep* her; ***a ~*** to her; ***com ~*** with her; ***para ~*** for her; ***~ mesma*** herself; ***~s*** → ***eles***
elã [e'lã] *m* enthusiasm
elaboração [elabora'sãw] *f* development; (*preparação*) preparation
elaboradamente [elaborada'mẽtʃi] *adv* elaborately
elaborado [elabo'radu] *adj* elaborate
elaborar [elabo'rar] ⟨1e⟩ *v/t* (*preparar*) prepare; (*fazer*) make
elasticidade [elastʃisi'dadʒi] *f* elasticity; *fig* suppleness
elástico [e'lastʃiku] **1** *adj* elastic; (*feito com elástico*) elasticated; (*flexível*) flexible; *colchão* springy; *tecido etc* stretchy **2** *m* elastic band
ele ['eli] *pron* he; *coisa* it; *com prep* him; ***a ~*** to him; ***com ~*** with him; ***para ~*** for him; ***~ mesmo*** himself
elect... *Port* → ***elet...***
elefante [ele'fãtʃi] *m* elephant; *fig* ***~ branco*** white elephant
elegância [ele'gãsja] *f roupa*: elegance; ***com ~*** smartly, elegantly
elegante [ele'gãtʃi] *adj* elegant
elegantemente [elegãtʃɪ'mẽtʃi] *adv* elegantly
eleger [ele'ʒer] ⟨2h⟩ *v/t* elect; (*escolher*) choose; ***~ para*** elect to
elegível [ele'ʒivew] *adj* eligible
eleição [elej'sãw] *f* election; (*escolha*) choice; ***eleições gerais*** general election; ***eleições municipais*** local elections
eleitor [elej'tor] *m*, **-a** *f* voter, elector
eleitoral [elejto'raw] *adj* electoral
eleitorado [elejto'radu] *m* electorate
elementar [elemẽ'tar] *adj* elementary; (*fundamental*) rudimentary
elemento [ele'mẽtu] *m* element *tb* QUÍM; (*parte*) component; (*recurso*) means *sg*; (*informação*) grounds; ***~s indesejáveis*** undesirable elements
elenco [e'lẽku] *m* list; TEAT cast; ***escolher o ~ de*** cast
eles ['elis], **elas** ['ɛlas] *pron pl* they; ***a ~***

to them; ***com ~*** with them; ***para ~*** for them
eletivo [ele'tʃivu] *adj* elective
eletrão [ele'trãw] *m* electron
eletricidade [eletrisi'dadʒi] *f* electricity; **~ *estática*** static electricity
eletricista [eletri'sista] *m/f* electrician
elétrico [e'lɛtriku] **1** *adj* electric; *fig agitado* worked up; ***cabo*** *m* **~** electric cable; ***rede*** *f* ***elétrica*** power grid **2** *m Port* streetcar, *Brit* tram
eletrificar [eletrifi'kar] ⟨1n⟩ *v/t* electrify *tb fig*
eletrocardiograma [elɛtrokardjo'grama] *m* MED electrocardiogram
eletrocutar [eletroku'tar] ⟨1a⟩ *v/t* electrocute
eletródio [ele'trɔdiu] *m*, **elétrodo** [e'lɛtrudu] *m* electrode
eletrodoméstico [elɛtrodo'mɛstʃiku] *m* **~*s*** *pl* (electrical) household appliances
eletrólito [ele'trɔlitu] *m* electrolyte
eletrônica, *Port* **electrónica** [ele'tronika] *f* electronics
eletrônico, *Port* **electrónico** [ele'troniku] *adj* electronic
elevação [eleva'sãw] *f* elevation; (*aumento*) rise; *ato* raising; (*altura*) height; (*promoção*) promotion; (*ponto elevado*) bump
elevado [ele'vadu] *adj* high; *pensamento*, *estilo* elevated; *luzes etc* overhead
elevador [eleva'dor] *m* elevator, *Brit* lift; **~ *de serviço*** service elevator
elevar [ele'var] ⟨1c⟩ *v/t* (*levantar*) lift up; *preço*, *voz* raise; (*promover*) promote; *efeito*, *tensão* heighten
eliminação [elimina'sãw] *f* elimination
eliminado [elimi'nadu] *adj* ESP ***ficar ~*** be eliminated, be knocked out
eliminar [elimi'nar] ⟨1a⟩ *v/t* eliminate; (*excluir*) rule out; ESP knock out; MED expel
eliminatória [elimina'tɔrja] *f concurso*: test; ESP heat, preliminary round
elite [e'litʃi] *f* élite
elo ['ɛlu] *m* link
elogiar [elo'ʒjar] ⟨1g⟩ *v/t* praise; **~ *alguém por algo*** praise s.o. on sth
elogio [elo'ʒiu] *m* praise
eloqüência, *Port* **eloquência** [elo'kwẽsja] *f* eloquence
eloqüente, *Port* **eloquente** [elo'kwẽtʃi] *adj* eloquent
elucidação [elusida'sãw] *f* elucidation
elucidar [elusi'dar] ⟨1a⟩ *v/t* elucidate, clarify
em [ẽ] *prep* ◊ *lugar*: in; (*sobre*) on; **~ *casa*** at home; **~ *Portugal*** in Portugal; ***na mesa*** on the table; ***de casa ~ casa*** from house to house; ***na esquina*** on the corner, at the corner; ***na mercearia*** at the grocery store, *Brit* at the grocer's; ***na pauta*** on the agenda; ***no andar acima*** on the floor above; ***no chão*** on the ground
◊ *tempo*: in; **~ *3 semanas*** in three weeks; ***no dia primeiro de …*** on the 1st of …; ***no final de julho*** at the end of July
◊ *modo*: in; **~ *português*** in Portuguese; ***ser bom / mau ~*** be good / bad at; ***crescer ~ 15%*** grow by 15%
emagrecer [emagre'ser] ⟨2g⟩ *v/i* lose weight, slim
emagrecimento [emagresi'mẽtu] *m* slimming
emancipação [emãsipa'sãw] *f* ⟨*sem pl*⟩ emancipation; (*atingir a maioridade*) coming of age; **~ *das mulheres*** women's liberation
emancipado [emãsi'padu] *adj* emancipated; *mulher etc* liberated
emancipar [emãsi'par] ⟨1a⟩ *v/t* emancipate; **emancipar-se** *v/r* become emancipated; *mulher* become liberated
embaçado [ẽba'sadu] *adj vidro* steamed up; *olhos* misty
embaçar [ẽba'sar] ⟨1b & 1p⟩ **1** *v/t* steam up **2** *v/i* steam up; *olhos* grow misty
embaixada [ẽbaj'ʃada] *f* embassy
embaixador [ẽbajʃa'dor] *m*, **-a** *f* ambassador *tb fig*
embaixatriz [ẽbajʃa'tris] *f* ambassador; *esposa* ambassador's wife
embaixo [ẽ'bajʃu] **1** *adv* below **2** *prep* **~ *de*** beneath, under
embalagem [ẽba'laʒẽ] *f* packing; (*in-*

E

vólucro) packaging
embalar [ẽba'lar] ⟨1b⟩ pack; *com invólucro* package; *bebê etc* rock; ***embalado a vácuo*** vacuum-packed
embaraçado [ẽbara'sadu] *adj* embarrassed; (*difícil*) difficult
embaraçar [ẽbara'sar] ⟨1p & 1b⟩ *v/t* (*dificultar*) complicate; (*constranger*) embarrass
embaraço [ẽba'rasu] *m* obstacle; (*constrangimento*) embarrassment
embaralhado [ẽbara'ʎadu] *adj* messy
embaralhar [ẽbara'ʎar] ⟨1a⟩ *v/t cartas* shuffle
embarcação [ẽbarka'sãw] *f* vessel
embarcar [ẽbar'kar] ⟨1n & 1b⟩ **1** *v/t* embark, take on board **2** *v/i* embark, go on board; ~ ***em*** *nova fase* embark on
embargar [ẽbar'gar] ⟨1o & 1b⟩ seize; ***a obra foi embargada*** building works have been stopped
embargo [ẽ'bargu] *m* (*confiscação*) seizure; COM embargo; DIR objection
embarque [ẽ'barki] *m* embarcation; AERO boarding; *mercadoria, bagagens*: loading; ***cartão*** *m* ***de*** ~ boarding card; ***sala*** *f* ***de*** ~ departure lounge; ***porta*** *f* ***de*** ~ boarding gate
embate [ẽ'batʃi] *m* clash; (*choque*) shock
embater [ẽba'ter] ⟨2b⟩ ~ ***em*** collide with
embebedar [ẽbebe'dar] ⟨1c⟩ *v/t* make drunk; **embebedar-se** *v/r* get drunk
embeber [ẽbe'ber] ⟨2c⟩ absorb, soak up
embelezar [ẽbele'zar] ⟨1c⟩ *v/t pessoa* make beautiful; *casa* do up
embevecer [ẽbeve'ser] ⟨2g⟩ enchant
emblema [ẽ'blema] *m* emblem
embocadura [ẽboka'dura] *f* mouth; MÚS mouthpiece
embolia [ẽbo'lia] *f* embolism
êmbolo ['ẽbulu] *m* piston
embolorado [ẽbolo'radu] *adj* moldy, *Brit* mouldy
embolsar [ẽbow'sar] ⟨1e⟩ *dinheiro* pocket; *dívidas, credores* pay off
embonecar-se [ẽbonɛ'karsi] ⟨1c & 1n⟩ *v/r fam* get dolled up
embora[1] [ẽ'bɔra] *adv* ***ir-se*** ~ go away; ***mandar*** ~ send away
embora[2] [ẽ'bɔra] *conj* although
emborrachar [ẽboha'ʃar] ⟨1b⟩ make drunk; **emborrachar-se** *v/r* get drunk
emboscada [ẽbos'kada] *f* ambush
emboscar [ẽbos'kada] ⟨1e⟩ *v/t* ambush
embraiagem [ẽbra'jaʒẽ] *f Port* clutch
embranquecer [ẽbrãke'ser] ⟨2g⟩ *v/i* go white
embreagem [ẽbre'aʒẽ] *f Bras* clutch
embrenhar-se [ẽbre'ɲarsi] ⟨1d⟩ penetrate
embriagar [ẽbria'gar] ⟨1o & 1b⟩ make drunk; *fig* intoxicate; **embriagar-se** *v/r* get drunk
embriaguez [ẽbria'ges] *f* drunkenness; (*êxtase*) intoxication
embrião [ẽbri'ãw] *m* embryo
embrionário [ẽbrio'nariu] *adj* embryonic
embrulhada [ẽbru'ʎada] *f* mess
embrulhar [ẽbru'ʎar] ⟨1a⟩ *presente* wrap; *pessoa* cheat; (*confundir*) confuse
embrulho [ẽ'bruʎu] *m* package; *fig* confusion, muddle; ***papel*** *m* ***de*** ~ wrapping paper
embrutecer [ẽbrute'ser] ⟨2g⟩ *v/t* brutalize
emburrado [ẽbu'hadu] *adj* sulky
embuste [ẽ'bustʃi] *m* swindle
embutido [ẽbu'tʃidu] **1** *adj armário* built-in, fitted **2** *m* inlay work
embutir [ẽbu'tʃir] ⟨3a⟩ *v/t* build in
emenda [e'mẽda] *f* (*correção*) amendment; *costura*: alteration
emendar [emẽ'dar] ⟨1a⟩ *erro* correct, amend; *dano, mal* put right; *vestuário* alter; *lei etc* amend; **emendar-se** *v/r fig* improve, change for the better
ementa [e'mẽta] *f Port* menu
emergência [emer'ʒẽsja] *f* (*incidente*) emergency; (*urgência*) urgency; (*surgir*) emergence; POL rise; ***estado*** *m* ***de*** ~ state of emergency; ***descida*** *f* ***de*** ~ emergency exit; ***saída*** *f* ***de*** ~ emergency exit
emergente [emer'ʒẽtʃi] *adj* ***país*** *m* ~ emerging country

emergir [emer'ʒir] ⟨3n & 3c⟩ *v/i* emerge
emigração [emigra'sãw] *f* ⟨*sem pl*⟩ emigration
emigrado [emi'gradu] *m*, **-a** *f* emigrant
emigrante [emi'grãtʃi] *m/f* emigrant
emigrar [emi'grar] ⟨1a⟩ emigrate
eminência [emi'nẽsja] *f* eminence
eminente [emi'nẽtʃi] *adj* eminent
emissão [emi'sãw] *f* emission; *ações*: issue; RÁDIO broadcast
emissário [emi'sariu] *m*, **-a** *f* emissary
emissor [emi'sor] **1** *m*, **-a** *f* transmitter **2** *adj* (***aparelho*** *m*) ~ transmitter; ***banco*** *m* ~ issuing bank
emissora [emi'sora] *f* transmitter, radio station
emitir [emi'tʃir] ⟨3a⟩ *v/t* send out; *cheiro* give off; RÁDIO broadcast; TECN emit; *ações, notas bancárias* issue; *opinião* express; *voto* cast
emoção [emo'sãw] *f* emotion
emocionado [emosjo'nadu] *adj* emotional
emocional [emosjo'naw] *adj* emotional
emocionante [emosjo'nãtʃi] *adj* moving; (*excitante*) exciting
emocionar [emosjo'nar] ⟨1f⟩ *v/t* (*comover*) move; (*excitar*) excite; **emocionar-se** *v/r* get emotional
emoldurar [emowdu'rar] ⟨1a⟩ *v/t* frame
emotivo [emo'tʃivu] *adj* emotive
empacotar [ẽpako'tar] ⟨1e⟩ *v/t* pack
empada [ẽ'pada] *f* pie
empadão [ẽpa'dãw] *m* GASTR pie
empalidecer [ẽpalide'ser] ⟨2g⟩ *v/i* go pale
empanar [ẽpa'nar] ⟨1a⟩ *v/t metal* tarnish; ***o carro está empanado*** the car has broken down
empanturrar [ẽpãtu'har] ⟨1a⟩ *v/t* cram; **empanturrar-se** *v/r* ~ ***de algo*** gorge oneself on sth
emparedar [ẽpare'dar] ⟨1c⟩ *v/t* wall up; *pessoa* close in
empatado [ẽpa'tadu] *adj* drawn; *xadrez*: in stalemate; *dinheiro* tied up
empatar [ẽpa'tar] ⟨1b⟩ **1** *v/t* (*impedir*) hinder; *número de votos* tie; COM *dinheiro* ~ ***em*** tie up in **2** *v/i* ESP *jogo* draw, tie; *gol de empate*: level the score, *Brit* equalize
empate [ẽ'patʃi] *m votos*: tie, tied vote; ESP draw, tie; *xadrez*: stalemate; ***gol*** *m* ***de*** ~ goal that levels the score, *Brit* equalizer
empatia [ẽpa'tʃia] *f* empathy; ***ter*** ~ ***com*** empathize with
empecilho [ẽpe'siʎu] *m* stumbling block
empedernido [ẽpeder'nidu] *adj* hard-hearted; (*inveterado*) inveterate
empena [ẽ'pena] *f* ARQUIT gable
empenar [ẽpe'nar] ⟨1d⟩ warp
empenhado [ẽpe'ɲadu] *adj* in pawn; (*obrigado*) indebted; (*endividado*) in debt; (*dedicado*) committed; ~ ***em uma causa*** commited to a cause
empenhar [ẽpe'ɲar] ⟨1d⟩ *v/t* pawn; (*dedicar*) commit; **empenhar-se** *v/r* put oneself in debt; ~ ***em*** commit onself to, get really involved in; ~ ***por*** support
empenho [ẽ'peɲu] *m* (*esforço*) input; *objeto*: pawning; ~ ***em uma causa*** commitment to a cause
empenhorar [ẽpeɲo'rar] ⟨1e⟩ *v/t* pawn
emperrar [ẽpe'har] ⟨1c⟩ **1** *v/t janela* jam **2** *v/i* jam; *motor* seize up
empestar [ẽpes'tar] ⟨1a⟩ *v/t* infect; *com cheiro* stink out
empilhadeira [ẽpiʎa'dejra] *f* fork-lift truck
empilhar [ẽpi'ʎar] ⟨1a⟩ pile up
empipocado [ẽpipo'kadu] *adj* spotty
empírico [ẽ'piriku] *adj* empirical
empobrecer [ẽpobre'ser] ⟨2g⟩ **1** *v/t* impoverish **2** *v/i* become impoverished
empobrecido [ẽpobre'sidu] *adj* impoverished
empobrecimento [ẽpobresi'mẽtu] *m* impoverishment
empoeirado [ẽpwe'radu] *adj* dusty
empoeirar [ẽpwe'rar] ⟨1a⟩ make dusty; **empoeirar-se** *v/r* get dusty
empolar [ẽpo'lar] ⟨1e⟩ *v/i* blister
empoleirado [ẽpolej'radu] *adj* ~ ***numa árvore*** high up in a tree; ~ ***numa função*** in an exalted position

E

empoleirar-se [ẽpolej'ɾaɾsi] ⟨1a⟩ *v/r galinha* perch; *fig* rise to high office
empolgação [ẽpowga'sãw] *f* excitement
empolgante [ẽpow'gãtʃi] *adj* exciting, thrilling
empolgar [ẽpow'gaɾ] ⟨1o & 1e⟩ *v/t* excite, thrill
empossar [ẽpo'saɾ] ⟨1e⟩ *cargo*: appoint; **empossar-se** *v/r* **~ de** take possession of
empreendedor [ẽpɾeẽde'doɾ] **1** *adj* enterprising; COM entrepreneurial **2** *m* entrepreneur
empreender [ẽpɾeẽ'deɾ] ⟨2a⟩ *v/t* undertake
empreendimento [ẽpɾeẽde'mẽtu] *m* undertaking; **~ *conjunto*** joint venture
empregado [ẽpɾe'gadu] **1** *adj* employed **2** *m*, **-a** *f* employee; *Port de mesa* waiter; waitress; *Port* **~ *de bar*** bartender, *Brit* barman; barmaid
empregar [ẽpɾe'gaɾ] ⟨1o & 1c⟩ employ; *algo, força, palavra* use; *dinheiro* invest; **empregar-se** *v/r* get a job
emprego [ẽ'pɾegu] *m* job; (*lugar de trabalho*) place of work; (*utilização*) use; ***sem* ~** out of work; **~ *remunerado*** paid employment; ***procurar* ~** seek employment, look for a job; ***pleno* ~** full employment; ***de* ~** instructions for use
empreiteiro [ẽpɾej'tejɾu] *m*, **-a** *f* contractor
empresa [ẽ'pɾeza] *f* company, firm; ***trabalhar na* ~** work in-house; **~ *de consultoria*** consultancy firm; **~ *matriz*** parent company
empresariado [ẽpɾeza'ɾjadu] *m* employers
empresarial [ẽpɾeza'ɾjaw] *adj* business *atr*, corporate
empresário [ẽpɾe'zaɾiu] *m* entrepreneur; MÚS *etc* impresario
emprestador [ẽpɾesta'doɾ] *m*, **-a** *f* lender
emprestar [ẽpɾes'taɾ] ⟨1c⟩ lend, loan
empréstimo [ẽ'pɾestʃimu] *m* loan; ***de* ~, *por* ~** on loan; **~ *bancário*** bank loan; **~ *sem juros*** interest-free loan
empurrão [ẽpu'hãw] *m* push; ***ela saiu da sala aos empurrões*** she pushed her way out of the room
empurrar [ẽpu'haɾ] ⟨1a⟩ push
emular [ẽpu'haɾ] ⟨1a⟩ *v/t* emulate
emulsão [emuw'sãw] *f* emulsion
enamorar-se [enamo'ɾaɾsi] ⟨1e⟩ *v/r* fall in love (***de*** with)
encabeçar [ẽkabe'saɾ] ⟨1p & 1c⟩ lead, head
encadeamento [ẽkadʒia'mẽtu] *m* chain; (*ligação*) link
encadear [ẽka'dʒiaɾ] ⟨1l⟩ chain; (*ligar*) chain together, link up; *idéias* link; (*enfileirar*) line up
encadernação [ẽkadeɾna'sãw] *f* binding
encadernar [ẽkadeɾ'naɾ] ⟨1c⟩ *v/t* bind
encaixar [ẽkaj'ʃaɾ] ⟨1a⟩ **1** *v/t* (*embalar*) pack; (*enfiar*) fit in; (*juntar*) fit together **2** *v/i* fit; **encaixar-se** *v/r* slot in, fit in
encaixe [ẽ'kajʃi] *m* fitting; (*ranhura*) groove; (*junção*) join
encaixilhar [ẽkajʃi'ʎaɾ] ⟨1a⟩ *v/t* frame
encaixotar [ẽkajʃo'taɾ] ⟨1e⟩ *v/t* put into boxes
encalhar [ẽka'ʎaɾ] ⟨1b⟩ *v/i barco* run aground; *fig* get stuck
encaminhar [ẽkami'ɲaɾ] ⟨1a⟩ put in motion; **~ *alguém para um lugar*** direct s.o. to a place; **~ *um pedido para outro departamento*** refer a request to another department
encanador [ẽkana'doɾ] *m*, **-a** *f* plumber
encantador [ẽkãta'doɾ] *adj* enchanting; *floresta* enchanted
encantamento [ẽkãta'mẽtu] *m* (*bruxedo*) spell; ***ter* ~ *por alguém*** hold a fascination for s.o.
encantar [ẽkã'taɾ] ⟨1a⟩ bewitch; *fig* enchant, delight
encanto [ẽ'kãtu] *m* charm; (*deleite*) delight
encaração [ẽkaɾa'sãw] *f* stare
encaracolado [ẽkaɾako'ladu] *adj* curly
encaracolar [ẽkaɾako'laɾ] ⟨1e⟩ *cabelo* curl; **encaracolar-se** *v/r cabelo* curl
encarado [ẽka'ɾadu] *adj* ***bem* ~** good-

looking; (*simpático*) nice; (*amável*) friendly; ***mal*** **~** ugly; (*doente*) ill-looking; (*de mau humor*) grumpy; (*sombrio*) gloomy

encarar [ẽka'ɾaɾ] ⟨1b⟩ stare at; (*olhar*) look at; *perigo*, *dificuldade* face up to; **~ *algo com tranqüilidade*** take sth in one's stride

encarcerar [ẽkaɾse'ɾaɾ] ⟨1c⟩ *v/t* imprison

encardido [ẽkaɾ'dʒidu] *adj* dirty

encarecer [ẽkaɾe'seɾ] ⟨2g⟩ **1** *v/t* make more expensive, raise the price of **2** *v/i* get more expensive

encarecidamente [ẽkaɾesida'mẽtʃi] *adv* fervently

encarecimento [ẽkaɾesi'mẽtu] *m* price increase

encargo [ẽ'kaɾgu] *m* job, task; (*obrigação*) responsibility; (*imposto*) burden

encarnação [ẽkaɾna'sãw] *f* incarnation

encarnado [ẽkaɾ'nadu] *adj* scarlet

encaroçado [ẽkaɾo'sadu] *adj* lumpy

encaroçar [ẽkaɾo'saɾ] ⟨1e⟩ *farinha etc* go lumpy; (*endurecer*) go hard; (*inchar*) swell up

encarregado [ẽkahe'gadu] *m*, **-a** *f* person in charge; *construção*, *fábrica*: foreman; POL **~ *de negócios*** chargé d'affaires

encarregar [ẽkahe'gaɾ] ⟨1o & 1c⟩ **~ *alguém de algo*** make s.o. responsible for sth; **~ *alguém de fazer algo*** give s.o. the job of doing sth; **encarregar-se** *v/r* **~ *de algo*** take sth on, deal with sth

encarte [ẽ'kaɾtʃi] *m* insert

encastrado [ẽkas'tɾadu] *adj* built-in, fitted; ***cozinha*** *f* ***encastrada*** fitted kitchen

encavacado [ẽkava'kadu] *adj fam* (*envergonhado*) embarrassed

encenação [ẽsena'sãw] *f* staging; (*representação*) production

encenador [ẽsena'doɾ] *m*, **-a** *f* TEAT director

encenar [ẽse'naɾ] ⟨1d⟩ *v/t* stage, put on

encerar [ẽse'ɾaɾ] ⟨1c⟩ *v/t* wax

encerramento [ẽseha'mẽtu] *m loja etc*: closure; COM close of business; ***ato*** *m* ***de*** **~**, *Port* ***acto*** *m* ***de*** **~** final act; ***balanço*** *m* ***de*** **~** closing balance

encerrar [ẽse'haɾ] ⟨1c⟩ *loja etc* close; *em cofre*, *gaveta etc* shut in; (*concluir*) conclude, close; (*conter*) contain; ***encerrado para férias*** closed for holidays

encetar [ẽse'taɾ] ⟨1c⟩ (*começar*) start

encharcar [ẽʃaɾ'kaɾ] ⟨1n & 1b⟩ (*inundar*) flood; *roupa* soak; **encharcar-se** *v/r* be flooded; *roupa* get soaked; *fig* **~ *em*** drown in

enchente [ẽ'ʃẽtʃi] *f* flood

encher [ẽ'ʃeɾ] ⟨2a⟩ **1** *v/t* fill; *balão* blow up; *pneu* inflate; **~ *alguém de elogios*** heap praises on s.o.; **~ *os bolsos*** line one's own pockets **2** *v/i maré* rise; *lua* wax; **encher-se** *v/r* fill up; *fam* get rich; **~ *de*** fill with; *esperança*, *coragem* take; *paciência etc* show; *fig ódio* feel

enchido [ẽ'ʃidu] *m* cured meat

enchimento [ẽʃi'mẽtu] *m* stuffing

enchova [ẽ'ʃova] *f* anchovy

enciclopédia [ẽsiklo'pɛdʒia] *f* encyclopedia

enciclopédico [ẽsiklo'pɛdʒiku] *adj* encyclopedic

encoberto [ẽko'bɛɾtu] *adj* (*velado*) concealed; *céu* overcast

encobrimento [ẽkobɾi'mẽtu] *m* cover-up

encobrir [ẽko'bɾiɾ] ⟨3f⟩ *v/t* conceal, hide; *crime*, *escândalo etc* cover up; **~ *alguém*** cover up for s.o.

encolher [ẽko'ʎeɾ] ⟨2d⟩ **1** *v/t membro* pull in; (*encurtar*) shorten; **~ *os ombros*** shrug one's shoulders **2** *v/i tecido* shrink; **encolher-se** *v/r de frio* hunch up; *em grupo* huddle together; *de vergonha* squirm

encomenda [ẽko'mẽda] *f* order; ***confirmação*** *f* ***de*** **~** order confirmation; **~ *postal*** postal parcel; ***de*** **~** to order; (*por medida*) made to order

encomendar [ẽkomẽ'daɾ] ⟨1a⟩ **~ *algo a alguém*** order sth from s.o.

encompridar [ẽkõpɾi'daɾ] ⟨1a⟩ *v/t* lengthen

encontrão [ẽkõ'tɾãw] *m* collision

encontrar [ẽkõ'tɾaɾ] ⟨1a⟩ *v/t coisa*

E

find; *idéia* hit on; (*ir de encontro*) come across; *pessoa* meet; *problemas* encounter; **encontrar-se** *v/r* meet; (*estar*) be; **~ com** meet; **encontrava-se à porta** he was standing by the door
encontro [ẽ'kõtru] *m* meeting; **ir / vir ao ~ de alguém** go / come to meet s.o.; **marcar ~** arrange a meeting; **~ às cegas** blind date
encorajador [ẽkoraʒa'dor] *adj* encouraging
encorajamento [ẽkoraʒa'mẽtu] *m* encouragement
encorajar [ẽkora'ʒar] ⟨1b⟩ *v/t* encourage
encorpado [ẽkor'padu] *adj* corpulent; *vinho* full-bodied
encosta [ẽ'kɔsta] *f* slope
encostar [ẽkos'tar] ⟨1e⟩ **1** *v/t* lean; *carro* park; *porta* leave ajar **2** *v/i motorista* pull over; **encostar-se** *v/r* lean; *na cadeira* lean back; *fig* **ela se encostou a mim** she got me to bail her out
encosto [ẽ'kostu] *m* back; (*apoio*) support
encravado [ẽkra'vadu] *adj unha* ingrowing; **estar ~** be stuck
encravar-se [ẽkra'varsi] ⟨1b⟩ *v/r* get stuck; *unha* grow in
encrenca [ẽ'krẽka] *f* mess, fix
encrencar [ẽkrẽ'kar] ⟨1n⟩ *v/t situação* complicate
encrenqueiro [ẽkrẽ'kejru] *m*, **-a** *f* troublemaker
encriptação [ẽkripta'sãw] *f* INFORM encryption; **~ de dados** data encryption
encriptar [ẽkrip'tar] ⟨1a⟩ *v/t dados* encrypt
encruzilhada [ẽkruzi'ʎada] *f* crossroads *sg*
encurralar [ẽkuha'lar] ⟨1a⟩ *v/t pessoa* corner
encurtar [ẽkur'tar] ⟨1a⟩ *v/t* shorten; **~ razões** be brief; **encurtar-se** *v/r* get shorter
encurvar [ẽkur'var] ⟨1a⟩ bend; **encurvar-se** *v/r* bend
endêmico [ẽ'demiku] *adj* endemic
endereçar [ẽdere'sar] ⟨1p & 1c⟩ (*dirigir*) direct; *carta* address; (*enviar*) send
endereço [ẽde'resu] *m esp Bras* address; **~ eletrônico** email address
endiabrado [ẽdʒia'bradu] *adj* devilish
endinheirado [ẽdʒiɲe'radu] *adj* well-off, monied
endireitar [ẽdʒirej'tar] ⟨1a⟩ *v/t* straighten; *fig* straighten out; **endireitar-se** *v/r* straighten up
endívia [ẽ'dʒivja] *f* endive
endividado [ẽdʒivi'dadu] *adj* in debt
endividamento [ẽdʒivida'mẽtu] *m* debt
endividar [ẽdʒivi'dar] ⟨1a⟩ put into debt; **endividar-se** *v/r* get into debt
endoidecer [ẽdojdʒi'ser] ⟨2g⟩ **1** *v/t* make mad **2** *v/i* go mad
endossar [ẽdo'sar] ⟨1e⟩ endorse
endosso [ẽ'dosu] *m* endorsement
endurecer [ẽdure'ser] ⟨2g⟩ harden
endurecimento [ẽduresi'mẽtu] *m* hardening
enegrecer [enegre'ser] ⟨2g⟩ **1** *v/t* darken; *fig* blacken **2** *v/i* darken; **enegrecer-se** *v/r* darken
energético [ener'ʒɛtʃiku] *adj* FÍS energy *atr*; **fonte** *f* **energética** source of energy
energia [ener'ʒia] *f* energy; **~ elétrica** energy, power; **~ eólica** wind power; **~ nuclear** nuclear energy; **~ solar** solar power; **~s** *pl* **renováveis** renewable energy, renewable energy sources
enérgico [e'nɛrʒiku] *adj* energetic; *caráter* forceful
enervar [ener'var] ⟨1c⟩ irritate; **enervar-se** *v/r* get irritated
enevoado [ene'vwadu] *adj* misty
enfadar [ẽfa'dar] ⟨1b⟩ *v/t* bore; (*irritar*) annoy
enfado [ẽ'fadu] *m* boredom; (*irritação*) annoyance
enfadonho [ẽfa'doɲu] *adj* boring; (*irritando*) annoying
enfarte [ẽ'fartʃi] *m* MED coronary; **~ do miocárdio** heart attack
ênfase ['ẽfazi] *f* emphasis
enfático [ẽ'fatʃiku] *adj* emphatic
enfatizar [ẽfatʃi'zar] ⟨1a⟩ *v/t* emphasize

enfeitar [ẽfej'taɾ] ⟨1a⟩ decorate
enfeite [ẽ'fejtʃi] *m* decoration
enfeitiçar [ẽfejtʃi'saɾ] ⟨1p⟩ put a spell on; *fig* bewitch
enfermagem [ẽfeɾ'maʒẽ] *f* nursing; *pessoal* nursing staff
enfermaria [ẽfeɾma'ɾia] *f* ward; *quartel militar*: infirmary
enfermeira [ẽfeɾ'mejɾa] *f* nurse
enfermeiro [ẽfeɾ'mejɾu] *m* (male) nurse
enfermo [ẽ'feɾmu] **1** *adj* ill, sick **2** *m*, **-a** *f* sick person, patient
enferrujado [ẽfehu'ʒadu] *adj* rusty
enferrujar [ẽfehu'ʒaɾ] ⟨1a⟩ *v/i* rust
enfezado [ẽfe'zadu] *adj* (*débil*) puny; (*mal disposto*) morose
enfiada [ẽ'fjada] *f* row; *pérolas*: string; ***de ~*** in a row
enfiar [ẽ'fjaɾ] ⟨1g⟩ **1** *v/t agulha* thread; *pérolas etc* string together; (*meter*) put; *vestuário*, *anel* put on; ***~ o nariz em*** stick one's nose in; ***~ mentiras*** tell lies **2** *v/i* ***enfia por essa rua*** take this street
enfileirar-se [ẽfilej'ɾaɾsi] ⟨1a⟩ *v/r* line up
enfim [ẽ'fĩ] **1** *adv* (*finalmente*) finally **2** *int* ***~!*** oh well!; ***até que ~!*** at last!
enfoque [ẽ'fɔki] *m* approach
enforcar [ẽfoɾ'kaɾ] ⟨1n & 1e⟩ *v/t* hang; **enforcar-se** *v/r* hang oneself
enfraquecer [ẽfɾake'seɾ] ⟨2g⟩ weaken
enfrascar [ẽfɾas'kaɾ] ⟨1n & 1b⟩ bottle
enfrentar [ẽfɾẽ'taɾ] ⟨1a⟩ confront; **enfrentar-se** *v/r exércitos* confront each other; *times* meet; *num debate* face each other
enfurecer [ẽfuɾe'seɾ] ⟨2g⟩ **1** *v/t* infuriate **2** *v/i* get furious; **enfurecer-se** *v/r* get furious; *vento*, *mar* grow wild
enfurecido [ẽfuɾe'sidu] *adj* furious
eng.o *abr* (***engenheiro***) engineer
enganado [ẽga'nadu] *adj* ***ser ~*** be deceived; ***estar ~*** be mistaken
enganador [ẽgana'doɾ] *adj* deceitful; *aparência* deceptive
enganar [ẽga'naɾ] ⟨1a⟩ deceive; *fig tempo*, *dor*, *fome* kill; ***~ alguém para que faça algo*** deceive s.o. into doing sth; **enganar-se** *v/r* be mistaken; (*iludir-se*) deceive oneself
engano [ẽ'ganu] *m* deceit, deception; (*erro*) error; (*ilusão*) deception; ***por ~*** by mistake
enganchar [ẽgã'ʃaɾ] ⟨1a⟩ hook up
engarrafado [ẽgaha'fadu] *adj* bottled; *trânsito* blocked
engarrafamento [ẽŋgahafa'mẽtu] *m* bottling; *fig* blockage; *trânsito*: traffic jam; COM bottleneck
engarrafar [ẽgaha'faɾ] ⟨1b⟩ bottle; *trânsito* block
engasgar-se [ẽgaʒ'gaɾsi] ⟨1b & 1o⟩ *v/r* choke; *fig* get tied up
engatador [ẽgata'doɾ] *m* TECN pawl; *fam* ladies' man
engatar [ẽga'taɾ] ⟨1b⟩ *cavalo* hitch up; FERROV couple; *fam mulher* pick up
engate [ẽ'gatʃi] *m* FERROV coupling; (*erro*) mistake; *fam* (*conquista*) pick-up
engatinhar [ẽgatʃi'ɲaɾ] ⟨1a⟩ crawl; *fig* be feeling one's way
engelhado [ẽʒe'ʎadu] *adj* wrinkled
engelhar [ẽʒe'ʎaɾ] ⟨1c⟩ *vestuário* wrinkle
engenharia [ẽʒeɲa'ɾia] *f* engineering; ***~ genética*** genetic engineering; ***~ mecânica*** mechanical engineering
engenheiro [ẽʒe'ɲejɾu] *m*, **-a** *f* engineer; ***~ agrônomo*** agricultural expert; ***~ civil*** civil engineer
engenho [ẽ'ʒaɲu] *m* ingenuity; (*gênio*) talent; (*máquina*) machine
engenhoca [ẽʒe'ɲɔka] *f* gadget; *pessoa* do-it-yourself whizzkid
engenhoso [ẽʒe'ɲozu] *adj* ingenious
engessar [ẽʒe'saɾ] ⟨1c⟩ *v/t* plaster; *membro* put in plaster
englobar [ẽglo'baɾ] ⟨1e⟩ include
englobável [ẽglo'bavew] *adj rendimento* taxable
engodar [ẽgo'daɾ] ⟨1e⟩ *v/t pesca*, *caça* bait; *pessoa* lure
engodo [ẽ'godu] *m peixe*, *caça*: bait; *pessoa*: lure
engolir [ẽgo'liɾ] ⟨3f⟩ swallow; *fig* ***~ em seco*** swallow it
engordar [ẽgoɾ'daɾ] ⟨1e⟩ **1** *v/t* fatten

E

up; *comida grassa etc* make fat; ~ ***5 kilos*** put on 5 kilos **2** *v/i* put on weight; ***o que não mata, engorda!*** it won't kill you
engraçado [ẽgɾa'sadu] *adj* (*cômico*) funny; (*giro*) cute
engrandecer [ẽgɾãdʒi'seɾ] ⟨2g⟩ (*elevar*) elevate; (*exagerar*) exaggerate
engravidar [ẽgɾavi'daɾ] ⟨1a⟩ **1** *v/t* make pregnant **2** *v/i* get pregnant
engraxador [ẽgɾaʃa'doɾ] *m* shoeshine boy / man
engraxar [ẽgɾa'ʃaɾ] ⟨1b⟩ *sapatos* polish; *cabedal* grease; *fam* ~ ***alguém*** soften s.o. up
engrenagem [ẽgɾe'naʒẽ] *f* gears; (*maquinismo*) machinery; ***roda*** *f* ***de*** ~ cog wheel
engrenar [ẽgɾe'naɾ] ⟨1d⟩ **1** *v/i rodas* engage **2** *v/t* AUTO engage; *fam* get on (***em*** with)
engrossar [ẽgɾo'saɾ] ⟨1e⟩ **1** *v/t* thicken; (*reforçar*) strengthen; (*aumentar*) increase **2** *v/i* thicken; (*inchar*) swell up
enguia [ẽ'gia] *f* eel
enguiçado [ẽgi'sadu] *adj Bras* broken down; *trânsito* stuck
enguiçar [ẽgi'saɾ] ⟨1p⟩ *Bras* **1** *v/t máquina* break **2** *v/i* break down
enguiço [ẽgi'su] *m Bras* breakdown
enigma [e'nigma] *m* enigma
enigmático [enig'matʃiku] *adj* enigmatic
enjeitar [ẽʒej'taɾ] ⟨1a⟩ (*recusar*) reject; *idéia, plano* abandon
enjoado [ẽ'ʒwadu] *adj mania* finicky; ***estou*** ~ I feel sick; (*estou cheio*) I'm fed up
enjoar [ẽ'ʒwaɾ] ⟨1f⟩ *v/t* ~ ***alguém*** make s.o. feel sick
enjôo, *Port* **enjoo** [ẽ'ʒou] *m* (*indisposição*) sickness; (*relutância*) reluctance; ~ ***matinal*** morning sickness
enlaçar [ẽla'saɾ] ⟨1p & 1b⟩ *v/t* (*ligar*) tie
enlace [ẽ'lasi] *m* (*ligação*) connection
enlameado [ẽla'mjadu] *adj* covered in mud
enlatado [ẽla'tadu] **1** *adj* canned **2** *m* canned food
enlatar [ẽla'taɾ] ⟨1b⟩ can
enlouquecer [ẽloke'seɾ] ⟨2g⟩ **1** *v/t* drive mad **2** *v/i* go mad
enluarado [ẽlua'ɾadu] *adj* moonlit
enlutado [ẽlu'tadu] **1** *adj* mourning; *papel* black-edged **2** *m* **-a** *f* mourner
enobrecer [enobɾe'seɾ] ⟨2g⟩ ennoble
enojar [eno'ʒaɾ] ⟨1e⟩ *v/t* disgust
enorme [e'nɔɾmi] *adj* enormous
enormemente [enoɾme'mẽtʃi] *adv* enormously
enormidade [enoɾmi'dadʒi] *f* enormity
enquadrar [ẽkwa'dɾaɾ] ⟨1b⟩ **1** *v/t* frame; (*compreender*) include; ~ ***em*** fit in with **2** *v/i fig* ~ ***em*** (*fazer parte de*) fit in with; (*aderir*) join
enquanto [ẽ'kwãtu] **1** *conj* while; ~ (***que***) whereas; ~ ***isso*** meanwhile **2** *adv* ***por*** ~ for the time being
enraivecer [ẽhajve'seɾ] ⟨2g⟩ **1** *v/t* infuriate **2** *v/i* go wild; **enraivecer-se** *v/r* go wild
enraizar [ẽhai'zaɾ] ⟨1q⟩ **1** *v/t* root **2** *v/i planta* take root; **enraizar-se** *v/r* put down roots
enrascar [ẽhas'kaɾ] ⟨1n & 1b⟩ *v/t coisas* jumble up; *pessoa* put in a difficult situation; *fam* ***estar enrascado*** be in a fix
enredo [ẽ'hedu] *m novela, filme*: plot; (*intriga*) intrigue
enregelar [ẽheʒe'laɾ] ⟨1c⟩ freeze
enrijecer [ẽhiʒe'seɾ] ⟨2g⟩ *v/i* stiffen; **enrijecer-se** *v/r* stiffen
enriquecer [ẽhike'seɾ] ⟨2g⟩ **1** *v/t* enrich **2** *v/i* get rich
enrolar [ẽho'laɾ] ⟨1e⟩ roll up; (*enredar*) wrap up; **enrolar-se** *v/r* curl up; ***a cobra se enrolou no meu braço*** the snake wound itself around my arm
enroscar [ẽhos'kaɾ] ⟨1n & 1e⟩ roll up; *lâmpada* screw in; **enroscar-se** *v/r fig* coil up
enrouquecer [ẽhoke'seɾ] ⟨2c⟩ *v/i* go hoarse
enrugado [ẽhu'gadu] *adj* wrinkled
enrugar [ẽhu'gaɾ] ⟨1o⟩ wrinkle; *vestuário* crease up
ensaboar [ẽsa'bwaɾ] ⟨1f⟩ *v/t* soap; ~ ***o juízo a alguém*** get on s.o.'s nerves
ensaiar [ẽsa'jaɾ] ⟨1b⟩ **1** *v/t* try out;

TEAT rehearse **2** *v/i* TEAT rehearse
ensaio [ẽ'saiu] *m* test, trial; TEAT rehearsal; LIT essay; ***proveta*** *f* (*ou* ***tubo*** *m*) ***de ~*** test tube; ***~ geral*** dress rehearsal
ensaísta [ẽsa'ista] *m/f* essayist
ensangüentado, *Port* **ensanguentado** [ẽsãgwẽ'tadu] *adj* bloodstained, bloody
enseada [ẽ'sjada] *f* bay
ensejo [ẽ'seʒu] *m* opportunity
ensinamento [ẽsina'mẽtu] *m* teaching
ensinar [ẽsi'naɾ] ⟨1a⟩ teach, (*mostrar*) show
ensino [ẽ'sinu] *m* teaching; ***~ secundário*** secondary education
ensolarado [ẽsola'ɾadu] *adj* sunny
ensopado [ẽso'padu] **1** *adj* soaked; ***estar ~ em água*** be soaking wet **2** *m* stew
ensopar [ẽso'paɾ] ⟨1e⟩ soak
ensurdecedor [ẽsuɾdese'doɾ] *adj* deafening
ensurdecer [ẽsuɾde'seɾ] ⟨2g⟩ **1** *v/t* deafen **2** *v/i* go deaf
ensurdecimento [ẽsuɾdesi'mẽtu] *m* deafness
entabular [ẽtabu'laɾ] ⟨1g⟩ *v/t* start
entalado [ẽta'ladu] *adj* ***estar*** (*ou* ***ver-se***) ***~*** be in a tight spot
entalar [ẽta'laɾ] ⟨1b⟩ wedge; *fig* put in a spot; **entalar-se** *v/r* get stuck; *fig* get into a fix
entalhar [ẽta'ʎaɾ] ⟨1b⟩ carve
entalhe [ẽ'taʎi] *m* (*fenda*) notch
entanto [ẽ'tãtu] *conj* ***no ~*** however
então [ẽ'tãw] *conj* then; ***desde ~*** since (then); ***até ~*** up to then; ***~?*** what's going on?; ***e ~?*** so what?; ***ou ~*** or else
ente ['ẽtʃi] *m* entity; (*ser*) being
enteado [ẽ'tʃiadu] *m*, **-a** *f* stepson; step daughter
entediado [ẽtʃi'dʒiadu] *adj* bored
entediante [ẽtʃi'dʒiãtʃi] *adj* boring, tedious
entender [ẽtẽ'deɾ] ⟨2a⟩ **1** *v/t* understand; (*crer, achar*) think; (*querer*) intend; ***~ de algo*** know about sth; ***~ mal*** misunderstand; ***fazer-se ~*** make oneself understood; ***entendido!*** understood! **2** *m* ***no meu ~*** in my opinion; **entender-se** *v/r* ***~*** get along (***com*** with); (*estar de acordo*) be in agreement (***com*** with); (*comunicar*) understand each other; (*perceber de*) be knowledgeable (***de, em*** about)
entendido [ẽtẽ'dʒidu] **1** *adj* knowledgeable; (*de acordo*) agreed **2** *m*, **-a** *f* expert; *fam* gay
entendimento [ẽtẽdʒi'mẽtu] *m* understanding; POL agreement
enternecedor [ẽteɾnese'doɾ] *adj* moving
enternecer [ẽteɾne'seɾ] ⟨2g⟩ move; **enternecer-se** *v/r* be moved
enterrar [ẽte'haɾ] ⟨1c⟩ bury; *fig pessoa, plano* do for; **enterrar-se** *v/r* sink (***em*** into)
enterro [ẽ'tehu] *m* burial
entidade [ẽtʃi'dadʒi] *f* entity; (*ser*) being; (*corporação*) body; ***~ pública*** pubic body
entontecer [ẽtõte'seɾ] ⟨2g⟩ **1** *v/t* make dizzy; (*tirar do sério*) drive mad **2** *v/i* go dizzy; (*ficar fora de si*) go mad
entornar [ẽtoɾ'naɾ] ⟨1e⟩ *v/t* knock over; (*derramar*) spill; *fig* waste; (*beber*) knock back; ***estar entornado*** be drunk
entorpecer [ẽtoɾpe'seɾ] ⟨2g⟩ **1** *v/t* numb **2** *v/i* go numb
entorpecimento [ẽtoɾpesi'mẽtu] *m* numbness
entorse [ẽ'tɔɾsi] *f* MED sprain
entortar [ẽtoɾ'taɾ] ⟨1e⟩ twist; ***~ os olhos*** squint
entrada [ẽ'trada] *f* entrance; *ato* entry; *hospital*: admission; *casa*: doorway; (*bilhete*) ticket; (*início*) start; GASTR starter; TEAT, MÚS entrance; *máquina*: inlet; (*sinal*) downpayment; INFORM input; AERO ***corredor*** *m* ***de ~*** approach path; ***visto*** *m* ***de ~*** entry visa ***200 de ~*** 200 down; ***ter ~s*** have a receding hairline; ***~ proibida*** keep out!; ESP ***~ da área*** goalmouth; ***~ de carro*** driveway; TEAT ***~ em cena*** entrance; ***~ franca*** admission free; ***~ da frente*** front entrance; ***~ grátis*** admission free; ***~ permanente*** season ticket

E

entranhas [ẽ'traɲas] *fpl* entrails
entranhado [ẽtra'ɲadu] *adj* deep; (*enraizado*) deep-rooted
entranhar-se [ẽtra'ɲarsi] ⟨1a⟩ *v/r* penetrate; ***isso se entranhou na minha vida*** this became part of my life
entrar [ẽ'trar] ⟨1d⟩ enter, go in; *de fora*: come in; *carro*: get in; TEAT enter; (*chegar*) arrive, get in; *barco* come in; ***deixar alguém ~*** let s.o. in; ***fazer alguém ~*** show s.o. in; ***entre!*** come in!; ***como eles entraram?*** how did they get in?; ***~ bem, ~ com o pé direito*** get off to a good start; ***~ em transe*** go into a trance; ***~ em vigor*** come into effect; ***~ com algo*** *quantia* put sth in
entravar [ẽtra'var] ⟨1b⟩ obstruct; (*impedir*) impede
entrave [ẽ'travi] *m* impediment
entre ['ẽtri] *prep dois*: between; *vários*: among; ***~ mim e você*** between you and me; ***~ outras coisas*** amongst other things
entreaberto [ẽtria'bɛrtu] *adj porta* ajar
entreabrir [ẽtria'brir] ⟨3b⟩ *v/t* half open
entrecosto [ẽtre'kostu] *m* GASTR entrecôte
entrega [ẽ'trɛga] *f* (*trespasse*) surrender; *mercadoria*: delivery; (*dedicação*) dedication; (*pagamento*) payment; ***~ de bagagem*** baggage reclaim; ***~ ao domicílio*** home delivery
entregador [ẽtrega'dor] *m* delivery man; ***~ de jornais*** paper boy
entregar [ẽtre'gar] ⟨1o & 1c⟩ surrender, hand over; *prêmio* present; *mercadoria* deliver; (*confiar*) entrust; ***~ uma decisão a alguém*** refer a decision to s.o.; **entregar-se** *v/r* ***~ a algo*** give oneself over to sth; ***~ à polícia*** give oneself up to the police
entrelinha [ẽtre'liɲa] *f* leading, line spacing; ***ler nas ~s*** read between the lines
entretanto [ẽtre'tãtu] *adv* meanwhile
entretenimento [ẽtreteni'mẽtu] *m* entertainment
entreter [ẽtre'ter] ⟨2xa⟩ *v/t* entertain; (*reter*) detain; *dor* relieve; *fome* stave off
entretido [ẽtre'ʧidu] *adj* ***estar ~ a fazer algo*** amuse oneself by doing sth
entrevista [ẽtre'vista] *f* interview
entrevistado [ẽtrevis'tadu] *m*, **-a** *f* interviewee
entrevistador [ẽtrevista'dor] *m*, **-a** *f* interviewer
entrevistar [ẽtrevis'tar] ⟨1a⟩ *v/t* interview
entristecer [ẽtriste'ser] ⟨2g⟩ **1** *v/t* sadden **2** *v/i* grow sad
entroncamento [ẽtrõka'mẽtu] *m* junction
entrouxar [ẽtrow'ʃar] ⟨1a⟩ *v/t* bundle up
entrudo [ẽ'trudu] *m* carnival
entulho [ẽ'tuʎu] *m* rubble
entupido [ẽtu'pidu] *adj* blocked
entupimento [ẽtupi'mẽtu] *m* blockage
entupir [ẽtu'pir] ⟨3a & 3h⟩ get blocked
entusiasmar [ẽtuzjaʒ'mar] ⟨1b⟩ enthuse; **entusiasmar-se** *v/r* get excited
entusiasmo [ẽtu'zjazmu] *m* enthusiasm
entusiasta [ẽtu'zjasta] **1** *m/f* enthusiast **2** *adj* enthusiastic
entusiástico [ẽtu'zjasʧiku] *adj* enthusiastic
enumeração [enumera'sãw] *f* enumeration; *custos etc*: breakdown
enumerar [enume'rar] ⟨1c⟩ *v/t* enumerate; *custos etc* break down
enunciar [enũ'sjar] ⟨1g⟩ state
envaidecer [ẽvajde'ser] ⟨2g⟩ make conceited; **envaidecer-se** *v/r* be conceited (**com** *ou* **de** about)
envasilhar [ẽvazi'ʎar] ⟨1a⟩ *v/t* bottle
envelhecer [ẽveʎe'ser] ⟨2g⟩ **1** *v/t* age **2** *v/i* age, grow old; (*passar de moda*) age
envelhecimento [ẽveʎesi'mẽtu] *m* ag(e)ing
envelope [ẽve'lɔpi] *m* envelope
envenenamento [ẽvenena'mẽtu] *m* poisoning; ***~ alimentar*** food poisoning
envenenar [ẽvene'nar] ⟨1d⟩ *v/t* poison; (*deturpar*) distort

enveredar [ẽvere'dar] ⟨1c⟩ **~ *por*** *caminho* take; (*entrar*) enter; (*optar*) opt for
envergadura [ẽverga'dura] *f* scale; *avião*: wingspan
envergonhar [ẽvergo'ɲar] ⟨1f⟩ shame; **envergonhar-se** *v/r* be ashamed
envernizado [ẽverni'zadu] *adj* varnished
envernizar [ẽverni'zar] ⟨1a⟩ *v/t* varnish
enviado [ẽ'vjadu] *m*, **-a** *f* envoy; **~ *especial*** special envoy
enviar [ẽ'vjar] ⟨1g⟩ send; *candidatura* send in
envidraçado [ẽvidra'sadu] *adj* glazed
envidraçar [ẽvidra'sar] ⟨1p & 1b⟩ glaze
envio [ẽ'viu] *m* shipment; (*remessa*) remittance
enviuvar [ẽviu'var] ⟨1q⟩ *v/i* be widowed
envolver [ẽvow'ver] ⟨2e⟩ wrap up; *fig* embrace; (*fazer participar*) involve; **envolver-se** *v/r* get involved
envolvimento [ẽvowvi'mẽtu] *m* involvement
enxada [ẽ'ʃada] *f* hoe
enxadrista [ẽʃa'drista] *m/f* chess player
enxaguar [ẽʃa'gwar] ⟨1m⟩ *v/t* rinse
enxaguatório [ẽʃagwa'tɔriu] *m* **~ *bucal*** mouthwash
enxame [ẽ'ʃami] *m* swarm
enxaqueca [ẽʃa'keka] *f* migraine
enxergar [ẽʃer'gar] ⟨1c⟩ see, notice; *momentariamente* catch sight of
enxertar [ẽʃer'tar] ⟨1c⟩ graft
enxerto [ẽ'ʃertu] *m* graft; *ação* grafting
enxofre [ẽ'ʃofri] *m* sulfur, *Brit* sulphur
enxotar [ẽʃo'tar] ⟨1e⟩ drive away
enxoval [ẽʃo'vaw] *m* trousseau; *bebé*: layette
enxovalhar [ẽʃova'ʎar] ⟨1b⟩ (*sujar*) dirty; (*enrugar*) crumple; *fig* sully; (*ofender*) insult
enxugar [ẽʃu'gar] ⟨1o⟩ dry
enxurrada [ẽʃu'hada] *f* deluge
enxuto [ẽ'ʃutu] *adj* dry; *fam* shapely
enzima [ẽ'zima] *m* enzyme
eólico [e'ɔliku] *adj* wind *atr*; ***turbina*** *f* ***eólica*** wind turbine
epicentro [epi'sẽtru] *m* epicenter, *Brit* epicentre
épico ['ɛpiku] **1** *adj* epic **2** *m* epic; (*autor*) epic poet
epidemia [epide'mia] *f* epidemic
epidêmico, *Port* **epidémico** [epi'demiku] *adj* epidemic
epiderme [epi'dɛrmi] *f* epidermis
epilepsia [epile'psia] *f* epilepsy
epilético [epi'lɛtʃiku] *adj* epileptic
epílogo [e'pilogu] *m* epilog, *Brit* epilogue
episcopal [episko'paw] *adj* episcopal
episódio [epi'zɔdiu] *m* episode
epitáfio [epi'tafiu] *m* epitaph
época ['ɛpuka] *f* epoch; ***naquela* ~** in those days; **~ *alta*** / ***baixa*** high / low season; **~ *balnear*** swimming season; ***fruta*** *f* ***da* ~** seasonal fruit
epopeia [epo'peja] *f* epic
equação [ekwa'sãw] *f* equation
equacionar [ekwasjo'nar] ⟨1f⟩ *fig* *problema* set out
equador [ekwa'dor] *m* equator
Equador [ekwa'dor] *m* Ecuador
equatorial [ekwato'rjaw] *adj* equatorial
equatoano [ekwato'rjanu] **1** *adj* Ecuadorian **2** *m*, **-a** *f* Ecuadorian
equilibrado [ekili'bradu] *adj* balanced
equilibrar [ekili'brar] ⟨1a⟩ *v/t* balance
equilíbrio [eki'libriu] *m* balance
equilibrista [ekili'brista] *m/f* tightrope walker
equinócio [eki'nɔsiu] *m* equinox
equipa [e'kipa] *f* *Port* team; **~ *de futebol*** football team
equipamento [ekipa'mẽtu] *m* equipment
equipar [eki'par] ⟨1a⟩ *v/t* equip
equiparar [ekipa'rar] ⟨1b⟩ *v/t* equate
equipe [e'kipi] *f* *Bras* team; **~ *de gerentes*** management team; **~ *de resgate*** rescue team
equitação [ekita'sãw] *f* horse riding
equivalência [ekiva'lẽsja] *f* equivalence; ***dar a* ~ *a*** recognize as equivalent
equivalente [ekiva'lẽtʃi] **1** *adj* equivalent **2** *m* equivalent

equivaler [ekiva'leɾ] ⟨2p⟩ *v/i* **~ a** be equivalent to
equívoco [e'kivuku] **1** *adj* equivocal **2** *m* (*erro*) error; (*mal-entendido*) misunderstanding
era[1] ['ɛɾa] *f* era
era[2] ['ɛɾa] *etc* → **ser**
ereção, *Port* **erecção** [eɾe'sãw] *f* erection *tb* ANAT
eremita [eɾe'mita] *m/f* hermit
ergonômico, *Port* **ergonómico** [eɾgo'nomiku] *adj* ergonomic
erguer [eɾ'geɾ] ⟨2i & 2c⟩ erect; *mão, voz etc* raise; **erguer-se** *v/r* **~ contra** stand up to
erguido [eɾ'gidu] *adj* upright
eriçar [eɾi'saɾ] ⟨1p⟩ *v/i* **fico com o cabelo eriçado** it makes my hair stand on end
erigir [eɾi'ʒiɾ] ⟨3n⟩ erect
erosão [eɾo'zãw] *f* ⟨*sem pl*⟩ erosion
erótico [e'ɾɔʧiku] *adj* erotic
erotismo [eɾo'ʧizmu] *m* eroticism
erradicação [ehadʒika'sãw] *f* eradication
errado [e'hadu] *adj* wrong; **estar ~** be wrong
errar [e'haɾ] ⟨1n⟩ *v/i* go wrong, make a mistake; *pontaria*: miss; (*vaguear*) wander around
erro ['ehu] *m* (*engano*) error, mistake; **salvo ~** if I am not mistaken; **~ de cálculo** miscalculation; **~ judicial** miscarriage of justice; **~ de julgamento** error of judgment
erroneamente [ehonja'mẽʧi] *adv* wrongly
erudição [eɾudʒi'sãw] *f* erudition
erudito [eɾu'dʒitu] *adj* erudite, learned
erupção [eɾu'psãw] *f* outbreak; *vulcão* eruption; MED rash
erva ['ɛɾva] *f* herb; *fam* dope; **~ daninha** weed
erva-cidreira [ɛɾvasi'dɾejɾa] *f* lemon balm
erva-doce [ɛɾva'dosi] *f* fennel
ervanária [ɛɾva'naɾja] *f shop selling natural health products*
ervilha [eɾ'viʎa] *f* pea
és [ɛs] → **ser**
esbanjador [ezbãʒa'doɾ] *m*, **-a** *f* spendthrift
esbanjar [ezbã'ʒaɾ] ⟨1a⟩ *v/t* squander
esbarrar [ezba'haɾ] ⟨1b⟩ *v/i* **~ em** bump into
esbelto [ez'bɛltu] *adj* slim, svelte
esboçar [ezbo'saɾ] ⟨1p & 1e⟩ sketch; *projeto* outline; *sorriso* give a hint of
esboço [ez'bosu] *m* sketch; *projeto*: outline; *sorriso*: hint
esbofetear [ezbofe'ʧiaɾ] ⟨1l⟩ hit, cuff
esborrachar [ezboha'ʃaɾ] ⟨1b⟩ squash
esborrifar [ezbohi'faɾ] ⟨1a⟩ *v/t* spray; **~ algo com algo** spray sth with sth
esburacar [ezbuɾa'kaɾ] ⟨1n & 1b⟩ make a hole in
escabeche [eska'bɛʃi] *m* marinade; **de ~** marinaded; *fig* **fazer** *ou* **armar um ~** make a scene
escabelo [eska'belu] *m* footstool
escabroso [eska'bɾozu] *adj* (*áspero*) rough; (*árduo*) difficult; (*indecente*) indecent, scabrous
escada [es'kada] *f* stairs; *na rua etc* steps; *de mão* ladder; **~ de caracol** spiral staircase; **~ de corda** rope ladder; **~ de emergência** fire escape; **~ de incêndio** fire escape; **~ de mão** ladder **~ rolante** escalator
escadaria [eskada'ɾia] *f* staircase
escadote [eska'dɔʧi] *m* step ladder
escafandrista [eskafã'dɾista] *m* diver
escafandro [eska'fãdɾu] *m* diving suit
escala [es'kala] *f* (*medida*), MÚS scale; (*sequência*) sequence; (*etapa*) stopover; NÁUT port of call; **em larga ~** on a large scale; **fazer ~ em** NÁUT put in at, AERO stop over at; **sem ~** non-stop
escalada [eska'lada] *f* ascent; ESP climbing; *fig* escalation; **~ de preços** price rise
escalador [eska'lada] *m*, **-a** *f* climber; **~ de montanhas** rock climber
escalão [eska'lãw] *m* step; *fig* level
escalar [eska'laɾ] ⟨1a⟩ *v/t* climb, scale; **muro** *m* **de ~** climbing wall
escaldadura [eskawda'duɾa] *f*, **escaldão** [eskaw'dãw] *m* scald; *sol*: sunburn
escaldar [eskaw'daɾ] ⟨1a⟩ scald; GASTR poach; **escaldar-se** *v/r* scald

oneself; *fig fam* get one's fingers burnt
escalonar [eskalo'naɾ] ⟨1f⟩ categorize; *pagamentos* schedule
escalope [eska'lɔpi] *m* GASTR escalope, cutlet
escalpelo [eskaw'pelu] *m* scalpel
escama [es'kama] *f* scale; *pele*: flake
escamado [eska'madu] *adj fig* angry
escamoso [eska'mozu] *adj* flaky
escamar [eska'maɾ] ⟨1a⟩ *v/t peixe* scale; **escamar-se** *v/r pele, pintura* flake (off); *fig fam* get angry
escanchado [eskã'ʃadu] *adj* **~ em** astride
escandalizar [eskãdali'zaɾ] ⟨1a⟩ scandalize; **escandalizar-se** *v/r* **~ com** be scandalized by
escândalo [es'kãdalu] *m* scandal; (*indignação*) indignation; **fazer ~** make a scene
escandaloso [eskãda'lozu] *adj* scandalous
Escandinávia [eskãdʒi'navja] *f* Scandinavia
escandinavo [eskãdʒi'navu] **1** *adj* Scandinavian **2** *m*, **-a** *f* Scandinavian
escanear [eskã'njaɾ] ⟨1h⟩ *v/t* scan
escangalhar [eskãga'ʎaɾ] ⟨1b⟩ take apart; *fam* break
escaninho [eskã'niɲu] *m* pigeonhole
escanteio [eskã'teju] *m* corner (kick)
escapada [eska'pada] *f*, **escapadela** [eskapa'dɛla] *f* escapade
escapamento *m gás*: escape; AUTO exhaust
escapar [eska'paɾ] ⟨1b⟩ *v/i* escape; *água* leak; *mão, pé* slip; **deixar ~** *peixe* let go; *detalhe* skip, leave out; **~ por pouco, ~ de boa** have a narrow escape; **~ à atenção de alguém** escape s.o.'s attention; **escapar-se** *v/r* escape; (*salvar-se*) get off
escape [es'kapi] *m* (*buraco*) leak; (*válvula*) escape valve; **gás** *m* **de ~** exhaust; **tubo** *m* **de ~** exhaust pipe; **ter um ~** leak; *fig* have a means of escape
escapismo [eska'pizmu] *m* escapism
escapulir [eskapu'liɾ] ⟨3h⟩ *v/i* escape
escaramuça [eskaɾa'musa] *f* MIL *fig* conflict
escaravelho [eskaɾa'veʎu] *m* beetle
escarcéu [eskaɾ'sɛu] *m* hullabaloo
escarlate [eskaɾ'latʃi] **1** *adj* scarlet **2** *m cor* scarlet
escarlatina [eskaɾla'tʃina] *f* MED scarlet fever
escarpado [eskaɾ'padu] *adj* steep
escárnio [es'kaɾniu] *m* mockery, scorn
escarola [eska'ɾɔla] *f* endive
escarrar [eska'haɾ] ⟨1b⟩ **1** *v/t* spit (out) **2** *v/i* spit
escarro [es'kahu] *m* spit
escassez [eska'ses] *f* shortage, scarcity
escasso [es'kasu] *adj* scarce; *renda* slender
escavação [eskava'sãw] *f* excavation, digging
escavadeira [eskava'dejɾa] *f* excavator, digger
escavador [eskava'doɾ] *m* excavator, digger
escavar [eska'vaɾ] ⟨1b⟩ excavate
esclarecedor [esklaɾese'doɾ] *adj* explanatory; (*interessante*) enlightening
esclarecer [esklaɾe'seɾ] ⟨2g⟩ explain, clarify; *consumidor* educate; *mistério* clear up; **~ alguém sobre algo** explain sth to s.o., clarify sth for s.o.
esclarecimento [esklaɾesi'mẽtu] *m* explanation, clarification; (*informação*) information
esclerose [eskle'ɾɔzi] *f* MED sclerosis; **~ múltipla** multiple sclerosis
escoadoiro [eskwa'dojɾu] *m* drain; *canal*: drainpipe
escoar [es'kwaɾ] ⟨1f⟩ drain; **escoar-se** *v/r* drain away; *tempo* go past; *fig* empty
escocês [esko'ses] **1** *adj* Scottish, Scots **2** *m*, **escocesa** [esko'seza] *f* Scot
Escócia [es'kɔsja] *f* Scotland
escola [es'kɔla] *f* school; **ir para a ~** go to school; *fig* **fazer ~** become the accepted thing; **~ de belas-artes** art school; **~ de línguas** language school; **~ noturna**, *Port* **~ nocturna** night school; **~ particular** private school, *Brit* public school; **~ politécnica** technical college; **~ primária**

elementary school, *Brit* primary school; ~ ***secundária*** high school, *Brit* secondary school; ~ ***superior*** college
escolar [esko'laɾ] *adj* school *atr*; ***férias*** *fpl* ~***es*** school holidays
escolaridade [eskolari'dadʒi] *f* schooling
escolha [es'koʎa] *f* choice
escolher [esko'ʎeɾ] ⟨2d⟩ choose, select
escolinha [esko'liɲa] *f* ~ ***particular*** playgroup
escolta [es'kɔlta] *f* escort
escoltar [eskow'taɾ] ⟨1e⟩ *v/t* escort
escombros [es'kõbɾus] *mpl* debris *sg*; *velho* ruins
esconde-esconde [es'kõdʒis'kõdʒi] *m* hide-and-seek
esconder [eskõ'deɾ] ⟨2a⟩ hide; **esconder-se** *v/r* hide; *sol* go in; *ladrão* go into hiding
esconderijo [eskõde'ɾiʒu] *m* hiding place
escondidas [eskõ'dʒidas] *fpl Port* hide-and-seek; ***às*** ~ secretly
escondido [eskõ'dʒidu] *adj* hidden
escorar [esko'ɾaɾ] ⟨1e⟩ *v/t* ARQUIT, *fig* support
escória [es'kɔɾja] *f* dross; *fig* scum; ***a*** ~ ***da sociedade*** the dregs of society
escoriação [eskoɾja'sãw] *f* graze
escorpião [eskoɾ'pjãw] *m* scorpion; ASTROL ***Ecorpião*** Scorpio
escorraçar [eskoha'saɾ] ⟨1p & 1b⟩ throw out
escorrega [esko'hɛga] *f/m* slide
escorregadela [eskohega'dɛla] *f* slip
escorregadio [eskohega'dʒiu] *adj* slippery
escorregador [eskohega'doɾ] *m* slide
escorregão [eskohe'gãw] *m* → ***escorregadela***
escorregar [eskohe'gaɾ] ⟨1o & 1c⟩ slip
escorreito [esko'hejtu] *adj* well; ***são e*** ~ fit and well
escorrendo [esko'hẽdu] *adj nariz* runny
escorrer [esko'heɾ] ⟨2d⟩ **1** *v/t* drain off; (*espremer*) squeeze out; *roupa* wring out; *salada* drain **2** *v/i* trickle; *pintura* run
escorrido [esko'hidu] *adj fig cabelo* smooth; *vestido* tight
escoteiro [esko'tejɾu] *m* boy scout
escotilha [esko'tʃiʎa] *f* NAUT hatch
escova [es'kova] *f* brush; ~ ***de cabelo*** hairbrush; ~ ***de chão*** scrubbing brush; ~ ***de dentes*** toothbrush; ~ ***de roupa*** clothes brush
escovar [esko'vaɾ] ⟨1e⟩ brush; *retirar* brush off
escravatura [eskɾava'tuɾa] *f* slave trade; (*escravidão*) slavery; ~ ***branca*** white slave trade
escravidão [eskɾavi'dãw] *f* ⟨*sem pl*⟩ slavery
escravo [es'kɾavu] **1** *adj* slave *atr* **2** *m*, **-a** *f* slave
escrever [eskɾe'veɾ] ⟨2c; *pp* escrito⟩ write; ~ ***à máquina*** type
escrevinhador [eskɾeviɲa'doɾ] *m*, **-a** *f* hack
escrita [es'kɾita] *f* writing
escrito [es'kɾitu] *m* piece of writing; ***por*** ~ in writing
escritor [eskɾi'toɾ] *m*, **-a** *f* writer
escritório [eskɾi'tɔɾiu] *m* office; *em casa* study
escritura [eskɾi'tuɾa] *f* (*documento*) deed; ***as Sagradas Escrituras*** the Holy Scriptures
escrituração [eskɾituɾa'sãw] *f* COM bookkeeping
escriturar [eskɾitu'ɾaɾ] ⟨1a⟩ enter in the books, record
escriturário [eskɾitu'ɾaɾiu] *m*, **-a** *f* bookkeeper
escrivaninha [eskɾiva'niɲa] *f* desk
escrivão [eskɾi'vãw] *m* ⟨*pl* -ães⟩, ~**vã** [eskɾi'vã] *f* clerk
escrúpulo [es'kɾupulu] *m* ~***s*** *pl* scruples; ***com*** ~ scrupulous; ***sem*** ~ unscrupulous
escrupuloso [eskɾupu'lozu] *adj* scrupulous
escrutínio [eskɾu'tʃiniu] *m* poll; (*contar*) count; (*apuração*) scrutiny
escudo [es'kudu] *m arma*: shield; *hist moeda* escudo
esculpir [eskuw'piɾ] ⟨3a⟩ *em pedra* sculpt; *em madeira* carve; *em barro* model; *inscrição* engrave

escultor [eskuw'toɾ] *m*, **-a** *f* sculptor
escultura [eskuw'tuɾa] *f* sculpture
escumadeira [eskuma'dejɾa] *f* skimmer
escuras [es'kuɾas] *fpl* ***às ~*** in the dark
escurecer [eskuɾe'seɾ] ⟨2g⟩ **1** *v/t* darken **2** *v/i* get dark; ***ao ~*** at nightfall
escuridão [eskuɾi'dãw] *f* ⟨*sem pl*⟩ darkness
escuro [es'kuɾu] **1** *adj* dark; (*triste*) gloomy **2** *m* dark
escusado [esku'zadu] *adj* unnecessary
escuta [es'kuta] **1** *m* → ***escuteiro*** **2** *f* bugging; ***aparelho*** *m* ***de ~*** bug, bugging device; ***encontrar-se sob ~*** be bugged; ***estar*** (*ou* ***ficar***) ***à ~*** listen in
escutar [esku'taɾ] ⟨1a⟩ **1** *v/i* hear; *às escondidas* eavesdrop, listen in; (*ouvir*) listen; ***escuta!*** listen! **2** *v/t música, ruídos etc* listen to; *às escondidas* eavesdrop on; *telefonema* bug, tap
escuteiro [esku'tejɾu] *m*, **-a** *f* (boy) scout
esfaquear [esfa'kjaɾ] ⟨1l⟩ *v/t* knife
esfarrapado [esfaha'padu] *adj* ragged
esfarrapar [esfaha'paɾ] ⟨1b⟩ rip to shreds
esfera [es'fɛɾa] *f* sphere *tb fig*
esférico [es'fɛɾiku] *adj* spherical
esferográfica [esfɛɾo'gɾafika] *f* ballpoint (pen)
esfinge [es'fĩʒi] *f* sphinx
esfolar [esfo'laɾ] ⟨1e⟩ skin; (*arranhar*) graze; (*pelar*) peel off; *cara* scratch; *fig* ***~ alguém*** fleece s.o.
esfomeado [esfo'mjadu] *adj* famished
esforçar-se [esfoɾ'saɾsi] ⟨1p & 1e⟩ make an effort (***por*** to)
esforço [es'foɾsu] *m* effort; ***não poupar ~s*** spare no effort
esfregão [esfɾe'gãw] *m* mop
esfregar [esfɾe'gaɾ] ⟨1o & 1c⟩ scrub; *sapatos* clean; *costas* scratch
esfriar [es'fɾjaɾ] ⟨1g⟩ *v/t* cool down
esfumar [esfu'maɾ] ⟨1a⟩ *v/t* smudge, smear
esgotado [ezgo'tadu] *adj* (*cansado*) exhausted; *livro* out of print; *bateria* dead; ***o tempo está ~*** time's up
esgotamento [ezgota'mẽtu] *m* (*exaustão*) exhaustion; ***~ nervoso*** nervous breakdown
esgotante [ezgo'tãtʃi] *adj* exhausting
esgotar [ezgo'taɾ] ⟨1e⟩ exhaust; *mantimentos* use up; *mercadoria* sell out of; ***gasolina esgotada*** sold out of gas; **esgotar-se** *v/r* (*cansar-se*) exhaust oneself; *mantimentos* run out; (*estar vendido*) sell out
esgoto [ez'gotu] *m* drain; ***~s*** *pl* sewers; ***águas*** *fpl* ***de ~*** sewage
esgrima [ez'gɾima] *f* fencing
esgrimir [ezgɾi'miɾ] ⟨3a⟩ *v/i* fence
esguichar [ezgi'ʃaɾ] ⟨1a⟩ **1** *v/t* squirt **2** *v/i* squirt out
esguicho [ez'giʃu] *m* squirt
esguio [ez'giu] *adj* slender
eslavo [ez'lavu] **1** *m*, **-a** *f* Slav **2** *adj* Slavic
eslovaco [ezlo'vaku] **1** *adj* Slovak(ian) **2** *m*, **-a** *f* Slovak
Eslováquia [ezlo'vakja] *f* Slovakia
Eslovênia, *Port* **Eslovénia** [ezlo'venja] *f* Slovenia
esloveno [ezlo'venu] **1** *adj* Slovene **2** *m*, **-a** *f* Slovene
esmagador [ezmaga'doɾ] *adj* crushing
esmagar [ezma'gaɾ] ⟨1o & 1b⟩ crush
esmalte [ez'mawtʃi] *m* enamel; *unhas*: nail polish
esmerado [ezme'ɾadu] *adj* careful; (*impecável*) impeccable
esmeralda [ezme'ɾawda] *f* emerald
esmero [ez'meɾu] *m* care; (*aperfeiçoamento*) perfection
esmola [ez'mɔla] *f* alms; ***pedir ~*** beg
esmigalhar [ezmiga'ʎaɾ] ⟨1b⟩ crumble
esmiuçar [ezmiu'saɾ] ⟨1p⟩ *v/t* investigate in detail
esmo ['ezmu] *m* ***a ~*** at random
esnobar [ezno'baɾ] ⟨1e⟩ **1** *v/i* be snobbish **2** *v/t* snub
esnobe [ez'nɔbi] **1** *adj* snobbish **2** *m/f* snob
esnobismo [ezno'bizmu] *m* snobbery
esófago [e'zɔfagu] *m* esophagus, *Brit* oesophagus
esotérico [ezo'tɛɾiku] *adj* esoteric
esp. *abr* (***especialmente***) esp (especially)

espaçado [espa'sadu] *adj* spaced out
espaçar [espa'saɾ] ⟨1p & 1b⟩ space out
espacial [espa'sjaw] *adj* spatial; ***estação*** *f* ~ space station; ***nave*** *f* ~ spaceship; ***ônibus*** *m* ~ space shuttle; ***roupa*** *f* ~ space suit
espaço [es'pasu] *m* space; *temporal*: period; (*distância*) gap; ***havia ~ para dois*** there was space *ou* room for two; ***é um ~ apertado*** it's a tight fit; ***~ aéreo*** airspace; ***~ livre*** *ponte*: headroom
espaçonave [espaso'navi] *f* spaceship
espaçoso [espa'sozu] *adj* spacious, roomy
espada [es'pada] *f* sword; *naipes*: ***~s*** *pl* spades; ***estar entre a ~ e a parede*** be between a rock and a hard place
espadarte [espa'daɾtʃi] *m* swordfish
espalhar [espa'ʎaɾ] ⟨1b⟩ scatter; *notícia, manteiga, doença* spread; **espalhar-se** *v/r* spread
espanador [espana'doɾ] *m* duster
espancar [espã'kaɾ] ⟨1n⟩ beat up
Espanha [es'paɲa] *f* Spain
espanhol [espa'ɲɔw] **1** *adj* Spanish **2** *m*, **-a** *f* Spaniard; ***os espanhoís*** the Spanish **3** *m lingua* Spanish
espantalho [espã'taʎu] *m* scarecrow
espantar [espã'taɾ] ⟨1a⟩ frighten; (*surpreender*) amaze, astonish; *caça* frighten away; **espantar-se** *v/r* be amazed; *cavalo* be frightened
espanto [es'pãtu] *m* amazement, astonishment
espantoso [espã'tozu] *adj* amazing
esparadrapo [espaɾa'dɾapu] *m* Band-Aid®, *Brit* sticking plaster
espargo [es'paɾgu] *m Port* asparagus
esparguete [espaɾ'gɛtʃi] *m* spaghetti
esparso [es'paɾsu] *adj* sparse
espartano [espaɾ'tanu] *adj* spartan
espasmo [es'pazmu] *m* spasm
espasmódico [espaʒ'mɔdʒiku] *adj* spasmodic
espatifar [espatʃi'faɾ] ⟨1a⟩ smash; *fortuna* squander
espátula [es'patula] *f* spatula
especial [espe'sjaw] *adj* special; ***em ~*** especially, in particular
especialidade [espesjali'dadʒi] *f* specialty, *Brit* speciality
especialista [espesja'lista] *m/f* specialist; ***médico ~*** specialist (***de*** for); UNIV ***~ em política*** politics major
especialização [espesjaliza'sãw] *f* specialization
especializado [espesjali'zadu] *adj* specialized
especializar-se [espesjali'zaɾsi] ⟨1a⟩ *v/r* specialize (***em*** in)
especialmente [espesjaw'mẽtʃi] *adv* especially
especiaria [espesja'ɾia] *f* spice
espécie [es'pɛsi] *f* sort; BIOL species *sg*; ***~ ameaçada*** endangered species; ***a ~ humana*** the human race; ***conservação*** *f* ***das ~s*** preservation of species; ***pagar em ~*** pay cash
especificação [espesifika'sãw] *f* (*levantamento*) specification; ***especificações*** specifications, specs
especificar [espesifi'kaɾ] ⟨1n⟩ specify; *fatura* itemize
específico [espe'sifiku] *adj* specific
espécime [es'pɛsimi] *m*, **espécimen** [es'pɛsimẽ] *m* specimen
espect... *Port* → ***espet...***
espectro [es'pɛktɾu] *m* specter, *Brit* spectre; *óptica*: spectrum
especulação [espekula'sãw] *f* speculation
especulador [espekula'doɾ] *m*, **-a** *f* speculator
especular [espeku'laɾ] ⟨1a⟩ *v/i* speculate
espedaçar [espeda'saɾ] ⟨1p⟩ *v/t* smash to pieces
espelhar [espe'ʎaɾ] ⟨1d⟩ mirror; **espelhar-se** *v/r* be mirrored
espelho [es'peʎu] *m* mirror; ***~ retrovisor*** rearview mirror
espelunca [es'pelunka] *f fam* joint, place; *bar etc* dive
espera [es'pɛɾa] *f* waiting; (*expectativa*) expectation; ***uma ~ de 2 horas*** a wait of 2 hours; ***estar*** *ou* ***ficar à ~*** (***de***) be waiting (for)
esperança [espe'ɾãsa] *f* hope; ***estar de ~s*** be hopeful
esperançosamente [espeɾãsoza'mẽtʃi] *adv* hopefully
esperar [espe'ɾaɾ] ⟨1c⟩ **1** *v/t* wait for;

(*desejar*) hope for; *bebê, chamada* expect **2** *v/i* wait; (*desejar*) hope; ***espere e verá!*** just you wait and see!; ***espero que sim*** I hope so; ***espero que não*** I hope not
esperma [es'pɛrma] *m* sperm
espertalhão [esperta'ʎãw] *fam* **1** *adj* crafty **2** *m*, **-ona** [esperta'ʎona] *f* crafty devil
esperteza [esper'teza] *f* shrewdness
espertinho [esper'ɲu] *adj* crafty, sneaky
esperto [es'pɛrtu] *adj* smart; (*inteligente*) intelligent; *fam* **xico ~** smart ass
espesso [es'pesu] *adj* thick
espessura [espe'sura] *f* thickness
espetacular [espetaku'lar] *adj* spectacular
espetáculo [espe'takulu] *m* show; ***armar um ~*** make a scene; *fam* ***ser um ~*** be great; ***~ de fogos de artifício*** fireworks display
espetada [espe'tada] *f* GASTR kabob, *Brit* kebab
espetador [espeta'dor] *m*, **-a** *f* onlooker; ESP spectator; TV viewer; TEAT member of the audience; TEAT ***~es*** audience
espetar [espe'tar] ⟨1c⟩ skewer; (*perfurar*) pierce; *fam* ***~ uma peta a alguém*** tell s.o. a lie; **espetar-se** *v/r* prick oneself; *fam* make a big mistake
espeto [es'petu] *m* skewer; *fig* beanpole
espezinhar [espezi'ɲar] ⟨1a⟩ *v/t* trample on
espião [es'pjãw] *m*, **-ã** *f* spy
espiar [es'pjar] ⟨1g⟩ **1** *v/t* spy on **2** *v/i* spy
espiga [es'piga] *f* ear
espinafre [espi'nafri] *m* BOT spinach; GASTR ***~s*** *pl* spinach
espinal [espi'naw] *adj* spinal
espingarda [espĩ'garda] *f* rifle
espinha [es'piɲa] *f* (fish)bone; *pele*: spot, zit; **~ (*dorsal*)** backbone
espinho [es'piɲu] *m* thorn; (*ferrão*) spike; *animal*: spine; *fig* snag
espinhoso [espi'ɲozu] *adj* prickly; *fig* tricky; *problema* thorny
espionagem [espjo'naʒẽ] *f* espionage, spying
espionar [espjo'nar] ⟨1f⟩ **1** *v/t* spy on **2** *v/i* spy
espiral [espi'raw] **1** *f* spiral; ***em ~*** spiral-shaped; ***escada*** *f* ***em ~*** spiral staircase **2** *adj* spiral-shaped
espírita [es'pirita] *m/f* spiritualist
espiritismo [espiri'tʃizmu] *m* spiritualism
espírito [es'piritu] *m* spirit; (*sentido*) sense; (*graça*) wit; (*álcool*) spirit; ***o Espírito Santo*** the Holy Spirit; ***com o ~ de amizade*** in a spirit of friendship
espiritual [espiri'twaw] *adj* spiritual; REL ***diretor*** *m* **~**, *Port* ***director*** *m* **~** father confessor
espirituoso [espiri'twozu] *adj* witty; ***bebida espirituosa*** spirit
espirrar [espi'har] ⟨1a⟩ **1** *v/i* sneeze **2** *v/t* (*salpicar*) spurt
espirro [es'pihu] *m* sneeze; ***dar um ~*** sneeze
esplanada [espla'nada] *f* street café; *dum restaurante* terrace
esplêndido [es'plẽdʒidu] *adj* splendid
esplendor [esplẽ'dor] *m* splendor, *Brit* splendour
espoleta [espo'leta] *f* fuse
espoliar [espo'ljar] ⟨1g⟩ *v/t* plunder
espólio [es'pɔliu] *m* estate; *de guerra* spoils
esponja [es'põʒa] *f* sponge
espontaneidade [espõtanej'dadʒi] *f* spontaneity
espontâneo [espõ'tʌniu] *adj* spontaneous
espora [es'pɔra] *f* spur
esporádico [espo'radʒiku] *adj* sporadic
esporte [es'pɔrtʃi] *m Bras* sport; ***~s de campo*** field events; ***~ espectador*** spectator sport; ***~s de inverno*** winter sports
esportista [espor'tʃista] *m/f Bras* sportsman; sportswoman
esportivo [espor'tʃivu] *adj Bras* athletic, sporty; *atitude* sporting
esposa [es'poza] *f* wife, *fml* spouse
esposo [es'pozu] *m* husband, *fml* spouse

E

esposos [es'pozus] *mpl* married couple
espreguiçadeira [espregisa'dejɾa] *f* deckchair, sun lounger
espreguiçar-se [espregi'sarsi] ⟨1p⟩ stretch out
espreitar [esprej'tar] ⟨1a⟩ **1** *v/t* (*observar*) watch; (*ver*) see; (*vigiar*) keep an eye on; *ocasião* watch for **2** *v/i pessoa, perigo* lurk; **~ através da neblina** peer through the mist
espremedor [espreme'dor] *m* press; **~ de alho** garlic press; **~ elétrico**, *Port* **~ eléctrico** juice extractor
espremer [espre'mer] ⟨2c⟩ squeeze (out); (*torcer*) wring (out); *tema* exhaust; *fig fam pessoa* bleed dry; **estar espremido entre dois ...** be sandwiched between two ...
espremida [espre'mida] *f* **dar uma ~** squeeze up
espuma [es'puma] *f* foam; *sabão*: lather; *cerveja*: froth; **~ de barbear** shaving foam; **~ de borracha** foam rubber
espumadeira [espuma'dejɾa] *f* skimmer
espumante [espu'mãtʃi] **1** *adj* sparkling **2** *m* sparkling wine
espumoso [espu'mozu] *adj* frothy
esquadra [es'kwadɾa] *f* squad; NÁUT fleet; *Port* police station
esquadrão [eskwa'drãw] *m* squadron; **~ especial** hit squad
esquadrilha [eskwa'driʎa] *f* NÁUT fleet; AERO squadron
esquadrinhar [eskwadri'ʎar] ⟨1a⟩ *v/t área* comb
esquecer [eske'ser] ⟨2g & 2a⟩ forget; **~ a alguém** slip s.o.'s mind; **esquecer-se** *v/r* **~ de** forget; *fig* **~ de si, ~ de quem é** forget oneself
esquecido [eske'sidu] *adj* forgotten; (*distraído*) forgetful
esquecimento [eskesi'mẽtu] *m* forgetfulness; **cair em ~** fall into oblivion
esquelético [eske'lɛtʃiku] *adj* scrawny, all skin and bones *pred*
esqueleto [eske'letu] *m* skeleton; *fig* framework
esquema [es'kema] *m* scheme; (*plano*) plan; **~ de cores** color scheme, *Brit* colour scheme
esquemático [eske'matʃiku] *adj* schematic
esquematizar [eskematʃi'zar] ⟨1a⟩ schematize
esquentado [eskẽ'tadu] *adj* fiery
esquentador [eskẽta'dor] *m* water heater
esquentar [eskẽ'tar] ⟨1a⟩ *v/t comida* warm up; *água* heat; **esquentar-se** *v/r pessoa* get annoyed
esquerda [es'kerda] *f* left *tb* POL; MIL **~!** left turn!; **à ~** on the left
esquerdismo [esker'dʒizmu] *m* POL left-wing politics; *tendência* leftism
esquerdista [esker'dʒista] **1** *adj* leftwing **2** *m/f* left-winger, *fam* leftie
esquerdo [es'kerdu] *adj* left; (*canhoto*) left-handed
esquete [es'kɛtʃi] *m* TEAT sketch
esqui [es'ki] *m* ski; *esporte* skiing; **fazer ~** ski; **~ alpino** downhill skiing; **~ aquático** water skiing
esquiador [eskja'dor] *m*, **-a** *f* skier
esquiar [es'kjar] ⟨1g⟩ *v/i* ski
esquife [es'kifi] *m* casket, coffin
esquilo [es'kilu] *m* squirrel
esquimó [eski'mɔ] *m* Eskimo
esquina [es'kina] *f* corner
esquisitão [eskizi'tãw] *m*, **-ona** *f* weirdo, oddball
esquisitice [eskizi'tʃisi] *f* quirk
esquisito [eski'zitu] *adj* odd, funny
esquivar-se [eski'varsi] ⟨1a⟩ *v/r* **~ de** *bola, carro* dodge; *tarefa* get out of; *policial* escape from
esquizofrenia [eskizofre'nia] *f* schizophrenia
esquizofrênico [eskizo'freniku] **1** *adj* schizophrenic **2** *m*, **-a** *f* schizophrenic
esse ['esi], **essa** ['ɛsa] *adj & pron Port* that; *plural* those; *Bras* this; *plural* these; **essa é boa!** that's a good one!
essência [e'sẽsja] *f* essence
essencial [esẽ'sjaw] **1** *adj* essential; (*principal*) main **2** *m* **o ~** the essential thing
Est. *abr* (**Estação**) station
esta ['ɛsta] *pron f* → **este**
estabelecer [estabele'ser] ⟨2g⟩ es-

tablish; *empresa* set up, establish; **estabelecer-se** *v/r pessoa* settle; (*ser fundado*) be set up, be established; *doença, idéia* gain a foothold; **~ como ...** establish oneself as ...; ***a empresa estabeleceu-se neste bairro ...*** the company set up in this area ...

estabelecimento [estabelesi'mẽtu] *m* establishment; **~ *comercial*** business; **~ *industrial*** industrial concern

estabilidade [estabili'dadʒi] *f* stability

estabilizador [estabiliza'doɾ] *m* stabilizer

estabilizar [estabili'zaɾ] ⟨1a⟩ *v/t* stabilize; **estabilizar-se** *v/r* stabilize

estábulo [es'tabulu] *m* stable; *vacas*: cowshed

estaca [es'taka] *f* post; *barraca*: pin, *Brit* peg; ***pegar de ~*** take root

estacada [esta'kada] *f* stockade

estação [esta'sãw] *f* (*paragem*) stop; FERROV, RÁDIO station; *do ano* season; *hospital*: room, *Brit* ward; **~ *de águas*** spa; **~ *alta*** high season; **~ *baixa*** low season; **~ *das chuvas*** rainy season; **~ *dos correios*** post office; **~ *espacial*** space station; **~ *de esqui*** ski resort; **~ *ferroviária*** railroad station, *Brit* railway station; **~ *final*** terminus; **~ *de rádio*** radio station; **~ *rodoviária*** bus station; *Port* AUTO **~ *de serviço*** service area; *Bras* **~ *telefônica*** telephone exchange; **~ *de trabalho*** work station; *Bras* **~ *de trem*** train station

estacionamento [estasjona'mẽtu] *m* AUTO parking; *Bras* parking lot, *Brit* car park

estacionar [estasjo'naɾ] ⟨1f⟩ *carro* park; ***lugar*** *m* ***de ~*** parking space

estacionário [estasjo'naɾiu] *adj* stationary; *preço etc* stable

estadia [esta'dʒia] *f* stay

estádio [es'tadiu] *m* stadium; **~ *de futebol*** football stadium

estadista [esta'dʒista] *m/f* statesman; stateswoman

estado [es'tadu] **1** *pp* → ***estar*** **2** *m* state; MED condition; *plano*: stage; ***qual é o ~ do tempo?*** what's the weather like?; ***em bom / mau ~*** in good / poor condition; **~ *civil*** marital status; **~ *de emergência*** state of emergency; **~ *policial*** police state; ***Estados*** *pl* ***Unidos da América*** United States of America

estadual [estadu'aw] *adj* state *atr*

estadunidense [estadoni'dẽsi] *adj* US *atr*

estafa [es'tafa] *f* exhaustion

estafante [esta'fãtʃi] *adj* exhausting

estafeta [esta'feta] **1** *f* relay (race) **2** *m/f* messenger

estagiar [esta'ʒjaɾ] ⟨1g⟩ *v/i* do a traineeship

estagiário [esta'ʒjaɾiu] *m*, **-a** *f* trainee; ***professor*** *m* **~** student teacher

estágio [es'taʒiu] *m* (*nível*) stage; *profissional* traineeship; **~ *probatório*** probation period

estagnação [estagna'sãw] *f* ⟨*sem pl*⟩ stagnation

estagnado [esta'gnadu] *adj* stagnant

estagnar [esta'gnaɾ] ⟨1b⟩ *v/i* stagnate

estalactite [estalak'tʃitʃi] *f* stalactite

estalada [esta'lada] *f* → ***bofetada***

estaladiço [estala'dʒisu] *adj comida, neve* crunchy

estalagem [esta'laʒẽ] *f* inn

estalagmite [estalag'mitʃi] *f* stalagmite

estalar [esta'laɾ] ⟨1b⟩ **1** *v/i vidro, gelo* crack; (*crepitar*) crackle; *guerra etc* break out **2** *v/t* crack; ***tenho a cabeça a ~*** I have a splitting headache

estaleiro [esta'lejɾu] *m* NÁUT shipyard

estampa [es'tãpa] *f* print; *tecido*: pattern; *fig* ***ser uma ~*** be good-looking

estampado [estã'padu] *adj tecido* patterned

estancado [estã'kadu] *adj* stagnant

estancar [estã'kaɾ] ⟨1n⟩ *v/t sangue* stop

estância [es'tãsja] *f* LIT stanza; **~ *balnear*** seaside resort; **~ *termal*** spa resort; **~ *de turismo*** tourist destination

estandardizar [estãdaɾdʒi'zaɾ] ⟨1a⟩ *v/t* standardize

estandarte [estã'daɾtʃi] *m* standard

estande [es'tãdʒi] *m* booth, *Brit* stand

estanho [es'taɲu] *m* tin; ***papel*** *m* ***de ~*** silver paper; ***folha*** *f* ***de ~*** tin foil

estanque [es'tãki] *adj* tight; (*hermético*) hermetically sealed; *líquido*: watertight
estante [es'tãtʃi] *f livros*: shelves; *leitura*, *música*: (music) stand; ~ ***para CD*** CD rack; ~ ***de livros*** bookcase
estar [es'taɾ] ⟨1s⟩ **1** *v/i* be; ***está bem!*** all right!; ***como está?*** what's the score?; ***a Claudia está? – não está*** is Claudia there - she's not here; *Port* TEL ***está*** hello **2** *v/aux Port* ~ ***a fazer algo***, *Bras* ~ ***fazendo algo*** be doing sth; ~ ***para fazer algo*** be about to do sth; ~ ***por fazer*** be still to be done
estatal [esta'taw] *adj* state *atr*
estática [es'tatʃika] *f* static
estático [es'tatʃiku] *adj* static
estatística [esta'tʃistʃika] *f* statistic; *ciência* statistics *sg*
estatisticamente [estatʃistʃika'mẽtʃi] *adv* statistically
estatístico [esta'tʃistʃiku] **1** *adj* statistical **2** *m*, **-a** *f* statistician
estatização [estatʃiza'sãw] *f* nationalization
estatizar [estatʃi'zaɾ] ⟨1a⟩ nationalize
estátua [es'tatwa] *f* statue
estatueta [esta'tweta] *f* statuette
estatura [esta'tuɾa] *f* stature
estatuto [esta'tutu] *m* statute
estável [es'tavew] *adj* stable; *tempo* settled
este[1] ['ɛstʃi] *m* east
este[2] ['estʃi], **esta** ['ɛsta] **1** *adj* this; *plural* these **2** *pron* this, this one; *plural* these
esteio [es'teiu] *m* support
esteira[1] [es'tejɾa] *f* mat
esteira[2] [es'tejɾa] *aeroporto*: carousel; ~ ***transportadora*** conveyor belt
esteira[3] [es'tejɾa] *f* NÁUT wake
esteja [es'teʒa] *etc* → ***estar***
estêncil [es'tẽsiw] *m* stencil
estendal [estẽ'daw] *para a roupa* clothes line; *estrutura* clothes horse
estender [estẽ'deɾ] ⟨2a⟩ *mão* hold out; (*desdobrar*) unfold; (*demorar, alargar*) extend; (*esticar*) tighten; *roupa etc* hang out; *sobre superfície*: spread; *massa* roll out; ***ele estendeu a mão ao irmão*** he helped his brother out; **estender-se** *v/r terra etc* extend; *pessoa* stretch out; ***estende-se por 161 quilômetros*** it stretches for 100 miles; ~ ***sobre um assunto*** dwell on a point
estenografia [estenogɾa'fia] *f* shorthand
estepe [es'tɛpi] *f* AUTO spare tire, *Brit* spare tyre
esterco [es'teɾku] *m* dung
estéreo [es'tɛɾiu] *adj* stereo
estereotipado [esteɾiotʃi'padu] *adj* stereotypical
estereótipo [esteɾi'ɔtʃipu] *m* stereotype
estéril [es'tɛɾiw] *adj* sterile
esterilidade [esteɾili'dadʒi] *f* sterility
esterilizador [esteɾiliza'doɾ] *m* sterilizer
esterilizar [esteɾili'zaɾ] ⟨1a⟩ *v/t* sterilize
esteróide [este'ɾɔjdʒi] *m* steroid; ~ ***anabolizante*** anabolic steroid
estética [es'tɛtʃika] *f* esthetics, *Brit* aesthetics
esteticista [estetʃi'sista] *m/f* beautician
estético [es'tɛtʃiku] *adj* esthetic, *Brit* aesthetic
estetoscópio [estetos'kɔpiu] *m* MED stethoscope
esteve [es'tevi] → ***estar***
estibordo [estʃi'bɔrdu] *m* starboard
esticão [estʃi'kãw] *m* tug
esticar [estʃi'kaɾ] ⟨1n⟩ (*estender*) stretch; *fam* ~ ***a canela***, ~ ***a perna***, ~ ***o pernil*** kick the bucket
estigma [es'tʃigma] *m* stigma; MED, BOT scar
estigmatizar [estʃigmatʃi'zaɾ] ⟨1a⟩ *v/t* stigmatize
estilhaçar [estʃiʎa'saɾ] ⟨1p & 1b⟩ *v/t* splinter
estilhaço [estʃi'ʎasu] *m* splinter
estilista [estʃi'lista] *m/f* designer; *cabelo*: stylist
estilística [estʃi'listʃika] *f* stylistics
estilístico [estʃi'listʃiku] *adj* stylistic
estilizar [estʃili'zaɾ] ⟨1a⟩ *v/t* stylize
estilo [es'tʃilu] *m* style
estima [es'tʃima] *f* esteem; ***ter*** ~ ***a alguém*** hold s.o. in high esteem

estimação [estʃima'sãw] *f* ***animal de ~*** pet; ***meus sapatos de ~*** my favorite shoes, *Brit* my favourite shoes
estimado [estʃi'madu] *adj* valued; ***preço*** *m* ~ estimated price; *correspondência*: ***~ Senhor, estimada Senhora*** Dear Sir, Dear Madam
estimar [estʃi'mar] ⟨1a⟩ *v/t* estimate; (*valorizar*) value; (*amar*) love
estimativa [estʃima'tʃiva] *f* estimate; ***fazer uma ~ para algo*** give an estimate for sth
estimulante [estʃimu'lãtʃi] **1** *m* stimulant **2** *adj* stimulating
estimular [estʃimu'lar] ⟨1a⟩ stimulate; *ódio etc* arouse; *pessoa, crença* encourage; *pej* stir up
estímulo [es'tʃimulu] *m* stimulus
estipulação [estʃipula'sãw] *f* stipulation
estipular [estʃipu'lar] ⟨1a⟩ *v/t* stipulate
estivador [estʃiva'dor] *m* stevedore
estive [es'tʃivi] *etc* → ***estar***
estocar [esto'kar] ⟨1e & 1n⟩ *v/t* stock; *gasolina* stockpile
estofador [estofa'dor] *m* upholsterer
estofar [esto'far] ⟨1e⟩ *v/t móveis* upholster; (*enchumaçar*) pad
estofo [es'tofu] *m* (*tecido*) material; (*chumaço*) padding, stuffing; ***ter ~ para fazer algo*** have what it takes to do sth
estoicismo [estoi'sizmu] *m* stoicism
estóico [es'tɔiku] *adj* stoical
estojo [es'toʒu] *m* case; *faca*: sheath; ***~ de costura*** needle box; ***~ de desenho*** pencil case; ***~ para guitarra*** guitar case
estômago [es'tomagu] *m* stomach
Estônia, *Port* **Estónia** [es'tonja] *f* Estonia
estontear [estõ'tʃiar] ⟨1l⟩ *v/t* stun
estoque [es'tɔki] *m* stock
estoquista [esto'kista] *m/f* stockist
estore [es'tɔri] *m* shade, *Brit* blind
estória [es'tɔrja] *f Bras* story
estorninho [estor'niɲu] *m* ZOOL starling
estorvar [estor'var] ⟨1e⟩ *v/t* hinder
estorvo [es'torvu] *m* hindrance
estou [es'to] → ***estar***
estouvado [esto'vadu] *adj* foolhardy
estourar [esto'rar] ⟨1a⟩ **1** *v/i* explode; *pneu, balão* burst; *gado* stampede; ***~ de rir*** howl with laughter **2** *v/t* explode; *vidro* shatter
estouro [es'toru] *m* explosion; *gado*: stampede
estrábico [es'trabiku] *adj* cross-eyed
estrabismo [estra'bizmu] *m* squint
estrada [es'trada] *f* road; *fig* way; *Bras* ***~ de ferro*** railroad, *Brit* railway; ***~ nacional*** national highway, *Brit* trunk road; ***~ principal*** main road
estrado [es'tradu] *m* podium
estragado [estra'gadu] *adj alimento* rotten; *aparelho etc* ruined
estragão [estra'gãw] *m* ⟨*sem pl*⟩ tarragon
estraga-prazeres [estragapra'zeris] *m/f* spoilsport
estragar [estra'gar] ⟨1o & 1b⟩ ruin; **estragar-se** *v/r alimentos* go bad
estrago [es'tragu] *m* damage; (*perda*) loss; (*desperdício*) waste
estrangeiro [estrã'ʒejru] **1** *adj* foreign; ***Ministério*** *m* ***dos Negócios Estrangeiros*** State Department, *Brit* Foreign Office; ***moeda*** *f* ***estrangeira*** foreign currency **2** *m país*: ***no ~*** abroad **3** *m*, **-a** *f* foreigner
estrangulamento [estrãgula'mẽtu] *m* strangulation
estrangular [estrãgu'lar] ⟨1a⟩ strangle
estranhar [estra'ɲar] ⟨1a⟩ *v/t* ***~ algo*** find sth unfamiliar; ***eu estranhei a cama*** I couldn't get used to the bed; ***o bebê estranhou o colo*** the baby didn't like being held by a stranger
estranho [es'traɲu] **1** *adj* strange; ***ser ~ para alguém*** be alien to s.o.; ***por mais ~ que pareça*** strange as it may seem **2** *m*, **-a** *f* stranger; *não pertence ao grupo* outsider
estratégia [estra'tɛʒja] *f* strategy
estratégico [estra'tɛʒiku] *adj* strategic
estrategista [estrate'ʒista] *m/f* strategist
estrato [es'tratu] *m* layer; (*classe*) (social) stratum

E

estratosfera [estratos'fɛra] *f* stratosphere
estrear [estre'ar] ⟨1l⟩ **1** *v/t* use for the first time, christen; *sapatos* wear for the first time, christen; TEAT perform for the first time; *filme* premiere; ***a ~*** unused **2** *v/i* make one's début; **estrear-se** *v/r* make one's début; (*começar*) begin
estreia [es'treja] *f* début; *peça*: first night; *filme*: premiere; ***~ mundial*** first performance; *filme*: world premiere
estreitamente [estrejta'mẽtʃi] *adv cooperar* closely
estreitar [estrej'tar] ⟨1a⟩ **1** *v/t relações* strengthen **2** *v/i* narrow
estreito [es'trejtu] **1** *adj* (*apertado*) narrow; *cooperação* close; *ordem* strict **2** *m* strait
estrela [es'trela] *f* star *tb fig*; ***~ cadente*** falling star; ***~ de rock*** rock star
estrelado [estre'ladu] *adj* starry; *Port* ***ovo*** *m* ***~*** fried egg; ***cavalo*** *m* ***~*** horse with a blaze
estrela-do-mar [estrelado'mar] *f* ⟨*pl* estrelas-do-mar⟩ starfish
estrelar [estre'lar] ⟨1c⟩ star; *Port ovos* fry; ***estrela Brad Pitt como …*** it stars Brad Pitt as …
estremecer [estreme'ser] ⟨2g⟩ **1** *v/t* (*sacudir*) shake; (*abalar*) shatter **2** *v/i* shake; *medo*: shudder; *susto*: give a start, jump; *som* rumble
estrépito [es'trɛpitu] *m* din
estressado [estre'sadu] *adj* stressed out
estressante [estre'sãtʃi] *adj* stressful
estressar [estre'sar] ⟨1c⟩ *v/t* stress; **estressar-se** *v/r* get stressed
estresse [es'trɛsi] *m* stress; ***estar com muito ~*** be totally stressed out
estribilho [estri'biʎu] *m* chorus
estribo [es'tribu] *m cavalo*: stirrup
estricnina [estrik'nina] *f* strychnine
estridente [estri'dẽtʃi] *adj* strident
estrito [es'tritu] *adj* strict
estrofe [es'trɔfi] *f* stanza
estrondo [es'trõdu] *m* crash, rumble; *motor, tráfico*: roar; *fig* ***fazer ~*** cause a sensation
estrondoso [estrõ'dozu] *adj sucesso* resounding; *aplauso* thunderous; (*sensacional*) sensational
estrume [es'trumi] *m* manure
estrutura [estru'tura] *f* structure
estrutural [estrutu'raw] *adj* structural
estruturar [estrutu'rar] ⟨1a⟩ *v/t* structure
estuário [es'twariu] *m rio*: estuary
estudante [estu'dãtʃi] *m/f* student; ***~ universitário(-a)*** university student
estudar [estu'dar] ⟨1a⟩ study
estúdio [es'tudʒiu] *m* study; *pintor*: CINE, RÁDIO studio; ***~ de gravações*** recording studio
estudioso [estu'djozu] *adj* studious
estudo [es'tudu] *m* study; ***~ de viabilidade*** feasibility study
estufa [es'tufa] *f* MED, AGR incubator; *plantas*: greenhouse
estufado [estu'fadu] **1** *adj* stewed **2** *m* stew
estufar [estu'far] ⟨1a⟩ *v/t* GASTR stew
estupefação, *Port* **estupefacção** [estupefa'sãw] *f* ⟨*sem pl*⟩ (*assombro*) amazement
estupefato, *Port* **estupefacto** [estupe'fatu] *adj* amazed, stupefied
estupendo [estu'pẽdu] *adj* stupendous
estupidez [estupi'des] *f* stupidity
estúpido [es'tupidu] *adj* stupid
estupor [estu'por] *m* stupor
estuprar [estu'prar] ⟨1a⟩ rape
estupro [es'tupru] *m* rape; ***~ coletivo*** gang rape
estuque [es'tuki] *m* stucco
esvaecer-se [ezva'sersi] ⟨2g⟩ *v/r* slip away
esvaído [ezva'idu] *adj* weak; (*desfalecido*) in a faint
esvair-se [ezva'irsi] ⟨3l⟩ *v/r* ***~ em sangue*** lose a lot of blood
esvanecer-se [ezvane'sersi] ⟨2g⟩ *v/r* melt away
esvaziar [ezva'zjar] ⟨1g⟩ *v/t* empty; **esvaziar-se** *v/r* empty
esvoaçar [ezvwa'sar] ⟨1p & 1b⟩ *v/i* flutter
etapa [e'tapa] *f* stage
éter ['ɛtɛr] *m* ether
eternidade [eterni'dadʒi] *f* eternity
eterno [e'tɛrnu] *adj* eternal

ética ['ɛtʃika] *f* ethics
ético ['ɛtʃiku] *adj* ethical
etíope [e'tʃiupi] **1** *adj* Ethiopian **2** *m/f* Ethiopian
Etiópia [e'tʃiɔpja] *f* ***a*** ~ Ethiopia
etiqueta [etʃi'keta] *f* label; *comportamento*: etiquette; ***faltar à*** ~ commit a breach of etiquette; ~ ***de preço*** price tag
etiquetar [etʃike'tar] ⟨1c⟩ *v/t* COM label
étnico ['ɛtniku] *adj* ethnic
etnografia [ɛtnogra'fia] *f* ethnography
etnologia [ɛtnolo'ʒia] *f* ethnology
eu [ew] **1** *pron* I; ~ ***também*** me too; ***sou*** ~ it's me; ***ele saiu sem*** ~ ***notar*** he left without me noticing **2** *m* self
EUA ['ɛwa] *mpl abr* (***Estados Unidos da América***) USA
eucalipto [ewka'liptu] *m* eucalyptus
eufemismo [ewfe'mizmu] *m* euphemism
euforia [ewfo'ria] *f* euphoria
eufórico [ewfɔ'riku] euphoric
euro ['ewro] *m* euro
eurocrata [ewro'krata] *m/f* Eurocrat
eurodeputado [ewrodepu'tadu] *m*, **-a** *f* MEP, member of the European Parliament
Europa [ew'rɔpa] *f* ***a*** ~ Europe
europeu [ewro'pew] **1** *adj* European **2** *m*, **européia**, *Port* **europeia** [ewro'peja] *f* European
eutanásia [ewta'nazja] *f* euthanasia
evacuação [evakwa'sãw] *f* evacuation
evacuar [eva'kwar] ⟨1g⟩ *v/t* evacuate
evadir [eva'dʒir] ⟨3b⟩ (*evitar*) evade; **evadir-se** *v/r* escape
Evangelho [evã'ʒɛʎu] *m* gospel
evaporação [evapora'sãw] *f* ⟨*sem pl*⟩ evaporation
evaporar [evapo'rar] ⟨1e⟩ evaporate; **evaporar-se** *v/r* evaporate; (*desaparecer*) vanish
evasão [eva'zãw] *f* evasion; *prisão etc*: escape; ~ ***de impostos*** tax avoidance
evasivo [eva'zivu] *adj* evasive
evento [e'vẽtu] *m* event
eventual [evẽ'twaw] *adj* possible; (*ocasional*) occasional; ***trabalho*** *m* ~ casual work
eventualidade [evẽtwali'dadʒi] *f* eventuality
eventualmente [evẽtwaw'mẽtʃi] *adv* possibly; ~ ***ele será promovido*** he might possibly be promoted
evidência [evi'dẽsja] *f* evidence; ***ceder à*** ~ accept the evidence; ***pôr em*** ~ show up
evidenciar [evidẽ'sjar] ⟨1g⟩ *v/t* show; (*comprobar*) prove
evidente [evi'dẽtʃi] *adj* obvious, evident
evidentemente [evidẽtʃi'mẽtʃi] *adv* evidently
evitar [evi'tar] ⟨1a⟩ *v/t* avoid; *crise* avert, avoid
evitável [evi'tavew] *adj* avoidable
evocar [evo'kar] ⟨1n & 1e⟩ *v/t* evoke; *espíritos* invoke; *recordação* evoke, bring back; *imagem* conjure up
evolução [evolu'sãw] *f* evolution
evolucionismo [evolusjo'nizmu] *m* theory of evolution
evoluir [evo'lwir] ⟨3i⟩ *v/i* evolve
ex [es] *m/f* ex
exact... *Port* → ***exat...***
exagerar [ezaʒe'rar] ⟨1c⟩ exaggerate
exagero [eza'ʒeru] *m* exaggeration
exalar [eza'lar] ⟨1b⟩ *cheiro etc* give off; *suspiro* let out
exaltação [ezawta'sãw] *f* ⟨*sem pl*⟩ exaltation; (*aumento*) increase; (*excitação*) excitement; (*entusiasmo*) enthusiasm
exaltado [ezaw'tadu] *adj* overexcited, (*exagerado*) exaggerated
exaltar [ezaw'tar] ⟨1a⟩ exalt; (*aumentar*) increase; (*glorificar*) glorify; (*entusiasmar*) enthuse; (*excitar*) excite; **exaltar-se** *v/r* get worked up
exame [e'zami] *m* examination, exam; MED examination; ***prestar um*** ~ take an exam; ***passar no*** ~ pass the exam; ~ ***de admissão*** entrance exam; ~ ***final*** final; ~ ***médico*** medical (examination); ~ ***de motorista*** driving test
examinador [ezamina'dor] *m*, **-a** *f* examiner

E

examinar [ezami'naɾ] ⟨1a⟩ *v/t* examine
exasperado [ezaspe'ɾadu] *adj* exasperated
exasperante [ezaspe'ɾãtʃi] *adj* exasperating
exatamente [ezata'mẽtʃi] *adv* exactly
exatidão [ezatʃi'dãw] *f* ⟨*sem pl*⟩ accuracy; (*correção*) correctness
exato [e'zatu] *adj* exact; (*certo*) right; (*cuidadoso*) precise
exaustivo [ezaws'tʃivu] *adj* exhaustive
exausto [e'zawstu] *adj* exhausted
exaustor [ezaws'toɾ] *m* extractor fan; AUTO exhaust pipe
exceção [ese'sãw] *f* exception; DIR objection
excedentário [esedẽ'taɾiu] *adj* surplus
excedente [ese'dẽtʃi] **1** *adj* surplus **2** *m* surplus
exceder [ese'deɾ] ⟨2c⟩ *v/t* exceed; **~ *as expectativas*** exceed expectations; **exceder-se** *v/r* (*exagerar*) go too far; (*esmerar-se*) exceed oneself
excelência [ese'lẽsja] *f* excellence; ***por* ~** par excellence
Excelência [ese'lẽsja] *f* Excellency; ***Vossa* ~** Your Excellency
excelente [ese'lẽtʃi] *adj* (*óptimo*) excellent
excêntrico [e'sẽtɾiku] **1** *adj* excentric **2** *m* excentric
excepção *Port* → ***exceção***
excepcional [esesjo'naw] *adj* exceptional
excepcionalmente [esesjonaw'mẽtʃi] *adv* exceptionally
excepto *Port* → ***exceto***
excerto [es'seɾtu] *m* excerpt
excessivamente [esisiva'mẽtʃi] *adv* excessively
excessivo [ese'sivu] *adj* excessive
excesso [es'sɛsu] *m* excess; **~*s*** (*transgressão*) excesses; **~ *de bagagem*** excess baggage; **~ *de peso*** overweight, excess weight; **~ *de trabalho*** overwork; **~ *de velocidade*** speeding
exceto [es'sɛtu] *prep* except
excitação [esita'sãw] *f* excitement; *sexual* arousal
excitante [esi'tãtʃi] *adj* exciting
excitar [esi'taɾ] ⟨1a⟩ *v/t* excite; *sexualmente* arouse; **excitar-se** *v/r* get excited
excitável [esi'tavew] *adj* excitable
exclamação [esklama'sãw] *f* exclamation; ***ponto** m **de* ~** exclamation point, *Brit* exclamation mark
exclamar [eskla'maɾ] ⟨1a⟩ *v/t* exclaim
excluir [esklu'iɾ] ⟨3i⟩ *v/t* exclude
exclusão [esklu'zãw] *f* exclusion
exclusivo [esklu'zivu] **1** *adj* exclusive **2** *m* DIR sole right; COM exclusivity
excomungar [eskomũŋ'gaɾ] ⟨1o⟩ *v/t* excommunicate
excremento [eskɾe'mẽtu] *m* excrement
excursão [eskuɾ'sãw] *f* excursion, outing
excursionista [eskuɾsjo'nista] *m/f* tripper
execução [ezeku'sãw] *f* execution; MÚS, TEAT performance
executar [ezeku'taɾ] ⟨1a⟩ *v/t* execute, carry out; *peça* perform; *papel* play; *sentença* carry out; *criminoso* execute
executivo [ezeku'tʃivu] **1** *adj* executive **2** *m*, **-a** *f* executive
executor [ezeku'toɾ] *m* executioner; **~ *judicial*** bailiff; **~ *testamentário*** executor
exemplar [ezẽ'plaɾ] **1** *adj* exemplary, model **2** *m* model; *livro*: copy
exemplo [e'zẽplu] *m* example; (*ideal*) ideal; ***dar o* ~** set an example; ***por* ~** for example
exercer [ezeɾ'seɾ] ⟨2g⟩ exercise; *desporto* do; *negócio* carry on; *direito*, *medicina* practice, *Brit* practise; *autoridade* exert; **~ *represália*** take reprisals
exercício [ezeɾ'sisiu] *m* (*treino*) exercise; *direito*, *medicina*: practice; COM fiscal year, *Brit* financial year; ESP **~ *livre*** freestyle section; ***em* ~** in office
exercitar [ezeɾsi'taɾ] ⟨1a⟩ practice, *Brit* practise; MIL drill
exército [e'zɛɾsitu] *m* army
exibição [ezibi'sãw] *f* exhibition; TEAT performance; ***em* ~** on show
exibicionista [ezibisjo'nista] *m/f* exhibitionist

exibir [ezi'biɾ] ⟨3a⟩ *papéis*, *filme*, *motivos* show; *mercadoria* display; *exposição*: exhibit; *talento etc* show off; **exibir-se** *v/r pej* show off; *tarado* expose oneself
exigência [ezi'ʒẽsja] *f* demand; DIR requirement
exigente [ezi'ʒẽtʃi] *adj* demanding
exigir [ezi'ʒiɾ] ⟨3n⟩ demand, require
exilado [ezi'ladu] *m*, **-a** *f* exile
exilar [ezi'laɾ] ⟨1a⟩ *v/t* exile
exílio [e'ziliu] *m* exile
existência [ezis'tẽsja] *f* existence; COM **~s** *pl* stock
existir [ezis'tʃiɾ] ⟨3a⟩ exist; ***passar a ~*** come into existence
êxito ['ezitu] *m* (*resultado*) result; (*sucesso*) success
exonerar [ezone'ɾaɾ] ⟨1c⟩ *v/t* exonerate
exorbitante [ezoɾbi'tãtʃi] *adj* exorbitant
exótico [e'zɔtʃiku] *adj* exotic
expandir [espã'dʒiɾ] ⟨3a⟩ **1** *v/t* expand; *asas* spread; (*divulgar*) spread **2** *v/i* expand; **expandir-se** *v/r* expand
expansão [espã'sãw] *f* expansion; (*difusão*) spread; ***uma cidade em ~*** an expanding city
expansivo [espã'sivu] *adj* outgoing, expansive
expatriação [espatria'sãw] *f* expatriation
expatriado [espatɾi'adu] *m*, **-a** *f* expatriate, *fam* expat
expatriar [espatɾi'aɾ] ⟨1g⟩ *v/t* expatriate
expectativa [espekta'tʃiva] *f* expectation; ***estar na ~ de*** expect; ***~ de vida*** life expectancy
expectorante [espekto'ɾãtʃi] *m* MED expectorant
expectoração [espektoɾa'sãw] *f* MED expectoration
expectorar [espekto'ɾaɾ] ⟨1e⟩ *v/t* cough up
expedição [espedʒi'sãw] *f carta*: sending, despatch; *mercadoria*: shipment; (*viagem*) expedition
expediente [espe'djẽtʃi] **1** *adj pessoa* resourceful **2** *m* (*dia de trabalho*) workday; (*tarefas*) workload; (*correspondência*) correspondence; ***ele vive de ~s*** he just has the odd job now and again; ***horas** fpl **de ~*** opening hours
expedir [espe'dʒiɾ] ⟨3r⟩ *v/t correio*, *mercadoria*, *tropas* send
expelir [espe'liɾ] ⟨3c⟩ *v/t* expel
experiência [espe'ɾjẽsja] *f* experience; (*tentativa*, *teste*) experiment
experiente [espe'ɾjẽtʃi] *adj* experienced
experimental [espeɾimẽ'taw] *adj* experimental
experimentar [espeɾimẽ'taɾ] ⟨1a⟩ **1** *v/t* try out; *roupa* try on; *comida* try; (*tentar*) *método* experiment with; (*sentir*) experience **2** *v/i* experiment
expiar [es'pjaɾ] ⟨1g⟩ *v/t* atone for
expiração [espiɾa'sãw] *f* ⟨*sem pl*⟩ exhalation; *prazo*: expiration, *Brit* expiry
expirar [espi'ɾaɾ] ⟨1a⟩ **1** *v/t* breathe out **2** *v/i* expire; *som*, *voz*, (*morrer*) die
explicação [esplika'sãw] *f* explanation; ***explicações** pl* private tuition
explicar [espli'kaɾ] ⟨1n⟩ explain
explicitamente [esplisita'mẽtʃi] *adv* explicitly
explícito [es'plisitu] *adj* explicit
explodir [esplo'dʒiɾ] ⟨3f⟩ explode, blow up
exploração [esploɾa'sãw] *f* exploration; *abuso* exploitation
explorador [esploɾa'doɾ] **1** *m*, **-a** explorer; *abuso*: exploiter **2** *adj* exploratory; (*abusador*) exploitative
explorar [esplo'ɾaɾ] ⟨1e⟩ explore; MIN exploit, work; COM *negócio* run; *fig possibilidades* explore; (*abusar*) exploit
explosão [esplo'zãw] *f* explosion *tb fig*; ***~ de violência*** outbreak of violence
explosivo [esplo'zivu] **1** *adj* explosive **2** *m* explosive
expoente [es'pwẽtʃi] *m tb* MAT exponent
expor [es'poɾ] ⟨2z⟩ *v/t* show, display; *quadros etc* exhibit; *pensamentos* reveal; *acontecimentos* present; *foto*, *cri-*

minoso expose; **~ *alguém a algo*** expose s.o. to sth; **expor-se** *v/r* show oneself; (*arriscar-se*) expose oneself (to risk)
exportação [esporta'sãw] *f* export; ***autorização*** *f* ***de ~*** export permit; ***imposto*** *m* ***de ~*** export duty
exportador [esporta'dor] *m*, **-a** *f* exporter
exportar [espor'tar] ⟨1e⟩ export
exposição [espozi'sãw] *f* exhibition; (*explicação*) exposition; *foto*: exposure; ***estar em ~*** be on display; **~ *de flores*** flower show
expositor [espozi'tor] *m*, **-a** *f* exhibitor; **~ *de vidro*** display case
expressamente [espresa'mẽtʃi] *adv* expressly
expressão [espre'sãw] *f* expression; ***liberdade*** *f* ***de ~*** freedom of speech
expressar [espre'sar] ⟨1c⟩ *v/t* express; **expressar-se** *v/r* express oneself
expressionismo [espresjo'nizmu] *m* expressionism
expressivo [espre'sivu] *adj* expressive; (*enérgico*) emphatic
expresso [es'prɛsu] **1** *adj* express, clear; (*pronunciado*) definite **2** *m* express; *correio*: express delivery
exprimir [espri'mir] ⟨3a⟩ *v/t* express
expropriação [espropria'sãw] *f* expropriation
expropriar [espropri'ar] ⟨1g⟩ expropriate
expulsão [espuw'sãw] *f* expulsion; *jogador*: sending off
expulsar [espuw'sar] ⟨1a⟩ expel; (*pôr na rua*) throw out; *jogador* send off
êxtase ['estazi] *m* ecstasy
extasiado ['estaziadu] *adj* ecstatic
extensão [estẽ'sãw] *f* extension; (*comprimento*) extent; (*duração*) length; *Port* TEL extension
extenso [es'tẽsu] *adj* extensive; (*comprido*) long; *som*: extended; ***por ~*** in full
extenuado [este'nwadu] *adj* weakened, worn out
extenuante [este'nwãtʃi] *adj* exhausting
extenuar [este'nwar] ⟨1g⟩ *v/t* exhaust; (*enfraquecer*) weaken
exterior [este'rior] **1** *adj* outside, exterior **2** *m* outside, exterior; (*estrangeiro*) foreign countries; ***viajar no ~*** travel abroad; ***do ~*** from abroad
exteriorizar [esteriori'zar] ⟨1a⟩ *v/t* show, display
exterminar [estermi'nar] ⟨1a⟩ exterminate
extermínio [ester'miniu] *m* extermination
externo [es'tɛrnu] **1** *adj* external; ***mercado*** *m* **~** overseas market; ***uso*** *m* **~** external use; ***aluno*** *m* **~** day pupil **2** *m*, **-a** *f* day pupil; CINE ***em externas*** on location
extinção [estʃĩ'sãw] *f* ⟨*sem pl*⟩ extinction
extinguir [estʃĩ'gir] ⟨3o⟩ *v/t fogo* put out, extinguish; (*exterminar*) eradicate; *lei* abolish; *empresa* wind up; *dívida* get rid off; **extinguir-se** *v/r* go out; *espécie* die out, become extinct
extintor [estʃĩ'tor] *m* fire extinguisher
extorquir [estor'kir] ⟨3o⟩ *v/t* extort
extorsão [estor'sãw] *f* extortion
extra ['estra] *m* extra
extração, *Port* **extracção** [estra'sãw] *f* extraction; *lotaria*: draw
extraconjugal [estrakõʒu'gaw] *adj* extramarital
extracto *Port* → ***extrato***
extradição [estradʒi'sãw] *f* extradition
extraditar [estradʒi'tar] ⟨1a⟩ *v/t* extradite
extrair [estra'ir] ⟨3l⟩ *v/t* extract
extraordinário [estraordʒi'nariu] *adj* extraordinary
extraterrestre [estrate'hɛstri] **1** *adj* extraterrestrial **2** *m/f* extraterrestrial
extrato [es'tratu] *m* extract; FIN **~ *bancário*** bank statement
extravagante [estrava'gãtʃi] *adj* extravagant
extraviar [estra'vjar] ⟨1g⟩ *v/t* mislay; *fraude*: embezzle; ***as mercadorias foram extraviadas*** the goods went missing
extremamente [estrema'mẽtʃi] *adv* extremely

extremidade [estremi'dadʒi] *f* extremity; (*ponta*) tip
extremismo [estre'mizmu] *m* extremism; **~ de direita / esquerda** right-wing / left-wing extremism
extremista [estre'mista] *m/f* POL extremist
extremo [es'tremu] **1** *adj* extreme; (*final*) last **2** *m* extreme; (*fim*) end; ***Extremo Oriente*** Far East
extremoso [estre'mozu] *adj* doting
extrovertido [estrover'tʃidu] **1** *adj* extrovert **2** *m*, **-a** *f* extrovert
exuberante [ezube'rãtʃi] *adj* exuberant
exultar [ezuw'tar] ⟨1a⟩ *v/i* exult

F

fá [fa] *m* MÚS F
fã [fã] *m/f* fan
fábrica ['fabrika] *f* factory, plant; ***~ de gás*** gas works; ***~ de montagem*** assembly plant
fabricação [fabrika'sãw] *f* manufacture
fabricante [fabri'kãtʃi] *m* manufacturer
fabricar [fabri'kar] ⟨1n⟩ *v/t* manufacture, make; ***fabricado no Japão*** made in Japan
fabrico [fa'briku] *m* production; (*produto*) product
fábula ['fabula] *f* fable; *Bras dinheiro*: fortune
fabuloso [fabu'lozu] *adj* fabulous
faca ['faka] *f* knife; *fam* ***ir à ~*** go under the knife; *fig* ***ter a ~ e o queijo na mão*** have things in hand; ***~ de pão*** breadknife
facada [fa'kada] *f* stab
faça ['fasa] → ***fazer***
façanha [fa'saɲa] *f* exploit
facção [fa'ksãw] *f* faction
faccioso [fa'ksjozu] *adj* factious; (*parcial*) biased
face ['fasi] *f* cheek; (*rosto*) face; (*frente*) front; ***em ~ de*** in view of; ***~ a ~*** face to face
faceta [fa'seta] *f* facet
fachada [fa'ʃada] *f* façade; *livro*: front; ***~ da loja*** storefront
facho ['faʃu] *m*, **-a** *f fam* fascist
facial [fa'sjaw] *adj* facial
fácil ['fasiw] easy; (*acessível*) accessible; (*estouvado*) rash
facilidade [fasili'dadʒi] *f* ease; (*amabilidade*) kindness; ***~s*** *pl de pagamento etc* facilities; ***com ~*** easily; ***ela tem ~ para línguas*** she has a gift for languages
facilitar [fasili'tar] ⟨1a⟩ *v/t* make easy, facilitate; (*conseguir*) provide, supply; (*apoiar*) support
facilmente [fasiw'mẽtʃi] *adv* easily
faço ['fasu] → ***fazer***
fact... *Port* → ***fat...***
faculdade [fakuw'dadʒi] *f* faculty, ability; (*direito*) right; DIR authority; ***Faculdade*** faculty; ***~s*** *pl* ***mentais*** mental faculties
facultativo [fakuwta'tʃivu] *adj* optional
fada ['fada] *f* fairy
fadiga [fa'dʒiga] *f* fatigue; (*trabalho*) effort; (*esforço*) strain; ***~ ocular*** eye strain
fadista [fa'dʒista] *m/f* fado singer
fado ['fadu] *m* (*sina*) fate, destiny; MÚS fado
fagote [fa'gɔtʃi] *m* MÚS bassoon
faia ['faja] *f* beech
faiança [fa'jãsa] *f* crockery
faina ['fajna] *f* work, task; (*azáfama*) grind, toil
faisão [faj'zãw] *m* pheasant
faísca [fa'iska] *f* spark; (*relâmpago*) flash
faiscar [fais'kar] ⟨1n & 1q⟩ *v/i* (*relam-*

pejar) flash; (*cintilar*) sparkle
faixa ['fajʃa] *f* sling, bandage; (*fita*) strip; (*banda*) band; (*tira*) strip; *uniforme*: sash; AUTO, ESP lane; (*passadeira*) crosswalk, *Brit* zebra crossing; *salarial*: bracket; *etária* group; **~ *anti--suor*** sweatband; **~ *de contribuição*** tax bracket; **~ *etária*** age group; ESP **~ *interna*** inside lane; **~ *de paragem de emergência*** berm, *Brit* hard shoulder; **~ *de ultrapassagem*** passing lane, *Brit* overtaking lane

F

fala ['fala] *f* speech; (*palavras*) words; (*linguagem*) language; ***sem* ~** speechless
falador [fala'doɾ] *adj* talkative
falante [fa'lãʧi] **1** *adj* speaking *atr*, talking *atr* **2** *m/f* **~ *nativo, -a*** native speaker
falar [fa'laɾ] ⟨1b⟩ speak, talk; (*dizer*) say; **~ *bem de alguém*** speak highly of s.o.; **~ *em nome de*** speak on behalf of; **~ *sobre algo*** talk about sth; **~ *inglês / português*** speak English / Portuguese; ***estou falando sério*** I'm serious
falatório [fala'tɔriu] *m* (*mexericos*) gossip; *mídia*: hype
falcão [faw'kãw] *m* falcon
falecer [fale'seɾ] ⟨2g⟩ die, pass away
falecido [fale'sidu] **1** *adj* dead **2** *m*, **-a** *f* deceased
falecimento [falesi'mẽtu] *m* death, demise
falência [fa'lẽsja] *f* COM bankruptcy; ***abrir* ~** go bankrupt
falésia [fa'lɛzja] *f* cliff
falha ['faʎa] *f* (*erro*) fault; (*racha*) crack; (*lasca*) splinter; *dum plano*, TECN flaw, malfunction; ELÉT fault; INFORM crash; **~ *humana*** human error
falhar [fa'ʎaɾ] ⟨1b⟩ **1** *v/i* fail; TECN malfunction; *computador* crash **2** *v/t* **~ *a meta*** fail to meet the goal; **~ *o jogo*** miss the game
falido [fa'lidu] *adj* ECON bankrupt
falir [fa'liɾ] ⟨3b⟩ COM go bankrupt, *fam* go bust
falível [fa'livew] *adj* fallible
falsidade [fawsi'dadʒi] *f* falsehood, deceit; (*mentira*) lie
falsificação [fawsifika'sãw] *f* fake, forgery; *ato* falsification
falsificado [fawsifi'kadu] *adj* fake; *dinheiro* counterfeit
falsificador [fawsifika'doɾ] *m*, **-a** *f dinheiro*: forger
falsificar [fawsifi'kaɾ] ⟨1n⟩ fake; *dinheiro* forge, (*alterar deliberadamente*) falsify
falso ['fawsu] *adj* (*errado, dissimulado*) false; (*imitado*) fake; ***ataque*** *m* **~** feint; ***chave*** *f* ***falsa*** skeleton key; ***juramento*** *m* **~** perjury, false evidence
falta ['fawta] *f* (*erro*) fault; (*carência*) lack (***de*** of); (*avaria*) failure; (*ausência*) absence; *futebol*: foul; ***sem* ~** without fail; ***sentir* ~ *de*** miss; ***estar com* ~ *de pessoal*** be short-staffed; ESP ***cometer* ~ *em alguém*** foul s.o.; **~ *de água*** water shortage; **~ *de educação*** rudeness; **~ *de gravidade*** weightlessness; **~ *de luz*** power outage, *Brit* power cut
faltar [faw'taɾ] ⟨1a⟩ *v/i* be lacking; (*não estar*) be missing; (*não vir*) be absent; *provisões* run out; *forças etc* give out; ***faltam ainda seis semanas para o Natal*** there are still six weeks to go to Christmas; ***ainda falta muito para acabar*** it's nowhere near finished; ***faltei à aula*** I missed the class; ***me falta arroz*** I don't have any rice
fama ['fama] *f* (*reputação*) reputation; (*celebridade*) fame; (*opinião pública*) public opinion; ***ter* ~** be famous; ***ter boa / má* ~** have a good / bad reputation; ***ter* ~ *de*** be said to be
família [fa'milja] *f* family; **~ *monoparental*** single-parent family
familiar [fami'ljaɾ] **1** *adj* family *atr*; (*à vontade*) familiar **2** *m* relative
familiaridade [familjaɾi'dadʒi] *f* familiarity
familiarizar [familjaɾi'zaɾ] ⟨1a⟩ familiarize; **familiarizar-se** *v/r* familiarize oneself (***com*** with)
faminto [fa'mĩtu] *adj* hungry; *fig tb* eager (***de*** for)
famoso [fa'mozu] *adj* famous; **~ *mundialmente*** world-famous
fanático [fa'naʧiku] **1** *adj* fanatical

2 *m*, **-a** *f* fanatic
fanatismo [fana'tʃizmu] *m* fanaticism
fanfarrão [fãfa'hãw] *m*, **-ona** [fãfa'hona] *f* show-off, poser
fanfarrice [fãfa'hisi] *f* swagger
fantasia [fãta'zia] *f* (*imaginação*) imagination; fantasy *tb* MÚS, ARTE; *Carnaval*: costume; ***de ~*** imaginary; *tecido* patterned
fantasiar [fãta'zjaɾ] ⟨1g⟩ **1** *v/t* imagine; (*inventar*) invent **2** *v/i* fantasize; **fantasiar-se** *v/r* dress up (***de*** as)
fantasma [fã'tazma] *m* ghost; (*quimera*) illusion
fantasmagórico [fãtazma'gɔriku] *adj* ghostly
fantasticamente [fãtastʃika'mẽtʃi] *adv* fantastically
fantástico [fã'tastʃiku] *adj* fantastic
fantoche [fã'tɔʃi] *m* glove puppet
faqueiro [fa'kejɾu] *m* set of cutlery
farda ['faɾda] *f* uniform
fardo ['faɾdu] *m* bundle; (*carga*) load, burden
farei [fa'ɾej] *etc* → ***fazer***
farejar [faɾe'ʒaɾ] ⟨1d⟩ **1** *v/t* (*perseguir*) sniff around **2** *v/i* sniff
farelento [faɾe'lẽtu] *adj* crumbly
faria [fa'ɾia] *etc*→ ***fazer***
faringe [fa'ɾĩʒi] *f* pharynx
faringite [faɾĩ'ʒitʃi] *f* MED pharyngitis
farinha [fa'ɾiɲa] *f* flour; ***~ de aveia*** oatmeal; ***~ de rosca*** breadcrumbs
farmacêutico [faɾma'sewtʃiku] **1** *adj* pharmaceutical **2** *m*, **-a** *f* pharmacist
farmácia [faɾ'masja] *f* pharmacy, *Brit tb* chemist's
faro ['faɾu] *m* sense of smell; (*sagacidade*) flair, *fam* nose
faroeste [faɾo'ɛstʃi] *m* western
farol [fa'ɾɔw] *m* lighthouse; AUTO headlight; ***~ alto*** high beam, *Brit* full beam; ***~ baixo*** dimmed beam, *Brit* dipped headlights; ***~ traseiro*** rear light; ***~ vermelho*** red light
farolete [faɾo'letʃi] *m*, **farolim** [faɾo'lĩ] *m* parking lights
farpa ['faɾpa] *f* barb; (*lasca*) splinter
farpado [faɾ'padu] *adj* ***arame m ~*** barbed wire
farra ['faha] *f fam* party; ***cair na ~***, ***fazer ~*** paint the town red
farrapo [fa'hapu] *m* rag
farsa ['faɾsa] *f* farce
farsante [faɾ'sãtʃi] *m/f* (*brincalhão*) joker
fartar [faɾ'taɾ] ⟨1b⟩ *v/t* satisfy, fill up; **fartar-se** *v/r* eat one's fill; *fig* ***~ de*** get fed up with
farto ['faɾtu] *adj* (*cheio*) full; *Port* (*aborrecido*) fed up; ***estar ~ de*** be fed up with
fartura [faɾ'tuɾa] *f* plenty, abundance
fascículo [fas'sikulu] *m* installment, *Brit* instalment
fascinador [fasina'doɾ] *adj*, **fascinante** [fasi'nãtʃi] *adj* fascinating
fascinar [fasi'naɾ] ⟨1a⟩ fascinate
fascínio [fas'siniu] *m* fascination
fascismo [fas'sizmu] *m* fascism
fascista [fas'sista] **1** *m/f* fascist **2** *adj* fascist
fase ['fazi] *f* phase
fastidioso [fastʃi'djozu] *adj* (*monótono*) tedious; (*irritante*) annoying
fastio [fas'tʃiu] *m* (*falta de apetite*) lack of appetite
fatal [fa'taw] *adj dia*, *decisão* fateful; (*inevitável*) inevitable; (*mortal*) fatal; ***é ~ como o destino*** it's as sure as fate
fatalidade [fatali'dadʒi] *f* fate; *acidente*: fatality
fatalismo [fata'lizmu] *m* fatalism
fatalista [fata'lista] *m/f* fatalist
fatalmente [fataw'mẽtʃi] *adv ferido* fatally
fatia [fa'tʃia] *f* slice; ***~ de mercado*** market share
fatídico [fa'tʃidʒiku] *adj* ***o navio ~*** the doomed ship
fatigado [fatʃi'gadu] *adj* tired
fatigante [fatʃi'gãtʃi] *adj* tiring
fatigar [fatʃi'gaɾ] ⟨1o⟩ tire; (*fartar*) bore
fato[1] ['fatu] *m* fact; ***de ~*** really, in fact; ***estar ao ~ de*** be informed about
fato[2] ['fatu] *m Port* suit; (*roupa*) clothes; ***~ de banho*** swimsuit; ***~ de treino*** sweats, *Brit* tracksuit
fato-macaco [fatoma'kaku] *m Port* coverall, *Brit* overalls
fator [fa'toɾ] *m* factor *tb* MAT; ***~ de proteção solar*** protection factor

fatura [fa'tuɾa] *f* invoice

faturamento [fatuɾa'mẽtu] *m* turnover; (*enviar faturas*) invoicing

faturar [fatu'ɾaɾ] ⟨1a⟩ invoice

fauna ['fawna] *f* fauna

fava ['fava] *f* (broad) bean

favela [fa'vɛla] *f Bras* slum

favo ['favu] *m* **~ *de mel*** honeycomb

favor [fa'voɾ] *m* favor, *Brit* favour; ***por ~, (se) faz ~, faça ~*** please; ***a ~ de*** in favor of; ***fazer um ~ a alguém*** do s.o. a favor; ***faça-me o ~!*** give me a break!

favorável [favo'ɾavew] *adj* favorable, *Brit* favourable; *cor, roupa* flattering

favorecer [favoɾe'seɾ] ⟨2g⟩ favor, *Brit* favour; *vestuário* suit

favorito [favo'ɾitu] **1** *adj* favorite, *Brit* favourite **2** *m*, **-a** *f* favorite, *Brit* favourite

fax [faks] *m* fax

faxineiro [faʃi'nejɾu] *m*, **-a** *f* cleaner

faz [fas] → ***fazer***

faz-de-conta [fazdʒi'kõta] *m* make-believe

fazenda [fa'zẽda] *f* AGR farm; *açucar*: plantation; *tecido*: cloth; *Bras* ***Ministério*** *m* ***da Fazenda*** Treasury Department, *Brit* Exchequer

fazendeiro [fazẽ'dejɾu] *m*, **-a** *f* farmer; *açucar*: plantation owner

fazer [fa'zeɾ] ⟨2v⟩ **1** *v/t* (*fabricar*) make; *trabalho, honra, cabelo, exame* do; *dinheiro* earn, make; *cama* make; *seguro* take out; *cheque* make out; *foto* take; *mala* pack; ***o que estás fazendo?*** what are you doing?; ***ser feito de*** be made of; ***ele foi feito para ser músico*** he's a natural musician; ***ela foi feita para mim*** she was made for me; *fig* ***é bem feito para você*** it serves you right; ***não faz diferença*** it doesn't make any difference, it doesn't matter; ***faz 50 dólares*** it comes to 50 dollars, it makes 50 dollars; **~ *algo brilhar*** make sth shine; **~ *mal a alguém*** hurt s.o.; **~ *anos*** have a birthday; ***faz 30 anos*** he's 30
2 *v/i* do; ***faça você mesmo*** do it yourself; ***vá em frente, faça!*** go on, do it!; **~ *bem / mal*** do the right / wrong thing; **~ *com que alguém faça algo*** make s.o. do sth; **~ *de conta que*** pretend that; ***tanto faz*** it's all the same, I don't mind
3 *v/impessoal* ***hoje faz calor*** it is hot today; ***faz uma semana*** a week ago; ***faz dois anos que eu o vi*** it's two years since I saw him, I haven't seen him in two years
4 ***fazer-se*** *v/r* **~ *entender*** make oneself understood; **~ *passar por*** pose as; ***isso não se faz*** that's not done; ***faz-se com arroz*** it's made with rice

fé [fɛ] *f* faith; (*confiança*) trust (***de, em*** in); ***de boa ~*** in good faith; ***de má ~*** in bad faith; ***dar ~ a*** have faith in

fealdade [fjaw'dadʒi] *f* ugliness

febre ['fɛbɾi] *f* fever; ***estar com ~*** have a temperature *ou* fever; **~ *do feno*** hay fever

febril [fe'bɾiw] *adj* feverish

fechadura [feʃa'duɾa] *f porta*: lock

fechamento [feʃa'mẽtu] *m* closure

fechar [fe'ʃaɾ] ⟨1d⟩ **1** *v/t* close, shut; *trabalho, contrato* conclude; *companhia* close down; *venda* close; *torneira* turn off; *dinheiro* lock away; *pessoa* lock up; **~ *à chave*** lock **2** *v/i* close, shut; **fechar-se** *v/r fig* shut oneself away

fecho ['feʃu] *m* fastening; *porta*: latch; *Bras* **~ *ecler***, *Port* **~ *éclair*** zip fastener, *Brit* zip

fécula ['fɛkula] *f* starch

fecundação [fekũda'sãw] *f* fertilization; **~ *artificial*** artificial fertilization

fecundar [fekũ'daɾ] ⟨1a⟩ *v/t* fertilize

fecundidade [fekũdʒi'dadʒi] *f* fertility

fecundo [fe'kũdu] *adj* fertile

feder [fe'deɾ] ⟨2c⟩ stink

federação [fedeɾa'sãw] *f* federation

federal [fede'ɾaw] *adj* federal

federalismo [fedeɾa'lizmu] *m* federalism

federalista [fedeɾa'lista] *adj* federalist

fedor [fe'doɾ] *m* stench

fedorento [fedo'ɾẽtu] *adj* stinking

feição [fej'sãw] *f* form, shape; (*aparência*) appearance; (*caráter*) nature; *fisionomia*: ***feições*** features; ***estar de ~*** be favorable, *Brit* be favourable

feijão [fej'ʒãw] *m* bean; **~ *roxo*** kidney

bean; ~ ***de soja*** soy bean; ~ ***verde*** green bean
feijão-da-espanha [fejʒãwdas'paɲa] *m Port* runner bean
feijoada [fej'ʒwada] *f dish made of black beans and pork*
feinho [fe'iɲu] *adj* homely, *Brit* plain
feio ['feiu] *adj* ugly; *futuro* grim; *tempo* foul
feira ['fejɾa] *f popular* fair; (*mercado*) market; (*exposição*) trade fair
feitiçaria [fejʧisa'ɾia] *f* witchcraft
feiticeiro [fejʧi'sejɾu] *m*, **-a** *f* wizard; *mulher* witch
feitiço [fej'ʧisu] *m* (magic) spell
feitio [fej'ʧiu] *m* shape; (*caráter*) nature; *vestido*: cut; ***não é de seu*** ~ it's not like him
feito ['fejtu] **1** *pp de* ***fazer***; finished; (*pronto*) ready; ~ ***em casa*** homemade **2** *adj* ***homem*** *m* ~ grown man **2** *m* feat
feixe ['fejʃi] *m* bundle; AGR sheaf
fel [fɛw] *m* gall
felicidade [felisi'dadʒi] *f* happiness; ~***s!*** good luck!; ***muitas*** ~ ***s!*** congratulations!
felicitação [felisita'sãw] *f* congratulations
felicitar [felisi'taɾ] ⟨1a⟩ congratulate (***por*** on)
felino [fe'linu] **1** *adj* feline; *fig* treacherous **2** *m* ZOOL ~***s*** *pl* cats, felines
feliz [fe'lis] *adj* happy; ***Feliz Ano Novo!*** Happy New Year!
felizmente [feliz'mẽʧi] *adv* fortunately
feltro ['fewtɾu] *m* felt
fêmea ['femja] *f* female
feminino [femi'ninu] *adj* feminine; (*para senhoras*) women's *atr*
feminismo [femi'nizmu] *m* feminism
feminista [femi'nista] **1** *m/f* feminist **2** *adj* feminist
fêmur, *Port* **fémur** ['femuɾ] *m* femur
fenda ['fẽda] *f* crack, split
fender [fẽ'deɾ] ⟨2a⟩ *v/t* crack, split
feno ['fenu] *m* hay
fenol [fe'nɔw] *m* phenol
fenomenal [fenome'naw] *adj* phenomenal
fenômeno, *Port* **fenómeno** [fe'nomenu] *m* phenomenon *tb fig*
fera ['fɛɾa] *f* wild animal; *fig pop* beast
feriado [fe'ɾjadu] **1** *adj* vacation *atr*, *Brit* holiday *atr*; ***dia*** *m* ~ public holiday **2** *m* public holiday; ~ ***nacional*** national holiday
férias ['fɛɾjas] *fpl* vacation, *Brit* holidays; *escola*: vacation; ***tirar*** ~***s*** take a vacation; ***tirar um dia / uma semana de*** ~ take a day / week off; ~***s*** *pl* ***de verão*** summer vacation, *Brit* summer holidays
ferida [fe'ɾida] *f* wound; (*ferimento*) injury
ferido [fe'ɾidu] **1** *m*, **-a** *f* casualty **2** *adj* injured; *fig* hurt; MIL wounded
ferimento [feɾi'mẽtu] *m* injury; MIL wound; ~ ***à bala*** gunshot wound
ferir [fe'ɾiɾ] ⟨3c⟩ *v/t* injure; *fig* hurt; MIL wound
fermentação [feɾmẽta'sãw] *f* fermentation
fermentar [feɾmẽ'taɾ] ⟨1a⟩ *v/i* ferment *tb fig*; *massa* rise
fermento [feɾ'mẽtu] *m* yeast; ~ ***em pó*** baking powder
feroz [fe'ɾɔs] *adj* fierce
ferradura [fehã'duɾa] *f* horseshoe
ferragens [fe'haʒẽs] *fpl* hardware; ***loja*** *f* ***de*** ~ hardware store
ferramenta [fehã'mẽta] *f* tool
ferrão [fe'hãw] *m inseto*: sting
ferrar [fe'haɾ] ⟨1c⟩ *cavalo etc* shoe; *gado etc* brand; ~ ***os dentes*** *ou* ***as unhas em*** get stuck into
ferreiro [fe'hejɾu] *m*, **-a** *f* blacksmith
férreo ['fɛhiu] *adj* iron; (*intransigente*) strict; ***rede*** *f* ***férrea*** railroad network, *Brit* railway network; ***via*** *f* ***férrea*** railroad, *Brit* railway; ***vontade*** *f* ***férrea*** iron will
ferro ['fɛhu] *m* iron; (*queimadura*) brand; ***passar a*** ~ *roupa* iron; ~ (***de engomar***) iron; ~ ***batido*** *ou* ***forjado*** wrought iron; ~ ***fundido*** cast iron
ferrolho [fe'hoʎu] *m* bolt
ferro-velho [fɛho'vɛʎu] *m* scrap metal; (*negociante*) scrap metal dealer; *lugar* junk yard
ferrovia [fɛho'via] *f* railroad, *Brit* railway
ferroviário [fɛho'vjaɾiu] **1** *adj* rail-

road *atr*, *Brit* railway *atr*; ***pessoal** m* **~** railroad workers **2** *m*, **-a** *f* railroad worker, *Brit* railwayman
ferrugem [fe'huʒẽ] *f* rust; AGR blight; ***criar* ~** go rusty *tb fig*
ferrugento [fehu'ʒẽtu] *adj* rusty
ferry ['fɛhi] *m*, **ferry-boat** [fɛhi'bot] *m* ferry
fértil ['fɛrʧiw] *adj* fertile
fertilidade [ferʧili'dadʒi] *f* fertility
fertilizante [ferʧili'zãʧi] *m* fertilizer
fertilizar [ferʧili'zaɾ] ⟨1a⟩ *v/t* fertilize
ferver [feɾ'ver] ⟨2c⟩ boil; **~ *de raiva*** seethe with rage; **~ *de insetos*** be crawling with insects; ***estar fervendo*** *raiva*: be seething
fervor [feɾ'voɾ] *m fig* fervor, *Brit* fervour
fervoso [fervo'rozu] *adj* (*veemente*) fervent; *aplausos* wild
fervura [feɾ'vura] *f* boiling; *fig* excitement; ***dar uma* ~** bring quickly to the boil
festa ['fɛsta] *f* party; (*festejo*) festival; ***boas* ~ *s!*** happy holidays!, Merry Christmas and a Happy New Year!; **~ *de aniversário*** birthday party; **~ *dançante*** dance, ball; **~ *de despedida*** leaving party; **~ *à fantasia*** fancy-dress party; ***festa junina*** *traditional Brazilian festival in June*; **~ *popular*** traditional festival
festejar [feste'ʒaɾ] ⟨1d⟩ celebrate
festejo [fes'teʒu] *m* celebration, festivity; **~ *popular*** traditional festival
festival [fesʧi'vaw] *m* festival
festivo [fes'ʧivu] *adj* festive
fétido ['fɛʧidu] *adj* foul, fetid
feto[1] ['fɛtu] *m* MED fetus
feto[2] ['fɛtu] *m Port* BOT fern
feudal [few'daw] *adj* feudal
feudalismo [fewda'lizmu] *m* feudalism
fevereiro [feve'rejɾu] *m* February; ***em* ~** in February
fez [fes] → ***fazer***
fezes ['fɛzis] *fpl* MED feces
fiação [fja'sãw] *f* TÊX spinning; (***fábrica** f **de***) **~** textile mill
fiado ['fjadu] *adj & adv* on credit; ***comprar* ~** buy on credit; *fig* ***conversa** f **fiada*** nonsense
fiador [fja'doɾ] *m*, **-a** *f* guarantor
fiambre ['fjãbɾi] *m* ham
fiança ['fjãsa] *f* guarantee; DIR bail; ***prestar* ~** stand bail; DIR ***sob* ~** on bail
fiar[1] ['fjaɾ] ⟨1g⟩ spin
fiar[2] ['fjaɾ] ⟨1g⟩ **1** *v/t* (*confiar*) entrust **2** *v/i* sell on credit; **fiar-se** *v/r* **~ *de, em*** trust; ***aqui não se fia*** no credit here
fiasco ['fjasku] *m* fiasco
fibra ['fibra] *f* fiber, *Brit* fibre; ***de* ~ *ótica***, *Port* ***de* ~ *óptica*** fiber-optic, *Brit* fibre-optic; **~ *de vidro*** fiberglass, *Brit* fibreglass
fibroso [fi'brozu] *adj* fibrous
ficar [fi'kaɾ] ⟨1n⟩ ◊ (*tornar-se*) get, become; **~ *entusiasmado com algo*** get *ou* become excited about sth; **~ *mareado*** get seasick; **~ *fora de controle*** get out of control; **~ *furioso*** go wild; **~ *louco*** go mad; **~ *amigo de alguém*** make friends with s.o.
◊ (*ser, estar*) be; ***fica muito longe*** it's a long way off; ***fique quieto!*** be quiet!
◊ *passivo* be; **~ *ofendido com algo*** be offended by sth:
◊ (*permanecer*) stay; **~ *calado*** stay silent; **~ *atrás*** stay behind; **~ *num hotel*** stay in a hotel; ***fique aqui!*** stay there!; ***como ficaram as coisas com ele?*** how did you leave things with him?; ***ficamos dentro do orçamento*** we kept within the budget; ***eu vou* ~ *na cerveja*** I'll stick with beer, I'll stay with beer
◊ (*sobrar*) be left; ***ficaram dois ovos*** there were two eggs left
◊ **~ *com*** keep; ***posso* ~ *com isto?*** can I keep it?; **~ *com a cara brava*** keep a straight face; *fam* **~ *com alguém*** make out with s.o.
◊ ***fiquei sem comida por três dias*** I went without food for three days; ***fiquei sem gás*** I ran out of gas
◊ ***fica bem?*** does that look ok?; ***o bolo ficou bom*** the cake looks good; *sabor*: the cake tastes good; ***o carro ficou bom agora*** *conserto*: the car feels good now
◊ **~ *de fazer algo*** arrange to do sth:

◊ ~ ***para*** be put back to; ***a reunião ficou para amanhã*** the meeting has been put back until tomorrow
ficção [fi'ksãw] *f* fiction; ***literatura*** *f* ***de*** ~ fiction; ~ ***científica*** science fiction, sci-fi
ficha ['fiʃa] *f jogo*: chip; (*cartão*) index card; *Port* ELÉT plug; ~ ***dupla*** two-way plug; ~ ***de inscrição*** application form; ~ ***médica*** medical record
fichário [fi'ʃaɾiu] *m*, *Port* **ficheiro** [fi'ʃejɾu] *m* card index; INFORM file; ***formato*** *m* ***de*** ~ file format
ficou [fi'ko] → ***ficar***
fictício [fik'ʧisiu] *adj* fictitious
fidalga [fi'dawga] *f* noblewoman
fidalgo [fi'dawgu] **1** *adj* noble **2** *m* nobleman
fidedigno [fide'dʒignu] *adj* trustworthy
fidelidade [fideli'dadʒi] *f* fidelity, loyalty; ***aparelho*** *m* ***de alta*** ~ hi-fi
fiduciário [fidu'sjaɾiu] **1** *adj* DIR trust *atr* **2** *m*, **-a** *f* trustee
fiel [fiɛw] **1** *adj* faithful, loyal; (*exato*) faithful; (*de confiança*) reliable **2** *m/f* REL believer; ***os fiéis*** *pl* REL the faithful
fig. *abr* (***figura***) fig. (figure)
figa ['figa] *f* talisman; *fig* ***fazer*** ~***s*** cross one's fingers
fígado ['figadu] *m* liver; *fig* character; ***ter maus*** ~***s*** be liverish, be bad-tempered
figo ['figu] *m* fig; ***eu chamei-lhe um*** ~ it was my lucky day
figueira [fi'gejɾa] *f* fig tree
figura [fi'gura] *f* figure; (*forma*) shape; (*reprodução*) reproduction; ***fazer boa*** ~ make a good impression; ***ele é uma verdadeira*** ~ he's a real character
figurado [figu'ɾadu] *adj* figurative
figurante [figu'ɾãʧi] *m/f* extra
figurão [figu'ɾãw] *m fam* big shot; ***fazer um*** ~ make a big impression
figurar [figu'ɾaɾ] ⟨1a⟩ *v/i* appear; ~ ***entre*** figure among
figurino [figu'ɾinu] *m fig* model; *costura*: pattern; (*revista*) fashion magazine
fila ['fila] *f* row; *pessoas* line, *Brit* queue; *Bras* ***fazer*** ~ get in line, *Brit* queue (up); ***fiquei na*** ~ ***por horas*** I stood in line for hours, *Brit* I queued (up) for hours; ~ ***da frente*** front row; ~ ***indiana*** single file
filantropia [filãtɾo'pia] *f* philanthropy
filantrópico [filã'tɾɔpiku] *adj* philanthropic
filantropo [filã'tɾopu] *m* philanthropist
filão [fi'lãw] *m* MIN seam
filar ['filaɾ] ⟨1a⟩ *v/t* scrounge; ~ ***algo de alguém*** scrounge sth from s.o.
filarmônica, *Port* **filarmónica** [filaɾ'monika] *f* philharmonic
filarmônico, *Port* **filarmónico** [filaɾ'moniku] *adj* philharmonic
filatelia [filate'lia] *f* stamp collecting, philately
filatelista [filate'lista] *m/f* stamp collector, philatelist
filete[1] [fi'lɛʧi] *m* GASTR fillet
filete[2] [fi'leʧi] *m parafuso*: thread
filha ['fiʎa] *f* daughter
filharada [fiʎa'ɾada] *f* horde of kids
filho ['fiʎu] *m* son; ~***s*** *pl* children; ~ ***de criação*** foster child; ***ele é como um*** ~ ***de criação*** he's like family; ~ ***único*** only child
filho-da-puta [fiʎoda'puta] *m pop* son-of-a-bitch
filhote [fi'ʎɔʧi] *m* cub; *cachorro*: pup
filiação [filja'sãw] *f* POL affiliation
filial [fi'ljaw] *f* branch; ***chefe*** *m* ***de*** ~ branch manager
filiar-se [fi'ljaɾsi] ⟨1g⟩ *v/r* join (***a algo*** sth)
Filipinas [fili'pinas] *fpl* Philippines
filisteu [filis'tew] *m* philistine
filmadora [filma'doɾa] *f* video camera
filmagem [fiw'maʒẽ] *f* filming, shooting
filmar [fiw'maɾ] ⟨1a⟩ film, shoot
filme ['filmi] *m* CINE movie, *Brit tb* film; FOT film; ~ ***colorido*** color film, *Brit* colour film; ~ ***de longa metragem*** feature-length movie; ~ ***negativo*** negative; ~ ***policial*** thriller
fílmico ['filmiku] *adj* cinematic
filó [fi'lɔ] *m* TÊX tulle
filologia [filolo'ʒia] *f* philology
filológico [filo'lɔʒiku] *adj* philological

filólogo [fi'lɔlogu] *m*, **-a** *f* philologist
filosofia [filozo'fia] *f* philosophy
filósofo [fi'lɔzufu] *m*, **-a** *f* philosopher
filtrar [fiw'trar] ⟨1a⟩ *v/t* filter; **filtrar-se** *v/r* seep, filter
filtro ['filtru] *m* filter
fim [fĩ] *m* end; (*intenção*) purpose; (*objetivo*) goal; ***a ~ de*** in order to; ***por ~*** finally
fim-de-semana [fĩdʒise'mana] *m* ⟨pl fins-de-semana⟩ weekend; ***no ~*** on the weekend

F

final [fi'naw] **1** *adj* final; ***exame** m* **~** final (examination); ***juízo** m* **~** Last Judgment **2** *m* end; MÚS finale; ***no ~ de contas*** at the end of the day; ***no ~ de julho*** at the end of July **3** *f* ESP final; ***~ da copa*** cup final
finalista [fina'lista] *m/f* ESP finalist; UNIV final year student
finalizar [finali'zar] ⟨1a⟩ *v/t* finish, end; **finalizar-se** *v/r* finish, end
finalmente [finaw'mẽtʃi] *adv* finally
finança [fi'nãsa] *f* finance; ***alta ~*** high finance; ***~s*** *pl* finances; ***Ministério** m* ***das Finanças*** Treasury Department, *Brit* Exchequer
financeiro [finã'sejru] **1** *adj* financial **2** *m*, **-a** *m* financier
financiamento [finãsja'mẽtu] *m* financing
financiar [finã'sjar] ⟨1g⟩ finance
financista [finã'sista] *m/f* financier
fincar [fĩ'kar] ⟨1n⟩ *v/t prego* drive in; (*apoiar*) lean (***em*** on)
findar [fĩ'dar] ⟨1a⟩ end
fineza [fi'neza] *f* fineness; (*atenção*) kindness; ***fazer a ~ de ...*** be so kind as to ...
fingido [fĩ'ʒidu] *adj* false; (*hipócrita*) hypocritical
fingimento [fĩʒi'mẽtu] *m* pretense, *Brit* pretence; (*falsidade*) falseness; (*hipocrisia*) hypocrisy
fingir [fĩ'ʒir] ⟨3n⟩ **1** *v/t* feign **2** *v/i* pretend; ***~ fazer*** pretend to do; ***~ que ...*** pretend that ...; **fingir-se** *v/r* pretend to be
finjo ['fĩʒu] *etc* → ***fingir***
finlandês [fĩlã'des] **1** *adj* Finnish **2** *m*, **finlandesa** [fĩlã'deza] *f* Finn **3** *m língua* Finnish
Finlândia [fĩ'lãdʒia] *f* Finland
fino ['finu] **1** *adj* fine; (*magro*) slim; (*sensível*) sensitive; (*delicado*) polite; (*afiado*) shrill; (*esperto*) clever **2** *m* beer
finura [fi'nura] *f* → ***fineza***
fiquei [fi'kej] → ***ficar***
fio ['fiu] *m* thread; *metal*: wire; *faca*: edge; ***um ~ de cabelo*** a (single) hair; ***de ~ a pavio*** from beginning to end; ***por um ~*** by the skin of one's teeth; ***~ de água*** trickle (of water); *fig* ***~ condutor*** connecting thread; ***~ corrido*** run, *Brit* ladder; ***~ dental*** dental floss; ***~ de terra*** ground lead, *Brit* earth lead
firma ['firma] *f* (*assinatura*) signature; (*sociedade*) firm
firmar [fir'mar] ⟨1a⟩ secure, make firm; (*confirmar*) confirm; (*reconhecer*) recognize; (*assinar*) sign
firme ['firmi] *adj* firm; (*forte*) strong; (*definitivo*) final; *namorado* steady; ***terra** f* **~** dry land, terra firma
fiscal [fis'kaw] **1** *adj* tax *atr*, fiscal; ***conselho** m* **~** supervisory board; ***dívida** f* **~** tax debt; ***fraude** m* **~** tax fraud; ***grupo** m* **~** tax bracket; ***indulto** m* **~** tax rebate; ***receita** f* **~** tax revenue **2** *m/f* tax inspector; *alfândega*: customs officer; (*controlador*) supervisor
fiscalização [fiskaliza'sãw] *f* supervision; (*controlo*) inspection
fiscalizar [fiskali'zar] ⟨1a⟩ supervise; (*verificar*) check
fisco ['fisku] *m* Internal Revenue Service, *Brit* Inland Revenue
física ['fizika] *f* physics
físico ['fiziku] **1** *adj* physical **2** *m* (*corpo*) physique **2** *m*, **-a** *f* physicist
fisiologia [fizjolo'ʒia] *f* physiology
fisionomia [fizjono'mia] *f* physiognomy; (*cunho*) character
fisioterapeuta [fizjotera'pewta] *m/f* physiotherapist, *fam* physio
fisioterapia [fizjotera'pia] *f* physiotherapy, *fam* physio
fissão [fi'sãw] *f* fission; ***~ nuclear*** nuclear fission
fissurado [fisu'radu] *adj* split, cracked; *fig* ***ser ~ em algo*** be hooked

on sth

fita ['fita] *f* band; *papel*: strip; *magnético* tape; *fig fam* ***fazer ~s*** make a fuss; ~ (***cinematográfica***) film(strip); ~ ***adesiva*** adhesive tape; ~ ***contínua*** conveyor belt; ~ ***isoladora*** friction tape, *Brit* insulating tape; ~ ***métrica*** tape measure; *Bras* ~ (***de vídeo***) (video)tape

fitar [fi'taɾ] ⟨1a⟩ *v/t* gaze at; (*fixar*) stare at

fivela [fi'vɛla] *f* buckle

fixação [fiksa'sãw] *f* fixing; PSICOL fixation

fixador [fiksa'doɾ] **1** *m* lacquer; ARTE fixative; FOT fixing bath **2** *adj* fixing *atr*

fixar [fi'ksaɾ] ⟨1a⟩ *v/t* fix; *data*, *regra* set; *poster* stick up; (*memorizar*) memorize; *pé* set (***em*** on); **fixar-se** *v/r* ~ ***em*** concentrate on; *lugar* settle in

fixe ['fiʃi] *adv Port fam* brilliant

fixo ['fiksu] *adj* fixed; *fig* (*estável*) stable; ***estrela*** *f* ***fixa*** fixed star; ***idéia*** *f* ***fixa*** idée fixe, obsession; ***preço*** *m* ~ fixed price

fiz [fis], **fizeste** [fi'zɛstʃi] *etc* → ***fazer***

flacidez [flasi'des] *f* flabbiness

flácido ['flasidu] *adj* flabby

flagrante [fla'gɾãtʃi] *adj* flagrant; ***pegar alguém em*** ~ (***delito***) catch s.o. red-handed

flama ['flama] *f* flame

flamengo [fla'mẽgu] **1** *adj* Flemish; ***queijo*** *m* ~ Edam **2** *m lingua* Flemish

flan [flã] *m* crème caramel

flanco ['flãku] *m* flank

flanela [fla'nɛla] *f* flannel

flanquear [flã'kjaɾ] ⟨1l⟩ flank

flash [flaʃ] *m* flash

flatulência [flatu'lẽsja] *f* flatulence

flauta ['flawta] *f* flute; ***tocar*** ~ play the flute; ~ ***doce*** recorder

flautista ['flawta] *m/f* flutist, *Brit* flautist

flecha ['flɛʃa] *f* arrow

flertar [fleɾ'taɾ] ⟨1c⟩ *v/i* flirt

flerte [fleɾ'tʃi] *m* flirt

fleuma ['flewma] *n* phlegm

fleumático [flew'matʃiku] *adj* phlegmatic

flexão [fle'ksãw] *f* GRAM inflection; ***fazer flexões*** do push-ups

flexibilidade [fleksibili'dadʒi] *f* flexibility

flexibilizar [fleksibili'zaɾ] ⟨1a⟩ *v/t* stretch

flexionar [fleksjo'naɾ] ⟨1a⟩ *v/t* flex

flexível [fle'ksivew] *adj* flexible

floco ['flɔku] *m* flake; ***~s*** *pl* ***de aveia*** oat flakes; ***~s*** *pl* ***de cereais*** cereals; ~ ***de neve*** snowflake

flor [floɾ] *f* blossom *tb fig*; *planta*: flower; ***a fina*** ~ the élite; *fig* ***à*** ~ ***de*** on the surface of

flora ['flɔra] *f* flora

floreado [flo'ɾjadu] *adj camisa* flowery; *fig* ornate; *estilo* flowery

florescer [flores'seɾ] ⟨2g⟩ *v/i flor* flower; *fig* flourish

floresta [flo'ɾɛsta] *f* forest; ~ ***pluvial*** rain forest; ~ ***virgem*** virgin forest

florestal [flores'taw] *adj* forest *atr*; ***guarda*** *m/f* ~ forest ranger

florir [flo'ɾiɾ] ⟨3f⟩ flower

florista [flo'ɾista] *m/f* florist

flotilha [flo'tʃiʎa] *f* NÁUT flotilla

fluência [flu'ẽsja] *f* fluency; ***ela fala espanhol com*** ~ she speaks fluent Spanish

fluente [flu'ẽtʃi] *adj* fluent

fluido ['fluidu] fluid

fluir [flu'iɾ] ⟨3i⟩ *v/i* flow

flúor ['fluoɾ] *m* fluoride

fluorescência [flwores'sẽsja] *f* fluorescence

fluorescente [flwores'sẽtʃi] *adj* fluorescent

flutuação [flutwa'sãw] *f* fluctuation

flutuador [flutwa'doɾ] *m* TECN float

flutuante [flu'twãtʃi] *adj* floating

flutuar [flu'twaɾ] ⟨1g⟩ (*boiar*) float; *preços etc* fluctuate

fluvial [flu'vjaw] *adj* river *atr*; ***porto*** *m* ~ river port

fluxo ['fluksu] *m* flow; MED flux

fluxograma [flukso'gɾama] *m* flowchart

FMI *m* (***Fundo Monetário Internacional***) *abr* IMF (International Monetary Fund)

fobia [fo'bia] *f* phobia

F

foca ['fɔka] *f* seal
focagem [fo'kaʒẽ] *f* FOT focus
focalizar [fokali'zaɾ] ⟨1a⟩ focus; **~ em** focus on
focar [fo'kaɾ] ⟨1n & 1e⟩ focus; *fig tema* focus on
focinho [fo'siɲu] *m* snout
foco ['fɔku] *m* focus; *fig* center, *Brit* centre; MED seat; ***profundidade** f* **de ~** depth of field; ***estar em ~ / fora de ~*** be in focus / out of focus; ***estar em ~*** be the focus of attention
foder [fo'deɾ] ⟨2d⟩ *v/t vulg* fuck
fodido [fo'dʒidu] *adj Bras pop, Port vulg* shitty; ***estar ~*** be in the shit, be fucked
fofo ['fofu] *adj* soft; *fig fam* cute
fofoca [fo'fɔka] *f fam* gossip; ***fazer ~*** gossip
fogão [fo'gãw] *m* cooker; (*forno*) oven
fogo ['fogu] *m* fire; NÁUT ***~s*** *pl* lights; ***em ~*** on fire; ***pegar ~*** catch fire; ***pôr ~ em algo*** set fire to sth; ***você tem ~?*** have you got a light?; ***~ de artilharia*** shellfire
fogo-de-artifício [fogudʒiaɾtʃi'fisiu] *m* ⟨*pl* fogos-de-artifício⟩ firework
fogoso [fo'gozu] *adj* fiery
fogueira [fo'gejɾa] *f* bonfire; (*lareira*) open fire
foguetão [foge'tãw] *m* rocket
foguete [fo'getʃi] *m* rocket; ***deitar um ~*** let off a rocket
foi [foj] → ***ir, ser***
folclore [fow'klɔɾi] *m* folklore
fole ['fɔli] *m* bellows
fôlego ['folegu] *m* breath; (*respiração*) breathing; (*pausa*) breathing space; ***estar sem ~*** be out of breath; ***tomar ~*** pause for breath
folga[1] ['fɔlga] *f* rest; (*lazer*) leisure; ***dia*** *m* ***de ~*** day off; ***estar de ~*** be off duty
folga[2] ['fɔlga] *f* TECN, *fig* play; ***dar ~*** leave some play
folgado [fow'gadu] *adj roupa* loose
folha ['foʎa] *f* BOT, *papel*: leaf; *carta*, *metal*: sheet; *faca*, *serra*: blade; ***novo em ~*** brand new; ***árvore** f* ***de ~ caduca*** deciduous tree; INFORM ***~ de cálculo*** spreadsheet; ***~ de chá*** tea leaf; ***~ de serviço*** service log
folhado [fo'ʎadu] **1** *adj* flaky; ***massa** f* ***folhada*** puff pastry **2** *m* puff pastry
folhagem [fo'ʎaʒẽ] *f* foliage
folhear [foʎi'aɾ] ⟨1l⟩ *v/t* leaf through
folheto [fo'ʎetu] *m* leaflet
folhinha [fo'ʎiɲa] *f* tear-off calendar
folho ['foʎu] *m* ruche, frill
folia [fo'lia] *f* revelry
folião [foli'ãw] *m*, **foliona** *f* Carnival reveler, *Brit* Carnival reveller
fome ['fɔmi] *f* hunger; ***estou com ~, tenho ~*** I'm hungry; ***estar a morrer de ~*** be starving; *fig* ***salário** m* ***de ~*** pittance, starvation wage
fomentar [fomẽ'taɾ] ⟨1a⟩ foment; *economia* boost; *ódio* incite; (*instigar*) instigate
fomos ['fomus] → ***ir, ser***
fone ['foni] *m* ***~ de ouvido*** headphones
fonética [fo'nɛtʃika] *f* phonetics
fonético [fo'nɛtʃiku] *adj* phonetic
fonte ['fõtʃi] *f* source *tb fig*; (*chafariz*) fountain; TIPO font
fontes ['fõtʃis] *fpl* temples
for [foɾ], **fora** ['foɾa] *etc* → ***ir, ser***
fora ['fɔɾa] **1** *adv* outside; ***~ de casa*** outdoors, outside; ***lá ~*** outside; *fam* (*no estrangeiro*) abroad; ***de ~*** from outside; ***deixar de ~*** leave out; ***estar ~*** be away **2** *prep* ◇ (*além de*) apart from, aside from
◇ ***~ de*** out of; ***estar ~ do assunto*** be missing the point; ***~ de jogo*** *adj futebol*: out of play; ***~ de ordem*** out of sequence; ***~ de moda*** out of fashion; ***~ da rodovia principal*** off the main road; ***ficar ~ de si*** go wild **3** *int* ***~!*** get out! **4** *m* ***dar o ~*** leave; ***dar o ~ em*** ditch; ***dê o ~!*** beat it!
foragido [foɾa'ʒidu] **1** *adj* fugitive **2** *m*, **-a** *f* fugitive
forasteiro [foɾas'tejɾu] **1** *adj* alien, foreign **2** *m*, **-a** *f* stranger; (*estrangeiro*) foreigner
forca ['foɾka] *f* gallows
força ['foɾsa] *f* strength; (*violência*) force; (*poder*) power; ***à ~*** by force; ***estar no fim das ~s*** be at one's wits' end; ***~ aérea*** air force; ***~ maior*** act of God; ***~ de trabalho*** workforce; ***~ de***

vontade willpower; **~*s*** *pl* ***armadas*** armed forces; **~*s*** *pl* ***de mercado*** market forces
forçado [for'sadu] *adj* forced
forçar [for'sar] ⟨1p & 1e⟩ force; **~ *alguém a fazer algo*** force s.o. to do sth
força-tarefa [forsata'rɛfa] *f* ⟨*pl* forças-tarefa⟩ task force
fórceps ['fɔrsɛps] *m* forceps
forçosamente [forsɔza'mẽtʃi] *adv* forcibly
forçoso [for'sozu] *adj* necessary, essential; (*obrigatório*) obligatory; (*violento*) violent; ***é* ~ *que ...*** (*conj*) it is essential that ...
forense [fo'rẽsi] *adj* forensic
forja ['fɔrʒa] *f* forge; *fig* ***estar na* ~** be in the pipeline
forjador [forʒa'dor] *m* blacksmith
forjar [for'ʒar] ⟨1e⟩ *v/t* forge *tb fig*
forma[1] ['fɔrma] *f* form; (*figura*) figure; (*modo*) way; ***desta* ~** in this way; ***de* ~ *nenhuma*** in no way; ***de outra* ~** otherwise; ***de*** (***tal***) **~ *que*** in such a way that; ***em* ~** *pessoa* fit; ***em devida* ~** in due form; **~ *de tratamento*** form of address
fôrma, *Port* **forma**[2] ['forma] *f* mold, *Brit* mould; *bolo*: baking pan; *sapato*: last; (***pão*** *m* ***de***) **~** loaf
formação [forma'sãw] *f* formation *tb* GEOL, MIL; (*educação*) training; (*geração*) background; **~ *profissional na empresa*** on-the-job training; ***em seus anos de* ~** in his formative years
formado [for'madu] **1** *adj* ***ser* ~ *em Medicina / Direito*** be a qualified doctor / lawyer **2** *m*, **-a** *f* graduate
formador [forma'dor] *adj* formative
formal [for'maw] *adj* formal; *inimigo* declared
formalidade [formali'dadʒi] *f* formality; ***por* ~** for form's sake
formalmente [formawmẽti] *adv* formally
formar [for'mar] ⟨1e⟩ **1** *v/t* form; (*instruir*) train; *plano* draw up **2** *v/i* MIL form up; **formar-se** *v/r* form; *faculdade, escola*: graduate
formatar [forma'tar] ⟨1b⟩ *v/t* format
formato [for'matu] *m* format
formatura [forma'tura] *f* *faculdade*: graduation
formidável [formi'davew] *adj fam* great, fantastic
formiga [for'miga] *f* ant
formigueiro [formi'gejru] *m* ant's nest; *fig* throng
formoso [for'mozu] *adj* beautiful
formosura [formo'zura] *f* beauty
fórmula ['fɔrmula] *f* formula
formular [formu'lar] ⟨1a⟩ *v/t* formulate; *pedido* voice
formulário [formu'lariu] *m Bras* form; INFORM **~ *contínuo*** continuous paper
fornecedor [fornese'dor] *m* supplier; ***indústria*** *f* ***fornecedora*** supply industry
fornecer [forne'ser] ⟨2g⟩ supply, provide (***de*** with)
fornecimento [fornesi'mẽtu] *m* supply; (*abastecimento*) provision
fornicar [forni'kar] ⟨1n⟩ fornicate
forno ['fornu] *m* GASTR oven *tb fig*; TECN furnace; **~ *de microondas*** microwave (oven)
forragem [fo'haʒẽ] *f* fodder
forrar [fo'har] ⟨1e⟩ *vestido etc* line; *com metal, madeira* clad; *parede* paper; *fig* ***forrado de*** *cheio* packed with
forro ['fohu] *m vestido*: lining; *madeira*: cladding; (*cobertura*) covering
fortalecer [fortale'ser] ⟨2g⟩ strengthen; (*encorajar*) encourage; MIL fortify; **fortalecer-se** *v/r* strengthen; (*refazer-se*) get better
fortalecimento [fortalesi'mẽtu] *m* strengthening
fortaleza [forta'leza] *f* strength; MIL fortress
forte ['fɔrtʃi] **1** *adj* strong; *chuva* heavy; *dor de cabeça etc* bad; (*firme*) firm; ***este é o seu ponto* ~** that's his strong point **2** *adv chuvar* heavily; *bater* hard **3** *m* fort
fortemente ['fɔrtʃimẽtʃi] *adv* strongly; *chover* heavily
fortuna [for'tuna] *f* fortune, (good) luck; (*êxito*) success; (*destino*) fate; (*riqueza*) wealth; ***fazer* ~** make a fortune
fórum ['fɔrũ] *m* forum

fosco ['fosku] *adj* dull; ***vidro*** *m* ~ frosted glass
fosforescência [fosfores'sẽsja] *f* phosphorescence
fosforescer [fosfores'ser] ⟨2g⟩ phosphoresce
fósforo ['fɔsfuru] *m* match; QUÍM phosphorus
fossa ['fɔsa] *f* pit; ANAT cavity; ***na ~*** down in the dumps; ~ ***comum*** mass grave
fosse ['fosi] *etc* → ***ir, ser***
fóssil ['fɔsiw] **1** *adj* fossilized **2** *m* fossil
fosso ['fosu] *m* ditch
foste ['fostʃi] *etc* → ***ir, ser***
foto ['fɔtu] *f* photo
fotocópia [foto'kɔpja] *f* photocopy; ***tirar uma ~ de algo*** make a photocopy of sth
fotocopiadora [fotokopja'dora] *f* photocopier
fotocopiar [fotoko'pjar] ⟨1g⟩ *v/t* photocopy
fotogênico, *Port* **fotogénico** [foto'ʒeniku] *adj* photogenic
fotografar [fotogra'far] ⟨1b⟩ photograph
fotografia [fotogra'fia] *f* photograph; *arte* photography; ***tirar uma ~*** take a photograph (***a*** of)
fotográfico [foto'grafiku] *adj* photographic; ***máquina*** *f* ***fotográfica*** camera
fotógrafo [fo'tɔgrafu] *m*, **-a** *f* photographer
fotômetro, *Port* **fotómetro** [fo'tometru] *m* light meter
foz [fɔs] *f rio*: river mouth
fracamente [fraka'mẽtʃi] *adv* faintly
fracassado [fraka'sadu] *m*, **-a** *f* loser, failure
fracassar [fraka'sar] ⟨1b⟩ *v/i* fail
fracasso [fra'kasu] *m* failure; (*ruído*) noise
fração, *Port* **fracção** [fra'sãw] *f* fraction; (*fragmento*) fragment
fracionar, *Port* **fraccionar** [frasjo'nar] ⟨1f⟩ break up, fragment
fraco ['fraku] **1** *adj* weak; *cheio*, *som* faint **2** *m* weakness; ***ter um ~ por algo*** have a weakness for sth **2** *m*, **-a** *f* weakling
fract... *Port* → ***frat...***
frade ['fradʒi] *m* monk
frágil ['fraʒiw] *adj* fragile; (*débil*) frail
fragilidade [fraʒili'dadʒi] *f* fragility; (*debilidade*) frailty
fragmentadora [fragmẽta'dora] *f* ~ ***de papel*** shredder
fragmentar [fragmẽ'tar] ⟨1a⟩ *v/t* break up, fragment; **fragmentar-se** *v/r* break up
fragmentário [fragmẽ'tariu] *adj* fragmentary
fragmento [frag'mẽtu] *m* fragment
fragrância [fra'grãsja] *f* fragrance
fralda ['frawda] *f* (shirt)tail; *bebé*: diaper, *Brit* nappy
framboesa [frã'bweza] *f* raspberry
França ['frãsa] *f* ***a ~*** France; ***em ~, na ~*** in France
francamente [frãka'mẽtʃi] *adv* frankly; *fig* ***~!*** honestly!
francês [frã'ses] **1** *adj* French **2** *m pessoa* Frenchman **3** *m lingua* French
francesa [frã'seza] *f* Frenchwoman; ***à ~*** French-style
franco ['frãku] *adj* frank
franco-atirador [frãkwatʃira'dor] *m* ⟨pl franco-atiradores⟩ sniper
frango ['frãgu] *m* GASTR chicken; *fig* little whippersnapper; *futebol*: sitter
franja ['frãʒa] *f* fringe; *cabelo*: bangs, *Brit* fringe
franquear [frã'kjar] ⟨1l⟩ *v/t carta etc* frank; (*abrir*) open
franqueza [frã'keza] *f* (*sinceridade*) frankness
franquia [frã'kia] *f* postage; (*isenção*) exemption; COM franchise
franzir [frã'zir] ⟨3a⟩ pleat; *pele* wrinkle; ***~ as sobrancelhas, ~ a testa*** frown
fraquejar [frake'ʒar] ⟨1d⟩ weaken
fraqueza [fra'keza] *f* weakness
frasco ['frasku] *m* bottle; *conserva*: jar
frase ['frazi] *f* sentence; (*oração*) phrase *tb* MÚS; ***~ feita*** set phrase
fraternal [frater'naw] *adj* fraternal
fraternidade [fraterni'dadʒi] *f* fraternity
fraterno [fra'tɛrnu] *adj* brotherly

fratura [fɾa'tuɾa] *f* MED fracture; **~ *múltipla*** multiple fracture
fraturar [fɾatu'ɾaɾ] ⟨1a⟩ fracture
fraude ['fɾawdʒi] *f* fraud
freada [fɾe'ada] *f* ***dar uma ~*** hit the brakes
frear [fɾe'aɾ] ⟨1h⟩ *v/i Bras* brake
freguês [fɾe'ges] *m*, **freguesa** [fɾe'geza] *f* customer; *habitual* regular
freguesia [fɾege'zia] *f* (*clientela*) customers; *Port* (*comunidade*) parish
freio ['fɾeiu] *m Bras* brake; ***~ de mão*** parking brake, *Brit* handbrake
freira ['fɾejɾa] *f* nun
freixo ['fɾejʃu] *m* ash (tree)
frenesi [fɾene'zi] *m*, **frenesim** [fɾene'zĩ] *m* frenzy
frenético [fɾe'nɛtʃiku] *adj* frenetic, frantic
frente ['fɾẽtʃi] *f* front *tb* MIL; ***~ a ~*** face to face; ***à ~ (de)*** at the front (of); ***em ~ (de)*** in front (of), across (from); ***de ~ para*** across from, *Brit* opposite; ***de ~*** *colidir* head-on; ***fazer ~ a alguém / /algo*** face s.o. / sth; ***levar à ~*** carry through; ***sempre em ~*** straight on; ***ir em ~ com*** *planos etc* go ahead with; ***~ fria*** cold front
freqüência, *Port* **frequência** [fɾe'kwẽsja] *f* frequency; *escola*: attendance; ***com ~*** frequently
freqüentar, *Port* **frequentar** [fɾekwẽ'taɾ] ⟨1a⟩ frequent; (*dar-se com*) go around with; *escola* attend
freqüente, *Port* **frequente** [fɾe'kwẽtʃi] *adj* frequent
freqüentemente, *Port* **frequentemente** [fɾekwẽtʃi'mẽtʃi] *adv* often, frequently
fresco ['fɾesku] **1** *adj* fresh; (*frio*) cool **2** *m* fresh air; ARTE fresco
frescor [fɾes'koɾ] *m*, **frescura** [fɾes'kuɾa] *f* freshness; (*frialdade*) coolness; ***ela é cheia de ~*** she's something of a prima donna
fresta ['fɾɛsta] *f* gap, slit
fretamento [fɾeta'mẽtu] *m* charter
fretar [fɾe'taɾ] ⟨1c⟩ *barco* charter; *meio de transporte* rent, *Brit tb* hire
frete ['fɾɛtʃi] *m* freight; (*aluguel*) rental, *Brit tb* hire; *avião*: charter; ***~ aéreo*** air freight; *fam* ***que ~!*** what a drag!
freudiano [fɾojdʒi'anu] *adj* Freudian
fricção [fɾi'ksãw] *f* friction
friccionar [fɾiksjo'naɾ] ⟨1f⟩ rub
frieira [fɾi'ejɾa] *f* chilblain
frigideira [fɾiʒi'dejɾa] *f* fry pan, *Brit* frying pan
frigidez [fɾiʒi'des] *f* coldness; MED frigidity
frígido ['fɾiʒidu] *adj* cold; MED frigid
frigorífico [fɾigo'ɾifiku] *m Port* refrigerator; *Bras* refrigerated warehouse
frincha ['fɾĩʃa] *f* slit
frio ['fɾiu] **1** *adj* cold *tb fig*; ***estar ~*** be cold; ***carnes*** *fpl* ***frias*** cold cuts **2** *m* coldness *tb fig*; ***instalação*** *f* ***de ~*** refrigeration plant; ***estou com ~*** I'm cold; ***faz ~*** it's cold; ***morrer de ~*** freeze to death
frisado [fɾi'zadu] *adj cabelo* curly; *caracóis apertados*: frizzy
frisar [fɾi'zaɾ] ⟨1a⟩ *v/t cabelo etc* curl; (*salientar*) emphasize; **frisar-se** *v/r* curl
fritadeira [fɾita'dejɾa] *f* deep fryer
fritar [fɾi'taɾ] ⟨1a⟩ fry
fritas ['fɾitas] *fpl* fries, *Brit tb* chips
frito ['fɾitu] *adj* fried; *fam fig* ***estar ~*** be done for
fritos ['fɾitus] *mpl*, **frituras** [fɾi'tuɾas] *fpl* fried food
frívolo ['fɾivulu] *adj* frivolous
fronha ['fɾoɲa] *f* pillow case
frontal [fɾõ'taw] *adj* frontal; ***choque ~*** head-on crash
fronte ['fɾõtʃi] *f* forehead; (*frente*) front
fronteira [fɾõ'tejɾa] *f* frontier, border; ***fazer ~ com*** *país* border
fronteiriço [fɾõtej'ɾisu] *adj* frontier *atr*; ***polícia*** *f* ***fronteiriça*** border guards
frota ['fɾɔta] *f* fleet
frouxo ['fɾoʃu] *adj* loose; (*fraco*) weak
frugal [fɾu'gaw] *adj* frugal
frustração [fɾustɾa'sãw] *f* frustration
frustrado [fɾus'tɾadu] *adj* frustrated; (*impedido*) thwarted
frustrante [fɾus'tɾãtʃi] *adj* frustrating
frustrar [fɾus'tɾaɾ] ⟨1a⟩ *v/t* frustrate; *planos etc* frustrate, thwart; **frustrar-se** *v/r planos* fall through, be thwarted

fruta ['fɾuta] *f* fruit; ~ ***da época*** seasonal fruit
fruta-pão [fɾuta'pãw] *f* breadfruit
fruteira [fɾu'tejɾa] *f* fruit bowl
frutífero [fɾu'ʧiferu] *adj* fruit-bearing; (*útil*) fruitful
fruto ['fɾutu] *m* fruit; (*resultado*) result; ***dar*** ~ *tb fig* bear fruit; ~***s do mar*** seafood
fubá [fu'ba] *m* cornmeal
fuga ['fuga] *f* flight; *gás etc*: leak; MÚS fugue; ***criminoso em*** ~ criminal on the run
fugaz [fu'gas] *adj* fleeting
fugir [fu'ʒiɾ] ⟨3n & 3h⟩ *v/i* run away; MIL, *ladrão* flee (***de, a*** from); *prisão*: escape (***de, a*** from); (*evitar*) avoid (***de algo*** s.o.); *tempo* fly; ***o ladão fugiu com o dinheiro*** the thief made off with the money
fugitivo [fuʒi'ʧivu] **1** *m*, **-a** *f* fugitive **2** *adj* fugitive
fui [fui] → ***ir, ser***
fulano [fu'lanu] *m*, **-a** *f* what's-his-name, what's-her-name, so-and-so; ~ ***perguntou ...*** the guy asked ...
fuligem [fu'liʒẽ] *f* soot
fulo ['fulu] *adj* furious
fumaça [fu'masa] *f Bras* smoke, fumes
fumador [fuma'doɾ] *m*, **-a** *f*, *Bras* **fumante** [fu'mãʧi] *m/f* smoker
fumar [fu'maɾ] ⟨1a⟩ **1** *v/t* smoke **2** *v/i* smoke; ***proibido*** ~ no smoking
fumigar [fumi'gaɾ] ⟨1o⟩ *v/t* fumigate
fumo ['fumu] *m Port* smoke; (*névoa*) fumes; *Bras* tobacco; (*fumar*) smoking
função [fũ'sãw] *f* function; (*cargo*) role; (*tarefa*) task; TECN ***em*** ~ working; ***em*** ~ ***de*** with regard to; ***na minha*** ~ ***de ...*** in my capacity as ...
funcho ['fũʃu] *m* fennel
funcional [fũsjo'naw] *adj* functional
funcionalismo *m* ~ ***público*** civil service
funcionamento [fũsjona'mẽtu] *m* functioning, operation; ***pôr em*** ~ put into operation
funcionar [fũsjo'naɾ] ⟨1f⟩ function, work; *software* run; ***não funciona!*** out of order; ***como isto funciona?*** how does this work?
funcionário [fũsjo'naɾiu] *m*, **-a** *f* official; POL civil servant; *museu*: attendant
fundação [fũda'sãw] *f* foundation
fundador [fũda'doɾ] **1** *adj* founding **2** *m*, **-a** *f* founder
fundamental [fũdamẽ'taw] *adj* fundamental
fundamentalista [fũdamẽta'lista] *m/f* fundamentalist
fundamentar [fũdamẽ'taɾ] ⟨1a⟩ ~ ***algo*** provide the basis for; (*justificar*) justify sth; (*apoiar*) support sth
fundamento [fũda'mẽtu] *m* foundation; (*base*) basis
fundar [fũ'daɾ] ⟨1a⟩ **1** *v/t* found **2** *v/i* ~ ***em*** be based on
fundear [fũ'dʒiaɾ] ⟨1l⟩ *v/i* NÁUT anchor
fundição [fũdʒi'sãw] *f* casting; (***fábrica*** *f* ***de***) ~ foundry; *siderurgia*: iron and steel works
fundilho [fũ'dʒiʎu] *m calças*: crotch
fundir [fũ'dʒiɾ] ⟨3a⟩ *v/t* melt down; *metal* cast; *minério* smelt; *fig* merge;
fundir-se *v/r* merge; ELÉT fuse
fundo ['fũdu] **1** *adj* deep; ***de olhos*** ~***s*** with deep-set eyes **2** *m* bottom; *vale*: floor; (*profundidade*) depth; *situação*: background; (*base*) basis; (*conteúdo*) content; FIN fund; ***no*** ~ in one's heart of hearts, inwardly; ***a*** ~ thoroughly; ***de*** ~ *corrida* long-distance; ~***s*** *pl* funds; ~ ***de aposentadoria*** pension fund; ~ ***de investimentos*** investment fund; ~***s*** *pl* ***públicos*** public money, public funds
fúnebre ['funebɾi] *adj* funeral *atr*; *fig* gloomy, funereal
funeral [fune'ɾaw] *m* funeral
funerário [fune'ɾaɾiu] *adj* funeral *atr*; ***agência*** *f* ***funerária*** undertakers
fungicida [fũʒi'sida] *m* fungicide
fungo ['fũgu] *m* BOT, MED fungus
funicular [funiku'laɾ] *m* funicular (railway)
funil [fu'niw] *m* funnel
furacão [fuɾa'kãw] *m* hurricane
furadeira [fuɾa'dejɾa] *f* drill
furador [fuɾa'doɾ] *m* punch
furar [fu'ɾaɾ] ⟨1a⟩ (*perfurar*) perforate; (*esburacar*) bore; *orelhas* pierce;

fig planos foil; **~ *a fila*** cut in line, *Brit* jump the queue
furgão [fur'gãw] *m* FERROV car, *Brit* van; **~ *de polícia*** patrol wagon, *Brit* police van
furgoneta [furgo'neta] *f* AUTO van
fúria ['furja] *f* fury
furioso [fu'rjozu] *adj* furious
furo ['furu] *m* hole; AUTO flat; ***abrir um ~*** bore a hole; ***ter um ~*** have a flat; **~ *de reportagem*** scoop
furor [fu'ror] *m* fury, rage; (*entusiasmo*) furore; ***fazer ~*** be all the rage
furtar [fur'tar] ⟨1a⟩ *v/t* steal; **furtar-se** *v/r* **~ *a*** dodge
furtivo [fur'tʃivu] *adj* furtive
furto ['furtu] *m* theft; *bens*: stolen goods; ***a ~*** secretly
furúnculo [fu'rũkulu] *m* boil
fusão [fu'zãw] *f* fusion; COM merger; **~ *nuclear*** nuclear fusion
fuselagem [fuze'laʒẽ] *f* AERO fuselage
fusionar [fuzjo'nar] ⟨1f⟩ *v/t* fuse; COM merge
fusível [fu'zivew] *m* ELÉT fuse
fuso ['fuzu] *m* spindle; **~ *horário*** time zone
futebol [futʃi'bɔw] *m* soccer, *Brit tb* football; **~ *americano*** American football
futebolista [futʃibo'lista] *m/f* soccer player, *Brit tb* footballer
fútil ['futʃiw] *adj* trivial; *pessoa* superficial; (*sem sentido*) futile
futurista [futu'rista] *adj* futuristic
futuro [fu'turu] **1** *adj* future **2** *m* future; ***de ~, para o ~*** in (the) future
fuzil [fu'ziw] *m* rifle
fuzilar [fuzi'lar] ⟨1a⟩ **1** *v/t* shoot **2** *v/i* flash

G

Gabão [ga'bãw] *m* ***o ~*** Gabon
gabar [ga'bar] ⟨1b⟩ *v/t* praise; **gabar-se** *v/r* boast, brag; **~ *de*** boast about
gabardine [gabar'dʒini], *Port* **gabardina** [gabar'dʒina] *f* gaberdine
gabinete [gabi'netʃi] *m em casa* study; (*escritório*) office; POL cabinet
gado ['gadu] *m* livestock; (*boi*) cattle
gafanhoto [gafa'ɲotu] *m* grasshopper
gafe ['gafi] *f fam* gaffe, faux-pas; ***cometer uma ~*** commit a faux-pas, make a gaffe
gagá [ga'ga] *adj fam* gaga; ***ele ficou ~*** he's gone gaga
gago ['gagu] **1** *adj* stuttering **2** *m*, **-a** *f* stutterer
gaguejar [gage'ʒar] ⟨1d⟩ **1** *v/i* stutter; *com algo na boca* splutter **2** *v/t frase* stutter
gaguez [ga'ges] *f* stutter
gaiato [ga'jatu] **1** *adj* mischievous **2** *m* rascal
gaiola [ga'jɔla] *f* cage
gaita ['gajta] *f* harmonica; *fam* cash; *fam* ***cheio da ~*** loaded; **~ *galega, ~ de foles*** bagpipes
gaivota [gaj'vɔta] *f* seagull
gajo ['gaʒu] *m Port pop pej* guy
gala ['gala] *f* gala; ***traje de ~*** black tie
galã [ga'lã] *m* beau; *cinema*: leading man, romantic lead
galantaria [galãta'ria] *f* gallantry, courtesy
galante [ga'lãtʃi] *adj* gallant; (*delicado*) polite, courteous
galanteador [galãtʃia'dor] **1** *m*, **-a** *f* admirer **2** *adj* flattering
galanteio [galã'teju] *m* flattery
galão[1] [ga'lãw] *m medida*: gallon; **~ *de metal*** canister; ***um quarto de ~*** a quart
galão[2] [ga'lãw] *m* MIL stripe
galão[3] [ga'lãw] *m Port milky coffee in a glass*

G

galáxia [ga'laksia] *f* galaxy
galeão [ga'ljãw] *m* NÁUT galleon
galego [ga'legu] **1** *adj* Galician **2** *m*, **-a** *f* Galician; *fam pej* Portuguese **3** *m lingua* Galician
galera [ga'lɛɾa] *f* NÁUT galley; *fam* gang; ***você vai sair com a ~?*** are you going out with the gang?
galeria [gale'ɾia] *f* gallery *tb* TEAT; NÁUT promenade deck; **~ *de arte*** art gallery; **~ *comercial*** shopping mall
galês [ga'les] **1** *adj* Welsh **2** *m*, **-esa** *f* Welshman; Welshwoman
galgar [gaw'gaɾ] ⟨1o⟩ *v/t* leap over; (*montar*) climb up; *rio* **~ *as margens*** burst its banks
galgo ['gawgu] *m* greyhound
galheteiro [gaʎe'tejɾu] *m* cruet
galho ['gaʎu] *m árvore*: branch; ***dá para quebrar um ~*** it's enough to get by with
galinha [ga'liɲa] *f* hen; GASTR, *fig* chicken; ***pele*** *f* ***de ~*** gooseflesh; ***pés*** *mpl* ***de ~*** crow's feet; **~ *assada na churrasqueira*** barbecued chicken
galinheiro [gali'ɲejɾu] *m* hen-house
galo ['galu] *m* rooster; *cabeça*: lump; ***missa*** *f* ***do Galo*** midnight mass; **~ *de briga*** fighting cock; *fig* troublemaker
galopante [galo'pãʧi] *adj inflação* rampant, galloping
galopar [galo'paɾ] ⟨1e⟩ *v/i* gallop
galope [ga'lɔpi] *m* gallop; ***a ~*** at a gallop; *fig* ***a todo o ~*** at full pace
galpão [gaw'pãu] *m* outbuilding; *menor* shed
galvanizar [gawvani'zaɾ] ⟨1a⟩ *v/t* galvanize *tb fig*
gama ['gama] *f produtos*: range; MÚS scale
gamba ['gãba] *f* prawn
gambá [gã'ba] *f* skunk
gana ['gana] *f* desire, craving; ***ter ~s de*** feel like, be in the mood for
Gana ['gana] *m* ***o ~*** Ghana
ganância [ga'nãsja] *f* greed
gananciosamente [ganãsjoza'mẽʧi] *adv* greedily
ganancioso [ganã'sjozu] *adj* greedy
gancho ['gãʃu] *m* hook; *Port cabelos*: hairclip, *Am* barrette; *calça*: crotch; TEL ***fora do ~*** off the hook
gânglio ['gãgliu] *m* ANAT ganglion
gangorra [gã'goha] *f* seesaw
gangrena [gã'gɾena] *f* MED gangrene
gângster ['gãgsteɾ] *m* gangster
ganha-pão [gaɲa'pãw] *m* ⟨*pl* -pães⟩ bread-winner
ganhar [ga'ɲaɾ] ⟨1a⟩ **1** *v/t* win; *com trabalho* earn; (*alcançar*) reach; (*adquirir*) get; *êxito* achieve; *consideração etc* gain; **~ *a vida*** earn a living **2** *v/i* win; **~ *por pontos*** win on aggregate
ganho ['gaɲu] *m* profit; *por trabalho* income, living; (*vantagem*) advantage; **~*s*** winnings; FIN **~ *de capital*** capital gain
ganir [ga'niɾ] ⟨3a⟩ *v/i* yelp, squeal
ganso ['gãsu] *m* goose; **~ *assado*** roast goose
garagem [ga'ɾaʒẽ] *f* garage
garantia [gaɾã'ʧia] *f* guarantee; (*fiança*) surety; ***estar na ~*** be under guarantee
garantir [gaɾã'ʧiɾ] ⟨3a⟩ *v/t* guarantee; **~ *algo a alguém*** guarantee sth to s.o.; **~ *que*** guarantee that
garça ['gaɾsa] *f* heron
garçom [gaɾ'sõ] *m Bras* waiter; *bar*: bartender, *Brit* barman; **~*, por favor!*** excuse me, waiter!
garçonete [gaɾso'nɛʧi] *f Bras* waitress; *bar*: bartender, *Brit* barmaid; **~*, por favor!*** excuse me, miss!
gardênia, *Port* **gardénia** [gaɾ'denja] *f* gardenia
garfo ['gaɾfu] *m* fork
gargalhada [gaɾga'ʎada] *f* burst of laughter; ***cair na ~*** burst out laughing
gargalo [gaɾ'galu] *m* bottleneck
garganta [gaɾ'gãta] *f* (*goela*) throat; GEOG ravine; *fam* ***ter ~*** boast
gargarejar [gaɾgaɾe'ʒaɾ] ⟨1d⟩ gargle
gargarejo [gaɾga'ɾeʒu] *m líquido* gargle; ***fazer ~*** gargle, have a gargle
gari [ga'ɾi] *m/f Bras* road sweeper
garota [ga'ɾota] *f Bras* girl; **~ *de programa*** call girl; **~ *prodígio*** whizzkid
garoto [ga'ɾotu] *m Bras* boy; *Port fam* coffee with milk; **~ *prodígio*** whizzkid

garoupa [ga'ropa] *f peixe* grouper
garra ['gaha] *f* claw; *ave*: talon; (*entusiasmo*) gusto, verve; ***nas ~s dela*** in her clutches
garrafa [ga'hafa] *f* bottle; ***~ térmica*** Thermos® flask
garrancho [ga'hãʃu] *m* scrawl
garrido [ga'hidu] *adj* (*animado*) lively; (*colorido*) colorful, *Brit* colourful; (*elegante*) elegant
gás [gas] *m* gas; ***com ~*** *bebida* carbonated, *Brit* fizzy; ***sem ~*** *bebida* still; ***estou com gases*** I've got wind; ***~ lacrimogêneo*** tear gas; ***~ natural*** natural gas; ***gases de escape*** exhaust fumes
gaseificar [gazejfi'kar] ⟨1n⟩ *v/t* vaporize
gasóleo [ga'zɔliu] *m Port* diesel; ***veículo*** *m* ***a ~*** diesel car
gasolina [gazo'lina] *f* gas(oline), *Brit* petrol; ***meter ~*** fill up; ***estar com pouca ~*** be low on gas; ***~ sem chumbo*** unleaded; ***bomba*** *f* ***de ~*** gas pump, *Brit* petrol pump; ***depósito*** *m* ***de ~*** gas tank, *Brit* petrol tank
gasômetro, *Port* **gasómetro** [ga'zometru] *m* (*contador*) gas meter
gasosa [ga'zɔza] *f* soda pop, *Brit* fizzy drink
gasoso [ga'zozu] *adj* carbonated, *Brit* fizzy; QUÍM gaseous
gastador [gasta'dor] **1** *adj* wasteful **2** *m/f* spendthrift
gastar [gas'tar] ⟨1b⟩ **1** *v/t dinheiro* spend (***em*** on); (*esbanjar*) waste; (*usar*) use; *vestuário* wear out; *salto* wear down; **gastar-se** *v/r* wear out; *salto* wear down
gasto ['gastu] **1** *adj sapato, tapete, pessoa* worn down; *dinheiro* spent **2** *m* (*consumo*) consumption; (*despesa*) expenditure; ***~s*** *pl* expenses
gástrico ['gastriku] *adj* gastric
gastrite [gas'tritʃi] *f* gastritis
gastronomia [gastrono'mia] *f* gastronomy
gastrônomo, *Port* **gastrónomo** [gas'tronumu] *m*, **-a** *f* gastronome
gata ['gata] *f* cat; *fam* sexy woman, sex kitten
gatilho [ga'tʃiʎu] *m espingarda*: trigger
gatinhar [gatʃi'ɲar] ⟨1a⟩ *v/i Port* crawl
gato ['gatu] *m* (tom)cat; *fam homem* hunk
gatuno [ga'tunu] *m*, **-a** *f* scoundrel; (*malandro*) crook
gaveta [ga'veta] *f* drawer; *impressora*: tray
gavião [ga'vjãw] *m* hawk
gaze ['gazi] *f* gauze
gazela [ga'zɛla] *f* gazelle
gazeta [ga'zeta] *f* newspaper; *Port* ***fazer ~*** cut classes, *Brit* play truant
gazeteiro [gaze'tejru] *m* truant
gazua [ga'zua] *f* skeleton key
geada ['ʒeada] *f* frost
gel [ʒew] *m cabelo, banho*: gel
geladeira [ʒela'dejra] *f Bras* refrigerator, fridge
gelado [ʒe'ladu] **1** *adj* frozen *tb fig*; *bebidas etc* chilled; *estrada* icy; ***estou ~!*** I'm frozen! **2** *m Port* ice cream
gelar [ʒe'lar] ⟨1c⟩ **1** *v/t* freeze; *bebida* chill **2** *v/i* freeze
gelatina [ʒela'tʃina] *f* gelatine; GASTR jello, *Brit* jelly
gelatinoso [ʒelatʃi'nozu] *adj* gelatinous
geléia [ʒe'lɛja] *f* jam; *carne*: jelly
geleira [ʒe'lejra] *f* glacier
gelo ['ʒelu] *m* ice; (*frio*) cold; *fig* frostiness; ***~ seco*** dry ice; ***com ~*** with ice, on the rocks
gema ['ʒema] *f ovo*: yolk; *pedra* gem; *fam* ***é da ~*** it's the genuine article; ***~ do ovo*** egg-yolk;
gêmeo, *Port* **gémeo** ['ʒemiu] **1** *adj* twin *atr* **2** ***~s*** *mpl*, **-as** *fpl* twins; ASTROL ***Gêmeos*** Gemini
gemer [ʒe'mer] ⟨2c⟩ **1** *v/i* moan, groan; (*chorar*) wail **2** *v/t canção* croon
gemido [ʒe'midu] *m* groan, moan; (*choro*) wail; *cachorro*: whine
gene ['ʒeni] *m* gene; ***está nos seus ~s*** it's in his genes
genealogia [ʒenealo'ʒia] *f* genealogy
genealógico [ʒenea'lɔʒiku] *adj* genealogical; ***árvore*** *f* ***genealógica*** family tree
Genebra [ʒe'nɛbra] *f* Geneva
general [ʒene'raw] *m* MIL general; ***~ de brigada*** major general; ***~ de divi-***

G

são lieutenant general
generalidade [ʒenerali'dadʒi] *f* generality; (*totalidade*) totality
generalização [ʒeneraliza'sãw] *f* generalization
generalizar [ʒenerali'zar] ⟨1a⟩ generalize
gênero, *Port* **género** ['ʒeneru] *m* (*espécie*) species *sg*; (*forma*) type; (*estilo*) style; GRAM gender; ***~s*** *pl* goods; ***~s*** *pl* ***alimentícios*** foodstuffs
generosidade [ʒenerozi'dadʒi] *f* generosity
generoso [ʒene'rozu] *adj* generous; *jantar* lavish
gênese, *Port* **génese** ['ʒenezi], **Gênesis** ['ʒenezis] **1** *f* origin **2** *m bíblia*: ***o*** (***livro do***) ***Gênesis*** (the Book of) Genesis
genética [ʒe'nɛtʃika] *f* genetics
genético [ʒe'nɛtʃiku] *adj* genetic; ***prova*** *f* ***genética*** DNA test
gengibre [ʒẽ'ʒibri] *m* ginger
gengiva [ʒẽ'ʒiva] *f* gum
genial [ʒe'njaw] *adj idéia* ingenious; *fam* terrific, brilliant
gênio, *Port* **génio** ['ʒeniu] *m* (*espírito*) temper; (*talento*) genius; ***ter bom ~*** be good-natured; ***ter mau ~*** be bad-tempered
genital [ʒeni'taw] *adj* genital; ***órgãos*** *mpl* ***genitais*** genitals
genitália [ʒeni'talia] *f* genitalia *pl*
genitivo [ʒeni'tʃivu] *m* GRAM genitive
genocídio [ʒeno'sidiu] *m* genocide
genoma [ʒe'noma] *m* genome
genro ['ʒẽhu] *m* son-in-law
gente ['ʒẽtʃi] *f* people; *fam* folk; ***a ~*** we; ***você vai sair com a ~?*** are you coming out with us?; ***ele é muito boa ~*** he's a good guy
gentil [ʒẽ'tʃiw] *adj* (*delicado*) polite; (*bondoso*) kind
gentileza [ʒẽtʃi'leza] *f* politeness; (*bondade*) kindness; ***por ~, pode …?*** would you kindly …?
gentilmente [ʒẽtʃiw'mẽtʃi] *adv* kindly
genuíno [ʒe'nwinu] *adj* genuine; (*inequívoco*) unmistakable
geografia [ʒeogra'fia] *f* geography
geográfico [ʒeo'grafiku] *adj* geographical
geógrafo [ʒe'ɔgrafu] *m*, **-a** *f* geographer
geologia [ʒeolo'ʒia] *f* geology
geólogo [ʒe'ɔlogu] *m*, **-a** *f* geologist
geometria [ʒeome'tria] *f* geometry
geométrico [ʒeo'mɛtriku] *adj* geometrical
Geórgia [ʒe'ɔrʒja] *f* Georgia
geração [ʒera'sãw] *f* generation
gerador [ʒera'dor] **1** *adj* ***o fator ~ dos problemas foi …*** the factor which caused the problems was … **2** ELÉT generator; (*produtor*) creator
geral [ʒe'raw] *adj* general; (*comum*) widespread; *declaração* sweeping; ***duma maneira ~*** on the whole; ***em ~*** in general
geralmente [ʒeraw'mẽtʃi] *adv* generally
gerânio [ʒe'rʌniu] *m* geranium
gerar [ʒe'rar] ⟨1c⟩ *v/t* produce; INFORM, ELÉT generate; (*causar*) cause
gerência [ʒe'rẽsja] *f* management
gerente [ʒe'rẽtʃi] **1** *adj atr* managing *atr* **2** *m/f* manager; (*diretor*) director; ***~ de banco*** bank manager; ***~ de vendas*** sales manager
gerir [ʒe'rir] ⟨3c⟩ *v/t* manage, run
germânico [ʒer'mʌniku] *adj* Germanic
germe ['ʒɛrmi] *m* germ; (*embrião*) embryo; *fig* origin; ***~ de trigo*** wheatgerm
germinar [ʒermi'nar] ⟨1a⟩ *v/i* germinate; *fig* develop
gesso ['ʒesu] *m* plaster; ***aparelho*** *m* ***de ~*** plaster cast
gestação [ʒesta'sãw] *f* pregnancy; *animais*: gestation
gestante [ʒes'tãtʃi] *f* pregnant woman
gestão [ʒes'tãw] *m* management
gesto ['ʒɛstu] *m* gesture; (*movimento*) movement; ***~ nobre*** sporting gesture, noble gesture
gestor [ʒes'tor] *m empresa*: manager
gibi [ʒi'bi] *m* comic book
gigabyte [ʒiga'bajtʃi] *m* gigabyte
gigante [ʒi'gãtʃi] **1** *m/f* giant **2** *adj* gigantic, huge
gigantesco [ʒigã'tesku] *adj* gigantic
gilete [ʒi'lɛtʃi] *m Bras* razor blade
ginásio [ʒi'naziu] *m* gymnasium; (*es-*

cola) high school, *Brit* secondary school
ginasta [ʒi'nasta] *m/f* gymnast
ginástica [ʒi'nastʃika] *f* gymnastics *sg*; ***fazer ~*** do gymnastics; *no ginásio* work out
ginecologia [ʒinekolo'ʒia] *f* gynecology, *Brit* gynaecology
ginecologista [ʒinekolo'ʒista] *m/f* gynecologist, *Brit* gynaecologist
gingar [ʒĩ'gaɾ] ⟨1a & 1o⟩ *v/i* sway
ginja ['ʒĩʒa] *f* morello cherry
ginjinha [ʒĩ'ʒiɲa] *f* cherry brandy
gira-discos [ʒiɾa'diskus] *m* ⟨*pl inv*⟩ *Port* record player
girafa [ʒi'ɾafa] *f* giraffe; *fam* beanpole
girar [ʒi'ɾaɾ] ⟨1a⟩ **1** *v/i* turn around; (*contornar*) go around; *roda* spin; *planeta terra* ***~ em torno de*** revolve around **2** *v/t* turn, rotate
girassol [ʒiɾa'sɔw] *m* ⟨*pl* -ssóis⟩ sunflower
giratório [ʒiɾa'tɔɾiu] *adj* revolving; (*rotativo*) rotating; *cadeira* swivel *atr*; ***ponte*** *f* ***giratória*** swing bridge; ***porta*** *f* ***giratória*** revolving door
gíria ['ʒiɾja] *f* slang; (*jargão*) jargon
girino [ʒi'ɾinu] *m* tadpole
giro ['ʒiɾu] **1** *m* turn; (*rotação*) revolution; ***vamos dar um ~?*** shall we go for a wander?; *num carro* shall we go for a spin? **2** *adj Port fam* great, terrific
giz [ʒis] *m* chalk
glacial [gla'sjaw] *adj* icy
glaciar [gla'sjaɾ] *m* glacier
gladiador [gladʒia'doɾ] *m* gladiator
glamouroso [glamo'ɾozu] *adj* glamorous
glândula ['glãdula] *f* gland; ***~ linfática*** lymph gland
glandular [glãdu'laɾ] *adj* glandular
glaucoma [glaw'koma] *m* MED glaucoma
glicerina [glise'ɾina] *f* glycerine
glicose [gli'kɔzi] *f* glucose
global [glo'baw] *adj* global; (*total*) overall
globalização [globaliza'sãw] *f* ⟨*sem pl*⟩ globalization
globo ['globu] *m* globe; ***~ terrestre*** globe; ***~ ocular*** eyeball
glóbulo ['glɔbulu] *m* globule; ANAT ***~ sanguíneo*** corpuscle
glória ['glɔɾja] *f* glory; (*esplendor*) splendor, *Brit* splendour
glorificar [glorifi'kaɾ] ⟨1n⟩ *v/t* glorify
glorioso [glo'ɾjozu] *adj* glorious
glossário [glo'saɾiu] *m* glossary
glutão [glu'tãw] *m*, **glutona** [glu'tona] *f* glutton
glúten ['gluten] *m proteína* gluten
gnomo ['gnomu] *m* gnome
goela ['gwɛla] *f* throat
goense ['gwẽsi], **goês** [gwes] **1** *adj* Goan **2** *m*, **goesa** ['gweza] *f* Goan
goiaba [goj'aba] *f* guava
gol [gow] *m Bras* goal; ***marcar um ~*** score a goal
gola ['gɔla] *f* collar; ***~ alta*** roll neck; ***~ redonda*** crew neck
gole ['gɔli] *m* gulp
goleador [go'ljadoɾ] *m* ESP scorer; *que marca muito* prolific scorer
golear [go'ljaɾ] ⟨1l⟩ *v/t* ESP hammer, trounce
goleiro [go'lejɾu] *m*, **-a** *f* goalkeeper
golfe ['gowfi] *m* golf; ***campo*** *m* ***de ~*** golf course
golfinho [gow'fiɲu] *m* dolphin
golfo ['gowfu] *m* gulf; ***corrente*** *f* ***do Golfo*** Gulf Stream
golinho [gɔ'liɲu] *m* sip
golo ['golu] *m Port* goal; ***marcar um ~*** score a goal
golpe ['gɔlpi] *m* blow *tb fig*; POL coup; *vento*: gust; ***dar um ~ em*** deal a blow to; ***~ de estado*** coup d'état; ***~ de caratê*** karate chop; ***~ mortal*** death blow; ***~ de sorte*** stroke of luck; ***~ sujo*** dirty trick
golpear [gow'pjaɾ] ⟨1h⟩ *v/t* hit; *com o punho* punch
golquíper [gow'kipɛɾ] *m* goalkeeper
goma ['goma] *f* (*cola*) gum, glue; *roupa*: starch
gôndola ['gõdula] *f* gondola
gongo ['gõgu] *m* gong
gonorreia [gono'heja] *f* MED gonorrhea
gonzo ['gõzu] *m porta*: hinge
gorar [go'ɾaɾ] ⟨1e⟩ **1** *v/t* frustrate; *plano* thwart **2** *v/i plano* go wrong
gordo ['goɾdu] **1** *adj* fat; *frango*

G

plump; (*gorduroso*) greasy; *carne* fatty; *fig* ample **2** *m*, **-a** *f* fat man / woman
gorducho [gor'duʃu] **1** *adj* plump, chubby **2** *m/f* plump person
gordura [gor'dura] *f* fat; *derretida* grease; **~ *animal* / *vegetal*** animal / vegetable fat; ***pobre em* ~** low-fat
gorgolejar [gor'goleʒar] ⟨1d⟩ *v/i* gurgle
gorila [go'rila] *m* gorilla
gorjear [gor'ʒjar] ⟨1l⟩ *v/i pássaros* chirp, twitter
gorjeta [gor'ʒeta] *f* gratuity, tip
gorro ['gohu] *m* woolen hat, *Brit* woollen hat
gostar [gos'tar] ⟨1e⟩ *v/i* **~ *de*** like; *viagem, passatempo* enjoy; (*amar*) love; **~ *de fazer algo*** like to do sth, enjoy doing sth; ***não* ~ *de*** dislike; ***eu gostaria de …*** I would like to …; **gostar-se** *v/r* like each other
gosto ['gostu] *m* taste; (*prazer*) pleasure; ***com muito* ~** willingly; ***com bom* ~** tastefully; ***a seu* ~** to your taste; ***mau* ~** bad taste
gostoso [gos'tozu] *adj* tasty; (*agradável*) pleasant; *pessoa* gorgeous
gota ['gota] *f* drop; MED gout; **~ *a* ~** drop by drop; ***essa é a* ~ *d'água!*** that's the last straw!; **~ *de chuva*** raindrop
goteira [go'tejra] *f* gutter; (*vazamento*) leak
gotejar [gote'ʒar] ⟨1d⟩ **1** *v/t* drip **2** *v/i* trickle; *telhado* leak
gótico ['gɔʧiku] *adj* Gothic
gotícula [go'ʧikula] *f* droplet
governador [governa'dor] *m* governor
governamental [governamẽ'taw] *adj* government *atr*; ***a política* ~** government policy
governanta [gover'nãta] *f* housekeeper; *crianças*: governess
governante [gover'nãʧi] **1** *m* POL ruler **2** *adj* ruling *atr*
governar [gover'nar] ⟨1c⟩ *v/t país* govern, rule; *casa* run; NÁUT steer
governo [go'vernu] *m* government; (*pilotagem*) steering, navigation; (*controle*) control; **~ *municipal*** local government; **~ *autônomo*** self-government
gozação [goza'sãw] *f* fun; (*desfrute*) enjoyment; ***foi só uma* ~** it was just a bit of fun
gozado [go'zadu] *adj* funny, amusing
gozar [go'zar] ⟨1e⟩ **1** *v/t* **~ (*de*)** enjoy; *fam* (*zombar de*) make fun of; ***pára de* ~ *de mim!*** stop making fun of me! **2** *v/i* enjoy oneself; (*ter orgasmo*) have an orgasm, come
gozo ['gozu] *m* pleasure; (*desfrute*) use; (*orgasmo*) orgasm
GPS [ʒepe'ɛse] *m* satnav
Grã-Bretanha [grãbre'taɲa] *f* Great Britain
graça ['grasa] *f* joke; REL, *dançarino*: grace; (*perdão*) pardon; (*charme*) charm; ***de* ~** for free; **~*s a*** thanks to; **~*s a Deus!*** thank God!; ***sem* ~** boring; ***isso não tem* ~** that's not funny; ***fazer* ~** joke, make a joke
gracejar [grase'ʒar] ⟨1d⟩ joke
gracejo [gra'seʒu] *m* joke
gracioso [gra'sjozu] *adj* gracious; (*charmoso*) charming; (*cómico*) funny
gradativo [grada'ʧivu] *adj* gradual
grade ['gradʒi] *f* grating, grille; (*tabique*) partition; *janela*: bars; (*cerca*) railings
gradeamento [gradʒia'mẽtu] *m* railing
gradear [gra'dʒiar] ⟨1l⟩ *v/t* fence in; *janela* bar
graduação [gradwa'sãw] *f* gradation; EDUC graduation; MIL rank; *álcool*: alcohol content; (*classificação*) grading
graduado [gra'dwadu] *adj escala* graduated; (*diplomado*) graduate; MIL high-ranking; (*respeitado*) respected
gradual [gra'dwaw] *adj* gradual
gradualmente [gradwaw'mẽʧi] *adv* gradually
graduar [gra'dwar] ⟨1g⟩ *v/t escala* graduate; (*escalonar*) schedule; (*regular*) regulate; (*classificar*) grade
gráfica ['grafika] *f* graphics; *lugar* print shop
gráfico ['grafiku] **1** *adj* graphic **2** *m* graph; INFORM graphic

grã-fino [grã'finu] *adj pessoa, lugar* grand
grafite [gra'fitʃi] *m* graphite; *lápis*: lead; (*pichação*) piece of graffiti
gralha ['graʎa] *f* ZOOL crow
grama[1] ['grama] *m peso*: gram
grama[2] ['grama] *f* BOT grass
gramado [gra'madu] *m Bras* lawn
gramática [gra'matʃika] *f* grammar
gramático [gra'matʃiku] *adj* grammatical
grampeador [gram'pjador] *m* stapler; **~ *industrial*** staple gun
grampear [gram'pjar] ⟨1l⟩ *v/t* staple; TEL bug, tap
grampo ['grampu] *m Bras cabelos*: hairclip, *Am* barrette; *papel*: staple
granada [gra'nada] *f* MIL shell; *pedra* garnet
grande ['grãdʒi] *adj* big, large; *autor, cientista, vinho, filme* great; (*alto*) tall; (*adulto*) grown-up; ***um ~ amor*** a great love
grandeza [grã'deza] *f* size; *autor, cientista, vinho, filme*: greatness; (*nobreza*) grandeur
grandiosidade [grãdjozi'dadʒi] *f* grandeur, magnificence
grandioso [grã'djozu] *adj* grand, magnificent
granel [gra'nɛw] *m* ***a ~*** in bulk; ***compra*** *f* ***a ~*** bulk buying
granito [gra'nitu] *m* granite
granizo [gra'nizu] *m* hailstone; ***chover ~*** hail
granja ['grãʒa] *f* farm; (*celeiro*) barn
granjear [grã'ʒjar] ⟨1l⟩ *v/t* win, gain
granulado [granu'ladu] *adj* grainy; *açúcar* granulated
grão [grãw] *m* ⟨*pl* grãos⟩ grain; *café*: bean
grão-de-bico [grãwdʒi'biku] *m* chickpea
grasnar [graz'nar] ⟨1b⟩ *pato* quack; *sapo* croak; *corvo* caw
gratidão [gratʃi'dãw] *f* ⟨*sem pl*⟩ gratitude
gratificação [gratʃifika'sãw] *f* gratuity; (*recompensa*) reward; *de partida* golden handshake
gratificante [gratʃifi'kãtʃi] *adj* gratifying
gratificar [gratʃifi'kar] ⟨1n⟩ *v/t* gratify; **~ *alguém*** reward s.o.; (*dar gorjeta*) give s.o. a gratuity
gratinado [gratʃi'nadu] **1** *m* gratin **2** *adj* au gratin
grátis ['gratʃis] *adj* free
grato ['gratu] *adj* (*agradável*) pleasant; (*reconhecido*) grateful; ***ser ~ a alguém*** be grateful to s.o.
gratuidade [gratui'dadʒi] *f* gratuity
gratuito [gra'tuitu] *adj* free; *sem razão* gratuitous
grau [graw] *m* degree; *fig tb* level; MIL rank; EDUC class; **~ *centígrado*** degree centigrade; ***primo em segundo ~*** second cousin
graúdo [gra'udu] *adj* big; *pessoa* important
gravação [grava'sãw] *f* (wood) carving; MÚS recording; **~ *em vídeo*** video recording
gravador [grava'dor] *m artesão* engraver; TECN recorder; **~ *de CD / DVD*** CD / DVD writer; **~ *de vôo***, *Port* **~ *de voo*** flight recorder
gravar [gra'var] ⟨1b⟩ *v/t* carve; *metal*: engrave; *memória*: etch; MÚS record; *CD* burn; **~ *em*** record onto
gravata [gra'vata] *f* tie; ***~-borboleta*** bow tie
grave ['gravi] *adj* serious, grave; (*importante*) important; *voz* deep; ***acento*** *m* **~** grave accent
gravemente [grave'mẽtʃi] *adv* seriously
grávida ['gravida] **1** *adj* pregnant **2** *f* pregnant woman
gravidade [gravi'dadʒi] *f* gravity; (*seriedade*) seriousness; ***centro*** *m* ***de ~*** center of gravity, *Brit* centre of gravity
gravidez [gravi'des] *f* pregnancy
gravitação [gravita'sãw] *f* gravitation
gravitar [gravi'tar] ⟨1a⟩ *v/t* (*rotar*) circle; **~ *em torno de*** gravitate toward *tb fig*
gravura [gra'vura] *f madeira*: carving; *metal*: engraving; (*ilustração em livro*) illustration; **~ *a água-forte*** etching
graxa ['graʃa] *f* grease; *sapatos*: polish
Grécia ['grɛsja] *f* Greece
grego ['gregu] **1** *adj* Greek **2** *m*, **-a** *f*

Greek **3** *m lingua* Greek
grelha ['greʎa] *f* broiler, *Brit* grill; ***frango na ~*** broiled chicken, *Brit* grilled chicken
grelhado [gre'ʎadu] *adj* broiled, *Brit* grilled
grelhar [gre'ʎar] ⟨1c⟩ *v/t* broil, *Brit* grill
grêmio, *Port* **grémio** ['gremiu] *m* guild; (*associação*) association, club
greta ['greta] *f* crack
gretar [gre'tar] ⟨1c⟩ *v/i*, **gretar-se** *v/r* crack
greve ['grɛvi] *f* strike; ***fazer ~*** (go on) strike; ***declarar ~***, ***ir para a ~*** go on strike; ***estar em ~*** be on strike; ***~ de braços caídos*** sit-down strike; ***~ geral*** general strike
grevista [gre'vista] *m/f* striker
grifado [gri'fadu] *adj* in italics *pred*, italicized
grifar [gri'far] ⟨1a⟩ *v/t* italicize; *fig* emphasize
griffe ['grifi] *m* designer label
grilado [gri'ladu] *adj fam* hung up (***em*** on)
grilar [gri'lar] ⟨1a⟩ *v/t fam* wind up; **grilar-se** *v/r* get wound up
grilo ['grilu] *m inseto* cricket; *fam de pessoa* hang-up; *fam* ***sem ~!*** no problem!
grinalda [gri'nawda] *f* garland
gringo ['grĩgu] *adj fam pej* foreigner
gripado [gri'padu] *adj* ***estar ~*** have flu
gripar-se [gri'parsi] ⟨1a⟩ *v/r* get the flu
gripe ['gripi] *f* flu; ***~ das aves*** bird flu; ***~ aviária*** avian; ***~ intestinal*** gastric flu; ***~ suína*** swine flu
grisalho [gri'zaʎu] *adj cabelo* gray, *Brit* grey
gritar [gri'tar] ⟨1a⟩ **1** *v/i* shout; *agudo* scream; (*chamar*) call; ***~ por auxílio*** call for help; ***~ com alguém*** shout at s.o. **2** *v/t* shout; (*chamar*) call
grito ['gritu] *m* shout; *agudo* scream; (*chamada*) call; ***aos ~s*** screaming; ***dar um ~*** cry out; ***dar ~s*** scream; ***~ de guerra*** war cry
groselha [gro'zeʎa] *f* gooseberry
grosseiro [gro'sejru] *adj* rude; (*vulgar*) crude; (*rude*) ignorant; *tecido* rough, coarse
grosseria [grose'ria] *f* rudeness; ***fazer ~*** do something rude
grossista [gro'sista] *m/f Port* wholesaler
grosso ['grosu] *adj* **1** *adj* (*gordo*) thick; (*volumoso*) bulky; (*áspero*) rough; *tom* deep; *pop* (*sexy*) hot; ***ser ~ com alguém*** be tough with s.o. **2** *adv* ***ele fala ~*** he speaks in a deep voice **3** *m* (*maioria*) large part; ***o ~ de*** the bulk of
grossura [gro'sura] *f* thickness; *modos*: roughness
grotesco [gro'tesku] *adj* grotesque
grua ['grua] *f construção*: crane
grudado [gru'dadu] *adj papel, plástico* stuck; *fig* ***ele ficou ~ em mim*** he stuck to me like glue
grudar [gru'dar] ⟨1a⟩ **1** *v/t* stick, glue **2** *v/i* stick
grude ['grudʒi] *m* glue
grunhido [gru'ɲidu] *m* grunt
grunhir [gru'ɲir] ⟨3a⟩ *v/i* grunt
grupo ['grupu] *m* group; *ferramentas*: set; POL ***~ dissidente*** splinter group; ***~ étnico*** ethnic group; ***~ de rock*** rock band; ***~ sangüíneo*** blood group; ***~ de trabalho*** team
gruta ['gruta] *f* grotto; (*caverna*) cave
guaraná [gwara'na] *m* guarana
guarda ['gwarda] **1** *m/f* (*sentinela*) guard; *polícia*: policeman / woman; ***~ costeiro*** coastguard; ***~ fiscal*** customs officer; ***~ florestal*** forest ranger; ***~ de segurança*** security guard **2** *f* (*vigia*) watch; (*vigilância*) guarding; (*proteção*) safekeeping
guarda-chuva [gwarda'ʃuva] *m* ⟨*pl* ~s⟩ umbrella
guarda-costas [gwarda'kɔstas] **1** *m/f* ⟨*pl inv*⟩ bodyguard **2** *m* NÁUT coastguard boat
guarda-lama [gwarda'lama] *m* ⟨*pl* ~s⟩ *bicicleta*: mudguard; AUTO fender, *Brit* wing
guarda-louça [gwarda'losa] *m* ⟨*pl* ~s⟩ hutch, *Brit* sideboard
guardanapo [gwarda'napu] *m* napkin, serviette
guarda-noturno, *Port* **guarda-nocturno** [gwardano'turnu] *m* ⟨*pl* guar-

das-nocturnos⟩ night watchman
guardar [gwaɾ'daɾ] ⟨1b⟩ *v/t* put away; (*vigiar*) guard; (*proteger*) protect; (*esconder*) hide; *lembrança, memória* keep; **~ *a distância*** keep one's distance; **~ *algo para si*** keep sth to oneself; **~ *à chave*** lock away; **~ *rancor*** bear *a* grudge
guarda-redes [gwaɾda'hedʒis] *m/f* ⟨*pl inv*⟩ *Port* goalkeeper
guarda-roupa [gwaɾda'hopa] *m* ⟨*pl* ~s⟩ closet, *Brit* wardrobe; *casacos*: checkroom, *Brit* cloakroom
guarda-sol [gwaɾda'sɔw] *m* ⟨*pl* -sóis⟩ sunshade
guarita [gwa'ɾita] *f* sentry box; (*torre*) watch tower
guarnecer [gwaɾne'seɾ] ⟨2g⟩ *v/t* GASTR garnish; MIL garrison; (*munir*) equip (***de*** with)
guarnição [gwaɾni'sãw] *f* MIL garrison; NÁUT crew; GASTR garnish
gude ['gudʒi] *m* ***bola de ~*** marble
guei [gej] **1** *adj* gay **2** *m/f* gay
guelra ['gɛlha] *f* ZOOL gill
guerra ['gɛha] *f* war; ***estar em ~*** be at war; **~ *biológica*** biological warfare; **~ *chímica*** chemical warfare; **~ *civil*** civil war; ***a Guerra Fria*** the Cold War; ***Guerra Mundial*** World War
guerreiro [ge'hejɾu] **1** *m*, **-a** *f* warrior **2** *adj* warlike; *espírito* fighting *atr*
guerrilha [ge'hiʎa] *f* guerrilla warfare
guerrilheiro [gehi'ʎejɾu] **1** *m*, **-a** *f* guerrilla **2** *adj* guerrilla *atr*
guia ['gia] **1** *f* guidance; COM bill of lading **2** *m/f* guide; **~ *turístico*** tour guide **3** *m* guidebook; **~ *de entretenimento*** listings magazine; **~ *de programas de televisão*** TV guide
Guiana ['gjana] *f* Guyana; **~ *Francesa*** French Guyana
guiar [gjaɾ] ⟨1g⟩ *v/t* guide; (*liderar*) lead; *cavalo, carroça* steer; *Port automóvel* drive; **guiar-se** *v/r* go (***por*** by)
guichê, *Port* **guiché** [gi'ʃe] *m* FERROV, TEAT *etc* window, counter
guidom [gi'dõ] *m Bras*, **guidão** [gi'dãw] *m Port* handlebars
guilhotina [giʎo'ʧina] *f* guillotine
guimba ['gĩba] *f* (cigarette) butt
guinada [gi'nada] *f* swerve; ***dar uma ~ com o carro*** swerve
guinchar [gĩ'ʃaɾ] ⟨1a⟩ **1** *v/t carro* tow **2** *v/i freios* screech
guincho ['gĩʃu] *m* squeal; *freios*: screech
guindar [gĩ'daɾ] ⟨1a⟩ *v/t* hoist, lift
guindaste [gĩ'dasʧi] *m* (*roldana*) hoist
Guiné [gi'nɛ] *f* Guinea
Guiné-Bissau [ginɛbi'saw] *f* Guinea-Bissau
guisado [gi'zadu] *m* stew
guisar [gi'zaɾ] ⟨1a⟩ *v/t* stew
guita ['gita] *f* twine
guitarra [gi'taha] *f* guitar; **~ *portuguesa*** Portuguese (*12-stringed*) guitar
guitarrista [gita'hista] *m/f* guitarist
guizo ['gizu] *m* bell
gula ['gula] *f* gluttony
gulodice [gulo'dʒisi] *f* greed
guloseima [gulo'zejma] *f* delicacy
guloso [gu'lozu] *adj* (*comilão*) greedy
gume ['gumi] *m* cutting edge; *fig* sharpness; ***de dois ~s*** double-edged
guri ['guɾi] *m*, **-a** *f* kid
guru [gu'ɾu] *m/f* guru
gutural [gutu'ɾaw] *adj* guttural

H

hábil ['abiw] *adj* (*habilidoso*) skillful, *Brit* skilful; (*desembaraçado*) efficient; (*capaz*) capable; (*autorizado*) entitled
habilidade [abili'dadʒi] *f* skill; (*competência*) ability

habilidoso [abili'dozu] *adj* skillful, *Brit* skilful
habilitação [abilita'sãw] *f* competence; (*direito*) entitlement; *profissional* qualification; ***habilitações literárias*** academic qualifications
habilitar [abili'taɾ] ⟨1a⟩ *v/t* enable; (*instruir*) instruct; (*autorizar*) entitle, qualify (***a*** to); **habilitar-se** *v/r* qualify
habitação [abita'sãw] *f* dwelling, residence; ***política** f **de ~*** housing policy
habitante [abi'tãtʃi] *m/f* inhabitant; *rua*: resident
habitar [abi'taɾ] ⟨1a⟩ **1** *v/t* inhabit **2** *v/i* live (***em*** in)
habitável [abi'tavew] *adj* (in)habitable
hábitat [abi'tatʃi] *m* habitat
hábito ['abitu] *m* habit
habitual [abi'twaw] *adj* usual; *fumador* habitual; ***cliente** m **~*** regular (customer)
habituar [abi'twaɾ] ⟨1g⟩ make used (***a*** to); **habituar-se** *v/r* ***~ a algo*** get used to sth
hacker ['hakeɾ] *m/f* hacker
hadoque [ha'dɔki] *m* haddock
haja ['aʒa] *etc* → ***haver***
hálito ['alitu] *m* (*bafo*) breath; ***mau ~*** bad breath
halogêneo, *Port* **halogéneo** [alo'ʒeniu] *m* halogen; ***lâmpada** f **de ~*** halogen lamp
halterofilismo [awtɛrofi'lizmu] *m* weightlifting
halterofilista [awtɛrofi'lista] *m/f* weightlifter
hambúrguer [ã'burger] *m* hamburger
handebol [hãdʒi'bɔw] *m Bras* handball
handebolista [hãdebo'lista] *m/f Bras* handball player
hangar [ã'gaɾ] *m* hangar
hão-de ['ãwndʒi] → ***haver***
hardware [haɾ'dwɛɾ] *m* INFORM hardware
harmonia [aɾmo'nia] *f* harmony
harmonioso [aɾmo'njozu] *adj* harmonious
harmonizar [aɾmoni'zaɾ] ⟨1a⟩ *vt & v/i* harmonize
harmonização [aɾmoniza'sãw] *f* harmonization
harpa ['aɾpa] *f* harp
hás-de ['aʒdʒi] *etc* → ***haver***
hashi ['haʃi] *mpl* chopsticks
hasta ['asta] *f **~ pública*** public auction; ***vender em ~ pública*** sell at public auction, auction off
haste ['astʃi] *f* shaft; *bandeira*: flagpole; *planta, copo*: stem; *touro*: horn; NÁUT masthead; ***meia ~*** half-mast
hastear [as'tʃiaɾ] ⟨1l⟩ *v/t* hoist, raise
haver [a'veɾ] ⟨2n⟩ **1** *v/aux* have **2** ◊ *impessoal*: ***há*** there is; *plural* there are; ***não havia ninguém em casa*** there was nobody at home ◊ *temporal*: ***há dois meses*** two months ago; ***estou aqui há horas*** I've been here for hours **3** *m* FIN credit; ***~es*** *pl* possessions; (*riqueza*) wealth
haxixe [a'ʃiʃi] *m* hashish
hebraico [e'bɾajku] *adj* → ***hebreu***
hebreu [e'bɾew] **1** *adj* Hebrew **2** *m*, **hebréia**, *Port* **hebreia** [e'bɾɛja] *f* Hebrew **3** *m lingua* Hebrew
hectare [ek'taɾi] *m* hectare
hegemonia [eʒemo'nia] *f* hegemony
hei de ['ejdʒi] *etc* → ***haver***
hélice ['ɛlisi] *f* helix; NÁUT, AERO propeller
helicóptero [eli'kɔpteɾu] *m* helicopter
hélio ['ɛliu] *m* QUÍM helium
heliporto [eli'poɾtu] *m* heliport
hematoma [ema'toma] *m* bruise
hemisfério [emis'fɛriu] *m* hemisphere
hemofilia [emofi'lia] *f* MED hemophilia, *Brit* haemophilia
hemofílico [emo'filiku] *m* hemophiliac, *Brit* haemophiliac
hemorragia [emoha'ʒia] *f* hemorrhage, *Brit* haemorrhage; ***~ nasal*** nosebleed
hemorróidas [emo'hɔidas], **hemorroídes** [emo'hɔidʒis] *fpl* hemorrhoids, *Brit* haemorrhoids
hepatite [epa'tʃitʃi] *f* MED hepatitis
hera ['ɛra] *f* ivy
herança [e'rãsa] *f* inheritance, heritage; ***deixar como ~*** bequeath

herbicida [erbi'sida] *m* weedkiller, herbicide
herbívoro [er'bivuru] *adj* herbivorous
herdade [er'dadʒi] *f* large farm
herdar [er'dar] ⟨1c⟩ inherit
herdeiro [er'dejru] *m*, **-a** *f* heir; heiress
hereditário [eredʒi'tariu] *adj* hereditary
herege [e'rɛʒi] **1** *m/f* heretic **2** *adj* heretical
heresia [ere'zia] *f* heresy
hermético [er'mɛtʃiku] *adj* airtight; *fig* impenetrable
hérnia ['ɛrnja] *f* MED hernia; **~ de disco** slipped disc
herói [e'rɔj]h *m* hero
heroicamente [eroika'mẽtʃi] *adv* heroically
heróico [e'rɔiku] *adj* heroic
heroína[1] [e'rwina] *f* heroine
heroína[2] [e'rwina] *f droga* heroin
heroísmo [e'rwizmu] *m* heroism
herpes ['ɛrpʃ] *m* herpes *sg*; **~ labial** cold sore
herpes-zoster [ɛrps'zɔster] *m* shingles *sg*
hesitação [ezita'sãw] *f* hesitation
hesitante [ezita'sãtʃi] *adj* hesitant
hesitar [ezi'tar] ⟨1a⟩ hesitate
heterogêneo, *Port* **heterogéneo** [etero'ʒeniu] *adj* heterogeneous
heterossexual [ɛterose'kswaw] **1** *adj* heterosexual **2** *m/f* heterosexual
hexágono [e'gzagunu] *m* hexagon
hibernar [iber'nar] ⟨1c⟩ *v/i* hibernate
híbrido ['ibridu] *adj* hybrid; **motor** *m* **~** hybrid engine
hidrante [i'drãtʃi] *f* hydrant
hidratante [idra'tãtʃi] *adj* moisturizing; **creme** *f* **~** moisturizing cream
hidratar [idra'tar] ⟨1b⟩ *pele* moisturize
hidráulica [i'drawlika] *f* hydraulics
hidráulico [i'drawliku] *adj* hydraulic
hidravião [idra'vjãw] *m* seaplane
hidrocarboneto [idrokarbo'netu] *m* hydrocarbon
hidroelétrico [idroe'lɛtriku] *adj* hydroelectric
hidrofólio [idro'fɔliu] *m* hydrofoil
hidrogênio, *Port* **hidrogénio** [idro'ʒeniu] *m* hydrogen
hidrovia [idro'vja] *f* waterway
hiena ['iena] *f* hyena
hierarquia [ierar'kia] *f* hierarchy
hierárquico [ie'rarkiku] *adj* hierarchical
hífen ['ifẽ] *m* hyphen
higiene [i'ʒieni] *f* hygiene
higiênico, *Port* **higiénico** [i'ʒieniku] *adj* hygienic; **penso** *m* **~** sanitary napkin, *Brit* sanitary towel
hilariante [ila'rjãtʃi] *adj* hilarious
hiléia [i'lɛja] *f* Amazon rainforest
hindu [ĩ'du] **1** *adj* Hindu **2** *m/f* Hindu; (*indiano*) Indian
hino ['inu] *m* hymn; **~ nacional** national anthem
hiper... [iper] hyper...
hiperativo, *Port* **hiperactivo** [ipera'tʃivu] *adj* hyperactive
hipérbole [i'pɛrbuli] *f* hyperbole
hiperligação [iperliga'sãw] *f* hyperlink
hipermercado [ipermer'kadu] *m* supermarket, *Brit* hypermarket
hipermetropia [ipermetro'pia] *f* MED far-sightedness, *Brit* long-sightedness
hipersensível [iperse͂'sivew] *adj* hypersensitive
hipertensão [iperte͂'saw] *f* MED high blood pressure
hipertexto [iper'testu] *m* hypertext
hipismo [i'pizmu] *m* (horse) riding
hipismo-salto [ipizmo'sawtu] *m* show jumping
hipnose [ipi'nɔzi] *f* hypnosis
hipnoterapia [ipinotera'pia] *f* hypnotherapy
hipnotizar [ipinotʃi'zar] ⟨1a⟩ hypnotize
hipocondria [ipokõ'dria] *f* hypochondria
hipocondríaco [ipokõ'driaku] **1** *adj* hypochondriac **2** *m*, **-a** *f* hypochondriac
hipocrisia [ipokri'zia] *f* hypocrisy
hipócrita [i'pɔkrita] **1** *adj* hypocritical **2** *m/f* hypocrite
hipódromo [i'pɔdrumu] *m* racecourse; *hipismo*: hippodrome, showing jumping arena

H

hipopótamo [ipo'pɔtamu] *m* hippopotamus, hippo
hipoteca [ipo'tɛka] *f* mortgage
hipotecar [ipote'kaɾ] ⟨1n & 1c⟩ *v/t* mortgage
hipotecário [ipote'kariu] *adj* mortgage *atr*
hipotenusa [ipote'nuza] *f* MAT hypotenuse
hipotermia [ipoteɾ'mia] *f* hypothermia
hipótese [i'pɔtʃizi] *f* (*suposição*) hypothesis; (*pressuposto*) assumption; ***na melhor das ~s*** at best; ***não ter ~*** not stand a chance
hipotético [ipo'tɛtʃiku] *adj* hypothetical

H

hirto ['iɾtu] *adj* stiff, rigid
hispânico [is'pʌniku] **1** *adj* Hispanic **2** *m*, **-a** *f* Hispanic
histerectomia [isteɾɛkto'mia] *f* hysterectomy
histeria [iste'ria] *f* hysteria
histérico [is'tɛriku] *adj* hysterical
história [es'tɔɾja] *f* history; *conto* story; ***~ do arco-da-velha*** yarn; ***~ de detetive*** whodunnit; ***~ em quadrinhos*** comic strip; ***~ universal*** world history; ***~ da vida*** life history
historiador [estoɾja'doɾ] *m*, **-a** *f* (*cronista*) historian; (*narrador*) storyteller
histórico [es'tɔriku] **1** *adj* historical; *significativo* historic **2** *m* history; ***~ médico*** medical history
historiografia [estoɾjogra'fia] *f* historiography
HIV positivo [agajvepozi'tʃivu] *adj* HIV-positive
hobby ['hɔbi] *m* hobby
hodômetro [o'dometɾu] *m* odometer, *Brit* mileometer
hoje ['oʒi] today; ***de ~*** modern, today's; ***~ em dia*** nowadays; ***~ à noite*** tonight
Holanda [o'lãda] *f* Holland
holandês [olã'des] **1** *adj* Dutch **2** *m*, **holandesa** [olã'deza] *f* Dutchman / woman **3** *m lingua* Dutch
holding ['howdĩ] *f* ***sociedade*** *f* ***~*** holding company
holocausto [olo'kawstu] *m* holocaust
holofote [olo'fɔtʃi] *m* searchlight, floodlight
holograma [olo'grama] *m* hologram
homem ['ɔmẽ] *m* man; ***uma conversa de ~ para ~*** a man to man talk; ***ele agora está um ~ feito*** he's a man now; ***~ da carrocinha*** dog catcher; ***~ de estado*** statesman; ***~ de negócios*** businessman; ***~ do tempo*** weatherman
homem-bomba [omẽ'bõba] *m* suicide bomber
homem-rã [omẽ'hã] *m* frogman
homenagear [omena'ʒjaɾ] ⟨1l⟩ honor, *Brit* honour, pay tribute to
homenagem [ome'naʒẽ] *f* tribute, homage
homeopatia [omjopa'tʃia] *f* homeopathy
homicida [omi'sida] **1** *m/f* murderer **2** *adj* homicidal
homicídio [omi'sidiu] *m* homicide, murder
homofobia [omofo'bia] *f* homophobia
homogêneo, *Port* **homogéneo** [omo'ʒeniu] *adj* homogeneous
homologar [omolo'gaɾ] ⟨1o & 1e⟩ recognize; DIR ratify
homólogo [o'mɔlogu] *m*, **-a** *f* opposite number, counterpart
homônimo, *Port* **homónimo** [o'monimu] *m* namesake; GRAM homonym
homossexual [omose'kswaw] **1** *adj* homosexual **2** *m/f* homosexual
homosexualidade [omosekswali'dadʒi] *f* homosexuality
honestamente [onɛsta'mẽtʃi] *adv* honestly
honestidade [onestʃi'dadʒi] *f* honesty; (*decência*) decency, integrity
honesto [o'nɛstu] *adj* honest; (*decente*) decent
honorário [ono'rariu] **1** *adj* honorary **2** *m* ***~s*** *pl* fees
honra ['õha] *f* honor, *Brit* honour; ***as ~s fúnebres*** the funeral rites; ***palavra*** *f* ***de ~*** word of honor
honradez [õha'des] *f* (*probidade*) honesty; (*decência*) decency
honrado [õ'hadu] *adj* (*honroso*) honorable, *Brit* honourable; (*íntegro*) upright

honrar [õ'haɾ] ⟨1a⟩ honor, *Brit* honour; **honrar-se** *v/r* **~ com** (*ou* **de**) be honored to, *Brit* be honoured to
honroso [õ'hozu] *adj* honorable, *Brit* honourable
hóquei ['hɔkej] *m* hockey
hora ['ɔɾa] *f* hour; (*tempo*) time; **meia ~** half an hour; **um quarto de ~** a quarter of an hour; **à ~** on time; **chegar a ~s** arrive on time; **de ~ em ~** every hour; **na última ~** at the last minute, at the eleventh hour; **a esta ~ amanhã** this time tomorrow; **que ~s são?** what time is it?; **a que ~ s?** at what time?; **às 4 ~s** at 4 o'clock; **dar ~s** *relógio*: strike; *fig estômago*: rumble; **~ de almoço** lunch hour; **~ de dormir** bed time; **~ de encerramento** closing time; **~ de entrada** *trabalho*: starting time; **~ da Europa Central** Central European time; **~ local** local time; **~ marcada** appointment; **~ de ponta** rush hour; **~ da refeição** meal time; **~ de saída** *trabalho*: finishing time; **~ de verão** summer time, daylight saving time; **~s** *pl* **extraordinárias** overtime; **~s** *pl* **de serviço** (*ou* **de expediente**) office hours, business hours; *Bras* **~s livres** free time
hora-homem [ɔɾa'ɔmẽ] *f* man-hour
horário [o'ɾariu] **1** *adj* hourly; **sinal** *m* **~** time signal **2** *m* schedule, *Brit* timetable; **estar no ~** be on schedule; **~ de abertura** opening hours; **~ do expediente** office hours; **~ flexível** flextime, *Brit* flexitime; **~ de ponta** rush hour; **~ de trabalho** working hours; **~ de visitas** visiting hours; **~ do vôo**, *Port* **~ do voo** flight time
horda ['ɔɾda] *f* horde
horizontal [oɾizõ'taw] *adj* horizontal
horizonte [oɾi'zõtʃi] *m* horizon
hormônio [oɾ'moniu] *m* hormone
hormonal [oɾmo'naw] *adj* hormonal
horóscopo [o'ɾɔskupu] *m* horoscope
horrendo [o'hẽdu] *adj* horrendous
horripilante [ohipi'lãtʃi] *adj* hair-raising
horrível [o'hivew] *adj* awful, horrible
horror [o'hoɾ] *m* horror; **~es** *pl* atrocities, horrors; **ter ~ a algo** hate sth; **que ~!** how awful!
horrorizar [ohoɾi'zaɾ] ⟨1a⟩ horrify; **horrorizar-se** *v/r* be horrified
horroroso [oho'ɾozu] *adj* horrible, awful
horta ['ɔɾta] *f* vegetable garden
hortaliça [oɾta'lisa] *f* vegetables, greens
hortelã [oɾ'telã] *f* mint
hortelã-pimenta [oɾtelãpi'mẽta] *f* peppermint
hortênsia [oɾ'tẽsja] *f* hydrangea
horticultor [oɾtʃikuw'toɾ] *m*, **-a** *f* truck farmer, *Brit* market gardener
horticultura [oɾtʃikuw'tuɾa] *f* horticulture
horto ['oɾtu] *m* truck farm, *Brit* market garden
hospedagem [ospe'daʒẽ] *f* lodging; (*residência*) accommodation
hospedar [ospe'daɾ] ⟨1c⟩ *v/t* put up; **hospedar-se** *v/r* stay, put up
hospedaria [ospeda'ɾia] *f* guest house
hóspede ['ɔspedʒi] *m* guest; *que aluga* lodger; **casa** *f* **de ~s** guest house; **quarto** *m* **de ~s** guest room
hospedeiro [ospe'dejɾu] **1** *adj* hospitable **2** *m*, **-a** *f* landlord; landlady; *Port* AERO steward; stewardess
hospital [ospi'taw] *m* hospital; **ir parar no ~** go into the hospital, *Brit* go into hospital
hospitalar [ospita'laɾ] *adj* hospital *atr*
hospitaleiro [ospita'lejɾu] *adj* hospitable
hospitalidade [ospitali'dadʒi] *f* hospitality
hospitalização [ospitaliza'sãw] *f* hospitalization
hospitalizado [ospitali'zadu] *adj* hospitalized; **ser / ficar ~** be hospitalized
hospitalizar [ospitali'zaɾ] ⟨1a⟩ *v/t* hospitalize, admit to hospital
hóstia ['ɔstʃia] *f* REL Host; wafer
hostil [os'tʃiw] *adj* hostile
hostilidade [ostʃili'dadʒi] *f* hostility
hotel [o'tɛw] *m* hotel
hotelaria [otela'ɾia] *f* hotel industry
hoteleiro [ote'lejɾu] **1** *m* hotelier **2** *adj* hotel *atr*
houve ['ovi] → ***haver***

H

hovercraft [hover'kraft] *m* hovercraft
humanidade [umani'dadʒi] *f* mankind; *comportamento*: humanity
humanitário [umani'tariu] *adj* humanitarian
humanitarismo [umanita'rizmu] *m* humanity
humano [u'manu] **1** *adj* human; (*bondoso*) humane; ***o ser ~*** man **2** *m* ***~s*** *pl* humans
humedecer *etc Port* → ***umedecer*** *etc*
humildade [umiw'dadʒi] *f* humility; *de origem* humbleness
humilde [u'mildʒi] *adj* humble
humilhação [umiʎa'sãw] *f* humiliation
humilhante [umi'ʎãtʃi] *adj* humiliating
humilhar [umi'ʎar] ⟨1a⟩ humiliate
humor [u'mor] *m* humor, *Brit* humour; (*disposição*) mood; ***estar de bom / mau ~*** be in a good / bad mood; ***perder o bom ~*** lose one's temper
humorista [umo'rista] *m/f* comedian
humorístico [umo'ristʃiku] *adj* humorous
húngaro ['ũgaru] **1** *adj* Hungarian **2** *m*, **-a** *f* Hungarian **3** *m lingua* Hungarian
Hungria [ũ'gria] *f* Hungary
hurra ['uha] *int* hooray

I

ia ['ia], **iam** ['iãw] *etc* → ***ir***
iate ['jatʃi] *m* NÁUT yacht
iatismo [ja'tʃizmu] *m* yachting
ibérico [i'bɛriku] *adj* Iberian; ***Península*** *f* ***Ibérica*** Iberian Peninsula
ibero [i'bɛru] **1** *m*, **-a** *f* Iberian **2** *adj* → ***ibérico***
içar [i'sar] ⟨1p⟩ hoist; (*guindar*) lift
ICM [ise'emi] *m Bras abr* (***Imposto de circulação de mercadorias***) sales tax, *Brit* VAT (value added tax)
ícone ['ikoni] *m* icon
icterícia [ikte'risja] *f* MED jaundice
ida ['ida] *f* going; (*viagem*) journey (***a*** to); (*partida*) departure; ***~s*** *pl* ***e voltas*** (*ou* ***vindas***) *pl* comings and goings; ***bilhete*** *m* ***de ~ e volta*** round trip ticket, *Brit* return (ticket)
idade [i'dadʒi] *f* age; ***que ~ tem?*** how old is he / she? ***com a ~ de*** at the age of; ***ter 6 anos de ~*** be 6 years old; ***~ adulta*** adulthood; ***na flor da ~*** in one's prime; ***maior de ~*** above age; ***de meia ~*** middle-aged; ***Idade Média*** Middle Ages
ideal [i'deaw] **1** *adj* ideal; (*de sonho*) imagined **2** *m* ideal; (*sonho*) dream; ***o ~ seria fazermos assim*** ideally, we would do it like this
idealismo [idea'lizmu] *m* idealism
idealista [idea'lista] **1** *adj* idealistic **2** *m/f* idealist
idealmente [ideaw'mẽtʃi] *adv* ideally
idéia, *Port* **ideia** [i'dɛja] *f* idea; ***fazer ~ de algo*** imagine sth; ***não fazer ~*** have no idea (***de*** about); ***boa ~!*** good idea!; ***mudar de ~*** change one's mind; ***não é uma boa ~ ...*** it's not a good idea to ...; ***não tenho a menor ~*** I haven't the slightest idea
idêntico [i'dẽtʃiku] *adj* identical
identidade [idẽtʃi'dadʒi] *f* identity; ***bilhete*** *m* ***de ~*** ID card
identificação [idẽtʃifika'sãw] *f* identification
identificar [idẽtʃifi'kar] ⟨1n⟩ identify
ideologia [ideolo'ʒia] *f* ideology
ideológico [ideo'lɔʒiku] *adj* ideological
idílico [i'dʒiliku] *adj* idyllic
idioma [i'djoma] *m* language
idiomático [idjo'matʃiku] *adj* idiomatic
idiota [i'djɔta] **1** *adj* idiotic **2** *m/f*

idiot
idiotice [idjo'ʧisi] *f* idiocy
ido ['idu] *pp* → ***ir***
ídolo ['idulu] *m* idol
idôneo, *Port* **idóneo** [i'doniu] *adj* suitable, fit
idoso [i'dozu] *adj* elderly, old; ***lar** m **de ~s*** old people's home
idiossincrasia [idjosĩkra'zia] *f* idiosyncrasy
Iêmen, *Port* **Iémen** ['iemen] *m* Yemen
iene ['ieni] *m* yen
ignição [igni'sãw] *f* ignition; ***chave** f **de ~*** ignition key
ignóbil [i'gnɔbiw] *adj* ignoble
ignomínia [igno'minja] *f* disgrace, ignominy
ignorância [igno'ɾãsja] *f* ignorance
ignorante [igno'ɾãʧi] **1** *adj* ignorant **2** *m/f* ignoramus
ignorar [igno'ɾaɾ] ⟨1e⟩ ignore; ***eu ignorava a existência de …*** I didn't know about the existence of …
igreja [i'gɾeʒa] *f* church
igual [i'gwaw] *adj* equal; (*inalterável*) even; ***exatamente ~ ao seu*** just like yours; ***parecer** / **soar ~*** look / sound the same
igualar [igwa'laɾ] ⟨1b⟩ **1** *v/t* equal; (*compensar*) even out, level out; (*aproximar*) bring into line, align (***a*** with); (*equiparar*) treat as equal **2** *v/i* be equal; **igualar-se** *v/r* ***~ a*** be equal to
igualdade [igwaw'dadʒi] *f* equality; ***~ de direitos*** equal rights
igualitário [igwali'taɾiu] *adj* egalitarian
igualmente [igwaw'mẽʧi] *adv* equally; ***Feliz Ano Novo – ~*** Happy New Year - and the same to you
iguaria [igwa'ɾia] *f* delicacy
ilegal [ile'gaw] *adj* illegal
ilegalidade [ilegali'dadʒi] *f* illegality
ilegítimo [ile'ʒiʧimu] *adj* illegitimate; DIR illegal; ***filho ~*** illegitimate son
ilegível [ile'ʒivew] *adj* illegible
ileso [i'lezu] *adj* unhurt
iletrado [ile'tɾadu] *adj* uneducated
ilha ['iʎa] *f* island; ***~ de tráfego**, **~ de trânsito*** traffic island
ilharga [i'ʎaɾga] *f* side, flank
ilhéu [i'ʎɛu] **1** *m* rocky island **2** *m*, **-oa** [i'ʎoa] *f* islander **3** *adj* island *atr*
ilhó [i'ʎɔ] *m/f sapato*: eyelet
ilícito [i'lisitu] *adj* illicit
ilimitado [ilimi'tadu] *adj* unlimited
ilógico [i'lɔʒiku] *adj* illogical
iludir [ilu'dʒiɾ] ⟨3a⟩ *v/t* deceive; *lei* evade; **iludir-se** *v/r* delude oneself
iluminação [ilumina'sãw] *f* lighting
iluminado [ilumi'nadu] *adj* illuminated, lit; ***~ por holofotes*** floodlit
iluminar [ilumi'naɾ] ⟨1a⟩ *v/t* light; *festividades* illuminate; *fig* enlighten
ilusão [ilu'zãw] *f* illusion; ***~ de ótica***, *Port* ***~ de óptica*** optical illusion
ilusório [ilu'zɔɾiu] *adj* illusory
ilustração [ilustɾa'sãw] *f* illustration
ilustrado [ilus'tɾadu] *adj livro* illustrated
ilustrar [ilus'tɾaɾ] ⟨1a⟩ illustrate
ilustre [i'lustɾi] *adj* illustrious
ímã [i'mã] *m* magnet
imaculado [imaku'ladu] *adj* immaculate
imagem [i'maʒẽ] *f* image; ***~ da marca*** brand image
imaginação [imaʒina'sãw] *f* imagination
imaginar [imaʒi'naɾ] ⟨1a⟩ imagine; ***obrigado – imagina!*** thank you - you're very welcome
imaginária [imaʒi'naɾja] *f* ARTE sculpture
imaginário [imaʒi'naɾiu] **1** *adj* imaginary **2** *m* imaginary world
imaginável [imaʒi'navew] *adj* imaginable
imaginoso [imaʒi'nozu] *adj* imaginative
íman ['iman] *m Port* magnet
imaterial [imate'ɾjaw] *adj* immaterial
imaturo [ima'tuɾu] *adj pessoa* immature
imbatível [ĩba'ʧivew] *adj time*, *recorde* unbeatable
imbecil [ĩbe'siw] **1** *adj* stupid **2** *m* imbecile, idiot
imediação [imedʒia'sãw] *f* directness; ***imediações*** *fpl* vicinity, surroundings
imediatamente [imedʒiata'mẽʧi] *adv* immediately

I

imediato [ime'dʒiatu] **1** *adj* immediate **2** *m* NÁUT mate
imensidade [imẽsi'dadʒi] *f* immensity
imensidão [imẽsi'dãw] *f* enormity
imenso [i'mẽsu] *adj* (*muito*) a lot of; (*colossal*) immense; ***tenho ~s sapatos*** I have a huge number of shoes
imerecido [imeɾe'sidu] *adj* undeserved
imergir [imeɾ'ʒiɾ] ⟨3n & 2c⟩ *v/t* immerse
imersão [imeɾ'sãw] *f* immersion
imigração [imigɾa'sãw] *f* immigration
imigrante [imi'gɾãtʃi] *m/f* immigrant
imigrar [imi'gɾaɾ] ⟨1a⟩ immigrate
iminência [imi'nẽsja] *f* imminence; ***está na ~ de caír*** it's threatening to fall down, it's in imminent danger of falling down
iminente [imi'nẽtʃi] *adj* imminent
imiscuir-se [imis'kwiɾsi] ⟨3i⟩ *v/r* meddle (***em*** in)
imitação [imita'sãw] *f* imitation; *comédia*: impersonation
imitador [imita'doɾ] *m*, **-a** *f* imitator
imitar [imi'taɾ] ⟨1a⟩ imitate; *comédia*: impersonate
imobiliária [imobi'ljaɾja] *f* realtor®, *Brit* estate agent's
imobiliário [imobi'ljaɾiu] **1** *adj* property *atr*; ***agente ~*** real estate agent; ***bens*** *mpl* ***~s*** real estate **2** *m* property
imobilização [imobiliza'sãw] *f* immobilization; (*suspensão*) stoppage; (*paralização*) paralysis
imobilizado [imobili'zadu] *adj* ***estar ~*** be immobilized, be at a standstill
imobilizador [imobiliza'doɾ] *m* AUTO immobilizer
imobilizar [imobili'zaɾ] ⟨1a⟩ *v/t* immobilize; (*paralizar*) bring to a standstill, paralyse; *dinheiro* tie up
imoderado [imode'ɾadu] *adj* immoderate
imolação [imola'sãw] *f* sacrifice
imolar [imo'laɾ] ⟨1e⟩ sacrifice *tb* REL
imoral [imo'ɾaw] *adj* immoral
imoralidade [imoɾali'dadʒi] *f* immorality
imortal [imoɾ'taw] *adj* immortal
imortalidade [imoɾtali'dadʒi] *f* immortality
imortalizar [imoɾtali'zaɾ] ⟨1a⟩ *v/t* immortalize
imóvel [i'mɔvew] *adj* motionless; ***bens*** *mpl* ***imóveis*** real estate
imóveis [i'mɔvejs] *mpl* real estate
impaciência [ĩpa'sjẽsja] *f* impatience
impaciente [ĩpa'sjẽtʃi] *adj* impatient
impacto [ĩ'paktu], *Port* **impacte** [ĩ'paktʃi] *m* impact; ***~ ambiental*** damage to the environment, environmental impact
ímpar ['ĩpaɾ] *adj número* odd; (*sem igual*) unique
imparcial [ĩpaɾ'sjaw] *adj* impartial
imparcialidade [ĩpaɾsjali'dadʒi] *f* impartiality
impasse [ĩ'pasi] *m fig* impasse, deadlock *tb fig*
impassibilidade [ĩpasibili'dadʒi] *f* impassivity
impassível [ĩpa'sivew] *adj* impassive
impávido [ĩ'pavidu] *adj* intrepid, fearless
impecável [ĩpe'kavew] *adj* impeccable
impedido [ĩpe'dʒidu] *adj rua* blocked; *Port telefone* busy; ESP offside
impedimento [ĩpedʒi'mẽtu] *m* impediment; ESP ***na posição de ~*** offside
impedir [ĩpe'dʒiɾ] ⟨3r⟩ obstruct; (*deter*) stop; *rua* block; (*vedar*) bar; *progresso* impede; ***~ alguém de fazer algo*** prevent s.o. from doing sth
impelir [ĩpe'liɾ] ⟨3c⟩ drive; (*empurrar*) push
impenetrável [ĩpene'tɾavew] *adj* impenetrable
impensável [ĩpẽ'savew] *adj* unthinkable
imperador [ĩpeɾa'doɾ] *m* emperor
imperar [ĩpe'ɾaɾ] ⟨1c⟩ **1** *v/t* rule, reign over **2** *v/i* reign
imperativo [ĩpeɾa'tʃivu] **1** *adj* imperative **2** *m* absolute necessity; GRAM imperative
imperatriz [ĩpeɾa'tɾis] *f* empress
impercetível, *Port* **imperceptível** [ĩpeɾse'tʃivew] *adj* imperceptible
imperdoável [ĩpeɾ'dwavew] *adj* unforgivable, inexcusable
imperfeição [ĩpeɾfej'sãw] *f* imperfec-

tion
imperfeito [ĩper'fejtu] **1** *adj* imperfect; (*incompleto*) incomplete; GRAM ***pretérito*** *m* **~** imperfect **2** *m* imperfect
imperial [ĩpe'rjaw] **1** *adj* imperial **2** *f cerveja*: draft beer, *Brit* draught beer
imperialismo [ĩperja'lizmu] *m* imperialism
imperialista [ĩperja'lista] *adj* imperialistic
império [ĩ'pɛriu] *m* (*domínio*) rule; (*reino*) empire *tb fig*
impermeável [ĩper'mjavew] **1** *adj* waterproof; ***~ a ...*** impervious to ... **2** *m* raincoat
impertinência [ĩpertʃi'nẽsja] *f* impertinence
impertinente [ĩpertʃi'nẽtʃi] *adj* impertinent
imperturbável [ĩpertur'bavew] *adj* imperturbable
impessoal [ĩpe'swaw] *adj* impersonal
ímpeto ['ĩpetu] *m* impetus
impetuosidade [ĩpetwozi'dadʒi] *f* impetuosity
impetuoso [ĩpe'twozu] *adj* impetuous
impiedoso [ĩpie'dozu] *adj* merciless, cruel
implacável [ĩpla'kavew] *adj* relentless
implantação [ĩplãta'sãw] *f* (*estabelecimento*) introduction; MED implant
implantar [ĩplã'tar] ⟨1a⟩ (*estabelecer*) introduce; MED implant
implante [ĩ'plãtʃi] *m* MED implant; ***~ de pele*** skin graft
implementar [ĩplemẽ'tar] ⟨1a⟩ implement
implemento [ĩple'mẽtu] *m* implement
implicação [ĩplika'sãw] *f* implication
implicar [ĩpli'kar] ⟨1n⟩ **1** *v/t* imply; (*enredar*) involve; ***~ alguém em algo*** implicate s.o. in sth **2** *v/i* ***~ com*** pick on
implícito [ĩ'plisitu] *adj* implicit
imploração [ĩplora'sãw] *f* begging
implorar [ĩplo'rar] ⟨1e⟩ implore; (*rogar*) ***~ algo*** plead for sth
imponderado [ĩpõde'radu] *adj* rash
imponderável [ĩpõde'ravew] **1** *adj* imponderable **2** *m* ***imponderáveis*** *pl* imponderables
imponente [ĩpo'nẽtʃi] *adj* impressive, imposing
impor [ĩ'por] ⟨2z⟩ *v/t pena, condição* impose; ***a lei impõe ...*** the law stipulates ...; **impor-se** *v/r* assert oneself
importação [ĩporta'sãw] *f* import; ***restrição*** *f* ***de ~*** import restriction
importatador [ĩporta'dor] **1** *adj* import *atr* **2** *m*, **-a** *f* importer
importância [ĩpor'tãsja] *f* importance; (*quantia*) sum, amount; ***não tem ~!*** it's not important, never mind!
importante [ĩpor'tãtʃi] *adj* important
importantíssimo [ĩportã'tʃiːsimu] *adj* very important
importar [ĩpor'tar] ⟨1e⟩ **1** *v/t* introduce; COM import **2** *v/i* matter, be important; ***~ em*** come to, add up to; *fig* amount to; ***não importa*** it doesn't matter; ***não me importa!*** I don't care!; ***não importa que sejam grandes*** no matter how big they are; ***não importa o que ela disser*** no matter what she says; **importar-se** *v/r* ***~ com*** take care of; ***se não se importa*** if you don't mind
importável [ĩpor'tavew] *adj* importable
importunar [ĩportu'nar] ⟨1a⟩ *v/t* annoy
imposição [ĩpozi'sãw] *f* imposition; *contrato*: requirement; (*obrigação*) obligation
impossibilidade [ĩposibili'dadʒi] *f* impossibility
impossibilitado [ĩposibili'tadu] *adj* ***estar ~ de fazer*** be unable to do
impossível [ĩpo'sivew] *adj* impossible
imposto [ĩ'postu] *m* tax; ***declaração*** *f* ***de ~s*** tax return; ***~ de circulação*** (***de mercadorias***) sales tax, *Brit* VAT; ***~ de renda*** income tax; ***~ sobre a venda*** sales tax, *Brit* VAT; ***~ de rendimento de capital*** capital gains tax; ***~ sobre os rendimentos*** income tax; ***~ sobre o valor acrescentado*** value-added tax; ***~ sobre veículos*** automobile tax
impostor [ĩpos'tor] *m*, **-a** *f* impostor
impotência [ĩpo'tẽsja] *f* powerlessness, impotence; MED impotence

I

impotente [ĩpo'tẽʧi] *adj* impotent, powerless; MED impotent
impregnar [ĩpre'gnaɾ] ⟨1c⟩ impregnate
imprensa [ĩ'prẽsa] *f* TIPO printing; (*prensa*) (printing) press; (*jornais etc*) press; ~ ***marrom*** gutter press
imprescindível [ĩpresĩ'dʒivew] *adj* essential, indispensable
impressão [ĩpre'sãw] *f* printing; INFORM printout; (*cópia*) copy, print; *fig* impression; ***tenho a ~ de que ...*** I get the impression that ...; ~ ***digital*** fingerprint; ~ ***genética*** genetic fingerprint
impressionante [ĩpresjo'nãʧi] *adj* impressive
impressionar [ĩpresjo'naɾ] ⟨1f⟩ impress, make an impression on; (*abalar*) affect
impressionável [ĩpresjo'navew] *adj* impressionable
impresso [ĩ'prɛsu] *m* form; (*panfleto*) leaflet
impressora [ĩpre'soɾa] *f* printing machine; INFORM printer; ~ ***a cores*** color printer, *Brit* colour printer; ~ ***jato de tinta*** inkjet (printer); ~ ***laser*** laser (printer)
imprestável [ĩpres'tavew] *adj* useless
imprevidência [ĩprevi'dẽsja] *f fig* short-sightedness
imprevidente [ĩprevi'dẽʧi] *adj* short-sighted
imprevisão [ĩprevi'zãw] *f* lack of foresight
imprevisível [ĩprevi'zivew] *adj* unforeseeable
imprevisto [ĩpre'vistu] **1** *adj* unforeseen, unexpected **2** *m* something unexpected; ***aconteceu um ~*** something came up
imprimir [ĩpri'miɾ] ⟨3a⟩ print; INFORM print (out)
improbabilidade [ĩprobabili'dadʒi] *f* improbability
improdutivo [ĩprodu'ʧivu] *adj* unproductive; (*inútil*) useless
impróprio [ĩ'prɔpriu] *adj* unsuitable; (*inconveniente*) improper
improvável *adj* improbable, unlikely; ***é ~ que*** it is unlikely that; ***é ~ que ganhe*** he is unlikely to win
improvisação [ĩproviza'sãw] *f* improvization
improvisadamente [ĩprovizada'mẽʧi] *adv* ad lib
improvisar [ĩprovi'zaɾ] ⟨1a⟩ *v/t & v/i* improvize
improviso [ĩpro'vizu] *m* ad-lib; ***de ~*** (*de repente*) suddenly; ***ele cantou de ~*** he ad-libbed a song
imprudência [ĩpru'dẽsja] *f* imprudence, rashness
imprudente [ĩpru'dẽʧi] *adj* rash, imprudent
impugnação [ĩpugna'sãw] *f* DIR contesting
impugnar [ĩpu'gnaɾ] ⟨1a⟩ contest
impulsionar [ĩpuwsjo'naɾ] ⟨1f⟩ drive, impel; *fig tb* urge
impulsionador [ĩpuwsjona'doɾ] *m* driving force
impulsivo [ĩpuw'sivu] *adj* impulsive
impulso [ĩ'puwsu] *m* impulse; TECN drive; ESP run-up
impune [ĩ'puni] *adj* unpunished; ***sair ~*** get off scot-free
impunidade [ĩpuni'dadʒi] *f* impunity
impureza [ĩpu'reza] *f* impurity
impuro [ĩ'puɾu] *adj* impure
imputação [ĩputa'sãw] *f* accusation
imputar [ĩpu'taɾ] ⟨1a⟩ ~ ***algo a alguém*** accuse s.o. of sth
imputável [ĩpu'tavew] *adj* punishable; (*atribuível*) attributable; (*responsável*) of sound mind
imundície [imũ'dʒisi] *f* dirt, filth
imundo [i'mũdu] *adj* dirty, filthy
imune [i'muni] *adj* MED, DIR immune; ~ ***de*** immune from; ~ ***contra*** immune to
imunidade [imuni'dadʒi] *f* POL, MED immunity; (*isenção*) exemption; ~ ***diplomática*** diplomatic immunity
imunizar [imuni'zaɾ] ⟨1a⟩ *v/t* immunize
imunodeficiência [imunodefi'sjẽsja] *f* immunodeficiency
inabalável [inaba'lavew] *adj* unshakeable
inabitado [inabi'tadu] *adj* uninhabited
inabitável [inabi'tavew] *adj* uninhabi-

table
inaceitável [inasej'tavew] *adj* unacceptable
inacessível [inase'sivew] *adj* unattainable; (*impenetrável*) inaccessible; *preço* prohibitive
inacreditável [inakredʒi'tavew] *adj* (*espantoso*) amazing; (*duvidoso*) dubious
inactivo [ina'ʧivu] *adj Port* inactive; *funcionário* retired; *máquina*, *fábrica* disused
inadequado [inade'kwadu] *adj* inadequate; (*impróprio*) unsuitable
inadimplência [inadʒĩ'plẽsja] *f* breach of contract
inadmissível *adj* → ***inaceitável***
inadvertência [inadʒiver'tẽsja] *f* oversight; ***por ~*** by mistake
inalação [inala'sãw] *f* inhalation
inalador [inala'dor] *m* inhaler
inalar [ina'lar] ⟨1b⟩ breathe in, inhale
inanimado [inani'madu] *adj*, **inânime** [i'nʌnimi] *adj* inanimate
inaptidão [inapʧi'dãw] *f* (*inabilidade*) unsuitability; unfitness *tb* MIL; (*incompetência*) incompetence
inapto [i'naptu] *adj* unsuited; (*incapaz*) incapable; MIL unfit
inativo [ina'ʧivu] *adj* inactive; *funcionário* retired; *máquina*, *fábrica* disused
inaudito [inaw'dʒitu] *adj* unheard-of
inauguração [inawgura'sãw] *f* opening; (*consagração*) inauguration
inaugurar [inawgu'rar] ⟨1a⟩ open; (*consagrar*) inaugurate; *estátua* unveil
incalculável [ĩkawku'lavew] *adj* incalculable
incansável [ĩkã'savew] *adj* tireless
incapacidade [ĩkapasi'dadʒi] *f* incompetence, inability
incapaz [ĩka'pas] *adj* incapable, incompetent
incendiar [ĩsẽ'dʒiar] ⟨1g & 1h⟩ set fire to; *fig* inflame
incendiário [ĩsẽ'dʒiariu] **1** *m*, **-a** *f* arsonist **2** *adj* incendiary; *fig* inflammatory
incêndio [ĩ'sẽdiu] *m* fire; ***~ forestal*** forest fire
incentivar [ĩsẽʧi'var] ⟨1a⟩ stimulate, encourage
incentivo [ĩsẽ'ʧivu] *m* incentive
incerteza [ĩser'teza] *f* uncertainty
incerto [ĩ'sɛrtu] *adj* uncertain
incesto [ĩ'sestu] *m* incest
incestuoso [ĩses'twozu] *adj* incestuous
inchaço [ĩ'ʃasu] *m* swelling; (*afetação*) pomposity
inchado [ĩ'ʃadu] *adj* swollen; (*afetado*) pompous
inchar [ĩ'ʃar] ⟨1a⟩ **1** *v/t* swell **2** *v/i* swell; *velas* billow; **inchar-se** *v/r* swell (up) (***de, com*** with); *velas* billow
incidência [ĩsi'dẽsja] *f* incidence; ***~ sobre o meio ambiente*** environmental impact
incidente [ĩsi'dẽʧi] **1** *adj* incidental **2** *m* incident
incineração [ĩsinera'sãw] *f* incineration
incinerar [ĩsine'rar] ⟨1e⟩ incinerate
incisão [ĩsi'zãw] *f* incision
incisivo [ĩsi'zivu] **1** *adj* cutting; (*agudo*) sharp; *estilo* incisive **2** *m* incisor
incitar [ĩsi'tar] ⟨1a⟩ *v/t* incite; (*impelir*) drive on; (*instigar*) urge
incivilizado [ĩsivili'zadu] *adj* uncivilized
inclinação [ĩklina'sãw] *f* inclination; GEOG slope; (*afeto*) preference; ***ângulo*** *m* ***de ~*** angle of inclination
inclinado [ĩkli'nadu] *adj* sloping; ***plano*** *m* ***~*** inclined plane
inclinar [ĩkli'nar] ⟨1a⟩ **1** *v/t* incline, tilt; (*baixar*) lower; (*dirigir*) turn **2** *v/i* ***~ para*** incline to; **inclinar-se** *v/r* bend; *fig* incline (***para*** to)
incluído [ĩklu'idu] *adj* included
incluir [ĩklu'ir] ⟨3i⟩ include; (*juntar*) enclose
inclusive [ĩklu'zivɛ] **1** *adv* inclusive; ***de segunda a quinta-feira ~*** from Monday to Thursday inclusive **2** *prep* including
incluso [ĩŋ'kluzu] *adj* included; *carta*: enclosed
incoerência [ĩkwe'rẽsja] *f* incoherence; *entre versões etc* inconsistency
incoerente [ĩkwe'rẽʧi] *adj* incoherent; *versões etc* inconsistent

I

incógnita [ĩŋ'kɔgnita] *f* MAT unknown
incógnito [ĩŋ'kɔgnitu] **1** *adj* unknown **2** *m* (*anonimato*) incognito
incomodado [ĩkomo'dadu] *adj* indisposed, unwell; ***estar ~ com algo*** not cope with sth
incomodar [ĩkomo'dar] ⟨1e⟩ bother, trouble; **incomodar-se** *v/r* (*maçar-se*) put oneself out; (*esforçar-se*) take trouble
incômodo, *Port* **incómodo** [ĩŋ'komudu] **1** *adj* uncomfortable; (*desagradável*) unpleasant; (*maçador*) troublesome; (*embaraçoso*) inconvenient **2** *m* trouble; (*indisposição*) inconvenience; ***causar ~*** cause trouble
incomparável [ĩkõpa'ravew] *adj* incomparable
incompatibilidade [ĩkõpatʃibili'dadʒi] *f* incompatibility
incompatível [ĩkõpa'tʃivew] *adj* incompatible
incompetência [ĩkõpe'tẽsja] *f* incompetence
incompetente [ĩkõpe'tẽtʃi] *adj* incompetent; (*não autorizado*) unauthorized
incompleto [ĩkõ'plɛtu] *adj* incomplete
incompreensão [ĩkõpriẽ'sãw] *f* ⟨*sem pl*⟩ incomprehension
incompreensível [ĩkõpriẽ'sivew] *adj* incomprehensible
incomum [iŋko'mũ] *adj* uncommon
incomunicável [iŋkomuni'kavew] *adj* TEL cut off (***com*** from); DIR in solitary confinement
inconcebível [ĩkõse'bivew] *adj* inconceivable
incondicional [ĩkõdʒisjo'naw] *adj* unconditional; (*ilimitado*) unlimited; *lealdade* unquestioning
inconfundível [ĩkõfũ'dʒivew] *adj* unmistakable
incongruente [ĩkõgro'ẽtʃi] *adj* incongruous; MAT non-congruent
inconsciência [ĩkõs'sjẽsja] *f* unconsciousness; (*irresponsabilidade*) irresponsibility
inconsciente [ĩkõs'sjẽtʃi] *adj* unconscious; (*irresponsável*) irresponsible
inconseqüência, *Port* **inconsequência** [ĩkõse'kwẽsja] *f* inconsistency
inconseqüente, *Port* **inconsequente** [ĩkõse'kwẽtʃi] *adj* inconsistent
inconsolável [ĩkõso'lavew] *adj* inconsolable
inconstância [ĩkõs'tãsja] *f* changeability, fickleness
inconstante [ĩkõs'tãtʃi] *adj* changeable, fickle
inconstitucional [ĩkõstʃitusjo'naw] *adj* unconstitutional
incontestável [ĩkõtes'tavew] *adj* undeniable
inconveniência [ĩkõve'njẽsja] *f* impoliteness; (*incômodo*) inconvenience; (*desvantagem*) disadvantage; (*dificuldade*) difficulty
inconveniente [ĩkõve'njẽtʃi] **1** *m* (*desvantagem*) disadvantage; (*dificuldade*) difficulty **2** *adj* rude; (*impróprio*) improper; (*inoportuno*) annoying; (*inadequado*) inconvenient
incorporar [ĩkorpo'rar] ⟨1e⟩ incorporate (***em*** into); (*ligar*) join
incorreção, *Port* **incorrecção** [ĩkohɛ'sãw] *f* inaccuracy; (*indelicadeza*) impoliteness, rudeness
incorrecto [ĩko'hɛtu] *adj Port* incorrect; (*grosseiro*) impolite, rude
incorrer [ĩko'her] ⟨2d⟩ *v/i* ***~ em erro*** make a mistake; ***~ em risco*** incur a risk
incorreto [ĩko'hɛtu] *adj* incorrect; (*grosseiro*) impolite, rude
incorrigível [ĩkohi'ʒivew] *adj* incorrigible
incredulidade [ĩkreduli'dadʒi] *f* incredulity
incrédulo [ĩŋ'krɛdulu] *adj* incredulous
incrementar [ĩkremẽ'tar] ⟨1a⟩ develop; (*multiplicar*) increase; COM boost
incremento [ĩkre'mẽtu] *m* increase; COM growth
incriminação [ĩkrimina'sãw] *f* incrimination
incriminar [ĩkrimi'nar] ⟨1a⟩ incriminate; ***~ de, ~ por*** accuse of
incrível [ĩŋ'krivew] *adj* incredible
incubadora [ĩkuba'dora] *f* incubator
inculto [ĩŋ'kuwtu] *adj* AGR uncultivated; (*ignorante*) uneducated

incumbência [ĩkum'bẽsja] *f* task, duty
incumbir [ĩkum'bir] ⟨3a⟩ ***~ alguém de algo*** put s.o. in charge of sth; **incumbir-se** *v/r* ***~ de algo*** undertake sth, take charge of sth
incurável [ĩku'ravew] *adj* incurable
incúria [ĩŋ'kurja] *f* negligence, carelessness
incutir [ĩku'tʃir] ⟨3a⟩ instill, *Brit* instil; *dúvida* sow; (*inculcar*) inculcate
indagação [ĩdaga'sãw] *f* investigation; (*pesquisa*) inquiry
indagar [ĩda'gar] ⟨1o & 1b⟩ **1** *v/t* investigate; (*averiguar*) inquire **2** *v/i* **~** (***acerca de***) inquire into, make inquiries about
indecência [ĩde'sẽsja] *f* indecency
indecente [ĩde'sẽtʃi] *adj* indecent; (*indecoroso*) rude
indeciso [ĩde'sizu] *adj* indecisive; (*pendente*) undecided; (*vago*) uncertain
indeferir [ĩdefe'rir] ⟨3c⟩ turn down, reject
indefeso [ĩde'fezu] *adj* defenseless, *Brit* defenceless
indefinido [ĩdefi'nidu] *adj* indefinite, undefined
indefinível [ĩdefi'nivew] *adj* undefinable
indelével [ĩde'lɛvew] *adj* indelible
indelicadeza [ĩdelika'deza] *f* impoliteness
indelicado [ĩdeli'kadu] *adj* rude; (*sem gosto*) tasteless
indenização, *Port* **indemnização** [ĩdeniza'sãw] *f* compensation; COM indemnity; *trabalho*: severance pay
indenizar, *Port* **indemnizar** [ĩdeni'zar] ⟨1a⟩ ***~ alguém por algo*** compensate s.o. for sth
independência [ĩdepẽ'dẽsja] *f* independence
independente [ĩdepẽ'dẽtʃi] *adj* independent
indescritível [ĩdeskri'tʃivew] *adj* indescribable
indesejável [ĩdeze'ʒavew] *adj* undesirable
indeterminado [ĩdetermi'nadu] *adj* indeterminate; (*indeciso*) undecided
indevido [ĩde'vidu] *adj* mistaken; (*imerecido*) unjust; (*impróprio*) inappropriate
Índia ['ĩdʒia] *f* India
indiano [ĩ'dʒianu] **1** *adj* Indian **2** *m*, **-a** *f* Indian
indicação [ĩdʒika'sãw] *f* indication; (*referência*) reference; (*sinal*) sign; (*alusão*) hint; (*instrução*) instruction
indicador [ĩdʒika'dor] **1** *adj* ***placa f ~ a*** sign **2** *m* (*ponteiro*) pointer; *pressão, nível de água etc*: gage, *Brit* gauge; *dedo*: index finger
indicar [ĩdʒi'kar] ⟨1n⟩ indicate; (*declarar*) declare; (*recomendar*) recommend; ***~ algo a alguém*** point sth out to s.o.; ***pode ~ -me o caminho?*** can you show me the way?
indicativo [ĩdʒika'tʃivu] *m* TEL area code; GRAM indicative
índice ['ĩdʒisi] *m* index; (*registro*) register; ***~ de audiência*** ratings
indício [ĩ'dʒisiu] *m* sign; DIR clue
indiferença [ĩdʒife'rẽsa] *f* indifference
indiferente [ĩdʒife'rẽtʃi] *adj* indifferent
indígena [ĩ'dʒiʒena] **1** *adj* (*nativo*) native **2** *m/f* native
indigente [ĩdʒi'ʒẽtʃi] *adj* destitute, indigent
indigestão [ĩdʒiʒes'tãw] *f* indigestion
indigesto [ĩdʒi'ʒɛstu] *adj* indigestible
indignação [ĩdʒigna'sãw] *f* indignation
indignar-se [ĩdʒi'gnarsi] ⟨1a⟩ *v/r* get indignant (***com*** about)
indigno [ĩ'dʒignu] *adj* unworthy
índio ['ĩdiu] *m*, **-a** *f* Indian
indireta, *Port* **indirecta** [ĩdʒi'rɛta] *f* insinuation
indireto, *Port* **indirecto** [ĩdʒi'rɛtu] *adj* indirect; *comentário* oblique
indiscernível [ĩdʒisir'nivew] *adj* indiscernible
indiscreto [ĩdʒis'krɛtu] *adj* indiscreet
indiscrição [ĩdʒiskri'sãw] *f* indiscretion
indiscriminado [ĩdʒiskrimi'nadu] *adj* indiscriminate
indispensável [ĩdʒispẽ'savew] *adj* (*imprescindível*) essential, indispensable

I

indisposição [ĩdʒispozi'sãw] *f* illness
indisposto [ĩdʒis'postu] *adj* unwell, indisposed
indissolúvel [ĩdʒiso'luvew] *adj* insoluble; *casamento* indissoluble
indistinto [ĩdʒis'tʃĩtu] *adj* indistinct
individual [ĩdʒivi'dwaw] *adj* individual; ***lições*** *fpl* ***individuais*** private lessons; ESP ***provas*** *fpl* ***individuais*** individual events
individualidade [ĩdʒividwali'dadʒi] *f* individuality
individualista [ĩdʒividwa'lista] **1** *adj* individualistic **2** *m/f* individualist
indivíduo [ĩdʒi'vidwu] *m* individual
indivisível [ĩdʒivi'zivew] *adj* indivisible
indo ['ĩdu] → ***ir***
índole ['ĩduli] *f* nature; (*peculiaridade*) characteristic; ***ter boa ~*** be good-natured
indolência [ĩdo'lẽsja] *f* indolence, laziness
indolente [ĩdo'lẽtʃi] *adj* indolent, lazy
indomável [ĩdo'mavew] *adj* untameable; *adolescente* wild; *alma* indomitable
Indonésia [ĩdo'nɛzja] *f* Indonesia
indonésio [ĩdo'nɛziu] **1** *adj* Indonesian **2** *m*, **-a** *f* Indonesian **3** *m lingua* Indonesian
indulgência [ĩduw'ʒẽsja] *f* leniency, indulgence
indulgente [ĩduw'ʒẽtʃi] *adj* lenient, indulgent
indultar [ĩduw'taɾ] ⟨1a⟩ *v/t pessoa* reprieve; *erro* forgive
indulto [ĩ'duwtu] *m* remission (of sentence)
indústria [ĩ'dustɾia] *f* industry; ***~ agrícola*** agriculture; ***~ automobilística*** automobile industry; ***~ básica, ~ de base*** primary industry; ***~ da construção*** construction industry; ***~ do turismo*** tourist industry
indústria-chave [ĩ'dustɾiaʃavi] *f* ⟨*pl* indústrias-chave⟩ key industry
industrial [ĩdustɾi'aw] **1** *adj* industrial **2** *m/f* industrialist
industrializar [ĩdustɾiali'zaɾ] ⟨1a⟩ industrialize
induzir [ĩdu'ziɾ] ⟨3m⟩ *v/t* induce (***a*** to); ***~ em erro*** mislead
inédito [i'nɛdʒitu] **1** *adj* unpublished; *fig* unheard of, rare **2** *m* unpublished work
ineficaz [inefi'kas] *adj* ineffective
inegável [ine'gavew] *adj* undeniable
inércia [i'nɛɾsja] *f* inertia; ***estado*** *m* / ***força*** *f* ***de ~*** state / force of inertia
inerte [i'nɛɾtʃi] *adj* inert; (*ocioso*) idle; (*mole*) lethargic
inescrupuloso [ineskɾupu'lozu] *adj* unscrupulous
inesgotável [inesgo'tavew] *adj* inexhaustible
inesperado [inespe'ɾadu] *adj* unexpected
inesquecível [ineske'sivew] *adj* unforgettable
inestimável [inestʃi'mavew] *adj* invaluable
inevitável [inevi'tavew] *adj* inevitable
inexatidão, *Port* **inexactidão** [inezatʃi'dãw] *f* inaccuracy
inexato, *Port* **inexacto** [ine'zatu] *adj* inaccurate
inexistente [inezis'tẽtʃi] *adj* non-existent
inexperiência [inespe'ɾjẽsja] *f* inexperience
inexperiente [inespe'ɾjẽtʃi] *adj* inexperienced; (*ingênuo*) naive
inexplicável [inespli'kavew] *adj* inexplicable
infalibilidade [ĩfalibili'dadʒi] *f* infallibility
infalível [ĩfa'livew] *adj* infallible
infame [ĩ'fami] *adj* awful, nasty
infâmia [ĩ'fʌmja] *f* disgrace; (*vileza*) vicious behavior, *Brit* vicious behaviour
infância [ĩ'fãsja] *f* childhood; *primeiros anos* infancy *tb fig*
infantaria [ĩfãta'ɾia] *f* infantry
infantário [ĩfã'taɾiu] *m* nursery
infanticida [ĩfãtʃi'sida] *m/f* child-killer
infanticídio [ĩfãtʃi'sidiu] *m* infanticide
infantil [ĩfã'tʃiw] *adj* childlike; *pej* childish; MED children's *atr*
infatigável [ĩfatʃi'gavew] *adj* untiring
infeção, *Port* **infecção** [ĩfe'sãw] *f* infection
infecioso, *Port* **infeccioso** [ĩfe'sjozu]

adj infectious
infectar [ĩfek'taɾ] ⟨1a⟩ infect; *fig* contaminate
infelicidade [ĩfelisi'dadʒi] *f* unhappiness
infeliz [ĩfe'lis] *adj* unhappy
infelizmente [ĩfeliʒ'mẽtʃi] *adv* unfortunately
inferior [ĩfe'ɾjoɾ] **1** *adj* inferior; (*mais baixo*) lower; (*subordinado*) subordinate **2** *m/f* subordinate
inferioridade [ĩfeɾjoɾi'dadʒi] *f* inferiority; ***complexo*** *m* ***de ~*** inferiority complex
inferiorizar [ĩfeɾjoɾi'zaɾ] ⟨1a⟩ put down, belittle
infernal [ĩfeɾ'naw] *adj* infernal
inferno [ĩ'fɛɾnu] *m* hell; *fam* ***vá pro ~!*** go to hell!; *fam* ***que ~!*** bloody hell!
infértil [ĩ'fɛɾtʃiw] *adj* infertile
infidelidade [ĩfideli'dadʒi] *f* infidelity; (*traição*) betrayal; (*inexatidão*) inaccuracy
infiel [ĩ'fiɛw] **1** *adj* disloyal; *marido etc* unfaithful **2** *m/f* REL non-believer
infiltração [ĩfiltɾa'sãw] *f* infiltration
infiltrar [ĩfiw'tɾaɾ] ⟨1a⟩ *v/t* permeate; **infiltrar-se** *v/r* permeate, infiltrate (***em algo*** sth)
ínfimo ['ĩfimu] *adj* lowest, poorest
infinidade [ĩfini'dadʒi] *f* infinity; ***uma ~ de*** countless
infinitivo [ĩfini'tʃivu] *m* infinitive
infinito [ĩfi'nitu] *adj* infinite
inflação [ĩfla'sãw] *f* COM inflation; ***taxa*** *f* ***de ~*** rate of inflation
inflacionário [ĩflasjo'naɾiu] *adj* inflationary
inflamação [ĩflama'sãw] *f* MED inflammation
inflamar [ĩfla'maɾ] ⟨1a⟩ set fire to; *fig* inflame
inflamável [ĩfla'mavew] *adj* (in)flammable
inflexível [ĩfle'ksivew] *adj* rigid; *pessoa, atitude* inflexible
influência [ĩflu'ẽsja] *f* influence
influenciar [ĩfluẽ'sjaɾ] ⟨1g⟩ influence
influenciável [ĩfluẽ'sjavew] *adj* easily influenced
influente [ĩflu'ẽtʃi] *adj* influential
influir [ĩflu'iɾ] ⟨3i⟩ *v/t* influence, have an influence (***em*** on)
informação [ĩfoɾma'sãw] *f* piece of information; (*participação*) announcement; (*notícia*) (piece of) news *sg*; ***informações*** *pl* information; TEL information, *Brit* directory enquiries; ***informações*** *pl* ***de trânsito*** traffic information; ***guichê*** *m* ***de informações*** information desk; ***pedido*** *m* ***de ~*** inquiry; ***tirar / tomar / colher informações*** make inquiries
informal [ĩfoɾ'maw] *adj* informal
informalidade [ĩfoɾmali'dadʒi] *f* informality
informante [ĩfoɾ'mãtʃi] *m/f* informant
informar [ĩfoɾ'maɾ] ⟨1e⟩ *v/t* inform; **informar-se** *v/r* find out, inquire (***sobre*** about)
informática [ĩfoɾ'matʃika] *f* computer science; ***não sei nada de ~*** I don't know anything about computers
informático [ĩfoɾ'matʃiku] **1** *adj* computing *atr*, IT **2** *m*, **-a** *f* IT specialist
informativo [ĩfoɾma'tʃivu] *adj* informative
informatizar [ĩfoɾmatʃi'zaɾ] ⟨1a⟩ *v/t* computerize
informe [ĩ'fɔɾmi] *m* report
infração [ĩfɾa'sãw] *f* infringement; AUTO violation
infra-estrutura(s) [ĩfɾastɾu'tuɾa(s)] *f(pl)* infrastructure
infravermelho [ĩfɾaveɾ'meʎu] *m* infrared
infringir [ĩfɾĩ'ʒiɾ] ⟨3n⟩ infringe, contravene
infrutífero [ĩfɾu'tʃifeɾu] *adj* fruitless
infundado [ĩfũ'dadu] *adj*, **infundamentado** [ĩfũdamẽ'tadu] *adj* unfounded, groundless
infusão [ĩfu'zãw] *f* infusion
ingenuidade [ĩʒenwi'dadʒi] *f* ingenuousness, naivety
ingênuo, *Port* **ingénuo** [ĩ'ʒenwu] **1** *adj* naive, ingenuous; (*natural*) childlike **2** *m*, **-a** *f* naive person
ingerir [ĩʒe'ɾiɾ] ⟨3c⟩ *v/t* ingest
Inglaterra [ĩgla'tɛha] *f* England
inglês [ĩ'gles] **1** *adj* English **2** *m* Englishman **3** *m língua* English
inglesa [ĩ'gleza] *f* Englishwoman

ingratidão [ĩgɾaʧi'dãw] *f* ingratitude
ingrato [ĩ'gɾatu] *adj* ungrateful; (*desagradável*) unpleasant
ingrediente [ĩgɾe'djẽʧi] *m* ingredient
íngreme ['ĩgɾemi] *adj* steep
ingresso [ĩ'gɾɛsu] *m* entry; *Bras* ticket
inibição [inibi'sãw] *f* inhibition
inibido [ini'bidu] *adj* inhibited
iniciação [inisja'sãw] *f* initiation; (*introdução*) introduction
iniciador [inisja'doɾ] *m*, **-a** *f* initiator
inicial [ini'sjaw] **1** *adj* initial **2** *f* initial
inicializar [inisjali'zaɾ] ⟨1a⟩ boot up; **incializar-se** *v/r* boot up
inicialmente [inisjaw'mẽʧi] *adv* initially
iniciar [ini'sjaɾ] ⟨1g⟩ begin, start; (*preparar*) initiate; **~ *em*** initiate into
iniciativa [inisja'ʧiva] *f* initiative; ***espírito*** *m* ***de* ~** initiative; ***ter* ~** have initiative; ***tomar a* ~** take the initiative
início [i'nisiu] *m* beginning, start; ***ter* ~** begin; ***dar* ~** open
inimigo [ini'migu] **1** *adj* enemy *atr* **2** *m*, **-a** *f* enemy
injeção, *Port* **injecção** [ĩʒe'sãw] *f* injection
injetar, *Port* **injectar** [ĩʒe'taɾ] ⟨1a⟩ inject
injúria [ĩ'ʒuɾja] *f* insult; ***fazer uma* ~ *a alguém*** insult s.o.
injuriar [ĩʒu'ɾjaɾ] ⟨1g⟩ insult
injurioso [ĩʒu'ɾjozu] *adj* insulting
injustiça [ĩʒus'ʧisa] *f* injustice
injustificado [ĩʒusʧifi'kadu] *adj* unjustified
injusto [ĩ'ʒustu] *adj* unjust; (*ilícito*) unauthorized
inocência [ino'sẽsja] *f* innocence
inocente [ino'sẽʧi] **1** *adj* innocent **2** *m/f* innocent person
inofensivo [inofẽ'sivu] *adj* harmless, inoffensive
inolvidável [inowvi'davew] *adj* unforgettable
inoportuno [inopoɾ'tunu] *adj* inconvenient
inovação [inova'sãw] *f* innovation
inovador [inova'doɾ] **1** *adj* innovative **2** *m*, **-a** *f* innovator
inovar [ino'vaɾ] ⟨1e⟩ *v/t* & *v/i* innovate
inoxidável [inoksi'davew] *adj* **aço** stainless
inquérito [ĩ'kɛɾitu] *m* inquiry; (*sondagem*) survey
inquietação [ĩkieta'sãw] *f* restlessness, uneasiness
inquietante [ĩkie'tãʧi] *adj* worrying, disturbing
inquietar [ĩkie'taɾ] ⟨1a⟩ worry, disturb
inquieto [ĩ'kiɛtu] *adj* anxious, restless
inquilino [ĩki'linu] *m*, **-a** *f* tenant
inquinação [ĩkina'sãw] *f* contamination
inquinar [ĩki'naɾ] ⟨1a⟩ contaminate; MED infect
inquirir [ĩki'ɾiɾ] ⟨3a⟩ (*pesquisar*) inquire; (*averiguar*) investigate
Inquisição [ĩkizi'sãw] *f* Inquisition
insatisfeito [ĩsaʧis'fejtu] *adj* dissatisfied, unhappy
inscrever [ĩskɾe'veɾ] ⟨2c; *pp* inscrito⟩ enroll, *Brit* enrol, register; (*escrever*) write (***em*** in *ou* on); (*gravar*) inscribe
inscrição [ĩskɾi'sãw] *f* inscription; *ato* entry; UNIV registration, enrollment, *Brit* enrolment
insect… *Port* → ***inset…***
insegurança [ĩsegu'ɾãsa] *f* insecurity
inseguro [ĩse'guɾu] *adj* insecure
inseminação [ĩsemina'sãw] *f* insemination; **~ *artificial*** artificial insemination
insensatez [ĩsẽsa'tes] *f* madness; (*disparate*) nonsense
insensato [ĩsẽ'satu] *adj* stupid; (*disparatado*) foolish; (*absurdo*) meaningless
insensibilidade [ĩsẽsibili'dadʒi] *f* insensitivity; (*frieza*) coldness
insensível [ĩsẽ'sivew] insensitive; (*indiferente*) indifferent; (*impercetível*) imperceptible
inseticida [ĩseʧi'sida] *m* insecticide
insetívoro [ĩse'ʧivuɾu] **1** *m* ZOOL insectivore **2** *adj* insect-eating, insectivorous
inseto [ĩ'sɛtu] *m* insect
insignificância [ĩsignifi'kãsja] *f* insignificance
insignificante [ĩsignifi'kãʧi] *adj* insig-

nificant
insinuação [ĩsinwa'sãw] *f* insinuation; (*dica*) hint
insinuante [ĩsi'nwãʧi] *adj* ingratiating
insinuar [ĩsi'nwar] ⟨1g⟩ hint, *pej* insinuate
insípido [ĩ'sipidu] *adj comida* insipid; *pessoa tb* dull
insistência [ĩsis'tẽsja] *f* insistence; (*persistência*) persistence
insistente [ĩsis'tẽʧi] *adj* insistent; (*que não desiste*) persistent; (*enérgico*) emphatic
insistir [ĩsis'ʧir] ⟨3a⟩ insist; **~ em** insist on; (*não desistir*) persist in; (*falar incessantemente sobre*) go on about
insociável [ĩso'sjavew] *adj* unsociable
insolação [ĩsola'sãw] *f* sunstroke
insolência [ĩso'lẽsja] *f* insolence
insolente [ĩso'lẽʧi] *adj* insolent
insólito [ĩ'sɔlitu] *adj* unusual
insolúvel [ĩso'luvew] *adj* insoluble
insolvência [ĩsow'vẽsja] *f* insolvency
insolvente [ĩsow'vẽʧi] *adj* insolvent
insônia, *Port* **insónia** [ĩ'sonja] *f* insomnia
insonorização [ĩsonoriza'sãw] *f* soundproofing
inspeção, *Port* **inspecção** [ĩspe'sãw] *f* inspection; *médica etc*: examination; (*verificação*) check
inspecionar, *Port* **inspeccionar** [ĩspesjo'nar] ⟨1f⟩ inspect; (*averiguar*) examine; (*verificar*) check
inspetor, *Port* **inspector** [ĩspe'tor] *m*, **-a** *f* inspector
inspiração [ĩspira'sãw] *f* inspiration; MED inhalation
inspirar [ĩspi'rar] ⟨1a⟩ inspire; MED inhale
instabilidade [ĩstabili'dadʒi] *f* instability
instalação [ĩstala'sãw] *f* installation; *elétrica*: wiring; *mecânica*: plant; **~ piloto** pilot plant; **instalações** *pl* **sanitárias** sanitary installations
instalado [ĩsta'ladu] *adj* **estar ~** have settled in
instalador [ĩstala'dor] *m*, **-a** *f* fitter
instalar [ĩsta'lar] ⟨1b⟩ *v/t* install; (*encastrar*) fit; **instalar-se** *v/r* settle in
instância [ĩs'tãsja] *f* DIR court; **com ~** urgently; *fig* **em última ~** as a last resort
instantâneo [ĩstã'tʌniu] *adj* instantaneous; (*passageiro*) momentary; **bebida** *f* **instantânea** instant drink; **bolo ~** cake made from a cake mix
instante [ĩs'tãʧi] **1** *adj* urgent; (*insistente*) insistent **2** *m* instant
instável [ĩs'tavew] *adj* unstable; METEO unsettled
instigar [ĩsʧi'gar] ⟨1o⟩ *v/t pessoa* provoke; *ato* incite; (*acirrar*) urge
instintivo [ĩsʧĩ'ʧivu] *adj* instinctive
instinto [ĩs'ʧĩtu] *m* instinct
instituição [ĩsʧitwi'sãw] *f* institution; (*colocação*) appointment; **~ de caridade** charity, charitable organization
instituto [ĩsʧi'tutu] *m* institute; **~ de beleza** beauty salon; **Instituto Industrial** (**Comercial**) commerical college; **Instituto Superior Técnico** technical college
instrução [ĩstru'sãw] *f* learning; (*diretiva*) instruction; (*regulamento*) regulation; *escolar*: education; **instruções** *pl* instructions
instruído [ĩstru'idu] *adj* educated
instruir [ĩstru'ir] ⟨3i⟩ teach; (*ordenar*) instruct; (*formar*) train
instrumentista [ĩstrumen'ʧista] *m f* instrumentalist
instrumento [ĩstru'mẽtu] *m* instrument *tb fig*; (*documento*) deed, document; **~ de corda** stringed instrument; **~ de sopro** wind instrument; **~s de sopro de madeira** woodwind
instrutivo [ĩstru'ʧivu] *adj* instructive
instrutor [ĩstru'tor] **1** *adj* **juiz**(**a**) *m*(*f*) **~** (**a**) examining magistrate **2** *m*, **-a** *f* instructor; **~ de autoescola** driving instructor
insuficiência [ĩsufi'sjẽsja] *f* insufficiency; (*carência*) lack; **~ cardíaca** heart failure
insuficiente [ĩsufi'sjẽʧi] *adj* insufficient
insuflar [ĩsu'flar] ⟨1a⟩ inflate, blow up; *ar* blow; (*injetar*) inject; *fig* instill, *Brit* instil; (*influenciar*) influence
insuflável [ĩsu'flavew] *adj* inflatable

insulina [ĩsu'lina] *f* insulin
insultar [ĩsuw'taɾ] ⟨1a⟩ insult
insulto [ĩ'suwtu] *m* insult
insuperável [ĩsupe'ravew] *adj* insuperable
insuportável [ĩsupoɾ'tavew] *adj* unbearable
insurgir-se [ĩsuɾ'ʒiɾsi] ⟨3n⟩ *v/r* revolt, rebel
insurreição [ĩsuhej'sãw] *f* insurrection
intacto [ĩ'taktu] *adj* intact; (*ileso*) unharmed
íntegra ['ĩtegɾa] *f* ***na ~*** in full
integração [ĩteɾa'sãw] *f* integration
integral [ĩte'gɾaw] **1** *adj* whole; MAT integral; ***pão*** *m* **~** wholewheat bread, *Brit* wholemeal bread **2** *f* MAT integral
integrar [ĩte'gɾaɾ] ⟨1c⟩ integrate; (*formar*) form, make up
íntegro ['ĩtegɾu] *adj* entire; (*ileso*) unharmed; ***um homem ~*** a man of integrity
inteirar [ĩtej'ɾaɾ] ⟨1a⟩ *v/t* (*completar*) complete; (*informar*) inform (***de*** of)
inteiro [ĩ'tejɾu] *adj* whole, complete; (*ileso*) unharmed; ***a tempo ~*** full-time
intelecto [ĩte'lɛktu] *m* intellect
intelectual [ĩtelek'twaw] **1** *adj* intellectual **2** *m/f* intellectual
inteligência [ĩteli'ʒẽsja] *f* intelligence; (*entendimento*) understanding; ***~ artificial*** artificial intelligence
inteligente [ĩteli'ʒẽtʃi] *adj* intelligent
inteligível [ĩteli'ʒivew] *adj* intelligible
intenção [ĩtẽ'sãw] *f* intention; ***segundas intenções*** *pl* ulterior motives; ***ter boas intenções*** have good intentions
intencional [ĩtẽsjo'naw] *adj* intentional, deliberate
intensidade [ĩtẽsi'dadʒi] *f* intensity
intensificar [ĩtẽsifi'kaɾ] ⟨1n⟩ intensify; **intensificar-se** *v/r* intensify
intensivo [ĩtẽ'sivu] *adj* intensive; *ruído* piercing; *sabor* strong; ***curso*** *m* **~** intensive course
intenso [ĩ'tẽsu] *adj* intense
intento [ĩ'tẽtu] *m* intention; ***de ~*** intentionally, on purpose; ***no ~ de fazer*** with the intention of doing
interativo, *Port* **interactivo** [ĩteɾa'tʃivu] *adj* interactive
intercalar [ĩteɾka'laɾ] ⟨1b⟩ *v/t* insert
intercâmbio [ĩteɾ'kãbiu] *m* exchange
interceder [ĩteɾse'deɾ] ⟨2c⟩ *v/i* intervene, intercede (***por*** on behalf of)
interceptar [ĩteɾsep'taɾ] ⟨1a⟩ intercept; *notícia* pick up; TEL listen in on; *trem* stop
inter-cidades [ĩteɾsi'dadʒis] *m* FERROV intercity
intercultural [ĩteɾkuwtu'ɾaw] *adj* intercultural
interdependência [ĩteɾdepẽ'dẽsja] *f* interdependence
interdependente [ĩteɾdepẽ'dẽtʃi] *adj* interdependent
interdição [ĩteɾdʒi'sãw] *f* ban; DIR *pessoa*: injunction
interditar [ĩteɾdʒi'taɾ] ⟨1a⟩ *v/t* ban; *acesso etc* close off; DIR *pessoa* interdict
interessado [ĩteɾe'sadu] **1** *adj* interested; (*egoísta*) self-seeking **2** *m*, **-a** *f* interested party
interessante [ĩteɾe'sãtʃi] *adj* interesting
interessar [ĩteɾe'saɾ] ⟨1c⟩ interest; ***~ a alguém por*** interest s.o. in; (***isso***) ***não interessa*** that's of no interest; **interessar-se** *v/r* ***~ por*** take an interest in, be interested in
interesse [ĩte'ɾesi] *m* interest (***em*** in)
interesseiro [ĩteɾe'sejɾu] *adj* self-seeking
interface [ĩteɾ'fasi] *f* INFORM interface; ***~ de utilizador*** user interface
interferência [ĩteɾfe'ɾẽsja] *f* interference
interferir [ĩteɾfe'ɾiɾ] ⟨3c⟩ ***~ em*** interfere in
interfone [ĩteɾ'fɔni] *m Bras* intercom
interino [ĩte'ɾinu] *adj* interim *atr*
interior [ĩte'ɾjoɾ] **1** *adj* inner, inside; *mercado, comércio* domestic **2** *m* inside, interior; *do país* interior; ***Ministério do Interior*** Department of the Interior
interlocutor [ĩteɾloku'toɾ] *m*, **-a** *f* ***meu ~*** the person I was speaking to
intermediário [ĩteɾme'dʒiaɾiu] **1** *adj*

intermediary **2** *m*, **-a** *f* (*mediador*) mediator; COM middleman
interminável [ĩtermi'navew] *adj* endless, interminable
intermitente [ĩtermi'tẽtʃi] *adj* intermittent
internacional [ĩternasjo'naw] *adj* international
internacionalmente [ĩternasjonaw'mẽtʃi] *adv* internationally
internamento [ĩterna'mẽtu] *m hospital*: admission
internar [ĩter'nar] ⟨1c⟩ *v/t* MIL intern; *hospital*: admit; *internato*: put into boarding school; **internar-se** *v/r* penetrate; *fig* become engrossed (***em*** in)
internato [ĩter'natu] *m* boarding school
internauta [ĩter'nawta] *m/f* (Internet) surfer
Internet [ĩter'nɛt] *f* Internet; (***navegar***) ***na ~*** (surf) the Internet
interno [ĩ'tɛrnu] *adj* internal; (*nacional*) domestic, internal
interpor [ĩter'por] ⟨2z⟩ put in (***entre*** between); *influência etc* assert; DIR *recurso* lodge; **interpor-se** *v/r* intervene
interpretação [ĩterpreta'sãw] *f* interpretation; TEAT performance
interpretar [ĩterpre'tar] ⟨1c⟩ interpret; *canção, dança* perform; ***quem interpreta o papel?*** who is playing the part?
intérprete [ĩ'tɛrpretʃi] *m/f* MÚS *etc* performer, artist; (*tradutor*) interpreter
interrogação [ĩtehoga'sãw] *f* interrogation; (*pergunta*) question; *testemunhas*: examination; ***ponto*** *m* ***de ~*** question mark
interrogar [ĩteho'gar] ⟨1o & 1e⟩ interrogate; *aluno* question; DIR cross-examine
interrogatório [ĩtehoga'tɔriu] *m* questioning; DIR cross-examination
interromper [ĩtehõ'per] ⟨2a⟩ interrupt; ELÉT break
interrupção [ĩtehu'psãw] *f* interruption; ELÉT breaking
interruptor [ĩtehup'tor] *m* ELÉT switch
interurbano [ĩterur'banu] *adj* long-distance; ***chamada*** *f* ***interurbana*** long-distance call
intervalo [ĩter'valu] *m* interval; ESP half time; ***~ de almoço*** lunch break; ***~ comercial*** commercial break
intervenção [ĩtervẽ'sãw] *f* intervention; MED operation
intervir [ĩteir'vir] ⟨3wa⟩ intervene; *litígio*: mediate
intestino [ĩtes'tʃinu] *m* intestine; ***~ delgado*** small intestine; ***~ grosso*** large intestine
intimação [ĩtʃima'sãw] *f* (*anúncio*) announcement; (*convite*) invitation; DIR summons *sg*; ***~ (judicial) de pagamento*** order to pay
intimar [ĩtʃi'mar] ⟨1a⟩ ask, invite; DIR summon; *sessão* convene
intimidação [ĩtʃimida'sãw] *f* intimidation; (*advertência*) deterrent
intimidade [ĩtʃimi'dadʒi] *f* (*privacidade*) private life; (*amizade*) intimacy; (*confiança*) confidence
intimidar [ĩtʃimi'dar] ⟨1a⟩ *v/t* intimidate
íntimo ['ĩtʃimu] **1** *adj* intimate; *amigo* close **2** *m*, **-a** *f amigo* close friend
intolerância [ĩtole'rãsja] *f* intolerance
intolerante [ĩtole'rãtʃi] *adj* intolerant
intolerável [ĩtole'ravew] *adj* unbearable, intolerable
intoxicação [ĩtoksika'sãw] *f* poisoning; ***~ alimentar*** food poisoning
intoxicado [ĩtoksi'kadu] *adj* (*bêbado*) intoxicated
intoxicar [ĩtoksi'kar] ⟨1n⟩ *v/t* poison
intraduzível [ĩtradu'zivew] *adj* untranslatable
intransitável [ĩtrãzi'tavew] *adj* impassable; *estrada* closed off
intransitivo [ĩtrãzi'tʃivu] *adj* GRAM intransitive
intransmissível [ĩtrãzmi'sivew] *adj* non-transferable
intratável [ĩtra'tavew] *adj pessoa* awkward, difficult to deal with; *doença* untreatable
intra-uterino [ĩtraute'rinu] *adj* MED intra-uterine
intravenoso [ĩtrave'nozu] *adj* intravenous

intriga [ĩ'triga] *f* intrigue
intrigar [ĩtri'gar] ⟨1o⟩ **1** *v/t* intrigue **2** *v/i* be intriguing
intriguista [ĩtri'gista] *m/f* schemer
introdução [ĩtrodu'sãw] *f* introduction (***a*** to); INFORM input
introduzir [ĩtrodu'zir] ⟨3m⟩ *v/t* introduce; *dados* input; **~ *algo numa conversa*** bring sth up in a conversation
intrometer [ĩtrome'ter] ⟨2c⟩ insert, put in between; **intrometer-se** *v/r* interfere
intromissão [ĩtromi'sãw] *f* interference; (*incômodo*) annoyance
intrujão [ĩtru'ʒãw] *m pop* swindler
intrujar [ĩtru'ʒar] ⟨1a⟩ *pop* swindle, rip off
intrujice [ĩtru'ʒisi] *f pop* swindle, ripoff
intruso [ĩ'truzu] *m* intruder
intuição [ĩtwi'sãw] *f* intuition
intuitivo [ĩtwi'tʃivu] *adj* intuitive
intuito [ĩ'tuitu] *m* aim, intention
inumerável [inume'ravew], **inúmero** [i'numeru] *adj* innumerable, countless
inundação [inũda'sãw] *f* flood
inundar [inũ'dar] ⟨1a⟩ flood; *fig* inundate
inusitado [inuzi'tadu] *adj* unusual
inútil [i'nutʃiw] *adj* useless; (*sem valor*) worthless
inutilidade [inutʃili'dadʒi] *f* uselessness
inutilizado [inutʃili'zadu] *adj* ***estar*** (*ou* ***ficar***) **~** be no more use, *fam* have had it
inutilizar [inutʃili'zar] ⟨1a⟩ make useless, ruin; (*desvalorizar*) devalue
invadir [ĩva'dʒir] ⟨3b⟩ invade; *luz* flood; *fig* overcome
inválido [ĩ'validu] **1** *adj* (*deficiente*) disabled; *bilhete* invalid; MED invalid **2** *m*, **-a** *f* invalid
invariável [ĩva'rjavew] *adj* invariable
invasão [ĩva'zãw] *f* invasion; *fig* onslaught
invasor [ĩva'zor] *m* invader
inveja [ĩ'vɛʒa] *f* envy
invejar [ĩve'ʒar] ⟨1c⟩ *v/t* envy
invejável [ĩve'ʒavew] *adj* enviable
invejoso [ĩve'ʒozu] **1** *adj* envious **2** *m*, **-a** *f* envious person
invenção [ĩvẽ'sãw] *f* invention
invencível [ĩvẽ'sivew] *adj* invincible; *obstáculo* insurmountable
inventar [ĩvẽ'tar] ⟨1a⟩ *v/t* invent; *história* make up
inventário [ĩvẽ'tariu] *m* inventory
inventor [ĩvẽ'tor] *m*, **-a** *f* inventor
inverno [ĩ'vɛrnu] *m* winter
inverossímil, *Port* **inverosímil** [ĩvero'zimiw] *adj* implausible, unlikely
inversão [ĩver'sãw] *f* reversal, inversion; **~ *de marcha*** reverse (gear)
inversível [ĩver'sivew] *adj* reversible
inverso [ĩ'vɛrsu] **1** *adj* inverse; (*contrário*) contrary; (*oposto*) opposite; ***na razão inversa de*** in inverse proportion to **2** *m* opposite
inversor [ĩver'sor] *m* ELÉT switch
invertebrado [ĩverte'bradu] **1** *adj* invertebrate **2** *m* invertebrate
inverter [ĩver'ter] ⟨2c⟩ invert, reverse; (*alterar*) alter
invés [ĩ'vɛs] *m* ***ao* ~ *de*** instead of
investigação [ĩvestʃiga'sãw] *f* research; (*inquérito*) inquiry; *polícia*: investigation
investida [ĩves'tʃida] *f* approach; ESP tackle
investigador [ĩvestʃiga'dor] **1** *adj* investigating *atr* **2** *m*, **-a** *f cientista* researcher; *polícia*: investigator
investigar [ĩvestʃi'gar] ⟨1o⟩ research; (*averiguar*) inquire, check; *polícia* investigate
investimento [ĩvestʃi'mẽtu] *m* investment
investir [ĩves'tʃir] ⟨3c⟩ **1** *v/t* invest **2** *v/i* **~ *com*** attack
invicto [ĩ'viktu] *adj* unbeaten
inviolável [ĩvjo'lavew] *adj* inviolable, sacrosanct
invisível [ĩvi'zivew] *adj* invisible
invocar [ĩvo'kar] ⟨1n & 1e⟩ invoke; (*rogar*) plead, beseech
invólucro [ĩ'vɔlukru] *m* covering, wrapping
involuntário [ĩvolũ'tariu] *adj* involuntary
invulgar [ĩvuw'gar] *adj* unusual
invulnerável [ĩvuwne'ravew] *adj for-*

taleza impregnable; *pessoa* invulnerable
iodo ['jodu] *m* iodine
ioga ['jɔga] *m* yoga
iogurte [jo'gurʧi] *m* yog(h)urt
ir [iɾ] ⟨3x⟩ *v/i* ◊ go; **~ buscar** *pessoa, coisa* fetch; **~ a pé** go on foot, walk; ***já vou!*** I'm coming!; ***vamos!*** let's go!
◊ ***como vai?*** how are you?, how's it going?; ***vou bem*** I'm well; ***vou indo*** I'm OK, not bad
◊ *futuro* ***eu vou fazer o jantar*** I'm going to make dinner; **ir-se** *v/r* **~ *embora*** go away, leave; **~ *abaixo*** *motor* flood
ira ['iɾa] *f* anger, rage
irá [i'ɾa] → ***ir***
Irã [i'ɾã] *m Bras* ***o ~*** Iran
iraniano [iɾa'njanu] **1** *adj* Iranian **2** *m*, **-a** *f* Iranian
Irão [i'ɾãw] *m Port* ***o ~*** Iran
Iraque [i'ɾaki] *m* ***o ~*** Iraq
iraquiano [iɾa'kjanu] **1** *adj* Iraqi **2** *m*, **-a** *f* Iraqi
irás [i'ɾas] → ***ir***
irascível [iɾas'sivew] *adj* irritable, irascible
irei [i'ɾej], **iria** [i'ɾia] *etc* → ***ir***
íris ['iɾis] *f* ⟨*pl inv*⟩ BOT, ANAT iris
Irlanda [iɾ'lãda] *f* ***a ~*** Ireland
irlandês [iɾlã'des] **1** *adj* Irish **2** *m*, **-esa** *f* Irishman; Irishwoman
irmã [iɾ'mã] *f* sister
irmão [iɾ'mãw] ⟨*mpl* -ãos⟩ **1** *m* brother; ***são todos ~s*** they are all brothers and sisters **2** *adj* brotherly
ironia [iɾo'nia] *f* irony
irônico, *Port* **irónico** [i'ɾoniku] *adj* ironic
irracional [ihasjo'naw] *adj* irrational
irradiação [ihadʒia'sãw] *f* radiation; (*propagação*) spreading
irradiador [ihadʒia'doɾ] *m* (*aquecimento*) radiator
irradiar [iha'dʒiaɾ] ⟨1g⟩ **1** *v/t* radiate; (*propagar*) spread **2** *v/i* radiate, spread
irreal [i'heaw] *adj* unreal
irrealizável [iheali'zavew] *adj* unrealizable
irreconciliável [ihekõsi'ljavew] *adj* irreconcilable
irreconhecível [ihekoɲe'sivew] *adj* unrecognizable
irrecuperável [ihekupe'ɾavew] *adj* irretrievable
irrefletido, *Port* **irreflectido** [iheflе'ʧidu] *adj* rash
irregular [ihegu'laɾ] *adj* irregular; (*desregrado*) erratic
irregularidade [ihegulaɾi'dadʒi] *f* irregularity
irremediável [iheme'dʒiavew] *adj* irremediable; (*incurável*) incurable
irrequieto [ihe'kiɛtu] *adj* restless
irresistível [ihezis'ʧivew] *adj* irresistible
irresoluto [ihezo'lutu] *adj* irresolute, indecisive
irresponsável [ihespõ'savew] *adj* irresponsible
irrevogável [ihevo'gavew] *adj* irrevocable
irrigação [ihiga'sãw] *f* irrigation
irrigar [ihi'gaɾ] ⟨1o⟩ irrigate; *grama* water
irritação [ihita'sãw] *f* irritation
irritante [ihi'tãʧi] **1** *adj* irritating **2** *m* irritant
irritar [ihi'taɾ] ⟨1a⟩ irritate
irritável [ihi'tavew] *adj* irritable
irrupção [ihu'psãw] *f* (sudden) emergence; (*invasão*) invasion; (*transbordo*) overflow
isca ['iska] *f* bait *tb fig*; (*bocado*) bite, morsel; GASTR **~s** *pl fried liver in a garlic and wine sauce*
isenção [izẽ'sãw] *f* exemption (**de** from)
isento [i'zẽtu] *adj* exempt, free; **~ *de impostos*** tax-free
Islã [iz'lã] *m* Islam
islâmico [iz'lʌmiku] *adj* Islamic
islamismo [izla'mizmu] *m* Islam
islandês [izlã'des] **1** *adj* Icelandic **2** *m*, **-esa** *f* Icelander **3** *m lingua* Icelandic
Islândia [iz'lãdʒia] *f* ***a ~*** Iceland
Islão [iz'lãw] *m Port* Islam
isolação [izola'sãw] *f* → ***isolamento***
isoladamente [izolada'mẽʧi] *adv* in isolation
isolado *adj* insulated; (*fechado*) iso-

lated; **~ pela neve** cut off by the snow

isolador [izola'doɾ] **1** *adj* insulating **2** *m* ELÉT insulator

isolamento [izola'mẽtu] *m* insulation; MED *etc* isolation; **~ térmico** (heat) insulation

isolante [izo'lãtʃi] *adj* insulating; ***material*** *m* **~** insulating material, insulation

isolar [izo'laɾ] ⟨1e⟩ insulate; (*fechar*) isolate; (*separar*) separate

isqueiro [is'kejɾu] *m* (cigarette) lighter

Israel [izha'ew] *m* Israel

israelense [izhae'lẽsi] **1** *adj* Israeli **2** *m/f* Israeli

isso ['isu] *pron* that; ***~!*** that's it!; ***é ~!***, (***é***) ***~ mesmo!*** that's right!, you've got it!; ***por ~*** therefore, so

isto ['istu] *pron* this; ***~ é*** that is, namely

Itália [i'talia] *f* ***a ~*** Italy

italiano [ita'ljanu] **1** *adj* Italian **2** *m*, **-a** *f* Italian **3** *m lingua* Italian

itálico [i'taliku] **1** *adj* italic; ***letra*** *f* ***itálica*** italics **2** *m* italics; ***em ~*** in italics

itinerário [itʃine'ɾaɾiu] *m* itinerary

IVA ['iva] *m Port abr* (***Imposto sobre o Valor Acrescentado***) sales tax, *Brit* VAT (value added tax)

J

J

já [ʒa] *adv* already; (*imediatamente*) right now, right away; (*agora*) now; *perguntas*: yet; ***~, ~!*** pronto!; ***~ chegou o trem?*** is the train in yet?; ***~ chega, acalme-se!*** that's enough now, calm down!; ***eu ~ estava quase saindo quando …*** I was just about to leave when …; *Port* ***até ~*** see you; ***~ está?*** alright?, are you done?; ***~ que*** since, seeing that

jaca ['ʒaka] *f* jackfruit

jacarandá [ʒakaɾã'da] *f* jacaranda

jacaré [ʒaka'ɾɛ] *m* caiman

jacinto [ʒa'sĩtu] *m* BOT hyacinth

jactância [ʒak'tãsja] *f* boasting; (*arrogância*) haughtiness

jacto *Port* → ***jato***

jade ['ʒadʒi] *m* jade

jaguar [ʒa'gwaɾ] *m* jaguar

jamais [ʒa'majs] *adv* never; (*nunca mais*) never again

janeiro [ʒa'nejɾu] *m* January; ***em ~*** in January

janela [ʒa'nɛla] *f* window; ***à ~*** by the window; *direção*: to the window; ***da ~ abaixo*** out of the window; ***~ e sacada*** bay window

jangada [ʒã'gada] *f* raft

janota [ʒa'nɔta] **1** *adj* chic, elegant **2** *m/f* fashionista

jantar [ʒã'taɾ] **1** ⟨1a⟩ *v/t* have for dinner **2** *m* dinner

jante ['ʒãtʃi] *f* AUTO (wheel) rim

Japão [ʒa'pãw] *m* ***o ~*** Japan

japonês [ʒapo'nes] **1** *adj* Japanese **2** *m*, **-esa** *f* Japanese **3** *m lingua* Japanese

jaqueta [ʒa'keta] *f* jacket

jardim [ʒaɾ'dĩ] *m* garden; ***~ de infância, ~ infantil*** kindergarten; ***~ de inverno*** winter garden; ***~ zoológico*** zoo

jardinagem [ʒaɾdʒi'naʒẽ] *f* gardening

jardineira [ʒaɾdʒi'nejɾa] *f* window box

jardineiro [ʒaɾdʒi'nejɾu] *m*, **-a** *f* gardener

jargão [ʒaɾ'gãw] *m* jargon

jarra ['ʒaha] *f* vase; ***~ de leite*** milk pitcher, *Brit* milk jug

jarro ['ʒahu] *m* pitcher, *Brit* jug

jasmim [ʒaz'mĩ] *m* BOT jasmine

jato ['ʒatu] *m* (*lance*) throw; (*golpe*) blow; (*jorro*) jet; ***de um ~*** suddenly; ***avião*** *m* ***a ~*** jet plane; ***~ de água / ar*** jet of water / air

jaula ['ʒawla] *f* cage
javali [ʒava'li] *m* ZOOL wild boar
javanês [ʒava'nes] **1** *adj* Javanese **2** *m*, **javanesa** [ʒava'neza] *f* Javanese
jazer [ʒa'zer] ⟨2b, 3rd pess sg ***jaz***⟩ *v/i* lie
jazigo [ʒa'zigu] *m* tomb; MIN deposit
jazz [ʒɛz] *m* jazz
jeans ['ʒĩs] *m* jeans *pl*
jeito ['ʒejtu] *m* (*propensão*) talent; (*habilidade*) skill, knack; (*modo*) manner; (*aparência*) appearance; *fam* ***dar um ~*** fix, sort out; ***ter ~ para*** have a knack for; ***a ~*** handy; ***com ~*** carefully; ***não tem ~*** it's a hopeless case; ***de ~ nenhum!*** no way!
jeitoso [ʒej'tozu] *adj* (*hábil*) skillful, *Brit* skilful; (*bem feito*) well made; (*formoso*) handsome
jejum [ʒe'ʒũ] *m* fast; ***dia*** *m* ***de ~*** day of fasting; ***em ~*** fasting
jerez [ʒe'res] *m* sherry
Jesus [ʒe'zus] *m* Jesus; ***~!*** heavens!
jibóia [ʒi'bɔja] *f* boa (constrictor)
jipe ['ʒipi] *m* jeep
joalharia [ʒwaʎa'ria] *f* jewelry store, *Brit* jeweller's
joalheiro [ʒwa'ʎejru] *m* jeweler, *Brit* jeweller
joaninha [ʒwa'niɲa] *f* lady bug, *Brit* lady bird
joelho ['ʒweʎu] *m* knee; ***de ~s*** kneeling
jogada [ʒo'gada] *f no jogo* move; *dados*: throw; *jogo de azar*: stake
jogador [ʒoga'dor] *m*, **-a** *f* player; *casino*: gambler; ***~ de beisebol*** baseball player; ***~ de futebol*** football player, footballer; ***~ de tênis*** tennis player
jogar [ʒo'gar] ⟨1o & 1e⟩ *v/t* play; (*atirar*) throw; *fig* gamble, put at stake; (*perder no jogo*) gamble away, lose
jogging ['ʒɔgĩ] *m* jogging; ***fato*** *m* ***de ~*** jogging suit
jogo ['ʒogu] *m* play; (*partida*) game; (*brincadeira*) fooling around; (*conjunto*) set; (*manobra*) trick; *fig* ***estar em ~*** be at stake; ***~ de azar*** game of chance; ***~ em casa*** home game; ***~ de chá*** tea service, tea set; ***~ de computador*** computer game; ***~ de palavras*** play on words, pun; ***~ de sofá*** three-piece suite; ***~s individuais*** singles; ***os Jogos*** *pl* ***Olímpicos*** the Olympic Games
jóia ['ʒɔja] *f* jewel; (*quota de entrada*) admission fee; *fig* gem; ***~s*** *pl* jewelry, *Brit* jewellery
jóquei ['ʒɔkej] *m/f* jockey
Jordânia [ʒor'dʌnja] *f* Jordan
jornada [ʒor'nada] *f trabalho*: day's work; *viagem*: day's journey
jornal [ʒor'naw] *m* newspaper; ***pôr no ~*** put in the paper
jornaleiro [ʒorna'lejru] *m*, **-a** *f* news vendor, *Brit* newsagent
jornalismo [ʒorna'lizmu] *m* journalism; ***~ investigativo*** investigative journalism
jornalista [ʒorna'lista] *m/f* journalist; ***~ esportivo(-a)*** sports journalist
jornalístico [ʒorna'listʃiku] *adj* journalistic
jorrar [ʒo'har] ⟨1e⟩ *v/i* spurt out, gush out; *plantas*, *edifícios* shoot up
jorro ['ʒohu] *m* jet, spurt; ***correr em ~*** spurt out, gush out
jovem ['ʒɔvẽ] **1** *adj* young; *aparência* youthful **2** *m/f* young person; ***para jovens*** for young people
jovial [ʒo'vjaw] *adj* jovial, cheerful
jovialidade [ʒovjali'dadʒi] *f* cheerfulness
juba ['ʒuba] *f* mane
jubileu [ʒubi'lew] *m* jubilee
júbilo ['ʒubilu] *m* rejoicing, joy
judeu [ʒu'dew] **1** *adj* Jewish **2** *m*, **-ia** [ʒu'dʒia] *f* Jew
judiação [ʒudʒia'sãw] *f* ***que ~!*** what a terrible thing to do!
judicial [ʒudʒi'sjaw] *adj* judicial
judiciário [ʒudʒi'sjariu] *adj* judicial; ***polícia*** *f* ***judiciária*** criminal investigation department
judô, *Port* **judo** ['ʒudo] *m* judo
jugo ['ʒugu] *m* yoke
juiz [ʒwis] *m*, **juíza** ['ʒwiza] *f* judge
juízo ['ʒwizu] *m* judgment; (*processo*) trial; ***o ~ final*** the Last Judgment; ***o dia do ~*** the Day of Judgment; ***ter ~*** be sensible; ***não ter ~*** be silly
julgamento [ʒuwga'mẽtu] *m* trial;

J

(*sentença*) judgment; ***levar alguém a ~*** take s.o. to court
julgar [ʒuw'gaɾ] ⟨1o⟩ **1** *v/t* judge; *pessoa* pass sentence on; *caso* try **2** *v/i* judge
julho ['ʒuʎu] *m* July; ***em ~*** in July
jumento [ʒu'mẽtu] *m* donkey
junção [ʒũ'sãw] *f* join, junction
junho ['ʒuɲu] *m* June; ***em ~*** in June
júnior ['ʒunjoɾ] *m* ⟨*pl* juniores⟩ junior
junta ['ʒũta] *f* joint; *bois*: yoke; (*administração*) board; *de saúde etc* commission; POL junta; TECN gasket; *Port* ***~ de freguesia*** district council
juntamente [ʒũta'mẽtʃi] *adv* together
juntar [ʒũ'taɾ] ⟨1a⟩ join; (*reunir*) bring together; (*ligar*) connect; (*colecionar*) collect; (*unir*) join together; (*acrescentar*) add
junto ['ʒũtu] **1** *adj* (*próximo*) near; *documento* enclosed; **(*todos*) *~s*** together **2** *adv* (*próximo*) near; *enviar* enclosed; ***~ com*** together with; ***ele está ~ com ela*** he's living together with her **3** *prep* ***~ a, ~ de*** near; (*ao lado de*) next to
jura ['ʒuɾa] *f* vow; ***fazer uma ~*** make a vow, swear
jurado [ʒu'ɾadu] *m*, **-a** *f* juror
juramento [ʒuɾa'mẽtu] *m* oath; ***~ falso*** perjury; ***sob ~*** under oath
jurar [ʒu'ɾaɾ] ⟨1a⟩ swear (***sobre, por*** by); ***jura?*** honest?
júri ['ʒuɾi] *m* jury; UNIV examining board
jurídico [ʒu'ɾidʒiku] *adj* legal
jurisdição [ʒuɾizdʒi'sãw] *f* ⟨*sem pl*⟩ jurisdiction
jurisprudência [ʒuɾispɾu'dẽsja] *f* jurisprudence, law
jurista [ʒu'ɾista] *m/f* lawyer
jururu [ʒuɾu'ɾu] *adj fam* gloomy
juros ['ʒuɾus] *mpl* interest; ***~ compostos*** compound interest
justamente [ʒusta'mẽtʃi] *adv* exactly, just; (*de direito*) rightly, justly
justapor [ʒusta'poɾ] ⟨2z⟩ *v/t* juxtapose
justiça [ʒus'tʃisa] *f* justice; DIR judicial system; (*jurisdição*) jurisdiction; ***Ministério*** *m* ***da Justiça*** Ministry of Justice
justificação [ʒustʃifika'sãw] *f* justification
justificar [ʒustʃifi'kaɾ] ⟨1n⟩ justify
justificável [ʒustʃifi'kavew] *adj* justifiable
justo ['ʒustu] **1** *adj* just, fair; (*exato*) exact; (*certo*) right; (*apertado*) tight, narrow; ***uma causa justa*** a worthy cause **2** *adv* just; ***~ quando eu …*** just as I …
juta ['ʒuta] *f* jute
juvenil [ʒuve'niw] **1** *adj* youthful **2** *m* ESP junior; ***Taça*** *f* ***Nacional de Juvenis*** national junior cup
juventude [ʒuvẽ'tudʒi] *f* youth; (*jovens*) young people, youth

K

K

kilobyte [kilo'bajtʃi] *m* kilobyte
ketchup [kɛ'tʃap] *m* ketchup
kit [kit] *m* kit; ***~ mãos-livres*** hands-free kit
kitchenette [kitʃi'nɛtʃi] *f* studio apartment
kiwi [ki'wi] *m* kiwi fruit
kleenex® [kli'nɛks] *m Bras* kleenex®, paper handkerchief
Kuwait [ku'waitʃi] *m* Kuwait

L

L. *abr* (***Largo***) Sq. (square)
l *abr* (***litro***) l (liter)
lá [la] **1** *adv* there; ***~ em cima / baixo*** up / down there; ***~ no Japão*** over in Japan **2** *m* MÚS A
lã [lã] *f* wool; ***~s*** *pl* woolens, *Brit* woollens; ***de ~*** woolen, *Brit* woollen
labareda [laba'ɾeda] *f* flame
lábia ['labja] *f pop* persuasiveness; (*astúcia*) cunning; ***ter ~*** have the gift of the gab
lábil ['labiw] *adj* unstable
lábio ['labiu] *m* lip; ***ler os ~s*** lipread
labirinto [labi'ɾĩtu] *m* labyrinth
laboral [labo'ɾaw] *adj* labor *atr*, *Brit* labour *atr*
laboratório [laboɾa'tɔɾiu] *m* laboratory, lab; ***~ lingüístico*** language lab
laboratorista [laboɾato'ɾista] *m/f* lab technician
labrego [la'bɾegu] **1** *m* country bumpkin **2** *adj* boorish
labuta [la'buta] *f* toil
laca ['laka] *f* lacquer
laço ['lasu] *m* bow; *acessório*: bow tie; (*armadilha*) snare; *fig* bond; ***armar um ~*** set a trap; ***cair no ~*** fall into the trap
lacrar [la'kɾaɾ] ⟨1b⟩ *v/t* seal
lacrau [la'kɾaw] *m* scorpion
lacrimejar [lakɾime'ʒaɾ] ⟨1d⟩ *v/i* water
lacrimogêneo, *Port* **lacrimogéneo** [lakɾimo'ʒeniu] *adj* ***gás*** *m* ***~*** tear gas
lactação [lakta'sãw] *f* ⟨*sem pl*⟩ breastfeeding; BIOL lactation
lacuna [la'kuna] *f* gap
lacustre [la'kustɾi] *adj* lake *atr*; ***habitação*** *f* ***~*** lake dwelling
ladear [la'dʒiaɾ] ⟨1l⟩ *v/t* accompany; MIL flank
ladeira [la'dejɾa] *f* slope; *rua* steep street; *fig* ***ir ~ abaixo*** go downhill
lado ['ladu] *m* side; (*direção*) direction; ***~ a ~*** side by side; ***ao ~*** nearby *casa etc*: next door; ***ao ~ de*** beside, next to; ***de ~*** from the side, sideways; ***do ~*** *casa* next-door; ***do ~ direito*** on the right-hand side; ***para o ~ lado de*** across, to the other side of; ***por um ~ …, por outro ~ …*** on the one hand …, on the other hand …; ***de um ~ para o outro*** to and fro, ***10m de um ~ a outro*** 10m across; ***estou do seu ~*** I'm on your side
ladra ['ladɾa] *f* thief
ladrão [la'dɾãw] *m* thief
ladrar [la'dɾaɾ] ⟨1b⟩ bark
ladrilhar [ladɾi'ʎaɾ] ⟨1a⟩ *v/t* tile
ladrilho [la'dɾiʎu] *m* tile
lagarta [la'gaɾta] *f* caterpillar; TECN caterpillar track
lagartixa [lagaɾ'ʧiʃa] *f* gecko
lagarto [la'gaɾtu] *m* lizard
lago ['lagu] *m* lake
lagoa [la'goa] *f* pool; *costeiro* lagoon
lagosta [la'gosta] *f* lobster
lagostim [lagos'ʧĩ] *m* crayfish
lágrima ['lagɾima] *f* tear; *fig* (*gota*) drop
laguna [la'guna] *f* lagoon
lama[1] ['lama] *f* mud
lama[2] ['lama] *m* ZOOL llama
lamacento [lama'sẽtu] *adj* muddy
lambada [lã'bada] *f* blow; *dança*: lambada
lamber [lã'beɾ] ⟨2a⟩ lick
lambiscar [lãbis'kaɾ] ⟨1n⟩ *v/i* nibble
lambreta [lã'bɾeta] *f* scooter
lamentação [lamẽta'sãw] *f* lamentation; (*lamúria*) lament
lamentar [lamẽ'taɾ] ⟨1a⟩ (*lastimar*) lament; ***lamento muito!*** I'm so sorry!; ***lamento ter que informar-lhe …*** I regret to have to inform you …; **lamentar-se** *v/r* moan, whine
lamentável [lamẽ'tavew] *adj* lamentable
lamento [la'mẽtu] *m* lament; ***~ (s)*** (*pl*) moan

lâmina ['lʌmina] *f* sheet; *faca*: blade; *microscópio*: slide; *Port* **~ de barbear** razor blade
laminado [lami'nadu] *adj* laminated
lâmpada ['lãpada] *f* lamp; *peça que atarracha* light bulb; **~ fluorescente** fluorescent lamp; **~ halógena** halogen lamp
lamparina [lãpa'ɾina] *f* lamp
lampejo [lã'peʒu] *m* glimmer; **~ de esperança** glimmer of hope
lamúria [la'muɾja] *f* whimper
lança ['lãsa] *f* lance, spear
lançamento [lãsa'mẽtu] *m bombas*: dropping; *foguete*: launch, blast-off; *alicerce*: laying; *produto*: launch; COM entry
lançar [lã'saɾ] ⟨1p⟩ throw; *bomba* drop; *rede* cast; *produto*, *moda* launch; (*expelir*) emit; *imposto* put; *pergunta* raise; **~ em pára-quedas** parachute, drop by parachute
lance ['lãsi] *m* throw; *xadrez*: move; *leilão*: bid; *casas*: row; *muro*: section; (*momento*) (deciding) moment; **tenho um ~** I'm having an affair; **~ de escada** flight of stairs; **~ mínimo** reserve price
lancha ['lãʃa] *f* launch; **~ a motor** motor boat
lanchar [lã'ʃaɾ] ⟨1a⟩ *pela tarde* have a snack
lanche ['lãʃi] *m* snack
lanchonete [lãʃo'nɛʧi] *m* snackbar, diner
lancinante [lãsi'nãʧi] *adj dor* stabbing; *fig* heart-rending
lânguido ['lãgidu] *adj* listless; (*fraco*) weak; (*negligente*) careless; (*langoroso*) languid
lanifício [lani'fisiu] *m* woolens, *Brit* woollens; **indústria** *f* **de ~s** wool industry
lanterna [lã'tɛɾna] *f* lantern; *com bateria* flashlight, *Brit* torch; **~ de furta-fogo** signaling lantern, *Brit* signalling lantern; **~ traseira** tail light
lanternagem [lãteɾ'naʒẽ] *f* bodyshop
lanterninha [lãteɾ'niɲa] *f* usherette
Laos [laws] *m* Laos
lapela [la'pɛla] *f casaco*: lapel
lapidar [lapi'daɾ] ⟨1a⟩ *v/t pedras* cut; *fig* polish
lápide ['lapidʒi] *f* tombstone
lápis ['lapis] *m* ⟨*pl inv*⟩ pencil; **~ de cera** wax crayon; **~ de cor** colored pencil, *Brit* coloured pencil
lapiseira [lapi'zejɾa] *f* mechanical pencil, *Brit* propelling pencil
lapso ['lapsu] *m* lapse; *em conversa* slip of the tongue; **~** (**de tempo**) interval
laptop [lap'tɔpi] *m* laptop
laquê [la'ke] *m* lacquer
lar [laɾ] *m* home; *estudantes etc*: dormitory, *Brit* hall of residence; **~ adotivo** foster home; **~ de terceira idade** old people's home
laranja [la'ɾãʒa] **1** *f* orange **2** *m cor* orange
laranjada [laɾã'ʒada] *f* orangeade
laranjeira [laɾã'ʒejɾa] *f* orange tree
lareira [la'ɾejɾa] *f* hearth
largada [laɾ'gada] *f* **fazer uma boa / má ~** get off to a good / bad start
largar [laɾ'gaɾ] ⟨1o & 1b⟩ **1** *v/t* let go of; (*deixar cair*) drop; *fig pessoa*, *pássaro* let go; *vela* set; **largue-me!** let me go! **2** *v/i* leave; NÁUT *tb* sail
largo ['laɾgu] **1** *adj* wide; (*grande*) extensive; *casa* spacious; *tempo* long; (*abundante*) ample **2** *m* NÁUT open sea; (*praça*) square
largura [laɾ'guɾa] *f* width, breadth; **ter um metro de ~** be one meter wide
laringe [la'ɾĩʒi] *f* larynx
laringite [laɾĩ'ʒiʧi] *f* laryngitis
larva ['laɾva] *f inseto*: larva
lasanha [la'zaɲa] *f* GASTR lasagna
lasca ['laska] *f* splinter; *porcelana*: chip; *fig* little bit
lascar [las'kaɾ] ⟨1n & 1b⟩ *v/t* & *v/i* splinter; *porcelana* chip
lascivo [las'sivu] *adj* lascivious
laser ['lejzaɾ] *m* laser; **raio** *m* **~** laser beam; **impressora** *f* **~** laser printer; **tecnologia** *f* **~** laser technology
laserterapia [lejzaɾtera'pia] *f* laser treatment, laser therapy
lassidão [lasi'dãw] *f* lassitude, weariness
lasso ['lasu] *adj* lax; (*exausto*) weary
lástima ['lasʧima] *f* compassion, pity; (*miséria*) misery; **é uma ~ que** it's a

pity that
lastimar [lasʧi'maɾ] ⟨1a⟩ lament
lastimável [lasʧi'mavew] *adj* lamentable
lastimoso [lasʧi'mozu] *adj* (*miserável*) pitiful
lastro ['lastɾu] *m* ballast
lata[1] ['lata] *f conserva*: can, *Brit tb* tin; *mais grande* cannister; *material*: tinplate; **~ de lixo** trash can, *Brit* dustbin; *na rua* litter bin
lata[2] ['lata] *f* boldness; ***ter a ~ de*** have the nerve to
latão [la'tãw] *m* brass
latejar [late'ʒaɾ] ⟨1d⟩ throb, beat
latejo [la'teʒu] *m* throb, beat; **~s** *pl* throbbing, beating
latente [la'tẽʧi] *adj* hidden, latent
lateral [late'ɾaw] **1** *adj* side *atr*, lateral **2** *f* ESP touch; *jogador* winger
lateralmente [lateɾaw'mẽʧi] *adv* sideways
laticínio [laʧi'siniu] *m* dairy product
latido [la'ʧidu] *m* bark; **~s** *pl* barking
latifundiário [laʧifũ'dʒiaɾiu] *m*, **-a** *f* landowner
latifúndio [laʧi'fũdiu] *m* large estate
latim [la'ʧĩ] *m* Latin; ***gastar / perder o seu ~*** waste one's breath
latino [la'ʧinu] **1** *adj* Latin; ***América*** *f* ***Latina*** Latin-American; ***língua*** *f* ***latina*** Romance language **2** *m*, **-a** *f* Roman
latino-americano [laʧinoameɾi'kanu] **1** *adj* Latin-American **2** *m*, **-a** *f* Latin-American, Latino
latitude [laʧi'tudʒi] *f* latitude
latrocínio [latɾo'siniu] *m* armed robbery
lava ['lava] *f* lava
lavabo [la'vabu] *m* washbowl; *Port* **~s** *pl* rest rooms, *Brit* toilets
lavadora [la'vabu] *f* ***~ automática*** washing machine; ***~ de louça*** dishwasher
lavagante [lava'gãʧi] *m* lobster
lavagem [la'vaʒẽ] *f* washing; AUTO ***~ automática*** carwash; ***~ ao cérebro*** brainwashing; ***~ e penteado*** shampoo and set
lava-loiça [lava'lojsa] *m*, **~ -louça** [lava'losa] *f* dishwasher
lavanderia [lavãde'ɾia] *f* laundry; ***~ a seco*** dry cleaner
lavar [la'vaɾ] ⟨1b⟩ wash; *fig* cleanse; ***~ loiça*** wash the dishes, *Brit tb* wash up; ***~ os dentes*** brush one's teeth; *fig* ***~ as mãos de algo*** wash one's hands of sth; ***~ a roupa*** do the washing; ***lavado em lágrimas*** bathed in tears; **lavar-se** *v/r* have a wash
lavatório [lava'tɔriu] *m Port* washbowl
lavável [la'vavew] *adj* washable
lava-vidros [lava'vidɾus] *m* AUTO windshield wipers, *Brit* windscreen wipers
lavoura [la'voɾa] *f* farming
lavradeira [lavɾa'dejɾa] *f*, **lavrador** [lavɾa'doɾ] *m* farmer
lavrar [la'vɾaɾ] ⟨1b⟩ **1** *v/t* work; *documento* draw up **2** *v/i* spread
laxante [la'ʃãʧi] *m* laxative
lazer [la'zeɾ] *m* leisure
L.da *abr* (***Sociedade de Responsabilidade Limitada***) Ltd (Limited Company)
lê [le] → ***ler***
leal [leaw] *adj* loyal
lealdade [leaw'dadʒi] *f* loyalty; ***~ à marca*** brand loyalty
leão [ljãw] *m* lion; ASTROL ***Leão*** Leo
leão-de-chácara [ljãwdʒi'ʃakaɾa] *m* bouncer
lebre ['lɛbɾi] *f* hare
lecionar, *Port* **leccionar** [lesjo'naɾ] ⟨1f⟩ teach
lectivo *Port* → ***letivo***
legação [lega'sãw] *f* legation
legado [le'gadu] *m* REL envoy, legate; (*herança*) bequest, legacy
legal [le'gaw] *adj* legal; (*válido*) valid; *Bras fam* great, cool
legalidade [legali'dadʒi] *f* legality
legalização [legaliza'sãw] *f* legalization; *certificado*: authentication
legalizar [legali'zaɾ] ⟨1a⟩ legalize; *certificado* authenticate
legar [le'gaɾ] ⟨1o & 1c⟩ delegate; *herança* bequeath
legenda [le'ʒẽda] *f mapa*, *tabela*: key; (*inscrição*) inscription; CINE subtitle; ***~ explicativa*** caption
legendário [leʒẽ'daɾiu] *adj* legendary

legião [le'ʒjãw] *f* legion; ***Legião Estrangeira*** Foreign Legion
legionário [leʒjo'nariu] *m* legionnaire; *romano* legionary
legislação [leʒizla'sãw] *f* legislation
legislador [leʒizla'dor] *m*, **-a** *f* legislator
legislativo [leʒizla'tʃivu] **1** *adj* legislative; ***poder*** *m* ~ legislative power **2** *m* legislature
legislatura [leʒizla'tura] *f* legislature; *período* term of office
legitimar [leʒitʃi'mar] ⟨1a⟩ *v/t* legitimize
legitimidade [leʒitʃimi'dadʒi] *f* legitimacy
legítimo [le'ʒitʃimu] *adj* legitimate; ***legítima defesa*** *f* self-defense, *Brit* self-defence
legível [le'ʒivew] *adj* legible
legume [le'gumi] *m* vegetable
lei [lej] *f* law; (*prescrição*) regulation, rule; ***de*** ~ real; *metal* standard; *diamante* high-carat
leia ['leja] *etc* → ***ler***
leilão [lej'lãw] *m* auction
leio ['leiu] *etc* → ***ler***
leitão [lej'tãw] *m*, **leitoa** [lej'toa] *f* piglet; GASTR ~ ***assado*** suckling pig
leitaria [lejta'ria] *f* dairy
leite ['lejtʃi] *m* milk; ~ ***magro*** skim milk, *Brit* skimmed milk; ~ ***em pó*** powdered milk; ***batido*** *m* ***de*** ~ milkshake
leito ['lejtu] *m* bed; TECN bearing; ~ ***do rio*** river bed
leitor[1] [lej'tor] *m*, **-a** *f* reader; *editora*: editor
leitor[2] [lej'tor] *m* ~ ***de CD / DVD*** CD / DVD player; ~ / ***gravador de cassetes*** cassette recorder
leitura [lej'tura] *f* reading; *livros* reading matter
lema ['lema] *m* motto; LING lemma
lembrança [lẽ'brãsa] *f* memory; *objeto* souvenir; ~***s*** *pl* regards
lembrar [lẽ'brar] ⟨1a⟩ *v/t* ~ ***algo a alguém*** remind s.o. of sth; ~ ***algo*** be reminiscent of sth; ***ele me lembra o João*** he reminds me of João; **lembrar-se** *v/r* remember; ~ ***de*** remember
leme ['lemi] *m* helm; AERO, NÁUT rudder; *fig* helm, control
lenço ['lẽsu] *m* scarf; headscarf; *pequeno*: handkerchief; ~ ***de papel*** tissue
lençol [lẽ'sɔw] *m* sheet; *água*: pool; ~ ***de banho*** bath towel; ~ ***freático*** water table
lenda ['lẽda] *f* legend
lendário [lẽ'dariu] *adj* legendary
lenha ['laɲa] *f* firewood
lenhador [leɲa'dor] *m*, **-a** *f* woodcutter
lenitivo [leni'tʃivu] *m* pain reliever
lente ['lẽtʃi] **1** *m/f* professor, *Brit* university lecturer **2** *f ótica*: lens *sg*
lentidão [lẽtʃi'dãw] *f* slowness
lentilha [lẽ'tʃiʎa] *f* BOT, GASTR lentil
lento ['lẽtu] *adj* slow
leoa ['ljoa] *f* lioness
leopardo [ljo'pardu] *m* leopard
lepra ['lɛpra] *f* leprosy
leque ['lɛki] *m* array
ler [ler] ⟨2k⟩ read; MÚS sight-read
lês [les] → ***ler***
lesão [le'zãw] *f* harm; *corporal* injury; ~ ***cardíaca*** heart defect
lesar [le'zar] ⟨1c⟩ injure; (*danificar*) damage
lésbica ['lɛzbika] **1** *adj* lesbian **2** *f* lesbian
lesma ['lezma] *f* slug; *fig fam* slowpoke, *Brit* slowcoach
leste[1] ['lɛstʃi] *m* east; *vento* east wind; ***ao*** ~ ***de*** east of; *fig* ***estar a*** ~ have no idea
leste[2] ['lestʃi] → ***ler***
letal [le'taw] *adj* lethal
letão [le'tãw] ⟨*mpl* -ãos⟩ **1** *adj* Latvian **2** *m*, **-ã** *f* Latvian **3** *m lingua* Latvian
letargia [letar'ʒia] *f* lethargy
letárgico [le'tarʒiku] *adj* lethargic
letivo [le'tʃivu] *adj* school *atr*; ***ano*** *m* ~ school year, academic year
Letônia, *Port* **Letónia** [le'tonja] *f* Latvia
letra ['letra] *f* letter; (*escrita*) writing; (*caligrafia*) handwriting; MÚS lyrics; *fig* (*teor*) literal meaning; UNIV ~***s*** *pl* languages and literature; ***a*** ~ ***da lei*** the letter of the law

letreiro [le'trejru] *m* inscription; (*rótulo*) label; (*sinal*) sign
levantamento [levãta'mẽtu] *m* (*elevação*) lifting; (*revolta*) uprising; (*inventário*) stocktaking; *dinheiro*: withdrawal; **~ cênico**, *Port* **~ cénico** (stage) set; **~ topográfico** survey
levantar [levã'tar] ⟨1a⟩ **1** *v/t* lift; *coisa do chão* pick up; (*erigir*) erect; (*puxar*) pull up; *dinheiro* withdraw; **~ a âncora** weigh anchor **2** *v/i* rise; *tempo* brighten
levar [le'var] ⟨1c⟩ take; (*carregar*) carry; (*dirigir*) lead; **~ a mal** take amiss; **~ boa vida** enjoy life
leve ['lɛvi] *adj* light; (*passageiro*) fleeting; *esperança* slight; **de ~** gently
levedar [leve'dar] ⟨1c⟩ **1** *v/t massa* leaven **2** *v/i* rise
levedura [leve'dura] *f* yeast
leveza [le'veza] *f* lightness; (*inconstância*) fickleness
leviandade [levjã'dadʒi] *f* frivolity
leviano [le'vjanu] *adj* frivolous
léxico ['lɛksiku] *m* lexicon; (*vocabulário*) vocabulary
lha, lhas [ʎa, ʎas] = *pron* **lhe**(**s**) + *pron* **a, as**
lhe [ʎi] *pron* him; *f* her; (*a você*) you; **mande- ~ minhas lembranças** send him / her my regards; **posso fazer- ~ uma pergunta?** can I ask you something?
lhes [ʎis] *pron pl* them; *tratamento cortês*: you; **mande- ~ minhas lembranças** send them my regards
lho, lhos [ʎu, ʎus] = *pron* **lhe**(**s**) + *pron* **o, os**
li [li], **lia** ['lia] *etc* → **ler**
libanês [liba'nes] **1** *adj* Lebanese **2** *m*, **~ esa** [liba'neza] *f* Lebanese
Líbano ['libanu] *m* Lebanon
libélula [li'bɛlula] *f* dragonfly
liberal [libe'raw] **1** *adj* liberal *tb* POL; (*generoso*) generous **2** *m/f* liberal
liberalidade [liberali'dadʒi] *f* liberality; (*generosidade*) generosity
liberalismo [libera'lizmu] *m* liberalism
liberalização [liberaliza'sãw] *f* ECON, POL liberalization
liberalizar [liberali'zar] ⟨1a⟩ liberalize
liberdade [liber'dadʒi] *f* freedom, liberty; (*franqueza*) frankness; **~ condicional** parole, probation; **~ de circulação** freedom of movement; **~ de expressão** free speech; **~ de imprensa** freedom of the press; **tomar a ~ de fazer** take the liberty of doing; **tomar ~s** take liberties
Libéria [li'bɛrja] *f* Liberia
libertação [liberta'sãw] *f* release; *país, cidade*: liberation
libertar [liber'tar] ⟨1c⟩ release (**de** from); *país, cidade* liberate
liberto [li'bɛrtu] *adj* free, released
Líbia ['libja] *f* Libya
líbio ['libiu] **1** *adj* Libyan **2** *m*, **-a** *f* Libyan
libra ['libra] *f medida, moeda* pound; ASTROL **Libra** Libra
libré [li'brɛ] *f* livery; *fig* uniform
libreto [li'bretu] *m* MÚS libretto
lição [li'sãw] *f* lesson; UNIV lecture; (*matéria*) subject; **aprendi uma ~** I've learned my lesson
licença [li'sẽsa] *f* license, *Brit* licence; (*permissão*) permission; (*documento*) permit, license; *caça*: permit; (*férias*) leave; **~ de parto** maternity leave; **dar ~** permit; **com ~!** excuse me
licenciado [lisẽ'sjadu] *m*, **-a** *f* graduate
licenciamento [lisẽsja'mẽtu] *m* MIL leave; (*permissão*) permission
licenciar [lisẽ'sjar] ⟨1g & 1h⟩ *v/t* license; **licenciar-se** *v/r* graduate
licenciatura [lisẽsja'tura] *f* UNIV degree
liceu [li'sew] *m* high school
licor [li'kor] *m* liqueur; **~ de laranja** orange liqueur
lida ['lida] *f* toil; *fig* trouble
lidar [li'dar] ⟨1a⟩ *v/i* deal (**com** with)
lide ['lidʒi] *f* lawsuit; (*luta*) fight; **~ da casa** household chores
líder ['lider] **1** *m/f* leader **2** *adj* leading, top
liderança [lide'rãsa] *f* leadership
liderar [lide'rar] ⟨1c⟩ lead
lido ['lidu] *pp* → **ler**
liga ['liga] *f* league; QUÍM alloy
ligação [liga'sãw] *f* connection; *Bras*

TEL call; INTERNET link; ELÉT **~ à corrente** mains connection
ligadura [liga'duɾa] *f Port* MED bandage
ligamento [liga'mẽtu] *m* bond; ANAT ligament
ligar [li'gaɾ] ⟨1o⟩ (*juntar*) connect; (*atar*) tie up; *eletricidade* switch on; *motor* start up; **~ à canalização** plumb in; TEL *fam* **~ (para)** call; **não ~ a** not listen to
ligeiramente [liʒejɾa'mẽtʃi] *adv* lightly; (*um pouco*) slightly
ligeireza [liʒe'reza] *f* lightness; (*agilidade*) nimbleness
ligeiro [li'ʒejɾu] *adj* light; (*destro*) nimble; (*pequeno*) slight
ligue ['ligi] → **ligar**
lilás [li'las] **1** *m* lilac **2** *adj* lilac
lima[1] ['lima] *f* BOT lime
lima[2] ['lima] *f* TECN file
limagem [ài'maʒẽ] *f* filing
limalha [li'maʎa] *f* filings
limão [li'mãw] *m* lemon
limar [li'maɾ] ⟨1a⟩ *v/t* file; *fig* fine-tune
limiar [li'mjaɾ] *m* threshold
limitação [limita'sãw] *f* limitation, restriction; (*moderação*) restraint; **~ de preços** price freeze
limitado [limi'tadu] *adj* limited; **Sociedade Limitada** *f* Limited Company
limitar [limi'taɾ] ⟨1a⟩ **1** *v/t* limit; restrict; (*reduzir*) reduce **2** *v/i* **~ com** border on; **limitar-se** *v/r* limit oneself (**a** to); (*contentar-se*) content oneself (**a** with)
limite [li'mitʃi] *m* boundary; COM price limit; **~ de velocidade** speed limit
limoal [li'moaw] *m* lemon grove
limoeiro [li'moejɾu] *m* lemon tree
limonada [limo'nada] *f* lemon soda
limpa-chaminés [lĩpaʃami'nɛs] *m/f* ⟨*pl inv*⟩ chimneysweep
limpa-neves [lĩpa'nɛvis] *m* ⟨*pl inv*⟩ snowplow, *Brit* snowplough
limpa-pára-brisas [lĩpapaɾa'brizas] *m* ⟨*pl inv*⟩ windshield wipers, *Brit* windscreen wipers
limpar [lĩ'paɾ] ⟨1a⟩ clean; *nódoa* wipe away; *pele* cleanse; **~ o pó** dust
limpa-vidros [lĩpa'vidrus] *m* ⟨*pl inv*⟩ windshield wipers, *Brit* windscreen wipers
limpeza [lĩ'peza] *f estado* cleanliness; *ação* cleaning; (*depuração*) purge *tb* POL; *virtude*: purity; **~ de pele** facial
limpidez [lĩpi'des] *f* clarity; (*transparência*) transparency
límpido ['lĩpidu] *adj* clear; (*transparente*) transparent; (*puro*) pure; (*sincero*) honest; *céu* clear
limpo ['lĩpu] *adj* clean *tb fig*; *céu* clear; (*isento*) **~ de** free from; **passar algo a ~** make a clean copy of sth; **tirar a ~** clear up
lince ['lĩsi] *m* lynx
lindo ['lĩdu] *adj* lovely, pretty; *Bras fam* great
lingote [lĩ'gɔtʃi] *m* ingot
língua ['lĩŋgwa] *f* tongue; (*idioma*) language; *fig* **debaixo da ~** on the tip of one's tongue; **~ materna** mother tongue; **~ de sinais** sign language; GEOG **~ de terra** promontory, spit
linguado [lĩ'gwadu] *m* ZOOL sole
linguagem [lĩ'gwaʒẽ] *f* speech; LING, INFORM language; **~ corporal** body language
lingüeta, *Port* **lingueta** [lĩ'gweta] *f balança*: pointer; *sapato*: tongue; *porta*: bolt; *chave*: bit; TECN, MÚS key
lingüista, *Port* **linguista** [lĩ'gwista] *m/f* linguist
lingüiça, *Port* **linguiça** [lĩ'gwisa] *f* sausage
lingüístico, *Port* **linguístico** [lĩ'gwistʃiku] *adj* linguistic
linha ['liɲa] *f* line; TÊX thread; **pescar à ~** angle; INFORM **em ~** on line; **~ aérea** airline; **~ de chegada** finish line; **~ lateral** sideline; **~ de montagem** assembly line
linhaça [li'ɲasa] *f* linseed; **óleo** *m* **de ~** linseed oil
linhagem [li'ɲaʒẽ] *f* lineage
linho ['liɲu] *m* BOT flax; TÊX linen
liofilizado [ljofili'zadu] *adj* freeze-dried
liquidação [likida'sãw] *f* liquidation; *fatura*, *dívida*: settlement; *saldos* sale; *empresa*: closure; *fig* liquidation; COM **~ provisória / definitiva** advance / final payment
liquidar [liki'daɾ] ⟨1a⟩ FIN liquidate;

fatura, dívida settle; *défice* make up; *empresa* wind up; *armazêm* sell off; *conflito* settle; *fig fam pessoa* liquidate
liquidatário [likida'tariu] *adj* liquidating
liquidável [liki'davew] *adj* COM realizable
liquidez [liki'des] *f* FIN liquidity
líquido ['likidu] **1** *adj* liquid; ECON net; ***produto*** *m* ~ net profit **2** *m* liquid
lírica ['lirika] *f* lyric poetry
lírico ['liriku] **1** *adj* lyrical **2** *m*, **-a** *f* lyric poet
Lisboa [liz'boa] *f* Lisbon
lisboeta [liz'bweta] **1** *adj* Lisbon *atr* **2** *m/f* inhabitant of Lisbon
liso ['lizu] *adj* smooth; (*uniforme*) plain; (*simples*) simple; (*honesto*) honest; *Port fam* (*duro*) broke
lisonja [li'zõʒa] *f* flattery
lisonjear [lizõ'ʒjar] ⟨1l⟩ *v/t* flatter
lista ['lista] *f* list; (*ementa*) menu; *vinhos, bebidas*: (wine / drinks) list; ***à ~, por ~*** à la carte; ***~ chamada*** roll call; ***~ de compras*** shopping list; ***~ de espera*** waiting list; ***~ negra*** blacklist; ***~ de preços*** price list; ***~ telefônica***, *Port* ***~ telefónica*** telephone directory, phonebook
listagem [lis'taʒẽ] *f* listing; INFORM printout (*on continuous paper*)
listrado [lis'tradu] *adj* striped
literal [lite'raw] *adj* literal
literário [lite'rariu] *adj* literary
literatura [litera'tura] *f* literature
litigante [litʃi'gãtʃi] *adj* litigant
litigar [litʃi'gar] ⟨1o⟩ go to court; (*disputar*) dispute
litígio [li'tʃiʒiu] *m* lawsuit, case; ***estar em ~*** *fig* be in conflict
litigioso [litʃi'ʒjozu] *adj* disputed
litoral [lito'raw] **1** *m* coast **2** *adj* coastal
litro ['litru] *m* liter, *Brit* litre
Lituânia [li'twʌnja] *f* Lithuania
lituano [li'twanu] **1** *adj* Lithuanian **2** *m*, **-a** *f* Lithuanian
livrar [li'vrar] ⟨1a⟩ ***~ de*** release from; (*preservar*) protect from
livraria [livra'ria] *f* bookstore, *Brit* bookshop
livre ['livri] *adj* free; ESP (***pontapé*** *m*) ~ *m* free kick
livre-câmbio [livre'kãbiu] *m* ⟨*sem pl*⟩ free trade
livreiro [li'vrejru] *m*, **-a** *f* bookseller; ***~ editor*** publisher
livrete [li'vretʃi] *m* booklet; AUTO ***~ de circulação do veículo*** vehicle registration document; ***~ de poupança*** savings book
livro ['livru] *m* book; ***~ de bolso*** pocket book; ***~ de consulta*** reference book; ***~ escolar*** school book, textbook; ***~ ilustrado*** picture book ***~ infantil*** children's book; ***~ de receitas*** cookbook
lixa[1] ['liʃa] *f* sandpaper
lixa[2] ['liʃa] *f peixe* dogfish
lixar [li'ʃar] ⟨1a⟩ sand; *fig fam* screw
lixeira [li'ʃejra] *f* garbage can
lixívia [li'ʃivja] *f* bleach
lixo ['liʃu] *m* garbage, *Brit* rubbish; ***~ doméstico*** *ou* ***urbano*** household garbage, *Brit* domestic rubbish; ***~ tóxico*** toxic waste; ***condução*** *f* ***de ~*** garbage collection, *Brit* rubbish collection; ***depósito*** *m* ***de ~, caixote*** *m* ***de ~*** garbage can, *Brit* rubbish bin; ***homem*** *m* ***do ~*** garbage man, *Brit* dustman
lobo ['lobu] *m*, **-a** *f* wolf; ***~ do mar*** old sea dog
lóbulo ['lɔbulu] *m* ANAT lobe
locação [loka'sãw] *f* rental, lease
local [lo'kaw] **1** *adj* local **2** *m* place, site; (*localidade*) locality; ***no próprio ~*** there **3** *f jornal*: ***locais*** *pl* local news *sg*
localidade [lokali'dadʒi] *f* (*aldeia*) village; (*lugar*) locality
localização [lokaliza'sãw] *f* location; *software*: localization
localizar [lokali'zar] ⟨1a⟩ locate; *software* localize
loção [lo'sãw] *f* lotion; ***~ capilar*** hair lotion; ***~ para o rosto*** face cream
locatário [loka'tariu] *m*, **-a** *f* hirer; AGR, COM tenant
locomoção [lokomo'sãw] *f* ⟨*sem pl*⟩ locomotion
locomotiva [lokomo'tʃiva] *f* locomotive

L

locução [loku'sãw] *f* phrase
locutor [loku'tor] *m*, **-a** *f* speaker; TV announcer
lodo ['lodu] *m* mud; ***banho*** *m* ***de ~*** mud-bath
loendro ['lwẽdru] *m* oleander
logaritmo [loga'ritmu] *m* logarithm
lógica ['lɔʒika] *f* logic; ***erro*** *m* ***de ~*** flaw in the logic
lógico ['lɔʒiku] *adj* logical; ***é ~!*** of course!, absolutely!
logística [lo'ʒistʃika] *f* logistics
logístico [lo'ʒistʃiku] *adj* logistical
logo ['lɔgu] **1** *adv* right away, at once; (*depois*) later; (*em breve*) soon; (*portanto*) so, therefore; ***até ~!*** see you later!; ***~ a seguir ao banco*** right next to the bank **2** *conj* ***~ que*** as soon as
logomarca [logo'marka] *f* logo
logotipo [logo'tʃipu] *m* logo
logradouro [logra'dowru] *m* public area
logro ['logru] *m* fraud
loira ['lojra] *f* blonde
loiro ['lojru] *adj* blond; GASTR golden
loiça ['lojsa] *f* dishes, tableware; ***lavar a ~*** wash the dishes, *Brit tb* wash up
loja ['lɔʒa] *f* store, *Brit* shop; ***~ franca*** duty-free shop; ***~ de brinquedos*** toy store, *Brit* toy shop; ***~ de conveniência*** convenience store
lombo ['lõbu] *m* loin *tb* GASTR; ***~ assado*** roast loin; ***~ de porco*** loin of pork
lombriga [lõ'briga] *f* roundworm
lona ['lona] *f* tarpaulin; *material* canvas
Londres ['lõdris] *f* London
longe ['lõʒi] *adv* far away; (***ao***) ***~*** in the distance; ***de ~*** from far away; ***de ~ o melhor*** far and away the best
longevidade [lõʒevi'dadʒi] *f* longevity
longínquo [lõ'ʒĩkwu] *adj* distant
longitude [lõʒi'tudʒi] *f* longitude
longo ['lõgu] *adj* (*demorado*) long; (*longínquo*) distant; ***ao ~ de*** along; *temporal*: alongside, during
lontra ['lõtra] *f* otter
losango [lo'zãgu] *m* MAT lozenge
lota ['lɔta] *f* fish auction
lotação [lota'sãw] *f* capacity; ***~ esgotada*** sold out
lote ['lɔtʃi] *m* (*cautela*) lot; (*parte*) portion; *mercadoria*: item; *terreno*: plot
loteria [lote'ria] *f* lottery
loto ['lɔtu] *m* lotto
louça ['losa] *f* → ***loiça***
louco ['loku] **1** *adj* crazy, mad; ***ficar ~*** go crazy, go mad; ***estar ~ para fazer algo*** be dying to do sth; ***deixar alguém ~*** drive s.o. crazy *ou* mad **2** *m*, **-a** *f* lunatic
loucura [lo'kura] *f* madness; (*maluquice*) crazy thing; ***levar alguém à ~*** drive s.o. mad; ***é uma ~*** it's madness; *ótimo* it's really cool
louro[1] ['loru] *adj* blond
louro[2] ['loru] *m* BOT laurel; ***folha*** *f* ***de ~*** bay leaf
louro[3] ['loru] *m pop* (*papagaio*) parrot
louva-a-deus [lova'dews] *m* ⟨*pl inv*⟩ ZOOL praying mantis
louvar [lo'var] ⟨1a⟩ praise
louvável [lo'vavew] *adj* praiseworthy
louvor [lo'vor] *m* praise; *discurso*: eulogy
lua ['lua] *f* moon; ***~ cheia / nova*** full / new moon; ***~ -de-mel*** honeymoon
luar [lwar] *m* moonlight
lubrificação [lubrifika'sãw] *f* lubrication
lubrificante [lubrifi'kãtʃi] **1** *adj* lubricating *atr* **2** *m* lubricant
lubrificar [lubrifi'kar] ⟨1n⟩ lubricate
lucidez [lusi'des] *f* lucidity, clarity
lúcido ['lusidu] *adj* lucid, clear
lúcio ['lusiu] *m* pike
lucrar [lu'krar] ⟨1a⟩ **1** *v/t* bring in; (*ganhar*) gain (***com*** from); (*aproveitar*) make use of **2** *v/i* ***~ com*** profit by
lucrativo [lukra'tʃivu] *adj* lucrative
lucro ['lukru] *m* profit; (*rendimento*) return
lufada [lu'fada] *f* gust (of wind)
lugar [lu'gar] *m* place; ***em ~ de*** instead of; ***em primeiro ~*** in the first place; *fig* ***dar ~ a algo*** give rise to sth; (*possibilitar*) facilitate sth; ***em todo ~*** everywhere; ***ter ~*** take place; ***~ comum*** commonplace; ***~ de nascimento*** birthplace; ***~ de pé*** standing room; ***~ sentado*** seat

L

lugarejo [luga'reʒu] *m* village
lúgubre ['lugubri] *adj* mournful; (*sombrio*) gloomy
lula ['lula] *f* squid
lume ['lumi] *m* fire; (*luz*) light; ***dá-me ~*** got a light?; ***fazer ~*** light a fire
luminescência [lumines'sẽsja] *f* luminescence
luminosidade [luminozi'dadʒi] *f* (*claridade*) brightness
luminoso [lumi'nozu] *adj* bright; (*claro*) light
lunar [lu'naɾ] **1** *adj* lunar **2** *m pele*: mole
lunático [lu'natʃiku] **1** *adj* moonstruck; *fig* strange **2** *m fam* madman, oddball
lupa ['lupa] *f* magnifying glass
lúpulo ['lupulu] *m* hop
Lusitânia [luzi'tʌnja] *f* Lusitania
lusitano [luzi'tanu] **1** *adj* Portuguese; *hist* Lusitanian **2** *m*, **-a** *f* Portuguese
luso- ['luzu] Portuguese
lusófono [lu'zɔfunu] *adj* Portuguese-speaking
lustre ['lustɾi] *m* shine; *sociedade*: standing; (*candeeiro*) chandelier; ***dar ~ a*** polish up
lustroso [lus'tɾozu] *adj* shiny
luta ['luta] *f* struggle, fight; ESP wrestling match; *fig* struggle; ***dar ~*** put up a fight; ***~ de boxe*** boxing match; ***~ de classes*** class struggle
lutador [luta'doɾ] *m*, **-a** *f* fighter *tb fig*; ESP wrestler
lutar [lu'taɾ] ⟨1a⟩ fight *tb fig*; ESP wrestle; (*brigar*) fight
luterano [lute'ɾanu] *adj* Lutheran
luto ['lutu] *m* mourning; ***de ~*** in mourning; ***andar de ~*** wear mourning; ***fazer ~*** mourn
luva ['luva] *f* glove; ***~s de boxe*** boxing gloves
luxação [luʃa'sãw] *f* sprain
Luxemburgo [luʃẽ'burgu] *m* Luxembourg
luxo ['luʃu] *m* luxury; ***de ~*** luxury; ***dar-se ao ~ de fazer algo*** allow oneself the luxury of doing sth
luxuoso [lu'ʃwozu] *adj* luxurious
luxúria [lu'ʃuria] *f* luxuriance; (*lascívia*) lust
luz [lus] *f* light; ***ligar / apagar a ~*** switch the light on / off; *fig* ***dar à ~*** give birth to; ***~ de estacionamento*** parking light; *Bras* ***~ de freio*** brake light; *Port* ***~ de marcha-atrás*** reversing light; *Bras* ***~ de ré*** reversing light; *Port* ***~ dos travões*** brake light; ***~es*** *pl* ***de prevenção*** hazard lights, hazards
luzente [lu'zẽtʃi] *adj* shining
luzes ['luzis] *fpl* knowledge; (*cultura*) culture; ***século*** *m* ***das ~*** (the) Enlightenment
luzidio [luzi'dʒiu] *adj* shining
luzir [lu'ziɾ] ⟨3m⟩ shine
Lx. *abr* (***Lisboa***) Lisbon

M

M

m *abr* (***metro***) m (meter); (***minutos***) min. (minutes)
ma [ma] = *pron* ***me*** + *pron* ***a***
má [ma] *f* → ***mau***
maca ['maka] *f* gurney, *Brit* stretcher
maçã [ma'sã] *f* apple; ***~ do rosto*** cheekbone
maçã-de-adão [masãdʒia'dãw] *f Port* ANAT Adam's apple
macabro [ma'kabru] *adj* macabre; ***dança*** *f* ***macabra*** dance of death
macacão [maka'kãw] *m Bras* coveralls, *Brit* overalls
macaco [ma'kaku] *m* monkey; TECN (*cabrestante*) winch; AUTO jack; *Port* (***fato*** *m*) ***~*** coveralls, *Brit* overalls
maçada [ma'sada] *f Port fig* nuisance; (*aborrecimento*) bore

maçador [masa'doɾ] *adj* troublesome; (*aborrecido*) boring
maçaneta [masa'neta] *f* knob
maçapão [masa'pãw] *m* ⟨*sem pl*⟩ marzipan
maçar [ma'saɾ] ⟨1p & 1b⟩ (*aborrecer*) bore; (*irritar*) irritate; (*cansar*) tire
macarrão [maka'hãw] *m* pasta
Macau [ma'kaw] *m* Macau, Macao
macedônia, *Port* **macedónia** [mase'donja] *f* GASTR fruit salad
machadada [maʃa'dada] *f* blow with an ax, *Brit* blow with an axe
machado [ma'ʃadu] *m* ax, *Brit* axe
machismo [ma'ʃizmu] *m* machismo
machista [ma'ʃista] *m pej* male chauvinist
macho ['maʃu] **1** *m* male **2** *adj* male; *homem* macho
machucar [maʃu'kaɾ] ⟨1n⟩ hurt; *contusão*: bruise
maciço [ma'sisu] **1** *adj* massive; *ouro etc* solid **2** *m* GEOG massif
macieira [ma'siejɾa] *f* apple tree
macilento [masi'lẽtu] *adj* emaciated
macio [ma'siu] *adj* soft; (*liso*) smooth; (*suave*) mild; (*brando*) gentle
maço ['masu] *m* mallet; *papel*, *cartas de jogar*: stack; *cigarros*: pack; *notas*: bundle, wad
maconha [ma'kõɲa] *f* cannabis
má-criação [makɾia'sãw] *f* rudeness
maçudo [ma'sudu] *adj* boring, tedious
mácula ['makula] *f* stain
madeira [ma'dejɾa] **1** *f* wood; ~ ***contraplacada*** plywood **2** *m* Madeira (wine)
Madeira [ma'dejɾa] *f* Madeira
madeiramento [madejɾa'mẽtu] *m* woodwork
madeirense [madej'rẽsi] **1** *adj* Madeiran **2** *m/f* Madeiran
madeixa [ma'dejʃa] *f* tuft, lock
madona [ma'dona] *f* Madonna
madrasta [ma'dɾasta] *f* stepmother
madre ['madɾi] *f* nun; (*título de freira*) mother superior
madrepérola [madɾe'pɛɾula] *f* mother of pearl
madrinha [ma'dɾiɲa] *f batismo*: godmother; *casamento*: witness
madrugada [madɾu'gada] *f* early morning; (*amanhecer*) daybreak; ***de*** ~ early in the morning
madrugador [madɾu'gadoɾ] *m*, **-a** *f* early riser, early bird
madrugar [madɾu'gaɾ] ⟨1o⟩ *v/i* get up early
madurar [madu'ɾaɾ] ⟨1a⟩ *v/i* ripen
maduro [ma'duɾu] *adj* ripe; (*sensato*) mature, sensible; (*refletido*) careful
mãe [mãj] *f* mother; ~ ***de aluguel***, *Port* ~ ***de aluguer*** surrogate mother; ~ ***de criação*** foster mother; ~ ***solteira*** single mother
maestro [ma'ɛstɾu] *m* MÚS conductor
mãezinha [mãj'ziɲa] *f* mom, *Brit* mum
magazine [maga'zini] *m Bras loja* department store
magia [ma'ʒia] *f* magic
mágico ['maʒiku] *adj* magic; *efeito* magical
magistério [maʒis'tɛɾiu] *m* teacher training
magistrado [maʒis'tɾadu] *m*, **-a** *f* magistrate, judge
magistratura [maʒistɾa'tuɾa] *f* magistracy; ~ ***judicial*** judicial office
magnânimo [ma'gnʌnimu] *adj* magnanimous
magnata [ma'gnata] *m* magnate, tycoon
magnésia [ma'gnɛzja] *f* magnesia
magnésio [ma'gnɛziu] *m* magnesium
magnete [ma'gnetʃi] *m* magnet
magnético [ma'gnɛtʃiku] *adj* magnetic; ***agulha*** *f* ***magnética*** magnetic needle
magnetismo [magne'tʃizmu] *m* magnetism
magnífico [ma'gnifiku] *adj* magnificent
magnitude [magni'tudʒi] *f* magnitude
mago ['magu] *m* magician
mágoa(s) ['magwa(s)] *f(pl) fig* grief, sorrow
magoado [ma'gwadu] *adj* hurt
magoante [ma'gwãtʃi] *adj* hurtful
magoar [ma'gwaɾ] ⟨1f⟩ bruise; (*doer*) hurt
magreza [ma'gɾeza] *f* thinness
magro ['magɾu] *adj* slim; *carne* lean
maio ['maju] *m* May; ***em*** ~ in May

M

maiô [ma'jo] *m Bras* swimsuit
maionese [majo'nɛzi] *f* mayonnaise, mayo; *fam* ***viajar na ~*** ramble on, *Brit* rabbit on
maior [ma'jɔr] **1** *adj comparativo*: bigger; (*mais velho*) older; *superlativo*: biggest; oldest; (*principal*) main; ***~ de idade*** of age **2** *m/f* adult
maioria [majo'ria] *f* majority; ***em ~*** in the majority; ***a ~ de …*** most of …, the majority of…
maioridade [majori'dadʒi] *f* DIR majority, adulthood; ***alcançar a ~*** come of age, reach the age of majority
maioritário [majori'tariu] *adj* majority *atr*; ***sistema*** *m* ***~*** majority vote system, *Brit* first-past-the-post system
mais [majs] **1** *adv* ◊ more; ***~ uma vez*** one more time; ***~ cinco*** five more; ***~ o menos*** more or less; ***mais ou menos 50*** 50 odd; ***você quer ~ uma cerveja?*** do you want another beer? ◊ *comparativo*: more; ***~ alto*** (***do***) ***que ela*** taller than her; ***~ inteligente*** (***do***) ***que ela*** more intelligent than her ◊ *superlativo*: most; ***a mulher ~ velha*** the oldest woman; ***a idéia ~ interessante*** the most interesting idea ◊ *negativo*: ***ele já não é ~ o mesmo*** he's not the same any more; ***não me ocorre ~ nada*** I can't think of anything more, I can't think of anything else; ***não vou ~ fazer isso*** I won't do it again ◊ ***por ~ difícil que seja*** however difficult it may be
2 *pron* more; ***~ chá?*** more tea?; ***que ~?*** what else?; ***sem ~ nem menos*** for no good reason
3 *prep* plus ***2 ~ 2*** 2 plus 2
4 *conj* ***por ~ que trabalhe*** however much he / she works
mais-que-perfeito [majskeper'fejtu] *m* pluperfect
mais-valia [majzva'lia] *f* COM added value
maître [mɛtr] *m Bras* head waiter, maitre d'
maiúscula [ma'iuskula] *f* capital (letter)
majestade [maʒes'tadʒi] *f* majesty
majestoso [maʒes'tozu] *adj* majestic
major [ma'ʒɔr] *m* major
mal [maw] **1** *adv* badly; (*errado*) wrongly; (*injusto*) unjustly; ***sentir-se ~*** feel bad; ***ele anda ~ de dinheiro*** he is badly off; ***~ pude acreditar*** I could hardly believe it; ***eu ~ cheguei*** I just got here; ***informar / pronunciar ~*** misinform / mispronounce; ***passar ~*** feel sick **2** *conj* hardly, as soon as; ***ele ~ mencionou o seu nome …*** hardly had he mentioned her name … **3** *m* evil; DIR wrong; (*doença*) illness; (*maldade*) harm; (*prejuízo*) damage; ***fazer ~ a*** harm; *comida* be bad for; ***não faria ~ algum*** it wouldn't do any harm at all; ***distinguir o bem do ~*** know the difference between right and wrong; ***levar a ~ algo*** take offense at sth; ***um vestido sem alças não tem nada de ~*** a strapless dress is perfectly harmless; ***ir de ~ a pior*** go from bad to worse
mala ['mala] *f* suitcase; *senhora*: purse, *Brit* handbag; AUTO trunk, *Brit* boot; ***~s*** baggage, luggage; ***fazer a ~, fazer as ~s*** pack; ***~ do correio*** (mail) sack; ***~ de mão*** hand luggage; ***~ térmica*** cool box
mal-afamado [mawafa'madu] *adj* disreputable
malabarismo [malaba'rizmu] *m* juggling; ***fazer ~*** juggle
malabarista [malaba'rista] *m/f* juggler
mal-agradecido [mawgrade'sidu] *adj* ungrateful
malandragem [malã'draʒẽ] *f*, **malandrice** [malã'drisi] *f* swindling
malandro [ma'lãdru] *m* scoundrel; (*perguiçoso*) loafer; (*gatuno*) crook
malar [ma'lar] *m* cheekbone
malária [ma'larja] *f* malaria
malcriado [mawkri'adu] **1** *adj* rude, ill-mannered **2** *m* slob
maldade [maw'dadʒi] *f* wickedness; (*baixeza*) meanness; *crianças*: naughtiness
maldição [mawdʒi'sãw] *f* curse
maldito [maw'dʒitu] *adj* damned
maldizer [mawdʒi'zer] ⟨2t⟩ curse
maleabilidade [maljabili'dadʒi] *f* malleability

M

maleável [ma'ljavew] *adj* malleable
mal-educado [mawedu'kadu] *adj* rude
maledicência [maledʒi'sẽsja] *f* slander
malefício [male'fisiu] *m* harm; (*maldade*) cruelty
maléfico [ma'lɛfiku] *adj* malicious; (*pernicioso*) harmful
mal-entendido [mawẽtẽ'dʒidu] *m* misunderstanding
mal-estar [mawes'taɾ] *m físico* discomfort; *psíquico* uneasiness
maleta [ma'leta] *f* briefcase
malevolência [malevo'lẽsja] *f* malice, spite
malfeitor [mawfej'toɾ] *m*, **-a** *f* wrongdoer
malformação [mawforma'sãw] *f* malformation
malha ['maʎa] *f* mesh; **~ *caída*** run, *Brit* ladder; *Port* **~*s*** *pl*, ***obras*** *fpl* ***de* ~** knitwear; *Port* ***fazer* ~** knit
malhado [ma'ʎadu] *adj* mottled; *cavalo* piebald
malhar [ma'ʎaɾ] ⟨1b⟩ **1** *v/i pop* fall; *exercício*: work out **2** *v/t grão* thresh; *ferro* beat; *fig* (*criticar*) run down
malho ['maʎu] *m* sledgehammer; (*maço*) mallet
mal-humorado [mawumo'ɾadu] *adj* moody
malícia [ma'lisja] *f* malice
malicioso [mali'sjozu] *adj* malicious; (*equívoco*) lewd
maligno [ma'lignu] *adj* MED malignant
mal-intencionado [mawĩtẽsjo'nadu] *adj* malicious
maljeitoso [mawʒej'tozu] *adj* awkward, clumsy
malograr-se [malo'gɾaɾsi] ⟨1e⟩ *v/r* fail
malogro [ma'logɾu] *m* failure
malpassado [mawpa'sadu] *adj* rare; (*mal cozinhado*) underdone
malsucedido [mawsuse'dʒidu] *adj* unsuccessful
malta ['mawta] *f Port pej* mob
malte ['mawtʃi] *m* malt
maltrapilho [mawtɾa'piʎu] **1** *adj* ragged **2** *m* ragamuffin
maltratar [mawtɾa'taɾ] ⟨1b⟩ ill-treat
maluco [ma'luku] **1** *adj fam* crazy, nuts **2** *m*, **-a** *f* madman / woman, nut
maluqueira [malo'kejɾa] *f* madness
maluquice [malu'kisi] *f* crazy idea; (*disparate*) nonsense
malvadez [mawva'des] *f* wickedness
malvado [maw'vadu] **1** *adj* (*pérfido*) wicked, malicious; (*criminoso*) criminal **2** *m*, **-a** *f* villain
Malvinas [maw'vinas] ***as*** (***ilhas***) **~** the Falkland Islands
mama ['mʌma] *f* breast; *vaca*: udder; (*teta*) teat
mamã [mʌ'mã] *f*, **mamãe** [mʌ'mãj] *f Bras* mom, *Brit* mum
mamadeira [mama'dejra] *f Bras* feeding bottle
mamão [ma'mãw] *m Bras* papaya
mamar [ma'maɾ] ⟨1a⟩ *v/i* suck; ***dar de* ~ *a*** breastfeed
mamífero [ma'mifeɾu] *m* mammal
mamilo [ma'milu] *m* nipple; (*teta*) teat
mana ['mʌna] *f fam* sister
manada [ma'nada] *f* herd
manancial [manã'sjaw] *m* spring; *fig* source
mancar [mã'kaɾ] ⟨1n⟩ *v/i* hobble
mancha ['mãʃa] *f* stain; (*defeito*) mark; **~ *de óleo*** oil slick; **~ *de sangue*** bloodstain
Mancha ['mãʃa] *f* (***Canal*** *m* ***da***) **~** English Channel
manchado [mã'ʃadu] *adj* stained
manchar [mã'ʃaɾ] ⟨1a⟩ stain *tb fig*; (*sujar*) soil; *fig* sully
manchete [mã'ʃɛtʃi] *f* headline
mandado [mã'dadu] *m* order; **~ *de busca*** search warrant; **~ *de prisão*** warrant; **~ *de segurança*** injunction
mandamento [mãda'mẽtu] *m* command; REL ***os dez* ~*s*** the ten commandments
mandante [mã'dãtʃi] *m/f* DIR client
mandão [mã'dãw], **-ona** *adj* bossy
mandar [mã'daɾ] ⟨1a⟩ **1** *v/t* order; (*enviar*) send; **~ *alguém fazer algo*** tell s.o. do sth; **~ *fazer algo*** have sth done; ***devias* ~ *lavar o casaco*** you should have your jacket cleaned; **~ *buscar alguém*** send for s.o.; **~ *chamar*** call in; ***ser mandado em-***

bora get the sack; ***~ de volta*** send back **2** *v/i* (*dirigir*) be in charge; **mandar-se** *v/r* ***se manda!*** get lost!
mandatário [mãda'tariu] *m* agent
mandato [mã'datu] *m* mandate
mandíbula [mã'dʒibula] *f* jaw(bone)
mandioca [mã'djɔka] *f* cassava; ***farinha*** *f* ***de ~*** cassava flour
mandrião [mãdri'ãw] **1** *adj* lazy **2** *m*, **-ona** [mãdri'ona] *f* idler, lazybones *sg*
mandriar [mãdri'ar] ⟨1g⟩ laze about
maneira [ma'nejra] *f* manner; (*modo*) way; (*possibilidade*) possibility; ***à ~ de*** like; ***de ~ alguma*** not at all; ***de qualquer ~*** anyway; ***de ~ que*** so that; ***de ~ diferente*** differently; ***de ~ irrefletida*** thoughtlessly; ***ok, vamos fazer da sua ~*** OK, we'll do it your way; ***~s*** *pl* manners; ***não ter ~s*** have no manners
maneirismo [manej'rizmu] *m* mannerism
maneiro [ma'nejru] *adj* manageable; (*cômodo*) easy; (*jeitoso*) capable; *fam* great, super
manejar [mane'ʒar] ⟨1d⟩ handle; *dispositivo* work; (*saber tratar com*) know how to handle; *barco, pessoa* steer
manejável [mane'ʒavew] *adj* manageable; (*dominável*) controllable
manejo [ma'neʒu] *m* handling; (*comando*) operation; (*tratamento*) treatment
manequim [mane'kĩ] *m* dummy; *pessoa* model
manga[1] ['mãga] *f* sleeve; ***de ~ comprida / curta*** long- / shortsleeved; ***dar ~s*** allow movement
manga[2] ['mãga] *f* BOT mango
mangueira[1] [mã'gejra] *f* hose(pipe)
mangueira[2] [mã'gejra] *f* BOT mango tree
manha ['maɲa] *f* trick; (*astúcia*) craftiness, guile
manhã [ma'ɲã] *f* morning; ***de ~, pela ~*** in the morning; ***amanhã de ~*** tomorrow morning
manhoso [ma'ɲozu] *adj* crafty; (*traiçoeiro*) sly
mania [ma'nia] *f* MED mania; *fig* craze
maníaco [ma'niaku] *adj* MED manic; *fig* obsessed; ***~ por*** obsessed with
manicômio, *Port* **manicómio** [mani'komiu] *m* asylum, mental hospital
manicure [mani'kuri] *f*, *Port* **manicura** [mani'kura] *f* manicure
manifestação [manifesta'sãw] *f* expression; POL rally: (*demonstração*) demonstration; (*sinal*) sign
manifestante [manifes'tãtʃi] *m/f* demonstrator
manifestar [manifes'tar] ⟨1c⟩ **1** *v/t* show, display; (*expressar*) express **2** *v/i* POL demonstrate; **manifestar-se** *v/r* manifest itself
manifesto [mani'fɛstu] **1** *adj* obvious, manifest **2** *m* manifesto
manipulação [manipula'sãw] *f* manipulation; (*manejo*) handling
manipular [manipu'lar] ⟨1a⟩ manipulate; (*utilizar*) handle
manipulador [manipula'dor] *adj* manipulative
manipulável [manipu'lavew] *adj* manipulable
manivela [mani'vɛla] *f* crank; ***~ de comando*** control lever
manjar [mã'ʒar] *m* delicacy
manjericão [mãʒeri'kãw] *m* basil
manjerona [mãʒe'rona] *f* marjoram
mano ['mʌnu] *m fam* brother; ***~s*** *pl* siblings
manobra [ma'nɔbra] *f* NÁUT, MIL maneuver, *Brit* manoeuvre; *quartel*: drill; FERROV shunting; TECN operation; (*conexão*) connection
manobrar [mano'brar] ⟨1e⟩ maneuver, *Brit* manoeuvre; FERROV shunt
manômetro, *Port* **manómetro** [ma'nometru] *m* pressure gage, *Brit* pressure gauge, manometer
mansão [mã'sãw] *f* mansion
mansarda [mã'sarda] *f* garret, attic
manso ['mãsu] *adj* gentle; (*suave*) mild; *caráter* gentle; *animal* tame; calm
manta ['mãta] *f* blanket; *roda*: rim
manteiga [mã'tejga] *f* butter
manteigueira [mãtej'gejra] *f* butter dish
manter [mã'ter] ⟨2xa⟩ keep; *família* support; *paz* keep, maintain; *ritmo* keep up, maintain; *opinião* stick to; ***~ algo para si mesmo*** keep sth

for oneself; **~ *alguém em dia*** keep s.o. up to date; **~ *contato com alguém*** keep *ou* stay in contact with s.o.; **manter-se** *v/r* **~ *calmo*** keep calm, stay calm; **~ *informado de algo*** keep oneself in the picture; **~ *unido*** stay together
mantilha [mã'tʃiʎa] *f* mantilla, veil
mantimento [mãtʃi'mẽtu] *m* maintenance; **~s** *pl* provisions
manto ['mãtu] *m* cloak
manual [ma'nwaw] **1** *adj* manual **2** *m* manual
manufatura, *Port* **manufactura** [manufa'tuɾa] *f* manufacture
manufaturar, *Port* **manufacturar** [manufatu'ɾaɾ] ⟨1a⟩ *v/t* manufacture
manuscrito [manus'kɾitu] **1** *adj* handwritten **2** *m* manuscript
manusear [manu'zjaɾ] ⟨1l⟩ *v/t* handle; ***fácil de ~*** user-friendly
manutenção [manutẽ'sãw] *f* maintenance; (*sustento*) upkeep; (*administração*) administration
mão [mãw] *f* ⟨*pl* ~s⟩ hand; *medida* handful; (*camada*) coat; *estrada*: lane; ***de primeira / segunda ~*** first- / second-hand; **~ *única*** one-way traffic, ***à ~ direita / esquerda*** right / left hand; ***dar uma ~ a alguém*** give s.o. a hand; ***~s ao alto!*** hands up!; ***~s à obra!*** let's go to work!; ***ter ~ em*** be in control of; ***abrir ~ de*** part with
mão-de-obra [mãw'dʒiɔbɾa] *f* labor, *Brit* labour; *pessoal* workforce
mão-francesa [mãwfɾã'seza] *f* ⟨*pl* mãos-francesas⟩ bracket
mapa ['mapa] *m* map; **~ *da cidade*** city map; **~ *das estradas*** road map; **~ *meteorológico*** weather chart
maqueta [ma'kɛta] *f*, **maquete** [ma'kɛtʃi] *f* model
maquiador [makia'doɾ] *m*, **-a** *f* beautician; TEAT, TV make-up artist
maquiagem [maki'aʒẽ] *f* make-up
maquiar [maki'ar] ⟨1a⟩ make up; **maquiar-se** *v/r* put one's make-up on
maquilh... *Port* → ***maqui...***
máquina ['makina] *f* machine; (*aparelho*) machinery; FERROV engine; *fam* car; ***à ~*** by machine; **~ *automática de bebidas*** drinks dispenser; **~ *de barbear*** electric razor; **~ *de costura*** sewing machine; **~ *de escrever*** typewriter; **~ *fotográfica*** camera; **~ *de lavar loiça*** dishwasher; **~ *de lavar roupa*** washing machine
maquinal [maki'naw] *adj* machine *atr*; *fig* mechanical; (*involuntário*) involuntary
maquinar [maki'naɾ] ⟨1a⟩ *v/t* plot
maquinaria [makina'ɾia] *f* plant, machinery
maquinismo [maki'nizmu] *m* mechanism; TEAT stage machinery
maquinista [maki'nista] *m/f* machinist; FERROV engineer, *Brit* engine driver
mar [maɾ] *m* sea; ***homem ao ~!*** man overboard!; ***Mar Morto*** Dead Sea; ***Mar Negro / Vermelho*** Black / Red Sea
maracujá [maɾaku'ʒa] *m* passion fruit
maratona [maɾa'tona] *f* marathon; **~ *de televisão*** telethon
maravilha [maɾa'viʎa] *f* wonder; ***à ~*** wonderfully
maravilhar-se [maɾavi'ʎaɾsi] ⟨1a⟩ *v/r* marvel (***com*** at)
maravilhoso [maɾavi'ʎozu] *adj* marvelous, *Brit* marvellous
marca ['maɾka] *f* mark; ECON brand; **~ *líder*** leading brand; **~ *do pênalti*** penalty spot; **~ *registrada***, *Port* **~ *registada*** registered trademark
marcação [maɾka'sãw] *f* marking; *rótulo*: label; NÁUT plotting; (*reserva*) reservation; *Port* TEL dialing, *Brit* dialling
marcador [maɾka'doɾ] *m caneta*: marker; *jogo*: scorer; **~ *fluorescente*** highlighter (pen), marker pen
marcapasso [maɾka'pasu] *m* MED pacemaker
marcar [maɾ'kaɾ] ⟨1n & 1b⟩ mark; (*rotular*) label; (*reservar*) reserve; *Port* TEL dial; *prazo, itinerário* fix; *hora, pontos etc* set; *golo* score; NÁUT plot; **~ *hora*** make an appointment; **~ *o placar*** keep the score; ***vou ~ a minha posição*** I'm going to make a stand on this
marceneiro [maɾse'nejɾu] *m*, **-a** *f* car-

M

penter
marcha ['marʃa] *f* march *tb fig*; TECN operation; AUTO gear; *fig* course; (*desenvolvimento*) progress, development; AUTO **~ *à re***, *Port* **~ *atrás*** reverse (gear); **~ *festiva*** procession; AUTO **~ *de força*** high, top
marchar [mar'ʃar] ⟨1b⟩ go; MIL, MÚS march; *máquina* run; *veículo* go; *fig* progress; (*desenvolver-se*) develop
marco ['marku] *m* boundary stone; *fig* milestone; *Port* **~ *postal*** mailbox, *Brit* letterbox
março ['marsu] *m* March; ***em* ~** in March
maré [ma'rɛ] *f* tide; *fig* ups and downs; **~ *alta*** high tide; **~ *baixa*** low tide; **~ *enchente*** flood tide, incoming tide; **~ *negra*** oil pollution; **~ *vazante*** ebb tide, outgoing tide
mareado [ma'rjadu] *adj* seasick
marechal [mare'ʃaw] *m* marshal; **~ *de campo*** field marshal
maremoto [mare'mɔtu] *m* (underwater) earthquake
marfim [mar'fĩ] *m* ivory
margarida [marga'rida] *f* BOT daisy
margarina [marga'rina] *f* margarine
margem ['marʒẽ] *f* edge; *rio*: bank; *lucro*, *documento*: margin; ***à* ~ *de*** alongside; ***dar* ~ *a algo*** permit sth; ***por uma pequena* ~** by a narrow margin; **~ *de lucro*** profit margin; **~ *do cais*** quayside; ***inundar suas margens*** burst its banks
marginal [marʒi'naw] **1** *adj* marginal; *costa*: coastal; ***homem*** *m* **~** outsider **2** *m/f* minor figure; PSICOL dropout; *pej* delinquent **3** *f* *estrada* coastal road
marginalidade [marʒinali'dadʒi] *f* delinquency
marginalizado [marʒinali'zadu] **1** *adj* marginalized **2** *m*, **-a** *f* outsider
marginalizar [marʒinali'zar] ⟨1a⟩ marginalize
maria-vai-com-as-outras [maria-vajkõa'zotras] *m/f* copycat
maricas [ma'rikas] *m* *Port fam* fairy, fag
marido [ma'ridu] *m* husband
marijuana [mari'hwana] *f* marijuana
marinha [ma'riɲa] *f* navy; *navíos* fleet
marinheiro [mari'ɲejru] *m*, **-a** *f* seaman, sailor
marinho [ma'riɲu], **marino** [ma'rinu] *adj* sea *atr*, marine *atr*
marionete [marjo'nɛtʃi] *f* puppet
mariposa [mari'poza] *f* moth
mariscos [ma'riskus] *m* shellfish *pl*; ***sopa*** *f* ***de* ~** shellfish soup
marital [ma'ritaw] *adj* marital
marítimo [ma'ritʃimu] *adj* maritime; ***milha*** *f* ***marítima*** nautical mile; ***pesca*** *f* ***marítima*** deep-sea fishing
marketing ['marketʃi] *m* marketing
marmelada [marme'lada] *f* quince jam
marmelo [mar'mɛlu] *m* quince; *pop* **~*s*** tits
marmita [mar'mita] *f* pot; *lancheira* lunch box; ***trazer* ~** brown-bag it
mármore ['marmuri] *m* marble
maroto [ma'rotu] **1** *m* good-for-nothing, rogue; (*gatuno*) crook **2** *adj* useless; (*manhoso*) sly, cunning; *criança* naughty
marquês [mar'kes] *m* marquis
marquesa[1] [mar'keza] *f* MED examining couch
marquesa[2] [mar'keza] *f* *nobreza*: marchioness
marquise [mar'kizi] *f* (*toldo*) canopy; (*varanda*) veranda
marrar [ma'har] ⟨1b⟩ butt
marreta [ma'heta] *f* sledgehammer
marta ['marta] *f* mink
Marrocos [ma'hɔkus] *mpl* Morocco
marrom [ma'hõ] *adj Bras* brown
marroquino [maho'kinu] **1** *adj* Moroccan **2** *m*, **-a** *f* Moroccan
Marte ['martʃi] *m* Mars
martelada [marte'lada] *f* blow (with a hammer); *ruído* hammering
martelar [marte'lar] ⟨1c⟩ hammer; (*moer*) wear down; *fig* ***vou* ~ *esta idéia*** I'm going to hammer this point home
martelo [mar'tɛlu] *m* hammer; (***peixe*** *m*) **~** hammerhead shark; **~ *pneumático*** pneumatic drill; *fig* ***a* ~** by force; ***ensinar alguém a* ~** hammer things into s.o
mártir ['martʃir] *m/f* martyr

martírio [mar'tʃiriu] *m* torment; REL martyrdom
martirizar [martʃiri'zar] ⟨1a⟩ torment
marujo [ma'ruʒu] *m* sailor
marulho [ma'ruʎu] *m* swell
marxismo [mar'ksizmu] *m* Marxism
marxista [mar'ksista] **1** *m/f* Marxist **2** *adj* Marxist
mas [mas] *conj* but
mascar [mas'kar] ⟨1n & 1b⟩ chew
máscara ['maskara] *f* mask; ***largar / deixar a ~*** drop / throw off the mask
mascote [mas'kɔtʃi] *f* mascot
masculino [masku'linu] *adj* masculine; *animal* male
másculo ['maskulu] *adj animal* male
masmorra [maz'moha] *f* dungeon
masoquismo [mazo'kizmu] *m* masochism
masoquista [mazo'kista] *m/f* masochist
massa ['masa] *f* mass *tb fig*; GASTR dough; (*esparguete etc*) pasta; TECN putty; *fam* ***que ~!*** that's really cool; *fam* ***ela é muito ~*** she's really cool; *fam* ***pôr a mão na ~*** get stuck in; ***turismo*** *m* ***de ~s*** mass tourism; ***as ~s*** the masses; ***~s*** *pl* ***alimentícias*** pasta; ***~ folhada*** puff pastry; ***~ de tomate*** tomato purée
massacrar [masa'krar] ⟨1b⟩ massacre; *pop* annoy
massacre [ma'sakri] *m* massacre
massagear [masa'ʒjar] ⟨1l⟩ *v/t* massage
massagem [ma'saʒẽ] *f* massage; ***dar ~ a*** give a massage
massagista [masa'ʒista] *m/f* masseur *m*, masseuse *f*
massivo [ma'sivu] *adj* massive
mastigar [mastʃi'gar] ⟨1o⟩ chew; (*murmurar*) murmur; *fig* think over, *fam* chew over
mastro ['mastru] *m* mast; ***~ de bandeira*** flagpole; ***~ grande*** mainmast
masturbação [masturba'sãw] *f* masturbation
masturbar-se [mastur'barsi] ⟨1a⟩ *v/r* masturbate
mata ['mata] *f* forest
mata-borrão [matabo'hãw] *m* blotting paper
matadouro [mata'doru] *m* slaughterhouse, *Brit* abattoir; *fig* bloodbath
matagal [mata'gaw] *m* wilderness, scrubland
matança [ma'tãsa] *f* massacre; *porco*: slaughter
matar [ma'tar] ⟨1b; *pp* morto⟩ *v/t* kill; *gado* slaughter; *tempo* kill; *fome etc* satisfy; *sede* quench; *aula* skip; **matar-se** *v/r* kill oneself
mate[1] ['matʃi] *adj* matt
mate[2] ['matʃi] *m xadrez*: (check)mate
mate[3] ['matʃi] *m chá* maté tea
matemática [mate'matʃika] *f* mathematics, math, *Brit* maths *sg*
matemático [mate'matʃiku] **1** *adj* mathematical **2** *m*, **-a** *f* mathematician
matéria [ma'tɛria] *f* matter, material; (*tema*) subject, topic; (*coisa*) matter; *exame*: subject
material [mate'riaw] **1** *adj* physical, material **2** *m* material; ***~ didático*** teaching aid; ***~ impresso*** printed matter; ***~ promocional*** promotional material
materialismo [materia'lizmu] *m* materialism
materialista [materia'lista] *adj* materialistic
materialização [materializa'sãw] *f* embodiment
materializar [materiali'zar] ⟨1a⟩ materialize; (*representar*) embody; **materializar-se** *v/r* materialize
matéria-prima [ma'tɛria'prima] *f* ⟨*pl* matérias-primas⟩ raw material
maternal [mater'naw] *adj*, **materno** [ma'tɛrnu] *adj* motherly, maternal; ***avô*** *m* ***materno*** maternal grandfather
maternidade [materni'dadʒi] *f* motherhood, maternity; *hospital* maternity hosptial
matilha [ma'tʃiʎa] *f* mob; *cães*: pack
matinal [matʃi'naw] *adj* morning *atr*
matiné [matʃi'ne] *f* CINE, TEAT matinée
matiz [ma'tʃis] *m* coloring, *Brit* colouring; (*tonalidade*) tone, shade
matizado [matʃi'zadu] *adj* colorful, *Brit* colourful; (*reluzente*) shimmer-

M

ing
mato ['matu] *m* bush; (*matagal*) scrubland
matriarca [matri'arka] *f* matriarch
matricídio [matri'sidiu] *m* matricide
matrícula [ma'trikula] *f* registration; (*registro*) register; UNIV matriculation, enrollment, *Brit* enrolment; *taxa*: enrollment fee; AUTO license plate, *Brit* registration plate
matricular [matriku'lar] ⟨1a⟩ enroll, *Brit* enrol, register; UNIV matriculate
matrimonial [matrimo'njaw] *adj* marriage *atr*, matrimonial
matrimônio, *Port* **matrimónio** [matri'moniu] *m instituição* marriage; *ato* wedding
matriz [ma'tris] *f* matrix; ANAT womb; TECN mold, *Brit* mould; COM head office; **~ *predial*** land register
maturação [matura'sãw] *f* maturing, ripening
maturidade [maturi'dadʒi] *f* maturity
matutino [matu'tʃinu] **1** *adj* morning *atr* **2** *m* morning paper
mau [maw] **1** *adj*, **má** *f* bad; *moralmente* evil; (*errado*) wrong **2** *m* ***o ~*** evil **3** *int* ***~!*** what the heck!
maxila [ma'ksila] *f* jawbone; ***~ inferior / superior*** lower / upper jaw
maxilar [maksi'lar] **1** *adj* jaw **2** *m* jawbone
máxima ['masima] *f* maxim
maximizar [maksimi'zar] ⟨1a⟩ *v/t* maximize
máximo ['masimu] **1** *adj* greatest; *o maior possível* maximum **2** *m* maximum; ***Eusébio é o ~*** Eusebio is the greatest; ***ao ~*** to the utmost; ***no ~*** at most; ***~s*** *pl* AUTO high beam
me [mi] *pron* me; *indireto* (to) me; ***~ dá isso*** give it (to) me
meada ['meada] *f* skein, hank
meado ['meadu] *m* middle; ***no ~ do mês*** in the middle of the month; ***no ~ de junho*** mid-June
mealheiro [mja'ʎejru] *m* money box
Meca ['mɛka] *f* Mecca
mecânica [me'kʌnika] *f* mechanics; (*mecanismo*) mechanism; ***~ de precisão*** precision engineering
mecânico [me'kʌniku] **1** *adj* mechanical **2** *m*, **-a** *f* mechanic; ***~ de automóveis*** motor mechanic
mecanismo [meka'nizmu] *m* mechanism; (*maquinaria*) machinery
mecanização [mekaniza'sãw] *f* ⟨*sem pl*⟩ mechanization
mecanizar [mekani'zar] ⟨1a⟩ mechanize
mecenas [me'senas] *m* patron
mecha ['mɛʃa] *f* wick; (*rastilho*) fuse; *bocado de cabelo* tuft; TECN stopper; ***~s no cabelo*** highlights
medalha [me'daʎa] *f* medal, medallion; ***~ de ouro / prata / bronze*** gold / silver / bronze medal
média ['mɛdʒia] *f* average; ***em ~*** on average; ***acima / abaixo da ~*** above / below average
mediação [medʒia'sãw] *f* mediation
mediador [medʒia'dor] **1** *adj* mediating **2** *m*, **-a** *f* mediator
mediano [me'dʒianu] *adj* average
mediante [me'dʒiãtʃi] *prep* by means of
medicação [medʒika'sãw] *f* medication
medicamento [medʒika'mẽtu] *m* medicine
medicamentoso [medʒikamẽ'tozu] *adj* healing, medicinal
medicar [medʒi'kar] ⟨1n⟩ treat; ***ela tem que ser medicada*** she needs medication
medicina [medʒi'sina] *f* medicine; ***~ legal*** forensic medicine
medicinal [medʒisi'naw] *adj* medicinal
médico ['mɛdʒiku] **1** *m*, **-a** *f* doctor; ***~-especialista*** specialist **2** *adj* medical
medida [me'dʒida] *f* measure; (*bitola*) scale *tb fig*; *vestido etc*: size; *fig* ***à ~ de*** according to; ***sem ~*** excessive, countless; ***sob ~*** bespoke; ***tomar ~s*** take measures, take steps
medieval [medie'vaw] *adj*, **medievo** [me'diɛvu] *adj* medieval
medidor [medʒi'dor] *m* gage, *Brit* gauge
médio ['mɛdiu] **1** *adj* middle, medium; (*regular*) average; ***classe*** *f* ***média*** middle class **2** *m futebol*: mid-

M

field player, midfielder **3** *m* AUTO **~s** *pl* dimmed headlights
medíocre [me'dʒiukri] *adj* mediocre
medir [me'dʒir] ⟨3r⟩ (*tirar medidas*) measure; (*calcular*) estimate; (*avaliar*) evaluate
meditação [medʒita'sãw] *f* meditation
meditar [medʒi'tar] ⟨1a⟩ (*refletir*) meditate
mediterrâneo [medʒite'hʌniu] **1** *adj* Mediterranean **2** *m* **Mediterrâneo** Mediterranean
mediterrânico [medʒite'hʌniku] *adj* → **mediterrâneo**
medo ['medu] *m* fear (**de** of); **com ~** afraid; **estar com ~** be afraid; **morrer de ~** be frightened to death
medroso [me'drozu] *adj* frightened
medula [me'dula] *f* marrow; *fig* core
medusa [me'duza] *f* jellyfish
megabyte [mɛga'bajtʃi] *m* megabyte
meia[1] ['meja] *f* stocking; *Bras curta* sock; **~ curta** sock; **fazer ~** knit
meia[2] ['meja] *f* half; **pagar a ~s** pay fifty-fifty
meia(s)-calça(s) [meja(s)'kawsa(s)] *f(pl)* pantihose, *Brit* tights
meia-estação [mejasta'sãw] *f* ⟨*pl* meias-estações⟩ spring; fall, *Brit* autumn
meia-idade [mejai'dadʒi] *f* middle age
meia-irmã [mejair'mã] *f* half-sister
meia-lua [meja'lua] *f* half-moon
meia-luz [meja'lus] *f* subdued light
meia-noite [meja'nojtʃi] *f* midnight
meigo ['mejgu] *adj* sweet; *criança*, *animal* trusting
meio ['meiu] **1** *adj* half; **um e ~, uma e meia** one and a half; **é ~ a ~** it's half and half; **meia hora** *f* half an hour; **meia pensão** *f* half board **2** *adv* half; **~ dormido** half asleep **3** *m* middle; (*auxílio*) means *sg*; (*instrumento*) tool; FÍS medium; **~s** *pl* means; **~s** *pl* **de comunicação** media; **~ ambiente** environment; **~ de transporte** means of transport
meio-bilhete [mejobi'ʎetʃi] *m* ⟨*pl* meios-bilhetes⟩ child's ticket
meio-dia [mejo'dʒia] *m* midday; **ao ~** midday
meio-fio [mejo'fiu] *m* curb, *Brit* kerb
meio-irmão [meiuir'mãw] *m* ⟨*pl* meios-irmãos⟩ half-brother
meio-termo [mejo'termu] *m* compromise
mel [mɛw] *m* honey
melancia [melã'sia] *f* watermelon
melancolia [melãko'lia] *f* melancholy, sadness
melancólico [melã'kɔliku] *adj* melancholy, sad
melão [me'lãw] *m* melon
meleca [me'lɛka] *m Bras pop* snot
melhor [me'ʎɔr] **1** *adj comparativo*: better; *superlativo*: **o / a ~** the best; **ser o / a ~** be the best; **levar a ~** come off best; **~ de vida** better off **2** *adv comparativo*: better; *superlativo*: best **3** *m* the best; **fazer o ~** do one's best **4** *int* **~!** so much the better!
melhora [me'ʎɔra] *f* improvement; **boas ~s!** get well soon!
melhoramento [meʎora'mẽtu] *m* improvement
melhorar [meʎo'rar] ⟨1e⟩ **1** *v/t* improve; (*refazer*) make better **2** *v/i* improve; *saúde*: get better
melhoria [meʎo'ria] *f saúde*: improvement; (*vantagem*) advantage; **ter ~** mend one's ways
melindrar [melĩ'drar] ⟨1a⟩ offend, hurt
melindre [me'lĩdri] *m* sensitivity
melindroso [melĩ'drozu] *adj assunto* tricky, delicate
meloa [me'loa] *f* cantaloupe melon
melodia [melo'dʒia] *f* melody, tune
melodioso [melo'djozu] *adj* melodic
melodramático [mɛlodra'matʃiku] *adj* melodramatic
melro ['mɛlhu] *m* blackbird
membrana [mẽ'brana] *f* membrane
membro ['mẽbru] *m* limb; (*sócio*) member
memorável [memo'ravew] *adj* memorable
memória [me'mɔrja] *f* memory; (*lembrança*) souvenir; **~s** *pl* memoirs
memorizar [memori'zar] ⟨1a⟩ *v/t* memorize
menção [mẽ'sãw] *f* mention

mencionar [mẽsjo'naɾ] ⟨1f⟩ mention
mendigar [mẽdʒi'gaɾ] ⟨1o⟩ **1** *v/t* beg for **2** *v/i* beg
mendigo [mẽ'dʒigu] *m*, **-a** *f* beggar
menina [me'nina] *f* (*criança*) (little) girl; ***a ~ quer sentar-se*** would you like to sit down, miss; ***~ do olho*** pupil; *fig* apple of one's eye
meningite [menĩ'ʒitʃi] *f* meningitis
meninice [meni'nisi] *f* childhood; (*infantilidade*) childishness
menino [me'ninu] *m* (little) boy
menopausa [mɛno'pawza] *f* menopause
menor [me'nɔɾ] **1** *adj tamanho*: smaller; *superlativo* smallest; *número, valor*: lower; *superlativo* lowest; DIR, MÚS minor; ***~ de idade*** under age; ***não tenho a ~ idéia*** I haven't the slightest idea **2** *m/f* juvenile; DIR minor
menoridade [menori'dadʒi] *f* ***por causa da ~ ele ...*** because he was under age, ...
menos ['menus] **1** *adj quantidade*: less; *número*: fewer; ***~ água*** less water; ***~ homens*** fewer men **2** *adv* less, ***~ interessante do que*** less interesting than; *superlativo*: ***o ~ interessante*** the least interesting; ***ao ~, pelo ~*** at least; ***se ao ~*** if only; ***muito ~*** much less, let alone; ***a ~ que*** unless **3** *prep* except; MAT minus; ***estava tudo ~ pronto*** it was anything but ready; *Port* ***são cinco ~ um quarto*** it's a quarter of five, *Brit* it's a quarter to five **4** *m* ***o ~*** the least
menosprezar [menospre'zaɾ] ⟨1c⟩ underrate; (*desprezar*) despise, scorn
menosprezo [menos'prezu] *m* disdain, contempt
mensageiro [mẽsa'ʒejɾu] *m*, **-a** *f* messenger
mensagem [mẽ'saʒẽ] *f* message; ***~ de erro*** error message; ***~ telefônica*** telephone message; ***~ de texto*** text (message); ***mandar uma ~ de texto a alguém*** text s.o., send s.o. a text
mensal [mẽ'saw] *adj* monthly; ***rendimento** m **~*** monthly income
mensalidade [mẽsali'dadʒi] *f* (*quantia*) monthly amount; (*pagamento*) monthly payment; (*ordenado*) monthly salary; ***pagamento** m **em ~s*** monthly payment
menstruação [mẽstɾua'sãw] *f* period, menstruation
menstruar [mẽstɾu'aɾ] ⟨1g⟩ *v/i* menstruate
menta ['mẽta] mint
mental [mẽ'taw] *adj* mental; ***cálculo** m **~*** mental arithmetic
mentalidade [mẽtali'dadʒi] *f* mentality
mente ['mẽtʃi] *f* mind; ***ter em ~*** bear in mind
mente[2] ['mẽtʃi] → ***mentir***
mentir [mẽ'tʃiɾ] ⟨3e⟩ lie
mentira [mẽ'tʃiɾa] *f* lie; ***parece ~!*** unbelievable!; ***~ branca*** white lie
mentiroso [mẽtʃi'rozu] **1** *adj* lying, deceitful **2** *m*, **-a** *f* liar
menu [me'nu] *m* menu *tb* INFORM; ***~ de atalho*** pull-down menu
mercado [meɾ'kadu] *m* market; ***~ Interno*** domestic market; ***~ mundial*** global market; ***~ negro*** black market; ***Mercado Único Europeu*** European Single Market
mercadoria [meɾkado'ɾia] *f* commodity; ***~s*** goods
mercantil [meɾkã'tʃiw] *adj* commercial, mercantile
mercearia [meɾsja'ɾia] *f* grocery store, *Brit* grocer's
merceeiro [meɾ'siejɾu] *m*, **-a** *f* grocer
mercenário [meɾse'naɾiu] *m* mercenary
mercúrio [meɾ'kuɾiu] *m* mercury
merda ['mɛɾda] *f vulg* shit; ***ir à ~*** fuck off
merdas ['mɛɾdas] *m vulg* jerk, asshole
merecer [mere'seɾ] ⟨2g⟩ *v/t* deserve; *gratidão etc* earn
merecido [mere'sidu] *adj* just, deserved
merecimento [meresi'mẽtu] *m* merit
merenda [me'ɾẽda] *f* snack
merengue [me'ɾẽŋgi] *m* GASTR meringue
meretriz [mere'tɾis] *f* prostitute
mergulhador [meɾguʎa'doɾ] *m*, **-a** *f* diver

M

mergulhar [mergu'ʎar] ⟨1a⟩ **1** *v/i* dive **2** *v/t* **~ *algo em algo*** dip sth in sth
mergulho [mer'guʎu] *m* dive; *atividade* diving; AERO nose-dive; **~ *autônomo*** scuba diving
meridiano [meri'dʒianu] **1** *m* meridian **2** *adj* midday; GEOG meridian
meridional [meridjo'naw] **1** *adj* southern **2** *m/f* southerner
mérito ['mɛritu] *m* merit
mero ['mɛru] *adj* mere
mês [mes] *m* month; ***por* ~** monthly, by the month; **(*no*) *fim do* ~** (at) the end of the month
mesa ['meza] *f* table; *de trabalho* desk; (*comissão*) board; ***pôr / levantar a* ~** set / clear the table; **~ *de jantar*** dining table
mesa-de-cabeceira [mezadʒikabe'sejra] *f* ⟨*pl* mesas-de cabeceira⟩ bedside table
mesinha [me'ziɲa] *f* **~ *de centro*** coffee table
mesmo ['mezmu], **mesma** ['mezma] **1** *adj* same; ***ele* ~** himself; ***ela mesma*** herself **2** *adv* even; (*muito*) really; ***agora* ~** just now; ***hoje* ~** this very day; ***isso* ~!** exactly!; **~ *assim*** even so; **~ *se*** even if; **~ *bom*** really good; ***isso* ~!** that's it!; ***é* ~?** is that so? **3** *m/f* ***o* ~, *a -a*** the same (***que*** as); ***dar no* ~** come to the same thing; ***o* ~, *por favor*** same again, please
mesocarpo [mezo'karpu] *m* pith
mesquinharia [meskiɲa'ria], **mesquinhez** [meski'ɲes] *f* meanness; (*insignificância*) trifle; (*pobreza*) wretchedness
mesquinho [mes'kiɲu] *adj* mean; petty; (*reles*) shabby; (*pobre*) wretched
mesquita [mes'kita] *f* mosque
mestiço [mes'tʃisu] *m*, **-a** *f* half-caste, person of mixed race
mestrado [mes'tradu] *m* master's (degree)
mestre ['mɛstri] **1** *m*, **-a** *f* master; (*professor*) teacher; **~ *de cerimônias*** master of ceremonies, MC **2** *adj* (*magistral*) masterly; (*principal*) main; *chave* master *atr*
mestre-cuca [mɛstre'kuka] *m* chef
mestre-de-obras [mɛstre'dʒiɔbras] *m* foreman
meta ['mɛta] *m* aim, goal; *produção etc*: target; ESP finish line
metabolismo [metabo'lizmu] *m* MED metabolism
metade [me'tadʒi] *f* half
metáfora [me'tafura] *f* metaphor
metafórico [meta'fɔriku] *adj* metaphorical
metal [me'taw] *m* metal
metálico [me'taliku] *adj* metallic
metalurgia [metalur'ʒia] *f* metallurgy
metalúrgico [meta'lurʒiku] **1** *adj* metallurgical **2** *m*, **-a** *f* metal worker
metamorfose [metamor'fɔzi] *f* metamorphosis
metástase [me'tastazi] *f* MED metastasis
meteórico [me'teɔriku] *adj fig* meteoric
meteorito [meteo'ritu] *m* meteorite
meteoro [me'teɔru] *m* meteor
meteorologia [meteorolo'ʒia] *f* meteorology
meteorológico [meteoro'lɔʒiku] *adj* meteorological; ***boletim*** *m* **~** weather report; ***serviço*** *m* **~** weather station
meteorologista [meteorolo'ʒista] *m/f* meteorologist; TV weatherman; weather girl
meter [me'ter] ⟨2c⟩ **1** *v/t* put; **~ *gasolina*** get some gas, fill up; *fam* **~ *a mão*** (*ou* ***unha***) pinch **2** *v/i* **~ *por*** go along; **meter-se** *v/r* get involved (***em*** in); **~ *a caminho*** set off; ***se eu fosse você, não me meteria*** I would keep out of it if I were you
meticuloso [metʃiku'lozu] *adj* meticulous
metido [me'tʃidu] *adj* curious, nosy
metódico [me'tɔdʒiku] *adj* methodical
método ['mɛtudu] *m* method
metralhadora [metraʎa'dora] *f* machine gun
métrico ['mɛtriku] *adj* metric; ***fita*** *f* ***métrica*** tape measure
metro[1] ['mɛtru] *m* meter, *Brit* metre
metrô[2] ['mɛtro] *m*, *Port* **metro**

[me'tru] *m* subway, *Brit* underground; ***estação** f **de ~*** subway station; ***rede** f **de ~*** subway network
metrópole [me'trɔpuli] *f* metropolis; (*capital*) capital
metropolitano [metropoli'tanu] *f* subway, *Brit* underground
meu [mew], **minha** ['miɲa] **1** *adj* my **2** *pron* mine **3** *m/f* ***o ~, a minha*** mine
mexer [me'ʃer] ⟨2c⟩ **1** *v/t* stir; (*mover*) move **2** *v/i* move; ***~ em*** (*tocar*) touch; *assunto* touch on; ***~ com*** fiddle around with; *mulher* mess around with; **mexer-se** *v/r* move; *irrequieto* fidget; (*apressar-se*) get a move on; ***mexe-te!*** get a move on!, move yourself!; ***ela mexe-se bem*** she's a doer
mexerico [meʃe'riku] *m* gossip
mexeriqueiro [meʃeri'kejru] *m*, **-a** *f* gossip
mexicano [meʃi'kanu] **1** *adj* Mexican **2** *m*, **-a** *f* Mexican
México ['mɛʃiku] *m* ***o ~*** Mexico
mexida [me'ʃida] *f* disorder, confusion
mexilhão [meʃi'ʎãw] *m* mussel
mi [mi] *m* MÚS E
miar [mjar] ⟨1g⟩ miaow
micro... [mikru-] micro...
micróbio [mi'krɔbiu] *m* microbe
microcomputador [mikrokõputa'dor] *m* microcomputer
microchip [mikro'ʃip] *m* microchip
microcosmo [mikro'kɔzmu] *m* microcosm
microempresa [mikroẽ'preza] *f* small business
microfibra [mikro'fibra] *f* microfiber, *Brit* microfibre
microfone [mikro'foni] *m* microphone
microondas [mikro'õdas] *m* microwave (oven)
microônibus [mikro'onibus] *m Bras* minibus
microprocessador [mikroprosesa'dor] *m* microprocessor
microrganismo [mikrorga'nizmu] *m* microorganism
microscópico [mikros'kɔpiku] *adj* microscopic
microscópio [mikros'kɔpiu] *m* microscope
mídia ['midʒia] *mpl* media
migalha [mi'gaʎa] *f* crumb; ***~ de pão*** breadcrumbs
migração [migra'sãw] *f* migration
migrar [mi'grar] ⟨1a⟩ *v/i* migrate
mijar [mi'ʒar] ⟨1a⟩ *v/i fam* piss
mijo ['miʒu] *m fam* piss
mil [miw] *num* thousand
milagre [mi'lagri] *m* miracle; *fam* ***fazer ~s*** work miracles
milagroso [mila'grozu] *adj* miraculous
milênio, *Port* **milénio** [mi'leniu] *m* millennium
milésimo [mi'lɛzimu] **1** *adj* thousandth **2** *m* thousandth
milha ['miʎa] *f* mile; ***~ marítima*** nautical mile
milhão [mi'ʎãw] *m* million
milhar [mi'ʎar] *m* thousand
milho ['miʎu] *m* corn; *fam* (*dinheiro*) dough; ***~ doce*** sweetcorn
milícia [mi'lisja] *f* militia
miligrama [mili'grama] *m* milligram
mililitro [mili'litru] *m* milliliter, *Brit* millilitre
milímetro [mi'limetru] *m* millimeter, *Brit* millilitre
milionário [miljo'nariu] *m*, **-a** *f* millionaire
militante [mili'tãtʃi] **1** *adj* militant **2** *m/f* militant
militar [mili'tar] **1** *adj* military **2** *m/f* soldier; ***os ~es*** the military
mim [mĩ] *pron* me; ***por ~ tudo bem*** that's ok by me
mimar [mi'mar] ⟨1a⟩ *v/t criança* spoil
mímica ['mimika] *f* mime
mimicar [mimi'kar] ⟨1n⟩ *v/t* mime
mímico ['mimiku] *m/f* mime artist, mimic
mimo ['mimu] *m* (*carícia*) caress; (*ternura*) tenderness; (*atenção*) attention; ***fazer ~s*** be tender; *fam* cuddle; ***dar ~ a*** spoil
mimosa [mi'mɔza] *f* mimosa
mimoso [mi'mozu] *adj* affectionate
mina[1] ['mina] *f* mine; *fig* gold mine; ***engenheiro** m **de ~s*** mining engineer; ***~ de carvão*** coalmine

mina[2] ['mina] *f* MIL mine
minar [mi'naɾ] ⟨1a⟩ *v/t* mine; *teoria etc* undermine
mineiro [mi'nejɾu] **1** *adj* mining *atr*; ***indústria*** *f* ***mineira*** mining **2** *m*, **-a** *f* miner
mineral [mine'ɾaw] **1** *adj* mineral; ***água*** *f* **~** mineral water **2** *m* mineral
minério [mi'nɛɾiu] *m* ore
minguante [mĩ'gwãtʃi] *adj* decreasing; ***quarto*** *m* **~** waning moon
minha ['miɲa] → ***meu***
minhoca [mi'ɲɔka] *f* earthworm; *pop* **~*s*** *pl* funny ideas
miniatura [minja'tuɾa] *f* miniature
minicarro [mini'kahu] *m* subcompact
minigolfe [mini'gowfi] *m* minigolf
minimalismo [minima'lizmu] *m* minimalism
minimizar [minimi'zaɾ] ⟨1a⟩ *v/t* minimize
mínimo ['minimu] **1** *m* minimum; *dedo* little finger, *fam* pinkie; **~** ***vital*** subsistence level; AUTO **~*s*** *pl* parking lights; ***no*** **~** at least **2** *adj* least, slightest; ***nos*** **~*s*** ***detalhes*** in minute detail
minissaia [mini'saja] *f* miniskirt
ministerial [ministe'ɾjaw] *adj* ministerial
ministério [minis'tɛɾiu] *m* ministry; (*serviço*) service; ***Ministério das Relações Exteriores*** State Department, *Brit* Foreign Office
ministro [mi'nistɾu] *m*, **-a** *f* minister; ***Primeiro Ministro*** *m* Prime Minister; ***Ministro das Relações Exteriores*** Secretary of State, *Brit* Foreign Secretary, foreign minister
mini-van [mini'vã] *f* minivan, MPV
minoria [mino'ɾia] *f* minority; ***estar em*** **~** be in the minority
minoritário [minoɾi'taɾiu] *adj* minority *atr*; ***governo*** *m* **~** minority government; **~** ***étnica*** ethnic minority
minto ['mĩtu] *etc* → ***mentir***
minúcia [mi'nusja] *f* detail
minucioso [minu'sjozu] *adj* exact, thorough; (*pormenorizado*) detailed
minúscula [mi'nuskula] *f* lower case letter
minúsculo [mi'nuskulu] *adj* minute, minuscule
minuta [mi'nuta] *f* rough draft; (*esboço*) sketch
minuto [mi'nutu] *m* minute
miocardite [miokaɾ'dʒitʃi] *f* myocarditis
miolo ['mjolu] *m pão*: *soft, inner part of a loaf*; *fruto*: pulp; *noz*: kernel; *fig* core; **~** (***s***) (*pl*) brains
míope ['miupi] *adj* short-sighted *tb fig*
miopia [mjo'pia] *f* short-sightedness
miosótis [mio'zɔtʃis] *m* forget-me-not
mira ['miɾa] *f espingarda*: sight; (*intenção*) purpose, aim; ***sob a*** **~** ***de uma arma*** at gunpoint
miradouro [miɾa'doɾu] *m* viewpoint
miragem [mi'ɾaʒẽ] *f* mirage *tb fig*
mirar [mi'ɾaɾ] ⟨1a⟩ **1** *v/t* look at **2** *v/i* aim at; **mirar-se** *v/r* look at oneself
mirtilo [miɾ'tʃilu] *m* blueberry
mirto ['miɾtu] *m* myrtle
misantropia [mizãtɾo'pia] *f* misanthropy
misantrópico [mizã'tɾɔpiku] *adj* misanthropic
misantropo [mizã'tɾopu] *m* misanthrope
mise ['mizi] *f fam cabelo*: shampoo and set; ***fazer uma*** **~** shampoo and set
miserável [mize'ɾavew] **1** *adj* wretched, miserable; (*reles*) mean; (*avarento*) miserly; (*patife*) despicable **2** *m/f* (*desgraçado*) wretch; (*avarento*) miser; (*patife*) scoundrel
miséria [mi'zɛɾja] *f* (*indigência*) misery, poverty; (*ninharia*) trifle; ***pagar uma*** **~** pay a pittance; ***ganhar uma*** **~** get paid peanuts
misericórdia [mizeɾi'kɔɾdʒia] *f* mercy; ***golpe*** *m* ***de*** **~** coup de grâce
mísero ['mizeɾu] *adj quantidade* miserly
missa ['misa] *f* mass; ***ir a*** **~** go to mass
missão [mi'sãw] *f* mission; (*incumbência*) job; ***ter por*** **~** ***de fazer*** have the task of doing
missionário [misjo'naɾiu] *m*, **-a** *f* missionary
míssil ['misiw] *m* MIL missile
mistério [mis'tɛɾiu] *m* mystery
misterioso [miste'ɾjozu] *adj* myster-

ious
místico ['mistʃiku] **1** *adj* mystic **2** *m*, **-a** *f* mystic
misto ['mistu] *adj* mixed
mistura [mis'tuɾa] *f* mixture
misturada [mistu'ɾada] *f* jumble, mixture
misturar [mistu'ɾaɾ] ⟨1a⟩ mix; (*confundir*) mix up, confuse
mítico ['mitʃiku] *adj* mythical
mito ['mitu] *m* myth
mitologia [mitolo'ʒia] *f* mythology
miudeza [miu'deza] *f* detail; (*exatidão*) precision; GASTR **~s** *pl* **de frango** chicken giblets
miúdo ['miudu] **1** *adj* small; (*delicado*) tender; *fig* exact, conscientious; (*mesquinho*) petty; **fazer algo a ~** do sth little by little **2** *m*, **-a** *f* youngster; (*rapaz*, *rapariga*) little boy; little girl **3** *mpl* **~s** small change; GASTR giblets
mo [mu] **= me + o**
mó [mɔ] *f* millstone; (*pedra de amolar*) grindstone
móbil ['mɔbiw] **1** *adj* mobile **2** *m* (*motivo*) motive
mobilar [mobi'laɾ] ⟨1a⟩ *Port* furnish
mobília [mo'bilja] *f* furniture
mobiliar [mobi'ljaɾ] ⟨1a⟩ *Bras* furnish
mobiliário [mobi'ljaɾiu] *m* furniture
mobilidade [mobili'dadʒi] *f* mobility; **~ social / profissional** social / professional mobility
mobilização [mobiliza'sãw] *f* mobilization
mobilizar [mobili'zaɾ] ⟨1a⟩ mobilize
moça ['mosa] *f Bras* girl, young woman
moçambicano [mosãbi'kanu] **1** *adj* Mozambican **2** *m*, **-a** *f* Mozambican
Moçambique [mosã'biki] *m* Mozambique
moção [mo'sãw] *f* POL motion
mochila [mo'ʃila] *f* backpack; **~ escolar** schoolbag
mochileiro [moʃi'lejru] *m*, **-a** *f* backpacker
mocidade [mosi'dadʒi] *f* youth
moço ['mosu] **1** *adj* young **2** *m* boy, young man; **~ de recados** messenger boy
moda ['mɔda] *f* fashion; **~ feminina / masculina / infantil** ladies' / men's / children's fashion; **à ~ de** in the style of, à la; **estar na ~** in fashion; **fora de ~** old-fashioned; **~ pronta** ready-to-wear clothing
modalidade [modali'dadʒi] *f* mode; ESP event
modelar [mode'laɾ] **1** *adj* model **2** *v/t* ⟨1c⟩ model; *barro* shape; **~ algo por algo** model sth on sth
modelo [mo'delu] **1** *m* model; *costura*: pattern; **~ exemplar** role model **2** *f* model
modem [mo'dem] *m* modem
moderação[1] [modeɾa'sãw] *f* ⟨*sem pl*⟩ moderation
moderação[2] [modeɾa'sãw] *f* TV *etc* presentation
moderado [mode'ɾadu] *adj* moderate
moderador [modeɾa'doɾ] *m*, **~ a** *f* TV presenter
moderar[1] [mode'ɾaɾ] ⟨1c ⟩ *v/t* TV present
moderar[2] [mode'ɾaɾ] ⟨1c⟩ *v/t* moderate; (*retardar*) reduce; **moderar-se** *v/r* control oneself
moderativo [modeɾa'tʃivu] *adj* moderating
modernismo [moder'nizmu] *m* modernism
modernista [moder'nista] **1** *adj* modernistic **2** *m/f* modernist
modernização [moderniza'sãw] *f* modernization
modernizar [moderni'zaɾ] ⟨1a⟩ *v/t* modernize; **modernizar-se** *v/r* modernize
moderno [mo'dɛrnu] *adj* modern; **à moderna** modern
modéstia [mo'dɛstʃia] *f* modesty
modesto [mo'dɛstu] *adj* modest
modificação [modʒifika'sãw] *f* modification
modificar [modʒifi'kaɾ] ⟨1n⟩ *v/t* modify
modista [mo'dʒista] *f* dressmaker
modo ['mɔdu] *m* way, manner; (*processo*) way; GRAM mood; MÚS mode; **~ de vida** way of life; **~s** *pl* (*trato*) manners; **de ~ algum** in no way; **de ~ que** so that

M

modulação [modula'sãw] *f* modulation
modular [modu'laɾ] ⟨1a⟩ modulate
módulo ['mɔdulu] *m* TECN module; (*bilhete*) ticket; ***~ espacial*** space module
moeda ['mwɛda] *f* coin; (*câmbio*) currency; ***~ forte*** hard currency
moer [mweɾ] ⟨2f⟩ *v/t* grind; (*triturar*) crush; ***~ alguém*** (*cansar*) wear s.o. down; **moer-se** *v/r* slave away
mofo ['mofu] *m* mold, *Brit* mould; (*bolor*) mildew; ***cheirar a ~*** smell musty
mogno ['mɔgnu] *m* mahogany
moinho ['mwiɲu] *m* mill; ***~ de vento*** windmill; ***levar a água ao seu ~*** line one's own pockets
moiro ['mojɾu] → ***mouro***
mola ['mɔla] *f* spring; *roupa etc*: clothes pin, *Brit* (clothes)peg; *fig* motivation; *fig* ***~ real*** mainspring; ***com / sem ~s*** sprung / unsprung
moldar [mow'daɾ] ⟨1e⟩ (*formar*) mold, *Brit* mould; (*criar*) form; (*fundir*) cast; *fig* shape
molde ['mɔldʒi] *m* mold, *Brit* mould; *alfaiate*: pattern; *fig* model; ***~ de gesso*** plaster cast
moldura [mow'duɾa] *f* frame; ARQUIT molding, *Brit* moulding
mole ['mɔli] *adj* soft; (*flácido*) limp; (*flexível*) pliable; (*preguiçoso*) lazy
moleca [mo'lɛka] *f* tomboy
molécula [mo'lɛkula] *f* molecule
moleiro [mo'lejɾu] *m*, **-a** *f* miller
molenga [mo'lẽga] *m/f* slowpoke, *Brit* slowcoach
moleque [mo'lɛki] *m* urchin
moléstia [mo'lɛstʃia] *f* unease; (*doença*) illness
molestar [moles'taɾ] ⟨1c⟩ bother; (*maçar*) pester; (*maltratar*) molest; (*irritar*) annoy
molhado [mo'ʎadu] *adj* wet
molhar [mo'ʎaɾ] ⟨1e⟩ wet; (*umedecer*) moisten; (*pôr de molho*) soak; (*ensopar*) dunk
molhe ['mɔʎi] *m* NÁUT pier
molho[1] ['mɔʎu] *m* bundle, bunch; ***~ de chaves*** bunch of keys; ***em ~s*** bundled
molho[2] ['moʎu] *m* sauce, gravy; ***pôr de ~*** soak; ***~ de salada*** salad dressing; ***~ de soja*** soy sauce
molusco [mo'lusku] *m* mollusk, *Brit* mollusc
momentâneo [momẽ'tʌniu] *adj* momentary
momentinho [mo'mẽtu] *m* moment; ***um ~!*** just a moment!
momento [mo'mẽtu] *m* moment; FÍS momentum; ***a cada ~*** any moment; ***de um ~ para o outro*** suddenly, from one moment to the next; ***~s depois*** just after; ***um ~, por favor!*** just a moment, please!
monarca [mo'naɾka] *m* monarch
monarquia [monaɾ'kia] *f* monarchy
monastério [monas'tɛɾiu] *m* monastery
monástico [mo'nastʃiku] *adj* monastic
monção [mõ'sãw] *f* monsoon
monda ['mõda] *f* AGR weeding
mondador [mõda'doɾ] *m ferramenta* hoe
mondar [mõ'daɾ] ⟨1a⟩ *campo, ervas* weed
monetário [mone'taɾiu] *adj* monetary
monge ['mõʒi] *m* monk
Mongólia [mõ'gɔlja] *f* Mongolia
monitor[1] [moni'toɾ] *m* INFORM monitor
monitor[2] [moni'toɾ] *m*, **-a** *f* monitor; (*instrutor*) instructor
monogamia [monoga'mia] *f* monogamy
monógamo [mo'nɔgamu] *adj* monogamous
monografia [monogɾa'fia] *f* monograph
monograma [mono'gɾama] *m* monogram
monólogo [mo'nɔlogu] *m* monologue
monopólio [mono'pɔliu] *m* monopoly
monopolista [monopo'lista] *adj* monopolistic
monopolizar [monopoli'zaɾ] ⟨1a⟩ monopolize
monossílabo [mono'silabu] *m* monosyllable
monotonia [monoto'nia] *f* monotony
monótono [mo'nɔtunu] *adj* monotonous
monstro ['mõstɾu] *m* monster

monstruosidade [mõstɾwozi'dadʒi] *f* monstrosity
monstruoso [mõstɾu'ozu] *adj* monstrous
montador [mõta'doɾ] *m*, **-a** *f* TECN fitter
montagem [mõ'taʒẽ] *f* TECN assembly; ELÉT wiring
montanha [mõ'taɲa] *f* mountain; **~ -russa** *f* roller coaster
montanhismo [mõta'ɲizmu] *m* mountaineering
montanhista [mõta'ɲista] *m/f* mountaineer
montanhoso [mõta'ɲozu] *adj* mountainous
montante [mõ'tãtʃi] **1** *m* amount, sum; ***no ~ de*** to the value of; ***a ~*** upstream **2** *adj* rising
montar [mõ'taɾ] ⟨1a⟩ **1** *v/t cavalo* mount, get on; (*cavalgar*) ride; *fábrica* set up; *máquina* assemble; *tenda*, *andaime* put up **2** *v/i* (*subir*) rise; (*cavalgar*) ride; ***~ a*** amount to
montão [mõ'tãw] *m* heap, pile
monte ['mõtʃi] *m* hill; ***um ~ de dívidas*** a mountain of debts
montículo [mõ'tʃikulu] *m* hillock; *beisebol*: mound
montra ['mõtɾa] *f Port* store window, *Brit* shop window
monumental [monumẽ'taw] *adj* monumental
monumento [monu'mẽtu] *m* monument
morada [mo'ɾada] *f* home, residence; *Port endereço* address; *fig* stay
moradia [moɾa'dʒia] *f* dwelling, house
moral [mo'ɾaw] **1** *adj* moral **2** *f* (*ética*) ethics **3** *m* (*ânimo*) morale; ***estar com a ~ alta / baixa*** be in good / poor spirits
moralidade [moɾali'dadʒi] *f* morality
moralista [moɾa'lista] *adj* moralistic
moranga [mo'ɾãga] *f* pumpkin
morango [mo'ɾãgu] *m* strawberry
morar [mo'ɾaɾ] ⟨1e⟩ *v/i* live; ***~ junto*** live together
moratória [moɾa'tɔɾja] *f* moratorium
morbidez [moɾbi'des] *f* morbidness
mórbido ['mɔɾbidu] *adj* morbid
morcego [moɾ'segu] *m* bat; *fig* night owl
morcela [moɾ'sɛla] *f* blood sausage, *Brit* black pudding
mordaça [moɾ'dasa] *f cão*: muzzle; *pessoa*: gag; TECN chuck
morador [moɾa'doɾ] **1 adj** resident **2** *m*, **-a** *f* resident; (*habitante*) inhabitant
mordaz [moɾ'das] *adj* scathing, biting
mordedela [moɾde'dɛla] *f*, **mordedura** [moɾde'duɾa] *f* bite
morder [moɾ'deɾ] ⟨2d⟩ **1** *v/t* bite; *ácido* corrode **2** *v/i* bite; (*arder*) burn; (*fazer comichão*) itch
mordiscar [moɾ'deɾ] *v/t* nibble
moreia [mo'ɾeja] *f peixe* Moray eel
morena[1] [mo'ɾena] *f* dark-skinned girl / woman; *cor de cabelo*: brunette
morena[2] [mo'ɾena] *f* GEOL moraine
moreno [mo'ɾenu] **1** *adj* dark brown, brunette; (*escuro*) dark **2** *m homem* dark-skinned man; *cor de cabelo*: dark-haired man
morfina [moɾ'fina] *f* morphine
morfologia [moɾfolo'ʒia] *f* morphology
morgue ['mɔɾgi] *f* morgue
moribundo [moɾi'bũdu] *adj* dying; *luz* fading
morno ['moɾnu] *adj* lukewarm, tepid
moroso [mo'ɾozu] *adj* sluggish, slow
morrer [mo'heɾ] ⟨2d; *pp* morto⟩ die; ***~ de*** die of; ***estar para ~*** be dying; ***fiquei para ~!*** I nearly died!; ***~ de rir*** kill oneself laughing, die laughing; ***um vestido que é lindo de ~*** a dress to die for
morro ['mohu] *m* hill
morsa ['mɔɾsa] *f* walrus
mortal [moɾ'taw] *adj* mortal; (*letal*) deadly; (*efêmero*) short-lived; ***pecado** m **~*** deadly sin
mortalidade [moɾtali'dadʒi] *f* mortality
morte ['mɔɾtʃi] *f* death; ***perigo** m **de ~*** danger of death; ***um olhar de ~*** a murderous look
morteiro [moɾ'tejɾu] *m* MIL mortar
mortificar [moɾtʃifi'kaɾ] ⟨1n⟩ (*flagelar*) castigate; (*humilhar*) humiliate; (*ofender*) offend
morto ['moɾtu] **1** *pp* (→ ***morrer***)

M

dead **2** *adj* dead; ***estar ~*** be dead; ***ser ~*** be killed; ***~ de frio / fome*** freezing / starving; ***~ de cansaço*** dead tired; *fig* ***estar ~ por*** be dying for

mosaico [mo'zajku] *m* mosaic

mosca ['moska] *f* fly

Moscou [mos'kow] *m Bras* Moscow

Moscovo [mos'kovu] *m Port* Moscow

mosquiteiro [moski'tejɾu] *m* mosquito net

mosquito [mos'kitu] *m* mosquito; *não venenoso* gnat, midge

mossa ['mosa] *f* dent

mostarda [mos'taɾda] *f* mustard

mosteiro [mos'tejɾu] *m* monastery; *freiras*: convent

mostra ['mɔstɾa] *f* display; *fig* sign; ***à ~*** visible

mostrador [mostɾa'doɾ] *m* face, dial; (*balcão*) store counter, *Brit* shop counter

mostrar [mos'tɾaɾ] ⟨1e⟩ show; *vitrina*: display

mostruário [mostɾu'aɾiu] *m* (*vitrina*) display case

mota ['mɔta] *f* motorbike

motel [mo'tɛw] *m* motel

motim [mo'ʧĩ] *m* revolt; POL riot; MIL mutiny

motivação [moʧiva'sãw] *f* motivation

motivar [moʧi'vaɾ] ⟨1a⟩ motivate; (*ocasionar*) cause

motivo [mo'ʧivu] *m* motive, cause; LIT, ARTE, MÚS motif

moto ['mɔtu] *f*, **motocicleta** [motosi'klɛta] *f* motorbike

motociclismo [motosi'klizmu] *m* motorcycling

motociclista [motosi'klista] *m/f* motorcyclist

motoneta [moto'neta] *f Bras* (motor) scooter

motor [mo'toɾ] *m* TECN motor, engine; *fig* driving force; ***~ a dois / quatro tempos*** two / four-stroke engine; ***~ de arranque*** starter motor; INFORM ***~ de busca*** search engine; ***~ de fora de borda*** outboard motor; INFORM ***~ de pesquisa*** search engine

motorista [moto'ɾista] *m/f* driver, motorist; *Bras camião*: truckdriver, *Brit* lorry driver; ***~ de táxi*** taxi driver; ***ser um bom ~*** be a good driver

motorizada [motoɾi'zada] *f Port* moped

mouro ['moɾu] **1** *adj* Moorish **2** *m*, **-a** *f* Moor; *Port fam* person from Lisbon; *fam* ***trabalhar como um ~*** work like a maniac

movediço [move'dʒisu] *adj* movable; *solo* loose; ***areia*** *f* ***movediça*** quicksand

móvel ['mɔvew] **1** *adj* movable; (*com rodas*) wheeled **2** *m* (*motivo*) motive; *mobília*: piece of furniture **3** *mpl* ***moveis*** furniture; DIR movables

mover [mo'veɾ] ⟨2d⟩ move *tb fig*; TECN drive; (*causar*) cause; **mover-se** *v/r* move

movimentação [movimẽta'sãw] *f* movement; (*mudança*) change; *mercadoria*: turnover

movimentado [movimẽ'tadu] *adj rua* busy

movimentar [movimẽ'taɾ] ⟨1a⟩ move; *atenção* direct; COM turn over; **movimentar-se** *v/r* move; (*girar*) turn

movimento [movi'mẽtu] *m* movement; *sentimentos*: stirring; (*trânsito*) traffic; *xadrez*: move; COM turnover; *fig tb* change; (*variedade*) variety; ***pôr em ~*** start moving; *motor* start up; ***pôr-se em ~*** get going; *veículo* start up

muco ['muku] *m* mucus

mucosa [mu'kɔza] *f* mucous membrane

mucosidade [mukozi'dadʒi] *f* mucus

muçulmano [musuw'manu] **1** *m*, **-a** *f* Muslim **2** *adj* Muslim

muda ['muda] *f* change; *pássaros*: molting, *Brit* moulting; *cobra, inseto*: sloughing

mudança [mu'dãsa] *f* change; *habitação*: move; AUTO ***~s*** *pl* gears; ***~ climática*** (*ou* ***de clima***) climate change; ***~ de óleo*** oil change; ***o João está no período de ~ da voz*** João's voice is breaking

mudar [mu'daɾ] ⟨1a⟩ **1** *v/t* change (***em*** into) **2** *v/i* change; *voz* break;

M

*~ **de*** change; *~ **de casa*** move; **mudar-se** *v/r* move (***para*** to); *transportes públicos*: change
mudez [mu'des] muteness; *fig* silence
mudo ['mudu] *adj* dumb; *fig* silent
mugido [mu'ʒidu] *m* mooing; *touro*: bellowing
mugir [mu'ʒiɾ] ⟨3n⟩ *vaca* moo; *touro* bellow
muito ['muĩtu] **1** *adj* a lot of, lots of; *negativo, interrogativo tb*: much; *negativo, interrogativo plural tb*: many; ~ (***tempo***) a long time **2** *pron* a lot, lots; *negativo, interrogativo tb*: much; *negativo, interrogativo plural tb*: many; ***há ~*** a long time ago; ***quando ~*** at the most **3** *adv* ◇ + *adj* very; *~ **bom*** very good; *~ **obrigado*** thanks a lot, thanks very much; *~ **pesado para carregar*** too heavy to carry
◇ + *verbo*: a lot; ***comer / beber ~*** eat / drink a lot
◇ + *comparativo*: a lot, much; *~ **mais fácil*** a lot easier, much easier
◇ *temporal*: a long time; *~ **antes disso*** a long time before that, long before that
mula ['mula] *f* (female) mule
mulato [mu'latu] *m*, **-a** [mu'lata] *f* mulatto
muleta [mu'leta] *f* crutch
mulher [mu'ʎɛɾ] *f* woman; (*esposa*) wife; *~ **a dias*** cleaning woman; *~ **-polícia*** policewoman; *pop ~ **da vida*** working girl
multa ['muwta] *f* fine; ***apanhar uma ~*** be fined
multar [muw'taɾ] ⟨1a⟩ fine
multi… [muwʧi] multi…
multi-banco [muwʧi'bãku] ATM, cash dispenser
multicolor [muwʧiko'loɾ] *adj*, **multicor** [muwʧi'koɾ] *adj* multicolored, *Brit* multicoloured
multicultural [muwʧikuwtu'ɾaw] *adj* multicultural
multidão [muwʧi'dãw] *f* crowd
multilateral [muwʧilate'ɾaw] *adj* multilateral
multimídia [muwʧi'midʒia] *f* multimedia
multinacional [muwʧinasjo'naw] **1** *adj* multinational; ***Estado** m ~* multinational state **2** *f* multinational
multipartidário [muwʧipaɾʧi'daɾiu] *adj* multiparty
multipartidarismo [muwʧipaɾʧida'ɾizmu] *m* multiparty system
multiplicação [muwʧiplika'sãw] *f* multiplication
multiplicador [muwʧiplika'doɾ] *m* multiplier
multiplicar [muwʧipli'kaɾ] ⟨1n⟩ (*reproduzir*) multiply; **multiplicar-se** *v/r* multiply *tb* BIOL
múltiplo ['muwʧiplu] *adj* multiple
múmia ['mumja] *f* mummy
mundano [mũ'danu] *adj* worldly, mundane
mundial [mũ'dʒiaw] **1** *adj* worldwide; ***recorde** m ~* world record; ***guerra** f ~* world war **2** *m* ESP world championship; *~ **de futebol*** World Cup
mundialmente [mũdʒiaw'mẽʧi] *adv* worldwide
mundo ['mũdu] *m* world; ***todo o ~*** everybody; ***Terceiro Mundo*** Third World; ***cidadão** m **do** ~* citizen of the world; *fam **no fim do** ~* in the boonies, *Brit* in the sticks
mungir [mũ'ʒiɾ] ⟨3n⟩ *v/t* milk
munição [muni'sãw] *f* MIL ammunition; (*alimentação*) supplies
municipal [munisi'paw] municipal; ***Câmara** f **Municipal*** town hall; ***eleições** fpl **municipais*** municipal elections
município [muni'sipiu] *m* municipality, district
munir [mu'niɾ] ⟨3a⟩ *v/t* equip, supply (***de*** with); (*fortificar*) fortify; **munir-se** *v/r ~ **de algo*** equip oneself with sth; *~ **de paciência*** bide one's soul in patience
muralha [mu'ɾaʎa] *f* (city) wall
murchar [muɾ'ʃaɾ] ⟨1a⟩ *v/i* wither; *cor* fade
murcho ['muɾʃu] *adj* wilted; (*mole*) listless
murmurar [muɾmu'ɾaɾ] ⟨1a⟩ **1** *v/t* murmur **2** *v/i* murmur; *folhas* rustle; *vento* whisper; *fig* grumble (***sobre*** about)
murmúrio [muɾ'muɾiu] *m* murmur-

M

ing; *folhas*: rustling; *vento*: whispering; (*resmungar*) grumbling
muro ['muɾu] *m* wall; **~ de escalada** climbing wall
murro ['muhu] *m* punch, blow
musa ['muza] *f* muse
muscular [musku'laɾ] *adj* muscular
musculatura [muskula'tuɾa] *f* musculature
músculo ['muskulu] *m* muscle; **ter ~** be muscular
musculoso [musku'lozu] *adj* muscular
museu [mu'zew] *m* museum; *arte*: gallery
musgo ['muzgu] *m* moss
música ['muzika] *f* music; (*canção*) song; *CD*: track; ***peça*** *f* ***de ~*** piece of music; **~ de câmara** chamber music; **~ folclórica** folk music; **~ pop** pop music; **~ sacra** sacred music; → **músico**
musical [muzi'kaw] *adj* musical
músico ['muziku] **1** *adj* musical **2** *m*, **-a** *f* musician
mutação [muta'sãw] *f* change; BIOL mutation
mutilação [mutʃila'sãw] *f* mutilation
mutilado [mutʃi'ladu] **1** *m* disabled person, cripple **2** *adj* mutilated; *pessoa* crippled
mutilar [mutʃi'laɾ] ⟨1a⟩ mutilate; *pessoa* maim
mutuamente [mutwa'mẽtʃi] *adv* mutually
mútuo ['mutwu] *adj* mutual

N

na [na] *prep* **em** *com art f* **a**
nabo ['nabu] *m* turnip
nação [na'sãw] *f* nation; ***as Nações*** *pl* ***Unidas*** the United Nations
nacional [nasjo'naw] *adj* national; ***mercado*** *m* **~** domestic market
nacionalidade [nasjonali'dadʒi] *f* nationality; **~ dupla** dual nationality
nacionalismo [nasjona'lizmu] *m* nationalism
nacionalista [nasjona'lista] **1** *adj* nationalist **2** *m/f* nationalist
nacionalização [nasjonaliza'sãw] *f* nationalization
nacionalizar [nasjonali'zaɾ] ⟨1a⟩ *indústria* nationalize
nada ['nada] **1** *pron* ◇ nothing; ***ele não faz ~*** he does nothing, he doesn't do anything; ***de ~!*** you're welcome!; ***~ disso!*** nonsense!, no chance!; **~ de novo** nothing new; **~ do chocolate** none of the chocolate **2** *adv* at all; **não é ~ mau** that's not bad at all; **não é ~ parvo** he's not stupid **3** *int* **~!** nonsense!; no chance! **4** *m* nothingness; (*insignificância*) trifle
nadadeira [nada'dejɾa] *f* flipper; *peixe*: fin
nadador [nada'doɾ] *m*, **-a** *f* swimmer
nadar [na'daɾ] ⟨1b⟩ swim
nádega ['nadega] *f* buttock; **~s** *pl* bottom, buttocks
nado ['nadu] *m* swimming; **~ de costas** backstroke; **~ livre** freestyle, crawl; **~ de peito** breaststroke
namorada [namo'ɾada] *f* girlfriend
namorado [namo'ɾadu] *m* boyfriend
namorador [namoɾa'doɾ]*adj* flirtatious
namorar [namo'ɾaɾ] ⟨1e⟩ (*cortejar*) date, go out with; (*desejar*) covet *tb fig*; **~ com alguém** date s.o., go out with s.o.; **namorar-se** *v/r* go out
namorico [namo'ɾiku] *m* flirtation
namoro [na'moɾu] *m* (*corte*) relationship
namori(s)car [namoɾi(s)'kaɾ] ⟨1n⟩ *v/t* flirt with
nanismo [na'nizmu] *m* dwarfism

não [nãw] **1** *adv* ◊ *resposta*: no; ***dizer que ~*** say no
◊ *negação*: not; ***~ trabalha*** he is not working, he isn't working; ***~ atire!*** don't shoot!; ***~ perturbe*** do not disturb; ***~ … nem …*** neither … nor …; ***ele é louco, ~ é?*** he's crazy, isn't he; ***está partido, ~ é?*** it's broken, isn't it?; ***vai correr, ~ é?*** you're going for a run, aren't you? **2** *m* no
não-alinhado [nãwali'ɲadu] *adj* POL non-aligned
não-alinhamento [nãwaliɲa'mẽtu] *m* non-alignment
não-fumador [nãwfuma'doɾ] *m*, **-a** *f* non-smoker; ***zona f reservada a ~es*** no-smoking area
não-intervenção [nãwĩtʃiɾvẽ'sãw] *f* ⟨*sem pl*⟩ non-intervention
não-violência [nãwvjo'lẽsja] *f* nonviolence
napa ['napa] *f* napa leather
naquela [na'kɛla], **naquele** [na'keli], **naquilo** [na'kilu] *prep+pron* = ***em*** + ***aquela*** *etc*
narciso [naɾ'sizu] *m* BOT narcissus; *pessoa* narcissist
narcótico [naɾ'kɔtʃiku] *m* narcotic
narcotraficante [naɾkotrafi'kãtʃi] *m/f* (drug) dealer
narcotráfico [naɾko'trafiku] *m* drug trade, drug trafficking
narina [na'ɾina] *f* nostril
nariz [na'ɾis] *m* nose; ***meter o ~*** stick one's nose in; *fig* ***torcer o ~*** turn one's nose up; ***tem ~ arrebitado*** he's stuck-up
narração [naha'sãw] *f* narration
narrador [naha'doɾ] *m*, **-a** *f* narrator
narrar [na'haɾ] ⟨1b⟩ narrate
narrativa [naha'tʃiva] *f* narrative
narrativo [naha'tʃivu] *adj* narrative
nasal [na'zaw] **1** *adj* nasal **2** *f* GRAM nasal (sound)
nascença [nas'sẽsa] *f* birth
nascente [nas'sẽtʃi] **1** *adj astro* rising; (*em começo*) nascent **2** *m* East, Orient **3** *f* spring
nascer [nas'seɾ] **1** *v/i* ⟨2g⟩ be born; *pássaro* hatch; *rio*, *sequência*, *astro* rise; *dia* break; *fig* come into being; *desejo*, *sentimento* awake; (*originar*) come (***de*** from) **2** *m* ***~ do sol*** sunrise
nascimento [nasi'mẽtu] *m* birth; (*formação*) descent; (*origem*) origin; ***data f de ~*** date of birth
nata ['nata] *f* cream
natação [nata'sãw] *f* ⟨*sem pl*⟩ swimming; ***de ~*** swimming *atr*
natal [na'taw] **1** *adj* native **2** *m* ***Natal*** Christmas; ***de ~*** Christmas *atr*
natalício [nata'lisiu] *adj* birth *atr*
natalidade [natali'dadʒi] *f* ***controlo m de ~*** birth control; ***taxa f de ~*** birth rate
natimorto [natʃi'moɾtu] *adj* stillborn
nativo [na'tʃivu] **1** *adj* native **2** *m*, **-a** *f* native; ***~ do leste*** easterner
natural [natu'ɾaw] **1** *adj* natural; (*inato*) native; ***~ de*** native of; ***é ~*** it's natural; ***água mineral ~*** mineral water not out of the fridge; GASTR ***ao ~*** fresh, uncooked **2** *m* (*caráter*) temperament **3** *m/f* (*nativo*) native
naturalidade [naturali'dadʒi] *f* naturalness; (*evidência*) self-evidence; (*origem*) descent, extraction; ***agir com ~*** act naturally
naturalista [natura'lista] **1** *adj* ARTE, LIT naturalist; MED natural **2** *m/f* naturalist
naturalização [naturaliza'sãw] *f* naturalization
naturalizar [naturali'zaɾ] ⟨1a⟩ naturalize; **naturalizar-se** *v/r* become naturalized
natureza [natu'ɾeza] *f* nature; (*caráter*) kind, type; ARTE ***~ morta*** still life
naufragar [nawfra'gaɾ] ⟨1o & 1b⟩ be shipwrecked
naufrágio [naw'fraʒiu] *m* shipwreck
náufrago ['nawfragu] **1** *adj* shipwrecked **2** *m*, **-a** *f* person who has been shipwrecked, castaway
náusea(s) ['nawzja(s)] *f(pl)* nausea; ***estou com nauseas*** I'm feeling nauseous
nauseabundo [nawzja'bũdu] *adj* nauseating, sickening
náutica ['nawtʃika] *f* seamanship
náutico ['nawtʃiku] nautical; ***associação f náutica*** watersports club
naval [na'vaw] *adj* naval
navalha [na'vaʎa] *f* pocket knife;

N

barbeiro: open razor; ***no fio da ~*** on the razor's edge
navalhada [nava'ʎada] *f* stab wound
nave ['navi] *f* nave; ***~ espacial*** spaceship
navegação [navega'sãw] *f* navigation, sailing; ***~ aérea*** air traffic; ***~ fluvial*** river traffic; AUTO ***sistema*** *m* ***de ~*** navigation system
navegador [navega'doɾ] *m* navigator; INTERNET browser
navegar [nave'gaɾ] ⟨1o & 1c⟩ *v/i* navigate, sail; *(dirigir)*, *computador*: navigate; *(voar)* fly; INTERNET surf
navegável [nave'gavew] *adj* navigable
navio [na'viu] *m* ship; ***~ cargueiro*** freighter; ***~ para cruzeiro*** cruise liner; ***~ de guerra*** warship; ***~ mercante*** merchant ship; ***~ de pesca*** fishing boat; ***~ porta-contêineres*** container ship; ***~ transatlântico*** liner
navio-escola [navios'kɔla] *m* ⟨*pl* navios-escola⟩ training ship
n/c *abr* (***nossa carta***) our letter; (***nossa conta***) our account
neblina [ne'blina] *f* fog, mist
nebuloso [nebu'lozu] *adj* misty; *(triste)* gloomy; *(enevoado)* foggy, hazy *tb fig*
necessário [nese'saɾiu] *adj* necessary
necessidade [nesesi'dadʒi] *f* necessity; *(aflição)* poverty, need; COM requirement; ***de primeira ~*** essential
necessitado [nesesi'tadu] *adj* poor, needy
necessitar [nesesi'taɾ] ⟨1a⟩ need; ***~ de algo*** need sth; ***~ de fazer algo*** need to do sth
necrológio [nekɾo'lɔʒiu] *m* obituary
necrotério [nekɾo'tɛɾiu] *m* mortuary, morgue
nectarina [nekta'ɾina] *f* nectarine
neerlandês [nieɾlã'des] **1** *adj* Dutch **2** *m*, **neerlandesa** [nieɾlã'deza] *f* Dutchman(woman) **3** *m lingua* Dutch
nefasto [ne'fastu] *adj* ominous
negação [nega'sãw] *f* negation; *(recusa)* refusal; *(rejeição)* denial; ***ser a ~ de*** be the total opposite of; ***ser uma ~ para*** be hopeless at
negar [ne'gaɾ] ⟨1o & 1c⟩ deny, refuse; ***~ algo a alguém*** *direito* deny s.o. sth; *comida etc* refuse s.o. sth; **negar-se** *v/r* refuse (***a*** to)
negativa [nega'tʃiva] *f* negative; *(recusa)* refusal
negativo [nega'tʃivu] **1** *adj* negative **2** *m* FOT negative
negligência [negli'ʒẽsja] *f* negligence, carelessness
negligente [negli'ʒẽtʃi] *adj* negligent, careless
negociação [negosja'sãw] *f* negotiation; ***ronda*** *f* ***de negociações*** round of negotiations
negociador [negosja'doɾ] *m*, **-a** *f* negotiator
negociante [nego'sjãtʃi] *m/f* merchant; *(grossista)* wholesaler; *(homem / mulher de negócios)* businessman / woman
negociar [nego'sjaɾ] ⟨1g & 1h⟩ **1** *v/i* negotiate; COM trade (***em*** with) **2** *v/t* trade with; *(discutir)* discuss
negociata [nego'sjata] *f* crooked deal
negócio [ne'gɔsiu] *m* *(comércio)* deal; *atividade* business; *(assunto)* matter, affair; ***casa*** *f* ***de ~*** firm; ***fazer ~*** do business; ***~ fechado!*** it's a deal!; ***a ~s*** on business; ***relações de ~*** business relations
negrito [ne'gɾitu] *adj texto* bold
negro ['negɾu] **1** *adj* black **2** *m*, **-a** *f* black man / woman
nela ['nɛla], **nele** ['neli] = ***em*** + ***ela, ele***
nem [nẽ] *conj* neither, nor; ***~ eu!*** nor do I! ***não sei nadar – ~ eu*** I can't swim - neither can I; ***~ ... ~ ...*** neither ... nor ...; ***~ um*** (***só***) not a single one; ***~ todos*** not all; ***~ sequer*** not even; ***~ um pouco surpreso*** not at all surprised
nenhum [ne'ɲũ], **~a** [ne'ɲuma] *adj & pron* none; *dos dois* neither; ***não tem ~ copo*** there aren't any glasses, there are no glasses; ***não sobrou ~*** there are none left, there aren't any left; ***em ~ lugar*** nowhere
néon ['neon] *m* neon
neozelandês [neozelan'des] *m*, **-esa** *f* New Zealander

nepotismo [nepo'ʧizmu] *m* nepotism
nervo ['nervu] *m* nerve; BOT, ARQUIT rib; ***isso me dá nos ~s*** it gets on my nerves
nervosismo [nervo'zizmu] *m* nervousness
nervoso [ner'vozu] *adj* nervous; (*inquieto*) on edge; ***sistema*** *m* **~** nervous system
nessa ['nɛsa], **nesse** ['nesi] = ***em*** + ***essa, esse***
nesta ['nɛsta], **neste** ['nesʧi] = ***em*** + ***esta, este***
neto ['nɛtu] *m*, **-a** *f* grandson / daughter; ***os ~s*** *pl* the grandchildren
neuralgia [newraw'ʒia] *f* neuralgia
neurocirurgia [newrosirur'ʒia] *f* brain surgery, neurosurgery
neurologista [newrolo'ʒista] *m/f* neurologist
neurose [new'rɔzi] *f* neurosis
neurótico [new'rɔʧiku] **1** *adj* neurotic **2** *m*, **-a** *f* neurotic
neutral [new'traw] *adj* neutral
neutralidade [newtrali'dadʒi] *f* neutrality
neutralizar [newtrali'zar] ⟨1a⟩ neutralize; (*tornar inofensivo*) counteract
neutrão [new'trãw] *m Port* neutron
neutro ['newtru] *adj* neutral; BOT, BIOL, GRAM neuter
nêutron ['newtrõ] *m Bras* neutron
nevão [ne'vãw] *m* snowstorm
nevar [ne'var] ⟨1c⟩ *v/i* snow
neve ['nɛvi] *f* snow; **~ *solta*** powder (snow)
névoa ['nɛvwa] *f* mist
nevoeiro [ne'vwejru] *m* thick fog
nevralgia [nevraw'ʒia] *f* neuralgia
nexo ['nɛksu] *m* connection, link
NIB [nib] *m abr* (***Número de Identificação Bancária***) BIC (Bank Identifier Code)
Nicarágua [nika'ragwa] *f* Nicaragua
nicho ['niʃu] *m* niche
nicotina [niko'ʧina] *f* nicotine
Nigéria [ni'ʒɛrja] *f* Nigeria
nigeriano [niʒe'rjanu] *adj* Nigerian **2** *m*, **-a** *f* Nigerian
niilismo [nii'lizmu] *m* nihilism
ninfa ['nĩfa] *f* nymph; ZOOL pupa
ninféia [nĩ'fɛja] *f* waterlily
ninguém [nĩ'gẽ] *pron* nobody, no-one; ***não havia lá ~*** there was nobody there, there wasn't anybody there
ninharia [niɲa'ria] *f* trifle; ***5000 é uma ~ para ele*** 5000 is peanuts for him
ninho ['niɲu] *m* nest
NIP *abr* (***número de identificação pessoal***) PIN (personal identification number)
nipônico, *Port* **nipónico** [ni'poniku] *adj* Japanese
niqueleira [nike'lejra] *f Bras* coin purse, *Brit* purse
nisei [ni'sej] *m/f Brazilian with Japanese parents*
nisso ['nisu], **nisto** ['nistu] = ***em*** + ***isso, isto***
nitidez [niʧi'des] *f fig* clarity; FOT sharpness
nítido ['niʧidu] clear, distinct; FOT sharp; ***pouco ~*** blurred
nitrato [ni'tratu] *m* nitrate
nítrico ['nitriku] *adj* nitric
nível ['nivew] *m* level; TECN spirit level; **~ *de vida*** standard of living; **~ *do mar*** sea level; ***passagem*** *f* ***de ~*** grade crossing, *Brit* level crossing
nivelamento [nivela'mẽtu] *m* leveling, *Brit* levelling
nivelar [nive'lar] ⟨1c⟩ level
no [nu] = *prep* ***em*** + *art/m* ***o***
nó [nɔ] *m* knot *tb* NÁUT; ANAT *dedo*: knuckle; *fig* crux
nobre ['nɔbri] noble
nobreza [no'breza] *f* nobility; *sentimentos*: nobleness
noção [no'sãw] *f* notion; ***ter noções*** have the basics
nocivo [no'sivu] *adj* harmful; **~ *ao meio ambiente*** environmentally unfriendly, harmful to the environment
nocturno *Port* → ***noturno***
nó-de-adão [nodʒia'dãw] *m* Adam's apple
nódoa ['nɔdwa] *f* spot; *fig* stain; **~ *negra*** bruise
nogueira [no'gejra] *f* walnut tree
noite ['nojʧi] *f* night; (*tardinha*) evening; (*escuridão*) darkness; ***uma ~*** one evening / night; ***à ~*** in the evening; ***de ~*** at night; ***boa ~!*** good

N

evening!; *antes de dormir* good night!; ***esta ~*** this evening, tonight
noiva ['nojva] *f* bride; *noivado*: fiancée
noivado [noj'vadu] *m* engagement
noivo ['nojvu] *m* bridegroom; *noivado*: fiancé; ***os ~s*** *pl* the bride and groom; *noivado*: the engaged couple
nojento [no'ʒẽtu] *adj* disgusting, nauseous
nojo ['noʒu] *m* disgust, nausea; ***causar ~*** disgust, nauseate; ***ter ~ de algo*** find sth disgusting / nauseating
no-lo [nulu], **no-la** [nula] = *pron* ***nos*** + *pron* ***o, a***
nômade, *Port* **nómade** ['nomadʒi] **1** *adj* nomadic **2** *m/f* nomad
nome ['nomi] *m* name; GRAM noun; ***de ~*** *pessoa*: by name; (*famoso*) famous, well-known; ***~ de batismo*** Christian name; ***~ próprio*** first name; ***~ de solteira*** maiden name; ***~ de utilizador*** user name
nomeação [nomja'sãw] *f* nomination; (*homologação*) appointment
nomeadamente [nomjada'mẽtʃi] *adv* namely
nomear [no'mjaɾ] ⟨1l⟩ (*designar*) name, appoint; (*chamar*) call
nominal [nomi'naw] *adj* nominal; ***valor*** *m* ***~*** nominal value
nono ['nonu] **1** *adj* ninth **2** *m* ninth
nora ['nɔra] *f pessoa* daughter-in-law
nordeste [noɾ'dɛstʃi] *m* northeast
nórdico ['nɔrdʒiku] **1** *adj* Nordic; Scandinavian **2** *m*, **-a** *f* Scandinavian
norma ['nɔrma] *f* standard, norm; (*regra*) rule; (*prescrição*) regulation; ***~ européia*** EU standard
normal [noɾ'maw] **1** *adj* normal; (*comum*) usual **2** *f* MAT normal
normalidade [noɾmali'dadʒi] *f* normality
normalização [noɾmaliza'sãw] *f* normalization; TECN standardization
normalizar [noɾmali'zaɾ] ⟨1a⟩ normalize; TECN standardize
normalmente [noɾmaw'mẽtʃi] *adv* normally, usually
normativo [noɾma'tʃivu] *adj* prescriptive, normative
noroeste [no'ɾwɛstʃi] *m* northwest
norte ['nɔɾtʃi] **1** *m* north; ***perder o ~*** lose one's bearings; ***ao ~ de*** to the north of **2** *adj* north, northern
norte-americano [nɔɾtʃiameri'kanu] **1** *adj* North American **2** *m*, **-a** *f* North American
norte-coreano [nɔɾtʃikor'jano] **1** *adj* North Korean **2** *m*, **-a** *f* North Korean
nortenho [noɾ'teɲu] **1** *adj* from northern Portugal **2** *m*, **-a** *f* Northern Portuguese
Noruega [no'ɾwɛga] *f* Norway; ***na ~*** in Norway
norueguês [noɾwɛ'ges] **1** *adj* Norwegian **2** *m*, **norueguesa** [noɾwɛ'geza] *f* Norwegian
nos [nus] **1** *pron* us; *relexivo* ourselves; ***nós ~ divertimos*** we enjoyed ourselves **2** = *prep* ***em*** + *art* ***os***
nós [nɔs] *pron* ◇ *sujeito* we ◇ *depois prep* us; ***a ~*** to us; ***de ~*** from us; ***para ~*** for us; ***por ~*** on our behalf
nosografia [nozogɾa'fja] *f* pathology
nosso, -a ['nɔsu, 'nɔsa] **1** *adj* our **2** *pron* ours; ***o ~, a nossa*** ours
nostalgia [nostaw'ʒia] *f* (*saudades*) nostalgia, longing
nota ['nɔta] *f* (*apontamento*) note; (*fatura*) check, *Brit* bill; *escola*: grade, *Brit* mark; MÚS, POL note; COM bill; ***digno de ~*** noteworthy; ***tomar ~ de*** take note of; (*apontar*) note
notação [nota'sãw] *f* notation
notar [no'taɾ] ⟨1e⟩ record; (*apontar*) note; (*observar*) notice; (*ter em conta*) pay attention to
notariado [nota'ɾjadu] *m* notary's office
notarial [nota'ɾjaw] *adj* notarial
notário [no'taɾiu] *m*, **-a** *f* notary public
notável [no'tavew] *adj* notable
notícia [no'tʃisja] *f* piece of news, some news *sg*; (*participação*) announcement; ***~s*** news *sg*; ***ter ~s de*** hear from, have word from; ***~s esportivas*** sports news
noticiar [notʃi'sjaɾ] *v/t* announce, report
noticiário [notʃi'sjaɾiu] *m* news bulletin

notificação [notʃifika'sãw] *f* announcement; *oficial* notification
notificar [notʃifi'kar] ⟨1n⟩ ~ ***alguém de algo*** notify s.o. of sth; DIR ~ ***alguém*** serve s.o. with a summons
notoriedade [notorie'dadʒi] *f* fame
notório [no'tɔriu] *adj* well-known, famous
noturno [no'turnu] **1** *adj* nocturnal, night *atr*; ***curso*** *m* ~ evening course; ***vida*** *f* ***noturna*** nightlife **2** *m* MÚS nocturne; ~***s*** *pl* ZOOL nocturnal animals
noutra ['notra], **noutro** ['notru] = ***em*** + ***outra, outro***
nova ['nɔva] **1** *adj* → ***novo*** **2** *f* piece of news; ***boa*** ~ good news *sg*
Nova Iorque [nɔva'jɔrki] *f* New York
Nova Zelândia [nɔvaze'lãdʒia] *f* New Zealand
novamente [nɔva'mẽtʃi] *adv* again
nove ['nɔvi] *num* nine
novecentos [nɔve'sẽtus] *num* nine hundred
novela [no'vɛla] *f* short novel, novella; TV soap (opera)
novelo [no'velu] *m* ~ ***de lã*** ball of wool
novembro [no'vẽbru] *m* November; ***em*** ~ in November
noventa [no'vẽta] *num* ninety
noviço [no'visu] *m*, **-a** *f* REL *fig* novice
novidade [novi'dadʒi] *f* novelty; *notícia* piece of news
novilho [no'viʎu] *m* young bull
novo ['novu] *adj* new; (*jovem*) young; (*outro*) further; (*fresco*) fresh; ***o que há de*** ~? what's new?; ***de*** ~ again; ***em*** ~ / ***nova*** when he / she was young
noz [nɔs] *f* walnut
noz-moscada [nɔzmos'kada] *f* nutmeg
nu [nu] **1** *adj* naked; (*mero*) mere; (*desfolhado*, *calvo*) bare; ***estar*** ~ be naked; *fig* ***pôr a*** ~ expose; ***a olho*** ~ with the naked eye **2** *m* ARTE nude
nublado [nu'bladu] *adj* cloudy; (*escuro*) overcast; ***pouco*** ~ slightly overcast
nubloso [nu'blozu] *adj* cloudy; *fig* hazy
nuca ['nuka] *f* nape (of the neck)
nuclear [nukle'ar] *adj* nuclear; ***central*** *f* ~ nuclear power station; ***energia*** *f* ~ nuclear energy
núcleo ['nukliu] *m* nucleus; *fig* center, *Brit* centre
nudez [nu'des] *f*, **nudeza** [nu'deza] *f* nakedness, nudity; *parede*, *ávore etc*: bareness
nudismo [nu'dʒizmu] *m* nudism, naturism; ***praia*** *f* ***de*** ~ nudist beach
nudista [nu'dʒista] *m/f* nudist, naturist
nulidade [nuli'dadʒi] *f* (*ninharia*) nullity; (*invalidade*) invalidity; *fig fam pessoa* dead loss
nulo ['nulu] *adj* null, void; *contribuição* zero; (*incapaz*) useless
num [nũ], **numa** ['numa] = *prep* ***em*** + *art* ***um, uma***
numeração [numera'sãw] *f* numbering; (*enumeração*) enumeration
numeral [nume'raw] *m* numeral
numerar [nume'rar] ⟨1c⟩ number; (*enumerar*) enumerate
numérico [nu'mɛriku] *adj* numerical
número ['numeru] *m* number; ***em grande*** ~ numerous; COM ~***s*** *pl* ***negativos*** / ***positivos*** negative / positive figures; ~ ***errado*** wrong number; ~ ***ímpar*** / ***par*** odd / even number; ~ ***da conta*** account number; ~ ***de contato*** contact number; ~ ***de identificação bancária*** → ***NIB***; ~ ***de série*** serial number; ~ ***de telefone*** telephone number; ~ ***do vôo***, *Port* ~ ***do voo*** flight number
numeroso [nume'rozu] *adj* numerous; ***família*** *f* ***numerosa*** large family
nunca ['nũka] *adv* never; (*jamais*) ever; ~ ***mais*** never again; ***mais do que*** ~ more than ever
nutrição [nutri'sãw] *f* nutrition
nutricionista [nutrisjo'nista] *m/f* nutritionist
nutrido [nu'tridu] *adj* well-nourished
nutritivo [nutri'tʃivu] *adj* nourishing; ***valor*** *m* ~ nutritional value
nuvem ['nuvẽ] *f* cloud *tb fig*

O

o [o] **1** *art/m* ◇ the; *pl* ***os*** the; ***com os cabelos curtos*** with short hair; ***vou cortar ~ cabelo*** I'm going to have my hair cut
◇ *omissão* ***~ medo é ...*** fear is ...
2 *pron* him; *animal, coisa* it; *Port tratamento cortês*: you; ***~ que*** what; ***~ qual*** that, which
oásis [o'azis] *m* oasis
obcecado [obse'kadu] *adj* obsessed
obcecar [obse'kaɾ] ⟨1n & 1c⟩ obsess
obedecer [obede'seɾ] ⟨2g⟩ obey
obediência [obe'djẽsja] *f* obedience; ***em ~ a*** in accordance with
obediente [obe'djẽʧi] *adj* obedient
obesidade [obezi'dadʒi] *f* obesity
obeso [o'bezu] *adj* obese
óbito ['ɔbitu] *m* death; ***certidão f de ~*** death certificate
objeção, *Port* **objecção** [obiʒe'sãw] *f* objection; ***pôr ~*** object
object... *Port* → ***objet***
objetar [obiʒe'taɾ] ⟨1a⟩ object (***a*** to)
objetiva [obiʒe'ʧiva] *f* FOT lens *sg*; MIL, *fig* objective
objetividade [obiʒeʧivi'dadʒi] *f* objectivity
objetivo [obiʒɛ'ʧivu] **1** *adj* objective **2** *m* objective, aim
objeto [obi'ʒɛtu] *m* object
oblíqua [o'blikwa] *f* oblique
oblíquo [o'blikwu] *adj* oblique; (*torto*) crooked
obliterar [oblite'ɾaɾ] ⟨1c⟩ obliterate; *bilhete* punch; MED close off
obra ['ɔbɾa] *f* work; (*ação*) action; (*efeito*) effect; TEAT play; ***~ de arte*** work of art; ***~ de consulta*** reference work; ***~ social*** social project; ***~s pl*** works; (*renovação*) renovation; ***está em ~s*** there are building works going on; *estrada* there are road repairs going on
obra-prima [obɾa'pɾima] *f* masterpiece
obrigação [obɾiga'sãw] *f* obligation, duty; (*promissória*) bond
obrigado [obɾi'gadu] **1** *int* **~** thank you **2** *adj* obliged; (*reconhecido*) thankful
obrigadinho [obɾiga'dʒiɲu] *int* ***~!*** thanks!
obrigar [obɾi'gaɾ] ⟨1o⟩ (*forçar*) compel, oblige; ***estar obrigado a*** be obliged to
obrigatório [obɾiga'tɔɾiu] *adj* obligatory
obscenidade [obiseni'dadʒi] *f* obscenity
obsceno [obi'senu] *adj* obscene
obscuro [obis'kuɾu] *adj* dark; (*escondido*) hidden; (*desconhecido*) obscure
obsequiar [obise'kjaɾ] ⟨1g⟩ treat kindly
obséquio [obi'sɛkiu] *m* kindness; (*atenção*) attention; (*favor*) favor, *Brit* favour; ***por ~*** *fml* please
observação [obiseɾva'sãw] *f* observation; (*cumprimento*) observance
observador [obiseɾva'doɾ] **1** *m*, **-a** *f* observer **2** *adj* (*cumpridor*) obedient; (*crítico*) observant; ***ter espírito ~*** be very observant
observar [obiseɾ'vaɾ] ⟨1c⟩ observe; (*reparar*) notice
obsessão [obise'sãw] *f* obsession
obsessivo [obise'sivu] *adj* obsessive
obsoleto [obiso'letu] *adj* obsolete
obstáculo [obis'takulu] *m* obstacle
obstante [obis'tãʧi] *adv* ***não ~*** nevertheless, however
obstar [obis'taɾ] ⟨1e⟩ ***~ a*** hinder
obstetra [obis'tɛtɾa] *m/f* obstetrician
obstetrícia [obste'tɾisja] *f* obstetrics
obstinação [obistina'sãw] *f* ⟨*sem pl*⟩ obstinacy
obstinado [obisti'nadu] *adj* obstinate, stubborn
obstipação [obisʧipa'sãw] *f* MED constipation

obstrução [obistru'sãw] *f* obstruction
obstruir [obistru'ir] ⟨3i⟩ block, obstruct
obtenção [obitẽ'sãw] *f* ⟨*sem pl*⟩ acquisition, attainment
obter [obi'ter] ⟨2xa⟩ obtain; (*conseguir*) get; **~ algo de alguém** get sth from s.o.
obturação [obitura'sãw] *f Bras* filling
obturador [obitura'dor] *m* FOT shutter
obturar [obitu'rar] ⟨1a⟩ plug; (*tapar*) block up; *dente* fill
obviamente [ɔbvja'mẽtʃi] *adv* obviously
óbvio ['ɔbviu] *adj* obvious
ocasião [oka'zjãw] *f* opportunity; (*ensejo*) occasion; **por ~ de** on the occasion of
ocasional [okazjo'naw] *adj* occasional; *namorado*, *trabalho* casual
oceânico [o'sjʌniku] *adj* oceanic, ocean *atr*
oceano [o'sjanu] *m* ocean; **Oceano Índico** Indian Ocean
oceanografia [osjanogra'fia] *f* oceanography
ocidental [osidẽ'taw] **1** *adj* GEOG western; POL *tb* Western **2** *m/f* westerner; POL *tb* Westerner
ocidente [osi'dẽtʃi] *m* west; POL *tb* West
ócio ['ɔsiu] *m* idleness; *tempo livre* leisure
ociosidade [osjozi'dadʒi] *f* idleness
ocioso [o'sjozu] *adj* idle; (*inútil*) superfluous
oco ['oku] *adj* hollow; *fig tb* empty; **cabeça** *f* **oca** empty head
ocorrência [oko'hẽsja] *f* incident, occurrence; (*coincidência*) coincidence; (*acaso*) chance; (*ocasião*) occasion
ocorrer [oko'her] ⟨2d⟩ (*ter lugar*) happen, occur; **ocorreu-lhe uma nova idéia** a new idea occurred to him
ocre ['ɔkri] **1** *m* ocher, *Brit* ochre **2** *adj* ocher, *Brit* ochre
ocular [oku'lar] *adj* eye *atr*, ocular; **testemunha ~** eye witness
oculista [oku'lista] *m/f* optometrist, *Brit* optician
óculos ['ɔkulus] *mpl* (eye)glasses, spectacles; **usar ~** wear glasses; **~s escuros** sunglasses; **~ de proteção** goggles
ocultar [okuw'tar] ⟨1a⟩ hide, conceal
oculto [o'kuwtu] *adj* hidden; (*secreto*) secret
ocupação [okupa'sãw] *f* occupation
ocupado [oku'padu] *adj Bras* TEL busy
ocupante [oku'pãtʃi] *m/f* occupant; MIL occupying force
ocupar [oku'par] ⟨1a⟩ occupy; (*reclamar*) claim; (*apropriar-se*) take possession of; *espaço* take up, occupy; *tempo* take up; (*habitar*) inhabit; **ocupar-se** *v/r* **~ com algo** busy oneself with sth; *tratar* deal with sth
odiar [o'dʒiar] ⟨1h⟩ hate
ódio ['ɔdiu] *m* hate, hatred
odioso [o'djozu] *adj* hateful; (*infame*) hated
odontologia [odõtolo'ʒia] *f* dentistry
odor [o'dor] *m* smell; **~ corporal** BO, body odor, *Brit* body odour
oeste [o'ɛstʃi] *m* west; **ao ~ de** to the west of
ofegante [ofe'gãtʃi] *adj* breathless, panting
ofegar [ofe'gar] ⟨1o & 1c⟩ pant, puff
ofender [ofẽ'der] ⟨2a⟩ offend; **ofender-se** *v/r* take offense, *Brit* take offence
ofensa [o'fẽsa] *f* offense, *Brit* offence; (*melindre*) insult; **~ corporal** physical assault; **sem ~** no offense meant
ofensiva [ofẽ'siva] *f* offensive; **ir para a ~** go on to the offensive
ofensivo [ofẽ'sivu] *adj* offensive; (*insultante*) insulting
oferecer [ofere'ser] ⟨2g⟩ offer; (*apresentar*) present; (*passar*) pass; *sacrifício* offer; (*dar*) give
oferta [o'fɛrta] *f* offer; COM bid; (*dádiva*) gift; (*prenda*) present; **estar em ~** be on special offer; **~ de emprego** job offer; **~ e procura** supply and demand; **~ pública de aquisição** takeover bid
office boy [ofise'bɔj] *m* biker, courier
oficial [ofi'sjaw] **1** *adj* official **2** *m/f* official; MIL officer; **~ comandante** commanding officer; **~ de diligências** bailiff

oficializar [ofisjali'zaɾ] ⟨1a⟩ make official
oficialmente [ofisjaw'mẽtʃi] *adv* officially
oficina [ofi'sina] *f* workshop; **~ *mecânica*** garage
ofício [o'fisiu] *m* trade, craft; (*profissão*) profession; (*cargo*) function, job; (*serviço*) service; (*incumbência*) duty; *escrito*: official letter; ***saber o seu ~*** know one's trade
oftalmologia [oftawmolo'ʒia] *f* ophthalmology
oftalmologista [oftawmolo'ʒista] *m/f* ophthalmologist
ofuscar [ofus'kaɾ] ⟨1n⟩ blot out; (*esconder*) conceal; *fig* (*deslumbrar*) dazzle; (*fazer sombra*) overshadow, eclipse
ogiva [o'ʒiva] *f* **~ *nuclear*** nuclear warhead
oi [oj] *int Bras* **~!** hi!
oiro ['ojɾu] *m Port etc* → **ouro** *etc*
oitavo [oj'tavu] **1** *adj* eighth **2** *m* eighth
oitenta [oj'tẽta] *num* eighty
oito ['ojtu] *num* eight
oitocentos [ojtu'sẽtus] *num* eight hundred
olá [o'la] *int* **~!** hello!, hi!
olaria [ola'ɾia] *f* pottery
óleo ['ɔliu] *m* oil; *Bras* **~ *diesel*** diesel (oil); **~ *de fígado de bacalhau*** cod-liver oil; **~ *mineral*** mineral oil; **~ *de motor*** engine oil; **~ *de proteção solar***, *Port* **~ *de protecção solar*** suntan oil
oleoduto [ɔljo'dutu] *m* (oil) pipeline
oleoso [o'ljozu] *adj* oily; (*gorduroso*) greasy
olfato, *Port* **olfacto** [ow'fatu] *m* sense of smell
olhadela [oʎa'dɛla] *f* glance; ***dar uma ~ a*** glance at
olhar [o'ʎaɾ] ⟨1d⟩ **1** *v/t* look at; (*observar*) watch; (*vigiar*) look after **2** *v/i* look; **~ *a***, **~ *para*** look at; **~ *pela janela*** look out of the window; ***olha, isto é sério*** look, this is serious **3** *m* look
olheiras [o'ʎejɾas] *fpl* (***grandes***) **~** (dark) rings under the eyes
olho ['oʎu] *m* eye; *queijo*, *pão*: hole; *salada*: heart; ***a ~ nu*** with the naked eye; ***não pregar ~*** not sleep a wink; **~ *mágico*** peephole; **~ *negro*** black eye; **~ *roxo*** black eye
oligarquia [oligaɾ'kia] *f* oligarchy
olimpíada [olĩ'piada] *f* Olympics
olímpico [o'lĩpiku] *adj* Olympic; ***Jogos*** *pl* ***Olímpicos*** Olympic Games
olival [oli'vaw] *m* olive grove
oliveira [oli'vejɾa] *f* olive tree
olmo ['owmu] *m* elm
ombreira [õ'brejɾa] *f vestuário*: shoulder pad; *porta*: doorpost; *fig* threshold
ombro ['õbɾu] *m* shoulder; ***encolher os ~s*** shrug one's shoulders; ***chorar no ~ de alguém*** cry on so.'s shoulder
omelete [ome'lɛtʃi] *f*, **omeleta** [ome'lɛta] *f Port* omelet, *Brit* omelette
omissão [omi'sãw] *f* omission
omitir [omi'tʃiɾ] ⟨3a⟩ omit
omni... *Port* → **oni...**
omoplata [omo'plata] *f* shoulder blade
onça[1] ['õsa] *f* COM ounce
onça[2] ['õsa] *f* ZOOL leopard; *Bras* jaguar; ***você é um amigo da ~!*** a fine friend you are!
onda ['õda] *f* wave; **~ *sonora*** sound wave; *fam* ***estar na ~*** be in fashion; **~ *curta* / *média* / *longa*** short / medium / long wave; **~ *de calor*** heatwave
onde ['õdʒi] **1** *adv* where; ***de ~?*** where from? ***de ~ é que você é?*** where are you from?; ***para ~*** where to **2** *pron* where; ***a cidade ~ moro*** the city where I live
ondulação [õdula'sãw] *f* undulation; **~ *permanente*** perm
ondulado [õdu'ladu] *adj* wavy; ***porta*** *f* ***ondulada*** corrugated iron door
ondulante [õdu'lãtʃi] *adj águas* undulating
ônibus ['onibus] *m Bras* bus
onipotência [onipo'tẽsja] *f* omnipotence
onipotente [onipo'tẽtʃi] *adj* omnipotent
onisciente [onis'sjẽtʃi] *adj* omniscient
online [on'lajn] *adv* on-line; ***serviço***

O

m ~ on-line service
ontem ['õtẽ] *adv* yesterday; ***de*** ~ yesterday's; ~ ***à noite*** last night; ~ ***de manhã*** yesterday morning
ONU [o'nu] *f abr* (***Organização das Nações Unidas***) UN (United Nations)
ônus, *Port* **ónus** ['onus] *m* onus, burden; (*tributo*) contribution; (*imposto*) tax burden; ~ ***da prova*** onus of proof
onze ['õzi] *num* eleven
oó [o'ɔ] *m fam* ***fazer*** ~ go bye-byes
opacidade [opasi'dadʒi] *f* opacity, opaqueness
opaco [o'paku] *adj* opaque
opala [o'pala] *f* opal
opção [o'psãw] *f* option; (*decisão*) decision
ópera ['ɔpeɾa] *f* opera; *edifício* opera (house)
operação [opeɾa'sãw] *f* operation; COM transaction; ***entrada*** *f* ***em*** ~ putting into operation, commissioning
operacional [opeɾasjo'naw] *adj* operational
operador [opeɾa'doɾ] *m*, **-a** *f* operator; ~ ***de câmara*** cameraman
operar [ope'ɾaɾ] ⟨1c⟩ **1** *v/t máquina* operate; MED operate on; (*causar*) effect; (*executar*) carry out, perform **2** *v/i* operate; (*agir*) act
operariado [opeɾa'ɾjadu] *m* workforce, workers
opinião [opi'njãw] *f* opinion; ~ ***pública*** public opinion; ***sondagem*** *f* ***de*** ~ opinion poll; ***na minha*** ~ in my opinion
ópio ['ɔpiu] *m* opium
oponente [opo'nẽtʃi] *m/f* opponent
opor [o'poɾ] ⟨2z⟩ oppose, resist; *dificuldade* raise; **opor-se** *v/r* object; ~ ***a algo*** object to sth, oppose sth
oportunidade [opoɾtuni'dadʒi] *f* opportunity
oportunista [opoɾtu'nista] **1** *m/f* opportunist **2** *adj* opportunistic
oportuno [opoɾ'tunu] *adj momento* opportune, right; (*a propósito*) convenient; (*favorável*) favorable, *Brit* favourable; (*adequado*) suitable
oposição [opozi'sãw] *f* opposition; (*contraste*) contrast; DIR objection; ***fazer*** ~ oppose
oposicionista [opozisjo'nista] **1** *m/f* member of the opposition **2** *adj* opposition *atr*
oposto [o'postu] **1** *adj* (*contraditório*) opposing; (*inverso*) opposite; (*em frente*) facing, opposite **2** *m* opposite
opressão [opɾe'sãw] *f* ⟨*sem pl*⟩ oppression
opressivo [opɾe'sivu] *adj* oppressive
opressor [opɾe'soɾ] *m* oppressor
oprimir [opɾi'miɾ] ⟨3a⟩ oppress
optar [opi'taɾ] ⟨1a⟩ choose; ~ ***por*** opt for; ~ ***por fazer algo*** opt to do sth
ópti..., opti... *Port* → ***óti..., oti...***
opulência [opu'lẽsja] *f* opulence
opulento [opu'lẽtu] *adj* opulent
ora ['ɔɾa] **1** *conj* (*pois*) well; (*no entanto*) however **2** *adv* now; ***por*** ~ for the time being; ~ ... ~ ... one moment … the next … **3** *int* ~ ***essa!*** oh, come on!; ~ ***bolas!*** for heaven's sake!; ~ ***viva!*** hi there!, hey!
oração [oɾa'sãw] *f* prayer; (*discurso*) speech; GRAM clause; ***fazer*** ~ say a prayer
oráculo [o'ɾakulu] *m* oracle
orador [oɾa'doɾ] *m*, **-a** *f* speaker
oral [o'ɾaw] *adj* oral; ***exame*** *m* ~ oral (exam)
orar [o'ɾaɾ] ⟨1a⟩ pray
oratória [oɾa'tɔɾja] *f* public speaking, oratory
oratório [oɾa'tɔɾiu] **1** *adj* oratorical **2** *m* oratory; MÚS oratorio
órbita ['ɔɾbita] *f* orbit; ANAT socket; *fig* sphere of influence
orçamental [oɾsamẽ'taw] *adj*, **orçamentário** [oɾsamẽ'taɾiu] *adj* budget *atr*; ***défice*** *m* ~ budget deficit
orçamento [oɾsa'mẽtu] *m* estimate; COM budget; ~ ***do Estado*** national budget; ~ ***para defesa*** defense budget, *Brit* defence budget
orçar [oɾ'saɾ] ⟨1p & 1e⟩ *v/t* estimate, value (***em*** at); ~ ***por*** come to around
ordem ['ɔɾdẽ] *f* order; *hierarquia*: tier; *advogados*, *médicos*: association; ***às ordens*** very well, as you wish; ***por*** ~ in order; ***dar uma*** ~ give an order ***até segunda*** ~, ***até segundas or-***

dens until further notice; **~ *jurídica*** warrant; **~ *de pagamento*** money order
ordenado [orde'nadu] **1** *m* salary, wage **2** *adj* orderly
ordenamento [ordena'mẽtu] *m* order
ordenar [orde'nar] ⟨1d⟩ put in order, order (*dispor*) arrange; (*mandar*) order; REL ordain
ordenhar [orde'ɲar] ⟨1d⟩ milk
ordinal [ordʒi'naw] *m* ordinal number
ordinário [ordʒi'nariu] *adj* ordinary; (*comum*) usual; *pej* vulgar; *coisa* cheap and nasty
orégano [o'rɛganu] *m* BOT oregano
orelha [o'reʎa] *f* ear; TECN flap
orelhão [ore'ʎãw] *m* phone booth, *Brit* phone box
órfã ['ɔrfã] *f* orphan
orfanato [orfa'natu] *m* orphanage
órfão ['ɔrfãw] ⟨*mpl* -ãos⟩ **1** *adj* orphaned **2** *m* orphan
orgânico [or'gʌniku] *adj* organic; ***lei*** *f* ***orgânica*** basic law
organismo [orga'nizmu] *m* ANAT, POL organism; (*corporação*) body, organization
organista [orga'nista] *m/f* organist
organização [organiza'sãw] *f* organization
organizador [organiza'dor] **1** *m*, **-a** *f* organizer **2** *adj* organizing *atr*
organizar [organi'zar] ⟨1a⟩ organize; *festa* hold
órgão ['ɔrgãw] *f* ⟨*pl* -ãos⟩ ANAT, MÚS organ; ***banco*** *m* ***de ~s*** organ bank; ***transplantação*** *f* ***de ~s*** organ transplant
orgasmo [or'gazmu] *m* orgasm
orgulhar-se [orgu'ʎarsi] *v/r* be proud (***de*** of)
orgulho [or'guʎu] *m* pride
orgulhoso [orgu'ʎozu] *adj* proud
orientação [orjẽta'sãw] *f* orientation; (*localização*) position; (*direção*) direction; (*instrução*) instruction; (*apoio*) guidance
orientador [orjẽta'dor] **1** *adj* guiding; (*dirigente*) supervising *atr* **2** *m*, **-a** *f* advisor; (*dirigente*) supervisor
oriental [orjẽ'taw] *adj* eastern, oriental
orientalista [orjẽta'lista] *m/f* orientalist
orientar [orjẽ'tar] ⟨1a⟩ orient; *fig* direct; (*aconselhar*) guide; **orientar-se** *v/r* get one's bearings; **~ *por*** (*guiar-se*) follow
oriente [o'rjẽtʃi] *m* east; ***a ~ de*** east of
Oriente [o'rjẽtʃi] *m* *Ásia*: East; ***Médio ~*** Middle East; ***Extremo / Próximo ~*** Far / Near East
orifício [ori'fisiu] *m* orifice
origem [o'riʒẽ] *f* origin; (*causa*) cause; ***país*** *m* ***de ~*** country of origin
original [oriʒi'naw] **1** *adj* original; (*particular*) strange, odd **2** *m* original; (*pessoa excêntrica*) eccentric
originalidade [oriʒinali'dadʒi] *f* originality
originar [oriʒi'nar] ⟨1a⟩ originate; (*causar*) give rise to; **originar-se** *v/r* originate
originário [oriʒi'nariu] *adj* native; ***ser ~ de*** come from
orla ['ɔrla] *f* edge, border; TÊX hem; **~ *marítima*** seafront
ornamentação [ornamẽta'sãw] *f* ornamentation
ornamentar [ornamẽ'tar] ⟨1a⟩ decorate, adorn
ornamento [orna'mẽtu] *m* decoration, adornment
ornitologia [ornitolo'ʒia] *f* ornithology
orquestra [or'kɛstra] *f* orchestra; **~ *de metais*** brass band; **~ *sinfônica*** symphony orchestra
orquestração [orkestra'sãw] *f* orchestration, arrangement
orquídea [or'kidʒia] *f* orchid
ortodoxia [ortodo'ksia] *f* orthodoxy
ortodoxo [orto'dɔksu] *adj* orthodox
ortografia [ortogra'fia] *f* spelling
ortográfico [orto'grafiku] *adj* spelling *atr*, orthographical
ortopedia [ortope'dʒia] *f* orthopedics
ortopedista [ortope'dʒista] *m/f* orthopedic specialist, orthopedist
orvalho [or'vaʎu] *m* dew
os [os] **1** *art mpl* the; **~ *livros*** the books **2** *pron mpl* them; *tratamento cortês*: you; ***eu ~ conheço*** I know them; → *tb* ***o***

O

oscilação [osila'sãw] *f* oscillation; *preços*: fluctuation
oscilar [osi'laɾ] ⟨1a⟩ oscillate; *preços* fluctuate
ósseo ['ɔsiu] *adj* bony
osso ['osu] *m* bone; **~ da sorte** wishbone
ostensível [ostẽ'sivew] *adj*, **ostensivo** [ostẽ'sivu] *adj* ostensible; (*claro*) apparent; (*vistoso*) ostentatious
ostentação [ostẽta'sãw] *f* display, exhibition; (*jactância*) ostentation
ostentar [ostẽ'taɾ] ⟨1a⟩ flaunt; (*mostrar*) show
ostentativo [ostẽta'ʧivu] *adj* ostentatious
ostra ['ostɾa] *f* oyster
OTAN [o'tã] *f abr* (***Organização do Tratado do Atlântico Norte***) NATO (North Atlantic Treaty Organization)
ótica ['ɔʧika] *f* optics
ótico ['ɔʧiku] **1** *adj* optical **2** *m*, **-a** *f* optician
otimismo [oʧi'mizmu] *m* optimism; (*confiança*) confidence
otimista [oʧi'mista] **1** *adj* optimistic **2** *m/f* optimist
ótimo ['ɔʧimu] *adj* excellent; **~!** great!
otorrinolaringologista [otohinolarĩgolo'ʒista] *m/f* ear, nose and throat doctor, ENT doctor
ou [ow] *conj* or; **~ … ~ …** either … or …
ouço ['owsu] *etc* → ***ouvir***
ouriço [o'ɾisu] *m* ZOOL hedgehog; BOT shell; **~ do mar** sea urchin
ourives [o'ɾivis] *m* goldsmith
ourivesaria [oɾiveza'ɾia] *f* goldsmith's art; *loja*: jewelry store, *Brit* jeweller's
ouro ['oɾu] *m* gold; **~s** *pl naipes*: diamonds; **de ~** golden
ousadia [owza'dʒia] *f* boldness; (*risco*) risk
ousado [ow'zadu] *adj* daring, bold; *decote* risqué
ousar [ow'zaɾ] ⟨1a⟩ dare
outdoor [awʧi'dɔɾ] *m* billboard
outonal [oto'naw] *adj* fall *atr*, *Brit* autumnal
Outono [o'tonu] *m* fall, *Brit* autumn; **no ~** in the fall
outorga [o'tɔɾga] *f* granting; (*doação*) awarding
outorgar [otoɾ'gaɾ] ⟨1o & 1e⟩ *v/t* DIR issue; (*aprovar*) approve; (*conceder*) grant; *diploma, título etc* award
outro ['otɾu], **outra** ['otɾa] *pron* other; (*mais um / uma*) another; **o ~, a outra** the other; ***outra cerveja, por favor*** another beer, please; ***outras duas cervejas*** two more beers, another two beers; ***eles se respeitam um ao ~*** they respect each other; ***vamos à ~ lugar*** let's go somewhere else; ***outra vez*** again
outrora [o'tɾɔɾa] *adv* formerly
outubro [o'tubɾu] *m* October; **em ~** in October
ouvido [o'vidu] **1** *m* hearing; ANAT ear; **~ *médio*** middle ear; ***dor** f **de ~*** earache; ***fora do alcance do ~*** out of earshot **2** *pp* → ***ouvir***
ouvinte [o'vĩʧi] *m/f* listener
ouvir [o'viɾ] ⟨3u⟩ hear; (*ter em conta*) listen; **~ *dizer*** hear it said that; ***ouviste?*** understood?
ovação [ova'sãw] *f* acclaim; (*aplausos*) ovation
ovacionar [ovasjo'naɾ] ⟨1f⟩ cheer
oval [o'vaw] *adj* oval
ovário [o'vaɾiu] *m* ovary
ovelha [o'veʎa] *f* sheep
OVNI ['ɔvni] *m abr* (***objecto voador não identificado***) UFO (unidentified flying object)
ovo ['ovu] *m* egg; ***pôr ~s*** lay eggs; **~ *cozido*** hard-boiled egg; **~ *estrelado*** fried egg; **~ *escalfado*** poached egg; **~ *mexido*** scrambled egg; GASTR **~s** *pl* ***moles*** *dessert made of eggs and sugar*; **~ *quente*** soft-boiled egg
óvulo ['ɔvulu] *m* egg, ovum
oxalá [oʃa'la] *adv* hopefully; **~!** let's hope so!; **~ *que*** (*subj*) let's hope
oxidação [oksida'sãw] *f* ⟨*sem pl*⟩ oxidation, rusting
oxidar [oksi'daɾ] ⟨1a⟩ oxidize
óxido ['ɔksidu] *m* oxide
oxigenado [oksiʒe'nadu] *adj* ***água** f **oxigenada*** peroxide
oxigenar [oksiʒe'naɾ] ⟨1d⟩ oxygenate; *cabelo* bleach

oxigênio, *Port* **oxigénio** [oksi'ʒeniu] *m* oxygen
ozônio, *Port* **ozónio** [o'zoniu] *m* ozone
ozono [o'zonu] *m* ozone; ***camada*** *f* ***de ~*** ozone layer

P

p. *abr* (***página***) p (page)
pá [pa] *f* shovel; TECN blade; ***~ de lixo*** dustpan
pacato [pa'katu] *adj* peaceful; *pessoa* easy-going
paciência [pa'sjẽsja] *f* patience; *jogo de cartas*: solitaire, *Brit* patience; (***não***) ***ter ~*** have (no) patience; ***perder a ~*** lose one's patience
paciente [pa'sjẽtʃi] **1** *adj* patient **2** *m/f* MED patient
pacífico [pa'sifiku] *adj* peaceful, peaceable; (***Oceano*** *m*) ***Pacífico*** Pacific (Ocean)
pacifista [pasi'fista] **1** *m/f* pacifist **2** *adj* pacifist
paço ['pasu] *m* palace; (*corte*) court; ***Paço***(***s***) (*pl*) ***do Concelho*** city hall
pacote [pa'kɔtʃi] *m* pack, packet; *turismo, ofertas*: package; ***~ de viagem*** package deal
pacotinho [pako'tʃiɲu] *m shampoo etc*: sachet
pacto ['paktu] *m* pact; (*contrato*) agreement; ***~ de suicídio*** suicide pact
pactuário [pak'twariu] *m*, **-a** *f* party to an / the agreement; (*aliado*) ally
padaria [pada'ria] *f* bakery
padeiro [pa'dejru] *m*, **-a** *f* baker
padrão [pa'drãw] *f* (*norma*) norm, standard; (*medida*) gage, *Brit* gauge; (*modelo, exemplo*) model; (*matriz*) template; *tecido*: pattern; ***aluno*** *f* ***~*** model pupil; ***estar fora do ~*** not be up to standard; ***~ de vida*** standard of living
padrasto [pa'drastu] *m* stepfather
padre ['padri] *m* priest; ***Padre Martin*** Father Martin
padrinho [pa'driɲu] *m batismo*: godfather; *casamento*: best man; UNIV *fam* supervisor
padroeiro [padro'ejru] *m*, **-a** *f* patron saint
padronização [padroniza'sãw] *f* standardization
padronizado [padroni'zadu] *adj* standardized
padronizar [padroni'zar] ⟨1a⟩ standardize
pág. *abr* (***página***) p (page)
paga ['paga] *f Port* pay
pagador [paga'dor] *m*, **-a** *f* payer
pagamento [paga'mẽtu] *m* payment; ***folha*** *f* ***de ~s*** pay check, *Brit* pay slip
pagão [pa'gãw] *m* ⟨*pl* -ãos⟩, **pagã** [pa'gã] *f* heathen
pagar [pa'gar] ⟨1o & 1b⟩ pay; *compra* pay for; *crédito* pay off; (*expiar*) pay for; *fig* pay back; ***~ uma bebida para alguém*** buy s.o. a drink
pagável [pa'gavew] *adj* payable
página ['paʒina] *f* page; ***~s*** *pl* ***amarelas*** Yellow Pages; ***virar a ~*** turn the page; *fig* make a new start; ***~ de esportes*** sports page; ***~ da web*** web page
paginação [paʒina'sãw] *f* page layout
paginar [paʒi'nar] ⟨1a⟩ *v/t* put into pages
pagode [pa'gɔdʒi] *m* pagoda; *fam* party
pai [paj] *m* father; ***meus ~s*** my parents; ***~ biológicos*** biological parents; ***~ de família*** family man
pai-nosso [paj'nɔsu] *m* ⟨*pl* ~ s⟩ REL Our Father, Lord's Prayer
painel [paj'nɛw] *m* panel; (*pintura*) picture; TECN instrument panel; AU-

P

TO dashboard; ***painéis*** *pl* paneling, *Brit* panelling; **~ *de especialistas*** panel of experts; **~ *solar*** solar panel
paio ['paiu] *m smoked pork sausage with garlic, white wine and paprika*
pairar [paj'raɾ]⟨1b⟩ *v/i* hover
país [pa'is] *m* country; ***País de Gales*** Wales; **~ *de origem*** country of origin
paisagem [paj'zaʒẽ] *f* scenery, landscape; *pintura* landscape
paisagista [pajza'ʒista] *m/f* landscape artist; ***arquiteto*** *m* **~**, *Port* ***arquitecto*** *m* **~** landscape architect
Países-Baixos [pa'isez'bajʃus] *pl* Netherlands
paixão [paj'ʃɐ̃w] *f* passion; ***Paixão de Cristo*** Christ's Passion; ***Semana*** *f* ***da Paixão*** Passion Week; ***Sexta-feira*** *f* ***da Paixão*** Good Friday
paixoneta [pajʃo'neta] *f Port*, **paixonite** [pajʃo'nitʃi] *f Bras* crush
pala ['pala] *f* peak; *pedra preciosa*: setting; *sapato*: tongue; *carro*: sun visor
palacete [pala'setʃi] *m* little palace
palácio [pa'lasiu] *m* palace; (*castelo*) castle
paladar [pala'daɾ] *m* ANAT palate; *fig* taste
palanque [pa'lɐ̃ki] *m* stand; **~ *das testemunhas*** witness stand, *Brit* witness box
palato ['palatu] *m* palate
palavra [pa'lavɾa] *f* word; ***em poucas* ~*s*** in a nutshell; INFORM **~ *-chave*** *f* key word; (*senha*) password; **~ *de honra*** word of honor, *Brit* word of honour; **~*s*** *pl* ***cruzadas*** crossword; **~*s*** *pl* ***de despedida*** parting words
palavrão [pala'vɾɐ̃w] *m* swearword
palco ['pawku] *m* stage; *circo*: ring
palerma [pa'lɛɾma] *fam* **1** *m/f* dope **2** *adj* dumb
Palestina [pales'tʃina] *f* Palestine
palestino [pales'tʃinu] **1** *adj* Palestinian **2** *m*, **-a** *f* Palestinian
palestra [pa'lɛstɾa] *f* lecture, talk
paletó [pale'tɔ] *m* jacket, coat
palha ['paʎa] *f* straw
palhaço [pa'ʎasu] *m* clown
palheiro [pa'ʎejɾu] *m* barn; ***procurar uma agulha num*** **~** be looking for a needle in a haystack
palhinha [pa'ʎiɲa] *f Port* straw; ***cadeira*** *f* ***de*** **~** cane chair
paliar [pa'ljaɾ] ⟨1g⟩ hide; (*suavizar*) mitigate
paliativo [palja'tʃivu] **1** *adj* palliative **2** *m* MED palliative
palidez [pali'des] *f* pallor
pálido ['palidu] *adj* pale
palito [pa'litu] *m* toothpick; *fam* ***pôr os* ~*s a alguém*** cheat on s.o.; **~ *de fósforo*** matchstick
palma[1] ['pawma] *f* BOT palm leaf; ***óleo*** *m* ***de*** **~** palm oil
palma[2] ['pawma] *f* **~ *da mão*** palm (of one's hand); **~*s*** *pl* applause; ***bater* ~*s*** applaud, put one's hands together
palmada [paw'mada] *f* slap
palmeira [paw'mejɾa] *f* palm (tree)
palmilha [paw'miʎa] *f* insole; ***em* ~*s*** in one's stockinged feet
palmito [paw'mitu] *m* palm heart
palmo ['pawmu] *m* span; (*mão*) hand's breadth
PALOP [pa'lɔp] *mpl abr* (***Países Africanos de Língua Oficial Portuguesa***) *African countries which have Portuguese as their official language*
palpável [paw'pavew] *adj* palpable
pálpebra ['pawpebɾa] *f* eyelid
palpitação [pawpita'sɐ̃w] *f* beat; ***palpitações*** palpitations
palpitar [pawpi'taɾ] ⟨1a⟩ (*coração*) beat, pound
palpite [paw'pitʃi] *m* hunch; *jogo*: tip; *fam* ***ter um*** **~** have a hunch
Panamá [pana'ma] *m* Panama; ***o canal do*** **~** the Panama Canal
pança ['pɐ̃sa] *f* belly; *irôn* paunch
pancada [pɐ̃'kada] *f* hit; *relógio*: stroke; *coração*: beat; **~ *de chuva*** shower (of rain)
pâncreas ['pɐ̃kɾias] *m* pancreas
pandeiro [pɐ̃'dejɾu] *m* MÚS tambourine
pane ['pani] *f* AUTO breakdown
panela [pa'nɛla] *f* pan; **~ *de pressão*** pressure cooker; *Port* AUTO **~ *de escape*** muffler, *Brit* silencer
paneleiro [pane'lejɾu] *m Port pop* fag, *Brit* queer
panfleto [pɐ̃'fletu] *m* pamphlet
pânico ['pʌniku] *m* panic; ***estar em*** **~**

P

be in a panic; ***entrar em ~*** panic
pano ['panu] *m* cloth; ***~ de limpeza*** cleaning cloth; ***~ de pó*** duster; ***~ de prato*** dishcloth
panorama [pano'rama] *m* panorama
panorâmico [pano'rʌmiku] *adj* panoramic
panqueca [pã'kɛka] *f* pancake
pantanal [pãta'naw] *m* swamp
pântano ['pãtanu] *m* swamp
pantanoso [pãta'nozu] *adj* swampy
pantera [pã'tɛra] *f* panther
pantufa [pã'tufa] *f* slipper
panturrilha [pãtu'hiʎa] *f* calf
pão [pãw] *m* ⟨*pl* pães⟩ bread; ***um ~*** a loaf (of bread); ***~ de alho*** garlic bread; ***~ de centeio*** rye bread; ***~ doce*** bun; ***~ fatiado*** sliced bread; ***~ de forma*** loaf; ***~ integral*** wholewheat bread, *Brit* wholemeal bread; GASTR ***~ de ló*** sponge cake; *Bras* ***~ de milho*** corn bread; ***~ preto*** black bread;*Port* ***~ ralado*** bread crumbs; ***~ sueco*** crispbread
pão-duro [pãw'duru] *adj* tight-fisted
pãozinho [pãw'ziɲu] *m* ⟨*pl* pãezinhos⟩ roll
papa[1] ['papa] *m* REL Pope
papa[2] ['papa] *f* GASTR mush; ***ele não tem ~s na língua*** he doesn't mince his words
papagaio [papa'gaiu] *m* parrot; *papel*: kite
papai [pa'paj] *m* pop, dad; ***Papai Noel*** Santa Claus, *Brit tb* Father Christmas
papaia [pa'paja] *f Port* papaya
papal [pa'paw] *adj* papal
paparicar [papari'kar] ⟨1n⟩ *v/t* pamper
papeira [pa'pejra] *f* MED mumps *sg*
papel [pa'pɛw] *m material*: paper; *nota*: piece of paper; TEAT part, role; ***lenço*** *m* ***de ~*** paper handkerchief; ***~ -aluminio*** kitchen foil, *Brit* tin foil; ***~ de carta*** note paper, writing paper; ***~ ecológico*** recycled paper; ***~ filtro*** filter paper; ***~ higiênico*** toilet paper; ***~ pardo*** wrapping paper; ***~ de parede*** wallpaper; ***~ de música*** (*ou* ***pautado***) music paper; ***~ usado*** wastepaper; ***~ vegetal*** greaseproof paper
papelada [pape'lada] *f* paperwork; (*documentos*) papers
papelão [pape'lãw] *m* cardboard
papelaria [papela'ria] *f* stationery store, *Brit* stationer's
papila [pa'pila] *f* ***~s gustativas*** taste buds
papo ['papu] *m pássaro*: crop; *macaco*: pouch; *pessoa*: double chin; *Bras* ***bater um ~*** have a chat; ***ele só tem ~*** he's all talk; *fam* ***está no ~*** it's in the bag
papo-seco [papo'seku] *m* roll
papoila [pa'pojla] *f Port*, **papoula** [pa'powla] *f Bras* poppy
paquerar [pake'rar] ⟨1c⟩ *v/t fam* hit on
paquete [pa'ketʃi] *m* steamship
paquistanês [pakista'nes] **1** *adj* Pakistani **2** *m*, **paquistanesa** [pakista'neza] *f* Pakistani
Paquistão [pakis'tãw] *m* Pakistan
par [par] **1** *adj número* even; (*semelhante*) similar **2** *m* pair; *pessoas*: couple; *dança*: partner; *golf*: par; ***encontrar seu ~*** meet one's match; ***ficar a ~ de*** keep abreast of
para ['para] **1** *prep* ◊ *local*: to; ***~ Chicago*** to Chicago; ***~ casa*** home; ***~ cá!*** over here!; ***~ cima / baixo*** upward / down

◊ *temporal*: for; ***um trabalho ~ uma semana*** a job for a week; ***~ sempre*** for ever; ***são quinze ~ as três*** it's a quarter of three, *Brit* it's quarter to three; ***~ já!*** coming up!

◊ *fim, destino*: for; ***~ mim não, obrigado*** not for me, thanks; ***~ que?*** what for?; ***~ que serve isto?*** what is this for?

◊ *relação*: ***~ mim, ele é ..*** as far as I'm concerned, he's … **2** *conj* to; ***~ terminar*** to conclude; ***~ variar*** to make a change; ***estar ~ fazer algo*** be about to do sth; ***era ~ ela ajudar*** she was supposed to help; ***~ que*** so that; ***~ que eu também viesse*** so that I could come too
parabenizar [parabeni'zar] ⟨1a⟩ *v/t* congratulate
parabéns [para'bẽs] *mpl* congratulations; ***muitos ~!*** *aniversário*: happy birthday!; ***dar os ~ a alguém*** con-

gratulate s.o.; *aniversário*: wish s.o. a happy birthday
parábola [pa'ɾabula] *f* parable; MAT parabola
parabólico [paɾa'bɔliku] *adj* ***antena f parabólica*** satellite dish
pára-brisas [paɾa'bɾizas] *m* ⟨*pl inv*⟩ windshield, *Brit* windscreen
pára-choques [paɾa'ʃɔkis] *m* ⟨*pl inv*⟩ AUTO bumper
parada [pa'ɾada] *f Bras* stop; (*desfile*) parade; ***~ nos boxes*** pitstop; ***~ cardíaca*** heart failure; ***~ de ônibus*** bus stop
paradeiro [paɾa'dejɾu] *m* whereabouts
paradigma [paɾa'dʒigma] *m* paradigm
paradoxo [paɾa'dɔksu] **1** *m* paradox **2** *adj* paradoxical
paráfrase [pa'ɾafɾazi] *f* paraphrase
parafuso [paɾa'fuzu] *m* screw; ***chave f de ~s*** screwdriver
paragem [pa'ɾaʒẽ] *f Port* stop; (*imobilização*) standstill; ***~ cardíaca*** heart failure; ***~ proibida*** no stopping; ***por estas paragens*** in these parts
parágrafo [pa'ɾagɾafu] *m* paragraph
Paraguai [paɾa'gwaj] *m* ***o ~*** Paraguay
paraguaio [paɾa'gwaiu] **1** *adj* Paraguayan **2** *m*, **-a** *f* Paraguayan
paraíso [paɾa'izu] *m* paradise
pára-lamas [paɾa'lamas] *m* fender, *Brit* wing; *bicicleta*: mudguard
paralela [paɾa'lɛla] *f* MAT parallel line; ***~s*** *pl* ESP parallel bars
paralelismo [paɾale'lizmu] *m fig* parallelism
paralelo [paɾa'lɛlu] **1** *adj* parallel *tb fig* **2** *m* GEOG parallel
paralisação [paɾaliza'sãw] *f* paralysis; (*suspensão*) stoppage; (*imobilidade*) standstill
paralisar [paɾali'zaɾ] ⟨1a⟩ *v/t* paralyze; *atividade* stop; *fábrica*, *trânsito* bring to a standstill; **paralisar-se** *v/r* be paralyzed; *trânsito*, *movimento* come to a standstill; *atividade* stop
paralisia [paɾali'zia] *f* paralysis
paralítico [paɾa'litʃiku] **1** *adj* paralytic **2** *m* MED paralytic
paramédico [paɾa'mɛdʒiku] *m*, **-a** *f* paramedic
parâmetro [pa'ɾʌmetɾu] *m* parameter
paramilitar [paɾamili'taɾ] *adj* paramilitary
paranóia [paɾa'nɔja] *f* paranoia
paranóico [paɾa'nɔjku] *adj* paranoid
parapeito [paɾa'pejtu] *m* parapet; *escadas*: landing; *janela*: windowsill
parapente [paɾa'pẽtʃi] *m* paraglider; *atividade* paragliding
paraplégico [paɾa'plɛʒiku] *adj* paraplegic
pára-quedas [paɾa'kɛdas] *m* ⟨*pl inv*⟩ parachute
pára-quedismo [paɾake'dʒizmu] *m* parachuting
pára-quedista [paɾake'dʒista] *m/f* ⟨*pl* ~ s⟩ parachutist
parar [pa'ɾaɾ] ⟨1b **3***rd pers. sg pres* pára⟩ **1** *v/t* stop **2** *v/i* stop; (*ficar*) stay, stop; ***~ de fazer algo*** stop doing sth; ***pare com isso!*** stop that!
pára-raios [paɾa'haius] *m* ⟨*pl inv*⟩ lightning rod, *Brit* lightning conductor
parasita [paɾa'zita] *m/f* parasite *tb fig*
parasitário [paɾazi'taɾiu] *adj* parasitic
pára-sol [paɾa'sɔw] *m* ⟨*pl* para-sóis⟩ parasol; FOT sun visor
parceiro [paɾ'sejɾu] *m*, **-a** *f* partner; *animal*: mate
parcela [paɾ'sɛla] *f terreno*: plot; (*pedaço*) piece; *fatura*: item
parcelar [paɾse'laɾ] ⟨1c⟩ *v/t* divide up
parceria [paɾse'ɾia] *f* partnership
parcial [paɾ'sjaw] *adj* partial; (*partidário*) biased
parcialidade [paɾsjali'dadʒi] *f* bias, partiality
parcialmente [paɾsjaw'mẽtʃi] *adv* partially
pardal [paɾ'daw] *m* sparrow
pardo ['paɾdu] *adj* gray, *Brit* grey; *cor*, *pele* dark; *pessoa* dark-skinned; ***ver-se em calças pardas*** be in a spot
parecer [paɾe'seɾ] ⟨2g⟩ **1** *v/i* seem, look; *bem*, *mal etc* look; ***você parece cansado*** you look tired; ***parece que*** it looks like, it look as if; ***parece que vai chover*** it looks like rain; ***parece-lhe bem se ...?*** is it ok with you if ...? **2** *v/t* (*dar a impressão*) appear to

be; ***parece seda*** it looks like silk; ***parece uma boa idéia*** that sounds like a good idea; ***parece-me*** it seem to me that **3** *m* (*aparência*) look, appearance; (*opinião*) opinion; (*relatório*) report; ***formar ~*** form an opinion; **parecer-se** *v/r* be alike; ***~ com alguém*** be like s.o.

parecido [paɾe'sidu] *adj* similar, alike; ***~ com*** similar to, like; ***bem ~*** nice; (*bonito*) pretty

parede [pa'ɾedʒi] *f* wall; ***na ~*** on the wall; *fig* ***estar entre a espada e a ~*** be between a rock and a hard place; ***~ de alpinismo*** climbing wall

parenta [pa'ɾẽta] *f* (female) relative, (female) relation

parente [pa'ɾẽtʃi] **1** *m/f* relative, relation; ***~ próximo*** next of kin **2** *adj* related

parentesco [paɾẽ'tesku] *m* degree of relationship

parêntese [pa'ɾẽtezi], **parêntesis** [pa'ɾẽtezis] *m* parenthesis, *Brit tb* bracket

paridade [paɾi'dadʒi] *f* parity

parir [pa'ɾiɾ] ⟨3y⟩ *v/t* give birth to

Paris [pa'ɾis] *sem art* Paris

parlamentar [paɾlamẽ'taɾ] **1** *adj* parliamentary **2** *m/f* member of parliament

parlamentarismo [paɾlamẽta'ɾizmu] *m* parliamentary system of democracy

parlamento [paɾla'mẽtu] *m* parliament

P

parmesão [paɾme'zãw] *adj/m* (***queijo*** *m*) ~ Parmesan (cheese)

pároco ['paɾuku] *m* parish priest

paródia [pa'ɾɔdʒia] *f* parody

parodiar [paɾo'dʒiaɾ] ⟨1g⟩ parody

paróquia [pa'ɾɔkja] *f* parish

paroquial [paɾo'kjaw] *adj* parish *atr*

parque ['paɾki] *m* park; *campismo*: site; *crianças*: playpen; ***~ de diversões*** amusement park; ***~ eólico*** wind farm; *Port* ***~ de estacionamento*** parking lot, *Brit* car park; ***~ de estacionamento subterrâneo*** underground parking garage, *Brit* underground carpark; ***~ infantil*** children's playground; ***~ nacional*** national park; ***~ natural*** nature reserve

parquímetro [paɾ'kimetɾu] *m* parking meter

parquinho [paɾ'kiɲu] *m* playground

parte ['paɾtʃi] *f* part; (*quota*) share; (*lado*) side; TEAT part, role; DIR party; ***~s do cenário*** scenes; *Port* ***em toda a ~*** everywhere; ***quinta / sétima ~*** fifth / seventh

parteira [paɾ'tejɾa] *f* midwife

participação [paɾtʃisipa'sãw] *f* participation; *filme*: appearance; (*notificação*) notification; ***~ obrigatória*** duty to notify

participante [paɾtʃisi'pãtʃi] **1** *adj* participating; ***não ~*** non-participating **2** *m/f* participant; *competição*: entrant

participar [paɾtʃisi'paɾ] ⟨1a⟩ **1** *v/t* notify of **2** *v/i* ***~ de, ~ em*** participate in, take part in; (*interessar-se*) take an interest in; (*compartilhar*) have a share in

particípio [paɾtʃi'sipiu] *m* participle; ***~ passado*** past participle

partícula [paɾ'tʃikula] *f* particle

particular [paɾtʃiku'laɾ] **1** *adj* particular; (*caraterístico*) peculiar; (*pessoal*) personal; (*privado*) private; ***em ~*** in private; (*especialmente*) particularly **2** *m* (private) individual; ***neste ~*** in this particular, in this matter; ***~es*** *pl* details

particularidade [paɾtʃikulaɾi'dadʒi] *f* peculiarity

particularmente [paɾtʃikulaɾ'mẽtʃi] *adv* particularly; *tratar etc* separately

partida [paɾ'tʃida] *f* departure; ESP start; *xadrez, tênis etc*: game; ***ponto*** *m* ***de ~*** departure point; ***~ anulada*** false start; ***~ internacional*** international

partidário [paɾtʃi'daɾiu] **1** *adj conferência etc* party *atr* **2** *m*, **-a** *f* supporter; POL party member

partido [paɾ'tʃidu] *m* party; *jogo*: handicap; *fig* advantage; ***tomar ~*** take sides (***por*** with)

partilha [paɾ'tʃiʎa] *f* (*parte*) share

partilhar [paɾtʃi'ʎaɾ] ⟨1a⟩ share out; ***~ de*** share

partir [paɾ'tʃiɾ] ⟨3b⟩ **1** *v/t* (*dividir*) divide; (*quebrar*) break; *noz* crack; *pão* cut; (*rasgar*) tear; (*distribuir*) distribute; **~ ao** (*ou* **pelo**) **meio** divide in two, halve **2** *v/i* break; (*viajar*) leave; **a ~ de** as of, from; **~ para cima de** go for; **partir-se** *v/r* come apart; *gelo* break up

parto ['partu] *m* birth; **~ prematuro** premature birth, premature delivery; **entrar em trabalho de ~** go into labor, *Brit* go into labour

part-time [part'tajm] *m Port* part time; **emprego** *m* **em ~** part-time job

parvo ['parvu] *adj Port* stupid, dumb; **seu ~!** you idiot!

Páscoa ['paskwa] *f* Easter; **domingo** *m* **de ~** Easter Sunday

pasmar [pas'mar] ⟨1b⟩ *v/t* dumbfound; **~ a vista em** stare at

passa ['pasa] *f* (*uva*) raisin; *fam cigarro*: puff

passadeira [pasa'dejra] *f* (*tapete*) carpet, runner; *Port* crosswalk, *Brit* zebra crossing

passadiço [pasa'dʒisu] *m* gangway

passado [pa'sadu] **1** *adj* past; (*anterior*) earlier; *fruta* dried; *fig de frio etc* stiff; GASTR **bem ~** well done; **mal ~** rare **2** *m* past

passador [pasa'dor] *m* GASTR sieve; (*contrabandista*) smuggler

passageiro [pasa'ʒejru] **1** *adj* passing **2** *m*, **-a** *f* passenger

passagem [pa'saʒẽ] *f tb texto, tempo*: passage; *entrada*: pass; *esp Bras* (*bilhete*) ticket; **de ~** passing; **preço da ~** fare; **~ de ida** one-way ticket, *Brit* single; **~ de ida e volta** round-trip ticket, *Brit* return; **~ de nível** grade crossing, *Brit* level crossing; **~ de ônibus** bus ticket; **~ de pedestres** crosswalk, *Brit* zebra crossing; **~ do século** turn of the century; **~ subterrânea** underpass

passaporte [pasa'pɔrtʃi] *m* passport

passar [pa'sar] ⟨1b⟩ **1** *v/t* (*atravessar*) cross, go across; *além*: go past; (*ultrapassar*) exceed; *bola* pass; *cartão de crédito* swipe; GASTR *sopa* strain; (*entregar*) pass (on); *recado* deliver; *pancada* give; *documento* issue; *tempo* spend; **~** (**a ferro**) iron; **~ algo a alguém** pass sth to s.o.; **passamos bons momentos** we had a lovely time; **~ a noite** spend the night **2** *v/i* pass, go past; *exame etc*: pass; *chuva*, *dor* ease up; *água*, *boato* get in; **~ bem** have a good time; **~ num exame** pass an exam; **~ de moda** go out of fashion; **fazer-se ~ por** pass oneself off as; **~ a conhecer** get to know; **~ a existir** come into existence; **~ sem** go without; **passar-se** *v/r* happen; *tempo* pass **3** *m tempo*: passage

passarela [pasa'rɛla] *f* footbridge; *modelos*: runway, *Brit* catwalk

pássaro ['pasaru] *m* bird

passatempo [pasa'tẽpu] *m* pastime

passe ['pasi] *m* (*autorização*), *futebol*: pass; **~ de calcanhar** backheeler

passeante [pa'sjãtʃi] *m/f* stroller

passear [pa'sjar] ⟨1l⟩ **1** *v/t* take out for a walk **2** *v/i* go for a stroll, walk around; *carro*: go for a drive, go for a ride; *cavalo*: go for a ride; **~ de barco** go for a sail; **~ pela loja** browse around the shop

passeio[1] [pa'seiu] *m* stroll, walk; *carro*: ride, drive; *cavalo*: ride; *barco*: sail; *Port* (*calçada*) sidewalk, *Brit* pavement; **~ de bicicleta** bike ride; **~ guiado** guided tour; **~ marítimo** sea front, promenade; **~ público** promenade

passeio[2] [pa'seiu] *etc* → **passear**

passional [pasjo'naw] *adj* passionate; **crime ~** crime of passion

passividade [pasivi'dadʒi] *f* passivity

passivo [pa'sivu] **1** *adj* passive; **voz** *f* **passiva** passive **2** *m* COM liabilities

passo ['pasu] *m* step; (*pegada*) footprint; (*modo de andar*) walk; *montanha*: pass; **~ a ~** step by step; **a dois ~s** a couple of minutes away; **a ~ de caracol** at a snail's pace; **dar um ~** take a step; **seguir os ~s de alguém** follow in s.o.'s footsteps

pasta[1] ['pasta] *f* paste; **~ de amendoim** peanut butter; **~ de dentes** toothpaste

pasta[2] ['pasta] *f atas*: folder; (*mala*) briefcase; INFORM folder, directory; POL portfolio

P

pastagem [pas'taʒẽ] *f* pasture
pastar [pas'taɾ] ⟨1b⟩ *v/i* graze
pastel [pas'tɛw] *m* GASTR (*pastelão*) pastry; ARTE pastel; **~ de bacalhau** cod croquette; **~ folhado** Danish (pastry); **~ de nata** (*ou* **de Belém**) *Portuguese custard tart*
pastelaria [pastela'ɾia] *f lugar* cake shop; *arte* pastry making
pastilha [pas'ʧiʎa] *f* pastille; MED tablet; INFORM chip; AUTO brake lining; *Port* **~ elástica** chewing gum
pasto ['pastu] *m gado*: feed; (*pastagem*) pasture; *fig* food; **casa** *f* **de ~** diner
pastor [pas'toɾ] *m* shepherd *tb fig*; (*padre protestante*) pastor; **~ alemão** German shepherd
pata[1] ['pata] *f* paw, foot; (*garra*) claw; *cavalo*: hoof; **à ~** on foot; **meter a ~ na poça** *fam* put one's foot in it
pata[2] ['pata] *f* duck
patamar [pata'maɾ] *m escadas*: landing
patente [pa'tẽʧi] **1** *adj* open; (*evidente*) obvious **2** *f* TECN patent; MIL commission; (*diploma*) diploma; (*documento*) pass
patentear [patẽ'ʧiaɾ] ⟨1l⟩ open; (*descobrir*) show; *invenção* patent
paternal [paʧiɾ'naw] *adj* paternal, fatherly
paternidade [pateɾni'dadʒi] *f* paternity
paterno [pa'tɛɾnu] *adj* paternal
pateta [pa'tɛta] *m/f* thickhead
patético [pa'tɛʧiku] **1** *adj* pathetic **2** *m* pathos
patim [pa'ʧĩ] *m* skate; *trenó*: runner; **patins** *pl* (**em linha**, *Bras* **in-line**) in-line skates; **hóquei** *m* **em patins** hockey, *Brit* ice hockey; **~ de rodas** roller skate
patinador [paʧina'doɾ] *m*, **-a** *f* skater
patinagem [paʧi'naʒẽ] *f* skating; **~ artística** figure skating
patinar [paʧi'naɾ] ⟨1a⟩ skate; AUTO skid
patinete [paʧi'neʧi] *f* scooter
pátio ['patiu] *m* patio; *prisão etc*: yard
pato ['patu] *m* ZOOL duck; *macho* drake; *fig fam* simpleton, dummy; **cair que nem um ~** fall for it
patologia [patolo'ʒia] *f* pathology
patológico [pato'lɔʒiku] *adj* pathological
patologista [patolo'ʒista] *m/f* pathologist
patrão [pa'tɾɐ̃w] *m* employer; (*chefe*) boss; (*estalajadeiro*, *senhorio*) landlord; NÁUT captain
pátria ['patɾia] *f* homeland, country
patriarca [patɾi'aɾka] *m* patriarch
patrimônio, *Port* **património** [patɾi'moniu] *m* inheritance; FIN asset
patriota [patɾi'ɔta] *m/f* patriot
patriotismo [patɾio'ʧizmu] *m* patriotism
patrocinador [patɾosina'doɾ] *m*, **-a** *f* patron; COM sponsor
patrocinar [patɾosi'naɾ] ⟨1a⟩ sponsor
patrocínio [patɾo'siniu] *m* (*proteção*) patronage; COM sponsorship; **sob o ~ de** under the auspices of
patronato [patɾo'natu] *m* patronage
patrulha [pa'tɾuʎa] *f* patrol
patrulhar [patɾu'ʎaɾ] ⟨1a⟩ *v/t* & *v/i* patrol
pau [paw] *m* wood; (*pedaço de madeira*) piece of wood; (*vara*) stick; (*cacete*) club; *chocolate*: bar; **~s** *pl naipes*: clubs; *Bras* **levar ~** fail
pau-brasil [pawbɾa'ziw] *m* Brazil wood
paupérrimo [paw'pɛhimu] *adj* poverty-stricken
pausa ['pawza] *f* pause, rest; EDUC recess, *Brit* break
pausado [paw'zadu] *adj* slow
pausar [paw'zaɾ] ⟨1a⟩ *v/i Bras* pause
pauta [paw'ta] *f* pattern
pavão [pa'vɐ̃w] *m* peacock
pavilhão [pavi'ʎɐ̃w] *m* pavillion; *jardim*: summerhouse; **~ de isolamento** isolation ward; **~ de maternidade** maternity ward
pavimentar [pavimẽ'taɾ] ⟨1a⟩ *v/t* pave
pavimento [pavi'mẽtu] *m* flooring; (*calçada*) sidewalk, *Brit* pavement
pavio [pa'viu] *m* wick
pavonear [pavo'niaɾ] ⟨1l⟩ *v/i* strut
pavor [pa'voɾ] *m* terror
pavoroso [pavo'ɾozu] *adj* terrible,

P

dreadful
paz [pas] *f* peace; ***fazer as ~es*** make up
pé [pɛ] *m* foot; (*tronco*) stalk; *couve*: head; ***a ~*** on foot; ***em ~*** standing; ***na ponta dos ~s*** on tippy-toe, *Brit* on tiptoe; *fam* ***meter os ~s pelas mãos*** screw up; ***perder o ~*** lose one's footing; ***fiquei de ~ o dia inteiro*** I've been on my feet all day; ***~ frio*** jinx; ***~ no saco*** pain in the neck; ***~s membranosos*** webbed feet
peão [pjãw] *m Port* pedestrian; MIL foot soldier; *xadrez*: pawn
peça ['pɛsa] *f* piece; TEAT play; (*móvel*) piece of furniture; (*assoalhada*) room; TECN part; *fam* trick
pecado [pe'kadu] *m* sin
pecador [peka'dor] **1** *adj* sinful **2** *m*, **-a** *f* sinner
pecar [pe'kar] ⟨1n & 1c⟩ sin
pechincha [pe'ʃĩʃa] *f* snip, bargain
pechinchar [peʃĩ'ʃar] ⟨1a⟩ *v/i* bargain, haggle
peço ['pɛsu] *etc* → ***pedir***
pecuária [pe'kwarja] *f* cattle-breeding; (*gado*) cattle
pecuário [pe'kwariu] **1** *adj* cattle *atr* **2** *m* cattle-breeder
pedaço [pe'dasu] *m* piece; *tempo*: while; *fam homem* hunk; ***fazer em ~s*** tear to pieces
pedágio [pe'daʒiu] *m Bras* toll
pedagogia [pedago'ʒia] *f* education
pedagógico [peda'gɔʒiku] *adj* educational, pedagogical
pedagogo [peda'gogu] *m*, **-a** *f* educationalist
pedal [pe'daw] *m* pedal; ***~ do acelerador*** gas pedal
pedalar [peda'lar] ⟨1b⟩ pedal
pedante [pe'dãtʃi] **1** *m/f* pedant; (*arrogante*) self-important person **2** *adj* pedantic; (*pomposo*) self-important
pé-de-cabra [pɛdʒi'kabra] *m* crowbar
pedestal [pedes'taw] *m* pedestal
pedestre [pe'dɛstri] *m/f Bras* pedestrian
pediatra [pe'dʒiatra] *m/f* pediatrician
pediatria [pedʒia'tria] *f* pediatrics
pedicure [pedʒi'kuri] *m/f pessoa* podiatrist, *Brit* chiropodist
pedido [pe'dʒidu] **1** *m* request; COM, *restaurante*: order; (*procura*) demand; *casamento*: proposal; ***a ~ de*** at the request of; ***fazer um ~ a alguém*** request sth from s.o.; COM order sth from s.o. **2** *pp* → ***pedir***
pedir [pe'dʒir] ⟨3r⟩ **1** *v/t* request, ask for; COM, *restaurante*: order; *tempo*, *esforço*, *etc* require; ***~ algo a alguém*** ask s.o. for sth; (*exigir*) demand sth from s.o.; (*encomendar*) order sth from s.o. **2** *v/i* ask; COM, *restaurante*: order; ***pede-se aos convidados que …*** guests are requested to …
pedra ['pɛdra] *f* stone; *maior* rock; *granizo*: hailstone; *xadrez*: piece, man; *açúcar etc*: lump; ***cair ~, chover ~*** hail; ***~ de calçamento*** paving stone; ***~ de gelo*** ice cube
pedrada [pe'drada] *f* stoning; *fam* ***estar com uma ~*** be stoned
pedra-pomes [pɛdra'pomis] *f* pumice stone
pedregoso [pedre'gozo] *adj* rocky, stony
pedregulho [pedre'guʎu] *m* big stone; (*cascalho*) gravel
pedreira [pe'drejra] *f* quarry
pedreiro [pe'drejru] *m* stonemason
pega[1] ['pega] *f* ZOOL mapgpie; *fig* gossip; *vulg* tart, whore
pega[2] ['pɛga] *f* (*cabo*) handle; (*pano*) hook; (*briga*) quarrel; *corrida de touros*: *attacking the bull without a weapon*
pegada [pe'gada] *f* footprint; (*pista*) track; *bola*: catch; ***ir nas ~s de alguém*** follow in s.o.'s footsteps
pegajoso [pega'ʒozu] *adj* sticky; *pessoa* clingy
pegar [pe'gar] ⟨1o & 1c⟩ **1** *v/t* (*colar*) stick; (*ligar*) stick together; (*agarrar*) grab; (*apanhar*) catch; *doença*, *trem etc* catch, get; *curva* take; *objeto caído*, *Bras homem*, *mulher*, *no carro*, *hábito* pick up; ***pegaste-me a gripe*** you've given me the flu; ***~ carona*** hitch a ride, get a ride; ***pegue qualquer um que quiser*** take any one you like **2** *v/i* stick; (*segurar*) hold; *moda* catch on, take off; *reclame* work; *motor* start; *doença* be catching; *planta*, *fogo* take; ***~ com*** border on; ***~ em algo***

P

take sth; *observação* pick sth up; (*tratar*) get going on sth; ~ ***no sono*** fall asleep; ***o carro não quer*** ~ the car won't start
peidar [pej'daɾ] *v/i pop* fart
peido ['pejdu] *m pop* fart
peito ['pejtu] *m* breast, chest; *fig* heart; (*alma*) soul; (*coragem*) courage; ***dar o*** ~ breastfeed; ~ ***de galinha*** chicken breast; ~ ***do pé*** instep
peitoril [pejto'riw] *m janela*: windowsill
peixe ['pejʃi] *m* fish; ~ ***frito*** fried fish; ***nem carne nem*** ~ neither one thing nor the other; ASTROL ***Peixes*** Pisces
peixe-espada [pejʃes'pada] *m* scabbard fish
peixeiro [pej'ʃejɾu] *m* fishmonger
peixe-vermelho [pejʃeveɾ'meʎu] *m* goldfish
pejorativo [peʒoɾa'tʃivu] *adj* pejorative
pela [pela, 'pela] = *prep* ***por*** *com art ou pron* ***a***
pelada [pe'lada] *f* game of soccer, *Brit* game of football
pelado [pe'ladu] *adj* hairless; (*despido*) naked
pelagem [pe'laʒẽ] *f dos animais* coat, skin
pele ['pɛli] *f* skin; *animal*: hide; *vestuário*: fur; ***casaco*** *m* ***de*** ~***s*** fur coat
peleiro [pe'lejɾu] *m* furrier
pelejar [pele'ʒaɾ] ⟨1d⟩ fight
pelica [pe'lika] *f* calfskin; ***luva*** *f* ***de*** ~ kid glove
pelicano [peli'kanu] *m* pelican; MED pliers
película [pe'likula] *f* film
pelo [pelu, 'pelu] *prep* ***por*** *com art ou pron* ***o***
pêlo ['pelu] *m* hair; *animal*: fur; (*penugem*) fluff; ***em*** ~ in the buff; ~***s púbicos*** pubic hair
pelotão [pelo'tãw] *m* MIL platoon
peludo [pe'ludu] *adj* hairy; *animal* furry
pena[1] ['pena] *f* (*castigo*) punishment, penalty; (*dó*) pity; (*sofrimento*) suffering; *inferno*: torment; ***sob*** ~ bei Strafe; ***cumprir uma*** ~ serve a prison sentence; ***vale a*** ~ it's worth it, it's worthwhile; ***é*** ~***!*** pity!; ***que*** ~***!*** what a pity!; ~ ***capital*** capital punishment; ~ ***máxima*** maximum penalty; ~ ***de morte*** death penalty
pena[2] ['pena] *f* feather
penal [pe'naw] *adj* penal; ***código*** *m* ~ penal code
penalidade [penali'dadʒi] *f* punishment; ESP penalty point
penalista [pena'lista] *m/f* criminologist
penalização [penaliza'sãw] *f* penalization
penalizar [penali'zaɾ] ⟨1a⟩ (*castigar*) penalize
pênalti [pe'nawtʃi] *m* ESP penalty
penar [pe'naɾ] ⟨1d⟩ pay for; (*sofrer*) suffer
pendência [pẽ'dẽsja] *f* dispute; DIR ***em*** ~ disputed
pendente [pẽ'dẽtʃi] **1** *adj* hanging; (*dependente*) dependent (***de*** on); (*iminente*) imminent; *fig* pending **2** *m* pendant
pender [pẽ'deɾ] ⟨2a⟩ *v/i* hang; (*tender*) tend (***a, para*** toward)
pêndulo ['pẽdulu] *m* pendulum
pendurado [pẽdu'ɾadu] *adj* hanging; ***estar*** ~ be left hanging
pendurar [pẽdu'ɾaɾ] ⟨1a⟩ hang (***por*** on)
peneira [pe'nejɾa] *f* sieve
peneirar [penej'ɾaɾ] ⟨1a⟩ sift
penetração [penetɾa'sãw] *f* penetration; *fig* perspicacity
penetrante [pene'tɾãtʃi] *adj* penetrating; (*agudo*) sharp; *ironia* caustic; *som* piercing; *sentimento* deep; *espírito* sharp, penetrating
penetrar [pene'tɾaɾ] ⟨1c⟩ **1** *v/t* penetrate; (*compreender*) understand **2** *v/i* get through; ~ ***em*** penetrate
penha ['peɲa] *f* cliff
penhasco [pe'ɲasku] *m* crag, cliff
penhor [pe'ɲoɾ] *m* pledge; ***casa*** *f* ***de*** ~***es*** pawnshop
penhora [pe'ɲɔɾa] *f casa*: repossession
penhorar [peɲo'ɾaɾ] ⟨1e⟩ pawn; (*garantir*) guarantee; (*prometer*) pledge; *fig* make grateful; *casa* repossess
penhorista [peɲo'ɾista] *m/f* pawnbroker

P

penicilina [penisi'lina] *f* penicillin
penico [pe'niku] *m* potty
península [pe'nĩsula] *f* peninsula
pênis, *Port* **pénis** ['penis] *m* penis
penitência [peni'tẽsja] *f* penitence; **~s** *pl* penance
penitenciar [penitẽ'sjaɾ] ⟨1g⟩ **~ alguém** make s.o. do penance; (*castigar*) punish s.o.; **~ algo** pay for sth
penitenciária [penitẽ'sjaɾja] *f* penitentiary, prison
penitenciário [penitẽ'sjaɾiu] **1** *n* prison *atr* **2** *m*, **-a** *f* prisoner, inmate **2** *m* REL confessor
penitente [peni'tẽtʃi] **1** *adj* repentant, contrite; REL penitent **2** *m/f* penitent
penoso [pe'nozu] *adj* painful; (*difícil*) difficult
pensador [pẽsa'doɾ] *m*, **-a** *f* thinker
pensamento [pẽsa'mẽtu] *m* thought; (*pensar*) thinking, thought; **vir ao ~ de alguém** occur to s.o.
pensão [pẽ'sãw] *f* pension; *casa* boarding house; **meia ~** half board; **~ alimentícia** maintenance; **~ completa** full board; **~ de velhice** old-age pension
pensar[1] [pẽ'saɾ] ⟨1a⟩ **1** *v/i* think (**em** of); **~ em, ~ sobre** think about **2** *v/t* **~ algo** think sth; (*considerar*) think about sth
pensar[2] [pẽ'saɾ] ⟨1a⟩ *v/t ferida* dress
pensativo [pẽsa'tʃivu] *adj* thoughtful, pensive
pensionato [pẽsjo'natu] *m* boarding school
pensionista [pẽsjo'nista] *m/f numa pensão* boarder
penso ['pẽsu] *Port* MED dressing; **~ higiênico** sanitary napkin, *Brit* sanitary towel; **~ rápido** Bandaid®, *Brit* plaster
pentágono [pẽ'tagunu] *m* pentagon
pente ['pẽtʃi] *m* comb; *fig* **passar a ~ fino** go through with fine-tooth comb
penteadeira [pẽtʃia'dejɾa] *f* dressing table
penteado [pẽ'tʃiadu] *m* hairstyle
pentear [pẽ'tʃiaɾ] ⟨1l⟩ comb; (*arranjar*) style
Pentecostes [pẽtʃi'kɔstʃis] *m* Pentecost, *Brit* Whitsun
penugem [pe'nuʒẽ] *f* fluff
penúltimo [pe'nuwtʃimu] *adj* penultimate
pepino [pe'pinu] *m* cucumber; *em conserva* gherkin; *fam* **~ choco** weakling; **salada** *f* **de ~** cucumber salad
pequenino [pe'kenu] *adj* tiny
pequeno [pe'kenu] *adj* little, small; *vitória* narrow
pequeno-almoço [pekenwaw'mosu] *m* ⟨*pl* pequenos-almoços⟩ *Port* breakfast; **tomar o ~** have breakfast
Pequim [pe'kĩ] *sem art* Beijing
pêra ['peɾa] *f* BOT pear; *fig* (*barba*) goatee; (*murro*) punch
perante [pe'ɾãtʃi] *prep* (*na presença de*) before; (*em vista de*) in view of
perca ['peɾka] *etc* → **perder**
perceber [peɾse'beɾ] ⟨2c⟩ perceive; *Port* (*entender*) understand; **percebeu?** do you understand?
percentagem [peɾsẽ'taʒẽ] *f* percentage
percentual [peɾsẽ'twaw] *adj* percentage *atr*
percepção [peɾsep'sãw] *f* perception
perceptível [peɾsɛ'tʃivew] *adj* perceptible
percevejo [peɾse'veʒu] *m* bug; *fig* thumbtack, *Brit* drawing pin
perco ['peɾku] → **perder**
percorrer [peɾko'heɾ] ⟨2d⟩ *distância* cover; *país* travel through; *mar* sail; *rio* cross; *fig* search through; **~ (com a vista)** scan
percurso [peɾ'kuɾsu] *m* route; (*via*) way; *rio*: course; (*viagem*) journey; **é um longo ~** it's a long way, it's a long distance
percussão [peɾ'kuɾsu] *f* percussion
perda ['peɾda] *f* loss; **é ~ de tempo / dinheiro** it's a waste of time / money
perdão [peɾ'dãw] *m* forgiveness; DIR pardon; **~, senhor** pardon me, I'm sorry
perdedor [peɾde'doɾ] *m*, **-a** *f* loser
perder [peɾ'deɾ] ⟨2o⟩ lose; *oportunidade*, *trem etc* miss; (*desperdiçar*) waste; **~ o poder** fall from power; **perder-se** *v/r* get lost; *fig* go astray

P

perdido [per'dʒidu] *adj* lost; *bala* stray; *apaixonado* head over heels in love (***por*** with); ***~s e achados*** *mpl* lost and found, *Brit* lost property
perdiz [per'dʒis] *f* partridge
perdoar [per'dwar] ⟨1f⟩ forgive; *castigo*, *dívida* cancel; DIR *pessoa* pardon; (*poupar*) spare
perecível [pere'sivew] *adj* perishable
peregrinação [peregrina'sãw] *f* REL pilgrimage
peregrino [pere'grinu] *m*, **-a** *f* REL pilgrim; *fig* pioneer
pereira [pe'rejra] *f* pear tree
perene [pe'reni] *adj* everlasting; BOT perennial
perfeccionismo [perfeksjo'nizmu] *m* perfectionism
perfeccionista [perfeksjo'nista] *m/f* perfectionist
perfeição [perfej'sãw] *f* ⟨*sem pl*⟩ perfection
perfeitamente [perfejta'mẽtʃi] *adv* perfectly
perfeito [per'fejtu] *adj* perfect
perfídia [per'fidʒia] *f* treachery
perfil [per'fiw] *m* profile; (*contorno*) outline; ***de ~*** in profile
perfilhar [perfi'ʎar] *v/t* DIR adopt
performance [per'fɔrmãsi] *f* TECN, ESP performance
perfumado [perfu'madu] *adj* fragrant; *pessoa* perfumed
perfumar [perfu'mar] ⟨1a⟩ *roupa* put perfume on; *ar* scent
perfumaria [perfuma'ria] *f* perfumery
perfume [per'fumi] *m* perfume; (*odor*) scent
perfuração [perfura'sãw] *f* drilling; (*brocagem*) drill hole; *esp* MED perforation; ***torre*** *f* ***de ~*** drilling platform
perfurado [perfu'radu] *adj linha* perforated
perfurador [perfura'dor] **1** *m*, **-a** *f* drill; *papel*: punch **2** *adj* ***máquina*** *f* ***~a*** *f* drill
perfurar [perfu'rar] ⟨1a⟩ puncture; *com perfurador* drill a hole in; *papel* punch a hole in
perfuratriz [perfura'tris] *f* drilling rig
pergaminho [perga'miɲu] *m* parchment
pergunta [per'gũta] *f* question; ***fazer uma ~ a alguém*** ask s.o. a question
perguntar [pergũ'tar] ⟨1a⟩ ask; (*interrogar*) question; ***~ a alguém*** ask s.o.; ***~ por*** ask after; **perguntar-se** *v/r* wonder
perícia [pe'risja] *f* (*experiência*) experience; (*habilidade*) expertise
periferia [perife'ria] *f* periphery; (*lado exterior*) outside; ***~s*** *pl de cidade* outskirts
periférico [peri'fɛriku] **1** *adj* peripheral **2** *m* INFORM peripheral
perigo [pe'rigu] *m* danger; ***pôr em ~*** put at risk; ***sem ~*** (***para***) safe (for); ***correr ~*** be at risk
perigosamente [perigoza'mẽtʃi] *adv* dangerously
perigoso [peri'gozu] *adj* dangerous
perímetro [pe'rimetru] *m* perimeter
periódico [pe'rjɔdʒiku] **1** *adj* periodical **2** *m* newspaper; (*revista*) periodical
período [pe'riudu] *m* period; ***~ de experiência*** trial period; ***~ de guerra*** wartime
periquito [peri'kitu] *m* budgerigar
periscópio [peris'kɔpiu] *m* periscope
perito [pe'ritu] **1** *adj* expert **2** *m*, **-a** *f* expert; *seguro*: assessor
perito-contador [pe'ritu] *m* certified public accountant, *Brit* chartered accountant
perjurar [perʒu'rar] ⟨1a⟩ *v/i* perjure oneself
perjúrio [per'ʒuriu] *m* perjury
permanecer [permane'ser] ⟨2g⟩ remain; (*durar*) last, remain
permanente [perma'nẽtʃi] **1** *adj* permanent; (*contínuo*) constant **2** *f* perm
permeável [per'mjavew] *adj* permeable
permissão [permi'sãw] *f* permission; (*licença*) permit; ***~ de trabalho*** work permit
permissível [permi'sivew] *adj* permissible
permissivo [permi'sivu] *adj* permissive
permitido [permi'tʃidu] *adj* permitted

P

permitir [permi'tʃir] ⟨3a⟩ permit, allow; ~ ***que alguém ...*** permit s.o. to ...

perna ['pɛrna] *f* leg; ~ ***de galinha*** chicken leg

pernicioso [perni'sjozu] *adj* pernicious

pernil [per'niw] *m* leg; ~ ***de porco*** leg of pork

pernilongo [perni'lõgu] *m* midge

pernoitar [pernoj'tar] ⟨1a⟩ spend the night

pérola ['pɛrula] *f* pearl *tb fig*

perpetuar [perpɛ'twar] *v/t* perpetuate

perpétuo [per'petwu] *adj* perpetual; ***pena*** ~ life (imprisonment)

perplexidade [perplɛksi'dadʒi] *f* perplexity

perplexo [per'plɛksu] *adj* perplexed; ***ficar*** ~ be taken aback; ***deixar*** ~ perplex, puzzle

perseguição [persegi'sãw] *f* chase, pursuit; REL, POL persecution

perseguidor [persegi'dor] *m*, **-a** *f* pursuer; REL, POL persecutor

perseguir [perse'gir] ⟨3o & 3c⟩ pursue, chase; (*importunar*) pester; REL, POL persecute; ***aquele homem anda a*** ~ ***-me*** that man has been stalking me

perseverança [perseve'rãsa] *f* perseverance

perseverante [perseve'rãtʃi] *adj* persevering

persiana [per'sjana] *f* shade, *Brit* blind

persistência [persis'tẽsja] *f* persistence

persistente [persis'tẽtʃi] *adj* persistent

persistir [persis'tʃir] ⟨3a⟩ persist; ~ ***em*** persist in

personagem [perso'naʒẽ] *f/m* personality; *romance etc*: character

personalidade [personali'dadʒi] *f* personality

personificar [personifi'kar] ⟨1n⟩ *v/t* personify

perspectiva [perspek'tʃiva] *f* perspective; *futuro*: prospect, outlook; ***um trabalho sem ~s*** a job with no prospects; ***pôr algo em*** ~ get sth into perspective

perspicácia [perspi'kasja] *f* perspicacity

perspicaz [perspi'kas] *adj* perspicacious, quick

persuadir [perswa'dʒir] ⟨3b⟩ ~ ***de*** persuade of; (*convencer*) persuade to

persuasão [perswa'zãw] *f* persuasion

persuasivo [perswa'zivu] *adj* persuasive

pertences [pertẽ'sis] *mpl* belongings

pertencer [pertẽ'ser] ⟨2g & 2a⟩ ~ ***a*** belong to; (*competir*) concern

pertinente [pertʃi'nẽtʃi] *adj* relevant

perto ['pɛrtu] **1** *adv* near, close; ***aqui*** ~ near here, nearby; ***de*** ~ *ouvir etc* closely **2** *prep* ~ ***de*** near, close to; *fig* near on; ***por*** ~ ***de $500*** near on $500, around $500

perturbação [perturba'sãw] *f* disturbance; (*preocupação*) perturbation

perturbado [pertur'badu] *adj* perturbed; (*desequilibrado*) unbalanced

perturbador [perturba'dor] **1** *adj* disruptive; (*preocupante*) disturbing **2** *m*, **-a** *f* troublemaker

perturbar [pertur'bar] ⟨1a⟩ *ordem, sossego* disturb, disrupt; (*preocupar*) perturb; ***não*** ~ do not disturb; **perturbar-se** *v/r* get agitated

Peru [pe'ru] *m* ***o*** ~ Peru; ***no*** ~ in Peru

peru [pe'ru] *m* turkey

perua [pe'rua] *f Bras* camper, van; ~ ***de entrega*** delivery van

peruano [pe'rwanu] **1** *adj* Peruvian **2** *m*, **-a** *f* Peruvian

peruca [pe'ruka] *f* wig

perversão [perver'sãw] *f* perversion

perversidade [perversi'dadʒi] *f* perversity

perverso [per'vɛrsu] **1** *adj* perverse **2** *m*, **-a** *f* pervert

perverter [perver'ter] ⟨2c⟩ pervert; *moralmente* corrupt, pervert

pesadelo [peza'delu] *m* nightmare

pesado [pe'zadu] **1** *adj* heavy; (*desagradável*) unpleasant; (*grave*) serious; ***ser*** (*ou* ***ficar***) ~ ***a alguém*** be a burden for s.o. **2** *m* ESP heavyweight

pêsames ['pezamis] *mpl* condolences

pesar [pe'zar] **1** *v/t* ⟨1c⟩ weigh; *fig* weigh up **2** *v/i* weigh **3** *m* grief;

(*remorso*) regret

pesca ['pɛska] *f* fishing; (*captura*) catch; **~ (*à linha*)** angling

pescada [pes'kada] *f type of cod*

pescador [peska'dor] **1** *m*, **-a** *f* fisherman; fisherwoman; *com anzol* angler; **~ *de águas turvas*** conman **2** *adj* fishing *atr*

pescar [pes'kar] ⟨1n & 1c⟩ **1** *v/i* fish **2** *v/t* catch; (*topar*) understand, get; *fam* ***não ~ nada*** not understand anything

pescoço [pes'kosu] *m* neck

peso ['pezu] *m* weight; *moeda* peso; *fig* burden; (*importância*) importance; **~ *bruto* / *liquido*** gross / net weight; **~ *médio*** ESP middleweight **~ *morto*** dead weight; **~ *pena*** ESP lightweight; **~ *pesado*** ESP heavyweight

pesquisa [pes'kiza] *f* research; (*inquérito*) investigation; ***fazer uma ~*** do research; ***centro*** *m* ***de ~*** research center, *Brit* research centre **~ *científica*** scientific research; **~ *e desenvolvimento*** research and development, R&D; **~ *de mercado*** market research; **~ *de opinião*** opinion poll

pesquisador [peskiza'dor] *m*, **-a** *f* researcher

pesquisar [peski'zar] ⟨1a⟩ **1** *v/t local* search; (*investigar*) investigate, research into **2** *v/i* research

pêssego ['pesegu] *m* peach

pessimismo [pesi'mizmu] *m* pessimism

pessimista [pesi'mista] **1** *m/f* pessimist **2** *adj* pessimistic

péssimo ['pɛsimu] *adj* very bad, terrible

pessoa [p(e)'soa] *f* person; ***em ~*** in person; **~*s*** people *pl*; ***outra ~*** someone else; **~ *da terceira idade*** senior citizen

pessoal [pe'swaw] **1** *adj* personal **2** *m* personnel, staff; ***falta*** *f* ***de ~*** staff shortage; ***seção*** *f* ***de ~***, *Port* ***secção*** *f* ***de ~*** personnel department; ***entra, ~*** *fam* come in, folks

pestana [pes'tana] *f* eyelash

pestanejar [pestane'ʒar] *v/i* wink; ***sem ~*** without batting an eyelid

peste ['pɛstʃi] *f* plague; (*epidemia*) epidemic; (*fedor*) stink; *fig* nuisance; *pessoa* pest, nuisance

pesticida [pestʃi'sida] *m* pesticide

peta ['peta] *f* lie; *fam* ***pregar uma ~ em alguém*** put s.o. on

pétala ['pɛtala] *f* petal

petição [petʃi'sãw] *f* petition; (*pedido*) request

petiscar [petʃis'kar] *v/i* nibble

petisco [pe'tʃisku] *m* snack

petroleiro [petro'lejru] *m* NÁUT oil tanker

petróleo [pe'trɔliu] *m* petroleum, oil; **~ *bruto*** crude (oil); ***manto*** *m* ***de ~*** oil slick

petroquímica [pɛtro'kimika] *f* petrochemicals

peúga ['piuga] *f Port* sock

p. ex. *abr* (***por exemplo***) eg

pia ['pia] *f* washbasin; *cozinha*: sink; *retrete*: toilet bowl; REL font

piaçaba [pja'saba] *f/m* toilet brush

piada [pja'da] *f* joke

pianista [pja'nista] *m/f* pianist

piano ['pjanu] **1** *m* piano; **~ *de cauda*** grand piano; **~ *de meia cauda*** baby grand; ***tocar ~*** play the piano **2** *adv* quietly

pião [pjãw] *m* top; AUTO ***fazer ~*** spin

piar [pjar] *v/i* peep; *coruja* hoot

PIB [pib] *m abr* (***Produto Interno Bruto***) GDP (gross domestic product)

pica ['pika] *f vulg* dick

picada [pi'kada] *f* sting *tb fig*; (*mordedela*) bite; AERO dive

picado [pi'kadu] **1** *adj mar* choppy; *fig* offended, piqued; (*irritado*) irritated; ***carne*** *f* ***picada*** ground meat, *Brit* minced meat; ***vôo*** *m* **~**, *Port* ***voo ~*** dive **2** *m* ground meat, *Brit* minced meat; MÚS pizzicato; AERO dive

picante [pi'kãtʃi] *adj* hot; (*excitante*) saucy; *piada* risqué

pica-pau [pika'paw] *m* ⟨*pl* ~ s⟩ woodpecker

picar [pi'kar] ⟨1n⟩ **1** *v/t* sting; (*morder*) bite; *bilhete* punch; *carne etc* chop up; *fig* provoke **2** *v/i vestuário* itch; *comida* be hot

picareta [pika'reta] *f* pickax, *Brit* pickaxe

P

pichação [piʃa'sãw] *f* graffiti
pichar [pi'ʃar] ⟨1g⟩ *v/t Bras parede* spray graffiti on; *fig* criticize, run down
pico ['piku] *m* point; *montanha*: peak; (*cume*) summit
pictórico [pik'tɔriku] *adj* pictorial
piedade [pie'dadʒi] *f* pity; ***sem ~*** pitiless
piedoso [pie'dozu] *adj* pious; (*compassivo*) merciful
piercing ['pirsĩ] *m* piercing
pifar [pi'far] **1** *v/t fam* pinch **2** *v/i* break down; *fam* (*morrer*) kick the bucket
pigarrear [piga'hjar] *v/i* clear one's throat
pijama [pi'ʒama] *m* pajamas, *Brit* pyjamas
pilão [pi'lãw] *m* mortar; ARQUIT pylon
pilar [pi'lar] *m* pillar
pilha ['piʎa] *f* pile; ELÉT battery; *fam* flashlight, *Brit* torch; ***~ de nervos*** bundle of nerves
pilhagem [pi'ʎaʒẽ] *f* pillaging; ***fazer pilhagens*** pillage
pilhar [pi'ʎar] ⟨1a⟩ *v/t* pillage; (*roubar*) steal; (*apanhar*) catch
pilotagem [pilo'taʒẽ] *f* steering; (*condução*) driving; (*voar*) flying
pilotar [pilo'tar] ⟨1e⟩ steer; AUTO drive; AERO fly
piloto [pi'lotu] *m* pilot; AUTO driver; ***projeto*** *m* ***~***, *Port* ***projecto*** *m* ***~*** pilot project; ***~ automático*** autopilot; ***~ de balão*** balloonist; ***~ de corrida*** race driver, *Brit* racing driver
pílula ['pilula] *f* pill; ***~ de fertilidade*** fertility drug; ***~ de vitamina*** vitamin pill
pimba ['pĩba] *adj Port pej* ***música*** *f* ***~*** cheesy pop (music)
pimenta [pi'mẽta] *f* pepper; ***~ malagueta*** chili pepper
pimentão [pimẽ'tãw] *m* chili pepper; *Bras tb* pepper; ***~ doce*** paprika
pimento [pi'mẽtu] *m Port* pepper
pinça ['pĩsa] *f* tweezers *pl*; ZOOL pincers *pl*
pincel [pĩ'sɛw] *m* brush
pincelada [pĩse'lada] *f* (brush) stroke
pincelar [pĩse'lar] ⟨1c⟩ paint
pinga ['pĩga] *f* drop *tb fig*; *Bras* white rum; *álcool* booze; *fam* ***entrar na ~*** get drunk; *fam* ***estar com a*** (*ou* ***tocado da***) ***~*** have had one too many; *fam* ***gostar da ~*** like the odd drink
pingar [pĩ'gar] ⟨1o⟩ drip; ***está pingando*** it's spitting with rain
pingente [pĩ'ʒẽtʃi] *m* pendant; ***~ de gelo*** icicle
pingo ['pĩgu] *m* drop; *fam* (*café*) espresso with a dash of milk
pingue-pongue ['pĩgpõg] *m* ping-pong
pingüim, *Port* **pinguim** [pĩ'gwĩ] *m* penguin
pinguinha [pĩ'giɲa] *f* quickie
pinha ['piɲa] *f* pine cone; *fam* (*cabeça*) nut, head; *fam* ***estar à ~*** be absolutely packed
pinheiro [pi'ɲejru] *m* pine tree
pino ['pinu] *m* pin; *fig* height; ESP handstand; ***a ~*** upright; *Port* ***~ do Verão*** high summer
pinta ['pĩta] *f* spot; *fig* look; ***às ~s*** spotted; ***ter*** (***muita***) ***~*** look (very) good
pintar [pĩ'tar] ⟨1a⟩ paint; *cabelo* dye; *rosto* put make-up on; *fig* portray; *pop* (*exagerar*) exaggerate; (*mentir*) lie
pinto ['pĩtu] *m* chick; *fam* ***como um ~*** soaking wet
pintor [pĩ'tor] *m*, **-a** *f* painter
pintura [pĩ'tura] *f* paint; (*ato*, *quadro*) painting; *fig* portrayal; ***~ brilhosa*** gloss paint; ***~ a óleo*** oil painting
piolho ['pjoʎu] *m* louse
pioneiro [pjo'nejru] **1** *adj* pioneering **2** *m*, **-a** *f* pioneer
pior [pjɔr] *adj* ⟨*comparativo de* ***mau*** *e* ***mal***⟩ worse; *superlativo* worst; (***tanto***) ***~!*** that makes it worse!
piorar [pjo'rar] ⟨1e⟩ **1** *v/i* get worse **2** *v/t* make worse
pipa ['pipa] *f vinho*: barrel; *Bras* kite
pipi [pi'pi] *m fam* pee; ***fazer ~*** do a pee
pipoca [pi'pɔka] *f* popcorn
piquenique [piki'niki] *m* picnic
piquete [pi'ketʃi] *m greve*: picket
pirado [pi'radu] *adj fam* crazy
pirâmide [pi'rʌmidʒi] *f* pyramid

piranha [pi'raɲa] *f* ZOOL piranha
pirar [pi'rar] *fam* go crazy; **pirar-se** *v/r fam* beat it
pirata [pi'rata] **1** *m* pirate; *fig* crook; **~ *do ar*** airplane hijacker **2** *adj* pirate *atr*; ***cópia** f* **~** pirate copy
pirataria [pirata'ria] *f* ECON piracy
piratagem [pira'taʒẽ] *f Port* ECON piracy
piratear [pira'ʧiar] *v/t* pirate
Pireneus [pire'neus] *mpl* Pyrenees
pires ['piris] *m* ⟨*pl inv*⟩ saucer
pirilampo [piri'lãpu] *m* glow-worm
piripíri [piri'piri] *m Port* chili (pepper)
piromaníaco [piroma'niaku] *m*, **-a** *f* arsonist
pirralho [pi'haʎu] *m*, **-a** *f* brat
pirueta [pi'rweta] *f* pirouette
pirulito [piru'litu] *m Bras* lollipop
pisar [pi'zar] ⟨1a⟩ step on, tread on; *local* enter; (*esmagar*) trample; (*calcar*) tread down; *uva* press; *fig* conquer; (*ofender*) offend; **~ *fundo*** put one's foot down; *Bras* ***não pise na grama!*** keep off the grass!
pisca-alerta [piska'lɛrta] *m* hazards, hazard lights
piscadela [piska'dɛla] *f* blink; *significativo* wink
pisca-pisca(s) [piska'piska(s)] *m(pl)* AUTO turn signal, *Brit* flasher, indicator
piscar [pis'kar] ⟨1n⟩ **~ *os olhos*** blink; **~ *o olho a alguém*** wink at s.o.
piscina [pis'sina] *f* (swimming) pool
piso ['pizu] *m* floor
pista ['pista] *f* (*trilho*) track; AUTO lane; AERO runway; *hipismo*: course; (*indicação*) clue; **~ *de aterrissagem*** runway; NÁUT flight deck; **~ *de boliche*** bowling alley; **~ *de descolagem*** runway; **~ *de esqui*** ski run, piste; **~ *de patinação*** ice rink; **~ *de pouso*** landing strip; **~ *para ônibus*** bus lane
pistache [pis'taʃi] *m Bras* pistachio
pistácio [pis'tasiu] *m Port* pistachio
pistão [pis'tãw] *m* piston
pistola [pis'tɔla] *f* pistol; ***pintar à* ~** spray; **~ *automática*** *ou* ***metralhadora*** submachine gun; **~ *de pintar*** paint gun
pitada [pi'tada] *f* GASTR pinch; ***uma* ~ *de sal*** a pinch of salt
pivô [pi'vo] *m*, **pivot** [pi'vo] *m* pivot; *fig*: *pessoa* anchor, news reader
pizza ['pitsa] *f* pizza
placa ['plaka] *f* sign; ELÉT circuit board; *Port* **~ *de aquecimento*** hotplate; **~ *comemorativa*** plaque; **~ *do carro*** license plate, *Brit* number plate; *Port* **~ *de desvio*** diversion sign; **~ *gráfica*** graphics card; **~ *-mãe*** motherboard; **~ *de som*** sound card; **~ *de video*** video card
placar [pla'kar] *m* scoreboard
placenta [pla'sẽta] *f* ANAT placenta
plácido ['plasidu] *adj* placid
plagiar [plaʒi'ar] *v/t* plagiarize
plágio ['plaʒiu] *m* plagiarism
plaina ['plajna] *f* plane
planalto [pla'nawtu] *m* plateau
planeador *etc Port* → ***planejador*** *etc*
planejador [planeja'dor] *m Bras* planner
planejamento [planeja'mẽtu] *m Bras* planning
planejar [pla'nejar] ⟨1l⟩ *Bras* plan; (*criar*) design; ***ter algo planejada*** have sth planned
planeta [pla'neta] *m* planet
planetário [plane'tariu] **1** *adj* planetary **2** *m* planetarium
planície [pla'nisi] *f* plain, lowlands
planificar [planifi'kar] ⟨1n⟩ plan; ***economia** f **planificada*** planned economy
planilha [pla'niʎa] *f* INFORM **~ *eletrônica*** spreadsheet
plano ['plʌnu] **1** *adj* level; (*baixo*) flat **2** *m* plan; MAT plane
planta[1] ['plãta] *f* BOT plant
planta[2] ['plãta] *f* ARQUIT plan, blueprint
planta[3] ['plãta] *f fig* **~ *do pé*** sole of one's foot
plantação [plãta'sãw] *f* plantation; (*cultura*) planting
plantar [plã'tar] ⟨1a⟩ plant; (*cultivar*) grow; *campo* sow (**de** with)
plasma ['plazma] *m* plasma; **~ *sanguíneo*** blood plasma; ***televisão** f **de*** **~** plasma television
plástica ['plasʧika] *f* plastic surgery

P

plasticidade [plastʃisi'dadʒi] *f* malleability; *fig* adaptability
plasticina [plastʃi'sina] *f* Plasticine®
plástico ['plastʃiku] **1** *adj* plastic **2** *m* plastic
plastificar [plastʃifi'kaɾ] ⟨1n⟩ *v/t* shrink-wrap
plataforma [plata'fɔrma] *f* platform; *Bras* FERROV platform; **~ *de lançamento*** launch pad; **~ *petrolífera*** oil rig
plátano ['platanu] *m* BOT plane tree
platéia [pla'tεja] *f* TEAT orchestra, *Brit* stalls; *fig* audience
platina [pla'tʃina] *f* platinum
platônico, *Port* **platónico** [pla'toniku] *adj* platonic
plausível [plaw'zivew] *adj* plausible
plebiscito [plebis'situ] *m* referendum, plebiscite
plenário [ple'naɾiu] **1** *adj* (*completo*) plenary **2** *m* plenary session
pleno ['plenu] *adj* full; (*inteiro*) complete; ***sessão** f **plena*** plenary session; DIR **~*s poderes*** *pl* full powers; ***em* ~ *inverno*** in the middle of winter
pluma ['pluma] *f* feather
plumagem [plu'maʒẽ] *f* plumage
plural [plu'ɾaw] *m* plural
pluralidade [pluɾali'dadʒi] *f* plurality; ***à* ~ (*de votos*)** with a majority (of votes)
pluralismo [pluɾa'lizmu] *m* pluralism
PNB *abr* (***produto nacional bruto***) GDP (gross domestic product)
pneu [pi'new] *m* tire, *Brit* tyre; **~ *radial*** radial tire; **~ *reserva*** spare tire
pneumático [pinew'matʃiku] **1** *adj* pneumatic; ***barco*** *m* **~** rubber dinghy **2** *m* tire, *Brit* tyre
pneumonia [pinewmo'nia] *f* pneumonia
pó [pɔ] *m* powder; (*poeira*) dust; ***leite*** *m* ***em* ~** powdered milk; **~ *compacto*** face powder; ***em* ~** powdered
p.o. *abr* (***por ordem***) *Port* pp
pobre ['pɔbɾi] **1** *adj* poor; (*miserável*) miserable; **~ *Tony!*** poor old Tony! **2** *m/f* poor person; ***os* ~*s*** the poor
pobreza [po'bɾeza] *f* poverty; (*miséria*) misery
poça ['pɔsa] *f* pool; *chuva*: puddle
pocilga [po'silga] *f* pigsty *tb fig*
poço ['posu] *m* well; MIN shaft; **~ *de ar*** air pocket; **~ *petrolífero*** oil well; **~ *de ventilação*** ventilation shaft
poda ['pɔda] *f árvores etc*: pruning; *Port fam* ***saber da* ~** know one's stuff
podar [po'daɾ] *v/t galhos* lop off; *sebe* trim; *planta* prune
pó-de-arroz [pɔdʒia'hos] *m* face powder
poder [po'deɾ] ⟨2l⟩ **1** *v/t* ◇ can, be able to; ***não posso andar*** I can't walk; ***podias me ter dito*** you could have told me; ***como é que pode?*** you can't be serious
◇ *autorização*: can, may; ***pode retirar-se*** you may go
◇ *suposição*: may, might; ***poderá já ser tarde*** it might be too late; ***pode ser que ...*** it might be that ...
◇ **~ *com algo / alguém*** be able to handle sth / s.o.; *peso* be able to carry sth **2** *m* power; **~ *de compra*** purchasing power
poderoso [pode'ɾozu] *adj* mighty, powerful
podia [po'dʒia] *etc*, **podido** [po'dʒidu] *pp* → ***poder***
pódio ['pɔdiu] *m* podium
podre ['podɾi] *adj* rotten; **~ *de rico*** filthy rich
podridão [podɾi'dãw] *f* ⟨*sem pl*⟩ rot, decay; (*corrupção*) corruption
põe [põj] *etc* → ***pôr***
poeira ['pwejɾa] *f* dust
poema ['pwema] *m* poem
poesia [pwe'zia] *f* poetry; *lírica*: poem
poeta ['pwεta] *m* poet
poética ['pwεtʃika] *f* poetics
poético ['pwεtʃiku] *adj* poetic *tb fig*
poetisa [pwe'tʃiza] *f* poet
pois [pojs] **1** *adv* so; (*claro*) of course **2** *int* **~*!*** exactly!; **~ *é!*** that's right!, of course! **2** *conj* as; **~ (*que*)** because
polaco [po'laku] *Port* **1** *adj* Polish **2** *m*, **-a** *f* Pole **3** *m língua* Polish
polar [po'laɾ] *adj* polar
polarizar [polaɾi'zaɾ] ⟨1a⟩ polarize
polegada [pole'gada] *f medida*: inch
polegar [pole'gaɾ] *m* thumb; *pé*: big toe
poleiro [po'lejɾu] *m* perch

polêmica, *Port* **polémica** [po'lemika] *f* controversy
polêmico, *Port* **polémico** [po'lemiku] *adj* controversial; *pessoa* argumentative
pólen ['pɔlẽ] *m* pollen
polícia [po'lisja] **1** *f* police; **~ *federal*** crime department, *Brit* CID; *Port* **~ *judiciária*** crime department, *Brit* CID; *Bras* **~ *rodoviária*** traffic police; **~ *secreta*** secret police; *Port* **~ *de trânsito*** traffic police **2** *m/f Port* policeman; policewoman
policial [poli'sjaw] **1** *adj* police *atr*; ***filme*** *m* **~** thriller; ***romance*** *m* **~** thriller, detective novel **2** *m/f Bras* policeman; policewoman
policlínica [poli'klinika] *f* general hospital
polido [po'lidu] *adj* polished; *fig* polite
poliomielite [pɔljome'litʃi] *f* poliomyelitis, polio
polir [po'lir] ⟨3g⟩ *v/t* polish *tb fig*
política [po'litʃika] *f* politics; ***uma* ~** a policy; **~ *de ambiente*, ~ *ambiental*** environmental policy
político [po'litʃiku] **1** *adj* political **2** *m*, **-a** *f* politician
politizar [politʃi'zar] ⟨1a⟩ *v/t* politicize
pólo ['pɔlu] GEOG pole; ESP polo; ***Pólo Norte*** North Pole; ***Pólo Sul*** South Pole
polonês [polo'nes] **1** *adj* Polish **2** *m*, **-esa** *f* Pole **3** *m lingua* Polish
Polônia, *Port* **Polónia** [po'lonja] *f* Poland
polpa ['powpa] *f* pulp
poltrão [pow'trãw] *Port* **1** *adj* cowardly **2** *m* coward
poltrona [pow'trona] *f* easy chair, armchair
poluente [po'lwẽtʃi] **1** *m* pollutant **2** *adj* polluting; ***não* ~** nonpolluting, environmentally friendly
poluição [polwi'sãw] *f* pollution; (*contaminação*) contamination; **~ *do meio ambiente*** environmental pollution
poluidor [polwi'dor] **1** *adj* polluting **2** *m* → ***poluente***
poluir [po'lwir] ⟨3i⟩ (*sujar*) pollute; (*contaminar*) contaminate; *fig* besmirch, sully
polvilhar [powvi'ʎar] ⟨1a⟩ (*espalhar*) sprinkle
polvilho [pow'viʎu] *m* powder; *farinha*: manioc flour
polvo ['powvu] *m* octopus
pólvora ['pɔlvora] *f* gunpowder
pomada [po'mada] *f* ointment
pomar [po'mar] *m* orchard
pomba ['põba] *f* pigeon, dove
pombo ['põbu] *m* pigeon, dove
pombo-correio ['põbuko'heiu] *m* ⟨*pl* pombos-correios⟩ carrier pigeon
pomo ['pomu] *m Bras* **~ *de Adão*** Adam's apple
pompa ['põpa] *f* pomp
pomposo [põ'pozu] *adj* pompous
ponderado [põde'radu] *adj* serious; (*refletido*) considered
ponderar [põde'rar] ⟨1c⟩ **1** *v/t* weigh up; (*considerar*) consider **2** *v/i* think (***sobre*** about)
ponho ['poɲu] *etc* → ***pôr***
pônei, *Port* **pónei** ['ponej] *m* ZOOL pony
ponta ['põta] *f* point; (*fim*) end; (*canto*) corner; *touro etc*: horn; *charuto, cigarro*: butt; ESP winger; ***tecnologia** f **de* ~** leading edge technology; ***agüentar as* ~*s*** stand firm
pontada [põ'tada] *f* twinge; prick
pontão [põ'tãw] *m* support; *ponte*: pontoon
pontapé [põta'pɛ] *m* kick; **~ *livre*** free kick
pontaria [põta'ria] *f* aim; *fig* goal; ***fazer* ~** take aim; ***ter boa* ~** be a good shot
ponte ['põtʃi] *f* bridge; *fig* ***fazer* ~** make a long weekend of it; **~ *pênsil*** suspension bridge; MED **~ *de safena*** bypass
ponteiro [põ'tejru] *m* pointer; *relógio*: hand; MÚS plectrum
pontiagudo [põtʃia'gudu] *adj* sharp; (*aguçado*) pointed
pontificado [põtʃifi'kadu] *m* pontificate; *papal*: papal office
pontífice [põ'tʃifisi] *m* pontiff; ***Sumo Pontífice*** Pope
ponto ['põtu] *m* point; *email*: dot; *pontuação*: period, *Brit* full stop; *costura*:

P

stitch; ***ganhar ~s*** earn brownie points; ***~ alto*** high point; ***~ cego*** blind spot; ***~ de controle*** checkpoint; ***~ de exclamação*** exclamation point, *Brit* exclamation mark; ***~ final*** period, *Brit* full stop; *ônibus*: terminus; ***~ de interrogação*** question mark; AUTO ***~ morto*** neutral; *Port* ***~ negro*** blackhead; ***~ de táxi*** cab stand, *Brit* taxi rank; ***~ turísticos*** sights; ***~ de venda*** point of sale; ***~ e vírgula*** semi-colon; ***~ de vista*** point of view, viewpoint

pontuação [põtwa'sãw] *f* punctuation; ESP score

pontual [põ'twaw] *adj* punctual, on time

pontualidade [põtwali'dadʒi] *f* punctuality

pontuar [põ'twaɾ] *v/t* punctuate

popa ['popa] *f* NÁUT stern; ***vento** m* ***em ~*** tail wind; *fig* ***correr de vento em ~*** go smoothly

população [popula'sãw] *f* population; *peixes etc*: stock

populacional [populasjo'naw] *adj* population *atr*

popular [popu'laɾ] *adj* popular; POL ***frente** f* ***~*** popular front

popularidade [populaɾi'dadʒi] *f* popularity

popularizar [populaɾi'zaɾ] ⟨1a⟩ *v/t* popularize, make popular

populoso [popu'lozu] *adj* populous

pôquer, *Port* **póquer** ['pokeɾ] *m* poker

por [poɾ] *prep* ◊ *distância*: for; ***~ três quilômetros*** for three kilometers
◊ (*através*) through; ***passar ~ São Paulo*** go through São Paulo
◊ (*em frente de*) ***passar ~ algo / alguém*** pass by sth / s.o.
◊ (*ao longo de*) along; ***passear pela praia*** walk along the beach
◊ *troca*: for; ***trocar algo ~ algo*** exchange sth for sth; ***tomar alguém ~ algo*** regard s.o. as sth; *engano*: take s.o. as sth
◊ *temporal*: for; ***é tudo ~ hoje*** that's everything for today; ***pela manhã / tarde*** in the morning / afternoon; ***pelas 2 horas*** at around two o'clock
◊ (*cerca*) about; ***~ aí / aqui*** over there / here
◊ *relação*: ***~ mim*** as far as I'm concerned; ***~ mim tudo bem*** that's fine by me; ***pelo que sei*** as far as I know; ***pelo que dizem*** according to what they say
◊ ***~ pessoa*** per person; ***~ ano*** per annum
◊ *motivo*, *causa*: out of; ***~ medo*** out of fear; ***~ alguma razão*** for some reason; ***~ engano*** by mistake
◊ *passivo*: by; ***ser atropelado ~ um carro*** be knocked down by a car
◊ MAT *divisão*: by
◊ *meio*, *instrumento*, *mediação*: by; ***~ acidente*** by accident; ***~ escrito*** in writing; ***~ mar*** by sea; ***~ terra*** by land; ***~ avião*** by plane
◊ *medida*: by; ***4 por 4*** metros 4 by 4 meters
◊ ***estar ~ fazer*** be still to be done

pôr [poɾ] ⟨2z⟩ **1** *v/t* put; (*colocar*) place; (*pendurar*) hang; (*plantar*) plant; *vestido etc* put on; ***~ a mesa*** set the table; ***~ na rua*** throw out; ***~ no prego*** pawn **2** *m* ***~ do sol*** sunset;

pôr-se *v/r astro* set; (*tornar-se*) turn; ***~ a fazer*** start to do

porão [po'ɾãw] *m* NÁUT hold; *Bras* cellar, basement

porca ['pɔɾka] *f* ZOOL sow; TECN nut

porção [poɾ'sãw] *f* part; (*pedaço*) piece; (*número*) number; (*dose*) portion

porcaria [poɾka'ɾia] *f* filth; (*sujeira*) dirt; ***uma ~*** a load of garbage

porcelana [poɾse'lana] *f* porcelain; ***~ chinesa*** china

porco ['poɾku] **1** *m* pig, hog *tb pop fig*; (*varrão*) boar; ***carne** f* ***de ~*** pork; ***~ bravo, ~ montês*** wild boar; ***~ chauvinista*** male chauvinist pig **2** *adj* (*sujo*) filthy

porco-espinho [poɾkos'piɲu] *m* ⟨*pl* porcos-espinhos⟩ porcupine

pôr-do-sol [poɾdo'sɔw] *m* ⟨*pl* pores--do-sol⟩ sunset

porei [po'ɾej] *etc* → ***pôr***

porém [po'ɾẽ] *conj* however

pormenor [poɾme'nɔɾ] *m* detail; ***em ~*** in detail

pormenorizadamente [pormenoriza'mẽtʃi] *adv* in detail
pormenorizado [pormenori'zadu] *adj* detailed
pormenorizar [pormenori'zar] ⟨1a⟩ *v/t* detail
pornografia [pornogra'fia] *f* pornography
pornográfico [porno'grafiku] *adj* pornographic
poro ['pɔru] *m* pore
poroso [po'rozu] *adj* porous
por que, porque ['porke] **1** *interr* why **2** *conj* because
porquê [por'ke] *adv* **~?** why? **2** *m fig* reason
porquinho-da-Índia [porkiɲoda'ĩdʒia] *m* guinea pig
porra ['poha] *int* **~!** *vulg* fucking hell!
porrada [po'hada] *f fam* beating; ***uma ~ de …*** a whole bunch of …
porreiro [po'hejru] *adj Port fam* great, super
porrete [po'hetʃi] *m* club
porta ['pɔrta] *f* door; (*portão*) gate *tb fig*; INFORM port; ***bater à ~*** knock on the door; ***~ corrediça*** sliding door; ***~ de embarque*** gate; ***~ de entrada*** front door; ***~ giratória*** revolving door; INFORM ***~ serial*** serial port; ***~ traseira*** back door
porta-aviões [pɔrta'vjõjs] *m* ⟨*pl inv*⟩ aircraft carrier
porta-bagagem [pɔrtaba'gaʒẽ] *m* ⟨*pl* porta-bagagens⟩ luggage rack
porta-chaves [pɔrta'ʃavis] *m* ⟨*pl inv*⟩ keyring
porta-copo [pɔrta'kɔpu] *m* coaster
portador [porta'dor] *m*, **-a** *f* bearer; *passaporte*: holder; MED carrier; ***pagável ao ~*** payable to bearer
portagem [por'taʒẽ] *f Port* toll
portal [por'taw] *m* gateway; INTERNET portal
porta-luvas [pɔrta'luvas] *m* AUTO glove compartment
porta-malas [pɔrta'malas] *m* AUTO trunk, *Brit* boot
porta-moedas [pɔrta'mwɛdas] *m Port* ⟨*pl inv*⟩ coin purse, *Brit* purse
portanto [por'tãtu] *conj* therefore
portão [por'tãw] *m* gate; *Bras* ***~ de embarque*** gate; ***~ de entrada*** gateway
portaria [porta'ria] *f* entrance hall; (*recepção*) reception desk; POL edict
portátil [por'tatʃiw] *adj* portable; ***computador m ~*** laptop, notebook
porta-voz [porta'vɔs] ⟨*pl* ~es⟩ **1** *m* megaphone; *tb fig* mouthpiece **2** *m/f* spokesperson *tb* POL
porte ['pɔrtʃi] *m* carriage; COM freight; *custos*: delivery charge; *fig* bearing; ***~ de arma*** carrying weapons
porteiro [por'tejru] *m* porter; (*guarda-portão*) doorman
porto ['portu] *m* port, harbor, *Brit* harbour; ***~ de mar*** seaport; ***~ fluvial*** river port; ***~ franco*** freeport
Porto ['portu] *m* ***vinho m do ~*** port
portuário [por'twariu] *adj* port *atr*; ***polícia f portuária*** harbor police, *Brit* harbour police; ***taxa f portuária*** port dues
Portugal [portu'gaw] *m* Portugal
português [portu'ges] **1** *adj* Portuguese **2** *m pessoa* Portuguese man / boy; *língua* Portuguese
portuguesa [portu'geza] *f* Portuguese woman / girl; ***a Portuguesa*** the Portuguese national anthem
porventura [porvẽ'tura] *adv* (*por acaso*) by chance
posar [po'zar] ⟨1e⟩ *v/i* pose
pós-datar [pɔsda'tar] ⟨1b⟩ *v/t* postdate
pose ['pozi] *f* pose
pôs [pos] → ***pôr***
pós-graduado [posgra'dwadu] *m*, **-a** *f* postgraduate
pós-guerra [pos'gɛha] *m* post-war period
posição [pozi'sãw] *f* position
posicionar [pozisjo'nar] ⟨1a⟩ *v/t* position
positivo [pozi'tʃivu] *adj* positive; (*real*) real; (*certo*) sure, certain
pós-modernismo [pɔzmoder'nizmu] *m* postmodernism
pós-moderno [pɔzmo'dɛrnu] *adj* postmodern
posologia [pozolo'ʒia] *f* MED dosage
possante [po'sãtʃi] *adj* (*poderoso*) powerful; (*robusto*) strong

possa ['pɔsa] *etc* → ***poder***
posse ['pɔsi] *f* ownership, possession; ***dar ~ a alguém*** install s.o. in office; ***tomar ~ de algo*** take possession of sth; *cargo* assume sth, take sth on; ***~s*** *pl* possessions *tb fig*
possessão [pose'sãw] *f* possession
possessivo [pose'sivu] **1** *adj* possessive *tb* GRAM **2** *m* possessive pronoun
possesso [po'sɛsu] *adj* possessed
possibilidade [posibili'dadʒi] *f* possibility
possibilitar [posibili'taɾ] ⟨1a⟩ *v/t* enable; ***o curso possibilita a entrada ...*** the course makes it possible to enter ...
possível [po'sivew] *adj* possible; ***tão ... quanto ~*** as ... as possible; ***fazer os possíveis*** do one's best
posso ['pɔsu] → ***poder***
possuidor [poswi'doɾ] **1** *adj* ***ser ~ de algo*** own sth, possess sth **2** *m*, **-a** *f* owner; *talentos etc*: possessor
possuir [po'swiɾ] ⟨3i⟩ possess, own; *talento etc* possess
posta ['pɔsta] *f peixe, carne*: slice; piece
postal [pos'taw] **1** *adj* postal; ***bilhete*** *m* ***~*** postcard **2** *m* postcard
postar [pos'taɾ] ⟨1e⟩ *v/t sentinela* post, station
poste ['pɔstʃi] *m* pole, post; ***~ de luz*** streetlight; ***~ telegráfico*** utility pole, *Brit* telegraph pole
pôster ['posteɾ] *m* poster
posteridade [posteɾi'dadʒi] *f* posterity
posterior [poste'ɾjoɾ] *adj temporal*: later, subsequent; *local*: rear *atr*, back *atr*
postiço [pos'tʃisu] *adj* artificial, false
posto[1] ['postu] **1** *m* post; (*lugar*) position; (*cargo*) job; *trabalho*: ***subir de ~*** be promoted; *Bras* ***~ de gasolina*** gas station, *Brit* petrol station; ***~ meteorológico*** weather station; ***~ de polícia*** police station; *Port* ***~ de socorros***, *Bras* ***~ de saúde*** first-aid post; ***~ de trabalho*** workplace, work station **2** *pp* → ***pôr*** **3** *Port adj* ***bem ~*** good-looking; (*vestido*) well-dressed; ***sol*** *m* ***~*** sunset
posto[2] ['postu] *conj* ***~ (que)*** although
postumamente [postuma'mẽtʃi] *adv* posthumously
póstumo ['pɔstumu] *adj* posthumous
postura [pos'tuɾa] *f* posture; *atitude* attitude; ***qual é a sua ~ em relação a ...*** what is his stance *ou* position on ...?; ***uma ~ profissional*** a professional attitude
potássio [po'tasiu] *m* potassium
potável [po'tavew] *adj* drinkable; ***água*** *f* ***~*** drinking water
pote ['pɔtʃi] *m* pot
potência [po'tẽsja] *f* power; MED potency; ELÉT energy; POL ***~ mundial*** world power; ***~ nuclear*** nuclear power
potencial [potẽ'sjaw] **1** *adj* potential; ELÉT ***energia*** *f* ***~*** potential energy **2** *m* potential
potencialmente [potẽsjaw'mẽtʃi] *adv* potentially
potente [po'tẽtʃi] *adj* potent; (*forte*) strong; (*poderoso*) powerful
potro ['potɾu] *m* colt
pouco ['poku] **1** *adj* little; *plural* few; *tempo* short; ***pouca gente sabe disso*** not many people know that **2** *m* ***um ~*** a little; ***um ~ de manteiga*** a little butter, a bit of butter; ***aos ~s*** bit by bit; ***um ~ mais*** a little more; ***o ~ que sei*** the little I know **3** *pron* little; ***~s ficaram*** not many were left; ***~ depois*** a little after; ***daqui a ~*** in a moment; ***há ~*** recently, a little while ago; ***~ a ~*** little by little; ***~ é melhor que nada*** a little is better than nothing; ***por ~*** *vencer etc* only just, narrowly; ***por ~ não perco o trem*** I almost missed the train **4** *adv negativo*: not very; ***~ convincente*** not very convincing; ***~ provável*** unlikely
poupado [po'padu] *adj* economical, thrifty
poupança [po'pãsa] *f fam* saving; ***~s*** *pl* savings
poupar [po'paɾ] ⟨1a⟩ *dinheiro* save; *vida* spare
pouquinho [po'kiɲu] *m* bit; ***um ~ de*** a little bit of
pousada [po'zada] *f* inn, bed and

breakfast; *Port an upscale hotel, often in an historic building*; ~ ***da juventude*** youth hostel

pousar [po'zaɾ] ⟨1a⟩ place; (*pôr*) put down; rest; (*aterrar*) land; *pássaro* settle

povo ['povu] *m* people

povoação [povwa'sãw] *f* population; (*aldeia*) village

povoado [po'vwadu] **1** *adj* populated; ~ ***de árvores*** wooded; ***pouco*** ~ sparsely populated **2** *m* settlement

povoar [po'vwaɾ] ⟨1f⟩ populate; (*encher*) stock (***de*** with)

praça ['pɾasa] *f* square; (*mercado*) marketplace; ~ ***de táxis*** cab stand, *Brit* taxi rank

prado ['pɾadu] *m* meadow, prairie

praga ['pɾaga] *f* plague; AGR pest; *fig* curse; ~***s domésticas*** vermin *pl*; ***rogar*** ~***s*** curse

pragmático [pɾag'maʧiku] *adj* pragmatic

pragmatismo [pɾagma'ʧizmu] *m* pragmatism

praguejar [pɾage'ʒaɾ] *v/i* curse

praia ['pɾaja] *f* beach; ***na*** ~ on the beach; ***férias*** *fpl* ***de*** ~ beach vacation, *Brit* beach holiday

praia-mar [pɾaja'maɾ] *f* high tide

prancha ['pɾãʃa] *f* plank; NÁUT gangplank; ESP board; ~ ***de skate*** skateboard; ~ ***de surf*** surfboard

prancheta [pɾã'ʃeta] *f* clipboard; ~ ***de desenho*** drawing board

pranto ['pɾãtu] *m* (*choro*) weeping; ***debulhado em*** ~ weeping bitterly

prata ['pɾata] *f* silver; ***de*** ~ silver

prateado [pɾa'ʧiadu] *adj* silver-plated

pratear [pɾa'ʧiaɾ] ⟨1l⟩ silver-plate

prateleira [pɾate'lejɾa] *f* shelf; ~ ***de livros*** bookshelf

prática ['pɾaʧika] *f* practice; (*experiência*) experience; (*costume*) custom, habit; ***pôr em*** ~ put into practice; ~ ***suspeita*** sharp practice

praticamente [pɾaʧika'mẽʧi] *adv* practically

praticante [pɾaʧi'kãʧi] **1** *m/f* apprentice **2** *adj* practicing, *Brit* practising

praticar [pɾaʧi'kaɾ] ⟨1n⟩ practice, *Brit* practise; *esporto* do; *crime* commit

praticável [pɾaʧi'kavew] *adj* workable, feasible; *caminho*, *estrada etc* passable

prático ['pɾaʧiku] **1** *adj* practical **2** *m*, **-a** *f* expert; NÁUT ~ ***costeiro*** pilot

prato ['pɾatu] *m* plate; GASTR dish; *parte da refeição* course; ~ ***do dia*** dish of the day; ~ ***feito*** prepared meal; ~ ***fundo*** soup plate; ~ ***principal*** main course; ~ ***raso*** dinner plate; ~ ***de sopa*** soup plate

praxe ['pɾaʃi] *f* custom; ***da*** ~ customary

prazer [pɾa'zeɾ] *m* pleasure; (*alegria*) delight; (*gozo*) enjoyment; (*vontade*) will; (***muito***) ~***!*** pleased to meet you!; ***com muito*** ~ with pleasure

prazo ['pɾazu] *m* period, term; ***qual é o*** ~ ***de construção?*** what's the building timescale?; ***a longo / curto*** ~ in the long / short term; ***trabalho*** *m* ***a*** ~ temporary work; ~ ***de entrega*** delivery period; ~ ***final*** deadline; ~ ***de teste*** trial period; ~ ***de validade*** sell-by date

preâmbulo [pɾɛ'ãbulu] *m* preamble

preaquecer [pɾɛakɛ'seɾ] *v/t* preheat

precariamente [pɾekaɾja'mẽʧi] *adv* precariously

precário [pɾe'kaɾiu] *adj* precarious

preçário [pɾe'saɾiu] *m Port* price list

precaução [pɾekaw'sãw] *f* precaution; ***a título de*** ~ as a precaution

precaver [pɾeka'veɾ] ⟨2b⟩ prevent; **precaver-se** *v/r* ~ ***contra*** guard against

precedência [pɾese'dẽsja] *f* precedence

precedente [pɾese'dẽʧi] **1** *adj* preceding; (*anterior*) previous **2** *m* precedent; ***sem*** ~ unprecedented

preceder [pɾese'deɾ] ⟨2c⟩ precede

preceito [pɾe'sejtu] *m* precept, ruling

preciosidade [pɾesjozi'dadʒi] *f* gem, treasure

precioso [pɾe'sjozu] *adj* precious

precipício [pɾesi'pisiu] *m* precipice

precipitação [pɾesipita'sãw] *f* haste; METEO precipitation; ***com*** ~ hastily, rashly

precipitado [pɾesipi'tadu] *adj* hasty,

P

rash

precipitar [presipi'tar] ⟨1a⟩ **1** *v/t* hurl; *fig* rush; *crise* precipitate **2** *v/i* QUÍM precipitate; **precipitar-se** *v/r* (*jogar-se*) throw oneself; ~ ***na água*** plunge into the water; ~ ***numa decisão*** rush into a decision

precisamente [presiza'mẽtʃi] *adv* precisely

precisão[1] [presi'zãw] *f* need; ***ter ~ de algo*** need sth

precisão[2] [presi'zãw] *f* (*exatidão*) precision; ***com ~*** precisely

precisar [presi'zar] ⟨1a⟩ *v/i* need; (*especificar*) specify; ~ ***de algo*** need sth; ~ (***de***) ***fazer algo*** need to do sth, have to do sth; ***preciso dizer algo mais?*** need I say more?; ***preciso falar com você*** I need to talk to you, I have to talk to you; ***precisa-se de vendedores*** sales personnel wanted

preciso [pre'sizu] *adj* necessary; (*exato*) precise; (*conciso*) concise

preço ['presu] *m* price; (*valor*) value, worth; ***de ~*** valuable; ***descer / subir de ~*** decrease / increase in price; ~ ***de compra*** purchase price; ~ ***de custo*** cost price; ~ ***da entrada*** entrance fee; ~ ***fixo*** fixed price; ~ ***do mercado*** market price; ~ ***de oferta*** asking price; ~ ***da passagem*** fare; ~ ***de rua*** street value; ~ ***de varejo*** retail price; ~ ***de venda*** selling price

precoce [pre'kɔsi] *adj* precocious; (*prematuro*) premature

preconcebido [prɛkõse'bidu] *adj* preconceived

preconceito [prekõ'sejtu] *m* prejudice

pré-cozinhado [prɛkozi'ɲadu] *adj* pre-cooked, ready

precursor [prekur'sor] *m* precursor; (*presságio*) harbinger

predador [preda'dor] *m* predator

predatório [preda'tɔriu] *adj* predatory

predecessor [predese'sor] *m* predecessor

predestinação [predestʃina'sãw] *f* ⟨*sem pl*⟩ predestination

predestinado [predestʃi'nadu] *adj* predestined

predial [pre'dʒiaw] *adj* real estate; ***registro m ~***, *Port* ***registo m ~*** land registry

predicado [predʒi'kadu] *m* characteristic; GRAM predicate

predição [predʒi'sãw] *f* prediction

predileção, *Port* **predilecção** [predʒile'sãw] *f* predilection, liking

predileto, *Port* **predilecto** [predʒi'lɛtu] *adj* favorite, *Brit* favourite

prédio ['prɛdiu] *m* building; ~ ***comercial*** office building

predizer [predʒi'zer] *v/t* predict

predominante [predomi'nãtʃi] *adj* predominant

predominantemente [predominãtʃi'mẽtʃi] *adv* predominantly

predominar [predomi'nar] ⟨1a⟩ *poder*: predominate; *número*: prevail

preencher [preẽ'ʃer] ⟨2a⟩ fill in; *dever* fulfill, *Brit* fulfil; *ordem* carry out; *lugar* fill

preenchimento [preẽʃi'mẽtu] *m impresso*: completion; *sonhos*, *desejos etc*: fulfillment, *Brit* fulfilment; *lugar*, *cargo*: occupation

pré-escola [prɛes'kɔla] *f* infant school

pré-estréia [prɛes'trɛja] *f filme etc*: preview

pré-fabricado [prɛfabri'kadu] *adj* prefabricated

prefácio [pre'fasiu] *m* preface, foreword

prefeito [pre'fejtu] *m*, **-a** *f Bras* mayor

prefeitura [prefej'tura] *f Bras* city hall; town hall

preferência [prefe'rẽsja] *f* preference; (*predileção*) predilection; (*prioridade*) priority, right of way; ***de ~*** preferably

preferencial [prefe'rẽsja] hh *adj* preferential

preferido [prefe'ridu] *adj* favorite, *Brit* favourite

preferir [prefe'rir] ⟨3c⟩ prefer; (*favorecer*) favor, *Brit* favour; ~ ***fazer algo*** prefer to do sth; ~ ***X a Y*** prefer X to Y

preferível [prefe'rivew] *adj* preferable

preferivelmente [preferivew'mẽtʃi] *adv* preferably

prefixo [pre'fiksu] *m* prefix
prega ['prɛga] *f saia*: pleat; *calças*: crease
pregador [prega'doɾ] *m* preacher; *roupa*: clothes pin, *Brit* clothes peg
pregar[1] [pre'gaɾ] ⟨1o & 1c⟩ *v/t* nail; *prego* knock in; *pregador* pin; *alfinete etc* put; (*colar*) stick on; *botão* sew on; *olhos* fix (***em*** on); **~ *um susto a alguém*** give s.o. a fright
pregar[1] [prɛ'gaɾ] *v/i* preach
prego ['prɛgu] *m* nail; *fig fam* pawn shop; ***pôr no ~*** pawn; ***dormir como um ~*** sleep like a log
preguiça [pre'gisa] *f* laziness; ZOOL sloth
preguiçar [pregi'saɾ] ⟨1p⟩ laze around
preguiçoso [pregi'sozu] **1** *adj* lazy; (*indolente*) idle **2** *m*, **-a** *f* lazybones *sg*
pré-história [prɛis'tɔɾja] *f* prehistory
pré-histórico [prɛis'tɔriku] *adj* prehistoric
preia-mar [preja'maɾ] *f* high tide
prejudicar [preʒudʒi'kaɾ] ⟨1n⟩ damage; (*desfavorecer*) prejudice; (*estorvar*) hinder
prejudicial [preʒudʒi'sjaw] *adj* damaging; (*desvantajoso*) prejudicial
prejuízo [pre'ʒwizu] *m* damage, harm (***em*** to); (*perda*) loss; (*desvantagem*) detriment; (*preconceito*) prejudice
prejulgar [preʒuw'gaɾ] *v/t* prejudge
preliminar [prelimi'naɾ] **1** *adj* preliminary **2** *m* preliminary; ***~es*** *pl* preliminaries **3** *f* ESP preliminary
prelúdio [pre'ludiu] *m* prelude
pré-marital [prɛmaɾi'taw] *adj* premarital
prematuro [prema'tuɾu] **1** *adj* premature **2** *m* premature birth; premature baby
premeditação [premedʒita'sãw] *f* premeditation; ***com ~*** premeditated
premeditado [premedʒi'tadu] *adj* premeditated
premeditar [premedʒi'taɾ] ⟨1a⟩ premeditate
premiado [pre'mjadu] **1** *adj* prizewinning; ***números*** *mpl* ***~s*** winning numbers **2** *m*, **-a** *f* prizewinner
premiar [pre'mjaɾ] ⟨1g & 1h⟩ award a prize to; (*recompensar*) reward
prêmio, *Port* **prémio** ['premiu] *m* prize; (*recompensa*) reward; COM premium; (*lotaria*) winnings; *seguro*: insurance premium; **~ *Nobel*** Nobel prize; ***levar um ~*** get a prize
premissa [pre'misa] *f* premise
premonição [premoni'sãw] *f* premonition
pré-natal [prɛna'taw] *adj* prenatal, *Brit* antenatal
prenda ['prẽda] *f* gift; (*oferta*) present; *Port* (*talento*) talent
prendado [prẽ'dadu] *adj* gifted, talented
prendedor [prẽde'doɾ] *m* fastener; **~ *de cabelo*** hairpin; **~ *de roupa*** clothes pin, *Brit* clothes peg
prender [prẽ'deɾ] ⟨2a; *pp* preso⟩ fasten; fix (***por*** to); (*atar*) tie; *ladrão etc* arrest; **~ *algo em algo*** fasten sth to sth; **~ *a respiração*** hold one's breath
prenome [pre'nomi] *m* first name
prensa ['prẽsa] *f* press
prensar [prẽ'saɾ] ⟨1a⟩ press
prenúncio [pre'nũsiu] *m* (*anúncio*) forewarning; *fig* (*presságio*) sign
preocupação [preokupa'sãw] *f* preoccupation; (*inquietação*) worry; ***estar com preocupações*** be worried
preocupado [preoku'padu] *adj* preoccupied (***com*** with); (*inquietado*) worried (***com*** about); **~ *com a imagem*** image-conscious
preocupante [preoku'pãtʃi] *adj* worrying
preocupar [preoku'paɾ] ⟨1a⟩ preoccupy; (*inquietar*) worry; **preocupar-se** *v/r* worry; **~ *com*** worry about; ***não se preocupe!*** don't worry!
pré-pago [prɛ'pagu] *adj* ***cartão*** *m* **~** prepaid card
preparação [prepara'sãw] *f* preparation
preparado [prepa'radu] *m* preparation
preparar [prepa'raɾ] ⟨1b⟩ prepare (***para*** for); (*aprestar*) get ready
preparativo [prepara'tʃivu] *m* preparation; ***~s*** *pl* preparations, arrangements
preposição [prepozi'sãw] *f* GRAM

P

preposition
prerrogativa [prehoga'tʃiva] *f* prerogative
pré-requisito [preheke'zitu] *m* prerequisite
presa ['preza] *f caça*: prey; (*dente*) fang; (*garra*) claw; *elefante*: tusk
prescindir [presĩ'dʒir] ⟨3a⟩ **~ de algo** dispense with sth, do without sth
prescrever [preskre'ver] ⟨2c; *pp* prescrito⟩ **1** *v/t* prescribe **2** *v/i* DIR lapse
prescrição [preskri'sãw] *f* prescription; DIR lapse; ***sob ~ médica*** on prescription
presença [pre'zẽsa] *f* presence; ***~ de espírito*** presence of mind; ***na ~ de*** in the presence of
presente [pre'zẽtʃi] **1** *adj* present; (*atual*) current **2** *m* present; (*prenda*) gift, present; GRAM ***tempo ~*** present tense; ***dar um ~*** give a present; ***~ de Natal*** Christmas present
presentear [prezẽ'tʃiar] ⟨1l⟩ present; ***~ alguém com algo*** present s.o. with sth, give s.o. sth
presépio [pre'zɛpiu] *m* REL creche, *Brit* crib
preservação [prezerva'sãw] *f* ⟨*sem pl*⟩ preservation; (*proteção*) protection
preservar [prezer'var] ⟨1c⟩ preserve, protect (***de*** from)
preservativo [prezerva'tʃivu] *m* condom
presidência [prezi'dẽsja] *f* POL presidency; *reunião*: chairmanship
presidencial [prezidẽs'jaw] *adj* presidential
presidente [prezi'dẽtʃi] *m*, **-a** *f* president; *empresa*: chairman, president; ***~ do conselho de administração*** chairman of the board of directors
presidiário [prezi'dʒiariu] *m*, **-a** *f* prisoner, inmate
presidir [prezi'dʒir] ⟨3a⟩ ***~ a*** preside over; (*dirigir*) chair
presilha [pre'ziʎa] *f* (*laço*) loop
preso ['prezu] **1** *m*, **-a** *f* prisoner **2** *adj* captured, under arrest; (*encarcerado*) imprisoned; (*fixo*) fastened; *cabelo* tied back; *fig* bound; ***~ a sete chaves*** safe and secure; ***ficar ~ a*** *emocionalmente* be attached to; ***ficar ~ por um fio*** hang by a thread
pressa ['prɛsa] *f* rush, hurry; (*rapidez*) speed; (*precipitação*) haste; ***estar com ~*** be in a hurry; ***à ~*** hurriedly
presságio [pre'saʒiu] *m* omen; (*indício*) sign; (*pressentimento*) premonition
pressão [pre'sãw] *f* pressure; ***~ arterial*** blood pressure; ***~ dos pneus*** tire pressure, *Brit* tyre pressure; ***cerveja f de ~*** draft beer, *Brit* draught beer; ***fazer ~*** apply pressure; ***zona f de alta / baixa ~*** high / low pressure area
pressentimento [presẽtʃi'mẽtu] *m* premonition
pressentir [presẽ'tʃir] ⟨3e⟩ foresee; (*notar*) sense
pressionar [presjo'nar] ⟨1f⟩ pressure; (*apertar*) press
pressupor [presu'por] ⟨2z⟩ presuppose
prestação [presta'sãw] *f* service; *pagamento* installment, *Brit* instalment; ***~ de serviço*** provision of services; ***a prestações*** in installments; ***compra f a prestações*** installment plan, *Brit* hire purchase
prestar [pres'tar] ⟨1c⟩ **1** *v/t* give; *auxílio, serviço, juramento etc* provide; *informação* supply; *honra, benefício* do; ***~ atenção*** pay attention **2** *v/i* be usable; ***isso não presta*** that's no use
prestativo [presta'tʃivu] *adj* obliging
prestável [pres'tavew] *adj* (*utilizável*) serviceable; (*zeloso*) eager
prestígio [pres'tʃiʒiu] *m* prestige
prestigioso [prestʃi'ʒjozu] *adj* prestigious
presumidamente [prezumida'mẽtʃi] *adv* smugly
presumido [prezu'midu] *adj* conceited, smug; ***estar ~ de algo*** be smug about sth
presumir [prezu'mir] ⟨3a⟩ presume
presunção [prezũ'sãw] *f* presumption; (*arrogância*) arrogance, conceit
presunçoso [prezũ'sozu] *adj* conceited, arrogant
presunto [pre'zũtu] *m* ham

pretendente [pretẽ'dẽtʃi] *m/f* (*candidato*) candidate; *ao trono* pretender
pretender [pretẽ'der] ⟨2a⟩ claim; (*aspirar*) aspire to, strive for; (*afirmar*) assert; (*tencionar*) intend; *em anúncios* ***pretende-se …*** … sought
pretensão [pretẽ'sãw] *f* claim; (*exigência*) demand; (*esforço*) effort; (*desejo*) aspiration; (*arrogância*) pretension
pretensioso [pretẽ'sjozu] *adj* pretentious
pretenso [pre'tẽsu] *adj* (*suposto*) supposed; (*falso*) alleged
pretérito [pre'tɛritu] **1** *adj* past **2** *m* GRAM preterite; ~ ***perfeito*** perfect
pretexto [pre'testu] *m* pretext
preto ['pretu] *adj* black
prevalecente [prevale'sẽtʃi] *adj* prevailing
prevalecer [prevale'ser] ⟨2g⟩ prevail; ~ ***sobre*** prevail over, triumph over
prevenção [prevẽ'sãw] *f* prevention; ***de*** ~ as a precaution; ***medida*** *f* ***de*** ~ preventive measure
prevenir [preve'nir] ⟨3d⟩ (*impedir*) prevent; (*avisar*) warn (***de*** about); (*informar*) inform
preventivo [prevẽ'tʃivu] *adj* preventive
prever [pre'ver] ⟨2m⟩ *v/t* predict, foresee; (*precaver-se*) provide for; ***prevê-se que …*** the forecast is that …
previdência [previ'dẽsja] *f* foresight; (*cautela*) caution; ***caixa*** *f* ***de*** ~ social security, *Brit* national insurance; ~ ***social*** welfare
previdente [previ'dẽtʃi] *adj* far-sighted; (*cauteloso*) prudent
prévio ['prɛviu] *adj* prior, previous
previsão [previ'zãw] *f* foresight; (*expectativa*) expectation; METEO ~ ***do tempo*** weather forecast
previsível [previ'zivew] *adj* predictable; ***num futuro*** ~ in the foreseeable future
prezado [pre'zadu] *adj* treasured, esteemed; ~ ***Senhor*** Dear Sir
prima ['prima] *f pessoa* (female) cousin
primário [pri'mariu] *adj* primary, (*inicial*) initial; (*básico*) basic, rudimentary; ***ensino*** *m* ~, ***instrução*** *f* ***primária*** elementary education, *Brit* primary education; ***escola*** *f* ***primária*** elementary school, *Brit* primary school; ***professor*** *m* ~ elementary school teacher, *Brit* primary school teacher
Primavera [prima'vɛra] *f* spring; BOT primrose
primeiramente [primejra'mẽtʃi] *adv* firstly
primeiro [pri'mejru] **1** *adj* first; ***em*** ~ ***lugar*** first of all **2** *adv* first; ~ ***que*** before
primeiro-ministro [primeromi'nistru] *m* ⟨*pl* primeiros-ministros⟩ prime minister; ~ ***de maio*** May Day; ~ ***plano*** foreground
primitivo [primi'tʃivu] *adj* (*original*) original; (*básico*) primitive; ***povos*** *mpl* ~***s*** primitive people
primo ['primu] **1** *m* cousin **2** *adj* first; ***número*** *m* ~ prime number
primogênito [primo'ʒenitu] *adj* first born
primordial [primor'dʒiaw] *adj* primordial; (*principal*) main
princesa [prĩ'seza] *f* princess
principal [prĩsi'paw] **1** *adj* principal, main; ***prato*** *m* ~ main course; ***refeição*** *f* ~ main meal **2** *m* principal
principalmente [prĩsipaw'mẽtʃi] *adv* mainly, principally
príncipe ['prĩsipi] *m* prince
principiante [prĩsi'pjãtʃi] *m/f* beginner; ***curso*** *m* ***para*** ~***s*** beginners' course
principiar [prĩsi'pjar] ⟨1g⟩ begin
princípio [prĩ'sipiu] *m* beginning; (*postulado*) principle; (*fundamento*) basis; ***a*** ~, ***ao*** ~ at the beginning; ***em*** ~ in principle; ***por*** ~ on principle
prioridade [priori'dadʒi] *f* priority; ***ceda a*** ~ yield, *Brit* give way; ***ter*** ~ ***sobre*** take priority over
prioritário [priori'tariu] *adj* overriding
prisão [pri'zãw] *f ato* arrest; *pena* imprisonment; *edifício* prison, jail; ~ ***perpétua*** life imprisonment; ***ordem*** *f* ***de*** ~ warrant for arrest; ~ ***solitária***

solitary confinement; MED **~ *de ventre*** constipation
prisioneiro [prizjo'nejɾu] *m*, **-a** *f* prisoner
prisma ['prizma] *m* prism; *fig* point of view, standpoint; ***por este ~*** in this light, from this angle
privação [priva'sãw] *f* deprivation
privacidade [privasi'dadʒi] *f* privacy
privada [pri'vada] *f* toilet
privado [pri'vadu] *adj* private; ***paciente** m* **~** private patient
privar [pri'vaɾ] ⟨1a⟩ *v/t* **~ *alguém de algo*** deprive s.o. of sth; **privar-se** *v/r* deprive oneself (***de*** of), do without (***de algo*** sth)
privativo [priva'tʃivu] *adj* private
privatizar [privatʃi'zaɾ] *v/t* privatize
privatização [privatʃiza'sãw] *f* privatization
privilegiado [privile'ʒjadu] *adj* privileged; (*excepcional*) exceptional
privilegiar [privile'ʒjaɾ] ⟨1g⟩ privilege; (*preferir*) favor, *Brit* favour; (*distinguir*) distinguish
privilégio [privi'lɛʒiu] *m* privilege
proa ['proa] *f* NÁUT bow, prow
probabilidade [probabili'dadʒi] *f* probability, likelihood
problema [pro'blema] *m* problem; (*dificuldade*) difficulty; **~ *de dicção*** speech defect
problemático [proble'matʃiku] *adj* problematic; (*incerto*) uncertain; (*duvidoso*) doubtful
procedência [prose'dẽsja] *f* origin
proceder [prose'deɾ] ⟨2c⟩ **1** *v/i* (*agir*) proceed, act; (*comportar-se*) behave; **~ *de*** originate from **2** *m* procedure
procedimento [prosedʒi'mẽtu] *m* (*comportamento*) conduct; (*modo de proceder*) procedure; DIR proceedings
processador [prosesa'doɾ] *m* INFORM processor
processamento [prosesa'mẽtu] *m* processing; INFORM **~ *de texto / dados*** word / data processing; ***sistema** m **de ~ de texto*** word processing system
processar [prose'saɾ] ⟨1c⟩ process; DIR take proceedings against, sue
processo [pro'sɛsu] *m* process, procedure; DIR *tb* lawsuit, legal proceedings; **~ *judicial*** court case; **~ *seletivo*** selection process
procissão [prosi'sãw] *f* procession
proclamação [proklama'sãw] *f* proclamation, declaration
proclamar [prokla'maɾ] ⟨1a⟩ proclaim, declare
procriar [prokri'aɾ] ⟨1g⟩ procreate
procura [pro'kuɾa] *f* search; COM demand; ***oferta e ~*** supply and demand
procuração [prokuɾa'sãw] *f* power of attorney; ***por ~*** by proxy
procurado [proku'ɾado] *adj* in demand, popular; *criminoso* wanted
procurador [prokuɾa'doɾ] *m*, **-a** *f* proxy; ***Procurador da República*** prosecuting attorney, *Brit* public prosecutor; **~ *geral*** Attorney General
procurar [proku'ɾaɾ] ⟨1a⟩ look for, seek; (*tentar*) try; **~ *alguém*** call on s.o., go and see s.o.; **~ *por*** check for, look for
prodígio [pro'dʒiʒiu] *m* prodigy; ***menino** m* **~** child prodigy
prodigioso [prodʒi'ʒjozu] *adj* prodigious
produção [produ'sãw] *f* production; LIT *etc* creation; (*produto*) product; ***custos** mpl **de ~*** production costs; ***linha** f **de ~*** production line; **~ *em massa*** mass production
produtividade [produtʃivi'dadʒi] *f* productivity
produtivo [produ'tʃivu] *adj* productive; *chão etc* fertile; *negócio* profitable
produto [pro'dutu] *m* product; (*rendimento*) proceeds; **~ *colateral*** spin-off; ***~s farmacêuticos*** pharmaceuticals; **~ *final*** end product; **~ *nacional bruto*** gross national product
produtor [produ'toɾ] **1** *adj* producing *atr* **2** *m*, **-a** *f* producer
produzir [produ'ziɾ] ⟨3m⟩ produce; **~ *em massa*** mass-produce; **produzir-se** *v/r* happen
proeminente [proemi'nẽtʃi] *adj* protruding; (*célebre*) prominent
proeza [pro'eza] *f* achievement, feat

P

profanação [profana'sãw] *f* desecration
profanar [profa'nar] ⟨1a⟩ desecrate
profano [pro'fʌnu] *adj* profane; *fig* inexperienced (***em*** in)
profecia [profe'sia] *f* prophecy
proferir [profe'rir] *v/t* utter; DIR *juízo* pronounce
professor [profe'sor] *m*, **-a** *f* teacher; UNIV professor, *Brit* lecturer; **~ *adjunto*** associate professor; **~ (*de*) *primária*** elementary school teacher, *Brit* primary school teacher
professorado [profeso'radu] *m* teaching staff, teachers
profeta [pro'fɛta] *m/f* prophet
profético [pro'fɛtʃiku] *adj* prophetic
profetizar [profetʃi'zar] *v/t* prophesy
profissão [profi'sãw] *f* profession
profissional [profisjo'naw] **1** *adj* professional; (*de profissão*) businesslike **2** *m/f* professional, *fam* pro
profissionalmente [profisjonaw'mẽtʃi] *adv* professionally
profundamente [profũda'mẽtʃi] *adv* profoundly, deeply
profundidade [profũdʒi'dadʒi] *f* depth
profundo [pro'fũdu] *adj* deep; *fig* profound
progenitor [proʒeni'tor] *m* progenitor; **~*es*** *pl* ancestors; *fig* parents
prognóstico [pro'gnɔstʃiku] *m* prediction, prognosis
programa [pro'grama] *m* program, *Brit* programme; INFORM program; *escola*: schedule, *Brit* timetable; **~ *antivírus*** antivirus program; INFORM **~ *de aplicação*** application (program); **~ *de televisão*** TV program; **~ *de treinamento*** training program
programação [programa'sãw] *f* programming; INFORM ***linguagem f de ~*** programming language
programador [programa'dor] *m*, **-a** *f* INFORM programmer
programar [progra'mar] ⟨1a⟩ plan; INFORM program
progredir [progre'dʒir] ⟨3d⟩ progress, make progress; (*continuar*) continue; (*avançar*) move forward
progressão [progre'sãw] *f* progression
progressivo [progre'sivu] *adj* progressive
progresso [pro'grɛsu] *m* progress
proibição [proibi'sãw] *f* prohibition, ban
proibido [proi'bidu] *adj* forbidden; **~ *estacionar*** no parking; **~ *fumar*** no smoking; **~ *parar*** no stopping
proibir [proi'bir] ⟨3s⟩ forbid, prohibit; *produto* ban; **~ *alguém de fazer algo*** forbid s.o. to do sth
proibitivo [proibi'tʃivu] *adj* prohibitive
projeção, *Port* **projecção** [proʒe'sãw] *f Port* MAT, PSICOL, CINE projection
project... *Port* → ***projet...***
projetar [proʒe'tar] ⟨1a⟩ throw; MAT, PSICOL, CINE project; *economia* plan; *carro*, *prédio* design
projétil [pro'ʒɛtʃiw] *m* projectile, missile
projeto [pro'ʒɛtu] *m* project; *economia*: plan; *carro*, *prédio*: design; (*intenção*) intention; **~ *de lei*** bill; **~ *de pesquisa***; research project **~ *piloto*** pilot project
projetor [proʒe'tor] *m* projector; (*luz*) floodlight
proletariado [proleta'rjadu] *m* proletariat
proletário [prole'tariu] **1** *adj* proletarian **2** *m*, **-a** *f* proletarian
prole ['prɔli] *f* offspring
prolixo [pro'liksu] *adj* longwinded, prolix
prólogo ['prɔlogu] *m* prolog, *Brit* prologue
prolongamento [prolõga'mẽtu] *m* extension; ESP stoppage time
prolongado [prolõ'gadu] *adj* protracted, prolonged
prolongar [prolõ'gar] ⟨1o⟩ lengthen, extend; (*dilatar*) prolong; (*protelar*) postpone
promessa [pro'mɛsa] *f* promise
prometedor [promete'dor] *adj* promising
prometer [prome'ter] ⟨2c⟩ **1** *v/t* promise **2** *v/i* **~ *muito*** be full of promise; **~ *pouco*** not hold out much promise

P

promiscuidade [promiskwi'dadʒi] *f* muddle; *sexual* promiscuity
promíscuo [pro'miskwu] *adj* mixed up; (*confuso*) muddled; *sexualmente* promiscuous
promissor [promi'sor] *adj* promising, hopeful
promoção [promo'sãw] *f* promotion; ***campanha*** *f* ***de ~*** promotional campaign; ***oferta*** *f* ***de ~*** promotional offer; ***preço*** *m* ***de ~*** promotional price
promontório [promõ'tɔriu] *m* headland, promontory
promotor [promo'tor] *m*, **-a** *f* promoter; DIR prosecutor
promover [promo'ver] ⟨2d⟩ promote, encourage; (*causar*) cause
promulgação [promuwga'sãw] *f* promulgation
promulgar [promuw'gar] ⟨1o⟩ *lei* enact, promulgate
pronome [pro'nɔmi] *m* GRAM pronoun; ***~ pessoal*** personal pronoun
prontidão [prõtʃi'dãw] *f* promptness; (*boa vontade*) readiness
pronto ['prõtu] *adj* ready; (*imediato*) prompt; (*solícito*) eager
pronto-a-comer [prõtwako'mer] *m* ⟨*pl* prontos-a-comer⟩ fastfood restaurant; *comida* prepared meal
pronto-socorro [prõtoso'kohu] *m* ⟨*pl* prontos-socorros⟩ first aid; (*lugar*) first aid post; *Port* (*reboque*) wrecker, *Brit* breakdown lorry
pronúncia [pro'nũsja] *f* pronunciation; DIR indictment
pronunciar [pronũ'sjar] ⟨1g⟩ pronounce; (*discurso*) make, deliver; *sentença* pass; DIR ***~ alguém*** charge s.o.; ***~ mal*** mispronounce; **pronunciar-se** *v/r* express one's opinion
propagação [propaga'sãw] *f* ⟨*sem pl*⟩ spread; (*reprodução*) propagation
propaganda [propa'gãda] *f* POL propaganda; (*publicidade*) advertising
propagar [propa'gar] ⟨1o & 1b⟩ propagate; *boato* spread; **propagar-se** *v/r* spread; *som* carry
propensão [propẽ'sãw] *f* inclination; tendency (***para*** to)
propício [pro'pisiu] *adj* auspicious; (*oportuno*) opportune; (*favorável*) favorable, *Brit* favourable
propina [pro'pina] *f* gratuity, tip
propor [pro'por] ⟨2z⟩ suggest; (*expor*) propose; *candidato* put forward
proporção [propor'sãw] *f* ratio, proportion; ***proporções*** *pl* proportions, dimensions
proporcional [proporsjo'naw] *adj* proportional
proporcionar [proporsjo'nar] ⟨1f⟩ provide; (*possibilitar*) enable; *ocasião etc* give
propositado [propozi'tadu] *adj* intentional
propósito [pro'pɔzitu] *m* purpose, point; ***a ~*** by the way; ***a ~ de*** as regards; ***a ~ do aniversário de …*** on the occasion of the birthday of …; ***de ~*** on purpose
proposta [pro'pɔsta] *f* proposal; *lei*: draft; DIR offer
propriamente [propria'mẽtʃi] *adv* properly
propriedade [proprie'dadʒi] *f* property; (*terras*) estate; (*terreno*) plot (of land)
proprietário [proprie'tariu] *m*, **-a** *f* owner; *terreno*: landowner
próprio ['prɔpriu] *adj* own; (*caraterístico*) characteristic, typical; (*exato*) exact; ***eu ~*** I myself; ***ser ~ de*** be typical of
propulsão [propuw'sãw] *f* TECN propulsion; ***~ a jato*** jet propulsion
propulsor [propuw'sor] *m* drive; AERO propeller
prorrogação [prohoga'sãw] *f* extension; FIN deferment; ESP overtime, *Brit* extra time
prorrogar [proho'gar] ⟨1o & 1e⟩ extend, prolong; FIN defer
prosa ['prɔza] *f* prose; *pej* chatter, gossip
prospecto [pros'pɛktu] *m* leaflet, brochure
prosperar [prospe'rar] ⟨1c⟩ prosper, thrive
prosperidade [prosperi'dadʒi] *f* prosperity
próspero ['prɔsperu] *adj* prosperous; (*favorável*) favorable, *Brit* favourable; *negócio* thriving

prosseguimento [prosegi'mẽtu] *m* continuation; ***dar ~ a*** *carta etc* follow up
prosseguir [prose'giɾ] ⟨3o & 3c⟩ **1** *v/t* continue; *intenção* pursue **2** *v/i* continue; (*insistir*) persist
próstata ['prɔstata] *f* ANAT prostate
prostíbulo [pros'ʧibulu] *m* brothel
prostituição [prosʧitwi'sãw] *f* ⟨*sem pl*⟩ prostitution
prostituta [prosʧi'tuta] *f* prostitute
prostituto [prosʧi'tutu] *m* male prostitute
protagonista [protago'nista] *m/f* protagonist
proteção, *Port* **protecção** [prote'sãw] *f* ⟨*sem pl*⟩ protection; (*padroado*) patronage, support; ***~ ao consumidor*** consumer protection; ***~ de dados*** data protection; ***~ do meio ambiente*** environmental protection
protecionismo, *Port* **proteccionismo** [protɛsjo'nizmu] *m* protectionism
protector *Port* → ***protetor***
proteger [prote'ʒeɾ] ⟨2h & 2c⟩ protect, shield (***de, contra*** from)
protegido [prote'ʒidu] **1** *adj* protected **2** *m*, **-a** *f* protégé(e)
proteína [prote'ina] *f* protein
protelar [prote'laɾ] ⟨1c⟩ put off, postpone
prótese ['prɔtezi] *f* MED prosthesis
protestante [protes'tãʧi] *m/f* Protestant
protestantismo [protestã'ʧizmu] *m* Protestantism
protestar [protes'taɾ] ⟨1c⟩ **1** *v/t* protest; *fidelidade etc* declare **2** *v/i* protest; ***~ contra*** protest; *testamento etc* contest
protesto [pro'tɛstu] *m* protest; (*asseveração*) declaration
protetor [prote'toɾ] **1** *adj* protective **2** *m*, **-a** *f* protector; (*patrono*) patron **3** *m* ***~ solar*** sunscreen; INFORM ***~ de tela*** screen saver
protocolo [proto'kɔlu] *m* protocol; ***~ de Quioto*** Kyoto protocol
protótipo [pro'tɔʧipu] *m* prototype
protuberância [protube'rãsja] *f* bulge, protuberance
prova ['prɔva] *f* proof, evidence; (*exame*) exam; (*amostra*) test; *vestido*: fitting; ESP event; FOT print; TIPO proof; ***à ~ d'água*** waterproof; ***à ~ de bala*** bullet-proof; ***à ~ de som*** soundproof; ***~ de vinhos*** wine tasting
provação [prova'sãw] *f* trial
provar [pro'vaɾ] ⟨1e⟩ prove, demonstrate; (*examinar*) test; *prato* sample, taste; *vestido* try on
provável [pro'vavew] *adj* probable
provavelmente [provavew'mẽʧi] *adv* probably
provedor [prove'doɾ] *m* INFORM provider; ***~ de Internet*** Internet service provider
proveito [pro'vejtu] *m* advantage; COM profit
proveitoso [provej'tozu] *adj* fruitful, useful; (*vantajoso*) advantageous
proveniência [prove'njẽsja] *f* (*origem*) origin; (*fonte*) source
proveniente [prove'njẽʧi] *adj* originating; ***~ de*** originating from
prover [pro'veɾ] ⟨2ma⟩ provide (***de*** with)
provérbio [pro'vɛrbiu] *m* proverb
proveta [pro'veta] *f* test tube
providência [provi'dẽsja] *f* (*precaução*) precaution; REL providence; ***tomar ~s*** take precautions
provido [pro'vidu] *pp* → ***prover***
província [pro'vĩsja] *f* province
provincial [provĩ'sjaw] *adj* provincial
provisão [provi'zãw] *f* provision; (*mantimentos*) supply; ***provisões*** *pl* provisions
provisório [provi'zɔriu] *adj* provisional
provocação [provoka'sãw] *f* provocation
provocador [provoka'doɾ] **1** *adj* provocative **2** *m* provoker
provocante [provo'kãʧi] *adj* → ***provocador***
provocar [provo'kaɾ] ⟨1n & 1e⟩ provoke, tease; (*causar*) cause
provocativo [provoka'ʧivu] *adj* provocative
proximidade [prosimi'dadʒi] *f* proximity; ***~s*** *pl* neighborhood, *Brit* neigh-

bourhood; (*imediações*) vicinity
próximo ['prɔsimu] **1** *adj* (*perto*) near; (*seguinte*) next; *amigo* close **2** *prep* **~ de, ~ a** near to, close to **3** *m*, **-a** *f* next person; (*ser humano*) fellow man
prudência [pru'dẽsja] *f* prudence, caution
prudente [pru'dẽtʃi] *adj* prudent, cautious
prudentemente [prudẽtʃi'mẽtʃi] *adv* prudently; *dirigir* safely
pseudônimo, *Port* **pseudónimo** [psew'donimu] *m* pseudonym
psicanálise [psika'nalizi] *f* psychoanalysis
psicanalista [psikana'lista] *m/f* psychoanalyst
psicanalizar [psikana'lista] *v/t* psychoanalyze
psicologia [psikolo'ʒia] *f* psychology
psicologicamente [psikoloʒika'mẽtʃi] *adv* psychologically
psicológico [psiko'lɔʒiku] *adj* psychological; ***ação*** *f* ***psicológica*** psychological warfare
psicólogo [psi'kɔlogu] *m*(*f*) psychologist
psicopata [psiko'pata] *m/f* PSICOL psychopath
psicossomático [psikoso'matʃiku] *adj* psychosomatic
psiquiatra [psi'kjatra] *m/f* psychiatrist
psiquiatria [psikja'tria] *f* psychiatry
psiquiátrico [psi'kjatriku] *adj* psychiatric
psíquico ['psikiku] *adj* psychic
puberdade [puber'dadʒi] *f* puberty
publicação [publika'sãw] *f* publication
publicar [publi'kar] ⟨1n⟩ publicize; *livro etc* publish
publicidade [publisi'dadʒi] *f* publicity; (*reclame*) advertising; ***agência*** *f* ***de ~*** advertising agency
publicista [publi'sista] *m/f* publicist
publicitário [publisi'tariu] **1** *adj* advertising *atr*, publicity *atr* **2** *m*, **-a** *f* advertising executive
público ['publiku] **1** *adj* public; ***relações*** *fpl* ***públicas*** public relations, PR *sg* **2** *m* public; (*audiência*) audience; (*espectadores*) spectators, crowd; (*leitores*) readership; ***~ alvo*** target audience; ***em ~*** in public
pude ['pudʒi] *etc* → ***poder***
pudim [pu'dĩ] *m* pudding; ***~ flan*** crème caramel
pudor [pu'dor] *m* ***atentado ao ~ público*** indecent exposure
pueril [pwe'riw] *adj* puerile
pugilismo [puʒi'lizmu] *m* boxing
pugilista [puʒi'lista] *m/f* boxer
pular [pu'lar] ⟨1a⟩ bounce, jump; ***~ a cerca*** play around
pulga ['puwga] *f* flea
pulmão [puw'mãw] *m* lung
pulmonar [puwmo'nar] *adj* pulmonary
pulo ['pulu] *m* jump, leap
pulôver [pu'lover] *m Bras* pullover
púlpito ['puwpitu] *m* pulpit
pulsação [puwsa'sãw] *f* pulsation
pulsar [puw'sar] ⟨1a⟩ pulsate; *coração* beat
pulseira [puw'sejra] *f* bracelet; *relógio*: strap
pulso ['puwsu] *m* MED pulse; ANAT wrist; *fig* energy, strength; ***tomar o ~ de alguém*** take s.o.'s pulse
pulverizador [puwveriza'dor] *m* spray, atomizer
pulverizar [puwveri'zar] ⟨1a⟩ pulverize; *líquido* spray; (*esmagar*) smash; *fig* destroy
pum [pũ] *m fam* fart; ***dar um ~*** fart
puma ['puma] *m* puma
punção [pũ'sãw] *f* puncture; TECN punch
punhado [pu'ɲadu] *m* ***um ~ de*** a handful of
punhal [pu'ɲaw] *m* dagger
punho ['puɲu] *m* fist; *camisa*: cuff; (*cabo*) grip
punição [puni'sãw] *f* punishment
punir [pu'nir] ⟨3a⟩ punish
punível [pu'nivew] *adj* punishable
pupila [pu'pila] *f* ANAT pupil
puramente [pura'mẽtʃi] *adv* purely
purê, *Port* **puré** [pu're] *m* purée, mash; ***~ de batata*** puréed potatoes, mashed potatoes; ***~ de maçã*** apple sauce

pureza [pu'reza] *f* purity; (*integridade*) integrity
purgante [pur'gãʧi] *m* purgative
purgar [pur'gar] *v/t* purge
purgatório [purga'tɔriu] *m* purgatory
purificar [purifi'kar] ⟨1n⟩ purify
puritano [puri'tanu] **1** *adj* puritanical **2** *m*, **-a** *f* puritan
puro ['puru] *adj* pure; *uísque* straight, neat
puro-sangue [puro'sãgi] *m* thoroughbred
púrpura ['purpura] **1** *f* purple **2** *adj* purple
pus[1] [pus] *m* pus
pus[2] [pus], **puser** [pu'zɛr] *etc* → **pôr**
puta ['puta] *f vulg* whore
puto ['putu] *m fam* kid
puxa ['puʃa] *int fam* wow!
puxador [puʃa'dor] *m Port porta*: handle, knob
puxão [pu'ʃãw] *m* tug, jerk; ***dar um ~*** (***a***) pull
puxa-puxa [puʃa'puʃa] *m Bras* taffy, *Brit* toffee
puxar [pu'ʃar] ⟨1a⟩ pull; (*arrancar*) pull out; *cadeira* pull up; *conversa* strike up; *freio de mão* put on; ***puxa ao pai*** he takes after his father; ***~ pela cabeça*** think hard; ***~ pela língua de alguém*** drag information out of s.o.

Q

QI [ke'i] *m abr* (***quociente de inteligência***) *m* IQ (intelligence quotient)
quadra ['kwadra] *f casas*: block; (*estação*) time; ***~ de esportes*** sports ground; ***~ de tênis*** tennis court
quadrado [kwa'dradu] **1** *adj* square; MAT ***ao ~*** squared; ***aos ~s*** checked **2** *m figura, potência*: square; *formulário*: box
quadrângulo [kwa'drãgulu] *m* quadrangle
quadril [kwa'driw] *m* hip
quadrigêmeos [kwadri'ʒemius] *mpl* quads, quadruplets
quadrilátero [kwadri'lateru] *adj* quadrilateral
quadrilha [kwa'driʎa] *f ladrões*: gang
quadrinhos [kwa'driɲus] *mpl* comics
quadro ['kwadru] *m* painting, picture; (*sinopse*) picture; *trabalho*: framework; (*tabela*) table; *bicicleta*: frame; ***~*** (***de pessoal***) staff, personnel; ***~ de avisos*** bulletin board, *Brit* notice board; ***~ clínico*** clinical picture
quadro-negro [kwadro'negru] *m* blackboard
quadrúpede [kwa'drupedʒi] *m* quadruped
quadruplicar [kwadrupli'kar] ⟨1n⟩ quadruple
quádruplo ['kwadruplu] *adj* quadruple
qual [kwaw] **1** *pron interr* which (one); ***~ é o seu?*** which (one) is yours?; ***~ é o problema?*** what's the problem?; ***~ é a distância até …?*** what's the distance to …? **2** *pron relativo* ***o*** / ***a ~*** that; ***os*** / ***as quais*** that **3** *conj* like; ***tal ~*** just like **4** *int* ***~ é!*** oh, come on!
qualidade [kwali'dadʒi] *f* quality; ***de primeira ~*** top quality; ***na sua ~ de …*** in his capacity as …
qualificação [kwalifika'sãw] *f* qualification
qualificado [kwalifi'kadu] *adj* qualified; (*apropriado*) suitable
qualificar [kwalifi'kar] ⟨1n⟩ qualify; **qualificar-se** *v/r* ESP qualify
qualitativo [kwalita'ʧivu] *adj* qualitative
qualquer [kwaw'kɛr] *adj & pron* any; (*nenhum*) no; ***~ um*** any one; ***~ pessoa*** anyone, anybody; ***~ coisa*** anything; ***~ dia*** any day; ***em ~ parte*** any-

Q

where; ***em ~ direção que você viaje*** in whichever direction you travel; ***você não tem motivo ~ …*** you have no reason whatever …
quando ['kwãdu] *adv & conj* when; ***de ~ em ~, de vez em ~*** now and again
quantia [kwã'ʧia] *f* sum, amount
quantidade [kwãʧi'dadʒi] *f* quantity; ***… em grande ~*** great quantities of …; ***uma ~ de*** a large amount of
quantificar [kwãʧifi'kaɾ] ⟨1b⟩ *v/t* quantify
quanto ['kwãtu] **1** *adj* how much; ***~s*** how many; (***tanto***) ***… ~*** as much / many … as **2** *adv* ***~ a*** with regard to; ***~ antes*** as soon as possible; ***~ mais cedo melhor*** the sooner the better
quarenta [kwa'rẽta] *num* forty
quarentena [kwarẽ'tena] *f* quarantine
quaresma [kwa'rɛzma] *f* REL Lent
quarta ['kwaɾta] *f fam* → ***quarta-feira***
quarta-de-final [kwaɾtadʒifi'naw] *f* quarter-final
quarta-feira [kwaɾta'fejɾa] *f* ⟨*pl* quartas-feiras⟩ Wednesday; ***na ~*** on Wednesday; ***às ~s*** on Wednesdays; REL ***~ de cinzas*** Ash Wednesday
quarteirão [kwaɾtej'rãw] *m casas*: block
quartel[1] [kwaɾ'tɛw] *m* MIL quarters, barracks; *bombeiros*: fire department, *Brit* fire station
quartel[2] [kwaɾ'tɛw] *m* quarter
quarteto [kwaɾ'tetu] *m* quartet
quarto[1] ['kwaɾtu] **1** *adj* fourth; ***quarta parte*** quarter **2** *m* quarter; ***~ de hora*** quarter of an hour; *Port* ***são três menos um ~*** it's a quarter of three, *Brit* it's quarter to three; *Port* ***são três e um ~*** it's a quarter after three, *Brit* it's quarter past three
quarto[2] ['kwaɾtu] *m* room; ***~ de banho*** bathroom; ***~ de casal*** double room; ***~ da criança*** (*ou* ***das crianças***) children's room; ***~ de dormir*** bedroom; ***~ de hóspedes*** guestroom; ***~ de hotel*** hotel room; ***~ individual*** single room; ***~ principal*** master bedroom
quartos-de-final [kwaɾtosdʒifi'naw] *mpl* quarter-finals
quartzo ['kwaɾtzu] *m* quartz
quase ['kwazi] *adv* almost, nearly; ***~ não houve tempo*** there was hardly time; ***~ nunca*** hardly ever
quati [kwa'ʧi] *m* ZOOL coati
quatro ['kwatɾu] *num* four; ***cair de ~ por*** fall head over heels in love with; ***de ~*** on all fours
que [ki] **1** *pron* ◊ *relativo*: that, which; *pessoa*: who, that; ***o carro ~ você esta vendo*** the car (that *ou* which) you see; ***a mulher ~ você esta vendo*** the woman (that *ou* who) you see
◊ *após prep*: which; ***em ~*** in which; ***com ~*** with which
◊ *interr*: what; ***~ é isto?*** what's that?; ***o ~ você tem contra ela?*** what do you have against her?
◊ *int* what; ***~ desastre!*** what a disaster!; ***~ bom vê-lo!*** how nice to see you!; ***~ triste!*** how sad!
2 *conj em frases subordinadas*: that; *após comparativo*: ***do ~*** than; ***para ~*** so that; ***não ~*** (*subj*) not that; ***~ eu saiba*** as far as I know
3 *adj* what; ***~ dia é hoje?*** what day is it today?; ***~ horas tem?*** what time do you make it?
quê [ke] **1** *pron* (***o***) ***~?*** what? **2** *m* ***tem um ~ de italiano*** it has something Italian about it; ***não tem de ~*** don't mention it; ***por ~?*** why?; ***para ~?*** what for?
quebra ['kɛbɾa] *f* break; COM bankruptcy; ELÉT power cut; ***~ da bolsa*** stockmarket crash; ***~ de contrato*** breach of contract
quebra-cabeças [kɛbɾaka'besas] *m* ⟨*pl inv*⟩ jigsaw (puzzle); *fig* teaser
quebradiço [kebɾa'dʒisu] *adj* fragile, breakable
quebrado [ke'bɾadu] *adj Bras* broken; *fam* (*cansado*) shattered; *sem dinheiro* broke; *ascensor, lavabos* out of order
quebra-gelo(s) [kɛbɾa'ʒelu(ʃ)] *m*(*pl*) NÁUT ice-breaker
quebra-luz [kɛbɾa'lus] *m* ⟨*pl ~ es*⟩ lampshade
quebra-mar [kɛbɾa'maɾ] *m* ⟨*pl ~ es*⟩ breakwater
quebra-molas [kɛbɾa'mɔlas] *m* ⟨*pl*

inv⟩ speed bump
quebra-nozes [kɛbra'nɔzis] *m* ⟨*pl inv*⟩ nutcrackers
quebra-quebra [kɛbra'kɛbra] *m* ⟨*pl quebras-quebras*⟩ street riot
quebrar [ke'brar] ⟨1c⟩ **1** *v/t* break; (*partir*) break off; *código* crack; **~ *a cabeça*** rack one's brains **2** *v/i* break; *bolsa* crash; *empresa, pessoa* go bankrupt, go bust
queda ['kɛda] *f* fall; *politico*: downfall; *preços, padrões etc*: drop, fall; *cabelo*: loss; AERO crash; (*preferência*) preference; (*habilidade*) skill, gift; ***ter ~ para matemática*** have a gift for math; ***sofrer uma ~*** *dolar etc* take a dive; **~ *de água*** waterfall; **~ *de avião*** plane crash; **~ *de energia*** power failure
quedê [ke'de] where is
queijada [kej'ʒada] *f* GASTR cheesecake
queijo ['kejʒu] *m* cheese; **~ *de cabra*** goat's cheese; **~ *ralado*** grated cheese
queima ['kejma] *f* burning
queimada [kej'mada] *f ação* burning; *lugar* burnt area
queimado [kej'madu] *adj* burnt; *lâmpada* dead; **~ *de sol*** sunburnt
queimadura [kejma'dura] *f* burn
queimar [kej'mar] ⟨1a⟩ **1** *v/t* burn; *água*: scald; (*chamuscar*) singe; ELÉT fuse, blow **2** *v/i* burn; (*estar quente*) be burning hot; ELÉT fuse, blow; **queimar-se** *v/r* get burnt; (*bronzear*) get a tan
queima-roupa [kejma'hopa] ***à ~*** at point-blank range
queira ['kejra] *etc* → ***querer***
queixa ['kejʃa] *f* lament; (*reclamação*) complaint; DIR charge; ***apresentar uma ~*** make a complaint (***contra*** about)
queixal [kej'ʃaw] *m* molar
queixar-se [kej'ʃarsi] ⟨1a⟩ *v/r* complain; **~ *de*** complain about; MED complain of
queixo ['kejʃu] *m* chin
queixoso [kej'ʃozu] **1** *adj* plaintive; (*descontente*) discontent **2** *m*, **-a** *f* DIR plaintiff
queixume [kej'ʃumi] *m* complaint; (*lamentação*) lament
quem [kẽ] *pron interr* who; ***de ~*** whose; ***o homem com ~ ela estava conversando*** the man she was speaking to; ***para ~ é isto?*** who's this for?; **~ *quer que seja*** whoever
Quênia, *Port* **Quénia** ['kenja] *m* ***o ~*** Kenya
quente ['kẽʧi] *adj* hot; *casaco* warm
quentíssimo [kẽ'ʧisimu] *adj* scorching hot
queque ['kɛki] **1** *adj fam* preppy **2** *m* GASTR tea cake
quer [kɛr] *conj* whether; **~ *você queira ~ não*** whether you like it or not; ***onde ~ que*** wherever; ***quem ~ que possa ser!*** whoever can that be!
querela [ke'rɛla] *f* DIR charge; *fig* dispute
querer [ke'rer] ⟨2s⟩ want; **~ *fazer algo*** want to do sth; ***querias!*** you'd like that, wouldn't you!; **~ *dizer*** mean; ***queria ...*** I would like ..., I'd like ...; ***como quiser*** as you wish; ***se Deus quiser*** God willing; ***sem ~*** unintentionally; *literário* **~ (*a*) *alguém*** love s.o.; **~ *bem a alguém*** be fond of s.o; **~ *mal a alguém*** have ill feelings toward s.o.
querido [ke'ridu] **1** *adj* dear; ***Querido / -a ...*** Dear ... **2** *m*, **-a** *f* darling
querubim [keru'bĩ] *m* cherub
questão [kes'tãw] *f* question; (*assunto*) issue; (*disputa*) dispute; *jurídica etc*: case; ***em ~*** at issue, in question; ***fazer ~ de*** insist on; ***a pessoa em ~*** the person in question
questionar [kesʧio'nar] ⟨1a⟩ *v/t* question
questionário [kesʧio'nariu] *m* questionnaire
questionável [kesʧio'navew] *adj* questionable
quicar [ki'kar] ⟨1g⟩ bounce
quieto ['kiɛtu] *adj* quiet; (*sossegado*) still; (*pacífico*) peaceful; ***ficar ~*** go quiet
quietude [kie'tudʒi] *f* (*sossego*) quiet; (*paz*) peace
quilate [ki'laʧi] *m ouro*: carat
quilha ['kiʎa] *f* NÁUT keel
quilo ['kilu] *m* kilo

quilocaloria [kilokalo'ria] *f* kilocalorie
quilograma [kilo'grama] *m* kilogram
quilometragem [kilome'traʒẽ] *f* mileage
quilômetro, *Port* **quilómetro** [ki'lometru] *m* kilometer, *Brit* kilometre
quilovátio [kilo'vatiu] *m*, **quilowatt** [kilo'wɔt] *m* kilowatt
quimera [ki'mɛra] *f* chimera
quimérico [ki'mɛriku] *adj* fantastic
química ['kimika] *f* chemistry
químico ['kimiku] **1** *adj* chemical **2** *m*, **-a** *f* chemist
quimioterapia [kimjotera'pia] *f* chemotherapy, chemo
quina [ki'na] *f* corner
quinhão [ki'ɲãw] *m* share
quinhentos [ki'ɲẽtus] *num* five hundred
quinina [ki'nina] *f* quinine
quinquilharias [kĩkiʎa'rias] *fpl* odds and ends
quinta ['kĩta] *f* estate; MÚS fifth; *fam* Thursday; ***estar nas suas sete ~s*** be in seventh heaven
quinta-essência [kĩtae'sẽsja] *f* quintessence
quinta-feira [kĩta'fejra] *f* ⟨*pl* quintas-feiras⟩ Thursday; ***na ~*** on Thursday; ***às ~s*** on Thursdays
quintal [kĩ'taw] *m* yard, back yard
quinteto [kĩ'tetu] *m* MÚS quintet
quinto ['kĩtu] **1** *adj* fifth **2** *m* fifth
quinze ['kĩzi] *num* fifteen; ***~ dias*** two weeks, *Brit* fortnight; ***são três e ~*** it's three fifteen, it's a quarter after three, *Brit* it's quarter past three; ***são ~ para as três*** it's a quarter of three, *Brit* it's quarter to three
quinzena [kĩ'zena] *f* two weeks, *Brit* fortnight; ***uma ~ de*** around fifteen
quiosque ['kjɔski] *m* kiosk; ***~ de jornais*** newspaper kiosk
quiromante [kiro'mãtʃi] *m/f* fortuneteller
quiroprático [kiro'pratʃiku] *m*, **-a** *f* chiropractor
quis [kis], **quiser** [ki'zɛr] *etc* → ***querer***
quisto ['kistu] *m* MED cyst
quitar [ki'tar] ⟨1a⟩ *v/t dívida* pay off
quite ['kitʃi] *adj* quits; ***ficar ~ com*** get even with; ***estar ~ com alguém*** be quits with s.o.
quitinete [kitʃi'nɛtʃi] *m fam* studio apartment
quitute [ki'tutʃi] *m* delicacy
quociente [kwo'sjẽtʃi] *m* MAT quotient
quota ['kɔta] *f* quota; (*parte*) share
quota-parte [kota'partʃi] *f* share
quotidiano [kotʃi'dʒianu] **1** *adj* everyday **2** *m* ***o ~*** everyday life
quotizar [kotʃi'zar] ⟨1a⟩ *curso* quote

R

rã [hã] *f* frog
rabanada [haba'nada] *f* gust of wind; GASTR cinnamon French toast
rabanete [haba'netʃi] *m* radish
rabiscar [habis'kar] ⟨1n⟩ **1** *v/i* scribble **2** *v/t* scribble on
rabisco [ha'bisku] *m* scribble
rabo ['habu] *m* tail; *fam* backside; ***~-de-cavalo*** ponytail
rabugento [habu'ʒẽtu] *adj* (*mal-humorado*) grumpy; *criança* whiney
raça ['hasa] *f* race; (*povo*) people; (*tribo*) tribe; ZOOL breed; ***~ humana*** human race
ração [ha'sãw] *f* ration; *animais*: feed
racha ['haʃa] *f*, **rachadela** [haʃa'dɛla] *f* crack; *vestido*: slit
rachado [ha'ʃadu] *adj* cracked; *mão* chapped
rachadura [haʃa'dura] *f* crack

rachar [ha'ʃaɾ] ⟨1b⟩ **1** *v/t* split; *xícara* crack **2** *v/i* split; *xícara* crack; ***calor*** *f* ***de ~*** searing heat; ***frio*** *m* ***de ~*** icy cold; ***vento*** *m* ***de ~*** cutting wind
racial [ha'sjaw] *adj* racial; ***integração*** *f* **~** racial integration; ***segregação*** *f* **~** racial segregation
raciocinar [hasjosi'naɾ] ⟨1a⟩ reason
raciocínio [hasjo'siniu] *m* reasoning
racionabilidade [hasjonabili'dadʒi] *f* rationality
racional [hasjo'naw] *adj* rational
racionalização [hasjonaliza'sãw] *f* rationalization
racionalizar [hasjonali'zaɾ] ⟨1a⟩ rationalize
racionalmente [hasjonaw'mẽtʃi] *adv* rationally
racionamento [hasjona'mẽtu] *m* rationing
racionar [hasjo'naɾ] ⟨1f⟩ ration
racismo [ha'sizmu] *m* racism
racista [ha'sista] **1** *adj* racist **2** *m/f* racist
racum [ha'kũ] *m* raccoon
radar [ha'daɾ] *m* radar
radiação [hadʒia'sãw] *f* radiation
radiactivo *Port* → ***radiativo***
radiador [hadʒia'doɾ] *m* radiator
radial [ha'dʒiaw] *adj* radial; ***pneu*** *m* **~** radial tire, *Brit* radial tyre
radiante [ha'dʒiãtʃi] *adj* radiant
radiativo [hadʒia'tʃivu] *adj* radioactive
radical [hadʒi'kaw] **1** *adj* radical **2** *m* radical; GRAM root **3** *m/f* POL radical
radicalismo [hadʒika'lizmu] *m* radicalism
radicalmente [hadʒikaw'mẽtʃi] *adv* radically
radicar [hadʒi'kaɾ] ⟨1n⟩ **1** *v/t* root **2** *v/i* take root; (*arreigar*) settle
rádio[1] ['hadiu] **1** *m* radio **2** *f* radio (station); ***programa*** *m* ***de ~*** radio program, *Brit* radio programme
rádio[2] ['hadiu] *m* QUÍM radium
radioact... *Port* → ***radioat...***
radioatividade [hadjoatʃivi'dadʒi] *f* radioactivity
radioativo [hadjoa'tʃivu] *adj* radioactive
rádio-despertador [hadjodʒisperta'doɾ] *m* radio alarm
radiodifusão [hadjodʒifu'zãw] *f* broadcast
radiofônico, *Port* **radiofónico** [hadjo'foniku] *adj* radio *atr*
radiografar [hadjogra'faɾ] ⟨1b⟩ X-ray
radiografia [hadjogra'fia] *f* X-ray
rádio-gravador [hadjograva'doɾ] *m* radio cassette
radiologia [hadjolo'ʒia] *f* radiology
radiológico [hadjo'lɔʒiku] *adj* radiological, X-ray *atr*
radiologista [hadjolo'ʒista] *m/f* radiologist
radioscopia [hadjosko'pia] *f* X-ray (examination)
radioso [ha'djozu] *adj* radiant
radioterapia [hadjotera'pia] *f* radiotherapy
radiouvinte [hadjo'vĩtʃi] *m/f* listener (to the radio)
rafeiro [ha'fejɾu] *m Port* mongrel
râguebi ['hʌgebi] *m Port* rugby
raia[1] ['haja] *f* line; (*faixa*) lane; (*risco*) dash; (*fronteira*) border; *fig* ***passar das ~s*** overstep the mark
raia[2] ['haja] *f* ZOOL ray
raiar [ha'jaɾ] ⟨1i⟩ *v/i sol* shine; *dia* break; **~ *por*** border on; **~ *pelos 20 anos*** be around 20 years old
rainha [ha'iɲa] *f* queen
raio ['haiu] *m* ray; MAT radius; (*circunferência*) circumference; *roda*: spoke; (*relâmpago*) flash (of lightning); ***um ~ de esperança*** a ray of hope; **~*s!*** blast!; **~ *de ação***, *Port* **~ *de acção*** range; **~ *visual*** line of sight; **~ *laser*** laser beam; AUTO **~ *de viragem*** turning circle; **~*s*** *pl* ***X*** X-rays
raiva ['hajva] *f* rabies *sg*; *fig* rage, fury; ***estar com*** (*ou* ***ter***) **~ *a algo / alguém*** be furious at sth / with s.o.
raivoso [haj'vozu] *adj* MED rabid; *fig* (*furioso*) furious, livid
raiz [ha'is] *f* root; ***cortar pela ~*** (*exterminar*) root out; ***lançar ~es*** take root; **~ *quadrada*** square root
rajada [ha'ʒada] *f* gust; *fig raiva*: fit; MIL burst of gunfire
ralador [hala'doɾ] *m* grater
ralar [ha'laɾ] ⟨1b⟩ grate; *fig* annoy;

(*atormentar*) torment; (*roer*) gnaw at; **ralar-se** *v/r* **~ com** *Port* get angry about

ralé [ha'lɛ] *f pej* scum

rali [ha'li] *m* rally

ralo[1] ['halu] *m pia*: drain

ralo[2] ['halu] **1** *m* → **ralador 2** *adj cabelo, caldo* thin; (*raro*) rare; (*intervalado*) few and far between

rama ['hʌma] *f* foliage; **em ~** raw

ramagem [ha'maʒẽ] *f* branches; (*floreado*) floral pattern; **de ~** flowery

ramal [ha'maw] *m* branch; FERROV branch line; *Bras* TEL extension

ramela [ha'mɛla] *f Port fam* sleep

ramificação [hamifika'sãw] *f problema*: ramification; (*bifurcação*) branching

ramificar [hamifi'kaɾ] ⟨1n⟩ branch out; (*dividir*) divide up; **ramificar-se** *v/r* branch out

ramo ['hamu] *m* branch *tb fig*; *flores*: bunch; (*seção*) section; *saber, profissional*: area; COM line; **domingo** *m* **de ~s** Palm Sunday; **~ da construção** construction trade

rampa ['hãpa] *f* ramp

rancheiro [hã'ʃejru] *m*, **-a** [hã'ʃejra] *f* rancher

rancho ['hãʃu] *m* ranch

ranço ['hãsu] *m* rancid smell; *fig* hackneyed; **ter ~** be rancid; *fig* be hackneyed

rançoso [hã'sozu] *adj* rancid

rancor [hã'koɾ] *m* rancor, *Brit* rancour; **guardar ~** bear a grudge

rancoroso [hãko'rozu] *adj* rancorous

ranger [hã'ʒeɾ] ⟨2h⟩ *porta* creak; *pneu* screech; **~ os dentes** grind one's teeth

ranho ['haɲu] *m Port pop* snot

ranhoso [ha'ɲozu] *adj Port pop* snotty; *fig* **ovelha** *f* **ranhosa** black sheep

ranhura [ha'ɲuɾa] *f* groove; *para moedas* slot

rap [hɛp] *m* MÚS rap; **cantar ~** rap

rapariga [hapa'ɾiga] *f Port* girl; *Bras* prostitute

rapaz [ha'pas] *m* boy

rapé [ha'pɛ] *m* snuff

rapidez [hapi'des] *f* speed; **com ~** speedily

rápido ['hapidu] **1** *adj* quick, fast; (*fugidio*) fleeting; **prato** *m* **~** fast food; **via** *f* **rápida** expressway **2** *m* rapids; FERROV express

rapina [ha'pina] *f* robbery; **ave** *f* **de ~** bird of prey

raposa [ha'poza] *f* fox; *fêmea* vixen

raptar [hapi'taɾ] ⟨1a⟩ abduct

rapto ['haptu] *m* abduction

raptor [hap'toɾ] *m*, **-a** *f* abductor

raqueta [ha'kɛta] *f Port*, **raquete** [ha'kɛtʃi] *f* raquet, racket; *pingue-pongue*: paddle, *Brit* bat; **~ de tênis** tennis racket

raquítico [ha'kitʃiku] *adj* suffering from rickets; (*enfezado*) puny

raquitismo [haki'tʃizmu] *m* rickets *sg*

rarear [ha'ɾjaɾ] ⟨1l⟩ *cabelo etc* thin out

raramente [haɾa'mẽtʃi] *adv* rarely, seldom

raridade [haɾi'dadʒi] *f* rarity

raro ['haɾu] **1** *adj* rare; **raras vezes** rarely, seldom **2** *adv* rarely, seldom

rascunho [has'kuɲu] *m* draft; (*esboço*) sketch; (*minuta*) rough

rasgado [haz'gadu] *adj* torn; *sorriso* big

rasgadura [hazga'duɾa] *f*, **rasgão** [haz'gãw] *m* rip, tear; (*racha*) slit; (*fenda*) gap; (*abertura*) opening

rasgar [haz'gaɾ] ⟨1o & 1b⟩ rip, tear; (*fender*) tear up, rip up; *caminho* open; *ondas* cut through; (*arrancar*) rip out

raso ['hazu] *adj* flat; (*plano*) level, smooth; *não profundo* shallow; (*nu*) bald; *cabelo* shorn; **soldado** *m* **~** enlisted man, private

raspa ['haspa] *f* shaving; *metal*: filing

raspadeira [haspa'dejɾa] *f Port* scraper

raspadura [haspa'duɾa] *f Port* shavings; *metal*: filings

raspagem [has'paʒẽ] *f* scrape, scratch

raspanete [haspa'netʃi] *m Port fam* **dar** *ou* **passar um ~ a alguém** give s.o. a bawling out

raspão [has'pãw] *m* scratch; **passar de ~** graze

raspar [has'paɾ] ⟨1b⟩ scratch; *cabeça* shave; (*rasurar*) erase

R

rasteira [has'tejra] *f* trip; ***dar uma ~ em alguém*** trip s.o. up
rastejar [haste'ʒar] ⟨1d⟩ **1** *v/t* track (down) **2** *v/i* crawl
rastilho [has'tʃiʎu] *m* fuse
rastro ['hastru], *Port* **rasto** ['hastu] *m Port* track; ***~ de carbono*** carbon footprint
rastrear [hastri'ar] ⟨1l⟩ *v/t* rake up
rastrilho [has'triʎu] *m* rake
ratazana [hata'zana] *f Port* rat
ratificação [hatʃifika'sãw] *f* POL ratification
ratificar [hatʃifi'kar] ⟨1n⟩ POL ratify
rato ['hatu] *m Port* mouse *tb* INFORM; *Bras* rat
rateira [ha'tejra] *f Port* mousetrap; *Bras* rat trap
ravina [ha'vina] *f* ravine
razão[1] [ha'zãw] *f* reason; (*direito*) right; (*explicação*) explanation; MAT ratio; ***com ~*** rightly; ***dar ~ a alguém*** agree with s.o.; ***ter ~*** be right; ***perder a ~*** lose one's mind
razão[2] [ha'zãw] *f* COM (***livro*** *m* ***de***) ~ ledger
razoável [ha'zwavew] *adj* reasonable
r/c *m abr* (***rés-do-chão***) first floor, *Brit* ground floor
ré[1] [hɛ] *f* DIR accused
ré[2] [hɛ] *f* NÁUT poop
ré[3] [hɛ] *m* MÚS D
ré[4] [hɛ] *m Bras* AUTO reverse
reabastecer [heabaste'ser] ⟨2g & 2c⟩ *avião* refuel
reabastecimento [heabastesi'mẽtu] *m avião*: refueling, *Brit* refuelling
reabilitação [heabilita'sãw] *f* rehab *tb* MED; ***clínica*** *f* ***de ~*** rehab clinic
reabilitar [heabili'tar] ⟨1a⟩ rehabilitate
reabrir [hea'brir] ⟨3b⟩ *v/t* & *v/i* reopen
reação, *Port* **reacção** [hea'sãw] *f* reaction; ***~ em cadeia*** chain reaction
reacionário, *Port* **reaccionário** [heasjo'nariu] *adj* reactionary
react... *Port* → ***reat...***
readaptação [headapta'sãw] *f* ***~ profissional*** retraining
reafirmar [heafir'mar] ⟨1a⟩ *v/t* reaffirm
reagir [hea'ʒir] ⟨3n⟩ ~ (***a*** *ou* ***contra***) react (to); (*defender-se*) defend oneself
reajustar [heaʒus'tar] ⟨1a⟩ readjust
reajuste [hea'ʒustʃi] *m* readjustment; ***~ de salário*** salary adjustment
real [he'aw] *adj* real; *de rei etc* royal; ***rendimento*** *m* ~ real income
Real [he'aw] *m moeda brasileira* Real
realçar [heaw'sar] ⟨1p⟩ highlight; (*embelezar*) enhance
realce ['heawsi] *m* emphasis
realeza [hea'leza] *f* royalty
realidade [heali'dadʒi] *f* reality; ***na ~*** in reality
realismo [hea'lizmu] *m* realism
realista [hea'lista] **1** *adj* realistic; *hist* royalist **2** *m/f* realist; *hist* royalist
realisticamente [healistʃika'mẽtʃi] *adv* realistically
realização [healiza'sãw] *f* realization; *de trabalho* execution; CINE direction; ***~ pessoal*** self-realization
realizador [healiza'dor] *m*, **-a** *f Port* CINE director
realizar [heali'zar] ⟨1a⟩ realize; *trabalho* execute; *concerto etc* put on; CINE make; **realizar-se** *v/r Bras* happen
realizável [heali'zavew] *adj* realizable
realmente [heaw'mẽtʃi] *adv* really
reanimação [heanima'sãw] *f* revival
reanimar [heani'mar] ⟨1a⟩ *v/t* revive
reaparecer [heapare'ser] ⟨2g⟩ *v/i* reappear
rearmamento [hearma'mẽtu] *m* rearmament
reatar [hea'tar] ⟨1b⟩ *v/t* retie; (*prosseguir*) carry on with; *discussões* renew; *namorada etc* get back
reativar [heatʃi'var] ⟨1a⟩ reactivate
reativo [hea'tʃivu] *adj* reactive
reator [hea'tor] *m* reactor; AERO jet engine; ***~ nuclear*** nuclear reactor; ***~ de rápido enriquecimento*** fast breeder reactor
reaver [hea'ver] ⟨2n⟩ *v/t* get back
reavivar [heavi'var] ⟨1a⟩ *v/t* freshen up
rebaixar [hebaj'ʃar] ⟨1a⟩ lower; *fig* humiliate; **rebaixar-se** *v/r* lower oneself
rebanho [he'baɲu] *m* herd; *ovelhas*: flock

rebatedor [hebate'doɾ] *m* batter

rebate[1] [he'batʃi] *m* alarm; ~ ***falso*** false alarm

rebate[2] [he'batʃi] *m* COM discount

rebater [heba'teɾ] ⟨2b⟩ *ataque* fend off; *acusação*, *motivos* refute

rebelde [he'bɛldʒi] **1** *adj* rebellious **2** *m/f* rebel

rebeldia [hebew'dʒia] *f* rebelliousness

rebelião [hebe'ljãw] *f* rebellion

rebentação [hebẽta'sãw] *f esp* MAR surf

rebentar [hebẽ'taɾ] ⟨1a⟩ **1** *v/i* burst (***de*** with); *onda*, *águas* break; *guerra* break out; *ruído*, *tempestade* start; *planta* open; ***ela rebentou em lágrimas*** she burst into tears **2** *v/t balão* burst; *porta* burst open

rebento [he'bẽtu] *m* BOT shoot; *fig* offspring

rebite [he'bitʃi] *m* rivet

rebobinagem [hebobi'naʒẽ] *f vídeo etc*: rewind

rebobinar [hebobi'naɾ] ⟨1a⟩ *vídeo etc* rewind

rebocador [heboka'doɾ] *m* NÁUT tug

rebocar [hebo'kaɾ] ⟨1n & 1e⟩ tow; *polícia etc* tow away; *parede* plaster

rebolar [hebo'laɾ] ⟨1e⟩ *v/t* swing; **rebolar-se** *v/r* swing, sway

reboque [he'bɔki] *m* tow; (*cabo*) towrope; *veículo*: wrecker, *Brit* tow truck; AUTO ***acoplamento*** *m* ***de*** ~ tow bar

rebuçado [hebu'sadu] *m Port* candy, *Brit* sweet

rebuliço [hebu'lisu] *m* commotion

recado [he'kadu] *m* errand; (*aviso*) message; ***dar um*** ~ give a message; ***deixar um*** ~ leave a message (***a alguém*** for s.o.); ***moço*** *m* ***de*** ~***s*** messenger

recaída [heka'ida] *f* relapse

recair [heka'iɾ] ⟨3l⟩ *v/i* relapse (***em*** into)

recalcado [hekaw'kadu] *adj* PSICOL repressed

recalcamento [hekawka'mẽtu] *m* repression

recalcar [hekaw'kaɾ] ⟨1n⟩ (*repetir*) repeat; *sentimentos* repress

recanto [he'kantu] *m* corner

recapitulação [hekapitula'sãw] *f* recapitulation; (*resume*) summary

recapitular [hekapitu'laɾ] ⟨1a⟩ *v/t* recap

recaptura [hekap'tuɾa] *f* recapture

recapturar [hekaptu'ɾaɾ] ⟨1a⟩ *v/t* recapture

recarregável [hekahe'gavew] *adj* ELÉT rechargeable

recatado [heka'tadu] *adj* reserved

recear [he'seaɾ] ⟨1l⟩ **1** *v/i* (*ter medo*) be afraid (***de*** of); ~ ***por*** fear for; ***receio que sim / não*** I'm afraid so / not **2** *v/t* fear

recebedor [hesebe'doɾ] *m*, **-a** *f* recipient; *tênis*: receiver

receber [hese'beɾ] ⟨2c⟩ *v/t* receive; (*aceitar*) accept; (*reconhecer*) recognize; *oposição* meet with; ~ ***de braços abertos*** welcome with open arms

receio [he'seiu] *m* fear; ***sem*** ~ without fear, without a thought

receita [he'sejta] *f* COM income; GASTR recipe; MED prescription; ***com / sem*** ~ ***médica*** prescription *atr* / over-the-counter; ***Receita Federal*** Internal Revenue Service, *Brit* Inland Revenue

receitar [hesej'taɾ] ⟨1a⟩ prescribe

recém-casados [hesẽka'zadus] *mpl* newly weds

recém-chegado [hesẽʃe'gadu] *m*, **-a** *f* newcomer

recém-nascido [hesẽnas'sidu] *m*, **-a** *f* new-born child

recenseamento [hesẽsja'mẽtu] *m* census

recensear [hesẽ'sjaɾ] ⟨1l⟩ *v/t* ~ ***a população*** carry out a census of the population

recente [he'sẽtʃi] *adj* recent

recentemente [hesẽtʃi'mẽtʃi] *adv* recently

receoso [he'seozu] *adj* afraid; (*preocupado*) fearful

recepção [hesep'sãw] *f* reception; ***acusar a*** ~ acknowledge receipt (***de*** of)

recepcionista [hesepsjo'nista] *m/f* receptionist

receptação [hesepta'sãw] *f* DIR receiving

receptador [hesepta'dor] *m*, **-a** *f* receiver, fence
receptividade [hesepʧivi'dadʒi] *f* receptiveness
receptivo [hesep'ʧivu] *adj* receptive
receptor [hesep'tor] *m* TECN receiver
recessão [hese'sãw] *f* recession
recesso [he'sɛsu] *m* recess
recheado [he'ʃjadu] *adj* GASTR filled; *carne* stuffed
rechear [he'ʃjar] ⟨1l⟩ fill; *carne* stuff
recheio [he'ʃeiu] *m* stuffing; *bolo*: filling; *casa*: contents
rechonchudo [heʃõ'ʃudu] *adj* plump
recibo [he'sibu] *m* receipt
reciclagem [hesi'klaʒẽ] *f* recycling; (*formação profissional*) retraining
reciclar [hesi'klar] ⟨1a⟩ *v/t* recycle
reciclável [hesi'klavew] *adj* recyclable
recife [he'sifi] *m* reef
recinto [he'sĩtu] *m* area; (*salão*) hall; (*pavilhão de exposições*) exhibition hall
recipiente [hesi'pjẽʧi] *m* container
reciprocidade [hesiprosi'dadʒi] *f* reciprocity
recíproco [he'sipruku] *adj* reciprocal
recitar [hesi'tar] ⟨1a⟩ recite
reclamação [heklama'sãw] *f* complaint; (*exigência*) claim
reclamar [hekla'mar] ⟨1a⟩ **1** *v/t* claim; (*exigir*) demand **2** *v/i* (*queixar-se*) complain; **~ *contra*** complain about
reclinar [hekli'nar] ⟨1a⟩ recline; (*pôr*) lay
recobrar [heko'brar] ⟨1e⟩ **1** *v/t saúde, ânimo, dinheiro* get back, recover **2** *v/i* recover
recolha [he'koʎa] *f* collection; *dinheiro, trigo etc*: bringing in; INFORM **~ *de dados*** data capture; **~ *do lixo*** garbage collection
recolher [heko'ʎer] ⟨2d⟩ collect; *pessoa* take in; (*guardar*) keep
recolhida [heko'ʎida] *f* round-up
recolocar [hekolo'kar] ⟨1n & 1e⟩ replace, put back
recomeçar [hekome'sar] ⟨ 1p & 1c⟩ *trabalho* recommence
recomeço [heko'mesu] *m* recommencement
recomendação [hekomẽda'sãw] *f* recommendation; ***carta** f **de** ~* letter of recommendation
recomendar [hekomẽ'dar] ⟨1a⟩ recommend
recomendável [hekomẽ'davew] *adj* recommendable
recompensa [hekõ'pẽsa] *f* reward, recompense; (*indenização*) compensation
recompensar [hekõpẽ'sar] ⟨1a⟩ reward (***de*** for); (*indenizar*) compensate
recompor [hekõ'por] ⟨2z⟩ restructure; **recompor-se** *v/r* recover
reconciliação [hekõsilja'sãw] *f* reconciliation
reconciliar [hekõsi'ljar] ⟨1g⟩ reconcile; **reconciliar-se** *v/r* become reconciled, make up (***com*** with)
reconfortante [hekõfor'tãʧi] *m* tonic
reconfortar [hekõfor'tar] ⟨1e⟩ invigorate; (*consolar*) comfort
reconhecer [hekoɲe'ser] ⟨2g⟩ recognize (***por*** by); DIR attest to; (*confessar*) admit; *serviço* be grateful for; MIL *terreno* reconnoiter, *Brit* reconnoitre
reconhecido [hekoɲe'sidu] *adj* grateful
reconhecimento [hekoɲesi'mẽtu] *m* recognition; (*homologação*) witnessing; (*gratidão*) gratitude; MIL reconnaissance; ***sinais** mpl **de** ~* distinguishing marks; ***~ de paternidade*** acknowledgement of paternity
reconhecível [hekoɲe'sivew] *adj* recognizable
reconquista [hekõ'kista] *f* reconquest; (*recuperação*) recovery
reconquistar [hekõkis'tar] ⟨1a⟩ reconquer; (*recuperar*) win back
reconsiderar [hekõside'rar] ⟨1c⟩ reconsider
reconstrução [hekõstru'sãw] *f* reconstruction
reconstruir [hekõstru'ir] ⟨3k⟩ reconstruct
recordação [hekorda'sãw] *f* memory; (*lembrança*) memento
recordar [hekor'dar] ⟨1e⟩ remember; ***~ algo a alguém*** remind s.o. of sth; **recordar-se** *v/r* ***~ de*** remember

recorde [he'kɔrdʒi] *m* record; ***bater um ~*** beat a record; ***~ mundial*** world record

recordista [hekor'dʒista] *m/f* record holder

recorrer [heko'her] ⟨2d⟩ **1** *v/t* (*percorrer*) go through again **2** *v/i* ***~ a*** turn to; *meios etc* fall back on; *violência* resort to; DIR ***~ de algo*** appeal against sth

recortar [hekor'tar] ⟨1e⟩ cut out

recorte [he'kɔrtʃi] *m* cutting; ***~ de jornal*** newspaper clipping

recostar [hekos'tar] ⟨1e⟩ lean; **recostar-se** *v/r* lean back

recreativo [hekria'tʃivu] *adj* recreational

recreio [he'kreiu] *m* recreation; *escola*: recess, *Brit* break; *trabalho*: break; *espaço*: school playground

recriminação [hekrimina'sãw] *f* recrimination

recriminar [hekrimi'nar] ⟨1a⟩ blame (***por*** for); (*acusar*) accuse; **recriminar-se** *v/r* blame oneself

recruta [he'kruta] *m/f* recruit

recrutamento [hekruta'mẽtu] *m* MIL, *tb* ECON recruitment

recrutar [hekru'tar] ⟨1a⟩ recruit

rect... *Port* → ***ret...***

recuar [he'kwar] ⟨1g⟩ **1** *v/i* move back; *fig* recoil (***de*** from) **2** *v/t* put back; *linha* indent

recuperação [hekupera'sãw] *f* recovery

recuperar [hekupe'rar] ⟨1c⟩ recover; **recuperar-se** *v/r* recover, recuperate

recurso [he'kursu] *m* resource; (*possibilidade*) possibility; (*expediente*) resort; DIR appeal; ***~s*** *pl* (*dinheiro*) resources; ***em último ~*** as a last resort; ***~s humanos*** human resources, HR; ***~ visual*** visual aid

recusa [he'kuza] *f* refusal; (*resposta negativa*) denial

recusar [heku'zar] ⟨1a⟩ (*rejeitar*) refuse; **recusar-se** *v/r* refuse (***a*** to)

redação, *Port* **redacção** [heda'sãw] *f* *texto*: writing; *escola*: essay; *jornal*: editorial office; ***chefe*** *m/f* ***de ~*** editor-in-chief

redator, *Port* **redactor** [heda'tor] *m*, **-a** *f* editor; ***~ de discursos*** speech writer; ***~ de propaganda*** copy writer

redator-chefe, *Port* **redactor-chefe** [heda'torʃɛfi] *m* ⟨*pl* redactores-chefes⟩ editor-in-chief

rede ['hedʒi] *f* net; ELÉT grid; INFORM network; ***a ~*** the Net; ***ligado à ~*** networked; ***cama*** *f* ***de ~*** hammock; ***~ ferroviária*** rail network; ***~ sem fio*** wireless network; TEL ***~ fixa*** fixed phone network; TEL ***~ móvel*** cell phone network, *Brit* mobile phone network; ***~ telefônica*** telephone network

rédea ['hɛdʒia] *f* rein

redemoinho [hede'mwiɲu] *m* → ***remoinho***

redenção [hedẽ'sãw] *f* ⟨*sem pl*⟩ redemption

redigir [hedʒi'ʒir] ⟨3n⟩ write

redobrar [hedo'brar] ⟨1e⟩ **1** *v/t* double; (*aumentar*) increase; (*repetir*) repeat; ***~ os esforços*** redouble one's efforts **2** *v/i* (*subir*) go up; (*aumentar*) increase

redondo [he'dõdu] *adj* round; *fig* well-rounded; (*liso*) smooth

redor [he'dɔr] *m* ***ao ~*** around; ***ao ~ de*** around

redução [hedu'sãw] *f* reduction; ***~ de despesas*** cost reduction

reduzir [hedu'zir] ⟨3m⟩ reduce (***a, para*** to); (*limitar*) restrict

reedição [heedʒi'sãw] *f* new edition

reedificação [heedʒifika'sãw] *f* rebuilding

reedificar [heedʒifi'kar] ⟨1n⟩ rebuild

reeditar [heedʒi'tar] ⟨1a⟩ bring out a new edition of

reeducar [heedu'kar] ⟨1n⟩ *v/t* reeducate

reembolsar [heẽbow'sar] ⟨1e⟩ pay back; *cheque* cash; ***~ alguém*** reimburse s.o.

reembolso [heẽ'bolsu] *m* repayment, reimbursement

reestruturação [heestrutura'sãw] *f* restructuring

reestruturar [heestrutu'rar] ⟨1a⟩ restructure

reexpedir [heespe'dʒiɾ] ⟨3r⟩ send on
ref. *abr* (***referência***) ref. (reference)
refazer [hefa'zeɾ] ⟨2v⟩ redo; (*restabelecer*) recreate; (*emendar*) repair, fix; (*reorganizar*) reorganize; *efetivos* restore; *perda* make up for
refeição [hefej'sãw] *f* meal
refeitório [hefej'tɔriu] *m* refectory, dining hall; *fábrica*: canteen
refém [he'fẽ] *m/f* hostage
referência [hefe'rẽsja] *f* reference; ***com ~ a*** with reference to
referendo [hefe'rẽdu] *m* POL referendum
referente [hefe'rẽtʃi] *adj* ***~ a*** referring to
referir [hefe'riɾ] ⟨3c⟩ relate; (*mencionar*) refer to; **referir-se** *v/r* refer to
refinado [hefi'nadu] *adj* refined; ***açúcar*** *m* **~** refined sugar
refinamento [hefina'mẽtu] *m* refinement
refinar [hefi'naɾ] ⟨1a⟩ refine
refinaria [hefina'ria] *f* refinery; ***~ de petróleo*** oil refinery
refletir, *Port* **reflectir** [hefle'tʃiɾ] ⟨3c⟩ *v/t* & *v/i* reflect
refletor, *Port* **reflector** [hefle'toɾ] *m* reflector
reflexão [hefle'ksãw] *f* reflection
reflexivo [hefle'ksivu] *adj* GRAM reflexive
reflexo [he'flɛksu] **1** *adj* reflected; GRAM reflexive **2** *m* reflection; MED reflex
reflorestamento [hefloresta'mẽtu] *m* reforestation
reflorestar [heflores'taɾ] *v/t* reforest
refogado [hefo'gadu] *m* GASTR *onions and garlic cooked in olive oil used as a basis for dishes*
refogar [hefo'gaɾ] ⟨1o & 1e⟩ *carne* stir-fry
reforçar [hefor'saɾ] ⟨1p & 1e⟩ reinforce
reforço [he'forsu] *m* reinforcement; MIL ***~s*** reinforcements
reforma [he'fɔrma] *f* POL *etc* reform; *gabinete*: shake up, *Brit* reshuffle; *edifício*: renovation; *Port* (*aposentação*) retirement; *hist* Reformation
reformação [heforma'sãw] *f* improvement; (*remodelação*) redesign
reformado [hefor'madu] **1** *adj* REL reformed; *Port* retired **2** *m*, **-a** *f Port* pensioner, retiree
reformar [hefor'maɾ] ⟨1e⟩ reform; *edifício* renovate; (*remodelar*) redesign; *gabinete* shake up, *Brit* reshuffle; (*melhorar*) improve; MIL retire
refratário, *Port* **refractário** [hefra'tariu] **1** *adj* fireproof; *prato* ovenproof; *fig* refractory **2** *m* conscientious objector
refrão [he'frãw] *m* chorus, refrain
refrear [hefri'aɾ] ⟨1l⟩ *v/t* curb, check
refrescante [hefres'kãtʃi] *adj* refreshing
refrescar [hefres'kaɾ] ⟨1n & 1c⟩ refresh; (*refrigerar*) cool; ***~ a memória de alguém*** refresh *ou* jog s.o.'s memory
refresco [he'fresku] *m* cold drink, soft drink
refrigeração [hefriʒera'sãw] *f* cooling; *alimentos*: refrigeration; ***água f de ~*** coolant
refrigerado [hefriʒe'radu] *adj* cooled; *alimentos* refrigerated; *casa* air-conditioned
refrigerador [hefriʒera'doɾ] *m* refrigerator
refrigerante [hefriʒe'rãtʃi] *m bebida* soft drink
refrigerar [hefriʒe'raɾ] ⟨1c⟩ cool; *alimentos* refrigerate; *edifício* air-condition
refugiado [hefu'ʒjadu] **1** *adj* refugee *atr* **2** *m*, **-a** *f* refugee
refugiar [hefuʒi'aɾ] ⟨1g⟩ *v/t* harbor, *Brit* harbour; **refugiar-se** *v/r* take refuge
refúgio [he'fuʒiu] *m* refuge
refugo [he'fugu] *m* COM reject; ***mercadoria*** *f* ***de ~*** rejects, seconds
rega ['hɛga] *f* irrigation; *com regador* watering
regador [hega'doɾ] *m* watering can
regalar [hega'laɾ] ⟨1b⟩ delight; (*amimar*) spoil; **regalar-se** *v/r* treat oneself
regalia [hega'lia] *f* (*privilégio*) privilege
regar [he'gaɾ] ⟨1o & 1c⟩ water

regata [he'gata] *f* regatta
regatear [hega'tʃiar] ⟨1l⟩ **1** *v/t* haggle over **2** *v/i* haggle
regato [he'gatu] *m* stream
regência [he'ʒẽsja] *f* regency; GRAM governing; MÚS conducting
regeneração [heʒenera'sãw] *f* regeneration
regenerar [heʒene'rar] ⟨1c⟩ regenerate
regente [he'ʒẽtʃi] *m/f* MÚS conductor
reger [he'ʒer] ⟨2h & 2c⟩ govern *tb* GRAM; *orquestra* conduct; *cadeira universitária* hold
reggae ['hɛgej] *m* MÚS reggae
região [he'ʒjãw] *f* region
regime [he'ʒimi] *m* POL regime; (*modo de vida*) lifestyle; MED diet; GRAM governing; **~ de trabalho** way of working
regimento [heʒi'mẽtu] *m* MIL regiment; (*regulamento*) rules
régio ['hɛʒiu] *adj* regal
regional [heʒjo'naw] *adj* regional; ***jornal** m* **~** local paper
regionalismo [heʒjona'lizmu] *m* regionalism
registado [heʒis'tadu] *etc Port* → ***registrado*** *etc*
registrado [heʒis'tradu] *adj Bras* COM registered; ***carta** f* ***registrada*** registered letter; ***marca** f* ***registrada*** registered trademark
registrar [heʒis'trar] ⟨1a⟩ *Bras* register; (*apontar*) record; **registrar-se** *v/r* (*dar-se*) happen; (*inscrever-se*) register; *hotel*: check in
registro [he'ʒistru] *m Bras* register; (*inscrição*) registration; *diário*, *contabilidade*: entry; *documento*, *base de dados*: record; *Bras vídeo etc*: recording; **~ *civil*** registry office; **~ *de patentes*** patent office; **~ *predial*** land register; ***certificado** m* ***do ~ criminal*** criminal record
regozijo [hego'ziʒu] *m* glee
regra ['hɛgra] *f* rule; (*diretiva*) guideline; (*régua*) rule, ruler; ***em ~ geral*** as a general rule; ***~s*** *pl menstruação* period
regredir [hegre'dʒir] ⟨3d⟩ regress
regressão [hegre'sãw] *f* PSICOL regression
regressar [hegre'sar] ⟨1c⟩ come / go back
regressivo [hegre'sivu] *adj* regressive; ***contagem** f* ***regressiva*** countdown
regresso [he'grɛsu] *m* return
régua ['hɛgwa] *f* rule
reguila [he'gila] *adj Port* impertinent
regulação [hegula'sãw] *f* regulation
regulador [hegula'dor] **1** *adj* regulatory **2** *m*, **-a** *f* regulator; **~ *de volume*** volume control
regulamentação [hegulamẽta'sãw] *f* regulation
regulamentar [hegulamẽ'tar] **1** *v/t* ⟨1a⟩ regulate **2** *adj* official
regulamento [hegula'mẽtu] *m* ruling; (*estatuto*) regulations; **~ *da casa*** house rules; **~ *de serviço*** offical regulations
regular [hegu'lar] **1** *v/t* ⟨1a⟩ regulate; (*ajustar*) adjust; (*ordenar*) straighten out **2** *v/i* work, function **3** *adj* regular; (*pontual*) punctual; *fig* tolerable, average
regularidade [hegulari'dadʒi] *f* regularity; (*ordem*) organization
regularização [hegulariza'sãw] *f* regularization
regularizar [hegulari'zar] ⟨1a⟩ regularize
rei [hej] *m* king
reimpressão [heĩpre'sãw] *f* reprint
reimprimir [heĩpri'mir] ⟨3a⟩ reprint
reinado [hej'nadu] *m* reign
reinar [hej'nar] ⟨1a⟩ rule
reiniciar [heinisi'ar] ⟨1g⟩ restart
reinicio [hei'nisiu] *m* resumption
reino ['hejnu] *m* kingdom; ***Reino Unido*** United Kingdom, UK
reintegrar [heĩte'grar] ⟨1c⟩ reintegrate
reinvestir [heĩves'tʃir] ⟨3c⟩ reinvest
reitor [hej'tor] *m*, **-a** *f* president, *Brit* vice-chancellor; REL rector
reivindicação [hejvĩdʒika'sãw] *f* (*reclamação*) claim; (*exigência*) demand (**de** for)
reivindicar [hejvĩdʒi'kar] ⟨1n⟩ (*reclamar*) claim; (*exigir*) demand
rejeição [heʒej'sãw] *f* rejection

rejeitar [heʒej'taɾ] ⟨1a⟩ reject; (*recusar*) refuse
rejuvenescer [heʒuvenes'seɾ] ⟨2g⟩ **1** *v/t* rejuvenate **2** *v/i* be rejuvenated
relação [hela'sãw] *f* relation; (*nexo*) connection; (*relatório*) report; (*descrição*) account; (*lista*) list; ***em ~ a*** in relation to; ***estabelecer relações com*** establish relations with; ***relações*** *pl* ***diplomáticas*** diplomatic relations; ***relações*** *pl* ***exteriores*** foreign affairs; ***relações*** *pl* ***públicas*** public relations *pl*
relacionado [helasjo'nadu] *adj* related, connected; ***bem ~*** well-connected
relacionamento [helasjona'mẽtu] *m* relationship; ***~ com clientes*** customer relations
relacionar [helasjo'naɾ] ⟨1f⟩ *v/t* ***~ com*** relate to; **relacionar-se** *v/r* be related; ***~ com*** mix with, associate with; *sexualmente* get off with
relâmpago [he'lãpagu] *m* flash of lightning
relampejar [helãpe'ʒaɾ] ⟨1d⟩ *v/i* flash
relance [he'lãsi] *m* ***~ de olhos, ~ de vista*** glance, quick look; ***de ~*** in a flash
relatar [hela'taɾ] ⟨1b⟩ recount
relatividade [helatʃivi'dadʒi] *f* relativity
relativamente [helatʃiva'mẽtʃi] *adv* relatively
relativo [hela'tʃivu] *adj* relative
relato [he'latu] *m* report, account; (*lista*) list
relator [hela'toɾ] *m*, **-a** *f* narrator
relatório [hela'tɔriu] *m* report
relaxado [hela'ʃadu] *adj* relaxed; *fig pej* sloppy, slack
relaxamento [helaʃa'mẽtu] *m* relaxation
relaxante [hela'ʃãtʃi] **1** *adj* relaxing **2** *m* sedative
relaxar [hela'ʃaɾ] ⟨1a⟩ relax; **relaxar-se** *v/r* relax
relembrar [helẽ'braɾ] ⟨1a⟩ recall
reles ['hɛlis] *adj* common, worthless
relevância [hele'vãsja] *f* relevance
relevante [hele'vãtʃi] *adj* relevant
relevo [he'levu] *m* relief; *fig* ***pôr em ~*** throw into relief, emphasize
religião [heli'ʒjãw] *f* religion
religiosa [heli'ʒjɔza] *f* nun
religiosidade [heliʒjozi'dadʒi] *f* holiness
religioso [heli'ʒjozu] **1** *adj* religious **2** *m* monk
relinchar [helĩ'ʃaɾ] ⟨1a⟩ neigh
relincho [he'lĩʃu] *m* neighing
relíquia [he'likja] *f* relic
relógio [he'lɔʒiu] *m* clock; ***funcionou como um ~*** it went like clockwork; ***~ de pé*** grandfather clock; ***~ de ponto*** time clock; ***~ de pulso*** wristwatch; ***~ de sol*** sundial
relojoaria [heloʒwa'ria] *f loja* watchmaker's; *mecanismo* clockwork
relojoeiro [helo'ʒwejru] *m*, **-a** *f* watchmaker
reluct... *Port* → ***relut...***
relutância [helu'tãsja] *f* reluctance
relutante [helu'tãtʃi] *adj* reluctant
relutar [helu'taɾ] ⟨1a⟩ *v/i* ***~ para fazer algo*** be reluctant to do sth
reluzir [helu'ziɾ] ⟨3m⟩ shine; (*cintilar*) glitter
relva ['hɛlva] *f*, **relvado** [hew'vadu] *m Port* grass, lawn
Rem. *abr* (***remetente***) sender, from
remador [hema'doɾ] *m* rower
remar [he'maɾ] ⟨1d⟩ row
rematar [hema'taɾ] ⟨1b⟩ **1** *v/t* finish **2** *v/i* finish; ESP score the winning goal
remate [he'matʃi] *m* end; ESP winning goal
remediar [heme'dʒiaɾ] ⟨1h⟩ remedy
remédio [he'mɛdiu] *m* remedy; DIR legal recourse
remela [ha'mɛla] *f Bras fam* sleep
remendar [hemẽ'daɾ] ⟨1a⟩ *roupa, pneu* mend; *fig* patch up
remendo [he'mẽdu] *m ação* mending; *material* patch; (*remédio*) makeshift
remessa [he'mɛsa] *f dinheiro*: remittance; *mercadoria*: shipment; COM ***guia*** *m* ***de ~*** shipping documents
remetente [heme'tẽtʃi] *m/f* sender
remeter [heme'teɾ] ⟨2c⟩ *v/t* send; *dinheiro* remit; **remeter-se** *v/r* ***~ a*** refer to
remexer [heme'ʃeɾ] ⟨2c⟩ *v/t gaveta*

search through, rummage through
reminiscência [heminis'sẽsja] *f* reminiscence
remissão [hemi'sãw] *f* (*remitência*) remission; LIT cross-reference
remissível [hemi'sivew] *adj pecado* redeemable
remo ['hemu] *m* oar
remoção [hemo'sãw] *f* removal; **~ do lixo** garbage disposal
remodelação [hemodela'sãw] *f* (*reorganização*) remodeling, *Brit* remodelling; POL shake-up, *Brit* reshuffle; ARQUIT conversion
remodelar [hemode'lar] ⟨1c⟩ remodel; ARQUIT convert; POL shake up, *Brit* reshuffle
remontar [hemõ'tar] ⟨1a⟩ **1** *v/t* raise **2** *v/i temporal*: date back (**a** to)
remorso [he'mɔrsu] *m* remorse
remoto [he'mɔtu] *adj* remote
removedor [hemove'dor] *m* remover; **~ de ferrugem** rust remover
remover [hemo'ver] ⟨2d⟩ move; (*retirar*) remove; *mancha* remove, get rid off; (*espantar*) chase away
removível [hemo'vivew] *adj* removable
remuneração [hemunera'sãw] *f* remuneration
remunerador [hemunera'dor] *adj* remunerative
remunerar [hemune'rar] ⟨1c⟩ remunerate
renascença [henas'sẽsa] *f*, **renascimento** [henasi'mẽtu] *m* rebirth *tb fig*; *hist* **Renascença** Renaissance
renda[1] ['hẽda] *f* COM income; *casa*: rent
renda[2] ['hẽda] *f* TÊX lace
rendeiro [hẽ'dejru] *m*, **-a** *f* tenant; TÊX lacemaker
render [hẽ'der] ⟨2a⟩ *v/t armas* surrender; *lucro* give, yield; *sentinela* relieve; **render-se** *v/r* MIL surrender; (*submeter-se*) submit; (*ceder*) yield
rendição [hẽdʒi'sãw] *f armas*: surrender; *sentinela*: changing; (*submissão*) submission
rendimento [hẽdʒi'mẽtu] *m* yield; (*lucro*) profit; (*renda*) income; ESP, TECN, *trabalho*: performance; (*rentabilidade*) profitability, efficiency; **~ sujeito à tributação** taxable income
rendoso [hẽ'dozu] *adj* profitable
renegado [hene'gadu] **1** *adj* renegade *atr* **2** *m*, **-a** *f* renegade
renegar [hene'gar] ⟨1o & 1c⟩ **1** *v/t* deny; (*abominar*) detest; (*amaldiçoar*) curse **2** *v/i* **~ de** reject
renitente [heni'tẽtʃi] *adj* obstinate
renome [he'nɔmi] *m* renown, fame
renomear [henomi'ar]⟨1l⟩ *v/t* rename
renovação [henova'sãw] *f* renewal; (*regeneração*) renovation
renovar [heno'var] ⟨1e⟩ *v/t contrato* renew; (*regenerar*) renovate; *sala* freshen up; *distrito* redevelop
renovável [heno'vavew] *adj* renewable
rentabilidade [hẽtabili'dadʒi] *f* profitability
rentabilizar [hẽtabili'zar] ⟨1a⟩ make profitable
rentável [hẽ'tavew] *adj* profitable
renúncia [he'nũsja] *f* renunciation (**a** of)
renunciar [henũ'sjar] ⟨1g⟩ **~ a** give up, renounce; *a um cargo* give up
reorganização [heorganiza'sãw] *f* reorganization
reorganizar [heorgani'zar] ⟨1a⟩ reorganize
reparação [hepara'sãw] *f* repair; (*satisfação*) making amends; *indenização*, POL reparation
reparar [hepa'rar] ⟨1b⟩ **1** *v/t* repair; (*remediar*) make amends for **2** *v/i* **~ em** notice
repartição [hepartʃi'sãw] *f* distribution; (*departamento*) department; **chefe** *m/f* **de ~** head of department
repartir [hepar'tʃir] ⟨3b⟩ distribute, divide up; *trabalho* **~ a alguém** allocate to s.o.
repassar [hepa'sar] ⟨1b⟩ (*rever*) go through again
repatriação [hepatria'sãw] *f* repatriation
repatriar [hepatri'ar] *v/t* repatriate
repavimentar [hepavimẽ'tar] ⟨1l⟩ *v/t* resurface
repelente [hepe'lẽtʃi] **1** *adj* repellent **2** *m* insect repellent

repelir [hepe'liɾ] ⟨3c⟩ repel
repensar [hepẽ'saɾ] ⟨1a⟩ rethink
repente [he'pẽtʃi] ***de ~*** suddenly
repentino [hepẽ'tʃinu] *adj* sudden
repercussão [heperku'sãw] *f* effect; ***repercussões*** *pl* repercussions
repercutir [heperku'tʃiɾ] ⟨3a⟩ **1** *v/t* echo **2** *v/i som* echo; **repercutir-se** *v/r* have repercussions
repertório [heperˈtɔriu] *m* repertoire
repetição [hepetʃi'sãw] *f* repetition
repetir [hepe'tʃiɾ] ⟨3c⟩ repeat; **repetir-se** *v/r* recur; ***estou me repetindo?*** am I repeating myself?
repetitivo [hepetʃi'tʃivu] *adj* repetitive
repisar [hepi'zaɾ] ⟨1a⟩ *passado* revisit
repleto [he'plɛtu] *adj* replete, full
réplica ['hɛplika] *f* retort; (*reprodução*) replica
replicar [hepli'kaɾ] ⟨1n⟩ retort; (*objetar*) object; (*contradizer*) answer back to
repolho [he'poʎu] *m* cabbage
repor [he'poɾ] ⟨2z⟩ put back; (*devolver*) give back; (*substituir*) replace; **repor-se** *v/r* recover
reportagem [hepoɾ'taʒẽ] *f* report; *ato* reporting
reportar [hepoɾ'taɾ] ⟨1e⟩ report; ***~ a*** refer to; *superior* report to; **reportar-se** *v/r* ***~ a*** refer to; *superior* report to
repórter [he'pɔrtɛɾ] *m/f* reporter
reposição [hepozi'sãw] *f* return; (*reinstalação*) reinstatement; TEAT, CINE re-run
repousado [hepo'zadu] *adj* refreshed, rested
repousar [hepo'zaɾ] ⟨1a⟩ rest
repouso [he'pozu] *m* (*pausa*) rest; AGR ***em ~*** lying fallow
repreender [hepreẽ'deɾ] ⟨2a⟩ reprimand
repreensão [hepreẽ'sãw] *f* reprimand
repreensível [hepreẽ'sivew] *adj* reprehensible
repreensivo [hepreẽ'sivu] *adj* reprehensive
represa [he'preza] *f* dam
represália [hepre'zalia] *f* reprisal; ***usar de ~ s, exercer ~s*** take reprisals; ***como / em ~ por*** in retaliation for
representação [heprezẽta'sãw] *f* representation; TEAT performance; ***~ proporcional*** proportional representation
representante [heprezẽ'tãtʃi] *m/f* representative
representar [heprezẽ'taɾ] ⟨1a⟩ represent; TEAT *papel* perform, put on
representatividade [heprezẽtatʃivi'dadʒi] *f* representativeness
representativo [heprezẽta'tʃivu] *adj* representative
repressão [hepre'sãw] *f* repression
repressivo [hepre'sivu] *adj* repressive
reprimenda [hepri'mẽda] *f* reprimand
reprimir [hepri'miɾ] ⟨3a⟩ repress
reprise [he'prizi] *f* TV repeat; ESP replay
reprocessamento [heprosesa'mẽtu] *m* TECN reprocessing; ***instalação f de ~*** reprocessing plant
reprocessar [heprose'saɾ] ⟨1c⟩ reprocess
reprodução [heprodu'sãw] *f* reproduction
reprodutivo [heprodu'tʃivu] *adj* reproductive
reprodutor [heprodu'toɾ] *adj* reproductive
reproduzir [heprodu'ziɾ] ⟨3m⟩ reproduce; **reproduzir-se** *v/r* reproduce
reprovação [heprova'sãw] *f* reproach; *exame*: failure
reprovador [heprova'doɾ] *adj* reproachful, disapproving
reprovar [hepro'vaɾ] ⟨1e⟩ reproach; *exame* fail
reprovável [hepro'vavew] *adj* reprehensible
réptil ['hɛptʃiw] *m* reptile
república [he'publika] *f* republic; ***República Popular*** People's Republic
republicano [hepubli'kanu] **1** *adj* republican **2** *m*, **-a** *f* republican
repudiar [hepu'dʒiaɾ] ⟨1g⟩ reject; *filho etc* disown; (*negar*) deny
repugnância [hepu'gnãsja] *f* repugnance
repugnante [hepu'gnãtʃi] *adj* disgusting
repulsa [he'puwsa] *f*, **repulsão** [he-

R

puw'sãw] *f* ⟨*sem pl*⟩ repulsion; (*rejeição*) rejection; ***causar ~ a alguém*** repel s.o.
repulsivo [hepuw'sivu] *adj* repulsive
reputação [heputa'sãw] *f* ⟨*sem pl*⟩ reputation
repuxão [hepu'ʃãw] *m* tug
repuxar [hepu'ʃaɾ] ⟨1a⟩ *v/t* tug, pull; (*esticar*) tighten
repuxo [he'puʃu] *m* fountain
requeijão [hekej'ʒãw] *f m* GASTR *type of cream cheese*
requentar [hekẽ'taɾ] ⟨1a⟩ *v/t* warm up
requerente [heke'rẽtʃi] *m/f* DIR claimant
requerer [heke'reɾ] ⟨2sa⟩ claim; (*solicitar*) apply for; (*exigir*) demand; (*desejar*) desire; (*reclamar*) require
requerido [heke'ɾidu] *adj* (*necessário*) requisite
requerimento [hekeri'mẽtu] *m* application; (*petição*) petition; (*exigência*) demand
requintado [hekĩ'tadu] *adj* refined
requinte [he'kĩtʃi] *m* refinement
requisição [hekizi'sãw] *f* request; (*confiscação*) requisitioning
requisitar [hekizi'taɾ] ⟨1a⟩ demand; (*requerer*) apply for; (*confiscar*) requisition
requisito [heki'zitu] *m* demand; (*condição*) requirement
rescindir [hesĩ'dʒiɾ] ⟨3a⟩ *contrato* cancel, terminate
rescisão [hesi'zãw] *f contrato*: cancellation, termination
rés-do-chão [hɛsdo'ʃãw] *m* ⟨*pl ~* s⟩ *Port* first floor, *Brit* ground floor
resenha [he'zẽɲa] *f* review, write-up
reserva [he'zɛɾva] *f* reserve; *bilhetes etc*: reservation; ***~ natural*** nature reserve; ***tanque*** *m* ***de ~*** reserve tank
reservado [hezeɾ'vadu] *adj lugar, pessoa* reserved
reservar [hezeɾ'vaɾ] ⟨1c⟩ *direito, bilhetes, lugar* reserve; (*guardar*) keep; *dinheiro* set aside; (*ter pronto*) keep ready
reservatório [hezeɾva'tɔriu] *m* reservoir
reservista [hezeɾ'vista] *m/f* reservist
resfriado [hesfri'adu] *Bras* **1** *adj* ***estar ~*** have a cold **2** *m* cold
resfriar [hesfri'aɾ] ⟨1g⟩ **1** *v/t* chill **2** *v/i* catch a cold; **resfriar-se** *v/r* cool; *Bras* MED catch a cold
resgatar [hezga'taɾ] ⟨1b⟩ pay off; (*libertar*) rescue; *reféns* ransom
resgate [hez'gatʃi] *m* redemption; (*libertação*) rescue; *reféns*: ransom
residência [hezi'dẽsja] *f* (*domicílio*) residence; ***autorização*** *f* ***de ~*** residence permit
residencial [hezidẽ'sjaw] **1** *adj* residential; ***bairro*** *m* ***~*** residential district **2** *m* guesthouse
residente [hezi'dẽtʃi] **1** *adj* resident **2** *m/f* resident
residir [hezi'dʒiɾ] ⟨3a⟩ live, reside
resíduo [he'zidwu] *m* residue; ***~s*** *pl* (industrial) waste; ***~ nuclear*** nuclear waste; ***~s*** *pl* ***tóxicos*** toxic waste
resignação [hezigna'sãw] *f* ⟨*sem pl*⟩ resignation
resignado [hezi'gnadu] *adj fig* resigned
resignar [hezi'gnaɾ] ⟨1a⟩ resign; **resignar-se** *v/r* resign oneself (***a*** to)
resina [he'zina] *f* resin
resistência [hezis'tẽsja] *f* resistance; (*perseverança*) stamina, endurance; (*estabilidade*) durability
resistente [hezis'tẽtʃi] *adj* tough; (*estável*) durable; ***~ ao calor*** heat resistant
resistir [hezis'tʃiɾ] ⟨3a⟩ hold out, last; (*opor-se*) resist (***a algo*** sth)
resmungar [hezmũŋ'gaɾ] ⟨1c⟩ *v/i* mumble; (*queixar-se*) grumble
resolução [hezolu'sãw] *f* resolution; *problema*: solution
resoluto [hezo'lutu] *adj* resolute, determined
resolver [hezow'veɾ] ⟨2e⟩ resolve; *problema* solve, clear up; *situação* clarify; *dúvida* dispel; (*decidir*) resolve; **resolver-se** *v/r* resolve, decide (***a fazer*** to do)
resolvido [hezow'vidu] *adj* determined, intent
respectivamente [hespektʃiva'mẽtʃi] *adv* respectively
respectivo [hespek'tʃivu] *adj* respective

respeitar [hespej'taɾ] ⟨1a⟩ **1** *v/t* respect; (*ter em conta*) bear in mind **2** *v/i* **~ *a alguém*** concern s.o.
respeitável [hespej'tavew] *adj* respectable; (*considerável*) considerable
respeito [hes'pejtu] *m* respect; ***falta** f **de*** **~** lack of respect; ***a*** **~ *de*** in respect of; ***dizer*** **~ *a*** concern
respeitoso [hespej'tozu] *adj* respectful
respiração [hespira'sãw] *f* breathing; ***fazer perder a*** **~ *a alguém*** take s.o.'s breath away; **~ *boca a boca*** mouth-to-mouth resuscitation, *Brit tb* kiss of life
respirar [hespi'ɾaɾ] ⟨1a⟩ **1** *v/i* breathe; (*descansar*) take a breather; **~ *fundo*** take a deep breath **2** *v/t* breathe (in / out)
resplandecer [hesplãde'seɾ] ⟨2g⟩ shine *tb fig*
responder [hespõ'deɾ] ⟨2a⟩ answer; **~ *a algo*** respond to sth; **~ *por*** be answerable for; **~ *afirmativamente*** answer in the affirmative
responsabilidade [hespõsabili'dadʒi] *f* responsibility; DIR liability; **~ *civil*** civil liability; ***responsabilidades** pl **da função*** job description
responsabilizar [hespõsabili'zaɾ] ⟨1a⟩ **~ *alguém*** hold s.o. responsible (***por*** for); **responsabilizar-se** answer (***por*** for)
responsável [hespõ'savew] **1** *adj* responsible; DIR liable **2** *m/f* person responsible
responsivo [hespõ'sivu] *adj* responsive
resposta [hes'pɔsta] *f* answer, reply
ressaca [he'saka] *f fig* hangover
ressaltar [hesaw'taɾ] ⟨1a⟩ **1** *v/t* emphasize **2** *v/i* jump; (*ricochetear*) ricochet; ARQUIT jut out; ***ressalta à vista*** it stands out
ressarcir [hesaɾ'siɾ] ⟨3q⟩ *v/t* reimburse
ressentido [hesẽ'tʃidu] *adj* resentful; (*sensível*) sensitive
ressentimento [hesẽtʃi'mẽtu] *m* resentment; (*sensibilidade*) sensitivity
ressentir [hesẽ'tʃiɾ] ⟨3e⟩ resent; **ressentir-se** *v/r* **~ *de algo*** suffer from sth; (*ofender-se*) be resentful about sth; (*sentir*) feel the effects of sth
ressoar [he'swaɾ] ⟨1f⟩ *v/i* echo; (*soar*) resound; *mexerico* be heard
ressonância [heso'nãsja] *f* resonance; (*eco*) echo; MÚS ***caixa** f **de*** **~** echo chamber
ressonante [heso'nãtʃi] *adj* resonant
ressonar [heso'naɾ] ⟨1f⟩ *v/i* snore
ressurgimento [hesuɾʒi'mẽtu] *m* resurgence
ressurgir [hesuɾ'ʒiɾ] ⟨3n⟩ (*renascer*) have a revival; (*reaparecer*) return; ***fazer*** **~** revive
ressurreição [hesuhej'sãw] *f* resurrection
ressuscitar [hesusi'taɾ] ⟨1a⟩ **1** *v/t* resuscitate **2** *v/i* be resuscitated
restabelecer [hestabele'seɾ] ⟨2g⟩ reestablish; **restabelecer-se** *v/r* recover, convalesce
restabelecimento [hestabelesi'mẽtu] *m* reestablishment; MED recovery, convalescence
restante [hes'tãtʃi] *adj* remaining
restar [hes'taɾ] ⟨1c⟩ be left, remain
restauração [hestawɾa'sãw] *f* restoration
restaurante [hestaw'ɾãtʃi] *m* restaurant
restaurar [hestaw'ɾaɾ] ⟨1a⟩ restore
restituição [hestʃitwi'sãw] *f* restitution, return
restituir [hestʃi'twiɾ] ⟨3i⟩ return; (*reconstituir*) restore
resto ['hɛstu] *m* rest; (*sobras*) remains; (*sobejo*) remnant; MAT remainder; ***de*** **~** for the rest; **~*s mortais*** mortal remains
restrição [hestɾi'sãw] *f* restriction
restringir [hestɾĩ'ʒiɾ] ⟨3n⟩ restrict; **restringir-se** *v/r* restrict oneself; ***vou me*** **~ *a …*** I'll restrict myself to …
restritivo [hestɾi'tʃivu] *adj* restrictive
resultado [hezuw'tadu] *m* result; ***dar*** **~** succeed, work
resultar [hezuw'taɾ] ⟨1a⟩ turn out to be; *consequência* result (***de*** from); **~ *em*** result in; ***não*** **~** not work out; ***resultou!*** it worked!

R

resumido [hezu'midu] *adj* summarized; (*curto*) concise
resumir [hezu'miɾ] ⟨3a⟩ summarize, sum up; ***resumindo*** in short; **resumir-se** *v/r* be brief; ***~ a*** limit oneself to; ***~ em*** boil down to
resumo [he'zumu] *m* summary; ***em ~*** in short
reta ['hɛta] *f* MAT straight line; ESP ***~ final*** home straight
retaguarda [hɛta'gwarda] *f* MIL rear guard; (*parte posterior*) rear; ***à ~*** at the rear
retalhista [heta'ʎista] *m/f Port* retailer
retalho [he'taʎu] *m* remnant; *Port* COM ***a ~*** retail; ***venda*** *f* ***a ~*** retail trade
retangular [hetãgu'laɾ] *adj* rectangular
retângulo [he'tãgulu] **1** *adj* rectangular **2** *m* rectangle
retardado [hetaɾ'dadu] *adj* late; PSICOL retarded
retardar [hetaɾ'daɾ] ⟨1b⟩ delay; (*reter*) hold up; (*adiar*) postpone; *relógio* put back
retardatário [hetaɾda'tariu] *m*, **-a** *f* straggler
retenção [hetẽ'sãw] *f* retention; DIR, *escola*: detention
reter [he'teɾ] ⟨2xa⟩ retain; *na memória* keep, hold; *lágrimas*, *informações* keep back; *alimentos* keep down; *respiração* hold; *pago* withhold; DIR detain
retesar [hete'zaɾ] ⟨1a⟩ *v/t* tighten
reticência [heʧi'sẽsja] *f* reticence; ***~s*** *pl* TIPO suspension points
retidão [heʧi'dãw] *f* ⟨*sem pl*⟩ straightness; (*probidade*) rectitude
retificação [heʧifika'sãw] *f* straightening; (*correção*) rectification
retificar [heʧifi'kaɾ] ⟨1n⟩ straighten; (*corrigir*) rectify
retina [he'ʧina] *f olho*: retina
retinir [heʧi'niɾ] ⟨3a⟩ jingle; (*ressoar*) echo
retirada [heʧi'ɾada] *f* withdrawal; MIL retreat, withdrawal; *náufragos*: rescue; MIL, *fig* ***bater em ~*** beat a retreat
retirar [heʧi'ɾaɾ] ⟨1a⟩ withdraw; *palavra* take back, withdraw; (*tirar*) take out; (*remover*) take away, remove; ***~ do mercado*** take off the market; ***~ gradualmente*** *produto etc* phase out; **retirar-se** *v/r* withdraw; MIL pull back, pull out
retiro [he'ʧiɾu] *m* retreat
reto ['hɛtu] *adj* straight; *fig pessoa* honest, upright
retocar [heto'kaɾ] ⟨1n & 1e⟩ touch up; AUTO soup up
retomar [heto'maɾ] ⟨1e⟩ take up again, resume; ***~ a posse de*** repossess
retoque [he'tɔki] *m* touch-up; ***dar os últimos ~s*** put the final *ou* finishing touches to
retórica [hɛ'tɔrika] *f* rhetoric
retórico [hɛ'tɔriku] *adj* rhetorical
retornado [hetoɾ'nadu] *m* homecomer
retornar [hetoɾ'naɾ] ⟨1e⟩ **1** *v/t* return; (*responder*) respond **2** *v/i* return
retorno [he'tornu] *m* return; ***fazer seu grande ~*** make a big comeback
retraído [hetɾa'idu] *adj* retracted; (*tímido*) withdrawn; *vida* secluded
retrair [hetɾa'iɾ] ⟨3l⟩ retract; (*puxar*) pull way; (*reter*) withdraw; **retrair-se** *v/r* contract
retratar [hetɾa'taɾ] ⟨1b⟩ portray, make a portrait of; (*descrever*) portray
retrato [he'tɾatu] *m* portrait
retribuição [hetɾibwi'sãw] *f* (*recompensa*) reward; (*réplica*) reciprocation
retribuir [hetɾi'bwiɾ] ⟨3i⟩ reciprocate; (*pagar*) recompense; (*recompensar*) reward
retroativo, *Port* **retroactivo** [hetɾoa'ʧivu] *adj* retroactive
retroceder [hetɾose'deɾ] ⟨2c⟩ retreat, withdraw; (*voltar para trás*) go back; *águas* recede; (*oposto a*: *desenvolver-se*) go backward
retrocesso [hetɾo'sɛsu] *m* retreat; (*diminuição*) decline, drop; *esp fig* backward move; ***tecla*** *f* ***de ~*** backspace key
retrógrado [he'tɾɔgradu] *adj* retrograde

R

retroprojetor, *Port* **retroprojector** [hɛtroproʒɛ'tor] *m* overhead projector

retrospeção, *Port* **retrospecção** [hetrospɛ'sãw] *f* retrospection

retrospect... *Port* → ***retrospet...***

retrospetiva [hetrospɛ'tʃiva] *f* retrospective

retrospetivo [hetrospɛ'tʃivu] *adj* retrospective

retrovisor [hetrovi'zor] *m* AUTO rear-view mirror

réu [hɛu] *m* accused, defendant

reumático [hew'matʃiku] *adj* rheumatic

reumatismo [hewma'tʃizmu] *m* rheumatism

reunião [heu'njãw] *f* reunion; (*união*) union; (*encontro*) meeting; (*sessão*) session; ***ele está em ~*** he's in a meeting; ***~ do conselho*** board meeting; ***~ de negócios*** business meeting; ***~ de vendas*** sales meeting

reunido [heu'nidu] *adj poemas* collected

reunificação [heunifika'sãw] *f* POL reunification

reunir [heu'nir] ⟨3t⟩ **1** *v/t* bring together; (*unir*) reunite; (*juntar*) combine (***a*** with) **2** *v/i* (*encontrar-se*) come together, gather; **reunir-se** *v/r* come together, meet; (*associar-se*) join (***com*** with)

reutilização [heutʃiliza'sãw] *f* re-use

revelação [hevela'sãw] *f* revelation; FOT development

revelador [hevela'dor] *adj* revealing

revelar [heve'lar] ⟨1c⟩ reveal; FOT develop

rever [he'ver] ⟨2m⟩ see again; (*estudar*) look through; (*examinar*) check over; (*corrigir*) go through again; (*repensar*) rethink; DIR review

reverência [heve'rẽsja] *f* reverence; (*vênia*) bow; *mulher*: curtsey

reverenciar [heverẽ'sjar] *v/t* revere

reverendo [heve'rẽdu] *m* Reverend

reversão [hever'sãw] *f* reversion

reversível [hever'sivew] *adj* reversible

reverso [he'vɛrsu] **1** *m* reverse **2** *adj* reverse

revés [he'vɛs] *m* reversal, setback; *tênis*: backhand; ***ao ~*** back to front

revestimento [hevestʃi'mẽtu] *m parede, chão*: covering; *interno* lining

revestir [heves'tʃir] ⟨3c⟩ cover; *interior* line (***de*** with); **revestir-se** *v/r fig* arm oneself (***de*** with)

revezar [heve'zar] ⟨1c⟩ *v/t & v/i* alternate; **revezar-se** *v/r* alternate, take turns

revirar [hevi'rar] ⟨1a⟩ turn around; (*fazer recuar*) turn back; *na cama* turn over; ***~ os olhos*** roll one's eyes

reviravolta [hevira'vɔlta] *f* about-turn

revisão [hevi'zãw] *f* revision; (*controlo*) check; AUTO service; ***~ de provas*** proofread

revisar [hevi'zar] ⟨1a⟩ *v/t opinião, texto* revise; *planos* overhaul; *carro, máquina* service; *para exame* review, *Brit* revise; *provas* check, proofread

revisor [hevi'zor] *m*, **-a** *f* inspector; TIPO proofreader

revista [he'vista] *f* inspection; (*busca*) search; DIR, TEAT review; LIT magazine; *profissional* journal; MIL parade; ***passar em ~*** inspect the troops; ***~ mensal*** monthly; ***~ de moda*** fashion magazine; ***~ em quadrinhos*** comic book

revistar [hevis'tar] ⟨1a⟩ search; DIR *processo* review; MIL inspect, review

reviver [hevi'ver] ⟨2a⟩ *v/t* relive

revogação [hevoga'sãw] *f* revoking; *lei*: repeal

revogar [hevo'gar] ⟨1o & 1e⟩ revoke; *lei* repeal

revolta [he'vɔlta] *f* revolt; (*indignação*) disgust

revoltado [hevow'tadu] *adj* (*indignado*) disgusted; POL rebellious

revoltante [hevow'tãtʃi] *adj fig* disgusting, revolting

revoltar [hevow'tar] ⟨1e⟩ **1** *v/t* revolt; POL stir up **2** *v/i* cause indignation; **revoltar-se** *v/r* revolt

revolução [hevolu'sãw] *f* revolution

revolucionar [hevolusjo'nar] ⟨1f⟩ (*transformar*) revolutionize

revolucionário [hevolusjo'nariu] **1** *adj* revolutionary **2** *m*, **-a** *f* revolutionary

revolver [hevow'veɾ] ⟨2e⟩ **1** *v/t* turn over; *gaveta* rummage through **2** *v/i* revolve
revólver [he'vɔwvɛɾ] *m* revolver
reza ['hɛza] *f* prayer
rezar [he'zaɾ] ⟨1c⟩ **1** *v/i* pray **2** *v/t* say
riacho ['hiaʃu] *m* creek, stream
ribanceira [hibã'sejɾa] *f* (*penedia*) steep riverbank
ribeira [hi'bejɾa] *f* riverbank
ribeiro [hi'bejɾu] *m* creek, stream
rico ['hiku] **1** *adj* rich; (*magnífico*) splendid; (*delicioso*) delicious; (*querido*) dear **2** *m/f* rich man / woman
ricochetear [hikoʃetʃi'aɾ] ⟨1l⟩ *v/i* ricochet
ricota [hi'kɔta] *f* cream cheese
ridícularizar [hidʒikulaɾi'zaɾ] ⟨1a⟩ *v/t* ridicule
ridículo [hi'dʒikulu] **1** *adj* ridiculous **2** *m* ridicule; ***cair no ~*** make oneself a laughing stock
rido ['hidu] *pp* → ***rir***
rifa ['hifa] *f* raffle
rifle ['hifli] *m* rifle
rigidez [hiʒi'des] *f* rigidity, stiffness; *cadáver*: *fig* strictness; (*dureza*) severity
rígido ['hiʒidu] *adj* rigid, stiff; (*severo*) strict; (*duro*) severe
rigor [hi'goɾ] *m* severity; (*severidade*) strictness; (*exatidão*) rigor, *Brit* rigour
rigoroso [higo'ɾozu] *adj professor* strict; *Inverno* severe; (*exato*) rigorous
rijo ['hiʒu] **1** *adj* hard; (*tenaz*) tough; *músculo* firm; *fig* strict **2** *m* ***o ~*** the majority
rim [hĩ] *m* kidney; ***rins*** *pl* small of the back
rima ['hima] *f* LIT rhyme
rimar [hi'maɾ] ⟨1a⟩ *v/t* & *v/i* rhyme
rímel ['himew] *m* mascara
ringue ['hĩgi] *m* ESP ring; ***~ de boxe*** boxing ring; ***~ de gelo*** ice rink; ***~ de patinagem*** skating rink
rinoceronte [hinose'ɾõtʃi] *m* rhinoceros, rhino
rio[1] ['hiu] *m* river; ***~ abaixo / acima*** downriver / upriver, downstream / upstream
rio[2] ['hiu] → ***rir***
ripa ['hipa] *f* slat
riqueza [hi'keza] *f* wealth; *de côr, sabor etc* richness
rir [hiɾ] ⟨3v⟩ laugh; ***~ de*** laugh at; ***~ para*** smile at
risada [hi'zada] *f* laughter
risca ['hiska] *f* stroke; *cabelo*: part, *Brit* parting; ***à ~*** precisely; ***às ~s*** striped
riscado [his'kadu] *m* striped material
riscar [his'kaɾ] ⟨1n⟩ (*corrigir*) strike out, cross out; (*esboçar*) sketch
risco[1] ['hisku] *m* risk; ***a todo o ~*** at all costs; ***correr ~ de fazer*** run the risk of doing; ***corra o ~*** take a risk; ***pôr em ~*** put at risk
risco[2] ['hisku] *m* stroke; (*esboço*) sketch; *cabelo*: part, *Brit* parting
riso ['hizu] *m* laugh; (*gargalhadas*) laughter, laughing
risonho [hi'zoɲu] *adj* smiling; (*alegre*) cheerful
risoto [hi'zotu] *m* GASTR risotto
rispidez [hispi'des] *f* harshness
ríspido ['hispidu] *adj* harsh
rissol [hi'sɔw] *m* ⟨*pl* rissóis⟩ GASTR *Port* ***~ de camarão*** *shrimps in a dough and batter wrapper*
rítmico ['hitʃimiku] *adj* rhythmical
ritmo ['hitʃimu] *m* rhythm; (*velocidade*) pace, speed; ***em um ~ veemente*** at a furious pace
rito ['hitu] *m* rite
ritual [hi'twaw] **1** *adj* ritual **2** *m* ritual
riu ['hiu] → ***rir***
rival [hi'vaw] **1** *adj* rival *atr* **2** *m/f* rival
rivalidade [hivali'dadʒi] *f* rivalry
rivalizar [hivali'zaɾ] ⟨1a⟩ ***~ com*** rival
rixa ['hiʃa] *f* fight
robô, *Port* **robot** [ho'bo] *m* robot
robustez [hobus'tes] *f* robustness
robusto [ho'bustu] *adj* robust
rocha ['hɔʃa] *f* rock
rochedo [ho'ʃedu] *m* crag; (*escolho*) cliff
rochoso [ho'ʃozu] *adj* craggy
rock [ho'ʃozu] *m* MÚS rock
roda ['hɔda] *f* wheel; (*círculo*), *pessoas*: circle; *saia*: width; (*lotaria*) lottery; *fig* turn; ***à ~ de*** around; ***a quatro ~s*** fourwheel; ***~ dentada*** cogwheel; ***~ de impressão*** print wheel; ***~ sobresselente*** spare wheel
rodada [ho'dada] *f bebidas*: round

rodagem [ho'daʒẽ] *f duma máquina*: cogwheels; ***faixa*** *f* ***de ~*** lane; ***fazer a ~ de*** run in
rodapé [hoda'pɛ] *m* baseboard, *Brit* skirting board; INFORM footer
rodar [ho'daɾ] ⟨1e⟩ **1** *v/t* turn; CINE shoot **2** *v/i* turn; (*rolar*) roll; *carro* run; *tempo* go past
rodear [ho'dʒiaɾ] ⟨1l⟩ surround; (*evitar, contornar*) go around *tb fig*; (*girar à volta*) circle around
rodeio [ho'deiu] *m* detour; (*subterfúgio*) excuse; ***sem ~s*** straight out
rodela [ho'dɛla] *f* slice
rodízio [ho'dʒiziu] *m Bras* GASTR all-you-can-eat; *cadeira*: caster
rodopio [hodo'piu] *m* ***andar num ~*** be in a spin
rodovia [hodo'via] *f* highway, *Brit* motorway
rodoviário [hodo'vjariu] *adj* road *atr*, traffic *atr*; ***empresa*** *f* ***rodoviária*** transport company; ***estação*** *f* ***rodoviária*** bus depot
roedor [hoe'doɾ] *m* rodent
roer [ho'eɾ] ⟨2f⟩ *v/t* gnaw; (*corroer*) corrode, eat away; (*desgastar*) gnaw at *tb fig*; **roer-se** *v/r* be eaten up (***de*** with)
rojão [ho'ʒãw] *m* rocket
rol [hɔw] *m* list; *roupa etc*: label
rolamento [hola'mẽtu] *m* TECN ball bearing
rolante [ho'lãtʃi] *adj* rolling; ***escada*** *f* ***~*** escalator
rolar [ho'laɾ] ⟨1e⟩ roll; *pomba* coo
roldana [how'dana] *f* pulley, block and tackle
roleta [ho'leta] *f* roulette
rolha ['hoʎa] *f* cork
roliço [ho'lisu] *adj* round; *pessoa* chubby
rolo ['holu] *m* roll; (*cilindro*) cylinder; *cabelo*: roller; *corda*: coil; GASTR rolling pin; GASTR ***~ de carne picada*** meatloaf; ***~ de papel higiênico*** toilet roll
Roma ['homa] *f* Rome
romã [ho'mã] *f* pomegranate
romance [ho'mãsi] *m* novel; *relações*: romance; ***~ policial*** detective novel
romancista [homã'sista] *m/f* novelist
romano [ho'manu] **1** *adj* Roman **2** *m*, **-a** *f* Roman
romântico [ho'mãtʃiku] **1** *adj* romantic **2** *m*, **-a** *f* romantic
romantismo [homã'tʃizmu] *m* romanticism
romaria [homa'ria] *f* pilgrimage
rombo ['hõbu] *m* rhombus, (*buraco*) hole
romeiro [ho'mejɾu] *m*, **-a** *f* pilgrim
Romênia, *Port* **Roménia** [ho'menja] *f* Romania
romeno [ho'menu] **1** *adj* Romanian **2** *m*, **-a** *f* Romanian **3** *m lingua* Romanian
romper [hõ'peɾ] ⟨2a⟩ **1** *v/t* break; *vestuário* tear; *silêncio* break; *segredo* give away; *caminho* make **2** *v/i* break out; *dia* break; *estrela* come out; (*surgir*) appear; **romper-se** *v/r* break; (*rebentar*) burst
roncar [hõ'kaɾ] ⟨1a⟩ *v/i* snore; *estômago* rumble
ronco [hõ'ku] *m* snoring
ronda ['hõda] *f* round; *polícia*: beat
rondante [hõ'dãtʃi] *m/f* prowler
rondar [hõ'daɾ] ⟨1a⟩ **1** *v/t* go on one's rounds in; (*vigiar*) patrol; (*circundar*) circle around; *tigre* prowl around **2** *v/i* ***~ em patrulha*** go on patrol; ***~ por $50*** come to around $50
ronronar [hõ'daɾ] *v/i* purr
rosa ['hɔza] **1** *f* BOT, ARQUIT rose; ***~-dos-ventos*** compass **2** *adj* pink
rosado [ho'zadu] *adj* rosy
rosário [ho'zariu] *m* rosary
rosbife [hoz'bifi] *m* roast beef
rosca ['hoska] **1** *f* coil; *parafuso*: thread; GASTR round loaf **2** *m/f* clever dick
roseira [ho'zejɾa] *f* rosebush
roseiral [hozej'ɾaw] *m* rose garden
rosnar [hoʒ'naɾ] ⟨1e⟩ mumble; *esp cão* growl
rosto ['hostu] *m* face
rota ['hɔta] *f* route; NÁUT course
rotação [hota'sãw] *f* rotation
rotar [ho'taɾ] ⟨1e⟩ rotate
rotativo [hota'tʃivu] *adj* rotary
rotatória [hota'tɔɾja] *f Bras* traffic circle, *Brit* roundabout
rotatório [hota'tɔriu] *adj* rotary

roteirista [hotej'rista] *m/f* scriptwriter
roteiro [ho'tejru] *m* (*plano*) streetmap; (*descrição*) itinerary; *filme etc*: script
rotina [ho'tʃina] *f* routine *tb* INFORM
rotineiro [hotʃi'nejru] *adj* routine
roto ['hotu] *adj* broken, bust; *vestuário* torn
rótula ['hɔtula] *f* ANAT kneecap
rotular [hotu'lar] ⟨1a⟩ label *tb fig* (**de** as)
rótulo ['hɔtulu] *m* label
rotunda [ho'tũda] *f Port* traffic circle, *Brit* roundabout; ARQUIT rotunda
roubar [ho'bar] ⟨1a⟩ steal; *pessoa, banco* rob
roubo ['hobu] *m* theft, robbery; ***seguro** m **contra** ~* theft insurance; ***~ de lojas*** shop-lifting
rouco ['hoku] *adj* hoarse
roulotte [ho'lɔtʃi] *f Port* trailer, *Brit* caravan
roupa ['hopa] *f* (*vestuário*) clothes; *suja* laundry, washing; ***estender a ~*** hang out the washing; ***tirar a ~*** undress; ***~ de cama*** bed linen, bedding; ***~ branca, ~ interior, ~ de baixo*** underwear; ***~ espacial*** spacesuit; ***~ esportiva*** sportswear; ***~ de malha*** knitwear; ***~ de mergulho*** wetsuit; ***~ de praia*** beachwear
roupão [ho'pãw] *m* bathrobe
rouquidão [hoki'dãw] *f* hoarseness
rouxinol [hoʃi'nɔw] *m* nightingale
roxo ['hoʃu] **1** *adj* violet **2** *m* violet
rua ['hua] *f* street; ***pôr na ~*** put out on the street; ***na ~*** in the street; ***~ lateral*** side street ***~ de mão única*** one-way street; ***~ principal*** main street
ruazinhas [hua'ziɲas] *fpl* back streets
rubéola [hu'bɛwla] *f* German measles *sg*
rubi [hu'bi] **1** *adj* ruby **2** *m* ruby
rubrica [hu'brika] *f* rubric, heading; (*assinatura*) initials
rubricar [hubri'kar] ⟨1n⟩ initial
rubro ['hubru] *adj* bright red
ruço ['husu] *adj animal* gray, *Brit* grey; (*louro*) blond; (*desbotado*) faded
rúcula ['hukula] *f* rocket
rude ['hudʒi] *adj maneiras* unsophisticated; *cara* harsh; (*bruto*) rough and ready; (*grosseiro*) rude
rudimentar [hudʒimẽ'tar] *adj* rudimentary
rudimento [hudʒi'mẽtu] *m* rudiment; ***~s** pl fig* rudiments
ruga ['huga] *f pele, vestuário*: crease, wrinkle
rúgbi ['hugbi] *m* rugby
ruge ['huʒi] *m* blusher, rouge
rugido [hu'ʒidu] *m* roar
rugir [hu'ʒir] ⟨3n⟩ roar
ruibarbo ['hwidu] *m* rhubarb
ruído ['hwidu] *m* noise
ruidoso [hwi'dozu] *adj* noisy; (*sensacional*) sensational
ruim [hwĩ] *adj* bad; (*inferior*) poor quality
ruína ['hwina] *f* ruin; ECON collapse; ***~s** pl* ruins
ruir [hwir] ⟨3i⟩ collapse, go to ruin
ruivo ['huivu] **1** *adj* red; *pessoa* red-haired **2** *m*, **-a** redhead
rum [hũ] *m* rum
ruminante [humi'nãtʃi] *m* ruminant
ruminar [humi'nar] ⟨1a⟩ ruminate *tb fig*
rumo ['humu] *m* NÁUT course, bearing; *fig* direction; *dos acontecimentos etc*: course; ***sem ~*** adrift; ***mudar de ~*** change course
rumor [hu'mor] *m* noise; *fig* rumor, *Brit* rumour
ruptura [hu'tura] *f* break, rupture; *fig* split
rural [ho'raw] *adj* rural
rush [haʃ] *m Bras* rush hour
Rússia ['husja] *f **a ~*** Russia
russo ['husu] **1** *adj* Russian **2** *m*, **-a** *f* Russian
rústico ['hustʃiku] *adj* rustic; (*primitivo*) simple, primitive

S

s/ *abr* (***sem***) without
S. *abr* (***Sul***) S (south)
S.A. [ɛsjˈa] *f abr* (***sociedade anônima***) Inc, *Brit* plc
sã [sã] → ***são***[2]
sábado [ˈsabadu] *m* Saturday; ***no ~*** on Saturday; ***aos ~s*** on Saturdays
sabão [saˈbãw] *m* soap; ***~ em pó*** soap powder, detergent
sabedor [sabeˈdoɾ] *adj* learned; (*competente*) knowledgeable; ***~ de*** well versed in
sabedoria [sabedoˈɾia] *f* wisdom; (*erudição*) learning
saber [saˈbeɾ] ⟨2r⟩ **1** *v/t* know; *comida etc* ***~ a*** taste of; (***vir a***) ***~*** find out; ***dar a ~, fazer ~*** make it known; ***~ ler / nadar**, etc* be able to read / swim etc, know how to read / swim etc; ***sei lá!*** who knows! **2** *m* knowledge
sabia [saˈbia] *etc*, **sabido** [saˈbidu] *pp* → ***saber***
sabichão [sabiˈʃãw] *m*, **-ona** [sabiˈʃona] *f fam* wiseguy, know-it-all
sábio [ˈsabiu] **1** *adj* wise; (*erudito*) learned **2** *m*, **-a** *f* wise person
sabonete [saboˈnetʃi] *m* soap
saboneteira [saboneˈtejɾa] *f* soap dish
sabor [saˈboɾ] *m* flavor, *Brit* flavour; (*paladar*) taste; ***não tem ~*** it has no taste
saborear [saboˈɾeaɾ] ⟨1l⟩ taste, try; (*apreciar*) enjoy, savor, *Brit* savour
saboroso [saboˈɾozu] *adj* delicious, tasty
sabotador [sabotaˈdoɾ] *m*, **-a** *f* saboteur
sabotagem [saboˈtaʒẽ] *f* sabotage
sabotar [saboˈtaɾ] ⟨1e⟩ sabotage
saca [ˈsaka] *f* sack; ***~ de compras*** shopping bag
sacada [saˈkada] *f Bras* balcony
sacador [sakaˈdoɾ] *m*, **-a** *f* server
sacana [saˈkʌna] *vulg m* son-of-a-bitch, bastard
sacanice [sakaˈnisi] *f pop* ***é uma ~!*** it's a dirty business!
sacar [saˈkaɾ] ⟨1n & 1b⟩ take out; *faca, pistola* pull; *fig proveito* get; *lucro* make; *esp* COM *letra de câmbio* draw up; *tênis*: serve
sacarina [sakaˈɾina] *f* saccharin
saca-rolhas [sakaˈhoʎas] *m* ⟨*pl inv*⟩ corkscrew
sacerdócio [saseɾˈdɔsiu] *m* priesthood
sacerdotal [saseɾdoˈtaw] *adj* priestly
sacerdote [saseɾˈdɔtʃi] *m* priest
sacerdotisa [saseɾdoˈtʃiza] *f* priestess; *atual* priest
saciar [saˈsjaɾ] ⟨1g⟩ *fome* quench; (*satisfazer*) satisfy
saco [ˈsaku] *m* bag; *vulg* balls; *fam* ***um pé no ~*** a pain in the neck; *fam* ***é um ~*** it sucks; ***~ de areia*** sandbag; ***~ de dormir*** sleeping bag; ***~ de mão*** handbag; ***~ de lixo*** garbage bag, *Brit* bin bag; ***~ de plástico*** plastic bag; ***~ de viagem*** travel bag
saco-cama [sakoˈkama] *m* ⟨*pl* sacos-cama⟩ sleeping bag
sacola [saˈkɔla] *f* bag; ***~ de compras*** shopping bag
sacramental [sakɾamẽˈtaw] *adj* sacramental
sacramento [sakɾaˈmẽtu] *m* sacrament; ***últimos ~s*** *pl* final sacraments
sacrificar [sakɾifiˈkaɾ] ⟨1n⟩ sacrifice; *cão etc* put away, *Brit* put down
sacrifício [sakɾiˈfisiu] *m* sacrifice; ***fazer ~s*** make sacrifices
sacrilégio [sakɾiˈlɛʒiu] *m* sacrilege
sacrílego [saˈkɾilegu] *adj* sacrilegious
sacristão [sakɾisˈtãw] *m* ⟨*pl* -ães, -ãos⟩ sacristan
sacristia [sakɾisˈtʃia] *f* sacristy
sacro [ˈsakɾu] **1** *adj* (*sagrado*) sacred, holy; ARTE sacred; ***música** f **sacra*** church music **2** *m* ANAT sacrum

sacudir [saku'dʒiɾ] ⟨3h⟩ shake; *pó* shake off; *ombros* shrug
sádico ['sadʒiku] **1** *m*, **-a** *f* sadist **2** *adj* sadistic
sadio [sa'dʒiu] *adj* healthy
sadismo [sa'dʒizmu] *m* sadism
safado [sa'fadu] **1** *adj* (*gasto*) worn out; (*vil*) mean; (*desavergonhado*) shameless **2** *m* rogue
safanão [safa'nãw] *m* tug
safar [sa'faɾ] *v/t* (*libertar*) free; (*salvar*) save; (*desgastar*) wear out; **safar-se** *v/r fam* save one's skin
safira [sa'fiɾa] *f* sapphire
sagacidade [sagasi'dadʒi] *f* (*perspicácia*) shrewdness
sagaz [sa'gas] *adj* shrewd
sagitário [saʒi'taɾiu] *m* ASTROL Sagittarius
sagrado [sa'gɾadu] *adj* holy; (*inviolável*) sacred
saguão [sa'gwãw] *m* (*pátio*) (court)-yard; *hotel*: lobby
saí [sa'i], **saia** ['saja] *etc* → ***sair***
saia ['saja] *f* skirt
saia-calça [saja'kawsa] *f* ⟨*pl* saias--calças⟩ culottes *pl*
saída [sa'ida] *f* exit; (*partida*) departure; *cano*: outlet; TEAT exit; COM outgoings; *fig* way out; (*piada*) witticism; ***estar de ~*** be on one's way out; ***vôo de ~***, *Port* ***voo de ~*** outgoing flight; *hotel*: ***hora de ~*** checkout time; ***~ de ar*** air vent; ***~ de emergência*** emergency exit; ESP ***pontapé*** *m* ***de ~*** kickoff
saído [sa'idu] *pp* → ***sair***
saiote [sa'jɔtʃi] *m* underskirt
sair [sa'iɾ] ⟨3l⟩ *v/i* come out; *da casa* go out; (*ir embora*) go away; TEAT exit; (*partir*) leave; (*mudar de casa*) move out; NÁUT, FERROV leave; AERO leave, take off (***de*** from); *livro* come out; *mancha* come out; ARQUIT jut out; INFORM quit, exit; (*deixar*) ***~ de*** leave; ***sai do meu caminho*** get out of my way; ***~ com alguém*** go out with s.o.; ***~ de moda*** go out of style; ***~ do trabalho*** leave work; **sair-se** *v/r* ***~ mal*** misfire, go wrong
saíste [sa'istʃi], **saiu** [sa'iu] *etc* → ***sair***
sal [saw] *m* salt; ***sem ~*** unsalted; *fig* dull
sala ['sala] *f grande* hall; *duma casa* room; ***~ de aula*** classroom; *Bras* ***~ de bate-papo*** chatroom; ***~ de conferência*** conference room; ***~ do conselho*** boardroom; ***~ de embarque*** departure lounge; ***~ de espera*** waiting room; ***~ de estar*** living room, lounge; ***~ de jantar*** dining room; ***~ de operações*** operating room, *Brit* operating theatre; ***~ do tribunal*** courtroom
salada [sa'lada] *f* salad; *fig* mess; ***~ de frutas*** fruit salad; ***~ mista*** mixed salad; ***~ russa*** Russian salad
saladeira [sala'dejɾa] *f* salad bowl
salamandra [sala'mãdɾa] *f* salamander
salame [sa'lami] *m* salami
salão [sa'lãw] *m* (big) room; ESP hall; ***futebol*** *m* ***de ~*** indoor soccer, *Brit* indoor football; ***~ de beleza*** beauty salon; ***~ de bilhar*** pool hall; ***~ de chá*** tearoom; ***~ de dança*** dance hall; ***~ de massagem*** massage parlor, *Brit* massage parlour; ***~ de jogo*** slot machine arcade; *em casa* games room
salarial [sala'ɾjaw] *adj* salary *atr*; ***grupo*** *m* ***~*** salary group, salary bracket
salário [sa'laɾiu] *m* salary, pay; ***~ mínimo*** minimum wage; ***~ líquido*** takehome pay; ***~ por peça*** (*ou* ***tarefa***) piecework rate
saldar [saw'daɾ] ⟨1a⟩ settle; *dívida* pay off, settle; ***~ contas*** settle (up) *tb fig*
saldo ['sawdu] *m* COM, FIN balance; *mercadoria*: surplus; ***~s*** *pl* sales; ***~ credor*** credit balance; ***~ positivo*** positive balance; COM surplus; ***~ negativo*** negative balance; COM shortfall
salgado [saw'gadu] **1** *adj* salted, salty; *comida* savory, *Brit* savoury; *fig* (*caro*) steep **2** GASTR ***~s*** *mpl pastries filled with meat or fish*
salgar [saw'gaɾ] ⟨1o⟩ salt; (*pôr demasiado sal*) put too much salt in
saliência [sa'ljẽsja] *f* projection
salientar [saljẽ'taɾ] ⟨1a⟩ point up, emphasize; **salientar-se** *v/r* stand out

saliente [sa'ljẽtʃi] *adj* prominent; (*excelente*) outstanding
saliva [sa'liva] *f* saliva; ***gastar ~*** *fam* waste one's breath
salivar [sali'var] ⟨1a⟩ *v/i* salivate
salmão [saw'mãw] *m* salmon; ***~ fumado*** smoked salmon
salmonelas [sawmo'nɛlas] *fpl* salmonella
salobre [sa'lobri] *adj*, **salobro** [sa'lobru] *adj* brackish
salpicão [sawpi'kãw] *m* pork sausage
salpicar [sawpi'kar] ⟨1n⟩ spray; (*polvilhar*) sprinkle
salsa ['sawsa] *f* BOT parsley (***música*** *f*) ~ salsa
salsicha [saw'siʃa] *f* sausage
salsichão [sawsi'ʃãw] *m* thick sausage
salsicharia [sawsiʃa'ria] *f* sausage factory; (*charcutaria*) delicatessen
saltada [saw'tada] *f* jump, leap; *fig* excursion; ***dar uma ~*** go on an excursion (***a*** to)
saltar [saw'tar] ⟨1a⟩ **1** *v/i* jump; (*pular*) hop; ***~ do ônibus*** get off the bus; ***~ aos olhos***, ***~ à vista*** be very obvious **2** *v/t* jump over
saltear [saw'tʃiar] *v/t* GASTR sauté
saltitar [sawtʃi'tar] ⟨1a⟩ jump around; ***ele anda a ~ de emprego em emprego*** he's always changing jobs
salto ['sawtu] *m* jump, leap; (*queda*) fall; *sapato*: heel; ***~ acrobático*** high diving; ***~ em altura*** high jump; ***~ em comprimento*** broad jump, *Brit* long jump; ***~ em distância*** broad jump, *Brit* long jump; ***~ com vara*** pole vault
salubre [sa'lubri] *adj* healthy
salutar [salu'tar] *adj* salutary
salva[1] ['sawva] *f* MIL salvo, volley; ***~ de palmas*** round of applause
salva[2] ['sawva] *f* tray
salva[3] ['sawva] *f* BOT sage
salvação [sawva'sãw] *f* salvation; ***exército*** *m* ***de ~*** Salvation Army
salvador [sawva'dor] *m* savior, *Brit* saviour; *fam* ***~ do mundo*** do-gooder
salvaguarda [sawva'gwarda] *f* safeguard; (*salvo-conduto*) safe-conduct; (*cautela*) precaution
salvaguardar [sawvagwar'dar] ⟨1b⟩ safeguard
salvamento [sawva'mẽtu] *m* rescue; *náufragos*: salvage
salvar [saw'var] ⟨1a⟩ **1** *v/t* save; (*resgatar*) rescue; (*proteger*) protect **2** *v/i* MIL fire a volley
salva-vidas [sawva'vidas] *m* ⟨*pl inv*⟩ *barco*: lifeboat; *cinto*: lifebelt; *bóia*: lifebuoy; *pessoa* lifeguard; ***colete*** *m* ~ life jacket
sálvia ['sawvja] *f* → ***salva***[3]
salvo ['sawvu] **1** *adj* safe **2** *prep* save, except; ***~ imprevistos*** barring accidents
salvo-conduto [sawvokõ'dutu] *m* safe-conduct
samambaia [samã'baja] *f Bras* fern
samba ['sãba] *m* samba
sambar [sã'bar] ⟨1a⟩ *v/i* samba, do the samba
sanar [sa'nar] ⟨1a⟩ → ***sarar***
sanatório [sana'tɔriu] sanatarium, *Brit* sanatorium
sanção [sã'sãw] *f* sanction; *de lei etc*: ratification; (*reconhecimento*) recognition; (*castigo*) sanction; ***sanções*** *pl* sanctions
sancionar [sãsjo'nar] ⟨1f⟩ sanction *lei* ratify; (*reconhecer*) recognize
sandália [sã'dalia] *f* sandal
sândalo ['sãdalu] *m* sandalwood
sande(s) ['sãdʒi(s)] *f Port* sandwich
sanduíche [sã'dwiʃi] *f Bras* sandwich; ***~ de queijo*** cheese sandwich
saneamento [sanja'mẽtu] *m* sanitation; (*canalização*) draining; POL, *bairro*: clean-up
sanear [sa'njar] ⟨1l⟩ *habitação* make habitable; (*canalizar*) drain; POL, *bairro* clean up
sangrar [sã'grar] ⟨1a⟩ *v/t & v/i* bleed
sangrento [sã'grẽtu] *adj* bloody
sangria [sã'gria] *f* MED blood letting; *perda*: bloodshed: *bebida* sangria
sangue ['sãgi] *m* blood; ***deitar ~*** bleed; ***retirar ~ a alguém*** take blood from s.o.
sangue-frio [sãge'friu] *m* ⟨*sem pl*⟩ cold-bloodedness; ***a ~*** in cold blood; MED without anesthetic
sanguessuga [sãge'suga] **1** *f* ZOOL

leech **2** *m/f fig* bloodsucker
sanguinário [sãg(w)i'nariu] *adj* bloodthirsty
sanguíneo [sã'g(w)iniu] *adj* blood *atr*; *cor*: blood-red; ***grupo*** *m* ~ blood group
sanita [sa'nita] *f* toilet
sanitário [sani'tariu] *adj* sanitary; ***instalações*** *fpl* ***sanitárias*** sanitary installations; ~ ***feminino*** ladies' room; ~ ***masculino*** men's room
santa ['sãta] *f* saint
santidade [sãʧi'dadʒi] *f* sanctity
santificar [sãʧifi'kaɾ] ⟨1n⟩ sanctify
santo ['sãtu] **1** *adj* holy; (*bondoso*) saintly; *pop meio* certain; ***todo o ~ dia*** all day long **2** *m* saint; ***Todos os Santos*** All Saints; ~ ***padroeiro*** patron saint
santuário [sã'twariu] *m* sanctuary
São [sãw] (+ *nome começado por consoante*) Saint
são[1] [sãw], *f* **sã** [sã] ⟨*mpl* sãos⟩ *adj* healthy; (*inteiro*) all in one piece; ~ ***e salvo*** safe and sound
são[2] [sãw] → ***ser***
sapataria [sapata'ɾia] *f* shoestore, *Brit* shoeshop
sapateado [sapa'ʧiadu] *m* tapdance
sapateiro [sapa'tejɾu] *m* shoemaker; *que conserta* shoe mender; *vendedor*: shoe seller
sapatilha [sapa'ʧiʎa] *f ballet*: ballet shoe
sapato [sa'patu] *m* shoe; ~ ***de tênis*** sneaker, *Brit* trainer
sapiência [sa'pjẽsja] *f* wisdom
sapo ['sapu] *m* toad
saque ['saki] *m* COM draft; (*pilhagem*) pillage; *tênis*: serve; ***meter*** (*ou* ***pôr***) ***a ~*** pillage
saqueador [sakja'doɾ] *m* pillager, looter
saquear [sa'kjaɾ] ⟨1l⟩ pillage, loot
saqueio [sa'keiu] *m* pillaging, looting
saquinho [sa'kiɲu] *m* (little) bag; ~ ***de chá*** teabag
saraiva [sa'ɾajva] *f*, **~da** [saɾaj'vada] *f* METEO, *fig* hail
sarampo [sa'ɾãpu] *m* MED measles *sg*
sarar [sa'ɾaɾ] ⟨1b⟩ **1** *v/t* heal **2** *v/i* get better
sarau [sa'ɾaw] *m* soirée; ~ ***musical / de arte*** musical / artistic evening
sarça ['saɾsa] *f* thornbush
sarcasmo [saɾ'kazmu] *m* sarcasm
sarcástico [saɾ'kasʧiku] *adj* sarcastic
sarcófago [saɾ'kɔfagu] *m* sarcophagus
sarda ['saɾda] *f* freckle
sardento [saɾ'dẽtu] *adj* freckled
sardinha [saɾ'dʒiɲa] *f* sardine; ~ ***de conserva*** canned sardines
sardônico, *Port* **sardónico** [saɾ'doniku] *adj* ***riso*** *m* ~ sardonic laugh
sargaço [saɾ'gasu] *m* seaweed
sargento [saɾ'ʒẽtu] *m* sergeant
sarjeta [saɾ'ʒeta] *f* gutter
S.A.R.L. [ɛsjaɛ'hiɛli] *f* (***sociedade de responsabilidade limitada***) Inc, *Brit* Ltd
sarna ['saɾna] *f* MED scabies *sg*
sarro ['sahu] *m* tartar
sasonal [sazo'naw] *adj* seasonal
sasonalmente [sazo'nawmẽʧi] *adv* ***ajustado*** ~ seasonally adjusted
Satanás [sata'nas] *m* Satan
satânico [sa'tʌniku] *adj* satanic
satélite [sa'tɛliʧi] *m* satellite; ~ ***de comunicações*** communications satellite
sátira ['saʧiɾa] *f* satire
satírico [sa'ʧiɾiku] **1** *adj* satirical **2** *m*, **-a** *f* satirist
satirista [saʧi'ɾista] *m/f* satirist
satisfação [saʧisfa'sãw] *f* satisfaction; ***pedir satisfações a alguém*** demand an explanation from s.o.; ***está tudo à sua ~?*** is everything to your satisfaction?
satisfatório [saʧisfa'tɔɾiu] *adj* satisfactory
satisfazer [saʧisfa'zeɾ] ⟨2v⟩ satisfy; *dívida* pay off; *condição etc* meet, satisfy; *sede* quench, satisfy; *dúvida* answer; ~ ***a alguém*** satisfy s.o.
satisfeito [saʧis'fejtu] *adj* satisfied
saturação [satuɾa'sãw] *f* saturation
saturar [satu'ɾaɾ] ⟨1a⟩ saturate
saudação [sawda'sãw] *f* greeting; ***saudações cordiais*** best wishes
saudade [saw'dadʒi] *f* longing; (*recordação*) nostalgia; ***~s*** *pl* best wishes; ***ter*** (*ou* ***sentir***) ***~s de*** long for

saudar [saw'daɾ] ⟨1q⟩ greet; (*aclamar*) acclaim; (*felicitar*) congratulate
saudável [saw'davew] *adj* healthy; ***pouco ~*** unhealthy
saúde [sa'udʒi] *f* health; (*brinde*) toast; ***atestado*** *m* ***de ~*** health certificate; ***fazer ~*** toast; ***à sua ~!*** your health!; ***~!*** cheers!; *espirro*: bless you!
sauna ['sawna] *f* sauna
saxofone [sakso'foni] *m* saxophone, sax
sazão [sa'zãw] *f* season
sazonal [sazo'naw] *adj* seasonal
sazonar [sazo'naɾ] *v/t & v/i* mature
scanear [ska'njaɾ] ⟨1l⟩ *v/t* INFORM scan
scâner ['skʌneɾ] *m*, **scanner** ['skʌneɾ] *m* scanner
scooter ['skutɛɾ] *f* (motor)scooter
se[1] [si] *pron* ◊ *reflexivo*: *ele*: himself; *ela*: herself; *coisa*, *animal*: itself; *você*: yourself; *eles*, *elas*: themselves; *vocês*: yourselves; *impessoal*: oneself; ***ela machucou-~*** she hurt herself; ***apresse-se*** hurry up!
◊ *recíproco*: each other, one another; ***eles não ~ parecem em nada*** they don't look at all like each other
◊ ***precisa-se ...*** we are looking for ...; ***vende-se*** for sale
se[2] [si] *conj* if; *pergunta indireta*: whether; ***~ o conheço!*** do I know him!; ***~ assim for*** if that is the case; ***~ bem que*** although
sé [sɛ] *f* REL cathedral; ***a Santa Sé*** the Holy See
sê [se] → ***ser***
sebe ['sɛbi] *f* hedge; (*muro*) fence
seca ['seka] *f* drought; *fam* ***estou a apanhar uma ~*** I'll be waiting here until the cows come home
secador [seka'doɾ] *m* dryer; ***~ de cabelo*** hair dryer
seção [se'sãw] *f* section
secar [se'kaɾ] ⟨1n & 1c⟩ **1** *v/t* dry **2** *v/i* dry; (*murchar*) dry up; *planta* wither; ***ficar a ~*** wait for an eternity
secção *Port* → ***seção***
seco ['seku] *adj* dry *tb vinho*; *fruta* dried; *planta* withered; (*magro*) thin, gaunt; ***ama*** *f* ***seca*** nanny; ***estou a ~*** I'm as dry as a bone; NÁUT ***dar*** (*ou* ***ficar***) ***em ~*** run aground; *fig fam* go wrong; ***limpeza*** *f* ***a ~*** dry cleaning
secreção [sekɾe'sãw] *f* secretion
secretaria [sekɾeta'ɾia] *f* office; POL department; ***~ eletrônica*** voicemail, answering machine
secretária [sekɾe'taɾja] *f* secretary; *móvel*: writing desk
secretário [sekɾe'taɾiu] *m* secretary
secreto [se'kɾɛtu] *adj* secret; ***serviço*** *m* ***~*** secret service
sectário [sek'taɾiu] *m*, **-a** *f* follower
sectarismo [sekta'ɾizmu] *m* sectarianism
sector *Port* → ***setor***
secular [seku'laɾ] *adj* centuries-old; REL secular
século ['sɛkulu] *m* century; (*era*) age; *fam* ***~s*** *pl* ages
secundário [sekũ'daɾiu] *adj* secondary; ***escola*** *f* ***secundária*** secondary school
seda ['seda] *f* silk
sedã [se'dã] *m* sedan, *Brit* saloon
sedativo [seda'tʃivu] **1** *adj* sedative **2** *m* sedative
sede[1] ['sedʒi] *f* thirst; ***estar com ~*** be thirsty
sede[2] ['sɛdʒi] *f* headquarters; *governo*: seat; *empresa* head office
sedentário [sedẽ'taɾiu] *adj* sedentary; ***vida*** *f* ***sedentária*** sedentary lifestyle
sedento [se'dẽtu] *adj* thirsty; (*ávido*) ***~ de*** thirsty for
sediar [sedʒi'aɾ] ⟨1g⟩ *v/t* host
sedimentar [sedʒimẽ'taɾ] ⟨1a⟩ silt up
sedimento [sedʒi'mẽtu] *m* sediment
sedoso [se'dozu] *adj* silky
sedução [sedu'sãw] *f* seduction
sedutor [sedu'toɾ] **1** *adj* seductive **2** *m*, **-a** *f* seducer
seduzir [sedu'ziɾ] ⟨3m⟩ seduce
segmento [seg'mẽtu] *m* segment
segredar [segɾe'daɾ] *v/i* whisper
segredo [se'gɾedu] *m* secret; (*sigilo*) secrecy; ***em ~*** in secret
segregação [segɾega'sãw] *f* segregation; ANAT secretion; ***~ racial*** racial segregation
segregar [segɾe'gaɾ] ⟨1o & 1c⟩ segregate; ANAT secrete
seguida [se'gida] *f* ***em ~*** next; ***5 dias***

S

em ~ 5 days in a row; ***trabalhar 6 horas de*** ~ work 6 hours without a break
seguido [se'gidu] *adj* following; (*ininterrupto*) consecutive; ***três horas -as*** three hours in a row, three consecutive hours
seguidor [segi'dor] *m*, **-a** *f* (*adepto*) follower
seguimento [segi'mẽtu] *m* following *tb fig*; (*perseguição*) persecution; (*continuação*) continuation; (*sequência*) sequence
seguinte [se'gĩʧi] *adj* following, next; ***o*** ~ the following
seguir [se'gir] ⟨3o & 3c⟩ **1** *v/t algo, exemplo, direção* follow; (*continuar*) continue; *curso* go to **2** *v/i* follow; (*continuar*) carry on; ***segue*** to be continued; ~ ***adiante*** push ahead, ~ ***destemido*** carry on undaunted; ~ ***em frente*** go straight ahead; ~ ***reto*** carry straight on; **seguir-se** *v/r* follow; ~ ***a*** follow on from; ~ ***de*** follow from
segunda-feira [segũda'fejra] *f* ⟨*pl* segundas-feiras⟩ Monday; ***na*** ~ on Monday; ***às ~s*** on Mondays
segundo [se'gũdu] **1** *adj* second; ~ ***prato*** *m* main course; ***em segunda mão*** secondhand; ***sem*** ~ unparalleled; ***não ter*** ~ be unique **2** *m* (*tempo*) second **3** *adv* secondly **4** *prep* according to
segurado [segu'radu] *m*, **-a** *f* insured; ***cartão*** *m* ***de*** ~ insurance card
segurador [segura'dor] **1** *adj* insurance *atr*; ***empresa*** *f* ~ ***a*** insurance company **2** *m*, **-a** *f empresa*: insurer
segurança [segu'rãsa] **1** *f* security; *inexistência de perigo* safety; (*certeza*) certainty; (*garantia*) guarantee; ***para*** ~ as a security measure; ***com*** ~ with certainty; (*sem perigo*) in safety; ~ ***do trânsito*** road safety; ~ ***social*** social security **2** *m* security guard; *bar*: bouncer
segurar [segu'rar] ⟨1a⟩ secure; (*pegar*) hold; COM insure
seguro [se'guru] **1** *adj* safe; (*certo*) certain; (*firme*) secure; (*de confiança*) reliable; ~ ***de si*** self-assured **2** *m* COM insurance; ~ ***contra todos os riscos*** all risks insurance, *Brit* comprehensive insurance; ~ ***parcial do veículo*** third-party insurance; ~ ***de saúde*** (*ou* ***médico***) health insurance; ~ ***social*** social insurance; ~ ***de viagem*** travel insurance; ~ ***de vida*** life insurance; ***companhia*** *f* ***de ~s*** insurance company
sei [sej] → ***saber***
seio ['seiu] *m* (*peito*) breast, bosom; *fig* heart
seis [sejs] *num* six
seiscentos [sejs'sẽtus] *num* six hundred
seita ['sejta] *f* sect
seiva ['sejva] *f* sap; *fig* vitality
seivoso [sej'vozu] *adj* full of vitality
seixo ['sejʃu] *m* pebble
seja ['seʒa] *etc* → ***ser***
sela ['sɛla] *f* saddle
selar [se'lar] ⟨1c⟩ seal; (*carimbar*) stamp, frank; *cavalo* saddle up
seleção, *Port* **selecção** [sele'sãw] *f* selection; ESP team; ~ ***nacional*** national team
selecionar, *Port* **seleccionar** [selesjo'nar] *v/t* select, choose
select... *Port* → ***selet...***
seletivo [selɛ'ʧivu] *adj* selective
seleto [se'lɛtu] *adj* select
self-service [sɛlf'sɛrvis] *m* ⟨*sem pl*⟩ self-service; ***restaurante*** *m* ~ self-service restaurant
selim [se'lĩ] *m* saddle
selo ['selu] *m* seal *tb fig*; (*carimbo*) stamp *tb fig*; ~ ***fiscal*** revenue stamp; ~ ***postal*** (postage) stamp
selva ['sɛlva] *f* jungle
selvagem [sew'vaʒẽ] **1** *adj* wild; (*feroz*) savage; (*bruto*) coarse **2** *m/f* savage
sem [sẽ] *prep* without; ~ ***chapéu*** without a hat; ~ ***filhos*** childless; ~ ***fôlego*** breathless; ~ ***perguntar / parar*** without asking / stopping; ~ ***que ele veja*** (*subj*) without him seeing
semáforo [se'mafuru] *m* traffic light, *Brit* traffic lights
semana [se'mana] *f* week; ***Semana Santa*** Holy Week
semanal [sema'naw] *adj* weekly

semanário [sema'nariu] **1** *m* weekly **2** *adj* → ***semanal***
semântica [se'mãtʃika] *f* semantics
semântico [se'mãtʃiku] *adj* semantic
semblante [sẽ'blãtʃi] *m* face, (*aparência*) appearance
semear [se'mjar] ⟨1l⟩ sow; (*espargir*) scatter; (*espalhar*) spread
semelhança [seme'ʎãsa] *f* resemblance, similarity; ***à ~ de*** like
semelhante [seme'ʎãtʃi] **1** *adj* similar **2** *m* ***o meu ~, meus ~s*** my fellow men
sêmen ['semẽ] *m* semen
semente [se'mẽtʃi] *f* seed *tb fig*
semestral [semes'traw] *adj* half-yearly
semestre [se'mɛstri] *m* half year; UNIV semester, *Brit* term; ***férias*** *pl* ***de ~*** vacation
sem-fim [sẽ'fĩ] *m* ***um ~ de tarefas*** an endless list of tasks
semi... [semi] semi...
semiaberto [semia'bɛrtu] *adj* half-open
semicírculo [semi'sirkulu] *m* semicircle
semicondutor [semikõdu'tor] *m* ELÉT semiconductor
semifinal [semifi'naw] *f* semifinal
semi-internato [semiĩter'natu] *m* day school
seminário [semi'nariu] *m* UNIV seminar; REL seminary
sem-par [sẽ'par] *adj* unique, unparalleled
sempre ['sẽpri] *adv* always; (*ainda*) still; ***ele ~ foi à praia?*** did he still go to the beach?; ***~ que*** (*subj*) whenever; ***para ~*** forever; ***nem ~*** not always; ***~ em frente*** straight on; ***o de ~, por favor*** the usual, please; ***está ~ chovendo aqui*** it's always *ou* forever raining here
sem-teto [sẽ'tɛtu] *mpl* streetpeople *pl*
senado [se'nadu] *m* senate
senador [sena'dor] *m*, **-a** *f* senator
senão [se'nãw] **1** *conj* otherwise **2** *prep* except, but **3** *m* but
senda ['sẽda] *f* path
senha ['seɲa] *f* sign; *palavra*: password; *cartão de crédito*: PIN (number); (*recibo*) receipt; (*cautela*) ticket
senhor [se'ɲor] *m* man, gentleman; (*proprietário*) owner; *tratamento cortês*: ***o ~*** you; ***o Senhor*** REL the Lord; ***sim senhor*** yes sir; ***~!*** sir!; ***~ Silva*** Mr Silva
senhora [se'ɲora] *f* lady; (*proprietária*) owner; *tratamento cortês*: ***a ~*** you; ***sim ~*** yes ma'am; ***~!*** ma'am!; ***~ Silva*** Mrs Silva
senhoria [seɲo'ria] *f* (*proprietária*) landlady
senhoril [seɲo'riw] *adj* distinguished
senhorio [seɲo'riu] *m* landlord
senhorita [seɲo'rita] *f* young lady; ***~!*** miss; ***~ Silva*** Miss Silva
senil [se'niw] *adj* senile
senilidade [senili'dadʒi] *f* senility
sênior, *Port* **sénior** ['senjɔr] ⟨*pl* seniores⟩ **1** *adj* senior **2** *m* ESP senior
sensação [sẽsa'sãw] *f* sensation, feeling; (*espetáculo*) sensation; ***de ~*** sensational; ***fazer ~*** cause a sensation
sensacional [sẽsasjo'naw] *adj* sensational
sensacionalismo [sẽsasjona'lizmu] *m* sensationalism
sensacionalista [sẽsasjona'lista] *adj* sensationalist
sensatez [sẽsa'tes] *f* good sense, sensibleness
sensato [sẽ'satu] *adj* sensible
sensibilidade [sẽsibili'dadʒi] *f* sensitivity
sensibilizar [sẽsibili'zar] ⟨1a⟩ move; (*alertar*) sensitize (***para*** to); **sensibilizar-se** *v/r* be moved
sensitivo [sẽsi'tʃivu] *adj* sensory; ***~ ao movimento*** sensitive to movement
sensível [sẽ'sivew] *adj* sensitive; (*perceptível*) perceptible
sensivelmente [sẽsivew'mẽtʃi] *adv* perceptibly; (*aproximadamente*) roughly
senso ['sẽsu] *m* sense; ***bom ~, ~ comum*** common sense
sensorial [sẽso'rjaw] *adj* sensory
sensual [sẽ'swaw] *adj* sensual
sensualidade [sẽswali'dadʒi] *f* sensuality
sentar-se [sẽ'tarsi] ⟨1a⟩ *v/r* sit down; ***~ direito*** sit (up) straight

sentença [sẽ'tẽsa] *f* sentence; ***proferir / proclamar a ~*** pass sentence
sentenciar [sẽtẽ'sjar] *v/t* sentence
sentido [sẽ'ʧidu] **1** *adj* sensitive; *dor, pena* deeply felt; (*ofendido*) hurt **2** *m* sense; (*significado*) meaning, sense; (*intenção*) intention; *movimento*: direction; ***os ~s*** the senses; ***no ~ dos ponteiros do relógio*** clockwise; *rua*: ***~ proibido*** no entrance; ***rua f de ~ único*** oneway street; ***não faz ~*** it doesn't make sense
sentimental [sẽʧimẽ'taw] *adj* sentimental; ***vida ~*** love life
sentimentalismo [sẽʧimẽta'lizmu] *m* sentimentality
sentimento [sẽʧi'mẽtu] *m* feeling, sentiment; ***~s*** *pl* (*pêsames*) condolences
sentinela [sẽʧi'nɛla] *f* sentry, guard
sentir [sẽ'ʧir] ⟨3e⟩ *v/t* feel; (*lamentar*) regret; (*levar a mal*) take amiss, be hurt by; ***sinto muito*** I'm very sorry; ***~ falta de*** miss; ***~ satisfação em algo*** get satisfaction out of sth; **sentir-se** *v/r* feel; ***~ fora de lugar*** feel out of place
separação [separa'sãw] *f* separation
separadamente [separada'mẽʧi] *adv* separately
separado [sepa'radu] *adj* separate; *mulher etc* separated
separar [sepa'rar] ⟨1b⟩ separate; ***~ algo de algo*** separate sth from sth; **separar-se** *v/r* separate, split
séptico ['sɛpʧiku] *adj* septic
sepulcro [se'puwkru] *m* tomb
sepultar [sepuw'tar] ⟨1a⟩ bury *tb fig*
sepultura [sepuw'tura] *f* burial; (*túmulo*) grave
sequência [se'kwẽsja] *f* sequence; (*seguimento*) continuation; ***~ de filme*** footage
sequer [se'kɛr] *adv* ***nem ~*** not even; ***sem ~*** without even
sequestração [sekestra'sãw] *f* seizure; *pessoas*: kidnapping
sequestrador [sekestra'dor] *m*, **-a** *f* kidnapper; *ônibus*: hijacker
sequestrar [sekes'trar] ⟨1c⟩ seize; *pessoa* kidnap; *ônibus* hijack
sequioso [se'kjozu] *adj* thirsty; (*seco*) dry
séquito ['sɛkitu] *m* retinue
ser [ser] ⟨2w⟩ **1** *v/i* be; (*ter lugar*) take place; ***~ de*** *origem*: be from; *propriedade*: ***~ de alguém*** belong to s.o.; ***quanto é?*** how much is it?; ***ser por algo*** be for sth; ***isto é*** that is; ***seja como for*** be that as it may; ***não é?*** isn't it?; ***pois é*** that's it **2** *v/aux passivo*: be; ***ser ~ de*** be accused of **3** *m* being; ***~ (vivo)*** being; ***~ humano*** human being
serão [se'rãw] *m trabalho*: night work; ***fazer ~*** work overtime
sereia [se'reja] *f* siren; NÁUT foghorn
serenar [sere'nar] ⟨1d⟩ (*acalmar-se*) calm down
serenata [sere'nata] *f* serenade
serenidade [sereni'dadʒi] *f* (*calma*) serenity
sereno [se'renu] *adj* (*calmo*) calm, serene
série ['sɛri] *f* series *sg*; EDUC grade, *Brit* year; ***produção f em ~*** mass production; ***fora da ~*** outstanding, amazing
seriedade [serie'dadʒi] *f* seriousness; (*retidão*) uprightness
seringa [se'rĩga] *f* syringe; ***~ descartável*** disposable syringe
sério ['sɛriu] **1** *adj* serious; (*reto*) trustworthy; (*de confiança*) reliable **2** *adv* ***a ~*** seriously; ***levar a ~*** take seriously **3** *m* seriousness
sermão [ser'mãw] *m* sermon
seronegativo [sɛronega'ʧivu] *adj* HIV-negative
seropositivo [sɛropozi'ʧivu] *adj* HIV-positive
serpente [ser'pẽʧi] *f* snake
serpentear [serpẽ'ʧiar] ⟨1l⟩ twist, wind
serpentina [serpẽ'ʧina] *f carnaval*: streamer
serra ['sɛha] *f* saw; GEOG mountain range; *montanha*: mountain; ***na ~*** in the mountains; ***~ circular*** circular saw; ***~ contínua, ~ de fita*** band saw
serração [seha'sãw] *f* → ***serraria***
serradura [seha'dura] *f* sawdust
serralheiro [seha'ʎejru] *m*, **-a** *f* locksmith

serrar [se'haɾ] ⟨1c⟩ saw; *separar* saw off
serraria [seha'ɾia] *f* sawmill; (*armação*) sawhorse
servente [seɾ'vẽtʃi] *m/f* servant
Sérvia ['sɛɾvja] *f* Serbia
serviçal [seɾvi'saw] **1** *adj* (*prestável*) helpful **2** *m/f* servant
serviço [seɾ'visu] *m* service; ***estar de ~*** be on duty; ***~ completo*** full service; ***~ doméstico*** domestic work; ***~ incluído*** service included; ***~ militar obrigatório*** (compulsory) military service; ***~ de quartos*** room service; ***~ de segurança*** security service; ***~s** pl **secretos*** sercret service; ***~s** pl **sociais*** social services; ***estação** f **de ~*** service station
servidão [seɾvi'dãw] *f* servitude
servidor [seɾvi'doɾ] *m* server
servil [seɾ'viw] *adj* servile
servilismo [seɾvi'lizmu] *m* servility
servir [seɾ'viɾ] ⟨3c⟩ **1** *v/t refeição* serve **2** *v/i* MIL serve; (*aproveitar*) be useful; *roupa*: fit; ***~ alguém*** serve s.o.; (*auxiliar*) help s.o.; **servir-se** *v/r* ***~ de*** make use of; *da comida etc*: help oneself to
servo ['sɛɾvu] **1** *m*, **-a** *f* servant, (*escravo*) slave **2** *adj* servile
sessão [se'sãw] *f* session; (*negociação*) negotiation; *cinema*: performance
sessenta [se'sẽta] *num* sixty
sesta ['sɛsta] *f* siesta
seta ['sɛta] *f* arrow
sete ['sɛtʃi] *num* seven
setecentista [sɛtʃisẽ'tʃista] *adj* 18th century
setecentos [sɛtʃi'sẽtus] *num* seven hundred
setembro [se'tẽbɾu] *m* September; ***em ~*** in September
setenta [se'tẽta] *num* seventy
setentrional [setẽtɾio'naw] **1** *adj* northern **2** *m/f* northerner
sétima ['sɛtʃima] *f* MÚS seventh
sétimo ['sɛtʃimu] **1** *adj* seventh **2** *m* seventh
setor [se'toɾ] *m* sector
seu [sew], **sua** ['sua] **1** *adj* (*dele*) his; (*dela*) her; *coisa*: its; (*deles*) their; (*de vôce*) your; ***seu idiota!*** you idiot! **2** *pron* (*dele*) his; (*dela*) hers; *coisa*: its; (*deles*) theirs; (*de vôce*) yours; *fig* ***uma das suas*** typical of him / her
severidade [seveɾi'dadʒi] *f* severity; (*precisão*) strictness
severo [se'vɛɾu] *adj* severe; (*exato*) strict
sevícia [se'visja] *f* abuse
sexagenário [seksaʒe'naɾiu] **1** *adj* sixty year-old **2** *m*, **-a** *f* sixty year-old
sexagésimo [seksa'ʒɛzimu] *adj* sixtieth
sexista [sek'sista] **1** *adj* sexist **2** *m*, **-a** *f* sexist
sexo ['sɛksu] *m* sex
sexta ['sesta] *f* MÚS sixth; *fam* Friday
sexta-feira [sesta'fejɾa] *f* ⟨*pl* sextas--feiras⟩ Friday; ***na ~*** on Friday; ***às ~s*** on Fridays; ***Sexta Feira Santa*** Good Friday
sextante [ses'tãtʃi] *m* sextant
sexteto [ses'tetu] *m* MÚS sextet
sexto ['sestu] **1** *adj* sixth **2** *m* six
sexual [se'kswaw] *adj* sexual
sexualidade [sekswali'dadʒi] *f* sexuality
short(s) [ʃɔrt(s)] *m*(*pl*) shorts
si[1] [si] *m* MÚS B
si[2] [si] *pron ele*: himself; *ela*: herself; *coisa*, *animal*: itself; *você*: yourself; *eles*, *elas*: themselves; *vocês*: yourselves; *impessoal*: oneself; ***voltar a ~*** come to; ***estar fora de ~*** be beside oneself
Sibéria [si'bɛɾja] *f* ***a ~*** Siberia
siberiano [sibe'ɾjanu] *adj* Siberian
sibilar [sibi'laɾ] ⟨1a⟩ hiss
Sida ['sida] *f* MED Aids *sg*; ***teste** m **da ~*** Aids test
siderurgia [sideɾuɾ'ʒia] *f* steel industry
siderúrgico [side'ɾuɾʒiku] *adj* steel *atr*; ***fundição** f **siderúrgica*** steelworks
sido ['sidu] *pp* → ***ser***
sidra ['sidɾa] *f* hard cider, *Brit* cider
sifão [si'fãw] *m* syphon
sífilis ['sifilis] *f* MED syphilis
sigilo [si'ʒilu] *m* secret; (*discrição*) secrecy
sigla ['sigla] *f* acronym; (*abreviatura*)

abbreviation
signatário [signa'taɾiu] *m*, **-a** *f* signatory
significado [signifi'kadu] *m* meaning; (*sentido*) sense
significar [signifi'kaɾ] ⟨1n⟩ mean; (*representar*) represent; (*insinuar*) signify
significativo [signifika'tʃivu] *adj* significant
signo ['signu] *m* sign; ASTROL (star) sign
sílaba ['silaba] *f* syllable
silenciador [silẽsja'doɾ] *m* TECN muffler, *Brit* silencer
silêncio [si'lẽsiu] *m* silence; ***impor ~*** call for silence; ***~!*** silence!
silencioso [silẽ'sjozu] *adj* (*calado*) silent; (*oposto a barulhento*) quiet
silhueta [si'ʎweta] *f* silhouet, *Brit* silhouette
silício [si'lisiu] *m* silicon
silicone [sili'koni] *m* silicone
silo ['silu] *m* silo
silvar [siw'vaɾ] ⟨1a⟩ hiss; (*assobiar*) whistle
silvestre [siw'vɛstɾi] *adj* wild
silvicultura [silvikuw'tuɾa] *f* forestry
silvo ['silvu] *m* hiss; (*assobio*) whistle
sim [sĩ] **1** *adv* yes; ***espero que ~*** I hope so; ***dizer que ~*** say yes **2** *m* yes
simbólico [sĩ'bɔliku] *adj* symbolic
simbolizar [sĩboli'zaɾ] ⟨1a⟩ symbolize
simbologia [sĩbolo'ʒia] *f* symbolism
símbolo ['sĩbulu] *m* symbol; ***~ de prestígio*** status symbol
simetria [sime'tɾia] *f* symmetry
simétrico [si'mɛtɾiku] *adj* symmetrical
similar [simi'laɾ] *adj* similar
similitude [simili'tudʒi] *f* similarity
símio ['simiu] *m* ZOOL monkey
simpatia [sĩpa'tʃia] *f* friendliness; (*compaixão*) sympathy; (*afeto*) liking; *fam* ***ser uma ~*** be nice
simpático [sĩ'patʃiku] *adj* friendly; (*agradável*) nice
simpatizante [sĩpatʃi'zãtʃi] *m/f* sympathizer
simpatizar [sĩpatʃi'zaɾ] ⟨1a⟩ *v/i* ***~ com*** take to; (*compreender*) sympathize with
simples ['sĩplis] *adj* simple; (*só*) single
simplicidade [sĩplisi'dadʒi] *f* simplicity
simplificação [sĩplifika'sãw] *f* simplification
simplificar [sĩplifi'kaɾ] ⟨1n⟩ simplify
simplista [sĩ'plista] *adj* simplistic
simplório [sĩ'plɔɾiu] *adj* simple-minded
simulação [simula'sãw] *f* simulation
simulador [simula'doɾ] *m* TECN, MED simulator
simular [simu'laɾ] ⟨1a⟩ simulate
simultaneidade [simuwtanej'dadʒi] *f* simultaneity
simultâneo [simuw'tʌniu] *adj* simultaneous
sinagoga [sina'gɔga] *f* synagogue
sinal [si'naw] *m* sign; (*gesto*) signal; *na pele*: mole; COM downpayment; AUTO (road) sign; ***deixar sinais*** leave something behind; *fig* leave a mark; ***~ de discagem*** dial tone; ***~ horário*** time signal; TEL ***~ de chamada*** ringing tone; ***~ de mais*** plus sign; *Port* ***~ de marcar*** dial tone; ***~ de menos*** minus sign; ***~ de ocupado*** busy tone; ***~ de perigo*** danger signal; ***~ de pontuação*** punctuation mark; ***~ de stop*** stop sign; ***~ de trânsito*** road sign
sinaleiro [sina'lejɾu] **1** *m* FERROV signalman; (***polícia*** *m*) **~** traffic policeman **2** *adj* traffic *atr*
sinalização [sinaliza'sãw] *f* road signs *pl*; ***placa*** *f* ***de ~*** road sign
sinalizar [sinali'zaɾ] ⟨1a⟩ *v/t* signal; (*anunciar*) announce
sinceridade [sĩseɾi'dadʒi] *f* sincerity
sincero [sĩ'sɛɾu] *adj* sincere; (*sério*) honest
sincronização [sĩkɾoniza'sãw] *f* synchronization; *bailarinor*: timing; CINE dubbing
sincronizar [sĩkɾoni'zaɾ] ⟨1a⟩ synchronize; CINE dub
sindical [sĩdʒi'kaw] *adj* union *atr*; ***associação*** *f* **~** association of labor unions, *Brit* association of trade unions; ***representante*** *m* **~** union representative
sindicalismo [sĩdʒika'lizmu] *m* labor

S

union movement, *Brit* trade unionism
sindicalista [sĩdʒika'lista] **1** *adj* union *atr* **2** *m/f* labor unionist, *Brit* trade unionist
sindicato [sĩdʒi'katu] *m de trabalhadores*: (labor) union, *Brit* (trade) union; ECON syndicate
síndrome ['sĩdromi] *m* syndrome
sinfonia [sĩfo'nia] *f* symphony
sinfônico, *Port* **sinfónico** [sĩ'foniku] *adj* symphonic
singelo [sĩ'ʒɛlu] *adj* simple
singular [sĩgu'lar] **1** *adj* singular; (*único*) unique; (*peculiar*) extraordinary; ***número*** *m* **~** singular **2** *m* singular
singularidade [sĩgulari'dadʒi] *f* peculiarity, singularity
sinistro [si'nistru] **1** *adj* sinister (*obscuro*) dark **2** *m* accident
sino ['sinu] *m* bell
sinônimo, *Port* **sinónimo** [si'nonimu] **1** *adj* synonymous **2** *m* synonym
sintático, *Port* **sintáctico** [sĩ'tatʃiku] *adj* syntactic
sintaxe [sĩ'taksi] *f* syntax
síntese ['sĩtezi] *f* synthesis
sintético [sĩ'tɛtʃiku] *adj* synthetic
sintetizador [sĩtetʃiza'dor] *m* synthesizer
sintetizar [sĩtetʃi'zar] ⟨1a⟩ synthesize
sinto ['sĩtu] *etc* → ***sentir***
sintoma [sĩ'toma] *m* symptom
sintomático [sĩto'matʃiku] *adj* symptomatic
sintonia [sĩto'nia] *f* signature tune
sintonizar [sĩtoni'zar] **1** *v/t* TECN tune **2** *v/i* tune in
sinuca [si'nuka] *f* snooker
sinuoso [si'nwozu] *adj* winding; *linha* wavy
sinusite [sinu'zitʃi] *f* MED sinusitis
Síria ['siria] *f* Syria
sírio ['siriu] **1** *adj* Syrian **2** *m*, **-a** *f* Syrian
sisal [si'zaw] *m* sisal
sismo ['sizmu] *m* earthquake
sísmico ['sizmiku] *adj* ***abalo*** *m* **~** seismic tremor
sismógrafo [siz'mɔgrafu] *m* seismograph
sismologia [sizmolo'ʒia] *f* seismology
siso ['sizu] *m* sense, intelligence; ***dente*** *m* ***do*** **~** wisdom tooth
sistema [sis'tema] *m* system; AUTO **~** ***antiblocagem*** antiblocking system, ABS; **~** ***decimal*** decimal system; **~** ***imunológico*** immune system; **~** ***multi-partidário*** multiparty system; **~** ***nervoso*** nervous system; **~** ***operacional***, **~** ***operativo*** operating system; **~** ***solar*** solar system
sistemático [siste'matʃiku] *adj* systematic
sistematizar [sistematʃi'zar] ⟨1a⟩ systematize
site ['sajtʃi] *m* site
sitiar [si'tʃiar] *v/t* besiege
sítio ['sitiu] *m* place; (*localização*) site; MIL siege; *Bras* farm
situação [sitwa'sãw] *f* situation; *social* standing
situado [si'twadu] *adj* ***estar*** **~** be situated
situar [si'twar] ⟨1g⟩ put; *novo edifício etc* site, locate; *num mapa* locate
skate ['skejtʃi] *m* skateboarding
skatista ['skejtʃista] *m/f* skateboarder
slip [slip] *m* briefs
slogan ['slogan] *m* slogan; **~** ***publicitário*** advertising slogan
smoking ['smokĩ] *m* tuxedo, *Brit* dinner jacket, DJ
SMS [ɛsie'miɛsi] *m abr* (***Short Message Service***) text; ***mandar um*** **~** ***a alguém*** send s.o. a text, text s.o.
só [sɔ] **1** *adj* alone; (*solitário*) lonely; (*único*) only; ***a*** **~*s*** alone **2** *adv* only; **~** ***de pensar nisso*** the very thought of it, just thinking about it; **~** ***o software custa ...*** the software alone costs ...; **~** ***que*** except that
soalho ['swaʎu] *m* floor
soar [swar] ⟨1f⟩ sound; *sino* ring; *hora* strike; *fig* be said
sob ['sobi] *prep* under; **~** ***sua liderança*** under his leadership; **~** ***pena de*** on pain of; **~** ***juramento*** on oath
sobe ['sɔbi] → ***subir***
sobejar [sobe'ʒar] ⟨1d⟩ be left; (*abundar*) abound; (*ser supérfluo*) not be needed
soberana [sobe'rana] *f* sovereign

soberania [sobera'nia] *f* POL sovereignty
soberano [sobe'ranu] **1** *adj* sovereign **2** *m* sovereign
soberba [so'berba] *f* arrogance, pride
soberbo [so'berbu] *adj* arrogant, proud
sobra ['sɔbra] *f* rest, remains; ***... de ~*** plenty of ...; ***~s*** *comida*: leftovers
sobrancelha [sobrã'seʎa] *f* eyebrow
sobrar [so'brar] ⟨1e⟩ be left over; ***sobraram 5*** there were 5 left over
sobre ['sobri] *prep* on; *por cima de* above; ***~ o que é?*** what's it about?
sobrecapa [sobre'kapa] *f* dust jacket
sobrecarregar [sobrekahe'gar] *v/t* overload
sobre-humano [sobriu'manu] *adj* superhuman
sobremarcha [sobre'marʃa] *f* overdrive
sobremesa [sobre'meza] *f* dessert
sobrenatural [sobrenatu'raw] *adj* supernatural
sobrenome [sobre'nɔmi] *m* family name, surname; *Port* (*alcunha*) nickname
sobrepor [sobre'por] ⟨2z⟩ ***~ a*** put on; (*juntar*) add to; *fig* put before; **sobrepor-se** *v/r* gain the ascendancy (***a*** over); (*suceder-se*) follow after one another
sobrescrever [sobreskre'ver] ⟨2c⟩ overwrite
sobrescrito [sobres'kritu] *m* envelope
sobressair [sobresa'ir] ⟨3l⟩ stand out; **sobressair-se** *v/r* ***~ em*** excel at
sobressaltar [sobresaw'tar] ⟨1a⟩ startle, surprise
sobressalto [sobre'sawtu] *m* scare; (*surpresa*) surprise; (*excitação*) excitement
sobressalente [sobresa'lẽtʃi] **1** *adj* spare; ***peça*** *f* ***~*** spare part; ***pneu*** *m* ***~*** spare wheel **2** *m/f* substitute
sobretaxa [sobre'taʃa] *f* surcharge, supplement
sobretudo [sobre'tudu] **1** *m* overcoat **2** *adv* above all
sobrevivente [sobrevi'vẽtʃi] **1** *adj* surviving **2** *m/f* survivor
sobreviver [sobrevi'ver] ⟨2a⟩ ***~ a algo*** survive sth; ***~ a alguém*** outlive s.o.
sobrevoar [sobre'vwar] ⟨1f⟩ fly over
sobriedade [sobrie'dadʒi] *f* soberness, sobriety
sobrinha [so'briɲa] *f* niece
sobrinho [so'briɲu] *m* nephew; ***~s*** *pl* nephews and nieces
sóbrio ['sɔbriu] *adj* sober; (*moderado*) moderate
socar [so'kar] ⟨1e⟩ punch, sock
sociabilidade [sosjabili'dadʒi] *f* sociability
social [so'sjaw] *adj* social; ***Carta*** *f* ***Social*** Social Charter; ***regime*** *m* ***~*** social order
social-democrata [sosjawdemo'krata] *m/f* social democrat
social-democrático [sosjawdemo'kratʃiku] *adj* social democratic
socialismo [sosja'lizmu] *m* socialism
socialista [sosja'lista] **1** *adj* socialist **2** *m/f* socialist
sociável [so'sjavew] *adj* sociable
sociedade [sosie'dadʒi] *f* society; (*companhia*) company; ***~ anônima*** incorporated company, *Brit* plc; ***~ por ações***, *Port* ***~ por acções*** company based on shares; ***~ de responsabilidade limitada*** limited liability company; ***~ recreativa*** leisure club
sócio ['sɔsiu] *m*, **-a** *f clube, partido, etc*: member; FIN shareholder; COM partner
sociocultural [sosjokuwtu'raw] *adj* sociocultural
socioeconômico, *Port* **socioeconómico** [sɔsjoeko'nomiku] *adj* socio-economic
sociologia [sosjolo'ʒia] *f* sociology
sociológico [sosjo'lɔʒiku] *adj* sociological
sociólogo [so'sjɔlogu] *m*, **-a** *f* sociologist
soco ['soku] *m* (*murro*) punch
socorrer [soko'her] ⟨2d⟩ ***~ alguém*** come to s.o.'s assistance
socorro [so'kohu] *m* help, assistance; ***número*** *m* (***nacional***) ***de ~*** emergency number; ***primeiros ~s*** *pl* first aid; ***~!*** help!

soda ['sɔda] *f* soda(water)
sofá [so'fa] *m* sofa
sofa-cama [sofa'kama] *m* ⟨*pl* sofas--camas⟩ sofa-bed
sofisticado [sofisʧi'kadu] *adj* sophisticated
sôfrego ['sofregu] *adj* greedy; (*impaciente*) impatient
sofreguidão [sofregi'dãw] *f* ⟨*sem pl*⟩ greed; (*impaciência*) impatience
sofrer [so'frer] ⟨2d⟩ **1** *v/t* suffer; (*suportar*) put up with **2** *v/i* suffer (***de*** from)
sofrimento [sofri'mẽtu] *m* suffering
sofrível [so'frivew] *adj* bearable; (*médio*) passable
software [sof'twɛr] *f* INFORM software; ~ ***para utilizador*** application software
sogro ['sogru] *m*, **-a** ['sɔgra] *f* stepfather; step-mother
sogros ['sogrus] *mpl* step-parents
soirée [swa'he] *f* evening
soja ['sɔʒa] *f* soy, *Brit* soya; ***molho*** *m* ***de*** ~ soy sauce
sol[1] [sɔw] *m* sun; (*luz do dia*) daylight
sol[2] [sɔw] *m* MÚS G
sola ['sɔla] *f* sole
solar[1] [so'lar] *adj* solar
solar[2] [so'lar] *m* manor house
solar[3] [so'lar] ⟨1e⟩ *v/t* sole, resole
solário [so'lariu] *m* solarium
solavanco [sola'vãku] *m* jolt, jerk; ***andar aos ~s*** *trem etc* jolt; *passageiro* be jolted about; *na vida* go from one thing to another
solda ['sɔlda] *f* solder; → ***soldadura***
soldado [sow'dadu] *m/f* soldier; ~ ***raso*** private
soldador [sowda'dor] *m*, **-a** *f pessoa* welder
soldadura [sowda'dura] *f* welding; *arame pequeno*: soldering; (*parte soldada*) weld
soldagem [sow'daʒẽ] *f* welding; *arame pequeno*: soldering
soldar [sow'dar] ⟨1e⟩ weld; *arame pequeno* solder
solene [so'leni] *adj* solemn
solenidade [soleni'dadʒi] *f* (*festividade*) celebration; (*formalismo*) solemnity
soletrar [sole'trar] ⟨1c⟩ spell
solicitação [solisita'sãw] *f* request; (*exigência*) demand
solicitar [solisi'tar] ⟨1a⟩ request; *passaporte etc* apply for; (*exigir*) demand
solícito [so'lisitu] *adj* eager; (*prestável*) helpful
solicitude [solisi'tudʒi] *f* eagerness; (*pressuroso*) helpfulness
solidão [soli'dãw] *f* ⟨*sem pl*⟩ loneliness, solitude
solidariedade [solidarie'dadʒi] *f* solidarity; DIR joint liability
solidário [soli'dariu] *adj* showing solidarity
solidez [soli'des] *f* solidity
solidificar [solidʒifi'kar] ⟨1n⟩ solidify; *fig* firm up; **solidificar-se** *v/r* solidify; *cola* set
sólido ['sɔlidu] **1** *adj* solid **2** *m* solid
solista [so'lista] *m/f* soloist
solitária [soli'tarja] *f* MED tapeworm
solitário [soli'tariu] **1** *adj* lonely, solitary; (*único*) sole, solitary **2** *m* (*diamante*) solitaire; ***é um ~*** he's lonely; (*prefere estar sozinho*) he's a loner
solo ['sɔlu] **1** *m* (*terra*) ground; MÚS solo *n* **2** *adj* solo
solstício [sols'ʧisiu] *m* solstice
soltar [sow'tar] ⟨1e⟩ *v/t som, cheiro etc* give off; *grito* let out; *prisioneiros* set free; *nó* untie, undo; *cabelo* let down; *corda* let go of; *freio de mão* release, put off; (*separar*) unfix; *fam dinheiro* cough up
solteiro [sow'tejru] **1** *adj* single **2** *m*, **-a** *f* single man, bachelor; single woman
solto ['sowtu] *adj* free; *vestuário, cabelo, arroz* loose
solução [solu'sãw] *f* solution *tb* QUÍM
soluçar [solu'sar] ⟨1p⟩ hiccup; (*chorar*) sob; *motor* stutter
solucionar [solusjo'nar] ⟨1f⟩ solve
soluço [so'lusu] *m* (*choro*) sob; ***~s*** *pl* hiccups
solúvel [so'luvew] *adj* solvable; QUÍM soluble; ***café*** *m* ~ instant coffee
solvente [sow'vẽʧi] **1** *m* solvent **2** *adj* COM solvent
solver [sow'ver] ⟨2e⟩ *dívida, conta* settle, pay

som [sõ] *m* sound; ***volume** m **de** ~* volume; ***ao ~ de*** to the music of
soma ['soma] *f* sum
somar [so'maɾ] ⟨1f⟩ **1** *v/t* add up; (*juntar*) add on (***a*** to) **2** *v/i* ***~ em*** add up to
somatório [soma'tɔriu] *m* sum
sombra ['sõbɾa] *f* shadow *tb fig*; (*escuridão*) shade; (*vestígio*) trace; *esperança etc*: glimmer; *maquiagem* eyeshadow
sombrinha [sõ'briɲa] *f* sunshade; *chuva*: umbrella
sombrio [sõ'bɾiu] *adj* shady; *fig* gloomy
somente [so'mẽtʃi] *adv* only, just; ***~ o melhor*** nothing but the best
sonâmbulo [so'nãbulu] **1** *adj* sleepwalking *atr* **2** *m*, **-a** *f* sleepwalker
sonata [so'nata] *f* MÚS sonata
sonda ['sõda] *f* MED, MIN probe; NÁUT sound
sondagem [sõ'daʒẽ] *f* sounding; (*investigação*) probe; ***~ de opinião pública*** opinion poll; ***~ do mercado*** market survey
sondar [sõ'daɾ] ⟨1a⟩ sound; (*investigar*) probe; *opinião* sound out
soneca [so'nɛka] *f fam* snooze
sonegação [sonega'sãw] *f* withholding; *impostos*: evasion
sonegar [sone'gaɾ] ⟨1o & 1c⟩ conceal; (*não declarar*) withhold; *imposto* withhold, evade paying
soneto [so'netu] *m* sonnet
sonhador [soɲa'doɾ] **1** *adj* dreamy **2** *m*, **-a** *f* dreamer
sonhar [so'ɲaɾ] ⟨1f⟩ **1** *v/i* dream (***com*** about) **2** *v/t* dream
sonho ['soɲu] *m* dream; GASTR donut, *Brit* doughnut
sono ['sonu] *m* sleep; (*sonolência*) sleepiness; ***estar com ~, ter ~*** be sleepy
sonolência [sono'lẽsja] *f* sleepiness
sonolento [sono'lẽtu] *adj* sleepy
sonoridade [sonori'dadʒi] *f* sound, sound quality; (*volume de som*) sound level
sonoro [so'nɔɾu] *adj* sonorous; *consoante* voiced
sopa ['sopa] *f* soup; ***~ do dia*** soup of the day; ***~ de feijão*** bean soup; ***~ de legumes*** vegetable soup; ***~ de lentilha*** lentil soup; ***~ de peixe*** fish soup; ***~ de tomate*** tomato soup
sopapo [so'papu] *m fam* slap
sopé [so'pɛ] *m montanha*: foot
sopeira [so'pejɾa] *f* soup bowl
soporífero [sopo'ɾifeɾu] **1** *adj* soporific *tb fig* **2** *m* sleeping drug
soprano [so'pɾanu] **1** *m* MÚS treble **2** *f* soprano
soprar [so'pɾaɾ] ⟨1e⟩ blow; *luz* blow out; *balão* blow up; *pó* blow off
sopro ['sopɾu] *m* blow; (*bafo*) puff, breath; (*aragem*) breath; *vento*: gust; ***instrumento** m **de** ~* wind instrument
soquete [so'ketʃi] *m/f* (*peúga*) ankle sock
sordidez [soɾdʒi'des] *f* filth; (*vileza*) sordidness
sórdido ['sɔɾdʒidu] *adj* filthy; (*repugnante*) sordid
soro ['soɾu] *m* whey; MED serum
sorridente [sohi'dẽtʃi] *adj* smiling
sorrir [so'hiɾ] ⟨3v⟩ smile; ***~ para*** smile at
sorriso [so'hizu] *m* smile; ***~ amarelo*** forced smile, cheesy grin
sorte ['sɔɾtʃi] *f* (*fortuna*) fate, destiny; (*acaso*) chance; (*ventura*) luck; ***boa ~!*** good luck!; ***má ~, pouca ~*** bad luck; ***à ~*** trusting to luck; ***ler a ~ de alguém*** tell s.o.'s fortune; ***tirar a ~ grande*** hit the jackpot; ***ter muita ~*** be very lucky, luck out; ***ele tem ~ de estar vivo*** he's lucky to be alive
sortear [soɾ'tʃiaɾ] ⟨1l⟩ draw lots for; (*rifar*) raffle
sorteio [soɾ'teiu] *m* draw; (*rifa*) raffle
sortido [soɾ'tʃidu] **1** *adj* assorted **2** *m* assortiment
sortir [soɾ'tʃiɾ] *v/t* mix; (*abastecer*) supply (***com, de*** with)
sorvedoiro [soɾve'dojɾu] *m*, **sorvedouro** [soɾve'doɾu] *m* whirlpool; *fig* abyss
sorver [soɾ'veɾ] ⟨2d⟩ sip; (*chupar*) soak up; (*engolir*) swallow
sorvete [soɾ'vetʃi] *m Bras* ice cream; ***~ de chocolate*** chocolate ice cream; ***~ de limão*** lemon ice cream

sorveteria [sorvete'ria] *f* ice cream parlor, *Brit* ice cream parlour
sorvo ['sorvu] *m* sip
sósia ['sɔzja] *m/f* double
sossegado [sose'gadu] *adj* calm
sossegar [sose'gar] ⟨1o & 1c⟩ calm down, quieten down; (*manter-se calmo*) keep calm
sossego [so'segu] *m* peace and quiet
sótão ['sɔtãw] *m* ⟨*pl* -ãos⟩ attic; *fam* ***ter macacos no ~*** have bats in the belfry
sotaque [so'taki] *m* accent
soterrar [sote'har] ⟨1c⟩ bury
soturno [so'turnu] *adj* gloomy
sou [sow] → ***ser***
soube ['sobi] *etc* → ***saber***
soutien [su'tʃiã] *m Port* brassière, *Brit* bra
sova ['sɔva] *f* thrashing; ***dar uma ~*** thrash; ***apanhar uma ~*** get a thrashing
sovaco [so'vaku] *m fam* armpit
sovaquinho [sova'kiɲu] *m fam* BO
soviético [so'viɛtʃiku] *adj hist* Soviet
sovina [so'vina] *adj* mean, stingy
sozinho [so'ziɲu] *adj* alone; ***nós … ~s*** we … by ourselves
spa [spa] *m* health club
squash [skwɔʃ] *m* squash
Sr. [se'ɲor] *abr* (***Senhor***) Mr
Sra. [se'ɲora] *abr* (***Senhora***) Mrs; Ms
stand [stãdʒ] *m* booth, *Brit* stand
stock [stɔk] *m* COM stock
sua ['sua] *pron f* → ***seu***
suado ['swadu] *adj* sweaty; *fig* hard earned
suar [swar] ⟨1g⟩ sweat
suave ['swavi] *adj* soft; (*tenro*) gentle; *sabor* mild, smooth
suavidade [swavi'dadʒi] *f* softness; (*ternura*) gentleness
suavizar [swavi'zar] ⟨1a⟩ soften
sub… [subi-] sub…, under…
subalimentação [subalimẽta'sãw] *f* ⟨*sem pl*⟩ undernourishment
subalimentado [subalimẽ'tadu] *adj* undernourished
subalterno [subaw'tɛrnu] **1** *adj* subordinate; (*inferior*) inferior **2** *m*, **-a** *f* subordinate
subalugar [subalu'gar] *v/t* sublet
subarrendar [subahẽ'dar] sublet
subarrendatário [subahẽda'tariu] *m*, **-a** *f* subtenant
subchefe [subi'ʃɛfi] *m* deputy boss
subcomissão [subikomi'sãw] *f* subcommittee
subconsciente [subikõs'sjẽtʃi] **1** *adj* subconscious **2** *m* subconscious
subcontratação [subikõtrata'sãw] *f* ⟨*sem pl*⟩ subcontracting
subcontratar [subikõtra'tar] *v/i* subcontract
subcutâneo [subiku'tʌniu] *adj* subcutaneous
subdesenvolvido [subidesẽvow'vidu] *adj* underdeveloped
subdesenvolvimento [subidesẽvowvi'mẽtu] *m* underdevelopment
subdiretor, *Port* **subdirector** [subidʒire'tor] *m*, **-a** *f* deputy director
súbdito ['sudʒitu] *m*, **-a** *f Port* subject
subdividir [subidʒivi'dʒir] *v/t* subdivide
subdivisão [subidʒivi'zãw] *f* subdivision
subempresário [subẽpre'zariu] *m*, **-a** *f* subcontractor
subentender [subẽtẽ'der] *v/t* (*compreender*) understand; (*dar a entender*) give to understand; **subentender-se** *v/r* be understood
subestimar [subestʃi'mar] ⟨1a⟩ underestimate
subexposto [subes'postu] *adj* underexposed
subgerente [subiʒe'rẽtʃi] *m/f* assistant manager, deputy manager
subida [su'bida] *f* rise; (*ascensão*) climb
subinspetor, *Port* **subinspector** [subĩspe'tor] *m*, **-a** *f* deputy inspector
subir [su'bir] ⟨3h⟩ **1** *v/i* go up; *árvore*: climb up; *no ônibus etc* get on; ***subimos até Recife*** we went up to Recife; ***~ no ônibus*** get on the bus **2** *v/t montanha* go up, climb; (*trazer*) bring up; (*levantar*) take up; *preço etc* put up
súbito ['subitu] **1** *adj* sudden **2** *adv* ***de ~*** suddenly
subjacente [subiʒa'sẽtʃi] *adj* underlying

S

subject... *Port* → ***subjet...***
subjetividade [subiʒetʃivi'dadʒi] *f* subjectivity
subjetivismo [subiʒetʃi'vizmu] *m* subjectivity
subjetivo [subiʒe'tʃivu] *adj* subjective
subjugar [subiʒu'gar] ⟨1o⟩ subjugate; (*forçar*) subdue; *animal* tame
subjuntivo [subiʒũ'tʃivu] *m* subjunctive
sublevação [subleva'sãw] *f* uprising
sublevar [suble'var] *v/t* incite to revolt; **sublevar-se** *v/r* rise up (in revolt); NÁUT mutiny
sublime [su'blimi] *adj* sublime; (*refinado*) noble
sublinhar [subli'ɲar] ⟨1a⟩ underline
sublocação [subloka'sãw] *f* subletting
sublocar [sublo'kar] ⟨1n & 1e⟩ sublet
sublocatário [subloka'tariu] *m*, **-a** *f* subtenant
submarino [subima'rinu] **1** *adj* underwater **2** *m* submarine
submergir [subimer'ʒir] ⟨3n & 2c⟩ submerge *tb fig*
submeter [subime'ter] ⟨2c⟩ subdue; (*mostrar*) submit
submetralhadora [subimetraʎa'dora] *f* submachine gun
submissão [subimi'sãw] *f* ⟨*sem pl*⟩ submission
submisso [subi'misu] *adj* submissive
submundo [subi'mũdu] *m* underworld
subnutrição [subinutri'sãw] *f* ⟨*sem pl*⟩ malnutrition
subnutrido [subinu'tridu] *adj* undernourished
subordinação [subordʒina'sãw] *f* subordination; (*obediência*) obedience
subordinada [subordʒi'nada] *f* GRAM subordinate clause
subordinado [subordʒi'nadu] **1** *adj* subordinate **2** *m*, **-a** *f* subordinate
subordinar [subordʒi'nar] ⟨1a⟩ subordinate
subornar [subor'nar] ⟨1e⟩ bribe
suborno [su'bornu] *m* bribery
subproduto [subipro'dutu] *m* by-product
subscrever [subiskre'ver] *v/t* subscribe to *tb fig*
subscrição [subiskri'sãw] *f* subscription
subseqüente, *Port* **subsequente** [subise'kwẽtʃi] *adj* subsequent
subsidiar [subisi'dʒiar] ⟨1g⟩ subsidize
subsídio [subi'sidiu] *m* subsidy; **~ *diário*** daily allowance; **~ *de férias*** holiday pay
subsistência [subisis'tẽsja] *f* continuance; (*sustento*) livelihood, subsistence
subsistir [subisis'tʃir] ⟨3a⟩ continue to exist; **~ *a base de*** subsist on
subsolo [subi'sɔlu] *m Bras* basement; GEOL subsoil
substabelecer [subistabele'ser] ⟨2g⟩ delegate; (*representar*) represent
substância [subis'tãsja] *f* substance; ***em* ~** in essence
substancial [subistã'sjaw] *adj* substantial
substantivo [subistã'tʃivu] *m* noun
substituição [subistʃitwi'sãw] *f* substitution
substituir [subistʃi'twir] ⟨3i⟩ substitute for, replace; **~ *Y por X*** substitute X for Y
substituto [subistʃi'tutu] **1** *adj* substitute; *gerente etc* acting **2** *m*, **-a** *f* substitute
subterfúgio [subiter'fuʒiu] *m* subterfuge
subterrâneo [subite'hʌniu] **1** *adj* underground, subterranean; ***água*(*s*)** *f*(*pl*) ***subterrânea*(*s*)** ground water **2** *m* basement; *galeria*: underground passage; (*caverna*) cave
subtil [sub'tʃiw] *adj Port* subtle; (*delicado*) delicate
subtileza [subtʃi'leza] *f*, **subtilidade** [subtʃili'dadʒi] *f Port* subtlety; (*delicadeza*) delicacy
subtítulo [subi'tʃitulu] *m* subheading
subtração, *Port* **subtracção** [subitra'sãw] *f* MAT subtraction; QUÍM, *fig* extraction
subtrair [subitra'ir] ⟨3l⟩ MAT subtract; *fig* extract
subtropical [subitropi'kaw] *adj* subtropical

suburbano [subur'banu] *adj* suburban
subúrbio [su'burbiu] *m* suburb
subvenção [subivẽ'sãw] *f* subsidy; (*auxílio*) grant
subvencionar [subivẽsjo'nar] ⟨1f⟩ subsidize
subversão [subiver'sãw] *f* subversion
subversivo [subiver'sivu] *adj* subversive
sucata [su'kata] *f* scrap metal
suceder [suse'der] ⟨2c⟩ succeed (***a algo*** sth); (*dar-se*) follow; (*acontecer*) happen (***a alguém*** to s.o.)
sucessão [suse'sãw] *f* succession
sucessivo [suse'sivu] *adj* successive
sucesso [su'sɛsu] *m* success; MÚS hit; ***fazer ~*** be a hit
sucessor [suse'sor] *m*, **-a** *f* successor
sucinto [su'sĩtu] *adj* succinct
suco ['suku] *m Bras* juice; ***~ de fruta*** fruit juice; ***~ gástrico*** gastric juices; ***~ de laranja*** orange juice
suculento [suku'lẽtu] *adj* succulent
sucumbir [sukũ'bir] ⟨3a⟩ succumb (***a*** to)
sucursal [sukur'saw] **1** *adj* branch *atr* **2** *f* branch
Sudão [su'dãw] *m* (the) Sudan
súdito ['sudʒitu] *m*, **-a** *f* subject
sudoeste [su'dwɛstʃi] *m* southwest
Suécia ['swɛsja] *f* Sweden
sueco ['swɛku] **1** *adj* Swedish **2** *m*, **-a** *f* Swede **3** *m lingua* Swedish
sueste ['swɛstʃi] *m* southeast
suéter ['swɛter] *m* sweater
suficiente [sufi'sjẽtʃi] *adj* enough, sufficient; *nota*: satisfactory; ***o ~*** enough
suficientemente [sufisjẽtʃi'mẽtʃi] *adv* enough, sufficiently; ***~ quente*** warm enough
sufocação [sufoka'sãw] *f* suffocation; (*repressão*) repression
sufocante [sufo'kãtʃi] *adj* oppressive, suffocating
sufocar [sufo'kar] ⟨1n & 1e⟩ **1** *v/t* suffocate; (*reprimir*) repress **2** *v/i* suffocate
sufrágio [su'fraʒiu] *m* (*voto*) vote; (*direito de voto*) suffrage, vote
sugar [su'gar] ⟨1o⟩ suck; *energia* sap
sugerir [suʒe'rir] ⟨3c⟩ suggest
sugestão [suʒes'tãw] *f* suggestion
sugestionar [suʒestʃio'nar] *v/t* influence
sugestionável [suʒestʃio'navew] *adj* suggestible
sugestivo [suʒes'tʃivu] *adj* suggestive
Suíça ['swisa] *f* Switzerland
suicida [swi'sida] **1** *m/f* suicide **2** *adj* suicidal
suicidar-se [swisi'darsi] ⟨1a⟩ *v/r* commit suicide
suicídio [swi'sidiu] *m* suicide
suíço ['swisu] **1** *adj* Swiss **2** *m*, **-a** *f* Swiss
suíno ['swinu] **1** *adj* ***gado*** *m* **~** hogs, pigs **2** *m* hog, pig; *fam pessoa* swine, pig
suíte ['switʃi] *f* suite; *banheiro*: en suite bathroom; ***~ nupcial*** bridal suite
sujar [su'ʒar] ⟨1a⟩ **1** *v/t* dirty **2** *v/i* make things dirty
sujeição [suʒej'sãw] *f* ⟨*sem pl*⟩ subjection
sujeira [su'ʒejra] *f* dirt
sujeitar [suʒej'tar] ⟨1a⟩ subject; **sujeitar-se** *v/r fig* ***~ a*** submit to
sujeito [su'ʒejtu] **1** *adj* subjected; ***~ a*** subject to; ***~ a imposto(s)*** liable to tax; ***~ a um risco*** subject to risk **2** *m* GRAM subject; *fam* character; ***um ~ muito legal*** one hell of a nice guy
sujidade [suʒi'dadʒi] *f Port* dirt *tb fig*
sujo ['suʒu] *adj* dirty
sul [suw] *m* south; ***ao ~ de*** south of; ***do ~*** south
sul-americano [sulameri'kanu] *adj* South American
sulcar [suw'kar] ⟨1n⟩ plow, *Brit* plough; *ondas etc* plow through; *mar* sail
sulco ['suwku] *m* furrow; NÁUT wake
sulfato [suw'fatu] *m* QUÍM sulfate, *Brit* sulphate
sulfuroso [suwfu'rozu] *adj* sulfurous, *Brit* sulphurous
sulista [su'lista] *m/f* southerner
sultão [suw'tãw] *m*, **-ana** [suw'tana] *f* sultan; sultana
sumamente [suma'mẽtʃi] *adv* extremely
sumarento [suma'rẽtu] *adj* juicy

sumário [su'mariu] **1** *adj* brief **2** *m* summary
sumição [sumi'sãw] *f*, **sumiço** [su'misu] *m* disappearance; ***levar ~*** disappear
sumido [su'midu] *adj* vanished; *olhos* sunken; *voz* quiet; *cor* faded; ***andar ~*** make oneself scarce; ***estar ~*** be all skin and bones
sumir [su'mir] ⟨3h⟩ *v/i* vanish, disappear; *fam* piss off; ***suma!*** piss off!; **sumir-se** *v/r* disappear; (*passar*) go away
sumo ['sumu] **1** *adj* highest, extreme **2** *m Port fruta*: juice; ***~ de maçã*** apple juice; ***~ de laranja*** orange juice
sumptuoso *Port* → ***suntuoso***
sunga ['sũga] *f Bras* swimming trunks
suntuoso [sũ'twozu] *adj* sumptuous
suor [swɔr] *m* sweat
super ['super] *adj* premium; ***gasolina*** *f* **~** premium
superar [supe'rar] ⟨1c⟩ overcome; *decepção* get over; (*suplantar*) exceed; (*transpor*) go beyond; ***~ em número*** outnumber
superável [supe'ravew] *adj* superable
superavit [supe'ravit] *m* FIN surplus
superestimar [superestʃi'mar] ⟨1a⟩ overestimate
superexpor [superes'por] ⟨2z⟩ overexpose
superficial [superfi'sjaw] *adj* superficial *tb fig*; MIN surface *atr*
superficialidade [superfisjali'dadʒi] *f* superficiality
superfície [super'fisi] *f* surface; MIN ***pessoal*** *m* ***da ~*** surface personnel
supérfluo [su'pɛrflwu] *adj* superfluous
superintendente [superĩtẽ'dẽtʃi] *m/f* superintendent; (*dirigente*) director
superior [supe'rjor] **1** *adj de cima* top, highest; (*maior*) greater; (*mais alto*) higher; (*melhor*) superior; ***instituto*** *m ou* ***escola*** *f* **~** college; ***a parte ~ de*** the top of **2** *m*, **-a** *f* superior
superioridade [superjori'dadʒi] *f* superiority
superlativo [superla'tʃivu] **1** *adj* superlative; ***grau*** *m* **~** superlative **2** *m* superlative
superlotado [superlo'tadu] *adj* overfull, overcrowded
supermercado [supermer'kadu] *m* supermarket
superpopulação [superpopola'sãw] *f* overpopulation
superpotência [superpo'tẽsja] *f* superpower
superpovoado [superpo'vwadu] *adj* overpopulated
superprodução [superprodo'sãw] *f* ECON overproduction; CINE blockbuster, mega-production
supersônico, *Port* **supersónico** [super'soniku] *adj* supersonic
superstição [superstʃi'sãw] *f* superstition
supersticioso [superstʃi'sjozu] *adj* superstitious
superstrutura [superstru'tura] *f* superstructure
supervalorizado [supervalori'zadu] *adj* overrated
supervisão [supervi'zãw] *f* supervision
supervisionar [supervizjo'nar] *v/t* supervise
supervisor [supervi'zor] *m*, **-a** *f de produção etc* supervisor
suplantar [suplã'tar] ⟨1a⟩ *pessoa* replace
suplementar [suplemẽ'tar] *adj* supplementary; ***horas*** *fpl* ***~es*** overtime
suplemento [suple'mẽtu] *m* supplement
suplente [su'plẽtʃi] **1** *adj* deputy, acting; (*sobresselente*) spare; ***pneu*** *m* **~** spare wheel **2** *m/f* deputy, stand-in; ESP sub
súplica ['suplika] *f* appeal; ***~s*** *pl* entreaties
suplicar [supli'kar] ⟨1n⟩ ***~ alguém*** beseech s.o.; ***~ algo*** beg for sth
supor [su'por] ⟨2z⟩ suppose; ***suponho que sim*** I suppose so
suportar [supor'tar] ⟨1e⟩ bear, put up with
suportável [supor'tavew] *adj* bearable
suporte [su'pɔrtʃi] *m* support; INFORM ***~ de informação*** data carrier
suposição [supozi'sãw] *f* supposition

supositório [supozi'tɔriu] *m* MED suppository
supostamente [suposta'mẽtʃi] *adv* supposedly
suposto [su'postu] **1** *adj* supposed; **~ *que*** supposing **2** *m* supposition
supra [supra] *adv* **~ *citado*** above-mentioned
supranacional [supranasjo'naw] *adj* transnational
supraregional [suprahezjo'naw] *adj* transregional
supremacia [suprema'sia] *f* supremacy
supremo [su'premu] *adj* supreme; (*final*) ultimate
supressão [supre'sãw] *f* suppression; (*omissão*) omission; (*eliminação*) elimination
suprimir [supri'mir] ⟨3a⟩ suppress; (*eliminar*) eliminate; (*omitir*) omit; (*afastar*) remove; INFORM delete
suprir [su'prir] ⟨3a⟩ **1** *v/t* complete; (*substituir*) replace; (*compensar*) make up for; (*abastecer*) supply; *necessidade* meet; **~ *a alguém*** take s.o.'s place **2** *v/i* help out; (*substituir*) act as a substitute
surdez [sur'des] *f* deafness; ***aparelho*** *m* ***de* ~** hearing aid
surdina [sur'dʒina] *f* MÚS mute; ***à* ~, *pela* ~** on the quiet
surdo ['surdu] *adj pessoa* deaf; *som* dull; (*silencioso*) quiet, silent
surdo-mudo [surdu'mudu] *adj* deaf and dumb
surfe ['surfi] *m* surfing; ***prancha*** *f* ***de* ~** surfboard
surfista [sur'fista] *m/f* surfer
surgir [sur'ʒir] ⟨3n⟩ appear; *problemas* arise, come up; AGR come up; ***surgiu um boato que ...*** a rumor got about that ...
surpreendente [surpreẽ'dẽtʃi] *adj* surprising
surpreendentemente [surpreẽdẽtʃi'mẽtʃi] *adv* surprisingly
surpreender [surpreẽ'der] ⟨2a⟩ surprise
surpresa [sur'preza] *f* surprise
surra ['suha] *f fam* thrashing; ***dar uma* ~ *em*** give a thrashing to; ***levar uma* ~** get a thrashing
surrado [su'hadu] *adj* worn-out, shabby
surrupiar [suhupi'ar] ⟨1g⟩ steal
surtir [sur'tʃir] ⟨3a⟩ **1** *v/t* bring about; **~ *efeito*** have an effect **2** *v/i bem, mal* end
surto ['surtu] *m* surge; (*epidemia*) outbreak; **~ *de crescimento*** growth spurt; **~ *econômico*** economic boom
suscept... *Port* → ***suscet...***
suscetibilidade [susetʃibili'dadʒi] *f* susceptibility
suscetível [suse'tʃivew] *adj* susceptible (***de*** to); **~ *de*** liable to
suscitar [susi'tar] ⟨1a⟩ *situação* give rise to; *dúvidas* raise; *revolta* cause
suspeição [suspej'sãw] *f* suspicion
suspeita [sus'pejta] *f* suspicion; ***lançar* ~*s sobre alguém*** cast suspicion on s.o.
suspeitar [suspej'tar] ⟨1a⟩ *v/t* suspect; **~ *de alguém*** be suspicious of s.o.
suspeito [sus'pejtu] **1** *adj* suspicious; ***andar* ~ *de*** be suspicious of **2** *m*, **-a** *f* suspect
suspeitoso [suspej'tozu] *adj* suspicious
suspender [suspẽ'der] ⟨2a⟩ suspend; (*adiar*) defer; (*interromper*) interrupt; (*pendurar*) hang
suspensão [suspẽ'sãw] *f* suspension; (*adiamento*) deferment; (*interrupção*) interruption; MÚS pause
suspensórios [suspẽ'sɔrius] *mpl* suspenders, *Brit* braces
suspirar [suspi'rar] ⟨1a⟩ sigh; **~ *por*** long for; ***suspirar de* ~** heave a sigh of relief
suspiro [sus'piru] *m* sigh; GASTR meringue
sussurrar [susu'har] ⟨1a⟩ **1** *v/t* whisper **2** *v/i* whisper; *vento, folhas* rustle; *fonte* murmur; *inseto* hum
sussurro [su'suhu] *pessoa*: whisper *vento*: rustling; *fonte*: murmuring; *inseto*: hum
sustentabilidade [sustẽtabili'dadʒi] *f* sustainability
sustentado [sustẽ'tadu] *adj* sustained

sustentar [sustẽ'taɾ] ⟨1a⟩ support; *ritmo* sustain
sustentável [sustẽ'tavew] *adj* sustainable
sustento [sus'tẽtu] *m* (*alimentação*) sustenance; (*apoio*) support
suster [sus'teɾ] ⟨2xa⟩ support; (*reter*) hold back
susto ['sustu] *m* scare; ***pregar um ~ a alguém*** give s.o. a scare
sutiã [su'ʧiã] *m Bras* brassière, *Brit* bra
sutil [su'ʧiw] *adj Bras* subtle; (*delicado*) delicate
sutileza [suʧi'leza] *f*, **sutilidade** [suʧili'dadʒi] *f Bras* subtlety; (*delicadeza*) delicacy
sutura [su'tuɾa] *f* MED suture
suturar [suto'ɾaɾ] ⟨1a⟩ *ferida* suture, put stiches in
suvenir [suve'niɾ] *m* souvenir

T

ta [ta] = *pron* ***te*** + *pron* ***a***
tabacaria [tabaka'ria] *f* tobacco store, *Brit* tobacconist
tabaco [ta'baku] *m* tobacco
tabagismo [taba'ʒizmu] *m* smoking; ***~ passivo*** passive smoking
tabefe [ta'bɛfi] *m fam* slap
tabela [ta'bɛla] *f* table; (*lista*) list; ***à ~*** according to plan
tabelado [tabe'ladu] *adj* price-controlled
tabelamento [tabela'mẽtu] *m* price list, pricing; POL price control
tabelar [tabe'laɾ] **1** *adj* tabular **2** *v/t preços* fix, control
tabelião [tabe'ljãw] *m*, **-ã** [tabe'ljã] *f Bras* notary
taberna [ta'bɛɾna] *f* bar, tavern
tabique [ta'biki] *m* partition
tablete [ta'blɛʧi] *f chocolate*: bar
tablier [tabli'e] *m* AUTO dashboard
tabu [ta'bu] *m* taboo
tábua ['tabwa] *f* board, plank; *fig* list; (*tabela*) table; ***~ de assoalho*** floorboard; ***~ de cortar*** chopping board; ***~ de passar roupa*** ironing board
tabuada [ta'bwada] *f* (*índice*) table of contents; ***~ de multiplicar*** multiplication table
tabuado [ta'bwadu] *m* wooden fence; *pavimento*: boardwalk
tabulador [tabula'doɾ] *m* tab
tabuleiro [tabu'lejɾu] *m* tray; *jogo*: board; ***~ de damas*** checkerboard, *Brit* draughts board; ***~ de xadrez*** chessboard
tabuleta [tabu'leta] *f* sign; (*mostrador*) display case
taça ['tasa] *f champanhe*: glass, ESP cup; ***Taça Europeia*** European Cup; ***~ de vinho*** wine glass
tacanho [ta'kaɲu] *adj* (*mesquinho*) mean; *fig fam* narrow-minded
tacão [ta'kãw] *m* heel
tacha ['taʃa] *f* tack
tacho ['taʃu] *m* small pan; *Port fam* ***ele arranjou um ~*** he got a nice little job through his connections
tácito ['tasitu] *adj* tacit
taciturno [tasi'tuɾnu] *adj* taciturn, monosyllabic; (*triste*) gloomy
taco ['taku] *m bilhar*: cue; *golfe*: club; *hoquei*: stick; TECN dowel
tacógrafo [ta'kɔgɾafu] *m* tachograph
tacômetro, *Port* **tacómetro** [ta'kometɾu] *m* speedometer
tact... *Port* → ***tat...***
tafetá [tafe'ta] *m* taffeta
tagarela [taga'ɾɛla] **1** *adj* talkative **2** *m/f* chatterbox **3** *f* chat; (*barulho*) chattering
tagarelice [tagare'lisi] *f* talkativeness
Tailândia [taj'lãdʒia] *f* Thailand
tal [taw] *adj* such; ***de ~ maneira*** in such a way; ***um ~ de João telefonou*** there was a João on the phone,

somebody called João called; ***e o ~ carro estava ...*** and that car was ...; ***a tua voz é ~ e qual ...*** your voice is just like ...; ***que ~?*** how's things?, how's it going?; ***sexta-feira é ruim, que ~ na quinta-feira?*** Friday's no good, how about Thursday?; ***~ pai, ~ filho*** like father, like son; ***~ e coisa*** this and that; ***... ~ e coisa*** ... and so on; ***Recife, ~ como Natal ...*** Recife, just like Natal, ...

tala ['tala] *f* MED splint

talão [ta'lãw] *m* heel; COM stub; ***~ de caixa*** receipt slip; ***~ de cheque*** checkbook, *Port* check stub

talco ['tawku] *m* taclum powder, talc

talento [ta'lẽtu] *m* talent

talentoso [talẽ'tozu] *adj* talented

talha ['taʎa] *f* carving

talhada [ta'ʎada] *f* (*pedaço*) chunk

talhar [ta'ʎar] ⟨1b⟩ cut; *em madeira* carve; *em cobre* engrave

talharim [taʎa'rĩ] *m* tagliatelle

talhe ['taʎi] *m* cut; (*forma*) shape, form

talher [ta'ʎɛr] *m* (*faca, garfo, colher*) flatware, cutlery; ***tens ~ (es)?*** do you have any cutlery?

talho ['taʎu] *m* cut; *da carne* slice; *Port loja*: butcher's

talo ['talu] *m* stem; *coluna*: shaft

taluda [ta'luda] *f pop* top lottery prize

talvez [taw'ves] *adv* perhaps, maybe

tamanho [ta'maɲu] **1** *adj* such; ***foi tamanha confusão*** it was such a mess **2** *m* size; ***~ econômico***, *Port* ***~ económico*** economy size; ***~ natural*** lifesized

tâmara ['tʌmara] *f* date

tamareira [tʌma'rejra] *f* date palm

também [tã'bẽ] *adv* too, also; ***eu também*** me too; ***~ não vou*** I won't go either; ***ele é músico, ela ~*** he's a musician, so is she

tambor [tã'bor] *m* MÚS, TECN drum; *músico* drummer; ANAT eardrum

tamborilar [tãbori'lar] ⟨1a⟩ *com dedos* tap; *chuva* patter

Tâmisa, *Port* **Tamisa** [tʌ'miza] *f* Thames

tampa ['tãpa] *f* lid; *garrafa*: stopper; *roda*: cap; *fogão*: hood; ***~ de rosca*** screw top; ***~ do radiador*** radiator cap

tampinha [tã'piɲa] *pia*: plug; ***~ de rosca*** screw top

tampão [tã'pãw] *m* plug; *de algodão* wad; MED tampon; ***zona*** *f* ***~*** buffer zone

tampo ['tãpu] *m* table top; *sanita*: lid

tampouco [tã'poku] *adv* ***eu ~*** me neither; ***não tenho dinheiro – eu ~*** I don't have any money - me neither, neither do I; ***eu não posso ir – eu ~*** I can't go - me neither, neither can I

tanga ['tãga] *f* tanga; *fam* lie

tangente [tã'ʒẽtʃi] *f* MAT tangent; ***à ~*** barely, just; ***passar à ~*** just scrape through

tangerina [tãʒe'rina] *f* BOT tangerine

tangerineira [tãʒeri'nejra] *f* tangerine tree

tangível [tã'ʒivew] *adj* tangible

tango ['tãgu] *m* tango

tanque ['tãki] *m* (*recipiente*), MIL tank; ***~ de água*** water tank; *lavar a roupa*: sink

tantalizante [tãtali'zãtʃi] *adj* tantalizing

tanto ['tãtu] **1** *adj quantidade*: so much; *plural* so many; *interr, negativo* as much; *plural* as many; ***esperei ~ tempo*** I waited so long; ***estava ~ calor*** it was so hot **2** *adv* so much; *temporal* so long; ***~ melhor / pior*** so much the better / worse; ***é um advogado e ~*** he's some lawyer; ***~ Rio como São Paulo*** both Rio and São Paulo **3** *pron* ***~ quanto pude*** as much as I could; ***~ (me) faz*** I don't mind; ***outro ~*** just as much; ***às tantas*** in the small hours

Tanzânia [tã'zʌnja] *f* Tanzania

tão [tãw] *adv* so, that; ***~ caro*** so expensive, that expensive; ***~ bonito quanto*** as pretty as

tão-pouco [tãw'poku] *adv Port* → ***tampouco***

tapa ['tapa] *f fam* slap

tapar [ta'par] ⟨1b⟩ cover; *erro* cover up; *garrafa* put the stopper in; *tacho* put the lid on; *buraco* fill in

tapeçaria [tapesa'ria] *f* tapestry

T

tapete [ta'peʧi] *m* carpet; (*passadeira*) rug; ESP mat; **~ *de banheiro*** bath mat; **~ *rolante*** conveyor belt
tapume [ta'pumi] *m* wooden fence
taquicardia [takikaɾ'dʒia] *f* MED palpitations
tara ['taɾa] *f* COM tare; MED hereditary defect; *doença* hereditary illness
tarado [ta'ɾadu] *adj fig* (*louco*) crazy; ***ser* ~ *por*** be crazy about
tarântula [ta'ɾɐ̃tula] *f* ZOOL tarantula
tardar [taɾ'daɾ] ⟨1b⟩ **1** *v/t* delay **2** *v/i* delay (***em*** to); (*ficar*) take one's time; (*atrasar-se*) be late; (*demorar*) take a long time; ***não* ~** be quick
tarde ['taɾdʒi] **1** *adv* late; ***cedo ou* ~** sooner or later **2** *f* afternoon; *fim da tarde* evening; ***à* ~, *de* ~** in the afternoon / evening
tardinha [taɾ'dʒiɲa] *f* late afternoon, early evening; ***pela* ~** toward evening
tardio [taɾ'dʒiu] *adj* AGR late
tarefa [ta'ɾɛfa] *f* task, job
tareia [ta'ɾeja] *f* thrashing
tarifa [ta'ɾifa] *f* tariff; **~ *aérea*** air fare; **~ *do correio*** postage; **~ *única*** flat rate
tarifário [taɾi'faɾiu] **1** *m* price list **2** *adj* price *atr*; ***aumento*** *m* **~** price increase
tarimba [ta'ɾĩba] *f* bunk
tarrafa [ta'hafa] *peixe*: haul
tartaruga [taɾta'ɾuga] *f* tortoise; *material* tortoise shell; **~ *marinha*** turtle
tasca ['taska] *f* bar
tatear [ta'ʧiaɾ] ⟨1l⟩ **1** *v/t* touch **2** *v/i* grope
tática ['taʧika] *f* tactics
tático ['taʧiku] **1** *adj* tactical **2** *m*, **-a** *f* tactician
tato ['tatu] *m* touch; *fig* tact, tactfulness; ***falta*** *f* ***de* ~** tactlessness
tatuagem [ta'twaʒẽ] *f* tattoo
tatuar [ta'twaɾ] ⟨1g⟩ tattoo
tauromaquia [tawɾoma'kia] *f* bullfighting
tauromáquico [tawɾo'makiku] *adj* bull-fighting *atr*
tautologia [tawtolo'ʒia] *f* tautology
taxa ['taʃa] *f televisão etc*: fee; (*imposto*) tax; FIN **~ *bancária*** bank rate; FIN **~ *básica de juros*** base rate; **~ *de admissão*** entrance fee; **~ *de aeroporto*** airport tax; **~ *de aumento*** growth rate; **~ *de câmbio*** exchange rate; **~ *de cancelamento*** cancellation fee; FIN **~ *de desconto*** base rate; **~ *de entrega*** delivery charge; **~ *extra*** extra charge; **~ *de inflação*** inflation rate; **~ *de juros*** interest (rate); **~ *de mortalidade infantil*** infant mortality rate; **~ *de natalidade*** birth rate; **~ *de proteção*** protection money; **~ *de serviço*** service charge
taxação [taʃa'sɐ̃w] *f* estimate; *impostos*: taxation; *preços*: fixing
taxar [ta'ʃaɾ] ⟨1b⟩ (*avaliar*) estimate (***em*** at); *preço etc* fix (***de*** of); *mercadoria* tax; *despesas* restrict
taxativo [taʃa'ʧivu] *adj* categorical; ***preço*** *m* **~** fixed price
táxi ['taksi] *m* taxi
taxímetro [ta'ksimetɾu] *m* taxi meter
taxista [ta'ksista] *m/f* taxi driver
tchau [ʧaw] *int* **~!** bye!
tcheco ['ʃɛku] *Bras* **1** *adj* Czech; ***República*** *f* ***Tcheca*** Czech Republic **2** *m*, **-a** *f* Czech **3** *m lingua* Czech
te [ʧi] *pron* you
teagem ['teaʒẽ] *f* TÊX cloth; ANAT tissue
tear ['ʧiaɾ] *m* loom; **~ *de malha*** knitting machine
teatral [ʧia'tɾaw] *adj* theatrical
teatro ['ʧiatɾu] *m* theater, *Brit* theatre; **~ *de revista*** vaudeville, *Brit* variety
teça ['tɛsa] *f* teak
tecedor [tese'doɾ] *m*, **-eira** [tese'dejɾa] *f* weaver; *fig* cause
tecelagem [tese'laʒẽ] *f* weaving; ***fábrica*** *f* ***de* ~** mill
tecelão [tese'lɐ̃w] *m*, **teceloa** [tese'loa] *f* weaver
tecer [te'seɾ] ⟨2g⟩ weave; *fig* think up; *intrigas* plot; **~ *louvores*** (*ou* ***hinos de louvor***) ***a alguém*, ~ *o elogio de alguém*** sing s.o.'s praises
tecido [te'sidu] *m* ANAT tissue; *fig* fabric; *vestuário*: material, cloth
tecla ['tɛkla] *f* key; INFORM **~ *de comando*** control (key); **~ *de escape*** escape (key); **~ *de enter*** enter (key); **~ *de função*** function key; **~ *de maiúscula*** shift key; **~ *de retor-***

T

no backspace key; ***~ de stop*** stop button
teclado [te'kladu] *m* keyboard; ***telefone*** *m* ***de ~*** keypad telephone
técnica ['tɛknika] *f* technique
técnico ['tɛkniku] **1** *adj* technical **2** *m*, **-a** *f* technician; (*especialista*) expert; ESP coach, trainer
tecnocrata [tɛkno'krata] *m/f* technocrat
tecnofobia [tɛknofo'bia] *f* technophobia
tecnologia [tɛknolo'ʒia] *f* technology; ***transferência*** *f* ***de ~*** technology transfer; ***de alta ~*** hitech; ***~ de informática*** information technology; ***~ de ponta*** leading-edge technology
tecnológico [tɛkno'lɔʒiku] *adj* technological; ***parque*** *m* ***~*** technology park
tecto *Port* → ***teto***
tédio ['tɛdiu] *m* tedium, boredom
teia ['teja] *f* web; *trama*: plot; ***~ de aranha*** spider's web, cobweb
Teerão [tee'rãw] *sem art* Tehran
teima ['tejma] *f* stubbornness
teimar [tej'maɾ] ⟨1a⟩ be stubborn; (*insistir*) insist (***em*** on)
teimosia [tejmo'zia] *f* stubbornness
teimoso [tej'mozu] *adj* stubborn
teixo ['tejʃu] *m* yew
tejadilho [teʒa'dʒiʎu] *m* cover; AUTO roof; ***~ de abrir*** sliding roof
tela ['tɛla] *f* material; ARTE canvas; CINE, INFORM screen; (*pintura*) painting; ***vir à ~*** be mentioned, come up; ***~ de ajuda*** help screen; ***~ de cristal líquido*** LCD-screen; ***~ de radar*** radar screen; ***~ sensível ao toque*** touch screen, touch-sensitive screen
tele... [tɛlɛ-, ʧile-] tele...
telecomando [tɛleko'mãdu] *m* remote control
telecomunicação [tɛlekomunika'sãw] *f* telecommunication; ***telecomunicações*** *pl* telecommunications *pl*
telefax [tɛle'faks] *m* fax
teleférico [tele'fɛriku] *m* cable car
telefilme [tɛle'filmi] *m* television film
telefonar [telefo'naɾ] ⟨1f⟩ telephone, phone; ***~ a alguém*** telephone s.o., call s.o.
telefone [tele'fɔni] *m* telephone, phone; ***atender o ~*** answer the phone; ***~ celular*** cell phone, *Brit* mobile phone; ***~ fixo*** fixed phone; ***~ móvel*** cell phone, *Brit* mobile phone; ***~ sem fio*** cordless (phone)
telefonema [telefo'nema] *m* phonecall; ***dar um ~ a alguém*** call s.o.; ***~ a pagar pelo destinatário*** collect call
telefonia [telefo'nia] *f* telephony; ***empresa*** *f* ***de ~*** telephone company
telefônico, *Port* **telefónico** [tele'foniku] *adj* telephone *atr*; ***chamada*** *f* ***telefônica*** telephone call; ***conversa*** *f* ***telefônica*** telephone conversation; ***lista*** *f* ***telefônica*** phonebook; ***rede*** *f* ***telefônica*** telephone network
telefonista [telefo'nista] *m/f* operator
teleguiado [tɛle'gjadu] *adj* remote controlled
telejornal [tɛleʒoɾ'naw] *m* TV news *sg*
telemóvel [tɛle'mɔvew] *m* cell phone, *Brit* mobile (phone)
telenovela [tɛleno'vɛla] *f* soap (opera)
teleobjetiva, *Port* **teleobjectiva** [tɛleobiʒe'ʧiva] *f* telephoto lens *sg*
telepatia [telepa'ʧia] *f* telepathy
telepático [tele'paʧiku] *adj* telepathic
telescópio [teles'kɔpiu] *m* telescope
telespectador [tɛlespekta'doɾ] **1** *adj* viewing *atr* **2** *m*, **-a** *f* viewer
telesqui [teles'ki] *m* ski tow
televisão [televi'zãw] *f* ⟨*sem pl*⟩ television; ***ver ~*** watch television; ***~ a cores*** color television, *Brit* colour television; ***~ digital*** digital television; ***~ por cabo*** cable (TV); ***~ por satélite*** satellite TV
televendas [tɛle'vẽdas] *fpl* telesales
televisivo [televi'zivu] *adj* television *atr*
televisionar [televizio'naɾ] ⟨1a⟩ *vt* televise
televisor [televi'zoɾ] *m* television, TV (set)
telha ['teʎa] *f* tile; *fam* ***estar com a ~*** be in a bad mood

T

telhado [te'ʎadu] *m* roof; ***área** f **de ~*** roof area
tem [tẽ], **têm** ['tẽẽ] *etc* → ***ter***
tema ['tema] *m* theme; *Bras* ***~ de casa*** homework
temático [te'matʃiku] *adj* thematic; GRAM root *atr*
temer [te'mer] ⟨2c⟩ be afraid of, fear
temerário [teme'rariu] *adj* reckless
temeridade [temeri'dadʒi] *f* recklessness
temível [te'mivew] *adj* dreadful, fearsome
temor [te'mor] *m* fear
têmpera ['tẽpera] *f metal*: tempering; (*cunha*) wedge; *fig* type; ***pintura** f **a ~*** distemper
temperado [tẽpe'radu] *adj* temperate *tb clima*; (*comedido*) measured; MÚS tuned; GASTR seasoned
temperamento [tẽpera'mẽtu] *m* temperament
temperar [tẽpe'rar] ⟨1c⟩ **1** *v/t metal* temper, harden; *fig* temper; GASTR season; *vinho* water down; MÚS tune **2** *v/i* ***~ com*** blend in with
temperatura [tẽpera'tura] *f* temperature; ***~ ambiente*** room temperature
tempero [tẽ'peru] *m* seasoning
tempestade [tẽpes'tadʒi] *f* storm
tempestuoso [tẽpes'twozu] *adj* tempestuous
templo ['tẽplu] *m* temple
tempo[1] ['tẽpu] *m* time; MÚS tempo, time; GRAM tense; ESP timeout; ***a ~*** on time; ***matar o ~*** kill time; ***ao mesmo ~*** at the same time; ***há muito ~*** a long time ago; ***quanto ~?*** how long?; ***emprego** m **em ~ parcial*** part-time job; TV ***~ de antena*** transmission time; ***~ de garantia*** guarantee period; INFORM ***~ real*** real time; ***~s** pl **livres*** free time
tempo[2] ['tẽpu] *m* (*atmosférico*) weather; ***bom / mau ~*** good / bad weather
têmpora ['tẽpora] *f* ANAT temple
temporada [tẽpo'rada] *f* period; (*estação*), TEAT season
temporal [tẽpo'raw] **1** *adj* worldly, GRAM tense *atr* **2** *m* (*borrasca*) storm
temporário [tẽpo'rariu] *adj* temporary
tenacidade [tenasi'dadʒi] *f* tenacity
tenaz [te'nas] **1** *adj* tenacious **2** *f* **~ (*es*)** (*pl*) tongs *pl*
tenção [tẽ'sãw] *f* intention
tencionar [tẽsjo'nar] ⟨1f⟩ intend
tenda ['tẽda] *f* tent; *mercado*: stall
tendão [tẽ'dãw] *m* ANAT tendon
tendência [tẽ'dẽsja] *f* tendency; *moda*: trend
tendencioso [tẽdẽ'sjozu] *adj* tendentious
tender [tẽ'der] ⟨2a⟩ *v/i* ***~ a, ~ para algo*** tend toward sth; (*tencionar*) aim at sth; ***~ a fazer algo*** tend to do sth
tenebroso [tene'brozu] *adj* dark
tenente [te'nẽtʃi] *m* lieutenant
tenente coronel [tenẽtʃikoro'nɛw] *m* lieutenant colonel
tenho ['teɲu] *etc* → ***ter***
tênia, *Port* **ténia** ['tenja] *f* tapeworm
tênis, *Port* **ténis** ['tenis] *m* tennis; **~** *pl* sneakers, *Brit* trainers; *Bras* ***~ de gramado*** lawn tennis; ***~ de mesa*** table tennis; *Port* ***~ de relvado*** lawn tennis
tenista [te'nista] *m/f* tennis player
tenor [te'nor] *m* MÚS tenor
tens [tẽs] → ***ter***
tensão [tẽ'sãw] *f* tension *tb fig*; ELÉT voltage; ***alta ~*** high tension; ***~ arterial*** blood pressure
tenso ['tẽsu] *adj* taught, tight; *fig* tense
tentação [tẽta'sãw] *f* temptation
tentáculo [tẽ'takulu] *m* tentacle *tb fig*
tentador [tẽta'dor] **1** *adj* tempting **2** *m*, **-a** *f* tempter; temptress
tentar [tẽ'tar] ⟨1a⟩ try; (*arriscar*) risk; ***~ fazer algo*** try to do sth; (*seduzir*) ***~ alguém*** lead s.o. into temptation
tentativa [tẽta'tʃiva] *f* attempt; ***~ de fazer algo*** attempt to do sth
tênue, *Port* **ténue** ['tenwi] *adj* tenuous; (*suave*) delicate; (*fino*) thin
teologia [teolo'ʒia] *f* theology
teológico [teo'lɔʒiku] *adj* theological
teólogo ['teɔlogu] *m*, **-a** *f* theologian
teor [teor] *m dum texto* gist; (*tipo*) type; ***~ de álcool no sangue*** blood alcohol level
teorema [teo'rema] *m* theorem
teoria [teo'ria] *f* theory
teorético [teo'rɛtʃiku] *adj* → ***teórico***

teoricamente [teɔrika'mẽtʃi] *adv* theoretically, in theory
teórico ['teɔriku] **1** *adj* theoretical **2** *m*, **-a** *f* theoretician
tépido ['tɛpidu] *adj* tepid, lukewarm
ter [teɾ] ⟨2x⟩ **1** *v/t* ◇ have; (*conter*) hold; ***tenho duas irmãs*** I have two sisters, I've got two sisters; ~ ***lugar*** take place; ***que idade tem?*** how old are you?; ~ ***que ver com*** have to do with; ~ ***vestido um …*** be wearing a …, have a … on; ***ir ~ com alguém*** go to meet s.o.; ***não tem de quê*** don't mention it
◇ ***ter que fazer algo*** have to do sth; ***eu tenho que …*** I must …, I have to …, I've got to …
◇ ***tem um carro lá fora*** there is a car outside; ***tem dois carros*** there are two cars; ***tinha dois carros*** there were two cars
2 *v/aux perfeito e mais-que-perfeito* have; ~ ***amado*** to have loved
terapeuta [teɾa'pewta] *m/f* therapist; ~ ***de linguagem*** speech therapist; ~ ***ocupacional*** occupational therapist
terapêutica [teɾa'pewtʃika] *f* therapy
terapêutico [teɾa'pewtʃiku] *adj* therapeutic; ***efeito*** *m* ~ therapeutic effect
terapia [teɾa'pia] *f* therapy; ~ ***genética*** gene therapy; ~ ***de grupo*** group therapy; ~ ***laser*** laser therapy; ~ ***de linguagem*** speech therapy; ~ ***ocupacional*** occupational therapy
terça ['teɾsa] **1** *adj* ~ ***parte*** *f* third **2** *f fam* → ***terça-feira***
terça-feira [teɾsa'fejɾa] *f* ⟨*pl* terças-feiras⟩ Tuesday; ***na*** ~ on Tuesday; ***às ~s*** on Tuesdays; ~ ***de carnaval*** Mardi Gras
terceira [teɾ'sejɾa] *f* MÚS third
terceiro [teɾ'sejɾu] **1** *adj* third **2** *m* third party; ***seguro*** *m* ***de ~s*** third party insurance
terceiro-mundista [teɾsejɾumũ'dʒista] *adj* Third World *atr*
terceto [teɾ'setu] *m* MÚS trio
terço ['teɾsu] *m parte*: third; REL rosary; ***rezar o*** ~ say a rosary
terebintina [terebĩ'tʃina] *f* turpentine
terei [te'ɾej] *etc* → ***ter***

termal [teɾ'maw] *adj* thermal
termas ['tɛɾmas] *fpl* spa
térmico ['tɛɾmiku] *adj* thermal; ***garrafa*** *f* ~ thermos® flask
terminação [teɾmina'sãw] *f* GRAM ending
terminado [teɾmi'nadu] *adj* finished
terminal [teɾmi'naw] **1** *m* INFORM, AERO, MAR terminal; *ônibus*: depot **2** *adj* terminal; ***doente*** *m/f* ~ terminally ill patient; ***estação*** *f* ~ terminus
terminantemente [teɾminãtʃi'mẽtʃi] *adv negar* flatly
terminar [teɾmi'naɾ] ⟨1a⟩ **1** *v/t* finish, end **2** *v/i* finish, end; (*acabar*) end (***em*** in); (*fechar*) close; ~ ***de fazer algo*** finish doing sth
terminologia [teɾminolo'ʒia] *f* terminology
termo[1] ['tɛɾmu] *m Port* thermos® flask
termo[2] ['teɾmu] *m* boundary; (*marco*) boundary marker; (*fim*) end; (*prazo*) deadline; (*expressão*) term; (*palavra*), MAT term; ***pôr ~ a algo*** put an end to sth; ~ ***de comparação*** point of comparison; ~ ***técnico*** technical term; ~ ***médio, meio ~*** compromise
termodinâmica [tɛɾmodʒi'nʌmika] *f* thermodynamics
termômetro, *Port* **termómetro** [teɾ'mometɾu] *m* thermometer
termonuclear [tɛɾmonukli'aɾ] *adj* thermonuclear
termóstato [teɾ'mɔstatu] *m*, **termostato** [tɛɾmos'tatu] *m* thermostat
terno[1] ['tɛɾnu] *adj* tender
terno[2] ['tɛɾnu] *m Bras* suit
ternura [teɾ'nuɾa] *f* tenderness
terra ['tɛha] *f* land; (*solo*) earth; (*pátria*) country; (*propriedade*) land; (*região*) region; ELÉT ground, *Brit* earth; ***~s*** *pl* land; ~ ***firme*** dry land; ~ ***natal*** native land; ***a Terra*** *planeta* the Earth; ***Terra do Fogo*** Tierra del Fuego; ***Terra Nova*** Newfoundland; AERO ***pessoal*** *m* ***de*** ~ ground staff
terra-a-terra [tɛha'tɛha] *adj* down-to-earth
terraço [te'hasu] *m* terrace
terramoto [teha'mɔtu] *m Port* earthquake

terra-nova [tɛha'nɔva] *m cão* Newfoundland
terraplenagem [tɛhaple'naʒẽ] *f* earthmoving
terreiro [te'hejɾu] *m (espaço)* open space
terremoto [tehe'mɔtu] *m Bras* earthquake
terreno [te'henu] **1** *adj* earth *atr*; REL earthly **2** *m* ground; (*propriedade, campo*) land; ***um ~*** a piece of land; ***~ para construção*** building site
térreo ['tɛhiu] *adj* ground level; ***andar m ~*** first floor, *Brit* ground floor
terrestre [te'hɛstɾi] *adj* terrestrial; *rota* overland; (*oposto a celeste*) earthly
terrificar [tehifi'kaɾ] ⟨1n⟩ terrify
terrífico [te'hifiku] *adj* terrifying
terrina [te'hina] *f* tureen
territorial [tehito'ɾjaw] *adj* territorial; POL ***águas** fpl **territoriais*** territorial waters
território [tehi'tɔɾiu] *m* territory
terrível [te'hivew] *adj* terrible
terror [te'hoɾ] *m* terror
terrorismo [teho'ɾizmu] *m* terrorism
terrorista [teho'ɾista] **1** *m/f* terrorist; ***~ suicida*** suicide bomber **2** *adj* terrorist *atr*
terrorizar [tehoɾi'zaɾ] ⟨1a⟩ terrorize
tese ['tɛzi] *f* thesis; ***em ~*** in theory
teso ['tezu] *adj* stiff, rigid; (*corajoso*) brave; *fam* ***estar ~*** be broke; *fam* ***ficar ~*** have a hard-on
tesoira *etc* → ***tesoura*** *etc*
tesoura [te'zoɾa] *f* scissors *pl*; *caranguejo*: pincers *pl*; ***uma ~*** a pair of scissors; ***~ de unha*** nail scissors
tesouraria [tezoɾa'ɾia] *f* treasury; ***Tesouraria da Fazenda Pública*** Treasury
tesoureiro [tezo'ɾejɾu] *m*, **-a** *f* treasurer
tesouro [te'zoɾu] *m* treasure; LIT treasury; ***~ público*** Treasury
testa ['tɛsta] *f* forehead
testamentário [testamẽ'taɾiu] *adj* of a / the will
testamenteiro [testamẽ'tejɾu] *m*, **-a** *f* executor
testamento [testa'mẽtu] *m* will; REL ***Velho** / **Novo Testamento*** Old / New Testament
testar [tes'taɾ] ⟨1a⟩ test
teste ['tɛstʃi] *m* test; ***~ de aptidão*** aptitude test; ***~ cinematográfico*** screen test; AUTO ***~ de emissões de tubo de escape*** emissions test; ***~ de inteligência*** IQ test; ***~ de múltipla escolha*** multiple choice question; ***~ de sangue*** blood test; ***~ da SIDA*** Aids test
testemunha [teste'muɲa] *f* witness; ***~s** pl **de acusação*** witnesses for the prosecution; ***~ ocular*** eye witness
testemunhar [testemu'ɲaɾ] ⟨1a⟩ **1** *v/t* testify as to, give evidence about; (*ver*) witness **2** *v/i* testify (***de*** as to)
testemunho [teste'muɲu] evidence, testimony; (*prova*) evidence
testículo [tes'tʃikulu] *m* testicle
testificar [testʃifi'kaɾ] ⟨1n⟩ testify to; (*assegurar*) maintain; (*atestar*) attest to
tesudo [tez'udu] *adj fam* horny
teta ['teta] *f* ZOOL teat; *vaca*: udder; *vulg* tit
tétano ['tɛtanu] *m* MED tetanus
tetina [te'tʃina] *f do biberão* teat
teto ['tɛtu] *m* ceiling; *fig* roof; (*abrigo*) shelter; ***~ solar*** sun roof
teu [tew] **1** *adj* your **2** *pron* yours
teve ['tevi] → ***ter***
têxtil ['testʃiw] **1** *adj* textile *atr*; ***indústria** f **~*** textile industry **2** *m* textile; ***têxteis*** *pl* textiles
texto ['testu] *m* text
textual [tes'twaw] *adj* textual; *significado* literal
textura [tes'tuɾa] *f* texture
texugo [te'ʃugu] *m* badger; ***ele está gordo que nem um ~*** he's a fatso
tez [tes] *f* complexion
TI *f abr* (***tecnologia informática***) IT (Information Technology)
tia ['tʃia] *f* aunt(y)
tia-avó [tʃia'vɔ] *f* ⟨pl tias-avós⟩ great aunt
tíbia ['tʃibja] *f* ANAT shinbone, tibia
ticar [tʃi'kaɾ] ⟨1a⟩ check, *Brit* tick
ticket [tʃi'ket] *m* ticket
tido ['tʃidu] *pp* → ***ter***
tiete [tʃi'ɛtʃi] *f fam* groupie

tifo ['ʧifu] *m* MED typhus
tifóide [ʧi'fɔidʒi] *adj* typhoid; ***febre f ~*** typhus
tigela [ʧi'ʒɛla] *f* bowl
tigelada [ʧiʒe'lada] *f* GASTR *sweet dish made from eggs and milk*
tigre ['ʧigɾi] *m* tiger
tijolo [ʧi'ʒolu] *m* brick
til [ʧiw] *m* tilde
tília ['ʧilja] *f* lime; ***chá m de ~*** lime blossom tea
tilintar [ʧilĩ'taɾ] ⟨1a⟩ jingle, tinkle
timão [ʧi'mãw] *m* NÁUT (*leme*) tiller, helm; ESP *fam* great team
timbrar [ʧĩ'bɾaɾ] *v/t* stamp
timbre ['ʧĩbɾi] *m* MÚS timbre; (*carimbo*) stamp; (*insígnia*) insignia; (*logotipo*) logo; (*cabeçalho*) letterhead
time ['ʧimi] *f Bras* team
timidez [ʧimi'des] *f* timidity, shyness
tímido ['ʧimidu] *adj* timid, shy
Timor-Leste [ʧimoɾ'lɛsʧi] *m* East Timor
timoneiro [ʧimo'nejɾu] *m* NÁUT, *fig* helmsman
tímpano ['ʧĩpanu] *m* MÚS kettledrum; ANAT (***membrana f do***) **~** eardrum
tímpanite [ʧĩpa'niʧi] *f* inflammation of the middle ear
tingir [ʧĩ'ʒiɾ] ⟨3n⟩ dye; ***papel tingido*** tinted paper
tinha ['ʧiɲa] *etc* → ***ter***
tinido [ʧi'nidu] *m* jingle
tinir [ʧi'niɾ] ⟨3a⟩ jingle; *sino, ouvidos* ring
tinta ['ʧĩta] *f de escrever* ink; *geral* paint; *para cabelo* dye; *fam* ***estou-me nas ~s*** I don't mind; ***~ plástica*** emulsion; ***~ fresca!*** wet paint!
tintim [ʧĩ'ʧĩ] *m* ***~ por ~*** blow by blow
tintura [ʧĩ'tuɾa] *f* dye; *ato* dyeing
tinto ['ʧĩtu] *adj vinho* red
tinturaria [ʧĩtura'ɾia] *f* (*limpeza a seco*) dry cleaner
tio ['ʧiu] *m* uncle
tio-avô [ʧioa'vo] *m* great uncle
típicamente [ʧipika'mẽʧi] *adv* typically
típico ['ʧipiku] *adj* typical
tipo ['ʧipu] *m* type; *imprensa*: print; *Port fam* guy
tipografia [ʧipogɾa'fia] *f* print works *sg*; *arte* printing
tipográfico [ʧipo'gɾafiku] *adj* printing *atr*
tipógrafo [ʧi'pɔgɾafu] *m*, **-a** *f* printer
tique[1] ['ʧiki] *m* checkmark, *Brit* tick
tique[2] ['ʧiki] *m* tick; ***~ nervoso*** nervous tick, twitch
tique-taque ['ʧiketaki] *m* ticking, tick-tock
tiquete [ʧi'keʧi] *m* ticket
tira ['ʧiɾa] *f* strip; ***fazer em ~s*** shred; ***~ cômica*** comic strip
tira-cápsulas [ʧiɾa'kapsulas] *m* ⟨*pl inv*⟩ bottle opener
tira-caricas [ʧiɾaka'ɾikas] *m* ⟨*pl inv*⟩ bottle opener
tiragem [ʧi'ɾaʒẽ] *f chaminé*: draft, *Brit* draught; TIPO printing; (*edição*) prinrun; *correio*: collection
tirânico [ʧi'ɾʌniku] *adj* tyrannical
tiranizar [ʧiɾani'zaɾ] ⟨1a⟩ tyrannize
tirano [ʧi'ɾanu] **1** *m*, **-a** *f* tyrant **2** *adj* tyrannical
tira-nódoas [ʧiɾa'nɔdwas] *m* ⟨*pl inv*⟩ stain-remover
tirar [ʧi'ɾaɾ] ⟨1a⟩ *v/t* take; (*sacar*) take away; *dente* take out, extract; *sapatos, casaco* take off; *mesa* clear; *dor* take away; *nódoa* remove, get rid off; MATH take away; *conclusão* draw; ***~ algo de algo*** take sth out of sth; ***~ o dia*** take the day off; **tirar-se** *v/r* (*afastar-se*) step aside; (*libertar-se*) get away; ***~ de apuros*** get out of trouble
tiritar [ʧiɾi'taɾ] ⟨1a⟩ *de frio* shiver
tiro ['ʧiɾu] *m* shot; (*tiroteio*) shooting; ***ela levou um ~*** she was shot; ***~ de meta*** goalkick
tiróide [ʧi'ɾɔidʒi] *f* thyroid gland
tiroteio [ʧiɾo'teiu] *m* ***escutar um ~*** hear gunfire, hear shooting; ***acabou num ~*** it ended in a shootout
tísica ['ʧizika] *f* MED consumption
tísico ['ʧiziku] *adj* consumptive
titubear [ʧitu'bjaɾ] ⟨1l⟩ stagger; (*vacilar*) hesitate; (*gaguejar*) stammer
titular [ʧitu'laɾ] **1** *v/t* ⟨1a⟩ title; (*registar*) register **2** *adj* titular … **3** *m/f* title holder; (*detentor*) holder
título ['ʧitulu] *m* title; (*cabeçalho*) heading; (*denominação*) denomina-

tion; FIN bond; ~ ***de campeão*** championship; ~ ***eletoral***, *Port* ~ ***electoral*** voting slip; ~ ***de propriedade*** title deed

tive ['tʃivi] *etc* → ***ter***

to [tu] = *pron* ***te*** + *pron* ***o***

toa ['toa] *adv* ***à*** ~ at random; ***rir à*** ~ laugh out loud; ***ficar à*** ~ lounge about, goof off

toalete [toa'lɛtʃi] *m* toilet, *Am* rest room

toalha ['twaʎa] *f mesa*: tablecloth; *mãos*: towel; *louça*: dishcloth; ~ ***de banho*** bath towel

toalheiro [twa'ʎejɾu] *m* towel rail

toca ['tɔka] *f* hole, den

toca-discos [tɔka'dʒiskus] *m* ⟨*pl inv*⟩ *Bras* record player

tocador [toka'doɾ] *m*, **-a** *f* player; ~ ***de guitarra*** guitar player

toca-fitas [tɔka'fitas] *m* ⟨*pl inv*⟩ cassette player

tocar [to'kaɾ] ⟨1n & 1e⟩ **1** *v/t* touch *tb fig*; (*roçar*) brush; (*acertar*) hit; *música* play **2** *v/i campaínha* ring; ~ ***em*** touch; ***toca a ti*** it's your turn

tocha ['tɔʃa] *f* torch; (*luz*) light

todavia [toda'via] *adv* still, yet

todo ['todu] **1** *adj* ◇ all; ~ ***o bolo*** all the cake, the whole cake; ~***s os bolos*** all the cakes ◇ *cada*: every; ~***s os dias*** every day; ***todas as vezes*** every time **2** *m* ◇ ***o*** ~ ***da humanidade*** all of humanity, the whole of humanity; ***ao*** ~ altogether ◇ ~***s*** everyone, everybody; ~***s nós / eles*** all of us / them

toldo ['towdu] *m* awning

tolerância [tole'rãsja] *f* tolerance *tb* TECN

tolerante [tole'rãtʃi] *adj* tolerant

tolerar [tole'raɾ] ⟨1c⟩ tolerate

tolerável [tole'ravew] *adj* tolerable

tolher [to'ʎeɾ] ⟨2d⟩ hinder; (*proibir*) forbid; ~ ***alguém de algo*** rob s.o. of sth; ~ ***o caminho a alguém*** bar s.o.'s way

tolice [to'lisi] *f* foolishness

tolo ['tolu] **1** *adj* foolish **2** *m*, **-a** *f* fool

tom [tõ] *m* tone; (*escala*) key; *cor*: shade; TEL ~ ***de toque*** ringtone

tomada [to'mada] *f* capture, taking; POL *poder*: takeover; ELÉT outlet, *Brit* socket; *Bras tb* plug; CINE take; ~ ***de posse*** taking office

tomar [to'maɾ] ⟨1f⟩ *v/t* take; *refeição, café, chá etc* have; *ar, peso* get; *temperatura* take; *altura* measure; *tempo, espaço etc* take (up); ***tomara que*** hopefully; ~ ***alguém por algo*** take s.o. for sth

tomate [to'matʃi] *m* tomato; ~ ***cereja*** cherry tomato; *vulg* ~***s*** balls, nuts

tombar [tõ'baɾ] ⟨1a⟩ **1** *v/t* knock over **2** *v/i* fall

tombo ['tõbu] *m* fall

tomilho [to'miʎu] *m* BOT thyme

tomo ['tomu] *m* volume

tomografia [tomogra'fia] *f* tomography; ~ ***computadorizada*** computer-aided tomography

tona ['tona] *f* surface; ***vir à*** ~ come to the surface

tonelada [tone'lada] *f* ton; ~ ***de arqueação*** registered tonnage

tonelagem [tone'laʒẽ] *f* NÁUT tonnage

toner ['toneɾ] *m* toner

tônica, *Port* **tónica** ['tonika] *f* MÚS tonic; *fig* main stress

tônico, *Port* **tónico** ['toniku] **1** *adj* tonic; ***acento*** *m* ~ stress; ***vogal*** *f* ***tônica*** stressed vowel; ***água*** *f* ***tônica*** tonic (water) **2** *m* MED tonic

tonto ['tõtu] **1** *adj* dizzy; (*aturdido*) light-headed; (*tolo*) silly **2** *m*, **-a** *f* silly billy

tontura [tõ'tuɾa] *f* dizzy spell

topar [to'paɾ] **1** *v/t fam* (*perceber*) get **2** *v/i* ~ ***com*** bump into

topázio [to'paziu] *m* topaz

tópico ['tɔpiku] **1** *adj* topical **2** *m* topic

topo ['topu] *m* top

toque ['tɔki] *m* touch; MÚS playing; *tambor*: beat; *sinos*: ringing; *corneta*: sound; *fig* touch, trace; ***os últimos*** ~***s*** the final touches; ***dar um*** ~ ***a alguém*** give s.o. a hint; TEL give s.o. a call, *Brit tb* give s.o. a ring

toranja [tuɾãʒa] *f* BOT grapefruit

tórax ['tɔraks] *m* ANAT thorax

torcedor [torse'doɾ] *m*, **-a** *f* supporter, fan

torcer [toɾ'seɾ] ⟨2g & 2d⟩ **1** *v/t* twist; (*dobrar*) bend; *braço etc* sprain; *roupa* wring out; *nariz* turn up; *sentido*, *palavras* twist; **~ os olhos** go cross-eyed **2** *v/i* **~ por** support; **vou ~ por ti** I'll keep my fingers crossed for you
torcicolo [toɾsi'kɔlu] *m* stiff neck
torcida [toɾ'sida] *f* cheering; (*torcedores*) fans
torcido [toɾ'sidu] *adj* (*teimoso*) strong-minded
tordo ['toɾdu] *m* thrush
tormenta [toɾ'mẽta] *f* storm; *fig* **que ~!** it's such a struggle!
tormento [toɾ'mẽtu] *m* torment
tormentoso [toɾmẽ'tozu] *adj* stormy
tornado [toɾ'nadu] *m* tornado
tornar [toɾ'naɾ] *v/i* go back; **~ a fazer algo** do sth again; **tomar-se** *v/r* become; **~ profissional** turn professional
tornedó [toɾne'dɔ] *m* GASTR tournedos
torneio [toɾ'neiu] *m* ESP tournament
torneira [toɾ'nejɾa] *f* faucet, *Brit* tap
torno ['toɾnu] *m* lathe; **em ~** around; **em ~ de** around
tornozelo [toɾno'zelu] *m* ANAT ankle
torpedeamento [toɾpedʒia'mẽtu] *m* torpedoing
torpedear [toɾpe'dʒiaɾ] ⟨1l⟩ torpedo
torpedeiro [toɾpe'dejɾu] *m* motor torpedo boat
torrada [to'hada] *f* (*tosta*) toast; **uma ~** a piece of toast
torradeira [toha'dejɾa] *f* toaster
torrado [to'hadu] *adj* roast
torrão [to'hãw] *m* lump of earth; *açúcar*: lump; GASTR *confection made from almonds, egg white and sugar*; **torrões** *pl* land
torrar [to'haɾ] ⟨1e⟩ roast; *pão* toast; (*chamuscar*) burn
torre ['tohi] *f* tower; **~ de televisão** television mast
torreão [to'hjãw] *m* MIL turret
torrefação, *Port* **torrefacção** [tohefa'sãw] *f* ⟨*sem pl*⟩ roasting; (**fábrica** *f* **de**) **~** roasting house
torrencial [tohẽ'sjaw] *adj* torrential; **chuva** *f* **~** torrential rain
torrente [to'hẽtʃi] *f* torrent *tb fig*; **a ~ s, em ~s** in torrents
tórrido ['tɔhidu] *adj* torrid
torta ['tɔɾta] *f* pie; *aberta* tart
torto ['toɾtu] **1** *adj* crooked **2** *adv* wrong; **a ~ e a direito** left, right and center
tortuoso [toɾ'twozu] *adj* crooked *tb fig*; (*sinuoso*) tortuous
tortura [toɾ'tuɾa] *f* torture; (*tormento*) torment
torturar [toɾtu'ɾaɾ] ⟨1a⟩ torture; (*tormentar*) torment
tosco ['tosku] *adj* raw; *pedra*, *fig* unpolished
tosquiar [tos'kjaɾ] ⟨1g⟩ *ovelha* shear
tosse ['tɔsi] *f* cough; **~ convulsa** whooping cough; **estar com ~** have a cough
tossicar [tosi'kaɾ] ⟨1n⟩ clear one's throat
tossidela [tosi'dɛla] *f* cough
tossir [to'siɾ] ⟨3f⟩ cough
tosta ['tɔsta] *f* toast; **~ mista** cheese and ham toastie
tostão [tos'tãw] *m hist* **um ~** 10 centavos; *fig* **não valer um ~** not be worth a red cent
tostar [tos'taɾ] ⟨1e⟩ roast; *pão* toast
total [to'taw] **1** *adj* total **2** *m* total; **no ~** in total
totalidade [totali'dadʒi] *f* totality; **na ~** altogether; **a ~ da ...** the entirety of the ...
totalitário [totali'taɾiu] *adj* POL totalitarian
totalmente [totaw'mẽtʃi] *adv* totally
Totobola [toto'bɔla] *m* football pools
Totoloto [toto'lɔtu] *m* lottery
touca ['toka] *f* cap; *natação*: swimming cap; **~ de banho** shower cap
toucinho [to'siɲu] *m* bacon; GASTR **~ do céu** *cake made from almonds, sugar and eggs*
toupeira [to'pejɾa] *f* mole
tourada [to'ɾada] *f* bullfight
toureio [to'ɾeiu] *m* bullfighting
toureiro [to'ɾejɾu] *m* bullfighter
touro ['toɾu] *m* bull; ASTROL **Touro** Taurus; **corrida** *f* **de ~s** bullfight
tóxico ['tɔksiku] **1** *adj* poisonous, toxic **2** *m* poison
toxicodependência [toksikodepẽ-

'dẽsja] *f* drug dependency
toxicodependente [toksikodepẽ'dẽʧi] **1** *adj* drug dependent **2** *m/f* drug addict
toxicomania [toksikoma'nia] *f* drug addiction
toxicômano, *Port* **toxicómano** [toksi'komanu] **1** *adj* drug addicted **2** *m*, **-a** *f* drug addict
toxina [to'ksina] *f* toxin
trabalhão [tɾaba'ʎãw] *m fam* ***um ~*** a lot of work, a big job
trabalhar [tɾaba'ʎaɾ] ⟨1b⟩ work
trabalho [tɾa'baʎu] *m* work; ***um ~*** a job; ***acidente*** *m* ***de ~*** industrial accident; ***autorização*** *f* ***de ~*** work permit; ***dar ~*** create work
trabalhoso [tɾaba'ʎozu] *adj* laborious
traça ['tɾasa] *f* ZOOL moth
traçado [tɾa'sadu] *m* sketch
tração [tɾa'sãw] *f* ⟨*sem pl*⟩ traction; TECN drive; AUTO ***~ à frente*** front-wheel drive; ***~ às quatro rodas*** four-wheel drive
traçar [tɾa'saɾ] ⟨1p & 1b⟩ *linha, círculo* draw; *caminho, limite* mark out; *papel* draw lines on; ***~ o limite em algo*** draw the line at sth
tracção *Port* → ***tração***
traço ['tɾasu] *m* line, dash; *rosto, caráter*: feature; (*vestígio*) trace
tract... *Port* → ***trator...***
tradição [tɾadʒi'sãw] *f* tradition
tradicional [tɾadʒisjo'naw] *adj* traditional
tradicionalismo [tɾadʒisjona'lizmu] *m* traditionalism
tradicionalista [tɾadʒisjona'lista] **1** *adj* traditional **2** *m/f* traditionalist
tradução [tɾadu'sãw] *f* translation
tradutor [tɾadu'toɾ] *m*, **-a** *f* translator
traduzir [tɾadu'ziɾ] ⟨3m⟩ translate (***para*** into)
tráfego ['tɾafegu] *m* traffic
traficante [tɾafi'kãʧi] *m/f* trafficker, dealer; ***~ de droga*** drug dealer
traficar [tɾafi'kaɾ] ⟨1n⟩ *v/t* deal in
tráfico ['tɾafiku] *m* trade; *ilegal* traffic; ***~ de armas*** arms dealing; ***~ de droga*** drug trafficking; ***~ de mulheres*** traffic in women, sex trafficking
tragar [tɾa'gaɾ] *v/t* swallow *tb fig*; (*aspirar*) inhale; *fig* tolerate
tragédia [tɾa'ʒɛdʒia] *f* tragedy *tb fig*
trágico ['tɾaʒiku] *adj* tragic
tragicomédia [tɾaʒiko'mɛdʒia] *f* tragicomedy
trago[1] ['tɾagu] *m* swallow; *fumo*: drag; ***de um só ~*** in one
trago[2] ['tɾagu] → ***trazer***
traição [tɾaj'sãw] *f* treason; ***alta ~*** high treason; ***~ de alguém / algo*** betrayal of s.o. / sth
traiçoeiro [tɾaj'swejɾu] *adj* treacherous; (*falso*) disloyal; (*enganador*) deceptive
traidor [tɾaj'doɾ] *m*, **-a** *f* traitor
trailer ['tɾejleɾ] *m* CINE trailer; AUTO (*atrelado*) trailer, *Brit* caravan
trair [tɾa'iɾ] ⟨3l⟩ betray; (*enganar*) be unfaithful to
trajar [tɾa'ʒaɾ] ⟨1b⟩ **1** *v/t* wear **2** *v/i* dress (***de*** as); ***~ de festa*** put on one's best clothes
traje ['tɾaʒi] *m* dress; (*fato*) suit; (*conjunto*) costume; ***~ de banho*** swimsuit; ***~ de cerimônia***, ***~ a rigor*** evening dress
traject... *Port* → ***trajet...***
trajeto [tɾa'ʒɛtu] *m* route; (*caminho*) path
trajetória [tɾaʒe'tɔɾja] *f* trajectory; *fig* course
trama ['tɾama] *f* plot
tramar [tɾa'maɾ] *v/t* weave; *fig* hatch
trâmite ['tɾʌmiʧi] *m* (official) procedure; ***~s*** *pl* ***de entrada*** entry formalities
trampolim [tɾãpo'lĩ] *m piscina*: diving board; *flexível* springboard; *ginástica*: trampoline
tranca ['tɾãka] *f* bolt; *dispositivo*: lock; AUTO ***~ central das portas*** central locking
trancafiar [tɾãka'fjaɾ] ⟨1g⟩ *v/t* lock in; *prisão*: lock up
trança ['tɾãsa] *f* braid, *Brit* plait
trancar [tɾã'kaɾ] ⟨1n⟩ lock
tranqüilamente, *Port* **tranquilamente** [tɾãkwila'mẽʧi] *adv* peacefully
tranqüilidade, *Port* **tranquilidade** [tɾãkwili'dadʒi] *f* tranquility, *Brit* tranquillity; (*silêncio*) silence

T

tranqüilizante, *Port* **tranquilizante** [trãkwili'zãtʃi] *m* tranquilizer, *Brit* tranquillizer
tranqüilizar, *Port* **tranquilizar** [trãkwili'zar] ⟨1a⟩ calm; ***a tua carta tranqüilizou-me*** your letter put my mind at rest
tranqüilo, *Port* **tranquilo** [trã'kwilu] *adj* peaceful, tranquil; (*calmo*) calm
transa ['trãza] *f Bras fam* deal; (*caso*) affair
transação, *Port* **transacção** [trãza'sãw] *f* COM transaction; ***ter transações com*** do business with
transacionar, *Port* **transaccionar** [trãzasjo'nar] ⟨1f⟩ trade; COM deal
transacto *Port* → ***transato***
transar [trã'zar] ⟨1a⟩ *v/i* **~ *com*** have sex with
transatlântico [trãza'tlãtʃiku] **1** *adj* transatlantic **2** *m* ocean liner
transato [trã'zatu] *adj* past, previous
transbordar [trãzbor'dar] **1** *v/i* overflow **2** *v/t mercadoria* transship
transbordo [trãz'bordu] *m mercadoria*: transshipment
transcender [trãsẽ'der] ⟨2a⟩ *v/t* transcend
transcrever [trãskre'ver] ⟨2c; *pp* transcrito⟩ transcribe
transcrição [trãskri'sãw] *f* transcription; **~ *fonética*** phonetic transcription
transcrito [trãs'kritu] **1** *pp* → ***transcrever*** **2** *m* transcript
transeunte [trã'zeũtʃi] *m/f* passer-by
transferência [trãsfe'rẽsja] *f* transfer
transferir [trãsfe'rir] ⟨3c⟩ transfer; *prazo* put back
transferível [trãsfe'rivew] *adj* transferable; *prazo* alterable
transfigurar [trãsfigu'rar] ⟨1a⟩ transfigure; (*deformar*) distort
transformação [trãsforma'sãw] *f* transformation
transformador [trãsforma'dor] *m* ELÉT transformer
transformar [trãsfor'mar] ⟨1e⟩ transform; (*converter*), TECN turn (***em*** into); **transformar-se** *v/r* be transformed; (*formar-se*) turn (***em*** into)
transfronteiriço [trãsfrõtej'risu] *adj* cross-border
transfusão [trãsfu'zãw] *f* transfusion; **~ *de sangue*** blood transfusion
transgredir [trãsgre'dʒir] ⟨3d⟩ *lei* break; (*infringir*) infringe against
transgressão [trãsgre'sãw] *f* transgression, infringement
transgressor [trãsgre'sor] *m*, **-a** *f lei*: law-breaker
transição [trãzi'sãw] *f* transition
transigência [trãzi'ʒẽsja] *f* flexibility
transigente [trãzi'ʒẽtʃi] *adj* flexible
transigir [trãzi'ʒir] ⟨3n⟩ **~ *com algo*** compromise on sth
transitar [trãzi'tar] ⟨1a⟩ pass through
transitável [trãzi'tavew] *adj* passable
transitivo [trãzi'tʃivu] *adj* GRAM transitive
trânsito ['trãzitu] *m* traffic; *passageiros, mercadoria*: transit; ***visto*** *m* ***de* ~** transit visa; ***em* ~** in transit
transitório [trãzi'tɔriu] *adj* transitory
translúcido [trãz'lusidu] *adj* translucent
transmissão [trãzmi'sãw] *f* transmission; TV *etc* broadcast; AUTO **~ *automática*** automatic transmission; INFORM **~ *de dados*** data transfer; RÁDIO, TV **~ *em direto***, *Port* **~ *em directo*** live broadcast
transmissível [trãzmi'sivew] *adj* transmittable
transmissor [trãzmi'sor] *m*, **-a** *f* transmitter
transmitir [trãzmi'tʃir] ⟨3a⟩ transmit; *programa* broadcast; *notícia* pass on, convey
transparecer [trãspare'ser] ⟨2g⟩ be visible
transparência [trãspa'rẽsja] *f* transparency
transparente [trãspa'rẽtʃi] **1** *adj* transparent *tb fig* **2** *m* transparency
transpiração [trãspira'sãw] *f* ⟨*sem pl*⟩ perspiration
transpirar [trãspi'rar] ⟨1a⟩ perspire; ***transpirou que ...*** it transpired that ...
transplantação [trãsplãta'sãw] *f* MED transplant; **~ *de órgãos*** organ transplant
transplantar [trãsplã'tar] ⟨1a⟩ BOT,

T

MED, *fig* transplant
transpor [trãs'por] ⟨2z⟩ transpose; (*galgar*) cross
transportadora [trãsporta'dora] *f* carrier; ~ ***aérea*** aircraft carrier
transportar [trãspor'tar] ⟨1e⟩ transport; MÚS transpose; *ônibus etc* carry
transporte [trãs'pɔrtʃi] *m* transportation, transport; *soma*: sum carried forward; (*entusiasmo*) delight; ***meio*** *m* ***de*** ~ means of transport; ~***s*** *pl* (***públicos***) mass transit, *Brit* public transport; ***Ministério*** *m* ***dos Transportes*** Transport Department; ***com*** ~***s à porta*** convenient for transport; ~ ***rodoviário*** road haulage
transposição [trãspozi'sãw] *f* transposition; (*travessia*) crossing
transsexual [trãse'kswaw] **1** *adj* transsexual **2** *m/f* transsexual
transtornar [trãstor'nar] ⟨1e⟩ upset; (*incomodar*) disrupt
transtorno [trãs'tornu] *m* upset; (*incómodo*) disruption
transversal [trãzver'saw] *adj* transverse; (*lateral*) side *atr*; ESP ***linha*** *f* ~ sideline; ***rua*** *f* ~ side street
transviar [trãʒ'vjar] ⟨1g⟩ lead astray; **transviar-se** *v/r* go astray
trapacear [trapa'sjar] ⟨1l⟩ *vt* cheat
trapalhada [trapa'ʎada] *f fig* confusion, mess
trapalhão [trapa'ʎãw] *m*, **-ona** [trapa'ʎona] *f* clumsy person, *fam* klutz
trapézio [tra'pɛziu] *m* trapeze
trapezista [trape'zista] *m/f* trapeze artist
trapo ['trapu] *m* rag
traque ['traki] *m* firecracker; *vulg* fart
traquéia [tra'kɛja] *f* windpipe
trarei [tra'rej], **traria** [tra'ria] *etc* → ***trazer***
trás [tras] **1** *adv* ***de*** ~ from behind; ***para*** ~ *olhar* behind, back; *andar* backwards; ***deixar para*** ~ leave behind; ***ficar para*** ~ lag behind **2** *prep* ***por*** ~ ***de*** behind
trasbordar [trazbor'dar] *v/i* → ***transbordar***
traseira(s) [tra'zejra(s)] *f(pl)* back
traseiro [tra'zejru] **1** *adj* back *atr*, rear **2** *m fam* backside, bottom
trasladar [trazla'dar] ⟨1b⟩ transfer
tratado [tra'tadu] *m* (*contrato*) treaty; ~ ***de extradição*** extradition treaty
tratamento [trata'mẽtu] *m* treatment; (*título*) title, form of address; ~ ***de choque*** shock therapy
tratante [tra'tãtʃi] *m/f* rogue
tratar [tra'tar] ⟨1b⟩ **1** *v/t* treat; (*manufaturar*) process; (*lidar*) deal with; ~ ***por tu / você*** use the familiar / polite form of address **2** *v/i* ~ ***de*** *livro* deal with; (*falar de*) talk about; (*cuidar de*) deal with, handle; ***de que se trata?*** what's it about?; ***trata da sua vida!*** mind your own business!; **tratar-se** *v/r* (*cuidar-se*) look after oneself; ~ ***de*** be about, deal with
trato ['tratu] *m* ***ele é de bom*** ~ he's well-mannered; ***maus*** ~***s*** ill-treatment
trator [tra'tor] *m* tractor
tratorista [trato'rista] *m/f* tractor driver
traumático [traw'matʃiku] *adj* traumatic
traumatismo [trawma'tʃizmu] *m* MED, PSICOL trauma
traumatizar [trawmatʃi'zar] ⟨1a⟩ MED, PSICOL traumatize
travagem [tra'vaʒẽ] *f Port* braking; ~ ***brusca*** emergency stop
travão [tra'vãw] *m Port* brake; ~ ***de estacionamento*** parking brake, *Brit* handbrake; ~ ***de pé*** footbrake
travar [tra'var] ⟨1b⟩ **1** *v/t carro, máquina* stop; *cavalo* rein in; (*impedir*) block; *conversa* strike up; *batalha* engage; *Port* ***o carro não está travado*** the car's brake isn't on; ~ ***conhecimento com alguém*** get to know s.o. **2** *v/i Port* AUTO brake
trave ['travi] *f* beam; *gol*: post
travessa [tra'vɛsa] *f* crossbeam; (*ruela*) side street; *loiça*: platter, dish; *pente*: *Am* barrette, *Brit* slide
travessão [trave'sãw] *m vento* cross wind; (*trave*) crossbar; MÚS bar line; GRAM dash
travesseiro [trave'sejru] *m* pillow
travessia [trave'sia] *f* crossing; ***fazer a*** ~ ***de*** cross
travesso[1] [tra'vɛsu] *adj* cross *atr*,

transverse; ***vento ~*** cross wind
travesso[2] [tra'vesu] *adj* naughty
travessura [trave'sura] *f* prank; ***~s*** mischief
travesti [traves'ʧi] *m/f* transvestite
traz [tras] → ***trazer***
trazer [tra'zer] ⟨2u⟩ bring; *intenção* have; *vestido* wear
trecho ['treʃu] *m caminho, tempo*: stretch; *música, texto*: passage
trégua ['trɛgwa] *f* pause; *fig* respite; MIL ***~s*** *pl* truce
treinador [trejna'dor] *m*, **-a** *f* coach
treinamento [trejna'mẽtu] *m* training; ***~ de incêndio*** fire drill
treinar [trej'nar] ⟨1a⟩ train
treino ['trejnu] *m* training
trela ['trɛla] *f* leash
trem [trẽ] *m Bras* train; AERO ***~ de aterragem*** undercarriage; *Port* ***~ de cozinha*** pots and pans
trema ['trema] *m* dieresis
tremendamente [tremẽda'mẽʧi] *adv* tremendously
tremendo [tre'mẽdu] *adj* tremendous
tremer [tre'mer] ⟨2c⟩ *v/i* shake; ***tremo só de pensar*** I shudder to think
tremoceiro [tremo'sejru] *m* BOT lupin
tremor [tre'mor] *m* shaking; ***~ de terra*** (earth) tremor
trêmulo, *Port* **trémulo** ['tremulu] **1** *adj* trembling, shaky; (*brilhante*) glittering **2** *m* MÚS tremolo
trenó [tre'nɔ] *m* sled, *Brit* sledge; ***~ dirigível*** bob(sleigh)
trepadeira [trepa'dejra] *f* (***planta*** *f*) ***~*** creeper
trepar [tre'par] ⟨1c⟩ **1** *v/t* climb; *vulg* lay **2** *v/i* climb up
trepidação [trepida'sãw] *f* shaking
trepidar [trepi'dar] ⟨1a⟩ shake; (*vacilar*) hesitate
três [tres] *num* three
trespasse [tres'pasi] *m* COM transfer
trevas ['trɛvas] *fpl* darkness
trevo ['trevu] *m* BOT clover; *estradas*: intersection
treze ['trezi] *num* thirteen
trezentos [tre'zẽtus] *num* three hundred
triagem [tri'aʒẽ] *f* (*escolha*) selection; (*separação*) sorting *tb* INFORM
triangular [triãgu'lar] *adj* triangular
triângulo [tri'ãgulu] *m tb* MÚS triangle; AUTO ***~ de sinalização*** warning triangle
triatlo [tri'atlu] *m* triathlon
tribo ['tribu] *f* tribe
tribulação [tribula'sãw] *f* tribulation
tribuna [tri'buna] *f* rostrum; ***~ principal*** grandstand
tribunal [tribu'naw] *m* court; ***~ de justiça*** law court; ***Supremo Tribunal*** Supreme Court
tributação [tributa'sãw] *f* taxation
tributar [tribu'tar] ⟨1a⟩ tax; *fig honra* pay
tributário [tribu'tariu] **1** *adj* taxable **2** *m*, **-a** *f* tax payer
tributo [tri'butu] *m* tax; *fig* tribute
triciclo [tri'siklu] *m* tricycle
tricô [tri'ko] *m* knitting; ***agulha*** *f* ***de ~*** knitting needle; ***artigos*** *mpl* ***de ~*** knitwear; ***trabalho*** *m* ***de ~*** knitting
tricotar [triko'tar] *v/i* knit
trigal [tri'gaw] *m* wheat field
trigésimo [tri'ʒɛzimu] **1** *adj* thirtieth **2** *m* thirtieth
trigo ['trigu] *m* wheat
trigonometria [trigonome'tria] *f* MAT trigonometry
trigueiro [tri'gejru] *adj* dark
trilha ['triʎa] *f* (*caminho*) path; ***~ de condensação*** vapor trail; *Bras* ***~ sonora*** soundtrack
trilhar [tri'ʎar] ⟨1a⟩ thresh; (*passar sobre*) tread on
trilho ['triʎu] *m* FERROV track
trimestral [trimes'traw] *adj* quarterly
trimestre [tri'mɛstri] *m* quarter
trincar [trĩ'kar] ⟨1n⟩ **1** *v/t* bite; *dentes* clench; NÁUT tie up **2** *v/i* crunch
trinchar [trĩ'ʃar] ⟨1a⟩ GASTR carve
trinco ['trĩku] *m* latch
trinta ['trĩta] *num* thirty
trintena [trĩ'tena] *f* ***uma ~*** (***de***) around thirty
trio ['triu] *m* trio
tripa ['tripa] *f* gut; GASTR ***~s*** *pl* tripe
tripa-forra [tripa'foha] *adv* ***à ~*** flat out
tripé [tri'pɛ] *m* tripod
triplicado [tripli'kadu] *m* ***em ~*** in triplicate
triplicar [tripli'kar] ⟨1n⟩ triple

T

tríplice ['triplisi] *adj*, **triplo** ['triplu] *adj* triple
tripulação [tripula'sãw] *f* crew
tripulante [tripu'lãtʃi] *m/f* crew member; ***os ~s*** the crew
tripular [tripu'lar] ⟨1a⟩ *v/t* crew, man
trisavô [triza'vo] *m* great-great-grandfather
trisavó [triza'vɔ] *f* great-great-grandmother
triste ['tristʃi] *adj* sad; (*insignificante*) pathetic little
tristeza [tris'teza] *f* sadness; (*luto*) mourning; ***~s*** *pl* sorrows; ***sofrer ~s*** be gloomy
tristonho [tris'toɲu] *adj* melancholy; (*escuro*) gloomy
triturador [tritura'dor] *m* grinder; *papel*: shredder; ***~ de lixo*** waste disposal unit
triturar [tritu'rar] ⟨1a⟩ grind; *papel*: shred
triunfador [triũfa'dor] **1** *adj* triumphant **2** *m*, **-a** *f* victor
triunfal [triũ'faw] *adj* triumphant
triunfante [triũ'fãtʃi] *adj* triumphant
triunfar [triũ'far] ⟨1a⟩ triumph (***de*** over)
triunfo [tri'ũfu] *m* triumph, victory
trivial [tri'vjaw] *adj* trivial
trivialidade [trivjali'dadʒi] *f* triviality
triz [tris] *m* ***eu não ganhei por um ~*** I only just lost; ***eu ganhei por um ~*** I only just won
troca ['trɔka] *f* exchange; ***em ~*** in exchange; ***em ~ de*** in exchange for; ***~ de idéias*** exchange of ideas; ***~ do óleo*** oil change
troça ['trɔsa] *f* mockery; ***fazer ~ de*** mock
trocado [tro'kadu] *m* (small) change
trocar [tro'kar] ⟨1n & 1e⟩ exchange; *palavras* twist; (*confundir*) confuse; ***~ as voltas a alguém*** thwart s.o.'s plans; ***~ de avião*** change planes; ***~ uma nota*** change a bill; **trocar-se** *v/r* change
troçar [tro'sar] ⟨1p & 1e⟩ mock; ***~ de*** mock
trocista [tro'sista] **1** *adj* mocking **2** *m/f* mocker
troco ['troku] *m* change; *fam* reply; ***dar o ~ a*** pay back
troço ['trosu] *m* part; *fam* (*coisa*) thing; *inútil* piece of junk; ***me deu um ~*** something came over me
troféu [tro'fɛu] *m* trophy
troleibus [trɔlej'bus] *m Port* trolley bus
tromba ['trõba] *f* trunk; *pop* mug; ***~ de água*** hosepipe; ***estar de ~s*** *fam* be in a huff
trombar [trõ'bar] ⟨1a⟩ *v/t* bump into
trombone [trõ'boni] *m* trombone; *músico* trombone player
trombose [trõ'bɔzi] *f* MED thrombosis
trompa ['trõpa] *f* MÚS horn; ANAT tube
trompete [trõ'pɛtʃi] *m/f* MÚS trumpet; *músico* trumpeter
tronco ['trõku] *m* trunk
trono ['tronu] *m* throne
tropa ['trɔpa] *f* troop; (*serviço militar*) military service
tropeçar [trope'sar] ⟨1p & 1c⟩ stumble (***em, com*** over); ***~ em dificuldades*** hit problems
tropical [tropi'kaw] *adj* tropical
trópico ['trɔpiku] *m* tropic; ***~s*** *pl* tropics
trotar [tro'tar] ⟨1e⟩ trot
trote ['trɔtʃi] *m* trot
trouxe ['trosi] *etc* → ***trazer***
trovão [tro'vãw] *m* thunder
trovejar [trove'ʒar] ⟨1d⟩ thunder
trovoada [tro'vwada] *f* thunderstorm
trufa ['trufa] *f* BOT truffle
trunfo ['trũfu] *m* trump
truque ['truki] *m* trick; *publicitário* publicity stunt
truste ['trustʃi] *m* trust
truta ['truta] *f* trout
tu [tu] *pron* you
tua ['tua] → ***teu***
tuba ['tuba] *f* MÚS tuba
tubarão [tuba'rãw] *m* shark
túbera ['tubera] *f* BOT truffle
tuberculose [tuberku'lɔzi] *f* MED tuberculosis
tubo ['tubu] *m* tube, pipe; ***~ de ensaio*** test tube; ***~ de escape*** tail pipe; ***~ de esgoto*** drainpipe; ***~ respirador*** snorkel

tudo ['tudu] *pron* everything; **~ *o que, ~ quanto*** everything (that)
tufão [tu'fãw] *m* typhoon
tule ['tuli] *m* tulle
tulipa [tu'lipa] *f* tulip
tumefação, *Port* **tumefacção** [tumefa'sãw] *f* MED swelling
tumefato, *Port* **tumefacto** [tume'fatu] *adj* swollen
tumor [tu'mor] *m* MED tumor, *Brit* tumour
túmulo ['tumulu] *m* grave
tumulto [tu'muwtu] *m* tumult; (*barulho*) uproar; (*agitação*) riot
túnel ['tunew] *m* tunnel
túnica ['tunika] *f* tunic
Tunísia [tu'nizja] *f* Tunisia
tunisino [tuni'zinu] **1** *adj* Tunisian **2** *m*, **-a** *f* Tunisian
turbante [tur'bãʧi] *m* turban
turbilhão [turbi'ʎãw] *m* whirlwind; (*redemoinho*) whirlpool
turbina [tur'bina] *f* turbine
turborreator, *Port* **turborreactor** [turbohea'tor] *m* AERO turbojet
turbulência [turbu'lẽsja] *f* turbulence
turbulento [turbu'lẽtu] *adj* turbulent; *criança* rowdy
turco ['turku] **1** *adj* Turkish **2** *m*, **-a** *f* Turk **3** *m lingua* Turkish
turismo [tu'rizmu] *m* tourism; ***agência f de ~*** tourist office; ***Junta f*** (*ou* ***Comissão*** *f*) ***de Turismo*** tourist office; ***~ ecológico*** ecotourism; ***~ sexual*** sex tourism
turista [tu'rista] *m/f* tourist
turístico [tu'risʧiku] *adj* tourist *atr*; *demais*: touristy
turma ['turma] *f* gang; *escola*: class
turno ['turnu] *m trabalho*: shift; (*vez*) turn; ***mudança f de ~*** change of shift; ***por ~s*** in shifts; ***trabalho m por ~s*** shiftwork; ***é o seu ~*** it's your turn; ***~ da noite*** nightshift
turquesa [tur'keza] *adj* turquoise
Turquia [tur'kia] *f* Turkey
turvo ['turvu] *adj* cloudy, murky
tusso ['tusu] *etc* → ***tossir***
tutela [tu'tɛla] *f* guardianship
tutelado [tute'ladu] *m* ward
tutor [tu'tor] *m*, **~ a** *f* guardian; UNIV tutor
TV [te've] *f abr* (***televisão***) TV; ***~ a cabo*** cable (TV)

U

úbere ['uberi] *m* udder
Ucrânia [u'krʌnja] *f* Ukraine
ucraniano [ukra'njanu] **1** *adj* Ukrainian **2** *m*, **-a** *f* Ukrainian
UE [u'e] *f abr* (***União Europeia***) EU (European Union)
ufano [u'fanu] *adj* proud (***com, de*** of); (*presunçoso*) conceited
uísque ['wiski] *m Bras* whiskey, *Brit* whisky
uivar [ui'var] ⟨1a⟩ howl
uivo ['uivu] *m* howling
úlcera ['uwsera] *f* ulcer
ulmeiro [uw'mejru] *m*, **ulmo** ['uwmu] *m* BOT elm
ulterior [uwte'rjor] *adj* later; (*seguinte*) further; (*último*) last
última ['uwʧima] *f* ***até à ~*** to the bitter end
ultimar [uwʧi'mar] *v/t* complete
ultimamente [uwʧima'mẽʧi] *adv* lately
ultimato [uwʧi'matu] *m* ultimatum
último ['uwʧimu] *adj* last; (*mais recente*) latest; (*extremo*) ultimate; (*inferior*) lowest; ***por ~*** finally; ***os ~s dias*** the past few days; ***em ~ caso*** as a last resort
ultra... [uwtra-] ultra...
ultracongelado [uwtrakõʒe'ladu] *adj* deep-frozen
ultrajante [uwtra'ʒãʧi] *adj* outrageous

ultrajar [uwtra'ʒar] ⟨1b⟩ insult
ultraje [uw'traʒi] *m* insult
ultramar [uwtra'mar] *m* overseas; (*tinta*) ultramarine
ultramarino [uwtrama'rinu] *adj* overseas; *cor* ultramarine
ultrapassado [uwtrapa'sadu] *adj* outdated
ultrapassagem [uwtrapa'saʒẽ] *f* passing, *Brit* overtaking; ***fazer uma ~*** pass, *Brit* overtake
ultrapassar [uwtrapa'sar] ⟨1b⟩ go beyond; *fig* exceed; *obstáculo* overcome; *carro* pass, *Brit* overtake; ***proibição** f **de ~*** passing ban; ***~ os limites*** overstep the mark
ultra-som [uwtra'sõ] *m* ultrasound
ultravioleta [uwtravjo'leta] *adj* ultraviolet
um [ũ], **uma** ['uma] **1** *art* a; *antes de vogal*: an; *pl* ***uns, umas*** some; (*por volta de*) around, some; ***umas 10 pinturas*** around 10 paintings, some ten paintings; ***mais ~ (a)*** another **2** *pron* one; ***~ ao outro*** one another, each other; ***cada ~ / ~ a*** every one; ***~ por ~*** one after the other **3** *m num* one
umbigo [ũ'bigu] *m* ANAT navel
umbilical [ũbili'kaw] *adj* umbilical
umbral [ũ'braw] *m* threshold
umedecer [umide'ser] ⟨2g⟩ *v/t Bras* moisten
umidade [umi'dadʒi] *f Bras* damp; *tropical* humidity
úmido ['umidu] *adj Bras* wet, damp; *tropical* humid; *bolo etc* moist
unânime [u'nʌnimi] *adj* unanimous
unanimidade [unanimi'dadʒi] *f* unanimity; ***por ~*** unanimously
ungüento, *Port* **unguento** [ũŋ'gwẽtu] *m* MED ointment
unha ['uɲa] *f pé*, *mão*: nail; (*garra*) claw; ***~ encravada*** ingrowing toenail; ***~ do pé*** toenail
união [u'njãw] *f* union; (*concórdia*) unity; (*ligação*) joining; POL union; ***União Européia***, *Port* ***União Europeia*** European Union; ***~ Soviética*** Soviet Union; ***traço** m **de ~*** hyphen
único ['uniku] *adj* only; (*excepcional*) unique; (*singular*) single; (*uniforme*) uniform; ***filho** m **~*** only child; ***Mercado** m **Único*** Single Market
unidade [uni'dadʒi] *f* unity; MAT, TECN, MIL unit; ***~ de CD / DVD*** CD- / DVD-drive; ***~ de disquete*** disk drive; COM ***100 ~s de*** 100 units of
unido [u'nidu] *adj* united; (*de acordo*) agreed
unificação [unifika'sãw] *f* unification
unificar [unifi'kar] ⟨1n⟩ unite
uniforme [uni'fɔrmi] **1** *adj* uniform **2** *m* uniform
uniformidade [uniformi'dadʒi] *f* uniformity
uniformização [uniformiza'sãw] *f* standardization
uniformizar [uniformi'zar] ⟨1a⟩ standardize
unilateral [unilate'raw] *adj* unilateral; (*partidário*) partisan
unir [u'nir] ⟨3a⟩ unite; (*ligar*) join; **unir-se** *v/r* unite; ***~ a*** join
uníssono [u'nisonu] *m* MÚS ***em ~*** in unison
unitário [uni'tariu] *adj* unit *atr*
universal [univer'saw] *adj* universal; (*geral*) general
universalidade [universali'dadʒi] *f* universality; (*totalidade*) totality
universalizar [universali'zar] ⟨1a⟩ universalize
universalmente [universaw'mẽtʃi] *adv* universally
universidade [universi'dadʒi] *f* university
universitário [universi'tariu] **1** *adj* university *atr* **2** *m*, **-a** *f* university student
universo [uni'vɛrsu] *m* universe
uno ['unu] *adj* one
uns [ũs] *pl* → ***um***
untar [ũ'tar] ⟨1a⟩ grease; *com óleo* oil; *fam* ***~ as mãos de alguém*** grease s.o.'s palm
unto ['ũtu] *m* grease; (*óleo*) lubricant; (*gordura*) fat
urânio [u'rʌniu] *m* uranium
urbanismo [urba'nizmu] *m* town planning
urbanização [urbaniza'sãw] *f* urbanization

urbanizar [urbani'zar] ⟨1a⟩ *bairro* develop, urbanize
urbano [ur'banu] *adj* urban, city *atr*
urbe ['urbi] *f* city
uréia [u'rɛja] *f* urine
uretra [u'rɛtra] *f* ANAT urethra
urgência [ur'ʒẽsja] *f* urgency; ***caso*** *m* ***de ~*** emergency; ***médico*** *m* ***de ~*** emergency doctor; MED ***serviço*** *m* ***de ~*** emergency service; ***de ~*** urgent; ***em caso de ~*** in an emergency
urgente [ur'ʒẽtʃi] *adj* urgent
urina [u'rina] *f* urine
urinar [uri'nar] ⟨1a⟩ **1** *v/i* urinate **2** *v/t* pass
urinol [uri'nɔw] *m* chamber pot
urna ['urna] *f* urn; POL ballot box
urologia [urolo'ʒia] *f* urology
urologista [urolo'ʒista] *m/f* urologist
urrar [u'har] ⟨1a⟩ *burro* bray
urro(s) ['uhu(s)] *m(pl) burro*: braying
urso ['ursu] *m* bear; ***~ branco*** *ou* ***polar*** polar bear; ***~ formigueiro*** anteater
urticária [urtʃi'karja] *f* MED nettle rash
urtiga [ur'tʃiga] *f* BOT nettle
urubu [uru'bu] *m* buzzard
Uruguai [uru'gwaj] *m* Uruguay
uruguaio [uru'gwaiu] **1** *adj* Uruguayan **2** *m*, **-a** *f* Uruguayan
urze ['urzi] *f* BOT heather
usado [u'zadu] *adj* (*comum*) common, usual; (*oposto a novo*) used
usar [u'zar] ⟨1a⟩ use; *vestuário* wear; (*gastar*) wear out; ***~ drogas*** be a drug user
usina [u'zina] *f* plant, factory; ***~ elétrica*** power plant
uso ['uzu] *m* use; (*gasto*) wear and tear; (*costume, hábito*) custom
USB [uɛsi'be] *abr* ***conexão*** *f* ***~*** USB-connection; ***memória*** *f* ***~*** memory stick
usual [u'zwaw] *adj* usual
usuário [u'zwariu] *m*, **-a** *f* user; ***~ final*** end user
usura [u'zura] *f* usury
usurpação [uzurpa'sãw] *f* usurpation
usurpador [uzurpa'dor] *m*, **-a** *f* usurper
usurpar [uzur'par] ⟨1a⟩ usurp
utensílio [utẽ'siliu] *m* utensil; (*ferramenta*) tool
utente [u'tẽtʃi] *m/f Port* user
útero ['uteru] *m* ANAT uterus, womb
útil ['utʃiw] *adj* useful; ***dia*** *m* ***~*** workday
utilidade [utʃili'dadʒi] *f* usefulness, utility; ***~ pública*** public utility
utilitário [utʃili'tariu] **1** *adj móvel* utilitarian **2** *m* AUTO utility vehicle
utilização [utʃiliza'sãw] *f* utilization, use
utilizador [utʃiliza'dor] *m*, **-a** *f* user *tb* INFORM
utilizar [utʃili'zar] ⟨1a⟩ utilize, use
utopia [uto'pia] *f* Utopia
utópico [u'tɔpiku] *adj* Utopian
uva ['uva] *f* grape; ***~ moscatel*** muscatel grape; ***~ passa*** raisin
uva-espim [uvas'pĩ] *f* gooseberry
úvula ['uvula] *f* ANAT uvula

V

v. *abr* (***ver***, ***veja***) see
vá [va] → ***ir***
vã [vã] → ***vão***[2]
vaca ['vaka] *f* cow; *Port* ***carne*** *f* ***de ~*** beef
vacância [va'kãsja] *f* job opening, *Brit* vacancy
vacante [va'kãtʃi] *adj* vacant
vacilação [vasila'sãw] *f* swaying; (*hesitação*) hesitation, vacillation
vacilar [vasi'lar] ⟨1a⟩ sway; (*hesitar*) hesitate, vacillate
vacina [va'sina] *f* vaccine
vacinação [vasina'sãw] *f* vaccination

vacinar [vasi'nar] ⟨1a⟩ vaccinate
vacuidade [vakwi'dadʒi] *f* emptiness
vácuo ['vakwu] **1** *adj* empty **2** *m* vacuum; AERO airpocket
vadiagem [va'dʒiaʒẽ] *f* vagrancy
vadiar [va'dʒiar] ⟨1g⟩ laze around, hang about
vadio [va'dʒiu] **1** *m*, **-a** *f* hobo, *Brit* tramp; *Port* ***vadia*** *mulher da vida* slut **2** *adj* (*errante*) vagrant, wandering; (*preguiçoso*) idle; *cão* stray
vaga[1] ['vaga] *f* wave; ***~ de emigração*** wave of emigration
vaga[2] ['vaga] *f* (*lugar*) opening; *para estacionar* gap, space; (*ausência*) absence
vagabundear [vagabũ'dʒiar] ⟨1l⟩ wander around
vagabundo [vaga'bũdu] **1** *adj* vagrant; *hotel etc* tacky, downscale **2** *m*, **-a** *f* hobo, *Brit* tramp, down-and-out; ***vagabunda*** *mulher da vida* slut
vagamente [vaga'mẽtʃi] *adv* vaguely
vagão [va'gãw] *m passageiros*: car; *carga*: wagon; ***~ -cama*** sleeping car; ***~ de carga*** freight car; ***~ dormitório*** sleeping car; *Bras* ***~ -leito*** sleeping car; *Bras* ***~ -restaurante*** dining car
vagar [va'gar] **1** *v/i* ⟨1o & 1b⟩ wander around; *quarto* be vacant; (*faltar*) be missing **2** *m* leisure; (*tempo*) time; (*lentidão*) slowness
vagoroso [vaga'rozu] *adj* slow
vagem ['vaʒẽ] *f Bras* green bean
vagina [va'ʒina] *f* ANAT vagina
vaginal [vaʒi'naw] *adj* vaginal
vago ['vagu] *adj* empty; *tempo* free; (*pouco claro*) vague
vaguear [va'gjar] ⟨1l⟩ *pessoa* wander; (*divagar*) ramble
vai [vaj] → ***ir***
vaia ['vaja] *f* hiss, boo
vaiar [va'jar] ⟨1i⟩ *v/i* hiss, boo
vaidade [vaj'dadʒi] *f* vanity
vaidoso [vaj'dozu] *adj* vain
vais [vajs] → ***ir***
vaivém [vaj'vẽ] *m* to-and-fro
vala ['vala] *f* ditch; ***~ comum*** common grave
vale[1] ['vali] *m* COM voucher; ***~ do correio*** postal order
vale[2] ['vali] *m* GEOG valley
vale-livro [vale'livru] *m* book token
valente [va'lẽtʃi] *adj* brave
valentia [valẽ'tʃia] *f* bravery; *ação* courageous deed
valentão [valẽ'tãw] *m*, **valentona** *f* bully
vale presente [valipre'zẽtʃi] *m* gift certificate, *Brt* gift voucher
valer [va'ler] ⟨2p⟩ *v/i* be worth; (*custar*) cost; (*servir*) be useful; (*ajudar*) help; ***~ a pena ler*** be worth reading; ***~ a pena*** be worthwhile; ***não vale a pena tentar*** it's no use trying, it's not worth trying; **valer-se** *v/r* ***~ de*** make use of
valho ['vaʎu], **vali** [va'li] *etc* → ***valer***
validade [vali'dadʒi] *f* validity
validar [vali'dar] ⟨1a⟩ make valid, validate
validez [vali'des] *f* validity
válido ['validu] **1** *adj* valid **2** *pp* → ***valer***
valioso [va'ljozu] *adj* valuable
valor [va'lor] *m* value; (*preço*) price; (*eficácia*) effectiveness; (*coragem*) valor, *Brit* valour; (*mérito*) worth; ***de ~*** valuable; ***sem ~*** of no value; ***~ assegurado*** sum insured; ***~ de mercado*** market value; ***~ meta*** target figure
valorização [valoriza'sãw] *f* valuation; (*revalorização*) increase in value
valorizar [valori'zar] ⟨1a⟩ value; (*revalorizar*) increase the value of, revalue; **valorizar-se** *v/r* increase in value
valoroso [valo'rozu] *adj* brave; (*valioso*) valuable
valsa ['vawsa] *f* waltz
valsar [vaw'sar] ⟨1a⟩ waltz
valva ['vawva] *f concha*: shell
válvula ['vawvula] *f* TECN, ANAT valve; ***~ de escape*** exhaust valve; ***~ de segurança*** safety valve
vampiro [vã'piru] *m*, **-a** *f* vampire
vamos ['vʌmus] → ***ir***
vandalismo [vãda'lizmu] *m* vandalism
vandalizar [vãdali'ʒar] ⟨1a⟩ *v/t* vandalize
vândalo ['vãdalu] *m*, **-a** *f* vandal
vangloriar-se [vãglo'rjarsi] *v/r* boast (***de*** about)

vanguarda [vã'gwaɾda] *f* vanguard; ***estar na ~*** be cutting edge
vantagem [vã'taʒẽ] *f* advantage; ESP lead
vantajoso [vãta'ʒozu] *adj* advantageous
vão[1] [vãw] → ***ir***
vão[2] [vãw] **1** *adj*, *f* **vã** [vã] (*vazio*) empty; (*oco*) hollow; (*inútil*) vain; (*fútil*) futile; ***em ~*** in vain **2** *m* gap
vapor [va'poɾ] *m* steam; *gas*: vapor, *Brit* vapour; NÁUT steamer; ***a ~*** steam *atr*; *fig* at full speed
vaporizador [vaporiza'doɾ] *m* vaporizer, atomizer
vaporizar [vapori'zaɾ] ⟨1a⟩ *v/t* vaporize; *perfume etc* spray
vaporoso [vapo'rozu] *adj* steamy; (*leve*) light; *vestido* diaphanous
vaqueiro [va'kejɾu] *m* cowboy
vaquinha [va'kiɲa] *f* kitty; ***fazer uma ~*** have a whipround
vara ['vaɾa] *f* rod; *remo etc*: shaft; *pau*: stick; (*circunscrição*) district; ***saltador com ~*** pole vaulter; ***~ de pesca*** fishing rod
varal ['vaɾaw] *m* clothes line
varanda [va'rãda] *f* verandah, stoop; (*balção*) balcony
varão [va'rãw] *m* man, male; ZOOL male; *fam* (*filho*) son and heir
varapau [vaɾa'paw] *m* beanpole
varejeira [vare'ʒejɾa] *f* bluebottle
varejista [vare'ʒista] *m/f Bras* retailer
varejo [va'reʒu] *Bras* ***a ~*** retail
vareta [va'reta] *f* rod
variabilidade [vaɾjabili'dadʒi] *f* variability
variação [vaɾja'sãw] *f* variation; (*variedade*) variety
variado [va'ɾjadu] *adj* varied
variante [va'ɾjãtʃi] *f* variant; (*alteração*) variation
variar [va'ɾjaɾ] ⟨1g⟩ **1** *v/t* vary **2** *v/i* vary; (*diferenciar-se*) be different, vary; ***para ~*** for a change
variável [va'ɾjavew] **1** *adj* variable; (*inconstante*) changeable **2** *f* MAT variable
varicela [vari'sɛla] *f* MED chickenpox
variedade [varie'dadʒi] *f* variety; (*mudança*) change
varinha [va'ɾiɲa] *f* ***~ mágica*** magic wand
vário ['vaɾiu] *adj* varied; (*colorido*) multicolored, *Brit* multicoloured; (*inconstante*) changeable, fickle; ***~s*** *pl* several, various
varíola [va'riula] *f* MED smallpox
variz [va'ɾis] *f* MED varicose vein
varrer [va'heɾ] ⟨2b⟩ sweep; *lixo* sweep up; *fig* sweep away; ***~ da memória*** erase from one's memory
várzea ['vaɾzja] *f* field
vás [vas] → ***ir***
vascular [vasku'laɾ] *adj* ANAT vascular; MED ***acidente*** *m* ***~ cerebral*** stroke
vasculhar [vasku'ʎaɾ] ⟨1a⟩ sweep; *gaveta* rummage through; *terreno* search
vasectomia [vazɛkto'mia] *f* vasectomy
vaselina [vaze'lina] *f* vaseline
vasilha [va'ziʎa] *f* container; (*garrafa*) bottle; (*barril*) barrel
vaso ['vazu] *m* vessel *tb* ANAT; *flores*: vase; ***~ sangüíneo*** blood vessel; ***~ sanitário*** toilet bowl
vassoura [va'soɾa] *f* broom; ***~ metálica*** (drum) brush; *fig* ***pau*** *m* ***de ~*** beanpole
vastidão [vastʃi'dãw] *f* vastness; (*dimensão*) extent
vasto ['vastu] *adj* vast
Vaticano [vatʃi'kanu] *m* Vatican
vaticinar [vatʃisi'naɾ] ⟨1a⟩ prophesy
vaticínio [vatʃi'siniu] *m* prophecy
vau [vaw] *m* ford
vazamento [vaza'mẽtu] *m* leak
vazante [va'zãtʃi] **1** *adj* ***maré*** *f* ***~*** ebb (tide) **2** *f* ebb (tide)
vazar [va'zaɾ] ⟨1b⟩ **1** *v/t* empty; (*despejar*) pour out; (*tornar oco*) hollow out; *buraco* make; *metal* smelt **2** *v/i* leak; *maré* ebb; *rio* empty, flow
vazio [va'ziu] **1** *adj* empty; (*oco*) idle, empty **2** *m* emptiness; (*aberta*) gap
vê [ve] → ***ver***
veado ['vjadu] *m* ZOOL stag
vedar [ve'daɾ] ⟨1c⟩ *v/t* (*cercar*) seal; *sangue* stem; (*proibir*) forbid
vedeta [ve'deta] *f* CINE, TEAT star

vedor [vɛ'doɾ] *m*, **-a** *f* supervisor; *inspeção*: inspector
veemência [vie'mẽsja] *f* vehemence
veemente [vie'mẽtʃi] *adj* vehement
vegano [ve'ganu] **1** *adj* vegan **2** *m*, **-a** *f* vegan
vegetação [veʒeta'sãw] *f* vegetation
vegetal [veʒe'taw] **1** *adj* vegetable *atr*, plant *atr*; ***gordura*** *f* **~** vegetable fat; ***papel*** *m* **~** parchment paper; ***seda*** *f* **~** artificial silk **2** *m* plant; GASTR ***vegetais*** *pl* vegetables
vegetar [veʒe'taɾ] ⟨1c⟩ vegetate
vegetariano [veʒeta'ɾjanu] **1** *adj* vegetarian **2** *m*, **-a** *f* vegetarian
veia ['veja] *f* vein; ***tem ~ para a música*** he has a gift for music
veículo [ve'ikulu] *m* vehicle; **~ *blindado*** armored vehicle, *Brit* armoured vehicle; **~ *motorizado*** motor vehicle
veio[1] ['veiu] *m* MIN seam; *pedra, metal*: vein; *madeira*: grain; TECN shaft; **~ *de água*** gutter
veio[2] ['veiu] → ***vir***
veja ['veʒa], **vejo** ['veʒu] → ***ver***
vela[1] ['vɛla] *f* (*cera*) candle; AUTO (spark) plug; **~ *perfumada*** scented candle
vela[2] ['vɛla] *f* sail; ***andar à ~*** sail
velar[1] [ve'laɾ] ⟨1c⟩ **1** *v/t* keep watch over; *noite* stay up throughout **2** *v/i* keep watch
velar[2] [ve'laɾ] ⟨1c⟩ *v/t* veil; (*tapar*) conceal
velcro® ['vɛlkɾu] *m* velcro
veleidade [velej'dadʒi] *f* (*capricho*) mood, whim; (*vontade*) fancy
veleiro [ve'lejɾu] *m* (*barco*) yacht, sailboat, *Brit* sailing boat
velejador [ve'leʒador] *m*, **-a** *f* yachtsman; yachtwoman
velejar [vele'ʒaɾ] ⟨1d⟩ sail
velha ['vɛʎa] *f* old woman
velhaco [ve'ʎaku] **1** *adj* crooked **2** *m*, **-a** *f* crook
velhice [ve'ʎisi] *f* old age
velhinho [vɛ'ʎiɲu] **1** *adj* elderly **2** *m*, **-a** *f* old man; old woman
velho ['vɛʎu] **1** *adj* old; ***chegar a ~*** grow old **2** *m*, **-a** *f* old man; old woman
velhote [ve'ʎɔtʃi] *m*, **-a** [ve'ʎɔta] *f fam* old man; old woman
velocidade [velosi'dadʒi] *f* speed; *Port* AUTO ***primeira / segunda ~*** first / second gear; *Port* ***alavanca*** *f* ***de ~s*** gear shift; ***limite*** *m* ***de ~*** speed limit; **~ *cruzeiro*** cruising speed
velocímetro [velo'simetɾu] *m* speedometer
velódromo [ve'lɔdrumu] *m* velodrome
velório [ve'lɔriu] *m* wake
veloz [ve'lɔs] *adj* quick, fast
veludo [ve'ludu] *m* velvet
veludo cotelê [ve'ludukote'le] *m* corduroy
vem [vẽ], **vêm** ['vẽẽ] *etc* → ***vir***
venal [ve'naw] *adj* venal
venatório [vena'tɔriu] *adj* hunting *atr*
vencedor [vẽse'doɾ] **1** *adj* winning *atr*, victorious **2** *m*, **-a** *f* winner, victor
vencer [vẽ'seɾ] ⟨2g & 2a⟩ **1** *v/t processo, competição* win; *medo* conquer **2** *v/i* win; FIN fall due; *prazo* expire; *apólice de seguro* mature; ***estar vencido*** be past its sell-by-date
vencimento [vẽsi'mẽtu] *m* COM maturity; (*caducidade*) due date; *prazo*: expiration, *Brit* expiry; *alimentícios*: sell-by date; **~*s*** *pl* earnings
venda[1] ['vẽda] *f* sale; (*loja*) store; COM **~*s*** *pl* sales; ***à ~*** for sale
venda[2] ['vẽda] *f para olhos* blindfold
vendar [vẽ'daɾ] ⟨1a⟩ *v/t* blindfold; ***de olhos vendados*** blindfold(ed)
vendaval [vẽda'vaw] *m* gale
vendedor [vẽde'doɾ] **1** *adj* sales *atr* **2** *m*, **-a** *f* seller; *loja*: sales clerk, *Brit* sales person; DIR vendor; **~ (*a*) *ambulante*** street seller
vender [vẽ'deɾ] ⟨2a⟩ sell; **vender-se** *v/r* be for sale; ***vende-se*** for sale; ***você tem que se vender*** you have to sell yourself; ***vendem-se pouco*** they're selling slowly
veneno [ve'nenu] *m* poison; *fig* venom; ***deitar ~ em*** poison
venenoso [vene'nozu] *adj* poisonous; *fig* venomous
veneração [veneɾa'sãw] *f* ⟨*sem pl*⟩ worship, veneration
venerador [veneɾa'doɾ] *adj* adoring
venerar [vene'ɾaɾ] ⟨1c⟩ worship, venerate

venerável [vene'ɾavew] *adj* venerable
venéreo [ve'nɛɾiu] *adj* venereal
Veneza [ve'neza] *f* Venice
veneziana [vene'zjana] *f* shade, *Brit* blind
Venezuela [vene'zwɛla] *f* Venezuela
venezuelano [venezwe'lanu] **1** *adj* Venezuelan **2** *m*, **-a** *f* Venezuelan
venha ['veɲa], **venho** ['veɲu] *etc* → ***vir***
vênia, *Port* **vénia** ['venja] *f* permission; (*perdão*) forgiveness
vens [vẽs] → ***vir***
venta ['vẽta] *f* nostril; ***~s*** *pl* nose
ventania [vẽta'nia] *f* gale
ventar [vẽ'taɾ] ⟨1a⟩ *v/i* ***está ventando muito*** it's really windy
ventilação [vẽtʃila'sãw] *f* ventilation
ventilador [vẽtʃila'doɾ] *m* ventilator, fan
ventilar [vẽtʃi'laɾ] ⟨1a⟩ ventilate; *fig* air
vento ['vẽtu] *m* wind; (*corrente de ar*) draft, *Brit* draught; ***~ contrário*** headwind; ***~ em popa*** tailwind
ventoinha [vẽ'twiɲa] *f* ventilator
ventoso [vẽ'tozu] *adj* windy
ventre ['vẽtɾi] *m* stomach, belly; (*bojo*) bulge
ventrículo [vẽ'tɾikulu] *m* ANAT ventricle
ventríloquo [vẽ'tɾiluku] *m*, **-a** *f* ventriloquist
ventura [vẽ'tuɾa] *f* fortune; ***por ~*** by chance
venturoso [vẽtu'ɾozu] *adj* happy
ver [veɾ] ⟨2m⟩ **1** *v/t* see; (*olhar para, observar, examinar*) look at; (***ir***) ***~*** have a look; ***veja acima / abaixo*** see above / below; *fig* ***não poder ~ alguém*** not be able to stand the sight of s.o.; ***depende de como você vê*** it depends on how you look at it; ***ele não terá nada a ~ com isso*** he won't have anything to do with it; **ver-se** *v/r* be seen, show
veracidade [veɾasi'dadʒi] *f* veracity, truthfulness
veraneante [veɾa'njãtʃi] *m/f* summertime vacationer, *Brit* summertime holidaymaker
verão [ve'ɾãw] *m* summer; ***no ~*** in summer; ***férias*** *fpl* ***de ~*** summer vacation, *Brit* summer holidays
verba ['vɛɾba] *f* (*quantia*) amount
verbal [veɾ'baw] *adj* verbal
verbalmente [veɾbaw'mẽtʃi] *adv* verbally
verbete [veɾ'betʃi] *m* entry
verbo ['vɛɾbu] *m* verb; (*palavra*) word
verdade [veɾ'dadʒi] *f* truth; ***em ~*** in fact; ***em boa ~, na ~*** in actual fact; ***é ~?*** really?; ***está calor, não é ~?*** it's hot, isn't it?; ***está linda, não é ~?*** she's pretty, isn't she?
verdadeiro [veɾda'dejɾu] *adj* true; (*verídico*) truthful; (*autêntico*) real
verde ['veɾdʒi] *adj* green; *fruta* unripe; ***~ de inveja*** green with envy; POL ***os Verdes*** the Greens; ***cintura*** *f* ***~*** green belt
verdejar [veɾde'ʒaɾ] ⟨1d⟩ turn green
verdugo [veɾ'dugu] *m* hangman, executioner
verdura [veɾ'duɾa] *f* green; (*planta*) greenery; (*legumes*) greens; *fig* greenness
vereação [veɾja'sãw] *f* town council
vereador [veɾja'doɾ] *m*, **-a** *f* counselman, *Brit* councillor
vereda [ve'ɾeda] *f* path
veredito, *Port* **veredicto** [veɾe'dʒitu] *m* verdict
verei [ve'ɾej] *etc* → ***ver***
verga ['veɾga] *f* stick; *metal*: rod; ***cadeira*** *f* ***de ~*** wicker chair
vergar [veɾ'gaɾ] ⟨1c⟩ bend
vergonha [veɾ'goɲa] *f* shame; ***ter ~*** be ashamed; *embaraço*: be embarrassed; ANAT ***~s*** *pl* genitals; ***isto é uma ~!*** it's a disgrace!
vergonhoso [veɾgo'ɲozu] *adj* shameful; (*envergonhado*) ashamed; (*desonroso*) disgraceful
verídico [ve'ɾidʒiku] *adj* true
verificação [veɾifika'sãw] *f* checking; (*confirmação*) verification
verificar [veɾifi'kaɾ] ⟨1n⟩ check; (*confirmar*) verify, **verificar-se** *v/r* come true
verificável [veɾifi'kavew] *adj* verifiable
verme ['vɛɾmi] *m* worm
vermelho [veɾ'meʎu] **1** *adj* red **2** *m*

V

red **3** *m*, **-a** *f pej* POL Red
vermute [veɾ'mutʃi] *m* vermouth
verniz [veɾ'nis] *m* varnish; *fig* finesse; ***ter falta de ~*** be rough and ready
verosímil [veɾo'zimiw] *adj* probable; (*plausível*) credible
verosimilhança [veɾozimi'ʎãsa] *f* probability; (*plausibilidade*) credibility
verruga [ve'huga] *f* wart; *pé*: verruca
versado [veɾ'sadu] *adj* versed
versão [veɾ'sãw] *f* version; *tradução* (prose) translation
versátil [veɾ'satʃiw] *adj* versatile
versatilidade [veɾsatʃili'dadʒi] *f* versatility
verso ['vɛɾsu] *m poesia*: verse; *objeto*: back, reverse
vértebra ['vɛɾtebɾa] *f* vertebra, spine
vertebrado [veɾte'bɾadu] **1** *m* vertebrate **2** *adj* vertebrate
vertebral [veɾte'bɾaw] *adj* spinal
vertente [veɾ'tẽtʃi] *f montanha*: slope; *telhado*: roof area
verter [veɾ'teɾ] ⟨2c⟩ **1** *v/t* pour (out); *lágrimas* shed; (*entornar*) spill; (*esvaziar*) empty; (*traduzir*) render **2** *v/i* flow; (*entornar-se*) overflow; (*deixar repassar*) leak
vertical [veɾtʃi'kaw] *adj* vertical; *fig* upright
vértice ['vɛɾtʃisi] *m* apex
vertigem [veɾ'tʃiʒẽ] *f* vertigo, dizziness
vertiginoso [veɾtʃiʒi'nozu] *adj* dizzy
verve ['vɛɾvi] *f* verve
vês [ves] → ***ver***
vesgo ['veʒgu] *adj* cross-eyed
vesícula [ve'zikula] *f* ANAT ~ **(*biliar*)** gall bladder
vespa ['vespa] *f* wasp
véspera ['vɛspeɾa] *f* eve, day before; REL **~*s*** *pl* vespers; ***Véspera de Natal*** Christmas Eve; ***Véspera de Ano Novo*** New Year's Eve
vespertino [vespeɾ'tʃinu] **1** *adj* evening *atr* **2** *m jornal* evening paper
vestiário [ves'tʃiaɾiu] *m* TEAT *etc* dressing room; ESP changing room, locker room
vestíbulo [ves'tʃibulu] *m* hallway, vestibule; TEAT lobby, foyer
vestido [ves'tʃidu] *m* dress; ***~ formal*** evening dress, evening gown; ***~ de gestante*** maternity dress; ***~ de noiva*** wedding dress;
vestígio [ves'tʃiʒiu] *m* vestige, trace
vestir [ves'tʃiɾ] ⟨3c⟩ **1** *v/t criança etc* dress; *roupa* put on; (*usar*) have on, wear; ***vestia sua melhor roupa*** he was wearing his best clothes **2** *v/i* fit; **vestir-se** *v/r* get dressed; ***ele se veste bem*** he dresses well
vestuário [ves'twaɾiu] *m* clothing
vetar [ve'taɾ] ⟨1c⟩ veto
veterano [vete'ɾanu] **1** *adj* veteran **2** *m*, **-a** *f* veteran
veterinária [veteɾi'naɾja] *f* veterinary medicine
veterinário [veteɾi'naɾiu] **1** *adj* veterinary **2** *m*, **-a** *f* veterinarian, vet
veto ['vɛtu] *m* veto
véu [vɛu] *m* veil
vexame [ve'ʃami] *m* shame, disgrace
vez [ves] *f* time; ***uma ~ / duas ~es*** once / twice; ***três ~es*** three times; ***cada ~*** each time; ***cada ~ mais*** more and more; ***outra ~*** again; ***a próxima / última ~*** next time / the last time; ***às vezes*** sometimes; ***muitas vezes*** often; ***de ~ em quando*** from time to time; ***em ~ de*** instead of; ***por sua ~*** on his part; ***é a ~ de João*** it's João's turn; ***fazer as ~es de*** stand in for; ***você já esteve alguma ~ em …?*** have you ever been to …?; ***era uma ~ …*** once upon a time there was …
vi [vi] → ***ver***
via ['via] **1** *f* way; (*rua*) road; FERROV track; *fig* means *sg*; (*cópia*) copy; ***~ rápida*** expressway; *correios*: ***~ aérea*** by airmail; ***por ~ legal*** through legal channels; **(*por*)** ***~ marítima / terrestre*** by sea / land; ***~ Láctea*** Milky Way **2** *prep* via; ***~ satélite*** via satellite
via[2] ['via] *etc* → ***ver***
viabilidade [vjabili'dadʒi] *f* viability; (*possibilidade*) feasibility
viação [vja'sãw] *f* road transport; (*rede rodoviária*) road network; (*transporte*) transport; ***acidente*** *m* ***de ~***

V

road accident; ***empresa*** *f* ***de ~*** bus company
viaduto [vja'dutu] *m* viaduct
viagem ['vjaʒẽ] *f* journey, trip; *barco*: voyage; ***~ com tudo incluído*** package tour; ***seguro*** *m* ***de ~*** travel insurance; ***boa ~!*** have a good journey!; ***~ de ida*** outward journey; ***~ de ida e volta*** round trip; ***~ inaugural*** maiden voyage; ***~ de negócios*** business trip; ***~ organizada*** package tour
viajante [vja'ʒãtʃi] *m/f* traveler, *Brit* traveller
viajar [vja'ʒaɾ] ⟨1b⟩ *v/t* & *v/i* travel
viatura [vja'tuɾa] *f* vehicle; ***~ de serviço*** company car
viável ['vjavew] *adj* viable; (*possível*) feasible
víbora ['viboɾa] *f* viper
vibração [vibɾa'sãw] *f* vibration; *fig* thrill, excitement
vibrador [vibɾa'doɾ] *m* vibrator; ***~ para betão*** cement mixer; ***~ para massagens*** vibrator
vibrar [vi'bɾaɾ] ⟨1a⟩ **1** *v/t* vibrate **2** *v/i* vibrate; (*ressoar*) echo
vice... [visi] vice...
vice-campeão [visekãpi'ãw] *m*, **-ã** *f* runner-up
vice-líder [vise'lideɾ] *m/f* deputy leader
vice-presidente [viseprezi'dẽtʃi] *m/f* vice-president
vice-versa [vise'vɛrsa] *adv* vice-versa
viciado [vi'sjadu] **1** *adj* (*adulterado*) tainted; *ar* stale; *drogas*: addicted **2** *m*, **-a** *f* addict; ***~ em heroína*** heroin addict
viciador [visja'doɾ] *adj* addictive
viciar [vi'sjaɾ] ⟨1g⟩ **1** *v/t* (*falsificar*) adulterate; *aposta* fix **2** *v/i droga* be addictive
vício ['visiu] *m* vice; (*mau hábito*) bad habit; *droga etc*: addiction
vicioso [vi'sjozu] *adj* defective; (*depravado*) depraved; ***círculo*** *m* ***~*** vicious circle
vicissitude [visisi'tudʒi] *f* vicissitude
viço ['visu] *m* vigor, *Brit* vigour; (*sumo*) sap; (*opulência*) lushness; (*ardor*) fire
viçoso [vi'sozu] *adj* (*vigoroso*) vigorous; *planta* lush
vida ['vida] *f* life; (*sustento*) living; (*vivacidade*) liveliness; ***é a ~*** that's life; ***em ~, ele ...*** in his lifetime he ...; ***ando a dizer mal da ~*** I'm feeling sorry for myself; ***~ noturna***, *Port* ***~ nocturna*** nightlife; ***ter muita ~*** be full of life
vide ['vidʒi] *f* vine
videira [vi'dejɾa] *f* grapevine
vidente [vi'dẽtʃi] *m/f* clairvoyant
vídeo ['vidʒju] *m* video; ***câmara*** *f* ***de ~*** video camera; ***gravador*** *m* ***de ~*** video recorder
videocâmara [vidʒjo'kʌmaɾa] *m Bras* video camera
videocassete [vidʒjoka'sɛtʃi] *m* video cassette
videoconferência [vidʒjokõfe'ɾẽsja] *f* video conference
videogravador [vidʒjoɡɾava'doɾ] *m* video recorder
videojogo [vidʒjo'ʒoɡu] *m* video game
videotexto [vidʒjo'testu] *m* videotext
videovigilância [vidʒjoviʒi'lãsja] *f* video surveillance
vidoeiro [vi'dwejɾu] *m* birch
vidraça [vi'dɾasa] *f* windowpane
vidraceiro [vidɾa'sejɾu] *m* glazier
vidrado [vi'dɾadu] **1** *adj olho* glazed; *barro etc* glass *atr* **2** *m* glazing
vidragem [vi'dɾaʒẽ] *f* glazing
vidrar [vi'dɾaɾ] ⟨1a⟩ glaze
vidraria [vidɾa'ɾia] *f* glassworks
vidreiro [vi'dɾejɾu] **1** *adj* glass *atr* **2** *m*, **-a** *f* glass blower
vidro ['vidɾu] *m* glass; AUTO window; ***um ~*** a pane of glass; ***~ fosco*** frosted glass
viela ['viɛla] *f* alley
vier [viɛɾ], **viesse** ['viɛsi] *etc* → ***vir***
Vietnã [viet'nã] *m*, *Port* **Vietname** [viet'nami] *m* Vietnam
vietnamita [vietna'mita] *adj* & *m/f* Vietnamese
viga ['viɡa] *f suporte* beam; *ferro*: girder
vigamento [viɡa'mẽtu] *m* beams; *ferro*: girders
vigarice [viɡa'ɾisi] *f* deception
vigário [vi'ɡaɾiu] *m* vicar
vigarista [viɡa'ɾista] **1** *m/f* crook

2 *adj* crooked
vigarizar [vigari'zar] *v/t* con, swindle
vigência [vi'ʒẽsja] *f* validity
vigente [vi'ʒẽtʃi] *adj* valid; *lei* in effect
vigésimo [vi'ʒɛzimu] **1** *adj* twentieth **2** *m* twentieth
vigia [vi'ʒia] **1** *f* watch, sentry; (*postigo*) peephole; NÁUT porthole; ***ficar de ~*** keep watch **2** *m/f* watchman, guard
vigiar [vi'ʒjar] ⟨1g⟩ **1** *v/i* keep a lookout, keep watch (***em*** over) **2** *v/t* guard; (*observar*) watch over
vigilância [viʒi'lãsja] *f* vigilance
vigilante [viʒi'lãtʃi] **1** *adj* vigilant **2** *m/f* watch, lookout
vigília [vi'ʒilja] *f* vigil; *segurança*: night watch
vigor [vi'gor] *m* vigor, *Brit* vigour; (*ênfase*) emphasis; DIR effect; ***com ~*** forcefully; ***estar em ~*** be in force; ***entrar / pôr em ~*** come / put into effect
vigoroso [vigo'rozu] *adj* vigorous; (*enérgico*) forceful
vil [viw] *adj* vile
vila ['vila] *f* small town; (*casa*) villa
vilania [vila'nia] *f* vileness
vilão [vi'lãw] *m*, **-ã** *f* villain
vim [vĩ] → ***vir***
vime ['vimi] *m* wicker; ***cesto*** *m* ***de ~*** wicker basket
vimeiro [vi'mejru] *m* BOT willow
vimos ['vimus] → ***ver, vir***
vinagre [vi'nagri] *m* vinegar; ***chegar o ~ ao nariz*** lose patience
vinagreta [vina'greta] *f* GASTR vinaigrette
vincar [vĩŋ'kar] ⟨1n⟩ crease; (*gravar*) furrow; *fig* stress
vinco ['vĩku] *m* crease; (*sulco*) furrow
vincular [vĩku'lar] ⟨1a⟩ link (***a*** to); (*determinar*) fix; (*obrigar*) bind (***a*** to); **vincular-se** *v/r* ***~ a algo*** be tied to sth
vínculo ['vĩkulu] *m* link, tie *tb fig*
vinda ['vĩda] *f* coming; (*chegada*) arrival; ***dar as boas ~s a alguém*** welcome s.o.
vindima [vĩ'dʒima] *f* grape harvest
vindo ['vĩdu] → ***vir***
vingança [vĩ'gãsa] *f* revenge
vingar [vĩ'gar] ⟨1o⟩ **1** *v/t* avenge; (*defender*) defend **2** *v/i* succeed; (*impor-se*) have one's way; (*desenvolver-se*) thrive; **vingar-se** *v/r* get one's revenge
vingativo [vĩga'tʃivu] *adj* vindictive
vinha[1] ['viɲa] *f* vineyard; *planta* vine
vinha[2] ['viɲa]', **vinhas** ['viɲas] → ***vir***
vinhedo [vi'ɲedu] *m* vineyard
vinho ['viɲu] *m* wine; ***~ branco*** white wine; ***~ da casa*** house wine; ***~ tinto*** red wine;; ***~ verde*** young white wine
vinícola [vi'nikula] *adj* wine-producing
vinicultor [vinikuw'tor] *m*, **-a** *f* winegrower, winemaker
vinicultura [vinikuw'tura] *f* winegrowing
vintavo [vĩ'tavu] *m* twentieth
vinte ['vĩtʃi] *num* twenty
vintena [vĩ'tena] *f* ***uma ~*** (***de***) around twenty
viola ['vjɔla] *f* MÚS guitar; ***~ de arco*** viola; ***tocar ~*** play the guitar / viola
violação [vjola'sãw] *f* violation; (*estupro*) rape
violar [vjo'lar] ⟨1e⟩ violate; (*estuprar*) rape
violão [vjo'lãw] *m* guitar
violência [vjo'lẽsja] *f* violence; *ato* act of violence
violentar [vjolẽ'tar] ⟨1a⟩ force
violento [vjo'lẽtu] *adj* violent
violeta [vjo'leta] **1** *f* BOT violet; MÚS viola **2** *adj* violet
violinista [vjoli'nista] *m/f* violinist
violino [vjo'linu] *m* violin; ***tocar ~*** play the violin
violoncelista [vjolõse'lista] *m/f* cellist
violoncelo [vjolõ'sɛlu] *m* cello
vir[1] [vir] ⟨3w⟩ come; ***~ de*** come from; ***mandar ~*** send for; ***~ buscar*** come and get; ***vem cá!*** come here!
vir[2] [vir] *etc* → ***ver***
vira-casaca(s) [viraka'zaka(s)] *m/f(pl) fig* turncoat
virada [vi'rada] *f* turning; *história*: twist; ***~ de 180 graus*** U-turn; ***~ em favor dos democratas*** swing to the Democrats
viragem [vi'raʒẽ] *f* AUTO turn; POL ***~ à direita / esquerda*** swing to the

right / left; ***ponto*** *m* ***de ~*** turning point

vira-lata [vira'lata] *m/f* ⟨*pl* ~ s⟩ mongrel

virar [vi'rar] ⟨1a⟩ **1** *v/t* (*voltar*) turn (around); NÁUT turn over; *página* turn (over); *rosto* turn away; *motorista* turn off; ~ ***as costas*** turn one's back on **2** *v/i* AUTO turn; ~ ***à direita / esquerda*** turn off to the right / left, take a right / left; **virar-se** *v/r pessoa* turn around; *objeto* turn over; *financeiramente etc* get by, manage

virei [vi'rej], **vires** ['viris] → ***vir, virar***

virgem ['virʒẽ] **1** *f* virgin **2** *adj* virgin; *fig* pure; *fita* blank; ***floresta*** *f* ~ virgin forest

Virgem ['virʒẽ] *f* ASTROL Virgo

vírgula ['virgula] *f* comma; ~ ***decimal*** point

viril [vi'riw] *adj* virile

virilha [vi'riʎa] *f* ANAT groin

virilidade [virili'dadʒi] *f* virility

virose [vi'rɔzi] *f* viral infection

virótico [vi'rɔtʃiku] *adj* viral

virtual [vir'twaw] *adj* virtual

virtualmente [vir'twaw] *adv* virtually

virtude [vir'tudʒi] *f* virtue; ***em ~ de*** by virtue of

virtuoso [vir'twozu] **1** *adj* virtuous; *artista* virtuoso **2** *m*, **-a** *f* virtuoso

virulência [viru'lẽsja] *f* virulence

virulento [viru'lẽtu] *adj* virulent

vírus ['virus] *m* virus

visão [vi'zãw] *f* sight, vision; (*percepção*) way of seeing; (*ponto de vista*) point of view; (*aspeto*) sight; (*aparição*) vision; ~ ***geral*** overview; ***de ~ limitada*** narrow-minded

visar [vi'zar] ⟨1a⟩ *v/t* aim at; ***visando fazer algo*** with a view to doing sth

vísceras ['viseras] *fpl* viscera

viscosidade [viskozi'dadʒi] *f* viscosity

viscoso [vis'kozu] *adj* viscous

viscose [vis'kɔzi] *f* TÊX viscose

viseira [vi'zejra] *f* visor

visibilidade [vizibili'dadʒi] *f* visibility; ~ ***atmosférica*** visibility

visita [vi'zita] *f* visit; *internet*: hit; ***estar de ~*** be visiting; ~ ***guiada*** guided tour; ~ ***oficial*** state visit

visitante [vizi'tãtʃi] *m/f* visitor

visitar [vizi'tar] ⟨1a⟩ visit; ~ ***o dentista*** pay a visit to the dentist

visível [vi'zivew] *adj* visible

visivelmente [vizivew'mẽtʃi] *adv* visibly

vislumbrar [vizlũ'brar] ⟨1a⟩ *v/t* glimpse

visor [vi'ʒor] *m* FOT viewfinder

visse ['visi], **viste** ['vistʃi] *etc* → ***ver***

vista ['vista] *f* sight; (*visão*) (eye)sight; (*opinião*), *paisagem*: view; ~ ***curta*** short-sightedness *tb fig*; ~ ***de olhos*** look; ~ ***para o mar*** sea view; ***ponto*** *m* ***de ~*** point of view; COM ***à ~*** sight; ***dar nas ~s*** stand out

visto ['vistu] **2** *pp* → ***ver*** **2** *m* visa; ~ ***turístico*** tourist visa; ***pelos ~s*** obviously, apparently **3** *adj* ~ ***que*** seeing (that)

vistoria [visto'ria] *f* inspection

vistoriar [visto'rjar] ⟨1g⟩ inspect

vistoso [vis'tozu] *adj* striking, eye-catching

visual [vi'zwaw] **1** *adj* visual **2** *m* look

visualizar [vizwali'zar] ⟨1a⟩ visualize; INFORM display

visualmente [vizwaw'mẽtʃi] *adv* visually

vital [vi'taw] *adj* vital; *fig* ***ponto*** *m* ~ essential point

vitalício [vita'lisiu] *adj* lifelong

vitalidade [vitali'dadʒi] *f* vitality

vitamina [vita'mina] *f* vitamin

vitela [vi'tɛla] *f* calf; GASTR veal; *couro*: calfskin

vitelo [vi'tɛlu] *m* calf

vítima ['vitʃima] *f* victim; ***ser ~ de*** be a victim of

vitimar [vitʃi'mar] *v/t* REL, *fig* sacrifice; (*matar*) kill; *discriminação*: victimize

vitória [vi'tɔrja] *f* victory; ESP POL *tb* win

vitorioso [vito'rjozu] *adj* victorious

vitral [vi'traw] *m* stained glass window

vítreo ['vitriu] *adj* glass

vitrina [vi'trina] *f*, **vitrine** [vi'trini] *f* (*montra*) store window, shop window; (*armário*) display case

vitríolo [vi'triulu] *m* vitriol

viu [viu] → ***ver***

viúva ['viuva] *f* widow
viuvez [viu'ves] *f* widowhood
viúvo ['viuvu] **1** *adj* widowed; *fig* abandoned **2** *m* widower
viva ['viva] *int* **~ *Brasil!*** *fam* come on Brazil!
vivacidade [vivasi'dadʒi] *f* vivacity, liveliness
vivaz [vi'vas] *adj* lively
viveiro [vi'vejɾu] *m aves*: aviary; *árvores*: nursery; *peixes*: fish farm
vivência [vi'vẽsja] *f* (*experiência*) experience; (*vida*) life
vivenda [vi'vẽda] *f* house
viver [vi'veɾ] ⟨2a⟩ live; **~ *com*** live with; **~ *de*** live on
víveres ['viveris] *mpl* provisions
viveza [vi'veza] *f* vivacity
vívido ['vividu] *adj* vivid
vivificar [vivifi'kaɾ] ⟨1n⟩ bring alive
vivo ['vivu] *adj* living; (*vivaz*) lively; (*esperto*) clever, bright; (*veemente*) heated; ***ao* ~** live
vizinhança [vizi'ɲãsa] *f* neighborhood. *Brit* neighbourhood
vizinho [vi'ziɲu] **1** *adj* neighboring, *Brit* neighbouring; (*próximo*) nearby; *fig* (*aparentado*) related **2** *m*, **-a** *f* neighbor, *Brit* neighbour
vô [vo] *m* grandpa
voador [vwa'doɾ] **1** *adj* flying; *fig* fleeting **2** *m* ZOOL flying fish
voar [vwaɾ] ⟨1f⟩ fly *tb fig*
vocabulário [vokabu'laɾiu] *m* vocabulary
vocábulo [vo'kabulu] *m* word
vocação [voka'sãw] *f* vocation
vocal [vo'kaw] *adj* vocal
vodca ['vɔdka] *f* vodka
voga ['vɔga] *f* (*moda*) vogue; ESP stroke; ***pôr em* ~** make fashionable; ***estar em* ~** be in vogue
vogal [vo'gaw] *f* vowel
volante [vo'lãtʃi] *m* AUTO steering wheel
volátil [vo'latʃiw] *adj* QUÍM volatile
volatilizar [volatʃili'zaɾ] ⟨1a⟩ QUÍM volatilize
vôlei ['volej] *m Bras*, **voleibol** [volej'bɔw] *m* volleyball; **~ *de praia*** beach volleyball
volt [volt] *m* ELÉT volt
volta ['vɔlta] *f* turn; (*retorno*) return; ESP lap; *museu, área*: tour; ***em* ~** (all) around; ***por* ~ *de*** around; ***estar às* ~*s com*** grapple with; ***dar uma* ~ *por*** go around; ***dar uma* ~ *no parque*** go for a walk in the park; ***dar uma* ~ *de carro*** go for a drive; ***estar de* ~** be back; ***eles escreveram / ligaram de* ~** they wrote / phoned back
voltagem [vow'taʒẽ] *f* ELÉT voltage
voltar [vow'taɾ] ⟨1e⟩ **1** *v/t* turn; (*virar*) turn around **2** *v/i* turn around; (*regressar*) go / come back; *dúvidas etc* come back (***a*** to); *cheque* bounce; **~ *atrás*** turn back, *fig* back out, backpedal; ***voltarei tarde*** I'll be back late; **~ *a dormir*** go back to sleep; **~ *a si*** come around; **voltar-se** *v/r* (*virar-se*) turn
vóltio ['vɔltiu] *m* → ***volt***
volubilidade [volubili'dadʒi] *f* fickleness
volume [vo'lumi] *m* volume; TECN cubic capacity; (*encomenda*) package; **~ *de pacientes*** caseload
volumoso [volu'mozu] *adj* bulky
voluntário [volũ'taɾiu] **1** *adj* voluntary **2** *m* volunteer
voluntarioso [volũta'ɾjozu] *adj* headstrong
volúpia [vo'lupja] *f*, **voluptuosidade** [voluptwozi'dadʒi] *f* voluptuousness
voluptuoso [volup'twozu] *adj* voluptuous
vomitar [vomi'taɾ] ⟨1a⟩ **1** *v/t* vomit; *fogo* spew out **2** *v/i* vomit
vômito, *Port* **vómito** ['vomitu] *m* vomit; ***dar* ~*s a alguém*** make s.o. want to throw up
vontade [võ'tadʒi] *f* will; (*desejo*) wish; (*apetite*) desire; ***contra a* ~** reluctantly; ***boa* ~** goodwill; ***de má* ~** grudgingly; ***estar com* ~ *de*** feel like, be in the mood for; ***perder a* ~** be put off; ***sentir muita* ~ *de fazer algo*** be keen to do sth; ***ele fez isso de livre e espontânea* ~** he did it of his own free will; ***à* ~** at ease
vôo, *Port* **voo** ['vou] *m* flight; ***levantar* ~** *pássaro* fly off; *avião* take off; *balão* fly up; **~ *direto***, *Port* **~ *directo*** direct

flight; ~ ***de carreira*** scheduled flight; ~ ***charter*** charter flight; ~ ***doméstico*** domestic flight; ~ ***de ida*** outward flight; ~ ***livre*** hang-gliding; ~ ***de volta*** return flight
voracidade [vorasi'dadʒi] *f* voraciousness
voraz [vo'ras] *adj* voracious
vos [vus] *pron* you
vós [vɔs] *pron* you
vosso, -a ['vɔsu, 'vɔsa] **1** *adj* your **2** *pron* yours; ***o ~, a nossa*** yours
votação [vota'sãw] *f* vote
votar [vo'tar] ⟨1e⟩ **1** *v/t* vote on; *alguém* vote for **2** *v/i* vote; ~ ***contra / a favor*** vote against / for
voto ['vɔtu] *m* vow; *fig* wish; POL vote; ***lançar o seu ~*** cast one's vote
vou [vo] → ***ir***
vovô [vo'vo] *m* grandpa
vovó [vo'vɔ] *f* gran(ny)
voz [vɔs] *f* voice; ***em ~ alta*** at the top of one's voice; *ler* aloud; ~ ***ativa***, *Port* ~ ***activa*** active voice; ~ ***passiva*** passive voice
vulcânico [vuw'kʌniku] *adj* volcanic
vulcão [vuw'kãw] *m* volcano
vulgar [vuw'gar] *adj* (*grosseiro*) vulgar
vulgaridade [vuwgari'dadʒi] *f* vulgarity
vulgarizar [vuwgari'zar] ⟨1a⟩ *v/t* popularize; **vulgarizar-se** *v/r* become well known
vulnerar [vuwne'rar] ⟨1c⟩ wound
vulnerável [vuwne'ravew] *adj* vulnerable
vulto ['vuwtu] *m* figure; (*volume*) extent; (*significado*) significance; ***de ~*** significant; ***tomar ~*** take shape; *fig* gain importance
vultoso [vuw'tozu] *adj* extensive; (*importante*) significant
vulva ['vuwva] *f* ANAT vulva

W

Web ['wɛb] *f* web; ***página ~*** web page
wellness ['wɛlnɛs] *f* wellness; ***centro*** *m* ~ wellness center, *Brit* wellness centre
whisky ['wiski] *m Port* whiskey, *Brit* whisky
windsurf [wĩd'surf] *m* windsurfing

X

X, x [ʃis] *m* X, x; ***raios X*** *mpl* X-rays
xá [ʃa] *m* shah
xadrez [ʃa'dres] **1** *m* chess; *tabuleiro* chessboard; *padrão*: checked pattern; *fam* clink **2** *adj* check *atr*, checked
xale ['ʃali] *m* shawl
xampu [ʃã'pu] *m Bras* shampoo
xarope [ʃa'rɔpi] *m* syrup; MED cough syrup
xenofobia [ʃenofo'bia] *f* xenophobia
xenófobo [ʃe'nɔfubu] *adj* xenophobic
xeque ['ʃɛki] *m pessoa* sheikh; *jogo* chess
xeque-mate [ʃɛke'matʃi] *m* checkmate
xereta [ʃe'reta] *adj* nosy

xerez [ʃɛ'ɾes] *m* sherry
xerife [ʃe'ɾifi] *m* sheriff
xexé [ʃe'ʃɛ] *adj* doddery, senile
xícara ['ʃikaɾa] *f Bras* cup; **~ de café** coffee cup; *bebida* cup of coffee
xico ['ʃiku] *m* guy
xilofone [ʃilo'foni] *m* MÚS xylophone
xilografia [ʃilogɾa'fia] *f* woodcut
xingar [ʃĩ'gaɾ] ⟨1o⟩ *v/t* swear at
xisto ['ʃistu] *m* GEOL slate
xixi [ʃi'ʃi] *m fam* pee, piddle; **fazer ~** have a pee

Z

zagueiro [za'gejɾu] *m* fullback
zambujeiro [zãbu'ʒejɾu] *m* wild olive tree
zanga ['zãga] *f* anger; (*briga*) fight
zangado [zã'gadu] *adj* angry, mad
zangar [zã'gaɾ] ⟨1o⟩ anger, annoy; ***estar zangado com alguém*** be angry with s.o.; **zangar-se** *v/r* get angry; (*brigar*) have a fight
zapping ['zapĩ] *m* **fazer ~** channel-hop
zarolho [za'ɾoʎu] *adj* cross-eyed; (*vesgo*) one-eyed
zarpar [zaɾ'paɾ] ⟨1b⟩ sail, depart; *fam* scram
zebra ['zebɾa] *f* zebra
zebrado [ze'bɾadu] *adj* striped
zelador [zela'doɾ] *m*, **-a** *f* super(intendent), *Brit* janitor
zelar [ze'laɾ] ⟨1c⟩ look after; (*ter ciúmes*) be jealous of
zelo ['zelu] *m* zeal; **~s** *pl* (*ciúmes*) jealousy; **greve** *f* **do ~** work-to-rule
zeloso [ze'lozu] *adj* zealous; (*ciumento*) jealous; (*cuidadoso*) careful
zé-ninguem [zɛnĩ'gẽ] *m fam* nobody, poor wretch
zênite, *Port* **zénite** ['zenitʃi] *m* zenith
zepelim [zepe'lĩ] *m* zeppelin
zero ['zɛɾu] *m* zero; *tênis*: love
zibelina [zibe'lina] *f* (**marta**) **~** sable
ziguezague [zige'zagi] *m* zigzag
ziguezaguear [zigezagi'aɾ] ⟨1l⟩ *v/i* zigzag
zinco ['zĩku] *m* zinc
zíngaro ['zĩŋgaɾu] *m*, **-a** *f pej* gypsy
zíper ['zipeɾ] *m* zipper, zip fastener, *Brit* zip; ***fechar o ~ de*** zip up
Zodíaco [zo'dʒiaku] *m* ASTROL zodiac; ***signo*** *m* **do ~** sign of the zodiac
zoeira [zo'ejɾa] *f* din
zombar [zõ'baɾ] ⟨1a⟩ *esp Bras* make fun, mock; **~ de** make fun of, mock
zombaria [zõba'ɾia] *f* mockery
zona ['zona] *f* zone; (*região*) region; MED shingles *sg*; *de prostituição* red light district; ***~ de baixa pressão*** low pressure area; ***~ de catástrofe*** disaster area; ***~ euro*** euro zone; ***~ industrial*** industrial zone; ***~ de peões*** pedestrian zone; AUTO ***~ de sombra*** blind spot; ***~ verde*** green area
zôo, *Port* **zoo** ['zow] *m* zoo
zoologia [zoolo'ʒia] *f* zoology
zoológico [zoo'lɔʒiku] *adj* zoological; ***jardim*** *m* **~** zoo
zoólogo [zo'ɔlogu] *m*, **-a** *f* zoologist
zoom [zum] *m* FOT zoom
zumbi ['zũbi] *m* zombie
zumbido [zũ'bidu] *m* buzzing, humming
zumbir [zũ'biɾ] ⟨3a⟩ buzz, hum; *vento* whistle
zunido [zu'nidu] *m* whistling; (*zumbido*) hum
zunir [zu'niɾ] ⟨3a⟩ *vento* whistle; (*zumbir*) hum
zunzum [zũ'zũ] *m* buzz, hum; (*rumor*) whisper
zurrapa [zu'hapa] *f fam* booze
zurrar [zu'haɾ] ⟨1a⟩ *burro* heehaw
zurros ['zuhus] *mpl* heehaw
zurzir [zuɾ'ziɾ] ⟨3a⟩ (*chicotear*) whip; (*castigar*) punish; (*criticar*) slate, slam

A

a [ə] *stressed* [eɪ] *art* um, uma; ***$50 ~ trip*** $50 por percurso
aback [ə'bæk] *adv* ***be taken ~*** estar tomado de surpresa
abandon [ə'bændən] *v/t object, plan* abandonar
abate [ə'beɪt] *v/i storm, flood waters* abrandar
abattoir ['æbətwɑːr] *Brit* abatedouro *m*
abbey ['æbɪ] abadia *f*
abbreviate [ə'briːvɪeɪt] *v/t* abreviar
abbreviation [əbriːvɪ'eɪʃn] abreviatura *f*, abreviação *f*
abdicate ['æbdɪkeɪt] *v/i* abdicar
abdication [æbdɪ'keɪʃn] abdicação *f*
abdomen ['æbdəmən] abdômen *m*
abdominal [æb'dɑːmɪnl] *adj* abdominal
abduct [əb'dʌkt] *v/t* raptar
abduction [əb'dʌkʃn] rapto *m*
♦ **abide by** [ə'baɪd] *v/t* cumprir
ability [ə'bɪlətɪ] capacidade *f*; ***the ~ to learn*** a capacidade para aprender
ablaze [ə'bleɪz] *adj* em chamas
able ['eɪbl] *adj* (*skillful*) capaz; ***be ~ to*** ser capaz de; ***I wasn't ~ to see / hear*** não consegui ver / ouvir
able-bodied ['eɪblbɒːdiːd] *adj* fisicamente capaz
abnormal [æb'nɔːrml] *adj* anormal
abnormally [æb'nɔːrməlɪ] *adv* de forma estranha; ***it has been ~ cold this month*** tem sido estranhamente frio esse mês
aboard [ə'bɔːrd] **1** *prep* a bordo de **2** *adv* ***be ~*** estar a bordo; ***go ~*** ir a bordo
abolish [ə'bɑːlɪʃ] *v/t* abolir
abolition [æbə'lɪʃn] abolição *f*
abort [ə'bɔːrt] *v/t also* COMPUT *program* abortar
abortion [ə'bɔːrʃn] aborto *m*; ***have an ~*** fazer um aborto
abortive [ə'bɔːrtɪv] *adj* fracassado
about [ə'baʊt] **1** *prep* (*concerning*) sobre; ***what's it ~?*** *book, movie* sobre o que é? **2** *adv* (*roughly*) cerca de; ***be ~ to ...*** (*be going to*) estar quase para ...; ***be ~*** *somewhere near* estar por perto; ***there are a lot of people ~*** há muita gente por perto
above [ə'bʌv] **1** *prep* acima de; ***~ all*** acima de tudo **2** *adv* acima; ***on the floor ~*** no andar acima
above-mentioned [əbʌv'menʃnd] *adj* acima mencionado
abrasion [ə'breɪʒn] abrasão *f*
abrasive [ə'breɪsɪv] *adj personality* abrasivo
abreast [ə'brest] *adv* lado a lado; ***keep ~ of*** ficar a par de
abridge [ə'brɪdʒ] *v/t* abreviar
abroad [ə'brɒːd] *adv live* no exterior; *go* ao exterior
abrupt [ə'brʌpt] *adj departure, manner* abrupto
abruptly [ə'brʌptlɪ] *adv* subitamente
abscess ['æbsɪs] abscesso *m*, *Port* abcesso *m*
absence ['æbsəns] ausência *f*
absent ['æbsənt] *adj* ausente
absentee [æbsən'tiː] absenteísta *m/f*
absenteeism [æbsən'tiːɪzm] absenteísmo *m*
absent-minded [æbsənt'maɪndɪd] *adj* distraído
absent-mindedly [æbsənt'maɪndɪdlɪ] *adv* distraidamente
absolute ['æbsəluːt] *adj power* absoluto; *idiot* completo
absolutely ['æbsəluːtlɪ] *adv* (*completely*) completamente; ***~ not!*** absolutamente não!; ***do you ~? – ~*** você concorda? - absolutamente
absolution [æbsə'luːʃn] REL absolvição *f*
absolve [əb'zɑːlv] *v/t* absolver
absorb [əb'sɔːrb] *v/t* absorver; ***~ed in ...*** absorvido em ...

absorbency [əb'sɔːrbənsɪ] absorvência *f*
absorbent [əb'sɔːrbənt] *adj* absorvente
absorbent 'cotton algodão *m* hidrófilo
absorbing [əb'sɔːrbɪŋ] *adj* absorvente
abstain [əb'steɪn] *v/i voting*: abster-se
abstention [əb'stenʃn] *voting*: abstenção *f*
abstract ['æbstrækt] *adj* abstrato
abstruse [əb'struːs] *adj* abstruso
absurd [əb'sɜːrd] *adj* absurdo
absurdity [əb'sɜːrdətɪ] absurdo *m*
absurdly [əb'sɜːrdlɪ] *adv* absurdamente
abundance [ə'bʌndəns] abundância *f*
abundant [ə'bʌndənt] *adj* abundante
abuse[1] [ə'bjuːs] *n* (*insults*) ofensa *f*; *of child, thing* abuso *m*
abuse[2] [ə'bjuːz] *v/t physically* abusar; *verbally* ofender
abusive [ə'bjuːsɪv] *adj language* abusivo; ***become ~*** tornar-se inconveniente
abysmal [ə'bɪʒml] *adj fam* (*very bad*) terrível
abyss [ə'bɪs] abismo *m*
AC ['eɪsiː] *abbr* (*of* ***alternating current***) corrente *f* alternada
academic [ækə'demɪk] **1** *n* acadêmico,-a *m,f* **2** *adj* acadêmico; *year* letivo
academy [ə'kædəmɪ] academia *f*
accelerate [ək'seləreɪt] *v/t & v/i* acelerar
acceleration [əkselə'reɪʃn] aceleração *f*
accelerator [ək'seləreɪtər] acelerador *m*
accent ['æksənt] *when speaking* sotaque *m*; (*emphasis*) acento *m*
accentuate [ək'sentjuːeɪt] *v/t* acentuar
accept [ək'sept] *v/t & v/i* aceitar
acceptable [ək'septəbl] *adj* aceitável
acceptance [ək'septəns] aceitação *f*
access ['ækses] **1** *n* acesso *m*; ***have ~ to*** *computer, child* ter acesso a **2** *v/t also* COMPUT acessar
'access code COMPUT código *m* de acesso
accessible [ək'sesəbl] *adj* acessível
accession [ək'seʃn] ascensão *f*
accessory [ək'sesərɪ] *for wearing* acessório *m*; LAW cúmplice *m/f*
'access road rodovia *f* de acesso
'access time COMPUT tempo *m* de acesso
accident ['æksɪdənt] acidente *m*; ***by ~*** por acidente
accidental [æksɪ'dentl] *adj* acidental
accidentally [æksɪ'dentlɪ] *adv* acidentalmente
acclaim [ə'kleɪm] **1** *n* aclamação *f* **2** *v/t* aclamar
acclamation [əklə'meɪʃn] aclamação *f*
acclimate, **acclimatize** [ə'klaɪmət, ə'klaɪmətaɪz] *v/t* aclimatizar
accommodate [ə'kɑːmədeɪt] *v/t* acomodar; *special requirements* suportar; (*bear*) comportar
accommodations [əkɑːmə'deɪʃnz] *npl Am* acomodações *fpl*
accompaniment [ə'kʌmpənɪmənt] MUS acompanhamento *m*
accompanist [ə'kʌmpənɪst] MUS acompanhante *m/f*
accompany [ə'kʌmpənɪ] *v/t* ⟨*pret & pp* ***accompanied***⟩ *also* MUS acompanhar
accomplice [ə'kʌmplɪs] cúmplice *m/f*
accomplish [ə'kʌmplɪʃ] *v/t task* cumprir; *goal* atingir
accomplished [ə'kʌmplɪʃt] *adj* talentoso
accomplishment [ə'kʌmplɪʃmənt] *of task* cumprimento *m*; (*achievement*) realização *m*; (*talent*) dom *m*
accord [ə'kɔːrd] concordância *f*; ***of one's own ~*** por iniciativa própria
accordance [ə'kɔːrdəns] acordo *m*; ***in ~ with*** de acordo com
according [ə'kɔːrdɪŋ] *adv* ***~ to*** conforme
accordingly [ə'kɔːrdɪŋlɪ] *adv* (*consequently*) conseqüentemente; (*appropriately*) adequadamente
accordion [ə'kɔːrdɪən] acordeão *m*
accordionist [ə'kɔːrdɪənɪst] acordeonista *m/f*
account [ə'kaʊnt] *financial* conta *f*; (*report, description*) relato *m*; ***give an ~ of*** fazer um relato de; ***on no***

~ de forma alguma; ***on ~ of*** por conta de; ***take ... into ~, take ~ of ...*** levar em conta
♦**account for** *v/t* (*explain*) explicar; (*make up, constitute*) responder por
accountability [əkaʊntə'bɪlətɪ] responsabilidade *f*
accountable [ə'kaʊntəbl] *adj* responsável; ***be held ~ for*** (*answer for*) ser considerado responsável por
accountant [ə'kaʊntənt] contador,a *m,f*, *Port* contabilista *m/f*
ac'count holder correntista *m/f*
ac'count number número *m* da conta
accounts [ə'kaʊnts] contabilidade *f*
ac'counts department departamento *m* financeiro
accumulate [ə'kju:mjʊleɪt] **1** *v/t* acumular **2** *v/i* acumular-se
accumulation [əkju:mjʊ'leɪʃn] acúmulo *m*
accuracy ['ækjʊrəsɪ] exatidão *f*
accurate ['ækjʊrət] *adj* exato
accurately ['ækjʊrətlɪ] *adv* com exatidão
accusation [ækju:'zeɪʃn] acusação *f*; *public* denúncia *f*
accuse [ə'kju:z] *v/t* acusar; *publicly* denunciar; ***he ~d me of lying*** ele me acusou de mentir; ***be ~d of ...*** LAW ser acusado de ...
accused [ə'kju:zd] *n* LAW acusado,-a *m,f*
accusing [ə'kju:zɪŋ] *adj look, tone* acusatório
accusingly [ə'kju:zɪŋlɪ] *adv* acusativamente
accustom [ə'kʌstəm] *v/t* ***get ~ed to*** acostumar-se a; ***be ~ed to*** estar acostumado a
ace [eɪs] *cards*: ás *m*; *tennis* (*shot*) ace *m*
ache [eɪk] **1** *n* dor *f* **2** *v/i* doer
achieve [ə'tʃi:v] *v/t* alcançar
achievement [ə'tʃi:vmənt] realização *f*
acid ['æsɪd] *n* ácido *m*
acidity [ə'sɪdətɪ] acidez *f*
acid 'rain chuva *f* ácida
'acid test *fig* teste *m* decisivo
acknowledge [ək'nɑ:lɪdʒ] *v/t truth, achievements* reconhecer; *presence, receipt* confirmar
acknowledgment, **acknowledgement** [ək'nɑ:lɪdʒmənt] *truth, achievements*: reconhecimento *m*; *presence, receipt*: confirmação *f*
acne ['æknɪ] MED acne *f*, *fam* espinha *f*
acorn ['eɪkɔ:rn] BOT bolota *f*
acoustics [ə'ku:stɪks] *npl* acústica *f*
acquaint [ə'kweɪnt] *v/t fml* ***be ~ed with*** conhecer
acquaintance [ə'kweɪntəns] *person* conhecido,-a *m,f*
acquiesce [ækwɪ'es] *v/i fml* aquiescer
acquiescence [ækwɪ'esns] *fml* aquiescência *f*
acquire [ə'kwaɪr] *v/t skill, knowledge, property* adquirir; *success* conseguir
acquisition [ækwɪ'zɪʃn] aquisição *f*
acquisitive [æ'kwɪzətɪv] *adj* aquisitivo
acquit [ə'kwɪt] *v/t* LAW inocentar
acquittal [ə'kwɪtl] LAW absolvição *f*
acre ['eɪkər] acre *m*
acreage ['eɪkrɪdʒ] área *f* medida em acres
acrimonious [ækrɪ'moʊnɪəs] *adj* acrimonioso
acrobat ['ækrəbæt] acrobata *m/f*
acrobatic [ækrə'bætɪk] *adj* acrobático
acrobatics [ækrə'bætɪks] *npl* acrobacia *f*
acronym ['ækrənɪm] acrônimo *m*
across [ə'krɑ:s] **1** *prep* (*on other side of*) do outro lado de; (*to other side of*) para o outro lado de; ***walk ~ the street*** atravessar a rua; ***he sailed ~ the Atlantic*** ele navegou pelo Oceano Atlântico; ***they live just ~ from us*** eles vivem logo ali de frente para nós **2** *adv* (*to other side*) para o outro lado; ***they swam ~*** eles atravessaram a nado; ***10 m ~*** 10m de um lado a outro
acrylic [ə'krɪlɪk] *adj* acrílico
act [ækt] **1** *v/i* THEA atuar; (*pretend*) fingir; ***~ as*** agir como; ***where did you learn to ~?*** onde você aprendeu a atuar? **2** *n* (*deed*) ato *m*; (*law*) lei *f*; *play*: ato *m*; *vaudeville*: número *m*; (*pretense*) farsa *f*
acting ['æktɪŋ] **1** *n* arte *f* dramática;

the ~ was terrible a atuação foi horrível **2** *adj* (*temporary*) interino; (*replacement*) substituto
action ['ækʃn] ação *f*; ***out of ~*** (*not functioning*) desativado; ***take ~*** agir; ***bring an ~ against*** LAW entrar com uma ação em juízo
action 'replay TV replay *m* instantâneo
active ['æktɪv] *adj* ativo; *party member* atuante; GRAM ***~ voice*** voz *f* ativa
activist ['æktɪvɪst] POL ativista *m/f*
activity [æk'tɪvətɪ] atividade *f*
act of 'God força *f* maior
actor ['æktər] ator *m*
actress ['æktrɪs] atriz *f*
actual ['æktʃʊəl] *adj* verdadeiro; *example* concreto; ***it is based on ~ facts*** baseado em fatos reais
actually ['æktʃʊəlɪ] *adv* (*in fact, to tell the truth*) na verdade; *expressing surprise* realmente; ***~ I do know him*** *stressing converse* de fato, eu o conheço
acupuncture ['ækjʊpʌŋktʃər] acupuntura *f*
acute [ə'kjuːt] *adj pain* agudo; *smell* forte; *sense* apurado
acutely [ə'kjuːtlɪ] *adv embarrassed, aware* extremamente
ad [æd] anúncio *m*
adamant ['ædəmənt] *adj* inflexível; ***she was ~ that she had seen it*** ela tinha toda a certeza que tinha visto isto
Adam's apple [ædəmz'æpəl] pomo *m* de Adão, *Port* maçã-de-Adão *f*
adapt [ə'dæpt] **1** *v/t* adaptar **2** *v/i person* adaptar-se
adaptability ['ədæptə'bɪlətɪ] adaptabilidade *f*
adaptable [ə'dæptəbl] *adj person, plant* adaptável; *vehicle etc* versátil
adaptation [ædæp'teɪʃn] *of play etc* adaptação *f*
adapter, **adaptor** [ə'dæptər] (*electrical*) adaptador *m*
add [æd] **1** *v/t* MATH somar; (*say, also include*) acrescentar **2** *v/i* MATH somar
♦**add on** *v/t 15% etc* adicionar
♦**add up** **1** *v/t* somar **2** *v/i fig* fazer sentido
adder ['ædər] cobra *f*
addict ['ædɪkt] viciado,-a *m,f*
addicted [ə'dɪktɪd] *adj* viciado; ***be ~ to*** ser viciado em
addiction [ə'dɪkʃn] *drugs, TV, chocolate etc*: vício *m*
addictive [ə'dɪktɪv] *adj drugs, TV, chocolate etc* viciador
addition [ə'dɪʃn] MATH adição *f*, *to list, company etc* inclusão *f*; ***in ~*** além disso; ***in ~ to*** além de; ***a new ~ to the family*** um novo membro da família
additional [ə'dɪʃnl] *adj* adicional
additive ['ædɪtɪv] aditivo *m*
add-on ['ædɑːn] extra *m*
address [ə'dres] **1** *n* endereço *m*; ***form of ~*** forma *f* de tratamento **2** *v/t letter* endereçar; *audience, person* dirigir-se a; *problem* tratar
ad'dress book agenda *f* de endereços
addressee [ædre'siː] destinatário,-a *m,f*
adept ['ædept] *adj* perito; ***be ~ at*** ser experiente em
adequate ['ædɪkwət] *adj* adequado; (*satisfactory*) satisfatório
adequately ['ædɪkwətlɪ] *adv* adequadamente
adhere [əd'hɪr] *v/i* aderir
♦**adhere to** *v/t surface, rules* aderir a
adhesive [əd'hiːsɪv] *n* cola *f*
adhesive 'plaster esparadrapo *m*
adhesive 'tape fita *f* adesiva
adjacent [ə'dʒeɪsnt] *adj* adjacente
adjective ['ædʒɪktɪv] adjetivo *m*
adjoin [ə'dʒɔɪn] *v/t* conjugar
adjoining [ə'dʒɔɪnɪŋ] *adj* conjugado
adjourn [ə'dʒɜːrn] *v/i court, meeting* adiar
adjournment [ə'dʒɜːrnmənt] adiamento *m*
adjust [ə'dʒʌst] *v/t* ajustar
adjustable [ə'dʒʌstəbl] *adj* ajustável
adjustment [ə'dʒʌstmənt] ajuste *m*
ad-lib [æd'lɪb] **1** *adj* improvisado **2** *adv* improvisadamente **3** *v/i* ⟨*pret & pp* ***ad-libbed***⟩ improvisar
administer [əd'mɪnɪstər] *v/t medicine, country* administrar
administration [ədmɪnɪ'streɪʃn] administração *f*

administrative [ədmɪnɪ'stətɪv] *adj* administrativo
administrator [əd'mɪnɪstreɪtər] administrador,a *m,f*
admirable ['ædmərəbl] *adj* admirável
admirably ['ædmərəblɪ] *adv* admiravelmente
admiral ['ædmərəl] MIL almirante *m*
admiration [ædmə'reɪʃn] admiração *f*
admire [əd'maɪr] *v/t* admirar
admirer [əd'maɪrər] admirador,a *m,f*
admiring [əd'maɪrɪŋ] *adj* admirado
admiringly [əd'maɪrɪŋlɪ] *adv* com admiração
admissible [əd'mɪsəbl] *adj* admissível
admission [əd'mɪʃn] (*confession*) confissão *f*; **~ *free*** entrada *f* grátis
admit [əd'mɪt] *v/t* ⟨*pret & pp* ***admitted***⟩ admitir; *school*: matricular; *hospital*: internar
admittance [əd'mɪtəns] entrada *f*; ***no ~*** entrada *f* proibida
admittedly [əd'mɪtedlɪ] *adv* reconhecidamente
admonish [əd'mɑːnɪʃ] *v/t fml* admoestar
ado [ə'duː] delonga *f*; ***without further ~*** sem mais delonga
adolescence [ædə'lesns] adolescência *f*
adolescent [ædə'lesnt] **1** *adj* adolescente **2** *n* adolescente *m/f*
adopt [ə'dɑːpt] *v/t child, plan* adotar
adoption [ə'dɑːpʃn] *child, plan*: adoção *f*
adoptive parents [ədɑːptɪv'perənts] pais *mpl* adotivos
adorable [ə'dɔːrəbl] *adj* adorável
adoration [ædə'reɪʃn] adoração *f*
adore [ə'dɔːr] *v/t* adorar
adoring [ə'dɔːrɪŋ] *adj expression* de adoração; *fans, parents* venerador
adrenalin [ə'drenəlɪn] adrenalina *f*; ***it gets the ~ going*** isso libera a adrenalina
adrift [ə'drɪft] *adj* à deriva; *fig* perdido
adulation [ædʊ'leɪʃn] adulação *f*
adult [ə'dʌlt] **1** *adj* adulto **2** *n* adulto,-a *m,f*
adult edu'cation educação *f* para adultos
adulterous [ə'dʌltərəs] *adj relationship* adulterino
adultery [ə'dʌltərɪ] adultério *m*
'adult movie *euph* filme *m* para adultos
advance [əd'væns] **1** *n* (*money*) adiantamento *m*; *in science etc*, MIL avanço *m*; ***in ~*** *money* adiantado; ***make ~s*** (*progress*) fazer progresso; (*sexually*) investir **2** *v/i* MIL avançar; (*make progress*) progredir **3** *v/t theory* desenvolver; *sum of money* adiantar; *human knowledge, a cause* avançar
advance 'booking reserva *f* com antecedência
advanced [əd'vænst] *adj country, level* avançado; *learner* adiantado
advance 'notice aviso *m* prévio
advance 'payment pagamento *m* adiantado
advantage [əd'væntɪdʒ] vantagem *f*; ***it's to your ~*** é para seu benefício; ***take ~ of*** *opportunity* aproveitar
advantageous [ædvən'teɪdʒəs] *adj* vantajoso
advent ['ædvent] *fig* chegada *f*
'advent calendar calendário *m* do advento
adventure [əd'ventʃər] aventura *f*
adventurous [əd'ventʃərəs] *adj* aventureiro
adverb ['ædvɜːrb] advérbio *m*
adversary ['ædvərserɪ] adversário,-a *m,f*
adverse ['ædvɜːrs] *adj* desfavorável
'advert *Brit* → ***advertisement***
advertise ['ædvərtaɪz] *v/t & v/i* anunciar
advertisement [əd'vɜːrtɪsmənt] anúncio *m*
advertiser ['ædvərtaɪzər] anunciante *m/f*
advertising ['ædvərtaɪzɪŋ] propaganda *f*; (*industry*) publicidade *f*
'advertising agency agência *f* de publicidade
'advertising campaign campanha *f* publicitária
advice [əd'vaɪs] conselho *m*; ***take s.o.'s ~*** aceitar o conselho de alguém; ***a good piece of ~*** um belo conselho

advisable [əd'vaɪzəbl] *adj* aconselhável

advise [əd'vaɪz] *v/t person* aconselhar; *caution etc* recomendar; **~ s.o. to ...** aconselhar alguém a ...

adviser [əd'vaɪzər] conselheiro,-a *m,f*

advocate ['ædvəkeɪt] *v/t* advogar

aerial ['erɪəl] *n Brit* antena *f*

aerial 'photograph fotografia *f* aérea

aerobics [e'roʊbɪks] aeróbica *f*

aerodynamic [eroʊdaɪ'næmɪk] *adj* aerodinâmico

aeronautical [eroʊ'nɒːtɪkl] *adj* aeronáutico

aeroplane ['eroʊpleɪn] *Brit* avião *m*

aerosol ['erəsɑːl] aerossol *m*

aerospace industry ['erəspeɪsɪndʌstrɪ] indústria *f* aeroespacial

aesthetic *Brit* → ***esthetic***

affable ['æfəbl] *adj* afável

affair [ə'fer] (*matter*) assunto *m*; (*business*) negócio *m*; *love*: caso *m*; ***foreign ~s*** assuntos internacionais; ***have an ~ with*** ter um caso com

affect [ə'fekt] *v/t* afetar

affection [ə'fekʃn] afeição *f*

affectionate [ə'fekʃnət] *adj* afetuoso

affectionately [ə'fekʃnətlɪ] *adv* afetuosamente

affinity [ə'fɪnətɪ] afinidade *f*

affirmative [ə'fɜːrmətɪv] *adj* afirmativo; ***answer in the ~*** responder afirmativamente

affluence ['æflʊəns] riqueza *f*

affluent ['æflʊənt] *adj* rico; ***~ society*** sociedade *f* rica

afford [ə'fɔːrd] *v/t* ***be able to ~ sth*** *financially* ter meios para pagar algo; ***it's a risk we can't ~ to take*** é um risco que não podemos correr; ***we can't ~ the time*** não temos tempo

affordable [ə'fɔːrdəbl] *adj price* razoável; ***it's not ~ for most people*** não é acessível para a maioria das pessoas

afloat [ə'floʊt] *adj boat* flutuante; ***keep the company ~*** manter a companhia solvente

afraid [ə'freɪd] *adj* ***be ~*** ter medo; ***be ~ of*** ter medo de; ***I'm ~ ...*** receio que ...; ***I'm ~ so / not*** receio que sim / não

afresh [ə'freʃ] *adv* de novo

Africa ['æfrɪkə] África *f*

African ['æfrɪkən] **1** *adj* africano **2** *n* africano,-a *m,f*

African-A'merican **1** *adj* afro-americano **2** *n* afro-americano,-a *m,f*

after ['æftər] **1** *prep* depois de; ***~ all*** além de tudo; ***~ that*** depois disso; ***it's ten ~ two*** *Am* são duas e dez **2** *adv* (*afterward*) depois; ***the day ~*** o dia seguinte

aftermath ['æftərmæθ] período *m* após

afternoon [æftər'nuːn] tarde *f*; ***in the ~*** à tarde; ***this ~*** esta tarde; ***good ~*** boa-tarde

'after sales service *Brit* serviço *m* pós-venda **'aftershave** loção *f* pós-barba **'aftertaste** sabor *m* residual

afterward ['æftərwərd] *adv Am* depois; após

again [ə'geɪn] *adv* novamente; ***can you try ~ later?*** você pode tentar novamente mais tarde?; ***I never saw him ~*** eu nunca mais o vi; ***don't do that ~!*** não faça isso outra vez!

against [ə'geɪnst] *prep* contra; ***~ the law*** contra a lei; ***I'm ~ the idea*** sou contra a idéia; ***what do you have ~ her?*** o que você tem contra ela?

age [eɪdʒ] **1** *n* idade *f*; (*era*) era *f*; ***at the ~ of 50*** com 50 anos; ***under ~*** menor de idade; ***she's five years of ~*** ela tem cinco anos; ***for ~s*** *fam* há séculos **2** *v/i* envelhecer

aged[1] [eɪdʒd] *adj* ***a girl ~ 16*** uma menina de 16 anos

aged[2] ['eɪdʒɪd] **1** *adj* envelhecido **2** *npl* ***the ~*** os idosos

'age group faixa *f* etária

'age limit limite *m* de idade

agency ['eɪdʒənsɪ] agência *f*

agenda [ə'dʒendə] agenda *f*; ***on the ~*** na pauta

agent ['eɪdʒənt] agente *m/f*

aggravate ['ægrəveɪt] *v/t* piorar, agravar; (*annoy*) piorar

aggregate ['ægrɪgət] *n* SPORT ***win on ~*** ganhar por pontos

aggression [ə'greʃn] agressão *f*

aggressive [ə'gresɪv] *adj* agressivo; (*dynamic*) dinâmico

aggressively [ə'gresɪvlɪ] *adv* agressivamente
aghast [ə'gæst] *adj* aterrorizado
agile ['ædʒaɪl] *adj* ágil
agility [ə'dʒɪlətɪ] agilidade *f*
agitate ['ædʒɪteɪt] *v/i* ~ ***for*** lutar por
agitated ['ædʒɪteɪtɪd] *adj* agitado
agitation [ædʒɪ'teɪʃn] agitação *f*
agitator [ædʒɪ'teɪtər] agitador,a *m,f*
AGM [eɪdʒiː'em] *Brit abbr* (*of* ***annual general 'meeting***) assembléia *f* geral anual
agnostic [æg'nɑːstɪk] *n* agnóstico,-a *m,f*
ago [ə'goʊ] *adv* atrás; ***2 days*** ~ dois dias atrás; ***long*** ~ há muito tempo; ***how long*** ~***?*** há quanto tempo?
agog [ə'gɑːg] *adj* ***be*** ~ ***at sth*** estar excitado sobre algo
agonize ['ægənaɪz] *v/i* agonizar; ~ ***over*** agoniar-se por
agonizing ['ægənaɪzɪŋ] *adj* angustiante
agony ['ægənɪ] agonia *f*
agree [ə'griː] **1** *v/i figures, accounts, also reach agreement* concordar; ***I*** ~ concordo; ***it doesn't*** ~ ***with me*** *food* isto me faz mal **2** *v/t price* concordar; ~ ***that sth should be done*** concordar que algo deve ser feito
agreeable [ə'griːəbl] *adj* (*pleasant*) agradável; ***be*** ~ (*in agreement*) estar de acordo
agreement [ə'griːmənt] (*consent, contract*) acordo *m*; ***reach*** ~ ***on*** chegar a um acordo sobre
agricultural [ægrɪ'kʌltʃərəl] *adj* agrícola
agriculture ['ægrɪkʌltʃər] agricultura *f*
ahead [ə'hed] *adv* na frente; ***be*** ~ ***of*** estar na frente de; ***plan / think*** ~ planejar / pensar antecipadamente; ***they are technologically*** ~ ***of us*** eles estão tecnologicamente mais avançados do que nós
aid [eɪd] **1** *n* ajuda *f*, auxílio *m*; ***humanitarian*** ~ ajuda humanitária **2** *v/t* auxiliar
aide [eɪd] assessor,a *m,f*
Aids [eɪdz] *nsg* Aids *f*, *Port* SIDA *f*
ailing ['eɪlɪŋ] *adj economy* enfraquecido
ailment ['eɪlmənt] doença *f*
aim [eɪm] **1** *n shooting*: mira *f*; (*objective*) meta *f* **2** *v/i shooting*: mirar; ~ ***at doing sth***, ~ ***to do sth*** ter o objetivo de fazer algo **3** *v/t* mirar; ***be*** ~***ed at*** *remark etc* ser dirigido para; *guns* estar apontado para
aimless ['eɪmlɪs] *adj* sem meta
air [er] **1** *n* ar *m*; ***by*** ~ *travel, mail* por avião; ***in the open*** ~ a céu aberto; ***on the*** ~ RADIO, TV no ar **2** *v/t room* arejar; *fig views* expressar
'airbag *in car* airbag *m* **'airbase** base *f* aérea **'air-conditioned** *adj* refrigerado **'air-conditioning** ar *m* condicionado **'aircraft** aeronave *f* **'aircraft carrier** transportadora *f* aérea **'air fare** tarifa *f* aérea **'airfield** campo *m* de aviação **'air force** força *f* aérea **'air hostess** comissária *f* de bordo, *Port* hospedeira *f* **'air letter** carta *f* aérea **'airline** companhia *f* aérea **'airliner** avião *m* de passageiros **'airmail** *n* ***by*** ~ via aérea **'airplane** avião *m* **'air pocket** poço *m* de ar **'air pollution** poluição *f* do ar **'airport** aeroporto *m* **'air rage** comportamento *m* agressivo em avião **'airsick** ***get*** ~ ficar enjoado **'airspace** espaço *m* aéreo **'air terminal** terminal *m* aéreo **'airtight** *adj container* hermético **'air traffic** tráfego *m* aéreo **'air-traffic control** controle *m* de tráfego aéreo **air-traffic con'troller** controlador,a *m,f* de vôo
airy ['erɪ] *adj room* arejado; *attitude* descontraído
aisle [aɪl] corredor *m*
'aisle seat assento *m* no corredor
alarm [ə'lɑːrm] **1** *n* alarme *m*; ***raise the*** ~ dar o alarme **2** *v/t* alarmar
a'larm clock despertador *m*
alarming [ə'lɑːrmɪŋ] *adj* alarmante
alarmingly [ə'lɑːrmɪŋlɪ] *adv* de modo alarmante
Alaska [ə'læskə] Alasca *m*
album ['ælbəm] *photographs*: álbum *m*; (*record*) disco *m*
alcohol ['ælkəhɑːl] álcool *m*
alcoholic [ælkə'hɑːlɪk] **1** *n* alcoólatra *m/f* **2** *adj* alcoólico

alert [ə'lɜːrt] **1** *n* (*signal*) alerta *m*; ***be on the ~*** ficar alerta **2** *v/t* alertar **3** *adj* atento
algebra ['ældʒɪbrə] álgebra *f*
algorithm ['ælgourɪðm] algoritmo *m*
alibi ['ælɪbaɪ] álibi *m*
alien ['eɪlɪən] **1** *n* (*foreigner*) estrangeiro,-a *m,f*; *from space* alienígena *m/f* **2** *adj* estranho; ***be ~ to s.o.*** ser estranho a alguém
alienate ['eɪlɪəneɪt] *v/t* alienar
alight [ə'laɪt] *adj* em chamas
align [ə'laɪn] *v/t* alinhar
alike [ə'laɪk] **1** *adj* ***be ~*** ser parecido **2** *adv* ***old and young ~*** jovens e idosos igualmente
alimony ['ælɪmənɪ] pensão *f* (*no caso de divórcio*)
alive [ə'laɪv] *adj* ***be ~*** estar vivo
all [ɔːl] **1** *adj* todo; ***~ the boys / ~ the girls*** todos os meninos / todas as meninas; ***~ the time*** o tempo todo; ***it rained ~ day*** choveu o dia todo **2** *pron* todo,-a; (*everything*) tudo; ***~ of us / them*** todos nós / eles; ***he ate ~ of it*** ele comeu tudo; ***that's ~, thanks*** isto é tudo, obrigado; ***for ~ I care*** por mim; ***for ~ I know*** que eu saiba; ***~ but*** (*except*) todos, com exceção de **3** *adv* todo, completamente; ***I'm ~ confused*** estou todo confuso; ***~ the better*** tanto melhor; ***they're not at ~ alike*** eles não são nem um pouco parecidos; ***not at ~!*** de jeito nenhum; ***two ~*** SPORT dois a dois; ***~ right*** tudo bem; ***~ but*** (*nearly*) praticamente
allay [ə'leɪ] *v/t* acalmar
allegation [ælɪ'geɪʃn] alegação *f*
allege [ə'ledʒ] *v/t* alegar
alleged [ə'ledʒd] *adj* alegado
allegedly [ə'ledʒɪdlɪ] *adv* supostamente
allegiance [ə'liːdʒəns] lealdade *f*
allergic [ə'lɜːrdʒɪk] *adj* alérgico; ***be ~ to*** ser alérgico a
allergy ['ælərdʒɪ] alergia *f*
alleviate [ə'liːvɪeɪt] *v/t* aliviar
alley ['ælɪ] alameda *f*
alliance [ə'laɪəns] aliança *f*
allocate ['æləkeɪt] *v/t* alocar
allocation [ælə'keɪʃn] *act* atribuição *f*; *amount* parte *f*
allot [ə'lɑːt] *v/t* ⟨*pret & pp* ***allotted***⟩ destinar
allow [ə'laʊ] *v/t* (*permit*) permitir; (*calculate for*) calcular; ***it's not ~ed*** não é permitido; ***~ s.o. to ...*** permitir que alguém ...; ***~ three hours for ...*** leve três horas em conta ...
♦ **allow for** *v/t* levar em conta
allowance [ə'laʊəns] *money* mesada *f*; (*pocket money*) diária *f*; ***make ~s*** *for weather etc* levar em consideração; *for person* dar um desconto
alloy ['ælɔɪ] liga *f* metálica
'all-purpose *adj* versátil
'all-round *adj* geral; (*versatile*) versátil
'all-time *adj* ***be at an ~ low*** estar mais baixo que nunca
♦ **allude to** [ə'luːd] *v/t* aludir a
alluring [ə'luːrɪŋ] *adj* atraente
all-wheel 'drive tração *f* nas quatro rodas
ally ['ælaɪ] *n* aliado,-a *m,f*
Almighty [ɔːl'maɪtɪ] ***the ~*** o Todo-Poderoso
almond ['ɑːmənd] amêndoa *f*
almost ['ɔːlmoʊst] *adv* quase
alone [ə'loʊn] *adj* sozinho; ***the software ~ costs ...*** só o software custa ...
along [ə'lɑːŋ] **1** *prep* (*moving forward*) ao longo de; (*situated beside*) ao lado de **2** *adv* junto; ***~ with*** juntamente com; ***all ~*** (*all the time*) todo o tempo
alongside [əlɑːŋ'saɪd] *prep* (*beside*) ao lado de; (*parallel to*) emparelhado com
aloof [ə'luːf] *adj* distante
aloud [ə'laʊd] *adv* em voz alta; ***I was thinking ~*** eu estava pensando em voz alta
alphabet ['ælfəbet] alfabeto *m*
alphabetical [ælfə'betɪkl] *adj* alfabético
already [ɔːl'redɪ] *adv* já
alright [ɔːl'raɪt] *adj* (*permitted*) tudo certo; (*not hurt*) bem; (*in working order*) funcionando; ***is it ~ with you if I ...?*** está bem para você se eu ...?; ***~, you can have one!*** está bem, você pode pegar um!; ***~, I heard you!*** está bem, eu ouvi!; ***everything is***

~ now between them agora está tudo bem entre eles; ***that's ~*** (*don't mention it*) de nada; ***that's ~*** (*I don't mind*) está bem

also ['ɔːlsoʊ] *adv* também

altar ['ɔːltər] altar *m*

alter ['ɔːltər] *v/t* alterar

alteration [ɔːltə'reɪʃn] alteração *f*

alternate ['ɔːltərneɪt] **1** *v/i* alternar **2** *adj* alternado

alternating current [ɔːltərneɪtɪŋ'kʌrənt] corrente *f* alternada

alternative [ɔːl'tɜːrnətɪv] **1** *n* alternativa *f* **2** *adj* alternativo

alternatively [ɔːl'tɜːrnətɪvlɪ] *adv* alternativamente

although [ɔːl'ðoʊ] *conj* embora

altitude ['æltɪtuːd] altitude *f*

altogether [ɔːltə'geðər] *adv* (*completely*) totalmente; (*in all*) no total

altruism ['æltruːɪzm] altruísmo *m*

altruistic [æltruː'ɪstɪk] *adj* altruísta

aluminium *Brit* → ***aluminum***

aluminum [ə'luːmɪnəm] *Am* alumínio *m*

always ['ɔːlweɪz] *adv* sempre

a.m. ['eɪem] *abbr* (*of* **ante meridiem**) da manhã

amalgamate [ə'mælgəmeɪt] *v/i companies* fusionar

amass [ə'mæs] *v/t* acumular

amateur ['æmətʃʊr] *n* amador,a *m,f*

amateurish ['æmətʃʊrɪʃ] *adj pej* amadorístico

amaze [ə'meɪz] *v/t* espantar

amazed [ə'meɪzd] *adj* espantado

amazement [ə'meɪzmənt] espanto *m*

amazing [ə'meɪzɪŋ] *adj* (*surprising*) surpreendente; *fam* (*very good*) incrível

amazingly [ə'meɪzɪŋlɪ] *adv* espantosamente

Amazon ['æməzɑːn] Amazonas *m*

Amazonian [æmə'zoʊnɪən] *adj region* amazônico; *of Amazonia* amazonense

ambassador [æm'bæsədər] embaixador,a *m,f*

amber ['æmbər] *adj* de cor âmbar; ***at ~*** no sinal amarelo

ambidextrous [æmbɪ'dekstrəs] *adj* ambidestro

ambience ['æmbɪəns] atmosfera *f*

ambiguity [æmbɪ'gjuːətɪ] ambigüidade *f*

ambiguous [æm'bɪgjʊəs] *adj* ambíguo

ambition [æm'bɪʃn] ambição *f*

ambitious [æm'bɪʃəs] *adj* ambicioso

ambivalent [æm'bɪvələnt] *adj* ambivalente

amble ['æmbl] *v/i* passear; ***he ~d to the door*** ele dirigiu-se lentamente até a porta

ambulance ['æmbjʊləns] ambulância *f*

ambush ['æmbʊʃ] **1** *n* emboscada *f* **2** *v/t* emboscar

amend [ə'mend] *v/t* corrigir

amendment [ə'mendmənt] emenda *f*

amends [ə'mendz] compensação *f*; ***make ~*** compensar por prejuízos

amenities [ə'miːnətɪz] encantos *mpl*

America [ə'merɪkə] América *f*

American [ə'merɪkən] **1** *adj* americano **2** *n* americano,-a *m,f*

amiable ['eɪmɪəbl] *adj* amável

amicable ['æmɪkəbl] *adj* amigável

amicably ['æmɪkəblɪ] *adv* amigavelmente

ammunition [æmjʊ'nɪʃn] munição *f*; *fig* arma *f*

amnesia [æm'niːzɪə] amnésia *f*

amnesty ['æmnəstɪ] anistia *f*

among, amongst [ə'mʌŋ(st)] *prep* dentre

amoral [eɪ'mɔːrəl] *adj* amoral

amount [ə'maʊnt] quantidade *f*; (*sum of money*) quantia *f*

◆ **amount to** *v/t* elevar-se a; (*be equivalent to*) equivaler a

amphibian [æm'fɪbɪən] anfíbio *m*

amphitheater ['æmfɪθiːətər] *Am* anfiteatro *m*

amphitheatre *Brit* → ***amphitheater***

ample ['æmpl] *adj* amplo

amplifier ['æmplɪfaɪr] amplificador *m*

amplify ['æmplɪfaɪ] *v/t* ⟨*pret & pp* ***amplified***⟩ *sound* amplificar

amputate ['æmpjʊːteɪt] *v/t* amputar

amputation [æmpjʊ'teɪʃn] amputação *f*

amuse [ə'mjuːz] *v/t* (*make laugh etc*) divertir; (*entertain*) entreter

amusement [ə'mju:zmənt] (*merriment*) divertimento *m*; (*entertainment*) entretenimento *m*; **~s** (*games*) jogos *mpl*; ***to our great* ~** para nosso grande deleite
a'musement arcade área *f* de lazer
a'musement park parque *m* de diversão
amusing [ə'mju:zɪŋ] *adj* divertido
an [æn, ən] um, uma → ***a***
anabolic steroid [ænəbɑ:lɪk'sterɔɪd] esteróide *m* anabolizante
anaemia *etc Brit* → ***anemia***
anaesthetic *etc Brit* → ***anesthetic***
analog ['ænəlɑ:g] *adj* COMPUT analógico
analogy [ə'nælədʒɪ] analogia *f*
analyse *Brit* → ***analyze***
analysis [ə'næləsɪs] ⟨*pl* ***analyses***⟩ análise *f*
analyst ['ænəlɪst] analista *m/f*; PSYCH psicanalista *m/f*
analytical [ænə'lɪtɪkl] *adj* analítico
analyze ['ænəlaɪz] *v/t* analisar
anarchy ['ænəkɪ] anarquia *f*
anatomy [ə'nætəmɪ] anatomia *f*
ancestor ['ænsestər] ancestral *m/f*
anchor ['æŋkər] **1** *n* NAUT âncora *f* **2** *v/i* NAUT ancorar
anchorman ['æŋkərmæn] TV âncora *m*
ancient ['eɪnʃənt] *adj* antigo
ancillary [æn'sɪlərɪ] *adj staff* auxiliar
and [ənd, *stressed* ænd] *conj* e
Andean ['ændɪən] *adj* andino
Andes ['ændi:z] ***the* ~** os Andes
anecdote ['ænɪkdoʊt] anedota *f*
anemia [ə'ni:mɪə] *Am* anemia *f*
anemic [ə'ni:mɪk] *adj Am* MED anêmico
anesthesiologist [ə'nəsθi:zi:ɑ:lədʒɪst] *Am* anestesista *m/f*
anesthetic [ænəs'θetɪk] *n Am* anestesia *f*
angel ['eɪndʒl] REL *also fig* anjo *m*
anger ['æŋgər] **1** *n* raiva *f* **2** *v/t* zangar
angina [æn'dʒaɪnə] angina *f*
angle ['æŋgl] *n* ângulo *m*
angry ['æŋgrɪ] *adj* zangado; ***be* ~ *with s.o.*** ficar zangado com alguém
anguish ['æŋgwɪʃ] angústia *f*
angular ['æŋgjʊlər] *adj* angular
animal ['ænɪml] animal *m*
animated ['ænɪmeɪtɪd] *adj* animado
animated car'toon desenho *m* animado
animation [ænɪ'meɪʃn] (*liveliness*) *also cartoon* animação *f*
animosity [ænɪ'mɑ:sətɪ] animosidade *f*
ankle ['æŋkl] tornozelo *m*
annex [ə'neks] **1** *n building* edifício *m* anexo **2** *v/t state* anexar
annexe *Brit* → ***annex***
annihilate [ə'naɪəleɪt] *v/t* aniquilar
annihilation [ənaɪə'leɪʃn] aniquilação *f*
anniversary [ænɪ'vɜ:rsərɪ] aniversário *m*
annotate ['ænəteɪt] *v/t book, report* anotar
announce [ə'naʊns] *v/t* anunciar
announcement [ə'naʊnsmənt] anúncio *m*
announcer [ə'naʊnsər] TV, RADIO locutor,a *m,f*
annoy [ə'nɔɪ] *v/t* incomodar; ***be* ~*ed*** ficar incomodado
annoyance [ə'nɔɪəns] (*anger*) irritação *f*; (*nuisance*) aborrecimento *m*
annoying [ə'nɔɪɪŋ] *adj* irritante
annual ['ænʊəl] *adj* anual
annuity [ə'nu:ətɪ] anuidade *f*
annul [ə'nʌl] *v/t* ⟨*pret & pp* ***annulled***⟩ *marriage* anular
annulment [ə'nʌlmənt] anulação *f*
anonymous [ə'nɑ:nɪməs] *adj* anônimo
anorexia [ænə'reksɪə] anorexia *f*
anorexic [ænə'reksɪk] *adj* anoréxico
another [ə'nʌðər] **1** *adj* outro **2** *pron* outro,-a; ***they respect one* ~** eles se respeitam (um ao outro)
answer ['ænsər] **1** *n letter, person*: resposta *f*; *problem, question*: solução *f* **2** *v/t letter, person, question* responder; **~ *the door*** atender a porta; **~ *the telephone*** atender o telefone
♦ **answer back** **1** *v/t person* responder a **2** *v/i* dar uma resposta malcriada
♦ **answer for** *v/t* responsabilizar-se por; ***such parents have a lot to answer for*** pais assim têm muito pelo

que responder
answering machine ['ænsərɪŋ] secretária *f* eletrônica
answerphone ['ænsərfoʊn] secretária *f* eletrônica
ant [ænt] formiga *f*
antagonism [æn'tægənɪzm] antagonismo *m*
antagonistic [æntægə'nɪstɪk] *adj* hostil
antagonize [æn'tægənaɪz] *v/t* antagonizar
Antarctic [ænt'ɑːrktɪk] *n* Antártica *f*
antenatal [æntɪ'neɪtl] *adj* pré-natal
antenna [æn'tenə] *of insect, TV* antena *f*
anthology [æn'θɑːlədʒɪ] antologia *f*
anthropology [ænθrə'pɑːlədʒɪ] antropologia *f*
antibiotic [æntaɪbaɪ'ɑːtɪk] *n* antibiótico *m*
antibody ['æntaɪbɑːdɪ] anticorpos *mpl*
anticipate [æn'tɪsɪpeɪt] *v/t* antecipar
anticipation [æntɪsɪ'peɪʃn] antecipação *f*
antics ['æntɪks] tolice *f*
antidote ['æntɪdoʊt] antídoto *m*
antifreeze ['æntaɪfriːz] anticongelante *m*
anti-globalist [æntaɪ'gloʊbəlɪst] **1** *adj* anti-globalista **2** *n* militante *m/f* anti-globalização
antipathy [æn'tɪpəθɪ] antipatia *f*
antiquated ['æntɪkweɪtɪd] *adj* antiquado
antique [æn'tiːk] *n* objeto *m* antigo
an'tique dealer antiquário *m*
antiquity [æn'tɪkwətɪ] antiguidade *f*
antiseptic [æntaɪ'septɪk] **1** *adj* anti-séptico **2** *n* anti-séptico *m*
antisocial [æntaɪ'soʊʃl] *adj* anti-social
antivirus program [æntaɪ'vaɪrəsproʊgræm] COMPUT programa *m* antivírus
anxiety [æŋ'zaɪətɪ] ansiedade *f*
anxious ['æŋkʃəs] *adj* (*apprehensive, eager*) ansioso; ***be ~ for ...*** *for news etc* ficar ansioso por ...
any ['enɪ] **1** *adj* qualquer; ***are there ~ glasses?*** tem algum copo?; ***is there ~ bread?*** tem pão?; ***is there ~ improvement?*** houve alguma melhora?; ***there aren't ~ glasses*** não tem nenhum copo; ***there isn't ~ improvement*** não há nenhuma melhora; ***there isn't ~ bread*** não tem pão; ***have you ~ idea at all?*** você tem alguma idéia?; ***take ~ one you like*** pegue qualquer um/uma que quiser **2** *pron* alguns, algumas; algum,a; ***do you have ~?*** você tem algum,a?; ***there aren't ~ left*** não sobrou nenhum; ***there isn't ~ left*** não sobrou nenhum; ***~ of them could be guilty*** qualquer um deles pode ser culpado **3** *adv* ***is that ~ easier?*** está mais fácil assim?; ***is that ~ better?*** está melhor assim?; ***I don't like it ~ more*** não gosto mais disto
anybody ['enɪbɒːdɪ] *pron* alguém; ***there wasn't ~ there*** não havia ninguém lá
anyhow ['enɪhaʊ] *adv in any case* em todo o caso; *in a haphazard way* de qualquer maneira
anyone ['enɪwʌn] → ***anybody***
anything ['enɪθɪŋ] *pron* qualquer coisa; *with negatives* nada; ***I didn't hear ~*** não ouvi nada; ***it was ~ but ready*** estava tudo menos pronto; ***~ else?*** algo mais?
anyway ['enɪweɪ] → ***anyhow***
anywhere ['enɪwer] *adv* em algum lugar; ***I can't find it ~*** não o encontro em nenhum lugar
apart [ə'pɑːrt] *adv* ***be X miles ~*** estar a X quilômetros; ***the two ends should be further ~*** as duas pontas deviam estar mais distantes; ***keep ~*** deixar separado; ***live ~*** *people* viver separado; ***~ from*** (*excepting*) com exceção de; (*in addition to*) além de
apartment [ə'pɑːrtmənt] apartamento *m*
a'partment block *Am* condomínio *m*
apathetic [æpə'θetɪk] *adj* apático
apathy ['æpəθɪ] apatia *f*
ape [eɪp] macaco,-a *m,f*
aperitif [ə'perɪtiːf] aperitivo *m*
aperture ['æpətʃər] PHOT abertura *f*
apiece [ə'piːs] *adv* por pessoa
apologetic [əpɑːlə'dʒetɪk] *adj person* que se desculpa constantemente;

she was very ~ about it ela desculpava-se muito pelo ocorrido
apologize [ə'pɑːlədʒaɪz] *v/i* desculpar-se; ***~ for sth*** desculpar-se por algo
apology [ə'pɑːlədʒɪ] desculpa *f*; ***I would like an ~*** quero um pedido de desculpas
apostle [ə'pɑːsl] REL apóstolo *m*
apostrophe [ə'pɑːstrəfɪ] GRAM apóstrofo *m*
appal *Brit* → ***appall***
Appalachians [æpə'leɪʧɪənz] montes *mpl* Apalaches
appall [ə'pɒːl] *v/t* horrorizar
appalling [ə'pɒːlɪŋ] *adj* espantoso; *language* horrível
apparatus [æpə'reɪtəs] aparelhagem *f*
apparent [ə'pærənt] *adj* aparente; ***become ~ that …*** tornou-se evidente que …
apparently [ə'pærəntlɪ] *adv* aparentemente
apparition [æpə'rɪʃn] (*ghost*) aparição *f*
appeal [ə'piːl] **1** *n* (*charm*) charme *m*; *funds etc*: apelo *m*; LAW apelação *f* **2** *v/i* LAW apelar
♦ **appeal for** *v/t* apelar por
♦ **appeal to** *v/t* (*be attractive to*) atrair a
appealing [ə'piːlɪŋ] *adj idea*, *offer* bom (boa); *look* suplicante
appear [ə'pɪr] *v/i in movie etc*, *new product* aparecer; *in court* comparecer; (*look*, *seem*) parecer; ***it ~s that …*** parece que …
appearance [ə'pɪrəns] (*arrival*) aparecimento *m*; *in movie etc* participação *f*; *in court* comparecimento *m*; (*look*) aparência *f*; ***put in an ~*** aparecer
appease [ə'piːz] *v/t* apaziguar
appendicitis [əpendɪ'saɪtɪs] apendicite *f*
appendix [ə'pendɪks] *of book*, MED apêndice *m*
appetite ['æpɪtaɪt] *also fig* apetite *m*
appetizer ['æpɪtaɪzər] aperitivo *m*
appetizing ['æpɪtaɪzɪŋ] *adj* apetitoso
applaud [ə'plɒːd] **1** *v/i* aplaudir **2** *v/t* aplaudir; *fig* admirar
applause [ə'plɒːz] *also fig* aplauso *m*
apple ['æpl] maçã *f*
apple 'pie torta *f* de maçã
apple 'sauce purê *m* de maçã
appliance [ə'plaɪəns] aparelho *m*; *household* (aparelho) eletrodoméstico *m*
applicable [ə'plɪkəbl] *adj* aplicável
applicant ['æplɪkənt] candidato,-a *m*,*f*
application [æplɪ'keɪʃn] *job*: candidatura *f*; *passport*, *visa*: requerimento *m*; *university*: matrícula *f*
appli'cation form formulário *m* de inscrição; *passport*, *visa*: formulário *m* de solicitação
apply [ə'plaɪ] ⟨*pret & pp* ***applied***⟩ **1** *v/t rules*, *ointment* aplicar **2** *v/i rule*, *law* aplicar-se
♦ **apply for** *v/t job*, *university* candidatar-se a; *passport* solicitar
♦ **apply to** *v/t* (*contact*) dirigir-se a; (*affect*) aplicar-se a
appoint [ə'pɔɪnt] *v/t to position* nomear
appointment [ə'pɔɪntmənt] *to position* nomeação *f*; ***make an ~*** *with doctor etc* marcar hora
ap'pointments diary agenda *f*
appraisal [ə'preɪz(ə)l] avaliação *f*
appreciable [ə'priːʃəbl] *adj* considerável
appreciate [ə'priːʃɪeɪt] **1** *v/t* (*value*) apreciar; (*be grateful for*) estimar; (*acknowledge*) reconhecer; ***thanks, I ~ it*** muito obrigado **2** *v/i* FIN valorizar
appreciation [əpriːʃɪ'eɪʃn] *of kindness etc* agradecimento *m*; *of music etc* apreciação *f*
appreciative [ə'priːʃətɪv] *adj* apreciativo
apprehensive [æprɪ'hensɪv] *adj* apreensivo
apprentice [ə'prentɪs] aprendiz *m*/*f*
approach [ə'prouʧ] **1** *n* aproximação *f*; (*with offer*, *proposal*) proposta *f*; *to problem* enfoque *m* **2** *v/t* (*get near to*) aproximar-se de; (*contact*) contatar
approachable [ə'preuʧəbl] *adj person* acessível
appropriate[1] [ə'prouprɪət] *adj clothing* apropriado; *behavior* adequado; ***delete as ~*** delete a vontade
appropriate[2] [ə'prouprɪeɪt] *v/t* apro-

priar
approval [ə'pru:vl] aprovação *f*
approve [ə'pru:v] *v/t & v/i* aprovar
♦**approve of** *v/t* aprovar
approximate [ə'prɑ:ksɪmət] *adj* aproximativo
approximately [ə'prɑ:ksɪmətlɪ] *adv* aproximadamente
approximation [əprɑ:ksɪ'meɪʃn] estimativa *f*
APR [eɪpi:'ɑ:r] *abbr* (*of* ***annual percentage rate***) Taxa *f* Real de Juros
apricot ['æprɪkɑ:t] damasco *m*
April ['eɪprəl] abril *m*
apt [æpt] *adj pupil* apto; *remark* certeiro; ***be ~ to …*** ser propenso a …
aptitude ['æptɪtu:d] aptidão *f*
'aptitude test teste *m* de aptidão
aqualung ['ækwəlʌŋ] aparelho *m* de mergulho
aquarium [ə'kwerɪəm] aquário *m*
Aquarius [ə'kwerɪəs] ASTROL Aquário *m*
aquatic [ə'kwætɪk] *adj* aquático
Arab ['ærəb] **1** *adj* árabe **2** *n* árabe *m/f*
Arabic ['ærəbɪk] **1** *n* árabe *m* **2** *adj* árabe; *numbers* arábico
arable ['ærəbl] *adj* arável
arbitrary ['ɑ:rbɪtrərɪ] *adj remark, attack* arbitrário
arbitrate ['ɑ:rbɪtreɪt] *v/i* arbitrar
arbitration [ɑ:rbɪ'treɪʃn] arbitragem *f*
arbitrator ['ɑ:rbɪtreɪtər] árbitro *m*
arch [ɑ:rtʃ] *n* abóboda *f*
archaeological *etc Brit* → ***archeological***
archaic [ɑ:r'keɪɪk] *adj* arcaico
archbishop [ɑ:rtʃ'bɪʃəp] arcebispo *m*
archeological [ɑ:rkɪə'lɑ:dʒɪkl] *adj Am* arqueológico
archeologist [ɑ:rkɪ'ɑ:lədʒɪst] *Am* arqueólogo,-a *m,f*
archeology [ɑ:rkɪ'ɑ:lədʒɪ] *Am* arqueologia *f*
archer ['ɑ:rtʃər] arqueiro *m*
architect ['ɑ:rkɪtekt] arquiteto,-a *m,f*
architectural [ɑ:rkɪ'tektʃərəl] *adj* arquitetônico
architecture ['ɑ:rkɪtektʃər] arquitetura *f*
archives ['ɑ:rkaɪvz] *npl* arquivo *m*
'archway arco *m*
Arctic ['ɑ:rktɪk] *n* Ártico *m*
ardent ['ɑ:rdənt] *adj* ardente
arduous ['ɑ:rdʊəs] *adj* árduo
area ['erɪə] área *f*; *activity; job, study etc*: campo *m*
'area code TEL código *m* de área
arena [ə'ri:nə] SPORT estádio *m*
Argentina [ɑ:rdʒən'ti:nə] Argentina *f*
Argentinian [ɑ:rdʒən'tɪnɪən] **1** *adj* argentino **2** *n* argentino,-a *m,f*
arguably ['ɑ:rgjʊəblɪ] *adv* provavelmente
argue ['ɑ:rgju:] **1** *v/i* (*quarrel*) discutir; (*reason*) argumentar **2** *v/t* ***~ that*** afirmar que
argument ['ɑ:rgjʊmənt] (*quarrel*) discussão *f*; (*reasoning*) argumento *m*
argumentative [ɑ:rgjʊ'mentətɪv] *adj* discutidor
aria ['ɑ:rɪə] MUS ária *f*
arid ['ærɪd] *adj land* árido
Aries ['eri:z] ASTROL Áries *m*
arise [ə'raɪz] *v/i* ⟨*pret* ***arose***, *pp* ***arisen***⟩ *situation, problem* surgir
arisen [ə'rɪzn] *pp* → ***arise***
aristocracy [ærɪ'stɑ:krəsɪ] aristocracia *f*
aristocrat ['ærɪstəkræt] aristocrata *m/f*
aristocratic [ærɪstə'krætɪk] *adj* aristocrático
arithmetic [ə'rɪθmətɪk] aritmética *f*
arm[1] [ɑ:rm] *n person, chair*: braço *m*
arm[2] [ɑ:rm] *v/t* armar
armaments ['ɑ:rməmənts] *npl* armamento *m*
'armchair cadeira *f* de braços
armed [ɑ:rmd] *adj* armado
armed 'forces *npl* Forças *fpl* Armadas
armed 'robbery assalto *m* à mão armada
armor ['ɑ:rmər] *Am* traje *m* de proteção
armored vehicle [ɑ:rmərd'vi:ɪkl] *Am* veículo *m* blindado
armour *Brit* → ***armor***
'armpit axila *f*
arms [ɑ:rmz] *npl* (*weapons*) arma *f*
army ['ɑ:rmɪ] exército *m*
aroma [ə'roʊmə] aroma *m*
arose [ə'roʊz] *pret* → ***arise***

around [ə'raʊnd] **1** *prep* (*in circle*) em volta de; *with expressions of time* por volta de; ***it's ~ the corner*** está na esquina **2** *adv* (*in the area*) por aí; (*encircling*) em torno; (*roughly*) aproximadamente; ***he lives ~ here*** ele vive por aqui; ***walk ~*** passear; ***she has been ~*** *has traveled, is experienced* ela já correu o mundo; ***he's still ~*** *fam alive* ele ainda anda por aí
arouse [ə'raʊz] *v/t sexually* despertar; *suspicion* levantar
arrange [ə'reɪndʒ] *v/t* (*put in order*) arrumar; *furniture* dispor; *flowers, music* fazer um arranjo de; *meeting, party etc* organizar; *time and place* marcar; ***~ to meet*** combinar um encontro; ***I've ~d to meet her*** eu marquei um encontro com ela
♦ **arrange for** *v/t* arranjar para
arrangement [ə'reɪndʒmənt] (*plan*) plano *m*; (*agreement*) acordo *m*; (*layout*) *of furniture etc* disposição *f*; *of flowers, music* arranjo *m*
arrears [ə'rɪərz] *npl* atrasos *mpl*; ***be in ~*** *person* estar em atraso
arrest [ə'rest] **1** *n* prisão *f*; ***be under ~*** estar detento **2** *v/t* prender
arrival [ə'raɪvl] chegada *f*; ***~s*** *sign* desembarque; *Port* chegadas
arrive [ə'raɪv] *v/i* chegar
♦ **arrive at** *v/t place, decision* chegar a
arrogance ['ærəgəns] arrogância *f*
arrogant ['ærəgənt] *adj* arrogante
arrogantly ['ærəgəntlɪ] *adv* arrogantemente
arrow ['æroʊ] flecha *f*
arse [ɑːrs] *Brit fam* bunda *f*
arsenic ['ɑːrsənɪk] arsênico *m*
arson ['ɑːrsn] incêndio *m* provocado
arsonist ['ɑːrsənɪst] piromaníaco,-a *m,f*
art [ɑːrt] arte *f*; ***the ~s*** as artes
artery ['ɑːrtərɪ] MED artéria *f*
'art gallery galeria *f* de arte
arthritis [ɑːr'θraɪtɪs] artrite *f*
artichoke ['ɑːrtɪtʃoʊk] alcachofra *f*
article ['ɑːrtɪkl] *also* GRAM artigo *m*
articulate [ɑːr'tɪkjʊlət] *adj* articulado
artificial [ɑːrtɪ'fɪʃl] *adj pearls, person* artificial
artificial in'telligence inteligência *f* artificial
artillery [ɑːr'tɪlərɪ] artilharia *f*
artisan ['ɑːrtɪzæn] artesão *m*, artesã *f*
artist ['ɑːrtɪst] artista *m/f*
artistic [ɑːr'tɪstɪk] *adj* artístico
'arts degree diploma *f* em ciências humanas
as [æz] **1** *conj* (*while, when*) quando; (*because, like*) como; ***~ if*** como se; ***~ usual*** como de costume; ***~ necessary*** como necessário **2** *adv* quanto; ***~ high ~ …*** tão alto quanto …; ***~ much ~ that?*** tanto assim? **3** *prep* como; ***~ a child*** como criança; ***work ~ a translator*** trabalhar como tradutor; ***~ for*** quanto a; ***~ Hamlet*** como Hamlet
asap ['eɪzæp] *abbr* (*of* ***as soon as possible***) o mais rápido possível
asbestos [æz'bestɑːs] asbesto *m*
Ascension [ə'senʃn] REL Ascensão *f*
ascent [ə'sent] escalada *f*
ash [æʃ] cinza *f*
ashamed [ə'ʃeɪmd] *adj* envergonhado; ***be ~ of*** estar envergonhado de; ***you should be ~ of yourself*** deveria estar envergonhado de si mesmo
'ash bin, **'ash can** lixeira *f*
ashore [ə'ʃɔːr] *adv* em terra firme; ***go ~*** desembarcar
'ashtray cinzeiro *m*
Asia ['eɪʃə] Ásia *f*
Asian ['eɪʃn] **1** *adj* asiático **2** *n* asiático,-a *m,f*
Asian-A'merican **1** *adj* asiático-americano **2** *n* asiático-americano,-a *m,f*
aside [ə'saɪd] *adv* de lado; ***~ from*** além de
ask [æsk] **1** *v/t person* perguntar; *question* fazer; (*invite*) convidar; *favor* pedir; ***can I ~ you something?*** posso fazer-lhe uma pergunta?; ***~ s.o. for sth*** pedir algo a alguém; ***~ s.o. to …*** pedir a alguém para …; ***~ s.o. about sth*** perguntar a alguém sobre algo **2** *v/i* perguntar
♦ **ask after** *v/t person* perguntar por
♦ **ask for** *v/t* pedir; *person* perguntar por; ***there's a man in reception asking for you*** há um homem na recepção perguntando por você

♦ **ask out** *v/t for drink, night out* convidar
asking price ['æskɪŋpraɪs] preço *m* de oferta
asleep [ə'sli:p] *adj* adormecido; ***be*** (***fast***) ~ estar num sono profundo; ***fall*** ~ adormecer
asparagus [ə'spærəgəs] aspargo *m*, *Port* espargo *m*
aspect ['æspekt] aspecto *m*
asphalt ['æsfælt] *n* asfalto *m*
asphyxiate [æ'sfɪksɪeɪt] *v/t* asfixiar
asphyxiation [əsfɪksɪ'eɪʃn] asfixia *f*
aspirations [æspə'reɪʃnz] *npl* aspirações *fpl*
aspirin ['æsprɪn] aspirina *f*
ass[1] [æs] (*idiot*) idiota *m/f*
ass[2] [æs] *fam* (*backside*) bunda *f*; (*sex*) sexo *m*
assailant [ə'seɪlənt] assaltante *m/f*
assassin [ə'sæsɪn] assassino,-a *m,f*
assassinate [ə'sæsɪneɪt] *v/t* assassinar
assassination [əsæsɪ'neɪʃn] assassinato *m*
assault [ə'sɒ:lt] **1** *n* agressão *f* **2** *v/t* agredir
assemble [ə'sembl] **1** *v/t parts* montar **2** *v/i people* reunir-se
assembly [ə'semblɪ] *of parts* montagem *f*, POL assembléia *f*
as'sembly line linha *f* de montagem
as'sembly plant fábrica *f* de montagem
assent [ə'sent] *v/i* consentir
assert [ə'sɜ:rt] *v/t* afirmar; ~ ***oneself*** impor-se
assertive [ə'sɜ:rtɪv] *adj person* determinado
assess [ə'ses] *v/t* avaliar
assessment [ə'sesmənt] avaliação *f*
asset ['æset] FIN patrimônio *m*; *fig* vantagem *f*
'asshole *Am vulg* cu *m*; (*idiot*) idiota *m/f*
assign [ə'saɪn] *v/t person* estipular; *thing* determinar
assignment [ə'saɪnmənt] (*task, study*) missão *f*
assimilate [ə'sɪmɪleɪt] *v/t information* assimilar; *person into group* integrar
assist [ə'sɪst] *v/t* assistir; ~***ed suicide*** suicídio *m* assistido
assistance [ə'sɪstəns] assistência *f*
assistant [ə'sɪstənt] assistente *m/f*
assistant di'rector diretor,a *m,f* assistente
assistant 'manager subgerente *m/f*
assistant refe'ree árbitro *m* auxiliar
associate [ə'soʊʃɪeɪt] **1** *v/t* associar **2** *v/i* associar-se; ~ ***with*** relacionar-se com **3** *n* colega *m/f*
associate pro'fessor professor *m* adjunto
association [əsoʊsɪ'eɪʃn] associação *f*; ***in*** ~ ***with*** em cooperação com
assorted [ə'sɔ:rtɪd] *adj* sortido
assortment [ə'sɔ:rtmənt] *food*: sortimento *m*; *people*: diversidade *f*
assume [ə'su:m] *v/t* (*suppose*) supor
assumption [ə'sʌmpʃn] suposição *f*
assurance [ə'ʃʊrəns] garantia *f*; (*confidence*) confiança *f*
assure [ə'ʃʊr] *v/t* (*reassure*) assegurar
assured [ə'ʃʊrd] *adj* (*confident*) confiante
asterisk ['æstərɪsk] asterisco *m*
asthma ['æsmə] asma *f*
asthmatic [æs'mætɪk] *adj* asmático
astonish [ə'stɑ:nɪʃ] *v/t* surpreender; ***be*** ~***ed*** estar surpreso
astonishing [ə'stɑ:nɪʃɪŋ] *adj* surpreendente
astonishingly [ə'stɑ:nɪʃɪŋlɪ] *adv* surpreendentemente
astonishment [ə'stɑ:nɪʃmənt] espanto *m*
astound [ə'staʊnd] *v/t* pasmar
astounding [ə'staʊndɪŋ] *adj* espantoso
astray [ə'streɪ] *adv* ***go*** ~ extraviar; *morally* perder-se
astride [ə'straɪd] **1** *adv* escanchadamente **2** *prep* escanchado em
astrologer [ə'strɑ:lədʒər] astrólogo *m/f*
astrology [ə'strɑ:lədʒɪ] astrologia *f*
astronaut ['æstrənɒ:t] autronauta *m/f*
astronomer [ə'strɑ:nəmər] astrônomo *m/f*
astronomical [æstrə'nɑ:mɪkl] *adj price etc* astronômico
astronomy [ə'strɑ:nəmɪ] astronomia *f*
astute [ə'stu:t] *adj* astuto

asylum [ə'saɪləm] *mental* manicômio *m*; *political* asilo *m*
at [ət, *stressed* æt] *prep* (*with places*) em; **~ *the cleaner's*** na lavanderia; **~ *Joe's*** na casa do Joe; **~ *the door*** na porta; **~ *10 dollars*** a 10 dólares; **~ *the age of 18*** aos 18 anos; **~ *5 o'clock*** às 5 horas; **~ *150 km/h*** a 150 km/h; ***be good / bad ~ sth*** ser bom (*ou* boa) / mau (*ou* má) em algo
atheism ['eɪθɪɪzm] ateísmo *m*
atheist ['eɪθɪɪst] ateu *m*, atéia *f*
athlete ['æθli:t] atleta *m/f*
athletic [æθ'letɪk] *adj* esportivo; (*strong, sporting*) atlético
athletics [æθ'letɪks] atletismo *m*
Atlantic [ət'læntɪk] *n* Oceano *m* Atlântico
atlas ['ætləs] atlas *m*
ATM [eɪti:'em] ATM *f*
atmosphere ['ætməsfɪr] *earth*: (*ambiance*) atmosfera *f*
atmospheric pollution [ætməsferɪkpə'lu:ʃn] poluição *f* atmosférica
atom ['ætəm] átomo *m*
'atom bomb bomba *f* atômica
atomic [ə'tɑ:mɪk] *adj* atômico
atomic 'energy energia *f* nuclear
atomic 'waste resíduo *m* radioativo
atomizer ['ætəmaɪzər] vaporizador *m*
atone [ə'toʊn] *v/i* **~ *for*** expiar
atrocious [ə'troʊʃəs] *adj* horrível
atrocity [ə'trɑ:sətɪ] atrocidade *f*
attach [ə'tætʃ] *v/t* fixar; *importance* atribuir; *to email* anexar; ***be ~ed to*** *thing, person* estar ligado a
attachment [ə'tætʃmənt] (*fondness*) apego *m*; *to email* anexo *m*
attack [ə'tæk] **1** *n* ataque *m* **2** *v/t* atacar
attempt [ə'tempt] **1** *n* intento *m* **2** *v/t* tentar
attend [ə'tend] *v/t meeting etc* comparecer a; *school* freqüentar
◆ **attend to** *v/t* ocupar-se de; *customer* atender a
attendance [ə'tendəns] *school*: freqüência *f*, *meeting etc*: comparecimento *m*; *assisting someone* atendimento *m*
attendant [ə'tendənt] *museum etc*: funcionário,-a *m,f*
attention [ə'tenʃn] atenção *f*; ***bring sth to s.o.'s ~*** informar a alguém de algo; ***your ~ please*** atenção, por favor; ***pay ~*** prestar atenção
attentive [ə'tentɪv] *adj listener* atento
attic ['ætɪk] sótão *m*
attitude ['ætɪtu:d] atitude *f*
attn *abbr* (*of* **for the attention of**) a/c (aos cuidados de)
attorney [ə'tɜ:nɪ] advogado,-a *m,f*; ***power of ~*** procuração *f*
attract [ə'trækt] *v/t* atrair; *attention* chamar; ***be ~ed to s.o.*** sentir-se atraído por alguém
attraction [ə'trækʃn] *of the city, romantic* atração *f*
attractive [ə'træktɪv] *adj* atraente
attribute[1] [ə'trɪbju:t] *v/t* atribuir; ***~ sth to ...*** atribuir algo a ...; *painting, poem* dedicar algo a ...
attribute[2] ['ætrɪbju:t] *n* atributo *m*
aubergine ['oʊbərʒi:n] *Brit* berinjela *f*
auction ['ɒ:kʃn] **1** *n* leilão *m* **2** *v/t* leiloar
◆ **auction off** *v/t* leiloar
auctioneer [ɒ:kʃə'nɪr] leiloeiro,-a *m,f*
audacious [ɒ:'deɪʃəs] *adj plan* audacioso
audacity [ɒ:'dæsətɪ] audácia *f*
audible ['ɒ:dəbl] *adj* audível
audibly ['ɒ:dəblɪ] *adv speak* em voz alta
audience ['ɒ:dɪəns] THEA espectadores *mpl*; *at show* público *m*; TV audiência *f*
audio ['ɒ:dɪoʊ] *adj* de áudio
audiovisual [ɒ:dɪoʊ'vɪʒʊəl] *adj* audiovisual
audit ['ɒ:dɪt] **1** *n* auditoria *f* **2** *v/t* fazer a auditoria de; *course* assistir a (*como ouvinte*)
audition [ɒ:'dɪʃn] **1** *n for part etc* audição *f* **2** *v/i* fazer uma audição
auditor ['ɒ:dɪtər] auditor,a *m,f*
auditorium [ɒ:dɪ'tɔ:rɪəm] THEA *etc* auditório *m*
August ['ɒ:gəst] agosto *m*
aunt [ænt] tia *f*
au pair [oʊ'per] *n* au pair *f*
aura ['ɒ:rə] aura *f*
auspices ['ɒ:spɪsɪz] ***under the ~ of*** sob o patrocínio de

auspicious [ɒːˈspɪʃəs] *adj* propício
austere [ɒːˈstiːr] *adj* austero
austerity [ɒːsˈterətɪ] austeridade *f*
Australia [ɑːˈstreɪlɪə] Austrália *f*
Australian [ɑːˈstreɪlɪən] **1** *adj* australiano **2** *n* australiano,-a *m,f*
Austria [ˈɑːstrɪə] Áustria *f*
Austrian [ˈɒstrɪən] **1** *adj* austríaco **2** *n* austríaco,-a *m,f*
authentic [ɒːˈθentɪk] *adj* autêntico
authenticity [ɒːθenˈtɪsətɪ] autenticidade *f*
author [ˈɒːθər] autor,a *m,f*
authoritarian [əθɑːrɪˈterɪən] *adj* autoritário
authoritative [əˈθɑːrɪtətɪv] *adj source* confiável; *manner* autoritário
authority [əˈθɑːrətɪ] autoridade *f*; (*permission*) autorização *f*; ***be an ~ on*** ser uma autoridade em; ***the authorities*** as autoridades
authorization [ɒːθəraɪˈzeɪʃn] autorização *f*
authorize [ˈɒːθəraɪz] *v/t* autorizar; ***be ~d to …*** estar autorizado a …
autistic [ɒːˈtɪstɪk] *adj* autista
autobiography [ɒːtoʊbaɪˈɑːgrəfɪ] autobiografia *f*
autocratic [ɒːtəˈkrætɪk] *adj* autocrático
autograph [ˈɒːtəgræf] autógrafo *m*
automate [ˈɒːtəmeɪt] *v/t* automatizar
automatic [ɒːtəˈmætɪk] **1** *adj* automático **2** *n car* câmbio *m* automático; *gun* arma *f* automática; *washing machine* lavadora *f* automática
automatically [ɒːtəˈmætɪklɪ] *adv* automaticamente
automation [ɒːtəˈmeɪʃn] automatização *f*
automobile [ˈɒːtəmoʊbiːl] automóvel *m*
ˈautomobile industry indústria *f* automobilística
autonomous [ɒːˈtɑːnəməs] *adj* autônomo
autonomy [ɒːˈtɑːnəmɪ] autonomia *f*
autopilot [ˈɒːtoʊpaɪlət] piloto *m* automático
autopsy [ˈɒːtɑːpsɪ] autópsia *f*
autumn [ˈɔːtəm] *Brit* outono *m*
auxiliary [ɒːgˈzɪljərɪ] *adj* auxiliar
avail [əˈveɪl] **1** *n* ***to no ~*** em vão **2** *v/t* ***~ oneself of*** aproveitar
available [əˈveɪləbl] *adj* disponível
avalanche [ˈævəlænʃ] avalanche *f*
avarice [ˈævərɪs] avareza *f*
avenue [ˈævənuː] avenida *f*; *fig* caminho *m*
average [ˈævərɪdʒ] **1** *adj* média; (*ordinary*) comum; (*of mediocre quality*) regular **2** *n* média *f*; ***above / below ~*** acima / abaixo da média; ***on ~*** em média **3** *v/t* ***I ~ six hours of sleep a night*** durmo em média 6 horas por noite
♦**average out** *v/t* calcular a média
♦**average out at** *v/t* sair numa média de
averse [əˈvɜːrs] *adj* adverso; ***not be ~ to*** não ter nada em contra
aversion [əˈvɜːrʃn] aversão *f*; ***have an ~ to*** ter aversão a
avert [əˈvɜːrt] *v/t one's eyes* desviar; *crisis* evitar
aviary [ˈeɪvɪrɪ] aviário *m*
aviation [eɪvɪˈaɪʃn] aviação *f*
avid [ˈævɪd] *adj* ávido
avocado [ɑːvəˈkɑːdoʊ] abacate *m*
avoid [əˈvɔɪd] *v/t* evitar
avoidable [əˈvɔɪdəbl] *adj* evitável
await [əˈweɪt] *v/t* aguardar
awake [əˈweɪk] *adj* acordado; ***it's keeping me ~*** isto me mantém acordado
award [əˈwɔːrd] **1** *n* (*prize*) prêmio *m* **2** *v/t* outorgar; *damages* conceder; ***~ damages to s.o.*** indenizar alguém
aware [əˈwer] *adj* consciente; ***be ~ of sth*** estar ciente de algo; ***become ~ of sth*** tomar consciência de algo
awareness [əˈwernɪs] conciência *f*
away [əˈweɪ] *adv* ***be ~*** (*traveling*) estar fora; (*sick*) não estar; ***walk / run ~*** ir embora; ***look ~!*** não olhe!; ***it's 3 kilometers ~*** fica a três quilômetros; ***Christmas is still six weeks ~*** faltam ainda seis semanas para o Natal; ***take sth ~ from s.o.*** tirar algo de alguém; ***put sth ~*** guardar algo
aˈway game SPORT jogo *m* fora de casa
awesome [ˈɒːsəm] *adj fam* (*terrific*) horrível

awful ['ɒːfʊl] *adj* horrível
awkward ['ɒːkwərd] *adj* (*clumsy*) acanhado; (*tricky*) difícil; (*embarrassing*) embaraçoso; ***feel ~*** sentir-se mal
awning ['ɒːnɪŋ] toldo *m*
ax [æks] *Am* **1** *n* machado *m* **2** *v/t project etc* cancelar; *budget, job* cortar
axe *Brit* → ***ax***
axle ['æksl] eixo *m*
Azores [ə'zɒːrz] *npl* Açores *mpl*

B

BA [biː'eɪ] *abbr* (*of* ***Bachelor of Arts***) Bacharelado *m* (*em Ciências Humanas*); *person* Bacharel *m/f* em Ciências Humanas
baby ['beɪbɪ] *n* bebê *m*
'baby boom baby boom *m*, explosão *f* demográfica
'baby carriage carrinho *m* de bebê
babyish ['beɪbɪɪʃ] *adj* infantil
'baby-sit *v/i* ⟨*pret & pp* ***baby-sat***⟩ fazer babysitting
'baby-sitter babá *f*
bachelor ['bæʧələr] bacharel *m/f*
back [bæk] **1** *n person*: costas *fpl*; *car, bus*: traseira *f*; *paper, book*: verso *m*; *clothes*: avesso *m*; *drawer*: fundo *m*; *chair*: encosto *m*; SPORT zagueiro *m*, *Port* defesa *m*; ***in ~*** *in store etc* lá atrás; lá dentro; ***in the ~*** (***of the car***) atrás no carro; ***at the ~ of the bus*** na parte de trás do ônibus; ***~ to front*** do avesso; ***at the ~ of beyond*** no fim do mundo **2** *adj* traseiro; ***~ road*** estrada *f* secundária **3** *adv* ***please move / stand ~*** por favor, vá para atrás; ***2 meters ~ from the edge*** a 2 metros da margem; ***~ in 1935*** em 1935; ***give X ~ to Y*** devolver algo a alguém; ***she'll be ~ tomorrow*** ela vai voltar amanhã; ***when are you coming ~?*** quando você voltará?; ***take sth ~ to the store*** *because unsatisfactory* devolver algo à loja; ***they wrote / phoned ~*** eles escreveram / ligaram de volta; ***he hit me ~*** ele me devolveu o golpe **4** *v/t* (*support*) apoiar; *car* dar ré; *horse* apostar **5** *v/i driver* dar ré, *Port* fazer marcha atrás; ***she ~ed into the garage*** ela entrou na garagem de marcha a ré
♦**back away** *v/i* recuar
♦**back down** *v/i* voltar atrás
♦**back off** *v/i* recuar; *from danger* afastar-se
♦**back onto** *v/t* ***our house backs onto a main road*** uma estrada passa nos fundos da nossa casa
♦**back out** *v/i of commitment* voltar atrás; ***they're trying to back out of our ~*** eles querem recuar no acordo
♦**back up 1** *v/t* (*support*) apoiar; *claim, argument* consolidar; *file* fazer backup de; ***be backed up*** *traffic* estar congestionado **2** *v/i in car* recuar; *drains* entupir
'backache dor *f* nas costas **'backbiting** fofoca *f* **'backbone** ANAT coluna *f* vertebral; *fig* (*courage*) coragem *f*; *fig* (*mainstay*) fonte *f* principal **'back-breaking** *adj* extenuante **back 'burner** *n* ***put sth on the ~ ~*** pôr algo de molho **'backdate** *v/t* antedatar **'backdoor** porta traseira *f*
backer ['bækər] financiador *m*
back'fire *v/i fig* sair o tiro pela culatra **'background** *n* fundo *m*; *person*: origem *f*, *situation*: contexto *m*; ***what sort of family ~ does he come from?*** de que tipo de ambiente familiar ele vem? **'backhand** *n tennis*: revés *m* **'backheeler** *soccer*: passe *m* de calcanhar
backing ['bækɪŋ] *n* (*support*) apoio *m*; MUS acompanhamento *m*

'backing group MUS banda *f* acompanhante
'backlash reação *f* violenta **'backlog** acúmulo *m* **'backpack 1** *n* mochila *f* **2** *v/i* viajar com mochila **'backpacker** mochileiro,-a *m,f* **'backpacking**: ***go ~*** viajar com mochila **'backpedal** *v/i fig* voltar atrás **'back seat** *car*: banco *m* traseiro **back-seat 'driver** *passageiro que dá palpites constantemente ao motorista* **'backspace**, **'backspace key** tecla *f* de retorno **'backstairs** *npl* escada *f* de serviço **'back streets** *npl* ruazinhas *fpl* **'backstroke** SPORT nado *m* de costas **'backtrack** *v/i* voltar **'backup** (*support*) reforço *m*; ***take a ~*** COMPUT fazer um back up
backward ['bækwərd] **1** *adj child* retardado; *society* retrógrado; *glance* para trás **2** *adv* para trás
back'yard *also fig* quintal *m* (dos fundos); ***the not in my ~ syndrome*** síndrome do NIMBY (não aqui no meu quintal)
bacon ['beɪkn] bacon *m*
bacteria [bæk'tɪrɪə] bactérias *fpl*
bad [bæd] *adj weather*, *condition* mau (má); *cold*, *headache etc* forte; *mistake*, *accident* grave; (*rotten*) deteriorado; ***it's not ~*** não é mau; ***that's really too ~*** (*shame*) é realmente uma pena; ***feel ~ about*** (*guilty*) sertir-se mal por; ***be ~ at*** não ser bom em; ***Friday's ~, how about Thursday*** sexta-feira é ruim, que tal na quinta-feira
bad 'debt dívida *f* incobrável
badge [bædʒ] crachá *m*
badger ['bædʒər] *v/t* cansar
bad 'language linguagem *f* obscena
badly ['bædlɪ] *adv work*, *behaved* mal; *damaged* seriamente; *injured* gravemente; ***he ~ needs a haircut / rest*** ele precisa urgentemente de um corte de cabelo / de descanso; ***he is ~ off*** (*poor*) ele anda mal de dinheiro
bad-mannered [bæd'mænərd] *adj* mal-educado
badminton ['bædmɪntən] badminton *m*
bad-tempered [bæd'tempərd] *adj* mal-humorado
baffle ['bæfl] *v/t* confundir; ***be ~d*** estar confuso
baffling ['bæflɪŋ] *adj mystery* insondável; *software etc* incompreensível
bag [bæg] (*plastic*, *paper*) saco *m*; *for school*, *traveling*, *also* (*handbag*) bolsa *f*, sacola *f*
baggage ['bægɪdʒ] bagagem *f*
'baggage car RAIL vagão *m* de cargas **'baggage check** controle *m* de bagagem **baggage reclaim** ['ri:kleɪm] entrega *f* de bagagem
baggy ['bægɪ] *adj pants* larga
Bahamas [bə'hɑ:məz] ***the ~*** as Bahamas
bail [beɪl] *n* LAW fiança *f*; (*money*) caução *f*; ***on ~*** sob fiança
♦ **bail out 1** *v/t* LAW libertar sob fiança; *fig* salvar *de situação difícil* **2** *v/i airplane* saltar de pára-quedas
bait [beɪt] *n* isca *f*
bake [beɪk] *v/t* assar
baked 'beans [beɪkt] *npl* feijão cozido (em molho de tomate)
baked po'tatoes *npl* batata *f* assada
baker ['beɪkər] padeiro *m*
bakery ['beɪkərɪ] padaria *f*
baking powder ['beɪkɪŋ] fermento *m* em pó
balance ['bæləns] **1** *n* equilíbrio *m*; (*remainder*) resto *m*; *bank account*: saldo *m* **2** *v/t* equilibrar; ***~ the books*** fazer o balanço **3** *v/i* equilibrar-se; *accounts* bater
balanced ['bælənst] *adj* (*fair*) objetivo; *personality*, *diet* equilibrado
balance of 'payments balança *f* de pagamento **balance of 'trade** balança *f* comercial **'balance sheet** balanço *m* geral
balcony ['bælkənɪ] *house*: sacada *f*; THEA balcão *m*
bald [bɒ:ld] *adj man* calvo; ***he's going ~*** ele está ficando calvo
balding ['bɒ:ldɪŋ] *adj* meio calvo
Balkan ['bɒ:lkən] *adj* balcânico
Balkans ['bɒ:lkənz] *npl* ***the ~*** *npl* os Bálcãs *mpl*
ball [bɒ:l] bola *f*; ***be on the ~*** estar atento; ***play ~*** *fig* cooperar; ***the ~'s in his court*** agora é com ele

B

ballad ['bæləd] balada *f*
ball 'bearing rolamento *m* de bolas
ballerina [bælə'riːnə] bailarina *f*
ballet [bæ'leɪ] balé *m*
'ballet dancer bailarino,-a *m,f* clássico,-a
'ball game (*baseball*) jogo *m* de beisebol; ***that's a different ~*** *fam* esta é uma outra questão
ballistic missile [bə'lɪstɪk] míssil *m* balístico
balloon [bə'luːn] *child's* bexiga *f*; *for flight* balão *m*
balloonist [bə'luːnɪst] piloto *m* de balão
ballot ['bælət] **1** *n* eleição *f* **2** *v/t members* fazer uma votação entre
'ballot box urna *f*
'ballot paper voto *m*
'ballpark (*baseball*) campo *m* de beisebol; ***be in the right ~*** *fam* estar no caminho certo; ***we're not in the same ~*** estamos falando de quantidades de dinheiro totalmente diferentes
'ballpark figure *fam* cifra *f* aproximada
'ballpoint, **'ballpoint pen** caneta *f* esferográfica
balls [bɒːlz] *npl vulg* saco *m*, *Port* tomates *mpl*; (*courage*) coragem *f*, (*nonsense*) asneira *f*
bamboo [bæm'buː] *n* bambu *m*
ban [bæn] **1** *n* proibição *f* **2** *v/t* ⟨*pret & pp* ***banned***⟩ proibir; ***be ~ned from a club*** ser proibido de entrar num clube
banal [bə'næl] *adj* banal
banana [bə'nænə] banana *f*
band [bænd] conjunto *m*; (*pop*) grupo *m*; (*material*) fita *f*
bandage ['bændɪdʒ] **1** *n* atadura *f*, *Port* ligadura *f* **2** *v/t* atar
'Band-Aid® band-aid *m*
bandit ['bændɪt] bandido,-a *m,f*
'bandwagon ***jump on the ~*** entrar na roda
bandy ['bændɪ] *adj legs* arqueado
bang [bæŋ] **1** *n* (*noise*) barulho *m*; (*blow*) golpe *m* **2** *v/t & v/i* bater
bangle ['bæŋgl] pulseira *f*
banisters ['bænɪstərz] *npl* corrimão *m*
banjo ['bændʒoʊ] banjo *m*
bank[1] [bæŋk] *n river*: margem *f*
bank[2] [bæŋk] **1** *n* FIN banco *m* **2** *v/i* ~ ***with*** ter uma conta com
♦ **bank on** *v/t* contar com; ***don't bank on it*** não conte com isso; ***bank on s.o. doing sth*** contar com alguém para fazer algo
'bank account conta *f* bancária
'bank balance saldo *m*
banker ['bæŋkər] banqueiro *m*
'banker's card cartão *m* bancário
banking ['bæŋkɪŋ] área *f* bancária; ***he's in ~*** ele trabalha na área bancária
'bank loan empréstimo *m* bancário
'bank manager gerente *m/f* de banco **'bank rate** taxa *f* bancária
'bankroll *v/t* financiar
bankrupt ['bæŋkrʌpt] **1** *adj person, company* falido; ***go ~*** ir a falência **2** *v/t person, company* levar a falência
bankruptcy ['bæŋkrʌpsɪ] falência *f*
'bank statement extrato *m* bancário
banner ['bænər] insígnia *f*
banns [bænz] *npl* anúncio *m* de casamento
banquet ['bæŋkwɪt] *n* banquete *m*
banter ['bæntər] *n* brincadeira *f*
baptism ['bæptɪzm] batismo *m*
baptize [bæp'taɪz] *v/t* batizar
bar[1] [bɑːr] *n iron, chocolate*, (*counter*) barra *f*, ***a ~ of soap*** uma barra de sabão; ***be behind ~s*** (*in prison*) estar atrás das grades
bar[2] [bɑːr] *v/t* ⟨*pret & pp* ***barred***⟩ barrar
bar[3] [bɑːr] *prep* (*except*) exceto
barbarian [bɑːr'berɪən] bárbaro *m*
barbaric [bɑːr'bærɪk] *adj* cruel
barbecue ['bɑːrbɪkjuː] **1** *n* churrasco *m*; *equipment* churrasqueira *f* **2** *v/t* assar na churrasqueira; ***~d chicken*** galinha assada na churrasqueira
barbed 'wire [bɑːrbd] arame *m* farpado
barber ['bɑːrbər] barbeiro *m*
barbiturate [bɑːr'bɪtjərət] barbiturato *m*
'bar code código *m* de barras
bare [ber] *adj* (*naked*) descoberto; *feet*

descalço; *floor* descoberto; *room* vazio; *mountainside* exposto
'barefoot *adj* ***be ~*** estar descalço
bare-'headed [ber'hedɪd] *adj* sem chapéu
barely ['berlɪ] *adv* quase não, apenas; ***there was ~ room for two*** quase não havia espaço para dois
bargain ['bɑːrgɪn] **1** *n* (*deal*) trato *m*; (*good buy*) pechincha *f*; ***it's a ~!*** *deal* é uma pechinha!; ***into the ~*** ainda por cima **2** *v/i* pechinchar
♦ **bargain for** *v/t* (*expect*) imaginar; ***you might get more than you bargained for*** é possível que você consiga mais do que imaginava
barge [bɑːrdʒ] *n* NAUT barcaça *f*
♦ **barge into** *v/t* trombar
baritone ['bærɪtoʊn] *n* barítono *m*
bark[1] [bɑːrk] *n dog*: latido *m*
bark[2] [bɑːrk] *n tree*: casca *f*
barley ['bɑːrlɪ] cevada *f*
'barmaid *Brit* garçonete *f*, *Port* empregada *f*
'barman *Brit* garçom *m*, *Port* empregado *m*
barn [bɑːrn] celeiro *m*
barometer [bə'rɑːmɪtər] *also fig* barômetro *m*
Baroque [bə'rɑːk] *adj* barroco
barracks ['bærəks] *npl* MIL quartel *m*
barrage [bə'rɑːʒ] MIL barreira *f* de fogo; *fig* chuva *f*
barrel ['bærəl] *container* barril *m*
barren ['bærən] *adj land* árido
barrette [bæ'ret] grampo *m*, *Port* gancho *m*
barricade [bærɪ'keɪd] *n* barricada *f*
barrier ['bærɪər] *also cultural* barreira *f*; ***language ~*** barreira *f* da língua
barring ['bɑːrɪŋ] *prep* salvo; ***~ accidents*** salvo imprevistos
barrow ['bæroʊ] carrinho *m* de mão
'bar tender barman *m*, *Port* empregado *m*; garçonete *f*, *Port* empregada *f*
barter ['bɑːrtər] **1** *n* troca *f* **2** *v/t* trocar
base [beɪs] **1** *n* (*bottom*) fundo *m*; (*center*), MIL base *f* **2** *v/t* basear; ***~ X on Y*** basear X em Y; ***be ~d on*** basear-se em; ***be ~d in*** *in city, country* estar estacionado em
'baseball (*ball*) bola *f* de beisebol; (*game*) beisebol *m*
'baseball bat bastão *m* de beisebol **'baseball cap** boné *m* **'baseball player** jogador *m* de beisebol
'baseboard *Am* rodapé *m*
baseless ['beɪslɪs] *adj* infundado
basement ['beɪsmənt] porão *m*
'base rate FIN taxa *f* básica de juros
bash [bæʃ] *fam* **1** *n* pancada *f* **2** *v/t* bater
basic ['beɪsɪk] *adj* (*rudimentary*) básico; (*fundamental*) fundamental
basically ['beɪsɪklɪ] *adv* basicamente
basics ['beɪsɪks] *npl* essencial *m*; ***the ~*** o básico; ***get down to ~*** ir direto ao assunto
basil ['bæzɪl] manjericão *m*
basilica [bə'zɪlɪkə] basílica *f*
basin ['beɪsn] *washing*: pia *f*
basis ['beɪsɪs] ⟨*pl* ***bases***⟩ *argument etc*: base *f*
bask [bæsk] *v/i* ***~ in the sun*** tomar sol
basket ['bæskɪt] cesto *m*; *basketball*: cesta *f*
'basketball basquetebol *m*
bass [beɪs] *n & adj* MUS baixo *m*
'bass clef clave *f* de fá
bastard ['bæstərd] *fam* canalha *m*; ***you stupid ~!*** seu idiota!
bat[1] [bæt] **1** *n baseball*: bastão *m* **2** *v/i* ⟨*pret & pp* ***batted***⟩ *baseball*: rebater
bat[2] [bæt] *v/t* ***he didn't ~ an eyelid*** ele não deu nem uma piscada
bat[3] [bæt] *n animal* morcego *m*
batch [bætʃ] *n students*: grupo *m*; *goods produced* lote *m*; *bread*: fornada *f*
bated ['beɪtɪd] *adj* ***watch with ~ breath*** assistir com ar de suspense
bath [bæθ] banheira *f*; ***have a ~, take a ~*** tomar um banho
bathe [beɪð] *v/i* (*swim*) nadar; (*have a bath*) tomar banho de banheira
'bathing costume traje *m* de banho
'bath mat tapete *m* de banheiro **'bathrobe** roupão *m* **'bathroom** *for bath* banheiro *m*, *Port* casa *f* de banho; *for washing hands* lavabo *m*; (*toilet*) toalete *m* **'bath towel** toalha *f* de banho **'bathtub** banheira *f*
baton [bə't ɑːn] *conductor*: batuta *f*

battalion [bə'tælıən] MIL batalhão *m*
batter ['bætər] *n* batedeira *f*; *baseball*: rebatedor *m*
battered ['bætərd] *adj* espancado
battery ['bætərı] *for toy*, *flashlight* pilha *f*; MOT bateria *f*
'battery charger carregador *m* de pilhas
battery-operated [bætərı'ɑːpəreıtıd] *adj toy* à pilha
battle ['bætl] **1** *n* batalha *f*; *fig* luta *f* **2** *v/i against illness etc* batalhar
'battlefield, **'battleground** campo *m* de batalha
'battleship couraçado *m*
bawdy ['bɒːdı] *adj* indecente
bawl [bɒːl] *v/i* (*shout*) gritar; (*weep*) chorar
♦**bawl out** *v/t fam* repreender
bay [beı] (*inlet*) baía *f*
bayonet ['beıənet] *n* baioneta *f*
bay 'window janela *f* de sacada
BC [biː'siː] *abbr* (*of* **before Christ**) antes de Cristo
be [biː] *v/i* ⟨*pret* **was** / **were**, *pp* **been**⟩
◊ *permanent characteristics*, *profession*, *nationality*: ser; *position*, *temporary condition*: estar; ***I'm 25*** tenho 25 anos; ***was she there?*** ela estava lá?; ***it's me*** sou eu; ***how much is / are …?*** quanto é / são …?; ***there is, there are*** há; ***~ careful!*** tenha cuidado!; ***don't ~ sad*** não fique triste; ***has the mailman been?*** o carteiro já veio?; ***I've never been to Japan*** eu nunca estive no Japão; ***I've been here for hours*** estou aqui há horas
◊ *in tags* ***that's right, isn't it?*** isso está certo, não está?; ***she's Chinese, isn't she?*** ela é chinesa, não é?
◊ *v/aux* ***I am thinking*** estou pensando; ***he was running*** ele estava correndo; ***you're being silly*** você está sendo tolo
◊ *obligation*: ***you are to do what I tell you*** você deve fazer o que eu digo; ***I was to tell you this*** eu deveria dizer-lhe isso; ***you were not to tell anyone*** o você não devia dizer a ninguém
◊ *passive*: ***he was killed*** ele foi morto; ***they have been sold*** foram vendidos
♦**be in for** *v/t* estar propenso a; ***he's in for a big disappointment*** ele está propenso a ter um grande desapontamento; ***he's in for trouble*** ele está procurando problema
beach [biːʧ] *n* praia *f*; ***on the ~*** na praia
'beach ball bola *f* de praia
'beachwear roupa *f* de praia
beads [biːdz] *npl* contas *fpl*
beak [biːk] bico *m* (*de aves*)
be-all *n* ***for her it's the ~ and end-all*** para ela é tudo que importa
beam [biːm] **1** *n ceiling etc*: viga *f* **2** *v/i* (*smile*) sorrir **3** *v/t* (*transmit*) transmitir
bean [biːn] feijão *m*; (*green bean*) vagem *f*; (*runner bean*) feijão-da-espanha *m*; (*coffee bean*) grão *m* de café; ***be full of ~s*** *fam* estar cheio de vida
'beanbag *seat* pufe *m*
bear[1] [ber] *n animal* urso *m*
bear[2] [ber] ⟨*pret* **bore**, *pp* **borne**⟩ **1** *v/t child* dar à luz; *weight* agüentar; ***she bore him six children*** ela deu-lhe seis filhos; ***I can't ~ to see that happen*** não suporto ver isso acontecendo **2** *v/i* ***bring pressure to ~ on*** fazer pressão sobre; ***~ left*** virar à esquerda
♦**bear out** *v/t* (*confirm*) comprovar
bearable ['berəbl] *adj* suportável
beard [bırd] barba *f*
bearded ['bırdıd] *adj* barbado
bearing ['berıŋ] *in machine* mancal *m*; (*ball bearing*) rolamento *m*; ***that has no ~ on the case*** isso não tem relação com a questão
'bear market FIN mercado *m* em baixa
beast [biːst] besta *f*
beat [biːt] **1** *n heart*, *music*: batida *f* **2** *v/i* ⟨*pret* **beat**, *pp* **beaten**⟩ *heart*, *rain*: bater; ***stop ~ing about the bush*** deixe de rodeios **3** *v/t* ⟨*pret* **beat**, *pp* **beaten**⟩ *in competition* derrotar; (*pound*) tamborilar; (*hit*) bater; (*spank*) espancar; ***~ it!*** *fam* dê o fora!; ***it ~s me*** não sei
♦**beat up** *v/t* dar uma surra

beaten[1] ['biːtən] *adj* ***he lives off the ~ track*** ele mora num lugar fora de mão
beaten[2] ['biːtən] *pp* → ***beat***
beating ['biːtɪŋ] *physical* surra *f*
'beat-up *adj fam* gasto
beautician [bjuː'tɪʃn] esteticista *m/f*
beautiful ['bjuːtəfʊl] *adj woman, house, day* bonito; *meal, vacation, story, movie* belo; ***thanks, that's just ~!*** obrigado, está ótimo!
beautifully ['bjuːtɪflɪ] *adv cooked, done* bem; *simple* maravilhosamente
beauty ['bjuːtɪ] beleza *f*
'beauty parlor salão *m* de beleza
beauty salon *Brit* → ***beauty parlor***
beaver ['biːvər] castor *m*
♦ **beaver away** *v/i fam* trabalhar duro
became [bɪ'keɪm] *pret* → ***become***
because [bɪ'kɑːz] *conj* porque; ***~ it was too expensive*** porque era muito caro; ***~ of*** por causa de
beckon ['bekn] **1** *v/i* acenar **2** *v/t* ***he ~ed us across to his table*** ele acenou nos chamando para a sua mesa
become [bɪ'kʌm] *v/i* ⟨*pret* ***became***, *pp* ***become***⟩ tornar-se; ***what's ~ of her?*** o que foi feito dela?; ***it's becoming evident that …*** está ficando evidente que …; ***he became a priest*** ele tornou-se padre
becoming [bɪ'kʌmɪŋ] *adj* apropriado
bed [bed] *n* cama *f*; *flowers*: canteiro *m*; *sea*: fundo *m*; *river*: leito *m*; ***go to ~*** ir para a cama; ***he's still in ~*** ele ainda está na cama; ***go to ~ with …*** ir para a cama com …
bed and 'breakfast pousada *f*
'bedclothes *npl* roupa *f* de cama
bedding ['bedɪŋ] roupa *f* de cama
bedlam ['bedləm] confusão *f*
bedridden ['bedrɪdən] *adj* acamado
'bedroom quarto *m* **'bedside** ***be at the ~ of*** estar ao lado da cama de **'bedspread** colcha *f* **'bedtime** hora *f* de dormir; ***it's your ~*** está na hora de ir para a cama
bee [biː] abelha *f*
beech [biːʧ] faia *f*
beef [biːf] **1** *n* bife *m*; *fam* ***what's your ~?*** qual é o seu problema? **2** *v/i fam* (*complain*) resmungar
♦ **beef up** *v/t* fortalecer
'beefburger hambúrguer *m* (de carne bovina)
'beehive colmeia *f*
'beeline: ***make a ~ for*** correr diretamente para
been [bɪn] *pp* → ***be***
beep [biːp] **1** *n* bipe *m* **2** *v/t & v/i* bipar
beer [bɪr] cerveja *f*
beetle ['biːtl] besouro *f*
before [bɪ'fɔːr] **1** *prep time, space, order*: antes **2** *adv* anteriormente; ***the week / day ~*** a semana / o dia anterior **3** *conj* antes que; ***~ we met him*** antes de nos encontrarmos; ***~ I go home*** antes de eu ir para casa, antes que eu vá para casa
be'forehand *adv* antecipadamente
befriend [bɪ'frend] *v/t* fazer amizade com
beg [beg] ⟨*pret & pp* ***begged***⟩ **1** *v/i* mendigar **2** *v/t* ***~ s.o. to …*** implorar a alguém para …
began [bɪ'gæn] *pret* → ***begin***
beggar ['begər] *n* mendigo *m*
begin [bɪ'gɪn] ⟨*pret* ***began***, *pp* ***begun***⟩ **1** *v/i* começar; ***to ~ with*** (*at first*) para começar; (*in the first place*) inicialmente **2** *v/t* começar
beginner [bɪ'gɪnər] iniciante *m/f*
beginning [bɪ'gɪnɪŋ] início *m*; (*origin*) começo *m*; ***at the ~ of the movie*** no começo do filme
begrudge [bɪ'grʌdʒ] *v/t* (*envy*) invejar; (*give reluctantly*) dar com relutância
begun [bɪ'gʌn] *pp* → ***begin***
behalf [bɪ'hæf] ***on my / his ~*** em meu / seu nome; ***on ~ of*** em nome de
behave [bɪ'heɪv] *v/i* portar-se; ***~ (oneself)*** comportar-se; ***~ (yourself)!*** comporte-se!
behavior [bɪ'heɪvjər] *Am* comportamento *m*
behaviour *Brit* → ***behavior***
behind [bɪ'haɪnd] **1** *prep position, progress, order*: atrás de; ***be ~ …*** (*responsible for*) estar por trás de …; (*support*) dar apoio … **2** *adv* (*at the back*) *also leave, stay, in match* atrás; ***be ~ with sth*** estar atrasado com algo

beige [beɪʒ] *adj* bege
being ['biːɪŋ] (*existence, creature*) ser
belated [bɪ'leɪtɪd] *adj* atrasado
belch [beltʃ] **1** *n* arroto *m* **2** *v/i* arrotar
Belgian ['beldʒən] **1** *adj* belga **2** *n* belga *m/f*
Belgium ['beldʒəm] Bélgica *f*
belief [bɪ'liːf] crença *f*
believe [bɪ'liːv] *v/t* acreditar
◆ **believe in** *v/t ghosts, person* acreditar em
believer [bɪ'liːvər] REL crente *m/f*; *fig* adepto,-a *m,f*
belittle [bɪ'lɪtl] *v/t* diminuir
Belize [bə'liːz] Belize *m*
bell [bel] sino *m*
'bellhop *Am* mensageiro *m*
belligerent [bɪ'lɪdʒərənt] *adj* beligerante
bellow ['beloʊ] **1** *n* berro *m*; *bull*: mugido *m* **2** *v/i* berrar; *bull* mugir
belly ['belɪ] *also* (*fat stomach*) pança *f*; *animal*: bucho *m*
'bellyache *v/i fam* resmungar
belong [bɪ'lɑːŋ] *v/i* ***where does this ~?*** aonde isto leva?; ***I don't ~ here*** aqui não é meu lugar
◆ **belong to** *v/t person, club, organization* pertencer a; ***who does this belong to?*** de quem é isso?
belongings [bɪ'lɑːŋɪŋz] *npl* pertences *mpl*
beloved [bɪ'lʌvɪd] *adj* adorado
below [bɪ'loʊ] **1** *prep amount, rate, level, position*: abaixo de **2** *adv* embaixo; *text*: abaixo; ***see ~*** ver abaixo; ***10 degrees ~*** 10 graus abaixo de zero
belt [belt] *n* cinto *m*; ***tighten one's ~*** *fig* apertar o cinto
bemoan [bɪ'moʊn] *v/t* lamentar
bench [bentʃ] (*seat*) banco *m*; (*workbench*) bancada *f*
'benchmark base *f* de referência
bend [bend] **1** *n* curva *f* **2** *v/t & v/i* ⟨*pret & pp* ***bent***⟩ dobrar
◆ **bend down** *v/i* abaixar-se
bender ['bendər] *fam* bebedeira *f*
beneath [bɪ'niːθ] **1** *prep* embaixo de; *status, value*: abaixo de **2** *adv* embaixo
benefactor ['benɪfæktər] benfeitor,a *m,f*
beneficial [benɪ'fɪʃl] *adj* benéfico
benefit ['benɪfɪt] **1** *n* benefício *m* **2** *v/t* beneficiar **3** *v/i* beneficiar-se; ***~ from sth*** ser beneficiado por algo
benevolence [bɪ'nevələns] benevolência *f*
benevolent [bɪ'nevələnt] *adj* benevolente
benign [bɪ'naɪn] *adj also* MED benigno
bent [bent] *pret & pp* → ***bend***
bequeath [bɪ'kwiːð] *v/t* legar; *fig* deixar como herança
bequest [bɪ'kwest] legado *m*
bereaved [bɪ'riːvd] *n* ***the ~*** a família do falecido / da falecida
beret [be'reɪ] boina *f*
berm [bɜːrm] acostamento *m*, *Port* berma *f*
berry ['berɪ] baga *f*
berserk [bə'sɜːrk] *adv* ***go ~*** ficar furioso
berth [bɜːrθ] *for sleeping* beliche *m*; *for ship* atracadouro *m*; ***give s.o. a wide ~*** evitar alguém
beseech [bɪ'siːtʃ] *v/t* ***~ s.o. to do sth*** suplicar a alguém para fazer algo
beside [bɪ'saɪd] *prep* ao lado de; ***be ~ oneself*** estar fora de si; ***that's ~ the point*** isto é irrelevante
besides [bɪ'saɪdz] **1** *adv* além do mais **2** *prep* (*apart from*) além de
besiege [bɪ'siːdʒ] *v/t fig* cercar
best [best] **1** *adj & adv* melhor; ***it would be ~ if ...*** seria melhor se ...; ***which did you like ~?*** de qual você gostou mais?; ***I like her ~*** eu gosto mais dela **2** *n* ***do one's ~*** fazer o melhor; ***the ~*** o/a melhor; ***make the ~ of*** fazer o melhor de; ***all the ~!*** tudo de bom!
best be'fore date data *f* de validade
best 'man *wedding*: padrinho *m*
best-'seller best-seller *m*
bet [bet] **1** *n* aposta *f* **2** *v/i* apostar; ***I ~ he doesn't come*** aposto que ele não vem; ***you ~!*** pode apostar!
betray [bɪ'treɪ] *v/t* trair
betrayal [bɪ'treɪəl] traição *f*
better ['betər] *adj & adv also health*: melhor; ***get ~*** melhorar; ***he's ~*** *health*: ele está melhor; ***you'd ~ ask permission*** seria melhor pedir

permissão; ***I'd really ~ not*** seria melhor não; ***all the ~ for us*** melhor para nós; ***I like her ~*** eu gosto mais dela
better 'off *adj* melhor de vida; ***you'll be ~ without me*** você vai ficar melhor sem mim; ***you'd be ~ selling it*** o melhor seria vendê-lo
between [bɪ'twiːn] *prep* entre; ***~ you and me*** entre mim e você
beverage ['bevərɪdʒ] *fml* bebida *f*
beware [bɪ'wer] *v/t* ***~ of*** cuidado com
bewilder [bɪ'wɪldər] *v/t* desconcertar
bewilderment [bɪ'wɪldərmənt] confusão *f*
beyond [bɪ'jɑːnd] **1** *prep time, place, degree*: além de; ***it's ~ me*** (*don't understand*) isto está além da minha compreensão; (*can't do it*) isto está além das possibilidades **2** *adv* além
bias ['baɪəs] *n* parcialidade *f*
biased, **biassed** ['baɪəst] *adj* parcial
bib [bɪb] *for baby* babador *m*
Bible ['baɪbl] Bíblia *f*
biblical ['bɪblɪkl] *adj* bíblico
bibliography [bɪblɪ'ɑːgrəfɪ] bibliografia *f*
bicarbonate of soda [baɪ'kɑːrbəneɪt] bicarbonato *m* de sódio
bicentenary *Brit* → ***bicentennial***
bicentennial [baɪsen'tenɪəl] *Am* bicentenário *m*
biceps ['baɪseps] *npl* bíceps *m*
bicker ['bɪkər] *v/i* brigar
bicycle ['baɪsɪkl] *n* bicicleta *f*
bid [bɪd] **1** *n auction*: lance *m*; (*attempt*) tentativa *f* **2** *v/i* ⟨*pret & pp* ***bid***⟩ *auction*: dar um lance
bidder ['bɪdər] licitante *m/f*
biennial [baɪ'enɪəl] *adj* bienal
bifocals [baɪ'foʊkəlz] *npl* óculos *mpl* bifocais
big [bɪg] **1** *adj* grande; ***my ~ sister*** minha irmã mais velha; ***my ~ brother*** meu irmão mais velho; ***~ name*** grande nome *m* **2** *adv* ***talk ~*** contar vantagem
bigamist ['bɪgəmɪst] bígamo,-a *m,f*
bigamous ['bɪgəməs] *adj* bígamo
bigamy ['bɪgəmɪ] bigamia *f*
'bighead *fam* convencido,-a *m,f*
big-headed [bɪg'hedɪd] *adj* convencido
bigot ['bɪgət] intolerante *m/f*
bike [baɪk] *n fam* bicicleta *f*; (*motorbike*) moto *f*
biker ['baɪkər] ciclista *m/f*; *motorbike*: motociclista *m/f*; (*for deliveries*) office boy *m*, *Port* estafeta *m*
bikini [bɪ'kiːnɪ] biquíni *m*
bilateral [baɪ'lætərəl] *adj* bilateral
bilingual [baɪ'lɪŋgwəl] *adj* bilíngüe
bill [bɪl] **1** *n* conta *f*; (*money*) nota *f*; POL projeto *m* de lei; (*poster*) cartaz *m* **2** *v/t* (*invoice*) mandar a conta
'billboard outdoor *m*
'billfold carteira *f*
billiards ['bɪljərdz] *nsg* bilhar *m*
billion ['bɪljən] bilhão *m*
bill of ex'change FIN letra *f* de câmbio
bill of 'sale nota *f* fiscal
bin [bɪn] *n storage*: caixa *f*; ***trash ~*** lata *f* de lixo
binary ['baɪnərɪ] *adj* binário
bind [baɪnd] *v/t* ⟨*pret & pp* ***bound***⟩ (*connect*) ligar; (*tie*) amarrar; LAW (*oblige*) obrigar
binding ['baɪndɪŋ] **1** *adj agreement* obrigatório **2** *n book*: encadernação *f*
binoculars [bɪ'nɑːkjʊlərz] *npl* binóculo *m*
biochemist ['baɪoʊkemɪst] bioquímico,-a *m,f*
biochemistry [baɪoʊ'kemɪstrɪ] bioquímica *f*
biodegradability [baɪoʊdɪgreɪdə'bɪlətɪ] biodegradabilidade *f*
biodegradable [baɪoʊdɪ'greɪdəbl] *adj* biodegradável
biofuel ['baɪoʊfjʊːəl] biocombustível *m*
biographer [baɪ'ɑːgrəfər] biógrafo,-a *m,f*
biography [baɪ'ɑːgrəfɪ] biografia *f*
biological [baɪoʊ'lɑːdʒɪkl] *adj* biológico; ***~ parents*** pais *mpl* biológicos; ***~ detergent*** detergente *m* biológico
biologist [baɪ'ɑːlədʒɪst] biólogo,-a *m,f*
biology [baɪ'ɑːlədʒɪ] biologia *f*
biometric [baɪoʊ'metrɪk] *adj* biométrico
biotechnology [baɪoʊtek'nɑːlədʒɪ]

B

biotecnologia *f*
biotope ['baɪoʊtoʊp] biótopo *m*
bird [bɜːrd] pássaro *m*
'birdcage gaiola *f* **bird of 'prey** ave *f* de rapina **'bird sanctuary** santuário *m* de aves **'bird's eye view** vista *f* aérea
birth [bɜːrθ] *child, country*: nascimento *m*; (*labor*) parto *m*; ***give ~ to*** *child* dar à luz a; ***date of ~*** data *f* de nascimento
'birth certificate certidão *f* de nascimento
'birth control controle *m* de natalidade
'birthday aniversário *m*, *Port* dia *m* de anos; ***happy ~!*** feliz aniversário! **'birthday party** festa *f* de aniversário **'birthday present** presente *m* de aniversário **'birthmark** marca *f* de nascença **'birthplace** local *m* de nascimento **'birthrate** taxa *f* de natalidade
biscuit ['bɪskɪt] *Am* pãozinho *m*; *Brit* bolacha *f*
bisexual ['baɪsekʃʊəl] **1** *adj* bissexual **2** *n* bissexual *m/f*
bishop ['bɪʃəp] bispo *m*
bit[1] [bɪt] *n* (*piece*) pedaço *m*; (*part*) parte *f*; COMPUT bit *m*; ***a ~*** (*a little*) um pouco; ***a ~ of*** (*a little*) um pouquinho de; ***a ~ of news / advice*** uma novidade / um conselho; ***~ by ~*** aos poucos; ***I'll be there in a ~*** estarei lá daqui a pouquinho
bit[2] [bɪt] *pret* → ***bite***
bitch [bɪtʃ] **1** *n dog* cadela *f*; *fam woman* chata *f* **2** *v/i* (*complain*) resmungar
bitchy ['bɪtʃɪ] *adj fam* maldoso
bite [baɪt] **1** *n* mordida *f*; *food*: pedaço *m*; ***I didn't get a ~*** *angler* eu não fisguei nada; ***let's have a ~ (to eat)*** vamos fazer uma boquinha **2** *v/t* ⟨*pret* ***bit***, *pp* ***bitten***⟩ morder **3** *v/i* ⟨*pret* ***bit***, *pp* ***bitten***⟩ *dog* morder; *mosquito, flea* picar; *fish* fisgar
bitten ['bɪtn] *pp* → ***bite***
bitter ['bɪtər] *adj taste, person* amargo; *argument* forte
bitterly ['bɪtərlɪ] *adv cold* cruelmente; *resent* amargamente
bizarre [bɪ'zɑːr] *adj* bizarro
blab [blæb] *v/i* ⟨*pret & pp* ***blabbed***⟩ *fam* alcagüetar
blabbermouth ['blæbərmaʊθ] *fam* dedo-duro *m*
black [blæk] **1** *adj coffee, tea, hair, dress, car* preto; *person, day* negro **2** *n color* preto *m*; *person* negro,-a *m,f*; ***in the ~*** FIN com saldo positivo; ***in ~ and white*** *fig* explicitamente
♦ **black out** *v/i* desmaiar
'blackberry amora *f* preta, *Port* amora silvestre **'blackbird** melro *m* **'blackboard** quadro-negro *m* **black 'box** caixa-preta *f* **black e'conomy** economia *f* informal
blacken ['blækn] *v/t fig person's name* difamar
black 'eye olho *m* roxo **'blackhead** pústula *f* **black 'ice** camada *f* de gelo **'blacklist 1** *n* lista *f* negra **2** *v/t* colocar na lista negra **'blackmail 1** *n* chantagem *f*; ***emotional ~*** chantagem *f* emocional **2** *v/t* chantagear **'blackmailer** chantagista *m/f* **black 'market** mercado *m* negro
blackness ['blæknɪs] negrume *m*
'blackout ELEC apagão *m*; MED perda *f* de consciência
bladder ['blædər] ANAT bexiga *f*
blade [bleɪd] *knife, sword*: lâmina *f*; *helicopter*: pá *f*; *grass*: folha *f*
blame [bleɪm] **1** *n* culpa *f* **2** *v/t* culpar; ***~ s.o. for sth*** culpar alguém de algo; ***I ~ myself for it*** eu ponho a culpa em mim mesmo por isto
bland [blænd] *adj* brando
blank [blæŋk] **1** *adj* (*not written on*) em branco; *tape* virgem; *look* vago **2** *n* (*empty space*) lacuna *f*; ***my mind's a ~*** me deu um branco
blank 'check *Am* cheque *m* assinado em branco
blank cheque *Brit* → ***blank check***
blanket ['blæŋkɪt] *n* cobertor *m*; ***a ~ of*** *fig* um tapete de
♦ **blare out** *v/i* retumbar
blaspheme [blæs'fiːm] *v/i* blasfemar
blasphemy ['blæsfəmɪ] blasfêmia *f*
blast [blæst] **1** *n* (*explosion*) explosão *f*; (*gust*) rajada *f* **2** *v/t* dinamitar; ***~!*** raios!

♦**blast off** *v/i rocket* ser lançado
'**blast furnace** alto-forno *m*
'**blast-off** lançamento *m*
blatant ['bleɪtənt] *adj* espalhafatoso
blaze [bleɪz] **1** *n (fire)* chama *f*; ***a ~ of color*** uma labareda de cores **2** *v/i fire* crepitar
♦**blaze away** *v/i with gun* metralhar
blazer ['bleɪzər] blazer *m*
bleach [bliːtʃ] **1** *n for clothes* alvejante *m* **2** *v/t hair* descolorir
bleak [bliːk] *adj countryside* deserto; *weather* gélido; *future* desolador
bleary-eyed ['blɪrɪaɪd] *adj* com olhos turvos
bleat [bliːt] *v/i sheep* balir
bled [bled] *pret & pp* → ***bleed***
bleed [bliːd] ⟨*pret & pp* ***bled***⟩ **1** *v/i* sangrar **2** *v/t fig* ***~ s.o. dry*** secar alguém financeiramente
bleeding ['bliːdɪŋ] *n* sangramento *m*
bleep [bliːp] **1** *n* bipe *m* **2** *v/i* bipar
blemish ['blemɪʃ] **1** *n* mancha *f* **2** *v/t reputation* manchar
blend [blend] **1** *n* mistura *f* **2** *v/t* misturar
♦**blend in 1** *v/i* misturar-se **2** *v/t cooking*: misturar
blender ['blendər] liquidificador *m*
bless [bles] *v/t* abençoar; ***(God) ~ you!*** Deus o abençoe!; *response to sneeze* saúde; ***be ~ed with*** ser abençoado com
blessing ['blesɪŋ] REL bênção *f*; *fig (approval)* aprovação *f*
blew [bluː] *pret* → ***blow***[2]
blind [blaɪnd] **1** *adj* cego; ***~ corner*** curva *f* cega; ***be ~ to*** *fig* ignorar **2** *npl* ***the ~*** os cegos **3** *v/t* cegar; *fig* ***this had ~ed him to the facts*** isso fez com que ele fechasse os olhos para os fatos
blind 'alley beco *m* sem saída **blind 'date** encontro *m* às cegas '**blindfold 1** *n* venda *f para olhos* **2** *v/t* vendar **3** *adv* de olhos vendados
blinding ['blaɪndɪŋ] *adj light* intenso; *headache* terrível
blindly ['blaɪndlɪ] *adv* às cegas; *fig* cegamente
'**blind spot** *road*: ponto *m* cego; *(ability that is lacking)* ponto *m* fraco
blink [blɪŋk] *v/i person, light* piscar
blinkered ['blɪŋkərd] *adj fig* estreito
blip [blɪp] *on radar screen* bipe *m*; *fig* pequeno hiato *m*
bliss [blɪs] êxtase *m*
blister ['blɪstər] **1** *n* bolha *f* **2** *v/i heel, paint* empolar
blizzard ['blɪzərd] nevasca *f*
bloated ['bloʊtɪd] *adj* inchado
blob [blɑːb] *liquid*: gota *f*
bloc [blɑːk] POL bloco *m*
block [blɑːk] **1** *n also shares*: bloco *m*; *town*: quadra *f*, *(blockage)* bloqueio *m*; ***he lives on the same ~*** ele vive na mesma quadra **2** *v/t* bloquear
♦**block in** *v/t with vehicle* bloquear
♦**block out** *v/t light* bloquear
♦**block up** *v/t sink etc* entupir
blockade [blɑː'keɪd] **1** *n* bloqueio *m* **2** *v/t* bloquear
blockage ['blɑːkɪdʒ] entupimento *m*
blockbuster ['blɑːkbʌstər] grande sucesso *m*
block 'letters *npl* letra *f* de fôrma
blog [blɑːg] *n* blog *m*
blogger ['blɑːgər] blogueiro,-a *m,f*
blond [blɑːnd] *adj* loiro
blonde [blɑːnd] *n woman* loira *f*
blood [blʌd] sangue *m*; ***in cold ~*** a sangue frio
'**blood alcohol level** teor *m* de álcool no sangue '**blood bank** banco *m* de sangue '**blood bath** banho *m* de sangue '**blood donor** doador,a *m,f* de sangue '**blood group** grupo *m* sangüíneo **bloodless** ['blʌdlɪs] *adj coup* sem derramamento de sangue
'**blood poisoning** septicemia *f* '**blood pressure** pressão *f* sangüínea '**blood relation**, '**blood relative** parente *m* consangüíneo '**blood sample** amostra *f* de sangue '**bloodshed** derramamento *m* de sangue '**bloodshot** *adj* injetado '**bloodstain** mancha *f* de sangue '**bloodstained** *adj* manchado de sangue '**bloodstream** corrente *f* sangüínea '**blood test** teste *m* de sangue '**bloodthirsty** *adj* sanguinolento '**blood transfusion** transfusão *f* de sangue '**blood vessel** vaso

m sangüíneo
bloody ['blʌdɪ] *adj hands, battle etc* sangrento; *Brit fam* maldito; **~ *hell!*** que inferno!
bloom [blu:m] **1** *n* flor *f*; ***in full ~*** em plena floração **2** *v/i also fig* florescer
blooper ['blu:pər] *Am fam* bobeira *f*
blossom ['blɑ:səm] **1** *n* flor *f* (*de árvore frutífera*) **2** *v/i* florescer; *fig* vicejar
blot [blɑ:t] **1** *n* rasura *f*; *fig* mancha *f* **2** *v/t* ⟨*pret & pp* ***blotted***⟩ *dry* secar
♦**blot out** *v/t* apagar
blotch [blɑ:ʧ] mancha *f*
blotchy ['blɑ:ʧɪ] *adj* manchado
blouse [blaʊz] blusa *f*
blow[1] [bloʊ] *n* golpe *m*
blow[2] [bloʊ] ⟨*pret* ***blew***, *pp* ***blown***⟩ **1** *v/t whistle* soprar; *smoke* bafejar; *fam* (*spend*) gastar; **~ *one's nose*** assoar o nariz **2** *v/i person* assoprar; *fuse, tire* estourar
♦**blow off** *v/t & v/i* levar
♦**blow out 1** *v/t candle* apagar **2** *v/i candle* apagar-se
♦**blow over 1** *v/t tree* derrubar **2** *v/i tree* cair; *argument* passar
♦**blow up 1** *v/t with explosives* explodir; *balloon* encher; *photograph* ampliar **2** *v/i* explodir; (*become angry*) explodir de raiva
'blow-dry *v/t* ⟨*pret & pp* ***blow-dried***⟩ secar com secador
'blowjob *vulg* chupada *f*
blown [bloʊn] *pp* → ***blow***[2]
'blow-out *tire*: pneu *m* furado; *fam* (*big meal*) banquete *m*
'blow-up *photo*: ampliação *f*
blue [blu:] **1** *adj* azul; *fam movie* obsceno **2** *n* azul *m*
'blueberry *Am* mirtilo *m* **blue 'chip** *adj* de primeira linha **blue-'collar worker** operário,-a *m,f* **'blueprint** planta *f* (arquitetônica); *fig* (*plan*) projeto *m*
blues [blu:z] *npl* MUS blues *m*; ***have the ~*** estar deprimido
'blues singer cantor,a *m,f* de blues
bluff [blʌf] **1** *n* (*deception*) blefe *m* **2** *v/i* blefar
blunder ['blʌndər] **1** *n* asneira *f* **2** *v/i* cometer uma asneira
blunt [blʌnt] *adj* cego; *person* direto
bluntly ['blʌntlɪ] *adv speak* asperamente
blur [blɜ:r] **1** *n* borrão *m* **2** *v/t* ⟨*pret & pp* ***blurred***⟩ borrar; ***~red vision*** visão *f* turva
blurb [blɜ:rb] *on book* sinopse *f*
♦**blurt out** [blɜ:rt] *v/t* falar sem pensar
blush [blʌʃ] **1** *n* rubor *m* **2** *v/i* ruborizar
blusher ['blʌʃər] *cosmetic* ruge *m*
bluster ['blʌstər] *v/i* vociferar
blustery ['blʌstərɪ] *adj* ventoso; ***~ wind*** ventania *f*
BO [bi:'oʊ] *abbr* (*of* ***body odor***) cê-cê *m*
board [bɔ:rd] **1** *n* tábua *f*; *for game* tabuleiro *m*; *for notices* quadro *m*; **~ (*of directors*)** conselho *m* de diretores; ***on ~*** *plane, train, boat*: a bordo; ***take on ~*** *comments etc* levar em consideração; (*fully realize truth of*) aceitar; ***across the ~*** geral **2** *v/t airplane etc* embarcar em **3** *v/i passengers* embarcar
♦**board up** *v/t* fechar com tábuas
♦**board with** *v/t* estar alojado em
board and 'lodging pensão *f* completa
boarder ['bɔ:rdər] pensionista *m/f*; EDUC aluno,-a *m,f* interno,-a
'board game jogo *m* de mesa
'boarding card cartão *m* de embarque **'boarding house** pensão *f* **'boarding pass** cartão *m* de embarque **'boarding school** internato *m*
'board meeting reunião *f* do conselho **'board room** sala *f* do conselho **'boardwalk** *Am* passarela *f* de madeira
boast [boʊst] **1** *n* ostentação *f* **2** *v/i* gabar-se
boat [boʊt] barco *m*; (*small, for leisure*) bote *m*; ***go by ~*** ir de barco
bob[1] [bɒ:b] *n haircut* cabelo *m* curto
bob[2] [bɒ:b] *v/i* ⟨*pret & pp* ***bobbed***⟩ *boat etc* balançar
♦**bob up** *v/i* erguer-se
bobsled → *esp. Am* ***bobsleigh***
'bobsleigh, **'bobsled** trenó *m* de corrida
bodice ['bɒ:dɪs] corpete *m*

bodily ['bɒːdɪlɪ] **1** *adj* físico **2** *adv eject* pessoalmente
body ['bɒːdɪ] corpo *m*; **~ *of water*** corpo *m* aquático
'body armor colete *m* à prova de balas **body armour** *Brit* → ***body armor*** **'body bag** saco *m* para transporte de cadáver **'bodyguard** guarda-costas *m/f* **'body language** linguagem *f* corporal **'body odor** odor *m* corporal **body odour** *Brit* → ***body odor*** **'body piercing** piercing *m* **'body shop** MOT lanternagem *f* **'body stocking** body *m* **'body suit** (*undergarment*) camiseta *f* **'bodywork** MOT carroceria *f*
boggle ['bɑːgl] *v/t* ***it ~s the mind!*** a cabeça roda!
bogus ['boʊgəs] *adj* falso
boil[1] [bɔɪl] *n swelling* furúnculo *m*
boil[2] [bɔɪl] **1** *v/t liquid* ferver; *egg, vegetables* cozinhar **2** *v/i* ferver
♦**boil down to** *v/t* resumir-se em
♦**boil over** *v/i milk etc* derramar
boiler ['bɔɪlər] caldeira *f*
boiling point ['bɔɪlɪŋ] ponto *m* de ebulição; ***reach ~*** *fig* chegar no limite
boisterous ['bɔɪstərəs] *adj* turbulento
bold [boʊld] **1** *adj* (*brave*) corajoso; *text* em negrito **2** *n print* negrito *m*; ***in ~*** em negrito
Bolivia [bə'lɪvɪə] Bolívia *f*
Bolivian [bə'lɪvɪən] **1** *adj* boliviano **2** *n* boliviano,-a *m,f*
bolster ['boʊlstər] *v/t confidence* aumentar
bolt [boʊlt] **1** *n door*: tranca *f*, *lightning*: raio *m*; ***like a ~ from the blue*** como um raio do céu **2** *adv* **~ *upright*** aprumado **3** *v/t* (*fix with bolts*) parafusar; (*close*) trancar **4** *v/i* (*run off*) fugir assustado; *prisoner* escapulir
bomb [bɑːm] **1** *n* bomba *f* **2** *v/t* MIL bombardear
bombard [bɑːm'bɑːrd] *v/t* (*attack*) bombardear; **~ *with questions*** bombardear com perguntas
'bomb attack ataque *m* de bomba
bomber ['bɑːmər] *airplane* bombardeiro *m*; *terrorist* bombardeador,a *m,f*
'bombproof *adj* à prova de bombas
'bomb scare suspeita *f* de bomba
'bombshell *fig news* surpresa *f* estarrecedora
bond [bɑːnd] **1** *n* (*tie*) laço *m*; FIN título *m* **2** *v/i glue* grudar; *two people* relacionar-se
bone [boʊn] **1** *n* osso *m* **2** *v/t meat, fish* desossar
bonfire ['bɑːnfaɪr] fogueira *f*
bonnet ['bɑːnɪt] *Brit* → ***hood***
bonus ['boʊnəs] bônus *m*
boo [buː] **1** *n* vaia *f* **2** *v/t & v/i* vaiar
boob [buːb] *n* (*fam breast*) teta *f*
booboo ['buːbuː] *n fam* bobeira *f*
book [bʊk] **1** *n* livro *m*; **~ *of matches*** caixa *f* de fósforos **2** *v/t* (*reserve*) reservar; *policeman* multar **3** *v/i* (*reserve*) reservar
'bookcase estante *f* para livros
booked up [bʊkt'ʌp] *adj* lotado; *person* com a agenda cheia
bookie ['bʊkɪ] *fam* corretor,a *m,f* de apostas
booking ['bʊkɪŋ] (*reservation*) reserva *f*
'bookkeeper técnico,-a *m,f* em contabilidade
'bookkeeping contabilidade *f*
booklet ['bʊklɪt] livreto *m*
'bookmaker corretor,a *m,f* de apostas, *Port* agenciador,a *m,f* de apostas
books [bʊks] *npl* (*accounts*) livros *mpl* contábeis; ***do the ~*** fazer a contabilidade; ***cook the ~*** falsificar os livros contábeis
'bookseller livreiro,-a *m,f* **'bookshelf** prateleira *f* de livros **bookshop** *Brit* → ***bookstore*** **'bookstall** banca *f* de livros **'bookstore** livraria *f* **'book token** vale-livro *m*
boom[1] [buːm] **1** *n* alta *f*, ***the postwar baby ~*** a explosão demográfica do pós-guerra **2** *v/i business* crescer
boom[2] [buːm] *n noise* bum *m*
boonies ['buːnɪz] *npl Am fam* fim *m* do mundo; ***out in the ~*** no mato
boor [bʊr] matuto,-a *m,f*
boorish ['bʊrɪʃ] *adj* rude
boost [buːst] **1** *n to sales, confidence* impulso *m*; *to economy* estímulo *m*

2 *v/t production, sales, morale* aumentar

boot [buːt] *n* bota *f*; *Brit car*: porta-malas *m*

♦**boot out** *v/t fam* expulsar

♦**boot up** COMPUT **1** *v/t* inicializar **2** *v/i* inicializar-se

booth [buːð] *at market, fair* estande *m*; *restaurant*: espaço *m* reservado

booze [buːz] *n fam* pinga *f*

border ['bɔːrdər] **1** *n between countries* fronteira *f*; *(edge)* borda *f* **2** *v/t country, river* limitar-se com

♦**border on** *v/i country* fazer fronteira com; *(be almost)* beirar a

'borderline *adj* limítrofe; ***a ~ case*** um caso dúbio

bore[1] [bɔːr] *v/t hole* perfurar

bore[2] [bɔːr] *n person* chato,-a *m,f*; ***it's such a ~*** é uma chatice

bore[3] [bɔːr] *pret* → ***bear***[2]

bored [bɔːrd] *adj* entediado; ***I'm ~*** estou entediado

boredom ['bɔːrdəm] tédio *m*

boring ['bɔːrɪŋ] *adj* chato

born [bɔːrn] *adj* ***be ~*** nascer; ***where were you ~?*** onde você nasceu?; ***she's a ~ teacher*** ela é uma professora nata

borne [bɔːrn] *pp* → ***bear***[2]

borrow ['bɑːroʊ] *v/t* pedir emprestado

bosom ['bʊzm] seio *m*

boss [bɑːs] chefe *m/f*

♦**boss about** *v/t* mandar em

bossy ['bɑːsɪ] *adj* mandão (mandona)

botanic → ***botanical***

botanical [bə'tænɪkl] *adj* botânico

botanic 'gardens, botanical 'gardens *npl* jardim *m* botânico

botanist ['bɑːtənɪst] botânico,-a *m,f*

botany ['bɑːtənɪ] botânica *f*

botch [bɑːtʃ] *v/t* fazer mal

both [boʊθ] **1** *adj & pron* ambos; ***I know ~ (of the) brothers*** conheço ambos os irmãos; ***~ (of the) brothers were there*** ambos os irmãos estavam lá; ***~ of them*** *(things, people)* ambos **2** *adv* ***he's ~ handsome and intelligent*** ele é tão bonito quanto inteligente; ***~ … and …*** tanto … como …

bother ['bɑːðər] **1** *n* incômodo *m*; ***it's no ~*** não é incômodo algum **2** *v/t (disturb, worry)* perturbar **3** *v/i* preocupar-se; ***don't ~!*** *(you needn't do it)* não se preocupe!; ***you needn't have ~ed*** não precisava ter se preocupado

bottle ['bɑːtl] **1** *n* garrafa *f*; *for baby* mamadeira *f*, *Port* biberão *m* **2** *v/t* engarrafar

♦**bottle up** *v/t feelings* reprimir

'bottle bank banco *m* de reciclagem de garrafas

bottled water ['bɑːtld] água *f* engarrafada

'bottleneck engarrafamento *m*; *production*: gargalo *m*

'bottle-opener abridor *m* de garrafas, *Port* abre-garrafas *m*

bottom ['bɑːtəm] **1** *adj* inferior **2** *n on the inside* fundo *m*; *hill*: sopé *m*; *page*: rodapé *m*; *pile*: embaixo; *(underside)* parte *f* de baixo; *street*: fim *m*; *garden*: fundo *m*; *(buttocks)* traseiro *m*; ***at the ~ of the screen*** na parte inferior da tela

♦**bottom out** *v/i* chegar ao fundo do poço

bottom 'line *fig (financial outcome)* resultado *m* final; *(the real issue)* questão *f* (principal)

bought [bɒːt] *pret & pp* → ***buy***

boulder ['boʊldər] pedregulho *m*

bounce [baʊns] **1** *v/t ball* quicar **2** *v/i ball* quicar; *on sofa etc* pular; *rain* bater; *check* voltar

bouncer ['baʊnsər] leão-de-chácara *m*

bouncy ['baʊnsɪ] *adj ball* saltante; *cushion, chair* macio

bound[1] [baʊnd] *adj* ***be ~ to do sth*** *(sure to)* estar a ponto de fazer algo; *(obliged to)* estar obrigado a fazer algo

bound[2] [baʊnd] *adj* ***to be ~ for*** *ship* com destino a

bound[3] [baʊnd] **1** *n (jump)* pulo *m* **2** *v/i* saltitar

bound[4] [baʊnd] *pret & pp* → ***bind***

boundary ['baʊndərɪ] limite *m*

boundless ['baʊndlɪs] *adj* ilimitado

bouquet [bʊ'keɪ] *flowers, wine*: buquê *m*

bourbon ['bɜːrbən] bourbon *m*

bout [baʊt] MED ataque *m*; *boxing*: luta *f*
boutique [buː'tiːk] b(o)utique *f*
bow[1] [baʊ] **1** *n as greeting* saudação *f* **2** *v/i* fazer uma mesura **3** *v/t head* abaixar
bow[2] [boʊ] *knot* laço *m*; MUS arco *m*
bow[3] [baʊ] *ship*: proa *f*
bowels ['baʊəlz] *npl* intestino *m*
bowl[1] [boʊl] *n container* bacia *f*; *rice, salad, soup*: tigela *f*
bowl[2] [boʊl] *n ball* bola *f* de boliche
◆ **bowl over** *v/t fig (astonish)* ficar perplexo; *romantically* impressionar
bowling ['boʊlɪŋ] boliche *m*; ***go ~*** jogar boliche
'bowling alley pista *f* de boliche
bowls → ***bowling***
bow tie [boʊ'taɪ] gravata-borboleta *f*
box[1] [bɑːks] *n* caixa *f*; *on form* quadrado *m*
box[2] [bɑːks] *v/i* boxear
boxer ['bɑːksər] boxeador,a *m,f*
'boxer shorts *npl* calção *m*
boxing ['bɑːksɪŋ] boxe *m*
'Boxing Day *Brit 26 de dezembro* **'boxing glove** luva *f* de boxe **'boxing match** luta *f* de boxe **'boxing ring** ringue *m*
'box number *post office*: caixa *f* postal
'box office bilheteria *f*, *Port* bilheteira *f*
boy [bɔɪ] rapaz *m*; *younger* garoto *m*, menino *m*; *(son)* garoto *m*
boycott ['bɔɪkɑːt] **1** *n* boicote *m* **2** *v/t* boicotar
'boyfriend namorado *m*
boyish ['bɔɪɪʃ] *adj* infantil
'boyscout escoteiro *m*
bra [brɑː] *Brit* sutiã *f*, *Port* soutien *m*
brace [breɪs] *on teeth* aparelho *m* ortodôntico
bracelet ['breɪslɪt] bracelete *m*
braces *Brit* → ***suspenders***
bracket ['brækɪt] *for shelf* mão-francesa *f*; *Brit in text* parêntese *m*; ***square ~*** colchete *m*
brag [bræg] *v/i* ⟨*pret & pp* ***bragged***⟩ gabar-se
braid [breɪd] *n hair*: trança *f*; *(trimming)* debrum *m*
braille [breɪl] braile *m*
brain [breɪn] cérebro *m*; ***use your ~*** use a cabeça
'brain dead *adj* MED cerebralmente morto
brainless ['breɪnlɪs] *adj fam* desmiolado
brains [breɪnz] *npl (intelligence)* inteligência *f*; ***she was the ~ of the operation*** ela era a cabeça da operação
'brainstorm *Am* idéia *f* brilhante **brainstorming** ['breɪnstɔːrmɪŋ] brainstorming *m* **'brain surgeon** neurocirurgião *m*, neurocirurgiã *f* **'brain surgery** neurocirurgia *f* **'brain tumor** tumor *m* cerebral **brain tumour** *Brit* → ***brain tumor*** **'brainwash** *v/t* fazer uma lavagem cerebral em **'brainwave** *(brilliant idea)* idéia *f* brilhante
brainy ['breɪnɪ] *adj fam* esperto
brake [breɪk] **1** *n* freio *m*, *Port* travão *m* **2** *v/i* frear, *Port* travar
'brake fluid MOT fluido *m* de freio, *Port* fluido *m* de travão **'brake light** MOT luz *f* de freio, *Port* luz *f* de travão **'brake pedal** MOT pedal *m* do freio, *Port* pedal *m* de travão*t*
branch [bræntʃ] *n tree*: galho *m*; *bank*: agência *f*
◆ **branch off** *v/i road* desviar
◆ **branch out** *v/i* diversificar-se
brand [brænd] **1** *n* marca *f* **2** *v/t* ***be ~ed a liar*** ser taxado de mentiroso
brand 'image imagem *f* da marca
brandish ['brændɪʃ] *v/t* brandir
brand 'leader marca *f* líder
brand 'loyalty lealdade *f* à marca
'brand name marca *f* registrada
brand-'new *adj* novíssimo
brandy ['brændɪ] conhaque *m*
brass [bræs] latão *m*; ***the ~*** MUS os instrumentos de sopro
brass 'band orquestra *f* de metais
brassière [brə'ziːr] sutiã *f*, *Port* soutien *m*
brat [bræt] *pej* pirralho,-a *m,f*
bravado [brə'vɑːdoʊ] bravata *f*
brave [breɪv] *adj* bravo
bravely ['breɪvlɪ] *adv* bravamente
bravery ['breɪvərɪ] bravura *f*
brawl [brɒːl] **1** *n* briga *f* **2** *v/i* brigar
brawny ['brɒːnɪ] *adj* forte

B

Brazil [brə'zɪl] Brasil *m*
Brazilian [brə'zɪlıən] **1** *adj* brasileiro **2** *n* brasileiro,-a *m,f*
Bra'zil nut castanha-do-pará *f*
breach [bri:tʃ] *n (violation)* quebra *f*; *party*: ruptura *f*
breach of 'contract LAW quebra *f* de contrato
bread [bred] *n* pão *m*
'breadcrumbs *npl* migalhas *fpl* de pão
'bread knife faca *f* de pão
breadth [bredθ] largura *f*
'breadwinner ganha-pão *m*
break [breɪk] **1** *n bone etc*: fratura *f*; *(rest)* descanso *m*; *relationship*: separação *f*; ***give s.o. a ~*** *fam (opportunity)* dar uma chance a alguém; ***take a ~!*** faça uma pausa!; ***without a ~*** *work, travel* sem escala **2** *v/t* ⟨*pret* **broke**, *pp* **broken**⟩ quebrar, *Port* partir; *news* dar; *record* bater **3** *v/i* ⟨*pret* **broke**, *pp* **broken**⟩ quebrar-se, *Port* partir-se; *news* dar; *storm* cair; *boy's voice* mudar
◆**break away** *v/i (escape)* fugir; *from family, tradition* desligar-se
◆**break down 1** *v/i vehicle, machine* enguiçar; *talks, marriage* fracassar; *in tears* desfazer-se **2** *v/t door* derrubar; *figures* discriminar
◆**break even** *v/i* COM manter-se
◆**break in** *v/i (interrupt)* interromper; *burglar* arrombar
◆**break off 1** *v/t* quebrar; *relationship* desmanchar; ***they've broken it off*** eles desmancharam o noivado **2** *v/i (stop talking)* interromper-se
◆**break out** *v/i (start up)* irromper; *prisoners* fugir; ***he broke out in a rash*** ele desenvolveu um exantema
◆**break up 1** *v/t (into component parts)* dividir em partes; *fight* parar **2** *v/i ice* partir-se; *couple, band* separar-se; *meeting* encerrar; ***you're breaking up*** *cell phone*: não consigo lhe ouvir
breakable ['breɪkəbl] *adj* quebrável
breakage ['breɪkɪdʒ] quebra *f*
'breakdown *vehicle, machine*: enguiço *m*; *talks*: fracasso *m*; *figures*: enumeração *f*; ***nervous ~*** colapso *m* nervoso
breakdown truck *Brit* → ***wrecker***
break-'even point ponto *m* de equilíbrio
breakfast ['brekfəst] *n* café *m* da manhã, *Port* pequeno almoço *m*; *first meal of day* desjejum *m*; ***have ~*** tomar café da manhã
'breakfast television programas *m* de TV matutinos
'break-in arrombamento *m*
'breakthrough *science, technology*: avanço *m*
'breakup *marriage, partnership*: dissolução *f*; *band*: separação *f*
breast [brest] peito *m*; *fml* mama *f*
'breastfeed *v/t* ⟨*pret & pp* **breastfed**⟩ amamentar
'breaststroke nado *m* de peito
breath [breθ] fôlego *m*; ***be out of ~*** ficar sem fôlego; ***take a deep ~*** respirar fundo
Breathalyzer®, breath analyzer ['breθəlaɪzər] *Am* bafômetro *m*
breathe [bri:ð] **1** *v/i* respirar **2** *v/t (inhale)* inalar; *(exhale)* exalar
◆**breathe in** *v/t & v/i* inspirar
◆**breathe out** *v/i* expirar
breathing ['bri:ðɪŋ] *n* respiração *f*
breathless ['breθlɪs] *adj* sem fôlego
breathlessness ['breθlɪsnɪs] falta *f* de fôlego
breathtaking ['breθteɪkɪŋ] *adj (exciting)* excitante; *view* de tirar o fôlego
bred [bred] *pret & pp* → ***breed***
breed [bri:d] **1** *n* raça *f* **2** *v/t* ⟨*pret & pp* **bred**⟩ criar; *fig* alimentar **3** *v/i* ⟨*pret & pp* **bred**⟩ *animals* criar
breeder ['bri:dər] criador,a *m,f*
breeding ['bri:dɪŋ] criação *f*; ***have ~*** *person* ter berço
'breeding ground *fig* meio *m* propício
breeze [bri:z] brisa *f*
breezily ['bri:zɪlɪ] *adv fig* jovialmente
breezy ['bri:zɪ] *adj* com brisa; *fig* jovial
brew [bru:] **1** *v/t beer* fermentar; *tea* fazer **2** *v/i storm, trouble* formar-se
brewer ['bru:ər] cervejeiro,-a *m,f*
brewery ['brʊərɪ] cervejaria *f*
bribe [braɪb] **1** *n* propina *f*, suborno *m* **2** *v/t* subornar
bribery ['braɪbərɪ] corrupção *f*
brick [brɪk] tijolo *m*

'bricklayer pedreiro *m*
bridal suite ['braɪdl] suíte *f* nupcial
bride [braɪd] noiva *f*
'bridegroom noivo *m*
'bridesmaid dama *f* de honra
bridge[1] [brɪdʒ] **1** *n* ponte *f*; *nose*: dorso *m*; *ship*: ponte *f* de comando **2** *v/t gap* fazer uma ponte entre
bridge[2] [brɪdʒ] *n card game* bridge *m*
brief[1] [bri:f] *adj* breve
brief[2] [bri:f] **1** *n* (*mission*) instruções *fpl* **2** *v/t* **~ s.o. on sth** dar instruções a alguém sobre algo
'briefcase maleta *f*
briefing ['bri:fɪŋ] reunião *f* de instruções
briefly ['bri:flɪ] *adv* (*for a short period of time*) brevemente; (*in a few words*) resumidamente; (*to sum up*) em resumo
briefs [bri:fs] *npl for women* calcinha *f*, *Port* cuecas *fpl*; *for men* cueca *f*, *Port* cuecas *fpl*
bright [braɪt] *adj* brilhante; (*sunny*) ensolarado; (*intelligent*) brilhante
◆**brighten up** ['braɪtn] **1** *v/t* alegrar **2** *v/i weather* clarear
brightly ['braɪtlɪ] *adv* alegremente; ***a ~ lit room*** uma sala intensamente iluminada
brightness ['braɪtnɪs] *weather*: claridade *f*; *smile*: brilho *m*; (*intelligence*) inteligência *f*
brilliance ['brɪljəns] *person*, *color*, *sun*: brilho *m*
brilliant ['brɪljənt] *adj also* (*very good*, *intelligent*) brilhante
brim [brɪm] *container*: borda *f*; *hat*: aba *f*
brimful ['brɪmfʊl] *adj* cheio
bring [brɪŋ] *v/t* ⟨*pret & pp* ***brought***⟩ trazer; ***~ it here, will you*** traga aqui, por favor; ***can I ~ a friend?*** posso trazer um amigo?
◆**bring about** *v/t* forjar
◆**bring around** *v/t from a faint* fazer voltar a si; (*persuade*) persuadir
◆**bring back** *v/t* (*return*) devolver; (*reintroduce*) reintroduzir; *memories* trazer de volta
◆**bring down** *v/t fence*, *tree*, *government* derrubar; *bird*, *airplane* abater; *inflation*, *price* diminuir
◆**bring in** *v/t interest*, *income* trazer; *legislation* apresentar; *verdict* declarar; (*involve*) envolver
◆**bring on** *v/t illness* provocar
◆**bring out** *v/t book* lançar; *video*, *CD*, *new product* produzir
◆**bring to** *v/t from a faint* fazer voltar a si
◆**bring up** *v/t child* educar; *subject* trazer à baila; *fam* (*vomit*) botar para fora
brink [brɪŋk] beira *f*; *fig* ***on the ~ of disaster*** à beira de um desastre
brisk [brɪsk] *adj person*, *walk*, *trade* animado
bristles ['brɪslz] *npl chin*: barba *f* curta; *brush*: cerdas *fpl*
bristling ['brɪslɪŋ] *adj* ***be ~ with*** estar cheio de
Brit [brɪt] *fam* britânico,-a *m*,*f*
Britain ['brɪtn] Grã-Bretanha *f*
British ['brɪtɪʃ] **1** *adj* britânico **2** *npl* ***the ~*** os britânicos
Briton ['brɪtn] britânico,-a *m*,*f*
brittle ['brɪtl] *adj* quebradiço
broach [broʊtʃ] *v/t subject* abordar
broad [brɒ:d] **1** *adj* largo; (*general*) geral; ***in ~ daylight*** em plena luz do dia **2** *n fam* (*woman*) mulher *f* qualquer
'broadband banda *f* larga
'broadcast **1** *n* transmissão *f* **2** *v/t* ⟨*pret & pp* ***broadcast***⟩ transmitir
'broadcaster transmissor *m*
'broadcasting radiodifusão *f*
broaden ['brɒ:dn] **1** *v/i* alargar-se **2** *v/t* alargar
'broadjump *Am* salto *m* em distância
broadly ['brɒ:dlɪ] *adv* ***~ speaking*** falando em termos gerais
broadminded [brɒ:d'maɪndɪd] *adj* mente aberta
broadmindedness [brɒ:d'maɪndɪdnɪs] liberalidade *f*
broccoli ['brɑ:kəlɪ] brócolis *mpl*, *Port* brócolos *mpl*
brochure ['broʊʃər] brochura *f*
broil [brɔɪl] *v/t Am* grelhar
broiler ['brɔɪlər] *on stove Am* grelha *f*; (*chicken*) *Am* frango *m*
broke[1] [broʊk] *adj fam temporarily* quebrado; *long term* arruinado; ***go***

B

~ falir
broke[2] [brouk] *pret* → ***break***
broken[1] ['broukn] *adj glass, window, neck, arm* quebrado; *home, marriage* desfeito; *English* imperfeito
broken[2] ['broukn] *pp* → ***break***
broken-hearted [broukn'hɑːrtɪd] *adj* de coração partido
broker ['broukər] corretor,a *m,f*
bronchitis [brɑːŋ'kaɪtɪs] bronquite *f*
bronze [brɑːnz] *n* bronze *m*
brooch [broutʃ] broche *m*
brood [bruːd] *v/i person* ruminar
broom [bruːm] vassoura *f*
broth [brɑːθ] *(soup)* sopa *f*; *(stock)* caldo *m*
brothel ['brɑːθl] prostíbulo *m*
brother ['brʌðər] irmão *m*
'brother-in-law ⟨*pl* ***brothers-in-law***⟩ cunhado *m*
brotherly ['brʌðərlɪ] *adj* fraternal
brought [brɒːt] *pret & pp* ***bring***
brow [brau] *(forehead)* testa *f*; *hill*: cumeada *f*
brown [braun] **1** *n* marrom *m* **2** *adj eyes, hair* castanho; *(tanned)* bronzeado **3** *v/t & v/i cooking*: dourar
'brownbag *v/t* ⟨*pret & pp* ***brownbagged***⟩ ***~ it*** *Am fam* trazer marmita; *with drink* embrulhar bebida alcoólica em papel
Brownie ['braunɪ] fadinha *f*
brownie ['braunɪ] *(cake)* brownie *m*
'Brownie points *npl fam* pontos *mpl* positivos; ***earn ~ ~*** ganhar pontos
'brown-nose *v/t pej Am* puxar o saco de **brown 'paper** papel *m* pardo **brown paper 'bag** saco *m* de papel **'brown sugar** açúcar *m* mascavo
browse [brauz] *v/i in store* passear pela loja; ***~ through a book*** folhear um livro; ***~ on the Web*** navegar na internet
browser ['brauzər] COMPUT navegador *m*, browser *m*
bruise [bruːz] **1** *n* contusão *f* **2** *v/t fruit, also (emotionally)* machucar **3** *v/i person, fruit* machucar-se
bruising ['bruːzɪŋ] *adj fig* doloroso
brunch [brʌntʃ] brunch *m*
brunette [bruː'net] *n* morena *f*
brunt [brʌnt] ***bear the ~ of …*** suportar a fúria de …
brush [brʌʃ] **1** *n* escova *f*; *(conflict)* escaramuça *f* **2** *v/t* escovar; *(touch lightly)* roçar; *(move away)* remover
♦**brush against** *v/t* esbarrar
♦**brush aside** *v/t* não levar em conta
♦**brush off** *v/t* espanar; *criticism* não reagir a; *fam* dar o contra
♦**brush up** *v/t* recapitular
'brushoff *get the ~* levar pau da testa
'brushwork traço *m* do pintor
brusque [brusk] *adj* brusco
Brussels ['brʌslz] Bruxelas
Brussels sprout [brʌsl'spraut] couve-de-bruxelas *f*
brutal ['bruːtl] *adj* brutal
brutality [bruː'tælətɪ] brutalidade *f*
brutally ['bruːtəlɪ] *adv* brutalmente; ***be ~ frank*** ser brutalmente franco
brute [bruːt] bruto,-a *m,f*
'brute force força *f* bruta
BSc [biːes'siː] *abbr* (*of* ***Bachelor of Science***) Bacharelado *m* (*em Ciências*); *person* Bacharel *m/f* em Ciências
bubble ['bʌbl] *n* bolha *f*, *Port* borbulha *f*
'bubble bath banho *m* de espuma **'bubble gum** goma *f* de mascar, *fam* chiclete *m*, *Port* pastilha *f* elástica **'bubble wrap** *n* plástico *m* bolha
bubbly ['bʌblɪ] *n fam (champagne)* champanha *m*
buck[1] [bʌk] *n fam (dollar)* dólar *m*
buck[2] [bʌk] *v/i horse* dar pinotes
buck[3] [bʌk] *n* ***pass the ~*** passar a bola
bucket ['bʌkɪt] *n* balde *m*
buckle[1] ['bʌkl] **1** *n* fivela *f* **2** *v/t belt* apertar
buckle[2] ['bʌkl] *v/i wood, metal* vergar-se
♦**buckle down** *v/i* começar a trabalhar
bud [bʌd] *n* BOT botão *m*
buddy ['bʌdɪ] *fam* camarada *m/f*; *form of address* amigo,-a *m,f*
budge [bʌdʒ] **1** *v/t* mexer; *(make reconsider)* fazer mudar de idéia **2** *v/i* mexer-se; *(change one's mind)* mudar de idéia
budgerigar ['bʌdʒərɪgɑːr] periquito *m*

budget ['bʌdʒɪt] **1** *n* orçamento *m*; ***be on a ~*** estar preso a um orçamento **2** *v/i* fazer orçamento
◆**budget for** *v/t* incluir no orçamento
budgie ['bʌdʒɪ] *fam* periquito *m*
buff[1] [bʌf] *adj* (*color*) pardo
buff[2] [bʌf] *n* grande admirador,a *m,f*; ***movie / jazz ~*** amante *m/f* de cinema / jazz
buffalo ['bʌfəloʊ] búfalo *m*
buffer ['bʌfər] RAIL pára-choque *m*; COMPUT buffer *m*; *fig* anteparo *m*
buffet[1] ['bʊfeɪ] *n* (*meal*) bufê *m*
buffet[2] ['bʌfɪt] *v/t wind* golpear
bug [bʌg] **1** *n insect* inseto *m*; (*virus*) micróbio *m*; (*spying device*) escuta *f*; COMPUT bug *m* **2** *v/t* ⟨*pret & pp* ***bugged***⟩ *room* colocar escuta em; *telephone* grampear; *fam* (*annoy*) incomodar
buggy ['bʌgɪ] *for baby* carrinho *m* de bebê
build [bɪld] **1** *n person*: estatura *f* **2** *v/t* ⟨*pret & pp* ***built***⟩ construir
◆**build up 1** *v/t strength* fortalecer; *relationship* construir; *collection* fazer **2** *v/i* acumular
builder ['bɪldər] construtor,a *m,f*
building ['bɪldɪŋ] edifício *m*; (*activity*) construção *f*
'**building blocks** *npl for child* jogo *m* de montar '**building site** terreno *m* '**building trade** indústria *f* da construção
'**build-up** (*accumulation*) aumento *m*; *publicity*: publicidade *f*
built [bɪlt] *pret & pp* → ***build***
'**built-in** *adj* embutido
built-up 'area área *f* urbana
bulb [bʌlb] BOT bulbo *m*; (*lightbulb*) lâmpada *f*
bulge [bʌldʒ] **1** *n* protuberância *f*; *wall*: abaulamento *m* **2** *v/i pocket* avolumar-se
bulimia [bʊ'lɪmɪə] bulimia *f*
bulk [bʌlk] maioria *f*; ***in ~*** a granel
bulky ['bʌlkɪ] *adj* volumoso
bull [bʊl] touro *m*
bulldoze ['bʊldoʊz] *v/t* (*demolish*) demolir; ***~ s.o. into doing sth*** *fig* coagir alguém a fazer algo
bulldozer ['bʊldoʊzər] escavadeira *f*
bullet ['bʊlɪt] bala *f*
bulletin ['bʊlɪtɪn] boletim *m*
'**bulletin board** *Am* quadro *m* de avisos; COMPUT BBS *f*
'**bullet-proof** *adj* à prova de bala
'**bull fight** tourada *f* '**bull fighter** toureiro *m* '**bull market** FIN mercado *m* em alta
bullock ['bʊlək] boi *m*
'**bull's-eye** centro *m* do alvo; ***hit the ~*** acertar na mosca
'**bullshit 1** *n vulg* besteira *f* **2** *v/i* ⟨*pret & pp* ***bullshitted***⟩ *vulg* falar besteira
bully ['bʊlɪ] **1** *n* brigão *m*, brigona *f*; (*child*) valentão *m*, valentona *f* **2** *v/t* ⟨*pret & pp* ***bullied***⟩ intimidar
bullying ['bʊlɪɪŋ] *n* assédio *m*
bum [bʌm] **1** *n Am fam* vagabundo,-a *m,f*; (*worthless person*) *Am* imprestável *m*; *Brit* (*backside*) bumbum *m* **2** *adj* (*useless*) *Am* inútil **3** *v/t* ⟨*pret & pp* ***bummed***⟩ *cigarette etc* filar
◆**bum around**, **bum about** *v/i fam* (*travel*) viajar sem rumo certo; (*be lazy*) ficar por aí
'**bumbag** *fam* pochete *f*
bumblebee ['bʌmblbi:] abelhão *m*
bump [bʌmp] **1** *n* (*swelling*) caroço *m*; *on road* saliência *f*; *to slow traffic* quebra-molas *m*; ***get a ~ on the head*** ficar com um galo na cabeça **2** *v/t* levar um baque
◆**bump into** *v/t table* colidir com; (*meet*) encontrar por acaso
◆**bump off** *v/t fam* (*murder*) matar
◆**bump up** *v/t fam* (*prices*) aumentar
bumper ['bʌmpər] **1** *n* MOT pára-choque *m*; ***the traffic was ~ to ~*** o tráfego estava pesado **2** *adj* (*extremely good*) farto
'**bump-start** *v/t car* empurrar; *fig* (*economy*) reanimar
bumpy ['bʌmpɪ] *adj road* esburacado; *flight* turbulento
bun [bʌn] *hairstyle*: coque *m*; *for eating* pão *m* doce, *Port* pãozinho *m*
bunch [bʌntʃ] *people*: punhado *m*; ***a ~ of flowers*** um ramalhete de flores; ***a ~ of keys*** um molho de chaves; ***a ~ of grapes*** um cacho de uvas; ***thanks a ~*** *ironic Am* muito obrigado; ***I still have a ~ of things to do*** eu ainda

tenho um monte de coisas para fazer

bundle ['bʌndl] *clothes*: trouxa *f*; *wood*: feixe *m*

♦**bundle up** *v/t clothes* entrouxar; (*dress warmly*) agasalhar

bung [bʌŋ] *v/t fam* jogar

bungee jumping ['bʌndʒɪdʒʌmpɪŋ] bundgee jump *m*

bungle ['bʌŋgl] *v/t* fazer mal-feito; ***a ~d attempt*** uma tentativa frustrada

bunk [bʌŋk] beliche *m*

'**bunk beds** *npl* beliches *mpl*

buoy [bɔɪ] *n* NAUT bóia *f*

buoyant ['bɔɪənt] *adj* animado

burden ['bɜːrdn] **1** *n* carga *f* **2** *v/t* ***~ s.o. with sth*** *fig* incomodar alguém com algo

bureau ['bjʊroʊ] (*chest of drawers*) *Am* cômoda *f*; (*office*) agência *f*

bureaucracy [bjʊ'rɑːkrəsɪ] burocracia *f*

bureaucrat ['bjʊrəkræt] burocrata *m/f*

bureaucratic [bjʊrə'krætɪk] *adj* burocrático

burger ['bɜːrgər] hambúrguer *m*

burglar ['bɜːrglər] arrombador,a *m,f*

'**burglar alarm** alarme *m* contra roubo

burglarize ['bɜːrgləraɪz] *v/t Am* arrombar

burglary ['bɜːrglərɪ] arrombamento *m*

burgle *Brit* → ***burglarize***

burial ['berɪəl] enterro *m*

burly ['bɜːrlɪ] *adj* robusto

burn [bɜːrn] **1** *n* queimadura *f* **2** *v/t* ⟨*pret & pp* ***burnt***⟩ *sun, house* queimar; *toast, meat* tostar; (*consume*) consumir **3** *v/i* ⟨*pret & pp* ***burnt***⟩ *sun* queimar; *toast* tostar; (*get sunburnt*) queimar-se; (*be on fire*) pegar fogo

♦**burn down 1** *v/t* incendiar **2** *v/i* queimar

♦**burn out** *v/t* ***burn oneself out*** esgotar-se (de trabalhar); ***a burned-out car*** um carro incinerado

'**burnout** *fam* (*exhaustion*) síndrome *f* de burnout

burnt [bɜːrnt] *pret & pp* ***burn***

burp [bɜːrp] **1** *n* arroto *m* **2** *v/i* arrotar **3** *v/t baby* fazer arrotar

burst [bɜːrst] **1** *n water pipe*: rompimento *m*; *gunfire*: rajada *f*; ***in a ~ of energy*** num rompente de energia **2** *adj tire* furado **3** *v/t* ⟨*pret & pp* ***burst***⟩ *balloon* estourar **4** *v/i* ⟨*pret & pp* ***burst***⟩ *balloon, tire* estourar; ***~ into a room*** irromper num quarto; ***~ into tears*** cair no choro; ***~ out laughing*** cair na gargalhada

bury ['berɪ] *v/t* ⟨*pret & pp* ***buried***⟩ *dead* enterrar; (*conceal*) esconder; ***be buried under*** (*covered by*) ser enterrado sob; ***~ oneself in work*** entregar-se inteiramente ao trabalho

bus [bʌs] **1** *n* ônibus *m*, *Port* autocarro *m* **2** *v/t* ⟨*pret & pp* ***bussed***⟩ ***they had to be ~sed to school*** eles tiverem que ir de ônibus para a escola

'**busboy** *Am* ajudante *m/f* de garçom

'**bus driver** motorista *m/f* de ônibus, *Port* motorista *m/f* de autocarro

bush [bʊʃ] *plant* arbusto *m*; *land* mato *m*

bushed [bʊʃt] *adj fam* (*tired*) exausto

bushy ['bʊʃɪ] *adj beard* cerrado

business ['bɪznɪs] (*trade, company*) negócio *m*; (*work*) trabalho *m*; (*sector*) setor *m*; (*affair, matter*) assunto *m*; (*as subject of study*) administração *f* de empresas; ***on ~*** a negócios; ***that's none of your ~!, mind your own ~!*** isto não é da sua conta

'**business card** cartão *m* de visita '**business class** classe *f* executiva '**business hours** *npl* horário *m* comercial '**businesslike** *adj* profissional '**business lunch** almoço *m* de negócios '**businessman** homem *m* de negócios '**business meeting** reunião *f* de negócios '**business school** escola *f* de administração '**business studies** *nsg* (*course*) curso *m* de administração '**business trip** viagem *f* de negócios '**businesswoman** mulher *f* de negócios

'**bus lane** pista *f* para ônibus '**bus shelter** ponto *m* de ônibus coberto '**bus station** estação *f* rodoviária '**bus stop** parada *f* de ônibus, *Port* paragem *f* de autocarro

bust[1] [bʌst] *n woman*: busto *m*

bust[2] [bʌst] **1** *adj fam* (*broken*) falido; ***go ~*** ir à falência **2** *v/t fam* fracassar
'bus ticket passagem *f* de ônibus
♦ bustle about ['bʌsl] *v/i* estar atarefado
'bust-up *fam* discussão *f*
busty ['bʌstɪ] *adj* peitudo
busy ['bɪzɪ] **1** *adj street etc* movimentado; (*full of people*) cheio; TEL ocupado, *Port* impedido; ***be ~ doing sth*** estar ocupado fazendo algo **2** *v/t* ⟨*pret & pp* ***busied***⟩ ***~ oneself with*** ocupar-se com
'busybody pessoa *f* metida
'busy signal *Am* sinal *m* de ocupado, *Port* sinal de impedido
but [bʌt] **1** *conj* mas; ***it's not me ~ my father you want*** não é a mim, mas ao meu pai que você quer; ***~ then*** (***again***) mas mesmo assim; ***~ that's not fair!*** mas isto não é justo! **2** *prep* ***all ~ him*** todos, exceto ele; ***the last ~ one*** o penúltimo; ***the next ~ one*** o antepenúltimo; ***~ for you*** se não fosse você; ***nothing ~ the best*** somente o melhor
butcher ['bʊtʃər] *n* açougueiro *m*, *Port* homem *m* do talho (*murderer*) assassino,-a *m,f*
butt [bʌt] **1** *n cigarette*: ponta *f*; *joke*: alvo *m*; *fam* (*buttocks*) *Am* bumbum *m* **2** *v/t* dar cabeçada; *goat*, *bull* marrar
♦ butt in *v/i* interromper
butter ['bʌtər] **1** *n* manteiga *f* **2** *v/t* passar manteiga em
♦ butter up *v/t fam* bajular
'buttercup botão-de-ouro *m*
'butterfly *insect*, *swimming*: borboleta *f*
buttocks ['bʌtəks] *npl* nádegas *fpl*
button ['bʌtn] **1** *n* botão *m*; (*badge*) broche *m* de lapela **2** *v/t* abotoar
♦ button up abotoar
'buttonhole *n* casa *f* de (botão)
buttress ['bʌtrɪs] esteio *m*
buxom ['bʌksəm] *adj* com curvas
buy [baɪ] **1** *n* compra *f* **2** *v/t* ⟨*pret & pp* ***bought***⟩ comprar; ***can I ~ you a drink?*** posso pagar-lhe uma bebida?; ***$5 doesn't ~ much*** com $5 não dá para comprar muito
♦ buy off *v/t* (*bribe*) comprar
♦ buy out *v/t* COM comprar a parte de
♦ buy up *v/t* comprar
buyer ['baɪr] comprador,a *m,f*
buzz [bʌz] **1** *n* zumbido *m*; *fam* ***get a ~ out of sth*** comprazer-se com algo **2** *v/i insect* zumbir; *with buzzer* tocar a campainha **3** *v/t with buzzer* chamar tocando a campainha
♦ buzz off *v/i fam* sumir
buzzard ['bʌzərd] urubu *m*
buzzer ['bʌzər] campainha *f* (*com som de cigarra*)
by [baɪ] **1** *prep agency*: por; (*near*, *next to*) perto de; (*no later than*) até; (*past*) por; *mode of transport*: de; ***side ~ side*** lado a lado; ***~ day / night*** durante o dia / a noite; ***~ bus / train*** de ônibus / trem; ***~ the hour / ton*** por hora / tonelada; ***~ my watch*** de acordo com meu relógio; ***a play ~ ...*** uma peça escrita por ...; ***~ oneself*** sozinho,-a; ***~ a couple of minutes*** por alguns minutos; ***2 ~ 4*** *measurement* por 4; ***~ this time tomorrow*** a esta hora amanhã **2** *adv* ***~ and ~*** (*soon*) logo
bye-bye ['baɪbaɪ] *int* tchau, *Port* adeus
bygone ['baɪgɑːn] coisa *f* do passado; ***you should let ~s be ~s*** o que passou, passou
'bypass 1 *n road* vía *f* circular; MED ponte *f* de safena **2** *v/t* evitar
'by-product subproduto *m*
bystander ['baɪstændər] espectador,a *m,f*
byte [baɪt] byte *m*
'byword ***be a ~ for*** ser sinônimo de

C

C

cab [kæb] (*taxi*) táxi *m*; *truck*: boléia *f*
cabaret ['kæbəreɪ] cabaré *m*
cabbage ['kæbɪdʒ] repolho *m*, couve *f*
'cab driver motorista *m/f* de táxi
cabin ['kæbɪn] *airplane*: cabine *f*, *ship*: camarote *m*
'cabin attendant comissário,-a *m,f* de bordo
'cabin crew tripulação *f* de cabine
cabinet ['kæbɪnɪt] armário *m*; POL gabinete *m*
'cabinet maker marceneiro,-a *m,f*
cable ['keɪbl] cabo *m*; **~ (*TV*)** TV *f* a cabo
'cable car teleférico *m*; *streetcar* bonde *m*
'cable television televisão *f* a cabo
'cab stand ponto *m* de táxi
cactus ['kæktəs] cacto *m*
cadaver [kə'dævər] cadáver *m*
caddie ['kædɪ] *n golf*: carregador,a *m,f* de tacos
cadet [kə'det] cadete *m*
cadge [kædʒ] *v/t* ***~ sth from s.o.*** filar algo de alguém
Caesarean *Brit* → ***Cesarean***
café ['kæfeɪ] café *m*
cafeteria [kæfɪ'tɪrɪə] lanchonete *f*
caffeine ['kæfiːn] cafeína *m*
cage [keɪdʒ] *bird*: gaiola *f*, *lion*: jaula *f*
cagey ['keɪdʒɪ] *adj* esquivo
cahoots [kə'huːts] *npl fam* ***be in ~ with*** *fam* agir em parceria com
cajole [kə'dʒoʊl] *v/t* ***~ s.o. into doing sth*** agradar alguém para conseguir algo
cake [keɪk] *n* bolo *m*; ***be a piece of ~*** *fam* ser uma moleza
calamity [kə'læmətɪ] calamidade *f*
calcium ['kælsɪəm] cálcio *m*
calculate ['kælkjʊleɪt] *v/t* calcular
calculating ['kælkjʊleɪtɪŋ] *adj* calculista
calculation [kælkjʊ'leɪʃn] cálculo *m*
calculator ['kælkjʊleɪtər] calculadora *f*
calendar ['kælɪndər] calendário *m*
calf[1] [kæf] ⟨*pl calves*⟩ bezerro *m*
calf[2] [kæf] ⟨*pl calves*⟩ *leg*: panturrilha *f*
'calfskin *n* pelica *f*
caliber ['kælɪbər] *Am gun*: calibre *m*; ***a man of his ~*** um homem de seu calibre
calibre *Brit* → ***caliber***
call [kɒːl] **1** *n* (*phonecall*) chamada *f* telefônica; (*shout*) grito *m*; (*demand*) exigência *f*, ***there's a ~ for you*** há uma chamada telefônica para você **2** *v/t* (*summon*) chamar; (*describe as*) chamar de; *on phone* telefonar; ***what have they ~ed the baby?*** que nome deram ao bebê?; ***but we ~ him Tom*** mas nós o chamamos de Tom; ***~ s.o. names*** insultar alguém **3** *v/i* (*shout*) gritar; (*visit*) visitar; *on phone* telefonar
♦**call at** *v/t* (*stop at*) parar em
♦**call back 1** *v/t on phone* ligar de volta; (*summon*) chamar de volta **2** *v/i on phone* ligar de volta; (*make another visit*) voltar
♦**call for** *v/t* (*collect*) apanhar; (*demand*) exigir; (*require*) requerer
♦**call in 1** *v/t* (*summon*) mandar chamar **2** *v/i on phone* telefonar; ***she called in sick*** telefonou para avisar que está doente
♦**call off** *v/t* (*cancel*) cancelar
♦**call on** *v/t* (*urge*) apelar; (*visit*) visitar
♦**call out** *v/t* (*shout*) gritar; (*summon*) convocar
♦**call up** *v/t* (*on phone*) dar uma ligada; COMPUT abrir
call box *Brit* → ***phone booth***
'call center call center *m*
'call centre → ***call center***
caller ['kɒːlər] *on phone* pessoa *f* que ligou; (*visitor*) visitante *m/f*
'call girl garota *f* de programa
callous ['kæləs] *adj* insensível

callously ['kæləslɪ] *adv* duramente
callousness ['kæləsnɪs] insensibilidade *f*
calm [kɑːm] **1** *adj* calmo **2** *n of countryside, person* calma *f*
◆ **calm down 1** *v/t* acalmar **2** *v/i sea, weather, person* acalmar-se
calmly ['kɑːmlɪ] *adv* calmamente
calorie ['kælərɪ] caloria *f*
camcorder ['kæmkɔːrdər] filmadora *f* portátil
came [keɪm] *pret* → ***come***
camera ['kæmərə] câmera *f*
'cameraman operador *m* de câmara
camisole ['kæmɪsoʊl] corpete *m*
camouflage ['kæməflɑːʒ] **1** *n* camuflagem *f* **2** *v/t* camuflar
camp [kæmp] **1** *n* acampamento *m* **2** *v/i* acampar
campaign [kæm'peɪn] **1** *n* campanha *f* **2** *v/i* fazer campanha
campaigner [kæm'peɪnər] ativista *m/f*
camper ['kæmpər] *person* campista *m/f*; *vehicle* caminhonete *f*, *fam* perua *f*
camping ['kæmpɪŋ] camping *m*, *Port* campismo *m*
'campsite área *f* de acampamento
campus ['kæmpəs] campus *m*
can[1] [kæn, *unstressed* kən] *v/aux* ⟨*pret* ***could***⟩ ◊ poder; ***~ you hear me?*** você está me ouvindo?; ***I ~ 't*** *ou* ***cannot see*** não posso enxergar; ***~ he call me back?*** ele pode me ligar de volta?; ***as fast / well as you ~*** o mais rápido / melhor que puder; ***~ I help you?*** posso ajudá-lo?; ***~ you help me?*** você pode me ajudar?; ***~ I have a coffee?*** eu queria um café; pode me dar um café; ***that ~'t be right*** isto não pode estar certo; ***the car ~ reach speeds of …*** o carro pode atingir uma velocidade de … ◊ *ability* saber; ***~ you speak French?*** você sabe falar francês?; ***~ you swim?*** você sabe nadar?
can[2] [kæn] **1** *n* lata *f* **2** *v/t* ⟨*pret & pp* ***canned***⟩ enlatar
Canada ['kænədə] Canadá *m*
Canadian [kə'neɪdɪən] **1** *adj* canadense **2** *n* canadense *m/f*
canal [kə'næl] canal *m*
canary [kə'nerɪ] canário *m*
cancel ['kænsl] *v/t* ⟨*pret & pp* ***-ed***, *Brit* ***-led***⟩ cancelar
cancel'lation fee taxa *f* de cancelamento
cancer ['kænsər] câncer *m*, *Port* cancro *m*
Cancer ['kænsər] ASTROL Câncer *m*
cancerous ['kænsərəs] *adj* canceroso
c and f *abbr* (*of* ***cost and freight***) custo e frete *m*
candid ['kændɪd] *adj* franco
candidacy ['kændɪdəsɪ] candidatura *f*
candidate ['kændɪdət] candidato,-a *m,f*
candidly ['kændɪdlɪ] *adv* francamente
candied ['kændiːd] *adj* cristalizado
candle ['kændl] vela *f*
'candlestick castiçal *m*
candor ['kændər] *Am* lisura *f*
candour *Brit* → ***candor***
candy ['kændɪ] *Am* doce *m*
candyfloss *Brit* → ***cotton candy***
cane [keɪn] taquara *f*; *walking*: bengala *f*
canister ['kænɪstər] galão *m* de metal
cannabis ['kænəbɪs] maconha *f*
canned [kænd] *adj fruit* enlatado; (*recorded*) gravado
cannibalize ['kænɪbəlaɪz] *v/t* canibalizar
cannot ['kænɑːt] → ***can***[1]
canny ['kænɪ] *adj* (*astute*) sagaz
canoe [kə'nuː] canoa *f*
'can opener abridor *m* de latas, *Port* abre-latas *m*
can't [kænt] → ***can***[1]
cantankerous [kæn'tæŋkərəs] *adj* intratável
canteen [kæn'tiːn] *factory etc*: cantina *f*
canvas ['kænvəs] *for painting* tela *f*; (*material*) lona *f*
canvass ['kænvəs] **1** *v/t* (*seek opinion of*) escrutinar **2** *v/i* POL fazer campanha
canyon ['kænjən] desfiladeiro *m*
cap [kæp] (*hat*) boné *m*; *bottle, jar, pen*: tampa *f*; *lens*: capa *f*
capability [keɪpə'bɪlətɪ] capacidade *f*; MIL poder *m*
capable ['keɪpəbl] *adj* (*efficient*) efici-

ente; ***be ~ of*** ser capaz de
capacity [kə'pæsətɪ] capacidade *f*; ***in my ~ as …*** na minha função de …
Cape Verde [keɪp'vɜːrdɪ] Cabo-Verde *m*
capital ['kæpɪtl] *n of country* capital *f*; (*money*) capital *m*; (*capital letter*) maiúscula *f*
capital ex'penditure investimento *m* em capital **capital 'gains tax** imposto *m* sobre ganhos de capital **capital 'growth** crescimento *m* de capital
capitalism ['kæpɪtəlɪzm] capitalismo *m*
'capitalist ['kæpɪtəlɪst] **1** *adj* capitalista **2** *n* capitalista *m/f*
♦ **capitalize on** ['kæpɪtəlaɪz] capitalizar em
capital 'letter letra *f* maiúscula
capital 'punishment pena *f* capital
capitulate [kə'pɪtʊleɪt] *v/i* capitular
capitulation [kæpɪtʊ'leɪʃn] capitulação *f*
Capricorn ['kæprɪkɔːrn] ASTROL Capricórnio *m*
capsize [kæp'saɪz] *v/t & v/i* emborcar
capsule ['kæpsʊl] *medicine, spaceship*: cápsula *f*
captain ['kæptɪn] *n ship, aircraft*: comandante *m*; *team*: capitão *m*, capitã *f*
caption ['kæpʃn] *n* título *m*
captivate ['kæptɪveɪt] *v/t* cativar
'captive ['kæptɪv] *adj* cativo; ***hold s.o. ~*** manter alguém em cativeiro
captive 'market mercado *m* cativo
captivity [kæp'tɪvətɪ] cativeiro *m*
capture ['kæptʃər] **1** *n* captura *f* **2** *v/t person, animal, city* capturar; *market share* conquistar; (*portray*) captar
car [kɑːr] carro *m*; *train*: vagão *m*; ***by ~*** de carro
carafe [kə'ræf] jarra *f*
carat ['kærət] quilate *m*
caravan *Brit* → ***trailer***
carbohydrate [kɑːrboʊ'haɪdreɪt] carboidrato *m*
'car bomb carro-bomba *m*
'carbon footprint rastros *mpl* de carbono
carbon monoxide [kɑːrbənmən'ɑːksaɪd] monóxido *m* de carbono
carbureter, **carburetor** [kɑːrbʊ'retər] carburador *m*
carburetor *Brit* → ***carbureter***
carcass ['kɑːrkəs] carcaça *f*
carcinogen ['kɑːrsɪnədʒen] carcinógeno *m*
carcinogenic [kɑːrsɪnə'dʒenɪk] *adj* cancerígeno
card [kɑːrd] (*to mark special occasion*) cartão *m*; (***post***) ~ cartão *m* postal; (***business***) ~ cartão *m* de visita; ***playing ~*** carta *f*
'cardboard papelão *m*
cardboard 'box caixa *f* de papelão
cardiac ['kɑːrdɪæk] *adj* cardíaco
cardiac ar'rest enfarte *m*
cardigan ['kɑːrdɪgən] cardigã *m*
cardinal ['kɑːrdɪnl] *n* REL cardeal *m*
'card index fichário *m* **'card key** chave *f* de cartão **'card phone** telefone *m* de cartão
care [ker] **1** *n of baby, elderly, sick* cuidado *m*; (***medical***) ~ assistência *f* médica; ***without a ~ in the world*** sem nenhuma preocupação; ***~ of*** aos cuidados de **2** *v/i* (*worry*) preocupar-se; ***take ~*** (*be cautious*) tomar cuidado; ***take ~*** (***of yourself***)***!*** (*goodbye*) cuide-se; ***take ~ of*** *baby, dog* tomar conta de; *tool, house, garden* cuidar; (*deal with*) encarregar-se; (***handle***) ***with ~!*** *on label* cuidado frágil; ***I don't ~!*** não me importa!; ***I could***(***n't***) ***~ less*** não dou a mínima importância
♦ **care about** *v/t* preocupar-se com
♦ **care for** *v/t* (*look after*) cuidar de; (*be fond of*) gostar de; ***would you care for …?*** você gostaria de …?
career [kə'rɪr] carreira *f*
ca'reers officer orientador,a *m,f* vocacional
'carefree *adj* despreocupado
careful ['kerfʊl] *adj* (*cautious*) cauteloso; (*thorough*) cuidadoso; (***be***) ***~!*** tome cuidado!
carefully ['kerfʊlɪ] *adv* (*with caution*), *worded etc* cuidadosamente
careless ['kerlɪs] *adj* descuidado
carelessly ['kerlɪslɪ] *adv* descuidadamente
carer ['kerər] acompanhante *m/f*

caress [kə'res] **1** *n* carícia *f* **2** *v/t* acariciar
caretaker ['kerteɪkər] caseiro,-a *m,f*
'careworn *adj* aflito
'car ferry balsa *f*
cargo ['kɑːrgoʊ] carga *f*
'car hire *Brit* aluguel *m* de carro, *Port* aluguer *m* de carros
Caribbean [kə'rɪbɪən] **1** *adj* caraíba **2** *n* ***the ~*** o Caribe
caricature ['kærɪkətʊər] *n* caricatura *f*
caring ['kerɪŋ] *adj* bondoso
'car mechanic mecânico *m* de automóveis
carnage ['kɑːrnɪdʒ] carnificina *f*
carnation [kɑːr'neɪʃn] BOT cravo *m*
carnival ['kɑːrnɪvl] festa *f* anual
carol ['kærəl] *n* cântico *m*
carousel [kærə'sel] *airport*: esteira *f*; *for slide projector, also* (*merry-go-round*) carrossel *m*
car park *Brit* → ***parking lot***
carpenter ['kɑːrpɪntər] carpinteiro,-a *m,f*
carpet ['kɑːrpɪt] carpete *m*; (*rug*) tapete *m*
'car phone telefone *m* de carro **'carpool 1** *n* revezamento *m* de carro **2** *v/i* fazer revezamento de carro **'car port** abrigo *m* **car 'radio** rádio *m* de carro **'car rental** aluguel *m* de carro, *Port* aluguer *m* de carros **'car rental company** locadora *f*
carrier ['kærɪər] (*company*) transportadora *f*; *of disease* portador,a *m,f*
carrot ['kærət] cenoura *f*
carry ['kærɪ] ⟨*pret & pp* ***carried***⟩ **1** *v/t in hand, from a place to another* levar; (*have on one's person*) andar com; *pregnant woman*: *baby* esperar; *disease* portar; *ship, plane, bus etc* transportar; *charge, load* carregar; *proposal* aprovar; ***get carried away*** deixar-se levar **2** *v/i sound* propagar
◆ **carry on 1** *v/i* (*continue*) continuar; (*make a fuss*) fazer alvoroço; (*have an affair*) ter um romance **2** *v/t* (*conduct*) manter
◆ **carry out** *v/t survey etc* conduzir; *orders etc* cumprir
cart [kɑːrt] carrinho *m*
cartel [kɑːr'tel] cartel *m*
carton ['kɑːrtn] *storage, transport*: caixa *f* de papelão; *milk, eggs etc*: caixa *f*; *cigarettes*: maço *m*
cartoon [kɑːr'tuːn] cartum *m*; *TV, movie*: desenho *m* animado
cartoonist [kɑːr'tuːnɪst] cartunista *m/f*
cartridge ['kɑːrtrɪdʒ] *gun*: cartucho *m*
carve [kɑːrv] *v/t meat* trinchar; *wood* entalhar
carving ['kɑːrvɪŋ] (*figure*) escultura *f*
'car wash lavagem *f* de carro
case[1] [keɪs] *n of Scotch, wine* caixa *f*; (*container*) estojo *m*; *Brit* (*suitcase*) mala *f*
case[2] [keɪs] *n for police, mystery, instance etc* caso *m*; (*argument*) argumento *m*; LAW causa *f*; ***in any ~*** em todo caso; ***in that ~*** neste caso
'case history MED histórico *m* (do paciente); *social work*: antecedentes *mpl*
'caseload volume *m* de pacientes
cash [kæʃ] **1** *n* dinheiro *m*; ***~ down*** pagamento à vista; ***pay*** (***in***) ***~*** pagar em dinheiro; ***~ in advance*** dinheiro adiantado; ***~ on delivery*** pagamento contra-entrega **2** *v/t check* descontar
◆ **cash in on** *v/t* fazer dinheiro com
'cash cow empresa *f* mais rentável **'cash desk** caixa *f* **cash 'discount** desconto *m* à vista **'cash dispenser** caixa *m* eletrônico **'cash flow** fluxo *m* de caixa
cashier [kæ'ʃɪr] *n in store etc* caixa *m/f*
'cash machine caixa *m* automático
cashmere ['kæʃmɪr] *n* casimira *f*
'cashpoint *Brit* caixa *m* automático
'cash register caixa *f* registradora
casino [kə'siːnoʊ] cassino *m*
casket ['kæskɪt] *Am* (*coffin*) esquife *m*
casserole ['kæsəroʊl] caçarola *f*
cassette [kə'set] cassete *m*
cas'sette player toca-fitas *m*
cas'sette recorder gravador *m*
cast [kæst] **1** *n of play* elenco *m*; (*mold*) fôrma *f* **2** *v/t* ⟨*pret & pp* ***cast***⟩ *doubt, suspicion* lançar; *metal* fundir; *play* escolher o elenco de; *actor* dar o papel a
◆ **cast off** *v/i ship* jogar para fora
caste [kæst] casta *f*

caster ['kæstər] *on chair etc* rodízio *m*
cast 'iron ferro *m* fundido
cast-'iron *adj* de ferro fundido; ***a ~ alibi*** um álibi irrefutável
castle ['kæsl] castelo *m*
castor *Brit* → ***caster***
castrate [kæ'streɪt] *v/t* castrar
castration [kæ'streɪʃn] castração *f*
casual ['kæʒʊəl] *adj* (*chance*) casual; (*offhand*) descuidado; (*not formal*) informal; (*not permanent*) temporário; ***~ sex*** sexo *m* casual
casually ['kæʒʊəlɪ] *adv dressed* informalmente; *say* casualmente
'casual wear roupa *f* informal
cat [kæt] gato *m*
catalog ['kætəlɑːg] *n Am* catálogo *m*
catalogue *Brit* → ***catalog***
catalyst ['kætəlɪst] *fig* catalisador,a *m,f*
catalytic con'verter [kætə'lɪtɪk] conversor *m* catalítico
catapult ['kætəpʌlt] **1** *v/t fig to fame, stardom* catapultar **2** *n Brit* catapulta *f*
cataract ['kætərækt] MED catarata *f*
catastrophe [kə'tæstrəfɪ] catástrofe *f*
catastrophic [kætə'strɑːfɪk] *adj* catastrófico
catch [kætʃ] **1** *n* pegada *f*; *fish*: pescaria *f*; (*locking device*) tranca *f*; (*problem*) problema *m* **2** *v/t* ⟨*pret & pp* ***caught***⟩ (*get on*) *bus, train* pegar, *Port* apanhar; (*not miss*) *bus, train* tomar; *fish* pescar; (*in order to speak to*) encontrar; (*hear*) compreender; *illness* pegar, *Port* apanhar; ***~ (a) cold*** pegar um resfriado; ***~ s.o.'s eye*** chamar a atenção de alguém; ***~ sight of, ~ a glimpse of*** ver de relance; ***~ s.o. doing sth*** apanhar alguém fazendo algo; ***it's a ~-22 situation*** é um beco sem saída
♦ **catch on** *v/i* (*become popular*) tornar-se popular; (*understand*) entender, *Port* perceber
♦ **catch up on** *v/t* pôr em dia
catcher ['kætʃər] *baseball*: apanhador,a *m,f*
catching ['kætʃɪŋ] *adj disease* contagioso
'catch-up ***I'm still playing ~*** ainda estou pondo as coisas em dia
catchy ['kætʃɪ] *adj tune* contagiante
categoric [kætə'gɑːrɪk] *adj* categórico
categorically [kætə'gɑːrɪklɪ] *adv* categoricamente
category ['kætəgɔːrɪ] categoria *f*
♦ **cater for** ['keɪtər] *v/t* (*meet the needs of*) atender a; (*provide food for*) fornecer refeições a
caterer ['keɪtərər] serviço *m* de bufê
caterpillar ['kætərpɪlər] lagarta *f*
cathedral [kə'θiːdrl] catedral *f*
Catholic ['kæθəlɪk] **1** *adj* católico **2** *n* católico,-a *m,f*
Catholicism [kə'θɑːlɪsɪzm] catolicismo *m*
'catnap 1 *n* soneca *f* **2** *v/i* ⟨*pret & pp* ***catnapped***⟩ tirar uma soneca
'CAT scan tomografia *f* axial computorizada
'cat's eyes *npl road*: olho-de-gato *m*
catsup ['kætsʌp] *Am* ketchup *m*
cattle ['kætl] gado *m*
catty ['kætɪ] *adj* ferino
'catwalk *in theater, factory etc* passadiço *m*; *Brit at fashion show* passarela *f*
caught [kɒːt] *pret & pp* → ***catch***
cauliflower ['kɒːlɪflaʊər] couve-flor *f*
cause [kɒːz] **1** *n* (*reason, objective*) causa *f*; (*grounds*) motivo *m* **2** *v/t* causar
caustic ['kɒːstɪk] *adj fig* cáustico
caution ['kɒːʃn] **1** *n* (*carefulness*) cautela *f*; ***~ is advised*** aconselha-se cautela **2** *v/t* (*warn*) advertir
cautious ['kɒːʃəs] *adj* cauteloso
cautiously ['kɒːʃəslɪ] *adv* cautelosamente
cave [keɪv] caverna *f*
♦ **cave in** *v/i roof* desabar
caviar ['kævɪɑːr] caviar *m*
cavity ['kævətɪ] cavidade *f*
cc 1 *abbr* (*of* ***cubic centimeters***) centímetro *m* cúbico **2** *v/t* enviar uma cópia a
CD [siː'diː] *abbr* (*of* ***compact disc***) CD *m*
C'D player CD player *m* **CD-ROM** [siːdiː'rɑːm] CD-ROM *m* **CD-'ROM drive** drive *m* de CD-ROM
cease [siːs] *v/t & v/i* cessar; ***~ doing sth*** parar de fazer algo

'cease-fire cessar-fogo *m*
ceiling ['si:lɪŋ] teto *m*, *Port* tecto *m*
celeb ['seleb] *fam* celebridade *f*
celebrate ['selɪbreɪt] **1** *v/i* celebrar **2** *v/t* festejar; (*observe*) celebrar
celebrated ['selɪbreɪtɪd] *adj* célebre; ***be ~ for*** ser celebrado por
celebration [selɪ'breɪʃn] celebração *f*
celebrity [sɪ'lebrətɪ] celebridade *f*; **~ *magazines*** revistas cor-de rosa
celery ['selərɪ] aipo *m*
celibacy ['selɪbəsɪ] celibato *m*
celibate ['selɪbət] *adj* celibatário
cell [sel] *for prisoner* cela *f*; BIOL célula *f*; *phone* celular *m*
cellar ['selər] porão *m*; *wine*: adega *f*
cellist ['tʃelɪst] violoncelista *m/f*
cello ['tʃeloʊ] violoncelo *m*
cellophane ['seləfeɪn] celofane *m*
'cell phone telefone *m* celular
cellulite ['selju:laɪt] celulite *f*
cement [sɪ'ment] **1** *n* cimento *m* **2** *v/t also friendship* cimentar
cemetery ['semətərɪ] cemitério *m*
censor ['sensər] *v/t* censurar
censorship ['sensəʃɪp] censura *f*
census ['sensəs] censo *m*
cent [sent] cento *m*
centenary [sen'ti:nərɪ] centenário *m*
center ['sentər] **1** *n Am* centro *m*; ***in the ~ of*** no centro de; ***~ of gravity*** centro de gravidade **2** *v/t* centrar
♦ **center on** *v/t Am* centralizar em
centigrade ['sentɪgreɪd] centígrado; ***10 degrees ~*** 10 graus centígrados
centimeter ['sentɪmi:tər] *Am* centímetro *m*
centimetre *Brit* → ***centimeter***
central ['sentrəl] *adj* central; (*main*) principal; ***be ~ to sth*** ser o centro de algo
Central A'merica América *f* Central
Central A'merican **1** *adj* centro-americano **2** *n* centro-americano,-a *m,f*
central 'heating aquecimento *m* central
centralize ['sentrəlaɪz] *v/t* centralizar
central 'locking MOT travamento *m* central
central 'processing unit unidade *f* central de processamento
centre *Brit* → ***center***
century ['sentʃərɪ] século *m*
CEO [si:i:'oʊ] *abbr* (*of* ***Chief Executive Officer***) diretor-presidente *m*
ceramic [sɪ'ræmɪk] *adj* cerâmico
ceramics [sɪ'ræmɪks] *nsg* cerâmica *f*; *npl objects* cerâmica *f*
cereal ['sɪrɪəl] (*grain*) cereal *m*; (***breakfast***) **~** cereal *m* em flocos
ceremonial [serɪ'moʊnɪəl] **1** *adj* cerimonial **2** *n* cerimonial *m*
ceremony ['serɪmənɪ] cerimônia *f*
certain ['sɜ:rtn] *adj* (*sure*, *particular*) certo; ***it's ~ that …*** é certo que …; ***a ~ Mr S.*** um certo Sr. S.; ***make ~*** certifique-se; ***know / say for ~*** saber / dizer ao certo
certainly ['sɜ:rtnlɪ] *adv* certamente; (*of course*) claro; ***~ not!*** (é) claro que não
certainty ['sɜ:rtntɪ] certeza *f*; ***it's / he's a ~*** isto / ele é uma certeza
certificate [sər'tɪfɪkət] (*qualification*) certificado *m*; (*official paper*) certidão *f*
certified public accountant ['sərtɪfaɪd] *Am* perito-contador *m*, *Port* contabilista *m/f*
certify ['sɜ:rtɪfaɪ] *v/t* ⟨*pret & pp* ***certified***⟩ certificar
Cesarean [sɪ'zerɪən] *n Am* cesariana *f*
cessation [se'seɪʃn] cessação *f*
c/f *abbr* (*of* ***cost and freight***) custo e frete *m*
CFC [si:ef'si:] *abbr* (*of* ***chlorofluorocarbon***) clorofluorcarboneto *m*
chain [tʃeɪn] **1** *n* corrente *f*; *stores*, *hotels*: cadeia *f* **2** *v/t* ***~ sth / s.o. to sth*** acorrentar algo / alguém a algo
chain re'action reação *f* em cadeia
'chain smoke *v/i* fumar um cigarro atrás do outro **'chain smoker** fumante compulsivo,-a *m,f* **'chain store** cadeia *f* de lojas
chair [tʃer] **1** *n also professorship* cadeira *f*; *at university* cátedra *f*; *at meeting* presidente *m*; (*armchair*) poltrona *f*; ***the*** (***electric***) **~** a cadeira elétrica; ***go to the ~*** ir para a cadeira elétrica; ***take the ~*** presidir **2** *v/t meeting* presidir
'chair lift teleférico *m*

C

'chairman presidente *m*
chairmanship ['ʧermənʃɪp] presidência *f*
'chairperson presidente *m/f*
'chairwoman presidenta *f*
chalet [ʃæ'leɪ] chalé *m*
chalice ['ʧælɪs] REL cálice *m*
chalk [ʧɒːk] *for writing* giz *m*; *in soil* calcário *m*
challenge ['ʧælɪndʒ] **1** *n* (*difficulty*), *in race* desafio *m* **2** *v/t* (*defy*) *to race, debate* desafiar; (*call into question*) questionar
challenger ['ʧælɪndʒər] desafiante *m/f*
challenging ['ʧælɪndʒɪŋ] *adj job, undertaking* desafiador
'chambermaid ['ʧeɪmbərmeɪd] arrumadeira *f* **'chamber music** música *f* de câmara **Chamber of 'Commerce** Câmara *f* de Comércio
chamois, **chamois leather** ['ʃæmɪ] camurça *f*
champagne [ʃæm'peɪn] champanha *m*
champion ['ʧæmpɪən] **1** *n* SPORT campeão *m*, campeã *f*; *of cause* defensor,a *m,f* **2** *v/t* (*cause*) defender
championship ['ʧæmpɪənʃɪp] (*event*) campeonato *m*; (*title*) título *m* de campeão
chance [ʧæns] (*possibility*) chance *f*; (*opportunity*) oportunidade *f*; (*risk*) risco *m*; (*luck*) sorte *f*; ***by ~*** por acaso; ***take a ~*** correr o risco; ***I'm not taking any ~s*** não vou correr nenhum risco
Chancellor ['ʧænsələr] *Brit* **~** (***of the Exchequer***) Ministro,-a *m,f* da Fazenda
chandelier [ʃændə'lɪr] candelabro *m*
change [ʧeɪndʒ] **1** *n* mudança *f*; (*small coins*) trocado *m*; *from purchase* troco *m*; ***for a ~*** para variar; ***a ~ of clothes*** uma muda de roupa **2** *v/t* (*alter*) mudar; *dollar bill* trocar; (*replace*) substituir; *trains, planes* trocar de; *one's clothes* mudar de **3** *v/i* mudar; (*put on different clothes*) trocar-se; (*take different train / bus*) fazer baldeação, *Port* mudar
changeable ['ʧeɪndʒəbl] *adj* instável
'changeover mudança *f*; *in relay race* passe *m* do bastão
changing room ['ʧeɪndʒɪŋ] SPORT vestiário *m*; *in shop* provador *m*
channel ['ʧænl] *on TV*, (*waterway*) canal *m*; *on radio* estação *f*
chant [ʧænt] **1** *n* coro *m* **2** *v/i* cantar
chaos ['keɪɑːs] caos *m*
chaotic [keɪ'ɑːtɪk] *adj* caótico
chap [ʧæp] *n Brit fam* cara *m*, *Port* tipo *m*
chapel ['ʧæpl] capela *f*
chapped [ʧæpt] *adj* rachado
chapter ['ʧæptər] capítulo *m*; *organization*: seção *f*
character ['kærɪktər] (*nature*) caráter *m*; (*person*) figura *f*; *in book, play* personagem *m/f*; (*personality*) personalidade *f*; *in writing* caractere *m*; ***he's a real ~*** ele é uma verdadeira figura
characteristic [kærɪktə'rɪstɪk] **1** *n* característica *f* **2** *adj* característico
characteristically [kærɪktə'rɪstɪklɪ] *adv* caracteristicamente
characterize ['kærɪktəraɪz] *v/t* caracterizar
charade [ʃə'rɑːd] *fig* charada *f*
charbroiled ['ʧɑːrbrɔɪld] *adj* assado na brasa
charcoal ['ʧɑːrkoʊl] carvão *m*; *drawing*: lápis *m* de carvão
charge [ʧɑːrdʒ] **1** *n* (*fee*) taxa *f*; LAW queixa *f*; ***free of ~*** de graça; ***will that be cash or ~?*** será à vista ou crédito?; ***be in ~*** ser encarregado; ***take ~*** tomar lugar **2** *v/t sum of money* cobrar; (*put on account*) debitar; *credit card* debitar em; LAW acusar; *battery* carregar **3** *v/i* (*attack*) atacar
'charge account conta *f*
'charge card cartão *m* de crédito emitido por uma loja
charisma [kə'rɪzmə] carisma *m*
charismatic [kærɪz'mætɪk] *adj* carismático
charitable ['ʧærɪtəbl] *adj institution* beneficente; *person* caridoso
charity ['ʧærətɪ] (*assistance*) caridade *f*; (*organization*) instituição *f* de caridade
charlatan ['ʃɑːrlətən] charlatão *m*, charlatã *f*

C

charm [tʃɑːrm] **1** *n* charme *m*; *on bracelet etc* pingente *m* **2** *v/t* (*delight*) encantar
charming ['tʃɑːrmɪŋ] *adj* encantador
charred [tʃɑːrd] *adj* carbonizado
chart [tʃɑːrt] (*diagram*) diagrama *m*; *sailing*: carta *f* de navegação; *airplane*: mapa *m*; MUS ***the ~s*** la parada
charter ['tʃɑːrtər] *v/t* fretar
'charter flight vôo *m* fretado
chase [tʃeɪs] **1** *n* perseguição *f* **2** *v/t* perseguir
♦ **chase away** *v/t* enxotar
chaser ['tʃeɪsər] ***a beer with a whiskey ~*** *uma cerveja com um copo de whiskey depois*
chassis ['ʃæsɪ] *of car* chassi *m*
chat [tʃæt] **1** *n* conversa *f*; *on line* bate-papo *m* online **2** *v/i* 〈*pret & pp* ***chatted***〉 conversar
'chatline linha de chat **'chat room** sala *f* de bate-papo **'chat show** programa *m* de entrevista **'chat show host** entrevistador,a *m,f*
chatter ['tʃætər] **1** *n* tagarelice *f* **2** *v/i* (*talk*) conversar; *teeth* bater
'chatterbox tagarela *m/f*
chatty ['tʃætɪ] *adj person* conversador; *letter* informal
chauffeur ['ʃoʊfər] *n* chofer *m*
'chauffeur-driven *adj* com chofer
chauvinist ['ʃoʊvɪnɪst] *n*, *also* ***male ~*** machista *m*
chauvinistic [ʃoʊvɪ'nɪstɪk] *adj* chauvinista; *male chauvinism*: machista
cheap [tʃiːp] *adj* barato; (*nasty*) desprezível; (*mean*) avarento
cheat [tʃiːt] **1** *n person* trapaceiro,-a *m,f* **2** *v/t* trapacear; ***~ s.o. out of sth*** enganar alguém em algo **3** *v/i exam*: colar, *Port* cabular; *cards etc*: trapacear; ***~ on one's wife*** trair sua mulher
check[1] [tʃek] **1** *adj shirt* xadrez **2** *n* xadrez *m*
check[2] [tʃek] *n* FIN cheque *m*; *in restaurant etc* conta *f*; ***the ~ please*** a conta, por favor
check[3] [tʃek] **1** *n* (*to verify sth*) inspeção *f*; ***keep in ~, hold in ~*** manter sob controle; ***keep a ~ on*** faça um controle de **2** *v/t* (*verify*) checar; *machinery* inspecionar; (*restrain*) refrear; (*stop*) conter; *with a checkmark* ticar; *coat, package etc* entregar **3** *v/i* verificar; ***~ for*** procurar por
♦ **check in** *v/i at airport* apresentar-se; *at hotel* registrar-se, *Port* registar-se
♦ **check off** *v/t on list* conferir
♦ **check on** *v/t* dar uma olhada em
♦ **check out 1** *v/i of hotel* pagar a conta e sair **2** *v/t* (*look into*) verificar; *club, restaurant etc* provar
♦ **check up on** *v/t* investigar; ***he's always checking up on me*** ele está sempre me controlando
♦ **check with** *v/t person* perguntar a; (*tally*: *information*) conferir com
'checkbook talão *m* de cheque, *Port* livro *m* de cheques
checked [tʃekt] *adj shirt* xadrez
checkerboard ['tʃekərbɔːrd] *Am* tabuleiro *m* de damas
checkered ['tʃekərd] *adj Am pattern* xadrez; *career* diversificado
checkers ['tʃekərz] *nsg Am* jogo *m* de damas
check-in balcão *m* da recepção
checking account ['tʃekɪŋ] conta *f* corrente
'check-in time hora *f* de entrada
'checklist lista *f* (de verificação)
'check mark *Am* tique *m* **'checkmate** *n* xeque-mate *m* **'check-out** caixa *m* **'check-out time** *hotel*: hora *f* de saída **'checkpoint** *military, police* posto *m* de controle; *in race etc* ponto *m* de controle **'checkroom** *Am for coats* guarda-roupa *m*; *for baggage* depósito *m* de bagagem
'checkup *medical, dental* check-up *m*
cheek [tʃiːk] bochecha *f*
'cheekbone maçã *f* do rosto
cheekily ['tʃiːkɪlɪ] *adv* descaradamente
cheeky *Brit* → ***fresh***
cheer [tʃɪr] **1** *n* grito *m* de júbilo; ***~s!*** (*toast*) saúde! **2** *v/t* aplaudir **3** *v/i* gritar com entusiasmo
♦ **cheer on** *v/t* torcer
♦ **cheer up 1** *v/i* animar-se; ***cheer up!*** anime-se! **2** *v/t* animar
cheerful ['tʃɪrfʊl] *adj* animado
cheering ['tʃɪrɪŋ] torcida *f*

cheerio [ʧɪrɪ'oʊ] *Brit fam* tchau, *Port* adeus
'cheerleader líder *m/f* de torcida
cheery ['ʧɪrɪ] *adj* alegre
cheese [ʧi:z] queijo *m*
'cheeseburger hambúrguer *m* com queijo
'cheesecake torta *f* de queijo
chef [ʃef] cozinheiro,-a *m,f*, *fam* mestre-cuca *m*
chemical ['kemɪkl] **1** *adj* químico **2** *n* produto *m* químico
chemical 'warfare guerra *f* química
chemist ['kemɪst] *in laboratory* químico,-a *m,f*
chemistry ['kemɪstrɪ] *also fig* química *f*
chemist's ['kemɪsts] *Brit* drogaria *f*
chemotherapy [ki:moʊ'θerəpɪ] quimioterapia *f*
cheque *Brit* → ***check***[2]
cherish ['ʧerɪʃ] *v/t memory* lembrar com carinho
cherry ['ʧerɪ] cereja *f*; (*tree*) cerejeira *f*
cherub ['ʧerəb] querubim *m*
chess [ʧes] xadrez *m*
'chessboard tabuleiro *m* de xadrez
'chesspiece peça *f* de xadrez
'chessplayer enxadrista *m/f*
chest [ʧest] peito *m*; (*box*) baú *m*; ***get sth off one's ~*** tirar um peso dos ombros
chestnut ['ʧesnʌt] castanha *f*; (*tree*) castanheiro *m*
chest of 'drawers cômoda *f*
chew [ʧu:] *v/t* mascar; *dog, rats* morder
◆ **chew out** *v/t fam* dar uma esculhambada
chewing gum ['ʧu:ɪŋ] goma *f* de mascar, *Port* pastilha *f* elástica
chic [ʃi:k] *adj* chique
chick [ʧɪk] pintinho *m*; *fam* (*girl*) garota *f*
chicken ['ʧɪkɪn] **1** *n* galinha *f*; (*food*) frango *m*; *fam* covarde *m/f* **2** *adj fam* (*cowardly*) frouxo
◆ **chicken out** *v/i fam* perder a coragem
'chickenfeed *fam* ninharia *f*
'chicken pox catapora *f*, *Port* varicela *f*
chief [ʧi:f] **1** *n* (*head*) chefe *m/f*; *of tribe* cacique *m* **2** *adj* principal
chiefly ['ʧi:flɪ] *adv* principalmente
chilblain ['ʧɪlbleɪn] frieira *f*
child [ʧaɪld] ⟨*pl children*⟩ criança *f*; *pej* bobo,-a *m,f*
'child abuse maus-tratos *mpl*
'childbirth parto *m*
childhood ['ʧaɪldhʊd] infância *f*
childish ['ʧaɪldɪʃ] *adj pej* infantil
childishly ['ʧaɪldɪʃlɪ] *adv pej* infantilmente
childishness ['ʧaɪldɪʃnɪs] *pej* infantilidade *f*
childless ['ʧaɪldlɪs] *adj* sem filhos
childlike ['ʧaɪldlaɪk] *adj* inocente
'childminder *pessoa que toma conta de crianças*
children ['ʧɪldrən] *pl* crianças *fpl*
Chile ['ʧɪlɪ] *n* Chile *m*
Chilean ['ʧɪlɪən] **1** *adj* chileno **2** *n* chileno,-a *m,f*
chill [ʧɪl] **1** *n in air* friagem *f*; (*illness*) resfriado *m* **2** *v/t wine* resfriar **3** *v/i fam* relaxar
◆ **chill out** *v/i fam* relaxar
chilli, chilli pepper ['ʧɪlɪ] pimenta *f* malagueta
chilly ['ʧɪlɪ] *adj weather, welcome* frio; ***I'm ~*** estou com frio
chime [ʧaɪm] *v/i* badalar
chimney ['ʧɪmnɪ] chaminé *f*
chimpanzee [ʧɪm'pænzɪ] chimpanzé *m*
chin [ʧɪn] queixo *m*
China ['ʧaɪnə] China *f*
china ['ʧaɪnə] porcelana *f* chinesa
Chinese [ʧaɪ'ni:z] **1** *adj* chinês,-esa **2** *n language* chinês *m*; *person* chinês,-esa *m,f*
chink [ʧɪŋk] (*gap*) buraco *m*; (*sound*) tinido *m*
chip [ʧɪp] **1** *n* (*fragment, damage*) lasca *f*; *gambling*: ficha *f*; COMPUT chip *m*; ***~s*** *Brit & Am* batata *f* frita **2** *v/t* ⟨*pret & pp* ***chipped***⟩ (*damage*) lascar
◆ **chip in** *v/i* (*interrupt*) intrometer-se; *with money* fazer uma contribuição, *fam* fazer uma vaquinha
chiropractor ['kaɪroʊpræktər] quiroprático,-a *m,f*
chirp [ʧɜ:rp] *v/i* gorjear
chisel ['ʧɪzl] *n* cinzel *m*

chitchat ['ʧɪʧæt] *fam* bate-papo *m*
chivalrous ['ʃɪvlrəs] *adj* cavalheiresco
chive [ʧaɪv] cebolinha *f*
chlorine ['klɔːriːn] cloro *m*
chloroform ['klɔːrəfɔːrm] clorofórmio *m*
chocaholic [ʧɑːkə'hɑːlɪk] *n fam* chocólatra *m/f*
chock-a-block [ʧɑːkə'blɑːk] *adj fam* abarrotado
chock-full [ʧɑːk'fʊl] *adj fam* cheio
chocolate ['ʧɑːkələt] chocolate *m*
'chocolate cake bolo *m* de chocolate
choice [ʧɔɪs] **1** *n* escolha *f*; (*selection*) seleção *f*; ***I had no ~*** não tive escolha **2** *adj* (*top quality*) selecionado
choir ['kwaɪr] coro *m*
'choirboy menino *m* de coro
choke [ʧoʊk] **1** *n* MOT afogador *m*, *Port* ar *m* **2** *v/i* engasgar; ***he ~d on a bone*** ele engasgou-se com um osso **3** *v/t* asfixiar
cholesterol [kə'lestəroʊl] colesterol *m*
choose [ʧuːz] *v/t & v/i* ⟨*pret* ***chose***, *pp* ***chosen***⟩ escolher
choosey ['ʧuːzɪ] *adj fam* exigente
chop [ʧɑːp] **1** *n* golpe *m*; (*meat*) costeleta *f* **2** *v/t* ⟨*pret & pp* ***chopped***⟩ *wood* cortar; *meat*, *vegetables* picar
♦**chop down** *v/t tree* derrubar
chopper ['ʧɑːpər] (*tool*) cortador *m*; *fam* (*helicopter*) helicóptero *m*
chopping board ['ʧɑːpɪŋ] tábua *f* de cortar
'chopsticks *n/pl* hashi *m*
choral ['kɔːrəl] *adj* coral
chord [kɔːrd] MUS acorde *m*
chore [ʧɔːr] tarefa *f*
choreograph ['kɔːrɪəgræf] *v/t* coreografar
choreographer [kɔːrɪ'ɑːgrəfər] coreógrafo,-a *m,f*
choreography [kɔːrɪ'ɑːgrəfɪ] coreografia *f*
chorus ['kɔːrəs] (*singers*) coral *m*; *of song* refrão *m*
chose [ʧoʊz] *pret* → ***choose***
chosen ['ʧoʊzn] *pp* → ***choose***
Christ [kraɪst] Cristo *m*; ***~!*** por Cristo!
christen ['krɪsn] *v/t* batizar
christening ['krɪsnɪŋ] batismo *m*
Christian ['krɪsʧən] **1** *n* cristão *m*, cristã *f* **2** *adj* cristão (cristã)
Christianity [krɪstɪ'ænətɪ] cristianismo *m*
'Christian name nome *m* de batismo
Christmas ['krɪsməs] Natal *m*; ***at ~*** no Natal; ***Merry ~!*** Feliz Natal!
'Christmas card cartão *m* de Natal **Christmas 'Day** Dia *m* de Natal **Christmas 'Eve** Noite *f* de Natal **'Christmas present** presente *m* de Natal **'Christmas tree** árvore *f* de Natal
chrome, **chromium** [kroʊm, 'kroʊmɪəm] cromo *m*
chromosome ['kroʊməsoʊm] cromossomo *m*
chronic ['krɑːnɪk] *adj* crônico
chronological [krɑːnə'lɑːdʒɪkl] *adj* cronológico; ***in ~ order*** em ordem cronológica
chrysanthemum [krɪ'sænθəməm] crisântemo *m*
chubby ['ʧʌbɪ] *adj* gordinho
chuck [ʧʌk] *v/t fam* jogar, *Port* deitar
♦**chuck out** *v/t fam object* jogar fora, *Port* deitar fora; *person* expulsar
chuckle ['ʧʌkl] **1** *n* risada *f* **2** *v/i* rir
chum [ʧʌm] camarada *m/f*
chummy ['ʧʌmɪ] *adj fam* íntimo; ***be ~ with*** ser íntimo de
chunk [ʧʌŋk] grande pedaço *m*
chunky ['ʧʌŋkɪ] *adj sweater* grosso; *person*, *build* corpulento
church [ʧɜːrʧ] igreja *f*
church 'hall átrio *m* **church 'service** serviço *m* religioso **'churchyard** pátio *m* de igreja
churlish ['ʧɜːrlɪʃ] *adj* rude
chute [ʃuːt] tubo *m* de transporte; *garbage*: tubo *m* de lixo
CIA [siːaɪ'eɪ] *abbr* (*of* ***Central Intelligence Agency***) Agência *f* Central de Inteligência
cider ['saɪdər] cidra *f*
CIF [siːaɪ'ef] *abbr* (*of* ***cost insurance freight***) custo, seguro e frete *m*
cigar [sɪ'gɑːr] charuto *m*
cigarette, **cigaret** [sɪgə'ret] cigarro *m*
ciga'rette end ponta *f* de cigarro **ciga'rette lighter** isqueiro *m* **ciga'rette paper** papel *m* de cigarro

cinema ['sɪnɪmə] cinema *m*
cinnamon ['sɪnəmən] canela *f*
circle ['sɜːrkl] **1** *n* círculo *m*; **~ *of friends*** círculo de amigos **2** *v/t* (*draw circle around*) assinalar **3** *v/i plane, bird* fazer círculos
circuit ['sɜːrkɪt] circuito *m*; (*lap*) volta *f*
'circuit board COMPUT placa *f* de circuitos **'circuit breaker** ELEC interruptor *m* **'circuit training** SPORT treinamento *m* de circuito
circular ['sɜːrkjʊlər] **1** *n* circular *f* **2** *adj* circular
circulate ['sɜːrkjʊleɪt] *v/t & v/i* circular
circulation [sɜːrkjʊ'leɪʃn] *also newspaper*: circulação *f*
circumference [sər'kʌmfərəns] circunferência *f*
circumstances ['sɜːrkəmstənsɪs] *n/pl* circunstâncias *fpl*; *financial* situação *f* financeira; ***under no*** **~** sob circunstância alguma; ***under the*** **~** nestas circunstâncias
circus ['sɜːrkəs] circo *m*
cirrhosis [sɪ'roʊsɪs] cirrose *f*
cistern ['sɪstərn] cisterna *f*
cite [saɪt] *v/t* citar
citizen ['sɪtɪzn] cidadão *m*, cidadã *f*
citizenship ['sɪtɪznʃɪp] cidadania *f*
city ['sɪtɪ] cidade *f*
city 'center centro *m* da cidade
city 'hall prefeitura *f*
civic ['sɪvɪk] *adj also pride, responsibilities* cívico
civil ['ʃɪvl] *adj* (*not military*) *also disobedience* civil; (*polite*) cortês
civil engi'neer engenheiro,-a *m,f* civil
civilian [sɪ'vɪljən] **1** *n* civil *m/f* **2** *adj clothes* civil
civility [sɪ'vɪlɪtɪ] civilidade *f*
civilization [sɪvəlaɪ'zeɪʃn] civilização *f*
civilize ['sɪvəlaɪz] *v/t person* civilizar
civil 'rights direitos *mpl* civis **civil 'servant** funcionário,-a *m,f* público,-a **civil 'service** função *f* pública
civil 'war guerra *f* civil
claim [kleɪm] **1** *n* (*request*) reivindicação *f*; (*right*) direito *m*; (*assertion*) alegação *f* **2** *v/t* (*ask for as a right*) reivindicar; (*assert*) alegar; *lost property* reclamar; ***they have ~ed responsibility for the attack*** eles alegaram ser os responsáveis pelo ataque
claimant ['kleɪmənt] requerente *m/f*
clairvoyant [kler'vɔɪənt] *n* vidente *m/f*
clam [klæm] mexilhão *m*
♦ **clam up** *v/i* ⟨*pret & pp* **clammed**⟩ *fam* calar-se
clamber ['klæmbər] *v/i* escalar
clammy ['klæmɪ] *adj* úmido
clamor ['klæmər] *Am* clamor *m*
♦ **clamor for** *v/t Am* clamar por
clamour *Brit* → ***clamor***
clamp [klæmp] **1** *n* (*fastener*) torno *m* **2** *v/t* (*fasten*) apertar; *car* atarraxar
♦ **clamp down** *v/i* reprimir
♦ **clamp down on** *v/t* reprimir
clan [klæn] clã *m*
clandestine [klæn'destɪn] *adj* clandestino
clang [klæŋ] **1** *n* clangor *m* **2** *v/i* retinir
clap [klæp] *v/t & v/i* ⟨*pret & pp* ***clapped***⟩ aplaudir
claret ['klærɪt] *wine* clarete *m*
clarification [klærɪfɪ'keɪʃn] esclarecimento *m*
clarify ['klærɪfaɪ] *v/t* ⟨*pret & pp* ***clarified***⟩ esclarecer
clarinet [klærɪ'net] clarinete *m*
clarity ['klærətɪ] clareza *f*
clash [klæʃ] **1** *n also of personalities* choque *m* **2** *v/i* chocar-se; *opinions, colors* chocar; *events* coincidir
clasp [klæsp] **1** *n* fecho *m* **2** *v/t in hand, to self* apertar
class [klæs] **1** *n* (*lesson*) aula *f*; (*group of people*) turma *f*; (*category*) classe *f*; ***social*** **~** classe *f* social **2** *v/t* classificar
classic ['klæsɪk] **1** *adj* clássico **2** *n* clássico *m*
classical ['klæsɪkl] *adj music* clássico
classification [klæsɪfɪ'keɪʃn] classificação *f*
classified ['klæsɪfaɪd] *adj information* confidencial
'classified ad, 'classified advertisement anúncio *m* classificado
classify ['klæsɪfaɪ] *v/t* ⟨*pret & pp* ***classified***⟩ (*categorize*) classificar

'classroom sala *f* de aula
'class warfare guerra *f* de classes
classy ['klæsɪ] *adj fam* de classe
clatter ['klætər] **1** *n* estrépito *m* **2** *v/i* tropeliar
clause [klɒːz] *in agreement* cláusula *f*; GRAM oração *f*
claustrophobia [klɔːstrə'foʊbɪə] claustrofobia *f*
claw [klɒː] **1** *n also fig* garra *f* **2** *v/t* (*scratch*) arranhar
clay [kleɪ] argila *f*
clean [kliːn] **1** *adj* limpo **2** *adv fam* (*completely*) totalmente **3** *v/t house, room* limpar; *teeth, shoes* escovar; *car, hands, face, clothes* lavar; ***have sth ~ed*** mandar lavar algo
◆**clean out** *v/t room, closet* esvaziar; *fig* deixar liso
◆**clean up 1** *v/t room, papers* pôr em ordem; *fig* limpar **2** *v/i* fazer limpeza; *spilt water* enxugar; (*wash*) lavar-se; *on stock market etc* ganhar muito dinheiro
cleaner ['kliːnər] faxineiro,-a *m,f*; (*drycleaner*) tinturaria *f*
'cleaning woman mulher *f* da limpeza
cleanse [klenz] *v/t skin* limpar
cleanser ['klenzər] *for skin* limpador,a *m,f*
cleansing cream ['klenzɪŋ] creme *m* de limpeza
clear [klɪr] **1** *adj also* (*easy to understand*) claro; (*obvious*) evidente; *water, skin, profit* limpo; *photograph* nítido; *conscience* tranqüilo; ***I'm not ~ about it*** não tenho muita clareza com relação a isso; ***I didn't make myself ~*** não fui claro **2** *adv* claramente; ***stand ~ of*** afastar-se de; ***steer ~ of*** evitar **3** *v/t roads* liberar; *closet* esvaziar; (*acquit*) inocentar; (*authorize*) autorizar; (*earn*) ganhar; ***~ the table*** tirar a mesa; ***~ one's throat*** pigarrear; ***the security guards ~ed everybody out of the room*** os guardas de segurança retiraram todos da sala **4** *v/i mist* dissipar-se; *sky* limpar-se; *face* iluminar-se
◆**clear away** *v/t* remover
◆**clear off** *v/i fam* cair fora
◆**clear out 1** *v/t closet* esvaziar **2** *v/i* ir embora
◆**clear up 1** *v/i* arrumar; *weather* melhorar; *illness, rash* desaparecer **2** *v/t* (*tidy*) arrumar; *mystery, problem* resolver
clearance ['klɪrəns] (*space*) espaço *m*; (*authorization*) permissão *f*
'clearance sale liquidação *f* total
clearing ['klɪrɪŋ] clareira *f*
clearly ['klɪrlɪ] *adv* (*with clarity*) claramente; (*evidently*) evidentemente
cleavage ['kliːvɪdʒ] fenda *f* entre os seios
cleaver ['kliːvər] cutelo *m*
clemency ['klemənsɪ] clemência *f*
clench [klentʃ] *v/t teeth* trincar; *fist* cerrar
clergy ['klɜːrdʒɪ] clero *m*
clergyman ['klɜːrdʒɪmæn] clérigo *m*
clerk [klɜːrk] *administrative* auxiliar administrativo,-a *m,f*; *Am in store* balconista *m/f*
clever ['klevər] *adj person, animal, idea* astucioso; *gadget, device* engenhoso
cleverly ['klevəlɪ] *adv* astuciosamente
cliché [kliː'ʃeɪ] clichê *m*
clichéd ['kliːʃeɪd] *adj* estereotipado
click [klɪk] **1** *n* COMPUT clique *m* **2** *v/i* clicar
◆**click on** *v/t* COMPUT clicar em
client ['klaɪənt] cliente *m/f*
clientele [kliːən'tel] clientela *f*
cliff [klɪf] penhasco *m*
climate ['klaɪmət] clima *m*
'climate change mudança *f* climática
climatic [klaɪ'mætɪk] *adj* climático
climax ['klaɪmæks] *n* clímax *m*
climb [klaɪm] **1** *n mountain*: subida *f* **2** *v/t & v/i* subir
◆**climb down** *v/i* descer; *fig* ceder
climber ['klaɪmər] *person* alpinista *m/f*
climbing ['klaɪmɪŋ] alpinismo *m*
'climbing wall parede *f* de escalar
clinch [klɪntʃ] *v/t deal* fechar; ***that ~es it*** isso decide o assunto
cling [klɪŋ] *v/i* ⟨*pret & pp* **clung**⟩ *clothes* apertar
◆**cling to** *v/t child, tradition* apegar-se a
'clingfilm *Brit* filme *m* de PVC

C

clingy ['klɪŋɪ] *adj child, boyfriend* pegajoso
clinic ['klɪnɪk] clínica *f*
clinical ['klɪnɪkl] *adj* clínico
clink [klɪŋk] **1** *n noise* tinir *m* **2** *v/i* tinir
clip[1] [klɪp] **1** *n (fastener)* grampeador *m*; *hair*: grampo *m*, *Port* grancho *m* **2** *v/t* ⟨*pret & pp* ***clipped***⟩ prender com clipe; ***~ sth to sth*** prender algo a algo
clip[2] [klɪp] **1** *n (extract)* trecho *m* **2** *v/t* ⟨*pret & pp* ***clipped***⟩ *hair, hedge, grass* aparar
'**clipboard** prancheta *f*; COMPUT área *f* de transferência
clippers ['klɪpərz] *npl hair*: prendedor *m* de cabelo; *nails*: alicate *m* de unhas; *gardening*: podadeira *f*
clipping ['klɪpɪŋ] *from newspaper* recorte *m* de jornal
clique [kli:k] grupo *m* exclusivo, *fam* panelinha *f*
cloak [kloʊk] *n* capa *f*
'**cloakroom** *for coats* guarda-roupa *m*
clock [klɑ:k] relógio *m*; *fam (odometer)* contador *m* de quilometragem
'**clock radio** rádio-relógio *m* '**clockwise** *adv* no sentido horário '**clockwork** mecanismo *m* de relógio; ***it went like ~*** funcionou como um relógio
♦ **clog up** [klɑ:g] *v/i, v/t* ⟨*pret & pp* ***clogged***⟩ entupir
clone [kloʊn] **1** *n* clone *m* **2** *v/t* clonar
cloning ['kloʊnɪŋ] clonagem *f*
close[1] [kloʊs] **1** *adj family, friend* próximo; *cooperation* estreito; *resemblance* forte; ***we were very ~*** éramos muito próximos **2** *adv* perto; ***~ at hand*** à mão; ***~ by*** por perto
close[2] [kloʊz] *v/t & v/i* fechar
♦ **close down 1** *v/t* fechar as portas de **2** *v/i (permanently)* fechar
♦ **close in** *v/i* aproximar-se
♦ **close up 1** *v/t building* trancar **2** *v/i (move closer)* aproximar-se
closed [kloʊzd] *adj store* fechado; *eyes* cerrado
closed-circuit 'television circuito *m* fechado de televisão
'**close-knit** *adj* unido
closely ['kloʊslɪ] *adv listen, watch* de perto; *cooperate* estreitamente
closet ['klɑ:zɪt] armário *m* embutido; *(walk-in)* closet *m*
close-up ['kloʊsʌp] close-up *m*
closing date ['kloʊsɪŋ] data *f* final
closing time ['kloʊzɪŋ] *museum, library*: hora *f* de encerramento
closure ['kloʊʒər] *permanent* encerramento *m*; *shop*: fechamento *m*; ***get ~ on sth*** ultrapassar algo
clot [klɑ:t] **1** *n blood*: coágulo *m* **2** *v/i* ⟨*pret & pp* ***clotted***⟩ *blood* coagular
cloth [klɑ:θ] *(fabric)* tecido *m*; *kitchen, cleaning*: pano *m*
clothes [kloʊðz] *npl* roupa *f*; ***she has a lot of ~*** tem muitas roupas; ***he was wearing his best ~*** vestia sua melhor roupa
'**clothes brush** escova *f* de roupa '**clothes hanger** cabide *m* '**clotheshorse** estendedor *m* de roupas '**clothesline** varal *m* '**clothes peg** *Brit*, '**clothespin** *Am* prendedor *m* de roupa
clothing ['kloʊðɪŋ] vestuário *m*
cloud [klaʊd] *n* nuvem *f*; ***a ~ of smoke / dust*** uma nuvem de fumaça / poeira
♦ **cloud over** *v/i sky* tornar-se nublado
'**cloudburst** aguaceiro *m*
cloudless ['klaʊdlɪs] *adj sky* claro
cloudy ['klaʊdɪ] *adj* nublado
clout [klaʊt] *fig (influence)* influência *f*
clove of garlic [kloʊv] dente *m* de alho
clown [klaʊn] *in circus, also pej* palhaço *m*; *(joker)* brincalhão *m*, brincalhona *f*
club [klʌb] *n weapon* cacetete *m*; *golf*: taco *m*; *organization* clube *m*
clue [klu:] pista *f*; ***I haven't a ~*** *fam* não faço idéia; ***he hasn't a ~*** *(is useless)* ele não tem noção
clued-up [klu:d'ʌp] *adj fam* mais bem informado
clump [klʌmp] *n earth*: monte *m*; *(group)* grupo *m*
clumsiness ['klʌmzɪnɪs] falta *f* de jeito
clumsy ['klʌmzɪ] *adj person* desajeitado

clung [klʌŋ] *pret & pp* → ***cling***
cluster ['klʌstər] **1** *n* aglomerado *m* **2** *v/i people, houses* aglomerar-se
clutch [klʌʧ] **1** *n* MOT embreagem *f*, *Port* embraiagem *f* **2** *v/t* agarrar
◆ **clutch at** *v/t* agarrar-se a
clutter ['klʌtər] **1** *n* amontoado *m* **2** *v/t also* (*clutter up*) amontoar
c/o *abbr* (*of* ***care of***) aos cuidados de
Co. *abbr* (*of* ***Company***) companhia *f*
coach [kouʧ] **1** *n* (*trainer*) técnico,-a *m,f*; *on train* vagão *m*; *Brit* (*bus*) ônibus *m*, *Port* autocarro *m* **2** *v/t* treinar
coaching ['kouʧɪŋ] treinamento *m*
coach station → ***bus station***
coagulate [kou'ægjuleɪt] *v/i blood* coagular
coal [koul] carvão *m*
coalition [kouə'lɪʃn] coalizão *f*
'coalmine mina *f* de carvão
coarse [kɔːrs] *adj* áspero; *hair* grosso; (*vulgar*) grosseiro
coarsely ['kɔːrslɪ] *adv* (*vulgarly*) grosseiramente; **~ *ground coffee*** café *m* moído grosso
coast [koust] *n* costa *f*; ***at the* ~** no litoral
coastal ['koustl] *adj* costeiro
coaster ['koustər] *for plate* descansa-prato *m*; *for glass* porta-copo *m*
'coastguard *organization* guarda *f* costeira; *person* guarda costeiro,-a *m,f*
'coastline litoral *m*
coat [kout] **1** *n* casaco *m*; (*overcoat*) sobretudo *m*; *suit*: paletó *m*; *animal*: pêlo *m*; *paint etc*: demão *f* **2** *v/t* (*cover*) cobrir
'coathanger cabide *m*
coating ['koutɪŋ] camada *f*
co-author ['kouɒːθər] **1** *n* co-autor,a *m,f* **2** *v/t* escrever em co-autoria
coax [kouks] *v/t* persuadir
cobbled ['kaːbld] *adj* pavimentado com paralelepípedos
cobblestone ['kaːblstoun] paralelepípedo *m*
cobweb ['kaːbweb] teia *f* de aranha
cocaine [kə'keɪn] cocaína *f*
cock [kaːk] *n* (*chicken*) galo *m*; *any male bird* pássaro *m*
cockeyed [kaːk'aɪd] *adj fam idea etc* absurdo
'cockpit *plane*: cockpit *m*
cockroach ['kaːkrouʧ] barata *f*
'cocktail coquetel *m*, *Port* cocktail *m*
'cocktail party coquetel *m*, *Port* cocktail *m*
'cocktail shaker coqueteleira *f*
cocky ['kaːkɪ] *adj fam* convencido
cocoa ['koukou] *drink* chocolate *m* quente
coconut ['koukənʌt] coco *m*
coconut palm coqueiro *m*
COD [siːou'diː] *abbr* (*of* ***collect on delivery***) frete *m* a cobrar
code [koud] *n* código *m*
coeducational [kouedu'keɪʃnl] *adj* co-educacional
coerce [kou'ɜːrs] *v/t* coagir
coexist [kouɪg'zɪst] *v/i* coexistir
coexistence [kouɪg'zɪstəns] coexistência *f*
coffee ['kaːfɪ] café *m*
'coffee bean grão *m* de café **'coffee break** intervalo *m* **'coffee cup** xícara *f* de café, *Port* chávena *f* de café **'coffee grinder** ['graɪndər] moedor *m* de café **'coffee maker** cafeteira *f* elétrica **'coffee plantation** plantação *f* de café **'coffee pot** cafeteira *f* **'coffee shop** café *m* **'coffee table** mesinha *f* de centro
coffin ['kaːfɪn] caixão *m*
cog [kaːg] dente *m* de roda dentada
cognac ['kaːnjæk] conhaque *m*
'cogwheel roda *f* dentada
cohabit [kou'hæbɪt] *v/i* coabitar
coherent [kou'hɪrənt] *adj* coerente
coil [kɔɪl] **1** *n rope*: rolo *m* **2** *v/t* **~ (*up*)** enrolar-se
coin [kɔɪn] *n* moeda *f*
coincide [kouɪn'saɪd] *v/i* coincidir
coincidence [kou'ɪnsɪdəns] coincidência *f*
Coke® [kouk] coca-cola *f*
coke [kouk] *pej* (*cocaine*) coca *f*
cold [kould] **1** *adj* frio; ***I'm* (*feeling*) ~** estou com frio; ***it's* ~** *weather* está frio; ***in* ~ *blood*** a sangue frio; ***get* ~ *feet*** *fam* ficar nervoso **2** *n* frio *m*; MED resfriado *m*, *Port* constipação *f*; ***I have a* ~** estou resfriado, *Port* estou constipado

C

cold-blooded [koʊld'blʌdɪd] *adj* de sangue frio; *fig* insensível
cold 'calling COM telemarketing *m*
'cold cuts frios *mpl*
coldly ['koʊldlɪ] *adv say, look* friamente
coldness ['koʊldnɪs] *fig* frieza *f*
'cold sore herpes *m* labial
coleslaw ['koʊlslɒː] salada *f* de repolho
colic ['kɑːlɪk] cólica *f*
collaborate [kə'læbəreɪt] *v/i with enemy, in research* colaborar
collaboration [kəlæbə'reɪʃn] colaboração *f*
collaborator [kə'læbəreɪtər] *with enemy, in writing* colaborador,a *m,f*
collapse [kə'læps] *v/i roof* desabar, *person etc* ter um colapso
collapsible [kə'læpsəbl] *adj* dobrável
collar ['kɑːlər] *of shirt, jacket* colarinho *m*; *for dog, cat* coleira *f*
'collar-bone clavícula *f*
collateral [kə'lætərəl] **1** *n loan*: garantia *f* **2** *adj* **~ damage** danos *mpl* colaterais
colleague ['kɑːliːg] colega *m/f*
collect [kə'lekt] **1** *v/t person, tickets, cleaning etc* apanhar; *as hobby* colecionar; (*gather*) coletar **2** *v/i* (*gather together*) reunir-se **3** *adv* **call ~** chamar a cobrar
col'lect call chamada *f* a cobrar
collected [kə'lektɪd] *adj works, poems* reunido; *person* sereno
collection [kə'lekʃn] coleção *f*; *in church* coleta *f*
collective [kə'lektɪv] *adj* coletivo
collective 'bargaining acordo *m* tarifário
collector [kə'lektər] colecionador,a *m,f*
college ['kɑːlɪdʒ] escola *f* superior
collide [kə'laɪd] *v/i* colidir
collision [kə'lɪʒn] colisão *f*
colloquial [kə'loʊkwɪəl] *adj* coloquial
Colombia [kə'lʌmbɪə] Colômbia *f*
Colombian [kə'lʌmbɪən] **1** *adj* colombiano **2** *n* colombiano,-a *m,f*
colon ['koʊlɑːn] *punctuation*: dois-pontos *mpl*; ANAT cólon *m*
colonel ['kɜːrnl] coronel *m*
colonial [kə'loʊnɪəl] *adj* colonial
colonize ['kɑːlənaɪz] *v/t country* colonizar
colony ['kɑːlənɪ] colônia *f*
color ['kʌlər] **1** *n Am* cor *f*, *in cheeks* rubor *m*; **in ~** *movie etc* a cores; MIL **~s** bandeira *f* **2** *v/t hair* tingir **3** *v/i* (*blush*) corar
'color-blind *adj Am* daltônico
colored ['kʌləd] *adj Am person* de cor
'color fast *adj Am* que não desbota
colorful ['kʌlərfʊl] *adj Am* colorido
coloring ['kʌlərɪŋ] *Am* tonalidade *f*
'color photograph *Am* fotografia *f* colorida **'color scheme** *Am* esquema *m* de cores **'color TV** *Am* televisão *f* a cores
colossal [kə'lɑːsl] *adj* colossal
colour *etc Brit* → ***color***
colt [koʊlt] potro *m*
Columbus [kə'lʌmbəs] Colombo
column ['kɑːləm] *also figures, people, text*: coluna *f*
columnist ['kɑːləmɪst] colunista *m/f*
coma ['koʊmə] coma *f*
comb [koʊm] **1** *n* pente *m* **2** *v/t* pentear; *area* esquadrinhar
combat ['kɑːmbæt] **1** *n* combate *m* **2** *v/t* combater
combination [kɑːmbɪ'neɪʃn] *of things, safe* combinação *f*
combine [kəm'baɪn] **1** *v/t* combinar **2** *v/i chemical elements* misturar
combine harvester [kɑːmbaɪn'hɑːrvɪstər] ceifadeira *f* debulhadora
combustible [kəm'bʌstɪbl] *adj* combustível
combustion [kəm'bʌstʃn] combustão *f*
come [kʌm] *v/i* ⟨*pret* ***came***, *pp* ***come***⟩ *toward speaker* vir; *toward listener* ir; *train, bus* chegar; ***you'll ~ to like it*** você passará a gostar; ***how ~?*** *fam* como?
♦ **come about** *v/i* (*happen*) acontecer
♦ **come across 1** *v/t* (*find*) encontrar **2** *v/i idea, humor* fazer-se entender; ***she comes across as …*** ela se passou por …
♦ **come along** *v/i* (*come too*) ir junto; (*turn up*) aparecer; (*progress*) andar
♦ **come apart** *v/i* partir-se; (*break*)

partir
♦**come around** *v/i to s.o.'s home* aparecer; (*regain consciousness*) voltar a si
♦**come away** *v/i* (*leave*) ir embora; *button etc* desprender-se
♦**come back** *v/i* voltar; ***it came back to me*** me lembrei
♦**come by 1** *v/i* visitar **2** *v/t* (*acquire*) conseguir
♦**come down** *v/i* descer; *in price, amount etc* baixar; *rain, snow* cair; ***he came down the stairs*** ele desceu a escada
♦**come for** *v/t* (*attack*) atacar; (*collect*) vir buscar
♦**come forward** *v/i* (*present oneself*) apresentar-se
♦**come from** *v/t* ser de; ***I come from New York, where do you come from?*** sou de Nova York, de onde você é?
♦**come in** *v/i person* entrar; *train, tide, in race* chegar; ***come in!*** entre!
♦**come in for** *v/t* ***come in for criticism*** ser criticado
♦**come in on** *v/t* fazer parte de; ***come in on a deal*** participar de um negócio
♦**come off** *v/i handle etc* desprender-se
♦**come on** *v/i* (*progress*) progredir; ***come on!*** vamos!; ***oh come on!*** *disbelief*: deixe disso!
♦**come out** *v/i person, sun, results, product, stain etc* sair; *gay* revelar-se
♦**come to 1** *v/t place, hair, dress, water etc* chegar a; ***that comes to 70*** isso chega a 70 **2** *v/i* (*regain consciousness*) voltar a si
♦**come up** *v/i* subir; *sun* nascer; ***something has come up*** algo aconteceu
♦**come up with** *v/t* ***he came up with a new idea*** ocorreu-lhe uma nova idéia
'comeback volta *f*; ***make a ~*** fazer seu grande retorno
comedian [kə'mi:dɪən] humorista *m/f*; *pej* engraçadinho,-a *m,f*
'comedown caída *f*
comedy ['kɑ:mədɪ] comédia *f*
come round → ***come around***
comet ['kɑ:mɪt] cometa *m*
comeuppance [kʌm'ʌpəns] *fam* reprimenda *f* merecida; ***he'll get his ~*** ele terá o que merece
comfort ['kʌmfərt] **1** *n* conforto *m* **2** *v/t* consolar
comfortable ['kʌmfərtəbl] *adj* confortável; (*financially*) descansado
comic ['kɑ:mɪk] **1** *n* (*to read*) revista *f* em quadrinhos, *Port* revista *f* de banda desenhada; (*comedian*) humorista *m/f* **2** *adj* cômico
comical ['kɑ:mɪkl] *adj* cômico
'comic book revista *f* em quadrinhos
comics ['kɑ:mɪks] *npl* quadrinhos *mpl*
'comic strip história *f* em quadrinhos, *Port* banda *f* desenhada
comma ['kɑ:mə] vírgula *f*
command [kə'mænd] **1** *n* ordem *f* **2** *v/t* mandar
commandeer [kɑ:mən'dɪr] *v/t* requisitar
commander [kə'mændər] comandante *m/f*
commander-in-'chief comandante-em-chefe *m/f*
commanding officer [kə'mændɪŋ] oficial *m/f* comandante
commandment [kə'mændmənt] REL ***the Ten Commandments*** Os Dez Mandamentos
commemorate [kə'meməreɪt] *v/t* comemorar
commemoration [kəmemə'reɪʃn] comemoração *f*; ***in ~ of*** em comemoração a
commence [kə'mens] *v/t & v/i* começar
commendable [kə'mendəbl] *adj* louvável
commendation [kəmen'deɪʃn] *for bravery* menção *f* honrosa
commensurate [kə'menʃərət] *adj* ***~ with*** compatível com
comment ['kɑ:ment] **1** *n* comentário *m*; ***no ~!*** sem comentários! **2** *v/i* comentar
commentary ['kɑ:məntərɪ] comentário *m*
commentate ['kɑ:mənteɪt] *v/i* comentar

C

commentator ['kɑːmənteɪtər] comentarista *m/f*
commerce ['kɑːmɜːrs] comércio *m*
commercial [kə'mɜːrʃl] **1** *adj firm, success* comercial **2** *n (advert)* comercial *m*
commercial 'break intervalo *m* comercial
commercialize [kə'mɜːrʃlaɪz] *v/t* comercializar
commercial 'television televisão *f* comercial
commercial 'traveler caixeiro-viajante *m*
commercial traveller *Brit* → ***commercial traveler***
commiserate [kə'mɪzəreɪt] *v/i* comiserar
commission [kə'mɪʃn] **1** *n (payment) also (committee)* comissão *f*, *(job)* encargo *m* **2** *v/t for a job* encarregar
Commissioner [kə'mɪʃənər] *in European Union* Comissário *m*
commit [kə'mɪt] *v/t* ⟨*pret & pp* ***committed***⟩ *crime* cometer; *money* destinar; ***~ oneself*** comprometer-se
commitment [kə'mɪtmənt] *relationship*: compromisso *m*; *(responsibility)* responsabilidade *f*
committee [kə'mɪtɪ] comitê *m*
commodity [kə'mɑːdətɪ] mercadoria *f*
common ['kɑːmən] *adj (not rare, shared)* comum; ***in ~*** em comum; ***have sth in ~ with s.o.*** ter algo em comum com alguém
commoner ['kɑːmənər] plebeu *m*, plebéia *f*
common 'law wife companheira *f*
commonly ['kɑːmənlɪ] *adv* comumente
Common 'Market Mercado Comum *m*
'commonplace *adj* lugar-comum *m*
Commons ['kɑːmənz] *npl Brit* ***the ~*** a Câmara Baixa (*ou* dos Comuns)
common 'sense bom *m* senso
commotion [kə'moʊʃn] comoção *f*
communal [kəm'juːnl] *adj* comum
communally [kəm'juːnəlɪ] *adv* comunalmente
communicate [kə'mjuːnɪkeɪt] **1** *v/i* comunicar-se **2** *v/t* comunicar
communication [kəmjuːnɪ'keɪʃn] comunicação *f*
communi'cations comunicações *fpl*
communi'cations satellite satélite *m* de comunicações
communicative [kə'mjuːnɪkətɪv] *adj person* comunicativo
Communion [kə'mjuːnjən] REL Comunhão *f*
communiqué [kə'mjuːnɪkeɪ] comunicado *m*
Communism ['kɑːmjʊnɪzəm] comunismo *m*
Communist ['kɑːmjʊnɪst] **1** *adj* comunista **2** *n* comunista *m/f*
community [kə'mjuːnətɪ] comunidade *f*
com'munity center centro *m* comunitário
community centre → ***community center***
com'munity service serviço *m* comunitário
commute [kə'mjuːt] **1** *v/i* ir e voltar; ***she ~s to New York four times a week*** ela viaja à trabalho para Nova Iorque quatro vezes por semana **2** *v/t* LAW comutar
commuter [kə'mjuːtər] viajante *m* habitual; ***the train was full of ~s*** o trem estava cheio de trabalhadores
com'muter traffic tráfego *m* de trabalhadores
com'muter train trem *m* para trabalhadores
compact [kəm'pækt] **1** *adj* compacto **2** *n also* MOT compacto *m*
compact 'disc disco *m* compacto; → ***CD***
companion [kəm'pænjən] companheiro,-a *m,f*
companionship [kəm'pænjənʃɪp] companhia *f*
company ['kʌmpənɪ] COM empresa *f*, *(companionship)* companhia *f*, *(guests)* convidado,-a *m,f*; ***keep s.o. ~*** fazer companhia a alguém
company 'car carro *m* da empresa
company 'law direito *m* empresarial
comparable ['kɑːmpərəbl] *adj (which can be compared)* comparável; *(simi-*

lar) semelhante

comparative [kəm'pærətɪv] **1** *adj* (*relative*) relativo; *study*, GRAM comparativo **2** *n* GRAM comparativo *m*

comparatively [kəm'pærətɪvlɪ] *adv* relativamente

compare [kəm'per] **1** *v/t* comparar; **~ *sth with sth / s.o. with s.o.*** comparar algo com algo / comparar alguém com alguém; **~*d with …*** em comparação com … **2** *v/i* comparar-se

comparison [kəm'pærɪsn] comparação *f*; ***there's no ~*** não há comparação

compartment [kəm'pɑːrtmənt] compartimento *m*

compass ['kʌmpəs] bússola *f*; MATH compasso *m*

compassion [kəm'pæʃn] compaixão *f*

compassionate [kəm'pæʃənət] *adj* compassivo

compassionate 'leave licensa *f* por motivo de morte

compatibility [kəmpætə'bɪlɪtɪ] compatibilidade *f*

compatible [kəm'pætəbl] *adj* compatível; ***we're not ~*** não somos compatíveis

compel [kəm'pel] *v/t* ⟨*pret & pp* ***compelled***⟩ forçar

compelling [kəm'pelɪŋ] *adj argument* convincente; *movie*, *book* entusiasmado

compensate ['kɑmpənseɪt] **1** *v/t with money* compensar **2** *v/i* **~ *for*** compensar por

compensation [kɑmpən'seɪʃn] (*money*) indenização *f*; (*reward*) compensação *f*; (*comfort*) conforto *m*

compete [kəm'piːt] *v/i in sports*, *prices etc* competir; **~ *for*** competir por

competence ['kɑːmpɪtəns] competência *f*

competent ['kɑːmpɪtənt] *adj person*, *work* competente; ***I'm not ~ to judge*** não sou competente para julgar

competently ['kɑːmpɪtəntlɪ] *adv* competentemente

competition [kɑːmpə'tɪʃn] (*contest*, *competitors*) *also* SPORT competição *f*; ***the government wants to encourage ~*** o governo deseja encorajar a competição

competitive [kəm'petətɪv] *adj person*, *price* competitivo

competitively [kəm'petətɪvlɪ] *adv* competitivamente; **~ *priced*** com preço competitivo

competitiveness [kəm'petətɪvnɪs] COM *also of person* competitividade *f*

competitor [kəm'petɪtər] *in contest* competidor,a *m*,*f*; COM concorrente *m*/*f*

compile [kəm'paɪl] *v/t* compilar

complacency [kəm'pleɪsənsɪ] convencimento *m*; *Port* complacência *f*

complacent [kəm'pleɪsənt] *adj* convencido; *Port* complacente

complain [kəm'pleɪn] *v/i* reclamar; *to shop*, *manager* queixar-se; **~ *of*** MED queixar-se de

complaint [kəm'pleɪnt] reclamação *f*; MED doença *f*

complement ['kɑːmplɪmənt] *v/t* complementar; ***they ~ each other*** eles se complementam

complementary [kɑːmplɪ'mentərɪ] *adj* complementar

complete [kəm'pliːt] **1** *adj* completo; (*finished*) terminado **2** *v/t task*, *building etc* terminar; *course* concluir; *form* completar

completely [kəm'pliːtlɪ] *adv* completamente

completion [kəm'pliːʃn] conclusão *f*

complex ['kɑːmpleks] **1** *adj* complexo **2** *n* PSYCH complexo *f*; *buildings*: conjunto *m*

complexion [kəm'plekʃn] (*facial*) tez *f*

complexity [kəm'plekʃɪtɪ] complexidade *f*

compliance [kəm'plaɪəns] cumprimento *m*

complicate ['kɑːmplɪkeɪt] *v/t* complicar

complicated ['kɑːmplɪkeɪtɪd] *adj* complicado

complication [kɑːmplɪ'keɪʃn] complicação *f*

compliment ['kɑːmplɪmənt] **1** *n* cumprimento *m* **2** *v/t* cumprimentar

complimentary [kɑːmplɪ'mentərɪ] *adj*

lisonjeiro; (*free*) grátis; *in restaurant, hotel* de cortesia
'compliments slip nota *f* de cortesia
comply [kəm'plaɪ] *v/i* 〈*pret & pp* ***complied***〉 consentir; **~ *with*** cumprir com
component [kəm'poʊnənt] componente *m*
compose [kəm'poʊz] *v/t also* MUS compor; ***be ~d of*** ser composto de; **~ *oneself*** acalmar-se
composed [kəm'poʊzd] *adj* (*calm*) calmo
composer [kəm'poʊzər] MUS compositor,a *m,f*
composition [kɑːmpə'zɪʃn] (*make-up*) *also* MUS composição *f*; (*essay*) redação *f*
composure [kəm'poʊʒər] compostura *f*
compound ['kɑːmpaʊnd] *n* CHEM composto *m*
compound 'interest juros *m* compostos
comprehend [kɑːmprɪ'hend] *v/t* (*understand*) compreender
comprehension [kɑːmprɪ'henʃn] compreensão *f*
comprehensive [kɑːmprɪ'hensɪv] *adj* amplo
comprehensive in'surance seguro *m* total
comprehensively [kɑːmprɪ'hensɪvlɪ] *adv* amplamente; *beaten* completamente
comprehensive school *Brit* → ***high school***
compress 1 ['kɑːmpres] *n* MED compressa *f* **2** [kəm'pres] *v/t air, gas* comprimir; *information* resumir
comprise [kəm'praɪz] *v/t* compreender; ***be ~d of*** ser composto por
compromise ['kɑːmprəmaɪz] **1** *n* acordo *m* **2** *v/i* ceder **3** *v/t principles, also* (*jeopardize*) comprometer; **~ *oneself*** comprometer-se
compulsion [kəm'pʌlʃn] PSYCH compulsão *f*
compulsive [kəm'pʌlsɪv] *adj behavior, reading* compulsivo
compulsory [kəm'pʌlsərɪ] *adj* compulsório; **~ *education*** educação *f* compulsória
computer [kəm'pjuːtər] computador *m*; ***have sth on ~*** ter algo no computador
computer-aided de'sign projetos e desenhos *mpl* assistidos por computador **computer-con'trolled** *adj* controlado por computador **com'puter game** jogo *m* de computador
computerize [kəm'pjuːtəraɪz] *v/t* informatizar
computer 'literate *adj* ***applicants must be ~*** candidatos devem ter conhecimentos em informática **computer 'science** ciência *f* da computação, informática *f* **computer 'scientist** cientista *m/f* da computação
computing [kəm'pjuːtɪŋ] *n* computação *f*
comrade ['kɑːmreɪd] *also* POL camarada *m/f*
comradeship ['kɑːmreɪdʃɪp] camaradagem *f*
con [kɑːn] **1** *n fam* trapaça *f* **2** *v/t* 〈*pret & pp* ***conned***〉 *fam* trapacear
conceal [kən'siːl] *v/t* ocultar
concealment [kən'siːlmənt] ocultação *f*
concede [kən'siːd] *v/t* (*admit*) admitir; ***they ~d a goal in the last minute*** tiveram um gol marcado contra no último minuto
conceit [kən'siːt] presunção *f*
conceited [kən'siːtɪd] *adj* presunçoso
conceivable [kən'siːvəbl] *adj* concebível
conceive [kən'siːv] *v/i woman* conceber; **~ *of*** (*imagine*) imaginar
concentrate ['kɑːnsəntreɪt] **1** *v/i* concentrar-se; **~ *on a job*** concentrar-se em um trabalho **2** *v/t one's attention, energies* concentrar
concentrated ['kɑːnsəntreɪtɪd] *adj juice etc* concentrado
concentration [kɑːnsən'treɪʃn] concentração *f*
concept ['kɑːnsept] conceito *m*
conception [kən'sepʃn] *of child* concepção *f*
concern [kən'sɜːrn] **1** *n* (*care*) cuidado *m*; (*business*) empresa *f* **2** *v/t* (*in-*

volve) dizer respeito a; (*worry*) preocupar; ~ ***oneself with*** preocupar-se com
concerned [kən'sɜːrnd] *adj* (*anxious*) *also* (*caring*) preocupado; (*involved*) envolvido; ***as far as I'm*** ~ no meu entender
concerning [kən'sɜːrnɪŋ] *prep* sobre
concert ['kɑːnsərt] concerto *m*
concerted [kən'sɜːrtɪd] *adj* (*joint*) conjunto
'concertmaster *Am* primeiro violino *m*
concerto [kən'ʧertoʊ] concerto *m*
concession [kən'seʃn] (*compromise*) concessão *f*
conciliatory [kən'sɪlɪətɔːrɪ] *adj* conciliatório
concise [kən'saɪs] *adj* conciso
conclude [kən'kluːd] **1** *v/t* (*deduce, end*) concluir; ~ ***sth from sth*** concluir algo de algo **2** *v/i* terminar
conclusion [kən'kluːʒn] (*deduction, end*) conclusão *f*; ***in*** ~ para terminar
conclusive [kən'kluːsɪv] *adj* conclusivo
concoct [kən'kɑːkt] *v/t meal, drink* preparar; *excuse, story* urdir
concoction [kən'kɑːkʃn] *food, drink* mistura *f*
concrete ['kɑːŋkriːt] **1** *adj* concreto **2** *n* concreto *m*, *Port* betão *m*
concur [kən'kɜːr] *v/i* ⟨*pret & pp* ***concurred***⟩ concordar
concussion [kən'kʌʃn] concussão *f*
condemn [kən'dem] *v/t* condenar
condemnation [kɑːndəm'neɪʃn] condenação *f*
condensation [kɑːnden'seɪʃn] condensação *f*
condense [kən'dens] **1** *v/t* (*make shorter*) condensar **2** *v/i steam* condensar-se
condensed milk [kən'densd] leite *m* condensado
condescend [kɑːndɪ'send] *v/i* ***he*** ~***ed to speak to me*** ele dignou-se a falar comigo
condescending [kɑːndɪ'sendɪŋ] *adj* (*patronizing*) condescendente
condition [kən'dɪʃn] **1** *n* (*state, requirement*) condição *f*, MED estado *m*; ***on*** ~ ***that …*** com a condição de que … **2** *v/t* PSYCH condicionar
conditional [kən'dɪʃnl] **1** *adj acceptance* condicional **2** *n* GRAM tempo *m* condicional
conditioner [kən'dɪʃnər] *hair*: condicionador *m*; *fabric*: amaciante *f*
conditioning [kən'dɪʃnɪŋ] PSYCH condicionamento *m*
condo ['kɑːndoʊ] *Am fam* condomínio *m* fechado
condolences [kən'doʊlənsɪz] condolências *fpl*
condom ['kɑːndəm] preservativo *m*
condominium [kɑːndə'mɪnɪəm] condomínio *m* fechado
condone [kən'doʊn] *v/t actions* justificar
conducive [kən'duːsɪv] *adj* ~ ***to*** condutivo a
conduct **1** ['kɑːndʌkt] *n* (*behavior*) conduta *f* **2** [kən'dʌkt] *v/t* (*carry out*) conduzir; ELEC condutor *m*; MUS reger; ~ ***oneself*** conduzir-se
conducted tour [kən'dʌktɪd] passeio *m* guiado
conductor [kən'dʌktər] MUS regente *m/f*, *Am on train, also* PHYS condutor,a *m,f*
cone [koʊn] cone *m*; *ice cream*: casquinha *f*, *pine tree*: pinha *f*, *highway*: cone *m* de sinalização
confectioner [kən'fekʃənər] confeiteiro,-a *m,f*, *Port* pasteleiro,-a *m,f*
confectionery [kən'fekʃənerɪ] (*candy*) doces *mpl*
confederation [kənfedə'reɪʃn] confederação *f*
confer [kən'fɜːr] **1** *v/t* (*bestow*) conceder **2** *v/i* ⟨*pret & pp* ***conferred***⟩ (*discuss*) conferenciar
conference ['kɑːnfərəns] conferência *f*
'conference room sala *f* de conferência
confess [kən'fes] **1** *v/t* confessar; ***I*** ~ ***I don't know*** confesso que não sei **2** *v/i to crime, to police, also* REL confessar; ~ ***to a weakness for sth*** confessar ter uma fraqueza por algo
confession [kən'feʃn] *also* REL confissão *f*

C

C

confessional [kən'feʃnl] REL confessionário *m*
confessor [kən'fesər] REL confessor *m*
confide [kən'faɪd] **1** *v/t* confiar **2** *v/i* ~ ***in s.o.*** confiar em alguém
confidence ['kɑːnfɪdəns] (*assurance, trust*) confiança *f*; (*secret*) confidência *f*; ***in ~*** em confidencial
confident ['kɑːnfɪdənt] *adj* (*self-assured, convinced*) confiante
confidential [kɑːnfɪ'denʃl] *adj* confidencial
confidentially [kɑːnfɪ'denʃlɪ] *adv* confidencialmente
confidently ['kɑːnfɪdəntlɪ] *adv* confiantemente
confine [kən'faɪn] *v/t* (*imprison*) confinar; (*restrict*) restringir; ***be ~d to one's bed*** estar confinado ao leito
confined [kən'faɪnd] *adj space* confinado
confinement [kən'faɪnmənt] (*imprisonment*) confinamento *m*; MED parto *m*
confirm [kən'fɜːrm] *v/t* confirmar
confirmation [kɑːnfər'meɪʃn] confirmação *f*
confirmed [kən'fɜːrmd] *adj* (*inveterate*) convicto
confiscate ['kɑːnfɪskeɪt] *v/t* confiscar
conflict 1 ['kɑːnflɪkt] *n* (*disagreement, war*) conflito *m* **2** [kən'flɪkt] *v/i* (*clash*) conflitar
conform [kən'fɔːrm] *v/i* conformar-se; *product* estar em conformidade; ***~ to government standards*** está em conformidade com os padrões do governo
conformist [kən'fɔːrmɪst] *n* conformista *m/f*
confront [kən'frʌnt] *v/t* (*face*) enfrentar; (*tackle*) confrontar
confrontation [kɑːnfrən'teɪʃn] confronto *m*
confuse [kən'fjuːz] *v/t* confundir; ***~ s.o. with s.o.*** confundir alguém com alguém
confused [kən'fjuːzd] *adj* confuso
confusing [kən'fjuːzɪŋ] *adj* confuso
confusion [kən'fjuːʒn] confusão *f*
congeal [kən'dʒiːl] *v/i* coagular
congenial [kən'dʒiːnɪəl] *adj* (*pleasant*) agradável
congenital [kən'dʒenɪtl] *adj* MED congênito
congested [kən'dʒestɪd] *adj roads* congestionado
congestion [kən'dʒestʃn] *roads*: congestionamento *m*; *in chest* congestão *f*; ***traffic ~*** congestionamento *m* de trânsito
congratulate [kən'grætʊleɪt] *v/t* parabenizar
congratulations [kəngrætʊ'leɪʃnz] *npl* congratulações *fpl*; ***~ on …*** parabéns por …
congratulatory [kəngrætʊ'leɪtərɪ] *adj* de congratulações
congregate ['kɑːŋgrɪgeɪt] *v/i* (*gather*) congregar-se
congregation [kɑːŋgrɪ'geɪʃn] REL congregação *f*
congress ['kɑːŋgres] (*conference*) congresso *m*; ***Congress*** *US* Congresso *m* Nacional
Congressional [kən'greʃnl] *adj* do Congresso
Congressman ['kɑːŋgresmən] membro *m* do congresso
conifer ['kɑːnɪfər] conífera *f*
conjecture [kən'dʒektʃər] *n* (*speculation*) conjectura *f*
conjugate ['kɑːndʒʊgeɪt] *v/t* GRAM conjugar
conjunction [kən'dʒʌŋkʃn] GRAM conjunção *f*; ***in ~ with*** em conjunto com
conjunctivitis [kəndʒʌŋktɪ'vaɪtɪs] conjuntivite *f*
◆ **conjure up** ['kʌndʒər] *v/t* (*produce*) preparar; (*evoke*) evocar
conjurer, **conjuror** ['kʌndʒərər] mágico *m*
conjuring tricks ['kʌndʒərɪŋ] *npl* truques *mpl* de mágica
conjuror → ***conjurer***
con man ['kɑːnmæn] *fam* trapaceiro,-a *m,f*
connect [kə'nekt] *v/t* conectar; (*link*) associar
connected [kə'nektɪd] *adj* ***be well-~*** ter bons contatos; ***be ~ with …*** estar relacionado com …

connecting flight [kə'nektɪŋ] vôo *m* de conexão
connection [kə'nekʃn] conexão *f*; (*personal contact*) contato *m*; ***in ~ with …*** com relação a …
connoisseur [kɑːnə'sɜːr] conhecedor,a *m,f*
conquer ['kɑːŋkər] *v/t* conquistar; *fig fear etc* vencer
conqueror ['kɑːŋkərər] conquistador,a *m,f*
conquest ['kɑːŋkwest] conquista *f*
conscience ['kɑːnʃəns] consciência *f*; ***a guilty ~*** uma consciência pesada; ***it has been on my ~*** isso está pesando na minha consciência
conscientious [kɑːnʃɪ'enʃəs] *adj* consciencioso
conscientiousness [kɑːnʃɪ'enʃəsnəs] consciência *f*
conscientious ob'jector *pessoa que se recusa a servir as forças armadas por convicção*
conscious ['kɑːnʃəs] *adj also* MED consciente; ***be ~ of …*** estar consciente de …
consciously ['kɑːnʃəslɪ] *adv* conscientemente
consciousness ['kɑːnʃəsnɪs] (*awareness*) *also* MED consciência *f*, ***lose / regain ~*** perder / recobrar a consciência
consecutive [kən'sekjʊtɪv] *adj* consecutivo
consensus [kən'sensəs] consenso *m*
consent [kən'sent] **1** *n* consentimento *m* **2** *v/i* consentir
consequence ['kɑːnsɪkwəns] (*result*) conseqüência *f*
consequently ['kɑːnsɪkwəntlɪ] *adv* (*therefore*) conseqüentemente
conservation [kɑːnsər'veɪʃn] conservação *f*
conservationist [kɑːnsər'veɪʃnɪst] conservacionista *m/f*
conservative [kən'sɜːrvətɪv] **1** *adj* conservador; ***Conservative*** *Brit* POL conservador **2** *n Brit* POL membro *m* do partido conservador
conservatory [kən'sɜːrvətɔːrɪ] *for plants* estufa *f*; MUS conservatório *m*
conserve 1 ['kɑːnsɜːrv] *n* (*jam*) geléia *f* **2** [kən'sɜːrv] *v/t energy* conservar
consider [kən'sɪdər] *v/t* (*regard*) considerar; (*show regard for*) levar em consideração; (*think about*) pensar em; ***it is ~ed to be …*** isto é considerado como …
considerable [kən'sɪdrəbl] *adj* considerável
considerably [kən'sɪdrəblɪ] *adv* consideravelmente
considerate [kən'sɪdərət] *adj* atencioso
considerately [kən'sɪdərətlɪ] *adv* atenciosamente
consideration [kənsɪdə'reɪʃn] consideração *f*, ***take sth into ~*** levar algo em consideração
consignment [kən'saɪnmənt] COM consignação *f*
◆ **consist of** [kən'sɪst] *v/t* consistir em
consistency [kən'sɪstənsɪ] (*texture, unchangingness*) consistência *f*
consistent [kən'sɪstənt] *adj* (*unchanging*) consistente
consistently [kən'sɪstəntlɪ] *adv* consistentemente
consolation [kɑːnsə'leɪʃn] consolo *m*
console [kən'soʊl] *v/t* consolar
consolidate [kən'sɑːlɪdeɪt] *v/t* consolidar
consonant ['kɑːnsənənt] *n* GRAM consoante *f*
consortium [kən'sɔːrtɪəm] consórcio *m*
conspicuous [kən'spɪkjʊəs] *adj* conspícuo
conspiracy [kən'spɪrəsɪ] conspiração *f*
conspirator [kən'spɪrətər] conspirador,a *m,f*
conspire [kən'spaɪr] *v/i* conspirar
constant ['kɑːnstənt] *adj* constante
constantly ['kɑːnstəntlɪ] *adv* constantemente
consternation [kɑːnstər'neɪʃn] consternação *f*
constipated ['kɑːnstɪpeɪtɪd] *adj* com prisão de ventre
constipation [kɑːnstɪ'peɪʃn] prisão *f* de ventre
constituency [kən'stɪtʊənsɪ] *Brit* POL distrito *m* eleitoral

C

constituent [kən'stɪtʊənt] *n* (*component*) constituinte *m/f*; *Brit* POL eleitor,a *m,f*
constitute ['kɑːnstɪtuːt] *v/t* constituir
constitution [kɑːnstɪ'tuːʃn] POL constituição *f*
constitutional [kɑːnstɪ'tuːʃənl] *adj* POL constitucional
constraint [kən'streɪnt] (*restriction*) restrição *f*
construct [kən'strʌkt] *v/t* construir
construction [kən'strʌkʃn] construção *f*; (*trade*) ramo *m* da construção; ***under ~*** em construção
con'struction industry indústria *f* da construção **con'struction site** local *m* da construção **con'struction worker** trabalhador *m* de construção
constructive [kən'strʌktɪv] *adj* construtivo
consul ['kɑːnsl] cônsul,esa *m,f*
consulate ['kɑːnsʊlət] consulado *m*
consult [kən'sʌlt] *v/t* consultar
consultancy [kən'sʌltənsɪ] (*company*) empresa *f* de consultoria; (*advice*) consultoria *f*
consultant [kən'sʌltənt] *n* consultor,a *m,f*
consultation [kɑːnsl'teɪʃn] consulta *f*
consume [kən'suːm] *v/t* (*eat, drink, use*) consumir
consumer [kən'suːmər] consumidor,a *m,f*
consumer 'confidence confiança *f* do consumidor **con'sumer goods** bens *mpl* de consumo **con'sumer society** sociedade *f* de consumo
consumption [kən'sʌmpʃn] *of energy, water etc* consumo *m*
contact ['kɑːntækt] **1** *n* contato *m*; ***keep in ~ with s.o.*** manter contato com alguém **2** *v/t* contatar
'contact lens *nsg* lente *f* de contato
'contact number número *m* de contato
contagious [kən'teɪdʒəs] *adj illness* contagioso; *fig* contagiante
contain [kən'teɪn] *v/t tears, laughter* conter; ***it ~ed my camera*** continha minha câmara; ***~ oneself*** conter-se
container [kən'teɪnər] (*recipient*) recipiente *m*; COM contêiner *m*
con'tainer ship navio *m* porta-contêineres
contaminate [kən'tæmɪneɪt] *v/t* contaminar
contamination [kəntæmɪ'neɪʃn] contaminação *f*
contemplate ['kɑːntəmpleɪt] *v/t* contemplar; ***~ the idea of*** contemplar a idéia de
contemporary [kən'tempərerɪ] **1** *adj* contemporâneo **2** *n* contemporâneo,-a *m,f*
contempt [kən'tempt] desprezo *m*; ***be beneath ~*** estar abaixo da crítica
contemptible [kən'temptəbl] *adj* desprezível
contemptuous [kən'temptʊəs] *adj* desprezível
contend [kən'tend] *v/i* ***~ for …*** lutar por …; ***~ with …*** lutar com …
contender [kən'tendər] *in sport, competition* competidor,a *m,f*; *against champion* oponente *m/f*; POL adversário,-a *m,f*
content[1] ['kɑːntent] *n* conteúdo *m*
content[2] [kən'tent] **1** *adj* contente **2** *v/t* contentar; ***~ oneself with …*** contentar-se com …
contented [kən'tentɪd] *adj* satisfeito
contention [kən'tenʃn] (*assertion*) asserção *f*; ***be in ~ for …*** estar competindo por …
contentious [kən'tenʃəs] *adj* controverso
contentment [kən'tentmənt] contentamento *m*
contents ['kɑːntents] *npl of house, letter, bag* conteúdo *m*
contest[1] ['kɑːntest] *n* (*competition*) concurso *m*; (*struggle, for power*) disputa *f*
contest[2] [kən'test] *v/t leadership etc* disputar; (*oppose*) contestar
contestant [kən'testənt] adversário,-a *m,f*
context ['kɑːntekst] contexto *m*; ***look at sth in ~ / out of ~*** ver algo dentro / fora do contexto
continent ['kɑːntɪnənt] *n* continente *m*; ***the ~*** *Brit* o continente
continental [kɑːntɪ'nentl] *adj* conti-

nental; **~ Portuguese** português europeu

continental 'breakfast *Brit* café *m* continental

contingency [kən'tɪndʒənsɪ] contingência *f*

continual [kən'tɪnʊəl] *adj* contínuo

continually [kən'tɪnʊəlɪ] *adv* continuamente

continuation [kəntɪnʊ'eɪʃn] continuação *f*

continue [kən'tɪnju:] **1** *v/t* continuar; **to be ~d** segue **2** *v/i* continuar

continuity [kɑ:ntɪ'nu:ətɪ] continuidade *f*

continuous [kən'tɪnju:əs] *adj* contínuo

continuously [kən'tɪnju:əslɪ] *adv* continuamente

contort [kən'tɔ:rt] *v/t face, body* contorcer

contour ['kɑ:ntʊr] contorno *m*

contraception [kɑ:ntrə'sepʃn] contracepção *f*

contraceptive [kɑ:ntrə'septɪv] *n* (*device*) contraceptivo *m*; (*pill*) anticoncepcional *m*

contract[1] ['kɑ:ntrækt] *n* contrato *m*

contract[2] [kən'trækt] **1** *v/i* (*shrink*) contrair-se **2** *v/t illness* contrair

contractor [kən'træktər] contratante *m/f*

contractual [kən'træktʊəl] *adj* contratual

contradict [kɑ:ntrə'dɪkt] *v/t* contradizer

contradiction [kɑ:ntrə'dɪkʃn] contradição *f*

contradictory [kɑ:ntrə'dɪktərɪ] *adj* contraditório

contraption [kən'træpʃn] *fam* geringonça *f*

contrary[1] ['kɑ:ntrərɪ] **1** *adj* contrário; **~ to ...** ao contrário de ... **2** *n* **on the ~** muito pelo contrário

contrary[2] [kən'trerɪ] *adj* (*perverse*) do contra

contrast 1 ['kɑ:ntræst] *n* contraste *m* **2** [kən'træst] *v/t & v/i* contrastar

contrasting [kən'træstɪŋ] *adj* contrastante

contravene [kɑ:ntrə'vi:n] *v/t* infringir

contribute [kən'trɪbju:t] *v/t & v/i* contribuir

contribution [kɑ:ntrɪ'bju:ʃn] contribuição *f*

contributor [kən'trɪbjʊtər] *of money* contribuinte *m/f*; *to magazine* colaborador,a *m,f*

contrived [kən'traɪvd] *adj* artificial

control [kən'troʊl] **1** *n of country, organization, emotion* controle *m*; *ball game, sport*: domínio *m*; **lose ~ of ...** perder o controle de ...; **lose ~ of oneself** perder o controle das próprias emoções; **circumstances beyond our ~** circunstâncias *fpl* além do nosso controle; **be in ~ of ...** estar no controle de ...; **get out of ~** ficar fora de controle; **the situation is under ~** a situação está sob controle; **bring a blaze under ~** controlar um incêndio; **~s** *aircraft, vehicle*: controles *mpl*; (*restrictions*) restrições *fpl* **2** *v/t* controlar; **~ oneself** controlar-se

con'trol center *Am* centro *m* de controle

control centre → ***control center***

con'trol freak *fam* controlador,a *m,f*

controlled 'substance [kən'troʊld] substância *f* controlada

controlling 'interest [kən'troʊlɪŋ] FIN controle *m* acionário

con'trol panel painel *m* de controle

con'trol tower torre *f* de controle

controversial [kɑ:ntrə'vɜ:rʃl] *adj* controvertido

controversy ['kɑ:ntrəvɜ:rsɪ] controvérsia *f*

convalesce [kɑ:nvə'les] *v/i* convalescer

convalescence [kɑ:nvə'lesns] convalescença *f*

convene [kən'vi:n] *v/t* convocar

convenience [kən'vi:nɪəns] conveniência *f*; **at your / my ~** quando lhe / me convier; **all (modern) ~s** todos os confortos da vida moderna

con'venience food comida *f* de preparo rápido

con'venience store loja *f* de conveniência

C

convenient [kən'vi:nɪənt] *adj* conveniente
conveniently [kən'vi:nɪəntlɪ] *adv* convenientemente
convent ['kɑ:nvənt] convento *m*
convention [kən'venʃn] (*tradition, conference*) convenção *f*
conventional [kən'venʃnl] *adj* convencional
con'vention center *Am* centro *m* de convenções
conventioneer [kənvenʃ'nɪr] *Am* convencionalista *m/f*
♦**converge on** [kən'vɜ:rdʒ] *v/t* convergir para
conversant [kən'vɜ:rsənt] *adj* ***be ~ with …*** estar familiarizado com …
conversation [kɑ:nvər'seɪʃn] conversa *f*
conversational [kɑ:nvər'seɪʃnl] *adj* coloquial
converse ['kɑ:nvɜ:rs] *n* (*opposite*) inverso *m*
conversely [kən'vɜ:rslɪ] *adv* inversamente
conversion [kən'vɜ:rʃn] conversão *f*
con'version table tabela *f* de conversão
convert 1 ['kɑ:nvɜ:rt] *n* convertido,-a *m,f* **2** [kən'vɜ:rt] *v/t* converter
convertible [kən'vɜ:rtəbl] *n* (*car*) conversível *m*
convey [kən'veɪ] *v/t* (*transmit*) transmitir; (*carry*) transportar
conveyor belt [kən'veɪr] esteira *f* transportadora
convict 1 ['kɑ:nvɪkt] *n* condenado,-a *m,f* **2** [kən'vɪkt] *v/t* LAW condenar; ***~ s.o. of sth*** condenar alguém por algo
conviction [kən'vɪkʃn] LAW condenação *f*; (*belief*) convicção *f*
convince [kən'vɪns] *v/t* convencer
convincing [kən'vɪnsɪŋ] *adj* convincente
convivial [kən'vɪvɪəl] *adj* (*friendly*) simpático
convoy ['kɑ:nvɔɪ] comboio *m*
convulsion [kən'vʌlʃn] MED convulsão *f*
cook [kʊk] **1** *n* cozinheiro,-a *m,f* **2** *v/t* cozinhar; ***a ~ed meal*** uma refeição quente; ***~ the books*** *fam* falsificar os livros contábeis **3** *v/i* cozinhar
'cookbook livro *m* de receitas
cooker → ***stove***
cookery ['kʊkərɪ] culinária *f*
cookery book → ***cookbook***
cookie ['kʊkɪ] *Am* biscoito *m*
cooking ['kʊkɪŋ] (*food*) comida *f*
cool [ku:l] **1** *n* calma *f*; ***keep one's ~*** manter-se calmo; ***lose one's ~*** perder a calma **2** *adj weather, breeze* frio; *drink* gelado; (*calm*) calmo; (*unfriendly*) frio; *fam* legal **3** *v/i food* esfriar; *tempers* acalmar-se; *interest* diminuir **4** *v/t fam* ***~ it!*** relaxe!
♦**cool down 1** *v/i also fig tempers* acalmar-se **2** *v/t food* esfriar; *fig* acalmar
cooling-'off period período *m* para pensar
cooperate [koʊ'ɑ:pəreɪt] *v/i* cooperar
cooperation [koʊɑ:pə'reɪʃn] cooperação *f*
cooperative [koʊ'ɑ:pərətɪv] **1** *n* COM cooperativa *f* **2** *adj* COM *also* (*helpful*) cooperativo
coordinate [koʊ'ɔ:rdɪneɪt] *v/t activities* coordenar
coordination [koʊɔ:rdɪ'neɪʃn] coordenação *f*
cop [kɑ:p] *n fam* policial *m/f*, *Port* polícia *m/f*
cope [koʊp] *v/i* agüentar; ***~ with …*** agüentar com …
copier ['kɑ:pɪər] (*machine*) copiadora *f*
copilot ['koʊpaɪlət] co-piloto *m*
copious ['koʊpɪəs] *adj* copioso
copper ['kɑ:pər] *n* (*metal*) cobre *f*
copy ['kɑ:pɪ] **1** *n* (*duplicate, imitation*) *also of record, CD* cópia *f*; (*photocopy*) fotocópia *f*; *of book* exemplar *m*; (*written material*) matéria *f*; ***make a ~ of a file*** COMPUT fazer cópia de um arquivo **2** *v/t* ⟨*pret & pp* ***copied***⟩ copiar; (*photocopy*) fotocopiar
'copy cat *fam* maria *f* vai com as outras **copycat 'crime** crime *m* induzido pela mídia **'copyright** *n* direitos *mpl* autorais **'copy-writer** redator,a *m,f* de propaganda

C

coral ['kɑːrəl] coral *m*
cord [kɔːrd] (*string*) corda *f*; (*cable*) cabo *m*
cordial ['kɔːrdʒəl] *adj* cordial
cordless phone ['kɔːrdlɪs] telefone *m* sem fio
cordon ['kɔːrdn] cordão *m* de isolamento
♦ **cordon off** *v/t* cercar (com cordão de isolamento)
cords [kɔːrdz] (*pants*) calça *f* de veludo (cotelê), *Port* calças *fpl* de veludo (cotelê)
corduroy ['kɔːrdərɔɪ] veludo *m* cotelê
core [kɔːr] **1** *n fruit*: caroço *m*; *problem*: âmago *m*; *organization*: centro *m* **2** *v/t fruit* descaroçar **3** *adj issue*, *meaning* central
cork [kɔːrk] *in bottle* rolha *f*; (*material*) cortiça *f*
'**corkscrew** *n* saca-rolhas *m*
corn [kɔːrn] (*grain*) *Am* milho *m*; *Brit* cereal *m*
corner ['kɔːrnər] **1** *n page*, *room*: canto *m*; *street*: esquina *f*; *table*: quina *f*; (*bend on road*) curva *f*; *soccer*: córner *m*; ***in the ~*** no canto; ***on the ~*** *of street* na esquina **2** *v/t person* encurralar; ***~ the market*** monopolizar o mercado **3** *v/i driver*, *car* fazer curva
'**corner kick** *soccer*: escanteio *m*
'**cornflakes** *n/pl* flocos *mpl* de milho
cornflour *Brit* → ***cornstarch***
'**cornstarch** *Am* amido *m* de milho
corny ['kɔːrnɪ] *adj fam* banal
coronary ['kɑːrənerɪ] **1** *adj* coronário **2** *n* ataque *m* cardíaco
coroner ['kɑːrənər] investigador,a *m,f* criminal
corporal ['kɔːrpərəl] *n* MIL cabo *m*
corporal 'punishment castigo *m* corporal
corporate ['kɔːrpərət] *adj* COM empresarial; ***~ image*** imagem *f* da empresa; ***sense of ~ loyalty*** senso *m* de lealdade corporativa
corporation [kɔːrpə'reɪʃn] (*business*) empresa *f*
corps [kɔːr] *nsg* corpo *m*
corpse [kɔːrps] cadáver *m*
corpulent ['kɔːrpjʊlənt] *adj* corpulento
corpuscle ['kɔːrpʌsl] *in blood* glóbulo *m*
corral [kə'ræl] *n* curral *m*
correct [kə'rekt] **1** *adj* correto **2** *v/t* corrigir
correction [kə'rekʃn] correção *f*
correctly [kə'rekktlɪ] *adv* corretamente
correspond [kɑːrɪ'spɑːnd] *v/i* (*match*) corresponder; (*write letters*) corresponder-se; ***~ to ...*** corresponder a ...; ***~ with ...*** corresponder com ...
correspondence [kɑːrɪ'spɑːndəns] (*matching*, *also letters*) correspondência *f*; (*exchange of letters*) troca *f* de correspondência
correspondent [kɑːrɪ'spɑːndənũt] (*letter writer*, *also reporter*) correspondente *m/f*
corresponding [kɑːrɪ'spɑːndɪŋ] *adj* (*equivalent*) correspondente
corridor ['kɔːrɪdɔːr] *in building* corredor *m*
corroborate [kə'rɑːbəreɪt] *v/t* corroborar
corrode [kə'roʊd] **1** *v/t* corroer **2** *v/i* corroer-se
corrosion [kə'roʊʒn] corrosão *f*
corrugated 'cardboard ['kɑːrəgeɪtɪd] papelão *m* ondulado
corrugated 'iron chapa *f* ondulada
corrupt [kə'rʌpt] **1** *adj* corrupto **2** *v/t* corromper
corruption [kə'rʌpʃn] corrupção *f*
cosmetic [kɑːz'metɪk] *adj also fig* cosmético
cosmetics [kɑːz'metɪks] cosméticos *mpl*
cosmetic 'surgeon cirurgião (cirurgiã) plástico,-a *m,f*
cosmetic 'surgery cirurgia *f* plástica
cosmonaut ['kɑːzmənɒːt] cosmonauta *m/f*
cosmopolitan [kɑːzmə'pɑːlɪtən] *adj city* cosmopolita
cost[1] [kɑːst] **1** *n* custo *m* **2** *v/t* ⟨*pret & pp* ***cost***⟩ custar; *time* custar a; ***how much does it ~?*** quanto custa?; ***it ~ me my health*** custou-me a saúde
cost[2] [kɑːst] *v/t* ⟨*pret & pp* ***costed***⟩ FIN *proposal*, *project* calcular os custos de

cost and 'freight COM com custo e frete
Costa Rica [kɑːstə'riːkə] Costa Rica *f*
Costa Rican [kɑːstə'riːkən] **1** *adj* costarriquenho **2** *n* costarriquenho,-a *m,f*
'cost-conscious *adj* consciente dos custos **'cost-effective** *adj* rentável **'cost, insurance and freight** COM com custo, seguro e frete
costly ['kɑːstlɪ] *adj mistake* caro
cost of 'living custo *m* de vida
'cost price preço *m* de custo
costume ['kɑːstuːm] traje *m*
costume jewellery → ***costume jewelry***
'costume jewelry bijuteria *f*
cosy *Brit* → ***cozy***
cot [kɑːt] *Am* (*camp-bed*) cama *f* de campanha; *Brit* berço *m*
cottage ['kɑːtɪdʒ] casa *f* de campo
cottage 'cheese ricota *f*, *Port* queijo *m* creme
cotton ['kɑːtn] **1** *n* algodão *m* **2** *adj* de algodão
♦**cotton on** *v/i fam* entender
♦**cotton on to** *v/t fam* perceber
♦**cotton to** *v/t fam* apegar-se a
cotton 'candy *Am* algodão *m* doce
cotton 'wool *Brit* algodão *m* hidrófilo
couch [kaʊtʃ] *n* divã *m*
couchette [kuː'ʃet] leito *m*
'couch potato *fam* viciado,-a *m,f* em televisão
cough [kɑːf] **1** *n* tosse *f*; *to get attention* pigarro *m* **2** *v/i* tossir; *to get attention* pigarrear
♦**cough up 1** *v/t blood etc* expectorar; *fam money* soltar **2** *v/i fam* (*pay*) pagar
'cough medicine, **'cough syrup** antitússico *m*
cough syrup → ***cough medicine***
could [kʊd] *pret* → ***can***[1]; ***~ I have my key?*** poderia pegar minha chave?; ***~ you help me?*** você poderia ajudar-me?; ***this ~ be our bus*** este poderia ser nosso ônibus; ***you ~ be right*** você pode estar certo; ***I ~n't say for sure*** não poderia dizer ao certo; ***he ~ have got lost*** ele pode ter se perdido; ***you ~ have warned me!*** você poderia ter me avisado!
council ['kaʊnsl] (*assembly*) concílio *m*; (*advisory body*) conselho *m*
councillor → ***councilor***
'councilman *Am* vereador *m*
councilor ['kaʊnsələr] *Am* vereador,a *m,f*
counsel ['kaʊnsl] **1** *n* (*advice*) conselho *m*; (*lawyer*) advogado,-a *m,f* **2** *v/t course of action, person* aconselhar
counseling ['kaʊnslɪŋ] *Am* aconselhamento *m*
counselling → ***counseling***
counsellor → ***counselor***
counselor ['kaʊnslər] *Am* (*adviser*), conselheiro,-a *m,f*, LAW advogado,-a *m,f*
count[1] [kaʊnt] **1** *n* (*number arrived at*) soma *f*; (*action of counting*) *also in baseball, boxing* contagem *f*; ***keep ~ of ...*** contar ...; ***lose ~ of ...*** perder a conta de ...; ***at the last ~*** na última contagem **2** *v/i to ten etc, also* (*be important, qualify*) contar; (*calculate*) fazer contas **3** *v/t* contar
count[2] [kaʊnt] *n noble* conde *m*
♦**count on** *v/t* contar com
'countdown contagem *f* regressiva
countenance ['kaʊntənəns] *v/t* tolerar
counter[1] ['kaʊntər] *n in shop, café* balcão *m*; *in game* peça *f*
counter[2] ['kaʊntər] **1** *v/t* contrariar **2** *v/i* (*retaliate*) rebater
counter[3] ['kaʊntər] *adv* contrariamente; ***run ~ to ...*** ser contrário a ...
'counteract *v/t* neutralizar
'counter-attack 1 *n* contra-ataque *m* **2** *v/i* contra-atacar
'counterbalance 1 *n* contrapeso *m* **2** *v/t* contrabalançar
counter'clockwise *adv Am* em sentido anti-horário
counter'espionage contra-espionagem *f*
counterfeit ['kaʊntərfɪt] **1** *v/t* falsificar **2** *adj* falsificado
'counterpart *person* homólogo,-a *m,f*
counterpro'ductive *adj* contraproducente
'countersign *v/t* autenticar

countess ['kaʊntes] condessa *f*
countless ['kaʊntlɪs] *adj* inumerável
country ['kʌntrɪ] *n* (*nation*) país *m*; *as opposed to town* campo *m*; ***in the ~*** no campo
country and 'western MUS country *m* **'countryman** (*fellow countryman*) compatriota *m* **'countryside** campo *m*
county ['kaʊntɪ] condado *m*
coup [ku:] POL *also fig* golpe *m*
couple ['kʌpl] *n* (*married, man & woman*) casal *m*; (*two people*) par *m*; ***just a ~*** apenas alguns; ***a ~ of …*** alguns …
coupon ['ku:pɑ:n] (*form*) cupom *m*, *Port* cupão *m*; (*voucher*) vale *m*
courage ['kʌrɪdʒ] coragem *f*
courageous [kə'reɪdʒəs] *adj* corajoso
courier ['kʊrɪr] (*messenger*) mensageiro,-a *m,f*; *with tourist party* guia *m/f*
course [kɔ:rs] *n* (*series of lessons*) *also ship, plane*: curso *m*; (*part of meal*) prato *m*; *for sports event* campo *m*; ***of ~*** (*certainly*) (é) claro; (*naturally*) naturalmente; ***of ~ not*** (é) claro que não; ***~ of action*** modo *m* de ação; ***~ of treatment*** transcurso *m* do tratamento; ***in the ~ of …*** no decurso de …
court [kɔ:rt] *n also* LAW corte *f*; (*courthouse*) tribunal *m* de justiça; SPORT quadra *f*; ***take s.o. to ~*** levar alguém a julgamento
'court case processo *m* judicial
courteous ['kɜ:rtɪəs] *adj* cortês,-esa
courtesy ['kɜ:rtəsɪ] cortesia *f*
'courthouse tribunal *m* de justiça **court 'martial 1** *n* corte *f* marcial **2** *v/t* levar à corte marcial **'court order** mandado *m* judicial **'courtroom** sala *f* do tribunal **'courtyard** pátio *m*
cousin ['kʌzn] primo,-a *m,f*
cove [koʊv] (*small bay*) enseada *f*
cover ['kʌvər] **1** *n* (*protective*) *also book, magazine*: capa *f*; *bed*: cobertor *m*; (*shelter, insurance*) cobertura *f*; (*shelter from rain*) abrigo *m* **2** *v/t things, journalist, also* (*hide*) cobrir; *insurance policy* dar cobertura; *30 miles etc* cobrir uma distância de
♦ **cover up 1** *v/t crime, scandal etc* encobrir **2** *v/i fig* encobrir; ***cover up for s.o.*** encobrir alguém
coverage ['kʌvərɪdʒ] *by media* cobertura *f*
covering letter ['kʌvrɪŋ] carta *f* de introdução
covert ['koʊvɜ:rt] *adj* secreto
'cover-up disfarce *m*
cow [kaʊ] vaca *f*
coward ['kaʊərd] covarde *m/f*
cowardice ['kaʊərdɪs] covardia *f*
cowardly ['kaʊərdlɪ] *adj* covarde
'cowboy vaqueiro *m*
cower ['kaʊər] *v/i* encolher-se
coy [kɔɪ] *adj* (*evasive*) evasivo; (*flirtatious*) tímido
cozy ['koʊzɪ] *adj Am* aconchegante
CPU [si:pi:'ju:] *abbr* (*of **central processing unit***) CPU *f* (unidade *f* central de processamento)
crab [kræb] *n* caranguejo *m*
crack [kræk] **1** *n wall, cup, glass*: rachadura *f*; (*joke*) piadinha *f* **2** *v/t cup, glass* rachar; *nut* partir; *code* quebrar; *fam* (*solve*) resolver; ***~ a joke*** contar uma piada **3** *v/i* rachar; ***get ~ing*** *fam* pegar no batente
♦ **crack down on** *v/t* ser duro com
♦ **crack up** *v/i* (*have breakdown*) ter um colapso nervoso; *fam* (*laugh*) cair na gargalhada
'crackbrained *adj fam* tolo
crack (co'caine) crack *m*
'crackdown ***have a ~ on*** fazer uma batida em
cracked [krækt] *adj cup, glass* rachado; *fam* (*crazy*) pirado
cracker ['krækər] *to eat* biscoito *m* cream cracker
crackle ['krækl] *v/i fire* crepitar
cradle ['kreɪdl] *n for baby* berço *m*
craft[1] [kræft] NAUT embarcação *f*
craft[2] [kræft] (*skill*) arte *f*; (*trade*) ofício *m*
craftsman ['kræftsmən] artesão *m*
crafty ['kræftɪ] *adj* astuto
crag [kræg] (*rock*) penhasco *m*
cram [kræm] *v/t* enfiar
cramp [kræmp] *n* cólica *f*
cramped [kræmpt] *adj room* apertado
cramps [kræmps] *Am* cólica *f*
cranberry ['krænberɪ] oxicoco *m*

crane [kreɪn] **1** *n machine* guindaste *m* **2** *v/t* **~ *one's neck*** estender o pescoço
'cranefly pernilongo *m*
crank [kræŋk] *n (strange person)* excêntrico,-a *m,f*
'crankshaft eixo *m* de manivelas
cranky ['kræŋkɪ] *adj Am (bad-tempered)* irritado
crash [kræʃ] **1** *n (noise)* estrondo *m*; *(accident)* colisão *f*; *(plane crash)* queda *f*; COM quebra *f*; COMPUT falha *f* geral **2** *v/i (make noise)* despedaçar-se; *thunder* bramir; *car* colidir; *airplane* cair; COM *market* quebrar; COMPUT travar; *fam (sleep)* dormir **3** *v/t car* bater
♦ **crash out** *v/i fam (fall asleep)* apagar
'crash barrier muro *m* de proteção **'crash course** curso *m* intensivo **'crash diet** dieta *f* intensiva **'crash helmet** capacete *m* **'crash-land** *v/i* fazer uma aterrissagen de emergência **'crash landing** aterrissagem *f* forçada, *Port* aterrissagem *f* forçosa
crate [kreɪt] *(packing case)* caixote *m*
crater ['kreɪtər] *volcano*: cratera *f*
crave [kreɪv] *v/t* desejar fortemente
craving ['kreɪvɪŋ] desejo *m* forte
crawl [krɒːl] **1** *n in swimming* nado *m* livre; ***at a ~*** *(very slowly)* muito lentamente **2** *v/i on floor* rastejar; *baby* engatinhar; *(move slowly)* arrastar-se
♦ **crawl with** *v/t* ferver de
crayon ['kreɪən] *n* lápis *m* de cera
craze [kreɪz] moda *f*; ***the latest ~*** a última moda
crazy ['kreɪzɪ] *adj* louco; ***be ~ about*** ser louco por
creak [kriːk] **1** *n* rangido *m* **2** *v/i* ranger
creaky ['kriːkɪ] *adj* rangente
cream [kriːm] **1** *n for skin, coffee, cake, also (color)* creme *m* **2** *adj* creme
cream 'cheese requeijão *m*, *Port* queijo *m* creme
creamer ['kriːmər] *Am (pitcher)* pote *m* de creme; *for coffee* creme *m*
creamy ['kriːmɪ] *adj (with lots of cream)* cremoso
crease [kriːs] **1** *n (accidental)* amassado *m*; *deliberate* vinco *m* **2** *v/t accidentally* amassar
create [kriː'eɪt] *v/t & v/i* criar
creation [kriː'eɪʃn] criação *f*
creative [kriː'eɪtɪv] *adj* criativo
creator [kriː'eɪtər] criador,a *m,f*; ***the Creator*** REL o Criador
creature ['kriːtʃər] criatura *f*
crèche [kreʃ] *n for children* creche *f*
creche [kreʃ] *n* REL presépio *m*
credibility [kredə'bɪlətɪ] credibilidade *f*
credible ['kredəbl] *adj (believable)* acreditável; *candidate etc* digno de crédito
credit ['kredɪt] **1** *n* FIN, *(honor, payment received)* crédito *m*; ***be in ~*** ter crédito; ***get the ~ for sth*** obter o crédito por **2** *v/t (believe)* acreditar; ***~ an amount to an account*** creditar um valor em uma conta
creditable ['kredɪtəbl] *adj* respeitável
'credit card cartão *m* de crédito **'credit crunch** crise *f* de crédito **'credit limit** limite *m* de crédito
creditor ['kredɪtər] credor,a *m,f*
'creditworthy *adj* que tem crédito
credulous ['kredʊləs] *adj* crédulo
creed [kriːd] *(beliefs)* crença *f*
creek [kriːk] *Am (stream)* riacho *f*
creep [kriːp] **1** *n pej* nojento,-a *m,f* **2** *v/i* ⟨*pret & pp* ***crept***⟩ deslizar
creeper ['kriːpər] BOT trepadeira *f*
creeps [kriːps] *fam* arrepios *mpl*; ***the house / he gives me the ~*** a casa / ele me dá arrepios
creepy ['kriːpɪ] *adj fam* assustador
cremate [krɪ'meɪt] *v/t* cremar
cremation [krɪ'meɪʃn] cremação *f*
crematorium [kremə'tɔːrɪəm] crematório *m*
crept [krept] *pret & pp* → ***creep***
crescent ['kresənt] *(shape)* crescente *m*
crest [krest] *hill*: topo *m*; *bird*: crista *f*
'crestfallen *adj* desapontado
crevasse → ***crevice***
crevice ['krevɪs] fenda *f*
crew [kruː] *n ship, airplane*: tripulação *f*; *repairmen etc*: equipe *f*; *(crowd, group)* turma *f*
'crew cut corte *m* à escovinha

'crew neck gola *f* redonda
crib [krɪb] *n baby*: berço *m*
crick [krɪk] **~ *in the neck*** torcicolo
cricket ['krɪkɪt] *insect* grilo *m*
crime [kraɪm] crime *m*
criminal ['krɪmɪnl] **1** *n* criminoso,-a *m,f* **2** *adj* criminoso; LAW (*not civil*) penal; (*shameful*) vergonhoso
crimson ['krɪmzn] *adj* carmesim
cringe [krɪndʒ] *v/i* envergonhar-se
cripple ['krɪpl] **1** *n* (*disabled person*) deficiente *m/f* **2** *v/t person* aleijar; *fig* arruinar
crisis ['kraɪsɪs] ⟨*pl crises*⟩ crise *f*
crisp [krɪsp] *adj weather, air* fresco; *lettuce, apple* estaladiço; *bacon, toast* tostado; *dollar bill* limpo
crisps [krɪsps] *npl Brit* batatinha *f* frita
criterion [kraɪ'tɪrɪən] critério *m*
critic ['krɪtɪk] crítico,-a *m,f*
critical ['krɪtɪkl] *adj* (*making criticisms, serious*) crítico; *moment etc* crucial; MED grave
critically ['krɪtɪklɪ] *adv speak etc* criticamente; **~ *ill*** gravemente doente
criticism ['krɪtɪsɪzm] crítica *f*
criticize ['krɪtɪsaɪz] *v/t* criticar
croak [kroʊk] **1** *n frog*: coaxo *m*; *person*: rouquidão *f* **2** *v/i frog* coaxar; *person* rouquejar
crochet ['kroʊʃeɪ] *n* crochê *m*
crockery ['krɑːkərɪ] louça *f*
crocodile ['krɑːkədaɪl] crocodilo *m*
crocus ['kroʊkəs] açafrão-da-primavera *m*
crony ['kroʊnɪ] *fam* compadre *m*
crook [krʊk] *n dishonest* vigarista *m/f*
crooked ['krʊkɪd] *adj* (*not straight*) torto; *fam* (*dishonest*) desonesto
crop [krɑːp] **1** *n* colheita *f*; *fig* safra *f* **2** *v/t* ⟨*pret & pp* ***cropped***⟩ *hair, photo* cortar
♦ **crop up** *v/i* surgir
cross [krɑːs] **1** *adj* (*angry*) zangado **2** *n* cruz *f* **3** *v/t* (*go across*) atravessar, cruzar; **~ *oneself*** REL fazer o sinal da cruz; **~ *one's legs*** cruzar as pernas; ***keep one's fingers ~ed*** manter os dedos cruzados; ***it never ~ed my mind*** isto jamais me passou pela cabeça **4** *v/i* (*go across*) atravessar; *lines* cruzar-se
♦ **cross off, cross out** *v/t* riscar
'crossbar *goal*: trave *f*; *bicycle*: barra *f*; *high jump*: barra *f* transversal **'crosscheck 1** *n* rechecagem *f* **2** *v/t* rechecar **cross-'country, cross-country 'skiing** esqui *m* cross-country
crossed 'check [krɑːst] *Am* cheque *m* cruzado
cross-exami'nation LAW repergunta *f* **cross-ex'amine** *v/t* LAW reperguntar **cross-eyed** ['krɑːsaɪd] *adj* vesgo
crossing ['krɑːsɪŋ] NAUT travessia *f*
cross out → ***cross off***
'crossroads *nsg* cruzamento *m*; *fig* encruzilhada *f* **'cross-section** *of people* corte *m* representativo **'crosswalk** *Am* faixa *f* de pedestres, *Port* passadeira *f* **'crossword puzzle** palavras *fpl* cruzadas
crotch [krɑːtʃ] *of person* virilha *f*, *of pants* fundilho *m*
crouch [kraʊtʃ] *v/i* agachar-se
crow [kroʊ] *n* (*bird*) corvo *m*; ***as the ~ flies*** pelo caminho mais curto
'crowbar pé-de-cabra *m*
crowd [kraʊd] *n also at sports event* multidão *f*
crowded ['kraʊdɪd] *adj* lotado
crown [kraʊn] **1** *n king, tooth*: coroa *f* **2** *v/t tooth* colocar uma coroa em
crucial ['kruːʃl] *adj* crucial
crucifix ['kruːsɪfɪks] crucifixo *m*
crucifixion [kruːsɪ'fɪkʃn] crucificação *f*
crucify ['kruːsɪfaɪ] *v/t* ⟨*pret & pp* ***crucified***⟩ *also fig* crucificar
crude [kruːd] **1** *adj* (*vulgar*) grosseiro; (*unsophisticated*) tosco **2** *n* **~ (*oil*)** petróleo *m* bruto
crudely ['kruːdlɪ] *adv speak, made* grosseiramente
cruel ['kruːəl] *adj* cruel
cruelty ['kruːəltɪ] crueldade *f*
cruise [kruːz] **1** *n* cruzeiro *f* **2** *v/i people* fazer um cruzeiro; *plane* voar a uma velocidade cruzeiro; ***I was cruising around in my new car*** estava passeando no meu carro novo
'cruise liner navio *m* para cruzeiro

C

cruising speed ['kru:zɪŋ] velocidade *f* cruzeiro; *fig project etc*: ritmo *m* normal
crumb [krʌm] migalha *f*
crumble ['krʌmbl] **1** *v/t* esmigalhar **2** *v/i bread, stonework* esmigalhar; *fig opposition etc* aniquilar
crumbly ['krʌmblɪ] *adj* farelento
crumple ['krʌmpl] **1** *v/t (crease)* amarrotar **2** *v/i (collapse)* desmoronar
crunch [krʌntʃ] **1** *n fam* momento *m* decisivo; ***when it comes to the ~*** ao chegar o momento decisivo **2** *v/i snow, gravel* ranger
crusade [kru:'seɪd] *n also fig* cruzada *f*
crush [krʌʃ] **1** *n (crowd)* aglomeração *f*; ***have a ~ on*** ter uma paixão por **2** *v/t* esmagar; *(crease)* amassar; ***they were ~ed to death*** eles morreram esmagados **3** *v/i (crease)* amarrotar
crust [krʌst] *on bread* casca *f*
crusty ['krʌstɪ] *adj bread* com casca
crutch [krʌtʃ] *for injured person* muleta *f*
cry [kraɪ] **1** *n (call)* grito *m*; *(weep)* choro *m* **2** *v/t* ⟨*pret & pp* ***cried***⟩ *(call)* gritar **3** *v/i* ⟨*pret & pp* ***cried***⟩ *(weep)* chorar
♦ **cry out** *v/t & v/i* berrar
♦ **cry out for** *v/t (need)* precisar desesperadamente
cryptic ['krɪptɪk] *adj* enigmático
crystal ['krɪstl] cristal *m*
crystallize ['krɪstlaɪz] **1** *v/t* cristalizar **2** *v/i thoughts etc* cristalizar-se
cub [kʌb] filhote *m*
Cuba ['kju:bə] Cuba
Cuban ['kju:bən] **1** *adj* cubano **2** *n* cubano,-a *m,f*
cube [kju:b] cubo *m*
cubic ['kju:bɪk] *adj* cúbico
cubic ca'pacity *engine*: cilindrada *f*
cubicle ['kju:bɪkl] *(changing room)* cubículo *m*
cucumber ['kju:kʌmbər] pepino *m*
cuddle ['kʌdl] **1** *n* afago *m* **2** *v/t* afagar
cuddly ['kʌdlɪ] *adj kitten etc* carinhoso; *(liking cuddles)* chameguento
cue [kju:] *n for actor* deixa *f*; *for pool* taco *m*
cuff [kʌf] **1** *n of shirt* punho *m*; *Am of pants* bainha *f*; *(blow)* bofetada *f*; ***off the ~*** de improviso **2** *v/t (hit)* esbofetear
'cuff link abotoadura *f*
cul-de-sac ['kʌldəsæk] beco *m* sem saída
culinary ['kʌlɪnerɪ] *adj* culinário
culminate ['kʌlmɪneɪt] *v/i* culminar; ***~ in ...*** terminar em ...
culmination [kʌlmɪ'neɪʃn] auge *m*
culprit ['kʌlprɪt] culpado,-a *m,f*
cult [kʌlt] *(sect)* culto *m*
cultivate ['kʌltɪveɪt] *v/t land* cultivar; *person* cultivar a amizade de
cultivated ['kʌltɪveɪtɪd] *adj person* culto
cultivation [kʌltɪ'veɪʃn] *of land* cultivo *m*
cultural ['kʌltʃərəl] *adj* cultural
culture ['kʌltʃər] *n* cultura *f*
cultured ['kʌltʃərd] *adj* culto
'culture shock choque *m* cultural
cumbersome ['kʌmbərsəm] *adj package* difícil de manusear; *method etc* complicado
cumulative ['kju:mjʊlətɪv] *adj* acumulativo
cunning ['kʌnɪŋ] **1** *n* astúcia *f* **2** *adj* astuto
cup [kʌp] *n* xícara *f*, *Port* chávena *f*; *(trophy)* taça *f*; ***a ~ of tea*** uma xícara de chá; ***World Cup*** copa *f* do mundo
cupboard ['kʌbərd] cristaleira *f*, *Brit larger* armário *m*
'cup final final *f* da copa
cupola ['kju:pələ] cúpula *f*
curable ['kjʊrəbl] *adj* curável
curator [kjʊ'reɪtər] curador,a *m,f*
curb [kɜ:rb] **1** *n on powers etc* restrição *f*; *Am street*: meio-fio *m*, *Port* bordo *m* do passeio **2** *v/t* refrear
curdle ['kɜ:rdl] *v/i milk* coalhar
cure [kjʊr] **1** *n* MED cura *f* **2** *v/t* MED *also meat, fish* curar
curfew ['kɜ:rfju:] toque *m* de recolher
curiosity [kjʊrɪ'ɑ:sətɪ] *(inquisitiveness)* curiosidade *f*
curious ['kjʊrɪəs] *adj (inquisitive)* curioso; *(strange)* estranho
curiously ['kjʊrɪəslɪ] *adv (inquisitively)* curiosamente; *(strangely)* estra-

nhamente; ~ ***enough*** por mais estranho que pareça
curl [kɜːrl] **1** *n hair*: cacho *m*; *smoke*: anel *m* **2** *v/t hair* encaracolar; (*wind*) enrolar **3** *v/i hair* encaracolar-se; *leaf, paper etc* enrolar-se
◆ **curl up** *v/i* enrolar-se
curly ['kɜːrlɪ] *adj hair* encaracolado; *tail* enrolado
currant ['kʌrənt] *dried fruit* passa *f*
currency ['kʌrənsɪ] (*money*) moeda *f*; ***foreign*** ~ moeda *f* estrangeira
current ['kʌrənt] **1** *n in sea, also* ELEC corrente *f* **2** *adj* (*present*) atual
current account *Brit* → ***checking account***
current af'fairs, **current e'vents** *npl* atualidades *fpl*
current af'fairs program programa *m* de atualidades
current affairs programme → ***current affairs program***
currently ['kʌrəntlɪ] *adv* atualmente
curriculum [kə'rɪkjʊləm] currículo *m*
curriculum vitae → ***résumé***
curry ['kʌrɪ] (*spice*) caril *m*
curse [kɜːrs] **1** *n* (*spell*) praga *f*; (*swearword*) palavrão *m*, *Port* baixo calão *m* **2** *v/t* amaldiçoar; (*swear at*) xingar **3** *v/i* (*swear*) praguejar
cursor ['kɜːrsər] COMPUT cursor *m*
cursory ['kɜːrsərɪ] *adj* superficial
curt [kɜːrt] *adj* brusco
curtail [kɜːr'teɪl] *v/t* encurtar
curtain ['kɜːrtn] *also* THEA cortina *f*
curve [kɜːrv] **1** *n* curva *f* **2** *v/i* (*bend*) encurvar
cushion ['kʊʃn] **1** *n* almofada *f* **2** *v/t blow, fall* amortecer
custard ['kʌstərd] pudim *m* de ovos
custody ['kʌstədɪ] *of children* guarda *f*; LAW *f* custódia
custom ['kʌstəm] (*tradition*) costume *m*; COM clientela *f*; ***as was his*** ~ conforme seu costume
customary ['kʌstəmerɪ] *adj* costumeiro; ***it is*** ~ ***to …*** é costume …
customer ['kʌstəmər] cliente *m/f*
customer re'lations *npl* relacionamento *m* com clientes
customer 'service serviço *m* de atendimento aos clientes
customs ['kʌstəmz] alfândega *f*
Customs and 'Excise *Brit* Alfândega *f*
'customs clearance despacho *m* alfandegário **'customs inspection** inspeção *f* alfandegária **'customs officer** agente *m* alfandegário
cut [kʌt] **1** *n also of garment, hair,* (*injury*), (*reduction*) corte *m*; ***my hair needs a*** ~ meu cabelo precisa de um corte **2** *v/t* ⟨*pret & pp* ***cut***⟩ cortar; ***get one's hair*** ~ cortar o cabelo
◆ **cut back 1** *v/i costs*: reduzir despesas **2** *v/t employees* cortar
◆ **cut down 1** *v/t tree* derrubar **2** *v/i in smoking etc* diminuir
◆ **cut down on** *v/t smoking etc* diminuir
◆ **cut off** *v/t also* TEL cortar; (*isolate*) isolar; ***we were cut off*** nossa linha foi cortada
◆ **cut out** *v/t with scissors* recortar; (*eliminate*) eliminar; ***cut that out!*** *fam* pare com isso!; ***be cut out for sth*** ser talhado para algo
◆ **cut up** *v/t meat etc* picar
'cutback corte *m*
cute [kjuːt] *adj* (*pretty*) bonito; (*sexually attractive*) atraente; (*smart, clever*) esperto
cuticle ['kjuːtɪkl] cutícula *f*
cutlery *Brit* → ***flatware***
'cutoff date prazo *m* final
'cut-price *adj* preço *m* reduzido
'cut-throat *adj competition* cruel
cutting ['kʌtɪŋ] **1** *n from newspaper etc* recorte *m* **2** *adj remark* cortante
CV → ***résumé***
cyberspace ['saɪbərspeɪs] ciberespaço *m*
cycle ['saɪkl] **1** *n* (*bicycle*) bicicleta *f*; (*series of events*) ciclo *m* **2** *v/i to work etc* ir de bicicleta
'cycle path ciclovia *f*
cycling ['saɪklɪŋ] ciclismo *m*
cyclist ['saɪklɪst] ciclista *m/f*
cylinder ['sɪlɪndər] *container* bujão *m*; *in engine* cilindro *m*
cylindrical [sɪ'lɪndrɪkl] *adj* cilíndrico
cynic ['sɪnɪk] cínico,-a *m,f*
cynical ['sɪnɪkl] *adj* cínico
cynically ['sɪnɪklɪ] *adv* cinicamente

cynicism ['sɪnɪsɪzm] cinismo *m*
cyst [sɪst] cisto *m*
cystitis [sɪs'taɪtɪs] cistite *f*
Czech [tʃek] **1** *adj* checo; ***the ~ Republic*** a República Checa **2** *n person, language* checo,-a *m,f*

D

DA *Am abbr* (*of* ***district attorney***) promotor,a *m,f* público,-a
dab [dæb] **1** *n* (*small amount*) pouquinho *m* **2** *v/t* ⟨*pret & pp* ***dabbed***⟩ (*remove*) tocar levemente; (*apply*) aplicar de leve
♦ **dabble in** *v/t* interessar-se um pouco por
dad [dæd] pai *m*
daddy ['dædɪ] papai *m*
daddy 'longlegs *Brit* pernilongo *m*
daffodil ['dæfədɪl] narciso *m*
dagger ['dægər] adaga *f*
daily ['deɪlɪ] **1** *n* (*paper*) diário *m* **2** *adj* diário
dainty ['deɪntɪ] *adj* delicado
dairy ['derɪ] *on farm* leiteria *f*
'dairy products *npl* laticínios *mpl*
dais ['deɪɪs] estrado *m*
daisy ['deɪsɪ] margarida *f*
dam [dæm] **1** *n for water* barragem *f* **2** *v/t* ⟨*pret & pp* ***dammed***⟩ *river* construir uma barragem em
damage ['dæmɪdʒ] **1** *n* dano *m*; *fig to reputation etc* prejuízo *m* **2** *v/t* danificar; *fig reputation etc* prejudicar
damages ['dæmɪdʒɪz] *npl* LAW indenização *f*
damaging ['dæmɪdʒɪŋ] *adj* prejudicial
dame [deɪm] *fam* (*woman*) dama *f*
damn [dæm] **1** *interj fam* porra **2** *n fam* ***I don't give a ~!*** estou me lixando! **3** *adj fam* danado **4** *adv fam* demais; ***it's ~ hot*** é quente demais **5** *v/t* (*condemn*) condenar; ***~ it!*** *fam* que porra!; ***I'm ~ed if …*** *fam* que um raio me parta se …
damned [dæmd] *adj* maldito; *adj, adv* → ***damn***
damning ['dæmɪŋ] *adj evidence* prejudicial; *report* censurável
damp [dæmp] *adj* úmido
dampen ['dæmpən] *v/t* umedecer
dance [dæns] **1** *n* dança *f*; *social event* baile *m* **2** *v/i* dançar; ***would you like to ~?*** gostaria de dançar?
dancer ['dænsər] dançarino,-a *m,f*; *performer* bailarino,-a *m,f*
dancing ['dænsɪŋ] dança *f*
dandelion ['dændɪlaɪən] dente-de--leão *m*
dandruff ['dændrʌf] caspa *f*
dandruff sham'poo xampu *m* anticaspa
Dane [deɪn] dinamarquês *m*, dinamarquesa *f*
danger ['deɪndʒər] perigo *m*; ***be in ~*** estar em perigo; ***out of ~*** *patient* fora de perigo
dangerous ['deɪndʒərəs] *adj place, person, assumption etc* perigoso
dangerous 'driving direção *f* perigosa
dangerously ['deɪndʒərəslɪ] *adv drive* perigosamente; ***~ ill*** gravemente doente
dangle ['dæŋgl] **1** *v/t* balançar **2** *v/i* balançar-se
Danish ['deɪnɪʃ] **1** *adj* dinamarquês (dinamarquesa) **2** *n language* dinamarquês *m*; ***~ (pastry)*** pastel *m* folhado
dare [der] **1** *v/i* atrever-se; ***~ to do sth*** atrever-se a fazer algo; ***how ~ you!*** como você se atreve? **2** *v/t* ***~ X to do Y*** desafiar X a fazer Y
daredevil ['derdevɪl] atrevido,-a *m,f*
daring ['derɪŋ] *adj* atrevido
dark [dɑːrk] **1** *n* escuro *m*; ***after ~*** depois de escurecer; ***keep s.o. in the ~***

fig manter alguém no escuro **2** *adj* escuro; **~ *green / blue*** verde / azul-escuro

darken ['dɑːrkn] *v/i sky* escurecer

dark 'glasses óculos *mpl* escuros

darkness ['dɑːrknɪs] escuridão *f*

'darkroom PHOT câmara *f* escura

darling ['dɑːrlɪŋ] **1** *n* querido,-a *m,f* **2** *adj* querido

darn[1] [dɑːrn] **1** *n* (*mend*) remendo *m* **2** *v/t* (*mend*) remendar

darn[2] [dɑːrn] *adj, adv* → ***damn***

dart [dɑːrt] **1** *n for throwing* dardo *m* **2** *v/i* precipitar-se

'dartboard, 'dartsboard alvo *m* para dardos

darts [dɑːrts] *n pl* (*game*) dardos *mpl*

dash [dæʃ] **1** *n punctuation*: hífen *m*; (*small amount*) pitada *f*; MOT (*dashboard*) painel *m* de instrumentos; ***a ~ of brandy*** uma pitada de conhaque; ***make a ~ for*** correr para; ***make a ~ for it*** fugir **2** *v/i* ir depressa; ***I must ~*** preciso ir depressa **3** *v/t hopes* frustrar

♦ **dash off 1** *v/i* sair apressado **2** *v/t* (*write quickly*) escrever apressadamente

'dashboard painel *m* de instrumentos

data ['deɪtə] dados *mpl*

'database banco *m* de dados **data 'capture** captura *f* de dados **data 'processing** processamento *m* de dados **data pro'tection** proteção *f* de dados **data 'storage** armazenamento *m* de dados

date[1] [deɪt] *n* (*fruit*) tâmara *f*

date[2] [deɪt] **1** *n* data *f*; (*meeting*) encontro *m*; *person* acompanhante *m/f*; ***what's the ~ today?*** que dia é hoje?; ***out of ~*** *clothes* antiquado; *passport* expirado; ***up to ~*** atualizado **2** *v/t letter, check* datar; (*go out with*) namorar; ***that ~s you*** (*shows your age*) isto revela sua idade

dated ['deɪtɪd] *adj* antiquado

daub [dɔːb] *v/t* borrar

daughter ['dɒːtər] filha *f*

'daughter-in-law nora *f*

daunt [dɔːnt] *v/t* deter

dawdle ['dɔːdl] *v/i* perder tempo

dawn [dɒːn] **1** *n* amanhecer *m*; *fig of new age* alvorecer *m* **2** *v/i* ***it ~ed on me that ...*** comecei a perceber que ...

day [deɪ] dia *m*; ***what ~ is it today?*** que dia é hoje?; ***~ off*** dia de folga; ***by ~*** durante o dia; ***~ by ~*** dia a dia; ***the ~ after*** o dia seguinte; ***the ~ after tomorrow*** depois de amanhã; ***the ~ before*** o dia anterior; ***the ~ before yesterday*** anteontem; ***~ in ~ out*** dia após dia; ***in those ~s*** naquele tempo; ***one ~*** um dia; ***the other ~*** (*recently*) um dia desses; ***let's call it a ~!*** chega por hoje!

'daybreak amanhecer *m* **'day care** creche *f* **'daydream 1** *n* devaneio *m* **2** *v/i* devanear **'day dreamer** sonhador,a *m,f* **'daytime** *n* ***in the ~*** de dia, durante o dia **'daytrip** viagem *f* de um dia

daze [deɪz] *n* ***in a ~*** aturdido

dazed [deɪzd] *adj by news* aturdido; *by a blow* entorpecido

dazzle ['dæzl] *v/t light* ofuscar; *fig* deslumbrar

DC[1] *abbr* (*of* ***direct current***) corrente *f* contínua

DC[2] *abbr* (*of* ***District of Columbia***) Distrito *m* de Colúmbia

dead [ded] **1** *adj also fam place* morto; *battery* descarregado; *phone* cortado; *light bulb* queimado **2** *adv fam* (*very*) bastante; ***~ beat, ~ tired*** morto de cansaço; ***that's ~ right*** isto está totalmente certo **3** *n* ***the ~*** (*dead people*) os mortos; ***in the ~ of night*** no meio da noite

deaden ['dedn] *v/t pain, sound* amortecer

dead 'end (*street*) beco *m* sem saída **dead-'end job** trabalho *m* sem perspectivas **dead 'heat** empate *m* **'deadline** prazo *m* final; *for newspaper* fechamento *m* **'deadlock** *in talks* impasse *m*

deadly ['dedlɪ] *adj* (*fatal*) *also fam boring* mortal

deaf [def] *adj* surdo

deaf-and-'dumb *adj* surdo-mudo

deafen ['defn] *v/t* ensurdecer

deafening ['defnɪŋ] *adj* ensurdecedor

deafness ['defnɪs] surdez *f*

deal [diːl] **1** *n* negócio *m*; ***it's a ~!*** (*we have reached an agreement*) negócio fechado!; (*it's a promise*) está combinado; ***a good ~*** (*bargain*) um bom negócio; (*a lot*) um bocado; ***a great ~ of*** (*lots*) bastante **2** *v/t* ⟨*pret & pp* ***dealt***⟩ *cards* dar; ***~ a blow to*** dar um golpe em
♦ **deal in** *v/t* (*trade in*) negociar com
♦ **deal out** *v/t cards* dar
♦ **deal with** *v/t* (*handle*) tratar de; (*do business with*) fazer negócios com
dealer ['diːlər] (*merchant*) negociante *m/f*; (*drug dealer*) fornecedor,a *m,f*; *card game*: jogador *m* que dá as cartas
dealing ['diːlɪŋ] (*drug dealing*) tráfico *m* de drogas
dealings ['diːlɪŋz] *npl* (*business*) negócios *mpl*
dealt [delt] *pret & pp* → ***deal***
dean [diːn] *college*: reitor,a *m,f*
dear [dɪr] *adj* (*also expensive*) caro; ***Dear Sir*** Prezado Senhor; ***Dear Richard / Margaret*** Caro Richard / Cara Margaret; (***oh***) ***~!, ~ me!*** ai, meu Deus!
dearly ['dɪrlɪ] *adv love* ternamente; ***I would ~ like to …*** eu gostaria imensamente de …
death [deθ] morte *f*
'**death certificate** certidão *f* de óbito
'**death penalty** pena *f* de morte
'**death toll** número *m* de mortos
debatable [dɪ'beɪtəbl] *adj* discutível
debate [dɪ'beɪt] **1** *n* debate *m* **2** *v/t & v/i* debater
debauchery [dɪ'bɔːʧərɪ] devassidão *f*
debit ['debɪt] **1** *n* débito *m* **2** *v/t account, amount* debitar
'**debit card** cartão *m* de débito
debris [də'briː] escombros *mpl*
debt [det] dívida *f*; ***be in ~*** estar com dívidas
debtor ['detər] devedor,a *m,f*
debug [diː'bʌg] *v/t* ⟨*pret & pp* ***debugged***⟩ *room* eliminar os grampos de; COMPUT eliminar erros de
début ['deɪbjuː] *n* estréia *f*
decade ['dekeɪd] década *f*
decadence ['dekədəns] decadência *f*
decadent ['dekədənt] *adj* decadente
decaffeinated [dɪ'kæfɪneɪtɪd] *adj* descafeinado
decanter [dɪ'kæntər] decanter *m*
decapitate [dɪ'kæpɪteɪt] *v/t* decapitar
decay [dɪ'keɪ] **1** *n* deterioração *f*; (*decayed matter*) matéria *f* em decomposição; *in teeth* cárie *f* **2** *v/i* deteriorar; *teeth* cariar
deceased [dɪ'siːst] falecido; ***the ~*** o falecido (a falecida); os falecidos
deceit [dɪ'siːt] engano *m*
deceitful [dɪ'siːtfʊl] *adj* enganador
deceive [dɪ'siːv] *v/t* enganar
December [dɪ'sembər] dezembro *m*
decency ['diːsənsɪ] decência *f*; ***he had the ~ to …*** ele teve a decência de …
decent ['diːsənt] *adj person, salary* decente; *meal, sleep* suficiente; (*adequately dressed*) decoroso
decentralize [diː'sentrəlaɪz] *v/t* descentralizar
deception [dɪ'sepʃn] engano *m*
deceptive [dɪ'septɪv] *adj* enganoso
deceptively [dɪ'septɪvlɪ] *adv* ***it looks ~ simple*** parece simples mas não é
decibel ['desɪbel] decibel *m*
decide [dɪ'saɪd] **1** *v/t* decidir; (*conclude*) concluir **2** *v/i* decidir; ***you ~*** você decide
decided [dɪ'saɪdɪd] *adj* (*definite*) decidido
decider [dɪ'saɪdər] *match etc* disputa *f* final
deciduous [dɪ'sɪdʊəs] *adj* decíduo
decimal ['desɪml] *n* decimal *m*
decimal 'point vírgula *f* decimal
decimate ['desɪmeɪt] *v/t* dizimar
decipher [dɪ'saɪfər] *v/t* decifrar
decision [dɪ'sɪʒn] decisão *f*; (*conclusion*) conclusão *f*; ***come to a ~*** chegar a uma decisão
de'cision-maker tomador *m* de decisões
decisive [dɪ'saɪsɪv] *adj* decisivo
deck [dek] *ship*: convés *m*; *cards*: baralho *m*
'**deckchair** espreguiçadeira *f*
declaration [deklə'reɪʃn] declaração *f*; *of independence* proclamação *f*
declare [dɪ'kler] *v/t* (*state*) *also war, at customs* declarar; *independence* proclamar

decline [dɪ'klaɪn] **1** *n* (*fall*) declínio *m*; *in standards* queda *f*; *in health* agravamento *m* **2** *v/t invitation* declinar; **~ *to comment / accept*** negar-se a comentar / aceitar **3** *v/i* (*refuse*) recusar; (*decrease*) diminuir; *health* agravar-se
declutch [diː'klʌtʃ] *v/i* desengatar
decode [diː'koʊd] *v/t* decodificar
decompose [diːkəm'poʊz] *v/i* decompor
décor ['deɪkɔːr] decoração *f*
decorate ['dekəreɪt] *v/t* decorar; *soldier* condecorar
decoration [dekə'reɪʃn] (*paint, paper*) decoração *f*; (*ornament*) ornamentação *f*
decorative ['dekərətɪv] *adj* decorativo
decorator ['dekəreɪtər] (*interior decorator*) decorador,a *m,f*
decorum [dɪ'kɔːrəm] decoro *m*
decoy ['diːkɔɪ] *n* chamariz *m*
decrease ['diːkriːs] **1** *n* diminuição *f* **2** *v/t & v/i* diminuir
decrepit [dɪ'krepɪt] *adj* decrépito
dedicate ['dedɪkeɪt] *v/t book etc* dedicar; **~ *oneself to …*** dedicar-se a …
dedicated ['dedɪkeɪtɪd] *adj* dedicado
dedication [dedɪ'keɪʃn] *in book* dedicatória *f*; *to cause, work* dedicação *f*
deduce [dɪ'duːs] *v/t* deduzir
deduct [dɪ'dʌkt] *v/t* descontar; **~ *X from Y*** descontar X de Y
deduction [dɪ'dʌkʃn] *from salary* desconto *m*; (*conclusion*) dedução *f*
deed [diːd] *n* (*act*) ato *m*; LAW título *m*
deejay ['diːdʒeɪ] *fam* disc-jóquei *m*
deem [diːm] *v/t* julgar
deep [diːp] *adj hole, water, shelf, thinker* profundo; *trouble* sério; *voice* grave; *color* forte
deepen ['diːpn] **1** *v/t* aprofundar **2** *v/i river, crisis, mystery* aprofundar-se
'deep freeze *n* congelador *m* **'deep-frozen food** comida *f* congelada **'deep-fry** *v/t* ⟨*pret & pp* ***deep-fried***⟩ fritar **deep 'fryer** panela *f* funda para fritura
deer [dɪr] ⟨*pl* ***deer***⟩ cervo *m*
deface [dɪ'feɪs] *v/t* desfigurar
defamation [defə'meɪʃn] difamação *f*
defamatory [dɪ'fæmətərɪ] *adj* difamatório
default ['diːfɒːlt] *adj* COMPUT default
defeat [dɪ'fiːt] **1** *n* derrota *f* **2** *v/t* derrotar; *task, problem* vencer
defeatist [dɪ'fiːtɪst] *adj attitude* derrotista
defect [dɪ'fekt] *n* defeito *m*
defective [dɪ'fektɪv] *adj* defeituoso
defence *etc Brit* → ***defense***
defend [dɪ'fend] *v/t* defender; (*justify*) justificar
defendant [dɪ'fendənt] defensor,a *m,f*; *in criminal case* réu *m*
defense [dɪ'fens] *Am* defesa *f*; ***come to s.o.'s ~*** ir em defesa de alguém
de'fense budget orçamento *m* para defesa
de'fense lawyer advogado *m* de defesa
defenseless [dɪ'fenslɪs] *adj* indefeso
de'fense player SPORT jogador *m* de defesa **De'fense Secretary** POL Secretário *m* de Defesa **de'fense witness** LAW testemunha *f* de defesa
defensive [dɪ'fensɪv] **1** *n* ***on the ~*** na defensiva; ***go on the ~*** estar na defensiva **2** *adj* defensivo
defensively [dɪ'fensɪvlɪ] *adv* defensivamente
defer [dɪ'fɜːr] *v/t* ⟨*pret & pp* ***deferred***⟩ adiar
deference ['defərəns] deferência *f*
deferential [defə'renʃl] *adj* deferente
defiance [dɪ'faɪəns] desafio *m*; ***in ~ of*** em desafio a
defiant [dɪ'faɪənt] *adj* desafiador
deficiency [dɪ'fɪʃənsɪ] (*lack*) deficiência *f*
deficient [dɪ'fɪʃənt] *adj* deficiente; ***be ~ in …*** ser deficiente em …
deficit ['defɪsɪt] déficit *m*
define [dɪ'faɪn] *v/t* definir
definite ['defɪnɪt] *adj date, time* definido; *answer, improvement, also* (*certain*) definitivo; ***are you ~ about that?*** você tem certeza?; ***nothing ~ has been arranged*** não foi feito nada definitivo
definite 'article GRAM artigo *m* definido
definitely ['defɪnɪtlɪ] *adv* definitivamente

D

D

definition [defɪ'nɪʃn] definição *f*
definitive [dɪ'fɪnətɪv] *adj* definitivo
deflect [dɪ'flekt] *v/t* desviar; ***be ~ed from*** ser desviado de
deforestation [dɪfɑːrɪs'teɪʃn] desflorestamento *m*
deform [dɪ'fɔːrm] *v/t* deformar
deformity [dɪ'fɔːrmɪtɪ] deformidade *f*
defraud [dɪ'frɒːd] *v/t* fraudar
defrost [diː'frɒːst] *v/t food, fridge* descongelar
deft [deft] *adj* destro
defuse [diː'fjuːz] *v/t bomb* desarmar; *situation* neutralizar
defy [dɪ'faɪ] *v/t* ⟨*pret & pp* ***defied***⟩ desafiar
degenerate [dɪ'dʒenəreɪt] *v/i* degenerar; ***~ into*** transformar-se em
degrade [dɪ'greɪd] *v/t* degradar
degrading [dɪ'greɪdɪŋ] *adj* degradante
degree [dɪ'griː] *university*: diploma *m*; *of temperature, latitude, also* (*amount*) grau *m*; ***by ~s*** pouco a pouco; ***get one's ~*** formar-se
dehydrated [diːhaɪ'dreɪtɪd] *adj* desidratado
de-ice [diː'aɪs] *v/t* descongelar
de-icer [diː'aɪsər] (*spray*) descongelante *m*
deign [deɪn] *v/i* ***~ to …*** dignar-se a …
deity ['diːɪtɪ] divindade *f*
dejected [dɪ'dʒektɪd] *adj* deprimido
delay [dɪ'leɪ] **1** *n* atraso *m* **2** *v/t* demorar; ***be ~ed*** estar atrasado **3** *v/i* demorar-se
delegate 1 ['delɪgət] *n* delegado,-a *m,f* **2** ['delɪgeɪt] *v/t task* delegar; *person* autorizar
delegation [delɪ'geɪʃn] *of task, also* (*people*) delegação *f*
delete [dɪ'liːt] *v/t* apagar; (*cross out*) riscar
deletion [dɪ'liːʃn] (*act*) eliminação *f*; (*that deleted*) apagamento *m*
deli ['delɪ] delicatessen *f*
deliberate 1 [dɪ'lɪbərət] *adj* deliberado **2** [dɪ'lɪbəreɪt] *v/i* deliberar
deliberately [dɪ'lɪbərətlɪ] *adv* deliberadamente
delicacy ['delɪkəsɪ] *also* (*tact*) delicadeza *f*; *of problem* dificuldade *f*; (*food*) iguaria *f*
delicate ['delɪkət] *adj* delicado
delicatessen [delɪkə'tesn] delicatessen *f*
delicious [dɪ'lɪʃəs] *adj* delicioso
delight [dɪ'laɪt] *n* prazer *m*
delighted [dɪ'laɪtɪd] *adj* encantado
delightful [dɪ'laɪtfʊl] *adj* encantador
delimit [diː'lɪmɪt] *v/t* delimitar
delinquency [dɪ'lɪŋkwənsɪ] delinqüência *f*
delinquent [dɪ'lɪŋkwənt] *n* delinqüente *m/f*
delirious [dɪ'lɪrɪəs] *adj* MED *also* (*ecstatic*) delirante
deliver [dɪ'lɪvər] *v/t* entregar; *message* passar; *baby* parir; *promises etc* cumprir; ***~ a speech*** fazer um discurso
delivery [dɪ'lɪvərɪ] *goods, mail*: entrega *f*; *baby*: parto *m*; *promises*: cumprimento *m*
de'livery charge taxa *f* de entrega
de'livery date data *f* de entrega
de'livery man entregador *m* **de'livery note** nota *f* de entrega **de'livery service** serviço *m* de entrega **de'livery van** perua *f* de entrega
delude [dɪ'luːd] *v/t* iludir; ***you're deluding yourself*** você está se iludindo
deluge ['deljuːdʒ] **1** *n* dilúvio *m*; *fig* enxurrada *f* **2** *v/t fig* inundar; ***be ~d with …*** ser inundado com …
delusion [dɪ'luːʒn] ilusão *f*
de luxe [də'lʌks] *adj* de luxo
♦**delve into** [delv] *v/t* investigar
demand [dɪ'mænd] **1** *n* exigência *f*; COM procura *f*; ***in ~*** em demanda **2** *v/t* (*claim, require*) exigir
demanding [dɪ'mændɪŋ] *adj person, job* exigente
demeaning [dɪ'miːnɪŋ] *adj* aviltante
demented [dɪ'mentɪd] *adj* demente
demise [dɪ'maɪz] falecimento *m*; *fig* fim *m*
demitasse ['demɪtæs] *Am* xícara *f* de cafezinho
demo ['demoʊ] (*protest*) passeata *f*; *video*: demonstração *f*
democracy [dɪ'mɑːkrəsɪ] democracia *f*
democrat ['deməkræt] democrata *m/f*; ***Democrat*** POL *m/f* democrata

democratic [demə'krætɪk] *adj* democrático
democratically [demə'krætɪklɪ] *adv* democraticamente
'demo disk disco *m* de demonstração
demographic [demoʊ'græfɪk] *adj* demográfico
demolish [dɪ'mɑːlɪʃ] *v/t building* demolir; *argument* destruir
demolition [demə'lɪʃn] *of building* demolição *f*; *of argument* destruição *f*
demon ['diːmən] demônio *m*
demonstrate ['demənstreɪt] **1** *v/t* (*prove*) provar; *machine* demonstrar **2** *v/i politically* fazer passeata
demonstration [demən'streɪʃn] (*show*), *also of machine* demonstração *f*; (*protest*) passeata *f*
demonstrative [dɪ'mɑːnstrətɪv] *adj* demonstrativo; ***be ~*** ser afetivo
demonstrator ['demənstreɪtər] (*protester*) manifestante *m/f*
demoralized [dɪ'mɒːrəlaɪzd] *adj* desmoralizado
demoralizing [dɪ'mɒːrəlaɪzɪŋ] *adj* desmoralizante
demote [diː'moʊt] *v/t* rebaixar
demure [dɪ'mjʊər] *adj* recatado
den [den] (*study*) estúdio *m*
denial [dɪ'naɪəl] *of rumor, accusation* negação *f*; *of request* recusa *f*
denim ['denɪm] brim *m*
denims ['denɪmz] *npl* (*jeans*) jeans *m*, *Port* jeans *mpl*
Denmark ['denmɑːrk] Dinamarca *f*
denomination [dɪnɑːmɪ'neɪʃn] *of money* nota *f*; (*religious*) denominação *f*
denounce [dɪ'naʊns] *v/t* denunciar
dense [dens] *adj* (*thick*), *also foliage, crowd* denso; (*stupid*) bronco
densely ['denslɪ] *adv* ***~ populated*** densamente habitado
density ['densɪtɪ] *population*: densidade *f*
dent [dent] **1** *n* amassado *m* **2** *v/t* amassar
dental ['dentl] *adj treatment* dentário; *hospital* odontológico
dented ['dentɪd] *adj* amassado
dentist ['dentɪst] dentista *m/f*
dentistry ['dentɪstrɪ] odontologia *f*
dentures ['dentʃəz] *npl* dentadura *f*
deny [dɪ'naɪ] *v/t* ⟨*pret & pp* ***denied***⟩ negar
deodorant [diː'oʊdərənt] desodorante *m*, *Port* desodorizante *m*
depart [dɪ'pɑːrt] *v/i* partir; ***~ from*** (*deviate from*) afastar-se de
department [dɪ'pɑːrtmənt] *company, university*: departamento *m*; *government*: Ministério *m*; *store*: seção *f*
Department of 'Defense *Am* Ministério *m* da Defesa **Department of the In'terior** *Am* Ministério do Interior **Department of 'State** *Am* Ministério das Relações Exteriores
de'partment store magazine *m*, *Port* grande armazém *m*
departure [dɪ'pɑːrtʃər] partida *f*, *train, bus*: saída *f*, *person from job*: demissão *f*, (*deviation*) desvio *m*; ***a new ~*** *for government, organization* uma nova orientação; *for company* uma nova atividade; *for actor, writer* um novo começo
de'parture lounge sala *f* de embarque
de'parture time hora *f* de saída
depend [dɪ'pend] *v/i* ***that ~s*** isso depende; ***it ~s on the weather*** depende do tempo; ***I ~ on you*** confio em você
dependable [dɪ'pendəbl] *adj* confiável
dependant → ***dependent***
dependence, dependency [dɪ'pendəns, dɪ'pendənsɪ] dependência *f*
dependent [dɪ'pendənt] **1** *n* dependente *m/f* **2** *adj* dependente
depict [dɪ'pɪkt] *v/t in painting, writing* retratar
deplete [dɪ'pliːt] *v/t* esgotar
deplorable [dɪ'plɔːrəbl] *adj* deplorável
deplore [dɪ'plɔːr] *v/t* deplorar
deploy [dɪ'plɔɪ] *v/t* dispor
depopulation [dɪpɑːpjə'leɪʃn] despovoamento *m*
deport [dɪ'pɔːrt] *v/t* deportar
deportation [diːpɔːr'teɪʃn] deportação *f*
depor'tation order ordem *f* de deportação

D

depose [dɪ'poʊz] *v/t* depor
deposit [dɪ'pɑːzɪt] **1** *n in bank, also of mineral* depósito *m*; *on purchase* sinal *m* **2** *v/t* depositar
deposit account *Brit* → ***savings account***
deposition [diːpoʊ'zɪʃn] *Am* LAW depoimento *m*
depot ['diːpoʊ] (*train station*) estação *f*; (*bus station*) terminal *m*; *storage*: depósito *m*
depraved [dɪ'preɪvd] *adj* depravado
depreciate [dɪ'priːʃieɪt] *v/i* FIN depreciar
depreciation [dɪpriːʃɪ'eɪʃn] FIN depreciação *f*
depress [dɪ'pres] *v/t person* deprimir
depressed [dɪ'prest] *adj person* deprimido
depressing [dɪ'presɪŋ] *adj* deprimente
depression [dɪ'preʃn] MED, *also economic, meteorological* depressão *f*
deprivation [deprɪ'veɪʃn] privação *f*
deprive [dɪ'praɪv] *v/t* **~ *X of Y*** privar X de Y
deprived [dɪ'praɪvd] *adj* carente
depth [depθ] *water, hole, shelf thought*: profundidade *f*; *voice, color*: tonalidade *f*; ***in ~*** (*thoroughly*) em profundidade; ***in the ~s of winter*** no meio do inverno; ***be out of one's ~*** *in water* perder o pé; *in discussion etc* perder o fio da meada
deputation [depjʊ'teɪʃn] delegação *f*
♦ **deputize for** ['depjʊtaɪz] *v/t* representar
deputy ['depʊtɪ] vice *m/f*
'deputy leader vice-líder *m/f*
derail [dɪ'reɪl] *v/t* ***be ~ed*** *train* descarrilar
deranged [dɪ'reɪndʒd] *adj* transtornado
deregulate [dɪ'regjʊleɪt] *v/t* desregulamentar
deregulation [dɪregjʊ'leɪʃn] desregulamentação *f*
derelict ['derəlɪkt] *adj* abandonado
deride [dɪ'raɪd] *v/t* zombar
derision [dɪ'rɪʒn] zombaria *f*
derisive [dɪ'raɪsɪv] *adj remarks, laughter* zombador
derisively [dɪ'raɪsɪvlɪ] *adv* zombeteiramente
derisory [dɪ'raɪsərɪ] *adj amount, salary* irrisório
derivative [dɪ'rɪvətɪv] *adj* (*not original*) derivado
derive [dɪ'raɪv] *v/t* obter; ***be ~d from*** *word* derivar de
dermatologist [dɜːrmə'tɑːlədʒɪst] dermatologista *m/f*
derogatory [dɪ'rɑːgətɔːrɪ] *adj* depreciativo
descend [dɪ'send] **1** *v/t* descer; ***be ~ed from*** ser descendente de **2** *v/i airplane, climber, road, mood, darkness* descer
descendant [dɪ'sendənt] descendente *m/f*
descent [dɪ'sent] *from mountain, of airplane* descida *f*; (*ancestry*) descendência *f*; ***of Chinese ~*** de descendência chinesa
describe [dɪ'skraɪb] *v/t* descrever; ***~ X as Y*** descrever X como Y
description [dɪ'skrɪpʃn] descrição *f*
desecrate ['desɪkreɪt] *v/t* profanar
desecration [desɪ'kreɪʃn] profanação *f*
desegregate [diː'segrəgeɪt] *v/t* dessegregar
desert[1] ['dezərt] *n also fig* deserto *m*
desert[2] [dɪ'zɜːrt] **1** *v/t* (*abandon*) abandonar **2** *v/i soldier* desertar
deserted [dɪ'zɜːrtɪd] *adj* deserto
deserter [dɪ'zɜːrtər] MIL desertor,a *m,f*
desertification [dɪzɜːrtɪfɪ'keɪʃn] desertificação *f*
desertion [dɪ'zɜːrʃn] (*abandoning*) abandono *m*; MIL deserção *f*
desert 'island ilha *f* deserta
deserve [dɪ'zɜːrv] *v/t* merecer
design [dɪ'zaɪn] **1** *n* design *m*; (*pattern*) padrão *m* **2** *v/t* desenhar; *building, car, ship, machine* projetar; ***not ~ed for heavy use*** não projetado para uso intensivo
designate ['dezɪgneɪt] *v/t person* designar; *area* destinar
designer [dɪ'zaɪnər] *car, garden*: projetista *m/f*; *clothes, fashion*: estilista *m/f*; (*interior designer*) decorador,a *m,f*

de'signer clothes roupa *f* de marca
de'sign fault defeito *m* de projeto
de'sign school escola *f* de design
desirable [dɪ'zaɪrəbl] *adj* desejável
desire [dɪ'zaɪr] *n* (*wish*) *also sexual* desejo *m*
desk [desk] mesa *f*; *hotel*: recepção *f*; *classroom*: carteira *f na escola*; (*writing-desk*) escrivaninha *f*
'desk clerk *Am* recepcionista *m/f*
'desk diary agenda *f* de mesa
'desktop mesa *f* de trabalho; (*computer*) desktop *m*; (*screen*) área *f* de trabalho **desktop 'publishing** editoração *f* eletrônica
desolate ['desələt] *adj place* desolado
despair [dɪ'sper] **1** *n* desespero *m*; ***in ~*** em desespero **2** *v/i* desesperar-se; ***~ of doing sth*** desesperar-se de fazer algo; ***I ~ of him*** ele me deixa em desespero
desperate ['despərət] *adj person*, *action*, *situation* desesperado; *situation* desesperador; ***be ~ for a drink / a cigarette*** estar desesperado por uma bebida / um cigarro
desperation [despə'reɪʃn] desespero *m*; ***an act of ~*** um ato de desespero
despicable [dɪs'pɪkəbl] *adj* desprezível
despise [dɪ'spaɪz] *v/t* desprezar
despite [dɪ'spaɪt] *prep* apesar de
despondent [dɪ'spɑːndənt] *adj* desanimado
despot ['despɑːt] déspota *m*
dessert [dɪ'zɜːrt] sobremesa *f*
destination [destɪ'neɪʃn] destino *m*
destined ['destɪnd] *adj* ***be ~ for*** *fig* estar destinado a
destiny ['destɪnɪ] destino *m*
destitute ['destɪtuːt] *adj* indigente
destroy [dɪ'strɔɪ] *v/t* destruir
destroyer [dɪ'strɔɪr] NAUT contratorpedeiro *m*
destruction [dɪ'strʌkʃn] destruição *f*
destructive [dɪ'strʌktɪv] *adj power*, *criticism* destrutivo; *child* destruidor
detach [dɪ'tætʃ] *v/t* destacar
detachable [dɪ'tætʃəbl] *adj* destacável
detached [dɪ'tætʃt] *adj* (*objective*) imparcial
detachment [dɪ'tætʃmənt] (*objectivity*) imparcialidade *f*
detail ['diːteɪl] *n* detalhe *m*; ***in ~*** em detalhe
detailed ['diːteɪld] *adj* detalhado
detain [dɪ'teɪn] *v/t* (*hold back*) deter; *as prisoner* prender
detainee [dɪteɪn'iː] detento,-a *m,f*
detect [dɪ'tekt] *v/t* perceber; *smoke etc* detectar
detection [dɪ'tekʃn] *criminal*, *crime*: descoberta *f*; *smoke etc*: detecção *f*
detective [dɪ'tektɪv] detetive *m/f*
de'tective novel romance *m* policial
detector [dɪ'tektər] detector *m*
détente ['deɪtɑːnt] POL distensão *f*
detention [dɪ'tenʃn] (*imprisonment*) detenção *f*; *after school* retenção *f*; ***he was given ~ for cheating in the test*** ficou de castigo na escola por ter colado na prova
deter [dɪ'tɜːr] *v/t* ⟨*pret & pp* ***deterred***⟩ dissuadir; ***~ X from doing Y*** dissuadir X de fazer Y
detergent [dɪ'tɜːrdʒənt] detergente *m*
deteriorate [dɪ'tɪrɪreɪt] *v/i* deteriorar-se
deterioration [dɪtɪrɪə'reɪʃn] deterioração *f*
determination [dɪtɜːrmɪ'neɪʃn] determinação *f*
determine [dɪ'tɜːrmɪn] *v/t* determinar
determined [dɪ'tɜːrmɪnd] *adj person*, *effort* determinado
deterrent [dɪ'terənt] *n* dissuasivo *m*; ***nuclear ~*** arma *f* nuclear
detest [dɪ'test] *v/t* detestar
detestable [dɪ'testəbl] *adj* detestável
detonate ['detəneɪt] *v/t & v/i* detonar
detonation ['detəneɪʃn] detonação *f*
detour ['diːtʊər] *n* desvio *m*
◆ **detract from** [dɪ'trækt] *v/t* diminuir
detriment ['detrɪmənt] detrimento *m*; ***to the ~ of*** em detrimento de
detrimental [detrɪ'mentl] *adj* prejudicial
deuce [duːs] *in tennis* deuce *m*
devaluation [diːvæljʊ'eɪʃn] *of currency* desvalorização *f*
devalue [diː'væljuː] *v/t currency* desvalorizar
devastate ['devəsteɪt] *v/t countryside*, *city* devastar; *fig person* arrasar

D

D

devastating ['devəsteɪtɪŋ] *adj* devastador
develop [dɪ'veləp] **1** *v/t film* revelar; *land, site* desenvolver; *activity, business* expandir; (*originate*) produzir; (*improve on*) progredir; *illness, cold* contrair **2** *v/i* (*grow*) evoluir; *country, business* desenvolver-se
developer [dɪ'veləpər] *of property* empresário *m* de imóveis
de'veloping country país *m* em desenvolvimento
development [dɪ'veləpmənt] *film*: revelação *f*; *land, site*: desenvolvimento *m*; *business, country*: expansão *f*; (*event*) acontecimento *m*; (*origination*) criação *f*; (*improving*) progresso *m*
device [dɪ'vaɪs] (*tool*) aparelho *m*
devil ['devl] diabo *m*
devious ['diːvɪəs] (*sly*) dissimulado
devise [dɪ'vaɪz] *v/t* criar
devoid [dɪ'vɔɪd] *adj* ***be ~ of*** ser destituído de
devolution [diːvə'luːʃn] POL descentralização *f*
devote [dɪ'voʊt] *v/t* dedicar (***to*** a)
devoted [dɪ'voʊtɪd] *adj son etc* dedicado; ***be ~ to a person*** ser dedicado a uma pessoa
devotee [dɪvoʊ'tiː] devotado,-a *m,f*
devotion [dɪ'voʊʃn] dedicação *f*
devour [dɪ'vaʊər] *v/t food, book* devorar
devout [dɪ'vaʊt] *adj* devoto
dew [duː] orvalho *m*
dexterity [dek'sterətɪ] destreza *f*
diabetes [daɪə'biːtiːz] diabetes *m/f*
diabetic [daɪə'betɪk] **1** *n* diabético,-a *m,f* **2** *adj* diabético
diagnose ['daɪəgnoʊz] *v/t* diagnosticar
diagnosis [daɪəg'noʊsɪs] ⟨*pl diagnoses*⟩ diagnóstico *m*
diagonal [daɪ'ægənl] *adj* diagonal
diagonally [daɪ'ægənlɪ] *adv* diagonalmente
diagram ['daɪəgræm] diagrama *m*
dial ['daɪl] **1** *n clock, meter*: mostrador *m*; TEL disco *m* do telefone **2** *v/t & v/i* ⟨*pret & pp* ***dialed****, Brit* ***dialled***⟩ TEL discar, *Port* marcar
dialect ['daɪəlekt] dialeto *m*
dialling code *Brit* → ***area code***
dialling tone *Brit* → ***dial tone***
dialog ['daɪəlɑːg] *Am* diálogo *m*
'dialog box COMPUT caixa *f* de diálogo
dialogue *Brit* → ***dialog***
'dial tone *Am* sinal *m* de discagem, *Port* sinal *m* de marcar
diameter [daɪ'æmɪtər] diâmetro *m*
diametrically [daɪə'metrɪkəlɪ] *adv* ***~ opposed*** diametralmente oposto (***to*** a)
diamond ['daɪmənd] *jewel, cards*: diamante *m*; *shape* losango *m*
diaper ['daɪpər] *Am* fralda *f*
diaphragm ['daɪəfræm] ANAT *also contraceptive* diafragma *m*
diarrhea [daɪə'riːə] *Am* diarréia *f*
diarrhoea *Brit* → ***diarrhea***
diary ['daɪrɪ] *thoughts*: diário *m*; *appointments*: agenda *f*
dice [daɪs] **1** *n* dado *m* **2** *v/t* (*cut*) cortar em cubos
dichotomy [daɪ'kɑːtəmɪ] dicotomia *f*
dick [dɪk] *vulg* (*penis*) pica *f*
dictate [dɪk'teɪt] *v/t letter, course of action* ditar
dictation [dɪk'teɪʃn] ditado *m*
dictator [dɪk'teɪtər] POL ditador,a *m,f*
dictatorial [dɪktə'tɔːrɪəl] *adj tone of voice, person* arrogante; *powers* ditatorial
dictatorship [dɪk'teɪtəʃɪp] ditadura *f*
dictionary ['dɪkʃənrɪ] dicionário *m*
did [dɪd] *pret* → ***do***
die [daɪ] *v/i* morrer; ***~ of cancer / AIDS*** morrer de câncer / AIDS; ***I'm dying to know / leave*** estou louco para saber / sair
♦**die away** *v/i noise* extinguir-se
♦**die down** *v/i excitement, noise* diminuir; *storm* abrandar; *fire* apagar-se
♦**die out** *v/i custom, species* desaparecer
diesel ['diːzl] diesel *m*
diet ['daɪət] **1** *n* dieta *f* **2** *v/i to lose weight* fazer dieta
dietitian [daɪə'tɪʃn] nutricionista *m/f*
differ ['dɪfər] *v/i* (*be different*) diferir; (*disagree*) divergir
difference ['dɪfrəns] diferença *f*; (*disagreement*) divergência *f*; ***it doesn't***

make any ~ *(doesn't change anything)* não faz diferença alguma
different ['dɪfrənt] *adj (dissimilar)* diferente; *(distinct)* distinto
differentiate [dɪfə'renʃɪeɪt] *v/i* ***~ between*** fazer diferença entre
differently ['dɪfrəntlɪ] *adv* de modo diferente
difficult ['dɪfɪkəlt] *adj* difícil
difficulty ['dɪfɪkəltɪ] dificuldade *f*; ***with ~*** com dificuldade
diffidence ['dɪfɪdəns] timidez *f*
diffident ['dɪfɪdənt] *adj* tímido
dig [dɪg] ⟨*pret & pp* **dug**⟩ **1** *v/t* cavar **2** *v/i* ***it was ~ging into me*** estava me esfolando
♦**dig out** *v/t (find)* desenterrar
♦**dig up** *v/t* escavar; *information* descobrir
digest [daɪ'dʒest] *v/t* digerir; *information* assimilar
digestible [daɪ'dʒestəbl] *adj food* digerível
digestion [daɪ'dʒestʃn] digestão *f*
digestive [daɪ'dʒestɪv] *adj* digestivo
digger ['dɪgər] *(machine)* escavadeira *f*
digit ['dɪdʒɪt] *(number)* dígito *m*; ***a 4 ~ number*** um número de 4 dígitos
digital ['dɪdʒɪtl] *adj* digital; ***~ camera*** câmara *f* digital
dignified ['dɪgnɪfaɪd] *adj* digno
dignitary ['dɪgnɪterɪ] dignitário,-a *m,f*
dignity ['dɪgnɪtɪ] dignidade *f*
digress [daɪ'gres] *v/i* divagar
digression [daɪ'greʃn] divagação *f*
dike [daɪk] *(wall)* dique *m*
dilapidated [dɪ'læpɪdeɪtɪd] *adj* dilapidado
dilate [daɪ'leɪt] *v/i pupils* dilatar-se
dilemma [dɪ'lemə] dilema *m*; ***be in a ~*** estar num dilema
dilettante [dɪle'tæntɪ] diletante *m/f*
diligent ['dɪlɪdʒənt] *adj* diligente
dilute [daɪ'lu:t] *v/t* diluir
dim [dɪm] **1** *adj room* escuro; *light, prospects* fraco; *outline* indistinto; *(stupid)* burro **2** *v/t* ⟨*pret & pp* **dimmed**⟩ ***~ the headlights*** baixar os faróis **3** *v/i* ⟨*pret & pp* **dimmed**⟩ *lights* diminuir
dime [daɪm] *Am* moeda *f* de 10 centavos
dimension [daɪ'menʃn] dimensão *f*
diminish [dɪ'mɪnɪʃ] *v/t & v/i* diminuir
diminutive [dɪ'mɪnʊtɪv] **1** *n* diminutivo *m* **2** *adj* diminuto
dimple ['dɪmpl] covinha *f*
din [dɪn] *n* zoeira *f*
dine [daɪn] *v/i fml* jantar
diner ['daɪnər] *person* comensal *m/f*; *(restaurant)* lanchonete *f*
dinghy ['dɪŋgɪ] *rubber* bote *m* de borracha
dingy ['dɪndʒɪ] *adj atmosphere* sombrio; *(dirty)* sujo
dining car ['daɪnɪŋ] RAIL vagão-restaurante *m* **'dining room** sala *f* de jantar **'dining table** mesa *f* de jantar
dinner ['dɪnər] *in the evening* jantar *m*; *at midday* almoço *m*
'dinner guest convidado,-a *m,f* **'dinner jacket** smoking *m* **'dinner party** jantar *m* **'dinner service** serviço *m* de mesa
dinosaur ['daɪnəsɔ:r] dinossauro *m*
dip [dɪp] **1** *n (swim)* mergulho *m*; *for food* molho *m* para salgadinhos; *in road* declive *m* **2** *v/t* ⟨*pret & pp* **dipped**⟩ mergulhar; ***~ the headlights*** baixar os faróis **3** *v/i road* baixar
diploma [dɪ'ploʊmə] diploma *m*
diplomacy [dɪ'ploʊməsɪ] *also (tact)* diplomacia *f*
diplomat ['dɪpləmæt] diplomata *m/f*
diplomatic [dɪplə'mætɪk] *adj also (tactful)* diplomático
diplomatically [dɪplə'mætɪklɪ] *adv* diplomaticamente
diplomatic im'munity imunidade *f* diplomática
dire ['daɪr] *adj* terrível
direct [daɪ'rekt] **1** *adj* direto **2** *v/t to a place* indicar o caminho; *play, movie, attention* dirigir
direct 'current ELEC corrente *f* contínua
direction [dɪ'rekʃn] *to a place, of movie, play* direção *f*; ***~s*** *(instructions)* instruções *fpl*; *for use* modo *m* de usar; *for medicine* posologia *f*
di'rection indicator MOT indicador *m* de direção

D

D

directive [dɪ'rektɪv] *of EU etc* diretoria *f*
directly [dɪ'rektlɪ] **1** *adv (straight)* diretamente; *(soon)* logo; *(immediately)* imediatamente **2** *conj* logo que
director [dɪ'rektər] *of company, play, movie* diretor,a *m,f*
directory [dɪ'rektərɪ] diretório *m*; TEL lista *f* telefônica
dirt [dɜːrt] sujeira *f*, *Port* sujidade *f*
'dirt cheap *adj fam* baratíssimo
dirty ['dɜːrtɪ] **1** *adj* sujo; *(pornographic)* indecente **2** *v/t* ⟨*pret & pp* ***dirtied***⟩ sujar
dirty 'trick golpe *m* sujo
disability [dɪsə'bɪlətɪ] deficiência *f*
disabled [dɪs'eɪbld] **1** *n* deficiente *m/f* **2** *adj* deficiente
disadvantage [dɪsəd'væntɪdʒ] desvantagem *f*; ***be at a ~*** estar em desvantagem
disadvantaged [dɪsəd'væntɪdʒd] *adj* desfavorecido
disadvantageous [dɪsədvən'teɪdʒəs] *adj* desvantajoso
disagree [dɪsə'griː] *v/i person* discordar
♦**disagree with** *v/t person* discordar de; *food* fazer mal
disagreeable [dɪsə'griːəbl] *adj* desagradável
disagreement [dɪsə'griːmənt] discordância *f*; *(argument)* desavença *f*
disappear [dɪsə'pɪr] *v/i* desaparecer; *(run away)* sumir
disappearance [dɪsə'pɪrəns] desaparecimento *m*
disappoint [dɪsə'pɔɪnt] *v/t* desapontar
disappointed [dɪsə'pɔɪntɪd] *adj* desapontado
disappointing [dɪsə'pɔɪntɪŋ] *adj* decepcionante
disappointment [dɪsə'pɔɪntmənt] desapontamento *m*
disapproval [dɪsə'pruːvl] desaprovação *f*
disapprove [dɪsə'pruːv] *v/i* desaprovar; ***~ of*** desaprovar
disapproving [dɪsə'pruːvɪŋ] *adj* reprovador
disapprovingly [dɪsə'pruːvɪŋlɪ] *adv* com desaprovação
disarm [dɪs'ɑːrm] **1** *v/t robber, militia* desarmar **2** *v/i* desarmar-se
disarmament [dɪs'ɑːrməmənt] desarmamento *m*
disarming [dɪs'ɑːrmɪŋ] *adj* irresistível
disaster [dɪ'zæstər] desastre *m*
di'saster area zona *f* de calamidade; *fig person* calamidade *f*
disastrous [dɪ'zæstrəs] *adj* desastroso
disband [dɪs'bænd] **1** *v/t* dissolver: **2** *v/i* dissolver-se
disbelief [dɪsbə'liːf] incredulidade *f*; ***in ~*** com incredulidade
disc [dɪsk] *(CD)* CD *m*
discard [dɪ'skɑːrd] *v/t* descartar
discern [dɪ'sɜːrn] *v/t* discernir
discernible [dɪ'sɜːrnəbl] *adj* discernível
discerning [dɪ'sɜːrnɪŋ] *adj* discernidor
discharge ['dɪstʃɑːrdʒ] **1** *n from hospital* alta *f*, *from army* baixa *f* **2** *v/t* cumprir; *from hospital* dar alta; *from army* dar baixa; *from job* demitir
disciple [dɪ'saɪpl] discípulo,-a *m,f*
disciplinary [dɪsɪ'plɪnərɪ] *adj* disciplinar
discipline ['dɪsɪplɪn] **1** *n* disciplina *f* **2** *v/t* disciplinar
'disc jockey disc-jóquei *m/f*
disclaim [dɪs'kleɪm] *v/t* negar
disclose [dɪs'kloʊs] *v/t* revelar
disclosure [dɪs'kloʊʒər] revelação *f*
disco ['dɪskoʊ] discoteca *f*
discolor [dɪs'kʌlər] *v/i Am* desbotar
discolour *Brit* → ***discolor***
discomfort [dɪs'kʌmfət] *n (pain)* desconforto *m*; *(embarrassment)* embaraço *m*
disconcert [dɪskən'sɜːrt] *v/t* desconcertar
disconcerted [dɪskən'sɜːrtɪd] *adj* desconcertado
disconnect [dɪskə'nekt] *v/t hose, appliance* desconectar; *supply, telephones* desligar
disconsolate [dɪs'kɑːnsələt] *adj* desconsolado
discontent [dɪskən'tent] descontentamento *m*
discontented [dɪskən'tentɪd] *adj* des-

contente
discontinue [dıskən'tınuː] *v/t product* suspender; *bus, train service, magazine* interromper
discord ['dıskɔːrd] MUS dissonância *f*; *in relations* discórdia *f*
discotheque ['dıskətek] discoteca *f*
discount 1 ['dıskaʊnt] *n* desconto *m* **2** [dıs'kaʊnt] *v/t* descontar; *goods* dar desconto em; *theory* ignorar
discourage [dıs'kʌrıdʒ] *v/t* (*dissuade*) desaconselhar; (*dishearten*) desencorajar
discouragement [dıs'kʌrıdʒmənt] desencorajamento *m*
discover [dı'skʌvər] *v/t* descobrir
discoverer [dı'skʌvərər] descobridor,a *m,f*
discovery [dı'skʌvərı] descoberta *f*
discredit [dıs'kredıt] *v/t person, theory* desacreditar
discreet [dı'skriːt] *adj person, restaurant* discreto
discreetly [dı'skriːtlı] *adv* discretamente
discrepancy [dı'skrepənsı] discrepância *f*
discretion [dı'skreʃn] discrição *f*; ***at your ~*** a seu critério
discriminate [dı'skrımıneıt] *v/i* ***~ against*** discriminar; ***~ between*** *red and green etc* distinguir entre
discriminating [dı'skrımıneıtıŋ] *adj* criterioso
discrimination [dı'skrımıneıʃn] *sexual, racial etc* discriminação *f*
discus ['dıskəs] SPORT disco *m*
discuss [dı'skʌs] *v/t* discutir; *article:* analisar
discussion [dı'skʌʃn] discussão *f*
'discus thrower arremessador,a *m,f* de disco
disdain [dıs'deın] *n* desdém *m*
disease [dı'ziːz] doença *f*
disembark [dısəm'bɑ;k] *v/i from plane, ship* desembarcar
disenchanted [dısən'ʧæntıd] *adj* desencantado; ***~ with*** desencantado com
disengage [dısən'geıdʒ] *v/t* soltar
disentangle [dısən'tæŋgl] *v/t* desembaraçar
disfigure [dıs'fıgər] *v/t* desfigurar
disgrace [dıs'greıs] **1** *n* desgraça *f*; ***it's a ~*** é uma desgraça; ***in ~*** na desgraça **2** *v/t* desgraçar
disgraceful [dıs'greısful] *adj behavior, situation* vergonhoso
disgruntled [dıs'grʌntld] *adj* descontente
disguise [dıs'gaız] **1** *n* disfarce *m* **2** *v/t voice, fear, anxiety* disfarçar; ***~ oneself as*** disfarçar-se de; ***he was ~d as*** ele estava disfarçado de
disgust [dıs'gʌst] **1** *n* repugnância *f* **2** *v/t* repugnar
disgusting [dıs'gʌstıŋ] *adj habit, smell, food* repugnante; ***it is ~ that ...*** é revoltante que ...
dish [dıʃ] prato *m*; ***do the ~es*** lavar a louça
'dishcloth pano *m* de prato
disheartened [dıs'hɑːrtnd] *adj* desanimado
disheartening [dıs'hɑːrtnıŋ] *adj* desanimador
disheveled [dı'ʃevld] *adj hair* despenteado; *clothes* amassado; *person* desalinhado
dishonest [dıs'ɑːnıst] *adj* desonesto
dishonesty [dıs'ɑːnıstı] desonestidade *f*
dishonor [dıs'ɑːnər] *n Am* desonra *f*; ***bring ~ on*** trazer desonra a
dishonorable [dıs'ɑːnərəbl] *adj Am* desonroso
dishonour *etc Brit* → ***dishonor***
'dishwasher *person* lavador,a *m,f* de louça; *machine* lava-louças *f*
'dishwashing liquid *Am* detergente *m*
disillusion [dısı'luːʒn] *v/t* desiludir
disillusionment [dısı'luːʒnmənt] desilusão *f*
disinclined [dısın'klaınd] *adj* indisposto
disinfect [dısın'fekt] *v/t* desinfetar
disinfectant [dısın'fektənt] desinfetante *m*
disinherit [dısın'herıt] *v/t* deserdar
disintegrate [dıs'ıntəgreıt] *v/i* desintegrar-se
disinterested [dıs'ıntərestıd] *adj* (*unbiased*) desinteressado

disjointed [dɪs'dʒɔɪntɪd] *adj* desconexo
disk [dɪsk] *also* COMPUT disco *m*; ***on ~*** em disco
'disk drive COMPUT unidade *f* de disco
diskette [dɪs'ket] disquete *m*
dislike [dɪs'laɪk] **1** *n* antipatia *f* **2** *v/t* não gostar de
dislocate ['dɪsləkeɪt] *v/t shoulder* deslocar
dislodge [dɪs'lɑːdʒ] *v/t* desalojar
disloyal [dɪs'lɔɪəl] *adj* desleal
disloyalty [dɪs'lɔɪəltɪ] deslealdade *f*
dismal ['dɪzməl] *adj weather, news,* (*sad*) deprimente; *person* (*negative*) pessimista; *failure* horrível
dismantle [dɪs'mæntl] *v/t object* desmontar; *organization* desmantelar
dismay [dɪs'meɪ] **1** *n* (*alarm*) espanto *m*; (*disappointment*) desapontamento *m* **2** *v/t* consternar
dismiss [dɪs'mɪs] *v/t employee* demitir; *suggestion* rejeitar; *idea, thought* esquecer; *possibility* descartar
dismissal [dɪs'mɪsl] *of employee* demissão *f*
dismount [dɪs'maʊnt] *v/i* desmontar
disobedience [dɪsə'biːdɪəns] desobediência *f*
disobedient [dɪsə'biːdɪənt] *adj* desobediente
disobey [dɪsə'beɪ] *v/t* desobedecer a
disorder [dɪs'ɔːrdər] (*untidiness*) desordem *f*; (*unrest*) tumulto *m*; MED distúrbio *m*
disorderly [dɪs'ɔːrdərlɪ] *adj room, desk* desordenado; *mob* incontrolável
disorganized [dɪs'ɔːrgənaɪzd] *adj* desorganizado
disorientated *Brit* → ***disoriented***
disoriented [dɪs'ɔːrɪəntɪd] *adj* desorientado
disown [dɪs'oʊn] *v/t* repudiar
disparaging [dɪ'spærɪdʒɪŋ] *adj* depreciativo
disparity [dɪ'spærətɪ] disparidade *f*
dispassionate [dɪ'spæʃənət] *adj* indiferente
dispatch [dɪ'spætʃ] *v/t* (*send*) despachar
dispensary [dɪ'spensərɪ] *in pharmacy* dispensário *m*
♦**dispense with** [dɪ'spens] *v/t* prescindir de
disperse [dɪ'spɜːrs] **1** *v/t crowd* dispersar **2** *v/i crowd* dispersar-se; *mist* dissipar-se
dispirited [dɪs'pɪrɪtɪd] *adj* desanimado
displace [dɪs'pleɪs] *v/t* (*supplant*) suplantar
display [dɪ'spleɪ] **1** *n* mostra *f*, *in store window* decoração *f*, COMPUT apresentação *f*; ***be on ~*** *at exhibition* ficar em exposição; (*be for sale*) estar à mostra para venda **2** *v/t emotion* manifestar; *at exhibition* exibir; *for sale* expor; COMPUT mostrar
di'splay cabinet mostrador *m*
displease [dɪs'pliːs] *v/t* desgostar
displeasure [dɪs'pleʒər] desgosto *m*
disposable [dɪ'spoʊzəbl] *adj* descartável
disposable 'income renda *f* líquida
disposal [dɪ'spoʊzl] eliminação *f*, *of pollutants, nuclear waste* depósito *m*; ***I am at your ~*** estou à sua disposição; ***put X at Y's ~*** colocar X à disposição de Y
♦**dispose of** [dɪ'spoʊz] *v/t* eliminar
disposed [dɪ'spoʊzd] *adj* ***be ~ to do sth*** (*willing*) estar disposto a fazer algo; ***be well ~ toward*** estar bastante propenso a
disposition [dɪspə'zɪʃn] (*nature*) índole *f*
disproportionate [dɪsprə'pɔːrʃənət] *adj* desproporcional
disprove [dɪs'pruːv] *v/t* refutar
dispute [dɪ'spjuːt] **1** *n between people, countries* disputa *f*, *industrial* conflito *m* **2** *v/t* questionar; (*fight over*) disputar
disqualification [dɪskwɑːlɪfɪ'keɪʃn] desclassificação *f*
disqualify [dɪs'kwɑːlɪfaɪ] *v/t* 〈*pret & pp* ***disqualified***〉 desclassificar
disregard [dɪsrə'gɑːrd] **1** *n* desconsideração *f* **2** *v/t* ignorar
disrepair [dɪsrə'per] mau estado *m*; ***in a state of ~*** em mau estado
disreputable [dɪs'repjʊtəbl] *adj person, area* mal-afamado

disrespect [dɪsrə'spekt] desrespeito *m*
disrespectful [dɪsrə'spektfʊl] *adj* desrespeitoso
disrupt [dɪs'rʌpt] *v/t train service, meeting, class* interromper; (*intentionally*) perturbar
disruption [dɪs'rʌpʃn] *train service, meeting, class*: interrupção *f*; (*intentional*) perturbação *f*
disruptive [dɪs'rʌptɪv] *adj* perturbador
dissatisfaction [dɪssætɪs'fækʃn] insatisfação *f*
dissatisfied [dɪs'sætɪsfaɪd] *adj* insatisfeito
dissension [dɪ'senʃn] dissensão *f*
dissent [dɪ'sent] **1** *n* discórdia *f* **2** *v/i* **~ *from*** discordar de
dissident ['dɪsɪdənt] *n* dissidente *m/f*
dissimilar [dɪs'sɪmɪlər] *adj* dessemelhante
dissociate [dɪ'soʊʃɪeɪt] *v/t* **~ *oneself from*** desassociar-se de
dissolute ['dɪsəluːt] *adj* dissoluto
dissolution ['dɪsəluːʃn] POL dissolução *f*
dissolve [dɪ'zɑːlv] **1** *v/t substance* dissolver **2** *v/i* dissolver-se
dissuade [dɪ'sweɪd] *v/t* dissuadir; **~ *X from doing Y*** dissuadir X de fazer Y
distance ['dɪstəns] **1** *n* distância *f*; ***in the ~*** à distância **2** *v/t* **~ *oneself from*** distanciar-se de
distant ['dɪstənt] *adj place, time, relative, also* (*aloof*) distante
distaste [dɪs'teɪst] desagrado *m*
distasteful [dɪs'teɪstfʊl] *adj* desagradável
distillery [dɪs'tɪlərɪ] destilaria *f*
distinct [dɪ'stɪŋkt] *adj* (*clear, different*) distinto; ***as ~ from*** ao contrário de
distinction [dɪ'stɪŋkʃn] (*differentiation*) distinção *f*; ***hotel / product of ~*** hotel / produto de qualidade
distinctive [dɪ'stɪŋktɪv] *adj* distinto
distinctly [dɪ'stɪŋktlɪ] *adv* distintamente; (*decidedly*) decididamente
distinguish [dɪ'stɪŋgwɪʃ] *v/t* (*see*) distinguir; **~ *between X and Y*** distinguir entre X e Y
distinguished [dɪ'stɪŋgwɪʃt] *adj* (*famous*) ilustre; (*dignified*) distinto
distort [dɪ'stɔːrt] *v/t* distorcer
distract [dɪ'strækt] *v/t person* distrair; *attention* desviar
distracted [dɪ'stræktɪd] *adj* (*worried*) perturbado
distraction [dɪ'strækʃn] *of attention, also* (*amusement*) distração *f*; **~ *s.o. to ~*** levar alguém à loucura
distraught [dɪ'strɔːt] *adj* perturbado
distress [dɪ'stres] **1** *n* (*mental suffering*) angústia *f*; (*physical pain*) dor *f*; ***in ~*** *ship, aircraft* em perigo **2** *v/t* (*upset*) angustiar
distressing [dɪ'stresɪŋ] *adj* angustiante
dis'tress signal sinal *m* de perigo
distribute [dɪ'strɪbjuːt] *v/t* distribuir
distribution [dɪstrɪ'bjuːʃn] distribuição *f*
distributor [dɪs'trɪbjuːtər] COM distribuidor,a *m,f*
district ['dɪstrɪkt] distrito *m*
district at'torney promotor,a *m,f* público,-a
distrust [dɪs'trʌst] **1** *n* desconfiança *f* **2** *v/t* desconfiar
disturb [dɪ'stɜːrb] *v/t* (*interrupt*) interromper; (*upset*) perturbar; ***do not ~*** não perturbe
disturbance [dɪ'stɜːrbəns] (*interruption*) interrupção *f*; **~*s*** *pl* (*civil unrest*) distúrbios *mpl*
disturbed [dɪ'stɜːrbd] *adj* (*concerned, worried*) perturbado; ***be mentally ~*** ter problemas mentais
disturbing [dɪ'stɜːrbɪŋ] *adj* perturbador
disused [dɪs'juːzd] *adj* fora de uso
ditch [dɪʧ] **1** *n* fosso *m* **2** *v/t fam* (*get rid of*) abandonar
dither ['dɪðər] *v/i* vacilar
dive [daɪv] **1** *n* mergulho *m*; *plane*: picada *f*; *fam* (*bar etc*) espelunca *f*; ***take a ~*** *fam dollar etc* sofrer uma queda **2** *v/i* ⟨*Am pret also* ***dove***⟩ mergulhar; *plane* descer a pique
diver ['daɪvər] *off board* saltador,a *m,f*; *underwater* mergulhador,a *m,f*
diverge [daɪ'vɜːrdʒ] *v/i* divergir-se
diverse [daɪ'vɜːrs] *adj* variado

diversification [daɪvɜːrsɪfɪ'keɪʃn] COM diversificação *f*
diversify [daɪ'vɜːrsɪfaɪ] *v/i* ⟨*pret & pp* ***diversified***⟩ COM diversificar
diversion [daɪ'vɜːrʃn] *traffic*: desvio *m*; *to distract attention* distração *f*
diversity [daɪ'vɜːrsətɪ] diversidade *f*
divert [daɪ'vɜːrt] *v/t traffic* desviar; *attention* distrair
divest [daɪ'vest] *v/t* ***~ X of Y*** despojar X de Y
divide [dɪ'vaɪd] *v/t* dividir
dividend ['dɪvɪdend] *also fig* dividendo *m*
divine [dɪ'vaɪn] *adj also fam* divino
diving ['daɪvɪŋ] *from board* salto *m*; *scuba* mergulho *m*
'diving board trampolim *m*
divisible [dɪ'vɪzəbl] *adj* divisível
division [dɪ'vɪʒn] divisão *f*; *company*: departamento *m*
divorce [dɪ'vɔːrs] **1** *n* divórcio *m*; ***get a ~*** obter um divórcio **2** *v/t* divorciar; ***get ~d*** divorciar-se **3** *v/i* divorciar-se
divorced [dɪ'vɔːrst] *adj* divorciado
divorcee [dɪvɔːr'siː] *Am* divorciada *f*; *Brit* divorciado,-a *m,f*
divulge [daɪ'vʌldʒ] *v/t* divulgar
DIY [diːaɪ'waɪ] *abbr* (*of* ***do it yourself***) *Brit* faça você mesmo
dizziness ['dɪzɪnɪs] vertigem *f*
dizzy ['dɪzɪ] *adj* tonto; ***feel ~*** sentir-se tonto
DJ[1] ['diːdʒeɪ] *abbr* (*of* ***disc jockey***) disc-jóquei *m/f*
DJ[2] [diː'dʒeɪ] *abbr* (*of* ***dinner jacket***) *Brit* smoking *m*
DNA [diːen'eɪ] *abbr* (*of* ***deoxyribonucleic acid***) ADN (ácido *m* desoxirribonucléico)
do [duː] ⟨*pret* ***did***, *pp* ***done***⟩ **1** *v/t one's work, hair, the beds, French, chemistry, 100 mph etc* fazer; ***what are you ~ing tonight?*** o que você vai fazer hoje à noite?; ***I don't know what to ~*** não sei o que fazer; ***no, I'll ~ it*** não, eu faço; ***~ it right now!*** faça agora mesmo!; ***have you done this before?*** você já fez isso antes?; ***have one's hair done*** fazer o cabelo **2** *v/i* (*be suitable, enough*) bastar; ***that will ~!*** basta!; ***~ well*** *person, business* ir bem; ***well done!*** (*congratulations!*) parabéns!; ***how ~ you ~?*** como vai? **3** *v aux* ***~ you know him?*** você o conhece?; ***I don't know*** não sei; ***~ be quick*** seja bem rápido; ***~ you like Washington? – yes I ~*** você gosta de Washington? - sim, gosto; ***he works hard, doesn't he?*** ele trabalha duro, não é?; ***don't you believe me?*** você acredita em mim?; ***you ~ believe me, don't you?*** você acredita em mim, não?; ***you don't know the answer, ~ you? – no I don't*** você não sabe a resposta, sabe? - não, não sei
♦**do away with** *v/t* (*abolish*) abolir
♦**do in** *v/t fam* (*exhaust*) ficar exausto; ***I'm done in*** estou exausto
♦**do out of** *v/t* ***do X out of Y*** *fam* lograr X em Y
♦**do up** *v/t* (*renovate*) renovar; (*fasten*) fechar; *buttons* abotoar; *laces* atar
♦**do with** *v/t* ***I could do with ...*** bem que eu gostaria de ...; ***he won't have anything to do with it*** (*won't get involved*) ele não terá nada a ver com isso
♦**do without** *v/t & v/i* ficar sem
docile ['doʊsaɪl] *adj person* dócil; *animal* manso
dock[1] [dɑːk] NAUT **1** *n* doca *f* **2** *v/i* entrar em doca
dock[2] [dɑːk] *n* LAW banco *m* dos réus
'dockyard estaleiro *m*
doctor ['dɑːktər] *n* doutor,a *m,f*
doctorate ['dɑːktərət] doutorado *m*
doctrine ['dɑːktrɪn] doutrina *f*
docudrama ['dɑːkjʊdrɑːmə] drama-documentário *m*
document ['dɑːkjʊmənt] *n* documento *m*
documentary [dɑːkjʊ'mentərɪ] *n* documentário *m*
documentation [dɑːkjʊmen'teɪʃn] documentação *f*
dodge [dɑːdʒ] *v/t blow* esquivar-se de; *person, issue* evitar; *question* furtar-se a
dodgems ['dɑːdʒəms] *npl* autopista *m*
doe [doʊ] (*deer*) corça *f*
dog [dɒːg] **1** *n* cão *m* **2** *v/t* ⟨*pret & pp* ***dogged***⟩ *bad luck* perseguir

'dog catcher homem *m* da carrocinha
dog-eared ['dɒːgɪrd] *adj book* com orelhas
dogged ['dɒːgɪd] *adj* obstinado
doggie ['dɒːgɪ] *children's language* cachorrinho *m*
doggy bag ['dɒːgɪbæg] *saquinho m para levar embora o que sobrou numa refeição*
'doghouse canil *m*; ***be in the ~*** *fam* estar em maus lençóis
dogma ['dɒːgmə] dogma *m*
dogmatic [dɒːg'mætɪk] *adj* dogmático
do-gooder ['duːgʊdər] *pej* salvador,a *m,f* do mundo
dogsbody ['dɒːgzbɒːdɪ] *fam* faz-tudo *m/f*
'dog tag *Am* MIL placa *f* de identificação usada no pescoço
'dog-tired *adj fam* esgotado
do-it-yourself [duːɪtjə'self] *Brit* faça você mesmo
doldrums ['doʊldrəmz] ***be in the ~*** *economy* estar estagnada; *person* ficar abatido
dole [doʊl] *Brit fam* seguro-desemprego *m*; ***be on the ~*** receber seguro-desemprego
♦ **dole out** *v/t* distribuir
dole money *Brit* → ***welfare***
doll [dɑːl] (*toy*) *also fam* (*woman*) boneca *f*
♦ **doll up** *v/t* ***get dolled up*** *fam* embonecar-se, *Port* ataviar-se
dollar ['dɑːlər] dólar *m*
dollop ['dɑːləp] *n fam* bocado *m*
dolphin ['dɑːlfɪn] golfinho *m*
domain [də'meɪn] COMPUT domínio *m*
dome [doʊm] *of building* cúpula *f*
domestic [də'mestɪk] *adj chores* doméstico; *news, policy* nacional
domestic 'animal animal *m* doméstico
domesticate [də'mestɪkeɪt] *v/t animal* domesticar; ***be ~d*** *person* ser prendado
do'mestic flight vôo *m* doméstico
dominant ['dɑːmɪnənt] *adj* predominante; *gene* dominante
dominate ['dɑːmɪneɪt] *v/t* dominar; *landscape* predominar em
domination [dɑːmɪ'neɪʃn] dominação *f*
domineering [dɑːmɪ'nɪrɪŋ] *adj* mandão (mandona)
Dominican [də'mɪnɪkən] *adj* ***the ~ Republic*** a República Dominicana
donate [doʊ'neɪt] *v/t money, time, also* MED doar
donation [doʊ'neɪʃn] *money, time, liver*: MED doação *f*
done [dʌn] *pp* → ***do***
donkey ['dɑːŋkɪ] burro *m*
donor ['doʊnər] *also* MED doador,a *m,f*
donut ['doʊnʌt] rosquinha *f*, *Port* bola *f* de Berlim
doodle ['duːdl] *v/i* rabiscar
doom [duːm] *n* (*fate*) destino *m*; (*ruin*) perdição *f*
doomed [duːmd] *adj project* condenado; ***we are ~*** (*bound to fail*) estamos condenados; ***the ~ ship / plane*** o navio / avião fatídico
door [dɔːr] porta *f*; (*entrance*) entrada *f*; ***there's someone at the ~*** há alguém na porta
'doorbell campainha *f* **'doorknob** maçaneta *f*, *Port* puxador *m* **'doorman** porteiro *m* **'doormat** capacho *m* **'doorstep** degrau *m*; (*area around the door*) soleira *f* **'doorway** entrada *f*
dope [doʊp] **1** *n* (*drugs*) droga *f*; (*idiot*) imbecil *m/f*; (*information*) detalhes *mpl* **2** *v/t* dopar
dormant ['dɔːrmənt] *adj* inativo; ***~ volcano*** vulcão *m* inativo
dormitory ['dɔːrmɪtɔːrɪ] dormitório *m*; *Am* moradia *f* universitária
dosage ['doʊsɪdʒ] dosagem *f*
dose [doʊs] *n* dose *f*
dot [dɑːt] *n over i, in email address* ponto *m*; ***on the ~*** (*exactly*) em ponto
♦ **dote on** [doʊt] *v/t* adorar
doting ['doʊtɪŋ] *adj* afetivo
dotted line ['dɑːtɪd] linha *f* pontilhada
dotty ['dɑːtɪ] *adj fam* caduco
double ['dʌbl] **1** *n amount* dobro *m*; *person* sósia *m/f*; *of movie star* dublê

m/f; *room* quarto *m* de casal **2** *adj* (*twice as much*) dobrado; *whiskey*, *sink*, *oven*, *doors*, *layer* duplo; ***in ~ figures*** de dois dígitos **3** *adv* o dobro; ***he paid ~*** ele pagou o dobro **4** *v/t* & *v/i* dobrar; ***it ~s as a bed*** isso funciona também como cama

♦**double back** *v/i* (*go back*) voltar

♦**double up** *v/i in pain* curvar-se; (*share*) dividir

double-'bass contrabaixo *m* **double 'bed** cama *f* de casal **double-'breasted** *adj* com duas fileiras de botões **double'check** *v/t* & *v/i* reverificar **double 'chin** papo *m* **double-'click** *v/i* fazer duplo clique **double'cross** *v/t* enganar **double 'glazing** janela *f* de vidro duplo **double'park** *v/i* estacionar em fila dupla **'double-quick** *adj* ***in ~ time*** num piscar de olhos **'double room** quarto *m* de casal

doubles ['dʌblz] *in tennis* duplas *fpl*

doubt [daʊt] **1** *n* dúvida *f*; (*uncertainty*) incerteza *f*; ***be in ~*** estar em dúvida; ***no ~*** sem dúvida **2** *v/t* duvidar

doubtful ['daʊtfʊl] *adj remark*, *look* duvidoso; ***be ~*** *person* ter dúvida; ***it is ~ whether*** não é certo que

doubtfully ['daʊtflɪ] *adv* duvidosamente

doubtless ['daʊtlɪs] *adj* sem dúvida

dough [doʊ] massa *f*; *fam* (*money*) grana *f*

doughnut ['doʊnʌt] sonho *m* doce, *Port* bola *f* de Berlim

dove[1] [dʌv] *n* pombo,-a *m,f*; *fig* cordeiro *m*

dove[2] [doʊv] *pret Am* → ***dive***

dowdy ['daʊdɪ] *adj* deselegante

Dow Jones Average [daʊdʒoʊnz'ævərɪdʒ] índice *m* Dow Jones

down[1] [daʊn] *n* (*feathers*) penugem *f*

down[2] [daʊn] **1** *adv* (*downward*) para baixo; ***cut / shoot ~*** derrubar; ***come ~*** descer; ***go ~ on one's knees*** ficar de joelhos; ***fall ~*** cair; ***die ~*** abrandar; ***200 ~*** *as deposit* 200 de entrada; ***they are two goals ~*** estão perdendo por dois gols **2** *prep* (*along*) ao longo de; ***he walked ~ the street*** ele andou ao longo da rua; ***they live ~ the hill*** moram para baixo da colina; ***it's ~ south*** é rumo ao sul; ***~ there*** lá embaixo **3** *adj* ***be ~*** *fam depressed* ficar deprimido **4** *v/t* (*destroy*) destruir; *drink* entornar

'down-and-out *n* vagabundo,-a *m,f*

'downcast *adj* (*dejected*) abatido

'downfall ruína *f*; *of politician* queda *f* **'downgrade** *v/t* rebaixar **downhearted** [daʊn'hɑːrtɪd] *adj* desanimado **'downhill** *adv* em declive; ***go ~*** *fig* ir ladeira abaixo **'downhill skiing** esqui *m* alpino **'download** COMPUT **1** *v/t* fazer um download de **2** *n* download *m*; **'downmarket** *adj Brit* serviço barato **'down payment** entrada *f* **'downplay** *v/t* minimizar **'downpour** aguaceiro *m* **'downright 1** *adj lie*, *idiot* patente **2** *adv dangerous*, *stupid etc* absolutamente **'downscale** *adj* serviço barato **'downside** desvantagem *f* **'downsize 1** *v/t car* reduzir **2** *v/i company* reduzir o quadro de funcionários **downstairs** ['daʊnsterz] **1** *adj* no andar de baixo **2** *adv* lá embaixo **down-to-'earth** *adj approach*, *person* realista **'down-town 1** *adj* do centro da cidade **2** *adv* no centro da cidade **'downturn** *in economy* declínio *m*

'downward 1 *adj* descendente **2** *adv* de cima a baixo

downwards *Brit* → ***downward***

doze [doʊz] **1** *n* cochilo *m* **2** *v/i* cochilar

♦**doze off** *v/i* adormecer

dozen ['dʌzn] dúzia *f*; ***~s of …*** *fam* dúzias de …

drab [dræb] *adj* sombrio

draft [dræft] **1** *n document*: rascunho *m*; MIL alistamento *m*; *Am air*: lufada *f*; ***~ beer, beer on ~*** chope *m* **2** *v/t document* rascunhar; MIL alistar

'draft dodger *pessoa que se recusa a prestar o serviço militar*

draftee [dræft'iː] *Am* incorporado *m* ao serviço militar

draftsman ['dræftsmən] *Am* desenhista técnico,-a *m,f*; *plan*: projetista *m/f*

drafty ['dræftɪ] *adj Am* ***it's ~*** faz corrente de ar

drag [dræg] **1** *n* ***it's a ~ having to ...*** *fam* é uma chatice ter que ...; ***he's a ~*** *fam* ele é um chato; ***the main ~*** *fam* a rua principal; ***in ~*** vestido de mulher **2** *v/t* ⟨*pret & pp* ***dragged***⟩ (*pull*) arrastar; (*search*) dragar **3** *v/i* ⟨*pret & pp* ***dragged***⟩ *time, show, movie* arrastar-se; ***~ X into Y*** (*involve*) envolver X em Y; ***~ X out of Y*** (*get information from*) arrancar X de Y

◆**drag away** *v/t* ***drag oneself away from the TV*** arrastar-se para longe da TV

◆**drag in** *v/t into conversation* pôr no meio de

◆**drag on** *v/i* (*last long time*) arrastar-se

◆**drag out** *v/t* (*prolong*) prolongar

◆**drag up** *v/t fam* (*mention*) meter no meio da conversa

dragon ['drægn] *also fig* dragão *m*

drain [dreɪn] **1** *n* (*pipe*) tubo *m* de escoamento; *under street* bueiro *m*; ***a ~ on resources*** um sorvedouro no orçamento **2** *v/t water, vegetables* escorrer; *oil* escoar; *land* drenar; *glass, tank* esvaziar; (*exhaust person*) exaurir **3** *v/i dishes* secar

◆**drain away** *v/i liquid* escoar-se

◆**drain off** *v/t water* escorrer

drainage ['dreɪnɪdʒ] (*drains*) drenos *mpl*; *of water from soil* drenagem *f*

'**drainpipe** tubo *m* de esgoto

drama ['drɑːmə] drama *m*; *art form* arte *f* dramática

dramatic [drə'mætɪk] *adj* dramático

dramatically [drə'mætɪklɪ] *adv* dramaticamente

dramatist ['dræmətɪst] dramaturgo,-a *m,f*

dramatization [dræmətaɪ'zeɪʃn] dramatização *f*

dramatize ['dræmətaɪz] *v/t story, also fig* dramatizar

drank [dræŋk] *pret* → ***drink***

drape [dreɪp] *v/t* ***~ X over Y*** jogar X sobre Y

drapery ['dreɪpərɪ] tecido *m*

drapes [dreɪps] *npl Am* cortinado *m*

drastic ['dræstɪk] *adj* drástico

draught ***etc*** *Brit* → ***draft***

draw [drɒː] **1** *n match, competition*: empate *m*; *lottery*: sorteio *m*; (*attraction*) atração *f* **2** *v/t* ⟨*pret* ***drew***, *pp* ***drawn***⟩ *picture* desenhar; *in lottery* sortear; *gun, knife, also from bank account* sacar; (*attract*) atrair; (*lead*) levar; *cart* puxar; *curtain* fechar; (*open*) abrir **3** *v/i* ⟨*pret* ***drew***, *pp* ***drawn***⟩ desenhar; *in match, competition* empatar; ***~ near*** aproximar-se

◆**draw back 1** *v/i* (*recoil*) encolher-se **2** *v/t* (*pull back*) puxar para trás

◆**draw on 1** *v/i* (*approach*) aproximar-se **2** *v/t* (*make use of*) basear-se em

◆**draw out** *v/t wallet* tirar; *money from bank* sacar

◆**draw up 1** *v/t document* redigir; *chair* puxar **2** *v/i vehicle* parar

'**drawback** desvantagem *f*

drawer[1] [drɒːr] *of desk etc* gaveta *f*

drawer[2] [drɒːr] *person* desenhista *m/f*

drawing ['drɒːɪŋ] desenho *m*

'**drawing board** prancheta *f* de desenho; ***go back to the ~*** voltar para a prancheta

drawing pin *Brit* → ***thumbtack***

drawl [drɒːl] *n* fala *f* arrastada

drawn [drɒːn] *pp* → ***draw***

dread [dred] *v/t* ter pavor de

dreadful ['dredfʊl] *adj* terrível

dreadfully ['dredflɪ] *adv fam* (*extremely*) terrivelmente; *behave* horrivelmente

dream [driːm] **1** *n* sonho *m* **2** *adj fam house etc* de sonhos **3** *v/t & v/i* sonhar

◆**dream up** *v/t* devanear

dreamer ['driːmər] sonhador,a *m,f*

dreary ['drɪrɪ] *adj* monótono

dredge [dredʒ] *v/t canal* dragar

◆**dredge up** *v/t fig* trazer à tona

dregs [dregz] *npl coffee*: borra *f*; ***the ~ of society*** a escória da sociedade

drench [drentʃ] *v/t* encharcar; ***get ~ed*** ficar encharcado

dress [dres] **1** *n woman*: vestido *m*; (*clothing*) vestuário *m* **2** *v/t person* vestir; *wound* fazer um curativo em **3** *v/i* (*get dressed*) vestir-se

◆**dress up** *v/i* vestir-se com elegância; (*wear a disguise*) fantasiar-se; ***dress up as*** fantasiar-se de

'dress circle balcão *m* acima da platéia
dresser ['dresər] (*dressing table*) penteadeira *f*, *Port* toucador *m*; *in kitchen* guarda-louças *m*
dressing ['dresɪŋ] *salad*: molho *m*; *wound*: curativo *m*
dressing 'down repreensão *f* **'dressing room** *in theater* camarim *m* **'dressing table** penteadeira *f*
'dressmaker costureiro,-a *m,f*
'dress rehearsal ensaio *m* geral
dressy ['dresɪ] *adj fam* chique
drew [dru:] *pret* → ***draw***
dribble ['drɪbl] *v/i person* salivar; *baby* babar; *water* pingar; SPORT driblar
dried [draɪd] *adj fruit etc* seco
drier → ***dryer***
drift [drɪft] **1** *n snow*: monte *m* **2** *v/i snow* amontoar-se; *ship* ficar à deriva; (*go off course*) derivar; *person* vaguear
♦**drift apart** *v/i couple* distanciar-se
drifter ['drɪftər] ***be a ~*** não ter rumo
drill [drɪl] **1** *n tool* furadeira *f*; (*exercise*) exercício *m*; MIL manobra *f* militar **2** *v/t hole* furar **3** *v/i for oil* perfurar; MIL fazer manobras de exercício
drilling rig ['drɪlɪŋrɪg] (*platform*) perfuratriz *f*
drily ['draɪlɪ] *adv remark* secamente
drink [drɪŋk] **1** *n* bebida *f*; ***a ~ of ...*** um copo de ...; ***go for a ~*** sair para tomar uma bebida **2** *v/t & v/i* ‹*pret* ***drank***, *pp* ***drunk***› beber
♦**drink up 1** *v/i* (*finish drink*) beber tudo **2** *v/t* (*drink completely*) beber todo,-a o/a
drinkable ['drɪŋkəbl] *adj* potável
drink driving → ***drunk driving***
drinker ['drɪŋkər] alcoólatra *m/f*
drinking ['drɪŋkɪŋ] *alcohol*: bebedeira *f*
'drinking water água *f* potável
'drinks machine máquina *f* de bebidas
drip [drɪp] **1** *n* (*liquid*) pingo *m*; *Brit* MED soro *m* **2** *v/i* ‹*pret & pp* ***dripped***› pingar
dripping ['drɪpɪŋ] *adv* ***~ wet*** pingando
drive [draɪv] **1** *n* trajeto *m*; (*outing*) passeio *m* de carro; (*energy*) energia *f*; COMPUT drive *m*; (*campaign*) campanha *f*; ***left- / right-hand ~*** MOT direção à esquerda / direita **2** *v/t* ‹*pret* ***drove***, *pp* ***driven***› *vehicle* dirigir, *Port* guiar; (*own*) ter; (*take in car*) levar de carro; TECH acionar; ***that noise / he is driving me mad*** esse barulho / ele está me deixando maluco **3** *v/i* ‹*pret* ***drove***, *pp* ***driven***› dirigir, *Port* guiar
♦**drive at** *v/t* ***what are you driving at?*** o que você está tentando dizer?
♦**drive away 1** *v/t* levar (de carro); (*chase off*) afugentar **2** *v/i* ir embora de carro
♦**drive in** *v/t nail* pregar
♦**drive off** → ***drive away***
'drive-by shooting tiro *m* em andamento
'drive-in *n* (*movie theater*) drive-in *m*
drivel ['drɪvl] *n* besteira *f*
driven ['drɪvn] *pp* → ***drive***
driver ['draɪvər] motorista *m/f*; *of train* condutor,a *m,f*; COMPUT driver *m*
'driver's license *Am* carteira *f* de motorista, *Port* carta *f* de condução
'drive-thru *restaurante onde se compra a comida sentado no carro*
'driveway entrada *f* de carro
driving ['draɪvɪŋ] **1** *n* direção *f*, *Port* condução *f* **2** *adj rain* violento
driving 'force força *f* propulsora **'driving instructor** instrutor,a *m,f* de direção, *Port* instrutor,a de condução **'driving lesson** aula *f* de direção, *Port* aula de condução **'driving licence** *Brit* carteira *f* de motorista, *Port* carta *f* de condução **'driving school** auto-escola *f* **'driving test** exame *m* de motorista
drizzle ['drɪzl] **1** *n* chuvisco *m* **2** *v/i* chuviscar
drone [droʊn] *n dull noise* zumbido *m*
droop [dru:p] *v/i* pender; *plant* murchar
drop [drɑ:p] **1** *n of rain*, *also* (*small amount*) gota *f*; *in price*, *temperature* queda *f*; *in number* diminuição *f* **2** *v/t* ‹*pret & pp* ***dropped***› *object* deixar cair; *person from car* deixar; *person from team* cortar; (*stop seeing*)

abandonar; *charges, demand etc* retirar; (*give up*) largar; **~ a line to** escrever um bilhete a **3** *v/i* ⟨*pret & pp* **dropped**⟩ (*fall out, get down*) cair; *wind* parar
◆**drop in** *v/i* (*visit*) aparecer
◆**drop off 1** *v/t person* deixar; (*deliver*) entregar **2** *v/i* (*fall asleep*) adormecer; (*decline*) diminuir
◆**drop out** *v/i* (*withdraw*) retirar-se; *of school* desistir
'**dropout** *from society* marginal *m/f*
drops [drɑːps] *npl for eyes* colírio *m*
drought [draʊt] seca *f*
drove [droʊv] *pret* → **drive**
drown [draʊn] **1** *v/i* afogar-se **2** *v/t person* afogar; *sound* abafar; **be ~ed** afogar-se
drowsy ['draʊzɪ] *adj* sonolento
drudgery ['drʌdʒərɪ] trabalho *m* penoso
drug [drʌg] **1** *n* MED medicamento *m*; (*illegal*) droga *f*; **be on ~s** usar drogas **2** *v/t* ⟨*pret & pp* **drugged**⟩ drogar
'**drug abuse** abuso *m* de drogas
'**drug addict** viciado,-a *m,f* em drogas
'**drug dealer** traficante *m/f* de drogas
druggist ['drʌgɪst] *Am* farmacêutico,-a *m,f*
'**drugstore** drogaria *f*
'**drug trafficking** tráfico *m* de drogas
drum [drʌm] *n* MUS tambor *m*; (*container*) barril *m*
◆**drum into** *v/t* ⟨*pret & pp* **drummed**⟩ incutir; **drum sth into s.o.** incutir algo em alguém
◆**drum up** *v/t* **drum up support** angariar apoio
drummer ['drʌmər] baterista *m/f*
'**drumstick** MUS baqueta *f*; *of poultry* coxinha *f*
drunk [drʌŋk] **1** *n* bêbado,-a *m,f* **2** *adj* bêbado; **get ~** embebedar-se **3** *pp* → **drink**
drunk 'driving direção *f* em estado de embriaguez
drunken ['drʌŋkn] *adj voices, laughter* de bêbado; *party* com bebedeira
dry [draɪ] **1** *adj* seco; (*ironic*) irônico; (*where alcohol is banned*) sujeito à lei seca **2** *v/t* ⟨*pret & pp* **dried**⟩ secar; *dishes* enxugar **3** *v/i* ⟨*pret & pp* **dried**⟩ secar
◆**dry out** *v/i* secar; *alcoholic* desintoxicar-se
◆**dry up** *v/i river* secar; *fam* (*be quiet*) ficar quieto
'**dryclean** *v/t* lavar a seco '**dry cleaner** tinturaria *f* '**drycleaning** (*clothes*) roupa *f* lavada a seco
dryer ['draɪr] (*machine*) secadora *f*
DTP [diːtiː'piː] *abbr* (*of* **desk-top publishing**) editoração *f* eletrônica
dual ['duːəl] *adj* duplo
dual carriageway *Brit* pista *f* dupla
dub [dʌb] *v/t* ⟨*pret & pp* **dubbed**⟩ *movie* dublar
dubious ['duːbɪəs] *adj* dubioso; (*having doubts*) em dúvida
duchess ['dʌtʃes] duquesa *f*
duck [dʌk] **1** *n male* pato *m*; *female* pata *f* **2** *v/i* abaixar-se **3** *v/t head* abaixar; *question* evitar
dud [dʌd] *n fam* (*false bill*) nota *f* falsa
due [duː] *adj* (*owed, also proper*) devido; **be ~** *train etc* ser esperado; **when is the baby ~?** quando nasce o bebê?; **be ~ to** (*be caused by*) ser devido a; **in ~ course** no devido tempo
dues [duːz] *npl* taxas *fpl*
duet [duː'et] MUS dueto *m*
dug [dʌg] *pret & pp* → **dig**
duke [duːk] duque *m*
dull [dʌl] *adj weather* nublado; *sound, pain* surdo; (*boring*) enfadonho
duly ['duːlɪ] *adv* (*as expected*) no devido tempo; (*properly*) devidamente
dumb [dʌm] *adj* (*mute*) mudo; *fam* (*stupid*) burro
dumbfounded [dʌm'faʊndɪd] *adj* pasmado
dummy ['dʌmɪ] *for clothes* manequim *m*; *Brit* chupeta *f*
dump [dʌmp] **1** *n for garbage* lixeira *f*; (*unpleasant place*) lixo *m* **2** *v/t* (*deposit*) descarregar; *waste* depositar; **he ~ed the body in the canal** ele se desfez do corpo no canal
dumpling ['dʌmplɪŋ] bolinho *m* cozido
dune [duːn] duna *f*
dung [dʌŋ] estrume *m*
dungarees [dʌŋgə'riːz] *npl* macacão *m*, *Port* fato *m* macaco

dunk [dʌŋk] *v/t in coffee etc* embeber
duo ['duːoʊ] MUS duo *m*
duplex, **duplex apartment** ['duːpleks] *Am* apartamento *m* duplex
duplicate 1 ['duːplɪkət] *n* duplicata *f*; ***in ~*** em duas vias **2** ['duːplɪkeɪt] *v/t* duplicar; (*copy*) copiar; (*repeat*) refazer
duplicate 'key duplicata *f* de chave
durable ['dʊrəbl] *adj material, relationship* durável
duration [dʊ'reɪʃn] duração *f*
duress [dʊ'res] coação *f*; ***under ~*** sob coação
during ['dʊrɪŋ] *prep* durante
dusk [dʌsk] crepúsculo *m*
dust [dʌst] **1** *n* poeira *f* **2** *v/t* tirar o pó de; ***~ X with Y*** (*sprinkle*) polvilhar X com Y
'dustbin *Brit* lata *f* de lixo
'dust cover *for book* sobrecapa *f*
duster ['dʌstər] (*cloth*) pano *m* de pó
'dust jacket *book*: sobrecapa *f* **'dustman** *Brit* lixeiro *m*, gari *m* **'dustpan** pá *f* de lixo
dusty ['dʌstɪ] *adj* empoeirado
Dutch [dʌʧ] **1** *adj* holandês,-esa; ***go ~*** *fam* dividir a conta **2** *n language* holandês *m*; ***the ~*** os holandeses
duty ['duːtɪ] dever *m*; (*task*) tarefa *f*; *on goods* taxa *f*; ***be on ~*** estar de serviço; ***be off ~*** estar de folga
duty'free 1 *adj* livre de impostos **2** *n* mercadoria *f* livre de impostos
duty free al'lowance montante *m* de isenção *f* de taxas
duty'free shop duty-free shop *m*
DVD [diːvi'diː] DVD *m*
dwarf [dwɔːrf] **1** *n* anão *m*, anã *f* **2** *v/t* fazer parecer menor
♦ **dwell on** [dwel] *v/t* estender-se sobre
dwindle ['dwɪndl] *v/i* diminuir
dye [daɪ] **1** *n* tintura *f* **2** *v/t* tingir
dying ['daɪɪŋ] *adj person* moribundo; *industry, tradition* em declínio
dynamic [daɪ'næmɪk] *adj* dinâmico
dynamism ['daɪnəmɪzm] dinamismo *m*
dynamite ['daɪnəmaɪt] *n* dinamite *f*
dynamo ['daɪnəmoʊ] TECH dínamo *m*
dynasty ['daɪnəstɪ] dinastia *f*
dyslexia [dɪs'leksɪə] dislexia *f*
dyslexic [dɪs'leksɪk] **1** *adj* disléxico **2** *n* disléxico,-a *m,f*

E

each [iːʧ] **1** *adj* cada **2** *adv* cada; ***they're 1.50 ~*** custam 1,50 cada **3** *pron* cada um/uma; ***we know ~ other*** (nós) nos conhecemos; ***they know ~ other*** eles se conhecem; ***we should be kind to ~ other*** nós deveríamos ser gentis um com o outro
eager ['iːgər] *adj* ávido
eagerly ['iːgərlɪ] *adv* avidamente
eagerness ['iːgərnɪs] ânsia *f*
eagle ['iːgl] águia *f*
eagle-eyed [iːgl'aɪd] *adj* perspicaz
ear[1] [ɪr] *person, animal*: orelha *f*
ear[2] [ɪr] *corn*: espiga *f*
'earache dor *f* de ouvido
'eardrum tímpano *m*
earl [ɜːrl] conde *m*
'earlobe lóbulo *m* da orelha
early ['ɜːrlɪ] **1** *adj* (*not late*) cedo; (*ahead of time*) antecipado; (*farther back in time*) primitivo; (*in the near future*) breve; ***I'm an ~ riser*** sou madrugador,a; ***~ stages*** etapas iniciais; ***in the ~ hours*** nas primeiras horas; ***in ~ September*** no início de setembro; ***an ~ variety of potato*** uma primitiva variedade de batata **2** *adv* (*not late*) cedo; (*ahead of time*) antecipadamente ***my roses bloomed ~ this year*** minhas rosas floresceram antecipadamente esse ano; ***it's too***

~ to say é muito cedo para dizer
'early bird madrugador,a *m,f*
earmark ['ɪrmɑːrk] *v/t* reservar; **~ sth for sth** reservar algo para algo
earn [ɜːrn] *v/t salary, holiday, drink etc* ganhar; *respect* merecer
earnest ['ɜːrnɪst] *adj* sério; **in ~** a sério
earnings ['ɜːrnɪŋz] *npl* lucro *m*
'earphones *npl* fone *m* de ouvido **'ear-piercing** *adj* estridente **'earring** brinco *m* **'earshot within ~** ao alcance do ouvido; **out of ~** fora do alcance do ouvido
earth [ɜːrθ] *(soil)* terra *f*; *(world, planet)* Terra *f*; **where on ~ …?** *fam* onde diabos …?
earthenware ['ɜːrθnwer] *n* louça *f* de barro
earthly ['ɜːrθlɪ] *adj* terreno; **it's no ~ use** *fam* é inútil
earthquake ['ɜːrθkweɪk] terremoto *m*, *Port* terramoto *f*
earth-shattering ['ɜːrθʃætərɪŋ] *adj* chocante
ease [iːz] **1** *n* facilidade *f*; **be at (one's) ~, feel at ~** estar / sentir-se à vontade; **be or feel ill at ~** ficar / sentir-se irrequieto **2** *v/t (relieve)* aliviar **3** *v/i pain* aliviar
♦**ease off 1** *v/t (remove)* tirar **2** *v/i pain, rain* passar
easel ['iːzl] cavalete *m*
easily ['iːzəlɪ] *adv (with ease)* facilmente; *(by far)* de longe
east [iːst] **1** *n* leste *m* **2** *adj* leste **3** *adv travel* para o leste
Easter ['iːstər] Páscoa *f*
Easter 'Day Dia *m* de Páscoa
'Easter egg ovo *m* de Páscoa
easterly ['iːstəlɪ] *adj (coming from the east)* do leste; *(eastbound)* em direção leste
Easter 'Monday segunda-feira *f* de Páscoa
eastern ['iːstərn] *adj* do leste; *(oriental)* oriental
easterner ['iːstərnər] nativo,-a *m,f* do leste
eastward, eastwards ['iːstwərd(z)] *adv* em direção leste
easy ['iːzɪ] *adj* fácil; *(relaxed)* cômodo; **take things ~** *(slow down)* levar as coisas com calma; **take it ~!** *(calm down)* tenha calma!
'easy chair poltrona *f*
easy-going ['iːzɪgoʊɪŋ] *adj* pacato
eat [iːt] *v/t & v/i* ⟨*pret* **ate**, *pp* **eaten**⟩ comer
♦**eat out** *v/i* comer fora
♦**eat up** *v/t food* comer todo; *fig* consumir
eatable ['iːtəbl] *adj* comestível
eaten ['iːtn] *pp* → **eat**
eau de Cologne [oʊdəkə'loʊn] água-de-colônia *f*
eaves [iːvz] *npl* beira *f*
eavesdrop ['iːvzdrɑːp] *v/i* ⟨*pret & pp* **eavesdropped**⟩ escutar às escondidas
ebb [eb] *v/i tide* vazar
♦**ebb away** *v/i fig courage, strength* declinar
'ebb tide maré *f* vazante
e-book ['iːbʊk] livro *m* eletrônico
eccentric [ɪk'sentrɪk] **1** *adj* excêntrico **2** *n* excêntrico,-a *m,f*
eccentricity [ɪksen'trɪsɪtɪ] excentricidade *f*
echo ['ekoʊ] **1** *n* eco *m* **2** *v/i* ecoar **3** *v/t words, views* repetir; *(agree with)* concordar com
eclipse [ɪ'klɪps] **1** *n* eclipse *m* **2** *v/t fig* eclipsar
'ecofriendly *adj* ecológico
ecological [iːkə'lɑːdʒɪkl] *adj* ecológico; **~ balance** equilíbrio *m* ecológico
ecologically [iːkə'lɑːdʒɪklɪ] *adv* ecologicamente
ecologically 'friendly *adj* ecologicamente correto
ecologist [iː'kɑːlədʒɪst] ecologista *m/f*
ecology [iː'kɑːlədʒɪ] ecologia *f*
e-commerce ['iːkɑːmɜːrs] comércio *m* electrónico
economic [iːkə'nɑːmɪk] *adj* econômico
economical [iːkə'nɑːmɪkl] *adj* econômico
economically [iːkə'nɑːmɪklɪ] *adv (in terms of economics)* economicamente; *(thriftily)* modestamente
economics [iːkə'nɑːmɪks] economia *f*

economist [ɪ'kɑːnəmɪst] economista *m/f*
economize [ɪ'kɑːnəmaɪz] *v/i* economizar
♦**economize on** *v/t* economizar em
economy [ɪ'kɑːnəmɪ] *also* (*saving*) economia *f*
e'conomy class classe *f* econômica **e'conomy drive** esforço *m* para economizar **e'conomy size** tamanho *m* econômico
ecosystem ['iːkousɪstm] ecossistema *m*
ecotourism ['iːkoʊtʊrɪzm] ecoturismo *m*
ecstasy ['ekstəsɪ] êxtase *m*
ecstatic [ɪk'stætɪk] *adj* extasiado
Ecuador ['ekwədɔːr] Equador *m*
Ecuadorian [ekwə'dɔːrɪən] **1** *adj* equatoriano **2** *n* equatoriano,-a *m,f*
eczema ['eksmə] eczema *m*
edge [edʒ] **1** *n knife*: fio *m*; *table*, *seat*: borda *f*; *lawn*, *road*, *cliff*: beira *f*; *in voice* aspereza *f*; ***on ~*** nervoso **2** *v/i* (*move slowly*) mover-se lentamente
edgewise ['edʒwaɪz] *adv* lateralmente; ***I couldn't get a word in ~*** não pude entrar na conversa
edgy ['edʒɪ] *adj* nervoso
edible ['edɪbl] *adj* comestível
edit ['edɪt] *v/t text*, *newspaper*, *TV program*, *movie*, *book* editar
edition [ɪ'dɪʃn] edição *f*
editor ['edɪtər] *text*, *newspaper*, *TV program*, *movie*, *book*: editor,a *m,f*; ***sports / political ~*** editor de esportes / política
editorial [edɪ'tɔːrɪəl] **1** *adj* editorial **2** *n* editorial *m*
EDP [iːdiː'piː] *abbr* (*of* ***electronic data processing***) processamento *m* eletrônico de dados
educate ['edʊkeɪt] *v/t child* educar; *consumers* esclarecer
educated ['edʊkeɪtɪd] *adj person* instruído
education [edʊ'keɪʃn] educação *f*; ***to complete one's ~*** completar seus estudos
educational [edʊ'keɪʃnl] *adj* educacional; (*informative*) educativo
eel [iːl] enguia *f*
eerie ['ɪrɪ] *adj* estranho
effect [ɪ'fekt] efeito *m*; ***take ~*** *medicine*, *drug* fazer efeito; ***come into ~*** *law* entrar em vigor
effective [ɪ'fektɪv] *adj* (*efficient*) eficiente; (*striking*) impressionante; ***~ May 1*** a partir de 1º de maio
effeminate [ɪ'femɪnət] *adj* efeminado
effervescent [efər'vesnt] *adj* efervescente; *personality* vibrante
efficiency [ɪ'fɪʃənsɪ] eficiência *f*; *apartment* apartamento *m* tipo estúdio
efficient [ɪ'fɪʃənt] *adj* eficiente
efficiently [ɪ'fɪʃəntlɪ] *adv* eficientemente
effluent ['eflʊənt] efluente *m*
effort ['efərt] (*struggle*) esforço *m*; (*attempt*) tentativa *f*; ***make an ~ to do sth*** fazer um esforço para fazer algo
effortless ['efərtlɪs] *adj* fácil
effrontery [ɪ'frʌntərɪ] descaramento *m*
effusive [ɪ'fjuːsɪv] *adj* efusivo
e.g. [iː'dʒiː] p. ex.
egalitarian [ɪgælɪ'terɪən] *adj* igualitário
egg [eg] ovo *m*
♦**egg on** *v/t* incitar
'eggcup oveiro *m* **'egghead** *fam* intelectual *m/f* **'eggplant** *Am* berinjela *f* **'eggshell** casca *f* de ovo
ego ['iːgoʊ] PSYCH, *also* (*self-esteem*) ego *m*
egocentric [iːgoʊ'sentrɪk] *adj* egocêntrico
egoism ['iːgoʊɪzm] egoísmo *m*
egoist ['iːgoʊɪst] egoísta *m/f*
Egypt ['iːdʒɪpt] Egito *m*
Egyptian [ɪ'dʒɪpʃn] **1** *adj* egípcio **2** *n* egípcio,-a *m,f*
eiderdown ['aɪdərdaʊn] (*quilt*) edredom *m*, *Port* edredão *m*
eight [eɪt] oito
eighteen [eɪ'tiːn] dezoito
eighteenth [eɪ'tiːnθ] *n & adj* décimo-oitavo (*m*)
eighth [eɪtθ] *n & adj* oitavo (*m*)
eightieth ['eɪtɪəθ] *n & adj* octogésimo (*m*)
eighty ['eɪtɪ] oitenta
either ['iːðər] **1** *adj* um ou outro;

(*both*) ambos **2** *pron* qualquer **3** *adv* também não; ***I won't go ~*** também não vou **4** *conj* ou; ***~ … or*** ou … ou
eject [ɪ'dʒekt] **1** *v/t* expulsar **2** *v/i from plane* ejetar
◆**eke out** [iːk] *v/t* virar-se; ***they manage to eke out a living*** conseguiram se virar para viver
el [el] *abbr* (*of* ***elevated railroad***) *Am* ferrovia *f* elevada
elaborate 1 [ɪ'læbərət] *adj* elaborado **2** [ɪ'læbəreɪt] *v/i* elaborar; detalhar melhor
elaborately [ɪ'læbəreɪtlɪ] *adv* elaboradamente
elapse [ɪ'læps] *v/i* transcorrer
elastic [ɪ'læstɪk] **1** *adj* elástico **2** *n* elástico *m*
elasticated [ɪ'læstɪkeɪtɪd] *adj* elástico
elastic band → ***rubber band***
elasticity [ɪlæs'tɪsətɪ] elasticidade *f*
elasticized [ɪ'læstɪsaɪzd] *adj* elástico
Elastoplast® *Brit*→ ***Band-Aid®***
elated [ɪ'leɪtɪd] *adj* exultante
elation [ɪ'leɪʃn] júbilo *m*
elbow ['elboʊ] **1** *n* cotovelo *m* **2** *v/t* ***~ s.o. out of the way*** acotovelar alguém para fora do caminho; ***~ one's way through*** abrir caminho às cotoveladas
elder ['eldər] **1** *adj* mais velho **2** *n* primogênito,-a *m,f*
elderly ['eldəlɪ] *adj* idoso
eldest ['eldəst] **1** *adj* o/a mais velho,-a **2** *n* ancião *m*, anciã *f*; ***the ~*** o/a mais velho,-a
elect [ɪ'lekt] *v/t* eleger; ***~ to*** eleger para
elected [ɪ'lektɪd] *adj* eleito
election [ɪ'lekʃn] eleição *f*
e'lection campaign campanha *f* eleitoral
e'lection day dia *m* de eleição
elective [ɪ'lektɪv] *adj* optativo
elector [ɪ'lektər] eleitor,a *m,f*
electoral system [ɪ'lektərəlsɪstm] sistema *m* eleitoral
electorate [ɪ'lektərət] eleitorado *m*
electric [ɪ'lektrɪk] *adj also fig* elétrico
electrical [ɪ'lektrɪkl] *adj* elétrico
electrical engi'neer engenheiro,-a *m,f* elétrico,-a
electrical engi'neering engenharia *f* elétrica
electric 'blanket cobertor *m* elétrico
electric 'chair cadeira *f* elétrica
electrician [ɪlek'trɪʃn] eletricista *m/f*
electricity [ɪlek'trɪsətɪ] eletricidade *f*
electric 'razor barbeador *m* elétrico
electrify [ɪ'lektrɪfaɪ] *v/t* ⟨*pret & pp* ***electrified***⟩ *also fig* eletrificar
electrocute [ɪ'lektrəkjuːt] *v/t* eletrocutar
electrode [ɪ'lektroʊd] eletrodo *m*
electron [ɪ'lektrɑːn] elétron *m*, *Port* electrão *m*
electronic [ɪlek'trɑːnɪk] *adj* eletrônico
electronic data 'processing processamento *m* eletrônico de dados
electronic 'mail mensagem *f* eletrônica
electronics [ɪlek'trɑːnɪks] eletrônica *f*
elegance ['elɪgəns] elegância *f*
elegant ['elɪgənt] *adj* elegante
elegantly ['elɪgəntlɪ] *adv* elegantemente
element ['elɪmənt] *also* CHEM elemento *m*
elementary [elɪ'mentərɪ] *adj* (*rudimentary*) elementar
ele'mentary school *Am* escola *f* primária
elephant ['elɪfənt] elefante *m*
elevate ['elɪveɪt] *v/t* elevar
elevated railroad [elɪveɪtɪd'reɪlroʊd] *Am* ferrovia *f* elevada
elevation [elɪ'veɪʃn] (*altitude*) elevação *f*
elevator ['elɪveɪtər] elevador *m*
eleven [ɪ'levn] onze
eleventh [ɪ'levnθ] *n & adj* décimo-primeiro (*m*); ***at the ~ hour*** na última hora
eligible ['elɪdʒəbl] *adj* apto; (*qualified to be voted for*) elegível
eligible 'bachelor bom *m* partido
eliminate [ɪ'lɪmɪneɪt] *v/t* (*get rid of, kill*) eliminar; (*rule out*) descartar; ***be ~d*** *from competition* ser eliminado
elimination [ɪ'lɪmɪneɪʃn] eliminação *f*
elite [eɪ'liːt] **1** *n* elite *f* **2** *adj* elitizado
elk [elk] alce *m*
ellipse [ɪ'lɪps] elipse *f*
elm [elm] olmo *m*
elope [ɪ'loʊp] *v/i* fugir

eloquence ['eləkwəns] eloqüência *f*
eloquent ['eləkwənt] *adj* eloqüente
eloquently ['eləkwəntlɪ] *adv* eloqüentemente
El Salvador [el'sælvədɔːr] El Salvador
else [els] *adv* mais; ***anything ~?*** algo mais?; ***if you've got nothing ~ to do*** se você não tem mais nada a fazer; ***no one ~*** ninguém mais; ***everyone ~ is going*** todos os demais estão indo; ***who ~ was there?*** quem mais estava lá?; ***someone ~*** outra pessoa; ***something ~*** algo mais; ***let's go somewhere ~*** vamos à outro lugar; ***or ~*** ou então
elsewhere ['elswer] *adv be* em outro lugar; *go* para outro lugar
elude [ɪ'luːd] *v/t (escape from)* escapar; *(avoid)* evitar
elusive [ɪ'luːsɪv] *adj* esquivo
emaciated [ɪ'meɪsɪeɪtɪd] *adj* macilento
e-mail ['iːmeɪl] **1** *n* correio *m* eletrônico, e-mail *m* **2** *v/t person* enviar um e-mail a; ***~ sth to s.o.*** enviar algo a alguém por e-mail
'e-mail address endereço *m* eletrônico
emancipated [ɪ'mænsɪpeɪtɪd] *adj woman* emancipado
emancipation [ɪmænsɪ'peɪʃn] emancipação *f*
embalm [ɪm'bɑːm] *v/t* embalsamar
embankment [ɪm'bæŋkmənt] *of river* dique *m*; RAIL aterrado *m*
embargo [em'bɑːrgoʊ] embargo *m*
embark [ɪm'bɑːrk] *v/i* embarcar
♦ **embark on** *v/t* embarcar em
embarrass [ɪm'bærəs] *v/t* constranger
embarrassed [ɪm'bærəst] *adj* constrangido
embarrassing [ɪm'bærəsɪŋ] *adj* embaraçoso
embarrassment [ɪm'bærəsmənt] constrangimento *m*
embassy ['embəsɪ] embaixada *f*
embellish [ɪm'belɪʃ] *v/t* embelezar; *story* florear
embers ['embərz] *npl* brasa *f*
embezzle [ɪm'bezl] *v/t* desviar
embezzlement [ɪm'bezlmənt] desvio *m*
embezzler [ɪm'bezlər] defraudador,a *m,f*
embitter [ɪm'bɪtər] *v/t* amargurar
emblem ['embləm] emblema *m*
embodiment [ɪm'bɑːdɪmənt] encarnação *f*
embody [ɪm'bɑːdɪ] *v/t* ⟨*pret & pp* ***embodied***⟩ representar
embolism ['embəlɪzm] embolia *f*
emboss [ɪm'bɑːs] *v/t metal* gravar em relevo; *paper* colocar em relevo; *fabric* decorar em relevo
embrace [ɪm'breɪs] **1** *n* abraço *m* **2** *v/t (hug)* abraçar; *(take in)* abranger **3** *v/i two people* abraçar-se
embroider [ɪm'brɔɪdər] *v/t* bordar; *fig* enfeitar
embroidery [ɪm'brɔɪdərɪ] bordado *m*
embryo ['embrɪoʊ] embrião *m*
embryonic [embrɪ'ɑːnɪk] *adj fig* embrionário
emerald ['emərəld] *stone* esmeralda *f*; *color* verde-esmeralda *m*
emerge [ɪ'mɜːrdʒ] *v/i (appear)* emergir; ***it has ~d that …*** veio à tona que …
emergency [ɪ'mɜːrdʒənsɪ] emergência *f*; ***in an ~*** em caso de emergência
e'mergency exit saída *f* de emergência **e'mergency landing** aterrissagem *f* de emergência, *Port* aterragem *f* forçosa **e'mergency services** serviços *mpl* de emergência
emery board ['emərɪbɔːrd] lixa *f* de unhas
emigrant ['emɪgrənt] emigrante *m/f*
emigrate ['emɪgreɪt] *v/i* emigrar
emigration [emɪ'greɪʃn] emigração *f*
Eminence ['emɪnəns] REL eminência *f*; ***His ~*** Sua Eminência
eminent ['emɪnənt] *adj* eminente
eminently ['emɪnəntlɪ] *adv* extremamente
emission [ɪ'mɪʃn] *of gases* emissão *f*
emit [ɪ'mɪt] *v/t* ⟨*pret & pp* ***emitted***⟩ emitir
emotion [ɪ'moʊʃn] emoção *f*
emotional [ɪ'moʊʃnl] *adj problems, development* emocional; *(full of emotion)* emocionado
empathize ['empəθaɪz] *v/i* ter empa-

tia; ~ ***with*** ter empatia com

emperor ['empərər] imperador *m*

emphasis ['emfəsɪs] ênfase *f*

emphasize ['emfəsaɪz] *v/t* enfatizar

emphatic [ɪm'fætɪk] *adj* enfático

empire ['empaɪr] império *m*

employ [ɪm'plɔɪ] *v/t* (*give work to*, *use*) empregar; ***he's ~ed as a ...*** ele está empregado como ...

employee [emplɔɪ'iː] empregado,-a *m,f*

employer [em'plɔɪər] empregador,a *m,f*

employment [em'plɔɪmənt] emprego *m*; (*work*) trabalho *m*; ***be seeking ~*** estar procurando emprego

em'ployment agency agência *f* de empregos

empress ['emprɪs] imperatriz *f*

emptiness ['emptɪnɪs] vazio *m*

empty ['emptɪ] **1** *adj box, drawer, room, street, promises* vazio **2** *v/t* ⟨*pret & pp* ***emptied***⟩ esvaziar **3** *v/i* ⟨*pret & pp* ***emptied***⟩ *room, street* esvaziar-se

emulate ['emjʊleɪt] *v/t* emular

emulsion [ɪ'mʌlʃn] *paint* tinta *f* plástica

enable [ɪ'neɪbl] *v/t* possibilitar; ***~ s.o. to do sth*** capacitar alguém a fazer algo

enact [ɪ'nækt] *v/t law* promulgar; THEA encenar

enamel [ɪ'næml] esmalte *m*

enc, **encl** *abbr of* ***enclosure***

enchant [ɪn'ʧænt] *v/t* (*delight*) encantar

enchanting [ɪn'ʧæntɪŋ] *adj* encantador

encircle [ɪn'sɜːrkl] *v/t* cercar

enclose [ɪn'kloʊz] *v/t in letter* anexar, *Port* enviar junto; *area* cercar; ***please find ~d ...*** segue em anexo ...

enclosure, *pl* **enclosures** [ɪn'kloʊʒər] anexo(s) *m*(*pl*); *with letter* anexo *m*

encore ['ɑːŋkɔːr] bis *m*

encounter [ɪn'kaʊntər] **1** *n* encontro *m* **2** *v/t person, problem, resistance* encontrar

encourage [ɪn'kʌrɪdʒ] *v/t* encorajar

encouragement [ɪn'kʌrɪdʒmənt] encorajamento *m*

encouraging [ɪn'kʌrɪdʒɪŋ] *adj* encorajador

♦**encroach on** [ɪn'kroʊʧ] *v/t land* invadir; *rights* usurpar; *time* ocupar

encyclopedia [ɪnsaɪklə'piːdɪə] enciclopédia *f*

end [end] **1** *n* (*extremity*) extremidade *f*; (*conclusion*) final *m*; (*purpose*) fim *m*; ***in the ~*** no final; ***for hours on ~*** por horas a fio; ***stand sth on ~*** segurar algo em pé; ***at the ~ of July*** no final de julho; ***put an ~ to*** pôr um fim em **2** *v/t* terminar **3** *v/i* terminar; ***it all ~ed in failure*** tudo terminou em fracasso

♦**end up** *v/i* terminar-se; ***he ended up rich*** ele terminou rico; ***I ended up doing it myself*** acabei eu mesma fazendo isso

endanger [ɪn'deɪndʒər] *v/t* pôr em perigo

endangered 'species *nsg* espécie *f* ameaçada

endearing [ɪn'dɪrɪŋ] *adj* simpático

endeavor [ɪn'devər] **1** *n* esforço *m* **2** *v/t* tentar

endeavour *Brit* → ***endeavor***

endemic [ɪn'demɪk] *adj* endêmico

ending ['endɪŋ] final *m*; GRAM terminação *f*

endless ['endlɪs] *adj* sem fim

endorse [ɪn'dɔːrs] *v/t check* endossar; *candidacy* apoiar; *product* dar o aval a

endorsement [ɪn'dɔːrsmənt] *check*: endosso *m*; *candidacy*: apoio *m*; *product*: aval *m*

end 'product produto *m* final

end re'sult resultado *m* final

endurance [ɪn'dʊrəns] resistência *f*

en'durance test teste *m* de resistência

endure [ɪn'dʊər] **1** *v/t* suportar **2** *v/i* (*last*) durar

enduring [ɪn'dʊrɪŋ] *adj* duradouro

end-user [end'juːzər] consumidor,a *m,f* final

enemy ['enəmɪ] inimigo,-a *m,f*

energetic [enə'dʒetɪk] *adj also fig measures* enérgico

energetically [enə'dʒetɪklɪ] *adv* energicamente

energy ['enədʒɪ] energia *f*

'energy-saving *adj device* econômico
'energy supply fornecimento *m* de energia
enforce [ɪn'fɔːrs] *v/t* fazer cumprir; ***laws have to be ~d*** as leis devem ser cumpridas
engage [ɪn'geɪdʒ] **1** *v/t* (*hire*) contratar **2** *v/i* TECH engrenar
♦ **engage in** *v/t* dedicar-se a
engaged [ɪn'geɪdʒd] *adj to be married* noivo; ***get ~*** ficar noivo
en'gaged tone *Brit* TEL sinal *m* de ocupado, *Port* sinal *m* de impedido
engagement [ɪn'geɪdʒmənt] (*appointment*) compromisso *m*; *to be married* noivado *m*; MIL batalha *f*
en'gagement ring anel *m* de noivado
engaging [ɪn'geɪdʒɪŋ] *adj smile, person* atraente
engine ['endʒɪn] motor *m*
engineer [endʒɪ'nɪr] **1** *n* engenheiro,-a *m,f*; NAUT engenheiro,-a naval *m,f*; RAIL maquinista *m/f* **2** *v/t fig meeting etc* maquinar
engineering [endʒɪ'nɪrɪŋ] engenharia *f*
England ['ɪŋglənd] Inglaterra *f*
English ['ɪŋglɪʃ] **1** *adj* inglês,-esa **2** *n language* inglês *m*; ***the ~*** os ingleses
English 'Channel Canal *m* da Mancha
Englishman ['ɪŋglɪʃmən] inglês *m*
Englishwoman ['ɪŋglɪʃwʊmən] inglesa *f*
engrave [ɪn'greɪv] *v/t* gravar
engraving [ɪn'greɪvɪŋ] (*drawing*) gravura *f*; (*design*) gravação *f*
engrossed [ɪn'groʊst] *adj* absorto; ***~ in*** absorto em
engulf [ɪn'gʌlf] *v/t* engolfar
enhance [ɪn'hæns] *v/t beauty* realçar; *reputation, performance* melhorar; *enjoyment* aumentar; *flavor* ressaltar
enigma [ɪ'nɪgmə] enigma *m*
enigmatic [enɪg'mætɪk] *adj* enigmático
enjoy [ɪn'dʒɔɪ] *v/t* gostar de; ***~ oneself*** divertir-se; ***~!*** *said to s.o. eating* bom apetite!; ***did you ~ the movie?*** você gostou do filme?
enjoyable [ɪn'dʒɔɪəbl] *adj* agradável
enjoyment [ɪn'dʒɔɪmənt] prazer *m*
enlarge [ɪn'lɑːrdʒ] *v/t* ampliar
enlargement [ɪn'lɑːrdʒmənt] ampliação *f*
enlighten [ɪn'laɪtn] *v/t* (*inform*) esclarecer; (*educate*) instruir; ***a very ~ed employer*** um empregador muito bem informado; ***a very ~ed person*** uma pessoa muito culta
enlist [ɪn'lɪst] **1** *v/i* MIL alistar-se **2** *v/t* ***~ the help of*** conseguir o apoio de
enliven [ɪn'laɪvn] *v/t* animar
enmity ['enmətɪ] inimizade *f*
enormity [ɪ'nɔːrmətɪ] enormidade *f*
enormous [ɪ'nɔːrməs] *adj* enorme
enormously [ɪ'nɔːrməslɪ] *adv* enormemente; *fat* excessivamente
enough [ɪ'nʌf] **1** *adj* suficiente; ***~ money*** dinheiro suficiente **2** *pron* suficiente; ***will 50 be ~?*** 50 é suficiente?; ***I've had ~!*** estou farto!; ***that's ~, calm down!*** já chega, acalme-se! **3** *adv* suficientemente; ***strangely ~*** por mais estranho que pareça
enquire *etc* → ***inquire***
enraged [ɪn'reɪdʒd] *adj* enfurecido
enrich [ɪn'rɪtʃ] *v/t vocabulary, life* enriquecer
enrol *etc* → *Brit* ***enroll***
enroll [ɪn'roʊl] *v/i* inscrever-se
enrollment [ɪn'roʊlmənt] inscrição *f*; *at school* matrícula *f*
ensue [ɪn'suː] *v/i* seguir-se
en suite ['ɑːnswiːt] *n* ~ (***bathroom***) suíte *f*
ensure [ɪn'ʃʊr] *v/t* assegurar
entail [ɪn'teɪl] *v/t* implicar
entangle [ɪn'tæŋgl] *v/t in rope* enrolar; ***become ~d in*** estar envolvido em; *in love affair* envolver-se com
enter ['entər] **1** *v/t room, house* entrar (em); *competition* inscrever-se em; *person, horse in race* inscrever; *write down* escrever; COMPUT entrar com **2** *v/i* entrar; THEA entrar em cena; *in competition* inscrever-se **3** *n* COMPUT enter *m*
enterprise ['entərpraɪz] (*initiative*) iniciativa *f*; (*venture*) empreendimento *m*
enterprising ['entərpraɪzɪŋ] *adj* empreendedor
entertain [entər'teɪn] **1** *v/t* (*amuse*)

entreter; (*consider*) *idea* pensar sobre **2** *v/i* (*have guests*) receber
entertainer [entər'teɪnər] artista *m/f*
entertaining [entər'teɪnɪŋ] *adj* divertido
entertainment [entər'teɪnmənt] entretenimento *m*; (*show*) espetáculo *m*
enthrall [ɪn'θrɔːl] *v/t* fascinar
enthusiasm [ɪn'θuːzɪæzəm] entusiasmo *m*
enthusiast [ɪn'θuːzɪ'æst] entusiasta *m/f*
enthusiastic [ɪnθuːzɪ'æstɪk] *adj* entusiasmado
enthusiastically [ɪnθuːzɪ'æstɪklɪ] *adv* com entusiasmo
entice [ɪn'taɪs] *v/t* atrair
entire [ɪn'taɪr] *adj* inteiro
entirely [ɪn'taɪrlɪ] *adv* totalmente
entitle [ɪn'taɪtld] *v/t* ***be ~d to*** ter o direito de; ***~ s.o. to*** dar a alguém o direito de
entitled [ɪn'taɪtld] *adj book* intitulado
entrance ['entrəns] entrada *f*; THEA entrada *f* em cena; (*admission*) admissão *f*
entranced [ɪn'trænst] *adj* arrebatado
'entrance exam, **'entrance examination** exame *m* de admissão
'entrance fee taxa *f* de admissão
entrant ['entrənt] *in exam* candidato,-a *m,f*, *in competition* participante *m/f*
entreat [ɪn'triːt] *v/t* suplicar; ***~ s.o. to do sth*** suplicar a alguém que faça algo
entrenched [ɪn'trenʧt] *adj attitudes* arraigado
entrepreneur [ɑːntrəprə'nɜːr] empresário,-a *m,f*
entrepreneurial [ɑːntrəprə'nɜːrɪəl] *adj* empreendedor
entrust [ɪn'trʌst] *v/t* ***~ X with Y*** confiar a X Y; ***~ Y to X*** confiar Y a X
entry ['entrɪ] entrada *f*, *for competition* participante *m/f*, *in diary*, *accounts* registro *m*, *Port* registo *m*
'entry form formulário *m* de inscrição **'entryphone** interfone *m* **'entry visa** visto *m* de entrada
enumerate [ɪ'nuːməreɪt] *v/t* enumerar
envelop [ɪn'veləp] *v/t* envelopar
envelope ['envəloʊp] envelope *m*
enviable ['envɪəbl] *adj* invejável
envious ['envɪəs] *adj* invejoso; ***be ~ of s.o.*** ter inveja de alguém
environment [ɪn'vaɪrənmənt] (*nature*) meio *m* ambiente; (*surroundings*) ambiente *m*
environmental [ɪnvaɪrən'məntl] *adj* ambiental
environmentalist [ɪnvaɪrən'məntəlɪst] ambientalista *m/f*
environmentally friendly [ɪnvaɪrənməntəlɪ'frendlɪ] *adj* ambientalmente correto
environmental pol'lution poluição *f* ambiental
environmental pro'tection proteção *f* ambiental
environs [ɪn'vaɪrənz] *npl* arredores *mpl*
envisage [ɪn'vɪzɪdʒ] *v/t* imaginar
envision [ɪn'vɪʒn] *v/t Am* imaginar; ***do you ~ any major alterations?*** você prevê alguma grande alteração?
envoy ['envɔɪ] enviado,-a *m,f*
envy ['envɪ] **1** *n* inveja *f*, ***be the ~ of*** ser alvo de inveja de **2** *v/t* ⟨*pret & pp* ***envied***⟩ ***~ s.o. sth*** invejar alguém por algo
ephemeral [ɪ'femərəl] *adj* efêmero
epic ['epɪk] **1** *n* épico *m*; (*epic poem*) epopéia *f* **2** *adj journey* épico; ***a task of ~ proportions*** uma tarefa de proporções monumentais
epicenter ['epɪsentr] epicentro *m*
epicentre *Brit* → ***epicenter***
epidemic [epɪ'demɪk] epidemia *f*
epilepsy ['epɪlepsɪ] epilepsia *f*
epileptic [epɪ'leptɪk] *n* epilético,-a *m,f*
epileptic 'fit ataque *m* epilético
epilog ['epɪlɑːg] *Am* epílogo *m*
epilogue *Brit* → ***epilog***
episode ['epɪsoʊd] episódio *m*
epitaph ['epɪtæf] epitáfio *m*
epoch ['iːpɑːk] época *f*
epoch-making ['iːpɑːkmeɪkɪŋ] *adj* de marcar época
equal ['iːkwl] **1** *adj* igual; ***be ~ to*** *task etc* estar à altura de **2** *n* igual *m/f* **3** *v/t* ⟨*pret & pp* ***equaled***, *Brit* ***equalled***⟩ *with numbers* ser igual a; (*be as good as*) igualar-se a

E

equality [ɪ'kwɑːlətɪ] igualdade *f*
equalize ['iːkwəlaɪz] **1** *v/t* igualar **2** *v/i* *Brit* SPORT empatar
equalizer ['iːkwəlaɪzər] *Brit* SPORT gol *m* de empate, *Port* golo *m* de empate
equally ['iːkwəlɪ] *adv* igualmente; **~, ...** da mesma forma, ...
equal 'rights igualdade *f* de direitos
equate [ɪ'kweɪt] *v/t* equiparar; ***~ X with Y*** equiparar X a Y
equation [ɪ'kweɪʒn] MATH equação *f*
equator [ɪ'kweɪtər] equador *m*
equilibrium [iːkwɪ'lɪbrɪəm] equilíbrio *m*
equinox ['iːkwɪnɑːks] equinócio *m*
equip [ɪ'kwɪp] *v/t* ⟨*pret & pp* ***equipped***⟩ equipar; ***he's not ~ped to handle it*** *fig* ele não está preparado para agüentar
equipment [ɪ'kwɪpmənt] equipamento *m*
equity ['ekwətɪ] FIN ações *fpl* ordinárias
equivalent [ɪ'kwɪvələnt] **1** *adj* equivalente; ***be ~ to*** ser equivalente a **2** *n* equivalente *m/f*
era ['ɪrə] era *f*
eradicate [ɪ'rædɪkeɪt] *v/t* erradicar
erase [ɪ'reɪz] *v/t* apagar
eraser [ɪ'reɪzər] borracha *f de apagar*
erect [ɪ'rekt] **1** *adj* ereto **2** *v/t* erguer
erection [ɪ'rekʃn] *of building etc* construção *f*; *of penis* ereção *f*
ergonomic [ɜːrgoʊ'nɑːmɪk] *adj* ergonômico
erode [ɪ'roʊd] *v/t* causar erosão em; *fig rights, power* desgastar; ***the cliff is being ~d by the action of the waves*** a rocha está sofrendo erosão pela ação das ondas
erosion [ɪ'roʊʒn] erosão *f*, *fig* corrosão *f*
erotic [ɪ'rɑːtɪk] *adj* erótico
eroticism [ɪ'rɑːtɪsɪzm] erotismo *m*
errand ['erənd] recado *m*; ***run ~s*** (*go shopping*) ir às compras; (*deliver messages*) levar recados
erratic [ɪ'rætɪk] *adj* imprevisível
error ['erər] erro *m*
'error message COMPUT mensagem *f* de erro
erupt [ɪ'rʌpt] *v/i volcano* entrar em erupção; *violence, also fig person* explodir
eruption [ɪ'rʌpʃn] *of volcano* erupção *f*; *of violence* explosão *f*
escalate ['eskəleɪt] *v/i* intensificar-se
escalation [eskə'leɪʃn] intensificação *f*
escalator ['eskəleɪtər] escada *f* rolante
escape [ɪ'skeɪp] **1** *n of prisoner, animal* fuga *f*; *of gas* escapamento *m*; ***have a narrow ~*** escapar por pouco **2** *v/i prisoner, animal* fugir; *gas* escapar **3** *v/t* ***the word ~s me*** a palavra me fugiu
es'cape chute rampa *f* de emergência
escapism [ɪ'skeɪpɪzm] escapismo *m*
escort 1 ['eskɔːrt] *n* acompanhante *m/f*; (*guard*) escolta *f* **2** [ɪ'skɔːrt] *v/t* levar; (*socially*) acompanhar; (*act as guard to*) escoltar
especial [ɪ'speʃl] *adj* especial
especially [ɪ'speʃlɪ] *adv* especialmente
espionage ['espɪənɑːʒ] espionagem *f*
espresso, **espresso coffee** [es'presoʊ] café *m* expresso
essay ['eseɪ] *n* ensaio *m*
essential [ɪ'senʃl] *adj* essencial
essentially [ɪ'senʃlɪ] *adv* essencialmente
establish [ɪ'stæblɪʃ] *v/t company* fundar; (*create*) criar; (*determine*) estabelecer; ***~ oneself as*** estabelecer-se como
establishment [ɪ'stæblɪʃmənt] (*firm, shop etc*) estabelecimento *m*; ***the Establishment*** a classe dominante
estate [ɪ'steɪt] (*area of land*) propriedade *f*, (*possessions of dead person*) bens *mpl*
es'tate agency *Brit* imobiliária *f*
es'tate agent *Brit* corretor,a *m,f* de imóveis, *Port* agente *m/f* imobiliário,-a
esthetic [ɪs'θetɪk] *adj Am* estético
estimate ['estɪmət] **1** *n* (*calculation*) estimativa *f*, (*assessment*) avaliação *f*, COM orçamento *m* **2** *v/t* estimar
estimation [estɪ'meɪʃn] estima *f*, ***he***

has gone up / down in my ~ ele subiu / desceu em meu conceito; ***in my ~*** (*opinion*) na minha opinião
estranged [ɪs'treɪndʒd] *adj wife, husband* separado
estuary ['estʃəwerɪ] estuário *m*
ETA [i:ti:'eɪ] *abbr* (*of* ***estimated time of arrival***) horário *m* previsto de chegada
etc [et'setrə] *abbr* (*of* ***et cetera***) et cetera
etching ['etʃɪŋ] água-forte *f*
eternal [ɪ'tɜ:rnl] *adj* eterno
eternity [ɪ'tɜ:rnətɪ] eternidade *f*
ethical ['eθɪkl] *adj* ético
ethics ['eθɪks] ética *f*
ethnic ['eθnɪk] *adj* étnico
ethnic 'cleansing genocídio *m* **ethnic 'group** grupo *m* étnico **ethnic mi'nority** minoria *f* étnica
e-ticket ['i:tɪkɪt] bilhete *m* eletrônico
EU [i:'ju:] *abbr* → ***European Union***
euphemism ['ju:fəmɪzm] eufemismo *m*
euphoria [ju:'fɔ:rɪə] euforia *f*
euro ['jʊroʊ] euro *m*
Eurocrat ['jʊroʊkræt] eurocrata *m/f*
'Euro MP parlamentar *m/f* europeu (européia)
Europe ['jʊrəp] Europa *f*
European [jʊrə'pɪən] **1** *adj* europeu (européia) **2** *n* europeu *m*, européia *f*
European Com'mission Comissão *f* Européia **European 'Parliament** Parlamento *m* Europeu **European 'Union** União *f* Européia
euthanasia [jʊθə'neɪzɪə] eutanásia *f*
evacuate [ɪ'vækjʊeɪt] *v/t* (*clear people from*) evacuar; (*leave*) sair de
evade [ɪ'veɪd] *v/t* evadir
evaluate [ɪ'væljʊeɪt] *v/t* avaliar
evaluation [ɪvælju'eɪʃn] avaliação *f*
evangelist [ɪ'vændʒəlɪst] evangelista *m/f*
evaporate [ɪ'væpəreɪt] *v/i water* evaporar; *confidence* desaparecer
evaporation [ɪvæpə'reɪʃn] *of water* evaporação *f*
evasion [ɪ'veɪʒn] *of person* evasão *f*, *of tax* sonegação *f*
evasive [ɪ'veɪsɪv] *adj* evasivo
eve [i:v] véspera *f*
even ['i:vn] **1** *adj* (*regular*) uniforme; (*level*) plano; (*number*) par; ***get ~ with …*** ficar quite com … **2** *adv* até mesmo; ***~ bigger / better*** ainda maior / melhor; ***not ~*** nem mesmo; ***~ so*** mesmo assim; ***~ if*** mesmo se **3** *v/t* ***~ the score*** igualar o placar
evening ['i:vnɪŋ] noite *f*, *early evening* tarde *f*, ***in the ~*** à noite / tarde; ***this ~*** esta noite / tarde; ***good ~*** boa-noite / boa-tarde
'evening class aula *f* noturna **'evening dress** *for woman* vestido *m* formal; *for man* traje *m* a rigor, *Port* traje *m* de cerimônia **evening 'paper** jornal *m* vespertino
evenly ['i:vnlɪ] *adv* (*regularly*) uniformemente
event [ɪ'vent] evento *m*; SPORT prova *f*, ***at all ~s*** de qualquer modo
eventful [ɪ'ventfl] *adj* movimentado
eventual [ɪ'ventʊəl] *adj* final
eventually [ɪ'ventʊəlɪ] *adv* finalmente
ever ['evər] *adv* sempre; ***have you ~ been to …?*** você já esteve alguma vez em …?; ***for ~*** para sempre; ***~ since*** desde então
evergreen ['evərgri:n] *n* sempre-viva *f*
everlasting [evər'læstɪŋ] *adj* perene
every ['evrɪ] *adj* (*each*) cada; (*all possible*) todo; ***~ other day*** a cada dois dias; ***~ now and then*** de vez em quando
everybody ['evrɪbɑ:dɪ] *pron* todos, todas
everyday ['evrɪdeɪ] *adj* cotidiano
everyone ['evrɪwʌn] *pron* todos, todas
everything ['evrɪθɪŋ] *pron* tudo
everywhere ['evrɪwer] *adv* (*in all places*) em todo lugar, *Port* em toda a parte; (*wherever*) em todo lugar que, *Port* em toda a parte que
evict [ɪ'vɪkt] *v/t* despejar
evidence ['evɪdəns] evidência *f*, LAW prova *f*, ***give ~*** prestar depoimento
evident ['evɪdənt] *adj* evidente
evidently ['evɪdəntlɪ] *adv* (*clearly*) evidentemente; (*apparently*) aparentemente
evil ['i:vl] **1** *adj* mau (má) **2** *n* mal *m*

evoke [ɪ'voʊk] *v/t image* evocar
evolution [iːvə'luːʃn] evolução *f*
evolve [ɪ'vɑːlv] *v/i animals* evoluir; (*develop*) desenvolver-se
ewe [juː] ovelha *f*
ex [eks] *fam* (*former wife / husband*) ex *m/f*
ex... [eks] ex...

E

exact [ɪg'zækt] *adj* exato
exacting [ɪg'zæktɪŋ] *adj* exigente
exactly [ɪg'zæktlɪ] *adv* exatamente; ***~!*** exatamente!; ***not ~*** não exatamente
exaggerate [ɪg'zædʒəreɪt] *v/t & v/i* exagerar
exaggeration [ɪgzædʒə'reɪʃn] exagero *m*
exam [ɪg'zæm] exame *m*; ***take an ~*** prestar um exame; ***pass / fail an ~*** passar / não passar em um exame
examination [ɪgzæmɪ'neɪʃn] *of facts, patient etc, also* EDUC exame *m*
examine [ɪg'zæmɪn] *v/t* (*study*) *also patient*, EDUC examinar
examiner [ɪg'zæmɪnər] EDUC examinador,a *m,f*
example [ɪg'zæmpl] exemplo *m*; ***for ~*** por exemplo; ***set a good / bad ~*** dar um bom / mau exemplo
exasperated [ɪg'zæspəreɪt] *adj* exasperado
exasperating [ɪg'zæspəreɪtɪŋ] *adj* exasperante
excavate ['ekskəveɪt] *v/t* escavar
excavation [ekskə'veɪʃn] escavação *f*
excavator ['ekskəveɪtər] escavadeira *f*
exceed [ɪk'siːd] *v/t* exceder
exceedingly [ɪk'siːdɪŋlɪ] *adj* extremamente
excel [ɪk'sel] ⟨*pret & pp* ***excelled***⟩ **1** *v/i* sobressair-se; ***~ at*** sobressair-se em **2** *v/t* ***~ oneself*** exceder-se a si mesmo
excellence ['eksələns] excelência *f*
excellent ['eksələnt] *adj* excelente
except [ɪk'sept] *prep* exceto; ***~ for*** exceto por; ***~ that*** só que
exception [ɪk'sepʃn] exceção *f*; ***with the ~ of*** com exceção de; ***take ~ to*** opor-se a
exceptional [ɪk'sepʃnl] *adj* (*very good, also special*) excepcional
exceptionally [ɪk'sepʃnlɪ] *adv* (*extremely*) excepcionalmente
excerpt ['eksɜːrpt] excerto *m*
excess [ɪk'ses] **1** *n* excesso *m*; ***eat / drink to ~*** comer / beber em excesso; ***in ~ of*** mais de **2** *adj* em excesso
excess 'baggage excesso *m* de bagagem
excess 'fare sobretaxa *f* de excesso
excessive [ɪk'sesɪv] *adj* excessivo
excessively [ɪk'sesɪvlɪ] *adv* excessivamente
exchange [ɪks'tʃeɪndʒ] **1** *n of views, information* troca *f*; *between schools* intercâmbio *m*; ***in ~*** em troca; ***in ~ for*** em troca de **2** *v/t in store, also addresses, currency* trocar; ***~ X for Y*** trocar X por Y
ex'change rate FIN taxa *f* de câmbio
excitable [ɪk'saɪtəbl] *adj* excitável
excite [ɪk'saɪt] *v/t* (*make enthusiastic*) entusiasmar
excited [ɪk'saɪtɪd] *adj* empolgado; ***get ~*** entusiasmar-se; ***get ~ about sth*** ficar entusiasmado com algo
excitement [ɪk'saɪtmənt] empolgação *f*
exciting [ɪk'saɪtɪŋ] *adj* empolgante
exclaim [ɪk'skleɪm] *v/t* exclamar
exclamation [eksklə'meɪʃn] exclamação *f*
exclamation mark → ***exclamation point***
excla'mation point *Am* ponto *m* de exclamação
exclude [ɪk'skluːd] *v/t* excluir; *possibility* descartar
excluding [ɪk'skluːdɪŋ] *prep* fora
exclusive [ɪk'skluːsɪv] *adj* exclusivo
excommunicate [ekskə'mjuːnɪkeɪt] *v/t* REL excomungar
excruciating [ɪk'skruːʃɪeɪtɪŋ] *adj pain* agonizante
excursion [ɪk'skɜːrʃn] excursão *f*
excuse 1 [ɪk'skjuːs] *n* desculpa *f* **2** [ɪk'skjuːz] *v/t* (*forgive, allow to leave*) desculpar; ***~ X from Y*** dispensar X de Y; ***~ me*** (*to get attention*) desculpe; (*to get past, interrupting s.o.*) com licença
ex-di'rectory *adj Brit* ***be ~*** estar fora de lista
execute ['eksɪkjuːt] *v/t criminal, plan* executar

execution [eksɪ'kjuːʃn] *of criminal, plan* execução *f*
executioner [eksɪ'kjuːʃnər] executor,a *m,f*
executive [ɪg'zekjʊtɪv] *n* executivo,-a *m,f*
executive as'sistant assistente *m/f* executivo,-a
executive 'briefcase pasta *f* executiva
exemplary [ɪg'zemplərɪ] *adj* exemplar
exempt [ɪg'zempt] *adj* isento; ***be ~ from*** ser isento de
exercise ['eksərsaɪz] **1** *n* (*physical*) *also* EDUC, MIL exercício *m*; MIL treinamento *m*; ***take ~*** fazer exercícios **2** *v/t muscle* exercitar; *dog* levar para passear; *caution, restraint* exercer **3** *v/i* exercitar-se
'exercise bike bicicleta *f* ergométrica **'exercise book** caderno *m* de exercícios **'exercise class** aula *f* de ginástica
exert [ɪg'zɜːrt] *v/t authority* exercer; ***~ oneself*** esforçar-se
exertion [ɪg'zɜːrʃn] esforço *m* físico
exhale [eks'heɪl] *v/t* expirar
exhaust [ɪg'zɒːst] **1** *n* (*fumes, pipe* escapamento *m* **2** *v/t* (*tire*) esgotar; (*use up*) exaurir
exhausted [ɪg'zɒːstɪd] *adj* (*tired*) exausto
ex'haust fumes *npl* gases *mpl* de escapamento
exhausting [ɪg'zɒːstɪŋ] *adj* fatigante
exhaustion [ɪg'zɒːstʃn] exaustão *f*
exhaustive [ɪg'zɒːstɪv] *adj* exaustivo
ex'haust pipe escapamento *m*
exhibit [ɪg'zɪbɪt] **1** *n in exhibition* objeto *m* exposto **2** *v/t* exibir; *artist* expor
exhibition [eksɪ'bɪʃn] exposição *f*; *of bad behavior* exibição *f*; *of skill* demonstração *f*
exhibitionist [eksɪ'bɪʃnɪst] exibicionista *m/f*
exhilarating [ɪg'zɪləreɪtɪŋ] *adj* estimulante
exile ['eksaɪl] **1** *n* exílio *m*; *person* exilado,-a *m,f* **2** *v/t* exilar
exist [ɪg'zɪst] *v/i* existir; ***~ on*** viver de
existence [ɪg'zɪstəns] existência *f*; ***in ~*** existente; ***come into ~*** passar a existir
existing [ɪg'zɪstɪŋ] *adj* existente
exit ['eksɪt] **1** *n* saída *f* **2** *v/i* COMPUT sair
exonerate [ɪg'zɑːnəreɪt] *v/t* exonerar
exorbitant [ɪg'zɔːrbɪtənt] *adj* exorbitante
exotic [ɪg'zɑːtɪk] *adj* exótico
expand [ɪk'spænd] **1** *v/t* expandir **2** *v/i* expandir-se; *metal* dilatar-se
♦**expand on** *v/t* detalhar
expanse [ɪk'spæns] extensão *f*
expansion [ɪk'spænʃn] expansão *f*; *of metal* dilatação *f*
expatriate [eks'pætrɪət] **1** *adj* expatriado **2** *n* expatriado,-a *m,f*
expect [ɪk'spekt] **1** *v/t phone call, baby, also* (*demand*) esperar; ***I ~ you want to know how much I spent?*** (*suppose*) suponho que você queira saber quanto gastei **2** *v/i* ***I ~ so*** suponho que sim; ***she's ~ing*** ela está grávida
expectant [ɪk'spektənt] *adj* expectante
expectant 'mother gestante *f*
expectation [ekspek'teɪʃn] expectativa *f*
expedient [ɪk'spiːdɪənt] *adj* conveniente
expedition [ekspɪ'dɪʃn] expedição *f*
expel [ɪk'spel] *v/t* ⟨*pret & pp* ***expelled***⟩ *person* expulsar
expend [ɪk'spend] *v/t energy* gastar
expendable [ɪk'spendəbl] *adj* dispensável
expenditure [ɪk'spendɪtʃər] gasto *m*
expense [ɪk'spens] despesa *f*; ***at the company's ~*** por conta da companhia; ***a joke at my ~*** uma piada às minhas custas; ***at the ~ of his health*** às custas de sua saúde
ex'pense account conta *f* de despesas reembolsáveis
expenses [ɪk'spensɪz] despesas *fpl*
expensive [ɪk'spensɪv] *adj* caro
experience [ɪk'spɪrɪəns] **1** *n* experiência *f* **2** *v/t pain, pleasure* sentir; *problem, difficulty* enfrentar
experienced [ɪk'spɪrɪənst] *adj* experiente

experiment [ɪk'sperɪmənt] **1** *n* experiência *f* **2** *v/i* experimentar; **~ *on** animals* fazer experiências em; **~ *with*** (*try out*) fazer experiências com
experimental [ɪksperɪ'mentl] *adj* experimental
expert ['ekspɜːrt] **1** *adj* perito **2** *n* especialista *m*/*f*
expert ad'vice opinião *f* de um especialista
expertise [ekspɜːr'tiːz] perícia *f*
expi'ration [ekspɪ'reɪʃn] *Am* vencimento *m*
expi'ration date *Am* data *f* de validade
expire [ɪk'spaɪr] *v/i* expirar
expiry [ɪk'spaɪrɪ] vencimento *m*
ex'piry date *Brit* data *f* de validade
explain [ɪk'spleɪn] *v/t* explicar
explanation [eksplə'neɪʃn] explicação *f*
explicit [ɪk'splɪsɪt] *adj instructions* explícito
explicitly [ɪk'splɪsɪtlɪ] *adv state, forbid* explicitamente
explode [ɪk'sploʊd] *v/t & v/i* explodir
exploit[1] ['eksplɔɪt] *n* feito *m*
exploit[2] [ɪk'splɔɪt] *v/t person, resources* explorar
exploitation [eksplɔɪ'teɪʃn] exploração *f*
exploration [eksplə'reɪʃn] exploração *f*
exploratory [ɪk'splɑːrətərɪ] *adj surgery* exploratório *talks* preliminar
explore [ɪk'splɔːr] *v/t country etc* explorar; *possibility* examinar
explorer [ɪk'splɔːrər] explorador,a *m,f*
explosion [ɪk'sploʊʒn] *of bomb, in population* explosão *f*
explosive [ɪk'sploʊsɪv] *n* explosivo *m*
export ['ekspɔːrt] **1** *n* exportação *f* **2** *v/t goods, also* COMPUT exportar
'export campaign campanha *f* de exportação
exporter ['ekspɔːrtər] exportador,a *m,f*
expose [ɪk'spoʊz] *v/t* (*uncover*) expor; *scandal* revelar; *person* taxar; **~ *X to Y*** expor X a Y
exposure [ɪk'spoʊʒər] exposição *f*; MED exposição *f* ao clima; *of dishonest behavior* desmascaramento *m*; (*part of film*) pose *f*
express [ɪk'spres] **1** *adj* (*fast, explicit*) expresso **2** *n* (*train, bus*) expresso *m* **3** *v/t* (*speak of, voice, feelings*) expressar; **~ *oneself well / clearly*** expressar-se bem / com clareza; **~ *oneself*** (*emotionally*) expressar-se
ex'press elevator *Am* elevador *m* expresso
expression [ɪk'spreʃn] (*on face, phrase, expressiveness*) expressão *f*
expressive [ɪk'spresɪv] *adj* expressivo
expressly [ɪk'spreslɪ] *adv* expressamente
expressway [ɪk'spresweɪ] via *f* rápida
expulsion [ɪk'spʌlʃn] expulsão *f*
exquisite [ek'skwɪzɪt] *adj* (*beautiful*) requintado
extend [ɪk'stend] **1** *v/t* ampliar; *runway, path* aumentar; *contract, visa* prolongar; *thanks, congratulations* estender **2** *v/i garden etc* estender-se
extension [ɪk'stenʃn] *to house* ampliação *f*; *of contract, visa* prolongamento *m*; TEL ramal *m*, *Port* extensão *f*
ex'tension cable cabo *m* de extensão
extensive [ɪk'stensɪv] *adj* extenso
extent [ɪk'stent] dimensão *f*; ***to such an* ~ *that*** a tal ponto que; ***to a certain* ~** até certo ponto
extenuating circumstances [ɪk'stenʊeɪtɪŋ] *npl* circunstâncias *fpl* atenuantes
exterior [ɪk'stɪrɪr] **1** *adj* externo **2** *n of building* exterior *m*; *of person* aspecto *m*
exterminate [ɪk'stɜːrmɪneɪt] *v/t vermin, race* exterminar
external [ɪk'stɜːrnl] *adj* externo
extinct [ɪk'stɪŋkt] *adj species* extinto
extinction [ɪk'stɪŋkʃn] *species*: extinção *f*
extinguish [ɪk'stɪŋgwɪʃ] *v/t fire* extinguir; *cigarette* apagar
extinguisher [ɪk'stɪŋgwɪʃər] extintor *m*
extort [ɪk'stɔːrt] *v/t* extorquir; **~ *money from*** extorquir dinheiro de
extortion [ɪk'stɔːrʃn] extorsão *f*
extortionate [ɪk'stɔːrʃənət] *adj prices* exorbitante

extra ['ekstrə] **1** *n* extra *m* **2** *adj & adv* extra; ***meals are ~*** (*cost more*) as comidas são pagas a parte; ***that's $1 ~*** custa um dólar a mais
extra 'charge taxa *f* extra
extract[1] ['ekstrækt] *n* extrato *m*
extract[2] [ɪk'strækt] *v/t* tirar; *coal, oil, tooth, information* extrair, arrancar
extraction [ɪk'strækʃn] *of oil, coal, tooth* extração *f*
extradite ['ekstrədaɪt] *v/t* extraditar
extradition [ekstrə'dɪʃn] extradição *f*
extra'dition treaty tratado *m* de extradição
extramarital [ekstrə'mærɪtl] *adj* extraconjugal
extraordinarily [ɪkstrə'ɔːrdn'erɪlɪ] *adv* extraordinariamente
extraordinary [ɪkstrə'ɔːrdnerɪ] *adj* extraordinário
extra 'time *Brit* SPORT prorrogação *f*
extravagance [ɪk'strævəgəns] extravagância *f*
extravagant [ɪk'strævəgənt] *adj* (*with money*) extravagante
extreme [ɪk'striːm] **1** *n* extremo *m* **2** *adj* extremo
extremely [ɪk'striːmlɪ] *adv* extremamente
extremism [ɪk'striːmɪzm] extremismo *m*
extremist [ɪk'striːmɪst] extremista *m/f*
extricate ['ekstrɪkeɪt] *v/t* libertar
extrovert ['ekstrəvɜːrt] *n* extrovertido,-a *m,f*
exuberant [ɪg'zuːbərənt] *adj* exuberante
exult [ɪg'zʌlt] *v/i* exultar
eye [aɪ] **1** *n* olho *m*; *of needle* buraco *m*; ***keep an ~ on*** (*look after*) ficar de olho em; (*monitor*) vigiar **2** *v/t* olhar
'eyeball globo *m* ocular **'eyebrow** sobrancelha *f* **'eyecatching** *adj* chamativo **'eyeglasses** *Am* óculos *mpl* **'eyelash** cílio *m* **'eyelid** pálpebra *f* **'eyeliner** delineador *m* **'eyeshadow** sombra *f* **'eyesight** visão *f* **'eyesore** monstruosidade *f* **'eye strain** fadiga *f* ocular **'eyewitness** testemunha *f* ocular

F

F *abbr* (*of* ***Fahrenheit***) Fahrenheit
fabric ['fæbrɪk] (*material*) tecido *m*
fabulous ['fæbjʊləs] *adj* fabuloso
fabulously ['fæbjʊləslɪ] *adv* fabulosamente
façade [fə'sɑːd] *building, person*: fachada *f*
face [feɪs] **1** *n* cara *f*, rosto *m*; ***~ to ~*** face a face; ***lose ~*** desonrar-se **2** *v/t* *person* encarar; *the sea* estar de frente para
◆**face up to** *v/t* enfrentar
'facecloth *Brit* toalha *f* de rosto **'facelift** operação *f* plástica (facial) **'face pack** creme *m* facial **face 'value** valor *m* aparente; *truth, discourse* ***take sth at ~*** comprar algo pela aparência
facial ['feɪʃl] *n* limpeza *f* de pele
facilitate [fə'sɪlɪteɪt] *v/t* facilitar
facilities [fə'sɪlətɪz] *npl* instalações *fpl*; ***the hostel has cooking ~*** o hostel tem uma cozinha equipada
fact [fækt] fato *m*; ***in ~, as a matter of ~*** de fato, na verdade
faction ['fækʃn] facção *f*
factor ['fæktər] fator *m*
factory ['fæktərɪ] fábrica *f*
faculty ['fækəltɪ] *hearing etc, at university* faculdade *f*
fad [fæd] modismo *m*
fade [feɪd] *v/i colors* desbotar
faded ['feɪdɪd] *adj color, jeans* desbotado
fag [fæg] *fam Am* (*homosexual*) bicha

f, Port maricas *m*; *Brit* (*cigarette*) cigarro *m*

Fahrenheit ['færənhaɪt] *adj* Fahrenheit

fail [feɪl] **1** *v/i* fracassar; *brakes* falhar; *in exam* não passar **2** *n* ***without ~*** sem falta

failing ['feɪlɪŋ] *n* falha *f*

failure ['feɪljər] fracasso *m*; *in exam* reprovação *f*; ***I feel such a ~*** eu me sinto um fracassado

faint [feɪnt] **1** *adj line* indistinto; *difference, smile* leve; *smell, noise* fraco **2** *v/i* desmaiar

faintly ['feɪntlɪ] *adv* levemente; *hear* fracamente

fair[1] [fer] *adj hair* louro; *complexion* branco

fair[2] [fer] *n* COM feira *f*; (*funfair*) festa *f* anual

fair[3] *adj* (*just*) justo; ***it's not ~*** não é justo

fairly ['ferlɪ] *adv treat* com justiça; (*quite*) bastante

fairness ['fernɪs] *of treatment* justiça *f*

fairy ['ferɪ] fada *f*

'fairy tale conto *m* de fadas

faith [feɪθ] confiança *f*, REL fé *f*

faithful ['feɪθfl] *adj* fiel; ***be ~ to one's partner*** ser fiel ao seu parceiro

faithfully ['feɪθflɪ] *adv* fielmente

fake [feɪk] **1** *n* falsificação *f* **2** *adj* falso **3** *v/t* (*forge*) falsificar; (*feign*) fingir

Falkland Islands ['fɒ:lklənd] ***the ~*** as (ilhas) Malvinas

fall[1] [fɒ:l] *n Am* outono *m*

fall[2] [fɒ:l] **1** *v/i* ⟨*pret* ***fell***, *pp* ***fallen***⟩ *person, government, prices, temperature, night* cair; ***it ~s on a Tuesday*** cai numa terça-feira; ***~ ill*** cair doente **2** *n person, government, price, temperature*: queda *f*

♦**fall back on** *v/t* recorrer a

♦**fall behind** *v/i with work, studies* atrasar-se

♦**fall down** *v/i* desabar

♦**fall for** *v/t person* enamorar-se de; (*be deceived by*) cair em

♦**fall out** *v/i hair* cair; (*argue*) brigar

♦**fall over** *v/i* derrubar

♦**fall through** *v/i plans* malograr

fallen ['fɒ:lən] *pp* → ***fall***[2]

fallible ['fæləbl] *adj* falível

falling star ['fɒ:lɪŋ] estrela *f* cadente

fallout ['fɒ:laʊt] chuva *f* radioativa

false [fɒ:ls] *adj* falso

false a'larm alarme *m* falso

falsely ['fɒ:lslɪ] *adv* ***be ~ accused of sth*** ser falsamente acusado de algo

false 'start *in race* partida *f* anulada

false 'teeth dentadura *f* postiça

falsify ['fɒ:lsɪfaɪ] *v/t* ⟨*pret & pp* ***falsified***⟩ falsificar

fame [feɪm] fama *f*

familiar [fə'mɪljər] *adj* (*intimate*) íntimo; *form of address* informal; (*well-known*) conhecido; ***be ~ with sth*** estar familiarizado com algo; ***that looks / sounds ~*** isto parece / soa familiar

familiarity [fəmɪlɪ'ærɪtɪ] *with subject etc* familiaridade *f*

familiarize [fə'mɪljəraɪz] *v/t* familiarizar; ***~ oneself with …*** familiarizar-se com …

family 'doctor médico *m* de família **'family man** pai *m* de família **'family name** sobrenome *m*, *Port* apelido *m* **family 'planning** planejamento *m* familiar **family 'planning clinic** clínica *f* de planejamento familiar **family 'tree** árvore *f* genealógica

famine ['fæmɪn] fome *f*

famished ['fæmɪʃt] *adj fam* esfomeado

famous ['feɪməs] *adj* famoso; ***be ~ for …*** ser famoso por …

fan[1] [fæn] *n* (*supporter*) fã *m/f*

fan[2] [fæn] **1** *n cooling, electric*: ventilador *m*; *handheld*: leque *m* **2** *v/t* ⟨*pret & pp* ***fanned***⟩ ***~ oneself*** abanar-se

fanatic [fə'nætɪk] *n* fanático,-a *m,f*

fanatical [fə'nætɪkl] *adj* fanático

fanaticism [fə'nætɪsɪzm] fanatismo *m*

'fan belt MOT correia *f* do ventilador, *Port* correia *f* da ventoinha

'fan club fã-clube *m*

fancy ['fænsɪ] **1** *adj design* luxuoso **2** *n* ***as the ~ takes you*** conforme seus caprichos; ***take a ~ to s.o.*** afeiçoar-se a alguém

fancy 'dress fantasia *f*

fancy-'dress party festa *f* à fantasia

fang [fæŋ] presa *f*
'fan mail cartas *fpl* dos fãs
fantasize ['fæntəsaɪz] *v/i* fantasiar
fantastic [fæn'tæstɪk] *adj* fantástico
fantastically [fæn'tæstɪklɪ] *adv* (*extremely*) fantasticamente
fantasy ['fæntəsɪ] fantasia *f*
fanzine ['fænziːn] revista *f* de fãs
far [fɑːr] *adv* longe; (*much*) muito; ***~ away*** muito longe; ***how ~ is it to …?*** qual é a distância até …?; ***as ~ as the corner / hotel*** até a esquina / hotel; ***as ~ as I can see*** até onde posso ver; ***as ~ as I know*** que eu saiba; ***you've gone too ~*** *in behavior* você foi longe demais; ***so ~ so good*** até agora tudo bem
farce [fɑːrs] farsa *f*
fare [fer] *n travel*: tarifa *f*, *trains*, *buses*: preço *m* da passagem
Far 'East Extremo *m* Oriente
fare'well *n* despedida *f*
fare'well party festa *f* de despedida
farfetched [fɑːr'fetʃt] *adj* forçado
farm [fɑːrm] *n* fazenda *f*, *Port* quinta *f*
♦ **farm out** *v/t* sub-contratar
farmer ['fɑːrmər] fazendeiro,-a *m,f*, *Port* agricultor,a *m,f*
'farmhouse casa *f* de fazenda, *Port* casa *f* da quinta
farming ['fɑːrmɪŋ] *n* agricultura *f*, ***cattle ~*** criação *f* de gado
'farmworker lavrador,a *m,f*
'farmyard curral *m*
far-'off *adj* longínquo
farsighted [fɑːr'saɪtɪd] *adj* sagaz; *Am optically* hipermetrope
fart [fɑːrt] *fam* **1** *n* peido *m* **2** *v/i* peidar
farther ['fɑːrðər] *adv* mais longe; ***it's 10 miles ~ than the crossroads*** fica a 16 kilometros além do cruzamento
farthest ['fɑːrðəst] *adv travel etc* mais longe
fascinate ['fæsɪneɪt] *v/t* fascinar; ***be ~d by …*** ser fascinado por …
fascinating ['fæsɪneɪtɪŋ] *adj* fascinante
fascination [fæsɪ'neɪʃn] *with subject* fascinação *f*
fascism ['fæʃɪzm] fascismo *m*
fascist ['fæʃɪst] **1** *n* fascista *m/f* **2** *adj* fascista
fashion ['fæʃn] *n* moda *f*, (*manner*) modo *m*; ***in ~*** na moda; ***out of ~*** fora de moda
fashionable ['fæʃnəbl] *adj clothes* em moda; *person*, *idea* moderno
fashionably ['fæʃnəblɪ] *adv dressed* na moda
'fashion-conscious *adj* atento à moda **'fashion designer** costureiro,-a *m,f* **'fashion magazine** revista *f* de moda **'fashion show** desfile *m* de moda
fast[1] [fæst] **1** *adj* rápido; ***be ~*** *clock* estar adiantado **2** *adv* rapidamente; ***stuck ~*** emperrado; ***~ asleep*** dormindo profundamente
fast[2] [fæst] *n* (*not eating*) jejum *m*
fasten ['fæsn] **1** *v/t* fechar; ***~ sth onto sth*** prender algo em algo **2** *v/i dress etc* fechar
fastener ['fæsnər] *for dress* fecho *m*; *for lid* prendedor *m*
'fast food fast-food *f* **fastfood 'restaurant** restaurante *m* fast-food **fast 'forward 1** *n on video etc* avanço *m* rápido **2** *v/i* avançar rapidamente **'fast lane** *on road* pista *f* de alta velocidade **'fast train** trem *m* rápido
fat [fæt] **1** *adj* gordo **2** *n meat*, *baking*: gordura *f*
fatal ['feɪtl] *adj illness*, *error* fatal
fatality [fə'tælətɪ] fatalidade *f*
fatally ['feɪtəlɪ] *adv* ***~ injured*** fatalmente ferido
fate [feɪt] destino *m*
fated ['feɪtɪd] *adj* ***be ~ to do sth*** estar destinado a fazer algo
'fat-free *adj* sem gordura
father ['fɑːðər] *n* pai *m*; ***Father Martin*** REL Padre *m* Martin
Father 'Christmas *Brit* Papai *m* Noel
fatherhood ['fɑːðərhʊd] paternidade *f*
'father-in-law ⟨*pl* ***fathers-in-law***⟩ sogro *m*
fatherly ['fɑːðərlɪ] *adj* paterno
fathom ['fæðəm] *n* NAUT braça *f*
♦ **fathom out** *v/t* compreender
fatigue [fə'tiːg] *n* fadiga *f*
fatso ['fætsoʊ] *fam* balofo,-a *m,f*

F

fatten ['fætn] *v/t animal* engordar
fatty ['fætɪ] **1** *adj* gorduroso **2** *n fam person* gorducho,-a *m,f*
faucet ['fɒːsɪt] *Am* torneira *f*
fault [fɒːlt] *n* (*defect*) defeito *m*; ***it's your / my ~*** é culpa sua / minha; ***find ~ with …*** colocar críticas em …
faultless ['fɒːltlɪs] *adj person, performance* impecável
faulty ['fɒːltɪ] *adj goods* defeituoso
favor ['feɪvər] **1** *n* favor *m*; ***do s.o. a ~*** fazer um favor a alguém; ***do me a ~!*** (*don't be stupid*) faça-me o favor!; ***in ~ of …*** *resign, withdraw* em favor de …; ***be in ~ of …*** estar a favor de … **2** *v/t* (*prefer*) favorecer
favorable ['feɪvərəbl] *adj Am* favorável
favorite ['feɪvərɪt] **1** *n Am* favorito,-a *m,f* **2** *adj* favorito
favoritism ['feɪvrɪtɪzm] *Am* favoritismo *m*
favour *etc Brit* → ***favor***
fax [fæks] **1** *n* fax *m*; ***send sth by ~*** enviar algo via fax **2** *v/t* enviar por fax; ***~ sth to s.o.*** enviar algo por fax a alguém
FBI [efbiː'aɪ] *abbr* (*of* ***Federal Bureau of Investigation***) Agência *f* Federal de Investigação
fear [fɪr] **1** *n* medo *m* **2** *v/t* ter medo de
fearless ['fɪrlɪs] *adj* destemido
fearlessly ['fɪrlɪslɪ] *adv* destemidamente
feasibility study [fiːzə'bɪlətɪ] estudo *m* de viabilidade
feasible ['fiːzəbl] *adj* viável
feast [fiːst] *n* festa *f*
feat [fiːt] feito *m*
feather ['feðər] pena *f*
feature ['fiːʧər] **1** *n face*: feição *f*; *city, building, plan, style*: característica *f*; (*article in paper*) reportagem *f*; (*movie*) longa-metragem *m*; ***make a ~ of …*** dar destaque a … **2** *v/t movie* estrelar
'feature film filme *m* de longa-metragem
February ['februərɪ] fevereiro *m*
fed [fed] *pret & pp* → ***feed***
federal ['fedərəl] *adj* federal
federation [fedə'reɪʃn] federação *f*
fed 'up *adj fam* cheio, *Port* farto; ***be ~ with s.o. / sth*** estar cheio de alguém / algo
fee [fiː] taxa *f*; *lawyer, doctor, consultant*: honorário *m*; *entrance*: preço *m* da entrada; *membership*: mensalidade *f*
feeble ['fiːbl] *adj person* frágil; *attempt* ineficaz; *laugh, excuse* fraco
feed [fiːd] *v/t* ⟨*pret & pp* ***fed***⟩ alimentar; *animal* dar comida a
'feedback retorno *m*
feel [fiːl] ⟨*pret & pp* ***felt***⟩ **1** *v/t* (*touch*) tocar; (*sense*), *also pain, pleasure* sentir; (*think*) achar **2** *v/i* sentir; ***it ~s like silk / cotton*** parece seda / algodão; ***your hand ~s hot / cold*** sua mão está quente / fria; ***I ~ hungry / tired*** estou com fome / cansado; ***how are you ~ing today?*** como você está se sentindo hoje?; ***how does it ~ to be rich?*** qual é a sensação de ser rico?; ***do you ~ like a drink / meal?*** você está com vontade de tomar um drinque / comer?; ***I ~ like going / staying*** quero ir / ficar; ***I don't ~ like it*** não quero
♦ **feel up to** *v/t* animar-se para; ***I don't feel up to going, I'm too tired*** não estou animado para ir, estou muito cansado
feeler ['fiːlər] *insect*: antena *f*
'feelgood factor fator *m* de satisfação
feeling ['fiːlɪŋ] sensação *f*; (*emotion*) sentimento *m*; (*sensation*) sensibilidade *f*; ***what are your ~s about it?*** o que você acha disso?; ***I have mixed ~s about him*** tenho sentimentos contraditórios em relação a ele; ***I have this ~ that …*** tenho a sensação de que …
feet [fiːt] *pl* → ***foot***
feline ['fiːlaɪn] *adj* felino
fell [fel] *pret* → ***fall***[2]
fellow ['feloʊ] *n* (*man*) sujeito *m*
fellow 'citizen concidadão *m*, concidadã *f* **fellow 'countryman** compatriota *m* **fellow 'man** semelhante *m*
felony ['felənɪ] crime *m*
felt[1] [felt] *pret & pp* → ***feel***

felt[2] [felt] *n* feltro *m*
felt 'tip, **felt tip 'pen** caneta *f* hidrográfica
female ['fiːmeɪl] **1** *adj animal, plant* fêmea; *relating to people* feminino **2** *n animal, plant*: fêmea *f*; *person also fam* (*woman*) mulher *f*
feminine ['femɪnɪn] **1** *adj* feminino **2** *n* GRAM feminino *m*
feminism ['femɪnɪzm] feminismo *m*
feminist ['femɪnɪst] **1** *n* feminista *m/f* **2** *adj group, ideas* feminista
fence [fens] *n* cerca *f*; *fam* (*criminal*) receptador,a *m,f*; ***sit on the ~*** *fig* ficar em cima do muro
♦**fence in** *v/t land* cercar
fencing ['fensɪŋ] SPORT esgrima *f*
fend [fend] *v/i* ***~ for oneself*** defender-se
fender ['fendər] MOT *Am* pára-lama *m*
ferment[1] [fər'ment] *v/i liquid* fermentar
ferment[2] ['fɜːrment] *n* (*unrest*) agitação *f*
fermentation [fɜːrmen'teɪʃn] fermentação *f*
fern [fɜːrn] samambaia *f*, *Port* feto *m*
ferocious [fə'roʊʃəs] *adj* feroz
ferry ['ferɪ] *n* balsa *f*
fertile ['fɜːrtl] *adj* fértil
fertility [fɜːr'tɪlətɪ] fertilidade *f*
fer'tility drug pílula *f* de fertilidade
fertilize ['fɜːrtəlaɪz] *v/t ovum* fertilizar
fertilizer ['fɜːrtəlaɪzər] *soil*: fertilizante *m*
fervent ['fɜːrvənt] *adj admirer* fervoroso
fervently ['fɜːrvəntlɪ] *adv* fervorosamente
fester ['festər] *v/i wound* inflamar-se
festival ['festɪvl] MUS festival *m*; REL festa *f*
festive ['festɪv] *adj* festivo; ***the ~ season*** a época do Natal
festivities [fe'stɪvətɪz] *npl* festividades *fpl*
fetal ['fiːtl] *adj* fetal
fetch [fetʃ] *v/t person, thing* apanhar; *price* alcançar
fetus ['fiːtəs] feto *m*
feud [fjuːd] **1** *n* rixa *f* **2** *v/i* estar em disputa
fever ['fiːvər] febre *f*
feverish ['fiːvərɪʃ] *adj also fig* febril
few [fjuː] **1** *adj* (*not many*) pouco; ***a ~*** alguns, algumas; ***quite a ~, a good ~*** (*a lot*) um bom número de **2** *pron* (*not many*) poucos,-as; ***a ~*** (*some*) alguns, algumas; ***quite a ~, a good ~*** (*a lot*) muitos,-as
fewer ['fjuːər] *adj* menos; ***~ than …*** menos de …
fiancé [fɪ'ɑːnseɪ] noivo *m*
fiancée [fɪ'ɑːnseɪ] noiva *f*
fiasco [fɪ'æskoʊ] fiasco *m*
fib [fɪb] *n* lorota *f*
fiber ['faɪbər] *n Am* fibra *f*
'fiberglass *n Am* fibra *f* de vidro
fiber 'optic *adj* de fibra óptica
fiber 'optics *npl Am* tecnologia *f* da fibra óptica
fibre *etc Brit* → ***fiber***
fickle ['fɪkl] *adj* inconstante
fiction ['fɪkʃn] ficção *f*
fictional ['fɪkʃnl] *adj* de ficção
fictitious [fɪk'tɪʃəs] *adj* fictício
fiddle ['fɪdl] **1** *n fam* (*violin*) violino *m*; ***it's a ~*** *fam* (*cheat*) é uma trapaça **2** *v/i* ***~ with …*** brincar com …; ***~ around with …*** mexer com … **3** *v/t accounts, results* falsificar
fidelity [fɪ'delətɪ] fidelidade *f*
fidget ['fɪdʒɪt] *v/i* mexer-se
fidgety ['fɪdʒɪtɪ] *adj* inquieto
field [fiːld] *also sport*: campo *m*; (*competitors in race*) competidores *mpl*; *research, knowledge etc*: área *f*; ***that's not my ~*** está não é a minha área; ***there's a strong ~ for the 1500m*** há fortes competidores nos 1500m
fielder ['fiːldər] *baseball*: interceptador,a *m,f*
'field events *npl* esportes *mpl* de campo
fierce [fɪrs] *adj animal* feroz; *wind, storm* violento
fiercely ['fɪrslɪ] *adv* ferozmente
fiery ['faɪrɪ] *adj personality, temperament* esquentado
fifteen [fɪf'tiːn] quinze
fifteenth [fɪf'tiːnθ] *n & adj* décimo quinto (*m*)
fifth [fɪfθ] *n & adj* quinto (*m*)
fifthly ['fɪfθlɪ] *adv* em quinto lugar

fiftieth ['fɪftɪəθ] *n & adj* qüinquagésimo (*m*)
fifty ['fɪftɪ] cinqüenta
fifty-'fifty *adv* meio a meio
fig [fɪg] figo *m*
fight [faɪt] **1** *n also fig for survival etc* luta *f*; *in war* combate *m*; (*argument*) discussão *f* **2** *v/t* ⟨*pret & pp* ***fought***⟩ *enemy, person, also in boxing, disease* lutar; *in war* combater **3** *v/i* ⟨*pret & pp* ***fought***⟩ lutar; (*argue*) discutir
♦**fight for** *v/t rights, cause* lutar por
fighter ['faɪtər] guerreiro,-a *m,f*; (*airplane*) caça *m*; (*boxer*) lutador,a *m,f*; ***she's a ~*** ela é uma lutadora
fighting ['faɪtɪŋ] *n physical* luta *f*; *verbal* discussão *f*
figurative ['fɪgjərətɪv] *adj use of word* figurado; *art* simbólico
figure ['fɪgjər] **1** *n* (*digit*) cifra *f*; *of person* forma *f*; (*form, shape*) figura *f* **2** *v/t Am fam* (*think*) achar
♦**figure on** *v/t fam* (*plan*) planejar
♦**figure out** *v/t* (*understand*) entender; *calculation* calcular
'**figure skater** patinador,a *m,f* artístico,-a
'**figure skating** patinação *f* artística
file[1] [faɪl] **1** *n of documents, also* COMPUT arquivo *m* **2** *v/t documents* arquivar
file[2] [faɪl] *n wood, fingernails*: lixa *f*
♦**file away** *v/t documents* arquivar
'**file cabinet** *Am* arquivo *m*
'**file manager** COMPUT gerenciador *m* de arquivos
filial ['fɪlɪəl] *adj duties* de filho
fill [fɪl] **1** *v/t* encher; *tooth* obturar **2** *n* ***eat one's ~*** fartar-se
♦**fill in** *v/t form* preencher; *hole* tapar; ***fill s.o. in*** colocar alguém a par
♦**fill in for** *v/t* substituir
♦**fill out 1** *v/t form* preencher **2** *v/i* (*get fatter*) engordar
♦**fill up 1** *v/t* encher completamente **2** *v/i stadium, theater* lotar
fillet ['fɪlɪt] *n* faixa *f*
fillet 'steak filé *m*
filling ['fɪlɪŋ] **1** *n sandwich*: recheio *m*; *tooth*: obturação *f*, *Port* chumbo *m* **2** *adj food* pesado
'**filling station** posto *m* de gasolina
film [fɪlm] **1** *n for camera, also* (*movie*) filme *m* **2** *v/t person, event* filmar
'**film-maker** cineasta *m/f*
'**film star** astro de cinema *m*, estrela de cinema *f*
filter ['fɪltər] **1** *n* filtro *m* **2** *v/t coffee, liquid* filtrar
♦**filter through** *v/i news* filtrar
'**filter paper** filtro *m* de papel
'**filter tip** *cigarette* cigarro *m* com filtro
filth [fɪlθ] sujeira *f*, *Port* sujidade *f*
filthy [fɪlθɪ] *adj* sujo; *language etc* obsceno
fin [fɪn] *of fish* barbatana *f*
final ['faɪnl] **1** *adj* final **2** *n* SPORT final *f*
finale [fɪ'nælɪ] final *m*
finalist ['faɪnəlɪst] finalista *m/f*
finalize ['faɪnəlaɪz] *v/t plans, design* finalizar
finally ['faɪnəlɪ] *adv* finalmente; (*at last*) afinal
finance ['faɪnæns] **1** *n* finanças *fpl* **2** *v/t* financiar
finances ['faɪnænsɪz] *npl* finanças *fpl*
financial [faɪ'nænʃl] *adj* financeiro
financially [faɪ'nænʃəlɪ] *adv* financeiramente
financier [faɪ'nænsɪr] financista *m/f*
find [faɪnd] *v/t* ⟨*pret & pp* ***found***⟩ encontrar; ***if you ~ it too hot / cold*** se você achar muito quente / frio; ***~ a person innocent / guilty*** LAW declarar uma pessoa inocente / culpada
♦**find out 1** *v/t* descobrir **2** *v/i* (*enquire*) indagar; (*discover*) descobrir
findings ['faɪndɪŋz] *npl of report* conclusões *f*
fine[1] [faɪn] *adj day, weather* bonito; *weather, wine, performance, city* bom; *distinction* sutil; *line* fino; ***how's that? – that's ~*** como está? - está ótimo; ***that's ~ by me*** está bom para mim; ***how are you? – ~*** como vai? - vou bem
fine[2] [faɪn] **1** *n* multa *f* **2** *v/t* multar
fine-'tooth comb ***go through sth with a ~*** passar algo o pente fino
fine-'tune *v/t fig* fazer um último ajuste em
finger ['fɪŋgər] **1** *n* dedo *m* **2** *v/t* cutucar

'fingernail unha *f* **'fingerprint 1** *n* impressão *f* digital **2** *v/t* tirar as impressões digitais de **'fingertip** ponta *f* do dedo; ***have sth at one's ~s*** ter algo na ponta dos dedos

finicky ['fɪnɪkɪ] *adj person* enjoado; *design, pattern* muito detalhado

finish ['fɪnɪʃ] **1** *v/t* terminar; ***~ doing sth*** terminar de fazer algo **2** *v/i* terminar **3** *n product*: acabamento *m*; *race*: chegada *f*

'finish line linha *f* de chegada

◆**finish off** *v/t* terminar

◆**finish up** *v/t food* acabar; ***he finished up liking it / living there*** ele acabou gostando / vivendo lá

◆**finish with** *v/t boyfriend etc* terminar com

Finland ['fɪnlənd] Finlândia *f*

Finn [fɪn] finlandês,-esa *m,f*

Finnish ['fɪnɪʃ] **1** *adj* finlandês,-esa **2** *n language* finlandês *m*

fir [fɜːr] abeto *m*

fire ['faɪr] **1** *n* fogo *m*; *electric, gas* aquecedor *m*; (*blaze*) incêndio *m*; (*bonfire, campfire etc*) fogueira *f*; ***be on ~*** estar de cabeça quente; ***catch ~*** pegar fogo; ***set sth on ~, set ~ to sth*** incendiar algo, pôr fogo em algo **2** *v/i* (*shoot*) atirar **3** *v/t fam* (*dismiss*) demitir

'fire alarm alarme *m* de incêndio **'firearm** arma *f* de fogo **fire brigade** *Brit* → ***fire department*** **'firecracker** traque *m* **'fire department** *Am* corpo *m* de bombeiros **'fire door** porta *f* corta fogo **'fire drill** treinamento *m* de incêndio **fire engine** → ***fire truck*** **'fire escape** escada *f* de incêndio **fire extinguisher** ['faɪrɪkstɪŋgwɪʃər] extintor *m* de incêndio **'fire fighter** bombeiro *m* **'fireguard** guarda-fogo *m* **'fireman** bombeiro *m* **'fireplace** lareira *f* **'fire station** posto *m* de bombeiros **'fire truck** *Am* caminhão *m* de bombeiros **'firewood** lenha *f* **'fireworks** *npl* fogos *mpl* de artifício; (*display*) espetáculo *m* de fogos de artifício

firm[1] [fɜːrm] *adj grip, voice, decision* firme; *flesh, muscles* rijo; ***a ~ deal*** um negócio fechado

firm[2] [fɜːrm] *n* COM firma *f*

first [fɜːrst] **1** *adj* primeiro; ***who's ~ please?*** quem é o primeiro, por favor? **2** *n* primeiro,-a *m,f*; ***~ of January*** primeiro de janeiro **3** *adv arrive, finish, also* (*beforehand*) primeiro; ***~ of all*** (*for one reason*) em primeiro lugar; ***at ~*** no início

first 'aid primeiros socorros *mpl* **first-'aid box, first-'aid kit** caixa *f* de primeiros socorros **'firstborn** *adj* primogênito **'first class 1** *adj ticket, seat* de primeira classe; (*very good*) de primeira categoria **2** *adv travel* de primeira classe **first 'floor** *Am* térreo *m*; *Brit* primeiro andar *m*, *Port* rés-do-chão *m* **first'hand** *adj* de primeira mão **First 'Lady** *of US* primeira dama *f*

firstly ['fɜːrstlɪ] *adv* primeiramente

first 'name prenome *m* **first 'night** noite *f* de estréia **first of'fender** delinqüente *m/f* primário,-a **first-'rate** *adj* de primeira qualidade **first-time 'buyer** *adj house*: comprador,a *m,f* de primeira vez

fiscal ['fɪskl] *adj* fiscal

fiscal 'year ano *m* fiscal

fish [fɪʃ] **1** *n* ⟨*pl* ***fish***⟩ peixe *m*; ***drink like a ~*** *fam* beber como um gambá; ***feel like a ~ out of water*** sentir-se como um peixe fora d'água **2** *v/i* pescar

fish and 'chips *npl Brit* peixe *m* com batatas

'fishbone espinha *f* de peixe

fisherman ['fɪʃərmən] pescador *m*

fish finger *Brit* → ***fish stick***

fishing ['fɪʃɪŋ] pesca *f*

'fishing boat barco *m* de pesca **'fishing line** linha *f* de pesca **'fishing rod** vara *f* de pesca

'fish stick *Am* filezinho *m* de peixe

fishy ['fɪʃɪ] *adj fam* (*suspicious*) suspeito

fist [fɪst] punho *m*

fit[1] [fɪt] *n* MED ataque *m*; ***a ~ of rage / jealousy*** um ataque de raiva / ciúme

fit[2] [fɪt] *adj physically* em boa forma; *morally* apropriado; ***keep ~*** manter

a forma; ***it's not ~ to eat*** já não está bom para comer; ***he's not ~ to be a father*** ele não serve para ser pai
fit[3] [fɪt] **1** *v/t* ⟨*pret & pp* ***fitted***⟩ (*attach*) colocar **2** *v/i* ⟨*pret & pp* ***fitted***⟩ *clothes* servir; *piece of furniture etc* caber **3** *n* ***it is a good ~*** é um bom tamanho; ***it's a tight ~*** é um espaço apertado
♦**fit in 1** *v/i person in group* dar-se bem; ***it fits in with our plans*** isto se encaixa em nossos planos **2** *v/t* ***fit s.o. in*** encaixar alguém
fitful ['fɪtfl] *adj sleep* interrompido
fitness ['fɪtnɪs] (*physical*) boa *f* forma
'fitness center *Am* academia *f* de ginástica
fitness centre *Brit* → ***fitness center***
fitted 'carpet ['fɪtɪd] *Brit* carpete *m*
fitted 'kitchen cozinha *f* planejada
fitted 'sheet lençol *m* com elástico
fitter ['fɪtər] *n* montador,a *m,f*
fitting ['fɪtɪŋ] *adj* apropriado
fittings ['fɪtɪŋz] *npl* instalações *fpl*
five [faɪv] cinco
fix [fɪks] **1** *n* (*solution*) solução *f*; ***be in a ~*** *fam* estar em apuros **2** *v/t* (*attach*) fixar; (*repair*) consertar; (*arrange*) *meeting etc* marcar; *lunch* preparar; *dishonestly, match etc* subornar; ***~ sth onto sth*** fixar algo em algo; ***I'll ~ you a drink*** vou preparar-lhe um drinque
♦**fix up** *v/t meeting* marcar; ***it's all fixed up*** está tudo combinado
fixed [fɪkst] *adj* fixo
fixings ['fɪksɪŋz] *npl Am* acompanhamento *m* tradicional
fixture ['fɪkstʃər] *in room* elemento *m* fixo
♦**fizzle out** ['fɪzl] *v/i fam* não dar certo
fizzy ['fɪzɪ] *adj Brit drink* com gás
flab [flæb] *on body* flacidez *f*
flabbergast ['flæbərgæst] *v/t fam* espantar; ***be ~ed*** ficar pasmado
flabby ['flæbɪ] *adj muscles, stomach* flácido
flag[1] [flæg] *n* bandeira *f*
flag[2] [flæg] *v/i* ⟨*pret & pp* ***flagged***⟩ (*tire*) afrouxar
'flagpole mastro *m* de bandeira
flagrant ['fleɪgrənt] *adj* flagrante
'flagship *fig* carro-chefe *m* **'flagstaff** mastro *m* de bandeira **'flagstone** laje *f*
flair [fler] (*talent*) talento *m*; ***have a natural ~ for*** ter um talento natural para
flake [fleɪk] *n* floco *m*; *plaster*: camada *f*; *skin*: escama *f*
♦**flake off** *v/i* descamar
flaky ['fleɪkɪ] *adj* escamoso
flaky 'pastry massa *f* folhada
flamboyant [flæm'bɔɪənt] *adj personality* espalhafatoso
flamboyantly [flæm'bɔɪəntlɪ] *adv dressed* espalhafatosamente
flame [fleɪm] *n* flama *f*; ***go up in ~s*** arder em chamas
flammable ['flæməbl] *adj* inflamável
flan [flæn] torta *f*
flank [flæŋk] **1** *n horse etc*:, *also* MIL flanco *m* **2** *v/t* ***be ~ed by*** estar flanqueado por
flannel *Brit* → ***washcloth***
flap [flæp] **1** *n envelope, pocket*: aba *f*; *table*: borda *f*; ***be in a ~*** *fam* ficar desatinado **2** *v/t* ⟨*pret & pp* ***flapped***⟩ *wings* bater **3** *v/i* ⟨*pret & pp* ***flapped***⟩ *flag etc* bater
flare [fler] **1** *n* (*distress signal*) sinal *m* incandescente; *in dress* folga *f* **2** *v/t nostrils* dilatar
♦**flare up** *v/i violence, illness, rash* irromper; *fire* inflamar-se; (*get very angry*) enfurecer-se
flash [flæʃ] **1** *n light, also* PHOT flash *m*; ***in a ~*** *fam* num instante; ***have a ~ of inspiration*** ter um lampejo de inspiração; ***~ of lightning*** relâmpago *m* **2** *v/i light* piscar **3** *v/t headlights* piscar
'flashback *n* flashback *m*
flasher ['flæʃər] MOT pisca-pisca *m*
'flashlight *Am* lanterna *f*; PHOT flash *m*
flashy ['flæʃɪ] *adj pej* berrante
flask [flæsk] (*hip flask*) frasco *m*
flat [flæt] **1** *adj surface, land* plano; *beer* insípido; *Brit battery* descarregado; *tire* furado; *shoes* baixo; ***and that's ~*** *fam* e assunto encerrado; ***A / B ~*** MUS lá / si bemol **2** *adv* MUS desafinadamente; ***~ out*** *work*,

run a todo vapor **3** *n Am* pneu *m* furado
flat² [flæt] *n Brit* (*apartment*) apartamento *m*
flat-chested [flæ'ʧestɪd] *adj* ***be ~*** ser de peito achatado
flatly ['flætlɪ] *adv refuse, deny* terminantemente
flatmate *Brit* → ***room mate***
'flat rate tarifa *f* única
'flat screen monitor monitor *m* de ecrã plano
flatten ['flætn] *v/t land, road* aplanar; *by bombing, demolition* arrasar
flatter ['flætər] *v/t* lisonjear
flatterer ['flætərər] lisonjeador,a *m,f*
flattering ['flætərɪŋ] *adj comments* lisonjeiro; *color, clothes* favorável
flattery ['flætərɪ] bajulação *f*
flatulence ['flætjʊləns] flatulência *f*
'flatware *Am* (*cutlery*) talher *m*
flaunt [flɔːnt] *v/t* ostentar
flautist ['flɔːtɪst] flautista *m/f*
flavor ['fleɪvər] *Am* **1** *n* sabor *m* **2** *v/t food*, condimentar
flavoring ['fleɪvərɪŋ] *Am* aromatizante *m*
flavour *etc Brit* → ***flavor***
flaw [flɒː] *n* falha *f*
flawless ['flɒːlɪs] *adj* impecável
flea [fliː] pulga *f*
fleck [flek] pinta *f*
fled [fled] *pret & pp* → ***flee***
flee [fliː] *v/i* ⟨*pret & pp* ***fled***⟩ fugir
fleece [fliːs] *v/t fam* explorar
fleet [fliːt] *n* NAUT esquadra *f*; *taxis, trucks*: frota *f*
fleeting ['fliːtɪŋ] *adj visit etc* muito rápido; ***catch a ~ glimpse of*** ver de relance
flesh [fleʃ] carne *f*; *of fruit* polpa *f*; ***meet / see a person in the ~*** encontrar / ver uma pessoa em carne e osso
flew [fluː] *pret* → ***fly³***
flex [fleks] *v/t muscles* flexionar
flexibility [fleksə'bɪlətɪ] flexibilidade *f*
flexible ['fleksəbl] *adj* flexível; ***I'm quite ~*** *about arrangements, timing* sou bastante flexível
'flextime *Am* horário *m* flexível
flick [flɪk] *v/t tail* dar uma pancadinha; ***he ~ed a fly off his hand*** ele espantou uma mosca com a mão; ***she ~ed her hair out of her eyes*** ela afastou os cabelos dos olhos
♦**flick through** *v/t magazine* folhear
flicker ['flɪkər] *v/i light, computer screen* tremular
flier ['flaɪr] (*circular*) panfleto *m*
flies [flaɪz] *npl Brit pants*: braguilha *f*
flight [flaɪt] vôo *m*; (*fleeing*) fuga *f*; **~ (*of stairs*)** lance *m* (de escada)
'flight attendant comissário,-a *m,f* de bordo **'flight crew** tripulação *f* de vôo **'flight deck** cabine *f* de comando; *aircraft carrier*: pista *f* de aterrisagem, *Port* pista *f* de aterragem **'flight number** número *m* do vôo **'flight path** rota *f* de vôo **'flight recorder** gravador *m* de vôo **'flight time** *departure* horário *m* do vôo; *duration* duração *f* do vôo
flighty ['flaɪtɪ] *adj* inconstante
flimsy ['flɪmzɪ] *adj structure, furniture* frágil; *dress, material* fino; *excuse* fraco
flinch [flɪnʧ] *v/i* encolher-se
fling [flɪŋ] **1** *v/t* ⟨*pret & pp* ***flung***⟩ lançar; ***~ oneself into a chair*** atirar-se em uma cadeira **2** *n fam* (*affair*) aventura *f*
♦**flip through** [flɪp] *v/t* ⟨*pret & pp* ***flipped***⟩ *book, magazine* folhear
flipper ['flɪpər] *swimming*: nadadeira *f*
flirt [flɜːrt] **1** *v/i* flertar **2** *n* flerte *m*
flirtatious [flɜːr'teɪʃəs] *adj* namorador
float [floʊt] *v/i* flutuar; *fam* oscilar
floating voter ['floʊtɪŋ] eleitor,a *m,f* indeciso,-a
flock [flɑːk] **1** *n sheep*: rebanho *m*; *birds*: bando *m* **2** *v/i* afluir
flog [flɑːg] *v/t* ⟨*pret & pp* ***flogged***⟩ (*whip*) chicotear
flood [flʌd] **1** *n* inundação *f* **2** *v/t river* inundar; ***~ its banks*** *river* inundar suas margens
♦**flood in** *v/i letters etc* chover
flooding ['flʌdɪŋ] inundação *f*
'floodlight *n* holofote *m* **floodlit** ['flʌdlɪt] *adj game* iluminado por holofotes **'flood waters** *npl* águas *fpl* da enchente
floor [flɔːr] *n* chão *m*; (*story*) andar *m*

F

'floorboard tábua *f* de assoalho **'floor cloth** pano *m* de chão **'floor lamp** abajur *m* de pé

flop [flɑːp] **1** *v/i* ⟨*pret & pp* ***flopped***⟩ cair pesadamente; *fam* (*fail*) fracassar **2** *n fam* (*failure*) fracasso *m*

floppy[1] ['flɑːpɪ] *adj* mole

'floppy[2], **floppy 'disk** ['flɑːpɪ] disquete *m*

florist ['flɔːrɪst] florista *m/f*

floss [flɑːs] **1** *n teeth*: fio *m* dental **2** *v/t* ~ ***one's teeth*** passar o fio dental

flour ['flaʊr] farinha *f*

flourish ['flʌrɪʃ] *v/i* florir

flourishing ['flʌrɪʃɪŋ] *adj business* florescente

flow [floʊ] **1** *v/i river* correr; *electric current* circular; *traffic, work* fluir **2** *n river*: corrente *f*; *information, ideas*: fluxo *m*

'flowchart fluxograma *m*

flower ['flaʊr] **1** *n* flor *f* **2** *v/i* florir

'flowerbed canteiro *m* **'flowerpot** vaso *m* de flores **'flower show** exposição *f* de flores

flowery ['flaʊrɪ] *adj pattern* florido; *style* floreado

flown [floʊn] *pp* → ***fly***[3]

flu [fluː] gripe *f*

fluctuate ['flʌktjuːeɪt] *v/i* flutuar; *moods, opinions* variar

fluctuation [flʌktʃʊ'eɪʃn] flutuação *f*; *moods, opinions*: variação *f*

fluency ['fluːənsɪ] fluência *f*

fluent ['fluːənt] *adj* fluente; ***he speaks ~ Portuguese*** ele fala português com fluência

fluently ['fluːəntlɪ] *adv speak, write* fluentemente

fluff [flʌf] ***a bit of ~*** um pouco de penugem

fluffy ['flʌfɪ] *adj material, hair* macio; *clouds* fofo; ~ ***toy*** bichinho *m* de pelúcia

fluid ['fluːɪd] *n* fluido *m*

flung [flʌŋ] *pret & pp* → ***fling***

flunk [flʌŋk] *v/t Am fam subject* bombar em

fluorescent [flʊ'resnt] *adj light* fluorescente

flurry ['flʌrɪ] *snow*: lufada *f*

flush [flʌʃ] **1** *v/t* ~ ***the toilet*** dar descarga; ~ ***sth down the toilet*** jogar algo no vaso sanitário **2** *v/i toilet* dar descarga; (*go red in the face*) ruborizar-se **3** *adj* (*level*) rente; ***be ~ with ...*** estar rente com …

♦ **flush out** *v/t rebels etc* desentocar

fluster ['flʌstər] *v/t* atrapalhar; ***get ~ed*** ficar atrapalhado

flute [fluːt] MUS flauta *f*; *glass* taça *f*

flutist ['fluːtɪst] *Am* flautista *m/f*

flutter ['flʌtər] *v/i bird, wings, flag* esvoaçar; *heart* palpitar

fly[1] [flaɪ] *n insect* mosca *f*

fly[2] [flaɪ] *n pants*: braguilha *f*

fly[3] [flaɪ] ⟨*pret* ***flew***, *pp* ***flown***⟩ **1** *v/i bird, airplane* voar; *in airplane* ir de avião; *flag* hastear; (*rush*) precipitar-se; ~ ***into a rage*** exaltar-se **2** *v/t airplane* pilotar; *airline* voar com; (*transport by air*) transportar via aérea

♦ **fly away** *v/i bird, airplane* voar

♦ **fly back** *v/i* (*travel back*) voar de volta; ***I fly back to Brazil tomorrow*** vôo de volta ao Brasil amanhã

♦ **fly in 1** *v/i airplane, passengers* chegar **2** *v/t supplies etc* transportar de avião

♦ **fly off** *v/i* ***her hat flew off in the wind*** o chapéu dela voou com o vento

♦ **fly out** *v/i* partir de avião

♦ **fly past** *v/i in formation* voar em formação; *time* voar

flying ['flaɪɪŋ] *n* vôo *m*; ***I hate ~*** odeio voar

flying 'saucer disco *m* voador

foam [foʊm] *n on liquid* espuma *f*

foam 'rubber espuma *f* de borracha

FOB [efoʊ'biː] *abbr* (*of* ***free on board***) frete à pagar

focus ['foʊkəs] **1** *n of attention, also* PHOT foco *m*; ***be in ~ / out of ~*** estar em foco / fora de foco **2** *v/t* ~ ***one's attention on*** focalizar a atenção em **3** *v/i* focalizar

♦ **focus on** *v/t problem, also* PHOT focalizar em

fodder ['fɑːdər] forragem *f*

fog [fɑːg] neblina *f*

♦ **fog up** *v/i* ⟨*pret & pp* ***fogged***⟩ embaçar-se

'fogbound *adj* impedido devido a neblina
foggy ['fɑːgɪ] *adj* enevoado; ***I haven't the foggiest idea*** não tenho a menor idéia
foible ['fɔɪbl] *eccentricity* idiossincrasia *f*
foil[1] [fɔɪl] *n* papel *m* laminado, *Port* papel-aluminio *m*
foil[2] [fɔɪl] *v/t* (*thwart*) frustrar
fold[1] [foʊld] **1** *v/t paper etc* dobrar; ***~ one's arms*** cruzar os braços **2** *v/i business* abrir falência **3** *n cloth etc*: dobra *f*
fold[2] [foʊld] *n sheep etc*: curral *m*
◆ **fold up 1** *v/t* dobrar **2** *v/i chair, table* dobrar
folder ['foʊlder] *for documents, also* COMPUT pasta *f*
folding ['foʊldɪŋ] *adj* dobrável; ***~ chair*** cadeira *f* dobrável
foliage ['foʊlɪɪdʒ] folhagem *f*
folk [foʊk] (*people*) gente *f*; ***my ~s*** (*family*) a minha família; ***come in, ~s*** *fam* entra, pessoal
'folk dance dança *f* folclórica **'folk music** música *f* folclórica **'folk singer** cantor,a *m,f* de música regional **'folk song** canção *f* folclórica
follow ['fɑːloʊ] **1** *v/t person, road, instructions* seguir; TV *series, news* acompanhar; (*understand*) entender; ***~ me*** siga-me **2** *v/i* seguir; *logically* fazer sentido; ***it ~s from this that ...*** disso resulta que ...; ***as ~*** como segue
◆ **follow up** *v/t letter, inquiry* dar prosseguimento a; *leads* seguir
follower ['fɑːloʊər] *politician etc*: partidário,-a *m,f*; *football team*: torcedor,a *m,f*; *TV program*: espectador,a *m,f*
following ['fɑːloʊɪŋ] **1** *adj day, night, points, pages* seguinte **2** *n people* adeptos *mpl*; ***the ~*** o seguinte (a seguinte)
'follow-up meeting reunião *f* de acompanhamento
'follow-up visit *to doctor etc* visita de retorno *f*
folly ['fɑːlɪ] (*madness*) loucura *f*
fond [fɑːnd] *adj* (*loving*) carinhoso; *memory* terno; ***be ~ of ...*** gostar de ...
fondle ['fɑːndl] *v/t* acariciar
fondness ['fɑːndnɪs] predileção *f*
font [fɑːnt] *printing*: fonte *f*; *church*: pia *f* batismal
food [fuːd] comida *f*
'food chain cadeia *f* alimentar
foodie ['fuːdɪ] *fam* gourmet *m/f*
'food mixer batedeira *f*
food poisoning ['fuːdpɔɪznɪŋ] intoxicação *f* alimentar
fool [fuːl] **1** *n* tolo,-a *m,f*; ***make a ~ of oneself*** fazer papel de bobo **2** *v/t* enganar
◆ **fool about, fool around** *v/i* brincar (***with*** com); *sexually* trair (***with*** com)
'foolhardy *adj* temerário
foolish ['fuːlɪʃ] *adj* tolo
foolishly ['fuːlɪʃlɪ] *adv* tolamente
'foolproof *adj* infalível
foot [fʊt] ⟨*pl feet*⟩ *also measurement* pé *m*; *animal*: pata *f*; ***on ~*** a pé; ***I've been on my feet all day*** fiquei de pé o dia inteiro; ***be back on one's feet*** estar de pé novamente; ***at the ~ of the page / hill*** no rodapé da página / no sopé da montanha; ***put one's ~ in it*** *fam* botar o dedo na ferida
footage ['fʊtɪdʒ] seqüência *f* de filme
'football futebol *m* americano; (*soccer*) futebol *m*; *ball* bola *f* de futebol
footballer ['fʊtbɒːlər] futebolista *m/f*
football hooligan *Brit* → ***soccer hooligan***
'football player jogador,a *m,f* de futebol **'footbridge** passarela *f* **foothills** ['fʊthɪlz] *npl* contraforte *m*
'foothold *climbing*: apoio *m* para os pés; ***gain a ~*** *fig* estabelecer-se
footing ['fʊtɪŋ] (*basis*) base *f*; ***lose one's ~*** escorregar; ***be on the same / a different ~*** estar em condições iguais / diferentes; ***be on a friendly ~ with ...*** ter boas relações com ...
footlights ['fʊtlaɪts] *npl* luzes *fpl* da ribalta **'footmark** pegada *f* **'footnote** nota *f* de rodapé **'footpath** caminho *m* **'footprint** pegada *f*; ***reduce your carbon ~!*** reduza os seus rastros de

F

carbono! 'footstep passo *m*; **follow in s.o.'s ~s** *fig* seguir os passos de alguém 'footstool banquinho *m* 'footwear calçados *mpl*

for [fər, fɔːr] *prep* ◊ *purpose, destination etc*: para; ***a train ~ ...*** um trem para ...; ***clothes ~ children*** roupas infantis; ***it's too big ~ you*** é muito grande para você; ***this is ~ you*** isto é para você; ***what is there ~ lunch?*** o que é que há para o almoço?; ***the steak is ~ me*** o bife é para mim; ***what is this ~?*** para que serve isto?; ***what ~?*** para quê?
◊ *time*: durante; ***I have been waiting ~ three hours*** estive esperando durante três horas; ***it will last ~ two days*** vai durar dois dias; ***please get it done ~ Monday*** por favor, termine até segunda-feira
◊ *distance*: por; ***I walked ~ a mile*** andei uma milha; ***it stretches ~ 100 miles*** se estende por 161 kilometros
◊ (*in favor of*) a favor de; ***I am ~ the idea*** sou a favor da idéia
◊ (*instead of, in behalf of*) por; ***let me do that ~ you*** deixe-me fazer isso por você; ***we are agents ~ ...*** somos agentes de ...
◊ (*in exchange for*) por; ***I bought it ~ 25*** comprei por 25; ***how much did you sell it ~?*** por quanto você vendeu?

forbade [fər'bæd] *pret* → ***forbid***

forbid [fər'bɪd] *v/t* 〈*pret* **forbade**, *pp* **forbidden**〉 proibir; ***~ s.o. to do sth*** proibir alguém de fazer algo

forbidden [fər'bɪdn] **1** *adj* proibido; ***smoking / parking ~*** proibido fumar / estacionar **2** *pp* → ***forbid***

forbidding [fər'bɪdɪŋ] *adj person, tone, look etc* severo; *prospect* sombrio

force [fɔːrs] **1** *n* força *f*; ***come into ~*** *of law etc* entrar em vigor; ***the ~s*** MIL as Forças Armadas **2** *v/t door, lock* forçar; ***~ s.o. to do sth*** forçar alguém a fazer algo; ***~ sth open*** arrombar algo

♦ **force back** *v/t* conter

forced [fɔːrst] *adj laugh, smile* forçado

forced 'landing aterrissagem *f* forçada, *Port* aterragem *f* forçosa

forceful ['fɔːrsfl] *adj argument* forte; *speaker* vigoroso; *character* enérgico

forcefully ['fɔːrsflɪ] *adv argue* vigorosamente

forceps ['fɔːrseps] *npl* MED fórceps *m*

forcible ['fɔːrsəbl] *adj entry* à força; *argument* forte

forcibly ['fɔːrsəblɪ] *adv restrain* forçosamente

ford [fɔːrd] *n* vau *m*

fore [fɔːr] *n* dianteira *f*; ***come to the ~*** vir à tona

'forearm antebraço *m* **forebears** ['fɔːrberz] *npl* ancestrais *mpl* **foreboding** [fər'boudɪŋ] mau presságio *m* **'forecast 1** *n result, weather*: previsão *f* **2** *v/t* 〈*pret & pp* **forecast**〉 prever **'forecourt** *garage*: área *f* de estacionamento **forefathers** ['fɔːrfɑːðərz] *npl* antepassados *mpl* **'forefinger** dedo *m* indicador **'forefront** vanguarda *f*; ***be in the ~ of*** estar na vanguarda em **'foregone** *adj* ***that's a ~ conclusion*** é uma conclusão inevitável **'foreground** primeiro plano *m* **'forehand** *tennis*: forehand *m* **'forehead** testa *f*

foreign ['fɑːrən] *adj* estrangeiro

foreign af'fairs *npl* relações *fpl* exteriores **foreign 'aid** assistência *f* internacional **foreign 'body** corpo *m* estranho **foreign 'countries** exterior *m* **foreign 'currency** moeda *f* estrangeira

foreigner ['fɑːrənər] estrangeiro,-a *m,f*

foreign ex'change câmbio *m* **foreign 'language** língua *f* estrangeira **'Foreign Office** *in UK* Ministério *m* das Relações Exteriores **foreign 'policy** política *f* externa **Foreign 'Secretary** *in UK* Ministro *m* das Relações Exteriores

'foreman encarregado *m*

'foremost 1 *adv* em primeiro lugar **2** *adj* (*leading*) principal

forensic 'medicine [fə'rensɪk] medicina *f* legal

forensic 'scientist cientista *m/f* forense

'forerunner predecessor,a *m,f*

fore'saw *pret* → ***foresee***

fore'see *v/t* ⟨*pret* ***foresaw***, *pp* ***foreseen***⟩ prever
foreseeable [fər'siːəbl] *adj* previsível; ***in the ~ future*** num futuro previsível
fore'seen *pp* → ***foresee***
'foresight clarividência *f*
forest ['fɑːrɪst] floresta *f*
forester ['fɑːrɪstər] guarda *m* florestal
forestry ['fɑːrɪstrɪ] silvicultura *f*
'foretaste amostra *f*
fore'tell *v/t* ⟨*pret & pp* ***foretold***⟩ predizer
fore'told *pret & pp* → ***foretell***
forever [fə'revər] *adv* para sempre; ***it is ~ raining here*** está sempre chovendo aqui
foreword ['fɔːrwɜːrd] prefácio *m*
forgave [fər'geɪv] *pret* → ***forgive***
forge [fɔːrdʒ] *v/t signature* falsificar
♦**forge ahead** *v/i* avançar
forger ['fɔːrdʒər] falsificador,a *m,f*
forgery ['fɔːrdʒərɪ] (*bank bill, document*) falsificação *f*
forget [fər'get] ⟨*pret* ***forgot***, *pp* ***forgotten***⟩ **1** *v/t* esquecer-se de; ***I forgot to bring my keys*** esqueci-me de minhas chaves; ***it's too late now, you might as well ~ it*** é tarde demais agora, você pode deixar isso para lá **2** *v/i* esquecer-se
forgetful [fər'getfl] *adj* esquecido
for'get-me-not *flower* miosótis *m*
forgive [fər'gɪv] *v/t & v/i* ⟨*pret* ***forgave***, *pp* ***forgiven***⟩ perdoar; ***~ s.o. for sth*** perdoar alguém por algo
forgiven [fər'gɪvn] *pp* → ***forgive***
forgiveness [fər'gɪvnɪs] perdão *m*
forgot [fər'gɑːt] *pret* → ***forget***
forgotten [fər'gɑːtn] *pp* → ***forget***
fork [fɔːrk] *n* garfo *m*; *road*: bifurcação *f*
♦**fork out** *v/i fam* (*pay*) desembolsar
forklift 'truck empilhadeira *f*
form [fɔːrm] **1** *n* (*shape*) forma *f*; (*document*) formulário *m*; ***be on / off ~*** estar em/fora de forma **2** *v/t in clay etc* moldar; *friendship, opinion, past tense* formar **3** *v/i* (*take shape, develop*) formar-se
formal ['fɔːrml] *adj language, recognition etc* formal; *dress* a rigor, *Port* de cerimônia
formality [fər'mælətɪ] formalidade *f*; ***it's just a ~*** é apenas uma formalidade; ***the formalities*** as formalidades
formally ['fɔːrməlɪ] *adv* formalmente
format ['fɔːrmæt] **1** *v/t* ⟨*pret & pp* ***formatted***⟩ *text, document* formatar **2** *n* (*size, makeup*) formato *m*
formation [fɔːr'meɪʃn] formação *f*
formative ['fɔːrmətɪv] *adj* formador; ***in his ~ years*** em seus anos de formação
former ['fɔːrmər] *adj* anterior; ***the ~*** o primeiro
formerly ['fɔːrmərlɪ] *adv* anteriormente
formidable ['fɔːrmɪdəbl] *adj* formidável
formula ['fɔːrmjʊlə] MATH, CHEM, *also for success etc* fórmula *f*
formulate ['fɔːrmjʊleɪt] *v/t* (*express*) formular
fornicate ['fɔːrnɪkeɪt] *v/i fml* fornicar
fornication [fɔːrnɪ'keɪʃn] *fml* fornicação *f*
fort [fɔːrt] MIL forte *m*
forth [fɔːrθ] *adv* ***back and ~*** de lá para cá; ***and so ~*** e assim por diante; ***from that day ~*** daquele dia em diante
forthcoming ['fɔːrθkʌmɪŋ] *adj* (*future*) próximo; *personality* comunicativo
'forthright *adj* franco
fortieth ['fɔːrtɪəθ] *n & adj* quadragésimo (*m*)
fortnight ['fɔːrtnaɪt] *Brit* quinzena *f*
fortress ['fɔːrtrɪs] MIL fortaleza *f*
fortunate ['fɔːrʧnət] *adj* sortudo
fortunately ['fɔːrʧnətlɪ] *adv* felizmente
fortune ['fɔːrʧən] sorte *f*, (*lot of money*) fortuna *f*; ***tell s.o.'s ~*** ler a sorte de alguém
'fortune-teller *cards*: cartomante *m/f*; *palm reading*: quiromante *m/f*; *crystal ball*: vidente *m/f*
forty ['fɔːrtɪ] quarenta; ***have ~ winks*** *fam* tirar uma soneca
forum ['fɔːrəm] *fig* fórum *m*
forward ['fɔːrwərd] **1** *adv* adiante **2** *adj pej person* presunçoso **3** *n* SPORT atacante *m/f* **4** *v/t letter* enviar

'forwarding address ['fɔːrwərdɪŋ] endereço *m* de remessa
'forwarding agent COM despachante *m/f*
forward-looking ['fɔːrwərdlʊkɪŋ] *adj* avançado
fossil ['fɑːsl] fóssil *m*
fossilized ['fɑːsəlaɪzd] *adj* fossilizado
foster ['fɑːstər] *v/t child* criar; *attitude, belief* estimular
'foster child filho,-a *m,f* de criação **'foster home** lar *m* adotivo **'foster parents** *npl* pais *mpl* adotivos
fought [fɒːt] *pret & pp* → ***fight***
foul [faʊl] **1** *n* SPORT falta *f* **2** *adj smell, taste* desagradável; *weather* feio **3** *v/t* SPORT *player* cometer falta em
found[1] [faʊnd] *v/t school etc* fundar
found[2] [faʊnd] *pret & pp* → ***find***
foundation [faʊn'deɪʃn] *of theory etc* fundamento *m*; (*organization*) fundação *f*
foundations [faʊn'deɪʃnz] *npl of building* alicerce *m*
founder ['faʊndər] *n* fundador,a *m,f*
founding ['faʊndɪŋ] *n* criação *f*
foundry ['faʊndrɪ] fundição *f*
fountain ['faʊntɪn] chafariz *m*
'fountain pen caneta-tinteiro *f*
four [fɔːr] **1** *adj* quatro **2** *n* ***on all ~s*** de quatro
four-letter 'word palavra *f* de baixo calão **'four-poster, four-poster 'bed** dossel *m* **'four-star** *adj hotel etc* de quatro estrelas
fourteen ['fɔːrtiːn] catorze, quatorze
fourteenth ['fɔːrtiːnθ] *n & adj* décimo-quarto (*m*)
fourth [fɔːrθ] *n & adj* quarto *m*
four-wheel 'drive MOT tração *f* nas quatro rodas; *vehicle* 4x4 *m or f*
fowl [faʊl] ave *f*
fox [fɑːks] **1** *n* raposa *f* **2** *v/t* (*puzzle*) deixar perplexo
foyer ['fɔɪər] saguão *m*
fraction ['frækʃn] *also* MATH fração *f*
fractionally ['frækʃnəlɪ] *adv* fracionariamente
fracture ['fræktʃər] **1** *n* fratura *f* **2** *v/t* fraturar
fragile ['frædʒəl] *adj* frágil
fragment ['frægmənt] *n* fragmento *m*
fragmentary [fræg'mentərɪ] *adj* fragmentário
fragrance ['freɪgrəns] fragrância *f*
fragrant ['freɪgrənt] *adj* perfumado
frail [freɪl] *adj* fraco
frame [freɪm] **1** *n* moldura *f*; *bike*: quadro *m*; *glasses*: armação *f*; ***~ of mind*** estado *m* de espírito **2** *v/t picture* emoldurar; *fam person* incriminar
'frame-up *fam* armação *f*
'framework estrutura *f*
France [fræns] França *f*
franchise ['fræntʃaɪz] *n business*: franquia *f*
frank [fræŋk] *adj* franco
frankfurter ['fræŋkfɜːrtər] salsicha *f* alemã frankfurter
frankly ['fræŋklɪ] *adv* francamente
frankness ['fræŋknɪs] franqueza *f*
frantic ['fræntɪk] *adj* frenético
frantically ['fræntɪklɪ] *adv* freneticamente
fraternal [frə'tɜːrnl] *adj* fraternal
fraud [frɒːd] fraude *f*; *person* impostor,a *m,f*
fraudulent ['frɒːdjʊlənt] *adj* fraudulento
fraudulently ['frɒːdjʊləntlɪ] *adv* fraudulentamente
frayed [freɪd] *adj cuffs* puído
freak [friːk] **1** *n* (*unusual event*) imprevisto *m*; (*two-headed person, animal etc*) anormal *m/f*; *fam* (*strange person*) esquisito,-a *m,f*; ***jazz ~*** *fam* (*fanatic*) fanático,-a *m,f* de jazz **2** *adj wind, storm etc* anômalo
freckle ['frekl] sarda *f*
free [friː] **1** *adj* (*at liberty*) livre; (*no cost*) grátis; (*not occupied*) livre; ***are you ~ this afternoon?*** você está livre hoje à tarde?; ***~ and easy*** livre e solto; ***for ~*** *travel, get sth* de graça **2** *v/t prisoners* libertar
freebie ['friːbɪ] *Brit fam* brinde *m*
freedom ['friːdəm] liberdade *f*
freedom of 'speech liberdade *f* de expressão
freedom of the 'press liberdade *f* de imprensa
free 'enterprise iniciativa *f* privada
free 'kick *in soccer* cobrança *f* de fal-

ta **freelance** ['fri:læns] **1** *adj* freelance **2** *adv work* como freelance **freelancer** ['fri:lænsər] freelancer *m/f* **'freeloader** ['fri:loʊdər] *Am fam* parasita *m/f*
freely ['fri:lɪ] *adv admit* livremente
free market e'conomy economia *f* livre de mercado **free-range 'chicken** frango *f* caipira **free-range 'eggs** *npl* ovo *m* caipira **free 'sample** amostra *f* grátis **free 'speech** liberdade *f* de expressão **'freeway** *Am* auto-estrada *f* **free'wheel** *v/i on bicycle* rodar livremente **free 'will** livre *f* arbítrio; ***he did it of his own ~*** ele fez isso de livre e espontânea vontade
freeze [fri:z] ⟨*pret* ***froze***, *pp* ***frozen***⟩ **1** *v/t food, river, also wages, video* congelar; *bank account* bloquear **2** *v/i water* congelar
♦ **freeze over** *v/i river* cobrir-se de gelo
'freeze-dried *adj* liofilizado
freezer ['fri:zər] freezer *m*
freezing ['fri:zɪŋ] **1** *adj* gelado; ***it's ~*** (***cold***) *weather, water* está muito frio; ***I'm ~*** (***cold***) estou congelando **2** *n* congelamento *m*; ***10 below ~*** 10 graus abaixo de zero
'freezing compartment congelador *m*
'freezing point ponto *m* de congelamento
freight [freɪt] *n* frete *m*; (*costs*) custo *m* do frete
'freight car *Am train*: vagão *m* de carga
freighter ['freɪtər] *ship* navio *m* cargueiro; *airplane* avião *m* de carga
'freight train *Am* trem *m* de carga
French [frentʃ] **1** *adj* francês,-esa **2** *n language* francês *m*; ***the ~*** os franceses
French 'bread pão *m* francês **French 'doors** *npl Am* portas *fpl* duplas **'French fries** *npl* batata *f* frita **French Guiana** [gi:'ɑ:nə] Guiana Francesa *f* **'Frenchman** francês *m* **'Frenchwoman** francesa *f*
frenzied ['frenzɪd] *adj attack, activity* frenético; *mob* desvairado
frenzy ['frenzɪ] frenesi *m*
frequency ['fri:kwənsɪ] *buses, visits, also radio*: freqüência *f*
frequent[1] ['fri:kwənt] *adj* freqüente
frequent[2] [frɪ'kwent] *v/t bar* freqüentar
frequently ['frɪkwentlɪ] *adv* freqüentemente
fresco ['freskoʊ] afresco *m*
fresh [freʃ] *adj fruit, meat etc* fresco; (*cold*) frio; (*new*) *start* novo; *Am* (*impertinent*) atrevido
fresh 'air ar *m* fresco
freshen ['freʃn] *v/i wind* refrescar-se
♦ **freshen up** **1** *v/i* lavar-se **2** *v/t room, paintwork* renovar
fresher → ***freshman***
freshly ['freʃlɪ] *adv painted, arrived* recentemente
'freshman calouro,-a *m,f*
freshness ['freʃnɪs] *fruit, climate, weather*: frescor *m*; *style, approach*: novidade *f*
fresh 'orange suco *m* natural de laranja, *Port* sumo *m* natural de laranja
'freshwater *adj* de água doce
fret [fret] *v/i* ⟨*pret & pp* ***fretted***⟩ preocupar-se
Freudian ['frɔɪdɪən] *adj* freudiano; ***~ slip*** ato *m* falho
friction ['frɪkʃn] fricção *m*; *between people* atrito *m*
'friction tape *Am* fita *f* isolante
Friday ['fraɪdeɪ] sexta-feira *f*
fridge [frɪdʒ] geladeira *f*, *Port* frigorífico *m*
fried 'egg [fraɪd] ovo *m* frito
fried po'tatoes *npl* batata *f* frita
friend [frend] amigo,-a *m,f*; ***make ~s*** *one person* fazer amigos; *two people* ficar amigos; ***make ~s with s.o.*** ficar amigo de alguém
friendliness ['frendlɪnɪs] amabilidade *f*
friendly ['frendlɪ] *adj atmosphere* amigável; *person* amável; (*easy to use*) prático; *argument, match, relations* amistoso; ***be ~ with s.o.*** estar em boas relações com alguém
'friendship ['frendʃɪp] amizade *f*
fries [fraɪz] *npl* fritas *fpl*
fright [fraɪt] susto *m*; ***give s.o. a ~*** *Brit*

F

dar um susto em alguém
frighten ['fraɪtn] *v/t* assustar; ***be ~ed*** ficar assustado; ***don't be ~ed*** não se assuste; ***be ~ed of*** ter medo de
♦**frighten away** *v/t* espantar
frightening ['fraɪtnɪŋ] *adj person, prospect* assustador
frigid ['frɪdʒɪd] *adj sexually* frígido
frill [frɪl] *on dress etc* babado *m*; (*fancy extra*) extra *m*
frilly ['frɪlɪ] *adj* enfeitado
fringe [frɪndʒ] *on dress, curtains etc* bainha *f*; *Brit in hair* franja *f*; (*edge*) orla *f*
'fringe benefits *npl* benefícios *mpl* adicionais
frisk [frɪsk] *v/t* revistar
frisky ['frɪskɪ] *adj puppy etc fig* animado
♦**fritter away** ['frɪtər] *v/t time, fortune* desperdiçar
frivolity [frɪ'vɑːlətɪ] frivolidade *f*
frivolous ['frɪvələs] *adj* frívolo
frizzy ['frɪzɪ] *adj hair* frisado
frog [frɑːg] rã *f*
'frogman homem-rã *m*
from [frɑːm] *prep* ◇ *time*: de; ***~ 9 to 5*** (***o'clock***) das 9 às 5 (horas); ***~ the 18th century*** do século XVIII; ***~ today on*** a partir de hoje; ***~ next Tuesday*** a partir da próxima terça-feira ◇ *in space* do; ***~ here to there*** daqui para lá; ***we drove here ~ Paris*** dirigimos até aqui desde Paris ◇ *origin*: de; ***a letter ~ Jo*** uma carta de Jo; ***a gift ~ the management*** um presente da gerência; ***it doesn't say who it's ~*** não diz de quem é; ***I am ~ New Jersey*** sou de Nova Jersey; ***made ~ bananas*** feito de bananas ◇ (*because of*) devido a; ***tired ~ the journey*** cansado da viagem; ***it's ~ overwork*** é devido ao trabalho excessivo
front [frʌnt] **1** *n building, book, also* (*cover organization*) fachada *f*; MIL front *m*; *weather*: frente *f*; ***in ~*** em frente; *in a race* na frente; ***in ~ of*** em frente de; ***at the ~ of*** na frente de **2** *adj wheel, seat* dianteiro **3** *v/t TV program* apresentar
front 'cover capa *f* frontal **front 'door** porta *f* de entrada **front 'entrance** entrada *f* da frente
frontier ['frʌntɪr] *also fig knowledge*: fronteira *f*
'front line MIL linha *f* de frente **front 'page** *newspaper*: primeira página *f* **front page 'news** *nsg* notícia *f* de primeira página **front 'row** fila *f* da frente **front seat 'passenger** *in car* passageiro,-a *m,f* do banco da frente **front-wheel 'drive** tração *f* dianteira
frost [frɑːst] *n* geada *f*
'frostbite *ulceração produzida pelo frio*
'frostbitten *adj* enregelado
frosted glass ['frɑːstɪd] vidro *m* fosco
frosting ['frɑːstɪŋ] *Am on cake* glacê *m*
frosty ['frɑːstɪ] *adj weather* gelado; *fig welcome* frio
froth [frɑːθ] *n* espuma *f*
frothy ['frɑːθɪ] *adj cream etc* espumoso
frown [fraʊn] **1** *n* carranca *f* **2** *v/i* franzir as sobrancelhas
froze [froʊz] *pret* → ***freeze***
frozen ['froʊzn] **1** *adj water, ground, food etc* congelado; *feet, wastes of Siberia etc* gelado; ***I'm ~*** *fam* estou gelado **2** *pp* → ***freeze***
frozen 'food comida *f* congelada
fruit [fruːt] fruta *f*
'fruit cake bolo *m* de frutas secas
fruitful ['fruːtfl] *adj discussions etc* proveitoso
'fruit juice suco *m* de fruta, *Port* sumo *m* de frutas
fruit 'salad salada *m* de fruta
frustrate [frʌ'streɪt] *v/t person, plans* frustrar
frustrated [frʌ'streɪtɪd] *adj look, sigh* frustrado
frustrating [frʌ'streɪtɪŋ] *adj* frustrante
frustratingly [frʌ'streɪtɪŋlɪ] *adv slow, hard* frustrantemente
frustration [frʌ'streɪʃn] frustração *f*; ***sexual ~*** frustração *f* sexual; ***the ~s of modern life*** as frustrações da vida moderna
fry [fraɪ] *v/t* ⟨*pret & pp* ***fried***⟩ fritar
'frypan *Am* frigideira *f*
fuck [fʌk] *v/t vulg* foder; ***~!*** caralho!; ***~***

him / that! foda-se!

♦**fuck off** *v/i vulg* ir à merda; ***fuck off!*** cai fora!

fucking ['fʌkɪŋ] *vulg* **1** *adj* porra de **2** *adv* ***don't be ~ stupid!*** não seja um porra de estúpido!

fuel ['fjʊːəl] **1** *n* combustível *m* **2** *v/t fig* atiçar

fugitive ['fjuːdʒətɪv] *n* fugitivo,-a *m,f*

fulfil *Brit* → ***fulfill***

fulfill [fʊl'fɪl] *v/t Am* realizar; ***feel ~ed*** *in job, life* sentir-se realizado

fulfilling [fʊl'fɪlɪŋ] *adj job* gratificante

fulfillment [fʊl'fɪlmənt] *Am of contract etc* cumprimento *m*; *moral, spiritual* realização *f*

fulfilment *Brit* → ***fulfillment***

full [fʊl] *adj bottle, schedule, day* cheio; *hotel, bus, disk* lotado; *account, report* completo; *life* pleno; ***~ of*** *water, tourists, errors etc* cheio de; ***~ up*** *hotel etc* completamente cheio; *with food* satisfeito; ***pay in ~*** pagar totalmente

'full back *in soccer* zagueiro *m*, *Port* defesa *m* **full 'board** diária *f* completa **'full-grown** *adj* maduro **'full-length** *adj dress* de tamanho normal; *movie* de longa-metragem **full 'moon** lua *f* cheia **full 'stop** *Brit* ponto *m* final **full-'time 1** *adj worker, job* de período integral **2** *adv work* em período integral

fully ['fʊlɪ] *adv booked, understand* completamente; *recovered* totalmente; *explain, describe* detalhadamente

fumble ['fʌmbl] *v/t catch* atrapalhar

♦**fumble about** *v/i* procurar desajeitadamente

fume [fjuːm] *v/i* ***be fuming*** *fam* (*be very angry*) estar com raiva

fumes [fjuːmz] *npl* gases *mpl*

fun [fʌn] divertimento *m*; ***it was great ~*** foi um grande divertimento; ***bye, have ~!*** tchau, divirta-se!; ***~ ~*** de brincadeira; ***what do you do for ~ around here?*** o que há para se divertir por aqui?; ***make ~ of*** zombar de

function ['fʌŋkʃn] **1** *n* (*purpose*) função *f*; (*reception etc*) evento *m* **2** *v/i* funcionar; ***~ as*** ter a função de

functional ['fʌŋkʃnl] *adj* funcional

fund [fʌŋd] **1** *n* fundo *m* **2** *v/t project etc* financiar

fundamental [fʌndə'mentl] *adj* (*basic, substantial*) fundamental; (*crucial*) essencial

fundamentalist [fʌndə'mentlɪst] *n* fundamentalista *m/f*

fundamentally [fʌndə'mentlɪ] *adv different, altered* fundamentalmente

funding ['fʌndɪŋ] (*money*) financiamento *m*

funeral ['fjuːnərəl] funeral *m*

'funeral director agente *m* funerário

'funeral home *Am* casa *f* funerária

fungus ['fʌŋgəs] fungo *m*; *mushroom* cogumelo *m*

funicular [fjuː'nɪkjʊlər] funicular *m*

funnel ['fʌnl] *n of ship* chaminé *f*

funnies ['fʌnɪz] *npl Am fam* seção *f* de passatempos

funnily ['fʌnɪlɪ] *adv* (*oddly*) estranhamente; (*comically*) de forma engraçada; ***~ enough*** surpreendentemente

funny ['fʌnɪ] *adj* (*comical*) engraçado; (*odd*) esquisito

'funny bone nervo *m* cubital

fur [fɜːr] pele *f*

furious ['fjʊrɪəs] *adj* (*angry*) furioso; (*intense*) intenso; ***at a ~ pace*** em um ritmo veemente

furnace ['fɜːrnɪs] fornalha *f*

furnish ['fɜːrnɪʃ] *v/t room* mobiliar, *Port* mobilar; (*supply*) fornecer

furniture ['fɜːrnɪtʃər] mobiliário *m*; ***a piece of ~*** um móvel

furry ['fɜːrɪ] *adj animal* peludo

further ['fɜːrðər] **1** *adj* (*additional*) adicional; (*more distant*) mais distante; ***until ~ notice*** até segunda ordem; ***have you anything ~ to say?*** você tem algo mais a dizer? **2** *adv walk, drive* mais; ***~, I want to say …*** além disso, quero dizer …; ***two miles ~ (on)*** três quilômetros mais à frente **3** *v/t cause etc* promover

further'more *adv* além do mais

furthest ['fɜːrðɪst] **1** *adj* mais longe **2** *adv* o mais longe

furtive ['fɜːrtɪv] *adj glance* furtivo

furtively ['fɜːrtɪvlɪ] *adv* furtivamente

fury ['fjʊrɪ] (*anger*) fúria *f*

fuse [fju:z] **1** *n* ELEC fusível *m* **2** *v/t & v/i* ELEC queimar
'fusebox caixa *f* de fusíveis
fuselage ['fju:zəlɑ:ʒ] fuselagem *f*
'fuse wire fio *m* de chumbo para fusível
fusion ['fju:ʒn] fusão *f*
fuss [fʌs] *n* estardalhaço *m*; ***make a ~*** (*complain*) criar caso; (*behave in exaggerated way*) fazer um drama; ***make a ~ of*** (*be very attentive to*) paparicar
fussy ['fʌsɪ] *adj person* exigente; *design etc* exagerado; ***be a ~ eater*** ser exigente com a comida
futile ['fju:tl] *adj* fútil
futility [fju:'tɪlətɪ] futilidade *f*
future ['fju:ʧər] **1** *n* futuro *m*; ***in ~*** no futuro **2** *adj* futuro
futures ['fju:ʧərz] *npl* FIN futuros *mpl*
'futures market FIN mercado *m* de commodities futuras
futuristic [fju:ʧə'rɪstɪk] *adj design* futurista
fuzzy ['fʌzɪ] *adj hair* crespo; (*out of focus*) indistinto

G

G

gab [gæb] *n* ***have the gift of the ~*** *fam* ter o dom da palavra
gabble ['gæbl] *v/i* tagarelar
gadget ['gædʒɪt] engenhoca *f*
gaffe [gæf] gafe *f*
gag [gæg] **1** *n* mordaça *f*; (*joke*) piada *f* **2** *v/t* ⟨*pret & pp* ***gagged***⟩ *person* amordaçar; *the press* silenciar
gaily ['geɪlɪ] *adv* (*blythely*) alegremente
gain [geɪn] *v/t* (*acquire*) ganhar; ***~ speed*** ganhar velocidade; ***~ 11 pounds*** engordar 5 kilos
gala ['gælə] gala *f*
galaxy ['gæləksɪ] galáxia *f*
gale [geɪl] ventania *f*
gallant ['gælənt] *adj* galante
gall bladder ['gɒ:lblædər] vesícula *f* biliar
gallery ['gælərɪ] galeria *f*
galley ['gælɪ] *on ship* cozinha *f*
♦ **gallivant around** ['gælɪvænt] *v/i* andar à toa
gallon ['gælən] galão *m*; ***~s of tea*** *fam* litrosde chá
gallop ['gæləp] *v/i* galopar
gallows ['gæloʊz] *npl* forca *f*
gallstone ['gɒ:lstoʊn] cálculo *m* biliar
galore [gə'lɔ:r] *adj* ... ~ ... à beça
galvanize ['gælvənaɪz] *v/t* TECH galvanizar; *fig* entusiasmar
gamble ['gæmbl] *v/i* jogar
gambler ['gæmblər] jogador,a *m,f*
gambling ['gæmblɪŋ] jogo *m* de azar
game [geɪm] *n sport*: jogo *m*; *children's*: brincadeira *f*; *tennis*: partida *f*
'game reserve reserva *f* de caça
gammon ['gæmən] *Brit* gamão *m*
gang [gæŋ] gangue *f*
♦ **gang up on** *v/t* conspirar contra
'gang rape *n* estupro *m* coletivo
gangrene ['gæŋgri:n] MED gangrena *f*
gangster ['gæŋstər] gângster *m*
'gang warfare guerra *f* de gangues
'gangway passadiço *m*
gaol [dʒeɪl] → ***jail***
gap [gæp] *wall*: fenda *f*; *time*, *conversation*: intervalo *m*; *parking*, *figures*: vaga *f*; *figures*: brecha *f*; *between two people's characters* diferença *f*; (*open space between structures*) vão *m*
gape [geɪp] *v/i person* ficar boquiaberto; *hole* abrir-se
♦ **gape at** *v/t* olhar boquiaberto
gaping ['geɪpɪŋ] *adj hole* aberto
garage ['gærɑ:ʒ] *n parking*: garagem *f*; *gas*: posto *m* de gasolina; *repairs*: oficina *f* mecânica
garbage ['gɑ:rbɪdʒ] *Am* lixo *m*; *fig* (*nonsense*) bobagem *f*

'garbage bag *Am* saco *m* de lixo **'garbage can** *Am* lata *f* de lixo **'garbage truck** *Am* caminhão *m* de lixo
garbled ['gɑːrbld] *adj message* confuso
garden ['gɑːrdn] jardim *m*
'garden center loja *f* de jardinagem
garden centre *Brit* → ***garden center***
gardener ['gɑːrdnər] jardineiro,-a *m,f*
gardening ['gɑːrdnɪŋ] jardinagem *f*
gargle ['gɑːrgl] *v/i* gargarejar
gargoyle ['gɑːrgɔɪl] gárgula *f*
garish ['gerɪʃ] *adj* extravagante
garland ['gɑːrlənd] *n* grinalda *f*
garlic ['gɑːrlɪk] alho *m*
garlic 'bread pão *m* de alho
garment ['gɑːrmənt] traje *m*
garnish ['gɑːrnɪʃ] *v/t* guarnecer
garret ['gærɪt] mansarda *f*
garrison ['gærɪsn] *n* guarnição *f* militar
garter ['gɑːrtər] liga *f*
gas [gæs] *n* gás *m*; (*gasoline*) gasolina *f*
gash [gæʃ] *n* corte *m*
gasket ['gæskɪt] junta *f*
gasoline ['gæsəliːn] gasolina *f*
gasp [gæsp] **1** *n* arquejo *m* **2** *v/i* ofegar; **~ *for breath*** ofegar
'gas pedal pedal *m* do acelerador **'gas pipeline** gasoduto *m* **'gas pump** *Am* bomba *f* de gasolina **'gas station** *Am* posto *m* de gasolina, *Port* bomba *f* de gasolina **'gas stove** fogão *m* a gás
gastric ['gæstrɪk] *adj* MED gástrico
gastric 'flu MED gripe *f* intestinal **gastric 'juices** *npl* suco *m* gástrico **gastric 'ulcer** MED úlcera *f* gástrica
'gas works *nsg* fábrica *f* de gás
gate [geɪt] *house, airport*: portão *m*
'gatecrash *v/t* entrar de penetra em
'gateway portão *m* de entrada; *fig* portal *m*; **~ *drug*** droga *f* leve
gather ['gæðər] **1** *v/t facts, information* colher; ***am I to ~ that …?*** eu deveria entender que …?; **~ *speed*** acelerar **2** *v/i* (*understand*) entender
♦ **gather up** *v/t possessions* juntar
gathering ['gæðərɪŋ] *n* (*group of people*) reunião *f*
gaudy ['gɒːdɪ] *adj* chamativo
gauge [geɪdʒ] **1** *n* medidor *m* **2** *v/t* medir; *opinion* avaliar
gaunt [gɒːnt] *adj* desolado
gauze [gɒːz] gaze *f*
gave [geɪv] *pret* → ***give***
gawky ['gɒːkɪ] *adj* desajeitado
gawp [gɒːp] *v/i fam* olhar com espanto
gay [geɪ] **1** *n* (*homosexual*) guei *m/f* **2** *adj* guei; **~ *marriage*** casamento *m* homossexual
gaze [geɪz] **1** *n* olhar *m* fixo **2** *v/i* fitar
♦ **gaze at** *v/t* fitar
GB [dʒiː'biː] *abbr* (*of **Great Britain***)
GDP [dʒiːdiː'piː] *abbr* (*of **gross domestic product***) BIP *m* (produto *m* interno bruto)
gear [gɪr] *n* (*equipment*) equipamento *m*; *vehicle*: marcha *f*, *Port* mudança *f*
'gearbox MOT caixa *f* de câmbio
'gear shift MOT alavanca *f* de câmbio
geese [giːs] *pl* → ***goose***
gel [dʒel] *hair, shower*: gel *m*
gelatine ['dʒelətiːn] gelatina *f*
gelignite ['dʒelɪgnaɪt] gelatina *f* explosiva
gem [dʒem] pedra *f* preciosa; *fig book, person etc* preciosidade *f*
Gemini ['dʒemɪnaɪ] ASTROL Gêmeos *m*
gender ['dʒendər] gênero *m*
gene [dʒiːn] gene *m*; ***it's in his ~s*** está em seus genes
general ['dʒenrəl] **1** *n* MIL general *m/f*; ***in ~*** em geral **2** *adj* geral
general e'lection eleições *fpl* gerais
generalization [dʒenrəlaɪ'zeɪʃn] generalização *f*; ***that's a ~*** isto é uma generalização
generalize ['dʒenrəlaɪz] *v/i* generalizar
generally ['dʒenrəlɪ] *adv* geralmente; **~ *speaking*** falando de um modo geral; (*usually*) normalmente
general prac'titioner clínico,-a *m,f* geral
generate ['dʒenəreɪt] *v/t* (*create*), *also electricity*, gerar
generation [dʒenə'reɪʃn] geração *f*
gene'ration gap diferença *f* de gerações
generator ['dʒenəreɪtər] gerador *m*
generic [dʒə'nerɪk] *adj* genérico; **~ *drug*** medicamento *m* genérico

G

generosity [dʒenə'rɑːsətɪ] generosidade *f*
generous ['dʒenərəs] *adj with money, also (not too critical), portion* generoso
'gene therapy terapia *f* genética
genetic [dʒɪ'netɪk] *adj* genético
genetically [dʒɪ'netɪklɪ] *adv* geneticamente; **~ *engineered*** geneticamente manipulado; **~ *modified*** geneticamente modificado
genetic 'code código *m* genético **genetic engi'neering** engenharia *f* genética **genetic 'fingerprint** impressão *f* genética
geneticist [dʒɪ'netɪsɪst] geneticista *m/f*
genetics [dʒɪ'netɪks] *nsg* genética *f*
genial ['dʒiːnjəl] *adj person, company* simpático
genitals ['dʒenɪtlz] *npl* genitália *f*
genius ['dʒiːnjəs] gênio *m*
genocide ['dʒenəsaɪd] genocídio *m*
gentle ['dʒentl] *adj* gentil; *detergent* delicado; *slope* leve
gentleman ['dʒentlmən] cavalheiro *m*; ***he's a real ~*** ele é um verdadeiro cavalheiro
gentleness ['dʒentlnɪs] gentileza *f*
gently ['dʒentlɪ] *adv* cuidadosamente; *blow, slope* suavemente
gents [dʒents] *nsg or npl Brit toilet* banheiro *m* masculino, *Port* casa *f* de banho dos homens
genuine ['dʒenʊɪn] *adj* genuíno
genuinely ['dʒenʊɪnlɪ] *adv* genuinamente
geographical [dʒɪə'græfɪkl] *adj* geográfico
geography [dʒɪ'ɑːgrəfɪ] geografia *f*
geological [dʒɪə'lɑːdʒɪkl] *adj* geológico
geologist [dʒɪ'ɑːlədʒɪst] geólogo,-a *m,f*
geology [dʒɪ'ɑːlədʒɪ] geologia *f*
geometric, **geometrical** [dʒɪə'metrɪk(l)] *adj* geométrico
geometrical → ***geometric***
geometry [dʒɪ'ɑːmətrɪ] geometria *f*
geranium [dʒə'reɪnɪəm] gerânio *m*
geriatric [dʒerɪ'ætrɪk] **1** *adj* geriátrico **2** *n* geriatra *m/f*
germ [dʒɜːrm] germe *m*; *of idea etc* origem *f*
German ['dʒɜːrmən] **1** *adj* alemão (alemã) **2** *n person* alemão *m*, alemã *f*; *language* alemão *m*
German 'measles *nsg* rubéola *f*
German 'shepherd pastor *m* alemão
Germany ['dʒɜːrmənɪ] Alemanha *f*
germinate ['dʒɜːrmɪneɪt] *v/i seed* germinar
germ 'warfare guerra *f* biológica
gesticulate [dʒe'stɪkjʊleɪt] *v/i* gesticular
gesture ['dʒestʃər] *n with hand* aceno *m*; *fig of friendship* gesto *m*
get [get] *v/t* ⟨*pret & pp* ***got***, *pp also* ***gotten***⟩ (*obtain*) obter; (*fetch*) pegar; (*receive*) *letter* receber; *knowledge, respect etc* conseguir; (*catch*) *bus, train etc* apanhar; (*become*) ficar; (*understand*) entender; ***~ sth done*** *have someone do it* mandar fazer algo; ***~ s.o. to do sth*** convencer alguém a fazer algo; ***~ to do sth*** (*have the opportunity*) ter a oportunidade de fazer algo; ***~ one's hair cut*** cortar o cabelo; ***~ sth ready*** preparar algo; ***~ going*** (*leave*) sair; ***have got*** ter; ***I have got to study / see him*** tenho que estudar / vê-lo; ***I don't want to, but I've got to*** não quero, mas tenho que; ***~ to know*** passar a conhecer
♦ **get about** *v/i* (*travel*) viajar; (*be mobile*) mover-se
♦ **get along** *v/i* (*progress*) progredir; (*come to party etc*) ir junto; *with s.o.* entender-se
♦ **get at** *v/t* (*criticize*) criticar; (*imply, mean*) querer dizer
♦ **get away** **1** *v/i* (*leave*) ir embora; *from robbery* fugir **2** *v/t* ***get sth away from s.o.*** tirar algo de alguém
♦ **get away with** *v/t* fazer impunemente; ***they shouldn't be allowed to get away with it*** não deviam se safar dessa
♦ **get back** **1** *v/i* (*return*) voltar; ***I'll get back to you on that*** darei uma resposta sobre isso **2** *v/t* (*obtain again*) recuperar; *old girlfriend* reatar
♦ **get by** *v/i* (*pass*) passar; (*financially*) virar-se

♦ **get down 1** *v/i from ladder etc* descer; (*duck etc*) abaixar-se **2** *v/t* (*depress*) deprimir

♦ **get down to** *v/t* (*start*) *work* pôr-se a; (*reach*) *real facts* alcançar

♦ **get in 1** *v/i* (*arrive*) *train, plane* chegar; (*come home*) chegar em casa; *to car* entrar; ***how did they get in?*** *thieves, mice etc* como eles entraram? **2** *v/t to suitcase etc* acomodar

♦ **get off 1** *v/i from bus etc* saltar, *Port* descer; (*finish work*) sair do trabalho; (*not be punished*) livrar-se **2** *v/t* (*remove*) *clothes, hat, footgear* tirar; ***get off the grass!*** saia de cima da grama!

♦ **get off with** *v/t fam* (*sexually*) relacionar-se com; ***he got off with a small fine*** ele escapou apenas com uma pequena multa

♦ **get on 1** *v/i to bike, bus, train* subir; (*be friendly with*) entender-se; (*advance*) *time* ficar tarde; (*become old*) envelhecer; (*make progress*) progredir; ***it's getting on*** está ficando tarde; ***he's getting on*** *becoming old* ele está envelhecendo; ***he's getting on for 50*** ele está chegando perto dos 50 **2** *v/t bus* subir em, *Port* subir para; ***get on one's bike*** montar na bicicleta; ***get one's hat on*** pôr o chapéu; ***I can't get these pants on*** não consigo tirar essas calças

♦ **get out 1** *v/i car, prison etc* sair; ***get out!*** saia!; ***let's get out of here*** vamos sair aqui; ***I don't get out much these days*** não tenho saído muito esses dias **2** *v/t* (*extract*) *nail, something jammed* arrancar; (*remove*) *stain* remover; (*pull out*) *gun, pen* tirar; *gun* sacar

♦ **get over** *v/t fence, disappointment etc* superar; *lover etc* esquecer

♦ **get over with** *v/t* terminar; ***let's get it over with*** vamos terminar com isso

♦ **get through** *v/i on telephone* completar a ligação; (*make oneself understood*) fazer-se entender; ***get through to s.o.*** (*make oneself understood*) fazer alguém entender

♦ **get to** *v/t* (*arrive at*) chegar a

♦ **get up 1** *v/i in morning, from chair etc* levantar-se; *wind* começar a soprar **2** *v/t hill* subir

'getaway car carro *m* de fuga

'get-together *n* encontro *m*

ghastly ['gæstlɪ] *adj color, experience, person etc* horrível; *look* medonho

gherkin ['gɜːrkɪn] pepino *m* em conserva

ghetto ['getoʊ] gueto *m*

ghost [goʊst] fantasma *m*

ghostly ['goʊstlɪ] *adj* fantasmagórico

'ghost town cidade *f* fantasma

ghoul [guːl] indivíduo *m* mórbido

ghoulish ['guːlɪʃ] *adj* abominável

giant ['dʒaɪənt] **1** *n* gigante *m* **2** *adj* gigante

gibberish ['dʒɪbərɪʃ] *fam* vozerio *m*

gibe [dʒaɪb] *n* deboche *m*

giblets ['dʒɪblɪts] *npl* miúdos *mpl*

giddiness ['gɪdɪnɪs] vertigem *f*

giddy ['gɪdɪ] *adj* tonto

gift [gɪft] presente *m*; ***have a ~ for sth*** ter jeito para algo

'gift card cartão-presente *m*

'gift certificate *Am* vale *m* presente

gifted ['gɪftɪd] *adj* talentoso

gift token *Brit* → ***gift certificate***

gift voucher *Brit* → ***gift certificate***

'giftwrap 1 *n* papel *m* de presente **2** *v/t* ⟨*pret & pp* ***giftwrapped***⟩ embrulhar para presente

gig [gɪg] *fam* show *m*

gigabyte ['gɪgəbaɪt] COMPUT gigabyte *m*

gigantic [dʒaɪ'gæntɪk] *adj* gigantesco

giggle ['gɪgl] **1** *v/i* dar uma risadinha **2** *n* risadinha *f*

gill [gɪl] *of fish* guelra *f*

gilt [gɪlt] *n* camada *f* de ouro; ***~s*** FIN obrigações *fpl* do tesouro nacional

gimmick ['gɪmɪk] artifício *m*

gimmicky ['gɪmɪkɪ] *adj* artificioso

gin [dʒɪn] gim *m*; ***~ and tonic*** gim-tônica *m*

ginger ['dʒɪndʒər] **1** *n* (*spice*) gengibre *m* **2** *adj hair* avermelhado; *cat* pardo

ginger 'beer gengibirra *f*

'gingerbread pão *m* de gengibre

gingerly ['dʒɪndʒərlɪ] *adv* cautelosamente

gipsy ['dʒɪpsɪ] cigano,-a *m,f*

giraffe [dʒɪ'ræf] girafa *f*
girder ['gɜːrdər] *n* viga *f*
girl [gɜːrl] garota *f*, menina *f*, *Port* rapariga *f*
'girlfriend *of boy* namorada *f*; *of girl* amiga *f*
girl guide *Brit* → ***girl scout***
girlie magazine ['gɜːrliː] revista *f* de mulher nua
girlish ['gɜːrlɪʃ] *adj* de menina
'girl scout *Am* bandeirante *f*
gist [dʒɪst] essência *f*
give [gɪv] *v/t* ⟨*pret* ***gave***, *pp* ***given***⟩ *present, cry, groan etc* dar; (*supply*) *electricity etc* fornecer; *talk, lecture* fazer; ***~ sth to s.o.***, ***~ s.o. sth*** dar algo a alguém; ***~ her my love*** mande-lhe minhas lembranças
◆**give away** *v/t as present* dar de presente; (*betray*) trair; ***give oneself away*** trair-se
◆**give back** *v/t* devolver
◆**give in 1** *v/i* (*surrender*) ceder **2** *v/t* (*hand in*) entregar
◆**give off** *v/t smell, fumes* soltar
◆**give onto** *v/t* (*open onto*) dar para
◆**give out 1** *v/t leaflets etc* distribuir **2** *v/i supplies, strength* esgotar-se
◆**give up 1** *v/t smoking etc* desistir de; ***give oneself up to the police*** entregar-se à polícia **2** *v/i* (*cease habit*) parar; (*stop making effort*) desistir
◆**give way** *v/i bridge etc* ceder
give-and-'take flexibilidade *f*
given ['gɪvn] **1** *adj* dado **2** *pp* → ***give***
'given name nome *m* de batismo
gizmo ['gɪzmoʊ] aparelhinho *m*
glacier ['gleɪʃər] geleira *f*
glad [glæd] *adj* contente
gladly ['glædlɪ] *adv* com muito prazer
glamor ['glæmər] *Am* glamour *m*
glamorize ['glæməraɪz] *v/t* exaltar
glamorous ['glæmərəs] *adj* glamouroso
glamour *etc Brit* → ***glamor***
glance [glæns] **1** *n* olhada *f* **2** *v/i* olhar de relance
◆**glance at** *v/t* olhar de relance para
gland [glænd] glândula *f*
glandular fever ['glændʒələr] febre *f* glandular
glare [gler] **1** *n sun, headlights*: luminosidade *f* **2** *v/i sun, headlights* brilhar
◆**glare at** *v/t* olhar furiosamente para
glaring ['glerɪŋ] *adj mistake* muito evidente
glaringly ['glerɪŋlɪ] *adv* ***be ~ obvious*** ser evidentemente óbvio
glass [glæs] *material* vidro *m*; *for drink* copo *m*
glass 'case expositor *m* de vidro
glasses *npl* óculos *mpl*
'glasshouse estufa *f*
glaze [gleɪz] *n* verniz *m*
◆**glaze over** *v/i eyes* vidrar
glazed [gleɪzd] *adj expression* vidrado
glazier ['gleɪzɪr] vidraceiro,-a *m,f*
glazing ['gleɪzɪŋ] envidraçamento *m*
gleam [gliːm] **1** *n* brilho *m* **2** *v/i* brilhar
glee [gliː] regozijo *m*
gleeful ['gliːfʊl] *adj* alegre
glib [glɪb] *adj* superficial
glibly ['glɪblɪ] *adv* superficialmente
glide [glaɪd] *v/i* planar
glider ['glaɪdər] planador *m*
gliding ['glaɪdɪŋ] *n sport* vôo *m* com planador
glimmer ['glɪmər] **1** *n light*: lampejo *m*; ***~ of hope*** lampejo de esperança **2** *v/i* cintilar
glimpse [glɪmps] **1** *n* vislumbre *m*; ***catch a ~ of ...*** dar uma olhada rápida em ... **2** *v/t* vislumbrar
glint [glɪnt] **1** *n* cintilação *f* **2** *v/i light* cintilar; *eyes* brilhar
glisten ['glɪsn] *v/i* brilhar
glitter ['glɪtər] *v/i* reluzir
glitterati *npl* famosos *mpl*
gloat [gloʊt] *v/i* exultar
◆**gloat over** *v/t* exultar com
global ['gloʊbl] *adj* (*worldwide*) mundial; (*without exceptions*) global
global e'conomy economia *f* mundial
globalization [gloʊbəlaɪ'zeɪʃn] globalização *f*
globalize ['gloʊbəlaɪz] globalizar
global 'market mercado *m* mundial
global navigation system sistema *m* global de navegação **global 'warming** aquecimento *m* global
globe [gloʊb] (*the earth*) globo *m*;

(*model of earth*) esfera *f* terrestre
gloom [gluːm] (*darkness*) escuridão *f*; *mood* tristeza *f*
gloomily ['gluːmɪlɪ] *adv* sombriamente
gloomy ['gluːmɪ] *adj room* escuro; *mood*, *person* sombrio
glorious ['glɔːrɪəs] *adj weather*, *day* magnífico; *victory* glorioso
glory ['glɔːrɪ] *n* glória *f*
gloss [glɑːs] *n* (*shine*) brilho *m*; *n* (*general explanation*) nota *f* explicativa
◆ **gloss over** *v/t* atenuar
glossary ['glɑːsərɪ] glossário *m*
'gloss paint pintura *f* brilhosa
glossy ['glɑːsɪ] **1** *adj paper* brilhoso **2** *n magazine* revista *f*
glove [glʌv] luva *f*
'glove compartment *in car* porta-luvas *m*
'glove puppet fantoche *m*
glow [gloʊ] **1** *n light*, *fire*: brilho *m*; *cheeks*: rubor *m* **2** *v/i light* brilhar; *fire* arder; *cheeks* ruborizar
glower ['glaʊr] *v/i* olhar furiosamente
glowing ['gloʊɪŋ] *adj description* ardente
glucose ['gluːkoʊs] glicose *f*
glue [gluː] **1** *n* cola *f* **2** *v/t* **~ *sth to sth*** colar algo em algo; ***be ~d to the TV*** *fam* ficar grudado na TV
glum [glʌm] *adj* abatido
glumly ['glʌmlɪ] *adv* tristemente
glut [glʌt] *n* fartura *f*
glutton ['glʌtən] glutão *m*, glutona *f*
gluttony ['glʌtənɪ] gula *f*
GMT [dʒiːem'tiː] *abbr* (*of* ***Greenwich Mean Time***) hora *f* média de Greenwich
gnarled [nɑːrld] *adj branch* nodoso; *hands* retorcido
gnat [næt] mosquito *m*
gnaw [nɒː] *v/t bone* roer
GNP [dʒiːen'piː] *abbr* (*of* ***gross national product***) PNB *m* (produto *m* nacional bruto)
go [goʊ] **1** *n* ***be on the ~*** estar na correria; ***in one ~*** *drink*, *write etc* de uma só vez **2** *v/i* ⟨*pret* ***went***, *pp* ***gone***⟩ ir; (*leave*) *train*, *plane* partir; (*leave*) *people* ir-se; (*work*, *function*) funcionar; (*become*) ficar; (*come out*) *stain etc* sair; (*cease*) *pain etc* passar; (*match*) *colors etc* combinar; ***~ shopping / jogging*** fazer compras / jogging; ***I must be ~ing*** tenho que ir; ***let's ~!*** vamos!; ***~ for a walk*** ir passear; ***~ to bed*** ir para a cama; ***~ to school*** ir para a escola; ***how's the work ~ing?*** como vai o trabalho?; ***they're ~ing for 50*** *being sold at* eles estão sendo vendidos por 50; ***hamburger to ~*** hambúrguer para viagem; ***be all gone*** *finished* estar acabado; ***be ~ing to do sth*** ir fazer algo; ***it's ~ing to snow*** vai nevar
◆ **go ahead** *v/i* ***he just went ahead and did it*** ele foi em frente e fez; ***go ahead!*** (*on you go*) vá em frente!
◆ **go ahead with** *v/t plans etc* ir em frente com
◆ **go along with** *v/t suggestion* concordar com
◆ **go at** *v/t* (*attack*) partir para cima de
◆ **go away** *v/i person*, *rain*, *pain*, *clouds etc* ir embora
◆ **go back** *v/i* (*return*) voltar; (*date back*) datar de; ***we go back a long way*** nós nos conhecemos de longa data; ***go back to sleep*** voltar a dormir
◆ **go by** *v/i car*, *people*, *time* passar
◆ **go down** *v/i* descer; *sun* pôr-se; *ship* afundar; *swelling* diminuir; ***go down well / badly*** *suggestion etc* ser aceito bem / mal
◆ **go for** *v/t* (*attack*) atacar; (*like*) gostar de
◆ **go in** *v/i to room*, *house* entrar; *sun* esconder-se; ***where does this go in?*** onde isto se encaixa?
◆ **go in for** *v/t competition*, *race* inscrever-se em; (*like*, *take part in*) gostar de
◆ **go off 1** *v/i* (*leave*) ir-se; *bomb* explodir; *gun*, *alarm* disparar; *milk etc* estragar **2** *v/t* (*stop liking*) deixar de gostar
◆ **go on** *v/i* (*continue*) continuar; (*happen*) acontecer; ***go on, do it!*** (*encouraging*) vá em frente, faça!; ***what's going on?*** o que está acontecendo?
◆ **go on at** *v/t* (*nag*) infernizar

G

♦**go out** *v/i person* sair; *light*, *fire* apagar
♦**go out with** *v/t romantically* sair com
♦**go over** *v/t* (*check*) verificar; (*do again*) revisar
♦**go through** *v/t illness*, *hard times* passar por; (*check*) revistar; (*read through*) examinar cuidadosamente
♦**go under** *v/i* (*sink*) afundar; *company* fechar
♦**go up** *v/i* (*climb*) subir; *prices* aumentar
♦**go without 1** *v/t food etc* ficar sem **2** *v/i* passar sem
goad [goʊd] *v/t* incitar
'go-ahead 1 *n* luz *f* verde; ***get the ~*** obter luz verde **2** *adj* (*enterprising*, *dynamic*) empreendedor
goal [goʊl] SPORT gol *m*, *Port* golo *m*, *structure* baliza *f*; (*objective*) meta *f*
goalie ['goʊlɪ] *fam* goleiro,-a *m,f*
'goalkeeper goleiro,-a *m,f* **'goal kick** tiro *m* de meta, *Port* pontapé *m* de baliza **'goalmouth** boca *f* do gol, *Port* boca *f* da baliza **'goalpost** trave *f* de baliza
goat [goʊt] cabra *f*
gobble ['gɑːbl] *v/t* comer rapidamente
♦**gobble up** *v/t* devorar
gobbledygook ['gɑːbldɪguːk] *fam* linguagem *f* incompreensível
'go-between intermediário,-a *m,f*
god [gɑːd] deus *m*; ***thank ~!*** graças a deus!; ***oh ~!*** que coisa!
'godchild afilhado,-a *m,f*
'goddaughter afilhada *f*
goddess ['gɑːdɪs] deusa *f*
'godfather padrinho *m*; *mafia*: chefão *m* **'godforsaken** *adj place*, *town* abandonado **'godmother** madrinha *m* **'godparent** padrinho *m*, madrinha *f* **'godsend** dádiva *f* do céu **'godson** afilhado *m*
gofer ['goʊfər] *fam* menino de recado *m*, menina de recado *f*
goggles ['gɑːgl] *npl* óculos *mpl* de proteção
going ['goʊɪŋ] *adj price etc* corrente; ***~ concern*** negócio *m* próspero
goings-on [goʊɪŋz'ɑːn] *npl* atividades *fpl*
gold [goʊld] **1** *n* ouro *m*; *medal* medalha *f* de ouro **2** *adj* de ouro
golden ['goʊldn] *adj sky*, *hair* dourado
golden 'handshake gratificação *f de demissão*
golden 'wedding, **golden 'wedding anniversary** bodas *fpl* de ouro
'goldfish peixe-vermelho *m* **'gold mine** *fig* mina *f* de ouro **'goldsmith** ourives *m/f*
golf [gɑːlf] golfe *m*
'golf ball bola *f* de golfe **'golf club** (*organization*, *stick*) clube *m* de golfe **'golf course** campo *m* de golfe
golfer ['gɑːlfər] golfista *m/f*
gone [gɑːn] *pp* → ***go***
gong [gɑːŋ] gongo *m*
good [gʊd] **1** *adj* bom (boa); ***a ~ many*** bastante; ***be ~ at …*** ser bom de …; ***be ~ for s.o.*** fazer bem para alguém **2** *n* bem *m*; ***it's no ~ getting angry*** não adianta ficar zangado; ***for the ~ of your health*** para o bem da sua saúde; ***for ~*** para sempre
goodbye [gʊd'baɪ] até logo, *Port* adeus; ***say ~ to s.o., wish s.o. ~*** despedir-se de alguém
good-for-nothing *n* inútil *m/f* **Good 'Friday** Sexta-Feira Santa *f* **good-humored** [gʊd'hjuːmərd] *adj Am* bem-humorado **good-humoured** *Brit* → ***good-humored*** **good-looking** [gʊd'lʊkɪŋ] *adj woman*, *man* bonito **good-natured** [gʊd'neɪʧərd] bondoso
goodness ['gʊdnɪs] *moral* bondade *f*; *fruit etc*: propriedades *fpl*; ***thank ~!*** graças a deus!
goods [gʊdz] *npl* COM mercadorias *fpl*
good'will boa vontade *f*
goody-goody ['gʊdɪgʊdɪ] *n fam* bonzinho *m*, boazinha *f*
gooey ['guːɪ] *adj* grudento
goof [guːf] *v/i fam* falhar
♦**goof off** *v/i fam* ficar à toa
goose [guːs] ⟨*pl* ***geese***⟩ ganso *m*
gooseberry ['gʊːsbərɪ] groselha *f*
'goose bumps *npl Am* arrepio *m*
'goose pimples *npl Brit* arrepio *m*
gorge [gɔːrdʒ] **1** *n* desfiladeiro *m* **2** *v/t* ***~ oneself on sth*** empanturrar-se de algo

gorgeous ['gɔːrdʒəs] *adj weather* magnífico; *dress* lindo; *woman, hair, smell* maravilhoso
gorilla [gə'rɪlə] gorila *m/f*
gosh [gɑːʃ] *int* credo
go-'slow operação *f* tartaruga
gospel ['gɑːspl] *in Bible* evangelho *m*
'gospel truth pura verdade *f*
gossip ['gɑːsɪp] **1** *n* fofocas *fpl*; *person* fofoqueiro,-a *m,f* **2** *v/i* fofocar
'gossip column coluna *f* social
'gossip columnist colunista *m/f* social
gossipy ['gɑːsɪpɪ] *adj letter etc* cheio de novidades
got [gɑːt] *pret & pp* → ***get***
gotten ['gɑːtn] *pp* → ***get***
gourmet ['gʊrmeɪ] *n* gourmet *m/f*
govern ['gʌvərn] *v/t country* governar
government ['gʌvərnmənt] governo *m*
governor ['gʌvərnər] governador,a *m,f*
gown [gaʊn] (*long dress*) vestido *m* longo; (*wedding dress*) vestido *m* de noiva; *academic, judge*: toga *f*; *priest, monk*: batina *f*; *surgeon*: avental *m*
GP [dʒiː'piː] *Brit abbr* (*of* ***General Practitioner***) médico *m* de família
grab [græb] *v/t* ⟨*pret & pp* ***grabbed***⟩ pegar
grace [greɪs] *dancer etc*: graça *f*; *before meals* oração *f*
graceful ['greɪsfʊl] *adj* gracioso
gracefully ['greɪsfʊlɪ] *adv move* graciosamente
gracious ['greɪʃəs] *adj person, style* cortês; *living* agradável; ***good ~!*** nossa!
grade [greɪd] **1** *n* (*quality*) grau *m*; EDUC série *f*; (*school grade*) nota *f* **2** *v/t* classificar
grade 'crossing *Am* passagem *f* de nível
'grade school *Am* escola *f* primária
gradient ['greɪdɪənt] declive *m*
gradual ['grædʒʊəl] *adj* gradual
gradually ['grædʒʊəlɪ] *adv* gradualmente
graduate ['grædʒʊət] **1** *n* formado,-a *m,f* **2** *v/i* formar-se
graduation [grædʒʊ'eɪʃn] formatura *f*
gradu'ation ceremony cerimônia *f* de graduação
graffiti [grə'fiːtiː] pichação *f*
graft [græft] **1** *n* BOT, MED enxerto *m*; *fam* (*hard work*) trabalho *m* pesado **2** *v/t* BOT, MED enxertar
grain [greɪn] grão *m*; *wood*: veio *m*; ***it goes against the ~ for me to …*** vai contra os meus princípios …
gram [græm] grama *m*
grammar ['græmər] gramática *f*
'grammar school *Brit* liceu *m*
grammatical [grə'mætɪkl] *adj* gramatical
grammatically *adv* gramaticalmente
grand [grænd] **1** *adj* formidável; (*very good*) ótimo **2** *n fam* (*$1000*) mil dólares
'grandad ['grændæd] vovô *m*
'grandchild neto,-a *m,f*
'granddaughter neta *f*
grandeur ['grændʒər] grandeza *f*
'grandfather avô *m*
'grandfather clock relógio *m* de pé
grandiose ['grændɪoʊs] *adj* grandioso
'grandma *fam* vovó *f* **'grandmother** avó *f* **'grandpa** *fam* vô *m* **'grandparents** *npl* avós *mpl* **grand 'piano** piano *m* de cauda **grand 'slam** *tennis*: grand slam *m* **'grandson** neto *m* **'grandstand** tribuna *f* principal
granite ['grænɪt] granito *m*
granny ['grænɪ] *fam* vovó *f*
grant [grænt] **1** *n money* subvenção *f* **2** *v/t wish, peace, visa* conceder; *request* deferir; ***take sth for ~ed*** tomar algo por certo; ***take s.o. for ~ed*** não dar valor a alguém
granulated sugar ['grænʊleɪtɪd] açúcar *m* granulado
granule ['grænuːl] grânulo *m*
grape [greɪp] uva *f*
'grapefruit toranja *f* **'grapefruit juice** suco *m* de toranja, *Port* sumo *m* de toranja **'grapevine** videira *f*; ***hear on the ~ that …*** ouvir um boato de que …
graph [græf] gráfico *m*
graphic ['græfɪk] **1** *adj* (*vivid*) gráfico **2** *n* COMPUT gráfico *m*; ***~s*** artes *fpl* gráficas

graphically ['græfɪklɪ] *adv describe* graficamente
graphic de'signer artista *m/f* gráfico,-a
♦ **grapple with** ['græpl] *v/t attacker* lutar com; *problem etc* estar às voltas com
grasp [græsp] **1** *n* (*physical*) aperto *m*; (*mental*) compreensão *f* **2** *v/t* (*physically*) apertar; (*understand*) compreender
grass [græs] *n* grama *f*, *Port* relva *f*
'**grasshopper** gafanhoto *m* '**grass roots** *npl people* base *f* **grass 'widow** esposa *f* de marido ausente **grass 'widower** marido *m* de esposa ausente
grassy ['græsɪ] *adj* gramado, *Port* relvado
grate[1] [greɪt] *n metal* grade *f*
grate[2] [greɪt] **1** *v/t in cooking* ralar **2** *v/i sound* ranger
grateful ['greɪtful] *adj* agradecido; ***be ~ to s.o.*** ser grato a alguém
gratefully ['greɪtfulɪ] *adv* agradecidamente
grater ['greɪtər] ralador *m*
gratify ['grætɪfaɪ] *v/t* ⟨*pret & pp* ***gratified***⟩ gratificar
grating ['greɪtɪŋ] **1** *n* ralo *m* **2** *adj sound, voice* rangente
gratitude ['grætɪtuːd] gratidão *f*
gratuitous [grə'tuːɪtəs] *adj* desnecessário
gratuity [grə'tuːətɪ] gratificação *f*
grave[1] [greɪv] *n* túmulo *m*
grave[2] [greɪv] *adj error, voice* grave; *face* sério
gravel ['grævl] *n* cascalho *m*
'**gravestone** lápide *f*
'**graveyard** cemitério *m*
♦ **gravitate toward** ['grævɪteɪt] *v/t* gravitar em torno de
gravity ['grævətɪ] PHYS gravidade *f*
gravy ['greɪvɪ] molho *m*
gray [greɪ] *adj Am* cinzento; ***be going ~*** ficar grisalho
gray-'haired [greɪ'herd] *adj Am* grisalho
graze[1] [greɪz] *v/i cow, horse* pastar
graze[2] [greɪz] **1** *v/t arm etc* esfolar **2** *n* escoriação *f*
grease [griːs] gordura *f*, (*lubricant*) graxa *f*
greaseproof 'paper papel *m* vegetal
greasy ['griːsɪ] *adj food* gorduroso; *hair, skin, plate* oleoso
great [greɪt] *adj* grande; *fam* (*very good*) ótimo; ***how was it? – ~!*** como foi? - ótimo!; ***~ to see you!*** que bom vê-lo!
Great 'Britain Grã-Bretanha *f*
great-'grandchild bisneto,-a *m,f* **great-'granddaughter** bisneta *f* **great-'grandfather** bisavô *m* **great-'grandmother** bisavó *f* **great-'grandparents** *npl* bisavós *mpl* **great-'grandson** bisneto *m*
greatly ['greɪtlɪ] *adv* muito
greatness ['greɪtnɪs] grandeza *f*
Greece [griːs] Grécia *f*
greed [griːd] ganância *f*
greedily ['griːdɪlɪ] *adv* ganânciosamente
greedy ['griːdɪ] *adj* ganancioso
Greek [griːk] **1** *n* grego,-a *m,f*, *language* grego *m* **2** *adj* grego
green [griːn] *adj* verde; *environmentally* ecológico
green 'beans *npl* vagem *f* '**green belt** cinturão *m* verde '**green card** *Am* (*work permit*) visto *m* de residência '**greenfield site** terreno *m* edificável no campo '**greenhorn** *fam* novato,-a *m,f* '**greenhouse** estufa *f* '**greenhouse effect** efeito *m* estufa '**greenhouse gas** gás-estufa *m*
greens [griːnz] *npl* verduras *fpl*
green 'thumb ***have a ~*** *Am* ter o dom da horticultura
greet [griːt] *v/t* cumprimentar
greeting ['griːtɪŋ] cumprimento *m*
'**greeting card** cartão *m* comemorativo
gregarious [grɪ'gerɪəs] *adj person* gregário
grenade [grɪ'neɪd] granada *f*
grew [gruː] *pret* → ***grow***
grey *Brit* → ***gray***
'**greyhound** galgo *m*
grid [grɪd] grade *f*; ELEC rede *f*
'**gridiron** *Am* SPORT campo *m* de futebol
'**gridlock** *traffic*: engarrafamento *m*

G

grief [gri:f] tristeza *f*
grief-stricken ['gri:fstrɪkn] *adj* pesaroso
grievance ['gri:vəns] *at work* reclamação *f*
grieve [gri:v] *v/i* enlutar-se; ***~ for s.o.*** enlutar-se por alguém
grill [grɪl] **1** *n window*: grade *f*; *cooking*: grelha *f* **2** *v/t* (*interrogate*) interrogar
grille [grɪl] grade *f*
grim [grɪm] *adj* desagradável; (*stern*) severo
grimace ['grɪməs] *n* careta *f*
grime [graɪm] sujeira *f*, *Port* sujidade *f*
grimly ['grɪmlɪ] *adv* severamente
grimy ['graɪmɪ] *adj* sujo
grin [grɪn] **1** *n* sorriso *m* largo **2** *v/i* ⟨*pret & pp* ***grinned***⟩ dar um sorriso zombador
grind [graɪnd] *v/t* ⟨*pret & pp* ***ground***⟩ *coffee*, *meat* moer; ***~ one's teeth*** ranger os dentes
grip [grɪp] **1** *n on rope etc* punho *m*; ***be losing one's ~*** (*losing one's skills*) perder a habilidade **2** *v/t* ⟨*pret & pp* ***gripped***⟩ apertar
gripe [graɪp] **1** *n* reclamação *f* **2** *v/i* reclamar
gripping ['grɪpɪŋ] *adj* emocionante
gristle ['grɪsl] nervo *m*
grit [grɪt] **1** *n* (*dirt*) areia *f*, *for roads* pedregulho *m* **2** *v/t* ⟨*pret & pp* ***gritted***⟩ ***~ one's teeth*** cerrar os dentes
gritty ['grɪtɪ] *adj fam book*, *movie etc* realista
groan [groʊn] **1** *n* gemido *m* **2** *v/i* gemer
grocer ['groʊsər] dono,-a *m,f* de mercearia; ***at the ~'s (shop)*** na mercearia
groceries ['groʊsərɪz] *npl* gêneros *mpl* alimentícios
grocery store ['groʊsərɪ] mercearia *m*
groggy ['grɑ:gɪ] *adj fam* grogue
groin [grɔɪn] ANAT virilha *f*
groom [gru:m] **1** *n bride*: noivo *m*; *horse*: cavalariço *m* **2** *v/t horse* tratar; (*train*, *prepare*) preparar; ***well ~ed*** *in appearance* bem arrumado
groove [gru:v] ranhura *f*
grope [groʊp] **1** *v/i in the dark* tatear **2** *v/t sexually* apalpar
◆**grope for** *v/t handle*, *right word* procurar às cegas
gross [groʊs] *adj* (*coarse*, *vulgar*) vulgar; *exaggeration* enorme; FIN bruto
gross 'national product produto *m* nacional bruto
ground[1] [graʊnd] **1** *n* chão *m*; (*reason*) motivo *m*; ELEC terra *f*; ***on the ~*** no chão **2** *v/t* ELEC aterrar
ground[2] *pret & pp* → ***grind***
'ground control controle *m* de terra **'ground crew** tripulação *f* de terra **'ground floor** *esp Brit* térreo *m*, *Port* rés-do-chão *m*
grounding ['graʊndɪŋ] *in subject* conhecimento *m* básico
groundless ['graʊndlɪs] *adj* infundado
'ground meat *Am* carne *f* moída **'groundnut** amendoim *m* **'ground plan** planta *f* baixa **'ground staff** SPORT pessoal *m* de manutenção; *at airport* pessoal *m* de terra **'groundwork** trabalho *m* de base
group [gru:p] **1** *n* grupo *m* **2** *v/t* agrupar
groupie ['gru:pɪ] *fam* tiete *f*
group 'therapy terapia *f* de grupo
grouse[1] [graʊs] ⟨*pl* ***grouse***⟩ tetraz *m*
grouse[2] [graʊs] **1** *n fam* resmungo *m* **2** *v/i fam* resmungar
grovel ['grɑ:vl] *v/i fig* rebaixar-se
grow [groʊ] **1** *v/i* ⟨*pret* ***grew***, *pp* ***grown***⟩ crescer; *number*, *amount* aumentar; ***~ old / tired*** (*become*) ficar velho / cansado **2** *v/t flowers* plantar
◆**grow up** *person*, *city* crescer; ***grow up!*** não seja criança!
growl [graʊl] **1** *n* rosnado *m* **2** *v/i* rosnar
grown [groʊn] *pp* → ***grow***
'grown-up **1** *n* adulto,-a *m,f* **2** *adj* adulto
growth [groʊθ] *person*, *company*: crescimento *m*; (*increase*) aumento *m*; MED abscesso *m*
grub [grʌb] *of insect* larva *f*
grubby ['grʌbɪ] *adj* encardido
grudge [grʌdʒ] **1** *n* rancor *m*; ***bear a***

~ guardar rancor **2** *v/t* ***~ s.o. sth*** invejar algo de alguém
grudging ['grʌdʒɪŋ] *adj* de má vontade
grudgingly ['grʌdʒɪŋlɪ] *adv* relutantemente
grueling ['gru:əlɪŋ] *adj Am climb, task* árduo
gruelling *Brit* → ***grueling***
gruff [grʌf] *adj* brusco; *voice* rouco
grumble ['grʌmbl] *v/i* resmungar
grumbler ['grʌmblər] resmungão *m*, resmungona *f*
grumpy ['grʌmpɪ] *adj* rabugento
grunt [grʌnt] **1** *n* grunhido *m* **2** *v/i* grunhir
guarantee [gærən'ti:] **1** *n* garantia *f*; ***~ period*** tempo *m* de garantia **2** *v/t* garantir
guarantor [gærən'tɔ:r] fiador,a *m,f*
guard [gɑ:rd] **1** *n* (*security guard*) guarda *m*; MIL sentinela *m*; *in prison* carcereiro,-a *m,f*; ***be on one's ~ against*** estar prevenido contra **2** *v/t* guardar
♦**guard against** *v/t* prevenir-se contra
'**guard dog** cão *m* de guarda
guarded ['gɑ:rdɪd] *adj reply* cauteloso
guardian ['gɑ:rdɪən] LAW tutor,a *m,f*
guardian 'angel anjo *m* da guarda
Guatemala [gwɑ:tə'mɑ:lə] Guatemala *f*
guerrilla [gə'rɪlə] guerrilheiro,-a *m,f*
guerrilla 'warfare guerrilha *f*
guess [ges] **1** *n* palpite *m* **2** *v/t the answer* adivinhar; ***I ~ so*** acho que sim; ***I ~ not*** acho que não **3** *v/i* adivinhar
'**guesswork** suposição *f*
guest [gest] *for lunch, dinner* convidado,-a *m,f*; *in a house* hóspede *m/f*
'**guesthouse** pensão *f*
'**guestroom** quarto *m* de hóspedes
guffaw [gʌ'fɔ:] **1** *n* gargalhada *f* **2** *v/i* gargalhar
guidance ['gaɪdəns] orientação *f*
guide [gaɪd] **1** *n person* guia *m/f*; *book* guia *m* **2** *v/t* guiar
'**guidebook** guia *f*
guided missile ['gaɪdɪd] míssil *m* teleguiado
'**guide dog** *Brit* cão *m* guia
guided 'tour *city*: passeio *m* guiado; *museum, art gallery*: visita *f* guiada
guidelines ['gaɪdlaɪnz] *npl* diretivas *fpl*
guilt [gɪlt] culpa *f*
guilty ['gɪltɪ] *adj* culpado; ***have a ~ conscience*** ter a consciência pesada
guinea pig ['gɪnɪpɪg] porquinho-da-Índia *m*; *fig* cobaia *f*
guise [gaɪz] aparência *f*; ***under the ~ of*** sob o pretexto de
guitar [gɪ'tɑ:r] violão *m*; *electric* guitarra *f*
gui'tar case estojo *m* para violão; *electric guitar*: estojo *m* para guitarra
guitarist [gɪ'tɑ:rɪst] violonista *m/f*; (*electric guitar player*) guitarrista *m/f*
gui'tar player tocador,a *m,f* de violão; (*electric guitar player*) tocador,a *m,f* de guitarra
gulf [gʌlf] golfo *m*; *fig* abismo *m*; ***the Gulf*** o Golfo; ***the Gulf of Mexico*** o Golfo do México
gull [gʌl] *n bird* gaivota *f*
gullet ['gʌlɪt] ANAT esôfago *m*
gullible ['gʌlɪbl] *adj* crédulo
gulp [gʌlp] **1** *n water etc*: gole *m* **2** *v/i in surprise* engolir em seco
♦**gulp down** *v/t drink, food* engolir
gum[1] [gʌm] *n mouth*: gengiva *f*
gum[2] [gʌm] *n* (*glue*) goma *f*; (*chewing gum*) goma *f* de mascar, *Port* pastilha *f* elástica
gumption ['gʌmpʃn] bom *m* senso
gun [gʌn] *pistol, revolver, rifle* arma *f*; *cannon* canhão *m*
♦**gun down** *v/t* ⟨*pret & pp* ***gunned***⟩ matar a tiro
'**gunfire** tiroteio *m* '**gunman** atirador,a *m,f*; *robber* ladrão *m* '**gunpoint *at ~*** sob a mira de uma arma '**gunshot** tiro *m* (de arma de fogo) '**gunshot wound** ferimento *m* à bala
gurgle ['gɜ:rgl] *v/i baby* balbuciar; *drain* gorgolejar
guru ['guru] *fig* guru *m/f*
gush [gʌʃ] *v/i liquid* jorrar
gushy ['gʌʃɪ] *adj fam* (*enthusiastic*) efusivo
gust [gʌst] rajada *f* de vento

gusto ['gʌstoʊ] ***with ~*** com entusiasmo
gusty ['gʌstɪ] *weather* tempestuoso; ***~ wind*** ventania *f*
gut [gʌt] **1** *n* tripa *f*; *fam* (*stomach*) barriga *f* **2** *v/t* ⟨*pret & pp* ***gutted***⟩ (*destroy*) destruir
guts [gʌts] *npl fam* (*courage*) coragem *f*
gutsy ['gʌtsɪ] *adj fam* (*brave*) corajoso
gutter ['gʌtər] *on sidewalk* sarjeta *f*; *on roof* calha *f*
'gutterpress imprensa *f* marrom
guv *Brit* → ***mac***
guy [gaɪ] *fam* cara *m*, *Port* tipo *m*; ***hey, you ~s*** ei, vocês
Guyana [gaɪ'ænə] Guiana *f*
♦ **guzzle down** ['gʌzl] *v/t drink* engolir avidamente
gym [dʒɪm] (*sports club*) academia *f* de ginástica; *school*: ginásio *m* de esportes; *activity* ginástica *f*
'gym class aula *f* de educação física
gymnasium [dʒɪm'neɪzɪəm] ginásio *m* de esportes
gymnast ['dʒɪmnæst] ginasta *m*/*f*
gymnastics [dʒɪm'næstɪks] ginástica *f*
'gym shoes tênis *mpl*
'gym teacher professor,a *m*,*f* de ginástica
gynaecologist *etc Brit* → ***gynecologist***
gynecologist [gaɪnɪ'kɑːlədʒɪst] *Am* ginecologista *m*/*f*
gynecology [gaɪnɪ'kɑːlədʒɪ] *Am* ginecologia *f*
gypsy ['dʒɪpsɪ] cigano,-a *m*,*f*

H

habit ['hæbɪt] hábito *m*; ***get into the ~ of doing sth*** criar o hábito de fazer algo
habitable ['hæbɪtəbl] *adj* habitável
habitat ['hæbɪtæt] hábitat *m*
habitual [hə'bɪtʃʊəl] *adj smoker, drinker* habitual
hack [hæk] *n* (*poor writer*) escrevinhador,a *m*,*f*
hacker ['hækər] COMPUT hacker *m*/*f*
hackneyed ['hæknɪd] *adj* corriqueiro
had [hæd] *pret & pp* → ***have***
haddock ['hædək] hadoque *m*, *Port* eglefim *m*
haemorrhage *Brit* → ***hemorrhage***
haggard ['hægərd] *adj* abatido
haggle ['hægl] *v/i* pechinchar
hail [heɪl] *n* granizo *m*
'hailstone pedra *f* de granizo
'hailstorm tempestade *f* de granizo
hair [her] cabelo *m*; *single* fio *m* de cabelo; ***by a ~ 's breadth*** por um fio de cabelo; ***be having a bad ~ day*** *fam* passar um dia terrível
'hairbrush escova *f* de cabelo **'haircut** corte *m* de cabelo **'hairdo** *fam* penteado *m* **'hairdresser** cabeleireiro,-a *m*,*f*; ***at the ~*** no salão de beleza **'hairdrier**, **'hairdryer** secador *m* de cabelo, *Port* gancho *m* de cabelo **hairdryer** → ***hairdrier*** **'hair gel** gel *m* de cabelo
hairless ['herlɪs] *adj* pelado
'hairpin grampo *m* de cabelo, *Port* gancho *m* de cabelo **hairpin 'curve** curva *f* fechada **hair-raising** ['herreɪzɪŋ] *adj* horripilante **hair remover** ['herrɪmuːvər] creme *m* depilatório
'hair's breadth *fig* distância *f* muito curta
hair-splitting ['hersplɪtɪŋ] *n* ***that's just ~*** são apenas pormenores **'hair spray** laquê *m*, *Port* laca *f* **'hairstyle** penteado *m* **'hairstylist** cabeleireiro,-a *m*,*f*
hairy ['herɪ] *adj arm, animal* peludo; *fam* (*frightening*) perigoso

Haiti ['heɪtiː] Haiti *m*
half [hæf] **1** *n* ⟨*pl* ***halves***⟩ metade *f*; ***~ past ten*** dez e meia; ***~ an hour*** meia hora; ***~ a pound*** meia libra; ***go halves with s.o. on sth.*** dividir os custos de algo com alguém **2** *adj* meio **3** *adv* meio
half-hearted [hæf'hɑːrtɪd] *adj* irresoluto **half 'time 1** *n* SPORT intervalo *m*; ***half-time score*** placar *m* do primeiro tempo **2** *adj* de meio período; ***half-time job*** trabalho *m* de meio expediente **half'way 1** *adj stage*, *point* na metade; ***we have reached the ~ stage*** chegamos na metade **2** *adv* a meio caminho
hall [hɒːl] *large room* salão *m*; (*hallway in house*) entrada *f*
Halloween [hæloʊ'wiːn] dia *m* das bruxas
hallucination [həluːsɪn'eɪʃn] alucinação *f ed*
halo ['heɪloʊ] auréola *f*
halt [hɔːlt] **1** *v/t & v/i* parar **2** *n* ***come to a ~*** parar
halve [hæv] *v/t apple* dividir ao meio; *input*, *costs*, *effort* reduzir à metade
ham [hæm] presunto *m*
hamburger ['hæmbɜːrgər] hambúrguer *m*
hammer ['hæmər] **1** *n* martelo *m* **2** *v/i* martelar; ***~ at the door*** bater à porta insistentemente
hammock ['hæmək] rede *f* (de descanso)
hamper[1] ['hæmpər] *n for food* cesto *m*
hamper[2] *v/t* (*obstruct*) atrapalhar
hamster ['hæmstər] hamster *m*
hand [hænd] **1** *n* mão *f*; *clock*: ponteiro *m*; (*worker*) mão-de-obra *f*; ***at ~***, ***to ~*** à mão; ***at first ~*** em primeira mão; ***by ~*** em mãos; ***on the one ~ ...***, ***on the other ~ ...*** por um lado ..., por outro lado ...; ***in ~*** (*being done*) sob controle; ***on your right ~*** à sua direita; ***~s off!*** tire as mãos daí!; ***~s up!*** mãos ao alto!; ***change ~s*** mudar de dono; ***give s.o. a ~*** dar uma mão a alguém
♦**hand down** *v/t* passar
♦**hand in** *v/t* entregar
♦**hand on** *v/t* passar adiante
♦**hand out** *v/t* distribuir
♦**hand over** *v/t* entregar
'handbag *Brit* bolsa *f* **'handbook** manual *m* **handbrake** *Brit* → ***parking brake*** **'handcuff** *v/t* algemar
handcuffs ['hæn(d)kʌfs] *npl* algemas *fpl*
handicap ['hændɪkæp] deficiência *f*
handicapped ['hændɪkæpt] *adj physically* deficiente; ***~ by lack of funds*** prejudicado por falta de fundos
handicraft ['hændɪkræft] artesanato *m*
handiwork ['hændɪwɜːrk] trabalho *m* manual
handkerchief ['hæŋkərtʃɪf] lenço *m*
handle ['hændl] **1** *n* trinco *m*; *suitcase*: alça *f* **2** *v/t goods* manusear; *case*, *deal* cuidar; *difficult person* lidar; ***let me ~ this*** deixe-me cuidar disso
handlebars ['hændlbɑːrz] *npl* guidom *m*, *Port* guidão *m*
'hand luggage bagagem *f* de mão **'handmade** *adj* feito à mão **'handrail** corrimão *m* **'handshake** aperto *m* de mão
hands-off [hændz'ɑːf] *adv* sem interferência
handsome ['hænsəm] *adj* bonito
hands-on [hændz'ɑːn] *adj approach*, *manager* participativo
hands-free [hændz'friː] *adj phone* com viva voz; ***~ kit*** kit *m* de mãos livres
'handwriting caligrafia *f*
handwritten ['hændrɪtn] *adj* escrito à mão
handy ['hændɪ] *adj tool*, *device* conveniente; ***it's ~ for the shops*** é conveniente para as lojas; ***it might come in ~*** pode ser útil
hang [hæŋ] **1** *v/t* ⟨*pret & pp* ***hung***⟩ *picture* pendurar; *person* enforcar **2** *v/i dress*, *hair* cair **3** *n* ***get the ~ of sth*** *fam* pegar o jeito de algo
♦**hang about** *v/i* vadiar; ***hang about a minute!*** *fam* espere um minuto!
♦**hang on** *v/i* (*wait*) esperar
♦**hang on to** *v/t* (*keep*) ficar com
♦**hang up** *v/i* TEL desligar
hangar ['hæŋər] hangar *m*
hanger ['hæŋər] *for clothes* cabide *m*

'hang glider *person, device* asa-delta *f*
'hang gliding vôo *m* livre
hangover ['hæŋoʊvər] ressaca *f*
'hang-up *fam* complexo *m*; (*obsession*) mania *f*
♦ **hanker after** ['hæŋkər] *v/t* ansiar por
hankie, **hanky** ['hæŋkɪ] *fam* lencinho *m*
haphazard [hæp'hæzərd] *adj* desorganizado
happen ['hæpn] *v/i* acontecer; ***what has ~ed to you?*** o que aconteceu com você?; ***if you ~ to see him*** se por acaso você o vir
♦ **happen across** *v/t* encontrar por acaso
happening ['hæpnɪŋ] acontecimento *m*
happily ['hæpɪlɪ] *adv* alegremente; (*luckily*) felizmente
happiness ['hæpɪnɪs] felicidade *f*
happy ['hæpɪ] *adj* feliz
happy-go-'lucky *adj* despreocupado
'happy hour happy hour *m*
harass [hə'ræs] *v/t* assediar
harassed [hər'æst] *adj* incomodado
harassment [hə'ræsmənt] perseguição *f*; ***sexual ~*** assédio *m* sexual
harbor ['hɑːrbər] **1** *n Am* porto *m* **2** *v/t criminal* refugiar; *grudge* guardar
harbour *Brit* → ***harbor***
hard [hɑːrd] **1** *adj* duro; (*difficult*) difícil; *facts, evidence* concreto; ***~ of hearing*** surdo **2** *adv work* duro; *rain* forte; *push* com esforço; ***you should try ~er*** você deveria se esforçar mais
'hardback *n* livro *m* capa dura **hard-boiled** [hɑːrd'bɔɪld] *adj egg* cozido **'hard copy** cópia *f* impressa **'hard core** *n pornography* pornografia *f* pesada **hard 'currency** moeda *f* forte **'hard disk** disco *m* rígido
harden ['hɑːrdn] *v/t & v/i* endurecer
'hard hat capacete *m*; (*construction worker*) trabalhador *m* braçal **hard-headed** [hɑːrd'hedɪd] *adj* prático **hardhearted** [hɑːrd'hɑːrtɪd] *adj* desumano **hard 'line** linha *f* dura; ***take a ~ on*** adotar uma linha dura com relação a **hardliner** [hɑːrd'laɪnər] linha-dura *m/f*
hardly ['hɑːrdlɪ] *adv* ***I ~ ever see him*** quase nunca o vejo; ***I have ~ any money*** eu quase não tenho mais dinheiro; ***you can ~ be serious*** você não pode estar falando sério; ***there was ~ time to finish*** quase não houve tempo de terminar; ***that's ~ likely, is it?*** isso é altamente improvável, não é?
hardness ['hɑːrdnɪs] dureza *f*, (*difficulty*) dificuldade *f*
'hard sell venda *f* agressiva
hardship ['hɑːrdʃɪp] dificuldade *f*
hard 'shoulder *Brit* acostamento *m*, *Port* berma *f*
hard 'up *adj* duro, *Port* liso **hardware** ['hɑːrdwer] ferragens *fpl*; COMPUT hardware *m* **'hardware store** loja *f* de ferragens **hard-working** [hɑːrd'wɜːrkɪŋ] *adj* trabalhador
hardy ['hɑːrdɪ] *adj* resistente
hare [her] lebre *f*
harebrained ['herbreɪnd] *adj* maluco
harm [hɑːrm] **1** *n* dano *m*; ***it wouldn't do any ~ to ...*** não faria mal algum ... **2** *v/t* causar dano a; *reputation* danificar
harmful ['hɑːrmfl] *adj* nocivo
harmless ['hɑːrmlɪs] *adj* inofensivo
harmonious [hɑːr'moʊnɪəs] *adj* harmonioso
harmonize ['hɑːrmənaɪz] *v/i* harmonizar
harmony ['hɑːrmənɪ] MUS, *also fig* harmonia *f*
harp [hɑːrp] *n* harpa *f*
♦ **harp on about** *v/t fam* bater sempre na mesma tecla sobre
harpoon [hɑːr'puːn] arpão *m*
harsh [hɑːrʃ] *adj* duro; *light, color* forte
harshly ['hɑːrʃlɪ] *adv* severamente
harvest ['hɑːrvɪst] *n* colheita *f*
hash [hæʃ] *fam* ***make a ~ of*** estragar
hashish ['hæʃiːʃ] haxixe *m*
'hash mark cerquilha *f*
haste [heɪst] *n* pressa *f*
hasten ['heɪsn] *v/i* ***~ to do sth*** apressar-se a fazer algo
hastily ['heɪstɪlɪ] *adv* apressadamente
hasty ['heɪstɪ] *adj* apressado
hat [hæt] chapéu *m*
hatch [hætʃ] *n serving food*: passa-pratos *m*; *ship*: escotilha *f*

H

♦**hatch out** *v/i eggs* chocar
hatchet ['hætʃɪt] machadinha *f*; ***bury the ~*** fazer as pazes
hate [heɪt] **1** *n* ódio *m* **2** *v/t* odiar
hatred ['heɪtrɪd] ódio *m*
haughty ['hɔːtɪ] *adj* arrogante
haul [hɒːl] **1** *n fish*: tarrafa *f* **2** *v/t* (*pull*) puxar
haulage ['hɒːlɪdʒ] transporte *m* rodoviário
'**haulage company** companhia *f* de transporte rodoviário
haulier ['hɒːlɪər] companhia *f* de transporte rodoviário
haunch [hɒːntʃ] anca *f*
haunt [hɒːnt] **1** *v/t* assombrar; ***this place is ~ed*** este lugar é assombrado **2** *n* lugar *m* preferido
haunting ['hɒːntɪŋ] *adj tune* de uma tristeza recorrente
have [hæv] **1** *v/t* ⟨*pret & pp* ***had***⟩ ◇ (*own*) ter; ***can I ~ more time?*** pode me dar mais tempo?; ***can I ~ a cup of coffee?*** *in restaurant* eu quero um café; *to friend* posso tomar uma xícara de café?; ***do you ~ …?*** você tem … ?; ***~ breakfast*** tomar café da manhã; ***~ lunch*** almoçar
◇ ***you've been had*** *fam* você foi enganado
◇ ***~ (got) to*** tenho que; ***do I ~ to pay?*** eu tenho que pagar?; ***no, you don't ~ to*** não, você não precisa
◇ (*causative*); ***~ sth done*** *by someone else* mandar fazer algo; ***I had my hair cut*** cortei o cabelo
◇ *past tense*: ***I ~ come*** eu vim; ***~ you seen her?*** você a viu?; ***I hadn't expected that*** eu não esperava por isso
♦**have back** *v/t* ***when can I have it back?*** quando pode devolver-me?
♦**have on** *v/t* (*wear*) vestir; ***do you have anything on tonight?*** *have planned* você tem algum plano para esta noite?
haven ['heɪvn] *fig* refúgio *m*
havoc ['hævək] caos *m*; ***play ~ with*** estragar
hawk [hɒːk] falcão *m*; *fig* abutre *m*
hay [heɪ] feno *m*
'**hay fever** febre *f* do feno
hazard ['hæzərd] *n* perigo *m*
'**hazard lights** *npl* MOT pisca-alerta *m*
hazardous ['hæzərdəs] *adj* perigoso; ***~ waste*** lixo *m* tóxico
haze [heɪz] névoa *f*
hazel ['heɪzl] *n tree* aveleira *f*
'**hazelnut** avelã *f*
hazy ['heɪzɪ] *adj view, image* difuso; *memories* confuso; ***I'm a bit ~ about it*** estou um pouco confuso em relação a isso
he [hiː] *pron* ele; ***~ is an American / a student*** é um americano / estudante
head [hed] **1** *n person, nail*: cabeça *f*; (*boss, leader*) chefe *m/f*; *Brit school*: diretor,a *m,f*; *beer*: colarinho *m*; *line*: início *m*; ***15 a ~*** 15 por cabeça; ***~s or tails?*** cara ou coroa?; ***at the ~ of the list*** no topo da lista; ***~ over heels*** *fall* de pernas para o ar; ***fall ~ over heels in love*** cair de cabeça no amor; ***lose one's ~*** (*go crazy*) perder a cabeça **2** *v/t* (*lead*) chefiar; *ball* cabecear
♦**head for** *v/t* rumar para
'**headache** dor *f* de cabeça
'**headband** faixa *f* (para cabelo)
header ['hedər] *soccer*: cabeçada *f*; *document*: cabeçalho *m*
'**headhunt** *v/t* COM convidar para trabalhar
'**headhunter** COM caçador,a *m,f* de profissionais especializados
heading ['hedɪŋ] *in list* título *m*
'**headlamp** farol *m* dianteiro '**headlight** farol *m* dianteiro '**headline** *n* manchete *f*; ***make the ~s*** fazer manchete '**headlong** *adv fall* de cabeça **head'master** *Brit* diretor *m* de escola **head'mistress** *Brit* diretora *f* de escola '**head office** matriz *f* **head-'on** **1** *adv crash* de frente **2** *adj crash* frontal '**headphones** *npl* fones *mpl* de ouvido '**headquarters** *npl* sede *f* '**headrest** apoio *m* de cabeça '**headroom** *under bridge* espaço *m* livre; *in car* espaço *m* para cabeça '**headscarf** lenço *m* de cabeça '**headstrong** *adj* teimoso **head 'teacher** professor,a *m,f* chefe **head 'waiter** maître *m*, *Port* chefe *m* de mesa '**headwind** vento *m* contrário

heady ['hedɪ] *adj drink, wine* que sobe
heal [hi:l] *v/t* curar
♦**heal up** *v/i* sarar
health [helθ] saúde *f*; ***your ~!*** à sua saúde!
'health club SPA *m* **'health food** comida *f* natural **'health food store** loja *f* de alimentos biológicos **'health insurance** seguro *m* de saúde **'health resort** estância *f* termal
healthy ['helθɪ] *adj person, food, lifestyle, economy* saudável
heap [hi:p] *n* pilha *f*
♦**heap up** *v/t* empilhar; *sand* amontoar
hear [hɪr] *v/t & v/i* ⟨*pret & pp* ***heard***⟩ ouvir
♦**hear about** *v/t* ouvir falar sobre
♦**hear from** *v/t* (*have news from*) ter notícias de
heard [hɜ:rd] *pret & pp* → ***hear***
hearing ['hɪrɪŋ] audição *f*; LAW audiência *f*; ***within ~*** ao alcance da audição; ***out of ~*** fora do alcance da audição
'hearing aid aparelho *m* de surdez
'hearsay ouvir falar; ***by ~*** de ouvir falar
hearse [hɜ:rs] carro *m* fúnebre
heart [hɑ:rt] coração *m*; *problem*: núcleo *m*; *city, organization*: centro *m*; ***know sth by ~*** saber algo de cor
'heart attack ataque *m* cardíaco **'heartbeat** batimento *m* cardíaco **heartbreaking** ['hɑ:rtbreɪkɪŋ] *adj* desolador **'heartbroken** *adj* desolado **'heartburn** azia *f* **'heart failure** parada *f* cardíaca **heartfelt** ['hɑ:rtfelt] *adj sympathy* sincero
hearth [hɑ:rθ] lareira *f*
heartless ['hɑ:rtlɪs] *adj* sem coração
heartrending ['hɑ:rtrendɪŋ] *adj plea, sight* de cortar o coração
hearts [hɑ:rts] *npl cards*: copas *fpl*
'heart throb *fam* queridinho,-a *m,f*
'heart transplant transplante *m* de coração
hearty ['hɑ:rtɪ] *adj appetite* bom (boa); *meal* substancial; *person* cordial
heat [hi:t] calor *m*
♦**heat up** *v/t* aquecer
heated ['hi:tɪd] *adj swimming pool* aquecido; *discussion* acalorado
heater ['hi:tər] aquecedor *m*
heathen ['hi:ðn] *n* pagão *m*, pagã *f*
heather ['heðər] urze *f*
heating ['hi:tɪŋ] calefação *f*
'heatproof, **'heat-resistant** *adj* à prova de calor
'heatstroke insolação *f*
'heatwave onda *f* de calor
heave [hi:v] *v/t* (*lift*) levantar; (*push*) içar; (*pull*) puxar
heaven ['hevn] céu *m*; ***good ~s!*** céus!
heavenly ['hevənlɪ] *adj fam* celestial
heavy ['hevɪ] *adj traffic* pesado; *cold, rain, accent, food, bleeding* forte; *smoker, drinker* inveterado; *loss* grande
heavy-'duty *adj* resistente
'heavyweight *adj* SPORT peso *m* pesado
heckle ['hekl] *v/t* apartear
hectic ['hektɪk] *adj* frenético
hedge [hedʒ] *n* sebe *f*
hedgehog ['hedʒhɑ:g] ouriço *m*
hedgerow ['hedʒroʊ] cerca *f* viva
heed [hi:d] *v/t* prestar atenção; ***pay ~ to …*** prestar atenção a …
heel [hi:l] *foot*: calcanhar *m*; *shoe*: salto *m*
'heel bar sapateiro *m*
hefty ['heftɪ] *adj person* robusto; *suitcase* pesado
height [haɪt] altura *f*; *airplane*: altitude *f*; *season*: auge *m*
heighten ['haɪtn] *v/t effect, tension* elevar
heir [er] herdeiro *m*
heiress ['erɪs] herdeira *f*
held [held] *pret & pp* → ***hold***
helicopter ['helɪkɑ:ptər] helicóptero *m*
hell [hel] inferno *m*; ***what the ~ are you doing / do you want?*** *fam* que diabos você está fazendo / quer?; ***go to ~!*** *fam* vá pro inferno!; ***a ~ of a lot*** *fam* um monte; ***one ~ of a nice guy*** *fam* um sujeito muito legal; ***it hurts like ~*** isso machuca pra cacete
hello [hə'loʊ] olá; TEL alô; ***say ~ to s.o.*** dizer olá a alguém
helm [helm] NAUT leme *m*
helmet ['helmɪt] capacete *m*

help [help] **1** *n* ajuda *f* **2** *v/t* ajudar; ~ ***oneself*** *to food* servir-se à vontade; ***I can't*** ~ ***it*** não posso evitar; ***I couldn't*** ~ ***laughing*** não pude deixar de rir; ~***!*** socorro!
helper ['helpər] ajudante *m/f*
helpful ['helpfl] *adj* útil
helping ['helpɪŋ] *of food* porção *f*
helpless ['helplɪs] *adj* (*unable to cope*) indefeso; (*powerless*) impotente
helplessly ['helplɪslɪ] *adv* inutilmente
helplessness ['helplɪsnɪs] impotência *f*
'help screen COMPUT tela *f* de ajuda
hem [hem] *n dress etc*: bainha *f*
hemisphere ['hemɪsfɪr] hemisfério *m*
'hemline comprimento *m* de roupa
hemorrhage ['hemərɪdʒ] **1** *n* hemorragia *f* **2** *v/i* ter hemorragia
hen [hen] galinha *f*
henchman ['hentʃmən] *pej* capanga *m*
'hen party despedida *f* de solteira
henpecked ['henpekt] *adj* dominado *m* pela esposa; ~ ***husband*** marido *m* submisso
hepatitis [hepə'taɪtɪs] hepatite *f*
her [hɜːr] **1** *adj* seu (sua), dela; ~ ***book*** o livro dela; ~ ***ticket*** a entrada dela **2** *direct object* a; *indirect object* lhe; ***I know*** ~ eu a conheço; ***I gave*** ~ ***the keys*** eu lhe dei as chaves; ***who do you mean?*** – ~ a quem você se refere? - a ela **3** *after prep* ela; ***this is for*** ~ isto é para ela
herb [ɜːrb] erva *f*
herb 'tea, herbal 'tea ['ɜːrb(əl)] chá *m* de ervas
herd [hɜːrd] *n* rebanho *m* bovino
here [hɪr] *adv* aqui; ~ ***'s to you!*** *as toast* à sua saúde!; ~ ***you are*** *giving sth* aqui está; ~ ***we are!*** *finding sth* aqui está
hereditary [hə'redɪterɪ] *adj* hereditário
heredity [hə'redɪtɪ] hereditariedade *f*
heritage ['herɪtɪdʒ] herança *f*
hermit ['hɜːrmɪt] eremita *m/f*
hernia ['hɜːrnɪə] MED hérnia *f*
hero ['hɪroʊ] herói *m*
heroic [hɪ'roʊɪk] *adj* heróico
heroically [hɪ'roʊɪklɪ] *adv* heroicamente
heroin ['heroʊɪn] heroína *f droga*
'heroin addict viciado,-a *m,f* em heroína
heroine ['heroʊɪn] heroína *f*
heroism ['heroʊɪzm] heroísmo *m*
heron ['herən] garça *f*
herpes ['hɜːrpiːz] MED herpes *m*
herring ['herɪŋ] arenque *m*
hers [hɜːrz] *adj* seu (sua), dela; ***a cousin of*** ~ um primo dela; ***that book is*** ~ este livro é seu *ou* dela; ~ ***are red*** os dela são vermelhos
herself [hɜːr'self] *pron* ela mesma; ***she hurt*** ~ ela machucou-se; ***by*** ~ sozinha
hesitant ['hezɪtənt] *adj* hesitante
hesitantly ['hezɪtəntlɪ] *adv* hesitantemente
hesitate ['hezɪteɪt] *v/i* hesitar
hesitation [hezɪ'teɪʃn] hesitação *f*
heterosexual [hetəroʊ'sekʃʊəl] *adj* heterossexual
heyday ['heɪdeɪ] auge *m*
hi [haɪ] *int* oi
hibernate ['haɪbəneɪt] *v/i* hibernar
hiccup ['hɪkʌp] *n* soluço *m*; (*minor problem*) pequeno *m* problema; ***have the*** ~***s*** estar com soluço
hick [hɪk] *pej fam* caipira *m/f*
'hick town *pej fam* cidade *f* interiorana
hid [hɪd] *pret* → ***hide***[1]
hidden ['hɪdn] **1** *adj meaning* oculto; *treasure* escondido **2** *pp* → ***hide***[1]
hidden a'genda *fig* motivo *m* oculto
hide[1] [haɪd] ⟨*pret* ***hid***, *pp* ***hidden***⟩ **1** *v/t* esconder **2** *v/i* esconder-se
hide[2] *n of animal* toca *f*
'hide-and-seek esconde-esconde *m*
'hideaway refúgio *m*
hideous ['hɪdɪəs] *adj* horrível; *crime*, *face* horrendo
hiding[1] ['haɪdɪŋ] (*beating*) surra *f*
hiding[2] ['haɪdɪŋ] ***be in*** ~ estar foragido; ***go into*** ~ esconder-se
'hiding place esconderijo *m*
hierarchy ['haɪrɑːrkɪ] hierarquia *f*
hi-fi ['haɪfaɪ] alta-fidelidade *f*
high [haɪ] **1** *adj building*, *mountain*, *temperature*, *price*, *salary*, *speed*, *society*, *quality* alto; *wind* forte; *opinion* bom (boa); *on drugs* drogado; ***it is*** ~ ***time he understood*** está na hora de

ele entender **2** *n* MOT marcha *f* de força; *in statistics* pique *m*; EDUC escola *f* secundária **3** *adv* alto; ***~ in the sky*** nas alturas; ***that's as ~ as we can go*** isto é o máximo que podemos oferecer

'highbrow *adj* erudito **'highchair** cadeira *f* alta para crianças **high-'class** *adj* de alta classe **High 'Court** corte *f* suprema **high 'diving** salto *m* acrobático **high-'frequency** *adj* de alta-freqüência **high-'grade** *adj* de alta qualidade **high-handed** [haɪ'hændɪd] *adj* despótico **high-heeled** [haɪ'hiːld] *adj* de salto alto **'high jump** salto *m* em altura **high-'level** *adj* de alto nível **'high life** vida *f* em alta sociedade **'highlight 1** *n* (*main event*) ponto *m* alto; *hair*: mecha *f* **2** *v/t with pen* destacar; COMPUT selecionar **'highlighter** *pen* marcador *m* de texto

highly ['haɪlɪ] *adv desirable, likely* muito; ***be ~ paid*** ser bem pago; ***think ~ of s.o.*** ter alguém em alta conta

high per'formance *adj drill, battery* de alta desempenho **high-pitched** [haɪ'pɪtʃt] *adj* agudo **'high point** *life, career*: ponto *m* alto **high-powered** [haɪ'paʊərd] *adj engine* de alta potência; *intellectual, salesman* dinâmico **high 'pressure 1** *n weather* alta pressão *f* **2** *adj* TECH de alta pressão; *salesman* incisivo; *job, lifestyle* estressante **high 'priest** sumo *m* sacerdote **'high school** escola *f* secundária **high so'ciety** alta *f* sociedade **high-speed 'train** trem *m* de alta velocidade **high 'strung** *adj* nervoso **high 'tech 1** *n* alta *f* tecnologia **2** *adj* de alta tecnologia **high-'tension** *adj cable* de alta tensão **high 'tide** maré *f* alta **high 'water** maré *f* alta **'highway** auto-estrada *f* **'high wire** *circus*: corda *f* bamba

hijack ['haɪdʒæk] **1** *v/t plane, bus* seqüestrar **2** *n plane, bus*: seqüestro *m*

hijacker ['haɪdʒækər] *plane, bus*: seqüestrador,a *m,f*

hike[1] [haɪk] **1** *n* caminhada *f* **2** *v/i* caminhar

hike[2] [haɪk] *n prices*: aumento *m*

hiker ['haɪkər] andarilho,-a *m,f*

hiking ['haɪkɪŋ] caminhadas *fpl*

'hiking boots botas *fpl* para caminhadas

hilarious [hɪ'lerɪəs] *adj* hilariante

hill [hɪl] colina *f*; (*slope*) ladeira *f*

hill-billy ['hɪlbɪlɪ] *fam* matuto,-a *m,f* **hillside** ['hɪlsaɪd] vertente *f* **hilltop** ['hɪltɑːp] cume *m*

hilly ['hɪlɪ] *adj* montanhoso

hilt [hɪlt] punho *m*

him [hɪm] *pron direct object* o; *indirect object* lhe; *after prep* ele; ***I know ~*** eu o conheço; ***I gave ~ the keys*** eu lhe dei as chaves; ***this is for ~*** isto é para ele; ***who do you mean? – ~*** a quem você se refere? – a ele

himself [hɪm'self] *pron* ele mesmo; ***he hurt ~*** ele machucou-se; ***by ~*** sozinho

hind [haɪnd] *adj* traseiro

hinder ['hɪndər] *v/t* retardar

hindrance ['hɪndrəns] estorvo *m*, obstáculo *m*

hindsight ['haɪndsaɪt] ***with ~*** em retrospecto

hinge [hɪndʒ] dobradiça *f*

♦**hinge on** *v/t* depender de

hint [hɪnt] *n* (*clue*) pista *f*; (*piece of advice*) conselho *m*; (*implied suggestion*) insinuação *f*; *of red, sadness etc* leve toque *m*

hip [hɪp] *n* quadril *m*

hip 'pocket bolso *m* de trás

hippopotamus [hɪpə'pɑːtəməs] hipopótamo *m*

hire ['haɪr] *v/t room* alugar; *workers, staff* contratar

hire purchase *Brit* → ***installment plan***

his [hɪz] **1** *adj* seu (sua), dele; ***~ ticket*** a entrada dele; ***~ book*** o livro dele **2** *pron* ***it's ~*** é dele; ***a cousin of ~*** um primo dele; ***~ are red*** os dele são vermelhos

Hispanic [hɪ'spænɪk] **1** *n* hispânico,-a *m,f* **2** *adj* hispânico

hiss [hɪs] **1** *v/i snake* silvar **2** *n audience*: vaia *f*, *animal*: silvo *m*

historian [hɪ'stɔːrɪən] historiador,a *m,f*

H

historic [hɪ'stɑːrɪk] *adj* histórico
historical [hɪ'stɑːrɪkl] *adj* histórico
history ['hɪstərɪ] história *f*
hit [hɪt] **1** *v/t ⟨pret & pp* ***hit****⟩* bater; *ball* rebater; (*collide with*) ir de encontro a; ***he was ~ by a bullet*** ele foi atingido por uma bala; ***it suddenly ~ me*** *I realized* de repente percebi; ***~ town*** (*arrive*) chegar à cidade **2** *n* (*blow*) golpe *m*; (*success*) *also* MUS sucesso *m*; *website*: visita *f*
◆**hit back** *v/i* dar o troco
◆**hit on** *v/t idea* encontrar; *fam girl, boy* paquerar
◆**hit out at** *v/t* (*criticize*) criticar
hit-and-run *adj* ***~ accident*** *acidente em que o motorista fugiu*; ***~ driver*** *motorista que atropela e foge*
hitch [hɪʧ] **1** *n* (*problem*) dificuldade *f*; ***without a ~*** sem dificuldade **2** *v/t* atar; ***~ sth to sth*** atar algo a algo; ***~ a ride*** pegar uma carona, *Port* arranjar uma boleia **3** *v/i* (*hitchhike*) viajar de carona
◆**hitch up** *v/t wagon, trailer* acoplar
'hitchhike *v/i* viajar de carona, *Port* andar à boleia
'hitchhiker *pessoa que viaja de carona*
'hitchhiking viagem *f* de carona, *Port* andar *m* à boleia
hi-'tech 1 *n* alta *f* tecnologia **2** *adj* de alta tecnologia
'hitlist lista *f* de alvos **'hitman** assassino *m* de aluguel, *Port* contratado *m* **hit-or-'miss** *adj* arbitrário **'hit squad** esquadrão *m* especial
HIV *abbr* (*of* ***human immunodeficiency virus***) HIV *m*
hive [haɪv] *for bees* colmeia *f*
◆**hive off** *v/t* COM (*separate off*) transferir
HIV-'positive [eɪʧaɪ'viː] *adj* HIV positivo
hoard [hɔːrd] **1** *n* provisão *f* **2** *v/t* acumular
hoarder ['hɔːrdər] juntador,a *m,f* de tralha
hoarse [hɔːrs] *adj* rouco
hoax [hoʊks] *n* trote *m*
hob [hɑːb] *cooker*: boca *f* do fogão
hobble ['hɑːbl] *v/i* mancar
hobby ['hɑːbɪ] hobby *m*
hobo ['hoʊboʊ] *fam* vagabundo,-a *m,f*
hockey ['hɑːkɪ] hóquei *m*
hog [hɑːg] *n* (*pig*) porco *m*
hoist [hɔɪst] **1** *n* guincho *m* **2** *v/t* (*lift*) levantar; *flag* hastear
hokum ['hoʊkəm] *n* (*nonsense*) disparate *m*; (*sentimental stuff*) sentimentalismo *m* trivial
hold [hoʊld] **1** *v/t ⟨pret & pp* ***held****⟩ in hand, also* (*support, keep in place*) segurar; *passport, license* portar; *prisoner, suspect* prender; (*contain*) conter; *job, post* ter; *course* manter; ***he held her in his arms*** ele a abraçou; ***~ one's breath*** prender a respiração; ***he can ~ his drink*** ele aguenta a bebedeira; ***~ s.o. responsible*** responsabilizar alguém; ***~ that …*** (*believe, maintain*) achar que …; ***~ the line*** TEL aguarde na linha **2** *n ship, plane*: compartimento *m* de cargas; ***catch*** *ou* ***take ~ of sth*** agarrar algo; ***lose one's ~ on sth*** *rope*: soltar algo; *reality*: agarrar-se a algo
◆**hold against** *v/t* ***hold sth against s.o.*** ter algo contra alguém
◆**hold back 1** *v/t crowds* controlar, conter; *facts, information* reter **2** *v/i* (*not tell all*) titubear
◆**hold on** *v/i* (*wait*) esperar; ***now hold on a minute!*** ora, espere um minuto!; ***hold on*** TEL não desligar
◆**hold on to** *v/t* (*keep*) ficar com; *belief* agarrar-se a
◆**hold out 1** *v/t hand* estender; *prospect* oferecer **2** *v/i supplies* perdurar; *trapped miners etc* resistir
◆**hold up** *v/t shelf etc* suportar; *hand* levantar; *bank etc* assaltar; (*make late*) atrasar; ***hold sth up as an example*** manter algo como exemplo
◆**hold with** *v/t* (*approve of*) aprovar
'holdall bolsa *f* de viagem
holder ['hoʊldər] (*container*) recipiente *m*; *passport, ticket etc*: portador,a *m,f*; *record*: detentor,a *m,f*
holding company ['hoʊldɪŋ] holding *f*
'holdup (*robbery*) assalto *m*; (*delay*) atraso *m*
hole [hoʊl] buraco *m*
holiday ['hɑːlədeɪ] *single day* feriado

m; *period* férias *fpl*; ***take a ~*** tirar um dia de folga; *Brit* tirar umas férias

Holland ['hɑːlənd] Holanda *f*

hollow ['hɑːloʊ] *adj object* oco; *cheeks* côncavo; *promise* vazio

holly ['hɑːlɪ] azevinho *m*

holocaust ['hɑːləkɒːst] holocausto *m*

hologram ['hɑːləgræm] holograma *m*

holster ['hoʊlstər] coldre *m*

holy ['hoʊlɪ] *adj* sagrado

Holy 'Spirit Espírito *m* Santo

'Holy Week Semana *f* Santa

home [hoʊm] **1** *n* casa *f*; (*native country*) pátria *f*; (*town, part of country*) terra *f* natal; *old people*: asilo *m*; ***at ~*** *also* SPORT em casa; (*in my country*) na terra natal; ***make oneself at ~*** sentir-se em casa; ***at ~ and abroad*** em casa ou fora dela; ***work from ~*** trabalhar em casa **2** *adv* em casa; (*in own country*) na terra natal; (*in own town, part of country*) no torrão natal; ***go ~*** ir para casa; (*to country*) ir para a terra natal; (*to town, part country*) ir para o seu lugar; ***go ~!*** vá para casa!

'home address endereço *m* residencial **home 'banking** home banking *m* **'homecoming** volta *f* ao lar **home com'puter** computador *m* doméstico **'home game** partida *f* em casa

homeless ['hoʊmlɪs] *adj* desabrigado; ***the ~*** os desabrigados

'homeloving *adj* doméstico

homely ['hoʊmlɪ] *adj* (*homeloving*) simples; *Am* (*not good-looking*) feio

home'made *adj* caseiro **home 'movie** filme *m* caseiro **Home Office** *Brit* Ministério do Interior

homeopathy [hoʊmɪ'ɑːpəθɪ] homeopatia *f*

'home page COMPUT home page *f* **'homesick** *adj* saudoso; ***be ~*** estar com saudade de casa **'home town** cidade *f* natal

homeward ['hoʊmwərd] *adv to own house* de volta à casa; *to own country* de volta à pátria

'homework EDUC dever *m* de casa

'homeworking COM trabalho *m* em casa

homicide ['hɑːmɪsaɪd] *crime* homicídio *m*; *police department* delegacia *f* de homicídios

homograph ['hɑːməgræf] homógrafo *m*

homophobia [hoʊmə'foʊbɪə] homofobia *f*

homosexual [hoʊmə'sekʃʊəl] **1** *adj* homossexual **2** *n* homossexual *m/f*

Honduras [hɒn'dʊrəs] Honduras

honest ['ɑːnɪst] *adj* honesto

honestly ['ɑːnɪstlɪ] *adv* honestamente; ***~!*** francamente!

honesty ['ɑːnɪstɪ] honestidade *f*

honey ['hʌnɪ] mel *m*; *fam* (*darling*) bem *m*; *to husband, wife* (meu) amor

'honeycomb favo *m* de mel

'honeymoon *n* lua *f* de mel

honk [hɑːŋk] *v/t* ***~ the horn*** buzinar

honky ['hɑːŋkɪ] *pej fam* branquelo,-a *m,f*

honor ['ɑːnər] *Am* **1** *n* honra *f* **2** *v/t* honrar

honorable ['ɑːnrəbl] *adj Am* honrado

honour *etc Brit* → ***honor***

hood [hʊd] *head*: capuz *m*; *cooker*: tampa *f*; MOT capô *m*

hoodlum ['huːdləm] valentão *m*, valentona *f*

hoof [huːf] casco *m*

hook [hʊk] *clothes*: cabide *m*; *fishing*: anzol *m*; ***off the ~*** TEL fora do gancho

hooked [hʊkt] *adj* fissurado; *on drugs* viciado; ***be ~ on sth*** ser fissurado em algo

hooker ['hʊkər] *fam* meretriz *f*

hooligan ['huːlɪgən] desordeiro,-a *m,f*

hooliganism ['huːlɪgənɪzm] desordem *f*

hoop [huːp] argola *f*

hoot [huːt] **1** *v/t horn* tocar **2** *v/i car* buzinar; *owl* piar

hoover ['huːvər] **1** *n* aspirador *m* de pó **2** *v/i* passar o aspirador

hop[1] [hɑːp] *n plant* lúpulo *m*

hop[2] [hɑːp] *v/i* ⟨*pret & pp* ***hopped***⟩ saltar

hope [hoʊp] **1** *n* esperança *f*; ***there's no ~ of that*** não há esperança disso **2** *v/i* esperar; ***~ for sth*** esperar por algo; ***I ~ so*** espero que sim; ***I ~ not*** espero que não **3** *v/t* ***~ that …*** espero

H

que …; ***I ~ you like it*** espero que você goste

hopeful ['hoʊpfl] *adj* esperançoso; (*promising*) promissor

hopefully ['hoʊpflɪ] *adv say, wait* esperançosamente; ***~ he hasn't forgotten*** espero / esperamos que ele não tenha esquecido

hopeless ['hoʊplɪs] *adj position, prospect* sem esperança; (*useless*) *person* inútil

horizon [hə'raɪzn] horizonte *m*

horizontal [hɑːrɪ'zɑːntl] *adj* horizontal

hormone ['hɔːrmoʊn] hormônio *m*

horn [hɔːrn] *animal*: chifre *m*; MOT buzina *f*

H

hornet ['hɔːrnɪt] marimbondo *m*

horn-rimmed spectacles [hɔːrnrɪmd'spektəklz] óculos *mpl* com aro de chifre

horny ['hɔːrnɪ] *adj sexually* excitado, com tesão

horoscope ['hɑːrəskoʊp] horóscopo *m*

horrible ['hɑːrɪbl] *adj* horrível

horrify ['hɑːrɪfaɪ] *v/t* ⟨*pret & pp* ***horrified***⟩ horrorizar; ***I was horrified*** fiquei horrorizado

horrifying ['hɑːrɪfaɪŋ] *adj experience, idea, prices* horroroso

horror ['hɑːrər] horror *m*; ***the ~s of war*** os horrores da guerra

'horror movie filme *m* de terror

hors d'oeuvre [ɔːr'dɜːrv] entrada *f refeição*

horse [hɔːrs] cavalo *m*

'horseback ***on ~*** a cavalo **horse 'chestnut** castanha-da-índia *f* **'horsepower** cavalo-vapor *m* **'horse race** corrida *f* de cavalos **'horseshoe** ferradura *f*

horticulture ['hɔːrtɪkʌltʃər] horticultura *f*

hose [hoʊz] *n* mangueira *f*

hospice ['hɑːspɪs] asilo *m*

hospitable ['hɑːspɪtəbl] *adj* hospitaleiro

hospital ['hɑːspɪtl] hospital *m*; ***go into the ~*** ir parar no hospital

hospitality [hɑːspɪ'tælətɪ] hospitalidade *f*

host [hoʊst] *n party, reception*: anfitrião *m*; *TV program*: apresentador *m*

hostage ['hɑːstɪdʒ] refém *m/f*; ***be taken ~*** ser mantido como refém

'hostage taker pessoa *f* que faz reféns

hostel ['hɑːstl] *students*: albergue *m*; ***youth ~*** albergue *m* da juventude

hostess ['hoʊstɪs] *party, reception*: anfitriã *f*; *airplane*: comissária *f* de bordo, *Port* hospedeira *f*; *bar*: hostess *f*

hostile ['hɑːstl] *adj* hostil

hostility [hɑː'stɪlətɪ] hostilidade *f*; ***hostilities*** *fpl* hostilidades

hot [hɑːt] *adj weather, water, food etc* quente; (*spicy*) picante; ***I'm ~*** estou com calor; ***it's ~*** está quente; ***she's pretty ~ at math*** *fam* (*good*) ela é excelente em matemática

'hot dog cachorro-quente *m*

hotel [hoʊ'tel] hotel *m*

'hotplate chapa *f*

'hot spot *military, political* área *f* perigosa; *wi-fi*: local *m* de acesso wi-fi à internet

hour ['aʊr] hora *f*

hourly ['aʊrlɪ] *adj* de hora em hora; ***at ~ intervals*** de hora em hora

house [haʊs] *n* casa *f*; ***at your ~*** em sua casa

'houseboat casa *f* flutuante **'housebreaking** arrombamento *m* **'household** moradores *mpl* de uma casa **household 'name** nome *m* conhecido **'house husband** dono *m* da casa **'housekeeper** governanta *f* **'housekeeping** *activity* trabalhos *mpl* domésticos; *money* dinheiro *m* para os gastos domésticos **House of Repre'sentatives** *npl* Câmara *f* dos Deputados **housewarming**, **housewarming party** ['haʊswɔːrmɪŋ] festa *f* de inauguração da nova casa **'housewife** dona *f* de casa **'housework** trabalho *m* doméstico

housing ['haʊzɪŋ] habitação *f*; TECH caixa *f*

'housing conditions *npl* condições *fpl* de habitação

hovel ['hɑːvl] casebre *m*

hover ['hɑːvər] *v/i* pairar

'hovercraft aerobarco *m*
how [haʊ] *adv* como; **~ *are you?*** como vai?; **~ *about …?*** que tal …?; **~ *much?*** quanto?; **~ *much is it?*** *cost* quanto custa?; **~ *many?*** quantos?; **~ *often?*** quantas vezes?; **~ *funny* / *sad!*** que divertido / triste!
how'ever *adv* no entanto, entretanto; **~, *the problems got worse*** porém, os problemas pioraram; **~ *big* / *rich* / *small they are*** não importa que sejam grandes / ricos / pequenos
howl [haʊl] *v/i dog* uivar; *person in pain* gritar; **~ *with laughter*** estourar de rir
howler ['haʊlər] *Brit* (*mistake*) grande erro *m*
HR *abbr* (*of* ***human resources***) Recursos *mpl* Humanos
hub [hʌb] *of wheel* mancal *m*
'hubcap calota *f*
◆**huddle together** ['hʌdl] *v/i* aconchegar-se
hue [hjuː] matiz *m*
huff [hʌf] ***be in a* ~** ficar mal-humorado
hug [hʌg] *v/t* ⟨*pret & pp* ***hugged***⟩ abraçar
huge [hjuːdʒ] *adj* enorme
hull [hʌl] casco *m*
hullabaloo tumulto *m*
hum [hʌm] ⟨*pret & pp* ***hummed***⟩ **1** *v/t song, tune* cantarolar **2** *v/i person* cantarolar; *machine* zumbir
human ['hjuːmən] **1** *n* ser *m* humano **2** *adj* humano; **~ *error*** falha *f* humana
human 'being ser *m* humano
humane [hjuː'meɪn] *adj* humano
humanitarian [hjuːmænɪ'terɪən] *adj* humanitário
humanity [hjuː'mænətɪ] humanidade *f*
human 'race raça *f* humana
human 'resources *npl department* recursos *mpl* humanos
humble ['hʌmbl] *adj attitude, origins, meal, house* humilde
humdrum ['hʌmdrʌm] *adj* monótono
humid ['hjuːmɪd] *adj* úmido
humidifier [hjuː'mɪdɪfaɪr] umidificador *m*
humidity [hjuː'mɪdətɪ] umidade *f*
humiliate [hjuː'mɪlɪeɪt] *v/t* humilhar
humiliating [hjuː'mɪlɪeɪtɪŋ] *adj* humilhante
humiliation [hjuːmɪlɪ'eɪʃn] humilhação *f*
humility [hjuː'mɪlətɪ] humildade *f*
humor ['hjuːmər] humor *m*; ***sense of* ~** senso *m* de humor
humorous ['hjuːmərəs] *adj* cômico; *language* humorístico
humour *Brit* → ***humor***
hump [hʌmp] **1** *n camel*: corcova *f*; *person*: corcunda *f*; *road*: elevação *f* **2** *v/t fam* (*carry*) carregar
hunch [hʌntʃ] (*idea*) pressentimento *m*
hundred ['hʌndrəd] cem
hundredth ['hʌndrədθ] *n & adj* centésimo (*m*)
'hundredweight *Am* peso de 100 libras; *Brit* peso de 112 libras
hung [hʌŋ] *pret & pp* → ***hang***
Hungarian [hʌŋ'gerɪən] **1** *adj* húngaro **2** *n person* húngaro,-a *m,f*; *language* húngaro *m*
Hungary ['hʌŋgərɪ] Hungria *f*
hunger ['hʌŋgər] fome *f*
hung-'over *adj* ressacado
hungry ['hʌŋgrɪ] *adj* faminto; ***I'm* ~** estou com fome
hunk [hʌŋk] *n* pedação *m*; *fam man* pedaço *m*
hunky-dorey [hʌŋkɪ'dɔːrɪ] *adj fam* maravilhoso
hunt [hʌnt] **1** *n animals*: caça *f*; *new leader, criminal, missing child*: procura *f* **2** *v/t animal* caçar
◆**hunt for** *v/t* procurar
hunter ['hʌntər] caçador,a *m,f*
hunting ['hʌntɪŋ] caçada *f*
hurdle ['hɜːrdl] SPORT barreira *f*, *fig* (*obstacle*) obstáculo *m*
hurdler ['hɜːrdlər] SPORT corredor,a *m,f* de barreira
hurdles *npl* SPORT corrida *fpl* com barreiras
hurl [hɜːrl] *v/t* arremessar
hurray [hʊ'reɪ] *int* hurra
hurricane ['hʌrɪkən] furacão *m*
hurried ['hʌrɪd] *adj* apressado
hurry ['hʌrɪ] **1** *n* pressa *f*; ***be in a* ~** es-

tar com pressa **2** *v/i* ⟨*pret & pp* ***hurried***⟩ apressar-se

◆**hurry up 1** *v/i* apressar-se; ***hurry up!*** apresse-se! **2** *v/t* apressar

hurt [hɜːrt] ⟨*pret & pp* ***hurt***⟩ **1** *v/i* doer; ***does it ~?*** isso dói? **2** *v/t physically* machucar; *emotionally* magoar

husband ['hʌzbənd] marido *m*

hush [hʌʃ] *n* quietude *f*; ***~!*** psiu!

◆**hush up** *v/t scandal etc* abafar

husk [hʌsk] *of peanuts etc* casca *f*

husky ['hʌskɪ] *adj voice* rouco

hustle ['hʌsl] **1** *n* correria *f*; ***~ and bustle*** o movimento e a animação **2** *v/t person* apressar

hut [hʌt] choupana *f*

hyacinth ['haɪəsɪnθ] jacinto *m*

hybrid ['haɪbrɪd] *n* híbrido *m*

hydrant ['haɪdrənt] hidrante *f*

hydraulic [haɪ'drɒːlɪk] *adj* hidráulico

hydroe'lectric [haɪdroʊɪ'lektrɪk] *adj* hidrelétrico

'hydrofoil ['haɪdrəfɔɪl] *boat* hidrofólio *m*

hydrogen ['haɪdrədʒən] hidrogênio *m*

'hydrogen bomb bomba *f* de hidrogênio

hygiene ['haɪdʒiːn] higiene *f*

hygienic [haɪ'dʒiːnɪk] *adj* higiênico

hymn [hɪm] hino *m*

hype [haɪp] *n* falatório *m*; ***there's so much ~ about it*** está dando muito falatório

hyperactive [haɪpər'æktɪv] *adj* hiperativo

hypermarket ['haɪpərmɑːrkɪt] *Brit* hipermercado *m*

hypersensitive [haɪpər'sensɪtɪv] *adj* hipersensível

hypertension [haɪpər'tenʃn] hipertensão *f*

hypertext ['haɪpərtekst] COMPUT hipertexto *m*

hyphen ['haɪfn] hífen *m*

hypnosis [hɪp'noʊsɪs] hipnose *f*

hypnotherapy [hɪpnoʊ'θerəpɪ] hipnoterapia *f*

hypnotize ['hɪpnətaɪz] *v/t* hipnotizar

hypochondriac [haɪpə'kɑːndrɪæk] *n* hipocondríaco,-a *m,f*

hypocrisy [hɪ'pɑːkrəsɪ] hipocrisia *f*

hypocrite ['hɪpəkrɪt] hipócrita *m/f*

hypocritical [hɪpə'krɪtɪkl] *adj* hipócrita

hypothermia [haɪpoʊ'θɜːrmɪə] hipotermia *f*

hypothesis [haɪ'pɑːθəsɪs] ⟨*pl* ***hypotheses***⟩ hipótese *f*

hypothetical [haɪpə'θetɪkl] *adj* hipotético

hysterectomy [hɪstə'rektəmɪ] histerectomia *f*

hysteria [hɪ'stɪrɪə] histeria *f*

hysterical [hɪ'sterɪkl] *adj person, laugh* histérico; *fam* (*very funny*) hilariante; ***become ~*** ficar histérico

hysterics [hɪ'sterɪks] *npl* crise *f* histérica; *laughter* ataque *m* de riso

I

I [aɪ] *pron* eu; ***~ am American / a student*** sou americano / estudante

ice [aɪs] gelo *m*; ***break the ~*** *fig* quebrar o gelo

◆**ice up** *v/i engine* congelar

iceberg ['aɪsbɜːrg] iceberg *m* **'icebox** *Am* refrigerador *m* **'icebreaker** *ship* quebra-gelos *m* **'ice cream** sorvete *m*, *Port* gelado *m* **'ice cream parlor** *Am* sorveteria *f*, *Port* gelataria *f* **'ice cream parlour** *Brit* → ***ice cream parlor*** **'ice cube** pedra *f* de gelo

iced [aɪst] *adj drink* gelado

iced 'coffee café *m* gelado

'ice hockey hóquei *m* sobre gelo **ice lolly** *Brit* → ***Popsicle®*** **'ice rink** rinque *m* de gelo **'ice skates** patins

mpl de gelo **'ice skating** patinação *f* no gelo
icicle ['aɪsɪkl] pingente *m* de gelo
icing *Brit* → ***frosting***
icon ['aɪkɑːn] *cultural, also* COMPUT ícone *m*
icy ['aɪsɪ] *adj road, surface* gelado; *welcome* frio
ID [aɪ'diː] *abbr* (*of* ***identity***) carteira *f* de identidade
idea [aɪ'diːə] idéia *f*; ***good ~!*** boa idéia!; ***I have no ~*** não faço idéia; ***it's not a good ~ to ...*** não é uma boa idéia ...
ideal [aɪ'diːəl] *adj* (*perfect*) ideal
idealistic [aɪdiːə'lɪstɪk] *adj* idealista
ideally [aɪ'diːəlɪ] *adv situated etc* idealmente; ***~, we would do it like this*** o ideal seria fazermos assim
identical [aɪ'dentɪkl] *adj* idêntico; ***~ twins*** gêmeos *mpl* idênticos
identification [aɪdentɪfɪ'keɪʃn] identificação *f*; (*papers etc*) documento *m* de identidade
identify [aɪ'dentɪfaɪ] *v/t* ⟨*pret & pp* ***identified***⟩ identificar
identity [aɪ'dentətɪ] identidade *f*; ***have you got any ~ on you?*** você tem algum documento de identidade com você?; ***~ card*** carteira *f* de identidade
ideological [aɪdɪə'lɑːdʒɪkl] *adj* ideológico
ideology [aɪdɪ'ɑːlədʒɪ] ideologia *f*
idiom ['ɪdɪəm] (*saying*) ditado *m*
idiomatic [ɪdɪə'mætɪk] *adj* (*natural*) idiomático
idiosyncrasy [ɪdɪə'sɪŋkrəsɪ] idiossincrasia *f*
idiot ['ɪdɪət] idiota *m/f*
idiotic [ɪdɪ'ɑːtɪk] *adj* idiota
idle ['aɪdl] **1** *adj person* (*not doing anything*) ocioso; (*lazy*) preguiçoso; *machinery* fora de funcionamento; *time* vago; *threat* vão (vã); ***in an ~ moment*** numa hora vaga **2** *v/i engine* funcionar em ponto morto
◆ **idle away** *v/t the time etc* desperdiçar
idol ['aɪdl] ídolo *m*
idolize ['aɪdəlaɪz] *v/t* idolatrar
idyllic [ɪ'dɪlɪk] *adj* idílico
if [ɪf] *conj* se; ***what ~ ...?*** e se ...?; ***~ not*** se não; ***~ so*** nesse caso; ***~ only*** se ao menos
ignite [ɪg'naɪt] *v/t* inflamar
ignition [ɪg'nɪʃn] *in car* ignição *f*; ***~ key*** chave *f* de ignição
ignorance ['ɪgnərəns] ignorância *f*
ignorant ['ɪgnərənt] *adj* ignorante; (*rude*) grosseiro
ignore [ɪg'nɔːr] *v/t* ignorar
ill [ɪl] *adj* doente; ***fall ~*** ficar doente; ***be taken ~*** ficar doente; ***I feel ~ at ease*** sinto-me constrangido
illegal [ɪ'liːgl] *adj* ilegal
illegible [ɪ'ledʒəbl] *adj* ilegível
illegitimate [ɪlɪ'dʒɪtɪmət] *adj child* ilegítimo
ill-fated [ɪl'feɪtɪd] *adj* malfadado
illicit [ɪ'lɪsɪt] *adj* ilícito
illiterate [ɪ'lɪtərət] *adj* analfabeto
ill-mannered [ɪl'mænərd] *adj* mal-educado
ill-natured [ɪl'neɪtʃərd] *adj* mal-humorado
illness ['ɪlnɪs] doença *f*
illogical [ɪ'lɑːdʒɪkl] *adj* ilógico
ill-tempered [ɪl'tempərd] *adj* mal-humorado
ill'treat *v/t* maltratar
illuminate [ɪ'luːmɪneɪt] *v/t building etc* iluminar
illuminating [ɪ'luːmɪneɪtɪŋ] *adj remarks etc* esclarecedor
illusion [ɪ'luːʒn] ilusão *f*
illustrate ['ɪləstreɪt] *v/t* ilustrar
illustration [ɪlə'streɪʃn] ilustração *f*
illustrator [ɪlə'streɪtər] ilustrador,a *m,f*
ill 'will animosidade *f*
image ['ɪmɪdʒ] *also politician, company*: imagem *f*
'image-conscious *adj* preocupado com a imagem
imaginable [ɪ'mædʒɪnəbl] *adj* imaginável; ***the biggest / smallest size ~*** o maior / menor tamanho imaginável
imaginary [ɪ'mædʒɪnərɪ] *adj* imaginário
imagination [ɪmædʒɪ'neɪʃn] imaginação *f*; ***it's all in your ~*** é tudo imaginação sua

I

imaginative [ɪ'mædʒɪnətɪv] *adj* imaginativo
imagine [ɪ'mædʒɪn] *v/t* imaginar; ***I can just ~ it*** posso imaginar; ***you're imagining things*** você está imaginando coisas
imbecile ['ɪmbəsiːl] **1** *n* imbecil *m/f* **2** *adj* imbecil
IMF [aɪem'ef] *abbr* (*of* ***International 'Monetary Fund***) IMF *m* (= Fundo *m* Monetário Internacional)
imitate ['ɪmɪteɪt] *v/t* imitar
imitation [ɪmɪ'teɪʃn] imitação *f*
immaculate [ɪ'mækjʊlət] *adj* imaculado
immaterial [ɪmə'tɪrɪəl] *adj* (*not relevant*) irrelevante
immature [ɪmə'tur] *adj* imaturo
immediate [ɪ'miːdɪət] *adj* imediato; ***the ~ family*** a família próxima; ***in the ~ neighborhood*** na vizinhança mais próxima
immediately [ɪ'miːdɪətlɪ] *adv* imediatamente; ***~ after the bank*** logo depois do banco
immense [ɪ'mens] *adj* imenso
immerse [ɪ'mɜːrs] *v/t* imergir; ***~ oneself in*** concentrar-se em
immigrant ['ɪmɪgrənt] *n* imigrante *m/f*
immigrate ['ɪmɪgreɪt] *v/i* imigrar
immigration [ɪmɪ'greɪʃn] imigração *f*
imminent ['ɪmɪnənt] *adj* iminente
immobilize [ɪ'moʊbɪlaɪz] *v/t factory* paralisar; *car, person* imobilizar
immobilizer [ɪ'moʊbɪlaɪzər] *on car* imobilizador *m*
immoderate [ɪ'mɑːdərət] *adj* imoderado
immoral [ɪ'mɒːrəl] *adj* imoral
immorality [ɪmɒː'rælɪtɪ] imoralidade *f*
immortal [ɪ'mɔːrtl] *adj* imortal
immortality [ɪmɔːr'tælɪtɪ] imortalidade *f*
immune [ɪ'mjuːn] *adj to illness, infection* imune; *from ruling, requirement* isento
im'mune system MED sistema *m* imunológico
immunity [ɪ'mjuːnətɪ] *to infection* imunidade *f*; *from ruling* isenção *f*; ***diplomatic ~*** imunidade *f* diplomática
impact ['ɪmpækt] *n meteorite, new manager etc*: impacto *m*, *Port* impacte *m*
♦ **impact on** *v/t* ***how will this impact on our plans*** qual vai ser o impacto disso nos nossos planos?
impair [ɪm'per] *v/t* prejudicar
impaired [ɪm'perd] *adj* comprometido
impartial [ɪm'pɑːrʃl] *adj* imparcial
impassable [ɪm'pæsəbl] *adj road* intransitável; *river, bridge* intransponível
impasse ['ɪmpæs] *negotiations etc*: impasse *m*
impassioned [ɪm'pæʃnd] *adj speech, plea* comovido
impassive [ɪm'pæsɪv] *adj* impassível
impatience [ɪm'peɪʃəns] impaciência *f*
impatient [ɪm'peɪʃənt] *adj* impaciente
impatiently [ɪm'peɪʃəntlɪ] *adv* impacientemente
impeach [ɪm'piːtʃ] *v/t President* destituir (por processo político-criminal)
impeccable [ɪm'pekəbl] *adj* impecável
impeccably [ɪm'pekəblɪ] *adv dressed, pronounce* impecavelmente
impede [ɪm'piːd] *v/t* impedir
impediment [ɪm'pedɪmənt] *in speech* defeito *m*; ***speech ~*** defeito *m* de fala
impending [ɪm'pendɪŋ] *adj* iminente
impenetrable [ɪm'penɪtrəbl] *adj* impenetrável
imperative [ɪm'perətɪv] **1** *adj* imperativo **2** *n* GRAM imperativo *m*
imperceptible [ɪmpɜːr'septɪbl] *adj* imperceptível
imperfect [ɪm'pɜːrfekt] **1** *adj* imperfeito **2** *n* GRAM imperfeito *m*
imperial [ɪm'pɪrɪəl] *adj* imperial
impersonal [ɪm'pɜːrsnl] *adj* impessoal
impersonate [ɪm'pɜːrsəneɪt] *v/t as a joke* imitar; (*illegally*) fazer-se passar por
impertinence [ɪm'pɜːrtɪnəns] impertinência *f*
impertinent [ɪm'pɜːrtɪnənt] *adj* impertinente
imperturbable [ɪmpər'tɜːrbəbl] *adj*

imperturbável
impervious [ɪm'pɜːrvɪəs] *adj* insensível; **~ to** insensível a
impetuous [ɪm'petʃʊəs] *adj* impetuoso
impetus ['ɪmpətəs] *of campaign etc* ímpeto *m*; ***the election campaign lost a lot of ~*** a campanha eleitoral perdeu bastante impulso
implement ['ɪmplɪmənt] **1** *n* implemento *m* **2** *v/t measures etc* implementar
implicate ['ɪmplɪkeɪt] *v/t* implicar; ***~ s.o. in sth*** implicar alguém em algo
implication [ɪmplɪ'keɪʃn] implicação *f*
implicit [ɪm'plɪsɪt] *adj* implícito; *trust* absoluto
implore [ɪm'plɔːr] *v/t* implorar
imply [ɪm'plaɪ] *v/i* ⟨*pret & pp* ***implied***⟩ implicar
impolite [ɪmpə'laɪt] *adj* indelicado
impoliteness [ɪmpə'laɪtnɪs] *n* falta *f* de educação
import ['ɪmpɔːrt] **1** *n* importação *f* **2** *v/t* importar
importance [ɪm'pɔːrtəns] importância *f*
important [ɪm'pɔːrtənt] *adj* importante
importer [ɪm'pɔːrtər] importador,a *m,f*
impose [ɪm'poʊz] *v/t tax* impor; ***~ oneself on s.o.*** impor-se a alguém
imposing [ɪm'poʊzɪŋ] *adj* imponente
impossibility [ɪmpɑːsɪ'bɪlɪtɪ] impossibilidade *f*
impossible [ɪm'pɑːsɪbəl] *adj* impossível; ***I find it ~ to believe*** eu acho muito difícil acreditar nisso
impostor [ɪm'pɑːstər] impostor,a *m,f*
impotence ['ɪmpətəns] impotência *f*
impotent ['ɪmpətənt] *adj* impotente
impoverished [ɪm'pɑːvərɪʃt] *adj* empobrecido
impractical [ɪm'præktɪkəl] *adj person* pouco prático; *suggestion* impraticável
impress [ɪm'pres] *v/t* impressionar; ***be ~ed by s.o. / sth*** ficar impressionado por alguém / algo; ***I'm not ~ed*** não estou impressionado
impression [ɪm'preʃn] impressão *f*; (*impersonation*) imitação *f*; ***make a good / bad ~ on s.o.*** causar uma boa / má impressão a alguém; ***I get the ~ that …*** tenho a impressão de que …
impressionable [ɪm'preʃənəbl] *adj* impressionável
impressive [ɪm'presɪv] *adj* impressionante
imprint ['ɪmprɪnt] *n credit card*: marca *f*
imprison [ɪm'prɪzn] *v/t* encarcerar
imprisonment [ɪm'prɪznmənt] prisão *f*
improbable [ɪm'prɑːbəbəl] *adj* improvável
improper [ɪm'prɑːpər] *adj behavior* impróprio
improve [ɪm'pruːv] *v/t & v/i* melhorar
improvement [ɪm'pruːvmənt] melhora *f*
improvization [ɪmprəvaɪ'zeɪʃn] *n* improvisação *f*
improvize ['ɪmprəvaɪz] *v/i* improvisar
impudent ['ɪmpjʊdənt] *adj* insolente
impulse ['ɪmpʌls] impulso *m*; ***do sth on an ~*** fazer algo por impulso
'impulse buy compra *f* por impulso
impulsive [ɪm'pʌlsɪv] *adj* impulsivo
impunity [ɪm'pjuːnətɪ] impunidade *f*; ***with ~*** com impunidade
impure [ɪm'pjʊr] *adj* impuro
in [ɪn] **1** *prep* em; ***~ Washington / Recife*** em Washington / Recife; ***~ the street*** na rua; ***~ the box*** na caixa; ***wounded ~ the leg / arm*** ferido na perna / no braço
◊ ***~ 1999*** em 1999; ***~ two hours*** *from now* daqui a duas horas; (*over period of*) em duas horas; ***~ the morning*** de manhã; ***~ the summer*** no verão; ***~ August*** em agosto
◊ ***~ English / Portuguese*** em inglês / português; ***~ a loud voice*** em voz alta; ***~ his style*** no seu estilo; ***~ yellow*** de amarelo
◊ ***~ crossing the road*** (*while*) ao cruzar a estrada; ***~ agreeing to this*** (*by virtue of*) ao concordar com isto
◊ ***~ his novel*** em seu romance; ***~ Faulkner*** em Faulkner
◊ ***three ~ all*** no total de três; ***one ~***

ten um em dez; ***is the express ~ yet?*** (*has the train arrived?*) já chegou o expresso?; ***when the key is ~*** *in its position* quando a chave estiver dentro; ***~ here*** aqui dentro
2 *adj* (*fashionable*, *popular*) na moda
inability [ɪnə'bɪlɪtɪ] incapacidade *f*
inaccessible [ɪnək'sesɪbl] *adj* inacessível
inaccurate [ɪn'ækjʊrət] *adj* inexato
inactive [ɪn'æktɪv] *adj* inativo
inadequate [ɪn'ædɪkwət] *adj* insuficiente
inadvisable [ɪnəd'vaɪzəbl] *adj* desaconselhável
inanimate [ɪn'ænɪmət] *adj* inanimado
inappropriate [ɪnə'proʊprɪət] *adj clothing* impróprio; *behavior* inadequado
inarticulate [ɪnɑːr'tɪkjʊlət] *adj* incapaz de expressar-se; *speech* inarticulado
inaudible [ɪn'ɒːdəbl] *adj* inaudível
inaugural [ɪ'nɒːgjʊrəl] *adj speech* inaugural
inaugurate [ɪ'nɒːgjʊreɪt] *v/t* inaugurar
inborn ['ɪnbɔːrn] *adj* inato
inbreeding ['ɪnbriːdɪŋ] endogamia *f*
inc. *abbr* (*of* ***incorporated***) incorporada
incalculable [ɪn'kælkjʊləbl] *adj damage* incalculável
incapable [ɪn'keɪpəbl] *adj* incapaz; ***be ~ of doing sth*** ser incapaz de fazer algo
incendiary de'vice [ɪn'sendɪərɪ] artefato *m* incendiário
incense[1] ['ɪnsens] *n* incenso *m*
incense[2] [ɪn'sens] *v/t* exasperar
incentive [ɪn'sentɪv] incentivo *m*
incessant [ɪn'sesnt] *adj* incessante
incessantly [ɪn'sesntlɪ] *adv* incessantemente
incest ['ɪnsest] incesto *m*
inch [ɪntʃ] polegada *f*
incident ['ɪnsɪdənt] incidente *m*
incidental [ɪnsɪ'dentl] *adj* sem importância; ***~ expenses*** despesas *fpl* diversas
incidentally [ɪnsɪ'dentlɪ] *adv* a propósito
incinerator [ɪn'sɪnəreɪtər] incinerador *m*
incision [ɪn'sɪʒn] incisão *f*
incisive [ɪn'saɪsɪv] *adj mind*, *analysis* incisivo
incite [ɪn'saɪt] *v/t* incitar; ***~ s.o. to do sth*** incitar alguém a fazer algo
inclement [ɪn'klemənt] *adj weather* inclemente
inclination [ɪnklɪ'neɪʃn] (*tendency*, *liking*) inclinação *f*; ***I have no ~ to see him again*** eu não tenho a menor vontade de vê-lo novamente
incline [ɪn'klaɪn] *v/t* ***be ~d to do sth*** estar propenso a fazer algo
inclose *etc* → ***enclose***
include [ɪn'kluːd] *v/t* incluir
including [ɪn'kluːdɪŋ] *prep* inclusive
inclusive [ɪn'kluːsɪv] **1** *adj price* total **2** *prep* ***~ of*** incluindo **3** *adv* tudo incluso; ***from Monday to Thursday ~*** de segunda a quinta-feira inclusive
incoherent *adj* incoerente
income ['ɪnkəm] renda *f*
'income tax imposto *m* de renda, *Port* imposto *m* sobre o rendimento
incoming ['ɪnkʌmɪŋ] *adj flight* de chegada; *tide* enchente; *phonecall*, *mail* de entrada; *president* que entra
incomparable [ɪn'kɑːmpərəbl] *adj* incomparável
incompatibility [ɪnkəmpætɪ'bɪlɪtɪ] incompatibilidade *f*
incompatible [ɪnkəm'pætɪbl] *adj* incompatível
incompetence [ɪn'kɑːmpɪtəns] incompetência *f*
incompetent [ɪn'kɑːmpɪtənt] *adj* incompetente
incomplete [ɪnkəm'pliːt] *adj* incompleto
incomprehensible [ɪnkɑːmprɪ'hensɪbl] *adj* incompreensível
inconceivable [ɪnkən'siːvəbl] *adj* inconcebível
inconclusive [ɪnkən'kluːsɪv] *adj* inconcludente
incongruous [ɪn'kɑːŋgrʊəs] *adj* incongruente
inconsiderate [ɪnkən'sɪdərət] *adj* inconsiderado
inconsistent [ɪnkən'sɪstənt] *adj* in-

consistente
inconsolable [ɪnkən'souləbl] *adj* inconsolável
inconspicuous [ɪnkən'spɪkjʊəs] *adj* discreto; ***make oneself ~*** fazer-se discreto
inconvenience [ɪnkən'viːnɪəns] *n* inconveniência *f*
inconvenient [ɪnkən'viːnɪənt] *adj* inconveniente
incorporate [ɪn'kɔːrpəreɪt] *v/t* incorporar
incorporated [ɪn'kɔːrpəreɪtɪd] *adj* COM incorporada
incorrect [ɪnkə'rekt] *adj* incorreto
incorrectly [ɪnkə'rektlɪ] *adv* incorretamente
incorrigible [ɪn'kɑːrɪdʒəbl] *adj* incorrigível
increase [ɪn'kriːs] **1** *v/t & v/i* aumentar **2** *n* aumento *m*
increasing [ɪn'kriːsɪŋ] *adj* crescente
increasingly [ɪn'kriːsɪŋlɪ] *adv* progressivamente
incredible [ɪn'kredɪbl] *adj* (*amazing, very good*) incrível
incredibly [ɪn'kredɪblɪ] *adv* incrivelmente; ***~, nobody was hurt*** incrivelmente ninguém se feriu
incriminate [ɪn'krɪmɪneɪt] *v/t* incriminar; ***~ oneself*** incriminar-se
incubator ['ɪŋkjʊbeɪtər] incubadora *f*
incur [ɪn'kɜːr] *v/t* ⟨*pret & pp* ***incurred***⟩ incorrer; *expenses, debts* contrair
incurable [ɪn'kjʊrəbl] *adj* incurável
indebted [ɪn'detɪd] *adj* ***be ~ to s.o.*** estar em dívida com alguém
indecent [ɪn'diːsnt] *adj* indecente
indecisive [ɪndɪ'saɪsɪv] *adj* indeciso
indecisiveness [ɪndɪ'saɪsɪvnɪs] indecisão *f*
indeed [ɪn'diːd] *adv* (*in fact*) de fato; (*yes, agreeing*) sem dúvida; ***very much ~*** muitíssimo
indefinable [ɪndɪ'faɪnəbl] *adj* indefinível
indefinite [ɪn'defɪnɪt] *adj* indefinido; ***~ article*** GRAM artigo *m* indefinido
indefinitely [ɪn'defɪnɪtlɪ] *adv* indefinidamente
indelicate [ɪn'delɪkət] *adj* indelicado
indent 1 ['ɪndent] *n in text* parágrafo *m* recuado **2** [ɪn'dent] *v/t line* recuar
independence [ɪndɪ'pendəns] independência *f*
Inde'pendence Day Dia *m* da Independência
independent [ɪndɪ'pendənt] *adj* independente
independently [ɪndɪ'pendəntlɪ] *adv deal with* independentemente; ***~ of*** independentemente de
indescribable [ɪndɪ'skraɪbəbl] *adj also* (*very bad*) indescritível
indescribably [ɪndɪ'skraɪbəblɪ] *adv bad, beautiful* indescritivelmente
indestructible [ɪndɪ'strʌktəbl] *adj* indestrutível
indeterminate [ɪndɪ'tɜːrmɪnət] *adj* indeterminado
index ['ɪndeks] *for book* índice *m*
'index card ficha *f* **'index finger** dedo *m* indicador **index-linked** *adj* indexado
India ['ɪndɪə] Índia *f*
Indian ['ɪndɪən] **1** *adj* indiano **2** *n* indiano,-a *m,f*; *American* índio,-a *m,f*
Indian 'summer últimos dias *mpl* quentes de outono
indicate ['ɪndɪkeɪt] **1** *v/t* indicar **2** *v/i Brit driving*: ligar o pisca-pisca
indication [ɪndɪ'keɪʃn] indicação *f*
indicator ['ɪndɪkeɪtər] *Brit car*: pisca-pisca *m*
indict [ɪn'daɪt] *v/t* indiciar
indifference [ɪn'dɪfrəns] indiferença *f*
indifferent [ɪn'dɪfrənt] *adj* indiferente; (*mediocre*) medíocre
indigestible [ɪndɪ'dʒestɪbl] *adj* indigesto
indigestion [ɪndɪ'dʒestʃn] indigestão *f*
indignant [ɪn'dɪgnənt] *adj* indignado
indignation [ɪndɪg'neɪʃn] indignação *f*
indirect [ɪndɪ'rekt] *adj* indireto
indirectly [ɪndɪ'rektlɪ] *adv* indiretamente
indiscreet [ɪndɪ'skriːt] *adj* indiscreto
indiscretion [ɪndɪ'skreʃn] indiscrição *f*
indiscriminate [ɪndɪ'skrɪmɪnət] *adj* indiscriminado
indispensable [ɪndɪ'spensəbl] *adj* indispensável

indisposed [ɪndɪ'spoʊzd] *adj* (*not well*) indisposto
indisputable [ɪndɪ'spjuːtəbl] *adj* incontestável
indisputably [ɪndɪ'spjuːtəblɪ] *adv* incontestavelmente
indistinct [ɪndɪ'stɪŋkt] *adj* indistinto
indistinguishable [ɪndɪ'stɪŋgwɪʃəbl] *adj* indistinguível
individual [ɪndɪ'vɪdʒʊəl] **1** *n* indivíduo *m* **2** *adj* (*separate*) individual; (*personal*) pessoal
individualist [ɪndɪ'vɪdʒʊəlɪst] *n* individualista *m/f*
individually [ɪndɪ'vɪdʒʊəlɪ] *adv* individualmente
indivisible [ɪndɪ'vɪzɪbl] *adj* indivisível
indoctrinate [ɪn'dɑːktrɪneɪt] *v/t* doutrinar
indolence ['ɪndələns] indolência *f*
indolent ['ɪndələnt] *adj* indolente
Indonesia [ɪndə'niːʒə] Indonésia *f*
Indonesian [ɪndə'niːʒən] **1** *adj* indonésio **2** *n* indonésio,-a *m,f*
indoor ['ɪndɔːr] *adj* interno; *arena* coberto; *games*, *sport* de salão; **~ athletics** atletismo de salão
indoors [ɪn'dɔːrz] *adv* em local fechado; **stay ~** ficar dentro de casa
indorse → **endorse**
indulge [ɪn'dʌldʒ] *v/t oneself*, *one's tastes* satisfazer; **~ in sth** entregar-se a algo
indulgence [ɪn'dʌldʒəns] *tastes etc*: satisfação *f*; (*laxity*) indulgência *f*
indulgent [ɪn'dʌldʒənt] *adj* (*not strict enough*) indulgente
industrial [ɪn'dʌstrɪəl] *adj* industrial; **~ action** ação *f* industrial
industrial 'dispute conflito *m* trabalhista
industrialist [ɪn'dʌstrɪəlɪst] industrial *m/f*
industrialize [ɪn'dʌstrɪəlaɪz] **1** *v/t* industrializar **2** *v/i* industrializar-se
industrial 'waste lixo *m* industrial
industrious [ɪn'dʌstrɪəs] *adj* trabalhador
industry ['ɪndəstrɪ] indústria *f*
ineffective [ɪnɪ'fektɪv] *adj* ineficaz
ineffectual [ɪnɪ'fektʃʊəl] *adj person* inútil
inefficient [ɪnɪ'fɪʃənt] *adj* ineficiente
ineligible [ɪn'elɪdʒɪbl] *adj* POL inelegível; **be ~ for sth** não ter o direito a algo
inept [ɪ'nept] *adj* inepto
inequality [ɪnɪ'kwɑːlɪtɪ] desigualdade *f*
inescapable [ɪnɪ'skeɪpəbl] *adj* inevitável
inestimable [ɪn'estɪməbl] *adj* inestimável
inevitable [ɪn'evɪtəbl] *adj* inevitável
inevitably [ɪn'evɪtəblɪ] *adv* inevitavelmente
inexcusable [ɪnɪk'skjuːzəbl] *adj* imperdoável
inexhaustible [ɪnɪg'zɒːstəbl] *adj supply* inesgotável
inexpensive [ɪnɪk'spensɪv] *adj* barato
inexperienced [ɪnɪk'spɪrɪənst] *adj* inexperiente
inexplicable [ɪnɪk'splɪkəbl] *adj* inexplicável
inexpressible [ɪnɪk'spresɪbl] *adj joy* indescritível
infallible [ɪn'fælɪbl] *adj* infalível
infamous ['ɪnfəməs] *adj* infame
infancy ['ɪnfənsɪ] *person*: infância *f*; *state*, *institution*: estágio *m* inicial
infant ['ɪnfənt] (*child*) criança *f*; (*baby*) bebê *m*; **~ mortality rate** taxa *f* de mortalidade infantil
infantile ['ɪnfəntaɪl] *adj pej* infantil
infantry ['ɪnfəntrɪ] infantaria *f*
infantry 'soldier soldado *m* de infantaria
'infant school pré-escola *f*
infatuated [ɪn'fætjuːeɪtɪd] *adj* apaixonado; **be ~ with s.o.** estar apaixonado por alguém
infect [ɪn'fekt] *v/t* infectar; *person* contagiar; **become ~ed** *wound* ficar infeccionado; *person* contagiar-se
infection [ɪn'fekʃn] infecção *f*
infectious [ɪn'fekʃəs] *adj disease* infeccioso; *fig laughter* contagiante
infer [ɪn'fɜːr] *v/t* ⟨*pret & pp* **inferred**⟩ deduzir; **~ X from Y** deduzir X de Y
inferior [ɪn'fɪrɪər] *adj quality* inferior; *rank*, *military*: subalterno
inferiority [ɪnfɪrɪ'ɑːrətɪ] inferioridade *f*

inferi'ority complex complexo *m* de inferioridade
infertile [ɪn'fɜːrtl] *adj* infértil; *woman, man* estéril
infertility [ɪnfər'tɪlɪtɪ] infertilidade *f*
infidelity [ɪnfɪ'delɪtɪ] infidelidade *f*
infiltrate ['ɪnfɪltreɪt] *v/t* infiltrar-se em
infinite ['ɪnfɪnət] *adj* infinito
infinitive [ɪn'fɪnətɪv] infinitivo *m*
infinity [ɪn'fɪnətɪ] infinito *m*
infirm [ɪn'fɜːrm] *adj* enfermo
infirmary [ɪn'fɜːrmərɪ] enfermaria *f*
infirmity [ɪn'fɜːrmətɪ] enfermidade *f*
inflame [ɪn'fleɪm] *v/t* inflamar
inflammable [ɪn'flæməbl] *adj* inflamável
inflammation [ɪnflə'meɪʃn] MED inflamação *f*
inflatable [ɪn'fleɪtəbl] *adj dinghy* inflável
inflate [ɪn'fleɪt] *v/t tire, dinghy* encher; *economy* inflar
inflation [ɪn'fleɪʃən] inflação *f*
inflationary [ɪn'fleɪʃənərɪ] *adj* inflacionário
inflection [ɪn'flekʃn] *of voice* inflexão *f*
inflexible [ɪn'fleksɪbl] *adj attitude, person* inflexível
inflict [ɪn'flɪkt] *v/t* **~ sth on s.o.** infligir algo a alguém
'in-flight *adj* **~ entertainment** entretenimento *m* durante o vôo
influence ['ɪnfluəns] **1** *n* influência *f*; **be a good / bad ~ on s.o.** ter uma boa / má influência sobre alguém **2** *v/t s.o.'s thinking, decision* influenciar
influential [ɪnflʊ'enʃl] *adj* influente
influenza [ɪnflʊ'enzə] gripe *f*
infomercial ['ɪnfoʊmɜːrʃl] anúncio *m* informativo
inform [ɪn'fɔːrm] **1** *v/t* informar; **~ s.o. about sth** informar alguém sobre algo; **please keep me ~ed** por favor, mantenha-me informado **2** *v/i* delatar; **~ on s.o.** delatar alguém
informal [ɪn'fɔːrməl] *adj* informal
informality [ɪnfɔːr'mælɪtɪ] informalidade *f*
informant [ɪn'fɔːrmənt] informante *m/f*
information [ɪnfər'meɪʃn] informação *f*
information 'science informática *f* **information 'scientist** cientista *m/f* em informática **information tech'nology** tecnologia *f* de informática
informative [ɪn'fɔːrmətɪv] *adj* informativo
informer [ɪn'fɔːrmər] denunciante *m/f*
infra-red [ɪnfrə'red] *adj* infravermelho *m*
infrastructure ['ɪnfrəstrʌktʃər] infra-estrutura *f*
infrequent [ɪn'friːkwənt] *adj* pouco freqüente
infuriate [ɪn'fjʊrɪeɪt] *v/t* enfurecer
infuriating [ɪn'fjʊrɪeɪtɪŋ] *adj* enfurecedor
infuse [ɪn'fjuːz] *v/i* **let the tea ~** deixar o chá em infusão
infusion [ɪn'fjuːʒn] (*herb tea*) infusão *f*
ingenious [ɪn'dʒiːnɪəs] *adj* engenhoso
ingenuity [ɪndʒɪ'nuːətɪ] engenhosidade *f*
ingot ['ɪŋgət] lingote *m*
ingratiate [ɪn'greɪʃɪeɪt] *v/t* **~ oneself with s.o.** cair nas boas graças de alguém
ingratitude [ɪn'grætɪtuːd] ingratidão *f*
ingredient [ɪn'griːdɪənt] *for cooking, also fig* ingrediente *m*
'in-group grupo *m* fechado
inhabit [ɪn'hæbɪt] *v/t* habitar
inhabitable [ɪn'hæbɪtəbl] *adj* habitável
inhabitant [ɪn'hæbɪtənt] habitante *m/f*
inhale [ɪn'heɪl] **1** *v/t* inalar **2** *v/i when smoking* tragar
inhaler [ɪn'heɪlər] inalador *m*
inherit [ɪn'herɪt] *v/t* herdar
inheritance [ɪn'herɪtəns] herança *f*
inhibit [ɪn'hɪbɪt] *v/t* inibir
inhibited [ɪn'hɪbɪtɪd] *adj* inibido
inhibition [ɪnhɪ'bɪʃn] inibição *f*
inhospitable [ɪnhɑː'spɪtəbl] *adj* inóspito
'in-house 1 *adj* da casa; **our ~ translators** nossos tradutores efetivos **2** *adv work* na empresa

I

inhuman [ɪn'hjuːmən] *adj* desumano
initial [ɪ'nɪʃl] **1** *adj* inicial **2** *npl* **~s** iniciais *fpl* **3** *v/t* (*write initials on*) rubricar
initially [ɪ'nɪʃlɪ] *adv* inicialmente
initiate [ɪ'nɪʃɪeɪt] *v/t* iniciar
initiation [ɪnɪʃɪ'eɪʃn] iniciação *f*
initiative [ɪ'nɪʃətɪv] iniciativa *f*; ***do sth on one's own ~*** fazer algo por iniciativa própria
inject [ɪn'dʒekt] *v/t medicine*, *fuel*, *capital* injetar
injection [ɪn'dʒekʃn] MED, *also of fuel*, *capital* injeção *f*
'in-joke ***it's an ~*** é uma piada particular
injure ['ɪndʒər] *v/t* ferir
injured ['ɪndʒərd] **1** *adj leg* machucado; *feelings* magoado **2** *npl* ***the ~*** os feridos *mpl*
injury ['ɪndʒərɪ] ferimento *m*
'injury time SPORT desconto *m*
injustice [ɪn'dʒʌstɪs] injustiça *f*
ink [ɪŋk] tinta *f*
inkjet, **inkjet 'printer** impressora *f* jato de tinta
inland ['ɪnlənd] *adj* do interior; *mail*, *trade* interno
in-laws ['ɪnlɒːz] *npl* parentes *mpl* por afinidade
inlay ['ɪnleɪ] *n* incrustação *f*
inlet ['ɪnlet] *sea*: enseada *f*, *machine*: entrada *f*
inmate ['ɪnmeɪt] *prison*: presidiário,-a *m,f*, *mental hospital*: interno,-a *m,f*
inn [ɪn] hospedaria *f*
innate [ɪ'neɪt] *adj* inato
inner ['ɪnər] *adj* interno
inner 'city centro *m* urbano; ***~ city decay*** degradação *f* dos centros urbanos
'innermost *adj* recôndito
'inner tube câmara *f* de ar
innocence ['ɪnəsəns] inocência *f*
innocent ['ɪnəsənt] *adj* inocente
innocuous [ɪ'nɑːkjʊəs] *adj* inócuo
innovation [ɪnə'veɪʃn] inovação *f*
innovative ['ɪnəvətɪv] *adj* inovador
innovator ['ɪnəveɪtər] inovador,a *m,f*
innumerable [ɪ'nuːmərəbl] *adj* inumerável
inoculate [ɪ'nɑːkjʊleɪt] *v/t* inocular
inoculation [ɪ'nɑːkjʊ'leɪʃn] inoculação *f*
inoffensive [ɪnə'fensɪv] *adj* inofensivo
inorganic [ɪnɔːr'gænɪk] *adj* inorgânico
'in-patient paciente *m/f* interno,-a
input ['ɪnpʊt] **1** *n into project etc* aporte *m*; COMPUT entrada *f* **2** *v/t* ⟨*pret & pp* ***inputted*** *or* ***input***⟩ *into project* contribuir; COMPUT introduzir
inquest ['ɪnkwest] inquérito *m*
inquire [ɪn'kwaɪr] *v/i* perguntar; ***~ into sth*** investigar algo
inquiry ['ɪnkwərɪ] pergunta *f*
inquisitive [ɪn'kwɪzətɪv] *adj* perguntador
insane [ɪn'seɪn] *adj* louco
insanitary [ɪn'sænɪterɪ] *adj* anti-higiênico
insanity [ɪn'sænɪtɪ] loucura *f*
insatiable [ɪn'seɪʃəbl] *adj* insaciável
inscription [ɪn'skrɪpʃn] inscrição *f*
inscrutable [ɪn'skruːtəbl] *adj* inescrutável
insect ['ɪnsekt] inseto *m*
insecticide [ɪn'sektɪsaɪd] inseticida *m*
'insect repellent repelente *m* de insetos
insecure [ɪnsɪ'kjʊr] *adj* inseguro
insecurity [ɪnsɪ'kjʊrɪtɪ] insegurança *f*
insensitive [ɪn'sensɪtɪv] *adj* insensível
insensitivity [ɪnsensɪ'tɪvɪtɪ] insensibilidade *f*
inseparable [ɪn'seprəbl] *adj two issues*, *two people* inseparável
insert **1** ['ɪnsɜːrt] *n magazine etc*: encarte *m* **2** [ɪn'sɜːrt] *v/t* inserir; ***~ sth into sth*** inserir algo em algo
insertion [ɪn'sɜːrʃn] inserção *f*
inside [ɪn'saɪd] **1** *n house*, *box*: interior *m*; ***somebody on the ~*** alguém de dentro; ***~ out*** do lado avesso; ***turn sth ~ out*** virar algo do avesso; ***know sth ~ out*** saber algo muito bem **2** *prep* dentro de; ***~ the house*** dentro da casa; ***~ of 2 hours*** em menos de 2 horas **3** *adv stay*, *remain* dentro; *go*, *carry* para dentro; ***we went ~*** fomos para dentro **4** *adj* interno; ***~ in-***

formation informação *f* privilegiada; ***~ pocket*** bolso *m* interno
'inside lane SPORT faixa *f* interna; *Brit road*: pista *f* da direita (*circulação pela direita*)
insider [ɪn'saɪdər] pessoa *f* com acesso a informações confidenciais
in'sider dealing FIN uso *m* de informação privilegiada
insides [ɪn'saɪdz] *npl* tripas *fpl*
insidious [ɪn'sɪdɪəs] *adj* insidioso
insight ['ɪnsaɪt] insight *m*
insignificant [ɪnsɪg'nɪfɪkənt] *adj* insignificante
insincere [ɪnsɪn'sɪr] *adj* insincero
insincerity [ɪnsɪn'serɪtɪ] insinceridade *f*
insinuate [ɪn'sɪnjʊeɪt] *v/t* (*imply*) insinuar
insist [ɪn'sɪst] *v/i* insistir; ***please keep it, I ~*** por favor, fique com isto, eu insisto
♦**insist on** *v/t* insistir em
insistent [ɪn'sɪstənt] *adj* insistente
insolent ['ɪnsələnt] *adj* insolente
insoluble [ɪn'sɑːljʊbl] *adj problem, substance* insolúvel
insolvent [ɪn'sɑːlvənt] *adj* insolvente
insomnia [ɪn'sɑːmnɪə] insônia *f*
inspect [ɪn'spekt] *v/t* inspecionar
inspection [ɪn'spekʃn] inspeção *f*
inspector [ɪn'spektər] *factory, buses*: fiscal *m*; *police, school*: inspetor,a *m,f*
inspiration [ɪnspə'reɪʃn] *also* (*very good idea*) inspiração *f*
inspire [ɪn'spaɪr] *v/t respect etc* inspirar; ***be ~d by s.o. / sth*** ficar inspirado por alguém / algo
instability [ɪnstə'bɪlɪtɪ] *of character, economy* instabilidade *f*
install [ɪn'stɒːl] *v/t computer, phones, software* instalar
installation [ɪnstə'leɪʃn] *new equipment, software*: instalação *f*; ***military ~*** instalação *f* militar
installment [ɪn'stɒːlmənt] *Am story, TV drama etc*: episódio *m*; (*payment*) prestação *f*; ***pay in ~s*** pagar em prestações
in'stallment plan *Am* plano *m* de pagamento a prazo
instalment *Brit* → ***installment***
instance ['ɪnstəns] (*example*) exemplo *m*; ***for ~*** por exemplo; ***in many ~s*** em muitos casos
instant ['ɪnstənt] **1** *adj* instantâneo **2** *n* instante *m*; ***in an ~*** num instante
instantaneous [ɪnstən'teɪnɪəs] *adj* instantâneo
instant 'coffee café *m* instantâneo
'instant message mensagem *f* instantânea
instantly ['ɪnstəntlɪ] *adv* instantaneamente
instead [ɪn'sted] *adv* invés; ***~ of*** em vez de; ***would you like coffee ~?*** você gostaria de um café em vez disso?; ***I'll take that one ~*** vou levar aquele em vez deste
instep ['ɪnstep] peito *m* do pé
instinct ['ɪnstɪŋkt] instinto *m*
instinctive [ɪn'stɪŋktɪv] *adj* instintivo
institute ['ɪnstɪtuːt] **1** *n* instituto *m*; (*special home*) asilo *m* **2** *v/t new law, inquiry* instituir
institution [ɪnstɪ'tuːʃn] instituição *f*; ***~ of an inquiry*** abertura *f* de um inquérito
instruct [ɪn'strʌkt] *v/t* (*order*) instruir; (*teach*) ensinar; ***~ s.o. to do sth*** (*order*) instruir alguém a fazer algo
instruction [ɪn'strʌkʃn] instrução *f*; ***~s for use*** instruções *fpl* de uso
in'struction manual manual *m* de instruções
instructive [ɪn'strʌktɪv] *adj* instrutivo
instructor [ɪn'strʌktər] instrutor,a *m,f*
instrument ['ɪnstrʊmənt] MUS, *also* (*gadget, tool*) instrumento *m*
insubordinate [ɪnsə'bɔːrdɪneɪt] *adj* insubordinado
insufficient [ɪnsə'fɪʃnt] *adj* insuficiente
insulate ['ɪnsəleɪt] *v/t* ELEC isolar; *against cold* isolar termicamente
insulating tape *Brit* → ***friction tape***
insulation [ɪnsə'leɪʃn] ELEC isolamento *m*; *against cold* isolamento *m* térmico
insulin ['ɪnsəlɪn] insulina *f*
insult 1 ['ɪnsʌlt] *n* insulto *m* **2** [ɪn'sʌlt] *v/t* insultar
insurance [ɪn'ʃʊrəns] seguro *m*
in'surance company companhia *f*

de seguro **in'surance policy** apólice *f* de seguro **in'surance premium** prêmio *m* de seguro
insure [ɪn'ʃʊr] *v/t* segurar
insured [ɪn'ʃʊrd] **1** *adj* segurado; ***be ~*** estar segurado **2** *n* ***the ~*** o/a assegurado,-a
insurmountable [ɪnsər'maʊntəbl] *adj* insuperável
intact [ɪn'tækt] *adj* (*not damaged*) intacto
intake ['ɪnteɪk] *of college etc* alunos *mpl* matriculados; *of food* ingestão *f*
integrate ['ɪntɪgreɪt] *v/t* integrar
integrated 'circuit ['ɪntɪgreɪtɪd] *adj* circuito *m* integrado
integrity [ɪn'tegrətɪ] (*honesty*) integridade *f*
intellect ['ɪntəlekt] intelecto *m*
intellectual [ɪntə'lektʊəl] **1** *adj* intelectual **2** *n* intelectual *m/f*
intelligence [ɪn'telɪdʒəns] inteligência *f*; (*information*) informações *fpl*
in'telligence officer agente *m* do serviço de inteligência
in'telligence service serviço *m* de inteligência
intelligent [ɪn'telɪdʒənt] *adj* inteligente
intelligible [ɪn'telɪdʒəbl] *adj* inteligível
intend [ɪn'tend] *v/i* pretender; ***~ to do sth*** (*do on purpose*) intencionar fazer algo; (*plan to do*) planejar fazer algo; ***that's not what I ~ed*** isto não é o que eu pretendia
intense [ɪn'tens] *adj sensation, pleasure, heat, pressure* intenso; *personality* emotivo; *concentration* profundo
intensify [ɪn'tensɪfaɪ] ⟨*pret & pp* ***intensified***⟩ **1** *v/t effect, pressure* intensificar **2** *v/i pain, fighting* intensificar-se
intensity [ɪn'tensətɪ] intensidade *f*
intensive [ɪn'tensɪv] *adj* intensivo
intensive 'care, intensive 'care unit MED UTI *f* (= unidade *f* de terapia intensiva)
in'tensive course *of language study* curso *m* intensivo
intent [ɪn'tent] *adj* resolvido; ***be ~ on doing sth*** (*determined to do*) estar decidido a fazer algo; (*concentrating on*) estar fazendo algo muito concentrado
intention [ɪn'tenʃn] intenção *f*; ***I have no ~ of …*** (*refuse to*) não tenho a intenção de …
intentional [ɪn'tenʃənl] *adj* intencional
intentionally [ɪn'tenʃnlɪ] *adv* intencionalmente
interact [ɪntər'ækt] *v/i* interagir
interaction [ɪntər'ækʃn] interação *f*
interactive [ɪntər'æktɪv] *adj* interativo
intercede [ɪntər'siːd] *v/i* interceder
intercept [ɪntər'sept] *v/t ball, message, missile* interceptar
interchange [ɪntər'ʧeɪndʒ] *n of highways* trevo *m*
interchangeable [ɪntər'ʧeɪndʒəbl] *adj* intercambiável
intercom ['ɪntərkɑːm] intercomunicador *m*
intercourse ['ɪntərkɔːrs] *sexual* relação *f* sexual
interdependent [ɪntərdɪ'pendənt] *adj* interdependente
interest ['ɪntrəst] **1** *n* interesse *m*; *financial* juros *mpl*; ***take an ~ in sth*** interessar-se por algo **2** *v/t* interessar; ***does that offer ~ you?*** esta oferta lhe interessa?
interested ['ɪntrəstɪd] *adj* interessado; ***be ~ in sth*** estar interessado em algo
interest-free 'loan empréstimo *m* sem juros
interesting ['ɪntrəstɪŋ] *adj* interessante
'interest rate FIN taxa *f* de juros
interface ['ɪntərfeɪs] **1** *n* interface *f* **2** *v/i* funcionar conjuntamente
interfere [ɪntər'fɪr] *v/i* interferir
♦**interfere with** *v/t controls* mexer com; *plans* interferir em
interference [ɪntər'fɪrəns] *also on radio* interferência *f*
interior [ɪn'tɪrɪər] **1** *adj* interno **2** *n house, country*: interior *m*; ***Department of the Interior*** *Am* Ministério *m* do Interior
interior 'decorator decorador,a *m,f* de interiores **interior de'sign** deco-

ração *f* de interiores **interior de'signer** arquiteto,-a *m,f* de interior
interlude ['ɪntərluːd] *at theater, concert* intervalo *m*; (*period*) interlúdio *m*
intermarry [ɪntər'mærɪ] *v/i* ⟨*pret & pp* ***intermarried***⟩ casar-se entre si
intermediary [ɪntər'miːdɪerɪ] *n* intermediário,-a *m,f*
intermediate [ɪntər'miːdɪət] *adj* intermediário
intermission [ɪntər'mɪʃn] *theater*: intervalo *m*
intern [ɪn'tɜːrn] *v/t* internar
internal [ɪn'tɜːrnl] *adj* interno; ***~ combustion engine*** motor *m* de combustão interna
internally [ɪn'tɜːrnəlɪ] *adv* internamente
Internal 'Revenue, **Internal 'Revenue Service** *Am* Receita *f* federal, *Port* fisco *m*
international [ɪntər'næʃnl] **1** *adj* internacional **2** *n* (*game*) partida *f* internacional; (*player*) jogador,a *m,f* internacional
International Court of 'Justice Corte *f* Internacional de Justiça
internationally [ɪntər'næʃnəlɪ] *adv* internacionalmente
Internet ['ɪntərnet] Internet *f*; ***on the ~*** na Internet
'Internet café cibercafé *m*
internist [ɪn'tɜːrnɪst] *Am* generalista *m/f*
interpret [ɪn'tɜːrprɪt] *v/t & v/i* interpretar
interpretation [ɪntɜːrprɪ'teɪʃn] interpretação *f*
interpreter [ɪn'tɜːrprɪtər] intérprete *m/f*
interrelated [ɪntərɪ'leɪtɪd] *adj facts* inter-relacionado
interrogate [ɪn'terəgeɪt] *v/t* interrogar
interrogation [ɪnterə'geɪʃn] *of suspects* interrogatório *m*
interrogative [ɪntə'rɑːgətɪv] *adj* GRAM interrogativo
interrogator [ɪn'terəgeɪtər] interrogador,a *m,f*
interrupt [ɪntə'rʌpt] *v/t & v/i* interromper
interruption [ɪntə'rʌpʃn] interrupção *f*
intersect [ɪntər'sekt] **1** *v/t* cruzar **2** *v/i* cruzar-se
intersection ['ɪntərsekʃn] (*crossroads*) cruzamento *m*
interstate ['ɪntərsteɪt] *n Am* estrada *f* interestadual
interval ['ɪntərvl] intervalo *m*
intervention [ɪntər'venʃn] intervenção *f*
interview ['ɪntərvjuː] **1** *n* TV, *paper, job*: entrevista *f* **2** *v/t* entrevistar
interviewee [ɪntərvjuː'iː] TV, *for job* entrevistado,-a *m,f*
interviewer ['ɪntərvjuːər] TV, *for paper, job* entrevistador,a *m,f*
intestine [ɪn'testɪn] intestino *m*
intimacy ['ɪntɪməsɪ] intimidade *f*; *sexual* relações *fpl* íntimas
intimate ['ɪntɪmət] *adj* íntimo
intimidate [ɪn'tɪmɪdeɪt] *v/t* intimidar
intimidation [ɪntɪmɪ'deɪʃn] intimidação *f*
into ['ɪntʊ] *prep* em; ***he put it ~ his suitcase*** ele colocou-o em sua mala; ***translate ~ English*** traduzir para o inglês; ***be ~ sth*** *fam* (*like*) gostar muito de algo; (*be involved with*) estar por dentro de algo; ***when you're ~ the job*** quando você estiver familiarizado com o trabalho
intolerable [ɪn'tɑːlərəbl] *adj* intolerável
intolerant [ɪn'tɑːlərənt] *adj* intolerante
intoxicated [ɪn'tɑːksɪkeɪtɪd] *adj* intoxicado
intransitive [ɪn'trænsɪtɪv] *adj* intransitivo
intravenous [ɪntrə'viːnəs] *adj* intravenoso
intrepid [ɪn'trepɪd] *adj* intrépido
intricate ['ɪntrɪkət] *adj* complexo
intrigue **1** ['ɪntriːg] *n* intriga *f* **2** [ɪn'triːg] *v/t* intrigar; ***I would be ~d to know …*** eu ficaria curioso em saber …
intriguing [ɪn'triːgɪŋ] *adj* intrigante
introduce [ɪntrə'duːs] *v/t* apresentar; *new technique etc* introduzir; ***may I ~ …?*** posso apresentar …?
introduction [ɪntrə'dʌkʃn] *to person*:

I

apresentação *f*; *to new food, sport etc* iniciação *f*; *in book, of new technique etc* introdução *f*
introvert ['ɪntrəvɜːrt] *n* introvertido,-a *m,f*
intrude [ɪn'truːd] *v/i* intrometer-se
intruder [ɪn'truːdər] intruso,-a *m,f*
intrusion [ɪn'truːʒn] intromissão *f*
intuition [ɪntuː'ɪʃn] intuição *f*
invade [ɪn'veɪd] *v/t* invadir
invalid[1] [ɪn'vælɪd] *adj* inválido
invalid[2] ['ɪnvəlɪd] *n* MED inválido,-a *m,f*
invalidate [ɪn'vælɪdeɪt] *v/t claim, theory* invalidar
invaluable [ɪn'væljʊbl] *adj help, contributor* inestimável
invariably [ɪn'veɪrɪəblɪ] *adv* (*always*) sempre
invasion [ɪn'veɪʒn] invasão *f*
invent [ɪn'vent] *v/t* inventar
invention [ɪn'venʃn] invenção *f*
inventive [ɪn'ventɪv] *adj* inventivo
inventor [ɪn'ventər] inventor,a *m,f*
inventory ['ɪnvəntoʊrɪ] inventário *m*
inverse [ɪn'vɜːrs] *adj order* inverso
invert [ɪn'vɜːrt] *v/t* inverter
invertebrate [ɪn'vɜːrtɪbrət] *n* invertebrado *m*
inverted 'commas [ɪn'vɜːrtɪd] *npl Brit* aspas *fpl*
invest [ɪn'vest] *v/t & v/i* investir
investigate [ɪn'vestɪgeɪt] *v/t* investigar
investigation [ɪnvestɪ'geɪʃn] investigação *f*
investigative 'journalism [ɪn'vestɪgətɪv] jornalismo *m* investigativo
investment [ɪn'vestmənt] investimento *m*
investor [ɪn'vestər] investidor,a *m,f*
invigorating [ɪn'vɪgəreɪtɪŋ] *adj climate* revigorante
invincible [ɪn'vɪnsəbl] *adj* invencível
invisible [ɪn'vɪzɪbl] *adj* invisível
invitation [ɪnvɪ'teɪʃn] convite *m*
invite [ɪn'vaɪt] *v/t* convidar; ***can I ~ you for a meal?*** posso convidá-lo para jantar / almoçar?
◆**invite in** *v/t* convidar para entrar
invoice ['ɪnvɔɪs] **1** *n* fatura *f* **2** *v/t customer* faturar
involuntary [ɪn'vɑːlənterɪ] *adj* involuntário
involve [ɪn'vɑːlv] *v/t hard work, expense* implicar; (*concern*) envolver; ***what does it ~?*** o que isto envolve?; ***get ~d with sth*** estar envolvido em algo; ***get ~d with s.o.*** *emotionally, romantically* estar envolvido com alguém
involved [ɪn'vɑːlvd] *adj* (*complex*) complexo
involvement [ɪn'vɑːlvmənt] *in project, crime, accident etc* envolvimento *m*
invulnerable [ɪn'vʌlnərəbl] *adj* invulnerável
inward ['ɪnwərd] **1** *adj movement* interior; *thoughts* íntimo **2** *adv* para dentro
inwardly ['ɪnwədlɪ] *adv* por dentro
iodine ['aɪoʊdiːn] iodo *m*
IOU [aɪoʊ'juː] *abbr* (*of* ***I owe you***) vale *m*
IQ [aɪ'kjuː] *abbr* (*of* ***intelligence quotient***) QI *m*
Iran [ɪ'rɑːn] Irã *m*, *Port* Irão *m*
Iranian [ɪ'reɪnɪən] **1** *adj* iraniano **2** *n* iraniano,-a *m,f*
Iraq [ɪ'ræːk] Iraque *m*
Iraqi [ɪ'rækɪ] **1** *adj* iraquiano **2** *n* iraquiano,-a *m,f*
Ireland ['aɪrlənd] Irlanda *f*
iris ['aɪrɪs] *eye, flower*: íris *f*
Irish ['aɪrɪʃ] *adj* irlandês,-esa
'Irishman irlandês *m*
'Irishwoman irlandesa *f*
iron ['aɪərn] **1** *n substance, clothes*: ferro *m* **2** *v/t shirts etc* passar a ferro
ironic, ironical [aɪ'rɑːnɪk(l)] *adj* irônico
ironing ['aɪrnɪŋ] *n* ***do the ~*** passar roupa
'ironing board tábua *f* de passar roupa
'ironworks *npl* siderúrgica *f*
irony ['aɪrənɪ] ironia *f*
irrational [ɪ'ræʃənl] *adj* irracional
irreconcilable [ɪrekən'saɪləbl] *adj* irreconciliável
irrecoverable [ɪrɪ'kʌvərəbl] *adj* irrecuperável
irregular [ɪ'regjʊlər] *adj intervals, behavior* irregular; *sizes* desigual

irrelevant [ɪ'reləvənt] *adj* irrelevante
irreparable [ɪ'repərəbl] *adj* irreparável
irreplaceable [ɪrɪ'pleɪsəbl] *adj* insubstituível
irrepressible [ɪrɪ'presəbl] *adj sense of humor* irrefreável; *person* irreprimível
irreproachable [ɪrɪ'proʊʧəbl] *adj* irrepreensível
irresistible [ɪrɪ'zɪstəbl] *adj* irresistível
irrespective [ɪrɪ'spektɪv] *adv* **~ of** independentemente de
irresponsible [ɪrɪ'spɑːnsəbl] *adj* irresponsável
irretrievable [ɪrɪ'triːvəbl] *adj* irrecuperável
irreverent [ɪ'revərənt] *adj* irreverente
irrevocable [ɪ'revəkəbl] *adj* irrevogável
irrigate ['ɪrɪgeɪt] *v/t* irrigar
irrigation [ɪrɪ'geɪʃn] irrigação *f*
irri'gation canal canal *m* de irrigação
irritable ['ɪrɪtəbl] *adj* irritável
irritate ['ɪrɪteɪt] *v/t* irritar
irritating ['ɪrɪteɪtɪŋ] *adj* irritante
irritation [ɪrɪ'teɪʃn] irritação *f*
IRS [aɪɑːr'es] *abbr* (*of* ***Internal Revenue Service***) *Am* Receita *f* Federal, *Port* fisco *m*
Islam ['ɪzlɑːm] islamismo *m*; (*the Muslim world*) Islã *m*
Islamic [ɪz'læmɪk] *adj* islâmico
island ['aɪlənd] ilha *f*; ***traffic ~*** ilha de tráfego
islander ['aɪləndər] ilhéu *m*, ilhoa *f*
isolate ['aɪsəleɪt] *v/t* isolar
isolated ['aɪsəleɪtɪd] *adj house, occurrence* isolado
isolation [aɪsə'leɪʃn] isolamento *m*; ***in ~*** isoladamente
iso'lation ward pavilhão *m* de isolamento
ISP [aɪes'piː] *abbr* (*of* ***Internet service provider***) provedor *m* (de serviços) de internet
Israel ['ɪzreɪl] Israel
Israeli [ɪz'reɪlɪ] **1** *adj* israelense **2** *n person* israelense *m/f*
issue ['ɪʃuː] **1** *n* (*matter*) assunto *m*; (*result*) resultado *m*; *magazine*: edição *f*; ***the point at ~*** o ponto em questão; ***take ~ with s.o. / sth*** discordar de alguém / algo **2** *v/t coins, passports, visa* emitir; *supplies* distribuir; *warning* dar
IT [aɪ'tiː] *abbr* (*of* ***information technology***) TI *f*
it [ɪt] *pron* ◊ *as subject*: ele, *f* ela; ***what color is ~? – ~'s red*** de que cor é? - é vermelho,-a
◊ *as direct object*: o, *f* a; *with no previous reference* isso; ***give ~ to me*** me dá isso
◊ *as indirect object*: ***give ~ some food*** dê um pouco de comida a ele/ela
◊ *impersonal*: ***~ 's raining*** está chovendo; ***~ 's me / him*** sou eu / é ele; ***~ 's Charlie here*** TEL aqui é o Charlie; ***~ 's your turn*** é sua vez; ***that's ~!*** (*that's right*) isso mesmo!; (*finished*) pronto!
◊ *after prepositions*: ***I got $5 for ~*** eu vendi por $5; ***he needs the stick, he can't walk without ~*** ele precisa da muleta, não consegue andar sem ela
Italian [ɪ'tæljən] **1** *adj* italiano **2** *n person* italiano,-a *m,f*; *language* italiano *m*
italic [ɪ'tælɪk] *adj* itálico
italics [ɪ'tælɪks] *npl* itálico *m*
Italy ['ɪtəlɪ] Itália *f*
itch [ɪʧ] **1** *n* coceira *f* **2** *v/i* coçar
item ['aɪtəm] item *m*
itemize ['aɪtəmaɪz] *v/t invoice* especificar
itinerary [aɪ'tɪnərerɪ] itinerário *m*
it'll [ɪtl] (**= it will**)
it's [ɪts] (**= it is, it has**)
its [ɪts] *poss adj* seu (sua), dele (dela); ***the dog hurt ~ leg*** o cachorro feriu a perna
itself [ɪt'self] *pron* ***the dog hurt ~*** o cachorro machucou-se; ***the hotel ~ is fine, but the town …*** o hotel em si é ótimo, mas a cidade …; ***by ~*** (*alone, automatically*) sozinho,-a
ivory ['aɪvərɪ] marfim *m*
ivy ['aɪvɪ] hera *f*

J

jab [dʒæb] *v/t* ⟨*pret & pp* ***jabbed***⟩ cravar
jabber ['dʒæbər] *v/i* tagarelar
jack [dʒæk] MOT macaco *m*; *cards*: valete *m*
♦**jack up** *v/t* MOT levantar com macaco
jacket ['dʒækɪt] (*coat*) jaqueta *f*, *suit*: paletó *m*; *book*: sobrecapa *f*
jacket po'tato batata *f* assada
'jack-knife *v/i* ***the truck ~d*** o caminhão deu uma guinada
'jackpot bolada *f*; ***hit the ~*** tirar a sorte grande
jade [dʒeɪd] *n* jade *m*
jaded ['dʒeɪdɪd] *adj* cansado
jagged ['dʒægɪd] *adj* recortado
jaguar ['dʒæguar] *n* onça *f*
jail [dʒeɪl] prisão *f*
jam[1] [dʒæm] *n* geléia *f*
jam[2] [dʒæm] **1** *n* MOT congestionamento *m*; *fam* (*difficulty*) apuro *m*; ***be in a ~*** estar num apuro **2** *v/t* ⟨*pret & pp* ***jammed***⟩ (*ram*) enfiar; (*cause to stick*) emperrar; *broadcast* bloquear; ***be ~med*** *roads* estar bloqueado; *door, window* estar emperrado; ***~ on the brakes*** dar uma freada **3** *v/i* ⟨*pret & pp* ***jammed***⟩ (*stick*) emperrar; (*squeeze*) apertar-se
Jamaica [dʒə'meɪkə] Jamaica *f*
Jamaican [dʒə'meɪkən] **1** *adj* jamaicano **2** *n* jamaicano,-a *m,f*
jam-'packed *fam* abarrotado
janitor ['dʒænɪtər] zelador,a *m,f*
January ['dʒænjuerɪ] janeiro *m*
Japan [dʒə'pæn] Japão *m*
Japanese [dʒæpə'niːz] **1** *adj* japonês,-esa **2** *n person* japonês,-esa *m,f*, *language* japonês *m*; ***the ~*** os japoneses
jar[1] [dʒɑːr] *n container* jarro *m*
jar[2] [dʒɑːr] *v/i* ⟨*pret & pp* ***jarred***⟩ *noise* chiar; *colors* chocar-se; ***~ on*** chiar em
jargon ['dʒɑːrgən] jargão *m*
jaundice ['dʒɒːndɪs] *n* icterícia *f*
jaundiced ['dʒɒːndɪst] *adj fig* desanimado
jaunt [dʒɒːnt] *n* excursão *f*
jaunty ['dʒɒːntɪ] *adj* jovial
javelin ['dʒævlɪn] (*spear*) dardo *m*; *event* arremesso *m* de dardo
jaw [dʒɒː] *n* mandíbula *f*
jaywalker ['dʒeɪwɔːkər] pedestre *m/f* imprudente, *Port* peão *m* imprudente
'jaywalking *n* cruzar *m* a rua de maneira imprudente
jazz [dʒæz] *n* jazz *m*
♦**jazz up** *v/t fam* avivar
jealous ['dʒeləs] *adj* ciumento; (*envious*) invejoso; ***be ~ s of …*** ter ciúme / inveja de …
jealously ['dʒeləslɪ] *adv* com ciúmes; (*enviously*) invejosamente
jealousy ['dʒeləsɪ] ciúme *m*; (*envy*) inveja *f*
jeans [dʒiːnz] *npl* jeans *m*, *Port* jeans *mpl*
jeep [dʒiːp] jipe *m*
jeer [dʒɪr] **1** *n* zombaria *f* **2** *v/i* zombar; ***~ at*** zombar de
Jello® ['dʒeloʊ] gelatina *f*
jelly ['dʒelɪ] geléia *f*
'jelly bean jujuba *f*
'jellyfish água-viva *f*
jeopardize ['dʒepərdaɪz] *v/t* colocar em risco
jeopardy ['dʒepərdɪ] perigo *m*; ***be in ~*** estar em perigo
jerk[1] [dʒɜːrk] **1** *n* solavanco *m* **2** *v/t* empurrar; ***he ~ed his arm free*** ele soltou seu braço com um puxão
jerk[2] [dʒɜːrk] *n Am fam* babaca *m*
jerky ['dʒɜːrkɪ] *adj movement* brusco; *ride* balançante
jersey ['dʒɜːrzɪ] (*sweater*) suéter *m/f*, *Port* camisola *f*; *fabric* jérsei *m*
jest [dʒest] **1** *n* gracejo *m*; ***in ~*** de brincadeira **2** *v/i* gracejar

Jesus ['dʒiːzəs] Jesus *m*
jet [dʒet] **1** *n water, airplane* jato *m*; (*nozzle*) bico *m* **2** *v/i* ⟨*pret & pp* ***jetted***⟩ *travel* viajar de avião a jato
jet-'black *adj* azeviche **'jet engine** motor *m* a jato **'jetlag** jet lag *m*
jettison ['dʒetɪsn] *v/t also fig* alijar
jetty ['dʒetɪ] cais *m*
Jew [dʒuː] judeu *m*, judia *f*
jewel ['dʒuːəl] jóia *f*; *fig person* preciosidade *f*
jeweler ['dʒuːlər] *Am* joalheiro,-a *m,f*
jeweller *Brit* → ***jeweler***
jewellery *Brit* → ***jewelry***
jewelry ['dʒuːlrɪ] *Am* jóias *fpl*
Jewish ['dʒuːɪʃ] *adj* judeu (judia)
jiffy ['dʒɪfɪ] *fam* ***in a ~*** num instante
jigsaw ['dʒɪgsɒː] **~ (*puzzle*)** quebra-cabeça *m*
jilt [dʒɪlt] *v/t* dar o fora em
jingle ['dʒɪŋgl] **1** *n song* jingle *m* **2** *v/i keys, coins* tilintar
jinx [dʒɪŋks] *n person* pé *m* frio; (*bad luck*) azar *m*; ***there's a ~ on this project*** este projeto está com má sorte
jitters ['dʒɪtərz] *fam* ***get the ~*** ficar muito nervoso
jittery ['dʒɪtərɪ] *adj fam* nervoso
job [dʒɑːb] (*employment*) emprego *m*; (*task*) trabalho *m*; ***out of a ~*** sem emprego; ***it's a good ~ you …*** ainda bem que você …; ***you'll have a ~*** isso vai dar um trabalhão; ***good ~!*** muito bem!
'job description responsabilidades *fpl* da função
job hunt *v/i* ***be job hunting*** estar procurando emprego
jobless ['dʒɑːblɪs] *adj* desempregado
job satis'faction satisfação *f* com o trabalho
jockey ['dʒɑːkɪ] *n* jóquei *m/f*
jog ['dʒɑːg] **1** *n* jogging *m*; ***go for a ~*** ir fazer jogging **2** *v/i* ⟨*pret & pp* ***jogged***⟩ *as exercise* fazer cooper **3** *v/t* ⟨*pret & pp* ***jogged***⟩ *elbow etc* empurrar; **~ *s.o.'s memory*** refrescar a memória de alguém
♦**jog along** *v/i fam* ir levando
jogger ['dʒɑːgər] *person* corredor,a *m,f*; *shoe* tenis *m* de jogging
jogging ['dʒɑːgɪŋ] jogging *m*; ***go ~*** fazer jogging
'jogging suit jogging *m*
john [dʒɑːn] *Am fam* (*toilet*) privada *f*, *Port* casa *f* de banho
join [dʒɔɪn] **1** *n* junção *f* **2** *v/i roads, rivers* juntar-se; (*become a member*) associar-se **3** *v/t* (*connect*) juntar; *road* desembocar em; **~ *us instead of eating on your own*** sente-se conosco em vez de comer sozinho; ***he ~ed the club*** ele tornou-se sócio do clube; ***I ~ed the company in 1992*** entrei na companhia em 1992
♦**join in** *v/i* participar
♦**join up** *v/i Brit* MIL alistar-se
joiner ['dʒɔɪnər] *Brit* marceneiro,-a *m,f*
joint [dʒɔɪnt] **1** *n* ANAT articulação *f*; *woodwork*: encaixe *m*; *meat*: quarto *m*; *fam* (*place*) espelunca *f*; *cannabis*: baseado *m* **2** *adj* (*shared*) conjunto
joint ac'count conta *f* conjunta
joint 'venture empreendimento *m* conjunto
joke [dʒoʊk] **1** *n story* piada *f*; (*practical joke*) peça *f*; ***play a ~ on*** pregar uma peça em; ***it's no ~*** é sério **2** *v/i* (*pretend*) brincar; (*having a joke*) pilheriar
joker ['dʒoʊkər] *person* brincalhão *m*, brincalhona *f*; *pej* palhaço *m*; *cards*: coringa *m*
joking ['dʒoʊkɪŋ] brincadeira *f*; ***~ apart*** brincadeiras à parte
jokingly ['dʒoʊkɪŋlɪ] *adv* de brincadeira
jolly ['dʒɑːlɪ] *adj* divertido
jolt [dʒoʊlt] **1** *n* (*jerk*) solavanco *m* **2** *v/t* sacudir; ***someone ~ed my elbow and I spilt the coffee*** alguém bateu em meu cotovelo e derramei o café
jostle ['dʒɑːsl] *v/t* empurrar
♦**jot down** [dʒɑːt] *v/t* ⟨*pret & pp* ***jotted***⟩ anotar
journal ['dʒɜːrnl] (*magazine*) revista *f*; (*diary*) diário *m*
journalism ['dʒɜːrnəlɪzm] jornalismo *m*
journalist ['dʒɜːrnəlɪst] jornalista *m/f*
journey ['dʒɜːrnɪ] *n* viagem *f*
jovial ['dʒoʊvɪəl] *adj* jovial

joy [dʒɔɪ] alegria *f*
'joystick COMPUT joystick *m*
jubilant ['dʒuːbɪlənt] *adj* jubiloso
jubilation [dʒuːbɪ'leɪʃn] júbilo *m*
judge [dʒʌdʒ] **1** *n* LAW juiz *m*, juíza *f*; *competition*: árbitro,-a *m,f* **2** *v/t* julgar; *competition* arbitrar **3** *v/i* julgar
judgment, **judgement** ['dʒʌdʒmənt] LAW julgamento *m*; (*opinion*) opinião *f*; ***bad ~*** mau juízo; ***an error of ~*** um erro de julgamento; ***the Last Judgment*** REL o Juízo Final
'Judgment Day, **'Judgement Day** dia *m* do juízo final
judicial [dʒuː'dɪʃl] *adj* judicial
judicious [dʒuː'dɪʃəs] *adj* judicioso
judo ['dʒuːdoʊ] judô *m*
jug [dʒʌg] *Brit* jarra *f*
juggle [dʒʌgl] *v/t also fig* fazer malabarismo
juggler ['dʒʌglər] malabarista *m/f*
juice [dʒuːs] *n* suco *m*, *Port* sumo *m*
juicy ['dʒuːsɪ] *adj* suculento; *news*, *gossip* escandaloso
jukebox ['dʒuːkbɑːks] juke-box *f*
July [dʒʊ'laɪ] julho *m*
jumble ['dʒʌmbl] *n* confusão *f*
♦**jumble up** *v/t* misturar
jumbo, **jumbo jet** ['dʒʌmboʊ] jumbo *m*
'jumbo-sized *adj* gigante; ***~ pizza*** pizza *f* tamanho família
jump [dʒʌmp] **1** *n* salto *m*, pulo *m*; ***an enormous ~ in inflation*** um enorme salto na inflação; ***give a ~*** *surprise* dar um pulo **2** *v/i* saltar, pular; (*increase*) aumentar; ***~ to one's feet*** levantar-se de um salto; ***~ to conclusions*** tirar conclusões precipitadas; ***you made me ~!*** *in surprise* você me deu um susto! **3** *v/t fence etc* pular, saltar; *fam* (*attack*) assaltar; ***~ the queue*** *Brit* furar a fila, *Port* pôr-se à frente; ***~ the lights*** passar o sinal (vermelho)
♦**jump at** *v/t opportunity* não deixar escapar
jumper[1] ['dʒʌmpər] *Am* avental *m*; *Brit* pullover *m*, *Port* camisola *f*
jumper[2] ['dʒʌmpər] SPORT saltador,a *m,f*; *horse* cavalo *m* de salto
jumpy ['dʒʌmpɪ] *adj* nervoso
junction ['dʒʌŋkʃn] *Brit of roads* cruzamento *m*
juncture ['dʒʌŋktʃər] *fml* conjuntura *f*; ***at this ~*** nesta conjuntura
June [dʒuːn] junho *m*
jungle ['dʒʌŋgl] selva *f*
junior ['dʒuːnjər] **1** *adj* (*subordinate*) subordinado; (*younger*) mais jovem; ***William Smith Junior*** William Smith Júnior **2** *n in rank* subalterno,-a *m,f*; ***she is ten years my ~*** ela é dez anos mais nova que eu
junior 'high *Am* escola *f* de ensino fundamental
junior school *Brit* → ***grade school***
junk [dʒʌŋk] traste *m*
'junk food junk food *f*, comida *f* de plástico
junkie ['dʒʌŋkɪ] *fam* drogado,-a *m,f*
'junk mail correspondência *f* não desejada **'junk shop** loja *f* de utensílios usados **'junkyard** ferro-velho *m*
jurisdiction [dʒʊrɪs'dɪkʃn] LAW jurisdição *f*
juror ['dʒʊrər] jurado,-a *m,f*
jury ['dʒʊrɪ] júri *m*
just [dʒʌst] **1** *adj law*, *cause* justo **2** *adv* (*only*) somente; ***I've ~ seen her*** acabo de vê-la; ***~ about*** (*almost*) quase; ***I was ~ about to leave when …*** eu já estava quase saindo quando …; ***~ like yours*** exatamente igual ao seu; ***~ like that*** (*abruptly*) de repente; ***~ now*** (*a few moments ago*) agora mesmo; (*at the moment*) no momento; ***I'm busy ~ now*** estou ocupado no momento; ***~ you wait!*** espere e verá!; ***~ be quiet!*** cale-se de uma vez!; ***I ~ got here*** eu mal cheguei; ***my son is ~ as intelligent as yours*** meu filho é tão inteligente quanto o seu; ***I heard a scream ~ as I turned the corner*** ouvi um grito justamente quando dobrei a esquina
justice ['dʒʌstɪs] justiça *f*
justifiable [dʒʌstɪ'faɪəbl] *adj* justificável
justifiably [dʒʌstɪ'faɪəblɪ] *adv* justificadamente
justification [dʒʌstɪfɪ'keɪʃn] justificativa *f*
justify ['dʒʌstɪfaɪ] *v/t* ⟨*pret & pp* ***justi-***

***fied*〉 *also text* justificar

justly ['dʒʌstlɪ] *adv* (*fairly*) com justiça; (*rightly*) com razão

◆**jut out** [dʒʌt] *v/i* 〈*pret & pp* ***jutted***〉 sobressair

juvenile ['dʒu:vənəl] **1** *adj* juvenil; *court* de menores; *pej* infantil **2** *n fml* menor *m/f* de idade

juvenile de'linquency delinqüência *f* juvenil

juvenile de'linquent delinqüente *m/f* juvenil

K

k [keɪ] **1** *abbr* (*of* ***kilobyte***) kilobyte *m* **2** *n* (*thousand*) mil; ***50K*** cinqüenta mil

kabob ['keɪbɑ:b] *Am* churrasquinho *m*

kangaroo ['kæŋgəru:] canguru *m*

karate [kə'rɑ:tɪ] caratê *m*

ka'rate chop golpe *m* de caratê

kebab [ke'bæb] *Brit* churrasquinho *m*

keel [ki:l] NAUT quilha *f*

◆**keel over** *v/i structure* desaprumar-se; *person* desmaiar

keen [ki:n] *adj* entusiasmado; ***there's a ~ competition for the job*** há uma acirrada disputa pelo emprego; ***be ~ on*** gostar muito de; ***be ~ to do sth*** sentir muita vontade de fazer algo

keep [ki:p] **1** *n* (*maintenance*) subsistência *f*; ***for ~s*** *fam* para sempre **2** *v/t* (*not lose*) manter; (*detain*) deter; *in specific place* guardar; *family* sustentar; *animals* criar; *promise* cumprir; ***~ s.o. company*** fazer companhia a alguém; ***~ s.o. waiting*** deixar alguém esperando; ***~ sth to oneself*** (*not tell*) guardar algo para si; ***~ sth from s.o.*** ocultar algo de alguém; ***~ trying!*** continue tentando!; ***don't ~ interrupting!*** não fique interrompendo!; ***you can ~ it*** você pode ficar com isso **3** *v/i* (*remain*) manter-se; *food, milk* conservar-se

keeper ['ki:pər] *futebol*: goleiro,-a *m,f*

◆**keep away 1** *v/i* manter-se afastado; ***keep away from …*** mantenha-se afastado de … **2** *v/t* manter afastado; ***keep s.o. away from sth*** manter alguém afastado de algo

◆**keep back** *v/t* (*hold in check*) conter; *information* ocultar

◆**keep down** *v/t voice, noise* abaixar; *costs, inflation etc* reduzir; *food* reter

◆**keep in** *v/t in hospital* manter em observação; ***the teacher kept me in*** *in school* a professora me deixou de castigo

◆**keep off 1** *v/t* (*avoid*) evitar; ***keep off the grass!*** não pise na grama! **2** *v/i* ***if the rain keeps off*** se não chover

◆**keep on 1** *v/i* continuar; ***keep on doing sth*** continuar fazendo algo **2** *v/t* in job manter; ***I'll keep my coat on*** não vou tirar o casaco

◆**keep on at** *v/t* (*nag*) infernizar; ***she kept on at him until he agreed*** ela o infernizou até que concordasse

◆**keep out 1** *v/t the cold* proteger de; *person* impedir de entrar **2** *v/i* ***I told you to keep out!*** eu lhe disse para não entrar!; ***I would keep out of it if I were you*** se eu fosse você, não me meteria; ***I always keep out of other people's arguments*** eu sempre fico de fora nas discussões alheias; ***keep out!*** *as sign* Entrada Proibida!

◆**keep to** *v/t path* seguir; *rules* cumprir

◆**keep up 1** *v/i when walking, running etc* acompanhar; ***keep up with*** acompanhar o ritmo de; (*stay in touch with*) manter contato com **2** *v/t pace, payments* continuar com; *bridge, pants* sustentar

K

keeping ['ki:pɪŋ] ***be in ~ with*** estar de acordo com; *decor etc* combinar com
'keepsake lembrança *f*
keg [keg] barril *m*
kennel ['kenl] *Brit* casa *f* de cachorro; *Am* canil *m*
kennels ['kenlz] *npl Brit* canil *m*
kept [kept] *pret & pp* → ***keep***
kerb *Brit* → ***curb***
kernel ['kɜ:rnl] semente *f*
kerosene ['kerəsi:n] *Am* querosene *m*
ketchup ['ketʃʌp] ketchup *m*
kettle ['ketl] chaleira *f*
key [ki:] **1** *n to door, drawer* chave *f*; COMPUT, MUS tecla *f*; *piece of music*: clave *f*; *on a chart* legenda *f* **2** *adj* (*vital*) chave **3** *v/t & v/i* COMPUT teclar
♦ **key in** *v/t data* digitar
'keyboard COMPUT, MUS teclado *m* **'keyboarder** COMPUT digitador,a *m,f* **'keycard** chave *f* de cartão
keyed-up [ki:d'ʌp] *adj* tenso
'keyhole buraco *m* da fechadura **'keynote speech** discurso *m* que dá a tônica **'keyring** chaveiro *m* **'keyword** palavra-chave *f*
khaki ['kækɪ] *adj* cáqui
kick [kɪk] **1** *n* chute *m*; *horse, mule*: coice *m*; ***get a ~ out of …*** *fam* sentir prazer em …; (***just***) ***for ~s*** *fam* (apenas) para curtir **2** *v/t* chutar; *fam habit* deixar **3** *v/i person* chutar
♦ **kick around** *v/t ball, also* (*treat harshly*) chutar; *fam* (*discuss*) discutir
♦ **kick in 1** *v/t pej* (*money*) contribuir **2** *v/i* (*start to operate*) entrar em funcionamento
♦ **kick off** *v/i* dar o chute inicial; *fam* (*start*) começar
♦ **kick out** *v/t* expulsar; ***be kicked out of the company / army*** ser expulso da companhia / do exército
♦ **kick up** *v/t* ***kick up a fuss*** fazer uma cena
'kickback *fam* (*bribe*) suborno *m*
'kickoff SPORT chute *m* inicial
kid [kɪd] **1** *n* criança *f*; ***~ brother / sister*** irmão / irmã menor **2** *v/t* ⟨*pret & pp* ***kidded***⟩ *fam* brincar com; (*deceive*) enganar; ***you're ~ding yourself if you think …*** você está se iludindo se você pensa que …; ***I was ~ding you*** eu estava brincando contigo **3** *v/i* ⟨*pret & pp* ***kidded***⟩ *fam* brincar; ***I was only ~ding*** eu só estava brincando
kidder ['kɪdər] *fam* brincalhão *m*, brincalhona *f*
kid 'gloves *npl* ***handle s.o. with ~*** tratar alguém com luvas de pelica
kidnap ['kɪdnæp] *v/t* ⟨*pret & pp* ***kidnapped***⟩ seqüestrar
kidnaper, **kidnapper** ['kɪdnæpər] seqüestrador,a *m,f*
kidnaping, **kidnapping** ['kɪdnæpɪŋ] seqüestro *m*
kidney ['kɪdnɪ] ANAT, *also in cooking* rim *m*; ***~ machine*** rim *m* artificial
'kidney bean feijão *m* roxo
kill [kɪl] *v/t person, plant, time* matar; ***be ~ed in a car crash*** ser morto em um acidente de carro; ***~ oneself*** suicidar-se; ***~ oneself*** (***laughing***) *fam* morrer de rir
killer ['kɪlər] (*murderer*) assassino,-a *m,f*; ***be a ~*** *disease* ser mortal
killing ['kɪlɪŋ] *n* assassinato *m*; ***make a ~*** *fam* (*lots of money*) faturar uma boa grana
killingly ['kɪlɪŋlɪ] *adv fam* ***~ funny*** para morrer de rir
kiln [kɪln] forno *m*
kilo ['ki:loʊ] quilo *m*
kilobyte ['kɪloʊbaɪt] kilobyte *m*
kilogram ['kɪloʊgræm] quilograma *m*
kilometer [kɪ'lɑ:mɪtər] *Am* quilômetro *m*
kilometre *Brit* → ***kilometer***
kind[1] [kaɪnd] *adj* gentil
kind[2] [kaɪnd] *n* (*sort*) tipo *m*; (*make, brand*) marca *f*; ***what ~ of …?*** que tipo de …?; ***all ~s of people*** todos os tipos de pessoas; ***nothing of the ~!*** nada parecido!; ***~ of sad / strange*** *fam* um pouco triste / estranho
kindergarten ['kɪndərgɑ:rtn] jardim *m* de infância
kind-hearted [kaɪnd'hɑ:rtɪd] *adj* amável
kindly ['kaɪndlɪ] **1** *adj* amável **2** *adv* gentilmente; ***would you ~ …*** você poderia, por favor …

kindness ['kaındnıs] gentileza *f*
king [kıŋ] rei *m*
kingdom ['kıŋdəm] reino *m*
king-size → ***king-sized***
king-sized ['kıŋsaızd] *adj fam* king size; *headache* monstruoso
kink [kıŋk] *hose etc*: torção *f*
kinky ['kıŋkı] *adj fam* excêntrico
kiosk ['kiːɑːsk] quiosque *m*
kiss [kıs] **1** *n* beijo *m* **2** *v/t* beijar **3** *v/i* beijar-se
kiss of 'life *Brit* respiração *f* boca a boca
kit [kıt] kit *m*
kitchen ['kıʧın] cozinha *f*
kitchenette [kıʧı'net] kitchenette *f*
kitchen 'sink pia *f* de cozinha; ***everything but the ~*** *fam* a casa toda
kite [kaıt] papagaio *m pipa*
kitten ['kıtn] gatinho *m*
kitty ['kıtı] *money* vaquinha *f*
klutz [klʌts] *Am fam* (*clumsy person*) desajeitado,-a *m,f*
knack [næk] jeito *m*; ***there's a special ~ to it*** tem um jeito especial de fazer isso
knead [niːd] *v/t dough* amassar
knee [niː] *n* joelho *m*
'kneecap *n* rótula *f*
kneel [niːl] *v/i* 〈*pret & pp* ***knelt***〉 ajoelhar-se
'knee-length *adj* até o joelho
knelt [nelt] *pret & pp* → ***kneel***
knew [nuː] *pret* → ***know***
knickers *Brit* → ***panties***
knick-knacks ['nıknæks] *npl fam* penduricalhos *mpl*
knife [naıf] **1** *n* 〈*pl* ***knives***〉 faca *f* **2** *v/t* esfaquear
knight [naıt] cavaleiro *m*
knit [nıt] 〈*pret & pp* ***knitted***〉**1** *v/t* tricotar, *Port* fazer; **2** *v/i* tricotar, *Port* fazer malha
♦ **knit together** *v/i broken bone* unir-se
knitting ['nıtıŋ] tricô *m*, *Port* malha *f*
'knitting needle agulha *f* de tricô, *Port* agulha *f* de malha
'knitwear roupa *f* de malha
knob [nɑːb] *door*: maçaneta *f*, ***a ~ of butter*** um pouquinho de manteiga
knock [nɑːk] **1** *n on door, also* (*blow*) batida *f* **2** *v/t* bater; *fam* (*criticize*) criticar; ***he was ~ed to the ground*** ele foi derrubado **3** *v/i on door* bater
♦ **knock around** *fam* **1** *v/t* (*beat*) bater **2** *v/i* (*travel*) viajar
♦ **knock down** *v/t pedestrian* atropelar; *object, building etc* derrubar; *fam* (*reduce the price of*) baixar
♦ **knock off** *fam* **1** *v/t* (*steal*) surripiar **2** *v/i* (*stop work for the day*) terminar
♦ **knock out** *v/t* (*make unconscious*) nocautear; *medicine* apagar; *power lines etc* destruir; (*eliminate*) eliminar
♦ **knock over** *v/t* derrubar; *pedestrian* atropelar
'knockdown *adj* ***a ~ price*** um preço bastante baixo **knock-kneed** [nɑːk-'niːd] que tem os joelhos para dentro
'knockout *n boxing*: nocaute *m*
knot [nɑːt] **1** *n* nó *m* **2** *v/t* 〈*pret & pp* ***knotted***〉 dar um nó em
'knotty ['nɑːtı] *adj problem* espinhoso
know [noʊ] **1** *v/t* 〈*pret* ***knew***, *pp* ***known***〉 *fact, language* saber; *person, place* conhecer; (*recognize*) reconhecer; ***~ how to do sth*** saber como fazer algo **2** *v/i* saber; ***I don't ~*** não sei; ***yes, I ~*** sim, eu sei; ***will you let him ~?*** você pode informar a ele? **3** *n* ***be in the ~*** estar inteirado
know-all → ***know-it-all***
'knowhow *fam* know-how *m*
knowing ['noʊıŋ] *adj* de cumplicidade
knowingly ['noʊıŋlı] *adv* (*wittingly*) de propósito; *smile etc* com cumplicidade
'know-it-all *Am fam* sabichão *m*, sabichona *f*
knowledge ['nɑːlıdʒ] conhecimento *m*; ***to the best of my ~*** pelo que sei; ***have a good ~ of …*** ter bons conhecimentos de …
knowledgeable ['nɑːlıdʒəbl] *adj* entendido
known [noʊn] *pp* → ***know***
knuckle ['nʌkl] nó *m* do dedo
♦ **knuckle down** *v/i fam* empenhar-se
♦ **knuckle under** *v/i fam* sujeitar-se
KO [keı'oʊ] (*knockout*) K.O. *m*
Koran [kə'ræn] Alcorão *m*

Korea [kə'riːə] Coréia *f*
Korean [kə'riːən] **1** *adj* coreano **2** *n* coreano,-a *m,f*; *language* coreano *m*
kosher ['kouʃər] *adj* REL kosher; *fam* certo
kowtow ['kautau] *v/i* **~ to** *fam* reverenciar
kudos ['kjuːdɑːs] créditos *mpl*

L

lab [læb] laboratório *m*
label ['leɪbl] **1** *n* etiqueta *f* **2** *v/t* ⟨*pret & pp* ***labeled***, *Brit* ***labelled***⟩ *baggage* etiquetar
labor ['leɪbər] *n* (*work*) trabalho *m*; *pregnancy*: trabalho *m* de parto; ***go into ~*** entrar em trabalho de parto
laboratory ['læbrətɔːrɪ] laboratório *m*
laboratory tech'nician laboratorista *m/f*
labored ['leɪbərd] *adj style, speech* elaborado
laborer ['leɪbərər] trabalhador,a *m,f*
laborious [lə'bɔːrɪəs] *adj* trabalhador
'labor union *Am* sindicato *m*
'labor ward MED sala *f* de parto
labour *etc Brit* → ***labor***
'Labour Party *Brit* POL Partido *m* Trabalhista
lace [leɪs] *n material* renda *f*, *shoe*: cadarço *m*, *Port* atacador *m*
♦ **lace up** *v/t shoes* amarrar
lack [læk] **1** *n* falta *f* **2** *v/t* faltar **3** *v/i* ***be ~ing*** faltar
lacquer ['lækər] *n for hair* fixador *m*
lad [læd] rapaz *m*
ladder ['lædər] escada *f* de mão
laden ['leɪdn] *adj* carregado
ladies room ['leɪdiːz] sanitário *m* feminino, *Port* casa *f* de banho de senhoras
ladle ['leɪdl] *n* concha *f de sopa*
lady ['leɪdɪ] senhora *f*
ladybird *Brit* → ***ladybug***
'ladybug *Am* joaninha *f*
'ladylike refinado
lag [læg] *v/t* ⟨*pret & pp* ***lagged***⟩ *pipes* revestir
♦ **lag behind** *v/i* ficar para trás
lager ['lɑːgər] *Brit* cerveja *f* lager
lagoon [lə'guːn] lagoa *f*
laid [leɪd] *pret & pp* → ***lay***[1]
laid'back *adj* descontraído
lain [leɪn] *pp* → ***lie***[2]
lake [leɪk] lago *m*
lamb [læm] *animal, meat* cordeiro *m*
lame [leɪm] *adj person* manco; *excuse* pouco convincente
lament [lə'ment] **1** *n* lamento *m* **2** *v/t* lamentar
lamentable ['læməntəbl] *adj* lamentável
laminated ['læmɪneɪtɪd] *adj* laminado
laminated 'glass cristal *m* laminado
lamp [læmp] lâmpada *f*
'lamppost poste *m*
'lampshade abajur *m*
land [lænd] **1** *n* terra *f*, (*estate*) propriedades *fpl*; ***by ~*** por terra; ***on ~*** em terra; ***work on the ~*** *as farmer* trabalhar na terra **2** *v/t airplane* pousar; *job* conseguir **3** *v/i airplane* pousar; *ball, sth thrown* cair
landing ['lændɪŋ] *n airplane*: pouso *m*; (*top of staircase*) patamar *m*
'landing field campo *m* de pouso **'landing gear** trem *m* de aterrissagem, *Port* trem *m* de aterragem **'landing strip** pista *f* de pouso
'landlady *rented room*: senhoria *f*, *Brit bar, hostel etc*: proprietária *f* **'landlord** *rented room*: senhorio *m*; *Brit bar, hostel etc*: proprietário *m* **'landmark** *also fig* marco *m* **'land owner** latifundiário,-a *m,f* **landscape** ['lændskeɪp] **1** *n also* (*painting*) paisagem *f* **2** *adv print* em formato paisagem **'landslide** desmoronamento

m **landslide 'victory** vitória *f* esmagadora
lane [leɪn] *country*: estrada *f* estreita; (*alley*) caminho *m*; MOT pista *f*; SPORT faixa *f*
language ['læŋgwɪdʒ] língua *f*; (*way of speaking, style etc*) linguagem *f*; ***she speaks three ~s*** ela fala três línguas
'language lab laboratório *m* lingüístico
lank [læŋk] *adj hair* liso, escorrido
lanky ['læŋkɪ] *adj person* alto e magricelo
lantern ['læntərn] lanterna *f*
lap[1] [læp] *n track*: volta *f*
lap[2] [læp] *n water*: marulho *m*
lap[3] [læp] *n person*: colo *m*
♦ **lap up** *v/t* ⟨*pret & pp* ***lapped***⟩ *drink, milk* lamber; *flattery* deleitar-se com
lapel [lə'pel] lapela *f*
lapse [læps] **1** *n* (*mistake*) *also time, memory*: lapso *m*; *attention*: falta *f* **2** *v/i* expirar; ***~ into*** cair em; ***~ into silence*** ficar em silêncio; ***~ into English*** começar a falar inglês
'laptop COMPUT laptop *m*
larceny ['lɑːrsənɪ] furto *m*
lard [lɑːrd] banha *f* (de porco)
larder ['lɑːrdər] despensa *f*
large [lɑːrdʒ] *adj* grande; ***at ~*** *criminal, animal* à solta
largely ['lɑːrdʒlɪ] *adv* (*mainly*) em grande parte
lark [lɑːrk] *bird* cotovia *f*
larva ['lɑːrvə] larva *f*
laryngitis [lærɪn'dʒaɪtɪs] laringite *f*
larynx ['lærɪŋks] laringe *m/f*
laser ['leɪzər] laser *m*
'laser beam raio *m* laser **'laser printer** impressora *f* a laser **'laser surgery** cirurgia a laser
lash[1] [læʃ] *v/t with whip* chicotear
lash[2] [læʃ] *n* (*eyelash*) cílio *m*
♦ **lash down** *v/t with rope* amarrar
♦ **lash out** *v/i with fists, words* atacar
lass [læs] moça *f*
last[1] [læst] **1** *adj* último; ***~ but one*** penúltimo; ***~ night*** ontem à noite **2** *adv arrive, leave* por último; ***at ~*** finalmente; ***~ but not least*** por último, mas não menos importante
last[2] [læst] *v/i* durar
lasting ['læstɪŋ] *adj* duradouro
lastly ['læstlɪ] *adv* finalmente
latch [lætʃ] tranca *f*
late [leɪt] **1** *adj* (*behind time*) atrasado; *in day* tarde; ***it's getting ~*** está ficando tarde; ***of ~*** recentemente; ***the ~ 19th century*** no final do século XIX **2** *adv arrive, leave* tarde
lately ['leɪtlɪ] *adv* ultimamente
later ['leɪtər] *adv* mais tarde; ***see you ~!*** até mais tarde!; ***~ on*** mais tarde
latest ['leɪtɪst] *adj news, developments* último
lathe [leɪð] *n* torno *m*
lather ['lɑːðər] *soap*: espuma *f*, *sweaty* suor *m*
Latin A'merica América *f* Latina
Latin A'merican 1 *adj* latino-americano **2** *n* latino-americano,-a *m,f*
Latino [læ'tiːnoʊ] *n* latino,-a *m,f*
latitude ['lætɪtuːd] *geographical* latitude *f*, (*freedom*) liberdade *f*
latter ['lætər] *adj* último
laugh [læf] **1** *n* riso *m*; ***it was a ~*** *fam* foi hilário **2** *v/i* rir
♦ **laugh at** *v/t* rir de
laughing stock ['læfɪŋ] ***make oneself a ~*** cair no ridículo; ***become a ~*** tornar-se alvo de risos
laughter ['læftər] risada *f*
launch [lɒːntʃ] **1** *n type of boat* lancha *f*, *rocket, ship, product*: lançamento *m* **2** *v/t rocket, ship, product* lançar
'launch ceremony cerimônia *f* de lançamento
'launchpad plataforma *f* de lançamento
launder ['lɒːndər] *v/t clothes* lavar e passar
launderette® *Brit* → ***Laundromat®***
Laundromat® ['lɒːndrəmæt] *Am* lavanderia *f* automática
laundry ['lɒːndrɪ] *place* lavanderia *f*; (*clothes*) roupa *f*, ***get one's ~ done*** lavar e passar a roupa
laurel ['lɒːrəl] loureiro *m*
lavatory ['lævətərɪ] *place* lavatório *m*, lavabo *m*, *Port* casa *f* de banho; *equipment* vaso *m* sanitário
lavender ['lævəndər] lavanda *f*

lavish ['lævɪʃ] *adj* generoso; *person* pródigo
law [lɒː] lei *f*; *as subject* direito *m*; ***against the ~*** contra a lei; ***forbidden by ~*** proibido por lei
law-abiding ['lɒːəbaɪdɪŋ] *adj* obediente à lei
'law court tribunal *m* de justiça
lawful ['lɒːfʊl] *adj wife* legítimo; *behavior* lícito
lawless ['lɒːlɪs] *adj* anárquico
lawn [lɒːn] gramado *m*, *Port* relvado *m*
'lawn mower cortador *m* de grama, *Port* cortador *m* de relva
'lawsuit ação *f* judicial
lawyer ['lɒːjər] advogado,-a *m,f*
lax [læks] *adj discipline* relaxado; *teacher* negligente
laxative ['læksətɪv] *n* laxante *m*
lay[1] [leɪ] *v/t* ⟨*pret & pp* ***laid***⟩ (*put down*) colocar; *eggs* pôr; *vulg sexually* trepar
lay[2] [leɪ] *pret* → ***lie***[2]
♦ **lay into** *v/t* (*attack*) atacar
♦ **lay off** *v/t workers* demitir
♦ **lay on** *v/t* (*provide*) oferecer
♦ **lay out** *v/t objects* dispor; *page* formatar
'layabout *fam* preguiçoso,-a *m,f*
'lay-by *Brit road*: acostamento *m*, *Port* berma *f*
layer ['leɪr] camada *f*
'layman leigo *m* **'lay-off** demissão *f*
'layout leiaute *m*
♦ **laze around** [leɪz] *v/i* vadiar
lazy ['leɪzɪ] *adj person* preguiçoso; *day* parado
lb *abbr* (*of* ***pound***) libra *f*
LCD [elsiː'diː] *abbr* (*of* ***liquid crystal display***) display *m* de cristal líquido
lead[1] [liːd] **1** *v/t* ⟨*pret & pp* ***led***⟩ *procession, race* encabeçar; *company, team* liderar; (*guide, take*) guiar **2** *v/i* ⟨*pret & pp* ***led***⟩ *in race, competition, also* (*provide leadership*) liderar; ***a street ~ing off the square*** uma rua que sai da praça; ***where is this ~ing?*** aonde isso vai chegar? **3** *n race*: liderança *f*; ***be in the ~*** estar na frente; ***take the ~*** tomar a dianteira; ***lose the ~*** perder a liderança
lead[2] [liːd] *n dog*: correia *f*, *Port* trela *f*
lead[3] [led] *n substance* chumbo *m*
♦ **lead on** *v/i* (*go in front*) ir na frente
♦ **lead up to** *v/t* conduzir a; ***I wonder what she's leading up to*** pergunto-me onde ela quer chegar
leaded ['ledɪd] *adj gas* com chumbo
leader ['liːdər] líder *m/f*
leadership ['liːdərʃɪp] liderança *f*; ***under his ~*** sob sua liderança
'leadership contest competição *f* pela liderança
lead-free ['ledfriː] *adj gas* sem chumbo
leading ['liːdɪŋ] *adj runner* primeiro; *company, product* principal
'leading-edge *adj company, technology* de vanguarda; ***a ~ company in ...*** uma empresa líder em ...
leaf [liːf] ⟨*pl* ***leaves***⟩ folha *f*
♦ **leaf through** *v/t* folhear
leaflet ['liːflət] folheto *m*
league [liːg] liga *f*
leak [liːk] **1** *n water, information*: vazamento *m* **2** *v/i* vazar; *boat* fazer água
♦ **leak out** *v/i air, gas, news* vazar
leaky ['liːkɪ] *adj pipe* com vazamento; *boat* furado
lean[1] [liːn] **1** *v/i* (*be at an angle*) inclinar-se; ***~ against sth*** apoiar-se em algo **2** *v/t* apoiar; ***~ sth against sth*** apoiar algo em algo
lean[2] [liːn] *adj meat* magro; *style, prose* conciso
leap [liːp] **1** *n* pulo *m*; ***a great ~ forward*** um grande salto para frente **2** *v/i* pular
'leap year ano *m* bissexto
learn [lɜːrn] **1** *v/t* aprender; (*hear*) ouvir dizer; ***~ how to do sth*** aprender a fazer algo **2** *v/i* aprender
learner ['lɜːrnər] aprendiz *m/f*
'learner driver aprendiz *m/f* de motorista
learning ['lɜːrnɪŋ] *n* (*knowledge*) saber *m*; *act* aprendizagem *f*
'learning curve curva *f* de aprendizagem; ***be on the ~*** estar na curva de aprendizagem
lease [liːs] **1** *n* arrendamento *m* **2** *v/t apartment, equipment* arrendar
♦ **lease out** *v/t apartment, equipment* arrendar

lease 'purchase arrendamento *m* com opção de compra

leash [liːʃ] *dog*: correia *f*, *Port* trela *f*

least [liːst] **1** *adj* (*slightest*) menor **2** *adv* menos; ***the ~ expensive laptop*** o laptop menos caro **3** *n* ***he drank the ~*** ele bebeu menos; ***not in the ~ suprised*** nem um pouco surpreso; ***at ~*** pelo menos

leather ['leðər] **1** *n* couro *m* **2** *adj* de couro

leave [liːv] **1** *n* (*vacation*) licença *f*; ***on ~*** de férias **2** *v/t* ⟨*pret & pp* ***left***⟩ *person, food, scar, memory, also* (*forget*) deixar; *city, place* sair de; *husband, wife* abandonar; ***let's ~ things as they are*** vamos deixar as coisas como estão; ***how did you ~ things with him?*** como ficaram as coisas com ele?; ***~ s.o. / sth alone*** (*not touch, not interfere with*) deixar alguém / algo em paz; ***be left*** sobrar; ***there is nothing left*** não sobrou nada **3** *v/i* ⟨*pret & pp* ***left***⟩ *person, plane, train, bus* partir

◆ **leave behind** *v/t intentionally, forget* deixar para trás

◆ **leave on** *v/t hat, coat* continuar usando; *TV, computer* deixar ligado

◆ **leave out** *v/t word, figure* omitir; (*not put away*) deixar de fora; ***leave me out of this*** deixe-me fora disso

'leaving party festa *f* de despedida

lecture ['lekʧər] **1** *n* palestra *f*, *Brit university*: aula *f* **2** *v/i Brit at university* lecionar **3** *v/t* dar palpite

'lecture hall *Brit* sala *f* de palestra

lecturer ['lekʧərər] palestrante *m/f*, *Brit university*: professor,a *m,f*

led [led] *pret & pp* → ***lead***[1]

LED [eliː'diː] *abbr* (*of* ***light-emitting diode***) diodo *m* emissor de luz

ledge [ledʒ] *window*: peitoril *m*; *rock-face*: saliência *f*

ledger ['ledʒər] COM livro-razão *m*

leek [liːk] alho-poró *m*

leer [lɪr] *n sexual* olhar *m* insinuante; *evil* mau olhado *m*

left[1] [left] **1** *adj* esquerdo **2** *n* esquerda *f*; ***on the ~*** à esquerda; ***on the ~ of sth*** à esquerda de algo; ***to the ~*** *turn, look* para a esquerda **3** *adv turn, look* à esquerda

left[2] [left] *pret & pp* → ***leave***

'left-hand *curve* à direita; ***on the ~ side*** à esquerda **left-hand 'drive** direção *f* do lado esquerdo **left-handed** [left'hændɪd] *adj* canhoto **'left-overs** *food* sobras *fpl* **'left-wing** *adj* POL de esquerda

leg [leg] perna *f*; ***pull s.o.'s ~*** fazer uma brincadeira com alguém

legacy ['legəsɪ] legado *m*

legal ['lːgl] *adj* legal

legal ad'viser assessor,a *m,f* jurídico,-a

legality [lɪ'gælətɪ] legalidade *f*

legalize ['liːgəlaɪz] *v/t* legalizar

legend ['ledʒənd] lenda *f*

legendary ['ledʒəndrɪ] *adj person* legendário; (*fictitious*) lendário

legible ['ledʒəbl] *adj* legível

legislate ['ledʒɪsleɪt] *v/i* legislar

legislation [ledʒɪs'leɪʃn] legislação *f*

legislative ['ledʒɪslətɪv] *adj powers, assembly* legislativo

legislature ['ledʒɪsləʧər] POL legislatura *f*

legitimate [lɪ'dʒɪtɪmət] *adj* legítimo

'leg room espaço *m* para as pernas

leisure ['liːʒər] lazer *m*; ***at your ~*** quando quiser

'leisure center *Am* centro *m* de lazer

leisure centre *Brit* → ***leisure center***

leisurely ['liːʒərlɪ] *adj pace, lifestyle* calmo

'leisure time tempo *m* livre

lemon ['lemən] limão *m*

lemonade [lemə'neɪd] limonada *f*

'lemon juice suco *m* de limão, *Port* sumo *m* de limão

'lemon tea chá *m* com limão

lend [lend] *v/t* ⟨*pret & pp* ***lent***⟩ emprestar; ***~ s.o. sth*** emprestar algo a alguém

length [leŋθ] comprimento *m*; (*piece*) *of material etc* peça *f*; ***at ~*** *describe, explain* detalhadamente; (*eventually*) finalmente

lengthen ['leŋθən] *v/t* encompridar

lengthy ['leŋθɪ] *adj speech, stay* comprido

lenient ['liːnɪənt] *adj* leniente

lens [lenz] *nsg* lente *f*

'lens cover *of camera* protetor *m* de lente
Lent [lent] REL Quaresma *f*
lent [lent] *pret & pp* → ***lend***
lentil ['lentl] lentilha *f*
lentil 'soup sopa *f* de lentilha
Leo ['liːoʊ] ASTROL Leão *m*
leopard ['lepərd] leopardo *m*
leotard ['liːoʊtɑːrd] collant *m*
lesbian ['lezbɪən] **1** *n* lésbica *f* **2** *adj* lésbico
less [les] *adv* menos; ***eat ~*** comer menos; ***~ interesting*** menos interessante; ***it cost ~*** custa menos; ***~ than 200*** menos de 200
lesson ['lesn] lição *f*
let [let] *v/t* ⟨*pret & pp* ***let***⟩ (*allow*) deixar; ***~ s.o. do sth*** deixar alguém fazer algo; ***~ me go!*** largue-me!; ***~ him come in!*** deixe-o entrar!; ***~ 's go / stay*** vamos embora / ficar; ***~ 's not argue*** não vamos discutir; ***~ alone*** muito menos; ***~ go of sth*** *rope, handle* soltar algo
♦ **let down** *v/t hair* soltar; *shades* baixar; (*disappoint*) decepcionar; *dress, pants* encompridar
♦ **let in** *v/t to house* deixar entrar; ***the court let him off with a small fine*** o tribunal liberou-o com o pagamento de uma pequena multa
♦ **let off** *v/t* (*not punish*) perdoar; *from car* deixar saltar
♦ **let out** *v/t of room, building* alugar; *jacket etc* alargar; *groan, yell* soltar
♦ **let up** *v/i* (*stop*) cessar
lethal ['liːθl] *adj* letal
lethargic [lɪ'θɑːrdʒɪk] *adj* letárgico
lethargy ['leθərdʒɪ] letargia *f*
letter ['letər] *of alphabet* letra *f*; *in mail* carta *f*
'letterbox *Brit* caixa *f* do correio, *Port* marco *m* do correio **'letterhead** (*heading*) cabeçalho *m*; (*headed paper*) papel *m* timbrado **letter of 'credit** COM carta *f* de crédito
lettuce ['letɪs] alface *f*
'letup ***without a ~*** sem descanso
leukemia [luː'kiːmɪə] leucemia *f*
levée ['levɪ] represa *f*
level ['levl] **1** *adj field, surface* nivelado; *in competition, scores* empatado; ***draw ~ with s.o.*** ficar à altura de alguém **2** *n on scale, hierarchy, also* (*amount, quantity*) nível *m*; ***on the ~*** (*on level ground*) no nível térreo; *fam* (*honest*) honesto
level crossing *Brit* → ***grade crossing***
level-headed [levl'hedɪd] *adj* sensato
lever ['levər] **1** *n* alavanca *f* **2** *v/t* ***~ sth open with a knife*** abrir algo com uma faca como alavanca
leverage ['liːvrɪdʒ] força *f* de alavanca; (*influence*) influência *f*
levy ['levɪ] *v/t* ⟨*pret & pp* ***levied***⟩ *taxes* arrecadar
lewd [luːd] *adj* obsceno
liability [laɪə'bɪlətɪ] (*responsibility*) responsabilidade *f*; (*likeliness*) propensão *f*
liable ['laɪəbl] *adj* (*answerable*) responsável; ***be ~ to*** (*likely*) estar propenso a
♦ **liaise with** [lɪ'eɪz] *v/t* cooperar com
liaison [lɪ'eɪzɑːn] (*contacts*) ligação *f*
liar ['laɪr] mentiroso,-a *m,f*
libel ['laɪbl] **1** *n* calúnia *f* **2** *v/t* caluniar
liberal ['lɪbərəl] *adj* (*broad-minded*), *also* POL liberal; (*generous*) *portion etc* generoso
liberate ['lɪbəreɪt] *v/t* liberar
liberated ['lɪbəreɪtɪd] *adj woman etc* emancipado
liberation [lɪbə'reɪʃn] libertação *f*
liberty ['lɪbərtɪ] liberdade *f*; ***at ~*** (*prisoner etc* em liberdade; ***be at ~ to do sth*** ficar livre para fazer algo
Libra ['liːbrə] ASTROL Libra *m*
librarian [laɪ'brerɪən] bibliotecário,-a *m,f*
library ['laɪbrərɪ] biblioteca *f*
Libya ['lɪbɪə] Líbia *f*
lice [laɪs] *pl* → ***louse***
licence *Brit* → ***license*** **1** *n*
license ['laɪsns] **1** *n Am car*: carteira *f* de motorista, *Port* carta *f* de condução; *import, export*: licença *f*, *TV*: concessão *f*, ***gun ~*** porte *m* de arma **2** *v/t* ***be ~d*** ter licença
'license number número *m* da licença

'license plate *Am* placa *m* do carro

lick [lɪk] **1** *n* lambida *f* **2** *v/t* lamber; **~ *one's lips*** lamber os lábios

licking ['lɪkɪŋ] *n* ***get a ~*** *fam* (*defeat*) levar uma surra

lid [lɪd] tampa *f*

lie¹ [laɪ] **1** *n* mentira *f* **2** *v/i* mentir

lie² [laɪ] *v/i* ⟨*pret* ***lay***, *pp* ***lain***⟩ *person* deitar-se; *object* encontrar-se; (*be situated*) estar situado

♦ **lie down** *v/i* deitar-se

'lie-in *Brit* ***have a ~*** dormir até tarde

lieu [lu:] ***in ~ of*** em lugar de

lieutenant [lʊ'tenənt] tenente *m/f*

life [laɪf] ⟨*pl* ***lives***⟩ vida *f*, *machine*: vida *f* útil; ***all her ~*** a vida inteira; ***that's ~!*** é a vida!

'life belt *Brit* cinto *m* de segurança **'lifeboat** bote *m* salva-vidas **'life expectancy** expectativa *f* de vida **'lifeguard** salva-vidas *m/f* **'life history** história *f* da vida **life im'prisonment** prisão *f* perpétua **'life insurance** seguro *m* de vida **'life jacket** colete *m* salva-vidas

lifeless ['laɪflɪs] *adj* inerte

lifelike ['laɪflaɪk] *adj* realista

'lifelong *adj* para toda a vida **'life preserver** *Am swimmer*: colete *m* salva-vidas; (*buoy*) bóia *f* salva-vidas **'life-saving** *adj medical equipment*, *drug* que salva vidas **lifesized** ['laɪfsaɪzd] *adj* tamanho natural **'lifestyle** estilo *m* de vida **'life-threatening** *adj* que pode levar à morte **'lifetime** vida *f* (inteira); ***in my ~*** durante toda minha vida; ***a once in a ~ chance*** uma chance única

lift [lɪft] **1** *v/t* levantar **2** *v/i fog* dissipar-se **3** *n Brit* (*elevator*) elevador *m*; *car*: carona *f*, *Port* boleia *f* ***give s.o. a ~*** dar uma carona a alguém

♦ **lift off** *v/i rocket* decolar

ligament ['lɪgəmənt] MED ligamento *m*

light¹ [laɪt] **1** *n also* (*lamp*) luz *f*; ***in the ~ of*** à luz de; ***have you got a ~?*** você tem fogo? **2** *v/t* ⟨*pret & pp* ***lit***⟩ *fire*, *cigarette* acender; (*illuminate*) iluminar **3** *adj* (*not dark*) claro

light² [laɪt] **1** *adj* (*not heavy*) leve **2** *adv* ***travel ~*** viajar com pouca bagagem

♦ **light up 1** *v/t* (*illuminate*) iluminar **2** *v/i* (*start to smoke*) acender

'light bulb lâmpada *f*

lighten¹ ['laɪtn] *v/t color* clarear

lighten² ['laɪtn] *v/t load* tornar mais leve

♦ **lighten up** *v/i person* animar-se

lighter ['laɪtər] *cigarette*: isqueiro *m*

light-headed [laɪt'hedɪd] *adj* (*dizzy*) aturdido **light-hearted** [laɪt'hɑ:rtɪd] *adj* alegre **'lighthouse** farol *m*

lighting ['laɪtɪŋ] iluminação *f*

lightly ['laɪtlɪ] *adv touch* levemente; ***get off ~*** sair levemente punido

lightness¹ ['laɪtnɪs] *room*, *color*: claridade *f*

lightness² ['laɪtnɪs] *weight*: leveza *f*

lightning ['laɪtnɪŋ] relâmpago *m*

'lightning conductor *Brit*, **'lightning rod** *Am* pára-raios *m*

'light pen caneta *f* ótica

'lightweight *boxing*: peso *m* pena

'light year ano-luz *m*

like¹ [laɪk] **1** *prep* como; ***be ~ s.o. / sth*** *in appearance*, *character* ser como alguém / algo; ***what's she ~?*** *in looks*, *character* como ela é?; ***he looks ~ my brother*** ele se parece com o meu irmão; ***it looks ~ rain*** parece que vai chover; ***it's not ~ him*** *not his character* não é de seu feitio; ***do it ~ this*** faça assim **2** *conj fam* (*as*) como; ***~ I said*** como eu disse

like² [laɪk] *v/t* gostar de; ***I ~ it*** eu gosto disso; ***I ~ her*** eu gosto dela; ***I would ~ …*** eu gostaria de …; ***I would ~ to …*** eu gostaria de …; ***would you ~ …?*** você gostaria de …?; ***would you ~ to …?*** você gostaria de …?; ***~ to do sth*** gostar de fazer algo; ***if you ~*** se você quiser

likeable ['laɪkəbl] *adj* simpático

likelihood ['laɪklɪhʊd] probabilidade *f*; ***in all ~*** com toda probabilidade

likely ['laɪklɪ] *adj* (*probable*) provável; ***not ~!*** de jeito nenhum!

likeness ['laɪknɪs] (*resemblance*) semelhança *f*

'likewise ['laɪkwaɪz] *adv* igualmente; ***to do ~*** fazer o mesmo

liking ['laɪkɪŋ] simpatia *f*; ***to your ~*** a

L

seu gosto; ***I took an instant ~ to him*** gostei dele à primeira vista
lilac ['laɪlək] *flower, color* lilás *m*
lily ['lɪlɪ] lírio *m*
lily of the 'valley lírio-do-vale *m*
limb [lɪm] membro *m* (*do corpo*)
lime[1] [laɪm] *fruit* lima *f*, *tree* limeira *f*
lime[2] [laɪm] *substance* cal *f*
lime'green *adj* verde-lima
'limelight ***be in the ~*** ser o foco das atenções
limit ['lɪmɪt] **1** *n* limite *m*; ***within ~s*** dentro do limite; ***off ~s*** proibido; ***that's off ~s to military personnel*** isto é proibido aos militares; ***that's the ~!*** *fam* é o cúmulo! **2** *v/t* limitar
limitation [lɪmɪ'teɪʃn] limitação *f*
limited 'company companhia *f* limitada
limo ['lɪmoʊ] *fam* limusine *f*
limousine ['lɪməzi:n] limusine *f*
limp[1] [lɪmp] *adj* frouxo
limp[2] [lɪmp] *n* ***he has a ~*** ele manca
line[1] [laɪn] *n paper, road, also* TEL, *text etc*: linha *f*; *people*: fila *f*, *Port* bicha *m*; *trees*: fileira *f*; *face*: ruga *f*; ***we're in the same ~ of business*** estamos no mesmo ramo de negócio; ***what ~ are you in?*** o que você faz?; ***the ~ is busy*** a linha está ocupada; ***hold the ~*** aguardar na linha; ***draw the ~ at sth*** traçar o limite em algo; ***~ of inquiry*** linha de investigação; ***~ of reasoning*** linha de raciocínio; ***stand in ~*** ficar na fila, *Port* fazer bicha; ***in ~ with …*** (*conforming with*) de acordo com …
line[2] [laɪn] *v/t with lining* forrar
♦ **line up** *v/i* enfileirar-se
linear ['lɪnɪr] *adj* linear
linen ['lɪnɪn] *material* linho *m*; *sheets etc* roupa *f* de cama
liner ['laɪnər] *ship* navio *m* transatlântico
linesman ['laɪnzmən] SPORT juiz *m* de linha
linger ['lɪŋgər] *v/i person* demorar-se; *pain* persistir
lingerie ['lænʒəri:] lingerie *f*
linguist ['lɪŋgwɪst] lingüísta *m/f*; ***she's a good ~*** ela tem facilidade para línguas
linguistic [lɪŋ'gwɪstɪk] *adj* lingüístico
linguistics [lɪŋ'gwɪstɪks] lingüística *f*
lining ['laɪnɪŋ] *clothes*: forro *m*; *pipe, brakes*: revestimento *m*
link [lɪŋk] **1** *n* (*connection*) ligação *f*; *chain*: elo *m* **2** *v/t* ligar
♦ **link up** *v/i* reunir-se; TV conectar-se
lion ['laɪən] leão *m*
lioness ['laɪənes] leoa *f*
lip [lɪp] lábio *m*
liposuction ['laɪpoʊsʌkʃn] lipoaspiração *f*
'lipread *v/i* ⟨*pret & pp* ***lipread*** [-red]⟩ ler os lábios
'lipstick batom *m*
liqueur [lɪ'kjʊr] licor *m*
liquid ['lɪkwɪd] **1** *n* líquido *m* **2** *adj* líquido
liquidate ['lɪkwɪdeɪt] *v/t assets, also fam* (*kill*) liquidar
liquidation [lɪkwɪ'deɪʃn] liquidação *f*; ***go into ~*** entrar em liquidação
liquidity [lɪ'kwɪdɪtɪ] FIN liquidez *m*
liquidize ['lɪkwɪdaɪz] *v/t* liquidificar
liquidizer ['lɪkwɪdaɪzər] liquidificador *m*
liquor ['lɪkər] bebida *f* alcoólica
'liquor store *Am* loja *f* de bebidas alcoólicas
lisp [lɪsp] **1** *n* ceceio *m* **2** *v/i* cecear
list [lɪst] **1** *n* lista *f* **2** *v/t* listar
listen ['lɪsn] *v/i* ouvir
♦ **listen in** *v/i* escutar
♦ **listen to** *v/t radio*, *person* escutar
listener ['lɪsnər] *radio*: ouvinte *m/f*; ***he's a good ~*** ele é um bom ouvinte
listings magazine ['lɪstɪŋz] guia *m* de entretenimento
listless ['lɪstlɪs] *adj* apático
lit [lɪt] *pret & pp* → ***light***[1]
liter ['li:tər] *Am* litro *m*
literal ['lɪtərəl] *adj* literal
literally ['lɪtərəlɪ] *adv* literalmente
literary ['lɪtərerɪ] *adj* literário
literate ['lɪtərət] *adj* alfabetizado; (*educated*) letrado; ***be ~*** ser alfabetizado
literature ['lɪtrətʃər] literatura *f*; *about a product* prospectos *mpl*
litre *Brit* → ***liter***
litter ['lɪtər] lixo *m*; *animal*: ninhada *f*
'litter bin *Brit* lata *f* de lixo

little ['lɪtl] **1** *adj* pequeno; ***the ~ ones*** os pequenos **2** *n* pouco *m*; ***the ~ I know*** o pouco que sei; ***a ~*** um pouco; ***a ~ bread / wine*** um pouco de pão / /vinho; ***a ~ is better than nothing*** pouco é melhor que nada **3** *adv* ***~ by ~*** pouco a pouco; ***a ~ better / bigger*** um pouco melhor / maior; ***a ~ before 6*** um pouco antes das 6
live[1] [lɪv] *v/i* (*reside*) morar; (*be alive*) viver
live[2] [laɪv] *adj broadcast* ao vivo; ***~ ammunition*** munição *f* de guerra
♦ **live on 1** *v/t rice, bread* viver de **2** *v/i* (*continue living*) continuar vivendo
♦ **live together** *v/i* morar junto
♦ **live up** *v/t* ***live it up*** cair na farra
♦ **live up to** *v/t* corresponder a
♦ **live with** *v/t* viver com
livelihood ['laɪvlɪhʊd] sustento *m*; ***earn one's ~ from …*** tirar o sustento de …
liveliness ['laɪvlɪnɪs] *person*: vivacidade *f*; *debate*: ânimo *m*
lively ['laɪvlɪ] *adj person* vivaz; *party, music, city* animado
liver ['lɪvər] ANAT, *as food* fígado *m*
livestock ['laɪvstɑːk] gado *m*
livid ['lɪvɪd] *adj* (*angry*) furioso
living ['lɪvɪŋ] **1** *adj* vivo **2** *n* vida *f*; ***earn one's ~*** ganhar a vida; ***standard of ~*** padrão *m* de vida
'**living room** sala *f* de estar
lizard ['lɪzərd] lagarto *m*
load [loʊd] **1** *n also* ELEC carga *f*; ***~s of*** *fam* um monte de **2** *v/t car, truck, gun, software* carregar; *camera* colocar filme em; ***~ sth onto sth*** carregar algo em algo
loaded ['loʊdɪd] *adj fam* (*very rich*) cheio da nota; (*drunk*) de cara cheia
loaf [loʊf] ⟨*pl* ***loaves***⟩ pão *m*; ***a ~ of bread*** um pão
♦ **loaf about** *v/i fam* vadiar
loafer ['loʊfər] *shoe* mocassim *m*
loan [loʊn] **1** *n* empréstimo *m*; ***on ~*** emprestado **2** *v/t* ***~ s.o. sth*** emprestar algo a alguém
loathe [loʊð] *v/t* detestar
loathing ['loʊðɪŋ] ódio *m*
lobby ['lɑːbɪ] *hotel*: saguão *m*; *theater*: vestíbulo *m*; POL lobby *m*
lobe [loʊb] *of ear* lóbulo *m*
lobster ['lɑːbstər] lagosta *f*
local ['loʊkl] **1** *adj* local; ***I'm not ~*** não sou daqui **2** *n* local *m*
'**local call** TEL chamada *f* local **local e'lections** eleições *fpl* municipais **local 'government** governo *m* municipal
locality [loʊ'kælətɪ] localidade *f*
localize ['loʊkəlaɪz] *v/t software* localizar
locally ['loʊkəlɪ] *adv live, work* na vizinhança
local 'produce produção *f* local
'**local time** hora *f* local
lo carb ['loʊkɑːrb] *adj fam* baixo em hidratos de carbono
locate [loʊ'keɪt] *v/t new factory etc* situar; (*identify position of*) localizar; ***be ~d*** estar localizado
location [loʊ'keɪʃn] (*siting*) posição *f*; (*identifying position of*) localização *f*; ***on ~*** *movie* em externas
lock[1] [lɑːk] *hair*: mecha *f*
lock[2] [lɑːk] **1** *n door*: fechadura *f* **2** *v/t door* trancar; ***~ sth in position*** prender algo na posição
♦ **lock away** *v/t* guardar à chave
♦ **lock in** *v/t person* trancafiar
♦ **lock out** *v/t of house* trancar do lado de fora; ***I locked myself out*** tranquei-me do lado de fora
♦ **lock up** *v/t in prison* trancafiar
locker ['lɑːkər] cacifo *m*
'**locker room** vestiário *m*
locket ['lɑːkɪt] medalhão *m*
locksmith ['lɑːksmɪθ] serralheiro,-a *m,f*
locust ['loʊkəst] gafanhoto *m*
lodge [lɑːdʒ] **1** *v/t complaint* apresentar **2** *v/i bullet, ball* alojar-se
lodger ['lɑːdʒər] hóspede *m/f*
loft [lɑːft] sótão *m*
lofty ['lɑːftɪ] *adj heights* elevado; *ideals* nobre
log [lɑːg] *wood*: tora *f*, (*written record*) registro *m*, *Port* registo *m*
♦ **log in** *v/i* conectar-se, fazer login
♦ **log off** *v/i* ⟨*pret & pp* ***logged***⟩ desconectar-se, fazer logoff
♦ **log on** *v/i* conectar-se, fazer logon
♦ **log on to** *v/t* conectar-se a

L

♦ **log out** *v/i* ⟨*pret & pp* ***logged***⟩ desconectar-se, fazer logout
'logbook *driver's* documentação *f* do veículo; *captain's* diário *m* de bordo; *flight*: diário *m* de vôo; *hotel etc*: livro *m* de registro, *Port* livro *m* do registo
log 'cabin cabana *f* de madeira
loggerheads ['lɑːgərhedz] ***be at ~*** estar às turras
logic ['lɑːdʒɪk] lógica *f*
logical ['lɑːdʒɪkl] *adj* lógico
logically ['lɑːdʒɪklɪ] *adv* logicamente
logistics [lə'dʒɪstɪks] logística *f*
logo ['loʊgoʊ] logomarca *f*
loiter ['lɔɪtər] *v/i* vadiar
lollipop ['lɑːlɪpɑːp] pirulito *m*, *Port* chupa-chupa *m*
lolly ['lɑːlɪ] *fam* (*money*) grana *f*
London ['lʌndən] Londres
loneliness ['loʊnlɪnɪs] *person*: solidão *f*, *place*: isolamento *m*
lonely ['loʊnlɪ] *adj person*, *place* solitário
loner ['loʊnər] solitário,-a *m,f*
long[1] [lɑːŋ] **1** *adj* longo; ***it's a ~ way*** é um longo percurso **2** *adv* muito tempo; ***don't be ~*** não demore muito; ***5 weeks is too ~*** cinco semanas é muito tempo; ***2 meters ~*** 2 metros de comprimento; ***will it take ~?*** vai demorar muito?; ***that was ~ ago*** isso foi há muito tempo; ***~ before then*** muito antes disso; ***before ~*** pouco depois; ***we can't wait any ~er*** não podemos esperar mais; ***he no ~er works here*** ele não trabalha mais aqui; ***so ~ as*** (*provided*) contanto que; ***so ~!*** até logo!, *Port* adeus!
long[2] [lɑːŋ] *v/i* ***~ for sth*** desejar algo; ***be ~ing to do sth*** estar ansioso para fazer algo
long-'distance *adj phonecall* interurbano; *race* de fundo; *flight* de longa distância
longevity [lɑːn'dʒevɪtɪ] longevidade *f*
longing ['lɑːŋɪŋ] *n* anseio *m*
longitude ['lɑːndʒɪtuːd] longitude *f*
'long jump salto *m* em distância
'long-range *missile* de longo alcance; *forecast* a longo prazo **long-sighted** [lɑːŋ'saɪtɪd] *adj* hipermetrope **long-sleeved** [lɑːŋ'sliːvd] *adj* de manga comprida **long-'standing** *adj* de muito tempo **'long-term** *adj* de longo prazo **'long wave** RADIO onda *f* longa **longwinded** [lɑːŋ'wɪndɪd] *adj* prolixo
loo *Brit* → ***john***
look [lʊk] **1** *n* (*appearance*) aparência *f*; (*glance*) olhar *m*; ***give s.o. / sth a ~*** dar uma olhada em alguém / algo; ***have a ~ at sth*** (*examine*) examinar algo; ***can I have a ~?*** posso ver?; ***can I have a ~ around?*** *in shop etc* posso dar uma olhada por aí?; ***~s*** (*beauty*) boa aparência **2** *v/i* olhar; (*search*) procurar; (*seem*) parecer; ***you ~ tired*** você parece cansado
♦ **look after** *v/t* cuidar de
♦ **look ahead** *v/i fig* olhar adiante
♦ **look around 1** *v/i* olhar em volta **2** *v/t museum*, *shop*, *city* dar uma olhada em
♦ **look at** *v/t* olhar para; (*examine*) examinar; ***it depends on how you look at it*** depende de como você vê
♦ **look back** *v/i* olhar para trás
♦ **look down on** *v/t* desdenhar
♦ **look for** *v/t* procurar
♦ **look forward to** *v/t* estar ansioso por; ***I look forward to hearing from you*** aguardo notícias suas
♦ **look in on** *v/t* (*visit*) fazer uma visita a
♦ **look into** *v/t* (*investigate*) investigar
♦ **look on 1** *v/i* (*watch*) ficar olhando **2** *v/t* ***look on s.o. / sth as*** (*consider*) considerar alguém / algo como
♦ **look onto** *v/t garden*, *street* dar vista para
♦ **look out** *v/i of window etc* olhar para fora; (*pay attention*) prestar atenção; ***look out!*** cuidado!
♦ **look out for** *v/t* procurar; (*be on guard against*) ter cuidado com
♦ **look out of** *v/t window* olhar por
♦ **look over** *v/t house* inspecionar; *translation* revisar
♦ **look through** *v/t magazine*, *notes* passar uma vista em
♦ **look to** *v/t* (*rely on*) contar com
♦ **look up 1** *v/i from paper etc* levantar os olhos; (*improve*) melhorar; ***things are looking up*** as coisas estão me-

lhorando **2** *v/t word, phone number* procurar; (*visit*) visitar

♦**look up to** *v/t* (*respect*) admirar

'**lookout** *person* vigia *m/f*; ***be on the ~ for*** estar procurando

♦**loom up** [luːm] *v/i* aparecer lentamente

loony ['luːnɪ] *fam* **1** *n* maluco,-a *m,f* **2** *adj* maluco

loop [luːp] *n* presilha *f*

'**loophole** *in law etc* brecha *f*

loose [luːs] *adj connection, wire, button* frouxo; *clothes* folgado; *morals* livre; *wording* impreciso; ***~ change*** trocado *m*; ***~ ends*** *of problem, discussion* pormenores *mpl*

loosely ['luːslɪ] *adv tied* frouxamente; *worded* vagamente

loosen ['luːsn] *v/t collar, knot* afrouxar

loot [luːt] **1** *n* despojo *m* **2** *v/i* saquear

looter [luːtər] saqueador,a *m,f*

♦**lop off** [lɑːp] *v/t* ⟨*pret & pp* ***lopped***⟩ *branches* podar; *hair* cortar

lop-sided [lɑːp'saɪdɪd] *adj* torto

Lord [lɔːrd] (*god*) Senhor *m*

Lord's 'Prayer pai-nosso *m*

lorry ['lɑːrɪ] *Brit* caminhão *m*, *Port* camião *m*

lose [luːz] ⟨*pret & pp* ***lost***⟩ **1** *v/t object, match* perder; ***~ weight*** emagrecer **2** *v/i* SPORT perder; *clock* atrasar-se; ***I'm lost*** estou perdido; ***get lost!*** *fam* se manda!

♦**lose out** *v/i* sair perdendo

loser ['luːzər] perdedor,a *m,f*; *fam in life* fracassado,-a *m,f*

loss [lɑːs] *of object, loved one* perda *f*; *in business* prejuízo *m*; ***make a ~*** ter prejuízo; ***be at a ~*** estar perplexo

lost [lɑːst] **1** *adj* perdido **2** *pret & pp* → ***lose***

lost-and-'found *Am* posto *m* de achados e perdidos

lost property office *Brit* → ***lost-and-found***

lot [lɑːt] *n* ***a ~, ~s*** muito, muitos; ***I read a ~*** eu leio muito; ***a ~ of, ~s of*** muito, muitos; ***a ~ better*** muito melhor; ***a ~ easier*** muito mais fácil; ***the ~*** tudo

lotion ['loʊʃn] loção *f*

lottery ['lɑːtərɪ] loteria *f*

loud [laʊd] *adj music, voice, noise* alto; *color* forte

loud'speaker alto-falante *m*

lounge [laʊndʒ] *house*: sala *f* de estar; *hotel, airport*: salão *m*

♦**lounge about** *v/i* ficar à toa

'**lounge suit** *Brit* terno *m*, *Port* fato *m*

louse [laʊs] ⟨*pl* ***lice***⟩ piolho *m*

lousy ['laʊzɪ] *adj fam* ruim; ***I feel ~*** sinto-me péssimo

lout [laʊt] rústico,-a *m,f*

lovable ['lʌvəbl] *adj* encantador

love [lʌv] **1** *n* amor *m*; ***be in ~*** estar apaixonado; ***fall in ~*** apaixonar-se; ***make ~*** fazer amor; ***make ~ to …*** fazer amor com …; ***yes, my ~*** sim, meu amor; ***15 ~*** *in tennis* quinze a zero **2** *v/t person, country, wine* amar; ***~ to do sth*** adorar fazer algo

'**love affair** caso *m* amoroso '**love letter** carta *f* de amor '**lovelife** vida *f* sentimental

lovely ['lʌvlɪ] *adj face, hair* adorável; *color, tune* lindo; *person, character* encantador; *holiday, weather, meal* maravilhoso; ***we had a ~ time*** passamos bons momentos

lover ['lʌvər] amante *m/f*

loving ['lʌvɪŋ] *adj* afetuoso

lovingly ['lʌvɪŋlɪ] *adv* carinhosamente

low [loʊ] **1** *adj wall, price, quality* baixo; *voice* grave; ***be feeling ~*** estar deprimido; ***be ~ on tea*** ter pouco chá; ***be ~ on gas*** estar com pouca gasolina **2** *n weather*: zona *f* de baixa pressão; *sales, statistics*: baixa *f*

lowbrow ['loʊbraʊ] *adj* pouco intelectual '**low carb** *adj* baixo em hidratos de carbono **low-'calorie** *adj* de baixa caloria '**low-cut** *adj dress* decotado

lower ['loʊər] *v/t to the ground, pressure, price* baixar; *flag, hemline* arriar

'**low-fat** *adj* pobre em gordura '**low-key** *adj* discreto '**lowlands** *npl* planície *f* **low-'pressure area** área *f* de baixa pressão '**low season** baixa estação *f* '**low tide** maré *f* baixa

loyal ['lɔɪəl] *adj* leal

loyally ['lɔɪəlɪ] *adv* lealmente

loyalty ['lɔɪəltɪ] lealdade *f*

lozenge ['lɑːzɪndʒ] *shape* losango *m*; *tablet* pastilha *f*

LP [el'pi:] *abbr* (*of* ***long-playing record***) LP *m*
Ltd *abbr* (*of* ***limited***) limitada
lubricant ['lu:brɪkənt] lubrificante *m*
lubricate ['lu:brɪkeɪt] *v/t* lubrificar
lubrication [lu:brɪ'keɪʃn] lubrificação *f*
lucid ['lu:sɪd] *adj* (*clear*) transparente; (*sane*) lúcido
luck [lʌk] sorte *f*; ***bad ~*** má sorte; ***hard ~!*** que azar!; ***good ~!*** boa sorte!
♦ **luck out** *v/i fam* ter muita sorte
luckily ['lʌkɪlɪ] *adv* felizmente
lucky ['lʌkɪ] *adj person* sortudo; *day, number* de sorte; *coincidence* feliz; ***you were ~*** você teve sorte; ***he's ~ to be alive*** ele tem sorte de estar vivo; ***that's ~!*** que sorte!
lucrative ['lu:krətɪv] *adj* lucrativo
ludicrous ['lu:dɪkrəs] *adj* ridículo
lug [lʌg] *v/t* ⟨*pret & pp* ***lugged***⟩ *fam* arrastar
luggage ['lʌgɪdʒ] bagagem *f*
lukewarm ['lu:kwɔ:rm] *adj water* morno; *reception* sem entusiasmo
lull [lʌl] **1** *n storm, fighting*: interrupção *f*, *conversation*: pausa *f* **2** *v/t* ***~ s.o. into a false sense of security*** acalmar alguém dando-lhe uma (falsa) sensação de segurança
lullaby ['lʌləbaɪ] cantiga *f* de ninar
lumbago [lʌm'beɪgoʊ] lumbago *m*
lumber ['lʌmbər] (*timber*) tábua *f*
luminous ['lu:mɪnəs] *adj* luminoso
lump [lʌmp] *sugar*: torrão *f*, (*swelling*) inchação *f*, *head*: galo *m*
♦ **lump together** *v/t* ajuntar
lump 'sum pagamento *m* único
lumpy ['lʌmpɪ] *adj* encaroçado
lunacy ['lu:nəsɪ] loucura *f*
lunar ['lu:nər] *adj* lunar
lunatic ['lu:nətɪk] *n* louco,-a *m,f*
lunch [lʌntʃ] almoço *m*; ***have ~*** almoçar
'lunch box marmita *f* **'lunch break** intervalo *m* de almoço **'lunch hour** hora *f* de almoço **'lunchtime** hora *f* do almoço
lung [lʌŋ] pulmão *m*
'lung cancer câncer *m* de pulmão, *Port* cancro *m* de pulmão
♦ **lunge at** [lʌndʒ] *v/t* arremeter contra
lurch [lɜ:rtʃ] *v/i* balançar
lure [lʊr] **1** *n* sedução *f* **2** *v/t* seduzir
lurid ['lʊrɪd] *adj color* horrível; *details* escabroso
lurk [lɜ:rk] *v/i person, doubt* espreitar; (*hide*) esconder-se
luscious ['lʌʃəs] *adj fruit, dessert* saboroso; *fam woman, man* atraente
lush [lʌʃ] *adj vegetation* luxuriante
lust [lʌst] *n* luxúria *f*, (*greed*) cobiça *f*
luxurious [lʌg'ʒʊrɪəs] *adj* luxuoso
luxuriously [lʌg'ʒʊrɪəslɪ] *adv* luxuosamente
luxury ['lʌkʃərɪ] **1** *n* luxo *m* **2** *adj* de luxo
lymph gland ['lɪmfglænd] glândula *f* linfática
lynch [lɪntʃ] *v/t* linchar
lyricist ['lɪrɪsɪst] letrista *m/f*
lyrics ['lɪrɪks] letra *f*

M

M [em] *abbr* → ***medium***
MA [em'eɪ] *abbr* (*of* ***Master of Arts***) *degree* Mestrado *m* em Ciências Humanas; *person* Mestre,-a *m,f* em Ciências Humanas
ma'am [mæm] senhora *f*
mac [mæk] *fam* (*mackintosh*) mac *m*
machine [mə'ʃi:n] **1** *n* máquina *f* **2** *v/t with sewing machine* costurar à máquina; TECH fazer à máquina
ma'chine gun *n* metralhadora *f*
machine-'readable *adj* compatível com leitura à máquina
machinery [mə'ʃi:nərɪ] (*machines*)

M

maquinaria *f*
machine trans'lation tradução *f* automática
machismo [mə'kɪzmoʊ] machismo *m*
macho ['mætʃoʊ] *adj* macho
mackintosh ['mækɪntɑːʃ] capa *f* de chuva
macro ['mækroʊ] COMPUT macro *m/f*
mad [mæd] *adj* (*insane*) louco; *fam* (*angry*) furioso; ***be ~ about*** *fam* (*keen on*) ser louco por; ***drive s.o. ~*** deixar alguém louco; ***go ~*** *also fam enthusiasm*: ficar louco; ***like ~*** *fam run, work* como louco
madden ['mædən] *v/t* (*infuriate*) exasperar
maddening ['mædnɪŋ] *adj* exasperante
made [meɪd] *pret & pp* → ***make***
'madhouse *fig* casa *f* de loucos
madly ['mædlɪ] *adv* loucamente; ***~ in love*** loucamente apaixonado
'madman louco *m*
madness ['mædnɪs] loucura *f*
Madonna [mə'dɑːnə] madona *f*
Mafia ['mɑːfɪə] *n* ***the ~*** a máfia
magazine ['mægəziːn] *printed* revista *f*
maggot ['mægət] larva *f*
Magi ['meɪdʒaɪ] REL Magos *mpl*
magic ['mædʒɪk] **1** *n* magia *f*; (*tricks*) mágica *f*; ***like ~*** como num passe de mágica **2** *adj* mágico
magical ['mædʒɪkl] *adj* mágico
magician [mə'dʒɪʃn] *performer* mágico,-a *m,f*
magic 'spell feitiço *m* **magic 'trick** truque *m* de mágica **magic 'wand** varinha *f* mágica
magnanimous [mæg'nænɪməs] *adj* magnânimo
magnet ['mægnɪt] ímã *m*
magnetic [mæg'netɪk] *adj also fig personality* magnético
magnetic 'stripe tarja *f* magnética
magnetism ['mægnətɪzm] *of person* magnetismo *m*
magnificence [mæg'nɪfɪsəns] magnificência *f*
magnificent [mæg'nɪfɪsənt] *adj* magnífico
magnify ['mægnɪfaɪ] *v/t* ⟨*pret & pp* ***magnified***⟩ aumentar; *difficulties* exagerar
'magnifying glass lente *f* de aumento
magnitude ['mægnɪtuːd] magnitude *f*
mahogany [mə'hɑːgənɪ] mogno *m*
maid [meɪd] empregada *f*; *hotel*: arrumadeira *f*
maiden name ['meɪdn] nome *m* de solteira
maiden 'voyage viagem *f* inaugural
mail [meɪl] **1** *n* correio *m*; ***put sth in the ~*** levar algo ao correio **2** *v/t letter* enviar pelo correio; ***~ sth to s.o.*** enviar algo para alguém pelo correio
'mailbox *Am* caixa *f* dos correios; *also Brit* COMPUT caixa *f* de entrada
'mailing list lista *f* de correio
'mailman *Am* carteiro *f* **'mail-order catalog** *Am* catálogo *m* de venda postal **mail-order catalogue** *Brit* → ***mail-order catalog*** **'mail-order firm** empresa *f* de venda pelo correio **'mailshot** postagem *f*
maim [meɪm] *v/t* mutilar
main [meɪn] *adj* principal
'main course prato *m* principal **main 'entrance** entrada *f* principal **'mainframe** mainframe *m* **'mainland** continente *m*; ***on the ~*** no continente
mainly ['meɪnlɪ] *adv* principalmente
main 'road estrada *f* principal
'main street rua *f* principal
maintain [meɪn'teɪn] *v/t peace, speed, relationship, family* manter; *machine, house* conservar; *innocence, guilt* declarar; ***~ that*** afirmar que
maintenance ['meɪntənəns] *machine, house, law and order*: manutenção *f*; (*money*) pensão *f*
'maintenance costs *npl* custo *m* de manutenção
'maintenance staff pessoal *m* da manutenção
majestic ['mədʒestɪ] *adj* majestoso
majesty [mə'dʒestɪk] *n* ***Her Majesty*** Sua Majestade
major ['meɪdʒər] **1** *adj* (*significant*) importante; ***in C ~*** MUS em sol maior **2** *n* MIL major *m/f*; ***a politics ~*** um especialista em política

M

♦**major in** *v/t Am* especializar-se em
majority [mə'dʒɑːrətɪ] *also* POL maioria *f*; ***be in the ~*** ser uma maioria
make [meɪk] **1** *n* (*brand*) marca *f* **2** *v/t* ⟨*pret & pp* ***made***⟩ fazer; (*earn*) ganhar; ***two and two ~ four*** dois e dois são quatro; ***~ s.o. do sth*** (*force to*) obrigar alguém a fazer algo; (*cause to*) fazer com que alguém faça algo; ***you can't ~ me do it!*** você não pode me obrigar!; ***~ s.o. happy*** fazer alguém feliz; ***~ s.o. angry*** fazer alguém ficar zangado; ***~ a decision*** tomar uma decisão; ***~ a telephone call*** dar um telefonema; ***made in Japan*** fabricado no Japão; ***~ it*** (*catch bus, train*) chegar a tempo; (*come*) ir; (*succeed*) ter sucesso; (*survive*) sobreviver; ***what time do you ~ it?*** que horas tem?; ***~ believe*** fazer de conta; ***~ do with*** contentar-se com; ***what do you ~ of it?*** o que você pensa disso?
♦**make for** *v/t* (*go toward*) dirigir-se a
♦**make off** *v/i* fugir
♦**make off with** *v/t* (*steal*) fugir com
♦**make out 1** *v/t list* elaborar; *check* fazer; (*see*) distinguir; (*imply*) dar a entender **2** *v/i fam* ***make out with s.o.*** ficar com alguém
♦**make over** *v/t*: ***make X over to Y*** transferir X para Y
♦**make up 1** *v/i woman, actor* maquiar-se; *after quarrel* reconciliar-se **2** *v/t story, excuse* inventar; *face* maquiar; (*constitute*) constituir; ***be made up of*** ser feito de; ***make up one's mind*** decidir-se; ***make it up*** *after quarrel* fazer as pazes
♦**make up for** *v/t* compensar
'make-believe *n* faz-de-conta *m*
maker ['meɪkər] criador,a *m,f*
makeshift ['meɪkʃɪft] *adj* provisório
'make-up (*cosmetics*) maquiagem *f*, *Port* maquilhagem *f*
'make-up bag bolsa *f* de maquiagem, *Port* bolsa *f* de maquilhagem
maladjusted [mælə'dʒʌstɪd] *adj* desajustado
male [meɪl] **1** *adj* (*masculine*) masculino; ***~ teachers*** professores do sexo masculino **2** *n man* homem *m*; *animal, bird, fish* macho *m*
male 'chauvinism machismo *m*
male chauvinist 'pig porco *m* chauvinista **male 'nurse** enfermeiro *m*
malevolent [mə'levələnt] *adj* malévolo
malfunction [mæl'fʌŋkʃn] **1** *n* pane *f* **2** *v/i* falhar
malice ['mælɪs] malícia *f*
malicious [mə'lɪʃəs] *adj* malicioso
malignant [mə'lɪgnənt] *adj tumor* maligno
mall [mɒːl] (*shopping mall*) shopping *m*
malnutrition [mælnuː'trɪʃn] desnutrição *f*
maltreat [mæl'triːt] *v/t* maltratar
maltreatment [mæl'triːtmənt] maus-tratos *mpl*
mammal ['mæml] mamífero,-a *m,f*
mammoth ['mæməθ] *adj* (*enormous*) gigantesco
man [mæn] **1** *n* ⟨*pl* ***men***⟩ homem *m*; *checkers*: pedra *f*; ***ever since ~ has lived here*** desde então o homem viveu aqui **2** *v/t* ⟨*pret & pp* ***manned***⟩ *telephones, front desk* atender; *spacecraft* tripular
manage ['mænɪdʒ] **1** *v/t business* gerenciar; *money* administrar; *suitcase* arrumar; ***~ to …*** conseguir … **2** *v/i* (*cope*) *also financially* virar-se; ***can you ~?*** você pode se virar?
manageable ['mænɪdʒəbl] *adj* manejável; (*feasible*) viável
management ['mænɪdʒmənt] (*managing*) administração *f*, (*managers*) direção *f*; ***under his ~*** sob sua direção
'management consultant consultor,a *m,f* administrativo,-a **'management studies** estudos *mpl* de administração **'management team** equipe *f* de gerentes
manager ['mænɪdʒər] gerente *m/f*, *soccer team*: técnico *m*
managerial [mænɪ'dʒɪrɪəl] *adj* gerencial
managing di'rector diretor-gerente *m*, diretora-gerente *f*
mandarin orange ['mændərɪn] tangerina *f*

M

mandate ['mændeɪt] *n* (*authority*) mandato *m*; (*task*) tarefa *f*
mandatory ['mændətɔːrɪ] *adj* obrigatório
mane [meɪn] *of horse* crina *f*
maneuver [mə'nuːvər] *Am* **1** *n* manobra *f* **2** *v/t* manobrar
mangle ['mæŋgl] *v/t* (*crush*) destroçar
manhandle ['mænhændl] *v/t person* maltratar; *object* mover à força; ***they ~d him into the back of the truck*** eles o jogaram na parte de trás do caminhão
manhood ['mænhʊd] *maturity* idade *f* adulta; (*virility*) virilidade *f*
'man-hour hora-homem *f*
'manhunt caçada *f* humana
mania ['meɪnɪə] (*craze*) mania *f*
maniac ['meɪnɪæk] *fam* louco,-a *m,f*
manicure ['mænɪkjʊr] manicure *f*, *Port* manicura *f*
manifest ['mænɪfest] **1** *adj* manifesto **2** *v/t* manifestar; ***~ itself*** manifestar-se
manipulate [mə'nɪpjəleɪt] *v/t person* manipular; *equipment* manejar
manipulation [mənɪpjə'leɪʃn] *of person* manipulação *f*
manipulative [mənɪpjə'lətɪv] *adj* manipulador
man'kind humanidade *f*
manly ['mænlɪ] *adj* másculo
'man-made *adj fibers, materials* sintético; *structure* artificial
manner ['mænər] *of doing sth* modo *m*; (*attitude*) maneira *f*
manners ['mænərz] *npl* modos *mpl*; ***good / bad ~*** boas / más maneiras *fpl*; ***have no ~*** não ter boas maneiras
manoeuvre *Brit* → ***maneuver***
'manpower mão-de-obra *f*
mansion ['mænʃn] mansão *f*
mantelpiece ['mæntlpiːs] cornija *f* de lareira
manual ['mænjʊəl] **1** *adj* manual **2** *n* manual *m*
manually ['mænjʊəlɪ] *adv* manualmente
manufacture [mænjʊ'fæktʃər] **1** *n* fabricação *f* **2** *v/t equipment* fabricar
manufacturer [mænjʊ'fæktʃərər] fabricante *m/f*
manufacturing [mænjʊ'fæktʃərɪŋ] *adj industry* manufatureira
manure [mə'nʊr] esterco *m*
manuscript ['mænjʊskrɪpt] manuscrito *m*
many ['menɪ] *adj & pron* muitos,-as; ***~ times*** muitas vezes; ***not ~ people / taxis*** não muitas pessoas / muitos táxis; ***too ~ problems / beers*** problemas / cervejas demais; ***as ~ as 200 are still missing*** há no mínimo 200 desaparecidos; ***how ~ do you need?*** de quantos você precisa?; ***a great ~, a good ~*** muitos
'man-year ano-homem
map [mæp] mapa *m*
♦ **map out** *v/t* ⟨*pret & pp* ***mapped***⟩ traçar
maple ['meɪpl] bordo *m*
mar [mɑːr] *v/t* ⟨*pret & pp* ***marred***⟩ estragar
marathon ['mærəθɑːn] maratona *f*
marble ['mɑːrbl] *material* mármore *m*
March [mɑːrtʃ] março *m*
march [mɑːrtʃ] **1** *n* marcha *f*; (*demonstration*) passeata *f* **2** *v/i also in protest* marchar
marcher ['mɑːrtʃər] manifestante *m/f*
Mardi Gras ['mɑːrdɪgrɑː] terça-feira *f* de carnaval
mare [mer] égua *f*
margarine [mɑːrdʒə'riːn] margarina *f*
margin ['mɑːrdʒɪn] *also* COM margem *f*; ***by a narrow ~*** por uma pequena margem
marginal ['mɑːrdʒɪnl] *adj* (*slight*) ligeiro
marginally ['mɑːrdʒɪnlɪ] *adv* (*slightly*) ligeiramente
marihuana, **marijuana** [mærɪ'hwɑːnə] maconha *f*
marina [mə'riːnə] marina *f*
marinade [mærɪ'neɪd] *n* marinada *f*
marinate ['mærɪneɪt] *v/t* marinar
marine [mə'riːn] **1** *adj* marinho; *engineer* naval **2** *n* MIL marinha *f*
marital ['mærɪtl] *adj* conjugal
'marital status estado *m* civil
maritime ['mærɪtaɪm] *adj* marítimo
mark [mɑːrk] **1** *n* (*stain*) mancha *f*; EDUC nota *f*; (*sign, token*) sinal *m*; ***leave one's ~*** deixar sua marca

2 *v/t* (*stain*) manchar; (*commemorate*) comemorar
◆ **mark down** *v/t goods* remarcar
◆ **mark out** *v/t with a line etc* marcar; *fig* (*set apart*) distinguir
◆ **mark up** *v/t price* subir; *goods* subir de preço
marked [mɑːrkt] *adj* (*definite*) marcante
marker ['mɑːrkər] (*highlighter*) marcador *m* de texto
market ['mɑːrkɪt] **1** *n* mercado *m*; (*stock market*) bolsa *f*; ***on the ~*** no mercado **2** *v/t* comercializar
marketable ['mɑːrkɪtəbl] *adj* comercializável
market e'conomy economia *f* de mercado
'market forces *npl* forças *fpl* de mercado
marketing ['mɑːrkɪtɪŋ] marketing *m*
'marketing campaign campanha *f* de marketing **'marketing department** departamento *m* de marketing **'marketing mix** marketing mix *m* **'marketing strategy** estratégia *f* de marketing
market 'leader líder *m/f* de mercado **'market-place** *in town, also for commodities* mercado *m* **market 'research** pesquisa *f* de mercado **market 'share** fatia *f* de mercado
'mark-up margem *f*
marmalade ['mɑːrməleɪd] geléia *f*
marquee [mɑːr'kiː] toldo *m*
marriage ['mærɪdʒ] casamento *m*; *institution* matrimônio *m*
'marriage certificate certidão *f* de casamento
marriage guidance counsellor *Brit* → ***marriage guidance counselor***
marriage 'guidance counselor conselheiro,-a *m,f* matrimonial
married ['mærɪd] *adj* casado; ***be ~ to ...*** ser casado com …
married 'life vida *f* de casado
marry ['mærɪ] *v/t* ⟨*pret & pp* ***married***⟩ *also priest* casar; ***get married*** casar-se
marsh [mɑːrʃ] *Brit* pântano *m*
marshal ['mɑːrʃl] *police officer* comissário,-a *m,f*; *official* marechal *m/f*
marshmallow ['mɑːrʃmæloʊ] marshmallow *m*
marshy ['mɑːrʃɪ] *adj Brit* pantanoso
martial arts [mɑːrʃl'ɑːrtz] *npl* artes *fpl* marciais
martial 'law lei *f* marcial
martyr ['mɑːrtər] mártir *m/f*
martyred ['mɑːrtərd] *adj fig* martirizado
marvel ['mɑːrvl] maravilha *f*
◆ **marvel at** *v/t* maravilhar-se com
marvellous *Brit* → ***marvelous***
marvelous ['mɑːrvələs] *adj Am* maravilhoso
Marxism ['mɑːrksɪzm] marxismo *m*
Marxist ['mɑːrksɪst] **1** *adj* marxista **2** *n* marxista *m/f*
marzipan ['mɑːrzɪpæn] maçapão *m*
mascara [mæ'skærə] rímel *m*
mascot ['mæskət] mascote *m*
masculine ['mæskjʊlɪn] *adj* masculino
masculinity [mæskjʊ'lɪnətɪ] (*virility*) masculinidade *f*
mash [mæʃ] *v/t* amassar
mashed po'tatoes [mæʃt] *npl* purê *m* de batatas
mask [mæsk] **1** *n* máscara *f* **2** *v/t feelings* mascarar
'masking tape fita crepe *f*
masochism ['mæsəkɪzm] masoquismo *m*
masochist ['mæsəkɪst] masoquista *m/f*
mason ['meɪsn] canteiro *m*
masonry ['meɪsnrɪ] alvenaria *f*
masquerade [mæskə'reɪd] **1** *n fig* disfarce *m* **2** *v/i* ***~ as*** passar-se por
mass[1] [mæs] **1** *n* (*great amount*) grande quantidade *f*; ***the ~es*** as massas; ***~es of*** *fam* um montão de **2** *v/i* reunir-se
mass[2] [mæs] REL missa *f*
massacre ['mæsəkər] **1** *n* massacre *m*; *fam sport*: surra *f* **2** *v/t* massacrar; *fam sport*: dar uma surra
massage [mæ'sɑːʒ] **1** *n* massagem *f* **2** *v/t* massagear; *figures* maquiar
'massage parlor *Am* salão *m* de massagem
massage parlour *Brit* → ***massage parlor***
masseur [mæ'sɜːr] massagista *m*

masseuse [mæ'sɜːz] massagista *f*
massive ['mæsɪv] *adj* maciço
mass 'media *npl* meios *mpl* de comunicação de massa **mass-pro'duce** *v/t* produzir em massa **mass pro'duction** produção *f* em massa
mast [mæst] *ship*: mastro *m*; *radio*: antena *f*
master ['mæstər] **1** *n dog*: dono *m*; *ship*: capitão *m*; ***be a ~ of*** ser um especialista em **2** *v/t skill, language* dominar; *situation* controlar
'master bedroom quarto *m* principal
'master key chave *f* mestra
masterly ['mæstərlɪ] *adj* magistral
'mastermind 1 *n* cabeça *m* **2** *v/t* planejar **'masterpiece** obra-prima *f*
'master's (degree) mestrado *m*
mastery ['mæstərɪ] domínio *m*
masturbate ['mæstərbeɪt] *v/i* masturbar
mat [mæt] *floor*: tapete *m*; *table*: descanso *m*
match[1] [mætʃ] *cigarette*: fósforo *m*
match[2] [mætʃ] **1** *n* (*competition*) partida *f*; ***be no ~ for s.o.*** não ser páreo para alguém; ***meet one's ~*** encontrar seu par **2** *v/t color, pattern* combinar com; (*be the same as*) ser igual a **3** *v/i colors etc* combinar-se
'matchbox caixa *f* de fósforos
matching ['mætʃɪŋ] *adj* que combina
'match stick palito *m* de fósforo
mate [meɪt] **1** *n animal*: parceiro,-a *m,f*; NAUT imediato *m* **2** *v/i* acasalar-se
material [mə'tɪrɪəl] **1** *n* (*fabric*) tecido *m*; (*substance*) material *m*; **~s** *pl* materiais *mpl* **2** *adj* material
materialism [mə'tɪrɪəlɪzm] materialismo *m*
materialist [mətɪrɪə'lɪst] materialista *m/f*
materialistic [mətɪrɪə'lɪstɪk] *adj* materialista
materialize [mə'tɪrɪəlaɪz] *v/i* materializar-se
maternal [mə'tɜːrnl] *adj* materno
maternity [mə'tɜːrnətɪ] maternidade *f*
ma'ternity dress vestido *m* de gestante **ma'ternity leave** licença-maternidade *f* **ma'ternity ward** pavilhão *m* de maternidade
math [mæθ] *Am* matemática *f*
mathematical [mæθə'mætɪkl] *adj* matemático
mathematician [mæθmə'tɪʃn] matemático,-a *m,f*
mathematics [mæθ'mætɪks] matemática *f*
maths *Brit* → ***math***
matinée ['mætɪneɪ] matinê *f*
matriarch ['meɪtrɪɑːrk] matriarca *f*
matrimony ['mætrəmoʊnɪ] matrimônio *m*
matt [mæt] *adj* fosco
matter ['mætər] **1** *n* (*affair*) assunto *m*; PHYS matéria *f*; ***as a ~ of course*** como de rotina; ***as a ~ of fact*** na realidade; ***what's the ~?*** qual é o problema?; ***no ~ what she says*** não importa o que ela disser **2** *v/i* importar; ***it doesn't ~*** não importa
matter-of-'fact prático; *tone of voice* impassível; *description* objetivo
mattress ['mætrɪs] colchão *m*
mature [mə'tur] **1** *adj* maduro **2** *v/i person* amadurecer; *insurance policy etc* vencer
maturity [mə'turətɪ] maturidade *f*
maul [mɒːl] *v/t animal* ferir; *critics* destroçar
maximize ['mæksɪmaɪz] *v/t* maximizar
maximum ['mæksɪməm] **1** *adj* máximo **2** *n* máximo *m*
May [meɪ] maio *m*
may [meɪ] ◇ (*possibility*) poder; ***it ~ rain*** pode ser que chova; ***you ~ be right*** pode ser que você esteja certo; ***it ~ not happen*** pode ser que não aconteça
◇ (*permission*) poder; ***~ I help / smoke?*** posso ajudar / fumar?; ***you ~ if you like*** você pode, se quiser
maybe ['meɪbiː] *adv* talvez
'May Day primeiro *m* de maio
mayo, mayonnaise ['meɪoʊ, meɪə'neɪz] maionese *f*
mayor ['meɪər] prefeito,-a *m,f*, *Port* presidente,-a *m,f* da câmara municipal
maze [meɪz] labirinto *m*

M

MB *abbr* (*of* ***megabyte***) COMPUT megabyte *m*

MBA [embiː'eɪ] *abbr* (*of* ***master of business administration***) Mestre *m/f* em Administração de Empresas

MBO [embiː'oʊ] *abbr* (*of* ***management buyout***) compra *f* de uma empresa por seus diretores

MC [em'siː] *abbr* (*of* ***master of ceremonies***) mestre *m/f* de cerimônias

MD [em'diː] *abbr* (*of* ***Doctor of Medicine***) doutor,a *m,f* em medicina

me [miː] *pron direct object* me; *indirect object* mim; *between a preposition and another verb* eu; ***did you see ~ on television?*** você me viu na televisão?; ***this is for ~ to decide*** isto é para eu decidir; ***without ~*** sem mim; ***it's ~*** sou eu; ***with ~*** comigo; ***give it to ~*** dê para mim

meadow ['medoʊ] prado *m*

meager ['miːgər] *adj Am* escasso

meagre *Brit* → ***meager***

meal [miːl] refeição *f*

'mealtime hora *f* da refeição

mean[1] [miːn] *adj* (*nasty*) cruel; *with money* pão-duro

mean[2] [miːn] ⟨*pret & pp* ***meant***⟩ **1** *v/t word, person* querer dizer; ***what do you ~?*** o que você quer dizer?; ***who do you ~?*** a quem você se refere?; ***do you really ~ it?*** você realmente está falando sério?; ***you weren't ~t to hear that*** não era para você ouvir isso; ***~ to do sth*** ter a intenção de fazer algo; ***be ~t for*** *remark* ser dirigido a; ***doesn't it ~ anything to you?*** (*doesn't it matter*) isso não significa nada para você? **2** *v/i* ***~ well*** ter boa intenção

meaning ['miːnɪŋ] *of word* significado *m*

meaningful ['miːnɪŋfʊl] *adj* significativo; (*constructive*) construtivo

meaningless ['miːnɪŋlɪs] *adj sentence, gesture etc* sem sentido

means [miːnz] *npl financial* condições *fpl*; *nsg* (*way*) meio *m*; ***~ of transportation*** meio de transporte; ***by all ~*** (*certainly*) claro que sim; ***by no ~ rich / poor*** de modo algum rico / pobre; ***by ~ of*** por meio de

meant [ment] *pret & pp of* ***mean***[2]

meantime ['miːntaɪm] **1** *adv* enquanto **2** *n* ***in the ~*** enquanto isso

meanwhile ['miːnwaɪl] **1** *adv* enquanto **2** *n* ***in the ~*** enquanto isso

measles ['miːzlz] *nsg* sarampo *m*

measure ['meʒər] **1** *n* (*step*) medida *f*; ***we've had a ~ of success*** tivemos um certo sucesso **2** *v/t & v/i* medir

♦ **measure out** *v/t* dosar

♦ **measure up to** *v/t* estar à altura de

measurement ['meʒərmənt] medida *f*; ***system of ~*** sistema *m* de medidas

measuring tape ['meʒərɪŋ] fita *f* métrica

meat [miːt] carne *f*

'meatball almôndega *f*

'meatloaf assado *m* de carne moída

mechanic [mɪ'kænɪk] mecânico,-a *m,f*

mechanical [mɪ'kænɪkl] *adj device, gesture* mecânico

mechanical engi'neer engenheiro,-a *m,f* mecânico,-a

mechanical engi'neering engenharia *f* mecânica

mechanically [mɪ'kænɪklɪ] *adv do sth* mecanicamente

mechanism ['mekənɪzm] mecanismo *m*

mechanize ['mekənaɪz] *v/t* mecanizar

medal ['medl] medalha *f*

medalist ['medəlɪst] *Am* ganhador,a *m,f* de medalha

medallist *Brit* → ***medalist***

meddle ['medl] *v/i* intrometer-se

media ['miːdɪə] *npl* mídia *f*; ***the ~*** a mídia

'media coverage cobertura *f* da mídia

mediaeval *Brit* → ***medieval***

'media event evento *m* de interesse da mídia

'media hype exagero *m* da mídia

median strip [miːdɪən'strɪp] *Am* canteiro *m* divisor

'media studies estudo *m* de mídia

mediate ['miːdɪeɪt] *v/i* mediar

mediation [miːdɪ'eɪʃn] mediação *f*

mediator ['miːdɪeɪtər] mediador,a *m,f*

medical ['medɪkl] **1** *adj* médico; ***~ student*** estudante *m/f* de medicina

2 *n* exame *m* médico

'medical certificate certificado *m* médico **'medical examination** exame *m* médico **'medical history** histórico *m* médico **'medical profession** profissão *f* médica; (*doctors*) médicos *mpl* **'medical record** ficha *f* médica

Medicare ['medɪker] *Am* sistema *m* nacional de seguro de saúde

medicated ['medɪkeɪtɪd] *adj* medicinal

medication [medɪ'keɪʃn] medicação *f*; ***are you on any ~?*** você está tomando alguma medicação?

medicinal [mɪ'dɪsɪnl] *adj* medicinal

medicine ['medsən] *science* medicina *f*; (*medication*) medicamento *m*

'medicine cabinet armário *m* de remédios

medieval [medɪ'iːvl] *adj* medieval

mediocre [miːdɪ'oʊkər] *adj* medíocre

mediocrity [miːdɪ'ɑːkrətɪ] *also person* mediocridade *f*

meditate ['medɪteɪt] *v/i* meditar

meditation [medɪ'teɪʃn] meditação *f*

Mediterranean [medɪtə'reɪnɪən] **1** *adj* mediterrâneo **2** *n* ***the ~*** o Mediterrâneo

medium ['miːdɪəm] **1** *adj* (*average*) médio; *steak* ao ponto **2** *n size*: médio *m*; (*vehicle*) meio *m*; (*spiritualist*) médium *m/f*

medium-sized ['miːdɪəmsaɪzd] *adj* de tamanho médio **'medium term** ***in the ~*** a médio prazo **'medium wave** RADIO onda *f* média

medley ['medlɪ] (*assortment*) mistura *f*

meek [miːk] *adj* dócil

meet [miːt] **1** *v/t* ⟨*pret & pp* ***met***⟩ encontrar; *be introduced to* conhecer; (*collect, at airport etc*) apanhar; *in competition* enfrentar(-se); *conditions etc* satisfazer; ***I'm going to ~ them in town tonight*** vou me encontrar com eles na cidade hoje à noite; ***come and ~ my brother*** venha conhecer o meu irmão; ***we met them in the finals*** nós os enfrentamos na final; ***a strange sight met his eyes*** uma estranha visão alcançou seus olhos; ***pleased to ~ you*** prazer em conhecê-lo **2** *v/i* ⟨*pret & pp* ***met***⟩ *also committee etc* reunir-se; *by accident, also eyes* encontrar-se; (*get to know each other*) conhecer-se; **3** *n sports*: competição *f*

♦ **meet with** *v/t person* reunir-se com; *opposition, approval etc* receber

meeting ['miːtɪŋ] encontro *m*; *committee, business*: reunião *f*; ***he's in a ~*** ele está em reunião

'meeting place local *m* de encontro

megabyte ['megəbaɪt] COMPUT megabyte *m*

melancholy ['melənkɑːlɪ] *adj* melancólico

mellow ['meloʊ] *adj* suave; ***I've ~ed with age*** amadureci com a idade

melodious [mɪ'loʊdɪəs] *adj* melodioso

melodramatic [melədrə'mætɪk] *adj* melodramático

melody ['melədɪ] melodia *f*

melon ['melən] melão *m*

melt [melt] **1** *v/i* derreter-se **2** *v/t* derreter

♦ **melt away** *v/i fig* esvanecer-se

♦ **melt down** *v/t metal* fundir

'meltdown dissolução *f*

melting pot ['meltɪŋpɑːt] *fig* cadinho *m*

member ['membər] membro *m*

Member of 'Congress *Am* deputado,-a *m,f*

membership ['membəʃɪp] afiliação *f*; (*number of members*) número *m* de sócios

'membership card carteira *f* de sócio

membrane ['membreɪn] membrana *f*

memento [me'mentoʊ] lembrança *f*

memo ['memoʊ] memorando *m*

memoirs ['memwɑːrz] *npl* memórias *fpl*

'memo pad bloco *m* de anotações

memorable ['memərəbl] *adj* memorável

memorial [mɪ'mɔːrɪəl] **1** *adj* comemorativo; ***~ service*** serviço *m* religioso **2** *n* memorial *m*

Me'morial Day *Am* dia *m* dos que tombaram em guerras

memorize ['meməraɪz] *v/t* memorizar

memory ['memərɪ] memória *f*, (*sth re-*

M

membered) lembrança *f*; ***have a good / bad ~*** ter boa / má memória; ***in ~ of*** em memória de
men [men] *pl* → ***man***
menace ['menɪs] **1** *n* ameaça *f* **2** *v/t* ameaçar
menacing ['menɪsɪŋ] *adj* ameaçador
mend [mend] **1** *v/t* consertar **2** *n* ***be on the ~*** *after illness* estar melhorando
menial ['mi:nɪəl] *adj* humilde
meningitis [menɪn'dʒaɪtɪs] meningite *f*
menopause ['menoʊpɒ:z] menopausa *f*
'men's room sanitário *m* masculino, *Port* casa *f* de banho de homens
menstruate ['menstrʊeɪt] *v/i* menstruar
menstruation [menstrʊ'eɪʃn] menstruação *f*
mental ['mentl] *adj* mental; *fam* (*crazy*) pirado
mental a'rithmetic cálculo *m* mental **mental 'cruelty** crueldade *f* mental **'mental hospital** hospital *m* psiquiátrico **mental 'illness** doença *f* mental
mentality [men'tælətɪ] mentalidade *f*
mentally ['mentəlɪ] *adv* mentalmente
mentally 'handicapped *adj* com disfunção mental
mentally 'ill *adj* doente mental
mention ['menʃn] **1** *n* menção *f* **2** *v/t* mencionar; ***don't ~ it*** de nada
mentor ['mentɔ:r] mentor,a *m,f*
menu ['menu:] *for food* cardápio *m*, *Port* ementa *f*, COMPUT menu *m*
mercenary ['mɜ:rsɪnərɪ] **1** *adj* mercenário **2** *n* MIL mercenário,-a *m,f*
merchandise ['mɜ:rʧəndaɪz] mercadoria *f*
merchant ['mɜ:rʧənt] comerciante *m/f*
merciful ['mɜ:rsɪfl] *adj* misericordioso
mercifully ['mɜ:rsɪflɪ] *adv* (*thankfully*) felizmente
merciless ['mɜ:rsɪlɪs] *adj* desumano
mercury ['mɜ:rkjʊrɪ] mercúrio *m*
mercy ['mɜ:rsɪ] misericórdia *f*; ***be at s.o.'s ~*** estar à mercê de alguém
mere [mɪr] *adj* mero
merely ['mɪrlɪ] *adv* somente
merge [mɜ:rdʒ] *v/i two lines etc* unir-se; *companies* fundir-se
merger ['mɜ:rdʒər] COM fusão *f*
merit ['merɪt] **1** *n* (*worth*) mérito *m*; (*advantage*) vantagem *f* **2** *v/t* merecer
merry ['merɪ] *adj* alegre; ***Merry Christmas!*** Feliz Natal!
'merry-go-round carrossel *m*
mesh [meʃ] malha *f*
mess [mes] (*untidiness*) bagunça *f*; (*trouble*) encrenca *f*, ***be a ~*** *room, desk, hair* estar uma bagunça; *situation, s.o.'s life* estar uma confusão
♦**mess about, mess around 1** *v/i* perder tempo; ***mess around with*** brincar com; *s.o.'s wife* mexer com **2** *v/t person* enrolar
♦**mess up** *v/t room, papers* desarrumar; *task* atrapalhar; *plans, marriage* arruinar
message ['mesɪdʒ] *also movie, book*: mensagem *f*
'message board mensageiro *m*
messenger ['mesɪndʒər] (*courier*) mensageiro,-a *m,f*
messy ['mesɪ] *adj room* bagunçado; *person, handwriting* embaralhado; *job* sujo; *divorce, situation* desagradável
met [met] *pret & pp* → ***meet***
metabolism [mətæ'bəlɪzm] metabolismo *m*
metal ['metl] **1** *adj* de metal **2** *n* metal *m*
metallic [mɪ'tælɪk] *adj* metálico
metaphor ['metəfər] metáfora *f*
meteor ['mi:tɪɔ:r] meteoro *m*
meteoric [mi:tɪ'ɑ:rɪk] *adj fig* meteórico
meteorite ['mi:tɪəraɪt] meteorito *m*
meteorological [mi:tɪərə'lɑ:dʒɪkl] *adj* meteorológico
meteorologist [mi:tɪə'rɑ:lədʒɪst] meteorologista *m/f*
meteorology [mi:tɪə'rɑ:lədʒɪ] meteorologia *f*
meter[1] ['mi:tər] *gas, electricity*: medidor *m*; (*parking meter*) parquímetro *m*
meter[2] ['mi:tər] (*unit of length*) metro *m*

M

method ['meθəd] método *m*
methodical [mə'θɑːdɪkl] *adj* metódico
methodically [mə'θɑːdɪklɪ] *adv* metodicamente
meticulous [mə'tɪkjʊləs] *adj* meticuloso
'meter reading leitura *f* do medidor
metre *Brit* → ***meter***[2]
metric ['metrɪk] *adj* métrico
metropolis [mɪ'trɑːpəlɪs] metrópole *f*
metropolitan [metrə'pɑːlɪtən] *adj* metropolitano
mew [mjuː] **1** *n* miado *m* **2** *v/i* miar
Mexican ['meksɪkən] **1** *adj* mexicano **2** *n* mexicano,-a *m,f*
Mexico ['meksɪkoʊ] México *m*
mezzanine ['mezəniːn] mezanino *m*
miaow [mɪaʊ] **1** *n* miado *m* **2** *v/i* miar
mice [maɪs] *pl* → ***mouse***
mickey mouse [mɪkɪ'maʊs] *adj fam pej course, qualification* reles
microbiology [maɪkroʊbaɪ'ɑːlədʒɪ] microbiologia *f* **'microchip** microchip *m* **'microclimate** microclima *m* **'microcosm** ['maɪkrəkɑːzm] microcosmo *m* **'micro electronics** microeletrônica *f* **'microfiber,** *Brit* **microfibre** microfibra *f* **'microfilm** microfilme *m* **'microorganism** micrsorganismo *m* **'microphone** microfone *m* **micro'processor** microprocessador *m* **'microscope** microscópio *m* **microscopic** [maɪkrə'skɑːpɪk] *adj* microscópico **'microwave** *oven* microondas *m*
midair [mɪd'er] ***in ~*** em pleno ar
midday [mɪd'deɪ] meio-dia *m*
middle ['mɪdl] **1** *adj* do meio **2** *n* meio *m*; ***in the ~ of*** *floor, room* no meio de; *period of time* em meados de; ***I was in the ~ of taking a shower*** estava no meio de um banho; ***the ~ class(es)*** a classe média **'middle-aged** *adj* de meia idade **'Middle Ages** Idade *f* Média **middle 'class 1** *adj* de classe média; **2** *n* classe *f* média **Middle 'East** Oriente *m* Médio **'middleman** intermediário *m* **middle 'management** gerência *f* intermediária **middle 'name** nome *m* do meio **'middleweight** *boxer* peso *m* médio
middling ['mɪdlɪŋ] *adj* mediano
'midfield *soccer*: meio *m* de campo
mid'fielder *soccer*: meio-campo *m/f*
midge [mɪdʒ] mosquito *m*
midget ['mɪdʒɪt] *adj* em miniatura
'midnight meia-noite *f*; ***at ~*** à meia-noite **'midsummer** alto verão *m* **'midway** *adv* na metade do caminho; ***coffee was served ~ through the meeting*** o café foi servido na metade da reunião **'midweek** *adv* no meio da semana **'Midwest** *Am* Meio-Oeste *m* **'midwife** parteira *f* **'midwinter** alto inverno *m*
might[1] [maɪt] *v/aux* poder; ***I ~ be late*** posso me atrasar; ***it ~ rain*** pode chover; ***it ~ never happen*** isso jamais pode acontecer; ***I ~ have lost it*** posso ter perdido; ***he ~ have left*** ele pode ter saído; ***you ~ as well spend the night here*** você também pode passar a noite aqui; ***you ~ have told me!*** você poderia ter me dito!
might[2] [maɪt] (*power*) poder *m*
mighty ['maɪtɪ] **1** *adj* poderoso **2** *adv fam* (*extremely*) incrivelmente
migraine ['miːgreɪn] enxaqueca *f*
migrant worker ['maɪgrənt] trabalhador *m* itinerante
migrate [maɪ'greɪt] *v/i* migrar
migration [maɪ'greɪʃn] migração *f*
mike [maɪk] *fam* microfone *m*
mild [maɪld] *adj weather, climate* ameno; *cheese, curry, voice* suave; *person* moderado
mildew ['mɪlduː] mofo *m*
mildly ['maɪldlɪ] *adv spicy* ligeiramente; *say sth* suavemente; ***to put it ~*** para não dizer coisa pior
mildness ['maɪldnɪs] *weather*: amenidade *f*; *voice*: suavidade *f*; *person*: moderação *f*
mile [maɪl] milha *f*; ***~s better / easier*** *fam* mil vezes melhor / mais fácil
mileage ['maɪlɪdʒ] milhagem *f*
'milestone *fig* marco *m*
militant ['mɪlɪtənt] **1** *adj* militante **2** *n* militante *m/f*
military ['mɪlɪterɪ] **1** *adj* militar **2** *n* ***the ~*** os militares
military a'cademy academia *f* militar **military po'lice** polícia *f* militar

M

military 'service serviço *m* militar
militia [mɪ'lɪʃə] milícia *f*
milk [mɪlk] **1** *n* leite *m* **2** *v/t* ordenhar
milk 'chocolate chocolate *m* ao leite
'milk jug jarra *f* de leite **'milkshake** milk-shake *m*
milky ['mɪlkɪ] *adj* com leite; **~ coffee** café com muito leite
Milky 'Way Via *f* Láctea
mill [mɪl] *for grain* moinho *m*; *for textiles* tecelagem *f*
♦ **mill around** *v/i* pulular
millennium [mɪ'lenɪəm] milênio *m*
milligram ['mɪlɪgræm] miligrama *m*
millimeter ['mɪlɪmi:tər] *Am* milímetro *m*
millimetre *Brit* → **millimeter**
million ['mɪljən] milhão *m*
millionaire [mɪljə'ner] milionário,-a *m,f*
mime [maɪm] *v/t* mimicar
mimic ['mɪmɪk] **1** *n* mímico *m* **2** *v/t* ⟨*pret & pp* **mimicked**⟩ imitar
mince [mɪns] *n Brit* carne *f* moída
'mincemeat recheio *m* de frutas secas, passas e nozes
mince 'pie empada *f* de frutas secas, passas e nozes
mind [maɪnd] **1** *n* mente *f*; ***it's all in your ~*** é tudo imaginação sua; ***be out of one's ~*** estar fora de si; ***bear*** *ou* ***keep sth in ~*** não esquecer de algo; ***I've a good ~ to ...*** estou pensando seriamente em ...; ***change one's ~*** mudar de idéia; ***it didn't enter my ~*** não me ocorreu; ***give s.o. a piece of one's ~*** dar uma chamada em alguém; ***make up one's ~*** decidir-se; ***have something on one's ~*** estar preocupado com algo; ***keep one's ~ on sth*** concentrar-se em algo **2** *v/t* (*look after*) cuidar de; (*heed*) ouvir com atenção; ***I don't ~ herbal tea*** não me importo em tomar chá de ervas; ***I don't ~ what we do*** não me importa o que vamos fazer; ***do you ~ if I smoke?, do you ~ my smoking?*** você se importa se eu fumar?; ***would you ~ opening the window?*** você se importaria de abrir a janela?; ***~ the step!*** cuidado com o degrau!; ***~ your own business!*** cuide da sua vida! **3** *v/i* **~!** (*be careful*) cuidado!; ***never ~!*** não tem importância!; ***I don't ~*** tanto faz
mind-boggling ['maɪndbɑ:glɪŋ] *adj* incrível
mindless ['maɪndlɪs] *adj violence* sem sentido
mine[1] [maɪn] *pron* meu (minha); ***that's ~*** isto é meu; ***this book is ~*** este é o meu livro; ***a female cousin of ~*** uma prima minha
mine[2] [maɪn] **1** *n coal etc*: mina *f* **2** *v/i for coal etc* minar
mine[3] [maɪn] **1** *n explosive* mina *f* **2** *v/t* minar
'minefield *also fig* campo *m* minado
miner ['maɪnər] minerador,a *m,f*
mineral ['mɪnərəl] *n* mineral *m*
'mineral water água *f* mineral
'minesweeper NAUT caça-minas *m*
mingle ['mɪŋgl] *v/i sounds, smells, at party* misturar-se
mini ['mɪnɪ] *skirt* minissaia *f*
miniature ['mɪnɪtʃər] *adj* em miniatura
'minibus microônibus *m*, *Port* minibus *m*
minimal ['mɪnɪməl] *adj* mínimo
minimalism ['mɪnɪməlɪzm] minimalismo *m*
minimize ['mɪnɪmaɪz] *v/t* minimizar
minimum ['mɪnɪməm] **1** *adj* mínimo **2** *n* mínimo *m*
minimum 'wage salário *m* mínimo
mining ['maɪnɪŋ] mineração *f*
'miniseries *nsg* TV minissérie *f*
'miniskirt minissaia *f*
minister ['mɪnɪstər] POL ministro,-a *m,f*; REL pastor *m*
ministerial [mɪnɪ'stɪrɪəl] *adj* ministerial
ministry ['mɪnɪstrɪ] POL ministério *m*
mink [mɪŋk] marta *f*; *coat* casaco *m* de martas
minor ['maɪnər] **1** *adj also* MUS menor **2** *n* LAW menor *m/f* de idade
minority [maɪ'nɑ:rətɪ] minoria *f*; ***be in the ~*** estar em minoria
mint [mɪnt] *n herb* hortelã *f*; *chocolate* chocolate *m* com menta; *hard candy* bala *f* de hortelã
minus ['maɪnəs] **1** *n* (*minus sign*) sinal *m* de menos **2** *prep* menos

minuscule ['mɪnəskjuːl] *adj* minúsculo
minute[1] ['mɪnɪt] *of time* minuto *m*; ***in a ~*** *(soon)* num minuto; ***just a ~*** um momentinho
minute[2] [maɪ'nuːt] *adj (tiny)* diminuto; *(detailed)* minucioso; ***in ~ detail*** nos mínimos detalhes
'minute hand ponteiro *m* dos minutos
minutely [maɪ'nuːtlɪ] *adv (in detail)* minuciosamente; *(very slightly)* minimamente
minutes ['mɪnɪts] *npl of meeting* ata *f*
miracle ['mɪrəkl] milagre *m*
miraculous [mɪ'rækjʊləs] *adj* milagroso
miraculously [mɪ'rækjʊləslɪ] *adv* milagrosamente
mirage ['mɪrɑːʒ] miragem *f*
mirror ['mɪrər] **1** *n* espelho *m*; MOT retrovisor *m* **2** *v/t* espelhar
misanthropist [mɪ'zænθrəpɪst] misantropo,-a *m,f*
misapprehension [mɪsæprɪ'henʃn] ***be under a ~*** estar equivocado
misbehave [mɪsbə'heɪv] *v/i* comportar-se mal
misbehavior [mɪsbə'heɪvɪər] *Am* mau comportamento *m*
misbehaviour *Brit* → ***misbehavior***
miscalculate [mɪs'kælkjʊleɪt] *v/t & v/i* calcular mal
miscalculation [mɪs'kælkjʊleɪʃn] erro *m* de cálculo
miscarriage ['mɪskærɪdʒ] MED aborto *m* espontâneo; ***~ of justice*** erro *m* judicial
miscarry ['mɪskærɪ] *v/i* ⟨*pret & pp **miscarried***⟩ *plan* fracassar
miscellaneous [mɪsə'leɪnɪəs] *adj* variado; ***put it in a file marked ~*** coloque-o em uma pasta marcada como miscelânea
mischief ['mɪstʃɪf] travessuras *fpl*
mischievous ['mɪstʃɪvəs] *adj (naughty)* travesso; *(malicious)* malicioso
misconception [mɪskən'sepʃn] concepção *f* errada
misconduct [mɪs'kɑːndʌkt] má conduta *f*
misconstrue [mɪskən'struː] *v/t* interpretar mal
misdemeanor [mɪsdə'miːnər] *Am* contravenção *f*
misdemeanour *Brit* → ***misdemeanor***
miser ['maɪzər] avaro,-a *m,f*
miserable ['mɪzrəbl] *adj (unhappy)* triste; *weather, performance* deprimente
miserly ['maɪzərlɪ] *adj person* mesquinho; *amount of money* mísero
misery ['mɪzərɪ] *(unhappiness)* tristeza *f*; *(wretchedness)* miséria *f*
misfire [mɪs'faɪr] *v/i joke, scheme* sair-se mal
misfit ['mɪsfɪt] *in society* inadaptado,-a *m,f*
misfortune [mɪs'fɔːrtʃən] desgraça *f*, infortúnio *m*
misgiving [mɪs'gɪvɪŋ] mau pressentimento *m*; ***I agreed but with some ~s*** concordei, porém com alguma desconfiança
misguided [mɪs'gaɪdɪd] *adj attempt* mal orientado; *person* equivocado
mishandle [mɪs'hændl] *v/t situation* manejar mal
mishap ['mɪshæp] contratempo *m*
misinform [mɪsɪn'fɔːrm] *v/t* informar mal
misinterpret [mɪsɪn'tɜːrprɪt] *v/t* interpretar mal
misinterpretation [mɪsɪntɜːrprɪ'teɪʃn] má interpretação *f*
misjudge [mɪs'dʒʌdʒ] *v/t* julgar mal
mislay [mɪs'leɪ] *v/t* ⟨*pret & pp **mislaid***⟩ extraviar
mislead [mɪs'liːd] *v/t* ⟨*pret & pp **misled***⟩ enganar
misleading [mɪs'liːdɪŋ] *adj* enganoso
mismanage [mɪs'mænɪdʒ] *v/t* administrar mal
mismanagement [mɪs'mænɪdʒmənt] má administração *f*
mismatch ['mɪsmætʃ] discrepância *f*
misplaced ['mɪspleɪst] *adj loyalty* imerecido; *enthusiasm* inoportuno
misprint ['mɪsprɪnt] erro *m* tipográfico
mispronounce [mɪsprə'naʊns] *v/t* pronunciar mal

mispronunciation [mɪsprənʌnsɪ'eɪʃn] má pronúncia *f*

misread [mɪs'ri:d] *v/t* ⟨*pret & pp* ***misread*** [-red]⟩ *word, figures* ler mal; *situation* interpretar mal

misrepresent [mɪsreprɪ'zent] *v/t* deturpar

miss[1] [mɪs] *n* ***Miss Smith*** senhorita Smith, *Port* senhora Smith; ***~!*** senhorita!, *Port* senhora!

miss[2] **1** *n* ***give sth a ~*** *meeting, party etc* deixar algo de lado **2** *v/t* (*not hit*) errar; (*emotionally*) sentir falta de; (*not meet*) desencontrar; ***we must have ~ed the turnoff*** devemos ter passado a saída; ***I ~ed the class*** faltei à aula; ***you don't ~ much!*** você não perde nada! **3** *v/i* (*not hit*) errar

misshapen [mɪs'ʃeɪpən] *adj* disforme

missile ['mɪsəl] míssil *m*; (*sth thrown*) projétil *m*

missing ['mɪsɪŋ] *adj* desaparecido; ***be ~*** *lost, in battle etc* estar desaparecido; *not in right place* estar faltando; ***one of the children is still ~*** uma das crianças ainda está faltando

mission ['mɪʃn] missão *f*

missionary ['mɪʃənrɪ] REL missionário,-a *m,f*

misspell [mɪs'spel] *v/t* escrever incorretamente

mist [mɪst] bruma *f*

♦ **mist over** *v/i eyes* turvar-se

♦ **mist up** *v/i mirror, window* embaçar

mistake [mɪ'steɪk] **1** *n* erro *m*; ***make a ~*** cometer um erro; ***by ~*** por engano **2** *v/t* ⟨*pret* ***mistook***, *pp* ***mistaken***⟩ ***~ X for Y*** confundir X com Y

mistaken [mɪ'steɪkən] **1** *adj* errado; ***be ~*** estar equivocado **2** *pp* → ***mistake***

mister ['mɪstər] senhor *m*

mistook [mɪ'stʊk] *pret* → ***mistake***

mistress ['mɪstrɪs] *lover* amante *f*; *servant*: senhora *f*; *dog*: dona *f*

mistrust [mɪs'trʌst] **1** *n* desconfiança *f* **2** *v/t* desconfiar de

misty ['mɪstɪ] *adj weather* nublado; *eyes* embaçado; *color* borrado

misunderstand [mɪsʌndər'stænd] *v/t* ⟨*pret & pp* ***misunderstood***⟩ entender mal

misunderstanding [mɪsʌndər'stændɪŋ] (*mistake*) mal-entendido *m*; (*argument*) desentendimento *m*

misuse **1** [mɪs'ju:s] *n* uso *m* impróprio **2** [mɪs'ju:z] *v/t* usar mal

mitigating circumstances ['mɪtɪgeɪtɪŋ] *npl* circunstâncias *fpl* atenuantes

mitt [mɪt] *baseball*: luva *f*

mitten ['mɪtən] mitene *f*

mix [mɪks] **1** *n* mistura *f* **2** *v/t cream, cement etc* misturar **3** *v/i* (*socially*) imiscuir-se

♦ **mix up** *v/t* confundir; ***mix X up with Y*** confundir X com Y; ***be mixed up*** *emotionally* ficar confuso; *of figures, papers* estar desordenado; ***get mixed up with*** envolver-se com

♦ **mix with** *v/t* (*associate with*) relacionar-se com

mixed [mɪkst] *adj feelings* contraditório; *reactions, reviews* variado

mixed 'marriage casamento *m* misto

mixer ['mɪksər] *for food* mixer *m*; *drink* refresco *m*; ***she's a good ~*** ela é muito sociável

mixture ['mɪkstʃər] mistura *f*; (*medicine*) preparado *m*

'mix-up confusão *f*

moan [moʊn] **1** *n pain*: gemido *m* **2** *v/i in pain* gemer

mob [mɑ:b] **1** *n* multidão *f*; ***the Mob*** a Máfia **2** *v/t* ⟨*pret & pp* ***mobbed***⟩ cercar

mobile ['moʊbəl] **1** *adj person* ativo; (*that can be moved*) móvel **2** *n decoration*: móbile *m*; *Brit phone* celular *m*

mobile 'home trailer *m*

mobile 'phone *Brit* telefone *m* celular

mobility [mə'bɪlətɪ] mobilidade *f*

mobster ['mɑ:bstər] gângster *m/f*

mock [mɑ:k] **1** *adj* falso; (*simulated*) simulado **2** *v/t* ridicularizar

mockery ['mɑ:kərɪ] (*derision*) zombaria *f*; (*travesty*) farsa *f*

'mock-up (*model*) maquete *f*

mod 'con ***with all ~s*** com todas as conveniências modernas

mode [moʊd] modo *m*; ***~ of transportation*** meio *m* de transporte

model ['mɑ:dl] **1** *adj employee, husband* modelo; ***a ~ boat*** um barco

de miniatura **2** *n* modelo *m*; *fashion*: modelo *f*; ***male*** **~** modelo *m* **3** *v/t* ***she ~s clothes for …*** ela trabalha como modelo para … **4** *v/i for designer* desfilar; *for artist*, *photographer* servir de modelo
modem ['moʊdem] modem *m*
moderate ['mɑːdərət] **1** *adj also* POL moderado **2** *n* POL moderado,-a *m,f* **3** ['mɑːdəreɪt] *v/t also voice*, *speed* moderar
moderately ['mɑːdərətlɪ] *adv* moderadamente
moderation [mɑːdə'reɪʃn] (*restraint*) moderação *f*, ***in*** **~** com moderação
modern ['mɑːdərn] *adj* moderno
modernization [mɑːdərnaɪ'zeɪʃn] modernização *f*
modernize ['mɑːdərnaɪz] **1** *v/t* modernizar **2** *v/i business*, *country* modernizar-se
modern 'languages línguas *fpl* modernas
modest ['mɑːdɪst] *adj person*, *apartment* modesto
modesty ['mɑːdɪstɪ] modéstia *f*
modification [mɑːdɪfɪ'keɪʃn] modificação *f*
modify ['mɑːdɪfaɪ] *v/t* ⟨*pret & pp* ***modified***⟩ modificar
modular ['mɑːdʒələr] *adj furniture* modular
module ['mɑːdʒuːl] *spacecraft*: módulo *m*
moist [mɔɪst] *adj* úmido, *Port* húmido
moisten ['mɔɪsn] *v/t* umedecer, *Port* humedecer
moisture ['mɔɪstʃər] umidade *f*, *Port* humidade *f*
moisturizer ['mɔɪstʃəraɪzər] *skin*: creme *m* hidratante
molar ['moʊlər] molar *m*
molasses [mə'læsɪz] *nsg* melado *m*
mold[1] [moʊld] *Am* bolor *m*
mold[2] [moʊld] *Am* **1** *n* molde *m* **2** *v/t clay*, *character* moldar
moldy ['moʊldɪ] *adj Am food* embolorado
mole [moʊl] *on skin* sinal *m*
molecular [mə'lekjʊlər] *adj* molecular
molecule ['mɑːlɪkjuːl] molécula *f*
molest [mə'lest] *v/t child*, *woman* molestar
mollycoddle ['mɑːlɪkɑːdl] *v/t fam* mimar
molten ['moʊltən] *adj* fundido
mom [mɑːm] *Am* mamãe *f*
moment ['moʊmənt] momento *m*; ***at the*** **~** no momento; ***for the*** **~** no momento
momentarily [moʊmən'terɪlɪ] *adv* (*for a moment*) momentaneamente; *Am* (*in a moment*) a qualquer momento
momentary ['moʊməntrɪ] *adj* momentâneo
momentous [mə'mentəs] *adj* importantíssimo
momentum [mə'mentəm] ímpeto *m*
monarch ['mɑːnərk] monarca *m/f*
monastery ['mɑːnəsterɪ] monastério *m*
monastic [mə'næstɪk] *adj* monástico
Monday ['mʌndeɪ] segunda-feira *f*
monetary ['mɑːnəterɪ] *adj* monetário
money ['mʌnɪ] dinheiro *m*; ***I'm not made of*** **~** não sou feito de dinheiro
'money belt algibeira *f* **'money-lender** emprestador,a *m,f* **'money market** mercado *m* monetário **'money order** ordem *f* de pagamento
mongrel ['mʌngrəl] vira-lata *m/f*
monitor ['mɑːnɪtər] **1** *n* COMPUT monitor *m* **2** *v/t* monitorar
monk [mʌŋk] monge *m*
monkey ['mʌŋkɪ] macaco *m*; *fam* (*child*) diabinho *m*
◆ **monkey about with** *v/t fam* mexer em
'monkey wrench chave *f* inglesa
monogram ['mɑːnəgræm] *Am* monograma *m*
monogrammed ['mɑːnəgræmd] *adj* com monograma
monolog ['mɑːnəlɑːg] *Am* monólogo *m*
monologue *Brit* → ***monolog***
monopolize [mə'nɑːpəlaɪz] *v/t also fig* monopolizar
monopoly [mə'nɑːpəlɪ] monopólio *m*
monotonous [mə'nɑːtənəs] *adj* monótono
monotony [mə'nɑːtənɪ] monotonia *f*

monsoon [mɑːn'suːn] monção *f*
monster ['mɑːnstər] *n* monstro,-a *m,f*
monstrosity [mɑːn'strɑːsətɪ] monstruosidade *f*
monstrous ['mɑːnstrəs] *adj* monstruoso; (*shocking*) escandaloso
month [mʌnθ] mês *m*
monthly ['mʌnθlɪ] **1** *adj* mensal **2** *adv* mensalmente **3** *n magazine* revista *f* mensal
monument ['mɑːnjʊmənt] monumento *m*
monumental [mɑːnjʊ'mentl] *adj fig* monumental
mood [muːd] (*frame of mind*) humor *m*; *of meeting, country* moral *f*; ***bad ~*** mau humor; ***be in a good / bad ~*** estar de bom / mau humor; ***be in the ~ for*** estar com vontade de
moody ['muːdɪ] *adj* temperamental; (*bad-tempered*) mal-humorado
moon [muːn] *n* lua *f*
'moonlight **1** *n* luar *m* **2** *v/i fam* trabalhar ilegalmente
'moonlit *adj* enluarado
moor [mʊr] *v/t boat* atracar
moorings ['mʊrɪŋz] *npl* ancoradouro *m*
moose [muːs] alce *m* americano
mop [mɑːp] **1** *n dishes*: esponja *f*; *floor*: esfregão *m* **2** *v/t* ⟨*pret & pp* ***mopped***⟩ *floor* esfregar; *eyes, face* limpar
♦ **mop up** *v/t* limpar; MIL eliminar
mope [moʊp] *v/i* ficar deprimido
moral ['mɔːrəl] **1** *adj* moral; *person, behavior* moralista **2** *n of story* moral *f*; ***~s*** *pl* moral *f*
morale [mə'ræl] moral *f*
morality [mə'rælətɪ] moralidade *f*
morbid ['mɔːrbɪd] *adj* mórbido
more [mɔːr] **1** *adj & pron* mais; ***~ and ~ students / time*** cada vez mais estudantes / tempo; ***some ~ tea?*** mais um chá?; ***do you want some ~?*** você quer mais?; ***a little ~*** um pouco mais **2** *adv* ***~ important*** mais importante; ***~ often*** mais freqüentemente; ***~ and ~*** cada vez mais; ***~ or less*** mais ou menos; ***once ~*** mais uma vez; ***~ than*** mais do que; ***I don't live there any ~*** eu não moro mais lá
moreover [mɔː'roʊvər] *adv* além disso
morgue [mɔːrg] necrotério *m*
morning ['mɔːrnɪŋ] manhã *f*; ***in the ~*** da manhã; (*tomorrow*) de manhã; ***this ~*** esta manhã; ***tomorrow ~*** amanhã de manhã; ***good ~*** bom dia
'morning sickness enjôo *m* matinal
moron ['mɔːrɑːn] *fam* idiota *m/f*
morose [mə'roʊs] *adj* mal-humorado
morphine ['mɔːrfiːn] morfina *f*
morsel ['mɔːrsl] pedacinho *m*
mortal ['mɔːrtl] **1** *adj blow, enemy* mortal **2** *n* mortal *m/f*
mortality [mɔːr'tælətɪ] mortalidade *f*
mortar[1] ['mɔːrtər] MIL morteiro *m*
mortar[2] ['mɔːrtər] (*cement*) argamassa *f*
mortgage ['mɔːrgɪdʒ] **1** *n* financiamento *m* (para aquisição de casa própria) **2** *v/t house, farm, land* hipotecar
mortician [mɔːr'tɪʃn] *Am* agente funerário,-a *m,f*
mortuary ['mɔːrtʃuerɪ] necrotério *m*
mosaic [moʊ'zeɪk] mosaico *m*
Moscow ['mɑːskaʊ] Moscou, *Port* Moscovo
mosquito [mɑːs'kiːtoʊ] mosquito *m*
mos'quito net mosquiteiro *m*
moss [mɑːs] musgo *m*
mossy ['mɑːsɪ] *adj* coberto de musgo
most [moʊst] **1** *adj* a maioria de; ***who had the ~ money?*** quem tinha mais dinheiro? **2** *adv* (*very*) muito; ***the ~ beautiful / interesting*** o mais bonito / interessante; ***that's the one I like ~*** este é o que eu mais gosto; ***~ of all*** sobretudo **3** *pron* a maioria; ***at*** (***the***) ***~*** no máximo; ***make the ~ of*** aproveitar ao máximo
mostly ['moʊstlɪ] *adv* principalmente
motel [moʊ'tel] motel *m*
moth [mɑːθ] mariposa *f*; (*clothes moth*) traça *f*
'mothball naftalina *f*
mother ['mʌðər] **1** *n* mãe *f* **2** *v/t* mimar
'motherboard COMPUT placa *f* mãe
'motherhood maternidade *f*
Mothering 'Sunday dia *m* das mães
'mother-in-law ⟨*pl* ***mothers-in-law***⟩ sogra *f*

motherly ['mʌðərlı] *adj* maternal
mother-of-'pearl madrepérola *f*
'Mother's Day dia *m* das mães
'mother tongue língua *f* materna
motif [moʊ'tiːf] motivo *m*
motion ['moʊʃn] **1** *n* movimento *m*; (*proposal*) proposta *f*; ***put** ou **set things in ~*** encaminhar as coisas **2** *v/t* ***he ~ed me forward*** ele me acenou para seguir adiante
motionless ['moʊʃnlıs] *adj* imóvel
motivate ['moʊtıveıt] *v/t person* motivar
motivation [moʊtı'veıʃn] motivação *f*
motive ['moʊtıv] motivo *m*
motor ['moʊtər] motor *m*
'motorbike moto *f*
'motorboat lancha *f*
motorcade ['moʊtərkeıd] desfile *m* de carros
'motorcycle motocicleta *f* **'motorcyclist** motociclista *m/f* **'motor home** trailer *m*
motorist ['moʊtərıst] motorista *m/f*
'motor mechanic mecânico *m* de automóveis **'motor racing** corrida *f* de carros **'motorscooter** scooter *m*, *Port* lambreta *f* **'motor vehicle** veículo *m* motorizado **'motorway** *Brit* auto-estrada *f*
motto ['mɑːtoʊ] lema *m*
mould *etc Brit* → ***mold***[1]; ***mold***[2] *etc*
mound [maʊnd] (*hillock*) colina *f*; *in baseball* montículo *m*; (*pile*) monte *m*
mount [maʊnt] **1** *n horse* montaria *f*; ***Mount Everest*** Monte *m* Everest **2** *v/t steps* subir; *horse, bicycle* montar em; *campaign* montar; *photo, painting* emoldurar **3** *v/i* (*increase*) aumentar
♦ **mount up** *v/i* (*grow*) acumular-se
mountain ['maʊntın] montanha *f*
'mountain bike mountain bike *f*
mountaineer [maʊntı'nır] alpinista *m/f*
mountaineering [maʊntı'nırıŋ] alpinismo *m*
mountainous ['maʊntınəs] *adj* montanhoso
mounted po'lice ['maʊntıd] polícia *f* montada
mourn [mɔːrn] *v/t* estar de luto por; *fig* chorar por
mourner ['mɔːrnər] enlutado,-a *m,f*
mournful ['mɔːrnfl] *adj* triste
mourning ['mɔːrnıŋ] luto *m*; ***be in ~*** estar de luto; ***wear ~*** usar luto
mouse [maʊs] ⟨*pl* ***mice***⟩ rato *m*; COMPUT mouse *m*; ***~ mat*** COMPUT mouse pad *m*
moustache *Brit* → ***mustache***
mouth [maʊθ] boca *f*; *river*: desembocadura *f*
mouthful ['maʊθfʊl] *of food* bocado *m*
'mouthorgan gaita *f* **'mouthpiece** *instrument*: bocal *m*; (*spokesperson*) porta-voz *m/f* **'mouthwash** enxaguatório *m* bucal **'mouthwatering** *adj* de dar água na boca
move [muːv] **1** *n* (*movement*) movimento *m*; *chess, checkers*: jogada *f*; (*step, action*) passo *m*; (*change of house*) mudança *f*; ***get a ~ on!*** *fam* anda logo!; ***don't make a ~!*** não se mova! **2** *v/t object* mover; (*transfer*) transferir; *emotionally* comover; ***~ house*** mudar-se de casa **3** *v/i* mudar-se; (*be transferred*) ser transferido; ***don't ~!*** não se mexa!
♦ **move around** *v/i in room etc* mover-se; *from town to town* mudar-se de lugar pra lugar
♦ **move away** *v/i* afastar-se; (*move house*) mudar-se
♦ **move in** *v/i* entrar na nova residência
♦ **move on** *v/i to another town* partir; *to another job* transferir-se; *to another subject* passar
♦ **move out** *v/i of house* mudar-se; *of area* retirar-se
♦ **move up** *v/i in league* subir; (*make room*) dar lugar
movement ['muːvmənt] *also* MUS, *organization* movimento *m*
movers ['muːvərz] *npl Am* empresa *f* de mudanças
movie ['muːvı] filme *m*; ***go to a ~ / the ~s*** ir ao cinema
moviegoer ['muːvıgoʊər] *Am* ***I'm a frequent ~*** eu vou muito ao cinema
'movie theater *Am* cinema *m*
moving ['muːvıŋ] *adj* (*which can move*) móvel; *emotionally* comovente

M

mow [moʊ] *v/t grass* cortar
♦ **mow down** *v/t* dizimar
mower ['moʊər] cortador *m* de grama, *Port* cortador *m* de relva
MP[1] [em'piː] *abbr* (*of* ***Member of Parliament***) *Brit* POL membro *m* do parlamento, deputado,-a *m,f*
MP[2] [em'piː] *abbr* (*of* ***Military Policeman***) policial *m* militar
mph [empiː'eɪtʃ] *abbr* (*of* ***miles per hour***) milhas por hora
MPV [empiː'viː] *abbr* (*of* ***multi-purpose vehicle***) mini-van *f*
Mr ['mɪstər] Sr. *m*
Mrs ['mɪsɪz] Sra. *f*
Ms [mɪz] Sra. *f utilizado para mulher solteira ou casada*
Mt *abbr* (*of* ***Mount***)
much [mʌtʃ] **1** *adj* muito; ***as ~ ... as ...*** tanto .... quanto **2** *adv* muito; ***very ~*** muito; ***too ~*** demais; ***as ~ as I could*** tanto quanto pude; ***I thought as ~*** eu deduzia isto **3** *pron* muito; ***nothing ~*** não muito
muck [mʌk] (*dirt*) sujeira *f*, *Port* sujidade *f*
mucus ['mjuːkəs] muco *m*
mud [mʌd] barro *m*
muddle ['mʌdl] **1** *n* desordem *f* **2** *v/t* confundir
♦ **muddle up** *v/t people*, *things* confundir
muddy ['mʌdɪ] *adj* lamacento
'mudguard para-lamas *m*
muesli ['muːzlɪ] cereais *mpl*
muffin ['mʌfɪn] *Am* muffin *m*
muffle ['mʌfl] *v/t* abafar
♦ **muffle up** *v/i* agasalhar-se
muffler ['mʌflər] *scarf* cachecol *m*; *Am* MOT silenciador *m*
mug[1] [mʌg] *tea*, *coffee*: caneca *f*; *fam* (*face*) careta *f*
mug[2] [mʌg] *v/t* ⟨*pret & pp* ***mugged***⟩ (*attack*) assaltar
mugger ['mʌgər] assaltante *m/f*
mugging ['mʌgɪŋ] assalto *m*
muggy ['mʌgɪ] *adj* abafado
mule [mjuːl] *animal* mula *f*; (*slipper*) mule *f*
♦ **mull over** [mʌl] *v/t* refletir sobre
multicultural ['mʌltɪkʌltʃərəl] *adj* multicultural
multilateral [mʌltɪ'lætərəl] *adj* POL multilateral
multilingual [mʌltɪ'lɪŋgwəl] *adj* multilíngüe
multimedia [mʌltɪ'miːdɪə] multimídia *f*
multinational [mʌltɪ'næʃnl] **1** *adj* multinacional **2** *n* COM multinacional *f*
multiple ['mʌltɪpl] *adj* múltiplo
multiple 'choice question teste *m* de múltipla escolha
multiple sclerosis [skle'rousɪs] esclerose *f* múltipla
multiplex ['mʌltɪpleks] multiplex *m*
multiplication [mʌltɪplɪ'keɪʃn] multiplicação *f*
multiply ['mʌltɪplaɪ] ⟨*pret & pp* ***multiplied***⟩ **1** *v/t* multiplicar **2** *v/i* multiplicar-se
multitasking ['mʌltɪtæskɪŋ] multitarefa *f*
mum [mʌm] *Brit* mamãe
mumble ['mʌmbl] **1** *n* murmúrio *m* **2** *v/t & v/i* murmurar
mumps [mʌmps] *nsg* caxumba *f*
mummy ['mʌmɪ] *Brit* → ***mum***
munch [mʌntʃ] *v/t & v/i* mascar
municipal [mjuː'nɪsɪpl] *adj* municipal
mural ['mjʊrəl] mural *m*
murder ['mɜːrdər] **1** *n* homicida *m* **2** *v/t person* assassinar; *song* acabar com
murderer ['mɜːrdərər] assassino,-a *m,f*
murderous ['mɜːrdrəs] *adj rage*, *look* de morte
murky ['mɜːrkɪ] *adj water* turvo; *fig* nebuloso
murmur ['mɜːrmər] **1** *n* murmúrio *m* **2** *v/t* murmurar
muscle ['mʌsl] músculo *m*
muscular ['mʌskjʊlər] *adj pain*, *strain* muscular; *person* musculoso
muse [mjuːz] *v/i* pensar
museum [mjuː'zɪəm] museu *m*
mushroom ['mʌʃrʊm] **1** *n* cogumelo *m* **2** *v/i* crescer rapidamente
music ['mjuːzɪk] música *f*; *written*: partitura *f*
musical ['mjuːzɪkl] **1** *adj person*, *voice* musical **2** *n* musical *m*

musical 'instrument instrumento *m* musical
'music box caixinha *f* de música
musician [mjuː'zɪʃn] músico,-a *m,f*
mussel ['mʌsl] mexilhão *m*
must [mʌst] ◊ *necessity*: ter que; ***I ~ be on time*** tenho que ser pontual; ***I ~*** tenho
◊ *with negative*: ***I ~n't be late*** não posso chegar atrasado; ***you ~n't cross this line*** você não deve cruzar esta linha
◊ *probability*: dever; ***it ~ be about 6 o'clock*** devem ser umas seis horas; ***they ~ have arrived by now*** eles devem ter chegado agora
◊ ***a ~-see movie*** um filme imperdível; ***the ~-have fashion accessory*** o acessório que todos devem ter
mustache ['mʌstæʃ] *Am* bigode *m*
mustard ['mʌstərd] mostarda *f*
musty ['mʌstɪ] *adj room* mofado; *smell* de bolor
mute [mjuːt] *adj animal* mudo
muted ['mjuːtɪd] *adj color* apagado; *opposition*, *criticism* fraco
mutilate ['mjuːtɪleɪt] *v/t* mutilar
mutiny ['mjuːtɪnɪ] **1** *n* motim *m* **2** *v/i* ⟨*pret & pp* ***mutinied***⟩ rebelar-se
mutter ['mʌtər] *v/i & v/t* balbuciar
mutton ['mʌtn] carne *f* de carneiro
mutual ['mjuːʧʊəl] *adj* mútuo; ***a ~ friend*** um amigo em comum
muzzle ['mʌzl] **1** *n animal*: focinho *m*; *for dog* focinheira *f* **2** *v/t* ***~ the press*** fazer calar a imprensa
my [maɪ] *adj* meu (minha); ***I had ~ hands in ~ pockets*** eu estava com as (minhas) mãos nos bolsos
myopic [maɪ'ɑːpɪk] *adj* míope
myself [maɪ'self] *pron* me; *emphatic* eu mesmo; ***I hurt ~*** eu me machuquei; ***by ~*** sozinho,-a
mysterious [mɪ'stɪrɪəs] *adj* misterioso
mysteriously [mɪ'stɪrɪəslɪ] *adv* misteriosamente
mystery ['mɪstərɪ] mistério *m*
mystify ['mɪstɪfaɪ] *v/t* ⟨*pret & pp* ***mystified***⟩ pasmar; ***I was mystified by her decision*** fiquei pasmo com sua decisão
myth [mɪθ] *also fig* mito *m*
mythical ['mɪθɪkl] *adj* mítico
mythology [mɪ'θɑːlədʒɪ] mitologia *f*

N

nab [næb] *v/t* ⟨*pret & pp* ***nabbed***⟩ *fam* (*take for oneself*) apanhar
nag [næg] ⟨*pret & pp* ***nagged***⟩ **1** *v/i* implicar **2** *v/t* implicar com; ***~ s.o. to do sth*** incomodar alguém para fazer algo
nagging ['nægɪŋ] *adj person* chato; *doubt* perturbante; *pain* irritante
nail [neɪl] *wood*: prego *m*; *finger, toe*: unha *f*
'nail clippers *npl* cortador *m* de unha **'nail file** lixa *f* de unhas **'nail polish** esmalte *m*, *Port* verniz *m* de unhas **'nail polish remover** removedor *m* de esmalte, *Port* acetona *f* **'nail scissors** *npl* tesoura *f* de unha **'nail varnish** *Brit* esmalte *m*, *Port* verniz *m* de unhas
naive [naɪ'iːv] *adj* ingênuo
naked ['neɪkɪd] *adj* nu; ***to the ~ eye*** a olho nu
name [neɪm] **1** *n* nome *m*; ***what's your ~?*** como você se chama?; ***call s.o. ~s*** insultar alguém; ***make a ~ for oneself*** ficar famoso **2** *v/t* chamar
◆ **name for** *v/t Am* ***name s.o. for s.o.*** nomear alguém para alguém
◆ **name after** → ***name for***
namely ['neɪmlɪ] *adv* a saber
'namesake homônimo *m*
'nametag *on clothing etc* etiqueta *f*
nanny ['nænɪ] babá *f*

nap [næp] *n* soneca *f*; ***have a ~*** tirar uma soneca
nape [neɪp] ~ (***of the neck***) nuca *f*
napkin ['næpkɪn] (*table napkin*) guardanapo *m*; (***sanitary***) ~ absorvente *m* higiênico
nappy ['næpɪ] *Brit* fralda *f*
narcotic [nɑːr'kɑːtɪk] *n* narcótico *m*
nar'cotics agent agente *m* da delegacia de entorpecentes
narrate ['næreɪt] *v/t* narrar
narration [næ'reɪʃn] relato *m*
narrative ['nærətɪv] **1** *n* (*story*) narrativa *f* **2** *adj poem*, *style* narrativo
narrator [næ'reɪtər] narrador,a *m,f*
narrow ['næroʊ] *adj street*, *bed etc* estreito; *views*, *mind* limitado; *victory* pequeno
narrowly ['næroʊlɪ] *adv win* por pouco; ~ ***escape sth*** escapar de algo por um fio
narrow-minded [næroʊ'maɪndɪd] *adj* de visão limitada
nasal ['neɪzl] *adj voice* nasal
nasty ['næstɪ] *adj person*, *thing to say* malvado; *smell*, *weather* ruim; *cut*, *wound*, *disease* grave
nation ['neɪʃn] nação *f*
national ['næʃənl] **1** *adj* nacional **2** *n* cidadão *m*, cidadã *f*
national 'anthem hino *m* nacional
national 'debt dívida *f* pública
nationalism ['næʃənəlɪzm] nacionalismo *m*
nationality [næʃə'nælətɪ] nacionalidade *f*
nationalize ['næʃənəlaɪz] *v/t industry etc* nacionalizar
national 'park parque *m* nacional
native ['neɪtɪv] **1** *adj* nativo; ~ ***language*** língua *f* nativa **2** *n* nativo,-a *m,f*
Native A'merican 1 *adj* americano nativo; **2** *n* americano,-a *m,f* nativo,-a **native 'country** terra *f* natal **native 'speaker** falante nativo,-a *m,f*
NATO ['neɪtoʊ] *abbr* (*of* ***North Atlantic Treaty Organization***) OTAN *f* (Organização *f* do Tratado do Atlântico Norte)
natural ['nætʃrəl] *adj* natural; ***a ~ blonde*** uma loira natural
natural 'gas gás *m* natural
naturalist ['nætʃrəlɪst] naturalista *m/f*
naturalize ['nætʃrəlaɪz] *v/t* ***become ~d*** naturalizar-se
naturally ['nætʃərəlɪ] *adv* (*of course*), *behave*, *speak* naturalmente; (*by nature*) por natureza
natural 'science ciências *fpl* naturais
natural 'scientist especialista *m/f* em ciências naturais
nature ['neɪtʃər] natureza *f*
'nature reserve reserva *f* natural
naughty ['nɔːtɪ] *adj* travesso; *photograph*, *word etc* malandro
nausea ['nɒːzɪə] náusea *f*
nauseate ['nɒːzɪeɪt] *v/t fig* (*disgust*) nausear
nauseating ['nɒːzɪeɪtɪŋ] *adj smell*, *taste*, *person* repugnante
nauseous ['nɒːʃəs] *adj* ***feel ~*** sentir náuseas
nautical ['nɒːtɪkl] *adj* náutico
'nautical mile milha *f* náutica
naval ['neɪvl] *adj* naval
'naval base base *f* naval
navel ['neɪvl] umbigo *m*
navigable ['nævɪgəbl] *adj river* navegável
navigate ['nævɪgeɪt] *v/i in ship*, *also* COMPUT navegar; *in airplane* pilotar; *in car* dirigir
navigation [nævɪ'geɪʃn] navegação *f*
navigator ['nævɪgeɪtər] navegador,a *m,f*
navy ['neɪvɪ] marinha *f*
navy 'blue 1 *n* azul-marinho *m* **2** *adj* azul-marinho
near [nɪr] **1** *adv* perto **2** *prep* perto de; ~ ***the bank*** perto do banco **3** *adj* próximo; ***in the ~ future*** num futuro próximo; ***the ~est bus stop*** a parada de ônibus mais próxima
nearby [nɪr'baɪ] *adv live* próximo
nearly ['nɪrlɪ] *adv* quase; ***I ~ dropped it*** eu quase deixei cair isso; ***he was ~ in tears*** ele estava quase chorando
near-sighted [nɪr'saɪtɪd] *adj* míope
neat [niːt] *adj room*, *desk* limpo; *person*, *solution* elegante; *whiskey* puro; *fam* (*terrific*) ótimo

necessarily ['nesəserəlɪ] *adv* necessariamente
necessary ['nesəserɪ] *adj* necessário; ***it is ~ to …*** é necessário …; ***you can, if ~, …*** você pode, se necessário …
necessitate [nɪ'sesɪteɪt] *v/t* necessitar
necessity [nɪ'sesɪtɪ] necessidade *f*
neck [nek] *person*, *animal*: pescoço *m*; *dress*, *sweater*: decote *m*
necklace ['neklɪs] colar *m* **'neckline** *of dress* decote *m* **'necktie** gravata *f*
née [neɪ] *adj* ***Susan Brown, ~ Masters*** Susan Brown, nascida Masters
need [ni:d] **1** *n* necessidade *f*; ***if ~ be*** se for necessário; ***in ~*** em necessidade; ***be in ~ of sth*** estar precisando de algo; ***there's no ~ to be rude / upset*** não precisa ser grosseiro / perder a calma **2** *v/t* precisar; ***you'll ~ to buy one*** você vai precisar comprar um/uma; ***you don't ~ to wait*** você não precisa esperar; ***I ~ to talk to you*** preciso falar com você; ***~ I say more?*** preciso dizer algo mais?
needle ['ni:dl] *sewing*, *injection*: agulha *f*; *dial*: ponteiro *m*
'needlework costura *f*
needy ['ni:dɪ] *adj* necessitado
negative ['negətɪv] **1** *adj also attitude* negativo; ***~ pole*** ELEC pólo *m* negativo **2** *n* ***answer in the ~*** dar uma resposta negativa
neglect [nɪ'glekt] **1** *n* negligência *f* **2** *v/t garden* abandonar; *one's health* descuidar de; ***~ to do sth*** esquecer-se de fazer algo
neglected [nɪ'glektɪd] *adj gardens* abandonado; *author* esquecido; ***feel ~*** sentir-se abandonado
negligence ['neglɪdʒəns] negligência *f*
negligent ['neglɪdʒənt] *adj* negligente
negligible ['neglɪdʒəbl] *adj quantity* insignificante
negotiable [nɪ'goʊʃəbl] *adj* negociável
negotiate [nɪ'goʊʃɪeɪt] **1** *v/i* negociar **2** *v/t deal*, *settlement* negociar; *obstacles* superar; *curve in road* pegar
negotiation [nɪgoʊʃɪ'eɪʃn] negociação *f*
negotiator [nɪ'goʊʃɪeɪtər] negociador,a *m,f*
Negro ['ni:groʊ] negro,-a *m,f*
neigh [neɪ] *v/i* relinchar
neighbor ['neɪbər] *Am* vizinho,-a *m,f*
neighborhood ['neɪbərhʊd] *Am town*: vizinhança *f*; ***in the ~ of …*** *fig* ao redor de …
neighboring ['neɪbərɪŋ] *adj Am house*, *state* vizinho
neighborly ['neɪbərlɪ] *adj Am* amigável
neighbour *etc Brit* → ***neighbor*** *etc*
neither ['ni:ðər], ['naɪðər] **1** *adj & pron* nenhum (nenhuma) **2** *adv* ***~ … nor …*** nem … nem … **3** *conj* nem; ***~ do I*** eu também não
neon light ['ni:ɑ:n] lâmpada *f* de neônio
nephew ['nefju:] sobrinho *m*
nerd [nɜ:rd] *fam* nerd *m*
nerve [nɜ:rv] nervo *m*; (*courage*) coragem *f*; (*impudence*) descaro *m*; ***it's bad for my ~s*** isso me deixa nervoso; ***he / it gets on my ~s*** ele / isso me dá nos nervos
nerve-racking ['nɜ:rvrækɪŋ] *adj* enervante
nervous ['nɜ:rvəs] *adj* nervoso; ***be ~ about sth*** estar nervoso em relação a algo
nervous 'breakdown esgotamento *m* nervoso
nervous 'energy vitalidade *f*
nervousness ['nɜ:rvəsnɪs] nervosismo *m*
nervous 'wreck ***be a ~*** estar com os nervos à flor da pele
nervy ['nɜ:rvɪ] *adj Am* (*fresh*) descarado
nest [nest] *n* ninho *m*
nestle ['nesl] *v/i* aconchegar-se
net[1] [net] *n* rede *f de pesca*, *etc*
net[2] [net] *adj price*, *amount*, *weight* líquido
net 'curtain cortina *f* de organza
net 'profit lucro *m* líquido
nettle ['netl] urtiga *f*
'network *also fig* rede *f*
'networking networking *m*
neurologist [nʊ'rɑ:lədʒɪst] neurologista *m/f*

neurosis [nʊ'roʊsɪs] neurose *f*
neurotic [nʊ'rɑːtɪk] *adj* neurótico
neuter ['nuːtər] *v/t animal* castrar
neutral ['nuːtrl] **1** *adj country, color* neutro **2** *n gear* ponto *m* morto; ***in ~*** em ponto morto
neutrality [nʊ'trælətɪ] neutralidade *f*
neutralize ['nʊtrəlaɪz] *v/t* neutralizar
never ['nevər] *adv also in disbelief* nunca; ***you're ~ going to believe this*** você nunca vai acreditar nisso; ***you ~ promised, did you?*** você nunca prometeu, não é mesmo?
never-'ending *adj* interminável
nevertheless [nevərðə'les] *adv* no entanto
new [nuː] *adj* novo; ***this system is still ~ to me*** este sistema ainda é novo para mim; ***I'm ~ to the job*** sou novo no trabalho; ***that's nothing ~*** não é nada novo
'newborn *adj* recém-nascido
newcomer ['nʊkʌmər] recém-chegado,-a *m,f*
newly ['nuːlɪ] *adv* (*recently*) recentemente
'newly weds [wedz] *npl* recém-casados *mpl*
new 'moon lua *f* nova
news [nuːz] *nsg on TV, radio* notícias *fpl*; ***that's ~ to me*** isto é novidade para mim; ***a piece of ~*** uma notícia
'news agency agência *f* de notícias **'newsagent** *Brit* jornaleiro *m* **'newscast** TV telejornal *m* **'newscaster** TV apresentador,a *m,f* **'news flash** notícia *f* de última hora **'newspaper** jornal *m* **'newsreader** TV *etc* apresentador,a *m,f* **'news report** reportagem *f* **'newsstand** banca *f* de jornal **'newsvendor** vendedor *m* de jornais
'new year Ano Novo *m*; ***Happy New Year!*** Feliz Ano Novo! **New Year's 'Day** Dia *m* de Ano Novo **New Year's 'Eve** Véspera *f* do Ano Novo **New Zealand** ['ziːlənd] Nova Zelândia *f* **New Zealander** ['ziːləndər] neozelandês,-esa *m,f*
next [nekst] **1** *adj in time, space* seguinte; ***the ~ week / month he came back again*** ele voltou na semana seguinte novamente / no mês seguinte novamente; ***who's ~?*** quem é o próximo? **2** *adv* depois; ***it's my turn ~*** é a minha vez depois; ***when shall we meet ~?*** quando nos vemos de novo?; ***~ to*** (*beside*) ao lado de; (*in comparison with*) em comparação com; ***there's ~ to nothing left*** não há quase mais nada
next 'door 1 *adj neighbor* do lado **2** *adv live* ao lado
next of 'kin parente próximo,-a *m,f*
nibble ['nɪbl] *v/t* mordiscar
Nicaragua [nɪkə'rægjʊə] Nicarágua
Nicaraguan [nɪkə'rægjʊən] **1** *adj* nicaragüense **2** *n* nicaragüense *m/f*
nice [naɪs] *adj appearance* bonito; (*likeable*) simpático; *meal, food* gostoso; *party, trip, vacation* agradável; ***be ~ to your sister!*** trate a sua irmã bem; ***that's very ~ of you*** é muito amável de sua parte
nicely ['naɪslɪ] *adv written, presented* bem; (*pleasantly*) agradavelmente
niceties ['naɪsətɪz] *npl* (***social***) ***~*** *npl* etiqueta *f*
niche [niːʃ] nicho *m*
nick [nɪk] *n* (*cut*) corte *m*; ***in the ~ of time*** na hora exata
nickel ['nɪkl] níquel *m*; *coin* moeda *f* de cinco centavos de dólar
'nickname *n* apelido *m*, *Port* alcunha *f*
niece [niːs] sobrinha *f*
niggardly ['nɪgərdlɪ] *adj amount, person* mísero
night [naɪt] noite *f*; ***tomorrow ~*** amanhã à noite; ***11 o'clock at ~*** onze horas da noite; ***travel by ~*** viajar de noite; ***during the ~*** durante a noite; ***stay the ~*** passar a noite; ***a room for 2 ~s*** um quarto para duas noites; ***work ~s*** trabalhar de noite; ***good ~*** boa noite; ***in the middle of the ~*** no meio da noite
'nightcap *drink* bebida *f* noturna **'nightclub** boate *f* **'nightdress** camisola *f*, *Port* camisa *f* de noite **'nightfall** *n* ***at ~*** ao anoitecer **'night flight** vôo *m* noturno **'nightgown** camisola *f*, *Port* camisa *f* de noite
nightie ['naɪtɪ] camisola *f*
nightingale ['naɪtɪŋgeɪl] rouxinol *m*

'nightlife vida *f* noturna
nightly ['naɪtlɪ] **1** *adj* noturno; ***his ~ walks*** suas caminhadas noturnas **2** *adv* toda noite; ***the band plays twice ~*** a banda toca duas vezes toda noite
'nightmare *also fig* pesadelo *m*
'night porter porteiro *m* noturno **'night school** escola *f* noturna **'night shift** turno *m* da noite **'nightshirt** pijama *m* **'nightspot** clube *m* noturno **'nighttime** *n* ***at ~*** à noite
nil [nɪl] *Brit* zero
nimble ['nɪmbl] *adj* ágil; *mind* inteligente
nine [naɪn] nove
nineteen [naɪn'tiːn] dezenove, *Port* dezanove
nineteenth [naɪn'tiːnθ] *n & adj* décimo nono (*m*)
ninetieth ['naɪntɪəθ] *n & adj* nonagésimo (*m*)
ninety ['naɪntɪ] noventa
ninth [naɪnθ] *n & adj* nono (*m*)
nip [nɪp] *n* (*pinch*) beliscão *m*; (*bite*) mordida *f*
nipple ['nɪpl] mamilo *m*
nitrogen ['naɪtrədʒn] nitrogênio *m*
no [noʊ] **1** *adv* não **2** *adj* ***there's ~ coffee / tea left*** não há mais café / chá; ***I have ~ family / money*** não tenho família / dinheiro; ***I'm ~ linguist / expert*** não sou lingüista / especialista; ***~ smoking / parking*** proibido fumar / estacionar; ***~ other survivor was found*** nenhum outro sobrevivente foi encontrado
nobility [noʊ'bɪlətɪ] nobreza *f*
noble ['noʊbl] *adj* nobre
nobody ['noʊbədɪ] *pron* ninguém; ***~ knows*** ninguém sabe; ***there was ~ at home*** não havia ninguém em casa
no-brainer [noʊ'breɪnər] ***it's a ~*** *fam* é lógico
nod [nɑːd] **1** *n* aceno *m* com a cabeça **2** *v/i* ⟨*pret & pp* ***nodded***⟩ acenar com a cabeça
♦**nod off** *v/i* (*fall asleep*) adormecer
no-hoper [noʊ'hoʊpər] *fam* inútil *m/f*
noise [nɔɪz] ruído *m*; *loud, unpleasant* barulho *m*
noisy ['nɔɪzɪ] *adj* barulhento
nominal ['nɑːmɪnl] *adj amount* simbólico
nominate ['nɑːmɪneɪt] *v/t* (*appoint*) nomear; ***~ s.o. for a post*** (*propose*) nomear alguém para um posto
nomination [nɑːmɪ'neɪʃn] nomeação *f*; (*proposal*) candidatura *f*
nominee [nɑːmɪ'niː] candidato,-a *m,f*
non... [nɑːn] não
nonalco'holic *adj* não alcoólico
nona'ligned *adj* não-alinhado
nonchalant ['nɑːnʃəlɑːnt] *adj* despreocupado
noncommissioned 'officer suboficial *m*
noncom'mittal *adj person, response* evasivo
nondescript ['nɑːndɪskrɪpt] *adj* indescritível; *color* indefinível
none [nʌn] *pron people*: ninguém; *things*: nada; ***~ of the students*** nenhum dos estudantes; ***~ of the chocolate*** nada do chocolate; ***there are ~ left*** não há nenhum sobrando; ***there is ~ left*** não sobra nada
non'entity pessoa *f* insignificante
nonetheless [nʌnðə'les] *adv* no entanto
nonex'istent *adj* inexistente
non'fiction não-ficção *f*
non'flammable, **nonin'flammable** *adj* não inflamável
noninter'ference, **noninter'vention** não-intervenção *f*
non-'iron *adj shirt* que não precisa passar
'no-no *n* ***that's a ~*** *fam* isto é impossível!
no-'nonsense *adj approach* direto
non'payment não pagamento *m*
nonpol'luting *adj* não poluente
non'resident *n* não residente *m/f*
nonre'turnable *adj* não retornável
nonsense ['nɑːnsəns] besteira *f*; ***don't talk ~*** não fale besteiras; ***~, it's easy!*** bobagem, isso é facil!
non'skid *adj tires* antiderrapante
non'slip *adj surface* antideslizante
non'smoker *person* não fumante *m/f*
non'standard *adj* não estandardizado
non'stick *adj pans* antiaderente

non'stop 1 *adj flight* sem escala; *train* direto **2** *adv fly, travel* diretamente
non'swimmer ***I'm a ~*** não sei nadar
non'union *adj* não sindicalizado
non'violence não-violência *f*
non'violent *adj* sem violência
noodles ['nu:dlz] *npl* macarrão *m*
nook [nʊk] cantinho *m*
noon [nu:n] meio-dia *m*; ***at ~*** ao meio--dia
noose [nu:s] nó *m* corrediço
nope [noʊp] *fam* não
nor [nɔ:r] *conj* nem; ***~ do I*** nem eu
norm [nɔ:rm] norma *f*
normal ['nɔ:rml] *adj* normal
normality [nɔ:r'mælətɪ] normalidade *f*
normalize ['nɔ:rməlaɪz] *v/t relationships* normalizar
normally ['nɔ:rməlɪ] *adv* normalmente
north [nɔ:rθ] **1** *n* norte *m*; ***to the ~ of*** ao norte de **2** *adj* norte **3** *adv travel* para o norte; ***~ of*** ao norte de
North Am'erica América *f* do Norte
North Am'erican 1 *adj* norte-americano **2** *n* norte-americano,-a *m,f*
north'east *n* nordeste *m*
northerly ['nɔ:rðərlɪ] *adj* norte
northern ['nɔ:rðərn] *adj* do norte
northerner ['nɔ:rðərnər] nortista *m/f*
North Ko'rea Coréia *f* do Norte
North Ko'rean 1 *adj* norte-coreano **2** *n* norte-coreano,-a *m,f* **'North Pole** Pólo *m* Norte
northward ['nɔ:rθwərd] *adv travel* em direção norte
'northwest *n* noroeste *m*
Norway ['nɔ:rweɪ] Noruega *f*
Norwegian [nɔ:r'wi:dʒn] **1** *adj* norueguês,-esa **2** *n person* norueguês,-esa *m,f*; *language* norueguês *m*
nose [noʊz] nariz *m*; ***it was right under my ~!*** estava debaixo do meu nariz
♦**nose about** *v/i fam* bisbilhotar
'nosebleed hemorragia *f* nasal
nostalgia [nɑ:'stældʒə] nostalgia *f*
nostalgic [nɑ:'stældʒɪk] *adj* nostálgico
nostril ['nɑ:strəl] narina *f*
nosy ['noʊzɪ] *adj fam* xereta
not [nɑ:t] *adv* não; ***~ now*** agora não; ***~ there*** não lá; ***~ like that*** assim não; ***~ for me, thanks*** para mim não, obrigado; ***~ a lot*** não muito; ***it's ~ allowed*** não é permitido; ***I don't know*** eu não sei; ***he's American, isn't he*** ele é americano, não é?; ***is he back? – ~ that I know of*** ele já voltou? - não que eu saiba
notable ['noʊtəbl] *adj* notável
notary ['noʊtərɪ] notário *m*, tabelião *m*
notch [nɑ:tʃ] entalhe *m*
note [noʊt] *n* nota *f*; ***take ~s*** tomar notas; ***take ~ of sth*** notar algo
♦**note down** *v/t* anotar
'notebook caderno *m*; COMPUT notebook *m*
noted ['noʊtɪd] *adj* famoso
'notepad bloco *m* de anotações
'notepaper papel *m* de carta
nothing ['nʌθɪŋ] *pron* nada; ***~ but*** somente; ***~ much*** não muito; ***for ~*** (*for free*) de graça; (*for no reason*) sem motivo; ***I'd like ~ better*** é o que eu mais gostaria
notice ['noʊtɪs] **1** *n* letreiro *m*; (*advance warning*) aviso *m*; *in newspaper* anúncio *m*; ***at short ~*** com pouca antecedência; ***until further ~*** até segundas ordens; ***give s.o. his / her ~*** *to quit job* dar o aviso prévio de demissão a alguém; *to leave house* dar o aviso de desocupação a alguém; ***hand in one's ~*** *to employer* apresentar a carta de demissão; ***four weeks' ~*** quatro semanas de aviso prévio; ***take ~ of sth*** prestar atenção em algo; ***take no ~ of s.o. / sth*** não fazer caso de alguém / algo **2** *v/t* notar
noticeable ['noʊtɪsəbl] *adj* perceptível
'notice board *Brit* quadro *m* de avisos
notify ['noʊtɪfaɪ] *v/t* ⟨*pret & pp* ***notified***⟩ avisar
notion ['noʊʃn] noção *f*
notions ['noʊsnz] *npl Am* aviamentos *mpl*
notorious [noʊ'tɔ:rɪəs] *adj* de má fama
nougat ['nu:gət] nougat *m*
nought [nɒ:t] *Brit* zero
noun [naʊn] substantivo *m*
nourishing ['nʌrɪʃɪŋ] *adj* nutritivo
nourishment ['nʌrɪʃmənt] nutriente *m*

novel ['nɑːvl] *n* romance *m*
novelist ['nɑːvlɪst] *Port* escritor,a *m,f*
novelty ['nɑːvəltɪ] novidade *f*
November [noʊ'vembər] novembro *m*
novice ['nɑːvɪs] (*beginner*) novato,-a *m,f*; REL noviço,-a *m,f*
now [naʊ] agora; ***~ and again, ~ and then*** de vez em quando; ***by ~*** já; ***from ~ on*** a partir de agora; ***right ~*** agora mesmo; ***just ~*** (*at this moment*) agora; ***he was here just ~*** (*a little while ago*) ele estava aqui até agora; ***~, ~!*** vamos! vamos!; ***~, where did I put it?*** e agora, aonde coloquei isto?
nowadays ['naʊədeɪz] *adv* hoje em dia
nowhere ['noʊwer] *adv* em nenhum lugar; ***it's ~ near finished*** ainda falta muito para acabar
nozzle ['nɑːzl] bocal *m*
nuclear ['nuːklɪər] *adj* nuclear
nuclear 'energy energia *f* nuclear **nuclear 'fission** fissão *f* nuclear **'nuclear-free** *adj* ***~ zone*** zona *f* livre de armas nucleares **nuclear 'physics** física *f* nuclear **nuclear 'power** *energy* energia *f* nuclear; POL potência *f* nuclear **nuclear 'power station** central *f* nuclear **nuclear re'actor** reator *m* nuclear **nuclear 'waste** resíduo *m* nuclear **nuclear 'weapon** arma *f* nuclear
nude [nuːd] **1** *adj* nu; ***in the ~*** nu **2** *n painting* nu *m* artístico
nudge [nʌdʒ] *v/t* acotovelar
nudist ['nuːdɪst] *n* nudista *m/f*
nuisance ['nuːsns] aborrecimento *m*; ***make a ~ of oneself*** importunar os outros; ***what a ~!*** que chato!
nuke [nuːk] *v/t fam* destruir com arma nuclear
null and 'void [nʌl] *adj* nulo e anulado
numb [nʌm] *adj* dormente; *emotionally* insensível
number ['nʌmbər] **1** *n* número *m*; (*quantity*) quantidade *f* **2** *v/t* (*put a number on*) numerar
'number plate *Brit* placa *m* do carro
numeral ['nuːmərəl] numeral *m*
numerate ['nuːmərət] *adj* bom em cálculos
numerical [nuː'merɪkl] *adj* numérico
numerous ['nuːmərəs] *adj* numeroso
nun [nʌn] freira *f*
nurse [nɜːrs] enfermeiro,-a *m,f*
nursery ['nɜːrsərɪ] *school* creche *f*; *for plants* viveiro *m*
'nursery rhyme canção *f* infantil **'nursery school** jardim *m* da infância **'nursery school teacher** professor,a *m,f* de jardim de infância
nursing ['nɜːrsɪŋ] enfermagem *f*
'nursing home *for old people* casa *f* de repouso
nut [nʌt] BOT fruto *m* seco; TECH porca *f*
'nutcrackers *npl* quebra-nozes *m*
nutrient ['nuːtrɪənt] *n* nutriente *m*
nutrition [nuː'trɪʃn] nutrição *f*
nutritious [nuː'trɪʃəs] *adj* nutritivo
nuts [nʌts] *adj fam* (*crazy*) louco; ***be ~ about s.o.*** estar louco por alguém
nutshell *n* ***in a ~*** em poucas palavras
nutty ['nʌtɪ] *adj fam* (*crazy*) louco
nylon ['naɪlɑːn] **1** *n* nylon *m* **2** *adj* de nylon

O

oak [oʊk] carvalho *m*
oar [ɔːr] remo *m*
oasis [oʊ'eɪsɪs] ⟨*pl* **oases**⟩ *also fig* oásis *m*
oath [oʊθ] LAW juramento *m*; (*swearword*) maldição *f*; ***on ~*** sob juramento
'oatmeal farinha *f* de aveia

oats [oʊts] aveia *f*
obedience [oʊ'bi:dɪəns] obediência *f*
obedient [oʊ'bi:dɪənt] *adj* obediente
obediently [oʊ'bi:dɪəntlɪ] *adv* obedientemente
obese [oʊ'bi:s] *adj* obeso
obesity [oʊ'bi:sɪtɪ] obesidade *f*
obey [oʊ'beɪ] *v/t* obedecer a
obituary [oʊ'bɪʧuerɪ] *n* obituário *m*
object[1] ['ɑ:bdʒɪkt] *n* (*thing*), GRAM objeto *m*; (*aim*) objetivo *m*
object[2] [əb'dʒekt] *v/i* fazer objeção
◆ **object to** *v/t* objetar a; ***I object to that!*** eu me oponho a isso!; ***do you object to them smoking?*** você objeta a que eles fumem?
objection [əb'dʒekʃn] objeção *f*
objectionable [əb'dʒekʃnəbl] *adj* (*unpleasant*) desagradável
objective [əb'dʒektɪv] **1** *adj* objetivo **2** *n* objetivo *m*
objectively [əb'dʒektɪvlɪ] *adv* objetivamente
objectivity [əbdʒek'tɪvətɪ] objetividade *f*
obligation [ɑ:blɪ'geɪʃn] obrigação *f*; ***be under an ~ to s.o.*** estar obrigado a alguém
obligatory [ə'blɪgətɔ:rɪ] *adj* obrigatório
oblige [ə'blaɪdʒ] *v/t* ***much ~d!*** muito obrigado,-a
obliging [ə'blaɪdʒɪŋ] *adj* prestativo
oblique [ə'bli:k] **1** *adj reference* indireto **2** *n punctuation*: barra *f*
obliterate [ə'blɪtəreɪt] *v/t city* destruir; *memory* apagar
oblivion [ə'blɪvɪən] esquecimento *m*; ***fall into ~*** cair em esquecimento
oblivious [ə'blɪvɪəs] *adj* ***be ~ to sth*** não estar consciente de algo
oblong ['ɑ:blɑ:ŋ] *adj* retangular
obnoxious [ɑ:b'nɑ:kʃəs] *adj* repugnante
obscene [ɑ:b'si:n] *adj* obsceno; *salary, poverty* escandaloso
obscenity [əb'senətɪ] obscenidade *f*
obscure [əb'skjʊr] *adj* (*hard to see*) escuro; (*hard to understand*) obscuro; (*little known*) anônimo
obscurity [əb'skjʊrətɪ] (*anonymity*) obscuridade *f*
observance [əb'zɜ:rvns] *of festival etc* prática *f*
observant [əb'zɜ:rvnt] *adj* observador
observation [ɑ:bzər'veɪʃn] observação *f*
observatory [əb'zɜ:rvətɔ:rɪ] observatório *m*
observe [əb'zɜ:rv] *v/t* observar
observer [əb'zɜ:rvər] observador,a *m,f*
obsess [ɑ:b'ses] *v/t* ***be ~ed by / with*** ser / estar obcecado por
obsession [ɑ:b'seʃn] obsessão *f*
obsessive [ɑ:b'sesɪv] *adj person, behavior* obsessivo
obsolete ['ɑ:bsəli:t] *adj* obsoleto
obstacle ['ɑ:bstəkl] obstáculo *m*
obstetrician [ɑ:bstə'trɪʃn] obstetra *m/f*
obstetrics [ɑ:b'stetrɪks] obstetrícia *f*
obstinacy ['ɑ:bstɪnəsɪ] obstinação *f*
obstinate ['ɑ:bstɪnət] *adj* obstinado
obstinately ['ɑ:bstɪnətlɪ] *adv* obstinadamente
obstruct [ɑ:b'strʌkt] *v/t road, investigation, police* obstruir
obstruction [əb'strʌkʧn] *on road etc* obstrução *f*
obstructive [əb'strʌktɪv] *adj behavior, tactics* obstrutivo
obtain [əb'teɪn] *v/t* obter
obtainable [əb'teɪnəbl] *adj products* obtenível
obtrusive [əb'tru:sɪv] *adj feature* desajustado
obtuse [əb'tu:s] *adj fig* lerdo
obvious ['ɑ:bvɪəs] *adj* óbvio; (*not subtle*) evidente
obviously ['ɑ:bvɪəslɪ] *adv* obviamente; ***~!*** é claro!, é óbvio; ***~ not!*** obviamente que não!
occasion [ə'keɪʒn] ocasião *f*
occasional [ə'keɪʒənl] *adj* ***I smoke the ~ cigar*** eu fumo um charuto de vez em quando
occasionally [ə'keɪʒnlɪ] *adv* de vez em quando; ***very ~*** raramente
occult [ə'kʌlt] **1** *adj* oculto **2** *n* ***the ~*** o oculto
occupant ['ɑ:kjʊpənt] *vehicle*: ocupante *m/f*; *apartment*: inquilino,-a *m,f*

occupation [ɑ:kjʊ'peɪʃn] ocupação *f*
occupational 'therapist [ɑ:kjʊ'peɪʃnl] terapeuta *m/f* ocupacional
occupational 'therapy terapia *f* ocupacional
occupy ['ɑ:kjʊpaɪ] *v/t* ⟨*pret & pp* ***occupied***⟩ ocupar; ***~ oneself with sth*** ocupar-se com algo
occur [ə'kɜ:r] *v/i* ⟨*pret & pp* ***occurred***⟩ ocorrer; ***it ~red to me that …*** me ocorreu que …
occurrence [ə'kʌrəns] ocorrência *f*
ocean ['oʊʃn] oceano *m*
oceanography [oʊʃn'ɑ:grəfɪ] oceanografia *f*
o'clock [ə'klɑ:k] ***at five / six ~*** às cinco / seis horas
October [ɑ:k'toʊbər] outubro *m*
octopus ['ɑ:ktəpəs] polvo *m*
OD [oʊ'di:] *fam* overdose *f*
odd [ɑ:d] *adj* (*strange*) estranho; (*not even*) ímpar; ***which is the ~ one out*** o que não pertence?; ***50 ~*** mais ou menos cinqüenta
'oddball *fam* esquisitão *m*
odds [ɑ:dz] *npl* ***be at ~ with*** estar em divergêcia com; ***the ~ are 10 to one*** as chances são de dez a um; ***the ~ are that …*** o mais provável é que …
odds and 'ends *npl* (*objects*) quinquilharias *fpl*; (*things to do*) coisas *fpl*
'odds-on *adj* ***he's the ~ favorite*** é o vencedor provável
odious ['oʊdɪəs] *adj* odioso
odometer [oʊ'dɑ:mətər] *Am* hodômetro *m*
odor ['oʊdər] *Am* odor *m*
odour *Brit* → ***odor***
of [ɑ:v] *unstressed* [əv] *prep* de; ***the name ~ the street / hotel*** o nome da rua / do hotel; ***the color ~ the car*** a cor do carro; ***the works ~ Dickens*** a obra de Dickens; ***five / ten minutes ~ twelve*** cinco / dez minutos para as doze; ***die ~ cancer*** morrer de câncer; ***love ~ money / adventure*** amor pelo dinheiro / pela aventura; ***~ the three this is …*** dos três este é …; ***that's good ~ you*** é bondade sua
off [ɑ:f] **1** *prep* ***~ the main road*** *away from* fora da rodovia principal; *leading off* saindo da rodovia principal; ***$20 ~ the price*** um desconto de 20 dólares no preço; ***he's ~ his food*** ele não come nada **2** *adv* ***be ~*** *light* estar apagado; *TV, machine* estar desligado; *brake, lid, top* não estar posto; *not at work* estar fora; (*canceled*) estar cancelado; ***we're ~ tomorrow*** *leaving* estaremos de partida amanhã; ***I'm ~ to New York*** estou indo para Nova Yorque; ***I must be ~*** tenho que ir; ***with his pants ~*** sem suas calças; ***take a day ~*** tirar o dia livre; ***it's 3 miles ~*** fica a 4,8 kilometros de distância; ***it's a long way ~*** *in distance* fica muito longe; *in future* está ainda muito distante; ***drive / walk ~*** ir embora de carro / ir embora; ***~ and on*** de vez em quando **3** *adj* ***the ~ switch*** o interruptor de desligar
offence *Brit* → ***offense***
offend [ə'fend] *v/t* (*insult*) ofender
offender [ə'fendər] LAW criminoso,-a *m,f*
offense [ə'fens] *Am* LAW delito *m*; ***take ~ at sth*** ficar ofendido com algo
offensive [ə'fensɪv] **1** *adj behavior, remark* ofensivo; *smell* repugnante **2** *n* (*MIL, attack*) ofensiva *f*; ***go onto the ~*** ir para a ofensiva
offer ['ɑ:fər] **1** *n* oferta *f* **2** *v/t* oferecer; ***~ s.o. sth*** oferecer algo a alguém
off'hand 1 *adj attitude* desinteressado **2** *adv say, estimate* de cabeça
office ['ɑ:fɪs] *building* prédio *m* comercial; *room* escritório *m*; *position* cargo *m*
'office block bloco *m* comercial
'office hours *npl* horário *m* do expediente
officer ['ɑ:fɪsər] MIL oficial *m*; *in police* agente *m* de polícia
official [ə'fɪʃl] **1** *adj* oficial **2** *n* funcionário,-a *m,f*
officially [ə'fɪʃlɪ] *adv* (*strictly speaking*) oficialmente
officious [ə'fɪʃəs] *adj* intrometido
off-licence *Brit* → ***liquor store***
'off-line *adv work* desconectado; ***go ~*** desconectar-se

'offpeak *adj rates* fora do auge; ***~ electricity*** energia *f* cobrada no nível mais barato

'off-ramp *from clearway etc* saída *f*

'off-season 1 *adj rates, vacation* fora de estação *or* temporada **2** *n* baixa temporada *f*

'offset *v/t* ⟨*pret & pp* ***offset***⟩ *losses, disadvantage* compensar

'offshore *adj drilling rig* em alto mar; *investment* no exterior

'offside 1 *adj Brit wheel etc* do lado do motorista **2** *adv* SPORT impedido, na posição de impedimento

'offspring prole *f*

'off-the-record *adj* inoficial

'off-white *adj* branco sujo

often ['ɑːfn] *adv* freqüentemente; ***how ~ do you go there?*** com que freqüência você vai lá?; ***that's ~ the way it goes*** é assim que acontece freqüentemente; ***it doesn't happen very ~*** isso não acontece freqüentemente; ***every so ~*** uma vez ou outra

oil [ɔɪl] **1** *n for machine, food, skin* óleo *m*; *from oil well* petróleo *m* **2** *v/t hinges, bearings* untar

'oil change troca *f* do óleo **'oil company** companhia *f* petrolífera **'oilfield** campo *m* petrolífero **'oil-fired** *adj central heating* a óleo **'oil painting** pintura *f* a óleo **'oil-producing country** país *m* produtor de petróleo **'oil refinery** refinaria *f* de petróleo **'oil rig** plataforma *f* petrolífera **'oilskins** *npl* roupa *f* impermeável **'oil slick** mancha *f* de óleo **'oil tanker** *ship* navio *m* petroleiro; *truck* carro-tanque *m* de petróleo **'oil well** poço *m* petrolífero

oily ['ɔɪlɪ] *adj* oleoso

ointment ['ɔɪntmənt] pomada *f*

ok [oʊ'keɪ] *adj & adv fam* ok; ***can I? – ~*** posso? - pode; ***is it ~ with you if …?*** parece-lhe bem se …?; ***does that look ~?*** fica bem?; ***that's ~ by me*** por mim tudo bem; ***are you ~?*** *well, not hurt* você está bem?; ***are you ~ for Saturday?*** está bem para você no sábado?; ***he's ~*** (*he is a good guy*) ele é um bom rapaz; ***is this bus ~ for …?*** este ônibus vai até …?; ***~, he was too aggressive, but …*** sim, ele era muito agressivo, mas …

old [oʊld] *adj* velho; (*previous*), *building, wine* antigo; ***how ~ are you / is he?*** quantos anos você / ele tem?; ***he's getting ~*** ele está ficando velho; ***~ people*** os velhos

old 'age velhice *f*

old-'fashioned *adj* antiquado

olive ['ɑːlɪv] azeitona *f*

'olive oil azeite *m*

Olympic 'Games [ə'lɪmpɪk] *npl* Jogos Olímpicos *mpl*

omelet ['ɑːmlət] *Am* omelete *f*, *Port* omeleta *f*

omelette *Brit* → ***omelet***

ominous ['ɑːmɪnəs] *adj signs, thunder* nefasto

omission [oʊ'mɪʃn] *act* exclusão *f*; (*that omitted*) omissão *f*

omit [ə'mɪt] *v/t* ⟨*pret & pp* ***omitted***⟩ *from team, list* tirar de; ***~ to do sth*** deixar de fazer algo

omnipotent [ɑːm'nɪpətənt] *adj* onipotente

omniscient [ɑːm'nɪsɪənt] *adj* onisciente

on [ɑːn] **1** *prep* em; ***~ the table*** na mesa; ***~ the bus / train*** no ônibus / no trem; ***~ a bus / train*** num ônibus / /num trem; ***~ TV / the radio*** na televisão / no rádio; ***~ Sunday*** no domingo; ***~ the 1st of …*** no dia primeiro de …; ***this is ~ me*** (*I'm paying*) isto é por minha conta; ***have you any money ~ you?*** você tem algum dinheiro (com você)?; ***~ his arrival / departure*** na sua chegada / partida; ***~ hearing this*** ao ouvir isto **2** *adv* ***be ~*** *light* estar aceso; *TV, computer etc* estar ligado; *brake, lid, top* estar posto; *program being broadcast* estar no ar; *meeting etc: be scheduled to happen* estar marcado; ***what's ~ tonight?*** qual é o programa desta noite?; ***with his jacket ~*** com sua jaqueta vestida; ***you're ~*** (*I accept your offer etc*) combinado; ***that's not ~*** *not allowed, not fair* isto é inadmissível; ***~ you go*** (*go ahead*) siga (adiante); ***walk / talk ~***

continuar andando / falando; ***and so ~*** etc.; ***~ and ~*** *talk etc* sem parar **3** *adj* ***the ~ switch*** o interruptor de ligar

once [wʌns] **1** *adv* (*one time*) uma vez; (*formerly*) antigamente; ***~ again, ~ more*** uma vez mais; ***at ~*** (*immediately*) imediatamente; ***all at ~*** (*suddenly*) todos de repente; (***all***) ***at ~*** (*together*) todos de uma vez; ***~ upon a time there was …*** era uma vez …; ***~ in a while*** de vez em quando; ***~ and for all*** de uma vez por todas; ***for ~*** somente desta vez **2** *conj* logo que, uma vez que; ***~ you have finished*** logo que você acabar

one [wʌn] **1** *number* um **2** *adj* um, uma; ***~ day*** um dia **3** *pron* ◊ um, uma; ***which ~?*** qual?; ***~ by ~*** *enter, deal with* um por um; ***the little ~s*** as criancinhas; ***I for ~ …*** eu pessoalmente …

◊ *fml* ***what can ~ say / do?*** o que se pode dizer / fazer?; ***~ has to admire …*** tem que se admirar …

one-'off *n* (*unique event*) acontecimento *m* único; (*exception*) exceção *f*; ***he is a ~*** ele é único

one-parent 'family família *f* monoparental

one'self *pron* ***hurt ~*** machucar-se; ***keep sth for ~*** manter algo para si mesmo; ***do sth by ~*** fazer algo sozinho

one-sided [wʌn'saɪdɪd] *adj discussion, fight* desigual **'one-track mind** *hum* ***have a ~*** só ter sexo na cabeça **'one-way street** rua *f* de mão única, *Port* rua *f* de sentido único **'one-way ticket** passagem *f* de ida

onion ['ʌnjən] cebola *f*

'on-line *adj & adv* online, em linha; ***go ~ to*** conectar com

'on-line service COMPUT serviço *m* online

onlooker ['ɑːnlʊkər] espectador,a *m,f*

only ['oʊnlɪ] **1** *adv* somente; ***not ~ X but also Y*** não somente X como também Y; ***~ just*** por pouco **2** *adj* único; ***~ son / ~ daughter*** filho único / filha única

'onset começo *m*

'onside *adv* SPORT ***be ~*** não estar na posição de impedimento

on-the-job 'training formação *f* profissional na empresa

onto '['ɑːntuː] *prep* ***put sth ~ sth*** pôr algo em cima de algo

onward ['ɑːnwərd] *adv* para a frente; ***from … ~*** a partir de …

onwards → ***onward***

ooze [uːz] **1** *v/i liquid, mud* ressumar **2** *v/t* ***he ~s charm*** ele esbanja charme

opaque [oʊ'peɪk] *adj glass* opaco

OPEC ['oʊpek] *abbr* (*of* ***Organization of Petroleum Exporting Countries***) OPEP *f* (Organização dos Países Exportadores de Petróleo)

open ['oʊpən] **1** *adj door, flower, file, countryside* aberto; ***in the ~ air*** ao ar livre **2** *v/t* abrir; *meeting* começar **3** *v/i door, shop* abrir; *flower* abrir-se

♦**open up** *v/i person* abrir-se

open-'air *adj meeting, concert* ao ar livre; *pool* descoberto **'open day** dia *m* das portas abertas **open-ended** [oʊpən'endɪd] *adj contract etc* aberto

opening ['oʊpənɪŋ] *in wall etc, of movie, novel etc* abertura *f*; (*job going*) vaga *f* aberta

'opening hours *npl* expediente *m*

openly ['oʊpənlɪ] *adv* (*honestly, frankly*) abertamente

open-minded [oʊpən'maɪndɪd] *adj* de cabeça aberta **'open plan office** escritório *m* aberto **'open ticket** ticket *m* aberto

opera ['ɑːpərə] ópera *f*

'opera glasses *npl* binóculo *m* (para teatro) **'opera house** casa *f* da ópera, teatro *m* lírico **'opera singer** cantor,a *m,f* de ópera

operate ['ɑːpəreɪt] **1** *v/i company, airline, bus service* operar **2** *v/t machine* funcionar; MED operar

♦**operate on** *v/t* MED operar

'operating instructions *npl* instruções *fpl* de funcionamento **'operating room** *Am* MED sala *f* de operações **'operating system** COMPUT sistema *m* operacional

operation [ɑːpə'reɪʃn] MED, *of machine* operação *f*; ***~s*** *of company* ati-

O

vidades *fpl*; MED ***have an ~*** ser operado
operator ['ɑːpəreɪtər] operador,a *m,f*
ophthalmologist [ɑːpθæl'mɑːlədʒɪst] *Am* oftalmologista *m/f*
opinion [ə'pɪnjən] opinião *f*; ***in my ~*** na minha opinião
o'pinion poll pesquisa *f* de opinião
opponent [ə'poʊnənt] oponente *m/f*
opportune ['ɑːpərtuːn] *adj fml* oportuno
opportunist [ɑːpər'tuːnɪst] oportunista *m/f*
opportunity [ɑːpər'tuːnətɪ] oportunidade *f*
oppose [ə'poʊz] *v/t* opor; ***be ~d to ...*** opor-se a ...; ***as ~d to ...*** ao contrário de ...
opposite ['ɑːpəzɪt] **1** *adj side, direction, views, characters* oposto; ***the ~ sex*** o sexo oposto **2** *n* contrário *m* **3** *prep Brit* de frente para; ***our house is ~ the church*** a nossa casa fica de frente para a igreja **4** *adv Brit* em frente de; ***he lives ~*** ele mora em frente daqui
opposite 'number homólogo,-a *m,f*
opposition [ɑːpə'zɪʃn] *to plan*, POL oposição *f*
oppress [ə'pres] *v/t the people* oprimir
oppressive [ə'presɪv] *adj rule* opressivo; *weather* sufocante
opt [ɑːpt] *v/t* ***~ to do sth*** optar por fazer algo
♦ **opt for** *v/t* optar por
optical illusion ['ɑːptɪkl] ilusão *f* de óptica
optician [ɑːp'tɪʃn] oculista *m/f*
optimism ['ɑːptɪmɪzəm] otimismo *m*
optimist ['ɑːptɪmɪst] otimista *m/f*
optimistic [ɑːptɪ'mɪstɪk] *adj* otimista
optimistically [ɑːptɪ'mɪstɪklɪ] *adv* com otimismo
optimum ['ɑːptɪməm] **1** *adj* ótimo **2** *n* melhor *m*
option ['ɑːpʃn] opção *f*
optional ['ɑːpʃnl] *adj* opcional
optional 'extras *npl* ítens *mpl* opcionais
or [ɔːr] *conj* ou; ***~ else*** senão
oral ['ɔːrəl] *adj* oral
orange ['ɔːrɪndʒ] **1** *adj color* laranja **2** *n fruit* laranja *f*
'orange juice suco *m* de laranja, *Port* sumo *m* de laranja
orange 'squash suco *m* de laranja concentrado, *Port* sumo *m* de laranja concentrado
orator ['ɔːrətər] orador,a *m,f*
orbit ['ɔːrbɪt] **1** *n of earth* órbita *f*; ***send sth into ~*** colocar algo em órbita **2** *v/t the earth* girar em torno de
orchard ['ɔːrtʃərd] pomar *m*
orchestra ['ɔːrkəstrə] orquestra *f*
orchid ['ɔːrkɪd] orquídea *f*
ordain [ɔːr'deɪn] *v/t priest* ordenar
ordeal [ɔːr'diːl] martírio *m*
order ['ɔːrdər] **1** *n* (*command, sequence, being well arranged*) ordem *f*; *goods, restaurant*: pedido *m*; ***in ~ to*** a fim de; ***out of ~*** (*not functioning*) fora de serviço; (*not in sequence*) fora de ordem; ***an ~ of fries*** uma porção de fritas **2** *v/t* (*put in sequence, proper layout*) ordenar; *goods* encomendar; *meal* pedir; ***~ s.o. to do sth*** mandar alguém fazer algo **3** *v/i in restaurant* pedir
orderly ['ɔːrdərlɪ] **1** *adj lifestyle* ordenado **2** *n hospital*: assistente *m/f*
ordinal number ['ɔːrdɪnl] número *m* ordinal
ordinarily [ɔːrdɪ'nerɪlɪ] *adv* (*as a rule*) normalmente
ordinary ['ɔːrdɪnerɪ] *adj* comum, normal
ore [ɔːr] minério *m*
organ ['ɔːrgən] ANAT, MUS órgão *m*
organic [ɔːr'gænɪk] *adj food, fertilizer* orgânico
organically [ɔːr'gænɪklɪ] *adv grown* organicamente
organism ['ɔːrgənɪzm] organismo *m*
organization [ɔːrgənaɪ'zeɪʃn] organização *f*
organize ['ɔːrgənaɪz] *v/t* organizar
organized 'crime crime *m* organizado
organizer ['ɔːrgənaɪzər] *person* organizador,a *m,f*
orgasm ['ɔːrgæzm] orgasmo *m*
Orient ['ɔːrɪənt] Oriente *m*
Oriental [ɔːrɪ'entl] **1** *adj* oriental **2** *n* oriental *m/f*

orientate ['ɔːrɪənteɪt] *v/t* (*direct*) direcionar; ~ ***oneself*** (*get one's bearings*) orientar-se
origin ['ɑːrɪdʒɪn] origem *f*
original [ə'rɪdʒənl] **1** *adj* original **2** *n painting etc* original *m/f*
originality [ərɪdʒə'nælətɪ] originalidade *f*
originally [ə'rɪdʒənəlɪ] *adv* originalmente; (*at first*) de início
originate [ə'rɪdʒɪneɪt] **1** *v/t scheme* criar **2** *v/i idea, belief* originar-se; *family* proceder
originator [ə'rɪdʒɪneɪtər] *of scheme etc* criador,a *m,f*; ***he's not an*** ~ ele não é um tipo criativo
ornament ['ɔːrnəmənt] ornamento *m*
ornamental [ɔːrnə'mentl] *adj* ornamental
ornate [ɔːr'neɪt] *adj style, architecture* ornamentado
orphan ['ɔːrfn] *n* órfão *m*, órfã *f*
orphanage ['ɔːrfənɪdʒ] orfanato *m*
orthodox ['ɔːrθədɑːks] *adj* ortodoxo
orthopedic [ɔːrθə'piːdɪk] *adj* ortopédico
ostensibly [ɑː'stensəblɪ] *adv* aparentemente
ostentation [ɑːsten'teɪʃn] ostentação *f*
ostentatious [ɑːsten'teɪʃəs] *adj* ostentativo
ostentatiously [ɑːsten'teɪʃəslɪ] *adv* ostentativamente
ostracize ['ɑːstrəsaɪz] *v/t* condenar ao ostracismo
other ['ʌðər] **1** *adj* outro; ***the*** ~ ***day*** (*recently*) o outro dia; ***every*** ~ ***day / person*** a cada dois dias / a cada duas pessoas **2** *n* outro,-a *m,f*; ***the*** ~***s*** os outros
otherwise ['ʌðərwaɪz] *adv* senão; (*differently*) de maneira diferente
otter ['ɑːtər] lontra *f*
ought [ɒːt] *v/aux* ***I / you*** ~ ***to know*** eu devo / você deve saber; ***you*** ~ ***to have done it*** você deveria ter feito isto
ounce [aʊns] onça *f*
our ['aʊr] *adj* nosso
ours ['aʊrz] *pron* nosso,-a; ***it's*** ~ é nosso
ourselves [aʊr'selvz] *pron* nós; *emphatic* nós mesmos, nós mesmas; ***we enjoyed*** ~ nós nos divertimos; ***by*** ~ sozinhos,-as
oust [aʊst] *v/t from office* depor
out [aʊt] *adv* ***be*** ~ *light, fire* estar apagado; *flower* florir; *sun* estar raiando; *not at home, not in building* estar fora; *be published* ser publicado; *calculations* estar errado; *secret* estar revelado; *no longer in competition* estar fora; *no longer in fashion* estar fora de moda; ~ ***here in Dallas*** aqui em Dallas; ***he's*** ~ ***in the garden*** ele está no jardim; (***get***) ~***!*** vá embora!; (***get***) ~ ***of my room!*** saia do meu quarto!; ***he's*** ~ ***to win*** ele está decidido a ganhar; ***that's*** ~***!*** isto, nem pensar!
outage ['aʊtɪdʒ] blecaute *m*, *Port* corte *m* de energia
outboard 'motor motor *m* externo
'outbreak explosão *f*; *of violence* erupção *f*
'outbuilding galpão *m*; *on a farm* celeiro *m*
'outburst (*emotional*) explosão *f*
'outcast *n* pária *m*
'outcome resultado *m*
'outcry protesto *m*
out'dated *adj* obsoleto
out'do *v/t* ⟨*pret* ***outdid***, *pp* ***outdone***⟩ ser superior a
out'door *adj toilet, activities, life* ao ar livre
out'doors *adv* fora
outer ['aʊtər] *adj wall etc* externo
outer 'space espaço *m*
'outfit *clothes* traje *m*; (*company, organization*) grupo *m*
'outgoing *adj flight* de saída; *personality* extrovertido
out'grow *v/t* ⟨*pret* ***outgrew***, *pp* ***outgrown***⟩ *old ideas* abandonar; ***he has*** ~***n those clothes*** ele esta muito grande para vestir estas roupas
outing ['aʊtɪŋ] (*trip*) excursão *f*
out'last *v/t* durar mais que
'outlet *pipe*: saída *f*, *sales*: ponto *m* de venda
'outline 1 *n person, building etc*: perfil *m*; *plan, novel*: esboço *m* **2** *v/t plans etc* esboçar

out'live *v/t* sobreviver a
'outlook (*prospects*) perspectiva *f*
'outlying *adj areas* afastado
out'number *v/t* superar em número; ***we were ~ed by the enemy*** fomos superados em número pelo inimigo
out of *prep* ◊ *motion* fora de; ***run ~ the house*** sair correndo de casa ◊ *position* de ***20 miles ~ Detroit*** a 32 kilometros de Detroit ◊ *cause* por; ***~ jealousy / curiosity*** por ciúme / curiosidade ◊ *without* sem; ***we're ~ gas / beer*** estamos sem gás / cerveja ◊ *from a group* ***5 ~ 10*** cinco de cada 10
out-of-'date *adj equipment* antiquado; *values* defasado
out-of-the-'way *adj place, restaurant* afastado
'outrage *n feeling* indignação *f*; *act* atrocidade *f*
outrageous [aʊt'reɪdʒəs] *adj acts* ultrajante, escandaloso; *prices* exorbitante
'outright 1 *adj winner* absoluto **2** *adv win* completamente; *kill* de imediato
out'run *v/t* ⟨*pret* ***outran***, *pp* ***outrun***⟩ (*run faster than*) correr mais rápido que; (*run for longer than*) correr mais que
'outset princípio *m*; ***from the ~*** desde o princípio
out'shine *v/t* ⟨*pret & pp* ***outshone***⟩ ser melhor que
'outside 1 *adj surface, wall, lane* exterior **2** *adv sit* fora; *go* para fora **3** *prep* fora de; (*apart from*) além de **4** *n* exterior *m*; ***at the ~*** no máximo
outside 'broadcast programa *m* externo; *sports* cobertura *f* externa
outsider [aʊt'saɪdər] estranho,-a *m,f*; *in election, race* temporão *m*
'outsize *adj clothing* de tamanho especial
'outskirts *npl* periferias *fpl*
out'smart *v/t* ser mais inteligente que
'outsource *v/t* subcontratar
out'standing *adj success, quality* fora de série; *writer, athlete* excelente; FIN *invoice, sums* em aberto
outstretched ['aʊtstretʃt] *adj hands* estendido
out'vote *v/t* vencer por votos
outward ['aʊtwərd] *adj appearance* exterior; ***~ journey*** viagem *f* de ida
outwardly ['aʊtwərdlɪ] *adv* aparentemente
out'weigh *v/t other considerations* pesar mais que
out'wit *v/t* ⟨*pret & pp* ***outwitted***⟩ ser mais esperto que
oval ['oʊvl] *adj* oval
ovary ['oʊvərɪ] ovário *m*
ovation [oʊ'veɪʃn] ovação *f*; ***give s.o. a standing ~*** aplaudir alguém de pé
oven ['ʌvn] forno *m*
'oven glove, 'oven mitt luva *f* térmica **'ovenproof** *adj* refratário **'oven-ready** *adj* pronto para forno
over ['oʊvər] **1** *prep* (*above*) acima de; (*across*) para o outro lado de; (*more than*) mais de; (*during*) durante; ***travel all ~ Brazil*** viajar por todo o Brasil; ***you find them all ~ Brazil*** você os encontra por todo o Brasil; ***let's talk ~ a drink*** vamos conversar enquanto comemos; ***we're ~ the worst*** o pior já passou; ***~ and above*** além de **2** *adv* ***be ~*** *finished* ter acabado; *left* restar; ***~ to you*** (*your turn*) é a sua vez; ***~ in Japan*** lá no Japão; ***~ here / there*** para cá / lá; ***it hurts all ~*** tenho dor por todos os lados; ***painted white all ~*** todo pintado de branco; ***it's all ~*** está tudo acabado; ***~ and ~ again*** mil vezes; ***do sth ~*** (***again***) refazer algo
overall ['oʊvərɒːl] **1** *adj length* total **2** *adv measure* no total; (*in general*) em geral
overalls ['oʊvərɒːlz] *npl* macacão *m*, *Port* fato *m* macaco
over'awe *v/t* intimidar; ***be ~d by s.o. / sth*** ser intimidado por alguém / algo
over'balance *v/i* perder o equilíbrio
over'bearing *adj* dominante
'overboard *adv* ***man ~!*** homem ao mar!; ***go ~ for s.o. / sth*** estar muito entusiasmado por alguém / algo
'overcast *adj day* escuro; *sky* nublado
over'charge *v/t customer* cobrar demais

'overcoat sobretudo *m*
over'come *v/t* ⟨*pret* **overcame**, *pp* **overcome**⟩ *difficulties*, *shyness* superar; **be ~ by emotion** ser tomado pela emoção
over'crowded *adj train* superlotado; *cities* superpovoado
over'do *v/t* ⟨*pret* **overdid**, *pp* **overdone**⟩ (*exaggerate*) exagerar; *in cooking* cozinhar demais; **you're ~ing things** você está exagerando
over'done *adj meat* mais do que pronto
'overdose *n* overdose *f*
'overdraft excedimento *m* do limite de crédito; **have an ~** estar em débito
over'draw *v/t* ⟨*pret* **overdrew**, *pp* **overdrawn**⟩ **be $800 ~n** estar com um débito de 800 dólares
over'dressed *adj* vestido muito formalmente; *too many clothes* vestido excessivamente
'overdrive MOT sobremarcha *f*
over'due *adj apology*, *alteration* atrasado
over'estimate *v/t abilities*, *value* superestimar
over'expose *v/t photograph* superexpor
'overflow[1] *n pipe* vazamento *m*
over'flow[2] *v/i water* inundar
over'grown *adj garden* coberto de mato; **he's an ~ baby** ele é um bebezão
over'haul *v/t engine*, *plans* revisar
'overhead 1 *adj lights*, *railway* elevado **2** *n Am* FIN, *Brit* **~s** despesas *fpl* gerais
over'hear *v/t* ⟨*pret & pp* **overheard**⟩ ouvir por acaso
over'heated *adj room*, *engine*, *economy* superaquecido
overjoyed [oʊvər'dʒɔɪd] *adj* contentíssimo
'overkill *n* **that's ~** é ir longe demais
'overland 1 *adj route* terrestre **2** *adv travel* via terrestre
over'lap *v/i* ⟨*pret & pp* **overlapped**⟩ *tiles etc* sobrepor-se; *periods of time* coincidir; *theories* ter pontos em comum
'overleaf *n* **see ~** veja página seguinte
over'load *v/t vehicle*, ELEC sobrecarregar
over'look *v/t tall building etc* ter vista para; (*not see*) não perceber; (*deliberately ignore*) deixar passar (em branco)
overly ['oʊvərlɪ] excessivamente; **not ~ ...** não excessivamente ...
'overnight *adv change*, *learn sth* da noite para o dia; **stay ~** passar a noite
'overnight bag bolsa de viagem
over'paid *adj* de salário muito alto
'overpass viaduto *m*
overpopulated [oʊvər'pɑːpjəleɪtɪd] *adj* superpovoado
over'power *v/t physically* dominar
overpowering [oʊvər'paʊrɪŋ] *adj smell* muito forte; *sense of guilt* insuportável
overpriced [oʊvər'praɪst] *adj* de preço exagerado
overrated [oʊvə'reɪtɪd] *adj* supervalorizado
overre'act *v/i* reagir de forma exagerada
over'ride *v/t* ⟨*pret* **overrode**, *pp* **overridden**⟩ anular; *technically* cancelar
over'riding *adj concern* prioritário
over'rule *v/t decision* anular
over'run *v/t* ⟨*pret* **overran**, *pp* **overrun**⟩ *country* invadir; *time* exceder; **be ~ with** estar cheio de
over'seas 1 *adv live*, *work*, *travel* no extrangeiro **2** *adj* extrangeiro
over'see *v/t* ⟨*pret* **oversaw**, *pp* **overseen**⟩ supervisionar
over'shadow *v/t fig* ofuscar
'oversight descuido *m*; (*control*) fiscalização *f*
oversimplifi'cation [oʊvərsɪmplɪfɪ'keɪʃn] simplificação *f* excessiva
over'simplify *v/t* ⟨*pret & pp* **oversimplified**⟩ simplificar demais
over'sleep *v/i* ⟨*pret & pp* **overslept**⟩ dormir demasiadamente
over'state *v/t* exagerar
over'statement exagero *m*
over'step *v/t* ⟨*pret & pp* **overstepped**⟩) *fig* **~ the mark** ultrapassar os limites
over'take *v/t* ⟨*pret* **overtook**, *pp* **over-**

O

taken⟩ *in work*, *development* alcançar; *Brit* MOT ultrapassar
over'throw[1] *v/t* ⟨*pret* ***overthrew***, *pp* ***overthrown***⟩ derrubar
'overthrow[2] *n* deposição *f*
'overtime horas *fpl* extras; *Am* SPORT prorrogação *f*; ***do ~*** fazer horas extras
'overture ['oʊvərtʃʊr] MUS abertura *f*; ***make ~s to*** *fig* estabelecer contatos com
over'turn 1 *v/t vehicle* capotar; *object*, *government* derrubar **2** *v/i vehicle* capotar
'overview visão *f* geral
over'weight *adj* obeso
over'whelm [oʊvər'welm] *v/t with work* sobrecarregar; *with emotion* comover; ***be ~ed by*** *by response* ficar muito comovido com
overwhelming [oʊvər'welmɪŋ] *adj feeling* arrebatador; *majority* devastador
over'work 1 *n* excesso *m* de trabalho **2** *v/i* trabalhar demais **3** *v/t* fazer trabalhar duro
owe [oʊ] *v/t* dever; ***~ s.o. $500*** dever a alguém 500 dólares; ***~ s.o. an apology*** dever desculpas a alguém; ***how much do I ~ you?*** quanto estou devendo a você?
owing to ['oʊɪŋ] *prep* devido a
owl [aʊl] coruja *f*
own[1] [oʊn] *v/t* possuir
own[2] [oʊn] **1** *adj* próprio **2** *pron* ***a car / an apartment of my ~*** meu carro / apartamento próprio; ***on my ~*** sozinho,-a
◆**own up** *v/i* confessar
owner ['oʊnər] dono,-a *m,f*, proprietário,-a *m,f*
ownership ['oʊnərʃɪp] posse *f*
ox [ɑːks] boi *m*
oxide ['ɑːksaɪd] óxido *m*
oxygen ['ɑːksɪdʒən] oxigênio *m*
oyster ['ɔɪstər] ostra *f*
oz *abbr* (*of* ***ounce***)
ozone ['oʊzoʊn] ozônio *m*
'ozone layer camada *f* de ozônio

P

p [piː] *abbr Brit* (*of* ***penny, pence***)
PA [piː'eɪ] *abbr* (*of* ***personal assistant***) secretário,-a *m,f* particular
pace [peɪs] **1** *n* (*step*) passo *m*; (*speed*) ritmo *m* **2** *v/i* ***~ up and down*** andar de um lado para o outro
'pacemaker MED marcapasso *m*; SPORT marcador *m* de ritmo de passadas
Pacific [pə'sɪfɪk] *n* ***the ~*** (***Ocean***) o oceano Pacífico
pacifier ['pæsɪfaɪər] *Am* chupeta *f*
pacifism ['pæsɪfɪzm] pacifismo *m*
pacifist ['pæsɪfɪst] *n* pacifista *m/f*
pacify ['pæsɪfaɪ] *v/t* ⟨*pret & pp* ***pacified***⟩ acalmar
pack [pæk] **1** *n cereal*, *food*: pacote *m*; (*backpack*) mochila *f*; *cigarettes*: maço *m*; *Brit cards*: baralho *m* **2** *v/t* (*put in bag*) pôr na mala; *goods*, *groceries* empacotar **3** *v/i* fazer a mala
package ['pækɪdʒ] **1** *n* (*parcel*), *offers etc*: pacote *m* **2** *v/t* empacotar, embalar; *for promotion* apresentar
'package deal *for vacation* pacote *m* de viagem
'package tour viagem *f* com pacote (de turismo)
packaging ['pækɪdʒɪŋ] *product*: embalagens *fpl*; *rock star etc*: apresentação *f*
packed [pækt] *adj* (*crowded*) lotado
packet ['pækɪt] pacote *m*
pact [pækt] pacto *m*
pad[1] *n writing*: bloco *m*
pad[2] *v/i* (*move quietly*) caminhar silenciosamente
◆**pad out** *v/t speech*, *report* extender

padded ['pædɪd] *adj jacket* acolchoado; *shoulders* com ombreira
padding ['pædɪŋ] *material* acolchoamento *m*; *in speech etc* enchimentos *mpl*
paddle[1] ['pædəl] **1** *n canoe*: remo *m*; *Am table tennis*: raquete *f* **2** *v/i in canoe, water* remar
paddock ['pædək] paddock *m*
padlock ['pædlɑːk] **1** *n* cadeado *m* **2** *v/t gate* trancar (com cadeado); **~ *X to Y*** trancar X com cadeado em Y
paediatric *Brit* → ***pediatric***
page[1] [peɪdʒ] *n book etc*: página *f*; **~ *number*** número *m* da página
page[2] [peɪdʒ] *v/t* (*call*) chamar
pager ['peɪdʒər] beeper *m*
paid [peɪd] *pret & pp* → ***pay***
paid em'ployment emprego *m* remunerado
pail [peɪl] balde *m*
pain [peɪn] dor *f*; ***be in ~*** estar com dor; ***take ~s to …*** fazer muitos esforços para …; ***a ~ in the neck*** *fam* um pé no saco, *Port* chato como o caraças
painful ['peɪnfʊl] *adj arm, leg etc* dolorido; (*distressing*) doloroso; (*laborious*) difícil
painfully ['peɪnflɪ] *adv* (*extremely, acutely*) extremamente
'painkiller analgésico *m*
painless ['peɪnlɪs] *adj* indolor
painstaking ['peɪnzteɪkɪŋ] *adj* meticuloso
paint [peɪnt] **1** *n* pintura *f* **2** *v/t & v/i* pintar
'paintbrush *wall, ceiling etc*: broxa *f*; *artist*: pincel *m*
painter ['peɪntər] pintor,a *m,f*
painting ['peɪntɪŋ] *activity, picture* pintura *f*
'paintwork pintura *f*
pair [per] par *m*; ***a ~ of shoes / sandals*** um par de sapatos / sandálias
pajama 'jacket camisa *f* do pijama
pajama 'pants calça *f* do pijama
pajamas [pə'dʒɑːməz] *npl* pijama *m*
Pakistan [pækɪ'stɑːn] Paquistão *m*
Pakistani [pækɪ'stɑːnɪ] **1** *adj* paquistanês,-esa **2** *n* paquistanês,-esa *m,f*
pal [pæl] *fam* amigo,-a *m,f*; ***hey ~, got a light?*** o amigo tem fogo?
palace ['pælɪs] palácio *m*
palate ['pælət] paladar *m*
palatial [pə'leɪʃl] *adj* suntuoso
pale [peɪl] *adj* pálido; **~ *pink / blue*** rosa / azul claro
Palestine ['pæləstaɪn] Palestina *f*
Palestinian [pælə'stɪnɪən] **1** *adj* palestino **2** *n* palestino,-a *m,f*
pallet ['pælɪt] palete *m*
pallor ['pælər] palidez *f*
palm[1] [pɑːm] *of hand* palma *f*
palm[2] [pɑːm] *tree* palmeira *f*
palpitations [pælpɪ'teɪʃnz] *npl* MED palpitações *fpl*
paltry ['pɔːltrɪ] *adj* miserável
pamper ['pæmpər] *v/t* mimar
pamphlet ['pæmflɪt] panfleto *m*
pan [pæn] **1** *n cooking*: panela *f*; *frying*: frigideira *f* **2** *v/t* ⟨*pret & pp* ***panned***⟩ *fam* (*criticize*) devastar
◆**pan out** *v/i* (*develop*) sair
Panama ['pænəmɑː] ***the ~ Canal*** o canal do Panamá
'pancake panqueca *f*
panda ['pændə] panda *m*
pandemonium [pændɪ'moʊnɪəm] pandemônio *m*
◆**pander to** ['pændər] *v/t* comprazer a
pane [peɪn] *glass*: folha *f*
panel ['pænl] *section* painel *m*; ***a ~ of experts*** uma comissão de especialistas
paneling ['pænəlɪŋ] painéis *mpl*
panelling *Brit* → ***paneling***
pang [pæŋ] *n* ***~ of remorse*** forte remorso *m*; ***~s of hunger*** a fome de contorcer
'panhandle *v/i fam* mendigar
panic ['pænɪk] **1** *n* pânico *m* **2** *v/i* ⟨*pret & pp* ***panicked***⟩ entrar em pânico; ***don't ~*** sem pânico
'panic buying FIN compra *f* motivada por pânico **'panic selling** FIN venda *f* motivada por pânico **'panic-stricken** *adj* apavorado
panorama [pænə'rɑːmə] panorama *m*
panoramic [pænə'ræmɪk] *adj view* panorâmico
pansy ['pænzɪ] *flower* amor-perfeito *m*
pant [pænt] *v/i* ofegar

P

panties ['pæntɪz] calcinhas *fpl*, *Port* cuecas *fpl*
pantihose, **pantyhose** meia-calça *f*, *Port* collants *mpl*
pants [pænts] *Am* calça *f*, *Port* calças *fpl*; *Brit* (*underpants*) calcinha *f*
pantyhose ['pæntɪhoʊz] meia-calça *f*, *Port* collants *mpl*
papal ['peɪpəl] *adj* papal
paparazzi ['pæpərætsiː] paparazzi *mpl*
paper ['peɪpər] **1** *n* papel *m*; (*newspaper*) jornal *m*; ***academic ~*** estudo *m*; ***examination ~*** exame *m*; ***~s*** *pl* (*documents*) documentos *mpl*; ***a piece of ~*** um pedaço de papel **2** *adj* de papel **3** *v/t room*, *walls* revestir com papel de parede
'paperback brochura *f* **paper 'bag** sacola *f* de papel **'paper boy** entregador *m* de jornais **'paper clip** clipe *m* **'paper cup** copo *m* de papel **'paperwork** papelada *f*
par [pɑːr] *in golf* par *m*; ***be on a ~ with*** ser comparável a; ***feel below ~*** não sentir-se bem
parachute ['pærəʃuːt] **1** *n* pára-quedas *m* **2** *v/i* saltar de pára-quedas **3** *v/t troops*, *supplies* lançar em pára-quedas
parachutist ['pærəʃuːtɪst] pára-quedista *m/f*
parade [pə'reɪd] **1** *n* (*procession*) parada *f* **2** *v/i* desfilar **3** *v/t knowledge*, *new car* exibir
paradise ['pærədaɪs] paraíso *m*
paradox ['pærədɑːks] paradoxo *m*
paradoxical [pærə'dɑːksɪkl] *adj* paradoxal
paradoxically [pærə'dɑːksɪklɪ] *adv* paradoxalmente
paragraph ['pærəgræf] parágrafo *m*
Paraguay ['pærəgwaɪ] Paraguai
Paraguayan [pærə'gwaɪən] **1** *adj* paraguaio **2** *n* paraguaio,-a *m,f*
parallel ['pærəlel] **1** *n geometry*: paralela *f*; GEOG, *also fig* paralelo *m*; ***do two things in ~*** fazer duas coisas ao mesmo tempo **2** *adj* paralelo; ***~ bars*** paralela *f* **3** *v/t* (*match*) igualar
paralyse *Brit* → ***paralyze***
paralysis [pə'ræləsɪs] paralisia *f*, *fig* paralização *f*
paralyze ['pærəlaɪz] *v/i also fig* paralizar
paramedic [pærə'medɪk] *n* paramédico,-a *m,f*
parameter [pə'ræmɪtər] parâmetro *m*
paramilitary [pærə'mɪlɪterɪ] **1** *adj* paramilitar **2** *n* paramilitar *m/f*
paramount ['pærəmaʊnt] *adj* mais importante; ***be of ~ importance*** ser de suma importância
paranoia [pærə'nɔɪə] paranóia *f*
paranoid ['pærənɔɪd] *adj* paranóico
paraphernalia [pærəfə'neɪlɪə] parafernália *f*
paraphrase ['pærəfreɪz] *v/t* parafrasear
paraplegic [pærə'pliːdʒɪk] *n* paraplégico,-a *m,f*
parasite ['pærəsaɪt] *also fig* parasita *m/f*
parasol ['pærəsɑːl] pára-sol *m*
paratrooper ['pærətruːpər] pára-quedista *m/f* (militar)
parcel ['pɑːrsl] *n* pacote *m*
♦ **parcel up** *v/t* empacotar
parch [pɑːrtʃ] *v/t* secar; ***be ~ed*** *person* estar morto de sede
pardon ['pɑːrdn] **1** *n* LAW absolvição *f*; ***I beg your ~?*** (*what did you say*) como, por favor?; (*I'm sorry*) perdão **2** *v/t* perdoar; LAW absolver; ***~ me?*** *Am* como, por favor?
pare [per] *v/t* (*peel*) descascar
parent ['perənt] *n* ***my ~s*** meus pais; ***as a ~ I...*** como pai / mãe eu …
parental [pə'rentl] *adj* dos pais
'parent company empresa *f* matriz
parent-'teacher association associação *f* de pais e mestres
parish ['pærɪʃ] paróquia *f*
park[1] [pɑːrk] *area* parque *m*
park[2] [pɑːrk] *v/t & v/i* MOT estacionar
parka ['pɑːrkə] parka *f*
parking ['pɑːrkɪŋ] MOT estacionamento *m*; ***no ~*** proibido estacionar
'parking brake freio *m* de mão, *Port* travão *m* de mão **'parking disc** bloco *m* de zona azul **'parking garage** *Am* estacionamento *m* fechado **'parking lot** *Am* estacionamento *m* **'parking meter** parquímetro *m*

P

'parking place vaga *f* (para estacionar) **'parking ticket** multa *f* de estacionamento
parliament ['pɑːrləmənt] parlamento *m*
parliamentary [pɑːrlə'mentərɪ] *adj* parlamentário
parole [pə'roʊl] **1** *n* liberdade *f* condicional; ***be on ~*** estar sob liberdade condicional **2** *v/t prisoner* pôr em liberdade condicional
parrot ['pærət] *n* papagaio *m*
parsley ['pɑːrslɪ] salsinha *f*
part [pɑːrt] **1** *n* (*portion, area*) parte *f*; (*section*) episódio *m*; *in play, movie* papel *m*; MUS voz *f*; *Am* (*in hair*) risca *f*; ***take ~ in*** participar de **2** *adv* (*partly*) em parte **3** *v/i* separar-se **4** *v/t* ***~ one's hair*** dividir o cabelo
◆**part with** *v/t* abrir mão de
part ex'change *n* ***take sth in ~*** levar algo como parte do pagamento
partial ['pɑːrʃl] *adj* (*incomplete*) parcial; ***be ~ to*** gostar de
partially ['pɑːrʃəlɪ] *adv* parcialmente
participant [pɑːr'tɪsɪpənt] participante *m/f*
participate [pɑːr'tɪsɪpeɪt] *v/i* participar; ***~ in sth*** participar de algo
participation [pɑːrtɪsɪ'peɪʃn] participação *f*
participle [pɑːr'tɪsɪpl] GRAM particípio *m*
particle ['pɑːrtɪkl] PHYS partícula *f*; (*small amount*) pingo *m*
particular [pər'tɪkjələr] *adj* (*specific*) específico; (*special*) especial; (*fussy*) sistemático; ***in ~*** em particular
particularly [pər'tɪkjələrlɪ] *adv* particularmente
parting ['pɑːrtɪŋ] *people*: separação *f*; *Brit hair*: risca *f*
partition [pɑːr'tɪʃn] **1** *n* (*screen*) biombo *m*; *of country* divisão *f* **2** *v/t country* dividir
◆**partition off** *v/t* separar
partly ['pɑːrtlɪ] *adv* em parte
partner ['pɑːrtnər] COM sócio,-a *m,f*; *relationship, particular activity*: parceiro,-a *m,f*
partnership ['pɑːrtnərʃɪp] COM sociedade *f*; *in particular activity* colaboração *f*
part of 'speech classe *f* gramatical
'part owner sócio,-a proprietário,-a *m,f* **'part-time 1** *adj job, worker* de meio período **2** *adv work* de meio período **part-'timer** trabalhador,a *m,f* de meio período
party ['pɑːrtɪ] **1** *n* (*celebration*) festa *f*; POL partido *m*; (*group of people*) grupo *m*; ***be a ~ to*** tomar parte em **2** *v/i* ⟨*pret & pp* ***partied***⟩ *fam* festejar
pass [pæs] **1** *n for getting into a place* passagem *f*; SPORT passe *m*; *mountains*: desfiladeiro *m*; ***make a ~ at*** dar uma cantada em **2** *v/t* (*hand*), SPORT passar; (*go past*) passar por; (*overtake, go beyond*) ultrapassar; (*approve*) aprovar; ***~ an exam*** passar num exame; ***~ sentence*** LAW promulgar uma sentença; ***~ the time*** passar o tempo **3** *v/i time, in exam*, SPORT, (*go away*) passar
◆**pass around** *v/t* distribuir
◆**pass away** *v/i euph* falecer
◆**pass by 1** *v/t* (*go past*) passar por **2** *v/i* (*go past*) passar
◆**pass on 1** *v/t information, book, costs, savings* passar **2** *v/i euph* (*die*) ir-se
◆**pass out** *v/i* (*faint*) desmaiar
◆**pass through** *v/t town* passar por
◆**pass up** *v/t opportunity* deixar passar
passable ['pæsəbl] *adj road* transitável; (*acceptable*) aceitável
passage ['pæsɪdʒ] (*corridor*) corredor *m*; *poem, book*: passagem *f*; *time*: passar *m*
'passageway passagem *f*
passenger ['pæsɪndʒər] passageiro,-a *m,f*
'passenger seat banco *m* de passageiro
passer-by [pæsər'baɪ] ⟨*pl* ***passers-by***⟩ transeunte *m*
passion ['pæʃn] paixão *f*
passionate ['pæʃnət] *adj lover* apaixonado; (*fervent*) fervoroso
passive ['pæsɪv] **1** *adj* passivo **2** *n* GRAM (voz *f*) passiva *f*; ***in the ~*** na passiva
passive 'smoking fumo *m* passivo

P

'pass mark EDUC nota *f* mínima para ser aprovado **'Passover** REL páscoa *f* judaica **'passport** passaporte *m* **'passport control** controle *m* de passaportes **'password** senha *f*

past [pæst] **1** *adj (former)* passado; ***the ~ few days*** os últimos dias; ***that's all ~ now*** isto tudo são águas passadas **2** *n* passado *m*; ***in the ~*** no passado **3** *prep in position* depois de; ***it's ~ your bedtime*** já passou da hora de você ir para a cama; ***it's half ~ two*** são duas e meia; ***she walked right ~ me*** ela passou bem en frente a mim **4** *adv* ***run / walk ~*** passar

pasta ['pæstə] macarrão *m*

paste [peɪst] **1** *n (adhesive)* cola *f* **2** *v/t (stick)* colar

pastel ['pæstl] **1** *n color* tom *m* pastel **2** *adj* pastel

pastime ['pæstaɪm] passatempo *m*

past par'ticiple GRAM particípio *m* passado

pastrami [pæ'strɑːmɪ] carne *f* defumada

pastry ['peɪstrɪ] *for pie* massa *f*; *(small cake)* tortinha *f*

'past tense GRAM passado *m*

pasty ['peɪstɪ] *adj complexion* pálido

pat [pæt] **1** *n* tapinha *m*; ***give s.o. a ~ on the back*** *fig* dar um tapinha nas costas de alguém **2** *v/t ⟨pret & pp **patted**⟩* dar uma palmadinha

patch [pætʃ] **1** *n on clothing* remendo *m*; *(period of time)* fase *f*; *(area)* área *f*; ***be not a ~ on*** *fig* não chegar aos pés de **2** *v/t clothing* remendar

◆ **patch up** *v/t (repair temporarily)* consertar provisoriamente; ***patch up a quarrel*** fazer as pazes

'patchwork 1 *n needlework* patchwork *m* **2** *adj* **~ *quilt*** colcha *f* de patchwork

patchy ['pætʃɪ] *adj quality* desigual; *work, performance* irregular

pâté [pɑː'teɪ] patê *m*

patent ['peɪtnt] **1** *adj* evidente **2** *n for invention* patente *f* **3** *v/t invention* patentear

'patent leather couro *m* envernizado

patently ['peɪtntlɪ] *adv (clearly)* evidentemente

paternal [pə'tɜːrnl] *adj relative, pride, love* paternal

paternalism [pə'tɜːrnlɪzm] paternalismo *m*

paternalistic [pətɜːrnl'ɪstɪk] *adj* paternalista

paternity [pə'tɜːrnɪtɪ] paternidade *f*

pa'ternity leave licença *f* de paternidade

path [pæθ] *also fig* caminho *m*

pathetic [pə'θetɪk] *adj (invoking pity)* patético; *fam (very bad)* lamentável

pathological [pæθə'lɑːdʒɪkl] *adj behavior, liar* patológico

pathologist [pə'θɑːlədʒɪst] patologista *m/f*

pathology [pə'θɑːlədʒɪ] *of a disease* nosografia *f*, *department* patologia *f*

patience ['peɪʃns] paciência *f*, ***she has the ~ of a saint*** ela tem uma paciência de santo

patient ['peɪʃnt] **1** *n* paciente *m/f* **2** *adj* paciente; ***just be ~!*** seja paciente!

patiently ['peɪʃntlɪ] *adv* pacientemente

patio ['pætɪoʊ] patio *m*

patriot ['peɪtrɪət] patriota *m/f*

patriotic [peɪtrɪ'ɑːtɪk] *adj* patriótico

patriotism ['peɪtrɪətɪzm] patriotismo *m*

patrol [pə'troʊl] **1** *n* patrulha *f*, ***be on ~*** rondar em patrulha **2** *v/t ⟨pret & pp **patrolled**⟩ streets, border* patrulhar

pa'trol car carro *m* de patrulha **pa'trolman** *Am* guarda *m* **pa'trol wagon** *Am* furgão *m* de polícia

patron ['peɪtrən] *store, movie theater*: cliente *m*; *artist, charity etc*: mecenas *m*

patronage ['peɪtrənɪdʒ] *store, movie theater*: patrocínio *m*; *artist, charity etc*: apoio *m*

patronize ['pætrənaɪz] *v/t shop* ser cliente de; *person* tratar com condescendência

patronizing ['pætrənaɪzɪŋ] *adj* condescendente

patron 'saint santo,-a *m,f* padroeiro,-a

patter ['pætər] **1** *n rain etc*: tamborilar *m*; *fam salesman*: tagarelice *f* **2** *v/i*

tamborilar
pattern ['pætərn] *n wallpaper, fabric*: estampa *f*; (*model*) *also for knitting, sewing*: modelo *m*; *behavior, events*: pauta *f*
patterned ['pætərnd] *adj* estampado
paunch [pɒːntʃ] barriga *f*
pause [pɒːz] **1** *n* pausa *f* **2** *v/i* fazer uma pausa **3** *v/t tape* pôr na pausa
pave [peɪv] *v/t* pavimentar; **~ *the way for*** *fig* preparar o terreno para
pavement ['peɪvmənt] *Am* (*roadway*) calçamento *m*; *Brit* (*sidewalk*) calçada *f*, *Port* passeio *m*
'pavement café *Brit* café *m* com mesas na calçada, *Port* esplanada *f*
paving stone ['peɪvɪŋ] pedra *f* de calçamento
paw [pɒː] **1** *n animal*: pata *f*; ***keep your ~s off that cake*** *fam* tire suas patas do bolo **2** *v/t fam* apalpar
pawn [pɒːn] **1** *n in chess* peão *m*; *fig* peça *f* de xadrez **2** *v/t* empenhorar
'pawnbroker penhorista *m/f*
'pawnshop casa *f* de penhores
pay [peɪ] **1** *n* pagamento *m*; *salary* salário *m*; ***in the ~ of*** pago por **2** *v/t* ⟨*pret & pp* **paid**⟩ *employee, sum, bill* pagar; **~ *attention*** prestar atenção; **~ *s.o. a compliment*** fazer um cumprimento a alguém **3** *v/i* ⟨*pret & pp* **paid**⟩ pagar; (*be profitable*) ser rentável; ***it doesn't ~ to ...*** não vale a pena ...; **~ *for*** *purchase* pagar; ***you'll ~ for this!*** *fig* você vai pagar por isto!
◆**pay back** *v/t person* devolver o dinheiro; *loan* reembolsar; (*get revenge on*) vingar-se de
◆**pay in** *v/t to bank* depositar
◆**pay off** **1** *v/t debt* saldar; *corrupt official* subornar **2** *v/i* (*be profitable*) valer a pena
◆**pay up** *v/i* pagar
payable ['peɪəbl] *adj* pagável
'pay check *Am* cheque *m* de pagamento
'payday dia *m* de pagamento
payee [peɪ'iː] beneficiário,-a *m,f*
'pay envelope *Am* envelope *m* de pagamento
payer ['peɪr] pagador *m*; ***they're good ~s*** eles são pagadores assíduos
payment ['peɪmənt] pagamento *m*
pay-per-'view pay-per-view *m* **'pay phone** telefone *m* público **'payroll** salários *mpl*; ***be on the ~*** estar na folha de pagamento **'payslip** *Brit* contracheque *m*
PC[1] [piː'siː] *abbr* (*of* ***personal computer***) PC *m*
PC[2] [piː'siː] *abbr* (*of* ***politically correct***) *adj* politicamente correto
PDA [piːdɪ'eɪ] *abbr* (*of* ***personal digital assistant***) palmtop *m*
pea [piː] ervilha *f*
peace [piːs] paz *f*, (*quietness*) tranqüilidade *f*
peaceable ['piːsəbl] *adj person* pacífico
'Peace Corps *Am* corpo *m* da paz
peaceful ['piːsfʊl] *adj* tranqüilo
peacefully ['piːsflɪ] *adv* tranqüilamente
peach [piːtʃ] pêssego *m*
'peacock pavão *m*
peak [piːk] **1** *n mountain*: cume *m*; *mountain itself* pico *m*; *fig* ponto *m* culminante **2** *v/i* chegar ao máximo
'peak consumption consumo *m* (de energia) no horário de pico
'peak hours *npl* horário *m* de pico
'peanut amendoim *m*; ***get paid ~s*** *fam* ganhar uma miséria; ***that's ~s to him*** *fam* isto é uma ninharia para ele
peanut 'butter pasta *f* de amendoim
pear [per] pêra *f*
pearl [pɜːrl] pérola *f*
peasant ['peznt] camponês,-esa *m,f*
pebble ['pebl] seixo *m*
pecan ['piːkən] noz *f* pecan
peck [pek] **1** *n* (*bite*) bicada *f*, (*kiss*) beijinho *m* **2** *v/t* (*bite*) bicar; (*kiss*) dar um beijinho
peculiar [pɪ'kjuːljər] *adj* (*strange*) peculiar; **~ *to*** característico de
peculiarity [pɪkjuːlɪ'ærətɪ] (*strangeness*) peculiaridade *f*, (*special feature*) característica *f*
pedal ['pedl] **1** *n* pedal *m* **2** *v/i* pedalar
pedantic [pɪ'dæntɪk] *adj* pedante
peddle ['pedl] *v/t drugs* traficar

pedestal ['pedəstl] pedestal *m*
pedestrian [pɪ'destrɪən] *n* pedestre *m/f*, *Port* peão *m*
pedestrian 'crossing *Brit* travessia *f* de pedestres, *Port* passadeira *f*
pediatric [piːdɪ'ætrɪk] *adj* pediátrico
pediatrician [piːdɪæ'trɪʃn] pediatra *m/f*
pediatrics [piːdɪ'ætrɪks] pediatria *f*
pedicure ['pedɪkjʊr] pedicure *f*
pedigree ['pedɪgriː] **1** *n* pedigree *m* **2** *adj* com pedigree
pee [piː] *v/i fam* fazer xixi
peek [piːk] **1** *n* olhadinha *f* **2** *v/i* dar uma olhadinha
peel [piːl] **1** *n* casca *f* **2** *v/t fruit, vegetables* descascar **3** *v/i nose, shoulders, paint* descascar-se
♦ **peel off** *v/t wrapper, jacket etc* tirar
peep [piːp] → ***peek***
'peephole olho *m* mágico
peer[1] [pɪr] *n* (*equal*) igual *m/f*; *in age* coetâneo,-a *m,f*
peer[2] [pɪr] *v/i* ~ ***through the mist*** tentar ver através da neblina; ~ ***at*** tentar ver
peeved [piːvd] *adj fam* irritado
peg [peg] *n hat, coat*: gancho *m*; *Brit tent*: estaca *f*; ***off the ~ clothing*** confecção *f*
pejorative [pɪ'dʒɑːrətɪv] *adj* pejorativo
pellet ['pelɪt] bolinha *f*; (*bullet*) chumbo *m*
pelt [pelt] **1** *v/t* ~ ***s.o. with sth*** atirar algo em alguém **2** *v/i* ***they ~ed along the road*** *fam* eles correram pela estrada; ***it's ~ing down*** *fam* está jorrando água
pelvis ['pelvɪs] pélvis *f*
pen[1] [pen] *n ballpoint pen* caneta *f* esferográfica; *fountain pen* caneta-tinteiro *f*
pen[2] [pen] *n* (*enclosure*) curral *m*
penalize ['piːnəlaɪz] *v/t* penalizar
penalty ['penltɪ] penalidade *f*; SPORT pênalti *m*; ***take the ~*** bater o pênalti
'penalty area SPORT área *f* de pênalti
'penalty clause LAW cláusula *f* de penalidades **'penalty kick** chute *m* do pênalti **penalty 'shoot-out** decisão *f* por pênalti **'penalty spot** marca *f* do pênalti
pencil ['pensɪl] lápis *m*
'pencil sharpener ['ʃɑːrpnər] apontador *m* de lápis, *Port* apara-lápis *m*
pendant ['pendənt] *necklace* pingente *m*
pending ['pendɪŋ] **1** *prep* até **2** *adj* ***be ~*** *awaiting a decision* estar pendente; *about to happen* estar iminente
penetrate ['penɪtreɪt] *v/t* penetrar; *market* entrar em
penetrating ['penɪtreɪtɪŋ] *adj stare, scream* penetrante; *analysis* minucioso
penetration [penɪ'treɪʃn] penetração *f*, *of market* infiltração *f*
'pen friend amigo,-a *m,f* de correspondência
penguin ['peŋgwɪn] pingüim *m*
penicillin [penɪ'sɪlɪn] penicilina *f*
peninsula [pə'nɪnsʊlə] península *f*
penis ['piːnɪs] pênis *m*
penitence ['penɪtəns] arrependimento *m*
penitent ['penɪtənt] *adj* arrependido
penitentiary [penɪ'tenʃərɪ] penitenciária *f*
'penknife *Brit* canivete *m*
'pen name pseudônimo *m*
pennant ['penənt] bandeirinha *f*
penniless ['penɪlɪs] *adj* sem um centavo
penny ['penɪ] pêni *m*
'pen pal amigo,-a *m,f* por correspondência
pension ['penʃn] pensão *f*
♦ **pension off** *v/t* aposentar
'pension fund fundo *m* de aposentadoria
'pension scheme plano *m* de aposentadoria
pensive ['pensɪv] *adj* pensativo
Pentagon ['pentəgɑːn] *n* ***the ~*** o Pentágono
pentathlon [pen'tæθlən] pentatlo *m*
Pentecost ['pentɪkɑːst] pentecostes *m*
penthouse ['penthaʊs] cobertura *f*
pent-up ['pentʌp] *adj* reprimido
penultimate [pe'nʌltɪmət] *adj* penúltimo

people ['piːpl] pessoas *fpl*; (*race, tribe*) povo *m*; ***there were a lot of ~ there*** havia muita gente lá; ***the American ~*** o povo americano; ***~ say ...*** estão dizendo que ...
pepper ['pepər] *spice* pimenta *f*, *vegetable* pimentão *m*
peppermint 1 *n sweet* bala *f* hortelã **2** *adj flavoring* de hortelã
pep talk ['peptɔːk] *n* conversa *f* de encorajamento
per [pɜːr] *prep* por; ***~ annum*** por ano
perceive [pər'siːv] *v/t with senses* perceber; (*view, interpret*) entender
percent [pər'sent] *adv* por cento
percentage [pər'sentɪdʒ] porcentagem *f*
perceptible [pər'septəbl] *adj* perceptível
perceptibly [pər'septəblɪ] *adv* visivelmente
perception [pər'sepʃn] *through senses, of situation* percepção *f*; (*insight*) perspicácia *f*
perceptive [pər'septɪv] *adj person, remark* perceptivo
perch [pɜːrtʃ] **1** *n for bird* poleiro *m* **2** *v/i bird* empoleirar-se; *person* sentar-se
percolate ['pɜːrkəleɪt] *v/i coffee* coar
percolator ['pɜːrkəleɪtər] cafeteira *f*
percussion [pər'kʌʃn] percussão *f*
per'cussion instrument instrumento *m* de percussão
perennial [pə'renɪəl] *n* BOT planta *f* perene
perfect ['pɜːrfɪkt] **1** *n* GRAM pretérito *m* perfeito **2** *adj* perfeito **3** [pər'fekt] *v/t* aperfeiçoar
perfection [pər'fekʃn] perfeição *f*; ***to ~*** à perfeição
perfectionist [pər'fekʃnɪst] perfeccionista *m/f*
perfectly ['pɜːrfɪktlɪ] *adv* perfeitamente; (*totally*) totalmente
perforated ['pɜːrfəreɪtɪd] *adj line* perfurado
perforations [pɜːrfə'reɪʃnz] *npl* perfurações *fpl*
perform [pər'fɔːrm] **1** *v/t* (*carry out*) realizar; *actor, musician etc* interpretar **2** *v/i actor, musician, dancer* atuar; *machine* funcionar
performance [pər'fɔːrməns] *actor, musician etc*: interpretação *f*, *employee, company etc*: atuação *f*, *machine*: funcionamento *m*; ***next ~: 7:30*** próximo show: 7:30
per'formance car carro *m* de alta potência
performer [pər'fɔːrmər] *musician, actor etc* artista *m/f*
perfume ['pɜːrfjuːm] perfume *m*
perfunctory [pər'fʌŋktərɪ] *adj* superficial
perhaps [pər'hæps] *adv* talvez
peril ['perəl] perigo *m*
perilous ['perələs] *adj* perigoso
perimeter [pə'rɪmɪtər] perímetro *m*
pe'rimeter fence cerca *f*
period ['pɪrɪəd] (*time*) período *m*; (*menstruation*) regras *fpl*; *punctuation*: ponto *m* final; ***I don't want to, ~!*** Am não quero e ponto final!
periodic [pɪrɪ'ɑːdɪk] *adj* periódico
periodical [pɪrɪ'ɑːdɪkl] *n* revista *f*
periodically [pɪrɪ'ɑːdɪklɪ] *adv* periodicamente
peripheral [pə'rɪfərəl] **1** *adj* (*not crucial*) secundário **2** *n* COMPUT periférico *m*
periphery [pə'rɪfərɪ] periferia *f*
perish ['perɪʃ] *v/i rubber* estragar; *person* falecer
perishable ['perɪʃəbl] *adj food* perecível
perjure ['pɜːrdʒər] *v/t* ***~ oneself*** perjurar
perjury ['pɜːrdʒərɪ] perjúrio *m*
perk [pɜːrk] *fam of job* vantagem *f*
♦ **perk up 1** *v/t* animar **2** *v/i* animar-se
perky ['pɜːrkɪ] *adj* (*cheerful*) animado
perm [pɜːrm] *n* permanente *f*
permanent ['pɜːrmənənt] *adj* permanente
permanently ['pɜːrmənəntlɪ] *adv* permanentemente
permeable ['pɜːrmɪəbl] *adj* permeável
permeate ['pɜːrmɪeɪt] *v/t* impregnar
permissible [pər'mɪsəbl] *adj* permissível
permission [pər'mɪʃn] permissão *f*
permissive [pər'mɪsɪv] *adj* permissivo

permissive so'ciety sociedade *f* permissiva
permit **1** ['pɜːrmɪt] *n* licença *f* **2** [pər'mɪt] *v/t* ⟨*pret & pp* ***permitted***⟩ ***I won't ~ it!*** não vou permitir isso!; ***~ s.o. to do sth*** dar permissão a alguém de fazer algo
perpendicular [pɜːrpən'dɪkjʊlər] *adj* perpendicular
perpetual [pər'petʃʊəl] *adj* eterno
perpetually [pər'petʃʊəlɪ] *adv* constantemente
perpetuate [pər'petjuːeɪt] *v/t* perpetuar
perplex [pər'pleks] *v/t* deixar perplexo
perplexed [pər'plekst] *adj* perplexo
perplexity [pər'pleksɪtɪ] perplexidade *f*
persecute ['pɜːrsɪkjuːt] *v/t* perseguir
persecution [pɜːrsɪ'kjuːʃn] perseguição *f*
persecutor [pɜːrsɪ'kjuːtər] perseguidor,a *m,f*
perseverance [pɜːrsɪ'vɪrəns] perseverança *f*
persevere [pɜːrsɪ'vɪr] *v/i* perseverar
persist [pər'sɪst] *v/i* persistir; ***~ in*** persistir em
persistence [pər'sɪstəns] persistência *f*
persistent [pər'sɪstənt] *adj* persistente
persistently [pər'sɪstəntlɪ] *adv* (*continually*) constantemente
person ['pɜːrsn] pessoa *f*; ***in ~*** em pessoa
personal ['pɜːrsənl] *adj* pessoal; ***don't make ~ remarks*** não faça observações pessoais
'personal column coluna *f* pessoal
personal 'hygiene higiene *f* pessoal
personality [pɜːrsə'nælətɪ] *also* (*celebrity*) personalidade *f*
personally ['pɜːrsənəlɪ] *adv* pessoalmente; ***don't take it ~*** não leve isso para o lado pessoal
personal 'organizer organizador *m* pessoal **personal 'pronoun** pronome *m* pessoal **personal 'stereo** walkman *m*
personify [pɜːr'sɑːnɪfaɪ] *v/t* ⟨*pret & pp* ***personified***⟩ personificar
personnel [pɜːrsə'nel] pessoal *m*
person'nel manager diretor *m* do departamento pessoal
perspective [pər'spektɪv] perspectiva *f*; ***get sth into ~*** pôr algo em perspectiva
perspiration [pɜːrspɪ'reɪʃn] suor *m*
perspire [pɜːr'spaɪr] *v/i* perspirar
persuade [pər'sweɪd] *v/t person* persuadir; ***~ s.o. to do sth*** persuadir alguém a fazer algo
persuasion [pər'sweɪʒn] persuasão *f*
persuasive [pər'sweɪsɪv] *adj* persuasivo
pertinent ['pɜːrtɪnənt] *adj fml* pertinente
perturb [pər'tɜːrb] *v/t* preocupar
perturbing [pər'tɜːrbɪŋ] *adj* preocupante
peruse [pə'ruːz] *v/t fml* ler atentamente
Peru [pə'ruː] Peru *m*
Peruvian [pə'ruːviən] **1** *adj* peruano **2** *n* peruano,-a *m,f*
pervasive [pər'veɪsɪv] *adj influence, ideas* dominante
perverse [pər'vɜːrs] *adj* perverso; (*awkward*) malvado
perversion [pər'vɜːrʃn] *sexual* perversão *f*
pervert ['pɜːrvɜːrt] *n sexual* perverso,-a *m,f*
pessimism ['pesɪmɪzm] pessimismo *m*
pessimist ['pesɪmɪst] pessimista *m/f*
pessimistic [pesɪ'mɪstɪk] *adj* pessimista
pest [pest] praga *f*; *fam person* peste *m/f*
pester ['pestər] *v/t* aborrecer; ***~ s.o. to do sth*** amolar alguém para fazer algo
pesticide ['pestɪsaɪd] pesticida *m*
pet [pet] **1** *n animal* animal *m* de estimação; (*favorite*) favorito,-a *m,f* **2** *adj* favorito **3** *v/i* ⟨*pret & pp* ***petted***⟩ *couple* trocar carícias íntimas
petal ['petl] pétala *f*
♦ **peter out** ['piːtər] *v/i rebellion* dissolver-se lentamente; *rain* parar pouco a pouco; *path* desaparecer gradualmente

petite [pə'tiːt] *adj* delicado
petition [pə'tɪʃn] *n* petição *f*
'pet name apelido *m* carinhoso
petrified ['petrɪfaɪd] *adj person* petrificado; *scream, voice* aterrorizado
petrify ['petrɪfaɪ] *v/t* ⟨*pret & pp* ***petrified***⟩ deixar petrificado
petrochemical [petroʊ'kemɪkl] *adj* petroquímico
petrol ['petrl] *Brit* gasolina *f*
petroleum [pɪ'troʊlɪəm] petróleo *m*
petrol pump *Brit* → ***gas pump***
'petrol station *Brit* posto *m* de gasolina, *Port* bomba *f* de gasolina
petting ['petɪŋ] troca *f* de carícias íntimas
petty ['petɪ] *adj person, behavior* mesquinho; *details, problem* trivial
petty 'cash dinheiro *m* para pequenas despesas
petulant ['petʃələnt] *adj person, remark* petulante
pew [pjuː] banco *m* de igreja
pewter ['pjuːtər] peltre *m*
pharmaceutical [fɑːrmə'suːtɪkl] *adj* farmacêutico
pharmaceuticals [fɑːrmə'suːtɪklz] *npl products* produtos *mpl* farmacêuticos
pharmacist ['fɑːrməsɪst] *in store* farmacêutico,-a *m,f*
pharmacy ['fɑːrməsɪ] farmácia *f*
phase [feɪz] fase *f*
◆**phase in** *v/t* introduzir gradualmente
◆**phase out** *v/t* retirar gradualmente
PhD [piːeɪtʃ'diː] *abbr* (*of* ***Doctor of Philosophy***) doutorado *m*
phenomenal [fə'nɑːmɪnl] *adj* fenomenal
phenomenally [fə'nɑːmɪnəlɪ] *adv* extraordinariamente
phenomenon [fə'nɑːmɪnən] fenômeno *m*
philanthropic [fɪlən'θrɑːpɪk] *adj* filantrópico
philanthropist [fɪ'lænθrəpɪst] filantropo,-a *m,f*
philanthropy [fɪ'lænθrəpɪ] filantropia *f*
Philippines ['fɪlɪpiːnz] *npl* ***the ~*** as Filipinas
philistine ['fɪlɪstaɪn] *n* filisteu *m*, filistéia *f*
philosopher [fɪ'lɑːsəfər] filósofo,-a *m,f*
philosophical [fɪlə'sɑːɒfɪkl] *adj* filosófico
philosophy [fɪ'lɑːsəfɪ] filosofia *f*
phobia ['foubɪə] fobia *f*
phone [foʊn] **1** *n* telefone *m*; ***be on the ~*** *have one* ter um telefone; *be talking* estar ao telefone **2** *v/t* telefonar para; ***I'll ~ you*** eu ligo para você **3** *v/i* ligar (por telefone)
'phone book lista *f* telefônica **'phone booth** orelhão *m* **'phone box** *Brit* orelhão *m* **'phone call** chamada *f* telefônica **'phone card** cartão *m* telefônico **'phone number** número *m* do telefone
phonetics [fə'netɪks] fonética *f*
phony, phoney ['foʊnɪ] *adj fam* falso
photo ['foʊtoʊ] *n* foto *f*
'photo album álbum *m* de fotos **'photocopier** copiadora *f* **'photocopy 1** *n* fotocópia *f* **2** *v/t* ⟨*pret & pp* ***photocopied***⟩ fotocopiar
photogenic [foʊtoʊ'dʒenɪk] *adj* fotogênico
photograph ['foʊtəgræf] **1** *n* fotografia *f* **2** *v/t* fotografar
photographer [fə'tɑːgrəfər] fotógrafo,-a *m,f*
photography [fə'tɑːgrəfɪ] fotografia *f*
phrase [freɪz] **1** *n* frase *f* **2** *v/t* expressar
'phrasebook livro *m* de expressões idiomáticas
physical ['fɪzɪkl] **1** *adj* físico **2** *n* MED exame *m* médico
physical 'handicap deficiência *f* física
physically ['fɪzɪklɪ] *adv* fisicamente
physically 'handicapped ***be ~ handicapped*** ser fisicamente deficiente
physician [fɪ'zɪʃn] médico,-a *m,f*
physicist ['fɪzɪsɪst] físico,-a *m,f*
physics ['fɪzɪks] física *f*
physiotherapist [fɪzɪoʊ'θerəpɪst] fisioterapeuta *m/f*
physiotherapy [fɪzɪoʊ'θerəpɪ] fisioterapia *f*
physique [fɪ'ziːk] físico *m*

P

pianist ['pɪənɪst] pianista *m/f*
piano [pɪ'ænoʊ] piano *m*
pick [pɪk] **1** *n* ***take your ~*** escolha um/uma **2** *v/t* (*choose*) escolher; *flowers* apanhar; *fruit* colher; ***~ one's nose*** cutucar o nariz **3** *v/i* ***~ and choose*** ser muito exigente
♦ **pick at** *v/t* ***pick at one's food*** comer como um passarinho
♦ **pick on** *v/t* (*treat unfairly*) implicar com; (*select*) eleger
♦ **pick out** *v/t* (*identify*) identificar
♦ **pick up 1** *v/t from ground*, (*collect*), *man, woman, in car, habit, illness* pegar; *from airport, school, etc* buscar; *language, skill* aprender; (*buy*) comprar; *criminal* prender; ***pick up the tab*** *fam* pagar a conta **2** *v/i* (*improve*) melhorar
picket ['pɪkɪt] **1** *n of strikers* piquete *m* **2** *v/t* fazer um piquete em
'picket fence cerca *f* estacas
'picket line piquete *m* de grevistas
pickle ['pɪkl] *v/t* pôr em conserva
pickles ['pɪklz] *npl* conserva *f*
pickpocket ['pɪkpɑːkɪt] batedor,a *m,f* de carteira, *Port* carteirista *m/f*
'pick-up, **pick-up truck** caminhonete *f*, pick up *f*
picky ['pɪkɪ] *adj fam* meticuloso
picnic ['pɪknɪk] **1** *n* piquenique *m* **2** *v/i* ⟨*pret & pp* **picnicked**⟩ fazer um piquenique
picture ['pɪktʃər] **1** *n* (*photo*) foto *f*; (*painting*) pintura *f*; (*illustration*) ilustração *f*; (*movie*) filme *m*; ***keep s.o. in the ~*** manter alguém em dia; ***go to the ~s*** *Brit* ir ao cinema **2** *v/t* imaginar
'picture book livro *m* ilustrado
picture 'postcard cartão *m* postal
picturesque [pɪktʃə'resk] *adj* pitoresco
pie [paɪ] torta *f*
piece [piːs] (*component*), *in board game* peça *f*; (*fragment*) pedaço *m*; ***a ~ of pie / bread*** um pedaço de torta / pão; ***a ~ of advice*** um conselho; ***go to ~s*** desmoronar; ***take to ~s*** desmontar
♦ **piece together** *v/t broken plate* juntar os pedaços de; *facts, evidence* reconstruir
'piecemeal *adv* aos poucos
'piecework trabalho *m* por tarefa
pier [pɪr] *at seaside* píer *m*
pierce [pɪrs] *v/t* perfurar; *ears* furar
piercing ['pɪrsɪŋ] **1** *adj noise, eyes* penetrante; *wind* cortante **2** *n* piercing *m*
pig [pɪg] *also fig* porco *m*
pigeon ['pɪdʒɪn] pombo,-a *m,f*
'pigeonhole 1 *n* escaninho *m* **2** *v/t person* rotular; *proposal* arquivar
piggybank ['pɪgɪbæŋk] cofrinho *m* (*em forma de porco*)
pigheaded ['pɪghedɪd] *adj* teimoso
'pigpen *also fig* chiqueiro *m* **'pigskin** couro *m* de porco **'pigtail** trança *f*
pile [paɪl] pilha *f*; *earth, sand, work*: monte *m*
♦ **pile up 1** *v/i work, bills* acumular **2** *v/t* empilhar
piles [paɪlz] *nsg* MED hemorróidas *fpl*
'pile-up MOT colisão *f* em cadeia
pilfering ['pɪlfərɪŋ] *adj* pequenos furtos *mpl*
pilgrim ['pɪlgrɪm] peregrino,-a *m,f*
pilgrimage ['pɪlgrɪmɪdʒ] peregrinação *f*
pill [pɪl] comprimido *m*; ***the ~*** a pílula (anticoncepcional); ***be on the ~*** tomar a pílula
pillar ['pɪlər] pilar *m*
pillion ['pɪljən] *motor bike*: garupa *f*
pillow ['pɪloʊ] *n* travesseiro *m*, *Port* almofada *f*
'pillowcase fronha *f*
pillowslip *Brit* → ***pillowcase***
pilot ['paɪlət] **1** *n airplane, port*: piloto *m* **2** *v/t airplane* pilotar
'pilot plant TECH instalação *f* piloto
'pilot scheme projeto *m* piloto
pimp [pɪmp] *n* cafetão *m*, *Port* cáften *m*
pimple ['pɪmpl] espinha *f*
PIN [pɪn] *abbr* (*of* ***personal identification number***) senha *f* pessoal
pin [pɪn] **1** *n sewing*: alfinete *m*; *bowling*: pino *m*; (*badge*) crachá *m*; ELEC pino *m* de conexão **2** *v/t* ⟨*pret & pp* ***pinned***⟩ (*hold down*) manter; (*attach*) pendurar

P

◆**pin down** *v/t* ***pin s.o. down to a date*** obrigar alguém a marcar uma data
◆**pin up** *v/t* (*notice*) pendurar
pincers ['pɪnsərz] *npl tool* pinça *f*; *crab*: tesouras *fpl*; ***a pair of ~*** uma pinça
pinch [pɪntʃ] **1** *n* beliscão *m*; *salt*, *sugar etc*: pitada *f*; ***at a ~*** se for realmente necessário **2** *v/t* beliscar; *fam* (*steal*) afanar **3** *v/i shoes* apertar
pine[1] [paɪn] *n tree* pinheiro *m*; *wood* pínus *m*
pine[2] [paɪn] *v/i* ***~ for*** sentir falta de
'pineapple abacaxi *m*, *Port* ananás *m*
ping [pɪŋ] **1** *n* toque *m* **2** *v/i* tilintar
ping-pong ['pɪŋpɑːng] pingue-pongue *m*
pink [pɪŋk] *adj* rosa
pinnacle ['pɪnəkl] *fig* topo *m*
'PIN number número *m* de código PIN
'pinpoint *v/t* determinar **pins and 'needles** formigamento *m* **'pinstripe** *adj* listrado
pint [paɪnt] quartilho *m*
'pin-up, **'pin-up girl** (garota) pinup *f*
pioneer [paɪə'nɪr] **1** *n fig* pioneiro,-a *m,f* **2** *v/t* ser pioneiro em
pioneering [paɪə'nɪrɪŋ] *adj work* pioneiro
pious ['paɪəs] *adj* piedoso
pip [pɪp] *n of fruit* semente *f*
pipe [paɪp] **1** *n smoking*: cachimbo *m*; *water*, *gas*, *sewage*: cano *m* **2** *v/t* encanar
◆**pipe down** *v/i fam* fechar o bico
'piped music [paɪpt] música *f* assoviada
'pipeline *gas*: gasoduto *m*; *oil*: oleoduto *m*; ***in the ~*** *fig* em andamento
piping hot ['paɪpɪŋ] *adj* muito quente
pirate ['paɪrət] *v/t software* piratear
Pisces ['paɪsiːz] ASTROL Peixes *m*
piss [pɪs] *fam* **1** *v/i* (*urinate*) mijar **2** *n* (*urine*) mijo *m*; ***take the ~*** tirar um sarro
◆**piss off** *v/i fam* sumir; ***piss off!*** suma!
pissed [pɪst] *adj fam* (*annoyed*) irritado; *Brit* (*drunk*) bêbado
pistol ['pɪstl] pistola *f*
piston ['pɪstən] pistom *m*
pit [pɪt] *n* (*hole*) buraco *m*; (*coal mine*) mina *f*
pitch[1] [pɪtʃ] *n* MUS tom *m*
pitch[2] [pɪtʃ] **1** *v/i in baseball* arremessar **2** *v/t tent* armar; *ball* lançar
'pitch black *adj* negro como piche
pitcher[1] ['pɪtʃər] *baseball*: arremessador *m*
pitcher[2] ['pɪtʃər] *container* jarra *f*
'pitfall *fig* dificuldade *f*
pith [pɪθ] *fruit*: mesocarpo *m*
pitiful ['pɪtɪfl] *adj sight* lastimável; *excuse*, *attempt* patético
pitiless ['pɪtɪləs] *adj* cruel
pits [pɪts] *npl motor racing*: boxes *mpl*
'pit stop *motor racing*: parada *f* nos boxes
pittance ['pɪtns] miséria *f*
pity ['pɪtɪ] **1** *n* piedade *f*; ***it's a ~ that*** é uma lástima que; ***what a ~!*** que pena!; ***take ~ on*** ficar com pena de **2** *v/t* ⟨*pret & pp* ***pitied***⟩ *person* ter pena de
pivot ['pɪvət] **1** *v/i* girar **2** *n* pivô *m*
pizza ['piːtsə] pizza *f*
placard ['plækɑːrd] cartaz *m*
place [pleɪs] **1** *n also in race*, *competition*, (*seat*) lugar *m*; *bar*, *restaurant* local *m*; *apartment* apartamento *m*; *house* casa *f*; ***at my / his ~*** na minha / na sua casa; ***in ~ of*** no lugar de; ***feel out of ~*** sentir-se fora de lugar; ***I've lost my ~*** *in book* não sei em que trecho do livro eu estava; ***take ~*** acontecer; ***in the first ~*** (*firstly*) em primeiro lugar; (*in the beginning*) no começo **2** *v/t* (*put*) pôr, colocar; ***I know you but I can't quite ~ you*** eu te conheço, mas não sei de onde; ***~ an order*** fazer um pedido
'place mat colchonete *m*
placid ['plæsɪd] *adj* calmo
plagiarism ['pleɪdʒərɪzm] plágio *m*
plagiarize ['pleɪdʒəraɪz] *v/t* plagiar
plague [pleɪg] **1** *n* praga *f* **2** *v/t* (*bother*) molestar
plain[1] [pleɪn] *n* planície *f*
plain[2] [pleɪn] **1** *adj* (*clear*, *obvious*) claro; (*not fancy*) simples; (*not pretty*) feinho; (*not patterned*) liso; (*blunt*) direto; ***~ chocolate*** chocolate *m*

P

meio-amargo **2** *adv* simplesmente; ***it's ~ crazy*** é uma verdadeira loucura
'plain-clothes *n* ***in ~*** à paisana
plainly ['pleɪnlɪ] *adv* (*obviously*) evidentemente; (*in a clear manner*) de modo claro; (*bluntly*) diretamente; ***~ dressed*** vestido com simplicidade
'plain spoken *adj* claro e direto
plaintiff ['pleɪntɪf] queixoso,-a *m,f*
plaintive ['pleɪntɪv] *adj voice* queixoso
plait *Brit* → ***braid***
plan [plæn] **1** *n* (*project, intention*) plano *m*; (*drawing*) planta *f* **2** *v/t* ⟨*pret & pp* ***planned***⟩ (*prepare, design*) planejar, *Port* planear; ***~ to do, ~ on doing*** estar planejando fazer **3** *v/i* ⟨*pret & pp* ***planned***⟩ planejar
plane[1] [pleɪn] *n* (*airplane*) avião *m*
plane[2] [pleɪn] *tool* plaina *f*
planet ['plænɪt] planeta *m*
plank [plæŋk] *wood*: tábua *f*; *fig policy*: plataforma *f*
planning ['plænɪŋ] planejamento *m*, *Port* planeamento *m*; ***at the ~ stage*** em fase de planejamento
plant[1] [plænt] **1** *n* planta *f* **2** *v/t* plantar
plant[2] [plænt] *n* (*factory*) fábrica *f*; (*equipment*) maquinário *m*
plantation [plæn'teɪʃn] plantação *f*
plaque [plæk] *wall, teeth*: placa *f*
plaster ['plæstər] **1** *n wall, ceiling*: reboco *m* **2** *v/t wall, ceiling* rebocar; ***be ~ed with*** estar estampado com
'plaster cast molde *m* de gêsso
plastic ['plæstɪk] **1** *n* plástico *m* **2** *adj* de plástico
plastic 'bag sacola *f* de plástico
'plastic money cartões *mpl* de crédito **plastic 'surgeon** cirurgião (cirurgiã) plástico,-a *m,f* **plastic 'surgery** cirurgia *f* plástica
plate [pleɪt] *n for food* prato *m*; *of metal* chapa *f* de metal
plateau [plæ'toʊ] planalto *m*
platform ['plætfɔːrm] (*stage*) palco *m*; *railroad station*: plataforma *f*, *Port* cais *m*; *fig political* programa *m*
platinum ['plætɪnəm] **1** *n* platina *f* **2** *adj* de platina
platitude ['plætɪtuːd] banalidade *f*
platonic [plə'tɑːnɪk] *adj relationship* platônico
platoon [plə'tuːn] *soldiers*: pelotão *m*
platter ['plætər] *meat, fish*: travessa *f*
plausible ['plɒːzəbl] *adj* plausível
play [pleɪ] **1** *n theater, TV, radio*: peça *f*; *of children*, SPORT, TECH jogo *m* **2** *v/i also children* brincar **3** *v/t* SPORT *perform, take part in* jogar; *music* tocar; *piece of music* interpretar; *opponent* jogar contra; (*perform*) *Macbeth etc* representar; ***she's ~ing Ophelia*** ela está atuando no papel de Ophélia; ***~ a joke on*** fazer uma brincadeira com
♦**play around** *v/i fam* (*be unfaithful*) pular a cerca
♦**play down** *v/t* minimizar
♦**play up** *v/i machine* dar problemas; *child* fazer escândalo; ***this tooth is playing up*** este dente está me incomodando
'playact *v/i* (*pretend*) fingir **'playback** playback *m* **'playboy** playboy *m*
player ['pleɪr] SPORT jogador,a *m,f*; (*musician*) musico,-a *m,f*; (*actor*) ator *m*, atriz *f*
playful ['pleɪfl] *adj punch etc* na brincadeira
'playground parquinho *m*
'playgroup escolinha *f* particular
playing card ['pleɪɪŋ] carta *f* de baralho
playing field ['pleɪɪŋ] quadra *f* de esportes, *Port* campo *m* de jogos
'playmate parceiro,-a *m,f* de jogo
playwright ['pleɪraɪt] autor,a *m,f* dramático,-a
plaza ['plɑːzə] *shopping*: centro *m* comercial
plc [piːel'siː] *abbr* (*of Brit* ***public limited company***) sociedade anônima *f*, S/A *f*
plea [pliː] *n* pedido *m*
plead [pliːd] *v/i* ***~ for*** pedir por; ***~ guilty / not guilty*** declarar-se culpado / inocente; ***~ with*** implorar
pleasant ['pleznt] *adj* agradável
please [pliːz] **1** *adv* por favor; ***more tea? – yes, ~*** mais chá? - sim, por favor; ***~ do*** fique a vontade **2** *v/t* agradar; ***~ yourself*** faça o que quizer

P

pleased [pliːzd] *adj* contente; **~ *to meet you*** muito prazer
pleasing ['pliːzɪŋ] *adj* agradável
pleasure ['pleʒər] prazer *m*; (*happiness, satisfaction*) satisfação *f*; ***it's a ~*** (*you're welcome*) é um prazer; ***with ~*** com prazer
pleat [pliːt] *n in skirt* prega *f*
pleated skirt ['pliːtɪd] saia *f* plissada
pledge [pledʒ] **1** *n* (*promise*) promessa *f*, ***Pledge of Allegiance*** juramento *m* de lealdade à bandeira dos Estados Unidos **2** *v/t* (*promise*) prometer
plentiful ['plentɪfl] *adj* abundante
plenty ['plentɪ] (*abundance*) fartura *f*, **~ *of people / of room*** muitas pessoas / muito espaço; ***that's ~*** é suficiente; ***there's ~ for everyone*** há suficiente para todos
pliable *adj* flexivel
pliers *npl* alicate *m*; ***a pair of ~*** um alicate
plight [plaɪt] situação *f* difícil
plod [plɑːd] *v/i* ⟨*pret & pp* ***plodded***⟩ *walk* arrastar-se
♦ **plod on** *v/i with a job* seguir laboriosamente
plodder ['plɑːdər] *work, school*: *sujeito lento mas persistente*
plot[1] [plɑːt] *n land*: terreno *m*
plot[2] [plɑːt] **1** *n* (*conspiracy*) complô *m*; *novel*: trama *f* **2** *v/t* ⟨*pret & pp* ***plotted***⟩ conspirar **3** *v/i* ⟨*pret & pp* ***plotted***⟩ tramar
plotter ['plɑːtər] conspirador,a *m,f*; COMPUT impressora *f* plotter
plough *Brit* → ***plow***
plow [plaʊ] *Am* **1** *n* arado *m* **2** *v/t & v/i* arar
♦ **plow back** *v/t Am profits* reinvestir
pluck [plʌk] *v/t eyebrows* tirar; *chicken* depenar
♦ **pluck up** *v/t* ***pluck up courage*** arranjar coragem
plug [plʌg] **1** *n sink, bath*: tampinha *f*, *electrical* tomada *f*, *Port* ficha *f*, *new book etc*: propaganda *f*, ***spark ~*** vela *f* de ignição **2** *v/t* ⟨*pret & pp* ***plugged***⟩ *hole* tampar; *new book etc* fazer propaganda de
♦ **plug away** *v/i fam* perseverar
♦ **plug in** *v/t* ligar na tomada
plum [plʌm] **1** *n fruit* ameixa *f*, *tree* ameixeira *f* **2** *adj* ***a ~ job*** um empregão
plumage ['pluːmɪdʒ] plumagem *f*
plumb [plʌm] *adj* vertical
♦ **plumb in** *v/t washing machine etc* conectar a rede de água e esgoto
plumber ['plʌmər] encanador,a *m,f*, *Port* canalizador,a *m,f*
plumbing ['plʌmɪŋ] *pipes* canos *mpl*
plume [pluːm] *n* pluma *f*
plummet ['plʌmɪt] *v/i airplane, share prices* cair vertiginosamente
plump [plʌmp] *adj* rechonchudo; *chicken* gordo
♦ **plump for** *v/t* decidir-se por
plunge [plʌndʒ] **1** *n also prices*: queda *f*, ***take the ~*** seguir em frente **2** *v/i* precipitar-se; *prices* cair; (*dive*) mergulhar **3** *v/t* meter; ***the city was ~d into darkness*** a cidade estava imersa na escuridão; ***the news ~d him into despair*** as notícias levaram-no ao desespero
plunging ['plʌndʒɪŋ] *adj neckline* decotado
pluperfect ['pluːpɜːrfɪkt] *n* GRAM pretérito *m* mais-que-perfeito
plural ['plʊrəl] **1** *n* plural *m* **2** *adj* plural
plus [plʌs] **1** *prep* mais **2** *adj* mais de; ***500 ~*** mais de 500 **3** *n symbol* sinal *m* de mais; (*advantage*) vantagem *f* **4** *conj* (*moreover, in addition*) além disso
plush [plʌʃ] *adj* luxuoso
'plus sign sinal *m* de mais
plywood ['plaɪwʊd] madeira *f* compensada
PM [piː'em] *Brit abbr* (*of* ***Prime Minister***) primeiro-ministro *m*, primeira-ministra *f*
p.m. [piː'em] *abbr* (*of* ***post meridiem***) ***at 2.00 p.m. / at 10.30 p.m.*** às 2:00 da tarde / às 10:30 da noite
pneumatic [nuː'mætɪk] *adj* pneumático
pneumatic 'drill martelo *m* pneumático
pneumonia [nuː'moʊnɪə] pneumonia *f*

poach[1] [poʊtʃ] *v/t cooking*: escaldar
poach[2] [poʊtʃ] *v/t pheasant, deer etc* caçar ilegalmente; *salmon etc* pescar ilegalmente
poached egg [poʊtʃt] ovo *m* poché, *Port* ovo *m* escalfado
poacher ['poʊtʃər] *salmon, game*: caçador,a *m,f* furtivo,-a
P.O. Box [piː'oʊbɑːks] caixa *f* postal
pocket ['pɑːkɪt] **1** *n* bolso *m*; ***line one's own ~s*** encher os bolsos; ***be out of ~*** estar sem dinheiro **2** *adj* (*miniature*) de bolso; ***out-of-~ expenses*** despesas *fpl* pequenas
'pocketbook (*handbag*) bolsa *f* de mão; (*wallet*) carteira *f*; *book* livro *m* de bolso **pocket 'calculator** calculadora *f* de bolso **'pocketknife** canivete *m*
podcast ['pɑːdkæst] podcast *m*
podiatrist [poʊ'daɪətrɪst] podólogo,-a *m,f*
podium ['poʊdɪəm] pódio *m*
poem ['poʊɪm] poema *m*
poet ['poʊɪt] poeta *m*, poetisa *f*
poetic [poʊ'etɪk] *adj* poético
poetic 'justice justiça *f* poética
poetry ['poʊɪtrɪ] poesia *f*
poignant ['pɔɪnjənt] *adj* comovente
point [pɔɪnt] **1** *n pencil, knife*: ponta *f*; *competition, exam, argument*: ponto *m*; (*purpose*) propósito *m*; (*moment*) momento *m*; *decimal*: ponto *m*; ***that's beside the ~*** isso não vem ao caso; ***be on the ~ of*** estar a ponto de; ***get to the ~*** ir direto ao ponto; ***the ~ is ...*** a questão é ...; ***there's no ~ in waiting*** não faz sentido esperar **2** *v/t & v/i also gun* apontar
♦**point at** *v/t with finger* apontar (com o dedo) para
♦**point out** *v/t sights* indicar; *advantages etc* ressaltar
♦**point to** *v/t with finger, also fig* indicar
'point-blank 1 *adj refusal, denial* categórico; ***at ~ range*** à queima-roupa **2** *adv refuse, deny* categoricamente
pointed ['pɔɪntɪd] *adj remark, question* mordaz
pointer ['pɔɪntər] *for teacher* bastão *m*; (*hint*) dica *f*; (*sign, indication*) indicador *m*
pointless ['pɔɪntləs] *adj* inútil; ***it's ~ trying*** é inútil tentar
'point of sale *place* ponto *m* de venda; *promotional material* material *m* promocional
'point of view ponto *m* de vista
poise [pɔɪz] autoconfiança *f*
poised [pɔɪzd] *adj person* autoconfiante
poison ['pɔɪzn] **1** *n* veneno *m* **2** *v/t* envenenar
poisonous ['pɔɪznəs] *adj* venenoso
poke [poʊk] **1** *n* empurrão *m* **2** *v/t* (*prod*) espetar; (*stick*) fincar, enfiar; ***~ fun at*** zombar de; ***~ one's nose into*** enfiar o nariz em
♦**poke around** *v/i* bisbilhotar
poker ['poʊkər] *card game* pôquer *m*
poky ['poʊkɪ] *adj* (*cramped*) minúsculo
Poland ['poʊlənd] Polônia *f*
polar ['poʊlər] *adj* polar
'polar bear urso *m* polar
polarize ['poʊləraɪz] *v/t* polarizar
Pole [poʊl] polonês,-esa *m,f*
pole[1] [poʊl] *wood, metal*: poste *m*
pole[2] [poʊl] *of the Earth* pólo *m*
'pole star estrela *f* polar **'polevault** salto *m* com vara **'pole-vaulter** saltador,a *m,f* com vara
police [pə'liːs] *n* polícia *f*
po'lice car carro *m* de polícia **po'liceman** policial *m*, *Port* polícia *m* **po'lice state** estado *m* policial **po'lice station** delegacia *f* de polícia, *Port* esquadra *f* **po'licewoman** policial *f*, *Port* mulher *f* polícia
policy ['pɑːləsɪ] política *f*; ***insurance ~*** apólice *f* de seguro
polio ['poʊlɪoʊ] pólio *f*
Polish ['poʊlɪʃ] **1** *adj* polonês,-esa **2** *n language* polonês *m*
polish ['pɑːlɪʃ] **1** *n* polidor *m*; *for shoes* graxa *f*; ***nail ~*** esmalte *m* **2** *v/t also fig speech* polir
♦**polish off** *v/t food* terminar
♦**polish up** *v/t skill* polir
polished ['pɑːlɪʃt] *adj performance* brilhante
polite [pə'laɪt] *adj* educado
politely [pə'laɪtlɪ] *adv* educadamente

P

politeness [pə'laɪtnɪs] educação *f*
political [pə'lɪtɪkl] *adj* político
politician [pɑːlɪ'tɪʃn] político,-a *m,f*
politics ['pɑːlɪtɪks] política *f*; ***what are his ~?*** quais são as suas convicções políticas?
poll [poʊl] **1** *n* (*survey*) pesquisa *f* de opinião; ***the ~s*** (*election*) as eleições; ***go to the ~s*** (*vote*) ir às urnas **2** *v/t people* sondar; *votes* obter
pollen ['pɑːlən] pólen *m*
'**pollen count** concentração *f* de pólen no ar
'**polling booth** ['poʊlɪŋ] cabine *f* eleitoral
'**polling day** dia *m* de eleição
pollster ['pɑːlstər] realizador,a *m,f* de pesquisas de opinião
pollutant [pə'luːtənt] poluente *m*
pollute [pə'luːt] *v/t* poluir
pollution [pə'luːʃn] poluição *f*
polo ['poʊloʊ] SPORT pólo *m*
'**polo neck** *sweater* cacharrel *m*
'**polo shirt** camisa *f* pólo
polyester [pɑːlɪ'estər] poliéster *m*
polyethylene [pɑːlɪ'eθɪliːn] polietileno *m*
polystyrene [pɑːlɪ'staɪriːn] poliestireno *m*
polyunsaturated [pɑːlɪʌn'sætʃəreɪtɪd] *adj* poliinsaturado
pompous ['pɑːmpəs] *adj* pomposo
pond [pɑːnd] laguinho *m*
ponder ['pɑːndər] *v/t* ponderar
pontiff ['pɑːntɪf] pontífice *m*
pony ['poʊnɪ] pônei *m*
'**ponytail** rabo-de-cavalo *m*
poodle ['puːdl] poodle *m*
pool[1] [puːl] *water, blood*: poça *f*; (*swimming pool*) piscina *f*
pool[2] [puːl] *game* pool *m*
pool[3] [puːl] **1** *n* (*common fund*) pote *m* comum **2** *v/t resources* unir
'**pool hall** salão *m* de bilhar
'**pool table** mesa *f* de bilhar
pooped [puːpt] *adj fam* acabado
poor [pʊr] **1** *adj* pobre; (*not good*) ruim, mau (má); ***be in ~ health*** estar doente; ***~ old Tony!*** pobre Tony! **2** *npl* ***the ~*** os pobres
poorly ['pʊrlɪ] **1** *adv* mal **2** *adj* ***feel ~*** sentir-se mal

pop[1] [pɑːp] **1** *n noise* barulho *m* **2** *v/i & v/t* ⟨*pret & pp* ***popped***⟩ *balloon etc* estourar
pop[2] [pɑːp] **1** *n* MUS música *f* pop **2** *adj* pop
pop[3] [pɑːp] *fam* (*father*) papai *m*
pop[4] [pɑːp] *fam* (*put*) pôr
♦ **pop in** *v/i fam* (*make a brief visit*) dar uma passadinha
♦ **pop out** *v/i fam* (*go out for a short time*) dar uma saidinha
♦ **pop up** *v/i fam* (*appear suddenly*) aparecer
'**pop concert** show *m* pop
'**popcorn** pipoca *f*
pope [poʊp] Papa *m*
'**pop group** grupo *m* pop
poppy ['pɑːpɪ] papoula *f*
Popsicle® ['pɑːpsɪkl] picolé *m*
'**pop song** canção *f* pop
popular ['pɑːpjələr] *adj* popular; *belief, support* geral
popularity [pɑːpjə'lærətɪ] popularidade *f*
populate ['pɑːpjəleɪt] *v/t* povoar
population [pɑːpjə'leɪʃn] população *f*
porcelain ['pɔːrsəlɪn] **1** *n* porcelana *f* **2** *adj* de porcelana
porch [pɔːrtʃ] varanda *f*
porcupine ['pɔːrkjʊpaɪn] porco-espinho *m*
pore [pɔːr] *of skin* poro *m*
♦ **pore over** *v/t* estudar minuciosamente
pork [pɔːrk] carne *f* de porco
porn [pɔːrn] *n fam* pornografia *f*
porn(**o**) [pɔːrn, 'pɔːrnoʊ] *adj fam* pornô
pornographic [pɔːrnə'græfɪk] *adj* pornográfico
pornography [pɔːr'nɑːgrəfɪ] pornografia *f*
porous ['pɔːrəs] *adj* poroso
port[1] [pɔːrt] *n town* cidade *f* portuária; *area* porto *m*
port[2] [pɔːrt] *adj side, bow etc* de bombordo
portable ['pɔːrtəbl] **1** *adj* portátil **2** *n* COMPUT portátil *m*; *TV* televisor *m* portátil
porter ['pɔːrtər] porteiro,-a *m,f*
'**porthole** NAUT escotilha *f*

P

portion ['pɔːrʃn] *n* parte *f*; *food*: porção *f*
portrait ['pɔːrtreɪt] **1** *n* (*painting, photograph*) retrato *m*; (*depiction*) descrição *f* **2** *adv print* em formato vertical
portray [pɔːr'treɪ] *v/t artist*, pintar; *photographer* retratar; *actor* interpretar; *author* descrever
portrayal [pɔːr'treɪəl] *actor*: interpretação *f*; *author*: descrição *f*
Portugal ['pɔːrʧəgl] Portugal *m*
Portuguese [pɔːrʧə'giːz] **1** *adj* português,-esa **2** *n person* português,-esa *m,f*; *language* português *m*
pose [poʊz] **1** *n* (*pretense*) pose *f* **2** *v/i for artist, photographer* posar; ***~ as*** fazer-se passar por **3** *v/t* ***~ a problem / a threat*** representar um problema / uma ameaça
posh [pɑːʃ] *adj Brit fam* chique
position [pə'zɪʃn] **1** *n* posição *f* **2** *v/t* posicionar
positive ['pɑːzətɪv] **1** *adj* positivo; ***be ~ sure*** ter certeza **2** *n* GRAM forma *f* positiva
positively ['pɑːzətɪvlɪ] *adv* (*decidedly*) sem dúvida; (*definitely*) definitivamente
possess [pə'zes] *v/t* possuir
possession [pə'zeʃn] posse *f*; ***~s*** posses *fpl*, bens *mpl*
possessive [pə'zesɪv] *adj person*, GRAM possessivo
possibility [pɑːsə'bɪlətɪ] possibilidade *f*
possible ['pɑːsəbl] *adj* possível; ***the shortest / quickest ~ route*** a rota mais curta / rápida; ***the best ~ …*** o melhor (a melhora) … possível
possibly ['pɑːsəblɪ] *adv* possivelmente; (*perhaps*) talvez; ***that can't ~ be right*** não há possibilidade disso estar certo; ***we're doing everything we ~ can*** estamos fazendo tudo que é possível; ***how could they ~ have known that?*** como é possível que pudessem saber disso?; ***could you ~ tell me …?*** o senhor / a senhora poderia me dizer …?
post[1] [poʊst] **1** *n wood, metal*: poste *m* **2** *v/t notice* colocar; *profits* apresentar; ***keep s.o. ~ed*** manter alguém informado
post[2] [poʊst] **1** *n* (*place of duty*) posto *m* **2** *v/t guards* postar; (*send*) *soldier, employee* transferir
post[3] [poʊst] *Brit* **1** *n* (*mail*) correio *m* **2** *v/t letter* pôr no correio
postage ['poʊstɪdʒ] tarifa *f* do correio
'postage stamp *fml* selo *m* postal
postal ['poʊstl] *adj* postal
'postal order *Brit* ordem *f* de pagamento
'postbox *Brit* caixa *f* dos correios, *Port* marco *m* do correio **'postcard** cartão *m* postal **'postcode** *Brit* CEP *m*, código *m* de endereçamento postal **'postdate** *v/t* pós-datar
poster ['poʊstər] pôster *m*
posterior [pɑː'stɪrɪər] *n hum* (*buttocks*) traseiro *m*
posterity [pɑː'sterətɪ] posteridade *f*
postgraduate ['poʊstgrædʒʊət] **1** *n* pós-graduado,-a *m,f* **2** *adj* de pós-graduação
posthumous ['pɑːsʧəməs] *adj* póstumo
posthumously ['pɑːsʧəməslɪ] *adv* postumamente
posting ['poʊstɪŋ] (*assignment*) transferência *f*
'postman *Brit* carteiro *f*
'postmark carimbo *m* do correio
postmortem [poʊst'mɔːrtəm] autópsia *f*
'post office correio *m*
postpone [poʊst'poʊn] *v/t* adiar
postponement [poʊst'poʊnmənt] adiamento *m*
posture ['pɑːsʧər] postura *f*
'postwar *adj* de após-guerra
pot[1] [pɑːt] *cooking*: panela *f*, *coffee, tea*: bule *m*; *plant*: vaso *m*
pot[2] [pɑːt] *fam* (*marijuana*) maconha *f*
potato [pə'teɪtoʊ] batata *f*
po'tato chips *Am* batata *f* frita
po'tato crisps *Brit* batata *f* frita
'potbelly pança *f*
potent ['poʊtənt] *adj* potente
potential [pə'tenʃl] **1** *adj* potencial **2** *n* potencial *m*
potentially [pə'tenʃəlɪ] *adv* potencialmente

'pothole *road*: buraco *m*
potter ['pɑːtər] *n* oleiro,-a *m,f*
pottery ['pɑːtərɪ] *n activity, items* cerâmica *f*; *place* olaria *f*
potty ['pɑːtɪ] *n baby*: penico *m*
pouch [paʊtʃ] (*bag*) bolsa *f*
poultry ['poʊltrɪ] *birds* aves *fpl* domésticas; *meat* aves *fpl*
pounce [paʊns] *v/i animal* saltar; *fig* efetuar um ataque
pound[1] [paʊnd] *n weight* libra *f*
pound[2] [paʊnd] *n strays*: canil *m*; *cars*: depósito *m*
pound[3] [paʊnd] *v/i heart* palpitar; **~ *on*** (*hammer on*) bater em
pound 'sterling Libra *f* esterlina
pour [pɔːr] **1** *v/t liquid* despejar; *tea, coffee* servir **2** *v/i* ***it's ~ing*** (***with rain***) está chovendo torrencialmente
♦**pour out** *v/t tea, coffee* servir; *troubles* revelar
pout [paʊt] *v/i* fazer cara zangada
poverty ['pɑːvərtɪ] pobreza *f*
poverty-stricken ['pɑːvərtɪstrɪkn] *adj* paupérrimo
powder ['paʊdər] **1** *n* pó *m*; *for face* pó *m* compacto **2** *v/t face* passar pó compacto em
'powder room *fam* toalete *m*
power ['paʊər] **1** *n argument, love, imagination, punch*: força *f*; *engine, explosion, drug*: potência *f*; (*authority*) poder *m*; (*energy*) energia *f*; (*electricity*) eletricidade *f*; ***in ~*** POL no poder; ***fall from ~*** POL perder o poder **2** *v/t* ***be ~ed by*** ser impulsionado por
'power-assisted steering *adj* direção *f* hidráulica **'power cut** blecaute *m*, *Port* corte *m* de energia **'power failure** queda *f* de energia
powerful ['paʊərfl] *adj* poderoso; *car, engine, drug, detergent* potente
powerless ['paʊərlɪs] *adj* impotente; ***be ~ to ...*** estar impotente para ...
'power line cabo *m* de energia elétrica **'power lunch** *fam* almoço *m* de negócios **'power outage** blecaute *m*, *Port* corte *m* de energia **'power station** usina *f* elétrica **'power steering** direção *f* hidráulica **'power unit** fonte *f* de alimentação
PR [piː'ɑːr] *abbr* (*of* ***public relations***) relações *fpl* públicas
practical ['præktɪkl] *adj* prático
practical 'joke brincadeira *f*
practically ['præktɪklɪ] *adv behave, think* de maneira prática; (*almost*) praticamente
practice ['præktɪs] **1** *n* (*not theory, repetition, training*) prática *f*; (*rehearsal*) ensaio *m*; (*custom*) costume *m*; ***in ~*** (*in reality*) na prática; ***be out of ~*** estar sem prática **2** *v/t piece of music, speech, shot* praticar; *law, medicine* exercer **3** *v/i musician, dancer* ensaiar; *soccer player* treinar
practise *Brit* → ***practice*** *v/t & v/i*
pragmatic [præg'mætɪk] *adj* pragmático
pragmatism ['prægmətɪzm] pragmatismo *m*
prairie ['prerɪ] prado *m*
praise [preɪz] **1** *n* elogio *m* **2** *v/t* elogiar
'praiseworthy *adj* elogiável
pram [præm] *Brit* carrinho *m* de bebê
prank [præŋk] travessura *f*
prattle ['prætl] *v/i* tagarelar
prawn [prɒːn] camarão *m*
pray [preɪ] *v/i* orar
prayer [prer] oração *f*
preach [priːtʃ] **1** *v/i in church* pregar; (*moralize*) dar um sermão **2** *v/t sermon* pregar
preacher ['priːtʃər] pregador,a *m,f*
preamble ['priːæmbl] preâmbulo *m*
precarious [prɪ'kerɪəs] *adj* precário
precariously [prɪ'kerɪəslɪ] *adv* precariamente
precaution [prɪ'kɒːʃn] precaução *f*
precautionary [prɪ'kɒːʃnerɪ] *adj measure* preventivo
precede [prɪ'siːd] *v/t in time* preceder; (*walk in front of*) ir à frente de
precedence ['presɪdəns] ***take ~ over*** ter prioridade sobre
precedent ['presɪdənt] *n* precedente *m*
preceding [prɪ'siːdɪŋ] *adj week, chapter* anterior
precinct ['priːsɪŋkt] distrito *m*
precious ['preʃəs] *adj* precioso
precipitate [prɪ'sɪpɪteɪt] *v/t crisis* precipitar

précis ['preɪsiː] *n* resumo *m*
precise [prɪ'saɪs] *adj* preciso
precisely [prɪ'saɪslɪ] *adv* precisamente
precision [prɪ'sɪʒn] precisão *f*
precocious [prɪ'koʊʃəs] *adj child* precoce
preconceived ['prɪkənsiːvd] *adj idea* preconcebido
precondition [prɪkən'dɪʃn] condição *f* prévia
predator ['predətər] predador *m*
predatory ['predətɔːrɪ] *adj* predatório
predecessor ['priːdɪsesər] *in job* predecessor,a *m,f*; *machine* modelo *m* anterior
predestination [priːdestɪ'neɪʃn] predestinação *f*
predestined [priː'destɪnd] *adj* ***be ~ to*** estar predestinado a
predicament [prɪ'dɪkəmənt] apuro *m*
predict [prɪ'dɪkt] *v/t* predizer, prognosticar
predictable [prɪ'dɪktəbl] *adj* previsível
prediction [prɪ'dɪkʃn] predição *f*
predominant [prɪ'dɑːmɪnənt] *adj* predominante
predominantly [prɪ'dɑːmɪnəntlɪ] *adv* predominantemente
predominate [prɪ'dɑːmɪneɪt] *v/i* predominar
prefabricated [priː'fæbrɪkeɪtɪd] *adj* pré-fabricado
preface ['prefɪs] *n* prefácio *m*
prefect ['priːfekt] *Brit* EDUC monitor,a *m,f*
prefer [prɪ'fɜːr] *v/t* ⟨*pret & pp* ***preferred***⟩ preferir; ***~ X to Y*** preferir X à Y; ***~ to do*** preferir fazer
preferable ['prefərəbl] *adj* preferível; ***be ~ to*** ser preferível a
preferably ['prefərəblɪ] *adv* preferivelmente
preference ['prefərəns] preferência *f*
preferential [prefə'renʃl] *adj* preferencial; ***they get ~ treatment*** eles têm tratamento favorecido
prefix ['priːfɪks] prefixo *m*
pregnancy ['pregnənsɪ] gravidez *f*
pregnant ['pregnənt] *adj* grávida
preheat ['priːhiːt] *v/t oven* preaquecer
prehistoric [priːhɪs'tɑːrɪk] *adj* pré-histórico
prejudge [priː'dʒʌdʒ] *v/t* prejulgar
prejudice ['predʒʊdɪs] **1** *n* preconceito *m* **2** *v/t person* influenciar; *chances* prejudicar
prejudiced ['predʒʊdɪst] *adj* parcial
prejudicial [predʒʊ'dɪʃl] *adj* ***be ~ to*** ser prejudicial a
preliminary [prɪ'lɪmɪnerɪ] *adj* preliminar
premarital [priː'mærɪtl] *adj* pré-marital
premature [priːmə'tʊr] *adj* prematuro
premeditated [priː'medɪteɪtɪd] *adj* premeditado
premier ['premɪr] *n* (*Prime Minister*) primeiro-ministro *m*, primeira-ministra *f*
première ['premɪer] *n* estréia *f*
premises ['premɪsɪz] *npl* local *m*
premium ['priːmɪəm] *n in insurance* prêmio *m*
premonition [premə'nɪʃn] premonição *f*
prenatal [priː'neɪtl] *adj* pré-natal
preoccupied [prɪ'ɑːkjʊpaɪd] *adj* preocupado
preparation [prepə'reɪʃn] preparação *f*; ***in ~ for*** como preparação para; ***~s*** preparativos *mpl*
prepare [prɪ'per] **1** *v/t* preparar; *room* arrumar; ***be ~d to do sth*** *willing* estar disposto a fazer algo; ***be ~d for sth*** *be expecting, ready* estar preparado para algo **2** *v/i* preparar-se
preposition [prepə'zɪʃn] preposição *f*
preposterous [prɪ'pɑːstərəs] *adj* absurdo
'prep school [prep] escola *f* primária preparatória
prerequisite [priː'rekwɪzɪt] pré-requisito *m*
prescribe [prɪ'skraɪb] *v/t doctor* prescrever
prescription [prɪ'skrɪpʃn] MED prescrição *f*
presence ['prezns] presença *f*; ***in the ~ of*** na frente de
presence of 'mind presença *f* de espírito

present[1] ['preznt] **1** *adj* presente; (*current*) atual; ***be ~*** estar presente **2** *n* ***the ~*** *also* GRAM o presente; ***at ~*** no momento
present[2] ['preznt] *n* (*gift*) presente *m*
present[3] [prɪ'zent] *v/t award, bouquet* entregar; *program* apresentar
presentation [prezn'teɪʃn] *to audience* apresentação *f*
present-day [preznt'deɪ] *adj* atual
presenter [prɪ'zentər] apresentador,a *m,f*
presently ['prezntlɪ] *adv* (*at the moment*) atualmente; (*soon*) logo
'present tense GRAM (tempo) presente *m*
preservation [prezə'veɪʃn] preservação *f*
preservative [prɪ'zɜːrvətɪv] *n wood, food*: conservante *m*
preserve [prɪ'zɜːrv] **1** *n* (*domain*) domínio *m* **2** *v/t standards, peace etc* manter; *wood etc* preservar; *food* conservar
preside [prɪ'zaɪd] *v/i at meeting* presidir; ***~ over*** *meeting* presidir
presidency ['prezɪdənsɪ] presidência *f*
president ['prezɪdnt] *of company*, POL presidente *m/f*
presidential [prezɪ'denʃl] *adj* presidencial
press [pres] **1** *n* ***the ~*** a imprensa *f* **2** *v/t button, person's hand* apertar; (*urge*) pressionar; (*squeeze*) espremer; *clothes* passar **3** *v/i* ***~ for*** *reform* reivindicar; *answer, payment* cobrar
'press agency agência *f* de notícias
'press conference conferência *f* de imprensa
pressing ['presɪŋ] *adj* urgente
'press-up *Brit gymnastics*: flexão *f*
pressure ['preʃər] **1** *n also of work, demands* pressão *f*; ***be under ~*** estar sob pressão **2** *v/t* pressionar
prestige [pre'stiːʒ] prestígio *m*
prestigious [pre'stɪdʒəs] *adj* prestigioso
presumably [prɪ'zuːməblɪ] *adv* provavelmente
presume [prɪ'zuːm] *v/t* presumir; ***~ to do sth*** *fml* tomar a liberdade de fazer algo
presumption [prɪ'zʌmpʃn] *of innocence, guilt* presunção *f*
presumptuous [prɪ'zʌmptʊəs] *adj* presunçoso
presuppose [priːsə'poʊs] *v/t* pressupor
pre-tax ['priːtæks] *adj* antes de impostos
pretence *Brit* → ***pretense***
pretend [prɪ'tend] *v/t & v/i* fingir; ***he's only ~ing to be annoyed*** ele está só fingindo que está aborrecido
pretense [prɪ'tens] *Am* fingimento *m*; ***it's all a ~*** é tudo fingimento; ***under false ~s*** sob falsas pretensões
pretentious [prɪ'tenʃəs] *adj* pretensioso
pretext ['priːtekst] pretexto *m*
pretty ['prɪtɪ] **1** *adj* bonito **2** *adv* (*quite*) muito
prevail [prɪ'veɪl] *v/i* (*triumph*) prevalecer
prevailing [prɪ'veɪlɪŋ] *adj* prevalecente
prevent [prɪ'vent] *v/t* impedir; ***~ s.o. from doing sth*** impedir alguém de fazer algo
prevention [prɪ'venʃn] prevenção *f*
preventive [prɪ'ventɪv] *adj medicine, measure* preventivo
preview ['priːvjuː] **1** *n movie, exhibition*: pré-estréia *f* **2** *v/t* fazer a apresentação prévia de
previous ['priːvɪəs] *adj* anterior
previously ['priːvɪəslɪ] *adv* anteriormente; ***six weeks ~*** seis semanas antes
pre-war ['priːwɔːr] *adj* de pré-guerra
prey [preɪ] *n* presa *f*
♦ **prey on** *v/t* caçar; *fig conman etc* aproveitar-se de
price [praɪs] **1** *n* preço *m* **2** *v/t* COM fixar o preço de; *in store* colocar o preço em
'price fixing fixação *f* de preços
priceless ['praɪslɪs] *adj* de valor inestimável; ***you ~ idiot!*** seu grande idiota!
'price tag etiqueta *f* de preço
'price war guerra *f* de preços
pricey ['praɪsɪ] *adj fam* caro

prick[1] [prɪk] **1** *n pain* pontada *f* **2** *v/t (jab)* espetar
prick[2] [prɪk] *n vulg (penis)* pica *f*; *person* filho-da-puta *m*
◆**prick up** *v/t* ***prick up one's ears*** *dog* aguçar as orelhas; *person* prestar atenção
prickle ['prɪkl] *on plant* espinho *m*
prickly ['prɪklɪ] *adj beard, plant* que pinica; *(irritable)* irritável
pride [praɪd] **1** *n* orgulho *m* **2** *v/t* **~ *oneself on*** orgulhar-se de
priest [pri:st] sacerdote *m*, sacerdotisa *f*
primarily [praɪ'merɪlɪ] *adv* principalmente
primary ['praɪmərɪ] **1** *adj reason, cause* principal **2** *n* POL eleição *f* primária
'primary school *Brit* escola *f* primária
prime [praɪm] **1** *n* ***be in one's*** **~** estar na flor da vida **2** *adj example, reason* primordial; ***of*** **~** ***importance*** de suma importância
prime 'minister primeiro-ministro *m*, primeira-ministra *f*
'prime time TV horário *m* de maior audiência
primitive ['prɪmɪtɪv] *adj* primitivo
prince [prɪns] príncipe *m*
princess ['prɪnses] princesa *f*
principal ['prɪnsəpl] **1** *adj* principal **2** *n of school* diretor,a *m,f*
principally ['prɪnsəplɪ] *adv* principalmente
principle ['prɪnsəpl] princípio *m*; ***on*** **~** por princípio; ***in*** **~** em princípio
print [prɪnt] **1** *n book, newspaper etc*: letra *f*; *(photograph)* impressão *f*; ***out of*** **~** *book* esgotado **2** *v/t book, newspaper, also* COMPUT imprimir; **~ *sth in block capitals*** *write* escrever algo com letras maiúsculas
◆**print out** *v/t* imprimir
printed matter ['prɪntɪd] material *m* impresso
printer ['prɪntər] *person* tipógrafo,-a *m,f*; *machine* impressora *f*
printing press ['prɪntɪŋ] imprensa *f*
'printout impressão *f*
prior ['praɪr] **1** *adj* prévio **2** *prep* **~ *to*** antes de
prioritize [praɪ'ɑ:rɪtaɪz] *v/t (put in order of priority)* priorizar; *(give priority to)* dar prioridade a
priority [praɪ'ɑ:rətɪ] prioridade *f*; ***have*** **~** ter prioridade
prison ['prɪzn] prisão *f*, cadeia *f*
prisoner ['prɪznər] prisioneiro,-a *m,f*; ***take s.o.*** **~** prender alguém
prisoner of 'war prisioneiro,-a *m,f* de guerra
privacy ['prɪvəsɪ] privacidade *f*
private ['praɪvət] **1** *adj* privado; *school, bathroom* particular; **~, *keep out*** *on sign* propriedade privada, mantenha-se fora **2** *n* MIL soldado *m* raso; ***in*** **~** em particular
privately ['praɪvətlɪ] *adv (in private)* em particular; *funded, owned* de iniciativa privada; *(inwardly)* no fundo
'private sector setor *m* privado
privatize ['praɪvətaɪz] *v/t* privatizar
privilege ['prɪvəlɪdʒ] *(special treatment)* privilégio *m*; *(honor)* honra *f*
privileged ['prɪvəlɪdʒd] *adj* privilegiado; *(honored)* honrado
prize [praɪz] **1** *n* prêmio *m* **2** *v/t* apreciar muito
'prizewinner premiado,-a *m,f*
'prizewinning *adj* premiado
pro[1] [proʊ] *n* ***the*** **~*s and cons*** os prós e os contras
pro[2] [proʊ] → ***professional***
pro[3] [proʊ] *prep (in favor of)* ***be*** **~ ...** estar a favor de ...
probability [prɑ:bə'bɪlətɪ] probabilidade *f*
probable ['prɑ:bəbl] *adj* provável
probably ['prɑ:bəblɪ] *adv* provavelmente
probation [prə'beɪʃn] *in job* probatório *m*; LAW liberdade *f* condicional
pro'bation officer encarregado,-a *m,f* pela liberdade condicional
pro'bation period *in job* estágio *m* probatório
probe [proʊb] **1** *n (investigation)* investigação *f*; *scientific* sondagem *f* **2** *v/t* examinar; *(investigate)* investigar
problem ['prɑ:bləm] problema *m*; ***no*** **~*!*** sem problema!

problematic ['prɑːbləmætɪk] *adj* problemático
procedure [prə'siːdʒər] procedimento *m*
proceed [prə'siːd] *v/i* (*go*) *people* dirigir-se; *work etc* correr; **~ *to do sth*** começar a fazer algo
proceedings [prə'siːdɪŋz] *npl* (*events*) evento *m*
proceeds ['prousiːdz] *npl* arrecadação *f*
process ['prɑːses] **1** *n* processo *m*; ***in the* ~** (*while doing it*) ao mesmo tempo **2** *v/t food, raw materials, data* processar; *application etc* tramitar
procession [prə'seʃn] desfile *m*
proclaim [prou'kleɪm] *v/t* declarar
prod [prɑːd] **1** *n* empurrãozinho *m* **2** *v/t* ⟨*pret & pp* ***prodded***⟩ *with elbow* cutucar
prodigy ['prɑːdɪdʒɪ] *n* (***infant***) ~ criança *f* prodígio
produce[1] ['prɑːduːs] *n* produtos *mpl* agrícolas
produce[2] [prə'duːs] *v/t* (*manufacture*) fabricar; *commodity, play, movie, TV program* produzir; (*bring about*) ocasionar; (*bring out*) tirar
producer [prə'duːsər] *commodity*: fabricante *m/f*; *rice, play, movie, TV program*: produtor,a *m,f*
product ['prɑːdʌkt] *also* (*outcome, result*) produto *m*
production [prə'dʌkʃn] *industry, play, movie, TV program*: produção *f*
pro'duction capacity capacidade *f* de produção
pro'duction costs custos *mpl* de produção
productive [prə'dʌktɪv] *adj factory, meeting* produtivo
productivity [prɑːdʌk'tɪvətɪ] produtividade *f*
profane [prə'feɪn] *adj language* profano
profess [prə'fes] *v/t* declarar
profession [prə'feʃn] profissão *f*
professional [prə'feʃnl] **1** *adj* profissional; ***turn* ~** tornar-se profissional; ***take* ~ *advice*** procurar ajuda profissional **2** *n doctor, lawyer etc* profissional *m/f*
professionally [prə'feʃnlɪ] *adv* profissionalmente
professor [prə'fesər] professor,a *m,f*
proficiency [prə'fɪʃnsɪ] competência *f*
proficient [prə'fɪʃnt] *adj* competente
profile ['proufaɪl] perfil *m*
profit ['prɑːfɪt] **1** *n* lucro *m* **2** *v/i* **~ *by,* ~ *from*** beneficiar-se de
profitability [prɑːfɪtə'bɪlətɪ] rentabilidade *f*
profitable ['prɑːfɪtəbl] *adj* lucrativo, rentável
'profit center *n* centro *m* de lucro
'profit margin margem *f* de lucro
profound [prə'faʊnd] *adj* profundo
profoundly [prə'faʊndlɪ] *adv* profundamente
prognosis [prɑːg'nousɪs] prognóstico *m*
program ['prougræm] *Am* **1** *n* RADIO, TV, *Brit also* COMPUT, THEA programa *m* **2** *v/t* ⟨*pret & pp* ***programmed***⟩ COMPUT programar
programme *Brit* → ***program***
programmer ['prougræmər] COMPUT programador,a *m,f*
progress 1 ['prɑːgres] *n* progresso *m*; ***make* ~** fazer progresso; ***in* ~** em andamento **2** [prə'gres] *v/i* (*advance in time*) avançar; (*move on*) passar; (*make progress*) ir; ***how is the work* ~*ing?*** como está indo o trabalho?
progressive [prə'gresɪv] *adj* (*enlightened*) progressista; (*which progresses*) progressivo
progressively [prə'gresɪvlɪ] *adv* progressivamente
prohibit [prə'hɪbɪt] *v/t* proibir
prohibition [prouhɪ'bɪʃn] proibição *f*; ***Prohibition*** a lei seca
prohibitive [prə'hɪbɪtɪv] *adj prices* proibitivo
project[1] ['prɑːdʒekt] *n* projeto *m*
project[2] [prə'dʒekt] **1** *v/t sales, movie, figures* projetar **2** *v/i* (*stick out*) sobressair
projection [prə'dʒekʃn] (*forecast*) previsão *f*
projector [prə'dʒektər] *slides*: retroprojetor *m*
prolific [prə'lɪfɪk] *adj writer, artist* prolífico

prolog ['proʊlɑːg] *Am* prólogo *m*
prologue *Brit* → ***prolog***
prolong [prə'lɑːŋ] *v/t* prolongar
prom [prɑːm] (*school dance*) baile *m* da escola
prominent ['prɑːmɪnənt] *adj nose, chin* proeminente; (*significant*) importante
promiscuity [prɑːmɪ'skjuːətɪ] promiscuidade *f*
promiscuous [prə'mɪskjʊəs] *adj* promíscuo
promise **1** *n* promessa *f* **2** *v/t* prometer; ***she ~d to help me*** ela prometeu me ajudar; ***~ X to Y*** prometer a X Y **3** *v/i* ***do you ~?*** você promete?
promising ['prɑːmɪsɪŋ] *adj* prometedor
promote [prə'moʊt] *v/t employee, good relations*, COM promover
promoter [prə'moʊtər] *sports event*: promotor,a *m,f*
promotion [prə'moʊʃn] *of employee, scheme*, COM promoção *f*
prompt [prɑːmpt] **1** *adj* (*on time*) pontual; (*speedy*) rápido **2** *adv* ***at two o'clock ~*** às duas horas em ponto **3** *v/t* (*cause*) provocar; *actor* dar a deixa **4** *n* COMPUT prompt *m*
promptly ['prɑːmptlɪ] *adv* (*on time*) na hora; (*immediately*) imediatamente
prone [proʊn] *adj* ***be ~ to*** ser propenso a
pronoun ['proʊnaʊn] pronome *m*
pronounce [prə'naʊns] *v/t word* pronunciar; (*declare*) declarar
pronounced [prə'naʊnst] *adj accent, views* forte
pronto ['prɑːntoʊ] *adv fam* já
pronunciation [prənʌnsɪ'eɪʃn] *n* pronúncia *f*
proof [pruːf] *n* prova *f*; *book*: prova *f* para revisão
prop [prɑːp] **1** *v/t* ⟨*pret & pp* ***propped***⟩ apoiar **2** *npl* THEA apetrechos *mpl*
◆ **prop up** *v/t also fig regime* apoiar
propaganda [prɑːpə'gændə] propaganda *f*
propel [prə'pel] *v/t* ⟨*pret & pp* ***propelled***⟩ propulsar
propellant [prə'pelənt] propelente *m*
propeller [prə'pelər] hélice *f*
proper ['prɑːpər] *adj* (*real*) de verdade; (*correct*) apropriado; (*fitting*) devido
properly ['prɑːpərlɪ] *adv* (*correctly*) corretamente; (*fittingly*) devidamente
property ['prɑːpərtɪ] propriedade *f*
'**property developer** corretor *m* imobiliário
prophecy ['prɑːfəsɪ] profecia *f*
prophesy ['prɑːfəsaɪ] *v/t* ⟨*pret & pp* ***prophesied***⟩ profetizar
proportion [prə'pɔːrʃn] proporção *f*; ***a large ~ of*** uma grande parte de
proportional [prə'pɔːrʃnl] *adj* proporcional
proportional represen'tation POL representação *f* proporcional
proposal [prə'poʊzl] (*suggestion*) proposta *f*; *of marriage* pedido *m*
propose [prə'poʊz] **1** *v/t* propor **2** *v/i* (*make offer of marriage*) propor casamento; ***~ to s.o.*** pedir alguém em casamento
proposition [prɑːpə'zɪʃn] **1** *n* proposta *f* **2** *v/t woman* fazer propostas a
proprietor [prə'praɪətər] proprietário,-a *m,f*
proprietress [prə'praɪətrɪs] proprietária *f*
prose [proʊz] prosa *f*
prosecute ['prɑːsɪkjuːt] *v/t* LAW processar
prosecution [prɑːsɪ'kjuːʃn] LAW acusação *f*
prosecutor [prɑːsɪ'kjuːtər] ***public ~*** promotor,a *m,f* público,-a
prospect ['prɑːspekt] **1** *n* (*chance, likelihood*) esperança *f*; *in the future* perspectiva *f*; ***~s*** perspectivas *fpl* **2** *v/i* ***~ for*** *gold* ir atrás de
prospective [prə'spektɪv] *adj* potencial
prosper ['prɑːspər] *v/i* prosperar
prosperity [prɑː'sperətɪ] prosperidade *f*
prosperous ['prɑːspərəs] *adj* próspero
prostitute ['prɑːstɪtuːt] *n* prostituta *f*; ***male ~*** prostituto *m*
prostitution [prɑːstɪ'tuːʃn] prostituição *f*

P

prostrate ['prɑːstreɪt] *adj* ***be ~ with grief*** estar prostrado pelo sofrimento
protection [prə'tekʃn] proteção *f*
pro'tection money taxa *f* de proteção
protective [prə'tektɪv] *adj* protetor
protective 'clothing roupa *f* protetora
protector [prə'tektər] protetor,a *m,f*
protein ['proʊtiːn] proteína *f*
protest 1 ['proʊtest] *n* protesto *m*; (*demonstration*) manifestação *f* **2** [prə'test] *v/t & v/i also* (*demonstrate*) protestar; *Am* (*object to*) protestar contra
Protestant ['prɑːtɪstənt] **1** *adj* protestante **2** *n* protestante *m/f*
protester [prə'testər] manifestante *m/f*
protocol ['proʊtəkɑːl] etiqueta *f*
prototype ['proʊtətaɪp] protótipo *m*
protracted [prə'træktɪd] *adj* prolongado
protrude [prə'truːd] *v/i* sobressair, sair
protruding [prə'truːdɪŋ] *adj ears, chin, teeth* proeminente
proud [praʊd] *adj* orgulhoso; (*independent*) arrogante; ***be ~ of*** estar orgulhoso de; ***we are ~ to announce that ...*** temos o orgulho de anunciar que ...
proudly ['praʊdlɪ] *adv* orgulhosamente
prove [pruːv] *v/t* provar
proverb ['prɑːvɜːrb] provérbio *m*
provide [prə'vaɪd] *v/t money, food, shelter, opportunity* fornecer; ***~ X with Y*** fornecer X com Y; ***~d (that)*** (*on condition that*) contanto que
♦ **provide for** *v/t family* manter; *law etc* prever
province ['prɑːvɪns] província *f*
provincial [prə'vɪnʃl] *adj city* provincial; *pej attitude* provinciano
provision [prə'vɪʒn] *food, water*: abastecimento *m*; *services*: fornecimento *m*; *law, contract*: provisão *f*; ***~s*** *pl* provisões *fpl*
provisional [prə'vɪʒnl] *adj* provisório
proviso [prə'vaɪzoʊ] condição *f*
provocation [prɑːvə'keɪʃn] provocação *f*
provocative [prə'vɑːkətɪv] *adj also sexually* provocativo
provoke [prə'voʊk] *v/t* (*cause, annoy*) provocar
prow [praʊ] *of ship* proa *f*
prowess ['praʊɪs] proeza *f*
prowl [praʊl] *v/i tiger, burglar* rondar
'prowl car carro *m* de patrulha
prowler ['praʊlər] rondante *m/f*
proximity [prɑːk'sɪmətɪ] proximidade *f*
proxy ['prɑːksɪ] (*authority*) procuradoria *f*; *person* procurador,a *m,f*
prude [pruːd] pudico,-a *m,f*
prudence ['pruːdns] prudência *f*
prudent ['pruːdnt] *adj* prudente
prudish ['pruːdɪʃ] *adj* pudico
prune[1] [pruːn] *n* ameixa *f* seca
prune[2] [pruːn] *v/t plant* podar; *fig* reduzir
pry [praɪ] *v/i* ⟨*pret & pp* ***pried***⟩ intrometer-se
♦ **pry into** *v/t* intrometer-se em
PS ['piːes] *abbr* (*of* ***postscript***) post scriptum (P.S.)
pseudonym ['suːdənɪm] pseudônimo *m*
psychiatric [saɪkɪ'ætrɪk] *adj* psiquiátrico
psychiatrist [saɪ'kaɪətrɪst] psiquiátra *m/f*
psychiatry [saɪ'kaɪətrɪ] psiquiatria *f*
psychic ['saɪkɪk] *adj* psíquico
psychoanalyse → ***psychoanalyze***
psychoanalysis [saɪkoʊən'æləsɪs] psicanálise *f*
psychoanalyst [saɪkoʊ'ænəlɪst] psicanalista *m/f*
psychoanalyze [saɪkoʊ'ænəlaɪz] *v/t* psicanalizar
psychological [saɪkə'lɑːdʒɪkl] *adj* psicológico
psychologically [saɪkə'lɑːdʒɪklɪ] *adv* psicologicamente
psychologist [saɪ'kɑːlədʒɪst] psicólogo,-a *m,f*
psychology [saɪ'kɑːlədʒɪ] psicologia *f*
psychopath ['saɪkoʊpæθ] psicopata *m/f*
psychosomatic [saɪkoʊsə'mætɪk] *adj* psicossomático

P

PTO [piːtiː'oʊ] *abbr* (*of* ***please turn over***) vire

pub [pʌb] *Brit* bar *m*

puberty ['pjuːbərtɪ] puberdade *f*

pubic hair ['pjuːbɪk] pêlos *mpl* púbicos; *single* pêlo *m* púbico

public ['pʌblɪk] **1** *adj* público **2** *n* ***the*** ~ o público; ***in*** ~ em público

publication [pʌblɪ'keɪʃn] publicação *f*

public 'holiday *Brit* feriado *m* público

publicity [pʌb'lɪsətɪ] publicidade *f*

publicize ['pʌblɪsaɪz] *v/t* (*make known*) publicar; COM fazer publicidade de

public 'library biblioteca *f* pública

public limited 'company *Brit* companhia limitada

publicly ['pʌblɪklɪ] *adv* publicamente

public 'prosecutor promotor,a *m,f* público **public re'lations** *npl* relações *fpl* públicas **'public school** *Am* escola *f* pública; *Brit* escola *f* particular **'public sector** setor *m* público

publish ['pʌblɪʃ] *v/t* publicar

publisher ['pʌblɪʃər] editor,a *m,f*

publishing ['pʌblɪʃɪŋ] área *f* editorial

'publishing company editora *f*

puddle ['pʌdl] *n* poça *f*

puff [pʌf] **1** *n of wind* rajada *f*; ***a ~ of smoke*** uma nuvenzinha de fumaça **2** *v/i* (*pant*) ofegar; ***~ on a cigarette*** dar uma baforada num cigarro

puffy ['pʌfɪ] *adj eyes, face* inchado

puke [pjuːk] *v/i fam* vomitar

pull [pʊl] **1** *n rope*: puxada *f*; *fam* (*appeal*) atração *f*; *fam* (*influence*) influência *f* **2** *v/t* (*drag*) puxar; (*tug*) arrastar; *tooth* arrancar; *muscle* estirar **3** *v/i* puxar

◆**pull ahead** *v/i in race, competition* levar a frente

◆**pull apart** *v/t* (*separate*) separar

◆**pull away 1** *v/t* ***pull sth away from s.o.*** afastar algo de alguém **2** *v/i vehicle* afastar-se

◆**pull down** *v/t* (*lower*) abaixar; (*demolish*) demolir

◆**pull in** *v/i bus, train* chegar

◆**pull off** *v/t leaves etc* tirar; *fam* conseguir; ***he pulled it off!*** ele conseguiu!

◆**pull out 1** *v/t also troops* retirar **2** *v/i of an agreement, a competition, troops* retirar-se; *ship* sair

◆**pull over** *v/i driver* encostar

◆**pull through** *v/i from an illness* recuperar-se

◆**pull together 1** *v/i* (*cooperate*) cooperar **2** *v/t* ***pull oneself together*** (*make an effort*) aplicar-se; (*calm down*) acalmar-se

◆**pull up 1** *v/t* (*raise*) tirar; *plant, weeds* arrancar **2** *v/i car etc* parar

pulley ['pʊlɪ] polia *f*

pullover ['pʊloʊvər] pulôver *m*

pulp [pʌlp] *also paper-making*: pasta *f*; *fruit*: polpa *f*

pulpit ['pʊlpɪt] púlpito *m*

pulsate [pʌl'seɪt] *v/i heart, blood* pulsar; *rhythm* vibrar

pulse [pʌls] pulso *m* (*batimento*)

pulverize ['pʌlvəraɪz] *v/t* pulverizar

pump [pʌmp] **1** *n* bomba *f* **2** *v/t* bombear

◆**pump up** *v/t* inflar

pumpkin ['pʌmpkɪn] moranga *f*

pun [pʌn] jogo *m* de palavras

punch [pʌntʃ] **1** *n blow* bofetão *m*, murro *m*; *implement* perfurador *m* **2** *v/t with fist* esbofetear, esmurrar; *hole, ticket* perfurar

'punch line graça *f*

punctual ['pʌŋktʃʊəl] *adj* pontual

punctuality [pʌŋktʃʊ'ælətɪ] pontualidade *f*

punctually ['pʌŋktʃʊəlɪ] *adv* pontualmente

punctuate ['pʌŋktjuːeɪt] *v/t* pontuar

punctuation [pʌŋktʃʊ'eɪʃn] pontuação *f*

punctu'ation mark sinal *m* de pontuação

puncture ['pʌŋktʃər] **1** *n* perfuração *f* **2** *v/t* perfurar

pungent ['pʌndʒənt] *adj* forte

punish ['pʌnɪʃ] *v/t* punir

punishing ['pʌnɪʃɪŋ] *adj pace, schedule* cansativo

punishment ['pʌnɪʃmənt] punição *f*, castigo *m*

punk [pʌŋk] MUS música *f* punk

puny ['pjuːnɪ] *adj person* raquítico

P

pup [pʌp] cachorrinho *m*
pupil[1] ['pju:pl] *eye*: pupila *f*
pupil[2] ['pju:pl] (*student*) aluno,-a *m,f*
puppet ['pʌpɪt] marionete *f*
'puppet government governo *m* fantoche
puppy ['pʌpɪ] cachorrinho *m*
purchase[1] ['pɜ:rtʃəs] **1** *n* aquisição *f* **2** *v/t* comprar
purchase[2] ['pɜ:rtʃəs] (*grip*) pega *f*
purchaser ['pɜ:rtʃəsər] comprador,a *m,f*
pure [pjʊr] *adj silk, air, water etc also* (*morally*) puro; *sound* nítido
purely ['pjʊrlɪ] *adv* puramente
purgatory ['pɜ:rgətɔ:rɪ] purgatório *m*
purge [pɜ:rdʒ] **1** *n political party*: expurgação *f* **2** *v/t* purgar
purify ['pjʊrɪfaɪ] *v/t* ⟨*pret & pp* ***purified***⟩ *water* depurar
puritan ['pjʊrɪtən] puritano,-a *m,f*
puritanical [pjʊrɪ'tænɪkl] *adj* puritano
purity ['pjʊrɪtɪ] (*moral*), *air, voice*: pureza *f*
purple ['pɜ:rpl] *adj* púrpura
Purple 'Heart *Am* MIL *medalha concedida a soldados americanos feridos em combate*
purpose ['pɜ:rpəs] objetivo *m*; ***on ~*** de propósito
purposeful ['pɜ:rpəsfʊl] *adj* decidido
purposely ['pɜ:rpəslɪ] *adv* de propósito
purr [pɜ:r] *v/i cat* ronronar
purse [pɜ:rs] *n Am* (*pocket book*) bolsa *f*; *Brit for money* carteira *f*
pursue [pər'su:] *v/t person* perseguir; *career* aspirar; *course of action* prosseguir
pursuer [pər'su:ər] perseguidor,a *m,f*
pursuit [pər'su:t] (*chase*) perseguição *f*; *of happiness etc* busca *f*; (*activity*) atividade *f*; ***those in ~*** os perseguidores
pus [pʌs] pus *m*
push [pʊʃ] **1** *n* (*shove*) empurrão *m*; ***at the ~ of a button*** apertando um botão **2** *v/t* (*shove*) empurrar; *button* apertar; (*pressurize*) pressionar; *fam drugs* vender; ***be ~ed for*** *fam* estar curto de; ***be ~ing 40*** *fam* estar chegando aos 40 **3** *v/i* empurrar
♦**push ahead** *v/i* seguir adiante
♦**push along** *v/t cart etc* empurrar
♦**push away** *v/t* afastar
♦**push off 1** *v/t lid* destampar **2** *v/i Brit fam* (*leave*) dar no pé; ***push off!*** vá embora!
♦**push on** *v/i* (*continue*) continuar
♦**push up** *v/t prices* aumentar
'pushchair *Brit* carrinho *m*
pusher ['pʊʃər] *fam of drugs* traficante *m*
'push-up *do ~s* fazer flexões *fpl*
pushy ['pʊʃɪ] *adj fam* controlador
pussy, pussy cat ['pʊsɪ (kæt)] *fam* gatinho,-a *m,f*
♦**pussyfoot about** ['pʊsɪfʊt] *v/i fam* ficar enrolando
put [pʊt] *v/t* ⟨*pret & pp* ***put***⟩ pôr; *question* fazer; ***~ the cost at …*** estimar os custos em …
♦**put across** *v/t idea etc* fazer chegar
♦**put aside** *v/t money* economizar; *work* deixar de lado
♦**put away** *v/t in closet etc* guardar; *in institution* encerrar; (*consume*) consumir; *money* economizar; *Am animal* sacrificar
♦**put back** *v/t* (*replace*) repor
♦**put by** *v/t money* economizar
♦**put down** *v/t* (*set down*), *deposit* deixar; *rebellion* reprimir; (*belittle*) *person* rebaixar; *in writing* escrever; ***put one's foot down*** *in car* pisar fundo; (*be firm*) bater o pé; ***put sth down to sth*** (*attribute*) atribuir algo a algo
♦**put forward** *v/t idea etc* propor
♦**put in** *v/t* colocar; *time* dedicar; *request, claim* apresentar; ***put it in your pocket*** coloque no seu bolso
♦**put in for** *v/t* (*apply for*) solicitar
♦**put off** *v/t radio, TV, machine* desligar; *light* apagar; (*postpone*) adiar; (*deter*) desanimar; (*repel*) fazer perder a vontade; ***put X off Y*** desencorajar X de Y
♦**put on** *v/t radio, TV* ligar; *light* acender; *tape, music, jacket, shoes, eye glasses* pôr; *parking brake* puxar; (*perform*) apresentar; (*assume*) fingir; ***put on makeup*** colocar maquiagem; ***put on weight*** engordar; ***she's just putting it on*** ela só está fingindo; ***you're***

putting me on! *fam* você está brincando!
◆**put out** *v/t hand* estender; *fire, light* apagar
◆**put through** *v/t on phone* passar
◆**put together** *v/t* (*assemble*) montar; (*organize*) organizar
◆**put up** *v/t hand, fence, building* levantar; *person* alojar; *prices* aumentar; *poster, notice* colocar; *money* disponibilizar; ***put up for sale*** pôr à venda
◆**put up with** *v/t* (*tolerate*) agüentar
putt [pʌt] *n* SPORT putt *m*
putty ['pʌtɪ] massa *f* de vidraceiro
puzzle ['pʌzl] **1** *n* (*mystery*) mistério *m*; ***jigsaw ~*** quebra-cabeças *m*; ***crossword ~*** palavras *fpl* cruzadas **2** *v/t* desconcertar
puzzling ['pʌzlɪŋ] *adj* dificíl de compreender
PVC [pi:vi:'si:] *abbr* (*of* ***polyvinyl chloride***) policloreto *m* de vinila (PVC *m*)
pyjamas *Brit* → ***pajamas***
pylon ['paɪlən] poste *m de fios elétricos*

Q

quack[1] [kwæk] **1** *n duck*: grasnido *m* **2** *v/i* grasnar
quack[2] [kwæk] *fam* (*bad doctor*) charlatão *m*
quadrangle ['kwɑ:dræŋgl] *figure* quadrângulo *m*; (*courtyard*) pátio *m*
quadruped ['kwɑ:drʊped] quadrúpede *m*
quadruple ['kwɑ:drʊpl] *v/i* quadruplicar
quadruplets ['kwɑ:drʊplɪts] *npl* quadrigêmeos *mpl*
quads [kwɑ:dz] *npl fam* quadrigêmeos *mpl*
quagmire ['kwɑ:gmaɪr] *fig* atoleiro *m*
quail [kweɪl] *v/i* ficar amedrontado
quaint [kweɪnt] *adj cottage* pitoresco; (*slightly eccentric*) *ideas etc* esquisito
quake [kweɪk] **1** *n* (*earthquake*) terremoto *m*, *Port* terramoto *f* **2** *v/i earth, with fear* tremer
qualification [kwɑ:lfɪ'keɪʃn] *university etc*: qualificação *f*; *of remark etc* restrição *f*; ***have the right ~s for a job*** estar bem qualificado para um trabalho
qualified ['kwɑ:lɪfaɪd] *adj doctor, engineer etc* capacitado; (*restricted*) limitado; ***I am not ~ to judge*** não estou na posição de poder julgar
qualify ['kwɑ:lɪfaɪ] ⟨*pret & pp* ***qualified***⟩ **1** *v/t degree, course etc* habilitar; *remark etc* restringir **2** *v/i* (*get degree etc*) habilitar-se; *in competition* ser qualificado; ***our team has qualified for the semi-final*** nosso time foi qualificado para a semi-final; ***that doesn't ~ as ...*** isto não pode ser considerado como ...
quality ['kwɑ:lətɪ] qualidade *f*
quality con'trol controle *m* de qualidade
qualm [kwɑ:m] adj escrúpulo *m*; ***have no ~s about doing sth*** não ter escrúpulos em fazer algo
quandary ['kwɑ:ndərɪ] dilema *m*
quantify ['kwɑ:ntɪfaɪ] *v/t* ⟨*pret & pp* ***quantified***⟩ quantificar
quantity ['kwɑ:ntətɪ] quantidade *f*
quantum physics ['kwɑ:ntəm] física *f* quântica
quarantine ['kwɑ:rənti:n] quarentena *f*
quarrel ['kwɑ:rəl] **1** *n* briga *f* **2** *v/i* ⟨*pret & pp* ***quarreled***, *Brit* ***quarrelled***⟩ brigar
quarrelsome ['kwɑ:rəlsʌm] *adj* brigalhão (brigalhona)
quarry[1] ['kwɑ:rɪ] *hunting*: caça *f*
quarry[2] ['kwɑ:rɪ] *mining*: pedreira *f*

quart [kwɔːrt] quarto *m* de galão
quarter ['kwɔːrtər] **1** *n* quarto *m*; (*25 cents*) quarto *m* de dólar; (*part of town*) bairro *m*; ***a ~ of an hour*** um quarto de hora; ***it's a ~ of 5*** são quinze para as cinco, *Port* são cinco menos um quarto; ***it's a ~ after 5*** são cinco e quinze, *Port* são cinco e um quarto **2** *v/t* dividir em quatro partes
'**quarterback** SPORT lançador *m*
quarter-'final quarta-de-final *f*
quarter-'finalist quarto-finalista *m*, quarta-finalista *f*
quarterly ['kwɔːrtərlɪ] **1** *adj* trimestral **2** *adv* trimestralmente
'**quarternote** *Am* MUS semínima *f*
quarters ['kwɔːrtərz] *npl* MIL quartel *m*
quartet [kwɔːr'tet] MUS quarteto *m*
quartz [kwɑːrts] quartzo *m*
quash [kwɑːʃ] *v/t rebellion* sufocar; *court decision* revogar
quaver ['kweɪvər] **1** *n voice*: tremor *m* **2** *v/i voice* estremecer
quay [kiː] cais *m*
'**quayside** cais *m*
queasy ['kwiːzɪ] *adj* enjoado
queen [kwiːn] rainha *f*
'**queen bee** abelha *f* rainha
queer [kwɪr] *adj* (*peculiar*) esquisito
queerly ['kwɪrlɪ] *adv* estranhamente
quell [kwel] *v/t* acalmar
quench [kwentʃ] *v/t thirst* saciar; *flames* apagar
query ['kwɪrɪ] **1** *n* (*question*) pergunta *f*; (*doubt*) dúvida *f* **2** *v/t* ⟨*pret & pp* ***queried***⟩ (*express doubt about*) questionar; (*check*) checar; ***~ sth with s.o.*** checar algo com alguém
quest [kwest] busca *f*
question ['kwestʃn] **1** *n also* (*matter*) questão *f*; ***in ~*** (*being talked about*) em questão; (*in doubt*) em dúvida; ***it's a ~ of money*** é uma questão de dinheiro; ***that's out of the ~*** isto está fora de cogitação **2** *v/t* questionar; LAW interrogar
questionable ['kwestʃnəbl] *adj honesty* duvidoso; *figures*, *statement* questionável
questioning ['kwestʃnɪŋ] **1** *adj look*, *tone* inquisitivo **2** *n* interrogatório *m*
'**question mark** ponto *m* de interrogação
questionnaire [kwestʃə'ner] questionário *m*
queue [kjuː] *Brit* **1** *n* fila *f*, *Port* bicha *f*; ***form a ~*** fazer uma fila, *Port* fazer bicha **2** *v/i* ***I ~d for hours*** fiquei na fila por horas
quibble ['kwɪbl] *v/i* discutir por tolices
quick [kwɪk] *adj* rápido; ***be ~!*** apresse-se!; ***let's have a ~ drink*** vamos tomar algo rapidinho?; ***can I have a ~ look?*** posso dar uma olhadinha?; ***that was ~!*** foi rapidíssimo!
quickie ['kwɪkɪ] *fam* (*quick drink*) pinguinha *f*
quickly ['kwɪklɪ] *adv* rapidamente
'**quicksand** areia *f* movediça '**quicksilver** mercúrio *m* **quickwitted** [kwɪk'wɪtɪd] *adj* perspicaz
quid [kwɪd] *Brit fam* libra *f*
quiet ['kwaɪət] *adj voice*, *music*, *street*, *life*, *town* tranqüilo; *engine* silencioso; ***keep ~ about sth*** não falar sobre algo; ***~!*** fique quieto!
♦ **quieten down** ['kwaɪətn] **1** *v/t children*, *class* acalmar **2** *v/i children*, *political situation* acalmar-se
quietness ['kwaɪətnɪs] tranqüilidade *f*
quilt [kwɪlt] *on bed* edredom *m*, *Port* edredão *m*
quilted ['kwɪltɪd] *adj* acolchoado
quinine ['kwɪniːn] quinina *f*
quintet [kwɪn'tet] MUS quinteto *m*
quip [kwɪp] **1** *n* piada *f*; *remark* indireta *f* **2** *v/i* ⟨*pret & pp* ***quipped***⟩ brincar
quirk [kwɜːrk] esquisitice *f*
quirky ['kwɜːrkɪ] *adj* estranho
quit [kwɪt] ⟨*pret & pp* ***quit***⟩ **1** *v/t job* abandonar; ***~ doing sth*** deixar de fazer algo **2** *v/i* (*leave job*) demitir-se; COMPUT sair; ***get one's notice to ~*** *from landlord* rescindir o contrato de arrendamento
quite [kwaɪt] *adv* (*fairly*) bastante; (*completely*) completamente; ***not ~ ready*** não totalmente pronto; ***I didn't ~ understand*** não entendi bem; ***is that right? – not ~*** isto está correto? - não totalmente; ***~!***

exatamente!; **~ a lot** muito; **~ a few** vários; ***it was ~ a surprise / change*** até que foi uma surpresa / mudança!

quits [kwɪts] *adj* ***be ~ with s.o.*** estar quite com alguém

quitter ['kwɪtər] *fam* ***she's not a ~*** ela não é uma desistente

quiver ['kwɪvər] *v/i* tremer

quiz [kwɪz] **1** *n TV*: programa *m* de perguntas e respostas; *magazine, newspaper*: jogo *m* de perguntas e respostas; *Am school*: prova *f* **2** *v/t* ⟨*pret & pp* **quizzed**⟩ interrogar

'quiz master apresentador,a *m,f* de programa de perguntas e respostas **'quiz program** *Am* programa *m* de perguntas e respostas **quiz programme** *Brit* → ***quiz program***

quota ['kwoʊtə] cota *f*

quotation [kwoʊ'teɪʃn] *from author* citação *f*; *commerce*: cotação *f*; ***give s.o. a ~ for sth*** dar a alguém uma cotação por algo

quo'tation marks *npl* aspas *fpl*

quote [kwoʊt] **1** *n author*: citação *f*; (*price*) cota *f*; **~s** (*quotation marks*) aspas *fpl*; ***in ~s*** entre aspas **2** *v/t text* citar; *price* dar **3** *v/i* ***~ from an author*** citar um autor

R

rabbi ['ræbaɪ] rabino *m*

rabbit ['ræbɪt] coelho *m*

rabble ['ræbl] multidão *f*

rabble-rouser ['ræblraʊzər] agitador,a *m,f*

rabies ['reɪbi:z] *nsg* raiva *f*

raccoon [rə'ku:n] racum *m*

race[1] [reɪs] *n people* raça *f*

race[2] [reɪs] **1** *n* SPORT corrida *f*; ***the ~s*** *horse races* a corrida de cavalos **2** *v/i* (*run fast*), SPORT correr; ***he ~d through his meal / work*** ele comeu / trabalhou correndo **3** *v/t* ***I'll ~ you!*** corrida!

'race car *Am* carro *m* de corrida **'racecourse** hipódromo *m* **'race driver** *Am* piloto,-a *m,f* de corrida **'racehorse** cavalo *m* de corrida **'race riot** tumulto *m* racial **'racetrack** autódromo *m*; *Am horses*: hipódromo *m*

racial ['reɪʃl] *adj* racial; ***~ equality*** igualdade *f* racial

racing ['reɪsɪŋ] corrida *f*

'racing car *Brit* carro *m* de corrida

'racing driver *Brit* piloto,-a *m,f* de corrida

racism ['reɪsɪzm] racismo *m*

racist ['reɪsɪst] **1** *adj* racista **2** *n* racista *m/f*

rack [ræk] **1** *n transporting bikes*: porta-bicicleta *m*; *bags on train*: porta-bagagem *m*; *CDs*: estante *f* para CD, rack *m* para CD **2** *v/t* ***~ one's brains*** quebrar a cabeça

racket[1] ['rækɪt] SPORT raquete *f*, *Port* raqueta *f*

racket[2] ['rækɪt] *noise* barulheira *f*; (*criminal activity*) fraude *f*

radar ['reɪdɑ:r] radar *m*

'radar screen tela *f* de radar

'radar trap radar *m* fixo

radial tire ['reɪdɪəl] *Am* pneu *m* radial

radial tyre *Brit* → ***radial tire***

radiance ['reɪdɪəns] brilho *m*

radiant ['reɪdɪənt] *adj smile, appearance* radiante

radiate ['reɪdɪeɪt] *v/i heat, light* irradiar

radiation [reɪdɪ'eɪʃn] PHYS radiação *f*

radiator ['reɪdɪeɪtər] *room, car*: radiador *m*

radical ['rædɪkl] **1** *adj* radical **2** *n* POL radical *m/f*

radicalism ['rædɪkəlɪzm] POL radicalismo *m*

radically ['rædɪklɪ] *adv* radicalmente

radio ['reɪdɪoʊ] rádio *f*; (*set*) rádio *m*; ***on the ~*** no rádio; ***by ~*** por radio
radio'active *adj* radioativo **radioactive 'waste** resíduos *mpl* radioativos **radioac'tivity** radioatividade *f* **'radio alarm** rádio-relógio *m*
radiographer [reɪdɪ'ɑːgrəfər] *n* radiologista *m/f*
radiography [reɪdɪ'ɑːgrəfɪ] radiografia *f*
'radio station estação *f* de rádio **'radio taxi** radiotáxi *m* **radio'therapy** radioterapia *f*
radish ['rædɪʃ] rabanete *m*
radius ['reɪdɪəs] raio *m*
raffle ['ræfl] *n* rifa *f*
raft [ræft] balsa *f*
rafter ['ræftər] viga *f*
rag [ræg] *n cleaning*: trapo *m*; ***in ~s*** com trapos
rage [reɪdʒ] **1** *n* raiva *f*; ***be in a ~*** estar furioso; ***be all the ~*** *fam* estar na moda **2** *v/i person* enfurecer-se; *storm* bramar
ragged ['rægɪd] *adj* esfarrapado
raid [reɪd] **1** *n troops*, FIN incursão *f*; *police*: batida *f* policial; *robbers*: assalto *m* **2** *v/t troops*, *police* fazer uma incursão em; *robbers* assaltar; *fridge*, *orchard* saquear
raider ['reɪdər] *bank*: assaltante *m/f*
rail [reɪl] *n track*: trilho *m*; (*handrail*) corrimão *m*; *towel*: grade *f*, ***by ~*** de trem
railings ['reɪlɪŋz] *around park etc* cerca *f*
'railroad *Am* estrada *f* de ferro, *Port* caminho *m* de ferro **'railroad station** *Am* estação *f* ferroviária, *Port* estação *f* de caminho de ferro **'railway** *Brit* estrada *f* de ferro, *Port* caminho *m* de ferro **'railway station** *Brit* estação *f* ferroviária, *Port* estação *f* de caminho de ferro
rain [reɪn] **1** *n* chuva *f*; ***in the ~*** na chuva; ***the ~s*** (*rainy season*) a estação chuvosa **2** *v/i* chover; ***it's ~ing*** está chovendo, *Port* está a chover
'rainbow arco-íris *m* **'raincheck *can I take a ~ on that?*** *Am fam* eu poderia adiar para uma outra data? **'raincoat** capa *f* de chuva **'raindrop** gota *f* de chuva **'rainfall** chuva *f* **'rain forest** floresta *f* pluvial **'rainproof** *adj fabric* à prova d'água **'rainstorm** tempestade *f*
rainy ['reɪnɪ] *adj* chuvoso; ***it's ~*** está chovendo muito
'rainy season estação *f* chuvosa
raise [reɪz] **1** *n salary*: aumento *m* **2** *v/t shelf etc* levantar; *offer* aumentar; *children* criar; *question* lançar; *money* arrecadar
raisin ['reɪzn] uva *f* passa
rake [reɪk] *n garden*: rastrilho *m*
♦ **rake up** *v/t leaves* rastrear; *fig* trazer à luz
rally ['rælɪ] *n* (*meeting*, *reunion*) comício *m*; MOT, *tennis*: rally *m*
♦ **rally around** ⟨*pret & pp* ***rallied***⟩ **1** *v/i* acudir **2** *v/t* ***rally around s.o.*** acudir alguém
RAM [ræm] *abbr* (*of* ***random access memory***) COMPUT memória *f* de acesso randômico, memória *f* RAM
ram [ræm] **1** *n* carneiro *m* **2** *v/t* ⟨*pret & pp* ***rammed***⟩ *ship*, *car* bater
ramble ['ræmbl] **1** *n walk* caminhada *f* **2** *v/i* caminhar; *speaking*: divagar
rambler ['ræmblər] caminhador,a *m,f*
rambling ['ræmblɪŋ] **1** *n* caminhadas *fpl*; *speech*: divagações *fpl* **2** *adj speech* divagante
ramp [ræmp] rampa *f*, *raising vehicle*: elevador *m* automotivo
rampage ['ræmpeɪdʒ] **1** *v/i* ***they ~d through the streets*** praticaram vandalismo pelas ruas **2** *n* ***go on the ~*** praticar vandalismo
rampant ['ræmpənt] *adj inflation* galopante
rampart ['ræmpɑːrt] muralha *f* (de defesa)
ramshackle ['ræmʃækl] *adj* acabado
ran [ræn] *pret* → ***run***
ranch [ræntʃ] rancho *m*
rancher ['ræntʃər] rancheiro,-a *m,f*
rancid ['rænsɪd] *adj* rançoso
rancor ['ræŋkər] rancor *m*
rancour *Brit* → ***rancor***
R & D [ɑːrən'diː] *abbr* (*of* ***research and development***) pesquisa *f* e desenvolvimento *m*

random ['rændəm] **1** *adj* aleatório; **~ sample** amostra *f* aleatória **2** *n* **at ~** a esmo
randy ['rændɪ] *adj Brit fam* tesudo; ***it makes me ~*** isso me deixa com tesão
rang [ræŋ] *pret* → ***ring***[2]
range [reɪndʒ] **1** *n products*: gama *f*; *voice, gun, airplane*: alcance *m*; *mountains*: cadeia *f*; ***at close ~*** de perto **2** *v/i* **~ *from X to Y*** ir de X até Y
ranger ['reɪndʒər] *Am* guarda *m* florestal
rank [ræŋk] **1** *n* MIL posto *f*; *society*: posição *f*; ***the ~s*** a tropa **2** *v/t* classificar
♦ **rank among** *v/t* figurar entre
rankle ['ræŋkl] *v/i* causar amargura
ransack ['rænsæk] *v/t* saquear
ransom ['rænsəm] *n* resgate *m*; ***hold s.o. to ~*** pedir resgate por alguém
'**ransom money** (dinheiro *m* do) resgate *m*
rant [rænt] *v/i* **~ *and rave*** desvairar
rap [ræp] **1** *n at door etc* batida *f*; MUS rap *m* **2** *v/t* ⟨*pret & pp* ***rapped***⟩ *table etc* bater
♦ **rap at** *v/t window etc* bater em
rape[1] [reɪp] **1** *n* estupro *m* **2** *v/t* estuprar
rape[2] [reɪp] *n* BOT colza *f*
'**rape victim** vítima *f* de estupro
rapid ['ræpɪd] *adj* rápido
rapidity [rə'pɪdətɪ] rapidez *f*
rapidly ['ræpɪdlɪ] *adv* rapidamente
rapids ['ræpɪdz] *npl* correntes *fpl*
rapist ['reɪpɪst] estuprador *m*
rapport [ræ'pɔːr] relacionamento *m*
rapture ['ræptʃər] ***go into ~s over*** entusiasmar-se com
rapturous ['ræptʃərəs] *adj* entusiasmado
rare [rer] *adj* raro; *steak* malpassado
rarely ['rerlɪ] *adv* raramente
rarity ['rerətɪ] raridade *f*
rash[1] [ræʃ] *n* MED eczema *m*
rash[2] [ræʃ] *adj action, behavior* precipitado
rashly ['ræʃlɪ] *adv* precipitadamente
raspberry ['ræzberɪ] framboesa *f*
rat [ræt] *n* rato *m*, *Port* ratazana *f*
rate [reɪt] **1** *n exchange*: taxa *f* (de câmbio); *pay*: tarifa *f*; (*price*) preço *m*; (*speed*) ritmo *m*; **~ *of interest*** FIN taxa *f* de juros; ***at this ~*** (*at this speed*) neste ritmo; (*carrying on like this*) deste jeito; ***at any ~*** em todo caso **2** *v/t* (*consider, rank*) considerar
rather ['ræðər] *adv* muito; ***I would ~ stay here*** eu preferiria ficar aqui; ***or would you ~ ...?*** ou você preferiria ...?
ratification [rætɪfɪ'keɪʃn] ratificação *f*
ratify ['rætɪfaɪ] *v/t* ⟨*pret & pp* ***ratified***⟩ ratificar
ratings ['reɪtɪŋz] *npl* índice *m* de audiência
ratio ['reɪʃɪoʊ] proporção *f*
ration ['ræʃn] **1** *n* ração *f* **2** *v/t supplies* racionar
rational ['ræʃənl] *adj* racional
rationality [ræʃə'nælɪtɪ] racionabilidade *f*
rationalization [ræʃənəlaɪ'zeɪʃn] racionalização *f*
rationalize ['ræʃənəlaɪz] *v/t & v/i* racionalizar
rationally ['ræʃənlɪ] *adv* racionalmente
'**rat race *he decided to get out of the ~*** decidiu livrar-se da competição da vida moderna
rattle ['rætl] **1** *n noise* tilintar *m*; *toy* chocalho *m* **2** *v/t chains etc* entrechocar **3** *v/i chains etc* entrechocar-se; *crates* bater
♦ **rattle off** *v/t poem, list of names* dizer rapidamente
♦ **rattle through** *v/t* fazer rapidamente
'**rattlesnake** cascavel *f*
raucous ['rɔːkəs] *adj laughter, party* estridente
ravage ['rævɪdʒ] **1** *n* ***the ~s of time*** as marcas do tempo **2** *v/t* **~*d by war*** destruído pela guerra
rave [reɪv] **1** *v/i* (*talk deliriously*) delirar; (*talk wildly*) desvairar; **~ *about sth*** (*be very enthusiastic*) estar muito entusiasmado com algo **2** *n party* festa *f* tecno
raven ['reɪvn] corvo *m*
ravenous ['rævənəs] *adj appetite* voraz
ravenously ['rævənəslɪ] *adv* vorazmente

'rave review crítica *f* entusiástica
ravine [rə'viːn] ravina *f*
raving ['reɪvɪŋ] *adj* **~ *mad*** doido varrido
ravioli [rævɪ'oʊlɪ] ravioli *m*
ravishing ['rævɪʃɪŋ] *adj* encantador
raw [rɒː] *adj meat, vegetable* cru; *sugar* não refinado; *iron* não tratado
raw ma'terials *npl* matéria-prima *f*
ray [reɪ] raio *m*; ***a ~ of hope*** um raio de esperança
raze [reɪz] *v/t* **~ *to the ground*** assolar
razor ['reɪzər] barbeador *m*
'razor blade lâmina *f* de barbear
re [riː] *prep* COM com referência a
reach [riːtʃ] **1** *n* ***within ~*** ao alcance; ***out of ~*** fora de alcance **2** *v/t city etc* chegar em; *decision, agreement* chegar a; ***can you ~ it?*** você alcança?
♦**reach out** *v/i* estender o braço
react [rɪ'ækt] *v/i* reagir
reaction [rɪ'ækʃn] reação *f*
reactionary [rɪ'ækʃnrɪ] POL **1** *adj* reacionário **2** *n* reacionário,-a *m,f*
reactor [rɪ'æktər] *nuclear* reator *m*
read [riːd] ⟨*pret & pp* ***read*** [red]⟩ **1** *v/t* ler **2** *v/i* ler; **~ *to s.o.*** ler para alguém
♦**read out** *v/t* (*read aloud*) ler em voz alta
♦**read up on** *v/t* estudar
readable ['riːdəbl] *adj handwriting* legível; *book* interessante
reader ['riːdər] *person* leitor,a *m,f*
readily ['redɪlɪ] *adv admit, agree* com prazer
readiness ['redɪnɪs] *for action, to agree* prontidão *f*
reading ['riːdɪŋ] *also from meter etc* leitura *f*
'reading matter leitura *f*
readjust [riːə'dʒʌst] **1** *v/t* reajustar **2** *v/i to conditions* readaptar-se
read-'only file COMPUT arquivo *m* somente para leitura
read-'only memory COMPUT memória *f* somente para leitura
ready ['redɪ] *adj prepared* pronto; (*willing*) disposto; ***get*** (***oneself***) **~** preparar-se; ***get sth ~*** preparar algo
ready 'cash dinheiro *m* vivo **ready-'made** *stew etc, solution* pronto
'ready-to-wear moda *f* pronta
real [riːl] *adj* verdadeiro
'real estate bens *mpl* imóveis
'real estate agent corretor,a *m,f* de imóveis, *Port* agente *m/f* imobiliário,-a
realism ['rɪəlɪzəm] realismo *m*
realist ['rɪəlɪst] realista *m/f*
realistic [rɪə'lɪstɪk] *adj* realista
realistically [rɪə'lɪstɪklɪ] *adv* realisticamente
reality [rɪ'ælətɪ] realidade *f*; ***in ~*** na realidade
re'ality TV reality shows *mpl*
realization [rɪəlaɪ'zeɪʃn] realização *f*; (*understanding*) percepção *f*
realize ['rɪəlaɪz] *v/t* perceber; FIN realizar; ***I ~ now that …*** agora eu percebi que …; ***I hadn't ~d that*** eu ainda não tinha percebido isso
really ['rɪəlɪ] *adv* realmente; **~?** é verdade?; ***not ~*** (*not much*) não muito
'real time *n* COMPUT tempo *m* real
'real-time *adj* COMPUT em tempo real
realtor ['riːltər] *Am* corretor,a *m,f* de imóveis, *Port* agente *m/f* imobiliário,-a
realty ['riːltɪ] *Am* bens *mpl* imóveis
reap [riːp] *v/t* colher
reappear [riːə'pɪr] *v/i* reaparecer
reappearance [riːə'pɪrəns] reaparição *f*
rear [rɪr] **1** *n* parte *f* de trás **2** *adj* traseiro
rear 'end *fam person* traseiro *m* **'rear-end** *v/t fam* ***be ~ed*** levar uma batida na traseira (do veículo) **'rear light** *car* farol *m* traseiro
rearm [riː'ɑːrm] **1** *v/t* rearmar **2** *v/i* rearmar-se
'rearmost *adj* último
rearrange [riːə'reɪnʒ] *v/t flowers, furniture* rearranjar; *schedule, meetings* reorganizar
rear-view 'mirror espelho *m* retrovisor
reason ['riːzn] **1** *n faculty, cause* razão *f*; ***listen to ~*** ouvir a voz da razão **2** *v/i* **~ *with s.o.*** conversar com alguém
reasonable ['riːznəbl] *adj person, behavior, price* razoável; ***a ~ number***

of people um número razoável de pessoas
reasonably ['riːznəblɪ] *adv act, behave* razoavelmente; (*quite*) bem
reasoning ['riːznɪŋ] raciocínio *m*
reassure [riːə'ʃʊr] *v/t* assegurar
reassuring [riːə'ʃʊrɪŋ] *adj* tranqüilizador
rebate ['riːbeɪt] (*money back*) reembolso *m*
rebel 1 ['rebl] *n* rebelde *m/f*; ***~ troops*** tropas *fpl* rebeldes **2** [rɪ'bel] *v/i* ⟨*pret & pp* ***rebelled***⟩ rebelar-se
rebellion [rɪ'belɪən] rebelião *f*
rebellious [rɪ'belɪəs] *adj* rebelde
rebelliously [rɪ'belɪəslɪ] *adv* com rebeldia
rebelliousness [rɪ'belɪəsnɪs] rebeldia *f*
rebound [rɪ'baʊnd] *v/i ball etc* bater e voltar
rebuff [rɪ'bʌf] *n* recusa *f*
rebuild ['riːbɪld] *v/t* ⟨*pret & pp* ***rebuilt***⟩ reconstruir
rebuke [rɪ'bjuːk] *v/t* repreender
recall [rɪ'kɒːl] *v/t* (*remember*) recordar; *goods* retirar do mercado
recap ['riːkæp] *v/i* ⟨*pret & pp* ***recapped***⟩ *fam* recapitular
recapture [riː'kæptʃər] *v/t* MIL reconquistar; *criminal* recapturar
recede [rɪ'siːd] *v/i flood waters* retroceder
receding [rɪ'siːdɪŋ] *adj forehead, chin* recuado; ***have a ~ hairline*** ter entradas
receipt [rɪ'siːt] *purchase*: recibo *m*; ***~s*** FIN renda *f*; ***acknowledge ~ of sth*** acusar o recebimento de algo
receive [rɪ'siːv] *v/t* receber
receiver [rɪ'siːvər] *letter*: destinatário,-a *m,f*; TEL auscultador *m*; *radio*: receptor *m*; *tennis*: recebedor,a *m,f*
receivership [rɪ'siːvərʃɪp] *n* ***be in ~*** estar insolvente
recent ['riːsnt] *adj* recente
recently ['riːsntlɪ] *adv* recentemente
reception [rɪ'sepʃn] *hotel, company, formal party*, (*welcome*), *phone*: recepção *f*
re'ception desk recepção *f*
receptionist [rɪ'sepʃnɪst] recepcionista *m/f*
receptive [rɪ'septɪv] *adj* ***be ~ to sth*** ser receptivo para algo
recess ['riːses] *wall etc*: nicho *m*; EDUC pausa *f*; *parliament*: recesso *m*
recession [rɪ'seʃn] *economic* recessão *f*
recharge [riː'tʃɑːrdʒ] *v/t battery* recarregar
recipe ['resəpɪ] receita *f*
'recipe book livro *m* de receitas
recipient [rɪ'sɪpɪənt] *parcel etc*: destinatário,-a *m,f*; *payment*: recebedor,a *m,f*
reciprocal [rɪ'sɪprəkl] *adj* recíproco
recital [rɪ'saɪtl] MUS recital *m*
recite [rɪ'saɪt] *v/t poem* recitar; *details, facts* enumerar
reckless ['reklɪs] *adj* imprudente
recklessly ['reklɪslɪ] *adv* imprudentemente
reckon ['rekən] *v/i* (*think, consider*) pensar, achar
♦**reckon on** *v/t* contar com
♦**reckon with** *v/t* ***have s.o. / sth to ~ with*** ter que contar com alguém / algo
reckoning ['rekənɪŋ] cálculos *mpl*
reclaim [rɪ'kleɪm] *v/t land from sea* recuperar; *from lost and found* reclamar
recline [rɪ'klaɪn] *v/i* reclinar-se
recliner [rɪ'klaɪnər] *chair* cadeira *f* reclinável
recluse [rɪ'kluːs] recluso,-a *m,f*
recognition [rekəg'nɪʃn] reconhecimento *m*; ***be changed beyond ~*** estar irreconhecível
recognizable [rekəg'naɪzəbl] *adj* reconhecível
recognize ['rekəgnaɪz] *v/t also* POL reconhecer
recoil [rɪ'kɔɪl] *v/i* recuar
recollect [rekə'lekt] *v/t* recordar
recollection [rekə'lekʃn] recordação *f*; ***to the best of my ~*** que eu me lembre
recommend [rekə'mend] *v/t* recomendar
recommendation [rekə'men'deɪʃn] recomendação *f*
recompense ['rekəmpens] *n fml* re-

compensa *f*; LAW indenização *f*
reconcile ['rekənsaɪl] *v/t people* reconciliar; *facts, differences* conciliar; ***~ oneself to …*** aceitar a idéia de …; ***be ~d*** *two people* estar reconciliados
reconciliation [rekənsɪlɪ'eɪʃn] *people*: reconciliação *f*, *facts, differences*: conciliação *f*
recondition [riːkən'dɪʃn] *v/t* recondicionar
reconnaissance [rɪ'kɑːnɪsəns] MIL reconhecimento *m*
reconsider [riːkən'sɪdər] *v/t & v/i* reconsiderar
reconstruct [riːkən'strʌkt] *v/t city, one's life, crime* reconstruir
record[1] ['rekərd] *n* MUS disco *m*; SPORT *etc* recorde *m*; (*written document etc*), *database*: registro *m*, *Port* registo *m*; ***say sth off the ~*** dizer algo inoficialmente; ***have a criminal ~*** ter antecedentes criminais; ***have a good ~ for sth*** ter um bom histórico em matéria de algo; ***I'll check in our ~s*** vou checar em nossos registros
record[2] [rɪ'kɔːrd] *v/t electronically* gravar; *in writing* registrar, *Port* registar
'record-breaking ['breɪkɪŋ] *adj* recorde
recorder [rɪ'kɔːrdər] MUS flauta *f* doce
'record holder recordista *m/f*
recording [rɪ'kɔːrdɪŋ] gravação *f*
re'cording studio estúdio *m* de gravações
'record player toca-discos *m*, *Port* gira-discos *m*
recount[1] [rɪ'kaʊnt] *v/t* (*tell*) relatar
recount[2] ['riːkaʊnt] **1** *n votes*: recontagem *f* **2** *v/t* (*count again*) recontar
recoup [rɪ'kuːp] *v/t financial losses* refazer-se de
recover [rɪ'kʌvər] **1** *v/t sth lost, stolen goods* recuperar; *composure* recobrar **2** *v/i from illness* recuperar-se
recovery [rɪ'kʌvərɪ] *sth lost, stolen goods, illness*: recuperação *f*; ***he has made a good ~*** ele se recuperou muito bem
recreation [rekrɪ'eɪʃn] recreação *f*
recreational [rekrɪ'eɪʃnl] *adj done for pleasure* recreacional
recruit [rɪ'kruːt] **1** *n* MIL recruta *m/f*; *company*: novo,-a trabalhador,a *m,f* **2** *v/t new staff* recrutar
recruitment [rɪ'kruːtmənt] recrutamento *m*
re'cruitment drive MIL campanha *f* de recrutamento
rectangle ['rektæŋgl] retângulo *m*
rectangular [rek'tæŋgjʊlər] *adj* retangular
rectify ['rektɪfaɪ] *v/t* ⟨*pret & pp* ***rectified***⟩ (*put right*) resolver
recuperate [rɪ'kuːpəreɪt] *v/i* recuperar-se
recur [rɪ'kɜːr] *v/i* ⟨*pret & pp* ***recurred***⟩ *error, event* repetir-se; *symptoms* reaparecer
recurrent [rɪ'kʌrənt] *adj* recorrente
recyclable [riː'saɪkləbl] *adj* reciclável
recycle [riː'saɪkl] *v/t* reciclar
recycling [riː'saɪklɪŋ] reciclagem *f*
red [red] *adj* vermelho; *wine* tinto; *hair* ruivo; ***in the ~*** no vermelho
Red 'Cross Cruz *f* Vermelha
redden ['redn] *v/i* (*blush*) corar
redecorate [riː'dekəreɪt] *v/t room, house* redecorar
redeem [rɪ'diːm] *v/t debt* amortizar; *sinners* redimir
redeeming [rɪ'diːmɪŋ] *adj* ***his one ~ feature is …*** a única coisa que se salva nele é …
redemption [rɪ'dempʃn] REL redenção *f*
redevelop [riːdɪ'veləp] *v/t part of town* renovar
red-handed [red'hændɪd] *adj* ***catch s.o. ~*** pegar alguém em flagrante
'redhead ruivo,-a *m,f* **red-'hot** *adj* vermelho-vivo **red-'letter day** dia *m* memorável **red 'light** *at traffic light* farol *m* vermelho **red 'light district** zona *f* (de prostituição) **'red meat** carne *f* vermelha **'redneck** *Am fam indivíduo reacionário, normalmente de classe baixa*
redouble [riː'dʌbl] *v/t* ***~ one's efforts*** redobrar os esforços
red 'pepper pimentão *m* vermelho
red 'tape burocracia *f*
reduce [rɪ'duːs] *v/t* reduzir
reduction [rɪ'dʌkʃn] redução *f*

redundancy *Brit* → ***lay-off***
redundant [rɪ'dʌndənt] *adj (unnecessary)* redundante; ***be made ~*** *Brit at work* ser demitido
reed [riːd] BOT cana *f*
reef [riːf] *in sea* recife *m*
'reef knot *Brit* nó *m* de rizos
reek [riːk] *v/i* feder; ***~ of …*** feder a …
reel [riːl] *n film, thread* rolo *m*
◆**reel off** *v/t* soltar de uma só vez
re-e'lect *v/t* reeleger
re-e'lection reeleição *f*
re-'entry *spacecraft*: reentrada *f*
ref [ref] *fam* árbitro *m*
refer [rɪ'fɜːr] ⟨*pret & pp* ***referred***⟩ **1** *v/t* ***~ a decision / problem to s.o.*** entregar uma decisão / um problema a alguém **2** *v/i* ***~ to*** *(allude to)* referir-se a; *dictionary etc* consultar
referee [refə'riː] SPORT árbitro *m*; *job*: referência *f*
reference ['refərəns] *(allusion)*, *job*: referência *f*; ***with ~ to*** com referência a
'reference book livro *m* de consulta **'reference library** biblioteca *f* de consulta **'reference number** número *m* de referência
referendum [refə'rendəm] referendo *m*
refill ['riːfɪl] *v/t tank, glass* reencher
refine [rɪ'faɪn] *v/t oil, sugar* refinar; *technique* aperfeiçoar
refined [rɪ'faɪnd] *adj manners, language* refinado
refinement [rɪ'faɪnmənt] *to process, machine* melhora *f*
refinery [rɪ'faɪnərɪ] refinaria *f*
reflation ['riːfleɪʃn] reflação *f*
reflect [rɪ'flekt] **1** *v/t light* refletir; ***be ~ed in …*** estar refletido em … **2** *v/i (think)* refletir
reflection [rɪ'flekʃn] *water, glass etc*: reflexão *f*
reflex ['riːfleks] *in body* reflexo *m*
reflex re'action reação *f* de reflexo
reform [rɪ'fɔːrm] **1** *n* reforma *f* **2** *v/t* reformar
reformer [rɪ'fɔːrmər] reformador,a *m,f*
refrain[1] [rɪ'freɪn] *v/i fml* abster-se; ***please ~ from smoking*** pede-se não fumar
refrain[2] [rɪ'freɪn] *n song, poem*: refrão *m*
refresh [rɪ'freʃ] *v/t person* refrescar; ***feel ~ed*** sentir-se como novo
refresher course [rɪ'freʃər] curso *m* de revisão
refreshing [rɪ'freʃɪŋ] *adj drink* refrescante; *experience* reconfortante
refreshments [rɪ'freʃmənts] *npl* salgadinhos *mpl* e bebidas *fpl*
refrigerate [rɪ'frɪdʒəreɪt] *v/t* refrigerar; ***keep ~d*** conservar sob refrigeração
refrigerator [rɪ'frɪdʒəreɪtər] refrigerador *m*, geladeira *f*, *Port* frigorífico *m*
refuel [riː'fjʊəl] *v/t & v/i* reabastecer
refuge ['refjuːdʒ] refúgio *m*; ***take ~*** *from storm etc* abrigar-se
refugee [refjʊ'dʒiː] refugiado,-a *m,f*
refu'gee camp acampamento *m* de refugiados
refund ['riːfʌnd] **1** *n* reembolso *m* **2** *v/t* reembolsar
refusal [rɪ'fjuːzl] recusa *f*
refuse[1] [rɪ'fjuːz] **1** *v/i* negar-se **2** *v/t help, food* recusar; ***~ to do sth*** recusar-se a fazer algo
refuse[2] ['refjuːs] *(garbage)* lixo *m*
regain [rɪ'geɪn] *v/t control, lost territory* recuperar; *the lead* retomar
regal ['riːgl] *adj* régio
regard [rɪ'gɑːrd] **1** *n* ***have great ~ for s.o.*** ter grande consideração por alguém; ***in this ~*** neste sentido; ***with ~ to*** com respeito a; ***(kind) ~s*** atenciosamente; ***give my ~s to Paula*** dê lembranças à Paula; ***with no ~ for …*** sem importar-se com … **2** *v/t* ***~ s.o. / sth as*** considerar alguém / algo como; ***as ~s …*** no que diz respeito a …
regarding [rɪ'gɑːrdɪŋ] *prep* com respeito a
regardless [rɪ'gɑːrdlɪs] *adv* apesar de tudo; ***~ of*** apesar de
regime [reɪ'ʒiːm] *(government)* regime *m*
regiment ['redʒɪmənt] *n* regimento *m*
region ['riːdʒən] região *f*; ***in the ~ of*** aproximadamente
regional ['riːdʒənl] *adj* regional

R

register ['redʒɪstər] **1** *n* registro *m*, *Port* registo *m*; *school*: matrícula *f* **2** *v/t birth*, *death*, *vehicle*, *letter* registrar, *Port* registar; *emotion* demonstrar; ***send a letter ~ed*** mandar uma carta registrada, *Port* mandar uma cara registada **3** *v/i university*: matricular-se; *course*: inscrever-se; *police*: registrar-se, *Port* registar-se

registered letter ['redʒɪstərd] carta *f* registrada, *Port* carta *f* registada

registration [redʒɪ'streɪʃn] registro *m*, *Port* registo *m*; *university*: matriculação *f*; *course*: inscrição *f*

registration number *Brit* → ***license number***

regret [rɪ'gret] **1** *v/t* ⟨*pret & pp* ***regretted***⟩ arrepender-se de; ***I ~ to inform you …*** lamento ter que informar-lhe … **2** *n* arrependimento *m*

regretful [rɪ'gretfəl] *adj* arrependido

regretfully [rɪ'gretfəlɪ] *adv* arrependidamente

regrettable [rɪ'gretəbl] *adj* lamentável

regrettably [rɪ'gretəblɪ] *adv* lamentavelmente

regular ['regjʊlər] **1** *adj* regular; (*normal*, *ordinary*) normal **2** *n at bar etc* freqüentador, a assíduo,-a *m,f*

regularity [regjʊ'lærətɪ] regularidade *f*

regularly ['regjʊlərlɪ] *adv* regularmente

regulate ['regʊleɪt] *v/t* regular

regulation [regʊ'leɪʃn] (*rule*) regra *f*, norma *f*

rehab ['ri:hæb] *fam* reabilitação *f*

rehabilitate [ri:hə'bɪlɪteɪt] *v/t ex-criminal* reabilitar

rehearsal [rɪ'hɜ:rsl] ensaio *m*

rehearse [rɪ'hɜ:rs] *v/t & v/i* ensaiar

reign [reɪn] **1** *n* reinado *m* **2** *v/i* reinar

reimburse [ri:ɪm'bɜ:rs] *v/t* reembolsar

rein [reɪn] redea *f*

reincarnation [ri:ɪnkɑ:r'neɪʃn] reincarnação *f*

reinforce [ri:ɪn'fɔ:rs] *v/t structure* reforçar; *beliefs* reafirmar

reinforced concrete [ri:ɪn'fɔ:rst] concreto *m* armado

reinforcements [ri:ɪn'fɔ:rsmənts] *npl* MIL reforços *mpl*

reinstate [ri:ɪn'steɪt] *v/t in office* reincorporar; *in text* reinserir

reiterate [ri:'ɪtəreɪt] *v/t* reiterar

reject [rɪ'dʒekt] *v/t* rejeitar

rejection [rɪ'dʒekʃn] rejeição *f*

relapse ['ri:læps] *n* MED recaída *f*; ***have a ~*** ter uma recaída

relate [rɪ'leɪt] **1** *v/t story* narrar; ***~ X to Y*** relacionar X com Y **2** *v/i* ***~ to*** (*be connected with*) estar relacionado com; ***he doesn't ~ to people*** ele não se relaciona facilmente com as pessoas

related [rɪ'leɪtɪd] *adj by family* aparentado; *events*, *ideas etc* relacionado

relation [rɪ'leɪʃn] *in family*, (*connection*) relação *f*; ***business / diplomatic ~s*** relações *fpl* de negócio / diplomáticas

relationship [rɪ'leɪʃnʃɪp] relação *f*; *sexual* relacionamento *m*

relative ['relətɪv] **1** *n* parente *m/f* **2** *adj* relativo; ***X is ~ to Y*** X é relativo a Y

relatively ['relətɪvlɪ] *adv* relativamente

relax [rɪ'læks] **1** *v/i* relaxar; ***~!, don't get angry*** relaxe!, não se aborreça **2** *v/t muscle* relaxar; *pace* diminuir

relaxation [ri:læk'seɪʃn] relaxamento *m*; *rules etc*: afrouxamento *m*

relaxed [rɪ'lækst] *adj* tranqüilo

relaxing [rɪ'læksɪŋ] *adj* relaxante

relay [ri:'leɪ] **1** *v/t message* passar; *radio*, *TV signals* transmitir **2** *n* ***~ (race)*** corrida *f* de revesamento

release [rɪ'li:s] **1** *n prison*: libertação *f*; *CD etc*: lançamento *m* **2** *v/t prisoner* libertar; *parking brake* soltar; *information* comunicar

relegate ['relɪgeɪt] *v/t* relegar

relent [rɪ'lent] *v/i* ceder

relentless [rɪ'lentlɪs] *adj* (*determined*) implacável; *rain etc* incessante

relentlessly [rɪ'lentlɪslɪ] *adv* implacávelmente; *rain etc* incessantemente

relevance ['reləvəns] relevância *f*

relevant ['reləvənt] *adj* relevante

reliability [rɪlaɪə'bɪlətɪ] *person*, *machine*: confiabilidade *f*

reliable [rɪ'laɪəbl] *adj person*, *machine* confiável

R

reliably [rɪ'laɪəblɪ] *adv* confiavelmente; ***I am ~ informed that …*** fui informado de fonte confiável que …
reliance [rɪ'laɪəns] confiança *f*; ***~ on s.o.*** / ***sth*** confiança em alguém / algo
reliant [rɪ'laɪənt] *adj* ***be ~ on*** depender de
relic ['relɪk] relíquia *f*
relief [rɪ'li:f] alívio *m*; ***that's a ~*** que alívio!; ***in ~*** *art*: em relevo
relieve [rɪ'li:v] *v/t pressure, pain* aliviar; (*take over from*) render; ***be ~d*** *at news etc* sentir-se aliviado
religion [rɪ'lɪdʒən] religião *f*
religious [rɪ'lɪdʒəs] *adj* religioso
religiously [rɪ'lɪdʒəslɪ] *adv* (*conscientiously*) conscientemente
relinquish [rɪ'lɪŋkwɪʃ] *v/t* renunciar a
relish ['relɪʃ] **1** *n sauce* molho *m*; (*enjoyment*) prazer *m* **2** *v/t idea, prospect* alegrar-se com
relive [ri:'lɪv] *v/t the past, event* reviver
relocate [ri:loʊ'keɪt] *v/i business, employee* mudar
relocation [ri:loʊ'keɪʃn] *business, employee*: mudança *f*
reluctance [rɪ'lʌktəns] relutância *f*
reluctant [rɪ'lʌktənt] *adj* relutante; ***be ~ to do sth*** relutar para fazer algo
reluctantly [rɪ'lʌktəntlɪ] *adv* relutantemente
♦ **rely on** [rɪ'laɪ] *v/t* ⟨*pret & pp* ***relied***⟩ confiar em; (*be dependent on*) depender de; ***rely on s.o. to do sth*** contar com alguém para fazer algo
remain [rɪ'meɪn] *v/i* (*be left*) ficar; MATH restar; (*stay*) permanecer
remainder [rɪ'meɪndər] **1** *n* (*rest*), MATH resto *m* **2** *v/t* vender como saldo
remaining [rɪ'meɪnɪŋ] *adj* restante
remains [rɪ'meɪnz] *npl body*: restos *mpl* mortais
remake ['ri:meɪk] *n movie*: refilmagem *f*
remand [rɪ'mænd] **1** *v/t* ***~ s.o. in custody*** decretar prisão preventiva de alguém **2** *n* ***be on ~*** estar cumprindo prisão preventiva
remark [rɪ'mɑ:rk] **1** *n* comentário *m*, observação *f* **2** *v/t* comentar
remarkable [rɪ'mɑ:rkəbl] *adj* notável
remarkably [rɪ'mɑ:rkəblɪ] *adv* notavelmente
remarry [ri:'marɪ] *v/i* ⟨*pret & pp* ***remarried***⟩ voltar a casar-se
remedy ['remədɪ] *n also fig* remédio *m*
remember [rɪ'membər] **1** *v/t* lembrar-se de; ***~ to lock the door*** lembre-se de trancar a porta; ***~ me to her*** mande lembranças minhas à ela **2** *v/i* lembrar; ***I don't ~*** eu não lembro
remind [rɪ'maɪnd] *v/t* ***~ s.o. of sth*** (*make remember*) lembrar algo a alguém; (*bring to their attention*) lembrar alguém de algo; ***he ~s me of João*** ele me lembra o João; ***that ~s me …*** isso me faz lembrar …
reminder [rɪ'maɪndər] lembrete *m*; *payment*: cobrança *f*
reminisce [remɪ'nɪs] *v/i* relembrar
reminiscent [remɪ'nɪsənt] *adj* ***be ~ of sth*** lembrar algo
remiss [rɪ'mɪs] *adj fml* negligente
remission [rɪ'mɪʃn] remissão *f*; ***go into ~*** MED entrar em remissão
remnant ['remnənt] resto *m*
remorse [rɪ'mɔ:rs] remorso *m*
remorseless [rɪ'mɔ:rslɪs] *adj person, demands* implacável; *pace* incansável
remote [rɪ'moʊt] *adj village, possibility* remoto; *ancestor*, (*aloof*) distante
remote 'access COMPUT acesso *m* remoto
remote con'trol controle *m* remoto
remotely [rɪ'moʊtlɪ] *adv related, connected* remotamente; ***it's just ~ possible*** é uma possibilidade remota
remoteness [rɪ'moʊtnəs] distância *f*
removable [rɪ'mu:vəbl] *adj* removível
removal [rɪ'mu:vl] *garbage, demonstrators*: retirada *f*; *home*: mudança *f*
remove [rɪ'mu:v] *v/t feet from table, suspicion* retirar; *top, lid, coat, doubt etc* tirar
remuneration [rɪmju:nə'reɪʃn] remuneração *f*
remunerative [rɪ'mju:nərətɪv] *adj* bem remunerado
Renaissance [rɪ'neɪsəns] Renascença *f*
rename [ri:'neɪm] *v/t* renomear

R

render ['rendər] *v/t service* prestar; ~ ***s.o. helpless / unconscious*** deixar alguém indefeso / inconsciente
rendering ['rendərɪŋ] *piece of music*: interpretação *f*
rendez-vous ['rɑːndeɪvuː] *romantic*, MIL encontro *m*
renew [rɪ'nuː] *v/t contract, license* renovar; *discussions* reatar; ***feel ~ed*** sentir-se renovado
renewable [rɪ'nuːəbl] *adj* renovável
renewal [rɪ'nuːəl] *contract etc*: renovação *f*, *discussions*: reatamento *m*
renounce [rɪ'naʊns] *v/t title, rights* renunciar a
renovate ['renəveɪt] *v/t* reformar
renovation [renə'veɪʃn] reforma *f*
renown [rɪ'naʊn] renome *m*
renowned [rɪ'naʊnd] *adj* renomado
rent [rent] **1** *n* aluguel *m*, *Port* aluguer *m*; ***for ~*** aluga-se **2** *v/t* alugar; ***~ out*** *apartment, car etc* alugar
rental ['rentl] aluguel *m*, *Port* aluguer *m*
'rental agreement contrato *m* de aluguel, *Port* contrato *m* de aluguer
'rental car carro *m* alugado
'rent-free *adv* livre de aluguel, *Port* livre de aluguer
reopen [riː'oʊpn] *v/t & v/i* reabrir
reorganization [riːɔːrgənaɪ'zeɪʃn] reorganização *f*
reorganize [riː'ɔːrgənaɪz] *v/t* reorganizar
rep [rep] COM representante *m/f*
repaint [riː'peɪnt] *v/t* repintar
repair [rɪ'per] **1** *v/t* consertar **2** *n* ***in a good / bad state of ~*** em bom / mau estado; ***~s*** *pl* conserto *m*
re'pairman técnico *m*
repatriate [riː'pætrɪeɪt] *v/t* repatriar
repatriation [riːpætrɪ'eɪʃn] repatriação *f*
repay [riː'peɪ] *v/t* ⟨*pret & pp* ***repaid***⟩ *money* devolver; *person* pagar (de volta)
repayment [riː'peɪmənt] reembolso *m*
repeal [rɪ'piːl] *v/t law* revogar
repeat [rɪ'piːt] **1** *v/t* repetir; ***am I ~ing myself?*** estou me repetindo? **2** *n TV program etc* reprise *f*
repeat 'business COM repetição *f* de negócios
repeated [rɪ'piːtɪd] *adj* repetido
repeatedly [rɪ'piːtɪdlɪ] *adv* repetidamente
re'peat order COM pedido *m* repetido
repel [rɪ'pel] *v/t* ⟨*pret & pp* ***repelled***⟩ repelir
repellent [rɪ'pelənt] **1** *n insects*: repelente *m* **2** *adj* repugnante
repent [rɪ'pent] *v/i* arrepender-se
repercussions [riːpər'kʌʃnz] *npl* repercussões *fpl*
repertoire ['repərtwɑːr] repertório *m*
repetition [repɪ'tɪʃn] repetição *f*
repetitive [rɪ'petɪtɪv] *adj* repetitivo
replace [rɪ'pleɪs] *v/t* (*put back*) recolocar; (*take the place of*) substituir
replacement [rɪ'pleɪsmənt] *n person, thing* substituto,-a *m,f*
replacement 'part peça *f* de reposição
replay ['riːpleɪ] **1** *n recording* replay *m*; *match* reprise *f* **2** *v/t match* reprisar
replenish [rɪ'plenɪʃ] *v/t container* encher; *supplies* repor
replica ['replɪkə] *n* réplica *f*
reply [rɪ'plaɪ] **1** *n* resposta *f* **2** *v/t & v/i* ⟨*pret & pp* ***replied***⟩ responder
report [rɪ'pɔːrt] **1** *n* (*account*) informe *m*; *journalist*: reportagem *f* **2** *v/t facts* informar; *to authorities* denunciar; ***~ one's findings to s.o.*** informar as descobertas a alguém; ***~ a person to the police*** denunciar alguém à polícia; ***he is ~ed to be in London*** disseram que ele está em Londres **3** *v/i* (*present oneself*) apresentar-se (***to*** a); ***~ing from Rio*** (falando) de Rio
♦ **report to** *v/t to an office etc* apresentar-se a; *business hierarchy*: reportar-se a
re'port card boletim *m* escolar
reporter [rɪ'pɔːrtər] repórter *m/f*
repossess [riːpə'zes] *v/t* COM retomar a posse de
reprehensible [reprɪ'hensəbl] *adj* repreensível
represent [reprɪ'zent] *v/t* representar
representative [reprɪ'zentətɪv] **1** *n* COM, POL representante *m/f* **2** *adj* representativo

repress [rɪ'pres] *v/t revolt, feelings* reprimir; *laugh* conter
repression [rɪ'preʃn] POL repressão *f*
repressive [rɪ'presɪv] *adj* POL repressivo
reprieve [rɪ'priːv] **1** *n* LAW suspensão *f* temporária; *fig* adiamento *m* **2** *v/t prisoner* indultar
reprimand ['reprɪmænd] *v/t* repreender
reprint ['riːprɪnt] **1** *n* reimpressão *f* **2** *v/t* reimprimir
reprisal [rɪ'praɪzl] represália *f*; ***take ~s*** tomar represálias; ***in ~ for*** em represália por
reproach [rɪ'proʊʧ] **1** *n* reprovação *f*; ***be beyond ~*** ser irreprochável **2** *v/t* reprovar
reproachful [rɪ'proʊʧfʊl] *adj* reprovador
reproachfully [rɪ'proʊʧfʊlɪ] *adv* com reprovação
reproduce [riːprə'duːs] **1** *v/t* reproduzir **2** *v/i* BIOL reproduzir-se
reproduction [riːprə'dʌkʃn] BIOL, *sound, furniture* reprodução *f*
reproductive [rɪprə'dʌktɪv] *adj* BIOL reprodutivo
reptile ['reptaɪl] réptil *m*
republic [rɪ'pʌblɪk] república *f*
republican [rɪ'pʌblɪkn] **1** *adj* republicano **2** *n* republicano,-a *m,f*
repudiate [rɪ'pjuːdɪeɪt] *v/t* (*deny*) repudiar
repulsive [rɪ'pʌlsɪv] *adj* repulsivo
reputable ['repjʊtəbl] *adj* respeitável
reputation [repjʊ'teɪʃn] reputação *f*; ***have a good / bad ~*** ter boa / má reputação
reputed [rep'jʊtəd] *adj* ***be ~ to be*** ter reputação de ser
reputedly [rep'jʊtədlɪ] *adv* pelo que dizem
request [rɪ'kwest] **1** *n* pedido *m*; ***on ~*** por encomenda **2** *v/t* pedir
requiem ['rekwɪəm] MUS réquiem *m*
require [rɪ'kwaɪr] *v/t* (*need*) necessitar; ***it ~s great care*** isto requer muito cuidado; ***as ~d by law*** como a lei prevê; ***guests are ~d to …*** pede-se aos convidados que …
required [rɪ'kwaɪrd] *adj* (*necessary*) necessário
requirement [rɪ'kwaɪrmənt] (*need*) necessidade *f*; (*condition*) requisito *m*
requisition [rekwɪ'zɪʃn] *v/t* requisitar
reroute [riː'ruːt] *v/t airplane etc* desviar
rerun ['riːrʌn] **1** *n TV program* reprise *f* **2** *v/t* ⟨*pret* ***reran***, *pp* ***rerun***⟩ *tape* tocar de novo
reschedule [riː'skedjuːl] *v/t* mudar a data / hora de
rescue ['reskjuː] **1** *n* resgate *m*; ***come to s.o.'s ~*** vir em socorro de alguém **2** *v/t* resgatar
'rescue party equipe *f* de resgate
research [rɪ'sɜːrʧ] *n* pesquisa *f*
♦ **research into** *v/t* pesquisar
re'search assistant assistente *m/f* de pesquisa
researcher [rɪ'sɜːrʧər] pesquisador,a *m,f*
re'search project projeto *m* de pesquisa
resemblance [rɪ'zembləns] semelhança *f*
resemble [rɪ'zembl] *v/t* parecer-se com; ***they don't ~ each other at all*** eles não se parecem em nada
resent [rɪ'zent] *v/t* ressentir
resentful [rɪ'zentfʊl] *adj* ressentido
resentfully [rɪ'zentfʊlɪ] *adv* ressentidamente
resentment [rɪ'zentmənt] ressentimento *m*
reservation [rezər'veɪʃn] *room etc*, (*special area*) reserva *f*; *mental* ressalva *f*; ***I have a ~*** *hotel, restaurant*: tenho uma reserva
reserve [rɪ'zɜːrv] **1** *n* (*store, aloofness*) reserva *f*; SPORT reserva *m/f*; FIN ***~s*** *pl* reservas *fpl*; ***keep sth in ~*** ter algo de reserva **2** *v/t seat, table, judgment* reservar
reserved [rɪ'zɜːrvd] *adj person, table* reservado
reservoir ['rezərvwɑːr] *for water* reservatório *m*
reshuffle ['riːʃʌfl] *Brit* POL **1** *n* reforma *f* **2** *v/t* reformar
reside [rɪ'zaɪd] *v/i fml* residir
residence ['rezɪdəns] *fml house etc* residência *f*; (*stay*) estadia *f*

'residence permit permissão *f* de residência
'resident ['rezɪdənt] **1** *n* residente *m/f* **2** *adj* residente
residential [rezɪ'denʃl] *adj district* residencial
residue ['rezɪduː] resíduo *m*
resign [rɪ'zaɪn] **1** *v/t position* demitir-se de; **~ oneself to** resignar-se a **2** *v/i from job* demitir-se
resignation [rezɪg'neɪʃn] *from job* demissão *f*; *mental* resignação *f*
resigned [re'zaɪnd] *adj* resignado; ***we have become ~ to the fact that ...*** nos resignamos ao fato de ...
resilient [rɪ'zɪlɪənt] *adj personality* forte; *material* resistente
resin ['rezɪn] resina *f*
resist [rɪ'zɪst] **1** *v/t enemy, temptation* resistir a; *new measures* opor-se a **2** *v/i* resistir
resistance [rɪ'zɪstəns] resistência *f*
resistant [rɪ'zɪstənt] *adj material* resistente; ***~ to heat / rust*** resistente ao calor / a oxidação
resolute ['rezəluːt] *adj* resoluto
resolution [rezə'luːʃn] (*decision*), *problem, image, New Year*: resolução *f*; (*determination*) determinação *f*
resolve [rɪ'zɑːlv] *v/t problem* resolver; *mystery* solucionar; ***~ to do sth*** resolver fazer algo
resort [rɪ'zɔːrt] *n* (*place*) resort *m*; ***as a last ~*** como último recurso
♦ **resort to** *v/t violence* recorrer a
♦ **resound with** [rɪ'zaʊnd] *v/t* ressoar com
resounding [rɪ'zaʊndɪŋ] *adj success, victory* estrondoso
resource [rɪ'sɔːrs] *material* recurso *m*; ***leave s.o. to his own ~s*** deixar alguém por conta própria
resourceful [rɪ'sɔːrsfʊl] *adj person, approach* engenhoso
respect [rɪ'spekt] **1** *n* (*consideration*) respeito *m*; ***show ~ to*** demonstrar respeito por; ***with ~ to*** com respeito a; ***in this / that ~*** com respeito a isso / aquilo; ***in many ~s*** em muitos aspectos; ***pay one's last ~s to s.o.*** prestar um último respeito a alguém **2** *v/t* respeitar
respectability [rɪspektə'bɪlətɪ] respeitabilidade *f*
respectable [rɪ'spektəbl] *adj* respeitável
respectably [rɪ'spektəblɪ] *adv* respeitavelmente
respectful [rɪ'spektfʊl] *adj* respeitoso
respectfully [rɪ'spektflɪ] *adv* respeituosamente
respective [rɪ'spektɪv] *adj* respectivo
respectively [rɪ'spektɪvlɪ] *adv* respectivamente
respiration [respɪ'reɪʃn] respiração *f*
respirator ['respɪreɪtər] MED respirador *m*
respite ['respaɪt] pausa *f* para respirar; ***without ~*** sem pausa; *storm* sem trégua
respond [rɪ'spɑːnd] *v/i* responder
response [rɪ'spɑːns] (*answer, reaction*) resposta *f*
responsibility [rɪspɑːnsɪ'bɪlətɪ] responsabilidade *f*; ***accept ~ for*** assumir a responsabilidade por; ***a job with more ~*** um trabalho de mais responsabilidade
responsible [rɪ'spɑːnsəbl] *adj* responsável
responsive [rɪ'spɑːnsɪv] *adj audience, brakes* responsivo
rest[1] [rest] **1** *n* descanso *m*; ***set s.o.'s mind at ~*** tranqüilizar alguém **2** *v/i* descansar; ***~ on*** (*be based on*) basear-se em; (*lean against*) estar encostado em; ***it all ~s with him*** tudo depende dele **3** *v/t* (*lean, balance*) encostar
rest[2] [rest] *n* ***the ~*** o resto
restart ['riːstɑːrt] **1** *v/t engine, car* religar; *work* reiniciar **2** *v/i school etc* recomeçar
restaurant ['restərɑːnt] restaurante *m*
'restaurant car vagão-restaurante *m*
'rest cure tratamento *m* de repouso
restful ['restfl] *adj* relaxante
'rest home casa *f* de repouso
restless ['restlɪs] *adj person* agitado; ***have a ~ night*** passar mal a noite
restoration [restə'reɪʃn] restauração *f*
restore [rɪ'stɔːr] *v/t building, law and order, self-esteem etc* restaurar; (*bring back*) restituir

restrain [rɪ'streɪn] *v/t dog, emotions* conter; ~ ***oneself*** conter-se
restraint [rɪ'streɪnt] (*moderation*) moderação *f*
restrict [rɪ'strɪkt] *v/t* restringir; ***I'll ~ myself to …*** vou me restringir a …
restricted [rɪ'strɪktɪd] *adj view* limitado
restricted 'area MIL área *f* restrita
restriction [rɪ'strɪkʃn] restrição *f*
'rest room *Am* toalete *m*, *Port* casa *f* de banho
result [rɪ'zʌlt] *n* resultado *m*; ***as a ~ of this*** como resultado disso
♦ **result from** *v/t* resultar de
♦ **result in** *v/t* resultar em
resume [rɪ'zuːm] **1** *v/t* retomar **2** *v/i* recomeçar
résumé ['rezʊmeɪ] *Am* currículo *m* (vitae)
resumption [rɪ'zʌmpʃn] reinício *m*
resurface [riː'sɜːrfɪs] **1** *v/t roads* repavimentar **2** *v/i* (*reappear*) reaparecer
resurrection [rezə'rekʃn] REL ressurreição *f*
resuscitate [rɪ'sʌsɪteɪt] *v/t* ressuscitar
resuscitation [rɪsʌsɪ'teɪʃn] ressuscitação *f*
retail ['riːteɪl] **1** *adv* no varejo, *Port* a retalho **2** *v/i* ~ ***at …*** ser vendido no varejo por …, *Port* ser vendido a retalho por …
retailer ['riːteɪlər] varejista *m/f*, *Port* retalhista *m/f*
'retail outlet ponto *m* de venda de varejo, *Port* ponto *m* de venda a retalho
'retail price preço *m* de varejo, *Port* preço *m* de venda a retalho
retain [rɪ'teɪn] *v/t* manter
retainer [rɪ'teɪnər] FIN adiantamento *m*
retaliate [rɪ'tælɪeɪt] *v/i* exercer represália
retaliation [rɪtælɪ'eɪʃn] retaliação *f*; ***in ~ for*** como represália por
retarded [rɪ'tɑːrdɪd] *adj mentally* retardado
rethink [riː'θɪŋk] *v/t* ⟨*pret & pp* ***rethought***⟩ repensar
reticence ['retɪsns] reserva *f*
reticent ['retɪsnt] *adj* reservado
retire [rɪ'taɪr] *v/i from work* aposentar-se, *Port also* reformar-se
retired [rɪ'taɪrd] *adj* aposentado, *Port also* reformado
retiree [rɪtaɪ'riː] aposentado,-a *m,f*, *Port also* reformado,-a *m,f*
retirement [rɪ'taɪrmənt] aposentadoria *f*, *Port also* reforma *f*
re'tirement age idade *f* para a aposentadoria, *Port also* idade *f* de reforma
retiring [rɪ'taɪrɪŋ] *adj* (*shy*) retraído
retort [rɪ'tɔːrt] **1** *n* réplica *f* **2** *v/t* replicar
retrace [rɪ'treɪs] *v/t footsteps* retraçar
retract [rɪ'trækt] *v/t claws* retrair; *undercarriage* recolher; *statement* retirar
re-train [riː'treɪn] *v/i worker* ser reciclado
retreat [rɪ'triːt] **1** *v/i* MIL retirar; *discussion: etc* recuar **2** *n* MIL retirada *f*; *place* retiro *m*
retrieve [rɪ'triːv] *v/t* recuperar
retriever [rɪ'triːvər] *dog* retriever *m*
retroactive [retroʊ'æktɪv] *adj law etc* retroativo
retroactively [retroʊ'æktɪvlɪ] *adv* com efeito retroativo
retrograde ['retrəgreɪd] *adj move, decision* retrógrado
retrospect ['retrəspekt] ***in ~*** em retrospectiva
retrospective [retrə'spektɪv] *n* retrospectiva *f*
return [rɪ'tɜːrn] **1** *n* retorno *m*, volta *f*; COMPUT tecla *f* return; (*giving back*) devolução *f*; *tennis*: retorno *m*; ***~s*** *pl* (*profit*) retorno *m*; ***by ~*** (***of post***) imediatamente (por correio); ***in ~ for*** em troca de; ***many happy ~s*** (***of the day***) feliz aniversário **2** *v/t* (*give back*), *favor, invitation* devolver; (*put back*) recolocar **3** *v/i* (*go back, come back*) retornar, voltar; *good times, doubts etc* voltar
re'turn flight vôo *m* de volta **re'turn journey** viagem *f* de volta **return ticket** *Brit* → ***round trip ticket***
reunification [riːjuːnɪfɪ'keɪʃn] reunificação *f*
reunion [riː'juːnjən] reunião *f*
reunite [riːjuː'naɪt] *v/t* reunir
reusable [riː'juːzəbl] *adj* reutilizável

reuse [riː'juːz] *v/t* reutilizar
rev [rev] *n* **~s per minute** revoluções *fpl* por minuto
♦ **rev up** *v/t* ⟨*pret & pp* **revved**⟩ *engine* pôr em aceleração
revaluation [riːvæljʊ'eɪʃn] revalorização *f*
reveal [rɪ'viːl] *v/t* revelar
revealing [rɪ'viːlɪŋ] *adj remark* revelador; *dress* insinuante
♦ **revel in** ['revl] *v/t* deleitar-se com
revelation [revə'leɪʃn] revelação *f*
revenge [rɪ'vendʒ] *n* vingança *f*; **take one's ~** vingar-se; **in ~ for** como vingança por
revenue ['revənuː] renda *f*
reverberate [rɪ'vɜːrbəreɪt] *v/i sound* ressoar
revere [rɪ'vɪr] *v/t* reverenciar
reverence ['revərəns] reverência *f*
Reverend ['revərənd] REL reverendo *m*
reverent ['revərənt] *adj* reverente
reverse [rɪ'vɜːrs] **1** *adj sequence* inverso; **in ~ order** em ordem inversa **2** *n* (*opposite*) contrário *m*; (*back*) verso *m*; MOT marcha *f* a ré, *Port* marcha *f* atrás **3** *v/t sequence* reverter; *vehicle* dar marcha a ré, *Port* fazer marcha atrás **4** *v/i* **~ into the garage** entrar de marcha a ré na garagem
revert [rɪ'vɜːrt] *v/i* **~ to** voltar a
review [rɪ'vjuː] **1** *n book, movie*: crítica *f*; *troops*: inspeção *f*; *situation*: análise *f* **2** *v/t book, movie* criticar; *troops* revistar; *situation etc* analisar; *Am* EDUC revisar
reviewer [rɪ'vjuːər] *book, movie*: crítico,-a *m,f*
revise [rɪ'vaɪz] *v/t opinion, text* revisar
revision [rɪ'vɪʒn] *opinion, text* revisão *f*
revival [rɪ'vaɪvl] *custom etc* ressurgimento *m*; *patient* reanimação *f*
revive [rɪ'vaɪv] **1** *v/t custom etc* fazer ressurgir; *patient* reanimar **2** *v/i business, exchange rate etc* reativar-se
revoke [rɪ'voʊk] *v/t law, license* revogar
revolt [rɪ'voʊlt] **1** *n* revolta *f* **2** *v/i* revoltar-se
revolting [rɪ'voʊltɪŋ] *adj* (*disgusting*) repugnante
revolution [revə'luːʃn] POL *etc* revolução *f*; (*turn*) giro *m*
revolutionary [revə'luːʃnərɪ] **1** *adj* revolucionário **2** *n* POL revolucionário,-a *m,f*
revolutionize [revə'luːʃnaɪz] *v/t* revolucionar
revolve [rɪ'vɑːlv] *v/i* girar; **~ around** girar em torno de
revolver [rɪ'vɑːlvər] revólver *m*
revolving door [rɪ'vɑːlvɪŋ] porta *f* giratória
revue [rɪ'vjuː] THEA revista *f*
revulsion [rɪ'vʌlʃn] náusea *f*
reward [rɪ'wɔːrd] **1** *n financial* recompensa *f*; (*benefit derived*) gratificação *f* **2** *v/t financially* recompensar
rewarding [rɪ'wɔːrdɪŋ] *adj experience* gratificante
rewind [riː'waɪnd] *v/t* ⟨*pret & pp* **rewound**⟩ *film, tape* rebobinar
rewrite [riː'raɪt] *v/t* ⟨*pret* **rewrote**, *pp* **rewritten**⟩ reescrever
rhetoric ['retərɪk] retórica *f*
rhetorical question [rɪ'tɑːrɪkl] pergunta *f* retórica
rheumatism ['ruːmətɪzm] reumatismo *m*
rhinoceros [raɪ'nɑːsərəs] rinoceronte *m*
rhubarb ['ruːbɑːrb] ruibarbo *m*
rhyme [raɪm] **1** *n* rima *f* **2** *v/i* rimar; **~ with ...** rimar com ...
rhythm ['rɪðm] ritmo *m*
rib [rɪb] ANAT costela *f*
ribbon ['rɪbən] fita *f*
rice [raɪs] arroz *m*
rich [rɪʧ] **1** *adj* rico; *food* saboroso **2** *n* **the ~** os ricos
richly ['rɪʧlɪ] *adv deserved* muito
rickety ['rɪkətɪ] *adj* que não está firme
ricochet ['rɪkəʃeɪ] *v/i* ricochetear
rid [rɪd] *v/t* ⟨*pret & pp* **rid**⟩ **get ~ of** desfazer-se de
riddance ['rɪdns] **good ~ to him!** *fam* que bom que nos livramos dele!
ridden ['rɪdn] *pp* → **ride**
riddle ['rɪdl] **1** *n* charada *f* **2** *v/t* **be ~d with** estar repleto de
ride [raɪd] **1** *n horse, vehicle*: passeio *m*; (*journey*) viagem *f*, *hitch-hiking*: carona *f*, *Port* boleia *f*; **do you want**

R

a ~ into town? você quer uma carona para a cidade? **2** *v/t* ‹*pret* ***rode***, *pp* ***ridden***› *bike* andar de; *horse* andar a **3** *v/i* ‹*pret* ***rode***, *pp* ***ridden***› *on horse* cavalgar; *on bike* pedalar; *in vehicle* ir

rider ['raɪdər] *horse*: cavaleiro *m*; *female* amazona *f*; *bike*: ciclista *m/f*

ridge [rɪdʒ] (*raised strip*) borda *f*; *mountain*: cume *m*; *roof*: cumeeira *f*

ridicule ['rɪdɪkju:l] **1** *n* ridículo *m* **2** *v/t* ridicularizar

ridiculous [rɪ'dɪkjʊləs] *adj* ridículo

ridiculously [rɪ'dɪkjʊləslɪ] *adv expensive*, *easy* irrisoriamente

riding ['raɪdɪŋ] *horseback*: equitação *f*

rifle ['raɪfl] *n* rifle *m*

rift [rɪft] *earth*: rachadura *f*; *party etc*: divergência *f*

rig [rɪg] **1** *n Am* (*truck*) caminhão *m*, *Port* camião *m*; **(*oil*) ~** plataforma *f* de petróleo **2** *v/t* ‹*pret & pp* ***rigged***› *elections* fraudar

right [raɪt] **1** *adj* (*correct*, *proper*, *just*) certo, correto; (*suitable*) adequado; (*not left*) direito; ***be ~*** *answer*, *clock*, *also person* estar certo; *person* ter razão; ***put things ~*** pôr as coisas em ordem, resolver o problema; ***that's ~!*** correto!; ***that's all ~*** (*doesn't matter*) está tudo bem; (*when s.o. says thank you*) de nada; (*is quite good*) está ótimo; ***I'm all ~*** (*not hurt*) estou bem; (*have got enough*) estou satisfeito, obrigado; ***all ~, that's enough!*** bom, agora chega! **2** *adv* (*directly*) justamente, diretamente; (*correctly*) corretamente; (*completely*) completamente; (*not left*) à direita; ***~ now*** (*immediately*) agora mesmo; (*at the moment*) no momento **3** *n civil*, *legal etc* direito *m*; (*not left*), POL direita *f*; ***on the ~*** à direita; POL de direita; ***turn to the ~, take a ~*** vire à direita, pegue à sua direita; ***be in the ~*** estar com razão; ***know ~ from wrong*** distinguir o bem do mal

'right-angle ângulo *m* reto; ***at ~s to ...*** formando um ângulo reto com ...

rightful ['raɪtful] *adj heir*, *owner etc* legal

'righthand *adj* à direita; ***on the ~ side*** à direita **righthand 'drive** MOT veículo *m* com o volante à direita **right-handed** [raɪt'hændɪd] *adj person* destro **righthand 'man** mão *f* direita **right of 'way** *across land* direito *m* de passagem; *in traffic* preferência *f* **'right wing** *n* POL ala *f* direita; SPORT ponta *m* direita **'right-wing** *adj* POL de direita **right 'winger** POL político *m* de direita **right-wing ex'tremism** POL extremismo *m* de direita

rigid ['rɪdʒɪd] *adj material*, *attitude* rígido

rigor ['rɪgər] *Am* rigor *m*

rigorous ['rɪgərəs] *adj discipline*, *tests* rigoroso

rigorously ['rɪgərəslɪ] *adv check* rigorosamente

rigour *Brit* → ***rigor***

rile [raɪl] *v/t fam* irritar

rim [rɪm] *wheel*: manta *f*; *cup*: beira *f*; *eyeglasses*: armação *f*

ring[1] [rɪŋ] (*circle*) círculo *m*; *finger*: anel *m*; *boxing*: ringue *m*; *circus*: palco *m*

ring[2] [rɪŋ] **1** *n bell*: tocar *m*; *voice*: tom *m* **2** *v/t* ‹*pret* ***rang***, *pp* ***rung***› *bell* tocar **3** *v/i bell* ‹*pret* ***rang***, *pp* ***rung***› tocar; *Brit* TEL ligar; ***please ~ for attention*** por favor, toque a campainha (para ser atendido)

'ringleader líder *m/f* **'ring-pull** argola *f* **'ring tone** *cell phone*: toque *m* do telefone

rink [rɪŋk] pista *f* de patinação

rinse [rɪns] **1** *n hair color*: shampoo *m* tonalizante **2** *v/t clothes*, *dishes*, *hair* enxaguar

riot ['raɪət] **1** *n* tumulto *m* **2** *v/i* tumultuar

rioter ['raɪətər] tumultuador,a *m,f*

'riot police polícia *f* anti-tumulto

rip [rɪp] **1** *n cloth etc*: rasgo *m* **2** *v/t* ‹*pret & pp* ***ripped***› *cloth etc* rasgar; ***~ open*** abrir rasgando

♦ **rip off** *v/t fam customers* roubar; *cheat* enganar

♦ **rip up** *v/t letter*, *sheet* rasgar

ripe [raɪp] *adj fruit* maduro

ripen ['raɪpn] *v/i fruit* amadurecer

ripeness ['raɪpnɪs] *fruit* amadurecimento *m*

R

'rip-off *n fam* roubo *m*; **~ *prices*** preços absurdos
ripple ['rɪpl] *water*: onda *f*
rise [raɪz] **1** *v/i* ⟨*pret* ***rose***, *pp* ***risen***⟩ *from chair etc* levantar-se; *sun* nascer; *price*, *temperature*, *water level* subir **2** *n price*, *temperature*, *salary*: aumento *m*; *water level*: subida *f*, ***give* ~ *to*** causar
risen ['rɪzn] *pp* → ***rise***
riser ['raɪzər] ***be an early* ~** ser um madrugador; ***be a late* ~** ser um dorminhoco
risk [rɪsk] **1** *n* risco *m*; ***take a* ~** arriscar-se **2** *v/t* arriscar; ***let's* ~ *it*** vamos arriscar
risky ['rɪskɪ] *adj* arriscado
risotto [rɪ'sɑːtoʊ] risoto *m*
risqué [rɪ'skeɪ] *adj* picante
ritual ['rɪtʊəl] **1** *adj* ritual **2** *n* ritual *m*
rival ['raɪvl] **1** *n* rival *m/f* **2** *v/t* rivalizar com, ***I can't* ~ *that*** não posso competir com isto
rivalry ['raɪvlrɪ] rivalidade *f*
river ['rɪvər] rio *m*
'riverbank margem *f* do rio **'riverbed** leito *m* (do rio) **'riverside** **1** *adj* beira-rio **2** *n* beira-rio *f*
rivet ['rɪvɪt] **1** *n* rebite *m* **2** *v/t* rebitar
riveting ['rɪvɪtɪŋ] *adj* fascinante
road [roʊd] estrada *f*, ***it's just down the* ~** fica bem perto daqui
'roadblock barreira *f* **'road hog** dono,-a *m,f* da estrada **'road holding** *vehicle*: aderência *f* **'road map** mapa *m* de estradas **'roadrage** *comportamento agressivo durante a condução de um veículo* **'road safety** segurança *f* no trânsito **'roadside *at the* ~** na beira da estrada **'roadsign** sinal *m* de trânsito **'roadway** estrada *f* **'roadworthy** *adj* em condições de circulação
roam [roʊm] *v/i* vagar
roar [rɔːr] **1** *n traffic*, *engine*: estrondo *m*; *lion*: rugido *m*; *person*: grito *m* **2** *v/i engine* estrondar; *lion* rugir; *person* gritar; **~ *with laughter*** gargalhar
roast [roʊst] **1** *n beef etc* assado *m* **2** *v/t* & *v/i food* assar; ***we're* ~*ing*** estamos cozinhando
roast 'beef rosbife *m*
roast 'pork assado *m* de porco
rob [rɑːb] *v/t* ⟨*pret* & *pp* ***robbed***⟩ *person* roubar; *bank* assaltar; ***I've been* ~*bed*** fui roubado
robber ['rɑːbər] ladrão *m*, ladra *f*, *bank*: assaltante *m/f*
robbery ['rɑːbərɪ] roubo *m*
robe [roʊb] *judge*: toga *f*, *priest*: batina *f*, (***bath***) **~** *Am* roupão *m* (de banho)
robin ['rɑːbɪn] pintarroxo *m*
robot ['roʊbɑːt] robô *m*
robust [roʊ'bʌst] *adj* robusto
rock [rɑːk] **1** *n* rocha *f*, *smaller* pedra *f*, *in sea* recife *m*; MUS rock *m*; ***on the* ~*s*** *drink* com gelo; *marriage* em crise **2** *v/t cradle* balançar; *baby* embalar, ninar; (*surprise*) surpreender **3** *v/i on chair*, *boat* balançar
'rock band grupo *m* de rock **rock 'bottom *reach* ~** chegar ao fundo do poço **'rock-bottom** *adj prices* mínimo **'rock climber** escalador,a *m,f* de montanhas **'rock climbing** alpinismo *m*
rocket ['rɑːkɪt] **1** *n* foguete *m*; *firework* rojão *m* **2** *v/i prices etc* subir como um rojão
rocking chair ['rɑːkɪŋ] cadeira *f* de balanço
'rocking horse cavalo *m* de pau
rock 'n 'roll rock-and-roll *m*
'rock star estrela *f* de rock
Rocky ['rɑːkɪ] ***the* ~ *Mountains*** as Montanhas Rochosas
rocky ['rɑːkɪ] *adj beach*, *path* pedregoso
rod [rɑːd] vareta *f*, *fishing*: vara *f*
rode [roʊd] *pret* → ***ride***
rodent ['roʊdnt] roedor *m*
rogue [roʊg] vigarista *m/f*
role [roʊl] *play*, *movie*: papel *m*; *company*: função *f*, cargo *m*
'role model modelo *m* exemplar
roll [roʊl] **1** *n bread*: pãozinho *m*; *film*: rolo *m*; *thunder*: estrondo *m*; (*list*, *register*) lista *f* **2** *v/i ball etc* rolar; *boat* balançar **3** *v/t* **~ *sth into a ball*** fazer uma bola com algo; **~ *sth along the ground*** fazer rolar algo no chão
◆**roll over 1** *v/i* virar-se **2** *v/t person*, *object* virar; (*renew*) renovar

R

♦**roll up** **1** *v/t sleeves* dobrar **2** *v/i fam* (*arrive*) chegar
'roll call lista *f* de chamada
roller ['roʊlər] *hair*: bob *m*
'roller blade® *n* patim *m* roller blade **'roller blind** persiana *f* **'roller coaster** montanha-russa *f* **'roller skate** *n* patim *m* de rodas
rolling pin ['roʊlɪŋ] rolo *m* de pastel
ROM [rɑːm] *abbr* (*of* ***read only memory***) COMPUT memória *f* somente para leitura, ROM
Roman ['roʊmən] **1** *adj* romano **2** *n* romano,-a *m,f*
Roman 'Catholic **1** *adj* católico romano **2** *n* REL católico,-a *m,f* romano,-a
romance [rə'mæns] (*affair*) romance *m*; *movie* filme *f* romântico
romantic [roʊ'mæntɪk] *adj* romântico
romantically [roʊ'mæntɪklɪ] *adv* ***be ~ involved with s.o.*** ter um caso com alguém
Rome [roʊm] Roma
roof [ruːf] telhado *m*; ***have a ~ over one's head*** ter um teto sobre a cabeça
'roof rack MOT bagageiro *m*
rookie ['rʊkɪ] *Am fam* novato,-a *m,f*
room [ruːm] sala *f*, *bedroom*, *hotel*: quarto *m*; (*space*) espaço *m*; ***there's no ~ for ...*** não há lugar para ...
'room clerk recepcionista *m/f* **'room mate** companheiro,-a *m,f* de quarto **'room service** serviço *m* de quarto **'room temperature** temperatura *f* ambiente
roomy ['ruːmɪ] *adj house*, *car etc* espaçoso; *clothes* folgado
root [ruːt] *n also word*: raiz *f*, ***~s*** *pl person*: raízes *fpl*
♦**root for** *v/t fam* apoiar
♦**root out** *v/t* (*get rid of*) expulsar; (*find*) achar
rope [roʊp] corda *f*, ***show s.o. the ~s*** *fam* pôr alguém a par das coisas
♦**rope off** *v/t* interditar
rosary ['roʊzərɪ] REL rosário *m*
rose[1] [roʊz] *n* BOT rosa *f*
rose[2] [roʊz] *pret* → ***rise***
rosemary ['roʊzmərɪ] alecrim *m*
rostrum ['rɑːstrəm] tribuna *f*
rosy ['roʊzɪ] *adj cheeks* rosado; *future* cor-de-rosa
rot [rɑːt] **1** *n wood*, *teeth*: podridão *f* **2** *v/i* ⟨*pret & pp* ***rotted***⟩ *wood*, *teeth* apodrecer; *food* estragar
rotate [roʊ'teɪt] **1** *v/i blades*, *earth* girar **2** *v/t crops* alternar
rotation [roʊ'teɪʃn] *around the sun etc* rotação *f*; ***do sth in ~*** fazer algo em turno rotatório
rotten ['rɑːtn] *adj wood etc* podre; *food* estragado; *trick* malvado; *thing to do* odioso; *weather*, *luck* horrível
rough [rʌf] **1** *adj surface* irregular; *hands*, *skin* áspero; *voice* rouco; *crossing* movimentado; *seas* bravo; (*violent*) bruto; (*approximate*) aproximado; ***~ draft*** rascunho *m* **2** *adv* ***sleep ~*** dormir ao ar livre **3** *n golf*: rough *m* **4** *v/t* ***~ it*** *fam* viver duramente
♦**rough up** *v/t fam* espancar
roughage ['rʌfɪdʒ] *in food* fibra *f*
roughly ['rʌflɪ] *adv* (*approximately*) aproximadamente; (*harshly*) brutalmente; ***~ speaking*** aproximadamente
roulette [ruː'let] roleta *f*
round [raʊnd] **1** *adj* redondo; ***in ~ figures*** em números arredondados **2** *n mailman*, *doctor*: ronda *f*; *toast*: fatia *f*; *drinks*, *competition*: rodada *f*; *boxing*: round *m* **3** *v/t corner* dobrar **4** *adv*, *prep* → ***around***
♦**round off** *v/t edges* arredondar; *meeting*, *night out* concluir
♦**round up** *v/t figure* arredondar; *suspects*, *criminals* deter
'roundabout **1** *adj route*, *way of saying sth* indireto **2** *n Brit road*: rotatória *f*, *Port* rotunda *f* **'round-the-world** *adj* ao redor do mundo **'round trip** *Am* viagem *f* de ida e volta **round trip 'ticket** *Am* ticket *m* de ida e volta **'round-up** *cattle*: recolhida *f*, *suspects*, *criminals*: captura *f*, *news*: resumo *m*
rouse [raʊz] *v/t from sleep*, *interest etc* despertar
rousing ['raʊzɪŋ] *adj speech*, *finale* emocionante
route [raʊt] rota *f*, caminho *m*
routine [ruː'tiːn] **1** *adj* rotineiro **2** *n*

R

rotina *f*; ***as a matter of ~*** como rotina
row[1] [roʊ] *n* (*line*) fileira *f*; ***5 days in a ~*** 5 dias em seguida
row[2] [roʊ] *v/t & v/i boat* remar
row[3] [raʊ] *n* (*quarrel*) briga *f*; (*noise*) barulho *m*
rowboat ['roʊboʊt] *Am* barco *m* a remo
rowdy ['raʊdɪ] *adj* barulhento
rowing boat *Brit* → ***rowboat***
royal ['rɔɪl] *adj* real
royalty ['rɔɪltɪ] (*royal persons*) realeza *f*; *book, recording*: direitos *mpl* autorais
rub [rʌb] *v/t* ⟨*pret & pp* ***rubbed***⟩ enxugar
◆ **rub down** *v/t to clean* raspar
◆ **rub in** *v/t ointment* aplicar massageando; ***don't rub it in!*** *fig* não ponha o dedo na ferida!
◆ **rub off 1** *v/t dirt* limpar esfregando; *paint etc* esfregar **2** *v/i* ***it rubs off on you*** está lhe contagiando
rubber ['rʌbər] **1** *n* borracha *f*; *fam* (*condom*) camisinha *f* **2** *adj* de borracha
rubber 'band elástico *m* de borracha
rubber 'glove luva *f* de borracha
rubbish ['rʌbɪʃ] *Brit* lixo *m*; (*poor quality*) porcaria *f*; (*nonsense*) tolice *f*; ***don't talk ~!*** não fale besteiras
rubbish bin *Brit* → ***garbage can***
rubble ['rʌbl] entulho *m*
ruby ['ru:bɪ] rubi *m*
rucksack ['rʌksæk] mochila *f*
rudder ['rʌdər] leme *m*
ruddy ['rʌdɪ] *adj* avermelhado
rude [ru:d] *adj* rude; ***it is ~ to …*** é falta de educação …; ***I didn't mean to be ~*** eu não quis ser rude
rudely ['ru:dlɪ] *adv* rudemente
rudeness ['ru:dnɪs] grosseria *f*
rudimentary [ru:dɪ'mentərɪ] *adj* rudimentar
rudiments ['ru:dɪmənts] *npl* rudimentos *mpl*
rueful ['ru:fl] *adj* arrependido
ruefully ['ru:fəlɪ] *adv* com arrependimento
ruffian ['rʌfɪən] bruto *m*
ruffle ['rʌfl] **1** *n dress*: babado *m* **2** *v/t person* irritar; *hair* despentear; *clothes* amarrotar; ***get ~d*** ficar irritado
rug [rʌg] tapete *m*; (*blanket*) manta *f* de viagem
rugby ['rʌgbɪ] rúgbi *m*, *Port* râguebi *m*
rugged ['rʌgɪd] *adj scenery, cliffs* escabroso; *face* de traços duros; *resistance* determinado
ruin ['ru:ɪn] **1** *n* ruína *f*; ***~s*** *pl* ruínas *fpl*; ***in ~s*** *city, building* em ruínas; *plans, marriage* arruinado **2** *v/t party, birthday, vacation, plans, reputation* arruinar; ***be ~ed*** *financially* estar arruinado
rule [ru:l] **1** *n club, game*: regra *f*; *monarch*: reinado *m*; *measuring*: régua *f*; ***as a ~*** em geral **2** *v/t country* governar; ***the judge ~d that …*** o juíz determinou que … **3** *v/i monarch* reinar
◆ **rule out** *v/t* excluir
ruler ['ru:lər] *measuring*: régua *f*; *state*: governante *m/f*
ruling ['ru:lɪŋ] **1** *n* veredicto *m* **2** *adj party* dominante
rum [rʌm] *drink* rum *m*
rumble ['rʌmbl] *v/i stomach* roncar; *train in tunnel* ressoar
◆ **rummage around** ['rʌmɪdʒ] *v/i* procurar por todas as partes
'rummage sale *Am* bazar *m*
rumor ['ru:mər] **1** *n* rumor *m* **2** *v/t* ***it is ~ed that …*** surgiu um boato que …
rumour *Brit* → ***rumor***
rump [rʌmp] *animal*: parte *f* traseira
rumple ['rʌmpl] *v/t clothes, paper* dobrar
'rumpsteak alcatra *f*
run [rʌn] **1** *n on foot* corrida *f*; *in car* viagem *f*; *Am tights*: fio *m* corrido; ***it has had a three year ~*** esteve tres anos em cartaz; ***go for a ~*** ir correr; ***go for a ~ in the car*** fazer um passeio de carro; ***make a ~ for it*** sair correndo; ***a criminal on the ~*** um criminoso em fuga; ***in the short / long ~*** a curto / longo prazo; ***a ~ on the dollar*** uma corrida pelo dólar **2** *v/i* ⟨*pret* ***ran***, *pp* ***run***⟩ *person, river* correr; *paint, makeup, nose, eyes* escorrer; *engine, machine, software* funcionar; *in election* concorrer; ***the trains ~***

R

every ten minutes os trens passam de 10 em 10 minutos; ***don't leave the faucet ~ning*** não deixe a torneira aberta; ***~ for President*** candidatar-se à presidência **3** *v/t* ⟨*pret* ***ran***, *pp* ***run***⟩ *race, 3 miles etc* correr; *business, hotel, project etc* dirigir; *software* usar; *car* ter; ***can I ~ you to the station?*** posso levá-lo à estação?; ***he ran his eye down the page*** ele deu uma olhada na página

♦**run across** *v/t* (*meet*) encontrar-se; (*find*) encontrar

♦**run away** *v/i* fugir; ***she ran away from home*** ela fugiu de casa

♦**run down 1** *v/t* (*knock down*) atropelar; (*criticize*) criticar; *stocks* reduzir **2** *v/i battery* descarregar

♦**run into** *v/t* (*meet*) encontrar-se com; *difficulties* encontrar-se em

♦**run off 1** *v/i* sair correndo **2** *v/t* (*print off*) tirar

♦**run out** *v/i contract, time* vencer; *supplies* esgotar-se

♦**run out of** *v/t time, patience, supplies* ficar sem; ***I ran out of gas*** fiquei sem gás

♦**run over 1** *v/t* (*knock down*) atropelar; ***can we run over the details again?*** podemos repassar os detalhes? **2** *v/i water etc* transbordar

♦**run through** *v/t* (*rehearse, go over*) repassar

♦**run up** *v/t debts* acumular; *clothes* costurar

'runaway pessoa *f* que fugiu de casa

run-'down *adj person* esgotado; *part town, building* decadente

rung[1] [rʌŋ] *ladder* degrau *m*

rung[2] [rʌŋ] *pp* → ***ring***[2]

runner ['rʌnər] corredor,a *m,f*

runner 'bean vagem *f*, *Port* feijão *m* verde

runner-'up vice-campeão *m*, vice-campeã *f*

running ['rʌnɪŋ] **1** *n* SPORT corrida *f*; *business*: administração *f* **2** *adj* ***for two days ~*** durante dois dias seguidos

running 'water água *f* corrente

runny ['rʌnɪ] *adj liquid* líquido; *nose* escorrendo

'run-up SPORT impulso *m*; ***in the ~ to the election*** no período pré-eleitoral

'runway pista *f* de decolagem; *fashion show*: passarela *f*

rupture ['rʌptʃər] **1** *n* ruptura *f* **2** *v/i pipe etc* romper-se

rural ['rʊrəl] *adj* rural

ruse [ru:z] artimanha *f*

rush [rʌʃ] **1** *n* pressa *f*; ***do sth in a ~*** fazer algo com pressa; ***be in a ~*** estar correndo; ***what's the big ~?*** porque a pressa? **2** *v/t person* apressar; *meal* comer depressa; ***~ s.o. to the hospital*** levar alguém depressa para o hospital **3** *v/i* apressar-se

'rush hour hora *f* do rush, *Port* hora *f* de ponta

Russia ['rʌʃə] Rússia *f*

Russian ['rʌʃən] **1** *adj* russo **2** *n* russo,-a *m,f*; *language* russo *m*

rust [rʌst] **1** *n* ferrugem *f* **2** *v/i* enferrujar

rustle ['rʌsl] **1** *n silk, leaves* cicio *m* **2** *v/i* ciciar

'rust-proof *adj* inoxidável

rust remover ['rʌstrɪmu:vər] removedor *m* de ferrugem

rusty ['rʌstɪ] *adj also French, math etc* enferrujado; ***I'm a little ~*** estou um pouco fora de prática

rut [rʌt] *road*: pista *f*; ***be in a ~*** *fig* estar numa rotina

ruthless ['ru:θlɪs] *adj* cruel

ruthlessly *adv* cruelmente

ruthlessness ['ru:θlɪsnɪs] crueldade *f*

rye [raɪ] centeio *m*

'rye bread pão *m* de centeio

S

sabbatical [sə'bætɪkl] *n academic* licença *f* de um ano
sabotage ['sæbətɑːʒ] **1** *n* sabotagem *f* **2** *v/t* sabotar
saboteur [sæbə'tɜːr] MIL sabotador,a *m,f*
saccharin ['sækərɪn] *n* sacarina *f*
sachet ['sæʃeɪ] *shampoo, cream etc*: pacotinho *m*
sack [sæk] **1** *n* (*bag*) saco *m*; *Am groceries*: saco *m* de papel; ***get the ~*** *fam* ser mandado embora **2** *v/t fam* demitir
sacred ['seɪkrɪd] *adj* sacro
sacrifice ['sækrɪfaɪs] **1** *n* sacrifício *m*; ***make ~s*** *fig* fazer sacrifícios **2** *v/t also fig* sacrificar
sacrilege ['sækrɪlɪdʒ] sacrilégio *m*
sad [sæd] *adj person, song, state of affairs* triste
saddle ['sædl] **1** *n* sela *f* **2** *v/t horse* selar; ***~ s.o. with sth*** *fig* encarregar alguém de algo
sadism ['seɪdɪzm] sadismo *m*
sadist ['seɪdɪst] sadista *m/f*
sadistic [sə'dɪstɪk] *adj* sádico
sadly ['sædlɪ] *adv look, sing etc* com tristeza; (*regrettably*) infelizmente
sadness ['sædnɪs] tristeza *f*
safe [seɪf] **1** *adj* seguro **2** *n* cofre *m*
'safeguard 1 *n* proteção *f*; ***as a ~ against*** como uma garantia contra **2** *v/t* salvaguardar
safe'keeping *n* ***give sth to s.o. for ~*** dar algo a alguém para cuidar
safely ['seɪflɪ] *adv arrive* são e salvo; *complete test etc* sem problemas; *drive* prudentemente; *look after* bem; *assume* com certeza
safety ['seɪftɪ] segurança *f*
'safety belt cinto *m* de segurança **'safety-conscious** consciente sobre a segurança **safety 'first** prevenção *f* de acidentes **'safety pin** alfinete *m* de segurança
sag [sæg] **1** *n ceiling etc*: afundamento *m*; (*sinking, fall*) caída *f* **2** *v/i rope* distender-se; *output, tempo* diminuir
saga ['sɑːgə] saga *f*
sage [seɪdʒ] *n herb* sálvia *f*
Sagittarius [sædʒɪ'terɪəs] ASTROL Sagitário *m*
said [sed] *pret & pp* → ***say***
sail [seɪl] **1** *n* vela *f*, *trip* viagem *f* de barco; ***go for a ~*** passear de barco **2** *v/t & v/i* velejar; (*depart*) zarpar
'sailboard 1 *n* prancha *f* de windsurf **2** *v/i* praticar windsurf **'sailboarding** windsurf *m* **'sailboat** *Am* barco a vela
sailing ['seɪlɪŋ] SPORT vela *f*
sailing boat *Brit* → ***sailboat***
'sailing ship veleiro *m*
sailor ['seɪlər] *navy*: marinheiro *m*; SPORT navegador,a *m,f*; ***be a good ~*** não ficar mareado facilmente; ***be a bad ~*** ficar mareado facilmente
'sailor's knot *Am* nó *m* de rizos
saint [seɪnt] santo *m*
sake [seɪk] *n* ***for my ~ / for your ~*** por mim / por você; ***for the ~ of*** por causa de
salad ['sæləd] salada *f*
'salad dressing molho *m* de salada
salary ['sælərɪ] salário *m*
'salary scale nível *m* salarial
sale [seɪl] venda *f*, *reduced prices*: liquidação *f*; ***for ~*** *sign* à venda; ***be on ~*** estar à venda; *reduced prices*: estar em liquidação
sales [seɪlz] *npl department* vendas *fpl*
sales assistant *Brit* → ***sales clerk***
'sales clerk *Am store*: vendedor,a *m,f* **'sales figures** cifras *fpl* de venda **'salesman** vendedor *m* **'sales manager** gerente *m/f* de vendas **'sales meeting** reunião *f* de vendas **'sales tax** *Am* ICM *m*, *Port* IVA *m* **'sales woman** vendedora *f*
salient ['seɪlɪənt] *adj* importante

saliva [sə'laɪvə] saliva *f*
salmon ['sæmən] ⟨*pl* ***salmon***⟩ salmão *m*
saloon [sə'luːn] (*bar*) bar *m*; *Brit* MOT sedã *m*
salt [sɒːlt] **1** *n* sal *m* **2** *v/t food* salgar
'saltcellar saleiro *m* **'salt water** água *f* salgada **'salt-water fish** peixe *m* de água salgada
salty ['sɒːltɪ] *adj* salgado
salutary ['sæljʊterɪ] *adj experience* benéfico
salute [sə'luːt] **1** *n* MIL continência *f*; ***take the ~*** presidir o desfile **2** *v/t* (*fig hail*) saudar **3** *v/i* MIL bater continência
salvage ['sælvɪdʒ] *v/t from wreck* resgatar
salvation [sæl'veɪʃn] salvação *f*
Salvation 'Army exército *m* da salvação
samba ['sæmbə] samba *m*; ***do the ~*** sambar
same [seɪm] **1** *adj* mesmo **2** *pron* ***the ~*** o/a mesmo,-a; ***Happy New Year – the ~ to you*** Feliz Ano Novo - igualmente; ***he's not the ~ any more*** ele já não é mais o mesmo; ***all the ~*** (*even so*) assim mesmo; ***men are all the ~*** os homens são todos iguais; ***it's all the ~ to me*** para mim tanto faz **3** *adv* igual; ***smell / look / sound the same*** cheirar / parecer / soar igual
sample ['sæmpl] *n* amostra *f*
sanatorium *Brit* → ***sanitarium***
sanctimonious [sæŋktɪ'moʊnɪəs] *adj* beato
sanction ['sæŋkʃn] **1** *n* (*approval*) consentimento *m*; (*penalty*) embargo *m* **2** *v/t* (*approve*) aprovar
sanctity ['sæŋktətɪ] santidade *f*
sanctuary ['sæŋktʃuerɪ] REL, *also wild animals*: santuário *m*
sand [sænd] **1** *n* areia *f* **2** *v/t with sandpaper* lixar
sandal ['sændl] sandália *f*
'sandbag saco *m* de areia **'sandblast** *v/t* limpar com jato de areia **'sand dune** duna *f* de areia
sander ['sændər] *tool* lixador *m*
'sandpaper **1** *n* lixa *f* **2** *v/t* lixar
'sandpit caixa *f* de areia **'sandstone** arenito *m*
sandwich ['sænwɪtʃ] **1** *n* sanduíche *m*, *Port* sandes *f* **2** *v/t* ***be ~ed between two …*** estar espremido entre dois …
sandy ['sændɪ] *adj* arenoso; *hair* loiro acinzentado
sane [seɪn] *adj* mentalmente são; ***no ~ person thinks …*** ninguém em perfeito juízo pensa que …
sang [sæŋ] *pret* → ***sing***
sanitarium [sænɪ'terɪəm] *Am* sanatório *m*
sanitary ['sænɪterɪ] *adj conditions* higiênico; ***~ installations*** instalações *fpl* sanitárias
'sanitary napkin *Am* absorvente *m* higiênico
sanitary towel *Brit* → ***sanitary napkin***
sanitation [sænɪ'teɪʃn] (*sanitary installations*) instalações *fpl* sanitárias; (*removal of waste*) saneamento *m*
sani'tation department departamento *m* de águas e esgotos
sanity ['sænətɪ] sanidade *f*
sank [sæŋk] *pret* → ***sink***
Santa Claus ['sæntəklɒːz] Papai *m* Noel
sap [sæp] **1** *n tree*: seiva *f* **2** *v/t* ⟨*pret & pp* ***sapped***⟩ *energy* sugar
sapphire ['sæfaɪr] *n jewel* safira *f*
sarcasm ['sɑːrkæzm] sarcasmo *m*
sarcastic [sɑːr'kæstɪk] *adj* sarcástico
sarcastically [sɑːr'kæstɪklɪ] *adv* sarcasticamente
sardine [sɑːr'diːn] sardinha *f*
sardonic [sɑːr'dɑːnɪk] *adj* cínico
sardonically [sɑːr'dɑːnɪklɪ] *adv* cinicamente
sash [sæʃ] *dress, uniform*: faixa *f*
Satan ['seɪtn] satanás *m*
satchel ['sætʃl] *schoolchild*: mochilinha *f*
satellite ['sætəlaɪt] satélite *m*
'satellite dish antena *f* parabólica
'satellite TV TV *f* por satélite
satin ['sætɪn] *n* cetim *m*
satire ['sætaɪr] sátira *f*
satirical [sə'tɪrɪkl] *adj* satírico
satirist ['sætərɪst] satirista *m/f*

satirize ['sætəraɪz] *v/t* satirizar
satisfaction [sætɪs'fækʃn] satisfação *f*; ***get ~ out of sth*** sentir satisfação em algo; ***a feeling of ~*** uma satisfação; ***is that to your ~?*** está tudo à sua inteira satisfação?
satisfactory [sætɪs'fæktərɪ] *adj* satisfatório; ***this is not ~*** não é satisfatório
satisfy ['sætɪsfaɪ] *v/t* ⟨*pret & pp* ***satisfied***⟩ *customers, needs* satisfazer; *conditions* cumprir; ***I am satisfied*** *enough to eat* estou satisfeito; ***I am satisfied that he …*** *convinced* estou convencido de que ele …; ***I hope you're satisfied!*** você está satisfeito agora?
satnav ['sætnæv] GPS *m*
Saturday ['sætərdeɪ] sábado *m*
sauce [sɒːs] molho *m*
'saucepan caçarola *f*
saucer ['sɒːsər] pires *m*
saucy ['sɒːsɪ] *adj person, dress* ousado
Saudi Arabia [saʊdɪə'reɪbɪə] Arábia *f* Saudita
sauna ['sɒːnə] sauna *f*
saunter ['sɒːntər] *v/i* passear tranqüilamente
sausage ['sɒːsɪdʒ] salsicha *f*
savage ['sævɪdʒ] **1** *adj animal, attack* selvagem; *criticism* feroz **2** *n* selvagem *m/f*
savagery ['sævɪdʒrɪ] brutalidade *f*
save [seɪv] **1** *v/t* (*rescue*) salvar; *money, time* economizar; (*collect*) guardar; COMPUT salvar; *goal* defender; ***you could ~ yourself a lot of effort*** você poderia economizar muito trabalho **2** *v/i* (*put money aside*) economizar; SPORT defender **3** *n* SPORT defesa *f*
♦**save up for** *v/t* economizar para
saver ['seɪvər] *person* economizador,a *m,f*
saving ['seɪvɪŋ] (*amount saved*) economia *f*; *activity* poupanças *fpl*
savings ['seɪvɪŋz] *npl* economias *fpl*
'savings account caderneta *f* de poupança **savings and 'loan** *Am* sociedade *f* de crédito imobiliário
'savings bank caixa *f* econômica
savior *Am*, **saviour** *Brit* ['seɪvjər] REL salvador *m*
savor ['seɪvər] *Am* **1** *n* sabor *m* **2** *v/t* saborear
savory ['seɪvərɪ] *adj Am* salgado
savour *etc Brit* → ***savor***
saw[1] [sɒː] *pret* → ***see***
saw[2] [sɒː] **1** *n tool* serra *f* **2** *v/t* serrar
♦**saw off** *v/t* serrar
'sawdust serradura *f*
saxophone ['sæksəfoʊn] saxofone *m*
say [seɪ] **1** *v/t* ⟨*pret & pp* ***said***⟩ dizer; *poem* recitar; ***can I ~ something?*** posso dizer uma coisa?; ***that is to ~*** ou seja; ***what do you ~ to that?*** o que você diz disso?; ***what does the note ~?*** o que essa nota diz? **2** *n* ***have one's ~*** dar sua opinião
saying ['seɪɪŋ] ditado *m*
scab [skæb] *on skin* crosta *f*
scaffolding ['skæfəldɪŋ] andaime *m*
scald [skɒːld] *v/t* queimar
scale[1] [skeɪl] *fish*: escama *f*
scale[2] [skeɪl] **1** *n* MUS, *thermometer etc, map*: escala *f*; (*size*) dimensão *f*; ***on a larger / smaller ~*** em maior / menor escala **2** *v/t cliffs etc* escalar
♦**scale down** *v/t* diminuir, reduzir
'scale drawing desenho *f* em escala
scales [skeɪlz] *npl weighing*: balança *f*
scallop ['skæləp] *n* marisco *m*
scalp [skælp] *n* couro *m* cabeludo
scalpel ['skælpl] bisturi *m*
scam [skæm] *fam* sacanagem *f*
scampi ['skæmpɪ] *nsg* camarões *mpl* fritos
scan [skæn] **1** *v/t* ⟨*pret & pp* ***scanned***⟩ *horizon, page* dar uma olhada em; MED, COMPUT escanear **2** *n* MED ecografia *f*
♦**scan in** *v/t* COMPUT escanear
scandal ['skændl] escândalo *m*
scandalize ['skændəlaɪz] *v/t* escandalizar
scandalous ['skændələs] *adj affair, price* escandaloso
Scandinavia [skændɪ'neɪvɪə] Escandinávia *f*
scanner ['skænər] MED, COMPUT scanner *m*
scant [skænt] *adj* pouco
scantily ['skæntɪlɪ] *adv* **~ *clad*** mini-

S

mamente vestido
scanty ['skæntɪ] *adj clothes* curtíssimo
scapegoat ['skeɪpgoʊt] bode *m* expiatório
scar [skɑːr] **1** *n* cicatriz *f* **2** *v/t* ⟨*pret & pp* ***scarred***⟩ cicatrizar
scarce [skers] *adj in short supply* escasso; ***make oneself ~*** desaparecer
scarcely ['skerslɪ] *adv* mal, quase não; ***I could ~ believe it*** mal pude acreditar
scarcity ['skersɪtɪ] escassez *f*
scare [sker] **1** *v/t* assustar; ***be ~d of*** ter medo de **2** *n* (*panic, alarm*) medo *m*; ***give s.o. a ~*** dar um susto em alguém
♦ **scare away** *v/t* espantar
'scarecrow espantalho *m*
scaremonger ['skermʌŋgər] alarmista *m/f*
scarf [skɑːrf] *neck, head*: lenço *m*; *winter*: cachecol *m*
scarlet ['skɑːrlət] *adj* escarlate
scarlet 'fever escarlatina *f*
scary ['skerɪ] *adj sight, music* horripilante; *movie* assustador
scathing ['skeɪðɪŋ] *adj* mordaz
scatter ['skætər] **1** *v/t leaflets* espalhar; *seeds* semear; ***be ~ed all over the room*** estar espalhado por toda a sala **2** *v/i people* dispersar-se
scatterbrained ['skætərbreɪnd] *adj* distraído
scattered ['skætərd] *adj showers, family, villages* disperso
scavenge ['skævɪndʒ] *v/i* vasculhar
scavenger ['skævɪndʒər] *animal, bird* carniceiro *m*; *person* catador *m* de lixo
scenario [sɪ'nɑːrɪoʊ] cenário *m*
scene [siːn] THEA, *of accident, novel etc*, (*argument*) cena *f*; ***make a ~*** fazer uma cena; ***~s*** THEA partes *fpl* do cenário; ***jazz / rock ~*** mundo *m* do jazz / rock; ***behind the ~s*** por trás dos bastidores
scenery ['siːnərɪ] THEA cenário *m*
scent [sent] *n* perfume *m*; *animal*: olfato *m*
sceptic *Brit* → ***skeptic***
schedule ['skedjuːl] **1** *n events*: programa *m*; *work, trains, lessons*: horário *m*; ***be on ~*** estar no horário; ***be behind ~*** estar atrasado **2** *v/t* (*put on schedule*) marcar; ***it's ~d for completion next month*** está previsto para ser completado no próximo mês
scheduled flight ['skedjuːld] vôo *m* regular
scheme [skiːm] **1** *n* (*plan*) plano *m*; (*plot*) complô *m* **2** *v/i* (*plot*) conspirar
scheming ['skiːmɪŋ] *adj* maquinador
schizophrenia [skɪtsə'friːnɪə] esquizofrenia *f*
schizophrenic [skɪtsə'frenɪk] **1** *adj* esquizofrênico **2** *n* esquizofrênico,-a *m,f*
scholar ['skɑːlər] estudioso,-a *m,f*
scholarly ['skɑːlərlɪ] *adj* erudito
scholarship ['skɑːlərʃɪp] (*scholarly work*) estudos *mpl*; *award* bolsa *f* de estudos
school [skuːl] escola *f*; *Am* (*university*) universidade *f*
'school bag mochila *f* escolar **'schoolboy** aluno *m* **'schoolchildren** *npl* alunos *mpl* **'school days** *npl* tempo *m* de escola **'schoolgirl** aluna *f* **'schoolmaster** professor *m* **'schoolmistress** professora *f* **'schoolteacher** professor,a *m,f*
sciatica [saɪ'ætɪkə] ciática *f*
science ['saɪəns] ciência *f*
science 'fiction ficção *f* científica
scientific [saɪən'tɪfɪk] *adj* científico
scientist ['saɪəntɪst] cientista *m/f*
scissors ['sɪzərz] *npl* tesoura *f*
scoff[1] [skɑːf] *v/t* (*eat fast*) devorar
scoff[2] [skɑːf] *v/i* zombar
♦ **scoff at** *v/t* zombar de
scold [skoʊld] *v/t* dar bronca
scoop [skuːp] **1** *n implement* colher *f*; *story* furo *m* de reportagem **2** *v/t* ***~ sth into sth*** recolher algo de volta a algo
♦ **scoop up** *v/t* pegar
scooter ['skuːtər] *with motor* scooter *m*, *Port* lambreta *f*; *child's* patinete *f*
scope [skoʊp] extensão *f*; (*freedom, opportunity*) oportunidade *f*
scorch [skɔːrtʃ] *v/t* queimar
scorching hot ['skɔːrtʃɪŋ] *adj* quentíssimo
score [skɔːr] **1** *n* SPORT placar *m*;

(*written music*) partitura *f*; *movie etc*: trilha *f* sonora; ***what's the ~?*** SPORT qual o placar?; ***have a ~ to settle with s.o.*** ter uma conta para acertar com alguém; ***keep (the) ~*** marcar o placar **2** *v/t goal, point, (cut) line* marcar **3** *v/i (keep the score)* marcar o placar; ***that's where he ~s*** este é o seu (ponto) forte

'scoreboard placar *m*

scorer ['skɔːrər] *goal* goleador,a *m,f*; *point* marcador,a *m,f*; (*score-keeper*) responsável *m/f* pela contagem

scorn [skɔːrn] **1** *n* desprezo *m*; ***pour ~ on sth*** desprezar algo **2** *v/t idea, suggestion* desprezar

scornful ['skɔːrnfʊl] *adj* depreciativo

scornfully ['skɔːrnfʊlɪ] *adv* com desprezo

Scorpio ['skɔːrpɪoʊ] ASTROL Escorpião *m*

Scot [skɑːt] escocês,-esa *m,f*

Scotch [skɑːtʃ] (*whiskey*) uísque *m* escocês, *Port* whisky *m* escocês

Scotch 'tape® *Am* durex® *m*

scot-'free *adv* ***get off ~*** sair impune

Scotland ['skɑːtlənd] Escócia *f*

Scotsman ['skɑːtsmən] escocês *m*

Scotswoman ['skɑːtswʊmən] escocesa *f*

Scottish ['skɑːtɪʃ] *adj* escocês,-esa

scoundrel ['skaʊndrəl] malvado,-a *m,f*

scour[1] ['skaʊr] *v/t (search)* explorar

scour[2] ['skaʊr] *v/t pans* esfregar

scout [skaʊt] *n (boy scout)* escoteiro *m*

scowl [skaʊl] **1** *n* cara *f* mau-humorada **2** *v/i* olhar com cara feia

scram [skræm] *v/i* ⟨*pret & pp* ***scrammed***⟩ *fam* sumir

scramble ['skræmbl] **1** *n (rush)* pressa *f* **2** *v/t message* codificar **3** *v/i (climb)* trepar; ***he ~d to his feet*** ele se levantou de um salto

scrambled eggs ['skræmbld] ovos *mpl* mexidos

scrap [skræp] **1** *n metal* ferro-velho *m*; (*fight*) briga *f*; (*little bit*) pedacinho *m*; ***not a ~ of evidence*** nem um pingo de evidência **2** *v/t* ⟨*pret & pp* ***scrapped***⟩ *plan, project etc* abandonar; *paragraph* apagar

'scrapbook álbum *m* de recortes

scrape [skreɪp] **1** *n paintwork etc*: raspagem *f* **2** *v/t paintwork, arm, vegetables etc* raspar; ***~ a living*** passar maus bocados

♦ **scrape through** *v/i in exam* passar raspando

'scrap heap ***good for the ~*** está bom para jogar fora **'scrap metal** sucata *f* **'scrap paper** papel *m* de rascunho

scrappy ['skræpɪ] *adj work* desorganizado; *Am person* brigão

scratch [skrætʃ] **1** *n mark* marca *f*; *paint*: raspagem *f*; ***have a ~*** *to stop itching* coçar-se; ***start from ~*** começar do zero; ***not be up to ~*** não ser bom o suficiente **2** *v/t (mark) skin, of cat, nails* arranhar **3** *v/i because of itch* coçar-se

scrawl [skrɒːl] **1** *n* garrancho *m* **2** *v/t* rabiscar

scrawny ['skrɒːnɪ] *adj* esquelético

scream [skriːm] **1** *n* grito *m*; ***~s of laughter*** gargalhadas *fpl* **2** *v/i* gritar

screech [skriːtʃ] **1** *n tires*: rangido *m*; (*scream*) berro *m* **2** *v/i tires* ranger; (*scream*) berrar

screen [skriːn] **1** *n room, hospital*: biombo *m*; *movie theater, television*: tela *f*, *Port* écran *m*; COMPUT monitor *m*; ***on (the) ~*** *movie* na tela; COMPUT no monitor **2** *v/t (protect, hide)* esconder; *movie* exibir; *security*: examinar

screening ['skriːnɪŋ] monitorização *f*; ***cancer ~*** monitorização do câncer

'screenplay roteiro *m* **'screen saver** COMPUT protetor *m* de tela **'screen test** *movie*: teste *m* cinematográfico

screw [skruː] **1** *n* parafuso *m*; *vulg sex*: transa *f* **2** *v/t* parafusar; *vulg* transar com; *fam (cheat)* trapacear; ***~ sth to sth*** parafusar algo em algo

♦ **screw up 1** *v/t eyes* fechar; *piece of paper* amassar; *fam (make a mess of)* arruinar **2** *v/i fam (make a bad mistake)* meter os pés pelas mãos

'screwdriver chave *f* de fenda

screwed up [skruːd'ʌp] *adj fam psychologically* complexado

'screw top *on bottle* tampinha *f* de rosca

screwy ['skru:ɪ] *adj fam* maluco
scribble ['skrɪbl] **1** *n* rabisco *m* **2** *v/t & v/i* (*write quickly*) rabiscar
script [skrɪpt] *movie, play*: roteiro *m*; (*form of writing*) caligrafia *f*
scripture ['skrɪptʃər] ***the (Holy) Scriptures*** as sagradas escrituras
'scriptwriter roteirista *m/f*
scroll [skroʊl] *n* (*manuscript*) pergaminho *m*
♦ **scroll down** *v/i* COMPUT mover para baixo
♦ **scroll up** *v/i* COMPUT mover para cima
scrounge [skraʊndʒ] *v/t* filar
scrounger ['skraʊndʒər] pidão *m*, pidona *f*
scrub [skrʌb] *v/t* ⟨*pret & pp* ***scrubbed***⟩ *floors, hands* esfregar
scrubbing brush ['skrʌbɪŋ] escova *f* de chão
scruffy ['skrʌfɪ] *adj* desleixado
♦ **scrunch up** [skrʌntʃ] *v/t plastic cup etc* esmagar
scruples ['skru:plz] *npl* escrúpulos *mpl*; ***have no ~ about doing sth*** não ter escrúpulos de fazer algo
scrupulous ['skru:pjʊləs] *adj with moral principles* escrupuloso; (*thorough*) meticuloso; *attention to detail* minucioso
scrupulously ['skru:pjʊləslɪ] *adv* (*meticulously*) meticulosamente
scrutinize ['skru:tɪnaɪz] *v/t* (*examine closely*) examinar
scrutiny ['skru:tɪnɪ] exame *m* detalhado; ***come under ~*** ser objeto de investigação
scuba diving ['sku:bə] mergulho *m* autônomo
scuffle ['skʌfl] *n* rixa *f*
sculptor ['skʌlptər] escultor,a *m,f*
sculpture ['skʌlptʃər] escultura *f*
scum [skʌm] *liquid*: espuma *f*; *pej people* ralé *f*
sea [si:] mar *m*; ***by ~*** por mar; ***by the ~*** perto do mar
'seabed fundo *m* do mar **'seabird** ave *f* marítima **'seafaring** ['si:ferɪŋ] *adj nation* marítimo **'seafood** frutos *mpl* do mar **'seafront** frente *f* do mar **'seagoing** *adj vessel* em condições de navegar **'seagull** gaivota *f*
seal[1] [si:l] *n animal* foca *f*
seal[2] [si:l] **1** *n document*: selo *m*; TECH lacre *m* **2** *v/t container* selar
♦ **seal off** *v/t area* interditar
'sea level *above / below ~* acima / abaixo do nível do mar
seam [si:m] *n garment*: costura *f*; *ore*: filão *m*
'seaman marinheiro *m*
seamstress ['si:mstrɪs] costureira *f*
'seaport porto *m* marítimo
'sea power *nation* potência *f* marítima
search [sɜ:rtʃ] **1** *n* busca *f*; ***be in ~ of*** estar procurando por **2** *v/t city, files* procurar em
♦ **search for** *v/t* procurar por
'search engine motor *m* de busca
searching ['sɜ:rtʃɪŋ] *adj look* crítico; *question* difícil
'searchlight holofote *m* **'search party** equipe *f* de resgate **'search warrant** mandado *m* de busca
'seashore litoral *m* **'seasick** *adj* mareado; ***get ~*** ficar mareado **'seaside** beira-mar *f*; ***at the ~*** à beira-mar; ***go to the ~*** ir à praia; ***~ resort*** resort *m* à beira-mar
season ['si:zn] *n winter, spring, for tourism etc* estação *f*; ***in / out of ~*** na / fora da estação
seasonal ['si:znl] *adj fruit, employment* sazonal
seasoned ['si:znd] *adj wood* seco; *traveler, campaigner etc* experiente
seasoning ['si:znɪŋ] condimento *m*
'season ticket entrada *f* permanente
seat [si:t] **1** *n* assento *m*; *pants*: parte *f* traseira; ***please take a ~*** por favor, sente-se **2** *v/t* (*have seating for*) ter lugar para; ***please remain ~ed*** permaneça sentado, por favor
'seat belt cinto *m* de segurança
'sea urchin ouriço *m* do mar
'seaweed algas *fpl*
secluded [sɪ'klu:dɪd] *adj* isolado
seclusion [sɪ'klu:ʒn] isolamento *m*
second[1] ['sekənd] **1** *n time* segundo *m*; ***just a ~*** (só) um momento **2** *adj* segundo **3** *adv come in* em segundo lugar **4** *v/t motion* apoiar

S

second[2] [sɪ'kɑːnd] *v/t* ***be ~ed to*** ser designado para
secondary ['sekənderɪ] *adj* secundário; ***of ~ importance*** de importância secundária
secondary edu'cation ensino *m* secundário
second 'best *adj* segundo melhor **second 'biggest** *adj* segundo maior **second 'class** *adj ticket* de segunda classe **second 'floor** segundo andar *m* **second 'gear** MOT segunda marcha *f* **'second hand** *on clock* ponteiro *m* de segundos **second-'hand, second'hand** *adj & adv* de segunda mão, *Port* em segunda mão
secondly ['sekəndlɪ] *adv* em segundo lugar
second-'rate *adj* de segunda categoria, inferior
second 'thoughts *npl* ***I've had ~*** mudei de idéia
secrecy ['siːkrəsɪ] sigilo *m*
secret ['siːkrət] **1** *n* segredo *m*; ***do sth in ~*** fazer algo em segredo **2** *adj* secreto
secret 'agent agente secreto,-a *m,f*
secretarial [sekrə'terɪəl] *adj tasks, job* de secretariado
secretary ['sekrəterɪ] secretário,-a *m,f*; POL ministro,-a *m,f*
Secretary of 'State *in USA* ministro,-a *m,f* do exterior
secrete [sɪ'kriːt] *v/t* (*give off*) segregar; (*hide away*) guardar
secretion [sɪ'kriːʃn] secreção *f*
secretive ['siːkrətɪv] *adj* reservado
secretly ['siːkrətlɪ] *adv* em segredo
secret po'lice polícia *f* secreta
secret 'service serviço *m* secreto
sect [sekt] seita *f*
section ['sekʃn] *apple, text, building, lung*: parte *f*; *company*: seção *f*
sector ['sektər] *society*: setor *m*; *city*: área *f*
secular ['sekjʊlər] *adj* secular
secure [sɪ'kjʊr] **1** *adj shelf, feeling etc* seguro **2** *v/t shelf etc* fixar; *help, job, contract* conseguir
se'curities market FIN mercado *m* de capitais
security [sɪ'kjʊrətɪ] *job, relationship, airport*: segurança *f*; *investment*: garantia *f*; *beliefs etc*: confiança *f*
se'curity alert alarme *m* de segurança **se'curity check** controle *m* de segurança **se'curity-conscious** *adj* consciente da segurança **se'curity forces** forças *fpl* de segurança **se'curity guard** garda *m/f* de segurança **se'curity risk** risco *m* de segurança
sedan [sɪ'dæn] *Am* sedã *m*
sedate [sɪ'deɪt] *v/t* dar um sedativo a
sedation [sɪ'deɪʃn] *n* ***be under ~*** estar sob sedativo
sedative ['sedətɪv] *n* sedativo *m*
sedentary ['sedənterɪ] *adj job* sedentário
sediment ['sedɪmənt] sedimento *m*
seduce [sɪ'duːs] *v/t sexually* seduzir
seduction [sɪ'dʌkʃn] *sexual* sedução *f*
seductive [sɪ'dʌktɪv] *adj* sedutor
see [siː] *v/t* ⟨*pret* ***saw***, *pp* ***seen***⟩ ver; (*understand*) entender; *romantically* encontrar-se com; ***I ~*** entendo; ***can I ~ the manager?*** chame o gerente, por favor; ***you should ~ a doctor*** o você deveria ir ao médico; ***~ s.o. home*** acompanhar alguém até sua casa; ***I'll ~ you to the door*** eu vou acompanhá-lo até a porta; ***~ you!*** *fam* tchau!; ***~ing that*** já que
♦ **see about** *v/t* (*look into*) tratar de
♦ **see off** *v/t at airport etc* despedir-se de; (*chase away*) espantar
♦ **see out** *v/t* ***see s.o. out*** acompanhar alguém até a porta
♦ **see to** *v/t* ***see to sth*** encarregar-se de algo; ***see to it that sth gets done*** certificar-se de que algo seja feito
seed [siːd] semente *f*; ***go to ~*** *person* descuidar-se; *district* decair
seedling ['siːdlɪŋ] muda *f*
seedy ['siːdɪ] *adj bar, district* decadente
seek [siːk] *v/t* ⟨*pret & pp* ***sought***⟩ *employment* procurar; *truth* buscar
seem [siːm] *v/i* parecer; ***it ~s that …*** parece que …
seemingly ['siːmɪŋlɪ] *adv* aparentemente
seen [siːn] *pp of* ***see***

seep [siːp] *v/i liquid* filtrar-se
◆**seep out** *v/i liquid* escorrer
seesaw ['siːsɒː] *n* gangorra *f*
seethe [siːð] *v/i fig* ferver de raiva
'see-through *adj dress, material* transparente
segment ['segmənt] segmento *m*; *orange*: gomo *m*
segregate ['segrɪgeɪt] *v/t* segregar
segregation [segrɪ'geɪʃn] segregação *f*
seismology [saɪz'mɑːlədʒɪ] sismologia *f*
seize [siːz] *v/t person, s.o.'s arm* agarrar; *opportunity* aproveitar; *contraband* confiscar
◆**seize up** *v/i engine* emperrar
seizure ['siːʒər] MED ataque *m*; *drugs etc*: apreensão *f*
seldom ['seldəm] *adv* raramente
select [sɪ'lekt] **1** *v/t* selecionar **2** *adj* (*exclusive*) seleto
selection [sɪ'lekʃn] (*choosing*) eleição *f*, escolha *f*; (*that / those chosen*) seleção *f*; (*assortment*) coleção *f*
se'lection process processo *m* seletivo
selective [sɪ'lektɪv] *adj* seletivo
self [self] ⟨*pl* ***selves***⟩ ego *m*
self-addressed envelope [selfə'drest] envelope *m* pré-endereçado **self-as'surance** auto-segurança *f* **self-assured** [selfə'ʃʊrd] *adj* seguro de si **self-'catering apartment** apartamento *m* sem serviço de refeições **self-centered** [self'sentərd] *adj Am* egocêntrico **self-centred** *Brit* → ***self-centered*** **self-'cleaning** *adj oven* autolimpante **self-confessed** [selfkən'fest] *adj* reconhecido **self-'confidence** autoconfiança *f* **self-'confident** *adj* autoconfiante **self-'conscious** *adj* inibido **self--'consciousness** inibição *f* **self-contained** [selfkən'teɪnd] *adj apartment* independente **self con'trol** autocontrole *m* **self-defence** *Brit* → ***self-defense*** **self-de'fense** *Am* autodefesa *f* **self-'discipline** autodisciplina *f* **self-'doubt** insegurança *f* **self-employed** [selfɪm'plɔɪd] *adj* autônomo **self-e'steem** auto-estima *f* **self-'evident** *adj* óbvio **self-ex'pression** auto-expressão *f* **self-'government** governo *m* autônomo **self-'interest** interesse *m* próprio
selfish ['selfɪʃ] *adj* egoísta
selfless ['selflɪs] *adj* altruísta
self-made 'man self-made man *m* **self-'pity** autocomiseração *f* **self-'portrait** auto-retrato *m* **self-pos'sessed** *adj* sereno **self-re'liant** *adj* auto-suficiente **self-re'spect** auto-respeito *m* **self-'righteous** [self'raɪtjəs] *adj pej* pretensioso **self-'satisfied** [self'sætɪsfaɪd] *adj pej* presunçoso **self-'service** *adj* self-service **self-service 'restaurant** restaurante *m* self-service **self-taught** [self'tɔːt] *adj* autodidata
sell [sel] *v/t & v/i* ⟨*pret & pp* ***sold***⟩ vender; ***you have to ~ yourself*** você tem que se vender
◆**sell out of** *v/t* vender todo o estoque de; ***it's sold out*** está esgotado
◆**sell up** *v/i* vender tudo
'sell-by date prazo *m* de validade; ***be past its ~*** estar vencido; ***he's past his ~*** ele já passou da data de validade
seller ['selər] vendedor,a *m,f*
selling point ['selɪŋ] COM ponto *m* forte
Sellotape® *Brit* → ***Scotch tape***®
semen ['siːmən] sêmen *m*
semester [sɪ'mestər] semestre *m*
semi ['semaɪ] *n Am truck* caminhão *m* de semi-reboque, *Port* camião *m* articulado
'semicircle ['semɪsɜːrkl] semicírculo *m* **semi'circular** *adj* semicircular **semi-'colon** ponto e vírgula **'semiconductor** ELEC semicondutor *m* **semide'tached** *Brit* casa *f* geminada **semi'final** semifinal *f*
seminar ['semɪnɑːr] seminário *m*
semi'skilled *adj* semiqualificado
senate ['senət] *Am* senado *m*
senator ['senətər] *Am* senador,a *m,f*
send [send] *v/t* ⟨*pret & pp* ***sent***⟩ mandar, enviar; ***~ sth to s.o.*** enviar algo a alguém; ***~ s.o. to s.o.*** mandar alguém para alguém; ***~ her my best***

wishes mande-lhe lembranças minhas

◆ **send back** *v/t person, letter* mandar de volta; *food in restaurant* devolver

◆ **send for** *v/t doctor, help* mandar buscar

◆ **send in** *v/t troops, application form* enviar

◆ **send off** *v/t letter, fax etc* enviar, mandar

sender ['sendər] *letter*: remetente *m/f*

senile ['si:naɪl] *adj* senil

senility [sɪ'nɪlətɪ] senilidade *f*

senior ['si:njər] *adj* (*older*) mais velho; *in rank* superior, sênior; ***be ~ to s.o.*** *in rank* ser superior a alguém

senior 'citizen pessoa *f* da terceira idade, idoso,-a *m,f*

sensation [sen'seɪʃn] *feeling, s.o. / sth very good* sensação *f*

sensational [sen'seɪʃnl] *adj* (*very good*) sensacional

sense [sens] **1** *n* (*meaning*) sentido *m*, significado *m*; (*purpose, point, sight, smell etc*) sentido *m*; (*common sense*) senso *m*; (*feeling*) sentimento *m*; ***in a ~*** em certo sentido; ***talk ~, man!*** não diga bobagens!; ***come to one's ~s*** cair em si; ***it doesn't make ~*** não faz sentido; ***there's no ~ in waiting*** não faz sentido esperar **2** *v/t s.o.'s presence* sentir

senseless ['senslɪs] *adj* (*pointless*) absurdo

sensible ['sensəbl] *adj person, decision, advice* sensato; *clothes, shoes* prático

sensibly ['sensəblɪ] *adv* com sensatez

sensitive ['sensətɪv] *adj skin, person* sensível

sensitivity [sensə'tɪvətɪ] *skin, person* sensibilidade *f*

sensor ['sensər] sensor *m*

sensual ['senʃʊəl] *adj* sensual

sensuality [senʃʊ'ælətɪ] sensualidade *f*

sensuous ['senʃʊəs] *adj* sensual

sent [sent] *pret & pp* → ***send***

sentence ['sentəns] **1** *n* GRAM frase *f*, LAW sentença *f* **2** *v/t* LAW sentenciar

sentiment ['sentɪmənt] (*sentimentality*) sentimentalismo *m*; (*opinion*) opinião *f*

sentimental [sentɪ'mentl] *adj* sentimental

sentimentality [sentɪmen'tælətɪ] sentimentalismo *m*

sentry ['sentrɪ] vigia *m/f*

separate[1] ['sepərət] *adj rooms, bills* separado; *problem* isolado; ***keep sth ~ from sth*** manter algo separado de algo

separate[2] ['sepəraɪt] **1** *v/t* separar; ***~ sth from sth*** separar algo de algo **2** *v/i couple* separar-se

separated ['sepəraɪtɪd] *adj couple* separado

separately ['sepərətlɪ] *adv pay* separadamente; *treat, deal with* particularmente

separation [sepə'reɪʃn] separação *f*

September [sep'tembər] setembro *m*

septic ['septɪk] *adj* séptico; ***go ~*** *wound* infeccionar-se

sequel ['si:kwəl] continuação *f*

sequence ['si:kwəns] *n* seqüência *f*; ***in ~*** em seqüência; ***out of ~*** fora de ordem; ***the ~ of events*** a ordem dos acontecimentos

serene [sɪ'ri:n] *adj* sereno

sergeant ['sɑ:rdʒənt] sargento *m*

serial ['sɪrɪəl] *n* série *f*

serialize ['sɪrɪəlaɪz] *v/t novel on TV* trasmitir em capítulos

'serial killer assassino,-a *m,f* em série

'serial number *product*: número *m* de série

series ['sɪri:z] *nsg numbers, events, errors*: série *f*

serious ['sɪrɪəs] *adj situation, company, person* sério; *illness, damage* grave; ***I'm ~*** estou falando sério; ***listen, this is ~*** olha, isto é sério; ***we'd better take a ~ look at it*** nós deveríamos dar uma boa olhada nisso

seriously ['sɪrɪəslɪ] *adv injured* gravemente; *understaffed* seriamente; ***~ intend to …*** estar realmente com a intenção de …; ***~?*** é sério?; ***take s.o. ~*** levar alguém a sério

seriousness ['sɪrɪəsnɪs] *person, situation*: seriedade *f*; *illness etc*: gravidade *f*

sermon ['sɜːrmən] sermão *m*
servant ['sɜːrvənt] empregado,-a *m,f*
serve [sɜːrv] **1** *n tennis*: saque *m* **2** *v/t food, meal* servir; *customer in shop* atender; *one's country, the people* servir a; ***it ~s you / him right*** é bem feito para você / ele **3** *v/i* (*give out food*) servir; *as politician etc* fazer parte; *in tennis* sacar
♦ **serve up** *v/t meal* servir
server ['sɜːrvər] *tennis*: sacador *m*; COMPUT servidor *m*
service ['sɜːrvɪs] **1** *n customers, community*: serviço *m*; *vehicle, machine*: revisão *f*; *tennis*: saque *m*; ***the ~s*** MIL as forças armadas **2** *v/t vehicle, machine* revisar
'**service area** posto *m* de serviço '**service charge** *restaurant, club*: taxa *f* de serviço '**service industry** indústria *f* do setor de prestação de serviços '**serviceman** MIL soldado *m* '**service provider** COMPUT provedor *m* (de serviços) de internet '**service sector** setor *m* de prestação de serviços '**service station** posto *m* de gasolina, *Port* estação *f* de serviço
serviette [sɜːrvɪ'et] guardanapo *m*
servile ['sɜːrvaɪl] *adj pej* servil
serving ['sɜːrvɪŋ] *n food*: porção *f*
session ['seʃn] *parliament, psychiatrist*: sessão *f*; (*meeting*) reunião *f*
set [set] **1** *n tools etc*: jogo *m*; *books*: coleção *f*; (*group of people*) grupo *m*; MATH conjunto *m*; THEA (*scenery*) cenário *m*; (*where a movie is made*) lugar *m* de filmagem; *tennis*: set *m*; ***television ~*** aparelho de TV **2** *v/t* 〈*pret & pp* ***set***〉 (*place*) pôr, colocar; *alarm clock* pôr; *limit, broken limb* fixar; *time, date* marcar; *mechanism* ajustar; *jewel* engastar; ***~ the table*** pôr a mesa; ***~ a task for s.o.*** dar uma tarefa para alguém; TECH ***~ in motion*** acionar; ***the movie is ~ in …*** o filme se ambienta em … **3** *v/i* 〈*pret & pp* ***set***〉 *sun* pôr-se; *glue* solidificar-se **4** *adj ideas* fixo; *views* rígido; (*ready*) pronto; ***be dead ~ on doing sth*** estar decidido a fazer algo; ***be very ~ in one's ways*** ser muito conservador em seu ponto de vista; ***~ meal*** prato *m* do dia
♦ **set apart** *v/t* ***set X apart from Y*** distinguir X de Y
♦ **set aside** *v/t for future use* deixar de reserva
♦ **set back** *v/t in plans etc* atrasar; ***it set me back 400 dollars*** isso acabou me custando 400 dólares
♦ **set off 1** *v/i on journey* partir **2** *v/t explosion, chain reaction* desencadear
♦ **set out 1** *v/i on journey* partir **2** *v/t ideas, proposal* expor; *put, place* colocar; *goods* pôr; ***set out to do sth*** *intend* ter a intenção de fazer algo
♦ **set to** *v/i* (*start on a task*) começar a trabalhar
♦ **set up 1** *v/t new company* estabelecer; *system, equipment, machine* instalar; *market stall* montar; *fam* (*frame*) pregar uma peça em **2** *v/i in business* começar
'**setback** contratempo *m*
settee [se'tiː] (*couch, sofa*) sofá *m*
setting ['setɪŋ] *n novel etc*: cenário *m*; *house*: localização *f*
settle ['setl] **1** *v/i bird* pousar; *liquid, dust* assentar-se; *building* afundar; *to live* estabelecer-se **2** *v/t dispute, uncertainty* resolver; *debts* saldar; *the bill* pagar; *nerves, stomach* acalmar; ***that ~s it!*** está decidido!
♦ **settle down** *v/i* (*stop being noisy*) acalmar-se; (*stop wild living*) assentar-se; *in an area* estabelecer-se
♦ **settle for** *v/t* (*take, accept*) contentar-se com
♦ **settle up** *v/i* (*pay*) acertar as contas
settled ['setld] *adj weather* estável
settlement ['setlmənt] *debt*: liquidação *f*; *dispute*: reconciliação *f*; (*payment*) pagamento *m*; *building* afundamento *m*; *village etc* povoado *m*
settler ['setlər] *in new country* colono,-a *m,f*
'**set-up** (*structure*) organização *f*; (*relationship*) relação *f*; *fam* (*frameup*) brincadeira *f*
seven ['sevn] sete
seventeen [sevn'tiːn] dezessete
seventeenth [sevn'tiːnθ] *n & adj* décimo sétimo (*m*)

seventh ['sevnθ] *n & adj* sétimo (*m*)
seventieth ['sevntɪəθ] *n & adj* septuagésimo (*m*)
seventy ['sevntɪ] setenta
sever ['sevər] *v/t cable, relations* cortar
several ['sevrl] **1** *adj* vários **2** *pron* vários,-as, diversos,-as
severe [sɪ'vɪr] *adj illness* grave; *teacher, face, penalty* severo; *winter, weather* rigoroso
severely [sɪ'vɪrlɪ] *adv punish* severamente; *speak, stare* com severidade; *injured, disrupted* gravemente
severity [sɪ'verətɪ] *illness*: gravidade *f*; *penalty, look etc*: severidade *f*; *winter*: rigorosidade *f*
sew [soʊ] *v/t & v/i* ⟨*pret* ***sewed***, *pp* ***sewn***⟩ costurar
♦ **sew on** *v/t button* pregar
sewage ['su:ɪdʒ] água *f* de esgoto
'sewage plant estação *f* de tratamento de águas residuais e esgoto
sewing ['soʊɪŋ] costura *f*
'sewing machine máquina *f* de costura
sewn [soʊn] *pp* → ***sew***
sex [seks] sexo *m*; ***have ~ with*** fazer sexo com
sexist ['seksɪst] **1** *adj* sexista **2** *n* sexista *m/f*
sexual ['sekʃʊəl] *adj* sexual
sexual as'sault agressão *f* sexual **sexual ha'rassment** assédio *m* sexual **sexual 'intercourse** relação *f* sexual
sexuality [sekʃʊ'ælətɪ] sexualidade *f*
sexually ['sekʃʊlɪ] *adv* sexualmente
sexually transmitted dis'ease [tranz'mɪtɪd] doença *f* sexualmente transmissível
sexy ['seksɪ] *adj person* sexy; *picture* excitante
shabbily ['ʃæbɪlɪ] *adv dressed* com desalinho; *treat* injustamente
shabbiness ['ʃæbɪnɪs] *coat etc*: desalinho *m*
shabby ['ʃæbɪ] *adj coat etc* surrado; *treatment* injusto
shack [ʃæk] cabana *f*
shade [ʃeɪd] **1** *n lamp*: cúpula *f*; *color* matiz *m*; *Am window*: persiana *f*; ***in the ~*** à sombra **2** *v/t from sun, light* proteger
shadow ['ʃædoʊ] *n* sombra *f*
shady ['ʃeɪdɪ] *adj spot* sombrio; *character, dealings* suspeito
shaft [ʃæft] *axle*: árvore *f*, eixo *m*; *mine*: poço *m*
shaggy ['ʃægɪ] *adj hair, dog* desgrenhado
shake [ʃeɪk] **1** *n* ***give sth a good ~*** agitar bem algo **2** *v/t* ⟨*pret* ***shook***, *pp* ***shaken***⟩ *bottle* agitar; *one's head* dizer não com a cabeça; (*emotionally*) comover; ***~ hands*** dar um aperto de mãos; ***~ hands with s.o.*** dar um aperto de mãos em alguém **3** *v/i* ⟨*pret* ***shook***, *pp* ***shaken***⟩ *hands, voice, building* estremecer
shaken[1] ['ʃeɪkən] *pp* → ***shake***
shaken[2] ['ʃeɪkən] *adj emotionally* abalado
'shake-up reestruturação *f*
shaky ['ʃeɪkɪ] *adj table etc* instável; *voice, hand* trêmulo; *after illness, shock* debilitado; *grasp, grammar etc* fraco
shall [ʃæl] *v/aux* ◇ *future* ***I ~ do my best*** farei tudo o que puder; ***I shan't see them*** não os verei ◇ *suggesting* ***~ we go now?*** vamos agora?
shallow ['ʃæloʊ] *adj water* raso; *person* superficial
shambles ['ʃæmblz] *nsg* caos *m*
shame [ʃeɪm] **1** *n* vergonha *f*; ***bring ~ on …*** causar vergonha a …; ***what a ~!*** que vergonha!; ***~ on you!*** tenha vergonha! **2** *v/t* envergonhar; ***~ s.o.into doing sth*** envergonhar alguém para que faça algo
shameful ['ʃeɪmfʊl] *adj* vergonhoso
shamefully ['ʃeɪmfʊlɪ] *adv* vergonhosamente
shameless ['ʃeɪmlɪs] *adj* sem vergonha
shampoo [ʃæm'pu:] **1** *n* shampoo *m*, *Port* champô *m*; ***a ~ and set*** uma lavagem e penteado **2** *v/t customer* lavar a cabeça de; *hair* lavar
shape [ʃeɪp] **1** *n* forma *f* **2** *v/t clay* modelar; *person's life, character* formar; *the future* dar forma a
shapeless ['ʃeɪplɪs] *adj dress etc* sem forma

shapely ['ʃeɪplɪ] *adv figure* esbelto
share [ʃer] **1** *n inheritance, work*: parte *f*; FIN ação *f*; ***do one's ~ of the work*** fazer sua parte do trabalho **2** *v/t* dividir; *s.o.'s feelings, opinions* compartilhar; (*discuss*) discutir **3** *v/i* repartir; ***do you mind sharing with Patrick?*** você se importa de dividir com Patrick?
♦**share out** *v/t* repartir
'**shareholder** acionista *m/f*
shark [ʃɑːrk] tubarão *m*
sharp [ʃɑːrp] **1** *adj knife* afiado; *mind, taste* aguçado; *pain* agudo **2** *adv* MUS desafinadamente; ***at 3 o'clock ~*** às 3 horas em ponto
sharpen ['ʃɑːrpn] *v/t knife* afiar; *skills* aperfeiçoar
sharp 'practice prática *f* suspeita
shat [ʃæt] *pret & pp* → ***shit***
shatter ['ʃætər] **1** *v/t glass* estilhaçar; *illusions* destruir **2** *v/i glass* estilhaçar
shattered ['ʃætərd] *adj fam* (*exhausted*) quebrado; (*very upset*) acabado
shattering ['ʃætərɪŋ] *adj news, experience* arrasador; *effect* impressionante
shave [ʃeɪv] **1** *v/t head* raspar; *legs, armpits* depilar **2** *v/i* barbear-se **3** *n* ***have a ~*** fazer a barba; ***that was a close ~*** foi por um fio
♦**shave off** *v/t beard* barbear; *from piece of wood* aplainar
shaven ['ʃeɪvn] *adj head* raspado
shaver ['ʃeɪvər] barbeador *m* elétrico
shaving brush ['ʃeɪvɪŋ] pincel *m* de barbear
'**shaving soap** espuma *f* de barbear
shawl [ʃɒːl] xale *m*
she [ʃiː] *pron* ela; ***~ is an American / a student*** é uma americana / estudante
shears [ʃɪrz] *npl* tesoura *f* de podar
sheath [ʃiːθ] *n for knife* estojo *m*; *contraceptive* camisinha *f*
shed[1] [ʃed] *v/t* ⟨*pret & pp* ***shed***⟩ *blood, tears* derramar; *leaves* perder; ***~ light on*** *fig* lançar uma luz sobre
shed[2] [ʃed] *n* barracão *m*
sheep [ʃiːp] ⟨*pl* ***sheep***⟩ ovelha *f*
'**sheepdog** cão *m* pastor
sheep-herder ['ʃiːphɜːrdər] *Am* pastor *m*
sheepish ['ʃiːpɪʃ] *adj* envergonhado
'**sheepskin** *adj lining* de pelica
sheer [ʃɪr] *adj madness, luxury* puro; *drop, cliffs* escarpado
sheet [ʃiːt] *bed*: lençol *m*; *paper*: folha *f*, *metal, glass*: chapa *f*
shelf [ʃelf] ⟨*pl* ***shelves***⟩ prateleira *f*; ***shelves*** *pl* estante *f*
'**shelflife** *product*: prazo *m* de validade
shell [ʃel] **1** *n mussel etc*: concha *f*; *egg*: casca *f*; *tortoise*: casco *m*; MIL granada *f*; ***come out of one's ~*** *fig* sair da concha **2** *v/t peas* descascar; MIL bombardear
'**shellfire** fogo *m* de artilharia; ***come under ~*** estar sob fogo de artilharia
'**shellfish** moluscos *mpl*
shelter ['ʃeltər] **1** *n* (*refuge*) refúgio *m*; (*construction*) cobertura *f* **2** *v/i from rain, bombing etc* refugiar-se **3** *v/t* (*protect*) proteger
sheltered ['ʃeltərd] *adj place* protegido; ***lead a ~ life*** levar uma vida protegida
shelve [ʃelv] *v/t fig* adiar
shelves [ʃelvz] *pl* estante *f*
shepherd ['ʃepərd] *n* pastor *m*
sheriff ['ʃerɪf] xerife *m*
sherry ['ʃerɪ] jerez *m*
shield [ʃiːld] **1** *n* MIL escudo *m*; (*sports trophy*) troféu *m*; TECH placa *f* protetora; *Am policeman* distintivo *m* **2** *v/t* (*protect*) proteger
shift [ʃɪft] **1** *n attitude, direction*: mudança *f*; (*switchover*) transição *f*; (*period of work*) turno *m* **2** *v/t* (*move*) deslocar; *stains etc* tirar; ***~ the emphasis onto*** transferir a ênfase para **3** *v/i* (*move*) mover-se; *in attitude, opinion, wind* mudar
'**shift key** COMPUT tecla *f* de maiúscula '**shift work** trabalho *m* em turnos '**shift worker** trabalhador,a *m,f* de turnos
shifty ['ʃɪftɪ] *adj pej* suspeito
shifty-looking ['ʃɪftɪlʊkɪŋ] *adj pej* de aparência suspeita
shilly-shally ['ʃɪlɪʃælɪ] *v/i* ⟨*pret & pp* ***shilly-shallied***⟩ *fam* hesitar, vacilar
shimmer ['ʃɪmər] *v/i* cintilar, brilhar

shin [ʃɪn] *n* canela *f*

shine [ʃaɪn] **1** *v/i* ⟨*pret & pp* ***shone***⟩ *sun, moon, also fig student etc* brilhar **2** *v/t* ⟨*pret & pp* ***shone***⟩ ***~ your flashlight here*** ilumina aqui **3** *n on shoes etc* brilho *m*

shingle ['ʃɪŋgl] *on beach* cascalhos *mpl*

shingles ['ʃɪŋglz] *nsg* MED herpes-zoster *m*

shiny ['ʃaɪnɪ] *adj surface* brilhante

ship [ʃɪp] **1** *n* navio *m* **2** *v/t* ⟨*pret & pp* ***shipped***⟩ (*send*) enviar; *by sea* enviar por navio

shipment ['ʃɪpmənt] (*consignment*) envio *m*

'shipowner armador *m*

shipping ['ʃɪpɪŋ] *n* (*sea traffic*) tráfego *f* marítimo; (*sending*) envio *m*; (*sending by sea*) envio *m* por navio

'shipping company companhia *f* de navegação

'shipshape *adj* em ordem **'shipwreck 1** *n* naufrágio *m* **2** *v/t* ***be ~ed*** naufragar **'shipyard** estaleiro *m*

shirk [ʃɜːrk] *v/t* evitar

shirker ['ʃɜːrkər] preguisoço,-a *m,f*

shirt [ʃɜːrt] camisa *f*; ***in his ~ sleeves*** em mangas de camisa

shit [ʃɪt] *fam* **1** *n* (*excrement, bad quality goods, work*) merda *f*; ***I need a ~*** preciso cagar **2** *v/i* ⟨*pret & pp* ***shat***⟩ cagar **3** *interj* merda

shitty ['ʃɪtɪ] *adj fam* ***be ~*** ser uma porcaria; ***I feel ~*** estou me sentindo um lixo

shiver ['ʃɪvər] *v/i* tremer

shock [ʃɑːk] **1** *n also* ELEC choque *m*; ***be in ~*** MED estar em estado de choque **2** *v/t* chocar; ***be ~ed by*** ficar chocado com

'shock absorber [əb'zɔːrbər] MOT amortecedor *m*

shocking ['ʃɑːkɪŋ] *adj behavior, poverty* escandaloso; *fam* (*very bad*) horrível

shockingly ['ʃɑːkɪŋlɪ] *adv behave* escandalosamente

shoddy ['ʃɑːdɪ] *adj goods* de baixa qualidade; *behavior* vergonhoso

shoe [ʃuː] sapato *m*

'shoehorn *n* calçadeira *f* **'shoe-lace** cadarço *m* **'shoemaker** sapateiro *m* **shoe mender** ['ʃuːmendər] sapateiro *m* **shoeshop** *Brit* → ***shoestore*** **'shoestore** *Am* sapataria *f*

'shoestring ***do sth on a ~*** fazer algo com uns poucos centavos

shone [ʃɑːn] *pret & pp* → ***shine***

◆ **shoo away** [ʃuː] *v/t children, chicken* espantar

shook [ʃuːk] *pret* → ***shake***

shoot [ʃuːt] **1** *n* BOT broto *m* **2** *v/t* ⟨*pret & pp* ***shot***⟩ balear; *movie* filmar; (*kill*) atirar para matar; ***~ s.o. in the leg*** atirar na perna de alguém **3** *v/i* ⟨*pret & pp* ***shot***⟩ *with gun* atirar; (*move quickly*) disparar; ***don't ~!*** não atire!; ***the car shot down the road*** o carro disparou rua abaixo

◆ **shoot down** *v/t airplane* derrubar; *fig suggestion* rejeitar

◆ **shoot off** *v/i* (*rush off*) andar depressa

◆ **shoot up** *v/i prices* disparar; *children* crescer em disparada; *new suburbs, buildings etc* jorrar; *fam drug addict* injetar

shooting star ['ʃuːtɪŋ] *Brit* estrela *f* cadente

shop [ʃɑːp] **1** *n* loja *f*; ***talk ~*** falar do trabalho **2** *v/i* ⟨*pret & pp* ***shopped***⟩ fazer compras; ***go ~ping*** ir fazer compras

shopaholic [ʃɑːpə'hɑːlɪk] *fam* viciado,-a *m,f* em comprar

'shop assistant *Brit* vendedor,a *m,f* **'shopkeeper** dono,-a *m,f* de loja **shoplifter** ['ʃɑːplɪftər] ladrão *m*, ladra *f* **shoplifting** ['ʃɑːplɪftɪŋ] *n* roubo *m* de lojas

shopper ['ʃɑːpər] comprador,a *m,f*

shopping ['ʃɑːpɪŋ] *activity, items* compras *fpl*; ***do one's ~*** fazer as compras

'shopping bag sacola *f* de compras **'shopping center** *Am* shopping center *m* **shopping centre** *Brit* → ***shopping center*** **'shopping list** lista *f* de compras **'shopping mall** centro *m* comercial

shop 'steward representante *m/f* sindical

shop 'window vitrina *f*, *Port* montra *f*

S

shore [ʃɔːr] margem *f*; ***on ~*** *not at sea* em terra
short [ʃɔːrt] **1** *adj in distance, time* curto; *in height* baixo; ***be ~ of*** ter pouco **2** *adv* ***cut a vacation / meeting ~*** interromper as férias / a reunião; ***stop a person ~*** fazer alguém parar de falar; ***go ~ of*** passar sem; ***in ~*** resumindo
shortage ['ʃɔːrtɪdʒ] escassez *f*, falta *f*
short 'circuit *n* curto-circuito *m*
shortcoming ['ʃɔːrtkʌmɪŋ] defeito *m* **'short cut** atalho *m*
shorten ['ʃɔːrtn] *v/t dress, hair, chapter etc* encurtar
shortening ['ʃɔːrtnɪŋ] *n cooking*: gordura *f* vegetal
'shortfall déficit *m* **'shorthand** *n* taquigrafia *f* **short-handed** [ʃɔːrt'hændɪd] *adj* ***be ~*** estar com falta de pessoal **short-lived** ['ʃɔːrtlɪvd] *adj* passageiro; *company* de curta existência
shortly ['ʃɔːrtlɪ] *adv* (*soon*) logo; ***~ after that*** logo depois
shortness ['ʃɔːrtnɪs] *visit*: brevidade *f*; *height*: baixa estatura *f*
shorts [ʃɔːrts] *npl* shorts *mpl*, *Port* calções *mpl*
shortsighted [ʃɔːrt'saɪtɪd] *adj also fig* míope **short-sleeved** ['ʃɔːrtsliːvd] *adj* de manga curta **short-staffed** [ʃɔːrt'stæft] *adj* com falta de pessoal **short 'story** história *f* curta **short-tempered** [ʃɔːrt'tempərd] *adj* impulsivo, de pavio curto **'short-term** *adj* de curto prazo **'short time** ***be on ~*** trabalhar com jornada reduzida **'short wave** onda *f* curta
shot[1] [ʃɑːt] *from gun* tiro *m*, disparo *m*; (*photograph*) foto *f*; (*injection*) injeção *f*; ***be a good / poor ~*** atirar bem / mal; ***like a ~*** *accept, run off* como um tiro
shot[2] [ʃɑːt] *pret & pp* → ***shoot***
'shotgun espingarda *f*
should [ʃʊd] ***what ~ I do?*** o que eu devo fazer?; ***you ~n't do that*** você não deveria fazer isso; ***that ~ be long enough*** deve ser longo o suficiente; ***you ~ have heard him!*** você deveria tê-lo ouvido

shoulder ['ʃoʊldər] *n* ombro *m*
'shoulder bag bolsa *f de ombro* **'shoulder blade** omoplata *f* **'shoulder strap** *bra, bag*: alça *f*
shout [ʃaʊt] **1** *n* grito *m* **2** *v/i & v/t* gritar; ***~ for help*** gritar por socorro
♦ **shout at** *v/t* gritar com
shouting ['ʃaʊtɪŋ] gritaria *f*
shove [ʃʌv] **1** *n* empurrão *m* **2** *v/t & v/i* empurrar
♦ **shove in** *v/i in line-up* entrar na frente empurrando
♦ **shove off** *v/i fam* (*go away*) ir embora
shovel ['ʃʌvl] *n* pá *f*
show [ʃoʊ] **1** *n* THEA espetáculo *m*; TV programa *m*; (*display*) mostra *f*; ***on ~*** *at exhibition* em exibição; ***it's all done for ~*** *pej* é tudo show **2** *v/t* ⟨*pret* ***showed***, *pp* ***shown***⟩ mostrar; *courage* demonstrar; *movie* exibir; ***~ s.o. sth, ~ sth to s.o.*** mostrar algo a alguém **3** *v/i* ⟨*pret* ***showed***, *pp* ***shown***⟩ ***what's ~ing this week?*** *movie* o que está passando esta semana?; ***does it ~?*** dá para notar?
♦ **show around** *v/t* ***show s.o. around sth*** mostrar algo a alguém
♦ **show in** *v/t* fazer entrar
♦ **show off** **1** *v/t skills* exibir **2** *v/i pej* exibir-se
♦ **show up** **1** *v/t s.o.'s shortcomings etc* pôr em evidência; ***don't show me up in public*** não me exponha ao ridículo em público **2** *v/i fam* (*arrive, turn up*) aparecer; (*be visible*) ver-se
'show business show business *m* **'showcase** *n* vitrina *f* **'showdown** confrontação *f*
shower ['ʃaʊər] **1** *n rain*: pancada *f* de chuva; *wash*: ducha *f*; ***baby ~*** *Am* chá *m* de bebê; ***take a ~*** tomar um banho **2** *v/i* tomar um banho **3** *v/t* ***~ s.o. with praise*** encher alguém de elogios
'shower cap touca *f* de banho **'shower curtain** cortina *f* de banho **'showerproof** *adj* impermeável
'showjumper cavaleiro *m*, amazona *f* **showjumping** ['ʃoʊdʒʌmpɪŋ] hipismo-salto *m* **'show-off** *pej* exibicionista *m/f* **'showroom** showroom

m; ***in ~ condition*** como novo
showy ['ʃoʊɪ] *adj jacket, behavior* chamativo
shrank [ʃræŋk] *pret* → ***shrink***[1]
shred [ʃred] **1** *n paper etc*: tira *f*; ***there isn't a ~ of evidence*** não há a mínima prova **2** *v/t* ⟨*pret & pp* ***shredded***⟩ *paper* triturar; *in cooking* cortar em tiras
shredder ['ʃredər] *for documents* fragmentadora *f* de papel
shrewd [ʃruːd] *adj person, investor* perspicaz; *judgment, investment* inteligente
shrewdly ['ʃruːdlɪ] *adv* com perspicácia
shrewdness ['ʃruːdnɪs] astúcia *f*
shriek [ʃriːk] **1** *n* berro *m* **2** *v/i* berrar
shrill [ʃrɪl] *adj* estridente
shrimp [ʃrɪmp] camarão *m*
shrine [ʃraɪn] santuário *m*
shrink[1] [ʃrɪŋk] *v/i* ⟨*pret* ***shrank***, *pp* ***shrunk***⟩ *material* encolher; *level of support etc* diminuir
shrink[2] [ʃrɪŋk] *n fam* (*psychiatrist*) psiquiatra *m/f*
'shrink-wrap plastificar
'shrink-wrapping *process* plastificação *f*; *material* plástico *m*
shrivel ['ʃrɪvl] *v/i skin* enrugar; *material* encolher; *leaves* murchar
Shrove 'Tuesday [ʃroʊv] terça-feira *f* de carnaval
shrub [ʃrʌb] arbusto *m*
shrubbery ['ʃrʌbərɪ] arbustos *mpl*
shrug [ʃrʌg] **1** *n* ***say sth with a ~*** dizer algo encolhendo os ombros **2** *v/i* ⟨*pret & pp* ***shrugged***⟩ encolher os ombros **3** *v/t* ⟨*pret & pp* ***shrugged***⟩ ***~ one's shoulders*** encolher os ombros
shrunk [ʃrʌŋk] *pp* → ***shrink***[1]
shudder ['ʃʌdər] **1** *n fear, disgust*: calafrio *m*; *earth etc*: tremor *m* **2** *v/i with fear, disgust, earth, building* estremecer; ***I ~ to think*** tremo só de pensar
shuffle ['ʃʌfl] **1** *v/t cards* embaralhar **2** *v/i walking*: arrastar-se
shun [ʃʌn] *v/t* ⟨*pret & pp* ***shunned***⟩ evitar
shut [ʃʌt] *v/t & v/i* ⟨*pret & pp* ***shut***⟩ fechar; ***they were ~*** está fechado
◆ **shut down** *v/t & v/i businesss* fechar; *computer* desligar
◆ **shut off** *v/t* cortar
◆ **shut up** *v/i fam* (*be quiet*) calar-se; ***shut up!*** cala a boca!
shutter ['ʃʌtər] *on window* persiana *f*; PHOT obturador *m*
'shutter speed PHOT tempo *m* de exposição
shuttle ['ʃʌtl] *v/i* trasladar
'shuttlebus ônibus *m* de traslado, *Port* autocarro *m* **'shuttlecock** SPORT peteca *f* **'shuttle service** serviço *m* de traslado
shy [ʃaɪ] *adj person, smile* tímido; *animal* arredio
shyness ['ʃaɪnɪs] timidez *f*
Siamese 'twins [saɪə'miːz] gêmeos *mpl* siameses
sick [sɪk] *adj also society* doente; *sense of humor* mórbido; ***feel ~*** *about to vomit* estar com náuseas; ***I'm going to be ~*** *vomit* vou vomitar; ***be ~ of*** *fed up with* estar farto de
sicken ['sɪkn] **1** *v/t* (*disgust*) enojar a **2** *v/i* ***be ~ing for*** estar incubando
sickening ['sɪknɪŋ] *adj stench, crime* repugnante
'sick leave ***be on ~*** estar de licença por motivo de saúde
sickly ['sɪklɪ] *adj person* doentio; *color* pálido
sickness ['sɪknɪs] doença *f*; (*vomiting*) náusea *f*
side [saɪd] *n* lado *m*; *mountain*: encosta *f*; SPORT time *m*, *Port* equipa *f*; ***take ~s*** (***with***) tomar partido a favor de; ***I'm on your ~*** estou do seu lado; ***~ by ~*** lado a lado; ***at the ~ of the road*** à beira da estrada; ***on the big / small ~*** no lado grande / pequeno
◆ **side with** *v/t* tomar partido a favor de
'sideboard aparador *m*, bufê *m* **'sideburns** *npl* costeletas *fpl* **'side dish** acompanhamento *m* **'side effect** efeito *m* colateral **'sidelight** MOT luz *f* de posição **'sideline** **1** *n* ocupação *f* secundária **2** *v/t* ***feel ~d*** sentir-se excluído **'sidestep** *v/t* ⟨*pret & pp* ***sidestepped***⟩ *fig* evitar **'side street** beco *m* **'sidetrack** *v/t*

S

distrair; ***get ~ed*** distrair-se **'sidewalk** *Am* calçada *f*, *Port* passeio *m* **sidewalk 'café** *Am* café *m* com mesas na calçada, *Port* esplanada *f* **sideways** ['saɪdweɪz] *adv* de lado
siege [siːdʒ] cerco *m*; ***lay ~ to*** sitiar
sieve [sɪv] *n* peneira *f*
sift [sɪft] *v/t corn, ore* peneirar; *data* analizar cuidadosamente
◆ **sift through** *v/t details, data* passar pela peneira
sigh [saɪ] **1** *n* suspiro *m*; ***heave a ~ of relief*** suspirar de alívio **2** *v/i* suspirar
sight [saɪt] *n* vista *f*; ***~s*** *city:* pontos *mpl* turísticos; ***catch ~ of*** avistar; ***know by ~*** conhecer de vista; ***within ~ of*** à vista de; ***out of ~*** fora de vista; ***what a ~ you are!*** que espetáculo!; ***lose ~ of*** *main objective etc* esquecer-se de
sightseeing ['saɪtsiːɪŋ] *n* turismo *m*; ***go ~*** visitar pontos turísticos
'sightseeing tour visita *f* de pontos turísticos
sightseer ['saɪtsiːər] turista *m/f*
sign [saɪn] **1** *n* (*indication*) sinal *m*; (*road sign*) placa *f* de trânsito; *outside shop, on building* placa *f*; ***it's a ~ of the times*** é um sinal dos tempos **2** *v/t & v/i document* assinar
◆ **sign in** *v/i* registrar-se, *Port* registar-se
◆ **sign up** *v/i Brit* (*join the army*) alistar-se
signal ['sɪgnl] **1** *n* sinal *m*; ***be sending out all the right / wrong ~s*** estar transmitindo uma mensagem correta / errada **2** *v/i* ⟨*pret & pp* ***signaled***, *Brit* ***signalled***⟩ *driver* sinalizar
signatory ['sɪgnətɔːrɪ] *n* signatário,-a *m,f*
signature ['sɪgnətʃər] *n* assinatura *f*
'signature tune sintonia *f*
signet ring ['sɪgnɪt] anel *m* com sinete
significance [sɪg'nɪfɪkəns] importância *f*
significant [sɪg'nɪfɪkənt] *adj* significante
significantly [sɪg'nɪfɪkəntlɪ] *adv larger, more expensive* consideravelmente
signify ['sɪgnɪfaɪ] *v/t* ⟨*pret & pp* ***signified***⟩ significar
'sign language língua *f* de sinais
'signpost placa *f*
silence ['saɪləns] **1** *n* silêncio *m*; ***in ~*** em silêncio; ***~!*** silêncio! **2** *v/t* silenciar
silencer ['saɪlənsər] *on gun* silenciador *m*
silent ['saɪlənt] *adj* silencioso; *movie* mudo; ***stay ~*** (*not comment*) ficar calado
silhouette [sɪluː'et] *n* silhueta *f*
silicon ['sɪlɪkən] silício *m*
silicon 'chip chip *m* de silício
silicone ['sɪlɪkoʊn] silicone *m*
silk [sɪlk] **1** *n* seda *f* **2** *adj shirt etc* de seda
silky ['sɪlkɪ] *adj hair, texture* sedoso
silliness ['sɪlɪnɪs] estupidez *f*
silly ['sɪlɪ] *adj* bobo
silo ['saɪloʊ] silo *m*
silver ['sɪlvər] **1** *n* prata *f*; (*silver objects*) prataria *f*; *medal* medalha *f* de prata **2** *adj ring* de prata; *hair* grisalho
silver-plated [sɪlvər'pleɪtɪd] *adj* prateado **silverware** ['sɪlvərwer] prataria *f* **silver 'wedding** bodas *fpl* de prata
similar ['sɪmɪlər] *adj* parecido
similarity [sɪmɪ'lærətɪ] semelhança *f*
similarly ['sɪmɪlərlɪ] *adv* da mesma maneira
simmer ['sɪmər] *v/i cooking*: cozinhar em fogo brando; *with rage* estar fervendo (de raiva)
◆ **simmer down** *v/i* acalmar-se
simple ['sɪmpl] *adj* (*easy*), *person, design* simples
simple-minded [sɪmpl'maɪndɪd] *adj pej* simplório
simplicity [sɪm'plɪsətɪ] (*easiness, plainness*) simplicidade *f*
simplify ['sɪmplɪfaɪ] *v/t* ⟨*pret & pp* ***simplified***⟩ simplificar
simplistic [sɪm'plɪstɪk] *adj* simplista
simply ['sɪmplɪ] *adv* (*absolutely*) simplesmente; (*in a simple way*) de forma simplificada; ***it is ~ the best*** é simplesmente o melhor
simulate ['sɪmjʊleɪt] *v/t* simular

simultaneous [saɪməl'teɪnɪəs] *adj* simultâneo
simultaneously [saɪməl'teɪnɪəslɪ] *adv* simultaneamente
sin [sɪn] **1** *n* pecado *m* **2** *v/i* ⟨*pret & pp* ***sinned***⟩ pecar
since [sɪns] **1** *prep* desde; ***~ last week*** desde a semana passada **2** *adv* desde então; ***I haven't seen him ~*** não o vejo desde então **3** *conj in expressions of time* desde que; (*seeing that*) já que; ***~ you left*** desde que você se foi; ***~ you don't like it*** já que você não gosta disso
sincere [sɪn'sɪr] *adj* sincero
sincerely [sɪn'sɪrlɪ] *adv speak, hope* sinceramente; ***Yours ~*** atenciosamente
sincerity [sɪn'serətɪ] sinceridade *f*
sinful ['sɪnfʊl] *adj* pecador
sing [sɪŋ] *v/t & v/i* ⟨*pret* ***sang***, *pp* ***sung***⟩ cantar
singe [sɪndʒ] *v/t* queimar
singer ['sɪŋər] cantor,a *m,f*
single ['sɪŋgl] **1** *adj* (*sole, not double*) único; (*not married*) solteiro; ***there wasn't a ~ …*** não havia somente um …; ***in ~ file*** em fila (indiana) **2** *n* MUS single *m*; (*single room*) quarto *m* de solteiro; *person* desimpedido,-a *m,f*; ***~s*** *tennis*: jogos *mpl* individuais
♦**single out** *v/t* (*choose*) escolher; (*distinguish*) distinguir
single-breasted [sɪŋgl'brestɪd] *adj jacket* com fileira simples de botões **single-handed** [sɪŋgl'hændɪd] *adj & adv attempts, rescue* sozinho **single-minded** [sɪŋgl'maɪndɪd] *adj* determinado **single 'mother** mãe *f* solteira **single 'parent** pai *m* solteiro; mãe *f* solteira **single parent 'family** família *f* monoparental **'single room** quarto *m* de solteiro
singular ['sɪŋgjʊlər] **1** *adj* GRAM singular **2** *n* GRAM singular *m*; ***in the ~*** no singular
sinister ['sɪnɪstər] *adj* sinistro
sink [sɪŋk] **1** *n* pia *f* **2** *v/i* ⟨*pret* ***sank***, *pp* ***sunk***⟩ *ship, object* afundar; *sun* pôr-se; *interest rates, pressure etc* baixar; ***he sank onto the bed*** ele caiu na cama **3** *v/t* ⟨*pret* ***sank***, *pp* ***sunk***⟩ *ship* afundar; *funds* investir
♦**sink in** *v/i liquid* penetrar; ***it still hasn't really sunk in*** *realization* ainda não caiu na realidade
sinner ['sɪnər] pecador,a *m,f*
sinus ['saɪnəs] *nasal* narinas *fpl*
sinusitis [saɪnə'saɪtɪs] MED sinusite *f*
sip [sɪp] **1** *n* golinho *m* **2** *v/t* ⟨*pret & pp* ***sipped***⟩ beberica r
sir [sɜːr] senhor
siren ['saɪrən] sirena *f*
sirloin ['sɜːrlɔɪn] lombo *m* de vaca
sister ['sɪstər] irmã *f*; *Brit hospital*: enfermeira-chefe *f*
'sister-in-law ⟨*pl* ***sisters-in-law***⟩ cunhada *f*
sit [sɪt] ⟨*pret & pp* ***sat***⟩ **1** *v/i* estar sentado; (*sit down*) sentar-se **2** *v/t exam* fazer
♦**sit down** *v/i* sentar-se
♦**sit up** *v/i in bed* ficar acordado; (*straighten back*) sentar-se direito; (*wait up at night*) esperar acordado
sitcom ['sɪtkɑːm] comédia *f* de situação
site [saɪt] **1** *n* lugar *m*; (*web~*) site *m* **2** *v/t new offices etc* situar
sitting ['sɪtɪŋ] *n committee, court, artist*: sessão *f*; *meals*: grupo *m*
'sitting room sala *f* de estar
situated ['sɪtjuːeɪtɪd] *adj* situado; ***be ~*** estar situado
situation [sɪtjuː'eɪʃn] situação *f*; *building etc*: localização *f*
six [sɪks] seis
sixteen [sɪks'tiːn] dezesseis
sixteenth [sɪks'tiːnθ] décimo sexto (*m*)
sixth [sɪksθ] *n & adj* sexto (*m*)
sixtieth ['sɪkstɪəθ] *n & adj* sexagésimo (*m*)
sixty ['sɪkstɪ] sessenta
six-'yard box *soccer*: pequena *f* área
size [saɪz] tamanho *m*; *loan*: quantia *f*
♦**size up** *v/t* avaliar
sizeable ['saɪzəbl] *adj* de tamanho considerável
sizzle ['sɪzl] *v/i* borbulhar
skate [skeɪt] **1** *n* patim *m* **2** *v/i* patinar

'skateboard *n* prancha *f* de skate **'skateboarder** skatista *m/f* **'skateboarding** skate *m*
skater ['skeɪtər] patinador,a *m,f*
skating ['skeɪtɪŋ] *n* patinação *f*
'skating rink pista *f* de patinação
skeleton ['skelɪtn] esqueleto *m*
'skeleton key chave *f* mestra
skeptic ['skeptɪk] *Am* céptico,-a *m,f*
skeptical ['skeptɪkl] *adj Am* céptico
skepticism ['skeptɪsɪzm] *Am* ceptismo *m*
sketch [sketʃ] **1** *n* esboço *m*; THEA esquete *m* **2** *v/t* esboçar
'sketchbook caderno *m* de desenho
sketchy ['sketʃɪ] *adj knowledge etc* superficial
skewer ['skjʊər] *n* espeto *m*
ski [ski:] **1** *n* esqui *m* **2** *v/i* esquiar
'ski boots botas *fpl* de esqui
skid [skɪd] **1** *n* derrapagem *f* **2** *v/i* ⟨*pret & pp* ***skidded***⟩ derrapar
skier ['ski:ər] esquiador,a *m,f*
skiing ['ski:ɪŋ] esqui *m*
'ski instructor instrutor,a *m,f* de esqui
skilful *Brit* → ***skillful***
'ski lift teleférico *m*
skill [skɪl] habilidade *f*
skilled [skɪld] *adj* habilidoso
skilled 'worker trabalhador *m* qualificado
skillful ['skɪlfʊl] *adj Am* habilidoso
skillfully ['skɪlfʊlɪ] *adv Am* habilmente
skim [skɪm] *v/t* ⟨*pret & pp* ***skimmed***⟩ *surface* resvalar; *milk* desnatar
♦ **skim off** *v/t the best* escolher
♦ **skim through** *v/t text* ler por cima
skimmed 'milk [skɪmd] leite *m* desnatado
skimpy ['skɪmpɪ] *adj account etc* superficial; *dress* curtíssimo
skin [skɪn] **1** *n* pele *f*; *fruit*: casca *f* **2** *v/t* ⟨*pret & pp* ***skinned***⟩ tirar a pele de; *fruit* descascar
'skin diving mergulho *m*
skinflint ['skɪnflɪnt] *fam* pão-duro *m/f*
'skin graft implante *m* de pele
skinny ['skɪnɪ] *adj* magricelo
'skin-tight *adj* justíssimo
skip [skɪp] **1** *n* (*little jump*) pulinho *m* **2** *v/i* ⟨*pret & pp* ***skipped***⟩ pular **3** *v/t* ⟨*pret & pp* ***skipped***⟩ (*omit*) pular
'ski pole bastão *m* de esqui
skipper ['skɪpər] NAUT comandante *m*; *team*: capitão *m*
'ski resort estação *f* de esqui
skirt [skɜ:rt] *n* saia *f*
'ski run pista *f* de esqui
'ski tow reboque *m*
skull [skʌl] crânio *m*
skunk [skʌŋk] gambá *m*
sky [skaɪ] céu *m*
'skylight clarabóia *f* **'skyline** horizonte *m* **skyscraper** ['skaɪskreɪpər] arranha-céu *m*
slab [slæb] *stone*: lousa *f*; *cake etc*: fatia *f* grossa
slack [slæk] *adj rope, discipline* frouxo; *person* relaxado; *work* descuidado; *period* tranqüilo
slacken ['slækn] *v/t rope* afrouxar; *pace* diminuir
♦ **slacken off** *v/i pace* diminuir
slacks [slæks] *npl* calças *fpl*
slain [sleɪn] *pp* → ***slay***
slam [slæm] *v/t & v/i* ⟨*pret & pp* ***slammed***⟩ *door* bater
♦ **slam down** *v/t* bater com força
slander ['slændər] **1** *n* difamação *f* **2** *v/t* difamar
slanderous ['slændərəs] *adj* difamatório
slang [slæŋ] gíria *f*; *of a specific group* jargão *m*
slant [slænt] **1** *v/i* inclinar-se **2** *n* inclinação *f*; *given to a story* enfoque *m*
slanting ['slæntɪŋ] *adj roof* inclinado; *eyes* amendoado
slap [slæp] **1** *n blow* bofetada *f* **2** *v/t* ⟨*pret & pp* ***slapped***⟩ dar um tapa em; ***she ~ped his face*** ela deu um tapa no rosto dele
'slapdash *adj* descuidado
slash [slæʃ] **1** *n* (*cut*) corte *m*; *in punctuation* barra *f* **2** *v/t skin, prices etc* cortar; ***~ one's wrists*** cortar o pulso
slate [sleɪt] *n* ardósia *f*
slaughter ['slɒ:tər] **1** *n animals*: abatimento *m*; *people, troops*: massacre *m* **2** *v/t animals* abater; *people, troops* massacrar
'slaughterhouse matadouro *m*

Slav [slɑːv] *adj* eslavo
slave [sleɪv] *n* escravo,-a *m,f*
'slave-driver *fam* capataz *m/f*
slay [sleɪ] *v/t* ⟨*pret* ***slew***, *pp* ***slain***⟩ assassinar
slaying ['sleɪɪŋ] *Am* (*murder*) assassinato *m*
sleaze [sliːz] POL corrupção *f*
sleazy ['sliːzɪ] *adj bar, character* sórdido
sled, sledge [sled, sledʒ] *n* trenó *m*
'sledge hammer marreta *f*
sleep [sliːp] **1** *n* sono *m*; ***go to ~*** ir dormir; ***I need a good ~*** preciso de um bom sono; ***I couldn't get to ~*** não consegui dormir **2** *v/i* ⟨*pret & pp* ***slept***⟩ dormir
◆**sleep in** *v/i* (*have a long lie*) dormir até tarde
◆**sleep on** *v/t proposal, decision* pensar sobre
◆**sleep with** *v/t* (*have sex with*) transar com, ir para a cama com
sleepily ['sliːpɪlɪ] *adv* meio dormindo
sleeping bag ['sliːpɪŋ] saco *m* de dormir **'sleeping car** RAIL vagão *m* dormitório, *Port* carruagem-camas *f* **'sleeping pill** sonífero *m*
sleepless ['sliːplɪs] *adj night* insone
'sleep walker sonâmbulo,-a *m,f*
'sleep walking sonambulismo *m*
sleepy ['sliːpɪ] *adj yawn, child* sonolento; *town* adormecido; ***I'm ~*** estou com sono
sleet [sliːt] *n* chuva *f* com neve
sleeve [sliːv] manga *f*
sleeveless ['sliːvlɪs] *adj* sem manga
sleigh [sleɪ] *n* trenó *m*
sleight of 'hand [slaɪt] truque *m* de mãos
slender ['slendər] *adj figure, arms* esbelto; *chance* remoto; *income, margin* escasso
slept [slept] *pret & pp* → ***sleep***
slew [sluː] *pret* → ***slay***
slice [slaɪs] **1** *n bread, also fig profits etc*: fatia *f* **2** *v/t loaf etc* cortar (em fatias)
sliced 'bread [slaɪst] pão *m* fatiado; ***the greatest thing since ~*** *fam* a coisa mais maravilhosa do mundo
slick [slɪk] **1** *adj performance* brilhante; *pej* (*cunning*) espertinho **2** *n oil*: mancha *f* de petróleo
slid [slɪd] *pret & pp* → ***slide***
slide [slaɪd] **1** *n for kids* escorregador *m*; PHOT slide *m* **2** *v/i* ⟨*pret & pp* ***slid***⟩ *person* escorregar; (*drop*) *exchange rate etc* diminuir **3** *v/t* ⟨*pret & pp* ***slid***⟩ *furniture* deslizar
sliding door ['slaɪdɪŋ] porta *f* corrediça
slight [slaɪt] **1** *adj person, figure* delicado; (*small*) leve; ***no, not in the ~est*** não, nem um pouco **2** *n* (*insult*) insulto *m*
slightly ['slaɪtlɪ] *adv* ligeiramente
slim [slɪm] **1** *adj* magro; *chance* remoto **2** *v/i* ⟨*pret & pp* ***slimmed***⟩ estar de dieta
slime [slaɪm] lodo *m*
slimy ['slaɪmɪ] *adj liquid* viscoso
sling [slɪŋ] **1** *n arm*: faixa *f* **2** *v/t* ⟨*pret & pp* ***slung***⟩ (*throw*) atirar
'slingshot *Am* catapulta *f*
slip [slɪp] **1** *n on ice etc* escorregão *m*; (*mistake*) lapso *m*; ***a ~ of paper*** um pedaço de papel; ***a ~ of the tongue*** um lapso; ***give s.o. the ~*** despistar alguém **2** *v/i* ⟨*pret & pp* ***slipped***⟩ *on ice etc* escorregar; (*decline*) *quality etc* decair; ***he ~ped out of the room*** saiu da sala fininho **3** *v/t* ⟨*pret & pp* ***slipped***⟩ ***he ~ped it into his briefcase*** ele o colocou sigilosamente em sua maleta; ***it ~ped my mind*** me esqueci
◆**slip away** *v/i time* passar; *opportunity* esvaecer-se; (*die quietly*) ir-se tranquilamente
◆**slip off** *v/t jacket etc* tirar
◆**slip on** *v/t jacket etc* vestir
◆**slip out** *v/i* (*go out*) sair de fininho
◆**slip up** *v/i* equivocar-se
slipped 'disc [slɪpt] hérnia *f* de disco
slipper ['slɪpər] mocassim *m*
slippery ['slɪpərɪ] *adj* escorregadiço
slipshod ['slɪpʃɑːd] *adj* desmazelado
'slip-up (*mistake*) equívoco *m*
slit [slɪt] **1** *n* (*tear*) rasgão *m*; (*hole*) brecha *f*; *in skirt* racha *f* **2** *v/t* ⟨*pret & pp* ***slit***⟩ abrir; *throat* cortar; ***~ s.o.'s throat*** cortar a garganta de alguém

slither ['slɪðər] *v/i* deslizar-se
sliver ['slɪvər] pedacinho *m*
slob [slɑːb] *pej* desleixado,-a *m,f*
slobber ['slɑːbər] *v/i* babar
slog [slɑːg] *n* trabalho *m* árduo
slogan ['sloʊgən] slogan *m*
slop [slɑːp] *v/t* ⟨*pret & pp* ***slopped***⟩ derramar
slope [sloʊp] **1** *n* inclinação *f*; *mountain*: declive *m*; ***built on a ~*** construido numa ladeira **2** *v/i* inclinar-se; ***the road ~s down to the sea*** a estrada desce para o mar
sloppy ['slɑːpɪ] *adj work, editing* malfeito; *in dressing* desleixado; (*too sentimental*) sentimentalista
slot [slɑːt] *n* abertura *f*, *schedule*: brecha *f*
♦ **slot in** ⟨*pret & pp* ***slotted***⟩ **1** *v/t* introduzir **2** *v/i* encaixar-se
'**slot machine** *vending*: máquina *f* automática de venda; *gambling*: máquina *f* caça-níqueis
slouch [slaʊʧ] *v/i* ficar em má postura
slovenly ['slʌvnlɪ] *adj* desmazelado
slow [sloʊ] *adj* lento; ***be ~*** *clock* estar atrasado
♦ **slow down** **1** *v/i driver* desacelerar; *walking*: andar mais devagar; *speaking*: falar mais devagar **2** *v/t traffic* acalmar
'**slowcoach** *Brit fam* molenga *m/f*
slowly ['sloʊlɪ] *adv* lentamente
slow 'motion ***in ~*** em câmera lenta
slowness ['sloʊnɪs] lentidão *f*
'**slowpoke** *Am fam* molenga *m/f*
slug [slʌg] *n animal* lesma *f*
sluggish ['slʌgɪʃ] *adj* lento
slum [slʌm] *n* favela *f*
slump [slʌmp] **1** *n trade*: queda *f* **2** *v/i economically* decair; (*collapse*) *person* tombar
slung [slʌŋ] *pret & pp* → ***sling***
slur [slɜːr] **1** *n on character* difamação *f* **2** *v/t* ⟨*pret & pp* ***slurred***⟩ *words* tartamudear
slurp [slɜːrp] *v/t* sorver
slurred [slɜːrd] *adj speech* com gaguejo
slush [slʌʃ] *n* neve *f* derretida; *pej sentimental* sentimentalismo *m*
'**slush fund** fundo *m* usado para propósitos dubiosos
slushy ['slʌʃɪ] *adj snow* derretido; *movie, novel* sentimental
slut [slʌt] *pej* vagabunda *f*
sly [slaɪ] *adj* astuto; ***on the ~*** às escondidas
smack [smæk] **1** *n* tapa *m* **2** *v/t child, bottom* dar um tapa em
small [smɒːl] **1** *adj* pequeno **2** *n* ***the ~ of the back*** o lombo
small 'change dinheiro *m* trocado
'**small hours** *npl* madrugada *f*
smallpox ['smɒːlpɑːks] varíola *f*
'**small print** letrinhas *fpl* '**small talk** conversa *f* banal
smart [smɑːrt] **1** *adj* (*elegant*) elegante; (*intelligent*) inteligente; *pace* rápido; ***get ~ with*** ser atrevido com **2** *v/i* (*hurt*) queimar
'**smart ass** *Am fam* sabichão *m*, sabichona *f*
'**smart card** cartão *m* eletrônico
♦ **smarten up** ['smɑːrtn] *v/t* melhorar
smartly ['smɑːrtlɪ] *adv dressed* com elegância
smash [smæʃ] **1** *n noise* estrondo *m*; (*car crash*) colisão *f*, *tennis*: smash *m* **2** *v/t & v/i* (*break*) quebrar; (*hit hard*) bater; ***~ sth to pieces*** espedaçar algo; ***the driver ~ed into ...*** o motorista colidiu contra ...
♦ **smash up** *v/t place* destruir
smash 'hit *fam* incrível sucesso *m*
smattering ['smætərɪŋ] *of a language* noções *fpl*
smear [smɪr] **1** *n ink etc*: mancha *f*, *character*: difamação *f*, MED exame *m* de papanicolau **2** *v/t* esfregar; *paint* esfumar; *character* difamar
'**smear campaign** campanha *f* de difamação
smell [smel] **1** *n* cheiro *m*; ***it has no ~*** não tem cheiro; ***sense of ~*** olfato *m* **2** *v/t* cheirar **3** *v/i unpleasantly* feder; (*sniff*) farejar; ***what does it ~ of?*** que cheiro é este?; ***you ~ of beer*** você está cheirando à cerveja; ***it ~s good*** está cheirando bem
smelly ['smelɪ] *adj* fedorento
smile [smaɪl] **1** *n* sorriso *m* **2** *v/i* sorrir
♦ **smile at** *v/t* sorrir para

smirk [smɜːrk] **1** *n* sorriso *m* falso **2** *v/i* dar um sorriso falso
smog [smɑːg] smog *m*
smoke [smoʊk] **1** *n* fumo *m*; ***have a ~*** fumar um cigarro **2** *v/t & v/i cigarettes* fumar; *bacon* defumar; ***I don't ~*** não fumo
'smokefree *adj zone* de não fumador
smoker ['smoʊkər] *person* fumante *m/f*
smoking ['smoʊkɪŋ] *n* ***~ is bad for the health*** fumar é prejucial à saúde; ***no ~*** proibido fumar
'smoking compartment RAIL compartimento *m* de fumantes
smoky ['smoʊkɪ] *adj room, air* enfumaçado
smolder ['smoʊldər] *v/i Am fire* arder; *fig with anger* arder de raiva; *fig with desire* arder de desejo
smooth [smuːð] **1** *adj surface, skin, sea* liso; *sea* calmo; *skin* macio; *ride* sem turbulência; *transition* sem problemas; *pej person* exageradamente educado **2** *v/t hair* alisar
♦ **smooth down** *v/t with sandpaper etc* lixar
♦ **smooth out** *v/t paper, cloth* alisar
♦ **smooth over** *v/t* ***smooth things over*** amenizar as coisas
smoothly ['smuːðlɪ] *adv* (*without any problems*) sem incidentes
smother ['smʌðər] *v/t flames* apagar; *person* asfixiar; ***~ s.o. with kisses*** cobrir alguém de beijos; ***bread ~ed with jam*** pão coberto de geléia
smoulder *Brit* → ***smolder***
smudge [smʌdʒ] **1** *n* mancha *f* **2** *v/t* manchar; *paint* esfumar
smug [smʌg] *adj* convencido
smuggle ['smʌgl] *v/t* contrabandear
smuggler ['smʌglər] contrabandista *m/f*
smuggling ['smʌglɪŋ] contrabando *m*
smugly ['smʌglɪ] *adv* presumidamente
smutty ['smʌtɪ] *adj joke, sense of humor* sujo
snack [snæk] *n* petisco *m*
'snack bar lanchonete *f*, *Port* snack-bar *m*
snag [snæg] *n* (*problem*) inconveniente *m*
snail [sneɪl] caracol *m*
'snail mail *hum* correio *m* normal
snake [sneɪk] *n* cobra *f*
snap [snæp] **1** *n* barulho *m seco*; PHOT foto *f* instantânea **2** *v/t & v/i* 〈*pret & pp* ***snapped***〉 (*break*) quebrar; (*say sharply*) dizer com severidade **3** *adj decision* súbito
♦ **snap up** *v/t bargains* comprar rapidamente
'snap fastener *Am* colchete *m*
snappy ['snæpɪ] *adj person, mood* irritável; *decision, response* rápido; (*elegant*) elegante
'snapshot foto *f* instantânea
snarl [snɑːrl] **1** *n dog*: rosnadura *f* **2** *v/i* rosnar
snatch [snætʃ] *v/t & v/i* arrebatar; (*steal*) roubar; (*kidnap*) raptar
snazzy ['snæzɪ] *adj fam* vistoso
sneak [sniːk] **1** *n* (*telltale*) mexeriqueiro,-a *m,f* **2** *v/t* (*remove, steal*) carregar; ***~ a glance at*** olhar disfarçadamente para **3** *v/i* (*tell tales*) mexericar; ***~ into the room / out of the room*** entrar / sair da sala de fininho
sneakers ['sniːkərz] *npl* tênis *mpl*, *Port* sapatilhas *fpl*
sneaking ['sniːkɪŋ] *adj* ***have a ~ suspicion that …*** tenho a leve suspeita de que …
sneaky ['sniːkɪ] *adj fam* (*crafty*) espertinho
sneer [snɪr] **1** *n* zombaria *f* **2** *v/i* zombar
sneeze [sniːz] **1** *n* espirro *m* **2** *v/i* espirrar
snicker ['snɪkər] **1** *n* risadinha *f* **2** *v/i* soltar uma risadinha
sniff [snɪf] **1** *v/i to clear nose* fungar; *dog* farejar **2** *v/t* (*smell*) cheirar
snip [snɪp] *n* (*bargain*) pechincha *f*
sniper ['snaɪpər] franco-atirador *m*
snivel ['snɪvl] *v/i* lamuriar
snob [snɑːb] esnobe *m/f*
snobbery ['snɑːbərɪ] esnobismo *m*
snobbish ['snɑːbɪʃ] *adj* esnobe
snooker ['snuːkər] sinuca *f*
snoop [snuːp] *n* bisbilhoteiro,-a *m,f*
♦ **snoop around** *v/i* bisbilhotar
snooty ['snuːtɪ] *adj* esnobe

snooze [snuːz] **1** *n* cochilo *m*; ***have a ~*** tirar um cochilo **2** *v/i* cochilar
snore [snɔːr] *v/i* roncar
snoring ['snɔːrɪŋ] *n* ronco *m*
snorkel ['snɔːrkl] snorkel *m*
snort [snɔːrt] *v/i horse* relichar; *bull, person, disdainfully* bufar
snout [snaʊt] *pig, dog*: focinho *m*
snow [snoʊ] **1** *n* neve *f* **2** *v/i* nevar
♦ **snow under** *v/t* ***be snowed under with …*** estar sobrecarregado de …
'snowball bola *f* de neve **'snowbound** *adj* isolado pela neve **'snow chains** *npl* MOT correntes *fpl* antiderrapantes **'snowdrift** monte *m* de neve (acumulada pelo vento) **'snowdrop** campânula *f* branca **'snowflake** floco *m* de neve **'snowman** boneco *m* de neve **'snowplough** *Brit*, **'snowplow** *Am* limpa-neves *m* **'snowstorm** tempestade *f* de neve
snowy ['snoʊɪ] *adj weather* nevoso; *roads, hills* nevado
snub [snʌb] **1** *n* desprezo *m* **2** *v/t* ⟨*pret & pp* ***snubbed***⟩ desprezar
snub-nosed ['snʌbnoʊzd] *adj* de nariz empinado
snug [snʌg] *adj* aconchegado; (*tight-fitting*) justo
♦ **snuggle down** ['snʌgl] *v/i* aconchegar-se
♦ **snuggle up to** *v/t* aconchegar-se a
so [soʊ] **1** *adv* ◇ (*in this way*) assim; ***and ~ on*** e assim por diante
◇ tão; ***~ hot / cold*** tão quente / frio; ***not ~ much*** não tanto; ***~ much better / easier*** muito melhor / mais fácil; ***eat / drink ~ much*** comer / beber muito; ***I miss you ~!*** sinto tanto a sua falta!
◇ também; ***~ am / do I*** eu também; ***~ is she / does she*** ela também
2 *pron* ***I hope / think ~*** espero / penso que sim; ***you didn't tell me – I did ~*** você não me disse - disse sim; ***50 or ~*** uns/umas 50
3 *conj* (*for that reason*) assim; (*in order that*) de maneira que; ***and ~ I missed the train*** e assim eu perdi o trem; ***~ (that) I could come too*** para que eu também pudesse vir; ***~ what?*** *fam* e daí?
soak [soʊk] *v/t* (*steep*) pôr de molho; *water, rain* ensopar
♦ **soak up** *v/t liquid* absorver; ***soak up the sun*** aquecer-se ao sol
soaked [soʊkt] *adj person, clothes* encharcado; ***be ~ to the skin*** estar molhado até os ossos
soaking ['soʊkɪŋ] *adj* **~ (*wet*)** encharcado
'so-and-so [soʊənsoʊ] *fam* (*unknown person*) fulano,-a *m,f*; (*annoying person*) chato,-a *m,f*
soap [soʊp] *n washing*: sabão *m*; *shower*: sabonete *m*
'soap opera novela *f*
soapy ['soʊpɪ] *adj water* com sabão
soar [sɔːr] *v/i rocket etc* subir; *prices* disparar
sob [sɑːb] **1** *n* soluço *m* **2** *v/i* ⟨*pret & pp* ***sobbed***⟩ soluçar
sober ['soʊbər] *adj* (*not drunk*) sóbrio; (*serious*) sério
♦ **sober up** *v/i* tornar-se sóbrio
so-called ['soʊkɒːld] *adj* assim chamado
soccer ['sɑːkər] futebol *m*
'soccer hooligan hooligan *m*, torcedor *m* violento
sociable ['soʊʃəbl] *adj* sociável
social ['soʊʃl] *adj* social
social 'democrat socialdemocrata
socialism ['soʊʃəlɪzm] socialismo *m*
socialist ['soʊʃəlɪst] **1** *adj* socialista **2** *n* socialista *m/f*
socialize ['soʊʃəlaɪz] *v/i* socializar
'social life vida *f* social **social 'science** ciências *fpl* sociais **social se'curity** *Brit* segurança *f* social **'social work** trabalho *m* social **'social worker** assistente *m/f* social
society [sə'saɪətɪ] sociedade *f*, (*organization*) associação *f*
sociologist [soʊsɪ'ɑːlədʒɪst] sociólogo,-a *m,f*
sociology [soʊsɪ'ɑːlədʒɪ] sociologia *f*
sock[1] [sɑːk] *foot*: meia *f*, *Port* peúga *f*
sock[2] [sɑːk] **1** *n punch* soco *m* **2** *v/t* (*punch*) socar
socket ['sɑːkɪt] *electrical* tomada *f*, *arm*: cavidade *f*, *eye*: órbita *f* ocular
soda ['soʊdə] (*soda water*) água *f* gaso-

S

sa; *Am* (*ice cream soda*) sorvete *m* com soda, *Port* gelado *m* com soda; *Am* (*soft drink*) refrigerante *m*; ***whiskey and ~*** uísque *m* (com) soda
sodden ['sɑːdn] *adj* encharcado
sofa ['soʊfə] sofá *m*
'sofa-bed sofá-cama *m*
soft [sɑːft] *adj voice, music, light, color, skin* suave; *pillow, chair* macio; (*lenient*) leniente; ***have a ~ spot for*** ter um fraco por
'soft drink refrigerante *m*
'soft drug droga *f* leve
soften ['sɑːfn] **1** *v/t position* abrandar; *impact, blow* amortecer **2** *v/i butter, ice cream* amolecer
softly ['sɑːftlɪ] *adv* delicadamente
soft 'toy bichinho *m* de pelúcia
software ['sɑːftwer] software *m*
soggy ['sɑːgɪ] *adj soil* encharcado; *pastry* mole
soil [sɔɪl] **1** *n* (*earth*) terra *f*, solo *m* **2** *v/t* sujar
solar 'energy ['soʊlər] energia *f* solar **'solar panel** painel *m* solar **'solar system** sistema *m* solar
sold [soʊld] *pret & pp* → ***sell***
soldier ['soʊldʒər] soldado *m*
♦**soldier on** *v/i* seguir adiante
sole[1] [soʊl] *n foot, shoe* sola *f*
sole[2] [soʊl] *adj* único
solely ['soʊlɪ] *adv* unicamente
solemn ['sɑːləm] *adj occasion, promise* solene
solemnity [sə'lemnətɪ] solenidade *f*
solemnly ['sɑːləmlɪ] *adv* solenemente
solicit [sə'lɪsɪt] *v/i prostitute* abordar o cliente
solicitor [sə'lɪsɪtər] *Brit* advogado,-a *m,f*
solid ['sɑːlɪd] *adj* (*hard*) duro; (*without holes*) massivo; *gold, silver* maciço; (*sturdy*) robusto; *evidence* consistente; *support* forte; ***a ~ hour*** uma hora inteira
solidarity [sɑːlɪ'dærətɪ] solidariedade *f*
solidify [sə'lɪdɪfaɪ] *v/i* ⟨*pret & pp* ***solidified***⟩ solidificar-se
solidly ['sɑːlɪdlɪ] *adv built* de maneira sólida; *in favor of sth* unanimemente
soliloquy [sə'lɪləkwɪ] *on stage* solilóquio *m*
solitaire ['sɑːlɪter] *card game* paciência *f*
solitary ['sɑːlɪterɪ] *adj life, activity* solitário; (*single*) único
solitary con'finement (prisão *f*) solitária *f*
solitude ['sɑːlɪtuːd] solidão *f*
solo ['soʊloʊ] **1** *n* MUS solo *m* **2** *adj performance, flight* solo
soloist ['soʊloʊɪst] solista *m/f*
soluble ['sɑːljʊbl] *adj substance, problem* solúvel
solution [sə'luːʃn] *also mixture* solução *f*
solve [sɑːlv] *v/t problem, crossword* resolver; *problem* solucionar; *mystery* esclarecer
solvent ['sɑːlvənt] *adj financially* solvente
somber ['sɑːmbər] *adj Am* (*dark*) escuro; (*serious*) sombrio
sombre *Brit* → ***somber***
some [sʌm] **1** *adj* ◇ (*a certain number, amount*) algum; *pl* alguns; (*a bit*) um pouco de; uns; ***~ people say that ...*** alguns dizem que ...; ***would you like ~ water / cookies?*** você quer um pouco de água / umas bolachinhas?
◇ *omitted*: ***there's ~ food in the fridge*** tem comida na geladeira; ***will you have ~ tea?*** vai querer chá? **2** *pron* um pouco, algum; *with plurals* alguns, algumas; ***would you like ~?*** *of this* você quer um pouco?; *of these* você quer alguns?; ***~ of the group*** parte do grupo **3** *adv* (*a bit*) um pouco; (*approximately*) uns, umas; ***we'll have to wait ~*** teremos que esperar um pouco; ***~ 10 paintings*** umas 10 pinturas
somebody ['sʌmbədɪ] *pron* alguém
'someday *adv* um dia
'somehow *adv* (*by one means or another*) de alguma maneira; (*for some unknown reason*) por alguma razão
'someone *pron* alguém
'someplace *adv* em algum lugar
somersault ['sʌmərsɒːlt] **1** *n* cambalhota *f* **2** *v/i* dar cambalhotas
'something *pron* algo; ***would you***

S

like ~ to drink / eat? você gostaria de algo para beber / comer; ***is ~ wrong?*** o que foi?
'sometime *adv* um dia destes; ***~ last year*** no ano passado
'sometimes ['sʌmtaɪmz] *adv* às vezes
'somewhat *adv* um tanto
'somewhere 1 *adv* em algum lugar **2** *pron* algum lugar
son [sʌn] filho *m*
sonata [sə'nɑːtə] MUS sonata *f*
song [sɑːŋ] música *f*
'songbird pássaro *m* canoro
'songwriter compositor,-a *m,f*
'son-in-law ⟨*pl* ***sons-in-law***⟩ genro *m*
sonnet ['sɑːnɪt] soneto *m*
soon logo; ***as ~ as*** assim que; ***as ~ as possible*** o quanto antes, o mais rápido possível; ***~er or later*** mais cedo ou mais tarde; ***the ~er the better*** quanto mais cedo melhor
soot [sʊt] fuligem *f*
soothe [suːð] *v/t* acalmar; *pain* aliviar
sophisticated [sə'fɪstɪkeɪtɪd] *adj person, machine* sofisticado
sophistication [səfɪstɪ'keɪʃn] *person, machine*: sofisticação *f*
sophomore ['sɑːfəmɔːr] *Am* estudante *m/f* do segundo ano
soppy ['sɑːpɪ] *adj fam* sentimental
soprano [sə'prɑːnoʊ] *n* soprano *f*
sordid ['sɔːrdɪd] *adj affair, business* sórdido
sore [sɔːr] **1** *adj* (*painful*) dolorido; *Am fam* (*angry*) zangado; ***is it ~?*** dói? **2** *n* ferida *f*
sorrow ['sɑːroʊ] *n* tristeza *f*
sorry ['sɑːrɪ] *adj* (*sad*) *day, sight* triste; (***I'm***) ***~!*** *apologizing* sinto muito; *regretting* lamento (muito); (***I'm***) ***~ but I can't help*** sinto muito, mas não posso ajudar; ***I won't be ~ to leave here*** não vou me arrepender de sair daqui; ***I feel ~ for her*** sinto pena dela
sort [sɔːrt] **1** *n* tipo *m*; ***~ of …*** *fam* um pouco …; ***is it finished? – ~ of*** *fam* já acabou? - mais ou menos **2** *v/t* classificar; *laundry* separar; COMPUT ordenar
♦ **sort out** *v/t papers* ordenar; *problem* resolver
SOS [esoʊ'es] *n* SOS *m*; *fig* pedido *m* de ajuda
so-'so *adv fam* mais ou menos
sought [sɒːt] *pret & pp* → ***seek***
soul [soʊl] REL, *fig* alma *f*; (*character*) personalidade *f*
sound[1] [saʊnd] **1** *adj* (*sensible*) sensato; (*healthy*) são (sã); *sleep* profundo **2** *adv* ***be ~ asleep*** estar dormindo profundamente
sound[2] [saʊnd] **1** *n* som *m*; (*noise*) barulho *m* **2** *v/t* (*pronounce*) pronunciar; MED auscultar; ***~ one's horn*** buzinar **3** *v/i* ***that ~s interesting*** parece interessante; ***that ~s like a good idea*** parece uma boa idéia; ***she ~ed unhappy*** parece triste
♦ **sound out** *v/t* sondar
'sound effects *npl* efeitos *mpl* sonoros
soundly ['saʊndlɪ] *adv sleep* profundamente; *beaten* decisivamente
'soundproof *adj* à prova de som
'soundtrack trilha *f* sonora
soup [suːp] sopa *f*
'soup bowl sopeira *f*
souped-up [suːp'tʌp] *adj fam* preparado
'soup plate prato *m* de sopa
'soup spoon colher *f* de sopa
sour ['saʊr] *adj apple, expression* azedo
source [sɔːrs] *n* fonte *f*; *river*: nascente *f*; *person* informante *m/f*
'source code código-fonte *m*
'source language língua *f* fonte
'sour cream creme *m* de leite azedo
south [saʊθ] **1** *adj* sul, do sul **2** *n* sul *m*; ***to the ~ of …*** ao sul de …
South 'Africa África *f* do sul **South 'African 1** *adj* sul-africano **2** *n* sul-africano,-a *m,f* **South A'merica** América *f* do Sul **South A'merican 1** *adj* sul-americano **2** *n* sul-americano,-a *m,f* **south'east 1** *n* sudeste *m* **2** *adj* sudeste **3** *adv* ao sudeste; ***it's ~ of …*** fica ao sudeste de … **south'eastern** *adj* sudeste
southerly ['sʌðərlɪ] *adj* sul
southern ['sʌðərn] *adj* sul
southerner ['sʌðərnər] sulista *m/f*
southernmost ['sʌðərnmoʊst] *adj*

S

mais ao sul
South 'Pole Pólo *m* Sul **southward** ['saʊθwərd] *adv Am* em direção sul **southwards** *Brit* → ***southward***
south'west 1 *n* sudoeste *m* **2** *adj* sudoeste **3** *adv* ao sudoeste; ***it's ~ of…*** ficar ao sudoeste de … **south-'western** *adj* do sudoeste
souvenir ['suːvənɪr] suvenir *m*
sovereign ['sɑːvrɪn] *adj state* soberano
sovereignty ['sɑːvrɪntɪ] soberania *f*
Soviet ['soʊvɪət] *adj* soviético
Soviet 'Union União *f* Soviética
sow[1] [saʊ] *n* (*female pig*) porca *f*
sow[2] [soʊ] ⟨*pret* ***sowed***, *pp* ***sown***⟩ *v/t seeds* semear
sown [soʊn] *pp* → ***sow***[2]
soya bean *Brit* → ***soy bean***
soy bean [sɔɪ] *Am* feijão *m* de soja
soy 'sauce molho *m* de soja
space [speɪs] *n* espaço *m*
♦ **space out** *v/t* espaçar
'space-bar COMPUT barra *f* de espaço **'spacecraft** nave *f* espacial **'spaceship** espaçonave *f* **'space shuttle** ônibus *m* espacial, *Port* space shuttle *m* **'space station** estação *f* espacial **'spacesuit** roupa *f* espacial
spacious ['speɪʃəs] *adj* espaçoso
spade [speɪd] pá *f*; ***~s*** *pl in cards* espadas *fpl*
'spadework *fig* trabalho *m* preliminar
spaghetti [spə'getɪ] espaguete *m*
Spain [speɪn] Espanha *f*
spam [spæm] spam *m*
span [spæn] *v/t* ⟨*pret & pp* ***spanned***⟩ abranger; *bridge* cruzar
Spaniard ['spænjərd] espanhol,-a *m,f*
Spanish ['spænɪʃ] **1** *adj* espanhol **2** *n language* espanhol *m*; ***the ~*** os espanhóis
spank [spæŋk] *v/t* dar umas palmadas (no traseiro)
spanking ['spæŋkɪŋ] palmada *f* no traseiro
spanner ['spænər] *Brit* chave *f* inglesa
spare [sper] **1** *v/t time, money* doar; *not execute* poupar; ***can you ~ the time?*** você tem tempo?; ***there were 5 to ~*** *left over, in excess* sobraram 5; ***the rebels ~d his life*** os rebeldes pouparam a vida dele; ***~ me the details*** poupe-me dos detalhes **2** *adj* de reserva **3** *n* reserva *f*
spare 'part peça *f* de reposição
spare 'ribs costelinha *f* de porco
spare 'room quarto *m* de visitas
spare 'time tempo *m* livre **spare 'tire** *Am* MOT pneu *m* reserva **spare tyre** *Brit* → ***spare tire***
sparing ['sperɪŋ] *adj* ***be ~ with*** ser econômico com
sparingly ['sperɪŋlɪ] *adv* com moderação
spark [spɑːrk] *n* faísca *f*
sparkle ['spɑːrkl] *v/i* cintilar
sparkling wine ['spɑːrklɪŋ] vinho *m* espumante
'spark plug MOT vela *f* (de ignição)
sparrow ['spæroʊ] pardal *m*
sparse [spɑːrs] *adj vegetation* esparso
sparsely ['spɑːrslɪ] *adv* ***~ populated*** pouco povoado
spartan ['spɑːrtn] *adj room* espartano
spasmodic [spæz'mɑːdɪk] *adj* intermitente
spat [spæt] *pret & pp* → ***spit***
spate [speɪt] *fig* onda *f*
spatial ['speɪʃl] *adj* espacial
spatter ['spætər] *v/t mud, paint* respingar
speak [spiːk] ⟨*pret* ***spoke***, *pp* ***spoken***⟩ **1** *v/i* falar; (*make a speech*) fazer um discurso; ***we're not ~ing (to each other)*** (*we've quarreled*) não estamos nos falando; ***~ing*** TEL é ele mesmo (ela mesma) (quem está falando) **2** *v/t foreign language* falar; ***~ one's mind*** dar sua opinião
♦ **speak for** *v/t* falar em nome de
♦ **speak out** *v/i* expressar-se
♦ **speak up** *v/i* (*speak louder*) falar mais alto
speaker ['spiːkər] *conference*: conferencista *m/f*; (*orator*) orador,a *m,f*; *sound system*: alto-falante *m*; ***a French ~*** um / uma falante de francês
spearmint ['spɪrmɪnt] menta *f*
special ['speʃl] *adj* especial; ***be on ~*** *Am* estar em oferta
special ef'fects *npl* efeitos *mpl* especiais

S

specialist ['speʃlɪst] especialista *m/f*
speciality *Brit* → ***specialty***
specialize ['speʃəlaɪz] *v/i* especializar-se; ~ ***in ...*** especializar-se em ...
specially ['speʃlɪ] *adv* especialmente
specialty ['speʃəltɪ] *Am* especialidade *f*
species ['spiːʃiːz] *nsg* espécie *f*
specific [spə'sɪfɪk] *adj* específico
specifically [spə'sɪfɪklɪ] *adv* especificamente
specifications [spesɪfɪ'keɪʃnz] *machine etc* especificações *fpl*
specify ['spesɪfaɪ] *v/t* ⟨*pret & pp* ***specified***⟩ especificar
specimen ['spesɪmən] amostra *f*
speck [spek] *dust, soot*: mancha *f*
specs [speks] *npl fam* (*spectacles*) óculos *mpl*
spectacle ['spektəkl] (*impressive sight*) espetáculo *m*; (***a pair of***) ~***s*** (um par de) óculos
spectacular [spek'tækjʊlər] *adj* espetacular
spectator [spek'teɪtər] espectador,a *m,f*
spec'tator sport esporte *m* espectador
spectrum ['spektrəm] *fig* espectro *m*
speculate ['spekjʊleɪt] *v/i also* FIN especular
speculation [spekjʊ'leɪʃn] *also* FIN especulação *f*
speculator ['spekjʊleɪtər] FIN especulador,a *m,f*
sped [sped] *pret & pp* → ***speed***
speech [spiːtʃ] (*address*) discurso *m*; *in play*, (*ability to speak*) fala *f*; (*way of speaking*) dicção *f*
'speech defect problema *m* de dicção
speechless ['spiːtʃlɪs] *adj shock, surprise*: sem fala
'speech therapist terapeuta *m/f* de linguagem **'speech therapy** terapia *f* de linguagem **'speech writer** redator,a *m,f* de discursos
speed [spiːd] **1** *n* velocidade *f*; ***at a ~ of ...*** a uma velocidade de ... **2** *v/i* ⟨*pret & pp* ***sped***⟩ (*go quickly*) ir a toda velocidade; (*drive too quickly*) ultrapassar o limite de velocidade
◆**speed by** *v/i* passar voando
◆**speed up** **1** *v/i* apressar-se **2** *v/t* acelerar
'speedboat lancha *f* **'speed bump** quebra-molas *m*, lombada *f* **'speed dial** marcação *f* rápida
speedily ['spiːdɪlɪ] *adv* rapidamente
speeding ['spiːdɪŋ] *n driving*: excesso *m* de velocidade
'speeding fine multa *f* por excesso de velocidade
'speed limit *on roads* limite *m* de velocidade
speedometer [spiː'dɑːmɪtər] velocímetro *m*
'speed trap radar *m* de controle de velocidade
speedy ['spiːdɪ] *adj* rápido
spell[1] [spel] *v/t & v/i word* soletrar
spell[2] [spel] *n period of time* temporada *f*; ***I'll sit here for a ~*** vou me sentar aqui por um tempo
'spellbound *adj* encantado **'spellcheck** COMPUT correção *f* ortográfica; ***do a ~ on ...*** fazer uma correção ortográfica em ... **'spellchecker** COMPUT corretor *m* ortográfico
spelling ['spelɪŋ] ortografia *f*
spend [spend] *v/t* ⟨*pret & pp* ***spent***⟩ *money* gastar; *time* passar
'spendthrift *n pej* esbanjador,a *m,f*
spent [spent] *pret & pp* → ***spend***
sperm [spɜːrm] espermatozóide *m*; (*semen*) esperma *m*
'sperm bank banco *m* de espermas
'sperm count contagem *f* espermática
sphere [sfɪr] esfera *f*; *fig* área *f*; ~ ***of influence*** área de influência
spice [spaɪs] *n* (*seasoning*) especiaria *f*
spicy ['spaɪsɪ] *adj food* temperado
spider ['spaɪdər] aranha *f*
'spiderweb teia *f* de aranha
spike [spaɪk] *n plant, animal*: espinho *m*; *running shoe*: trava *f*
spill [spɪl] **1** *v/t* derramar **2** *v/i* derramar-se **3** *n* derramamento *m*
spin[1] [spɪn] **1** *n* (*turn*) giro *m* **2** *v/t & v/i* ⟨*pret & pp* ***spun***⟩ girar; ***my head is ~ning*** minha cabeça está girando
spin[2] [spɪn] *v/t wool, cotton, web* fiar

S

♦**spin around** *v/i person, car* virar
♦**spin out** *v/t* prolongar
spinach ['spɪnɪdʒ] espinafre *m*
spinal ['spaɪnl] *adj* vertebral
spinal 'column coluna *f* vertebral
spinal 'cord medula *f* espinhal
'spin doctor *fam* assessor *m* de mídia
'spin-dry *v/t* centrifugar **'spin-dryer** centrifugadora *f*
spine [spaɪn] *person, animal*: coluna *f* vertebral; *book*: lombada *f*; *plant, hedgehog*: espinho *m*
spineless ['spaɪnlɪs] *adj* (*cowardly*) covarde
'spin-off produto *m* colateral
spinster ['spɪnstər] solteirona *f*
spiny ['spaɪnɪ] *adj* espinhoso
spiral ['spaɪrəl] **1** *n* espiral *f* **2** *v/i* ⟨*pret & pp* ***spiraled****, Brit* ***spiralled***⟩ (*rise quickly*) subir rapidamente
spiral 'staircase escada *f* caracol
spire ['spaɪr] *n* pináculo *m*
spirit ['spɪrɪt] *n not body, dead person*, (*attitude*) espírito *m*; (*courage*) coragem *f*; ***we did it in a ~ of cooperation*** o fizemos com o espírito de cooperação
spirited ['spɪrɪtɪd] *adj* (*energetic*) enérgico
'spirit level nível *m* de bolha de ar
spirits[1] ['spɪrɪts] *npl alcohol* destilados *mpl*
spirits[2] ['spɪrɪts] *npl* (*morale*) moral *f*; ***be in good / poor ~*** estar com a moral alta / baixa
spiritual ['spɪrɪtʊəl] *adj* espiritual
spiritualism ['spɪrɪtʊəlɪzm] espiritismo *m*
spiritualist ['spɪrɪtʊəlɪst] *n* espírita *m/f*
spit [spɪt] *v/i* ⟨*pret & pp* ***spat***⟩ *person* cuspir; ***it's ~ting with rain*** está pingando
♦**spit out** *v/t food, liquid* cuspir
spite [spaɪt] *n* maldade *f*; ***in ~ of*** apesar de
spiteful ['spaɪtfl] *adj* malicioso
spitefully ['spaɪtflɪ] *adv* com maldade
spitting 'image ['spɪtɪŋ] ***be the ~ of s.o.*** ser a cara de alguém
splash [splæʃ] **1** *n noise* barulho *m*; (*small amount of liquid*) pingada *f*; *color*: mancha *f* **2** *v/t person, water, mud* respingar **3** *v/i water* bater
♦**splash down** *v/i spacecraft* amerissar
♦**splash out** *v/i spending*: gastar uma fortuna (***on*** em)
'splashdown amerissagem *f*
splendid ['splendɪd] *adj* esplêndido
splendor ['splendər] *Am* pompa *f*
splendour *Brit* → ***splendor***
splint [splɪnt] *n* MED tala *m*
splinter ['splɪntər] **1** *n* estilhaço *m* **2** *v/i* estilhaçar
'splinter group grupo *m* dissidente
split [splɪt] **1** *n damage* rachadura *f*; *fabric*: rasgão *m*; *disagreement* ruptura *f*; *division, share* divisão *f* **2** *v/t & v/i* ⟨*pret & pp* ***split***⟩ *damage* rachar; *fabric* rasgar; *logs* partir em dois; (*cause disagreement in, divide*) dividir **3** *v/i* ⟨*pret & pp* ***split***⟩ (*disagree, divide*) dividir-se
♦**split up** *v/i couple* separar-se
split person'ality PSYCH personalidade *f* dividida
splitting ['splɪtɪŋ] *adj* ***~ headache*** dor *f* de cabeça forte
splutter ['splʌtər] *v/i* gaguejar
spoil [spɔɪl] *v/t child* estragar com mimos; *surprise, party etc* arruinar
'spoilsport *fam* desmancha-prazeres *m/f*
spoilt [spɔɪlt] *adj child* mimado; ***be ~ for choice*** ter muito o que escolher
spoke[1] [spoʊk] *wheel* raio *m*
spoke[2] [spoʊk] *pret* → ***speak***
spoken ['spoʊkən] *pp* → ***speak***
spokesman ['spoʊksmən] porta-voz *m*
spokesperson ['spoʊkspɜːrsən] porta-voz *m*
spokeswoman ['spoʊkswʊmən] porta-voz *f*
sponge [spʌndʒ] *n* esponja *f*
♦**sponge off, sponge on** *v/t fam* viver às custas de
'sponge cake bolo *m* fofo
sponger ['spʌndʒər] *fam* parasita *m/f*
sponsor ['spɑːnsər] **1** *n* patrocinador,a *m,f* **2** *v/t* patrocinar
sponsorship ['spɑːnsərʃɪp] patrocínio *m*

spontaneous [spɑːn'teɪnɪəs] *adj* espontâneo
spontaneously [spɑːn'teɪnɪəslɪ] *adv* espontaneamente
spooky ['spuːkɪ] *adj fam* assombrado
spool [spuːl] *n thread*: carretel *m*; *film*: bobina *f*
spoon [spuːn] *n* colher *f*
'spoonfeed *v/t* ⟨*pret & pp* ***spoonfed***⟩ *fig* dar tudo mastigado para
spoonful ['spuːnfʊl] colherada *f*
sporadic [spə'rædɪk] *adj* esporádico
sport [spɔːrt] *n* esporte *m*, *Port* desporto *m*
sporting ['spɔːrtɪŋ] *adj event* esportivo; (*fair, generous*) gentil; ***a ~ gesture*** um gesto nobre
'sports car [spɔːrts] carro *m* esportivo, *Port* carro *m* desportivo **'sports center**, *Brit* **'sports centre** centro *m* esportivo, *Port* centro *m* desportivo **'sportscoat** *Am* blazer *m* esportivo, *Port* blazer *m* desportivo **sports 'journalist** jornalista *m/f* esportivo,-a, *Port* jornalista *m/f* desportivo,-a **'sportsman** esportista *m*, *Port* desportista *m* **'sports medicine** medicina *f* esportiva, *Port* medicina *f* desportiva **'sports news** *nsg* notícias *fpl* esportivas, *Port* notícias *fpl* de desporto **'sports page** página *f* de esportes, *Port* página *f* desportiva **'sportswear** moda *f* esporte, *Port* moda *f* desportiva **'sportswoman** esportista *f*, *Port* desportista *f*
sporty ['spɔːrtɪ] *adj person* esportivo, *Port* desportivo
spot[1] [spɑːt] *n* (*pimple*) espinha *f*; *measles etc*: bolha *f*; *in pattern* bolinha *f*; ***a ~ of ...*** (*a little*) um pouco de ...
spot[2] [spɑːt] *n* (*place*) lugar *m*; ***on the ~*** *in the place in question* no local; (*immediately*) na mesma hora; ***put s.o. on the ~*** pôr alguém numa situação embaraçosa
spot[3] [spɑːt] *v/t* ⟨*pret & pp* ***spotted***⟩ (*notice*) procurar; (*identify*) ver
'spot check controle *m* aleatório; ***carry out ~s*** fazer controles aleatórios
spotless ['spɑːtlɪs] *adj* impecável
'spotlight *n* holofote *m*
spotted ['spɑːtɪd] *adj fabric* de bolinha colorida
spotty ['spɑːtɪ] *adj with pimples* empipocado
spouse [spaʊs] *fml* esposo,-a *m,f*
spout [spaʊt] **1** *n* bico *m bule etc* **2** *v/i liquid* jorrar **3** *v/t fam* discorrer
sprain [spreɪn] **1** *n* distorção *f* **2** *v/t* torcer
sprang [spræŋ] *pret* → ***spring***[3]
sprawl [sprɒːl] *v/i* esparramar-se; *city* expandir-se; ***send s.o. ~ing*** *punch* estender alguém com um murro
sprawling ['sprɒːlɪŋ] *adj city, suburbs* de crescimento desenfreado
spray [spreɪ] **1** *n sea water, fountain*: borrifo *m*; *hair*: spray *m* **2** *v/t* esborrifar; ***~ X with Y*** esborrifar X com Y
'spraygun pistola *f* pulverizadora
spread [spred] **1** *n disease, religion etc*: propagação *f*; *fam* (*big meal*) banquete *m* **2** *v/t* ⟨*pret & pp* ***spread***⟩ (*lay*), *arms, legs* estender; *butter, jam, news, rumor, disease* espalhar **3** *v/i* ⟨*pret & pp* ***spread***⟩ *rumor, news, butter* espalhar-se
'spreadsheet COMPUT planilha *f* eletrônica
spree [spriː] farra *f*; ***go*** (***out***) ***on a ~*** sair à farra; ***go on a shopping ~*** fazer uma orgia de compras
sprig [sprɪg] raminho *m*
sprightly ['spraɪtlɪ] *adj* cheio de energia
spring[1] [sprɪŋ] *n season* primavera *f*
spring[2] [sprɪŋ] *n device* mola *f*
spring[3] [sprɪŋ] **1** *n* (*jump*) pulo *m*; (*stream*) nascente *f* **2** *v/i* ⟨*pret* ***sprang***, *pp* ***sprung***⟩ pular; ***~ from*** proceder de
'springboard trampolim *m* **spring 'chicken** *hum* ***she's no ~*** ela não é (mais) uma garotinha **spring-'cleaning** limpeza *f* a fundo **'springtime** primavera *f*
springy ['sprɪŋɪ] *adj mattress, ground* flexível; *walk* ligeiro; *piece of elastic* elástico
sprinkle ['sprɪŋkl] *v/t* borrifar; ***~ sth with sth*** borrifar algo com algo
sprinkler ['sprɪŋklər] *garden*: aspersor

S

m; *ceiling*: (chuveiro) sprinkler *m*

sprint [sprɪnt] **1** *n* corrida *f* (de velocidade); ***the 100m ~*** a corrida dos 100m **2** *v/i* correr

sprinter ['sprɪntər] SPORT corredor,a *m,f*

sprout [spraʊt] **1** *v/i seed* brotar **2** *n* ***(Brussels) ~s*** couve *f* de bruxelas

spruce [spruːs] *adj* bem-arrumado, elegante

sprung [sprʌŋ] *pp* → ***spring***[3]

spry [spraɪ] *adj* cheio de energia

spun [spʌn] *pret & pp* → ***spin***[1]

spur [spɜːr] *n* espora *f*; *fig* incentivo *m*; ***on the ~ of the moment*** espontaneamente

♦ **spur on** *v/t* ⟨*pret & pp* ***spurred***⟩ (*encourage*) encorajar

spurt [spɜːrt] **1** *n race*: arrancada *f*; ***put on a ~*** dar uma arrancada **2** *v/i liquid* jorrar

sputter ['spʌtər] *v/i engine* crepitar

spy [spaɪ] **1** *n* espião *m*, espiã *f* **2** *v/i* ⟨*pret & pp* ***spied***⟩ espionar **3** *v/t* ⟨*pret & pp* ***spied***⟩ *fam* espiar

♦ **spy on** *v/t* espionar

squabble ['skwɑːbl] **1** *n* disputa *f* **2** *v/i* brigar

squalid ['skwɒːlɪd] *adj* sujo

squalor ['skwɒːlər] imundícia *f*

squander ['skwɒːndər] *v/t money* desperdiçar

square [skwer] **1** *adj in shape* quadrado; ***~ mile*** milha *f* quadrada **2** *n* (*shape*), *also* MATH quadrado *m*; *town*: praça *f*, *board game*: casa *f*; ***we're back to ~ one*** voltamos ao ponto de partida

♦ **square up** *v/i* (*settle up*) fazer as contas

square 'root raiz *f* quadrada

squash[1] [skwɑːʃ] *n vegetable* abóbora *f*

squash[2] [skwɑːʃ] *n game* squash *m*

squash[3] [skwɑːʃ] *v/t* (*crush*) amassar

squat [skwɑːt] **1** *adj in shape* baixo **2** *v/i* ⟨*pret & pp* ***squatted***⟩ (*sit*) agachar-se; *illegally* ocupar

squatter ['skwɑːtər] ocupante *m/f* ilegal

squeak [skwiːk] **1** *n mouse*: chiado *m*; *hinge*: rangido *m* **2** *v/i mouse* chiar; *hinge, shoes* ranger

squeaky ['skwiːkɪ] *adj hinge, shoes* rangente; *voice* estridente

squeal [skwiːl] **1** *n* grito *m*; *brakes*: rangido *m* **2** *v/i* gritar; *brakes* ranger

squeamish ['skwiːmɪʃ] *adj* nauseento

squeeze [skwiːz] **1** *n hand*: aperto *m* **2** *v/t* (*press*) apertar; (*remove juice from*) espremer

♦ **squeeze in 1** *v/i to a car etc* apertar--se **2** *v/t* enfiar

♦ **squeeze up** *v/i to make space* dar uma espremida, *Port* dar um jeitinho

squid [skwɪd] lula *f*

squint [skwɪnt] *n* estrabismo *m*; ***a man with a ~*** um homem estrábico

squirm [skwɜːrm] *v/i* (*wriggle*) esquivar-se; *in embarrassment* contorcer-se

squirrel ['skwɪrl] *n* esquilo *m*

squirt [skwɜːrt] **1** *v/t* esguichar **2** *n fam pej* moleque *m*, moleca *f*

stab [stæb] **1** *n fam* tentativa *f*; ***have a ~ at doing sth*** fazer uma tentativa de realizar algo **2** *v/t* ⟨*pret & pp* ***stabbed***⟩ *person* apunhalar

stability [stə'bɪlətɪ] estabilidade *f*

stabilize ['steɪbɪlaɪz] **1** *v/t prices, currency, boat* estabilizar **2** *v/i prices etc* estabilizar-se

stable[1] ['steɪbl] *n horses*: estábulo *m*

stable[2] ['steɪbl] *adj* estável

stack [stæk] **1** *n* (*pile*) pilha *f*; (*smokestack*) chaminé *f*; ***~s of*** *fam* um montão de; ***~s of time*** um tempão **2** *v/t* empilhar

stadium ['steɪdɪəm] estádio *m*

staff [stæf] *npl employees* pessoal *m*; *teachers* professorado *m*

staffer ['stæfər] *n* funcionário,-a *m,f*, colarinho-branco *m/f*

'staffroom *Brit school*: sala *f* dos professores

stag [stæg] *n* veado *m*

stage[1] [steɪdʒ] *n life, project, journey etc*: etapa *f*

stage[2] [steɪdʒ] **1** *n* THEA cenário *m*; ***go on the ~*** tornar-se ator / atriz **2** *v/t play* encenar; *demonstration* organizar

stage 'door entrada *f* dos artistas

'stage fright medo *m* do palco

'stage hand ajudante *m/f* de palco

stagger ['stægər] **1** *v/i* cambalear **2** *v/t* (*amaze*) surpreender; *coffee breaks etc* revezar
staggering ['stægərɪŋ] *adj* surpreendente
stagnant ['stægnənt] *adj water* estancado; *fig economy* estagnado
stagnate [stæg'neɪt] *v/i fig person, mind* estagnar
stagnation [stæg'neɪʃn] estagnação *f*
'stag party despedida *f* de solteiro
stain [steɪn] **1** *n* (*dirty mark*) mancha *f*; *wood*: tinta *f* **2** *v/t* (*dirty*) manchar; *wood* tingir **3** *v/i wine etc* deixar mancha; *fabric* manchar
stained-glass 'window [steɪnd] janela *f* de vitrais
stainless steel ['steɪnlɪs] **1** *m* aço *m* inoxidável **2** *adj* de aço inoxidável
'stain remover removedor *m* de manchas
stair [ster] degrau *m*; ***the ~s*** os degraus *mpl*
'staircase escadaria *f*
stake [steɪk] **1** *n wood*: estaca *f*; *gambling*: aposta *f*; *investment* investimento *m*; ***be at ~*** estar em jogo **2** *v/t tree* estacar; *money* apostar; *Am person* apoiar
stale [steɪl] *adj bread, fig news* velho; *air* viciado
'stalemate *chess*: empate *m*; *fig* beco *m* sem saída
stalk[1] [stɔːk] *n fruit, plant*: talo *m*
stalk[2] [stɔːk] *v/t* (*follow*) espreitar; *person* perseguir
stalker ['stɔːkər] *person* perseguidor,a *m,f*
stall[1] [stɒːl] *n market*: barraca *f*, *cow, horse*: estábulo *m*
stall[2] [stɒːl] **1** *v/i vehicle, engine* ir-se abaixo; *plane* adiar; (*play for time*) tentar ganhar tempo **2** *v/t engine* enguiçar; *people* deter
stallion ['stæljən] garanhão *m*
stalls [stɒːlz] *npl* platéia *f*
stalwart ['stɒːlwərt] *adj support, supporter* leal
stamina ['stæmɪnə] resistência *f*
stammer ['stæmər] **1** *n* gaguez *f* **2** *v/i* gaguejar
stamp[1] [stæmp] **1** *n letter*: selo *m*; *device, mark made with device* carimbo *m* **2** *v/t letter* selar; *document, passport* carimbar; ***~ed addressed envelope*** envelope *m* pré-endereçado e selado
stamp[2] [stæmp] *v/t* ***~ one's feet*** sapatear
◆ **stamp out** *v/t* (*eradicate*) erradicar
'stamp collecting filatelia *f* **'stamp collection** coleção *f* de selos **'stamp collector** colecionador,a *m,f* de selos
stampede [stæm'piːd] **1** *n cattle etc*: estouro *m*; *people*: correria *f* **2** *v/i cattle etc* estourar; *people* correr
stance [stæns] (*position*) postura *f*
stand [stænd] **1** *n* (*witness stand*) banco *m* das testemunhas; (*support, base*) suporte *m*; *Brit exhibition*: estande *m*; ***take the ~*** LAW testemunhar **2** *v/i* ⟨*pret & pp* ***stood***⟩ *as opposed to sit, also* (*rise*) ficar em pé, ficar de pé; (*be situated*) estar, ficar; ***he was ~ing by the door*** encontrava-se à porta; ***~ still!*** fique parado!; ***where do I ~ with you?*** qual é a nossa relação? **3** *v/t* ⟨*pret & pp* ***stood***⟩ (*tolerate*) suportar; (*put*) colocar; ***you don't ~ a chance*** você não tem chance; ***~ s.o. a drink*** pagar uma bebida para alguém; ***~ one's ground*** manter-se firme
◆ **stand back** *v/i* ficar atrás
◆ **stand by 1** *v/i* (*not take action*) ficar sem fazer nada; (*be ready*) ficar alerta **2** *v/t person* apoiar; *decision* ater-se a
◆ **stand down** *v/i* (*withdraw*) retirar-se
◆ **stand for** *v/t* (*tolerate*) tolerar; (*represent*) significar
◆ **stand in for** *v/t* substituir
◆ **stand out** *v/i* destacar-se
◆ **stand up 1** *v/i* levantar-se **2** *v/t fam date* dar o bolo
◆ **stand up for** *v/t* defender
◆ **stand up to** *v/t* erguer-se contra
standard ['stændərd] **1** *adj* (*usual*) habitual **2** *n* (*level of excellence*) nível *m*; (*expectation*) padrão *m* de exigência; TECH padrão *m*; ***be up to ~*** estar dentro do padrão; ***not be up to ~*** estar fora do padrão
standardize ['stændərdaɪz] *v/t* padronizar

S

standard of 'living padrão *m* de vida
'standby 1 *n* (*ticket*) passagem *f* stand by; ***on ~*** em stand by, em lista de espera **2** *adv fly* com passagem stand by
standing ['stændɪŋ] *n society etc*: posição *f*; (*repute*) reputação *f*; ***a politician of some ~*** um político renomado; ***a friendship of long ~*** um relacionamento de muito tempo
'standing room área *f* sem assentos
standoffish [stænd'ɑːfɪʃ] *adj* distante
'standpoint ponto *m* de vista
'standstill ***be at a ~*** estar paralisado; ***bring to a ~*** paralisar
stank [stæŋk] *pret* → ***stink***
stanza ['stænzə] estrofe *f*
staple[1] ['steɪpl] *n foodstuff* alimento *m* básico
staple[2] ['steɪpl] **1** *n fastener* grampo *m* **2** *v/t* grampear
staple 'diet dieta *f* básica
'staple gun grampeador *m* industrial
stapler ['steɪplər] grampeador *m*
star [stɑːr] **1** *n also fig* estrela *f* **2** *v/t & v/i* 〈*pret & pp* ***starred***〉 estrelar; ***it ~s Brad Pitt as ...*** estrela Brad Pitt como ...
'starboard estibordo *m*
starch [stɑːrʧ] fécula *f*
stare [ster] **1** *n* encaração *f* **2** *v/i* encarar; ***~ at*** encarar, olhar fixamente para
'starfish estrela *f* do mar
stark [stɑːrk] **1** *adj landscape* desolado; *reminder, contrast etc* severo **2** *adv* ***~ naked*** completamente nu
starling ['stɑːrlɪŋ] estorninho *m*
starry ['stɑːrɪ] *adj night* estrelado
starry-eyed [stɑːrɪ'aɪd] *adj person* ingênuo
Stars and 'Stripes bandeira *f* americana
start [stɑːrt] **1** *n* (*beginning*) começo *m*; ***get off to a good / bad ~*** *race*: fazer uma boa / má largada; *marriage, career*: ter um bom / mau começo; ***from the ~*** desde o começo; ***well, it's a ~!*** bom, já é pelo menos um começo **2** *v/i & v/t* começar; *engine, car* dar a partida; *business* montar; ***~ to do sth, ~ doing sth*** começar a fazer algo; ***~ing from tomorrow*** a partir de amanhã
starter ['stɑːrtər] *meal*: entrada *f*; *car*: motor *m* de arranque
'starting point *walk, thesis etc*: ponto *m* de partida
'starting salary salário *m* inicial
startle ['stɑːrtl] *v/t* assustar
startling ['stɑːrtlɪŋ] *adj* surpreendente
'start-up nova empresa *f*
starvation [stɑːr'veɪʃn] fome *f*
starve [stɑːrv] *v/i* passar fome; ***~ to death*** morrer de fome; ***I'm starving*** *fam* estou morrendo de fome
state[1] [steɪt] **1** *n* (*condition, part of country, country*) estado *m*; ***the States*** os Estados Unidos **2** *adj banquet etc* de estado; *capital etc* estadual, estatal
state[2] [steɪt] *v/t* declarar
'State Department *Am* ministéro *m* do exterior
statement ['steɪtmənt] *to police* depoimento *m*; (*announcement*) enunciado *m*; ***bank ~*** extrato *m* bancário
state of e'mergency estado *m* de emergência
state-of-the-'art *adj* avançado
statesman ['steɪtsmən] homem *m* de estado
state 'trooper *Am* polícia *f* estadual
state 'visit visita *f* oficial
static, static elec'tricity ['stætɪk] eletricidade *f* estática
station ['steɪʃn] **1** *n* RAIL estação *f*; RADIO emissora *f*; TV canal *m* **2** *v/t guard etc* postar; ***be ~ed at*** *soldier* estar estacionado em
stationary ['steɪʃnerɪ] *adj* estacionário
stationer's ['steɪʃənərz] papelaria *f*
stationery ['steɪʃənərɪ] artigos *mpl* de escritório
station 'manager chefe *m* da estação
'station wagon *Am* carro *m* de família
statistical [stə'tɪstɪkl] *adj* estatístico
statistically [stə'tɪstɪklɪ] *adv* estatisticamente
statistician [stætɪs'tɪʃn] estatístico,-a *m,f*

statistics [stə'tɪstɪks] *nsg science* estatística *f*; *npl figures* estatísticas *fpl*
statue ['stætʃuː] estátua *f*
Statue of 'Liberty Estátua *f* da Liberdade
status ['steɪtəs] status *m*, prestígio *m*; ***women want equal ~ with men*** as mulheres querem igualdade de direitos
'status bar COMPUT barra *f* de status
'status symbol símbolo *m* de prestígio
statute ['stætʃuːt] estatuto *m*
staunch [stɒːntʃ] *adj* leal
stay [steɪ] **1** *n* estadia *f* **2** *v/i in a place, in a condition* ficar; ***~ in a hotel*** ficar num hotel; ***~ right there!*** fique aqui!; ***~ put*** ficar
♦ **stay away** *v/i* ficar longe
♦ **stay away from** *v/t* ficar longe de
♦ **stay behind** *v/i* ficar atrás
♦ **stay up** *v/i* (*not go to bed*) ficar acordado
steadily ['stedɪlɪ] *adv improve etc* continuamente
steady ['stedɪ] **1** *adj* (*not shaking*), *also boyfriend* firme; (*regular*) constante; (*continuous*) contínuo **2** *adv* ***be going ~*** estar saindo; ***~ on!*** espera aí! **3** *v/t* ⟨*pret & pp* ***steadied***⟩ firmar
steak [steɪk] *n* bife *m*
steal [stiːl] *v/t & v/i* ⟨*pret* ***stole***, *pp* ***stolen***⟩ roubar; (*move quietly*) andar furtivamente
stealthy ['stelθɪ] *adj* furtivo
steam [stiːm] **1** *n* vapor *m* **2** *v/t food* cozinhar no vapor
♦ **steam up 1** *v/i window* embaçar-se **2** *v/t* ***be steamed up*** *fam* estar azedo
steamer ['stiːmər] *cooking*: panela *f* de pressão
'steam iron ferro *m* à vapor
steel [stiːl] **1** *n* aço *m* **2** *adj* de aço
'steelworker metalúrgico *m*
steep[1] [stiːp] *adj hill etc* escarpado; *fam prices* excessivo
steep[2] [stiːp] *v/t* (*soak*) pôr de molho
steeple ['stiːpl] torre *f*
'steeplechase corrida *f* de obstáculos
steeply ['stiːplɪ] *adv* ***climb ~*** *path* subir; *prices* subir em disparada
steer[1] [stɪr] *v/t car* dirigir; *boat* pilotar; *person* guiar; *conversation* levar
steer[2] [stɪr] *n animal* touro *m*
steering ['stɪrɪŋ] *vehicle* direção *f*
'steering wheel volante *m*
stem[1] [stem] *n plant*: caule *m*; *glass*: haste *f*, *pipe*: tubo *m*; *word*: raiz *f*
stem[2] [stem] *v/t* (*block*) conter
♦ **stem from** *v/t* ⟨*pret & pp* ***stemmed***⟩ proceder de
'stem cell célula-tronco *f*
stemware ['stemwer] *Am* taça *f*
stench [stentʃ] fedor *m*
stencil ['stensɪl] *n* estêncil *m*
step [step] **1** *n* (*pace*) passo *m*; (*stair*) degrau *m*; (*measure*) medida *f*; ***~ by ~*** passo a passo **2** *v/i* ⟨*pret & pp* ***stepped***⟩ ***she ~ped carefully over the cat*** ela passou cuidadosamente por cima do gato
♦ **step down** *v/i from post etc* demitir-se
♦ **step on** *v/t person's foot etc* pisar
♦ **step up** *v/t* (*increase*) aumentar
'stepbrother meio-irmão *m* **'stepdaughter** enteada *f* **'stepfather** padrasto *m* **'stepladder** escadote *m* **'stepmother** madrasta *f*
stepping stone ['stepɪŋ] degrau *m*; *fig* trampolim *m*
'stepsister meia-irmã *f*
'stepson enteado *m*
stereo ['sterɪoʊ] *n* estéreo *m*; (*sound system*) aparelho *m* de som
stereotype ['sterɪoʊtaɪp] *n* estereótipo *m*
sterile ['sterəl] *adj* estéril
sterilize ['sterəlaɪz] *v/t woman, equipment* esterilizar
sterling ['stɜːrlɪŋ] *n* Libra *f* (esterlina)
stern[1] [stɜːrn] *adj* severo
stern[2] [stɜːrn] *n* NAUT popa *f*
sternly ['stɜːrnlɪ] *adv* com severidade
steroid ['sterɔɪd] esteróide *m*
stethoscope ['steθəskoʊp] estetoscópio *m*
Stetson® ['stetsn] chapéu *m* de vaqueiro
stevedore ['stiːvədɔːr] estivador *m*
stew [stuː] *n* cozido *m*
steward ['stuːərd] *n plane, ship*: co-

missário *m* de bordo; *demonstration, meeting*: organizador *m*

stewardess ['stu:ərdes] *plane, ship*: comissária *f* de bordo

stewed [stu:d] *adj apples, plums* em compota

stick[1] [stɪk] *n wood*: pau *m*; *policeman*: cacetete *m*; (*walking stick*) bengala *f*; ***the ~s*** *fam* o fim do mundo

stick[2] [stɪk] ⟨*pret & pp* **stuck**⟩ **1** *v/t with adhesive* colar; *fam* (*put*) pôr **2** *v/i* (*jam*) emperrar; (*adhere*) colar

♦**stick around** *v/i fam* ficar (por perto)

♦**stick by** *v/t fam* apoiar; ***stick by s.o.*** apoiar alguém

♦**stick out** *v/i* (*protrude*) sobressair; (*be noticeable*) chamar a atenção

♦**stick to** *v/t* (*adhere to*) colar em; *fam* (*keep to*) continuar com; *fam* (*follow*) seguir; ***I'll stick to beer*** eu vou ficar na cerveja

♦**stick together** *v/i fam* manter-se unido

♦**stick up** *v/t poster, leaflet* fixar

♦**stick up for** *v/t fam* defender

sticker ['stɪkər] adesivo *m*

sticking plaster ['stɪkɪŋ] *Brit* band-aid *m*

'stick-in-the-mud *fam* quadrado,-a *m,f*

sticky ['stɪkɪ] *adj hands, surface* pegajoso; *label* adesivo

stiff [stɪf] **1** *adj brush, cardboard, muscle, body, competition* duro; *mixture, paste* consistente; *in manner* forçado; *drink* forte; *fine* severo **2** *adv* ***be scared ~*** *fam* estar morrendo de medo; ***be bored ~*** *fam* estar morrendo de tédio

stiffen ['stɪfn] *v/i* enrijecer-se

♦**stiffen up** *v/i muscle* enrijecer

stiffly ['stɪflɪ] *adv* com esforço; *fig* forçadamente

stiffness ['stɪfnəs] *muscles*: rigidez *f*; *fig manner*: dureza *f*

stifle ['staɪfl] *v/t yawn, laugh* conter; *criticism, debate* reprimir

stifling ['staɪflɪŋ] *adj* sufocante

stigma ['stɪgmə] estigma *m*

stilettos [stɪ'letoʊz] *Brit shoes* sapatos *mpl* de salto agulha

still[1] [stɪl] **1** *adj* quieto **2** *adv* ***keep ~!*** fique quieto!; ***stand ~!*** fique quieto!

still[2] [stɪl] *adv* (*yet*) ainda; (*nevertheless*) de todas as maneiras; ***do you ~ want it?*** você ainda quer isso?; ***she ~ hasn't finished*** ela ainda não terminou; ***she might ~ come*** pode ser que ainda venha; ***they are ~ my parents*** eles continuam sendo meus pais; ***~ more*** (*even more*) ainda mais

'stillborn *adj* natimorto; ***be ~*** nascer morto

still 'life natureza *f* morta

stilted ['stɪltɪd] *adj* forçado

stilts [stɪlts] *npl* andas *fpl*; *house*: estacas *fpl*

stimulant ['stɪmjʊlənt] estimulante *m*

stimulate ['stɪmjʊleɪt] *v/t person, demand* estimular

stimulating ['stɪmjʊleɪtɪŋ] *adj* estimulante

stimulation [stɪmjʊ'leɪʃn] estimulação *f*

stimulus ['stɪmjʊləs] estímulo *m*

sting [stɪŋ] **1** *n bee, jellyfish*: picada *f* **2** *v/t* ⟨*pret & pp* **stung**⟩ *bee, jellyfish* picar **3** *v/i* ⟨*pret & pp* **stung**⟩ *eyes, scratch* queimar

stinging ['stɪŋɪŋ] *adj remark, criticism* magoante

stingy ['stɪndʒɪ] *adj fam* pão-duro

stink [stɪŋk] **1** *n* (*bad smell*) fedor *m*; *fam* (*fuss*) auê *m*; ***kick up a ~*** *fam* rodar a baiana **2** *v/i* ⟨*pret* **stank**, *pp* **stunk**⟩ (*smell bad*) feder; *fam* (*be very bad*) ser nojento

stint [stɪnt] *n* temporada *f*; ***do a ~ in the army*** servir o exército

♦**stint on** *v/t fam* economizar

stipulate ['stɪpjʊleɪt] *v/i* estipular

stipulation [stɪpjʊ'leɪʃn] condição *f*

stir [stɜ:r] **1** *n* ***give the soup a ~*** dar uma mexida na sopa; ***cause a ~*** causar agitação **2** *v/t* ⟨*pret & pp* **stirred**⟩ mexer **3** *v/i* ⟨*pret & pp* **stirred**⟩ *sleeping person* mexer-se

♦**stir up** *v/t crowd* instigar; *bad memories* trazer à tona

stir-'crazy *adj fam* doido varrido

'stir-fry *v/t* ⟨*pret & pp* **stir-fried**⟩ refogar

stirring ['stɜːrɪŋ] *adj music, speech* emocionante

stitch [stɪʧ] **1** *n sewing*: ponto *m*; MED **~es** *pl* pontos *mpl*; ***be in ~es*** *laughing* morrer de rir; ***have a ~*** sentir uma pontada **2** *v/t sew* costurar

♦ **stitch up** *v/t wound* dar pontos, suturar

stitching ['stɪʧɪŋ] *(stitches)* costura *f*

stock [stɑːk] **1** *n (reserves)* reserva *f*; COM *store* estoque *m*; *animals* rebanho *m*; FIN ações *fpl*; *for soup etc* caldo *m*; ***in ~ / out of ~*** em estoque / em falta; ***take ~*** ponderar **2** *v/t* COM ter em estoque

♦ **stock up on** *v/t* estocar

'stockbroker corretor,a *m,f* de títulos **'stock cube** *beef* caldo *m* de carne em cubinhos **'stock exchange** bolsa *f* de valores **'stockholder** *Am* acionista *m/f*

stocking ['stɑːkɪŋ] meia-calça *f*

stockist ['stɑːkɪst] estoquista *m/f*

'stock market mercado *m* de ações **stockmarket 'crash** quebra *f* da bolsa **'stockpile 1** *n food, weapons*: estoque *m* **2** *v/t* estocar **'stockroom** depósito *m* **stock-'still** *adv* imóvel; ***stand ~*** ficar imóvel **'stocktaking** inventário *m*

stocky ['stɑːkɪ] *adj* atarracado

stodgy ['stɑːdʒɪ] *adj food* indigesto

stoical ['stoʊɪkl] *adj* estóico

stoicism ['stoʊɪsɪzm] estoicismo *m*

stole [stoʊl] *pret* → ***steal***

stolen ['stoʊlən] *pp* → ***steal***

stomach ['stʌmək] **1** *n insides* estômago *m*; *(abdomen)* barriga *f* **2** *v/t (tolerate)* suportar

'stomach-ache dor *f* de estômago

stone [stoʊn] *n* pedra *f*; *fruit*: caroço *m*

stoned [stoʊnd] *adj fam on drugs* drogado

stone-'deaf *adj* completamente surdo

'stonewall *v/i fam* subterfugir

stony ['stoʊnɪ] *adj ground, path* pedregoso

stood [stʊd] *pret & pp* → ***stand***

stool [stuːl] *seat* banqueta *f*

stoop[1] [stuːp] **1** *n* corcunda *f* **2** *v/i (bend down)* abaixar-se

stoop[2] [stuːp] *n Am (porch)* varanda *f*

stop [stɑːp] **1** *n train, bus*: parada *f*, *Port* paragem *f*; ***come to a ~*** parar; ***put a ~ to*** pôr fim a **2** *v/i* ⟨*pret & pp* ***stopped***⟩ *person, bus, train etc* parar; ***it has ~ped raining*** parou de chover **3** *v/t* ⟨*pret & pp* ***stopped***⟩ parar; *(put an end to)* pôr fim a; *(prevent)* impedir; ***~ talking immediately!*** pare de falar imediatamente; ***I ~ped her from leaving*** eu a impedi de ir; ***~ a check*** bloquear um cheque

♦ **stop by** *v/i (visit)* fazer uma visita rápida

♦ **stop off** *v/i* fazer uma parada

♦ **stop over** *v/i* fazer escala

♦ **stop up** *v/t sink* entupir

'stopgap solução *f* temporária **'stoplight** *(traffic light)* semáforo *m*; *(brake light)* luz *f* de freio, *Port* farol *m* de stop **'stopover** *n* parada *f*, *air travel*: escala *f*

stopper ['stɑːpər] *for basin, bottle* tampa *f*

stopping ['stɑːpɪŋ] ***no ~*** proibido parar

'stop sign placa *f* de pare

'stopwatch cronômetro *m*

storage ['stɔːrɪdʒ] armazenamento *m*; ***put sth in ~*** armazenar algo; ***be in ~*** estar guardado

'storage capacity COMPUT capacidade *f* de armazenamento

'storage space espaço *m* para guardar coisas

store [stɔːr] **1** *n Am* loja *f*; *(stock)* estoque *m*; *(storehouse)* depósito *m* **2** *v/t* guardar; COMPUT armazenar

'storefront *Am* fachada *f* da loja **'storehouse** *Am* armazém *m*, depósito *m* **'storekeeper** *Am* lojista *m/f* **'storeroom** armazém *m*

storey *Brit* → ***story***[2]

stork [stɔːrk] cegonha *f*

storm [stɔːrm] *n* tempestade *f*, temporal *m*

'storm drain *Am* valeta *f* **'storm warning** alerta *m* tempestade **'storm window** *Am* janela *f* externa

stormy *adj weather* tempestuoso; *relationship* tormentoso

story[1] ['stɔːrɪ] *(tale, account)* história *f*;

S

newspaper article artigo *m*; *fam* (*lie*) lorota *f*
story² ['stɔːrɪ] *Am building*: andar *m*
stout [staʊt] *adj person* corpulento; *boots* robusto; *defender* forte
stove [stoʊv] *cooking*: fogão *m*; *heating*: fogareiro *m*
stow [stoʊ] *v/t* guardar
♦ **stow away** *v/i* viajar clandestinamente
'stowaway *n* passageiro,-a *m,f* clandestino,-a
straight [streɪt] **1** *adj line*, *back*, *knees* reto; *hair* liso; (*honest*, *direct*) franco; (*not criminal*) honesto; *whiskey etc* puro; (*tidy*) em ordem; (*conservative*) correto; (*not homosexual*) heterossexual; ***be a ~ A student*** ser um estudante com excelente notas; ***keep a ~ face*** ficar com a cara brava **2** *adv* (*in a straight line*) diretamente; (*directly*, *immediately*) imediatamente; (*clearly*) claramente; ***stand up ~!*** fique reto!; ***look s.o. ~ in the eye*** olhar alguém diretamente nos olhos; ***go ~*** *fam criminal* rehabilitar-se; ***give it to me ~*** *fam* diga-me a verdade; ***~ ahead*** *be situated* adiante; *walk*, *drive* sempre em frente; *look* para a frente; ***carry ~ on*** *driver etc* seguir reto; ***~ off*** imediatamente; ***~ out*** diretamente; ***~ up*** *without ice* puro
straighten ['streɪtn] *v/t* endireitar
♦ **straighten out 1** *v/t situation* resolver; *fam person* endireitar **2** *v/i road* ficar reta
♦ **straighten up** *v/i* endireitar-se
'straightaway *adv* imediatamente
straight'forward *adj* (*honest*, *direct*) franco; (*simple*) simples
strain¹ [streɪn] **1** *n rope*, *heart*: tensão *f*, *engine*: carga *f*, *person*: estresse *m* **2** *v/t* (*injure*) prejudicar; *fig finances* apertar
strain² [streɪn] *v/t vegetables* escorrer; *oil*, *fat etc* filtrar
strain³ [streɪn] *n virus* cepa *f*
strained [streɪnd] *adj relations* tenso
strainer ['streɪnər] *vegetables etc*: peneira *f*
strait [streɪt] GEOG estreito *m*
straitlaced [streɪt'leɪst] *adj* puritano
strand¹ [strænd] *n hair*, *wool*: mecha *f*
strand² [strænd] *v/t* ***be ~ed*** ficar preso
strange [streɪndʒ] *adj* estranho
strangely ['streɪndʒlɪ] *adv* estranhamente; ***~ enough*** mesmo que pareça estranho
stranger ['streɪndʒər] (*person you don't know*) estranho,-a *m,f*; ***I'm a ~ here myself*** eu também não sou daqui
strangle ['stræŋgl] *v/t person* estrangular
strap [stræp] *n purse*, *brassiere*, *dress*: alça *f*, *watch*: pulseira *f*, *shoe*: correia *f*
♦ **strap in** *v/t* ⟨*pret & pp* ***strapped***⟩ pôr o cinto de segurança em
♦ **strap on** *v/t* pôr
strapless ['stræplɪs] *adj* sem alça
strategic [strə'tiːdʒɪk] *adj* estratégico
strategy ['strætədʒɪ] estratégia *f*
straw¹ [strɒː] palha *f*, ***that's the last ~!*** essa é a gota d'água
straw² [strɒː] *drink*: canudinho *m*
strawberry ['strɒːberɪ] morango *m*
stray [streɪ] **1** *adj animal* vadio; *bullet* perdido **2** *n dog* cão *m* vadio; *cat* gato *m* vadio **3** *v/i animal*, *child* perder-se; *fig eyes*, *thoughts* desviar-se
streak [striːk] **1** *n dirt*, *paint*: listra *f*, *hair*: mecha *f*, *fig nastiness etc*: veia *f* **2** *v/i* passar em disparada **3** *v/t* ***be ~ed with*** estar manchado de
streaky ['striːkɪ] *adj* manchado
stream [striːm] **1** *n* córrego *m*; *fig people*, *complaints*: chuva *f*, ***come on ~*** entrar em funcionamento **2** *v/i* afluir; *tears* derramar-se; ***sunlight ~ed into the room*** a luz do sol inundou a sala
streamer ['striːmər] serpentina *f*
streamline *v/t fig* racionalizar
'streamlined *adj car*, *plane* aerodinâmico; *fig organization* racionalizado
street [striːt] rua *f*
'streetcar *Am* bonde *m*, *Port* eléctrico *m* **'street kids** *npl* crianças *fpl* de rua **'streetlight** poste *m* (de luz) **'streetpeople** *npl* sem-teto *mpl* **'street value** *drugs*: preço *m* de rua **'streetwalker** *fam* prostituta *f* **'streetwise** *adj* que sabe se virar

strength [streŋθ] *physical, wind, current, currency etc*: força *f*; *fig (strong point)* ponto *m* forte; *emotion, friendship etc*: intensidade *f*
strengthen ['streŋθn] **1** *v/t muscles, currency* fortalecer; *bridge, foundations* reforçar; *bonds, relationship* consolidar **2** *v/i bonds, ties* consolidar-se; *currency* fortalecer-se
strenuous ['strenjʊəs] *adj* extenuante
strenuously ['strenjʊəslɪ] *adv deny* veementemente
stress [stres] **1** *n (emphasis)* ênfase *f*; *syllable*: acento *m* tônico; *(tension)* estresse *m*; ***be under ~*** estar estressado **2** *v/t (emphasize) syllable* acentuar; *importance etc* ressaltar; ***I must ~ that ...*** tenho que ressaltar que ...
stressed 'out [strest] *adj* estressado
stressful ['stresfl] *adj* estressante
stretch [stretʃ] **1** *n land, water*: trecho *m*; ***at a ~*** *(non-stop)* sem parar **2** *adj fabric* elástico **3** *v/t material, small income* esticar; *fam rules* flexibilizar; ***he ~ed out his hand*** ele estendeu a mão; ***a job that ~es me*** um trabalho que requere tudo de mim **4** *v/i to relax muscles* alongar-se; *to reach sth, fabric (give)* esticar-se; *(spread)* estender-se; *fabric (sag)* perder a forma; ***~ from X to Y*** estender-se de X até Y
stretcher ['stretʃər] maca *f*
strict [strɪkt] *adj person* rígido; *instructions, rules* estrito
strictly ['strɪktlɪ] *adv* com severidade; ***it is ~ forbidden*** é terminantemente proibido
strictness ['strɪktnəs] severidade *f*
stridden ['strɪdn] *pp* → ***stride***
stride [straɪd] **1** *n* passo *m* largo; ***take sth in one's ~*** encarar algo com tranqüilidade; ***make great ~s*** *fig* dar grandes passos **2** *v/i* ⟨*pret* ***strode***, *pp* ***stridden***⟩ andar rápido com passos largos
strident ['straɪdnt] *adj* estridente; *fig demands* estrondoso
strike [straɪk] **1** *n workers*: greve *f*; *baseball*: strike *m*; *oil*: descoberta *f*; ***be on ~*** estar em greve; ***go on ~*** entrar em greve **2** *v/i* ⟨*pret & pp* ***struck***⟩ *workers* fazer greve; *(attack)* atacar; *disaster* sobrevir; *clock* bater **3** *v/t* ⟨*pret & pp* ***struck***⟩ *(hit)* bater; *match* riscar; *idea, thought* ocorrer a; *oil* descobrir; ***she struck me as being ...*** ela me deu a impressão de ser ...
♦ **strike out** *v/t (delete)* riscar
'strikebreaker fura-greve *m/f*
striker ['straɪkər] grevista *m/f*; *soccer*: atacante *m*
striking ['straɪkɪŋ] *adj (marked)* impressionante; *(eye-catching)* deslumbrante
string [strɪŋ] *n (cord)* barbante *m*, *Port* cordel *m*; *violin, cello, tennis racket etc*: corda *f*; ***~s*** *pl musicians* cordas *fpl*; ***pull ~s*** usar de influência; ***a ~ of*** uma série de
♦ **string along** ⟨*pret & pp* ***strung***⟩ **1** *v/i fam* ir também **2** *v/t* ***string s.o. along*** *fam* enganar alguém
♦ **string up** *v/t fam* pendurar
stringed 'instrument [strɪŋd] instrumento *m* de corda
stringent ['strɪndʒnt] *adj* severo
'string player instrumentista *m/f* de cordas
strip [strɪp] **1** *n land*: faixa *f*, *cloth*: tira *f*, *(comic strip)* tira *f* cômica **2** *v/t* ⟨*pret & pp* ***stripped***⟩ *(remove)* tirar; *(undress)* despir; ***~ s.o. of sth*** despojar algo de alguém **3** *v/i* ⟨*pret & pp* ***stripped***⟩ *(undress)* despir-se; *stripper* fazer striptease
'strip club clube *m* de striptease
stripe [straɪp] listra *f*
striped [straɪpt] *adj* listrado
'strip joint *fam* clube *m* de striptease
'strip mall *Am rua comercial fora da cidade*
stripper ['strɪpər] stripper *m/f*
'strip show show *m* de striptease
'striptease striptease *m*
strive [straɪv] *v/i* ⟨*pret* ***strove***, *pp* ***striven***⟩ ***~ to do sth*** esforçar-se para fazer algo; ***~ for*** lutar por
striven ['strɪvn] *pp* → ***strive***
strobe, strobe light luz *f* estroboscópica
strode [stroʊd] *pret* → ***stride***
stroke [stroʊk] **1** *n* MED derrame *m*; *writing*: traço *m*; *painting*: pincelada

f; *swimming*: estilo *m*; **~ of luck** golpe *m* de sorte; **she never does a ~** (**of work**) ela nunca faz nada **2** *v/t* acariciar
stroll [stroʊl] **1** *n* passeio *m* **2** *v/i* caminhar
stroller ['stroʊlər] *Am* carrinho *m* de bebê
strong [strɑːŋ] *adj person, candidate, wind, drink, taste, smell, currency* forte; *structure* resistente; *support, supporter* sólido; *views, objections* concreto; **~ language** linguagem *f* grosseira
'stronghold *fig* fortaleza *f*
strongly ['strɑːŋlɪ] *adv deny* categoricamente; *advise* fortemente; **she feels very ~ about it** ela tem uma opinião muito forte a respeito disso
strong-minded [strɑːŋ'maɪndɪd] *adj* firme **'strong point** (ponto *m*) forte *m* **'strongroom** caixa-forte *f*
strong-willed [strɑːŋ'wɪld] *adj* **be ~** ter força de vontade
strove [stroʊv] *pret* → **strive**
struck [strʌk] *pret & pp* → **strike**
structural ['strʌktʃərl] *adj damage, fault, problems, steel* estrutural
structure ['strʌktʃər] **1** *n something built* edificação *f*; *novel, society etc*: estrutura *f* **2** *v/t* estruturar
struggle ['strʌgl] **1** *n* (*fight, hard time*) luta *f* **2** *v/i with a person* brigar; (*have a hard time*) lutar
strum [strʌm] *v/t* ⟨*pret & pp* **strummed**⟩ arranhar
strung [strʌŋ] *pret & pp* → **string**
strut [strʌt] *v/i* ⟨*pret & pp* **strutted**⟩ pavonear
stub [stʌb] **1** *n cigarette*: ponta *f*; *check, ticket*: canhoto *m* **2** *v/t* ⟨*pret & pp* **stubbed**⟩ **~ one's toe** bater o dedão do pé
♦ **stub out** *v/t* apagar
stubble ['stʌbl] *on man's face* barba *f* por fazer
stubborn ['stʌbərn] *adj* teimoso; *defense* obstinado
stubby ['stʌbɪ] *adj* curto e grosso
stuck[1] [stʌk] *pret & pp* → **stick**[2]
stuck[2] [stʌk] *adj fam* grudado; **be ~ on s.o.** estar fixado em alguém
stuck-'up *adj fam* esnobe
student ['stuːdnt] *high school*: aluno,-a *m,f*; *college, university*: estudante *m/f*
student 'nurse estudante *m/f* de enfermaria
student 'teacher estudante *m/f* de magistério
studio ['stuːdɪoʊ] *artist, sculptor, film, TV*: estúdio *m*
studious ['stuːdɪəs] *adj* estudioso
study ['stʌdɪ] **1** *n room* escritório *m*; *learning, investigation* estudo *m* **2** *v/t & v/i* ⟨*pret & pp* **studied**⟩ estudar
stuff [stʌf] **1** *n* coisas *fpl* **2** *v/t turkey* rechear; **~ sth into sth** enfiar algo em algo
stuffed 'toy [stʌft] brinquedo *m* de pelúcia
stuffing ['stʌfɪŋ] *turkey*: recheio *m*; *chair, teddy bear*: enchimento *m*
stuffy ['stʌfɪ] *adj room* abafado; *person* enfadonho
stumble ['stʌmbl] *v/i* tropeçar
♦ **stumble across** *v/t* deparar-se com
♦ **stumble over** *v/t also words* tropeçar em
stumbling-block ['stʌmblɪŋ] empecilho *m*
stump [stʌmp] **1** *n tree*: toco *m* **2** *v/t question, questioner* desconcertar; **that question really has me ~ed** aquela pergunta me deixou realmente desnorteado
♦ **stump up** *v/t fam* arranjar
stun [stʌn] *v/t* ⟨*pret & pp* **stunned**⟩ *blow* deixar sem sentidos; *news* ficar em estado de choque
stung [stʌŋ] *pret & pp* → **sting**
stunk [stʌŋk] *pp* → **stink**
stunning ['stʌnɪŋ] *adj* (*amazing*) espantoso; (*very beautiful*) maravilhoso
stunt [stʌnt] *n publicity*: truque *m*; *movie*: cena *f* arriscada
'stuntman *in movie* dublê *m/f*
stupefy ['stuːpɪfaɪ] *v/t* ⟨*pret & pp* **stupefied**⟩ estupefazer
stupendous [stuː'pendəs] *adj* estupendo
stupid ['stuːpɪd] *adj* estúpido
stupidity [stuː'pɪdətɪ] estupidez *f*
stupor ['stuːpər] estupor *m*

sturdy ['stɜːrdɪ] *adj* robusto
stutter ['stʌtər] *v/i* gaguejar
sty [staɪ] *pig*: chiqueiro *m*
style [staɪl] *n* estilo *m*; (*fashion*) moda *f*; ***go out of ~*** sair de moda
stylish ['staɪlɪʃ] *adj* elegante
stylist ['staɪlɪst] (*hair stylist, interior designer*) desenhador,a *m,f*
subcommittee ['sʌbkəmɪtɪ] subcomitê *m*
subcompact, **subcompact car** [sʌb'kɑːmpakt] *Am* minicarro *m*
subconscious [sʌb'kɑːnʃəs] *adj* subconsciente; ***the ~*** (***mind***) o subconsciente
subconsciously [sʌb'kɑːnʃəslɪ] *adv* subconscientemente
subcontract [sʌbkən'trakt] *v/t* subcontratar
subdivide [sʌbdɪ'vaɪd] *v/t* subdividir
subdue [səb'duː] *v/t rebellion, mob* subjugar
subheading ['sʌbhedɪŋ] subtítulo *m*
subhuman [sʌb'hjuːmən] *adj* desumano
subject ['sʌbdʒɪkt] **1** *n country*: cidadão *m*, cidadã *f*; (*topic*) tema *m*; (*branch of learning*) matéria *f*; GRAM sujeito *m*; ***change the ~*** mudar de tema **2** *adj* ***be ~ to*** *liable* ser propenso a; ***~ to availability*** segundo disponibilidade **3** [səb'dʒekt] *v/t* sujeitar
subjective [səb'dʒektɪv] *adj* subjetivo
subjunctive [səb'dʒʌŋktɪv] *n* GRAM subjuntivo *m*
sublet ['sʌblet] *v/t* ⟨*pret & pp* ***sublet***⟩ sublocar
subma'chine gun submetralhadora *f*
submarine ['sʌbməriːn] submarino *m*
submerge [səb'mɜːrdʒ] *v/t & v/i* submergir
submission [səb'mɪʃn] (*surrender*) submissão *f*; *to committee etc* proposta *f*
submissive [səb'mɪsɪv] *adj* submisso
submit [səb'mɪt] ⟨*pret & pp* ***submitted***⟩ **1** *v/t plan, proposal* apresentar **2** *v/i* render-se
subordinate [sə'bɔːrdɪneɪt] **1** *adj employee, position* subordinado **2** *n* subordinado,-a *m,f*
subpoena [sə'piːnə] **1** *n* intimação *f* judicial **2** *v/t person* intimar
♦ **subscribe to** [səb'skraɪb] *v/t magazine etc* assinar; *theory* apoiar
subscriber [səb'skraɪbər] *magazine*: assinante *m/f*
subscription [səb'skrɪpʃn] assinatura *f*
subsequent ['sʌbsɪkwənt] *adj* subseqüente
subsequently ['sʌbsɪkwəntlɪ] *adv* subseqüentemente
subside [səb'saɪd] *v/i flood waters* baixar; *high winds* acalmar-se; *building* afundar; *fears, panic* diminuir
subsidiary [səb'sɪdɪrɪ] *n* subsidiário,-a *m,f*
subsidize ['sʌbsɪdaɪz] *v/t* subsidiar
subsidy ['sʌbsɪdɪ] subsídio *m*
♦ **subsist on** [sʌb'sɪst] *v/t* subsistir a base de
subsistence farmer [səb'sɪstəns] agricultor *m* de subsistência
sub'sistence level nível *m* de subsistência
substance ['sʌbstəns] (*matter*) substância *f*
substandard [sʌb'stændərd] *adj* de qualidade inferior
substantially [səb'stænʃlɪ] *adv* (*considerably*) consideravelmente; (*in essence*) substancialmente
substantiate [səb'stænʃɪeɪt] *v/t* confirmar
substantive [səb'stæntɪv] *adj* significativo
substitute ['sʌbstɪtuːt] **1** *n* substituto,-a *m,f*; SPORT reserva *m/f* **2** *v/t* substituir; ***~ X for Y*** substituir Y por X **3** *v/i* ***~ for s.o.*** substituir por alguém
substitution [sʌbstɪ'tuːʃn] substituição *f*; ***make a ~*** SPORT fazer uma substituição
subtitle ['sʌbtaɪtl] *n* legenda *f*
subtle ['sʌtl] *adj* sutil
subtlety ['sʌtltɪ] sutileza *f*
subtract [səb'trækt] *v/t* subtrair
suburb ['sʌbɜːrb] subúrbio *m*; ***the ~s*** os subúrbios
suburban [sə'bɜːrbən] *adj* suburbano
subversive [səb'vɜːrsɪv] **1** *adj* subversivo **2** *n* subversivo,-a *m,f*

subway ['sʌbweɪ] *Am* metrô *m*, *Port* metro *m*
sub'zero *adj* abaixo de zero
succeed [sək'siːd] **1** *v/i* ter sucesso; **~ *in doing sth*** conseguir fazer algo **2** *v/t to throne*, (*come after*) suceder a
succeeding [sək'siːdɪŋ] *adj* seguinte
success [sək'ses] sucesso *m*; ***be a ~*** ser um sucesso
successful [sək'sesfl] *adj* bem-sucedido; ***be ~ in doing sth*** conseguir fazer algo
successfully [sək'sesflɪ] *adv* com êxito
succession [sək'seʃn] (*sequence*) série *f*; *throne*: sucessão *f*; ***in ~*** em sucessão
successive [sək'sesɪv] *adj* sucessivo
successor [sək'sesər] sucessor,a *m,f*
succinct [sək'sɪŋkt] *adj* sucinto
succulent ['sʌkjʊlənt] *adj meat*, *fruit* suculento
succumb [sə'kʌm] *v/i* (*give in*) sucumbir; **~ *to temptation*** sucumbir à tentação
such [sʌtʃ] **1** *adj* (*of that kind*) tal; **~ *a*** (*so much of a*) tamanho; ***it was ~ a ~*** foi uma tamanha surpresa; **~ *as*** como; ***there is no ~ word*** não existe tal palavra **2** *adv* tão; **~ *an easy question*** uma pergunta tão fácil; ***that's not ~ a good idea*** essa não é uma idéia tão boa; ***as ~*** como tal
suck [sʌk] **1** *v/t candy etc* chupar; **~ *one's thumb*** chupar o dedo **2** *v/i* ***it ~s*** *fam* é um saco
♦**suck up 1** *v/t* sugar **2** *v/i* ***suck up to s.o.*** *fam* puxar o saco de alguém
sucker ['sʌkər] *fam person* tonto,-a *m,f*; *Am fam* (*lollipop*) pirulito *m*, *Port* chupa-chupa *m*
suction ['sʌkʃn] sucção *f*
sudden ['sʌdn] *adj* repentino; ***all of a ~*** de repente
suddenly ['sʌdnlɪ] *adv* de repente
suds [sʌdz] *pl* (*soap suds*) espuma *f*
sue [suː] *v/t* processar
suede [swed] *n* camurça *f*
suffer ['sʌfər] *v/i & v/t* (*be in great pain*), *loss*, *setback* sofrer; (*deteriorate*) piorar; ***be ~ing from*** estar sofrendo de
suffering ['sʌfərɪŋ] *n* sofrimento *m*
sufficient [sə'fɪʃnt] *adj* suficiente
sufficiently [sə'fɪʃntlɪ] *adv* suficientemente
suffocate ['sʌfəkeɪt] *v/i & v/t* sufocar
suffocation [sʌfə'keɪʃn] asfixia *f*
sugar ['ʃʊgər] **1** *n* açúcar *m* **2** *v/t* adoçar *com açúcar*
'sugar bowl açucareiro *m*
suggest [sə'dʒest] *v/t* sugerir; ***I ~ that we stop now*** sugiro que paremos agora
suggestion [sə'dʒestʃən] sugestão *f*
suicide ['suːɪsaɪd] suicídio *m*; ***commit ~*** cometer suicídio
'suicide bomber terrorista *m/f* suicida
'suicide pact pacto *m* de suicídio
suit [suːt] **1** *n* terno *m*, *Port* fato *m*; *cards*: naipe *m* **2** *v/t clothes*, *color* cair bem; ***red ~s you*** vermelho combina contigo; **~ *yourself!*** *fam* faça como quiser; ***be ~ed for sth*** ser feito para algo
suitable ['suːtəbl] *adj* adequado
suitably ['suːtəblɪ] *adv* adequadamente; ***they were ~ impressed*** eles estavam devidamente impressionados
'suitcase mala *f*
suite [swiːt] *rooms*, *also* MUS suíte *f*; *furniture*: jogo *m* de sofá
sulfur ['sʌlfər] *Am* enxofre *m*
sulfuric acid [sʌl'fjuːrɪk] *Am* ácido *m* sulfúrico
sulk [sʌlk] *v/i* estar de mau humor
sulky ['sʌlkɪ] *adj* emburrado
sullen ['sʌlən] *adj* mal-humorado
sulphur *Brit* → ***sulfur***
sultry ['sʌltrɪ] *adj climate* sufocante; *sexually* sensual
sum [sʌm] (*total*) soma *f*, (*amount*) montante *m*; *arithmetic*: cálculo *m*; ***a large ~ of money*** uma grande quantia de dinheiro; **~ *insured*** valor *m* assegurado; ***the ~ total of his efforts*** a soma total dos seus esforços
♦**sum up** ⟨*pret & pp* ***summed***⟩ **1** *v/t* (*summarize*) resumir; (*assess*) estimar **2** *v/i* LAW recapitular
summarize ['sʌməraɪz] *v/t* resumir
summary ['sʌmərɪ] *n* resumo *m*

S

summer ['sʌmər] verão *m*
summit ['sʌmɪt] *mountain*: cume *m*; POL conferência *f* cimeira
'summit meeting → ***summit***
summon ['sʌmən] *v/t staff, ministers* reunir; *meeting* convocar
♦ **summon up** *v/t strength* empenhar
summons ['sʌmənz] *nsg* LAW intimação *f* judicial
sump [sʌmp] *for oil* cárter *m* (de óleo)
sun [sʌn] sol *m*; ***in the ~*** no sol; ***out of the ~*** fora do sol; ***he has had too much ~*** ele tomou muito sol
'sunbathe *v/i* tomar sol **'sunbed** cama *f* de bronzeamento artificial **'sunblock** bloqueador *m* solar **'sunburn** queimadura *f* de sol **'sunburnt** *adj* queimado de sol
Sunday ['sʌndeɪ] domingo *m*
'sundial relógio *m* de sol
sundries ['sʌndrɪz] *npl* diversos *mpl*
sung [sʌŋ] *pp* → ***sing***
'sunglasses *npl* óculos *mpl* de sol
sunk [sʌŋk] *pp* → ***sink***
sunken ['sʌnkn] *adj cheeks* afundado
sunny ['sʌnɪ] *adj day* ensolarado; *disposition* radiante; ***it's ~*** está fazendo sol
'sunrise nascer *m* do sol **'sunroof** *car* teto *m* solar **'sunset** pôr *m* do sol **'sunshade** *handheld* sombrinha *f*; *over table* guarda-sol *m* **'sunshine** luz *f* do sol **'sunstroke** insolação *f* **'suntan** bronzeado *m*; ***get a ~*** bronzear-se
super ['suːpər] **1** *adj fam* ótimo **2** *n Am* (*janitor*) zelador,a *m,f*
superb [suː'pɜːrb] *adj* maravilhoso
superficial [suːpər'fɪʃl] *adj* superficial
superfluous [sʊ'pɜːrfluəs] *adj* supérfluo
super'human *adj efforts* sobre-humano
superintendent [suːpərɪn'tendənt] *Am apartment block*: zelador,a *m,f*; *Brit police*: chefe *m* de polícia
superior [suː'pɪrɪər] **1** *adj* (*better*) superior; *pej attitude* arrogante **2** *n in organization* superior *m*
superlative [suː'pɜːrlətɪv] **1** *adj superb* excelente **2** *n* GRAM superlativo *m*
'supermarket supermercado *m*
'supermodel top model *m/f*, supermodelo *m/f*
super'natural 1 *adj powers* sobrenatural **2** *n* ***the ~*** forças *fpl* sobrenaturais
'superpower POL superpotência *f*
supersonic [suːpər'sɑːnɪk] *adj aircraft* supersônico
superstition [suːpər'stɪʃn] superstição *f*
superstitious [suːpər'stɪʃəs] *adj person* supersticioso
supervise ['suːpərvaɪz] *v/t* supervisionar
supervisor ['suːpərvaɪzər] *at work* supervisor,a *m,f*
supper ['sʌpər] jantar *m*
supple ['sʌpl] *adj person* ágil; *limbs, material* flexivel
supplement ['sʌplɪmənt] (*extra payment*) sobretaxa *f*
supplier [sə'plaɪr] COM fornecedor *m*
supply [sə'plaɪ] **1** *n* fornecimento *m*; ***~ and demand*** oferta e procura; ***supplies*** *pl* suprimentos *mpl* **2** *v/t* ⟨*pret & pp* ***supplied***⟩ *goods* fornecer; ***~ s.o. with sth*** abastecer alguém com algo
support [sə'pɔːrt] **1** *n for structure* suporte *m*; (*backing*) apoio *m* **2** *v/t building, structure* sustentar; *financially* manter; (*back*) apoiar
supporter [sə'pɔːrtər] partidário,-a *m,f*; *football team etc*: torcedor,a *m,f*
supportive [sə'pɔːrtɪv] *adj* apoiador
suppose [sə'poʊz] *v/t* (*imagine*) supor; ***I ~ so*** suponho que sim; ***be ~d to …*** (*be meant to*) estar destinado a …; (*be said to be*) ser supostamente …; ***you are not ~d to …*** (*not allowed to*) você não deve …
supposedly [sə'poʊzɪdlɪ] *adv* supostamente
suppository [sə'pɑːzɪtɔːrɪ] MED supositório *m*
suppress [sə'pres] *v/t rebellion etc* reprimir
suppression [sə'preʃn] repressão *f*
supremacy [suː'preməsɪ] supremacia *f*
supreme [suː'priːm] *adj* supremo;

commander superior
surcharge ['sɜːrtʃɑːrdʒ] *n* sobrecarga *f*
sure [ʃʊr] **1** *adj* claro, seguro, certo; ***I'm ~*** tenho certeza; ***I'm not ~*** não tenho certeza; ***be ~ about sth*** ter certeza de algo; ***make ~ that …*** assegurar-se de que … **2** *adv* obviamente; ***~ enough*** efetivamente; ***it is ~ hot today*** *Am fam* hoje está fazendo realmente muito calor; ***~!*** *fam* é claro (que sim)!
surely ['ʃʊrlɪ] *adv* certamente; (*gladly*) com prazer
surety ['ʃʊrətɪ] *loan*: fiança *f*
surf [sɜːrf] **1** *n sea*: arrebentação *f* **2** *v/t* ***~ the Net*** navegar na Net
surface ['sɜːrfɪs] **1** *n table, object, water*: superfície *f*; ***on the ~*** *fig* à primeira vista **2** *v/i swimmer, submarine* subir à superfície; (*appear*) aparecer
'surface mail correio *m* terrestre
'surfboard prancha *f* de surfe
surfer ['sɜːrfər] *on sea* surfista *m/f*
surfing ['sɜːrfɪŋ] surfar; ***go ~*** ir surfar
surge [sɜːrdʒ] *n electric current*: sobrecarga *f*; *demand, growth etc*: aumento *m* repentino
♦**surge forward** *v/i crowd* avançar empurrando
surgeon ['sɜːrdʒən] cirurgião *m*, cirurgiã *f*
surgery ['sɜːrdʒərɪ] cirurgia *f*; ***undergo ~*** passar por uma cirurgia
surgical ['sɜːrdʒɪkl] *adj* cirúrgico
surgically ['sɜːrdʒɪklɪ] *adv* através de cirurgia
surly ['sɜːrlɪ] *adj* grosseiro
surmount [sər'maʊnt] *v/t difficulties* superar
surname ['sɜːrneɪm] sobrenome *m*, *Port* apelido *m*
surpass [sər'pæs] *v/t* superar
surplus ['sɜːrpləs] **1** *n* excedente *m* **2** *adj* excedente
surprise [sər'praɪz] **1** *n* surpresa *f*; ***it'll come as no ~ to me to hear that …*** não me surpreenderia ouvir que … **2** *v/t* surpreender; ***be / look ~d*** estar / parecer surpreso
surprising [sər'praɪzɪŋ] *adj* surpreendente
surprisingly [sər'praɪzɪŋlɪ] *adv* surpreendentemente
surrender [sə'rendər] **1** *v/i army* capitular **2** *v/t* (*hand in*) *weapons etc* entregar **3** *n* capitulação *f*; (*handing in*) entrega *f*
surrogate 'mother ['sʌrəgət] mãe *f* de aluguel, *Port* mãe *f* de aluguer
surround [sə'raʊnd] **1** *v/t* cercar; ***be ~ed by …*** estar rodeado de … **2** *n picture*: moldura *f*
surrounding [sə'raʊndɪŋ] *adj* circundante
surroundings [sə'raʊndɪŋz] *npl* imediações *fpl*
survey 1 ['sɜːrveɪ] *n modern literature etc*: estudo *m*; *building*: inspeção *f* **2** [sər'veɪ] *v/t* (*look at*) contemplar; *building* inspecionar
surveyor [sɜːr'veɪr] perito *m*
survival [sər'vaɪvl] sobrevivência *f*
survive [sər'vaɪv] **1** *v/i species, patient* sobreviver; ***how are you? – I'm surviving*** como vai? – vou levando; ***his two surviving daughters*** suas duas filhas sobreviventes **2** *v/t accident, operation, also* (*outlive*) sobreviver a
survivor [sər'vaɪvər] sobrevivente *m/f*; ***he's a ~*** *fig* é duro na queda
susceptible [sə'septəbl] *adj emotionally* suscetível; ***be ~ to the cold / heat*** ser sensível ao frio / calor
suspect 1 ['sʌspekt] *n* suspeito,-a *m,f* **2** [sə'spekt] *v/t person* suspeitar; (*suppose*) supor
suspected [sə'spektɪd] *adj murderer* suspeito; *cause etc* suposto
suspend [sə'spend] *v/t* (*hang*) pendurar; *from office, duties* suspender
suspenders [sə'spendərz] *npl Am for pants* liga *f*
suspense [sə'spens] suspense *m*
suspension [sə'spenʃn] *in vehicle, from duty* suspensão *f*
sus'pension bridge ponte *f* pênsil
suspicion [sə'spɪʃn] suspeita *f*
suspicious [sə'spɪʃəs] *adj* (*causing suspicion*) suspeito; (*feeling suspicion*) desconfiado; ***be ~ of*** suspeitar de
suspiciously [sə'spɪʃəslɪ] *adv act* de maneira suspeita; *say* com desconfiança

sustain [sə'steɪn] *v/t* sustentar
sustainable [sə'steɪnəbl] *adj* sustentável
SUV [esjuː'viː] *abbr* (*of* ***sports utility vehicle***) SUV *m*
swab [swɑːb] lavar
swagger ['swægər] *n* fanfarrice *f*
swallow[1] ['swɑːloʊ] *v/t & v/i liquid, food* engolir
swallow[2] ['swɑːloʊ] *n bird* andorinha *f*
swam [swæm] *pret* → ***swim***
swamp [swɑːmp] **1** *n* pântano *m* **2** *v/t* ***be ~ed with*** ser inundado por
swampy ['swɑːmpɪ] *adj ground* pantanoso
swan [swɑːn] cisne *m*
swap [swɑːp] ⟨*pret & pp* ***swapped***⟩ **1** *v/t* ***~ sth for sth*** trocar algo por algo **2** *v/i* trocar
swarm [swɔːrm] **1** *n bees, tourists*: enxame *m* **2** *v/i ants etc* fervilhar; ***the town was ~ing with …*** a cidade estava abarrotada de …
swarthy ['swɔːrðɪ] *adj face, complexion* escuro
swat [swɑːt] *v/t* ⟨*pret & pp* ***swatted***⟩ *insect, fly* matar
sway [sweɪ] **1** *n* (*influence, power*) domínio *m* **2** *v/i* balançar
swear [swer] ⟨*pret* ***swore***, *pp* ***sworn***⟩ **1** *v/i* (*use swearword*) xingar; LAW, *on oath* prestar juramento; ***~ at s.o.*** xingar alguém **2** *v/t* (*promise*) prometer
♦**swear in** *v/t witnesses etc* ajuramentar
'**swearword** palavrão *m*
sweat [swet] **1** *n* suor *m*; ***covered in ~*** coberto de suor **2** *v/i* suar
'**sweat band** faixa *f* anti-suor
sweater ['swetər] suéter *m*, *Port* camisola *f*
sweats [swets] *npl Am* agasalho *m* esportivo, *Port* fato *m* de treino
'**sweatshirt** blusa *f* de moletom
sweaty ['swetɪ] *adj hands, smell* suado
Swede [swiːd] sueco,-a *m,f*
Sweden ['swiːdn] Suécia *f*
Swedish ['swiːdɪʃ] **1** *adj* sueco **2** *n* sueco *m*
sweep [swiːp] **1** *v/t* ⟨*pret & pp* ***swept***⟩ *floor, leaves* varrer **2** *n* (*long curve*) curva *f*
♦**sweep up** *v/t mess, crumbs* varrer
sweeping ['swiːpɪŋ] *adj generalization, statement* geral; *changes* radical
sweet [swiːt] *adj taste, tea* doce; *fam* (*cute*) engraçadinho; *fam* (*kind*) amável
sweet and 'sour *adj* agridoce
'**sweetcorn** milho *m* doce
sweeten ['swiːtn] *v/t drink, food* adoçar
sweetener ['swiːtnər] adoçante *m*
'**sweetheart** querido,-a *m,f*
swell [swel] **1** *v/i* ⟨*pret* ***swelled***, *pp* ***swollen***⟩ *wound, limb* inchar **2** *adj fam* (*good*) ótimo **3** *n sea*: marulho *m*
swelling ['swelɪŋ] *n* MED inchaço *m*
sweltering ['sweltərɪŋ] *adj heat, day* sufocante
swept [swept] *pret & pp* → ***sweep***
swerve [swɜːrv] *v/i driver, car* desviar
swift [swɪft] *adj* rápido
swim [swɪm] **1** *v/i* ⟨*pret* ***swam***, *pp* ***swum***⟩ nadar; ***go ~ming*** ir nadar; ***my head is ~ming*** minha cabeça está girando **2** *n* ***go for a ~*** ir nadar
swimmer ['swɪmər] nadador,a *m,f*
swimming ['swɪmɪŋ] natação *f*
swimming baths → ***swimming pool*** '**swimming costume** traje *m* de natação '**swimming pool** piscina *f*
'**swimsuit** maiô *m*, *Port* fato *m* de banho
swindle ['swɪndl] **1** *n* embuste *m* **2** *v/t* trapacear; ***~ s.o. out of sth*** roubar numa trapaça algo de alguém
swine [swaɪn] *fam person* suíno *m*
'**swine flu** gripe *f* suína
swing [swɪŋ] **1** *n pendulum, child*: balanço *m*; ***~ to the Democrats*** virada *f* em favor dos democratas **2** *v/t & v/i* ⟨*pret & pp* ***swung***⟩ balançar; (*turn*) virar; *public opinion etc* mudar
'**swing-door** porta *f* de vaivém
swipe [swaɪp] *v/t credit card* passar
Swiss [swɪs] **1** *adj* suíço **2** *n person* suíço,-a *m,f*; ***the ~*** os suíços
switch [swɪʧ] **1** *n light*: interruptor *m*; (*change*) mudança *f* **2** *v/t* (*change*) trocar **3** *v/i* (*change*) mudar
♦**switch off** *v/t lights, engine, PC, TV* desligar

S

♦ **switch on** *v/t lights, engine, PC, TV* ligar
'switchboard painél *m* de ligações
'switchover *n* mudança *f*
Switzerland ['swɪtsərlənd] Suíça *f*
swivel ['swɪvl] *v/i chair, monitor* girar
swollen ['swoʊlən] *adj* inchado
swoop [swu:p] *v/i bird* descer a pique
♦ **swoop down on** *v/t prey* mergulhar em vôo picado
♦ **swoop on** *v/t police etc* fazer uma batida em
sword [sɔ:rd] espada *f*
swore [swɔ:r] *pret* → ***swear***
sworn [swɔ:rn] *pp* → ***swear***
swum [swʌm] *pp* → ***swim***
swung [swʌŋ] *pret & pp* → ***swing***
sycamore ['sɪkəmɔ:r] sicômoro *m*
syllable ['sɪləbl] sílaba *f*
syllabus ['sɪləbəs] currículo *m*
symbol ['sɪmbəl] símbolo *m*
symbolic [sɪm'bɑ:lɪk] *adj* simbólico
symbolism ['sɪmbəlɪzm] simbolismo *m*
symbolist ['sɪmbəlɪst] simbolista *m/f*
symbolize ['sɪmbəlaɪz] *v/t* simbolizar
symmetric [sɪ'metrɪk] *adj* simétrico
symmetry ['sɪmətrɪ] simetria *f*
sympathetic [sɪmpə'θetɪk] *adj* (*showing pity*) compassivo; (*understanding*) compreensivo; ***be ~ toward a person / an idea*** simpatizar com uma pessoa / idéia
♦ **sympathize with** ['sɪmpəθaɪz] *v/t person, views* condoer-se de
sympathizer ['sɪmpəθaɪzər] POL simpatizante *m/f*
sympathy ['sɪmpəθɪ] (*pity*) pena *f*; (*understanding*) compreensão *f*; ***don't expect any ~ from me!*** não espere nenhuma compaixão de minha parte
symphony ['sɪmfənɪ] sinfonia *f*
'symphony orchestra orquestra *f* sinfônica
symptom ['sɪmptəm] MED, *also fig* sintoma *m*
symptomatic [sɪmptə'mætɪk] *adj* ***be ~ of*** *fig* ser sintomático de
synchronize ['sɪŋkrənaɪz] *v/t watches, operations* sincronizar
synonym ['sɪnənɪm] sinônimo *m*
synonymous [sɪ'nɑ:nɪməs] *adj* sinônimo; ***be ~ with*** *fig* ser sinônimo de
syntax ['sɪntæks] sintaxe *f*
synthesizer ['sɪnθəsaɪzər] MUS sintetizador *m*
synthetic [sɪn'θetɪk] *adj* sintético
syphilis ['sɪfɪlɪs] sífilis *f*
Syria ['sɪrɪə] Síria *f*
Syrian ['sɪrɪən] **1** *adj* sírio **2** *n* sírio,-a *m,f*
syringe [sɪ'rɪndʒ] seringa *f*
syrup ['sɪrəp] xarope *m*
system ['sɪstəm] (*method*) método *m*; (*orderliness*) ordem *f*; *computer* sistema *m*; ***the fuel injection / digestive ~*** o sistema de injeção de combustível / digestivo
systematic [sɪstə'mætɪk] *adj* sistemático
systematically [sɪstə'mætɪklɪ] *adv study, destroy* sistematicamente
systems 'analyst ['sɪstəmz] COMPUT analista *m/f* de sistemas

T

tab [tæb] *n for pulling* lingüeta *f*; *in text* tabulador *m*
table ['teɪbl] *n* mesa *f*; *figures*: tabela *f*
'tablecloth toalha *f* de mesa **'table lamp** luminária *f* de mesa, *Port* candeeiro *m* **table of 'contents** índice *m* **'tablespoon** colher *f* de sopa
tablet ['tæblɪt] MED comprimido *m*
'table tennis tênis *m* de mesa

tabloid ['tæblɔɪd] *n newspaper* tablóide *m*
taboo [tə'buː] *adj* tabu
tacit ['tæsɪt] *adj* tácito
taciturn ['tæsɪtɜːrn] *adj* calado
tack [tæk] **1** *n nail* tachinha *f* **2** *v/t sew* alinhavar **3** *v/i yacht* mudar de direção
tackle ['tækl] **1** *n* (*equipment*) equipamento *m*; SPORT investida *f*; ***sliding ~*** carrinho *m* **2** *v/t* SPORT dar uma investida; *problem* abordar; *intruder* enfrentar
tacky ['tækɪ] *adj paint, glue* pegajoso; *fam* (*cheap, poor quality*) vagabundo; *behavior* insolente
tact [tækt] tato *m*
tactful ['tæktfʊl] *adj* diplomático
tactfully ['tæktflɪ] *adv* diplomaticamente
tactical ['tæktɪkl] *adj* tático
tactics ['tæktɪks] *npl* tática *f*
tactless ['tæktlɪs] *adj person, remark* indiscreto
tadpole ['tædpoʊl] girino *m*
taffy ['tæfɪ] *Am* bala *f* de caramelo
tag [tæg] (*label*) etiqueta *f*
♦ **tag along** *v/i* ⟨*pret & pp* ***tagged***⟩ ir junto
tail [teɪl] *n* rabo *m*
'tailback *Brit* congestionamento *m*
'tail light lanterna *f* traseira
tailor ['teɪlər] alfaiate *m*
'tailor-made *adj suit, solution* sob medida
'tail pipe *car* tubo *m* de escape
'tailwind vento *m* em popa
tainted ['teɪntɪd] *adj food* contaminado; *reputation, atmosphere* estragado
Taiwan [taɪ'wɑn] Taiwan *m*
Taiwanese [taɪwɑn'iːz] **1** *adj* taiwanês,-esa **2** *n* taiwanês,-esa *m,f*; *dialect* taiwanês *m*

take [teɪk] *v/t* ⟨*pret* ***took***, *pp* ***taken***⟩ (*remove*), *s.o.'s temperature* tirar; (*grab*) pegar; *drink* tomar; (*steal*) roubar; (*transport, accompany*) levar; (*accept*) *money, gift, credit cards* aceitar; (*study*) *maths, French, exam, degree* fazer; *photograph* fazer; *stroll* dar; (*endure*) agüentar; (*require*) requerer; ***how long does it ~?*** quanto tempo demora?; ***I'll ~ it*** *shopping*: vou levar este; ***~ a shower*** tomar um banho
♦ **take after** *v/t* puxar a
♦ **take apart** *v/t dismantle* desmontar; *fam* (*criticize*) acabar com; *fam* (*reprimand*) dar uma bronca; *fam in physical fight* massacrar
♦ **take away** *v/t pain*, (*remove*) *object*, MATH tirar; ***take sth away from s.o.*** tirar algo de alguém
♦ **take back** *v/t* (*return*) *object* devolver; *person* buscar; (*accept back*) *husband etc* aceitar de volta; ***that takes me back*** *music, thought etc* me traz lembranças
♦ **take down** *v/t from shelf* descer; *scaffolding* desmontar; *pants* abaixar; (*write down*) anotar
♦ **take in** *v/t* (*take indoors*) recolher; (*give accommodation*) acomodar; (*make narrower*) apertar; (*deceive*) enganar; (*include*) incluir
♦ **take off 1** *v/t clothes, hat* tirar; *10% etc* descontar; (*mimic*) imitar; ***can you take a bit off here?*** *to barber* pode tirar um pouquinho aqui?; ***take a day / week off*** tirar um dia / uma semana de férias **2** *v/i airplane* decolar; (*become popular*) pegar
♦ **take on** *v/t job* aceitar; *staff* contratar
♦ **take out** *v/t from bag, pocket, text* tirar; *appendix, tooth* extrair; *money from bank* retirar; *to dinner etc* levar; *insurance policy* fazer; ***take sth out on s.o.*** descontar algo em alguém, *Port* descarregar algo em alguém
♦ **take over 1** *v/t company etc* adquirir; ***tourists take over the town*** os turistas invadem a cidade **2** *v/i new management etc* assumir; (*do sth in s.o.'s place*) continuar
♦ **take to** *v/t* (*like*) simpatizar com; (*form habit of*) começar a
♦ **take up** *v/t carpet etc* levantar; (*carry up*) carregar; (*shorten*) *dress etc* encurtar; *hobby, new job* começar; *judo, Spanish* começar a fazer; *offer* aceitar; *space, time* tomar; ***I'll take you up on your offer*** aceitarei sua oferta
'takeaway *Brit meal* comida *f* pronta (para levar); *restaurant* lanchonete *f*
'take-home pay salário *m* líquido

taken ['teɪkən] *pp* → ***take***
'takeoff *airplane*: decolagem *f*; (*impersonation*) imitação *f* **'takeover** COM aquisição *f* **'takeover bid** oferta *f* pública de aquisição
takings ['teɪkɪŋz] *npl* rendimento *m*
talcum powder ['tælkəm] talco *m*
tale [teɪl] conto *m*
talent ['tælənt] talento *m*
talented ['tæləntɪd] *adj* talentoso
'talent scout caça-talentos *m*
talk [tɒːk] **1** *v/i* falar; ***can I ~ to ...?*** posso falar com ...?; ***I'll ~ to him about it*** vou conversar com ele sobre isso **2** *v/t English etc* falar; *business, politics* falar de; ***~ s.o. into sth*** convencer alguém a fazer algo **3** *n* (*conversation*) conversa *f*; (*lecture*) palestra *f*; ***~s*** *pl* (*negotiations*) negociações *fpl*; ***he's all ~*** *pej* ele só tem papo
♦**talk back** *v/i* responder
♦**talk down to** *v/t* falar com ares de superioridade com
♦**talk over** *v/t* conversar sobre
talkative ['tɒːkətɪv] *adj* falador
talking-to ['tɒːkɪŋtuː] sermão *m*
'talk show programa *m* de entrevistas
tall [tɒːl] *adj* alto; ***how ~ are you?*** qual é a sua altura?; ***I'm ... ~*** tenho ... de altura
tall 'order ***that's a ~*** isso é uma tarefa muito difícil
tall 'story conto *m* da carochinha
tally ['tælɪ] **1** *n* conta *f* **2** *v/i* ⟨*pret & pp* ***tallied***⟩ *of amounts, stories* conferir
♦**tally with** *v/t* corresponder com
tame [teɪm] *adj animal* manso, domesticado; *joke etc* inocente
♦**tamper with** ['tæmpər] *v/t lock* forçar; *brakes* mexer em
tampon ['tæmpɑːn] tampão *m*
tan [tæn] **1** *n sun*: bronzeado *m* **2** *v/i* ⟨*pret & pp* ***tanned***⟩ *in sun* bronzear-se **3** *v/t* ⟨*pret & pp* ***tanned***⟩ *leather* curtir
tandem ['tændəm] *bike* bicicleta *f* de dois lugares
tangent ['tændʒənt] MATH tangente *f*
tangerine [tændʒə'riːn] tangerina *f*
tangible ['tændʒɪbl] *adj* tangível
tangle ['tæŋgl] *n* nó *m*; ***get into a ~*** *string etc* ficar emaranhado
tango ['tæŋgoʊ] *n* tango *m*
tank [tæŋk] *water*: depósito *m*; *fish*: aquário *m*; MOT, MIL, *skin diver*: tanque *m*
tanker ['tæŋkər] *truck* caminhão-tanque *m*, *Port* camião-tanque *m*; *ship* petroleiro *m*
'tank top camiseta *f* de alcinha
tanned [tænd] *adj* bronzeado
Tannoy® ['tænɔɪ] sistema *m* de alto-falantes público
tantalizing ['tæntəlaɪzɪŋ] *adj* tantalizante
tantamount ['tæntəmaʊnt] *adj* ***be ~ to*** equivaler a
tantrum ['tæntrəm] ataque *m* de raiva
tap [tæp] **1** *n Brit* torneira *f* **2** *v/t* ⟨*pret & pp* ***tapped***⟩ (*knock*) bater; *phone* interceptar
♦**tap into** *v/t resources* explorar
'tap dance *n* sapateado *m*
tape [teɪp] **1** *n recording*: fita *f*, *sticky* fita *f* adesiva **2** *v/t conversation etc* gravar; *with sticky tape* colar
'tape deck gravador *m* **'tape drive** COMPUT tape *m* drive **'tape measure** fita *f* métrica
taper ['teɪpər] *v/i* estreitar-se
♦**taper off** *v/i production, figures* diminuir
'tape recorder gravador *m*
'tape recording gravação *f*
tapestry ['tæpɪstrɪ] tapeçaria *f*
'tapeworm tênia *f*
tar [tɑːr] *n cigarettes*: alcatrão *m*; *road*: piche *m*
tardy ['tɑːrdɪ] *adj Am* atrasado
target ['tɑːrgɪt] **1** *n shooting*: alvo *m*; *sales, production*: meta *f* **2** *v/t market* direcionar a
target 'audience público *m* alvo **'target date** data *f* fixada **'target figure** valor *m* meta **'target group** COM grupo *m* estratégico **'target language** língua *f* alvo **'target market** mercado *m* alvo
tariff ['tærɪf] (*price*) tarifa *f*, (*tax*) imposto *m*
tarmac ['tɑːrmæk] *airport*: pista *f* de decolagem
tarnish ['tɑːrnɪʃ] *v/t metal* empanar; *reputation* manchar

tarpaulin [tɑːr'pɒːlɪn] lona *f*
tart[1] [tɑːrt] *n* torta *f*
tart[2] [tɑːrt] *n fam (prostitute)* biscate *f*
tartan ['tɑːrtn] tartã *m*
task [tæsk] tarefa *f*
'task force força-tarefa *f*
tassel ['tæsl] franja *f*
taste [teɪst] **1** *n food etc*: sabor *m*; *in clothes, art etc*: gosto *m*; *sense* paladar *m*; ***he has no ~*** ele tem mau gosto **2** *v/t food* provar; *(experience) freedom etc* experimentar **3** *v/i* ***it ~s like honey*** tem gosto de mel
'taste buds *npl* papilas *fpl* gustativas
tasteful ['teɪstfl] *adj* de bom gosto
tastefully ['teɪstflɪ] *adv arranged, decorated* com bom gosto
tasteless ['teɪstlɪs] *adj food* sem sabor; *remark, person* sem graça
tasting ['teɪstɪŋ] *wine*: degustação *f*
tasty ['teɪstɪ] *adj* saboroso
tattered ['tætərd] *adj clothes, book* rasgado
tatters ['tætərz] ***in ~*** *clothes* em trapos; *reputation, career* arruinado
tattoo [tə'tuː] *n* tatuagem *f*
tatty ['tætɪ] *adj* surrado
taught [tɔːt] *pret & pp* → ***teach***
taunt [tɔːnt] **1** *n* escárnio *m* **2** *v/t* zombar de
Taurus [tɔːrus] ASTROL Touro *m*
taut [tɔːt] *adj skin* firme; *rope* tenso
tawdry ['tɔːdrɪ] *adj* barato
tax [tæks] **1** *n* imposto *m*; ***before / after ~*** sem / com imposto **2** *v/t people* cobrar impostos de; *product* lançar impostos em
taxable 'income rendimento *m* sujeito à tributação
taxation [tæk'seɪʃn] *(act of taxing)* cobrança *f* de impostos; *(taxes)* impostos *mpl*
'tax avoidance evasão *f* de impostos **'tax bracket** faixa *f* de contribuição **'tax code** código *m* tributário **'tax deductible** *adj* dedutível de imposto **'tax evasion** fraude *f* fiscal **'tax free** *adj* isento de impostos
taxi ['tæksɪ] táxi *m*
'taxi driver motorista *m/f* de táxi
taxing ['tæksɪŋ] *adj* exigente
'tax inspector fiscal *m* tributário
'taxi stand ponto *m* de táxi
'taxpayer contribuinte *m/f* **'tax return** *form* formulário *m* de solicitação de devolução de imposto **'tax year** ano *m* fiscal
TB [tiː'biː] *abbr* → ***tuberculosis***
tea [tiː] *drink* chá *m*; *meal* chá *m* da tarde
teabag ['tiːbæg] saquinho *m* de chá
teach [tiːʧ] *v/t & v/i ⟨pret & pp* ***taught****⟩ person, subject* ensinar; ***~ s.o. to do sth*** ensinar alguém a fazer algo
teacher ['tiːʧər] professor,a *m,f*
teacher 'training magistério *m*
teaching ['tiːʧɪŋ] *profession* educação *f*
'teaching aid material *m* didático
'tea cloth pano *m* de prato **'teacup** xícara *f* de chá **'tea drinker** bebedor,a *m,f* de chá
teak [tiːk] teca *f*
'tea leaf folha *f* de chá
team [tiːm] time *m*, *Port* equipa *f*
'team mate colega *m/f* de time, *Port* colega *m/f* de equipa
team 'spirit espírito *m* de equipe, *Port* espírito *m* de equipa
teamster ['tiːmstər] *Am* caminhoneiro *m*, *Port* camionista *m*
'teamwork trabalho *m* de equipe
teapot ['tiːpɑːt] bule *m* de chá
tear[1] [ter] **1** *n cloth etc*: rasgadura *f* **2** *v/t ⟨pret* ***tore****, pp* ***torn****⟩ paper, cloth* rasgar; ***be torn between two alternatives*** estar dividido entre duas alternativas **3** *v/i ⟨pret* ***tore****, pp* ***torn****⟩ (run fast, drive fast)* ir a toda velocidade
tear[2] [tɪr] *eye*: lágrima *f*; ***burst into ~s*** começar a chorar; ***be in ~s*** estar chorando
♦**tear down** *v/t (remove)* arrancar; *building* demolir
♦**tear out** *v/t* arrancar
♦**tear up** *v/t paper* rasgar; *agreement* desfazer
teardrop ['tɪrdrɑːp] lágrima *f*
tearful ['tɪrfl] *adj* choroso
'tear gas gás *m* lacrimogêneo
'tearoom salão *m* de chá
tease [tiːz] *v/t* provocar

'tea service, **'tea set** jogo *m* de chá **'teaspoon** colher *f* de chá **'tea strainer** coador *m* de chá
teat [tiːt] *animal*: teta *f*; *woman*: mamilo *m*
'tea towel *Brit* pano *m* de prato
techie ['tekiː] *fam* técnico,-a *m,f*
technical ['teknɪkl] *adj* técnico
technicality [teknɪ'kælətɪ] detalhe *m* técnico; ***that's just a ~*** é só um detalhe técnico
technically ['teknɪklɪ] *adv* (*strictly speaking*) tecnicamente; *written* em linguagem técnica
technician [tek'nɪʃn] técnico,-a *m,f*
technique [tek'niːk] técnica *f*
technological [teknə'lɑːdʒɪkl] *adj* tecnológico
technology [tek'nɑːlədʒɪ] tecnologia *f*
technophobia [teknə'foʊbɪə] tecnofobia *f*
teddy bear ['tedɪber] ursinho *m* de pelúcia
tedious ['tiːdɪəs] *adj* entediante
tee [tiː] *n golf*: tee *m*
teem [tiːm] *v/i* ***be ~ing with tourists / ants*** estar cheio de turistas / formigas; ***be ~ing with rain*** estar chovendo torrencialmente
teenage ['tiːneɪdʒ] *adj fashions* adolescente; ***a ~ boy / girl*** um / uma adolescente
teenager ['tiːneɪdʒər] adolescente *m/f*
teens [tiːnz] *npl* adolescência *f*; ***be in one's ~*** estar na adolescência; ***reach one's ~*** entrar na adolescência
teeny ['tiːnɪ] *adj fam* pequenino
teeth [tiːθ] *pl* → ***tooth***
teethe [tiːð] *v/i* nascer os (primeiros) dentes
'teething problems *npl* primeiros problemas *mpl*
teetotal [tiː'toʊtl] *adj person, party* abstinente
teetotaler [tiː'toʊtlər] abstêmio *m*
teetotaller *Brit* → ***teetotaler***
telecommunications [telɪkəmjuːnɪ'keɪʃnz] telecomunicações *fpl*
teleconference ['telɪkɑːnfərəns] teleconferência *f*
telegraph pole ['telɪgræfpoʊl] *Brit* poste *m* telegráfico
telepathic [telɪ'pæθɪk] *adj* telepático; ***you must be ~!*** você deve ser dotado de telepatia
telepathy [tɪ'lepəθɪ] telepatia *f*
telephone ['telɪfoʊn] **1** *n* telefone *m*; ***be on the ~*** *speaking* estar ao telefone; (*possess a phone*) ter um telefone **2** *v/t & v/i person* telefonar
'telephone bill conta *f* do telefone
'telephone book lista *f* telefônica
'telephone booth orelhão *m* **'telephone box** *Brit* cabine *f* telefônica
'telephone call chamada *f* telefônica **'telephone conversation** conversa *f* telefônica **'telephone directory** lista *f* telefônica **'telephone exchange** central *f* telefônica **'telephone message** mensagem *f* telefônica **'telephone number** número *m* do telefone
telephoto lens ['telɪfoʊtoʊ] *nsg* teleobjetiva *f*
telesales ['telɪseɪlz] televendas *fpl*
telescope ['telɪskoʊp] telescópio *m*
telescopic [telɪ'skɑːpɪk] *adj* telescópico
telethon ['telɪθɑːn] maratona *f* de televisão
televise ['telɪvaɪz] *v/t* televisionar
television ['telɪvɪʒn] *also* (*set*) televisão *f*; ***on ~*** na televisão; ***watch ~*** assistir televisão
'television audience audiência *f* televisiva **'television program** programa *m* de televisão **television programme** *Brit* → ***television program*** **'television set** aparelho *m* de televisão **'television studio** estúdio *m* de televisão
tell [tel] ⟨*pret & pp* ***told***⟩ **1** *v/t story, lie* contar; ***~ s.o. sth*** contar algo a alguém; ***don't ~ Ma*** não conte para a mãe; ***who told you that?*** quem te contou isso?; ***could you ~ me the way to ...?*** poderia me dizer o caminho para ...?; ***I can't ~ the difference between them*** não consigo distinguir a diferença entre eles; ***~ s.o. to do sth*** dizer a alguém para fazer algo; ***you're ~ing me!*** *fam* eu que o diga! **2** *v/i* (*have effect*) ter efei-

T

to; ***the heat is ~ing on him*** o calor o está consumindo; ***time will ~*** o tempo irá dizer
teller ['telər] caixa *m/f*
telling ['telɪŋ] *adj* significativo
telling 'off repreensão *f*
'telltale *adj signs* revelador
telly ['telɪ] *Brit fam* TV *f*
temp [temp] **1** *n employee* temporário,-a *m,f* **2** *v/i* exercer trabalho temporário
temper ['tempər] (*bad temper*) mau humor *m*; ***be in a ~*** estar mal-humorado; ***keep one's ~*** manter o bom humor; ***lose one's ~*** perder o bom humor
temperament ['temprəmənt] temperamento *m*
temperamental [temprə'mentl] *adj* (*moody*) temperamental
temperate ['tempərət] *adj* temperado
temperature ['temprətʃər] temperatura *f*; (*fever*) febre *f*; ***have a ~*** estar com febre
temple[1] ['templ] REL templo *m*
temple[2] ['templ] ANAT têmpora *f*
tempo ['tempoʊ] MUS, *of work* ritmo *m*
temporarily [tempə'rerɪlɪ] *adv* temporariamente
temporary ['tempərerɪ] *adj* temporário
tempt [tempt] *v/t* tentar
temptation [temp'teɪʃn] tentação *f*
tempting ['temptɪŋ] *adj* tentador
ten [ten] dez
tenacious [tɪ'neɪʃəs] *adj* tenaz
tenacity [tɪ'næsɪtɪ] tenacidade *f*
tenant ['tenənt] *building*: morador,a *m,f*; *farm, land*: arrendatário,-a *m,f*
tend [tend] *v/t* (*look after*) cuidar de; ***~ to do sth*** tender a fazer algo; ***~ toward sth*** tender a algo
tendency ['tendənsɪ] tendência *f*
tender[1] ['tendər] *adj* (*sore*) dolorido; (*affectionate*) carinhoso; *steak* tenro
tender[2] ['tendər] *n* COM proposta *f*
tenderness ['tendərnɪs] (*soreness*) dor *f*; *of kiss etc* carinho *m*; *of steak* tenrura *f*
tendon ['tendən] tendão *m*
tennis ['tenɪs] tênis *m*
'tennis ball bola *f* de tênis **'tennis court** quadra *f* de tênis **'tennis player** jogador,a *m,f* de tênis **'tennis racket** raquete *f* de tênis
tenor ['tenər] *n* MUS tenor *m*
tense[1] [tens] *n* GRAM tempo *m*
tense[2] [tens] *adj muscle, voice, person* tenso; *moment* crítico
♦**tense up** *v/i muscles* tensionar; *person* ficar tenso
tension ['tenʃn] *rope, atmosphere, voice*: tensão *f*; *movie, novel*: suspense *m*
tent [tent] barraca *f*
tentacle ['tentəkl] tentáculo *m*
tentative ['tentətɪv] *adj move, offer* provisório
tenterhooks ['tentərhʊks] ***be on ~*** estar muito ansioso
tenth [tenθ] *n & adj* décimo (*m*)
tepid ['tepɪd] *adj* morno
term [tɜːrm] (*period of time*) período *m*; EDUC semestre *m*; (*condition, word*) termo *m*; ***be on good / bad ~s with s.o.*** entender-se bem / mal com alguém; ***in the long / short ~*** a longo / curto prazo; ***come to ~s with sth*** conseguir conviver com algo
terminal ['tɜːrmɪnl] **1** *n airport, bus, also* ELEC, COMPUT terminal *m*; *containers*: depósito *m* **2** *adj illness* terminal
terminally ['tɜːrmɪnəlɪ] *adv* ***~ ill*** em fase terminal
terminate ['tɜːrmɪneɪt] **1** *v/t contract* rescindir; *pregnancy* interromper **2** *v/i* terminar
termination [tɜːrmɪ'neɪʃn] *contract*: rescisão *f*; *pregnancy*: interrupção *f*
terminology [tɜːrmɪ'nɑːlədʒɪ] terminologia *f*
terminus ['tɜːrmɪnəs] *buses*: ponto final *m*; *trains*: estação *f* final
terrace ['terəs] (*patio*), *on hillside*, *Brit houses*: terraço *m*
terraced house ['terəst] *Brit* casa *f* germinada
terra cotta [terə'kɑːtə] *adj* de terracota
terrain [te'reɪn] terreno *m*
terrestrial [te'restrɪəl] **1** *n* terrestre

T

m/f **2** *adj television* de transmissão via terrestre
terrible ['terəbl] *adj* terrível
terribly ['terəblɪ] *adv* (*very*) terrivelmente
terrific [tə'rɪfɪk] *adj* ótimo
terrifically [tə'rɪfɪklɪ] *adv* (*very*) tremendamente
terrify ['terɪfaɪ] *v/t* ⟨*pret & pp* ***terrified***⟩ aterrorizar; ***be terrified*** ficar aterrorizado
terrifying ['terɪfaɪɪŋ] *adj* aterrador
territorial [terə'tɔːrɪəl] *adj* territorial
territorial 'waters águas *fpl* territoriais
territory ['terɪtɔːrɪ] *also fig* território *m*
terror ['terər] terror *m*
terrorism ['terərɪzm] terrorismo *m*
terrorist ['terərɪst] terrorista *m/f*
'terrorist attack atentado *m* terrorista
'terrorist organization organização *f* terrorista
terrorize ['terəraɪz] *v/t* aterrorizar
terse [tɜːrs] *adj* curto e grosso
test [test] **1** *n* prova *f* **2** *v/t* testar
testament ['testəmənt] *to s.o.'s life* testemunho *m*; REL ***Old / New Testament*** Velho / Novo Testamento *m*
'test-drive *v/t* ⟨*pret* ***test-drove***, *pp* ***test-driven***⟩ *car* fazer um test-drive em
testicle ['testɪkl] testículo *m*
testify ['testɪfaɪ] *v/i* ⟨*pret & pp* ***testified***⟩ LAW testemunhar
testimonial [testɪ'mounɪəl] *n* carta *f* de recomendação
testimony ['testɪmənɪ] LAW testemunho *m*
'test tube tubo *m* de ensaio, proveta *f*
'test tube baby bebê *m* de proveta
testy ['testɪ] *adj* irascível
tetanus ['tetənəs] tétano *m*
tether ['teðər] **1** *v/t horse* amarrar **2** *n* ***be at the end of one's ~*** estar a ponto de perder a paciência
text [tekst] **1** texto *m*; *message* mensagem *f* de texto, SMS *m*; **2** *v/t person* mandar uma mensagem de texto a
'textbook livro *m* escolar
textile ['tekstaɪl] tecido *m*
'text message mensagem *f* de texto
texture ['tekstʃər] textura *f*
Thai [taɪ] **1** *adj* tailandês,-esa **2** *n person* tailandês,-esa *m,f*; *language* tailandês *m*
Thailand ['taɪlænd] Tailândia *f*
than [ðæn] *adv* (do) que; ***bigger / faster ~ me*** maior / mais rápido (do) que eu; ***more ~ 50*** mais de 50
thank [θæŋk] *v/t* agradecer; ***~ you*** obrigado,-a; ***no ~ you*** não, obrigado,-a
thankful ['θæŋkful] *adj* grato
thankfully ['θæŋkfulɪ] *adv* com gratidão; (*luckily*) felizmente
thankless ['θæŋklɪs] *adj task* ingrato
thanks [θæŋks] agradecimento *m*; ***~!*** obrigado,-a!; ***~ to*** graças a
Thanksgiving, **Thanksgiving Day** [θæŋks'gɪvɪŋ] *Am* Dia *m* de Ação de Graças
that [ðæt] **1** *adj* esse, isso, *further away* aquele; ***~ one*** esse,-a **2** *pron* ◇ isso; *individuating* esse,-a; *further away* aquele,-a; ***what is ~?*** o que é isso?; ***who is ~?*** quem é aquele,-a?; ***~'s mine*** esse é meu; ***~'s my tea*** esse é meu chá; ***~'s very kind*** isto é muito gentil ◇ *relative*: que; ***the person / car ~ you see*** a pessoa / o carro que você esta vendo **3** *conj* que; ***I think ~ …*** penso que … **4** *adv* (*so*) tão; ***~ expensive*** tão caro
thaw [θɒː] *v/i snow* derreter; *frozen food* descongelar
the [ðə] o, a *m,f*; *with plural* os, as; ***~ sooner ~ better*** quanto antes melhor
theater ['θɪətər] teatro *m*
'theater critic crítico,-a *m,f* de teatro
theatre *Brit* → ***theater***
theatrical [θɪ'ætrɪkl] *adj also* (*overdone*) teatral
theft [θeft] roubo *m*
their [ðer] *adj* o seu / a sua, dele / dela; (*his or her*) o seu / a sua; ***everyone has ~ favorite*** todos tem o seu favorito
theirs [ðerz] *pron* o seu, a sua, deles, delas; ***a friend of ~*** um amigo deles; ***~ was easier*** o deles era mais fácil
them [ðem] *pron* ◇ *object* eles, elas; os,

as; ***I know*** ~ eu os conheço; ***he lives with*** ~ ele mora com eles; ***see the trees?, it's behind*** ~ está vendo aquelas árvores? é atrás delas
◊ *indirect object* a eles, a elas; ***I sent*** ~ ***an email*** eu mandei um email a eles
◊ (*him or her*) ***if someone loses, it's hard for*** ~ ***to …*** se alguém perder, ser-lhe-á difícil …; ***everyone took their camera with*** ~ todos levaram as suas câmeras com eles
theme [θi:m] tema *m*
'theme park parque *m* temático
'theme song música *f* tema
themselves [ðem'selvz] *pron* ◊ *reflexive* se; ***they hurt*** ~ eles se machucaram
◊ *after prep* si mesmos,-as; ***they were very pleased with*** ~ eles estavam muito satisfeitos com si mesmos
◊ *emphasizing* mesmos,-as; ***they did it*** ~ eles próprios fizeram isso; ***by*** ~ (*alone*) sozinhos,-as
then [ðen] *adv* então; ***by*** ~ até então
theologian [θɪə'loʊdʒɪən] teólogo,-a *m,f*
theology [θɪ'ɑ:lədʒɪ] teologia *f*
theoretical [θɪə'retɪkl] *adj* teórico
theoretically [θɪə'retɪklɪ] *adv* teoricamente
theory ['θɪrɪ] teoria *f*; ***in*** ~ teoricamente
therapeutic [θerə'pju:tɪk] *adj* terapêutico
therapist ['θerəpɪst] terapeuta *m/f*
therapy ['θerəpɪ] terapia *f*
there [ðer] *adv* lá; ***over*** ~ / ***down*** ~ lá / lá embaixo; ~ ***is*** / ***are …*** há …; ~ ***is*** / ***are not …*** não há …; ~ ***you are*** *giving, finding*: aqui está; *completing*: pronto; ~ ***and back*** ida e volta; ~ ***he is!*** lá está ele!; ~, ~, ***don't cry!*** não foi nada, não chore!
thereabouts [ðerə'baʊts] *adv* aproximadamente
therefore ['ðerfɔ:r] *adv* portanto
thermometer [θər'mɑ:mɪtər] termômetro *m*
thermos flask ['θɜ:rməs] garrafa *f* térmica, *Port* termo *m*
thermostat ['θɜ:rməstæt] termostato *m*
these [ði:z] *adj & pron* estes,-as
thesis ['θi:sɪs] ⟨*pl* ***theses***⟩ tese *f*
they [ðeɪ] *pron* ◊ eles, elas
◊ *impersonal* eles; ~ ***say that …*** eles disseram que; ~ ***are going to change the law*** vão mudar a lei
◊ (*he or she*) ele, ela; ***if anyone looks at this,*** ~ ***will see that …*** se alguém olhar para isso, vai ver que …
thick [θɪk] *adj hair, soup, wall, book etc* grosso; *fam* (*stupid*) estúpido
thicken ['θɪkən] *v/t sauce* engrossar
'thickset *adj* atarracado
thickskinned ['θɪkskɪnd] *adj fig* insensível
thief [θi:f] ⟨*pl* ***thieves***⟩ ladrão *m*, ladra *f*
thigh [θaɪ] coxa *f*
thimble ['θɪmbl] dedal *m*
thin [θɪn] *adj coat, line* fino; *person* magro; *hair, soup* ralo
thing [θɪŋ] coisa *f*; ~***s*** (*belongings*) pertences *mpl*; ***how are*** ~***s?*** como vão as coisas?; ***it's a good*** ~ ***you told me*** foi bom você ter me falado; ***what a*** ~ ***to do*** / ***say!*** que barbaridade!
thingumajig ['θɪŋʌmədʒɪg] *fam object* coisa *f*; *person* fulano,-a *m,f*
think [θɪŋk] *v/i* ⟨*pret & pp* ***thought***⟩ pensar; ***I*** ~ ***so*** penso que sim; ***I don't*** ~ ***so*** penso que não; ***I*** ~ ***so too*** penso o mesmo; ***what do you*** ~***?*** o que você acha?; ***what do you*** ~ ***of it?*** o que você pensa disto?; ***I can't*** ~ ***of anything more*** não me ocorre mais nada; ~ ***hard!*** pense bem!; ***I'm*** ~***ing about emigrating*** estou pensando em emigrar
♦**think over** *v/t* pensar sobre
♦**think through** *v/t* pensar bem sobre
♦**think up** *v/t plan* inventar
'think tank grupo *m* de especialistas
thin-skinned ['θɪnskɪnd] *adj* sensível
third [θɜ:rd] **1** *adj* terceiro **2** *n* terceiro,-a *m,f*; *fraction* terço *m*
thirdly ['θɜ:rdlɪ] *adv* em terceiro lugar
third-party in'surance seguro *m* de terceiros **third 'person** GRAM terceira *f* pessoa **'third-rate** *adj* de terceira qualidade **'Third World** terceiro *m* mundo

thirst [θɜːrst] sede *f*
thirsty ['θɜːrstɪ] *adj* sedento; ***be ~*** estar com sede
thirteen [θɜːr'tiːn] treze
thirteenth [θɜːr'tiːnθ] *n & adj* décimo terceiro (*m*)
thirtieth ['θɜːrtɪəθ] *n & adj* trigésimo (*m*)
thirty ['θɜːrtɪ] trinta
this [ðɪs] **1** *adj* este,-a; ***~ one*** este,-a **2** *pron* isto; ***~ is good*** isto é bom; ***~ is …*** *introducing s.o.* este,-a é …; TEL aqui quem fala é … **3** *adv* ***~ big*** grande assim
thorn [θɔːrn] espinho *m*
thorny ['θɔːrnɪ] *adj plant, also fig problem* espinhoso
thorough ['θɜːroʊ] *adj search, person* minucioso; *knowledge* profundo
thoroughbred ['θʌrəbred] *horse* puro sangue *m*
thoroughly ['θʌrəlɪ] *adv spoilt* totalmente; *search* minuciosamente
those [ðoʊz] *adj & pron* esses,-as; *further away* aqueles,-as
though [ðoʊ] **1** *conj* (*although*) apesar de que; ***~ he is your brother*** apesar dele ser seu irmão; ***as ~*** como se **2** *adv* não obstante; ***it's not finished ~*** mas não está acabado
thought[1] [θɒːt] *single* idéia *f*; *collective* pensamento *m*
thought[2] [θɒːt] *pret & pp* → ***think***
thoughtful ['θɒːtfʊl] *adj look, face, person* pensativo; *book* sério; (*considerate*) atencioso
thoughtfully ['θɒːtflɪ] *adv* (*pensively*) pensativamente; (*considerately*) atenciosamente
thoughtless ['θɒːtlɪs] *adj behavior* impensado; *driving, person* irresponsável
thoughtlessly ['θɒːtlɪslɪ] *adv* de maneira irrefletida
thousand ['θaʊznd] mil; ***~s of times*** mil vezes
thousandth ['θaʊzndθ] *adj & n* milésimo,-a *m,f*
thrash [θræʃ] *v/t* bater; SPORT dar uma surra em
♦**thrash around** *v/i with arms etc* debater-se
♦**thrash out** *v/t solution* elaborar
thrashing ['θræʃɪŋ] *also* SPORT surra *f*
thread [θred] **1** *n* fio *m*; *screw*: rosca *f* **2** *v/t needle, beads* enfiar
'**threadbare** *adj jacket, sleeves* surrado
threat [θret] ameaça *f*
threaten ['θretn] *v/t* ameaçar
threatening ['θretnɪŋ] *adj gesture, sky* ameaçador
three [θriː] três
three 'quarters três quartos
thresh [θreʃ] *v/t corn* trilhar
threshold ['θreʃhoʊld] *house*: soleira *f*; *new age*: limiar *m*; ***on the ~ of*** no limiar de
threw [θruː] *pret* → ***throw***
thrift [θrɪft] economia *f*
thrifty ['θrɪftɪ] *adj person, habits* econômico
thrill [θrɪl] **1** *n* emoção *f* **2** *v/t* ***be ~ed*** estar emocionado
thriller ['θrɪlər] *movie* filme *m* de suspense
thrilling ['θrɪlɪŋ] *adj* emocionante
thrive [θraɪv] *v/i plant* crescer; *business, economy* prosperar
throat [θroʊt] garganta *f*
'**throat lozenge** pastilha *f* para a garganta
throb [θrɑːb] **1** *n heart, music*: batida *f* **2** *v/i* ⟨*pret & pp* ***throbbed***⟩ *heart* palpitar; *music* vibrar
thrombosis [θrɑːm'boʊsɪs] trombose *f*
throne [θroʊn] trono *m*
throng [θrɑːŋ] *n* multidão *f*
throttle ['θrɑːtl] **1** *n motorbike, boat*: acelerador *m* **2** *v/t* (*strangle*) estrangular
♦**throttle back** *v/i* desacelerar
through [θruː] **1** *prep* ◇ (*across*) através de; ***go ~ the city*** atravessar a cidade
◇ (*during*) durante; ***~ the winter / summer*** durante o inverno / verão; ***Monday ~ Friday*** *Am* de segunda a sexta-feira
◇ (*thanks to*) graças a; ***arranged ~ him*** organizado por ele **2** *adv* ***wet ~*** completamente molhado; ***watch a movie ~*** assistir um filme até o fi-

T

nal; ***read a book*** ~ ler um livro até o fim **3** *adj* ***be*** ~ *couple* estar tudo acabado; (*have arrived*) *news etc* ter chegado; ***you're*** ~ TEL você já pode falar; ***I'm*** ~ ***with …*** (*finished with*) terminei com …
through'out **1** *prep* durante todo **2** *adv* (*in all parts*) por todas as partes
'through train trem *m* direto
throw [θroʊ] **1** *v/t* ⟨*pret* ***threw***, *pp* ***thrown***⟩ jogar; *rider* atirar; (*disconcert*) desconcertar; *party* dar; ~ ***oneself*** precipitar-se **2** *n* lançamento *m*
♦ **throw away** *v/t* jogar fora
♦ **throw off** *v/t jacket etc* tirar apressadamente; *cold etc* livrar-se de
♦ **throw on** *v/t clothes* vestir correndo
♦ **throw out** *v/t old things*, jogar fora; *from bar, husband, country etc* expulsar; *plan* rejeitar
♦ **throw up** **1** *v/t ball* arremessar; ***throw up one's hands*** levar as mãos à cabeça **2** *v/i* (*vomit*) vomitar
'throw-away *adj remark* à toa; (*disposable*) descartável
'throw-in SPORT arremesso *m*
thrown [θroʊn] *pp* → ***throw***
thru *Am* → ***through***
thrush [θrʌʃ] *bird* tordo *m*
thrust [θrʌst] *v/t* ⟨*pret & pp* ***thrust***⟩ (*push hard*) empurrar; ~ ***sth into s.o.'s hands*** pôr algo nas mãos de alguém; ~ ***one's way through the crowd*** abrir caminho através da multidão
thud [θʌd] *n* pancada *f* surda
thug [θʌg] brutamontes *m*
thumb [θʌm] **1** *n* polegar *m* **2** *v/t* ~ ***a ride*** pegar carona
'thumbtack *Am* percevejo *m*
thump [θʌmp] **1** *n blow* bofetada *f*; *noise* pancada *f* surda **2** *v/t person* espancar; ~ ***one's fist on the table*** dar um murro na mesa **3** *v/i heart* bater com força; ~ ***on the door*** espancar a porta
thunder ['θʌndər] *n* trovão *m*
thunderous ['θʌndərəs] *adj applause* estrondoso
'thunderstorm temporal *m*
'thunderstruck *adj* atônito
thundery ['θʌndərɪ] *adj weather* tormentoso
Thursday ['θɜːrzdeɪ] quinta-feira *f*
thus [ðʌs] *adv* (*in this way*) assim
thwart [θwɔːrt] *v/t person, plans* frustrar
thyme [taɪm] tomilho *m*
thyroid gland ['θaɪrɔɪd] tiróide *f*
tick [tɪk] **1** *n clock*: tique-taque *m*; *text*: sinal *m* de visto **2** *v/i clock* fazer tique-taque
ticket ['tɪkɪt] *bus, train, airplane*: passagem *f*, *Port* bilhete *m*; *theater, concert, museum*: entrada *f*, *Port* bilhete *m*; *lottery*: bilhete *m*
'ticket inspector controlador,a *m,f*
'ticket machine máquina *f* automática de bilhetes **'ticket office** *station*: guichê *m*; THEA bilheteria *f*, *Port* bilheteira *f*
ticking ['tɪkɪŋ] *noise* tique-taque *m*
tickle ['tɪkl] **1** *v/t person* fazer cócegas em **2** *v/i material* coçar; *person* fazer cócegas
ticklish ['tɪklɪʃ] *adj person* coceguento
♦ **tick off** → ***check off***
tidal wave ['taɪdl] onda *f* gigantesca
tide [taɪd] maré *f*; ***high*** ~ maré *f* alta; ***low*** ~ maré *f* baixa; ***the*** ~ ***is in / out*** a maré está alta / baixa
♦ **tide over** *v/t* auxiliar; ***$40 to tide you over*** $40 para você se manter
tidiness ['taɪdɪnɪs] *person*: asseio *m*; *room, desk*: ordem *f*
tidy ['taɪdɪ] *adj person, habits* asseado; *room, house* arrumado
♦ **tidy away** *v/t* ⟨*pret & pp* ***tidied***⟩ guardar
♦ **tidy up** **1** *v/t room, shelves* arrumar; ***tidy oneself up*** arrumar-se **2** *v/i* arrumar
tie [taɪ] **1** *n* (*necktie*) gravata *f*; SPORT (*even result*) empate *m*; ***he doesn't have any*** ~***s*** ele não tem nenhum vínculo **2** *v/t knot, hands* atar; ~ ***two ropes together*** atar duas cordas **3** *v/i* SPORT empatar
♦ **tie down** *v/t* (*restrict*) amarrar
♦ **tie up** *v/t person, laces* atar; *hair* amarrar; *boat* atracar; ***I'm tied up tomorrow*** *busy* amanhã estarei ocupado

tier [tɪr] *hierarchy*: nível *m*; *stadium*: fileira *f*
tiger ['taɪgər] tigre *m*
tight[1] [taɪt] *adj clothes* justo; *security* estrito; (*hard to move*) duro; (*properly shut*) trancado; (*not leaving much time*) curto; *fam* (*drunk*) chumbado
tight[2] [taɪt] *adv hold* fortemente; ***shut ~*** bem-fechado
tighten ['taɪtn] *v/t screw* apertar; *control* aumentar; *security* intensificar; ***~ one's grip on sth*** ter mais pulso com algo
♦ **tighten up** *v/i discipline*, *security*: ser mais rigoroso
tight-fisted [taɪt'fɪstɪd] *adj* pão-duro
tightly *adv* → ***tight***[2]
'**tightrope** corda *f* fina
tights [taɪts] *npl Brit* meia-calça *f*, *Port* collants *mpl*
tile [taɪl] *floor, wall*: ladrilho *m*; *roof*: telha *f*
till[1] [tɪl] *prep* (*until*) até
till[2] [tɪl] *n* (*cash register*) caixa *f* registradora
till[3] [tɪl] *v/t soil* lavrar
tilt [tɪlt] **1** *v/t* inclinar **2** *v/i* inclinar-se
timber ['tɪmbər] *n* madeira *f* de construção
time [taɪm] *n* tempo *m*; (*occasion*) vez *f*; ***~ is up*** acabou o tempo; ***for the ~ being*** nesse meio tempo; ***have a good ~*** passar bem; ***have a good ~!*** divirta-se!; ***what's the ~?, what ~ is it?*** que horas são?; ***the first ~*** a primeira vez; ***four ~s*** quatro vezes; ***~ and again*** várias vezes; ***all the ~*** todo o tempo; ***two / three at a ~*** de dois em dois / de três em três; ***at the same ~*** *speak, reply etc* ao mesmo tempo; (*however*) porém; ***in ~*** com tempo; ***on ~*** pontual; ***in no ~*** num piscar de olhos
'**time bomb** bomba-relógio *f* '**time clock** *in factory* relógio *m* de ponto
time-consuming ['taɪmkənsuːmɪŋ] *adj* demorado '**time difference** diferença *f* de horário '**time-lag** diferença *f* de tempo '**time limit** limite *m* de tempo
timely ['taɪmlɪ] *adj* na hora certa
'**time out** *Am* SPORT tempo *m*
timer ['taɪmər] *device* cronômetro *m*; *person* cronometrador,a *m,f*
'**timesaving** *n* economia *f* de tempo '**timescale** *project*: prazo *m* '**time switch** timer *m* programável '**timetable** *Brit* horário *m*; *school*: programa *m* '**timewarp** timewarp *m* '**time zone** fuso *m* horário
timid ['tɪmɪd] *adj person, smile* tímido; *animal* arredio
timidly ['tɪmɪdlɪ] *adv* timidamente
timing ['taɪmɪŋ] (*choice of a time*) momento *m*; *dancer*: sincronização *f*; *actor*: timing *m*; ***the ~ of the announcement was perfect*** o momento escolhido para o anúncio foi perfeito
tin [tɪn] *metal* estanho *m*; *Brit can* lata *f*
'**tinfoil** papel-alumínio *m*
tinge [tɪndʒ] *n color, sadness*: matiz *m*
tingle ['tɪŋgl] *v/i skin, hands* formigar
♦ **tinker with** ['tɪŋkər] *v/t* mexer com
tinkle ['tɪŋkl] *n bell*: tinido *m*
tinned [tɪnd] *adj Brit* enlatado
'**tin opener** *Brit* abridor *m* de latas, *Port* abre-latas *m*
tinsel ['tɪnsl] enfeite *m* prateado; enfeite *m* dourado
tint [tɪnt] **1** *n color*: tom *m*; *hair*: tonalidade *f* **2** *v/t hair* tingir
tinted ['tɪntɪd] *glasses* com tonalidade; *paper* tingido
tiny ['taɪnɪ] *adj* pequeno
tip[1] [tɪp] *n finger*: ponta *f*; *cigarette*: filtro *m*
tip[2] [tɪp] **1** *n* (*piece of advice*) dica *f*; (*money*) gorjeta *f* **2** *v/t* ⟨*pret & pp* ***tipped***⟩ *waiter etc* dar gorjeta
♦ **tip off** *v/t police, authorities* avisar
♦ **tip over** *v/t pitcher, liquid* entornar; ***he tipped water all over me*** ele derramou água em cima de mim
'**tip-off** dica *f*
tipped [tɪpt] *adj cigarettes* com filtro
'**Tipp-Ex**® *n Brit* líquido *m* corretor
tippy-toe ['tɪpɪtoʊ] *n* ***on ~*** na ponta dos pés
tipsy ['tɪpsɪ] *adj* bêbado
tiptoe ['tɪptoʊ] *n* ***on ~*** na ponta dos pés
tire[1] ['taɪr] *Am* pneu *m*
tire[2] ['taɪr] **1** *v/t* cansar **2** *v/i* cansar-

T

se; ***he never ~s of it*** ele nunca se cansa disso
tired ['taɪrd] *adj* cansado; ***be ~ of s.o. / sth*** estar cansado de alguém / algo
tiredness ['taɪrdnɪs] cansaço *m*
tireless ['taɪrlɪs] *adj efforts* incansável
tiresome ['taɪrsəm] *adj (annoying)* chato
tiring ['taɪrɪŋ] *adj* cansativo
tissue ['tɪʃuː] ANAT tecido *m*; *(handkerchief)* lenço *m* de papel
'tissue paper lenço *m* de papel
tit[1] [tɪt] *bird*: abelharuco *m*
tit[2] [tɪt] ***give ~ for tat*** pagar na mesma moeda
tit[3] [tɪt] *vulg (female breast)* teta *f*
title ['taɪtl] *novel, person etc*: título *m*; LAW título *m* de propriedade
'titleholder SPORT campeão *m*, campeã *f*
'title role *play, movie*: papel *m* principal
titter ['tɪtər] *v/i* rir amarelo
to [tuː] *unstressed* [tə] **1** *prep* para; ***~ Japan*** para o Japão; ***~ Chicago*** para Chicago; ***let's go ~ my place*** vamos à minha casa; ***walk ~ the station*** andar para a estação; ***~ the north / south of …*** para o norte / sul de …; ***give sth ~ s.o.*** dar algo a alguém; ***from Monday ~ Wednesday*** de segunda a quarta-feira; ***from 10 ~ 15 people*** de 10 a 15 pessoas **2** *with verbs*: ***~ speak*** falar; ***~ shout*** gritar; ***learn ~ drive*** aprender a dirigir; ***nice ~ eat*** saboroso; ***too heavy ~ carry*** muito pesado para carregar; ***~ be honest with you …*** para ser sincero com você … **3** *adv* ***~ and fro*** *walk, pace* de um lado para o outro
toad [toʊd] sapo *m*
'toadstool amanita *m*
toast [toʊst] **1** *n* torrada *f*, *drinking*: brinde *m*; ***propose a ~ to s.o.*** fazer um brinde a alguém **2** *v/t drinking* brindar
tobacco [tə'bækoʊ] tabaco *m*, fumo *m*
tobacconist [tə'bækənɪst] *Brit* negociante *m* de fumo
toboggan [tə'bɑːgən] *n* tobogã *m*
today [tə'deɪ] hoje
toddle ['tɑːdl] *v/i child* dar os primeiros passos
toddler ['tɑːdlər] *criança na idade em que aprende a andar*
todo [tə'duː] *fam* alvoroço *m*
toe [toʊ] **1** *n foot*: dedo *m* do pé; *shoe*: ponta *f* **2** *v/t* ***~ the line*** seguir a linha
'toenail unha *f* do pé
toffee ['tɑːfɪ] *Brit* bala *f* de caramelo
together [tə'geðər] *adv* juntos,-as
toil [tɔɪl] *n* trabalho *m* árduo
toilet ['tɔɪlɪt] *place* toalete *m*, banheiro *m*, *Port* casa *f* de banho; *equipment* vaso *m* sanitário; ***go to the ~*** ir a toalete
'toilet paper papel *m* higiênico
toiletries ['tɔɪlɪtrɪz] *npl* artigos *mpl* de uso pessoal
'toilet roll rolo *m* de papel higiênico
token ['toʊkən] *(sign)* sinal *m*; *gambling*: ficha *f*, *Brit (gift token)* vale-presente *m*
told [toʊld] *pret & pp* → ***tell***
tolerable ['tɑːlərəbl] *adj pain etc* suportável; *(quite good)* aceitável
tolerance ['tɑːlərəns] tolerância *f*
tolerant ['tɑːlərənt] *adj* tolerante
tolerate ['tɑːləreɪt] *v/t noise, person* tolerar; ***I won't ~ it!*** não vou tolerar isso!
toll[1] [toʊl] *v/i bell* tocar
toll[2] [toʊl] *n (deaths)* número *m* de mortos
toll[3] [toʊl] *n bridge, road*: pedágio *m*, *Port* portagem *f*, TEL tarifa *f*
'toll booth guichê *m* do pedágio, *Port* portagem *f* **'toll-free** *adj Am* TEL gratuito **'toll road** estrada *f* com pedágio, *Port* estrada *f* com portagem
tomato [tə'meɪtoʊ] tomate *m*
tomato 'ketchup ketchup *m*
tomato 'sauce *(ketchup)* molho *m* de tomate
tomb [tuːm] tumba *f*
tomboy ['tɑːmbɔɪ] moleca *f*
'tombstone lápide *f*
tomcat ['tɑːmkæt] gato *m*
tomorrow [tə'mɔːroʊ] amanhã; ***the day after ~*** depois de amanhã; ***~ morning*** amanhã de manhã

ton [tʌn] tonelada *f*
tone [toʊn] *color, conversation etc*: tom *m*; *musical instrument*: tonalidade *f*; *neighborhood*: nível *m*; ***~ of voice*** tom *m* de voz
◆ **tone down** *v/t demands, criticism* suavizar
toner ['toʊnər] toner *m*
tongs [tɑːŋz] *npl* alicate *m*; *hair*: tesoura *f*
tongue [tʌŋ] *n* língua *f*
tonic ['tɑːnɪk] MED tônico *m*; ***~ water*** água *f* tônica
tonight [tə'naɪt] *adv* esta noite, hoje à noite
tonsil ['tɑːnsl] amígdala *f*
tonsillitis [tɑːnsə'laɪtɪs] amigdalite *f*
too [tuː] *adv* (*also*) também; (*excessively*) demais; ***me ~*** eu também; ***~ big / hot*** grande / quente demais; ***~ much rice*** arroz demais; ***eat ~ much*** comer demais
took [tʊk] *pret* → ***take***
tool [tuːl] ferramenta *f*
toot [tuːt] *v/t & v/i* ~ (***the horn***) buzinar
tooth [tuːθ] 〈*pl* ***teeth***〉 dente *m*
'toothache dor *f* de dente **'toothbrush** escova *f* de dentes **toothless** ['tuːθlɪs] *adj* banguela **'toothpaste** pasta *f* de dentes **'toothpick** palito *m* de dentes
top [tɑːp] **1** *n mountain, list, page*: topo *m*; *tree*: copa *f*; (*upper part*) parte *f* superior; (*lid*) *bottle etc*: tampa *f*; *class, league*: primeiro,-a *m,f*; *clothing* top *m*; MOT *gear* marcha *f* rápida; ***on ~ of*** em cima de; ***at the ~ of*** *list, page, mountain* no topo de; ***get to the ~*** *company, mountain etc*: chegar ao topo; ***be over the ~*** *exaggerated* passar dos limites **2** *adj branches, floor, official* superior; *management, player* principal; *speed, note* máximo; ***a ~ model*** uma top-model **3** *v/t* 〈*pret & pp* ***topped***〉 ***~ped with cream*** coberto com creme
◆ **top up** *v/t glass, tank* encher
top 'hat cartola *f*
top 'heavy *adj structure* sobrecarregado na parte superior
topic ['tɑːpɪk] tópico *m*
topical ['tɑːpɪkl] *adj remarks, events* atual
topless ['tɑːplɪs] *adj* de topless
'topmost *adj branches, floor* superior
topping ['tɑːpɪŋ] *pizza*: cobertura *f*
topple ['tɑːpl] **1** *v/i* desabar **2** *v/t government* derrubar
top 'secret *adj* altamente confidencial
topsy-turvy [tɑːpsɪ'tɜːrvɪ] *adj* (*in disorder*) desordenado; *world* ao revés
torch [tɔːrtʃ] *with flame* tocha *f*; *Brit* lanterna *f*
tore [tɔːr] *pret* → ***tear***[1]
torment ['tɔːrment] **1** *n* tormento *m* **2** [tɔːr'ment] *v/t person, animal* atormentar; ***~ed by doubt*** atormentado pela dúvida
torn [tɔːrn] *pp* → ***tear***[1]
tornado [tɔːr'neɪdoʊ] tornado *m*
torpedo [tɔːr'piːdoʊ] **1** *n* torpedo *m* **2** *v/t fig* torpedear
torrent ['tɑːrənt] *water, lava, words*: torrente *f*
torrential [tə'renʃl] *adj rain* torrencial
tortoise ['tɔːrtəs] tartaruga *f*
torture ['tɔːrtʃər] **1** *n* tortura *f* **2** *v/t* torturar
toss [tɑːs] **1** *v/t ball* arremessar; *rider* derrubar; *salad* misturar; ***~ a coin*** tirar cara ou coroa **2** *v/i* ***~ and turn*** revirar
total ['toʊtl] **1** *n* total *m* **2** *adj sum, amount, disaster, stranger* total; *idiot* completo **3** *v/t* 〈*pret & pp* ***totaled***, *Brit* ***totalled***〉 *Am fam car* destruir
totalitarian [toʊtælɪ'terɪən] *adj* totalitário
totally ['toʊtəlɪ] *adv* totalmente
tote bag ['toʊtbæg] *Am* sacola *f*
totter ['tɑːtər] *v/i person* cambalear
touch [tʌtʃ] **1** *n* (*act of touching, little bit*) toque *m*; *sense* tato *m*; SPORT lateral *f*; ***lose ~ with s.o.*** perder o contato com alguém; ***keep in ~ with s.o.*** manter contato com alguém; ***we kept in ~*** continuamos em contato; ***be out of ~*** *with news, developments* estar desligado; *with language etc* estar fora de contato **2** *v/t also emotionally* tocar **3** *v/i* tocar; *two lines etc* tocar-se

♦**touch down** *v/i airplane* aterrissar; SPORT conquistar o touchdown
♦**touch on** *v/t* (*mention*) mencionar
♦**touch up** *v/t photo* retocar; (*sexually*) apalpar
touch-and-'go ***it was ~*** estava crítico
'touchdown *airplane*: aterrissagem *f*, *Port* aterragem *f*; SPORT touchdown *m*
touching ['tʌtʃɪŋ] *adj* emocionante
'touchline SPORT linha *f* lateral
'touch screen tela *f* sensível ao toque, monitor *m* touch screen
touchy ['tʌtʃɪ] *adj person* muito sensível
tough [tʌf] *adj person, meat, punishment* duro; *question, exam* difícil; *material* resistente
♦**toughen up** ['tʌfn] *v/t person* deixar mais independente
'tough guy *fam* cara *m* durão, *Port* tipo *m* durão
tour [tʊr] **1** *n museum, area*: volta *f* **2** *v/t area* dar uma volta em **3** *v/i* fazer excursão; *band* fazer uma turnê
'tour guide guia *m/f* turístico,-a
tourism ['tʊrɪzm] turismo *m*
tourist ['tʊrɪst] turista *m/f*
'tourist attraction atração *f* turística **'tourist industry** indústria *f* do turismo **'tourist office, tourist infor'mation office** centro *m* de informações turísticas **'tourist season** temporada *f* turística
tournament ['tʊrnəmənt] torneio *m*
'tour operator operador,a *m,f* de turismo
tousled ['taʊzld] *adj hair* desgrenhado
tow [toʊ] **1** *v/t car, boat* rebocar **2** *n* ***give s.o. a ~*** rebocar alguém
♦**tow away** *v/t car* rebocar
toward [tɔːrd] *prep* em direção a; ***my feelings ~ him*** meus sentimentos em relação a ele
towards *Brit* → ***toward***
towel ['taʊl] toalha *f*
tower ['taʊr] *n* torre *f*
♦**tower over** *v/t* dominar
town [taʊn] cidade *f*
town 'center centro *m* da cidade **town centre** *Brit* → ***town center*** **town 'council** conselho *m* municipal **town 'hall** prefeitura *f*, *Port* câmara *f* municipal
'towrope cabo *m* de reboque
toxic ['tɑːksɪk] *adj* tóxico
toxic 'waste resíduo *m* tóxico
toxin ['tɑːksɪn] BIOL toxina *f*
toy [tɔɪ] brinquedo *m*
♦**toy with** *v/t object, idea* brincar com
'toy store loja *f* de brinquedos
trace [treɪs] **1** *n substance*: vestígio *m* **2** *v/t* (*find*) achar; (*follow*) *footsteps* seguir; (*draw*) traçar
track [træk] *n* (*path*) trilho *m*; *on race course* circuito *m*; (*race course itself*) pista *f*; RAIL ferrovia *f*; *on CD* faixa *f*; ***~ 10*** RAIL plataforma 10; ***keep ~ of sth*** manter-se informado de algo
♦**track down** *v/t* localizar
'tracksuit agasalho *m* esportivo, *Port* fato *m* de treino
tractor ['træktər] trator *m*
trade [treɪd] **1** *n* (*commerce*) comércio *m*; (*profession, craft*) ofício *m* **2** *v/i* (*do business*) fazer negócios; ***~ in sth*** comercializar algo **3** *v/t* (*exchange*) trocar; ***~ sth for sth*** trocar algo por algo
♦**trade in** *v/t buying*: dar como parte do pagamento
'trade fair feira *f* comercial **'trademark** marca *f* registrada, *Port* marca *f* registada **'trade mission** representante *m* comercial
trader ['treɪdər] comerciante *m/f*
trade 'secret segredo *m* comercial
trade 'union sindicato *m*
tradition [trə'dɪʃn] tradição *f*
traditional [trə'dɪʃnl] *adj* tradicional
traditionally [trə'dɪʃnlɪ] *adv* tradicionalmente
traffic ['træfɪk] *n roads, airport*: tráfego *m*; *drugs*: tráfico *m*
♦**traffic in** *v/t* ⟨*pret & pp* ***trafficked***⟩ *drugs* traficar
'traffic circle rotatória *f*, *Port* rotunda *f* **'traffic cop** *fam* policial *m* de trânsito **'traffic island** ilha *f* de trânsito **'traffic jam** engarrafamento *m* **'traffic light** semáforo *m* **'traffic lights** *Brit* → ***traffic light*** **'traffic police** polícia *f* rodoviária **'traffic sign** placa *m* de trânsito
tragedy ['trædʒədɪ] tragédia *f*

T

tragic ['trædʒɪk] *adj* trágico

trail [treɪl] **1** *n* (*path*) caminho *m*; *blood*: rastro *m* **2** *v/t* (*follow*) seguir a pista de; (*tow*) rebocar **3** *v/i* (*lag behind*) ficar para trás

trailer ['treɪlər] *pulled by vehicle* reboque *m*, *Port* rulote *m*; (*mobile home*) trailer *m*, *Port* rulote *m*; *movie*: trailer *m*

train[1] [treɪn] *n* trem *m*, *Port* comboio *m*; ***go by ~*** ir de trem

train[2] [treɪn] **1** *v/t team, athlete, employee, dog* treinar **2** *v/i team, athlete* treinar; *teacher etc* instruir-se

trainee [treɪ'niː] estagiário,-a *m,f*

trainer ['treɪnər] SPORT treinador,a *m,f*; *of dog* adestrador,a *m,f*

trainers ['treɪnərz] *npl Brit shoes* tênis *mpl*, *Port* sapatilhas *fpl*

training ['treɪnɪŋ] *new staff*: treinamento *m*; SPORT treino *m*; ***be in ~*** SPORT estar treinando; ***be out of ~*** SPORT estar destreinado

'training course *educational, for job* curso *m* de preparação

'training scheme programa *m* de treinamento

'train station estação *f* de trem, *Port* estação *f*

trait [treɪt] traço *m*

traitor ['treɪtər] traidor,a *m,f*

tram *Brit* → ***streetcar***

tramp [træmp] *n Brit* (*vagabond*) vagabundo,-a *m,f*; *Am* puta *f*

trample ['træmpl] *v/t* ***be ~d to death*** morrer pisoteado; ***be ~d underfoot*** ser pisoteado

♦**trample on** *v/t person, object* pisotear

trampoline ['træmpəliːn] trampolim *m*

trance [træns] transe *m*; ***go into a ~*** entrar em transe

tranquil ['træŋkwɪl] *adj* tranqüilo

tranquility [træŋ'kwɪlətɪ] tranqüilidade *f*

tranquilizer ['træŋkwɪlaɪzər] tranqüilizante *m*

tranquillity *Brit* → ***tranquility***

tranquillizer *Brit* → ***tranquilizer***

transact [træn'zækt] *v/t deal, business* negociar

transaction [træn'zækʃn] transação *f*

transatlantic [trænzət'læntɪk] *adj* transatlântico

transcendental [trænsen'dentl] *adj* transcendental

transcript ['trænskrɪpt] transcrição *f*

transfer [træns'fɜːr] **1** *v/t* ⟨*pret & pp* ***transferred***⟩ transferir **2** *v/i in traveling* trasladar; *from one language to another* passar **3** ['trænsfɜːr] *n also money*: transferência *f*, *travel*: traslado *m*

transferable [træns'fɜːrəbl] *adj ticket* transferível

'transfer fee *football player*: passe *m* de tranferência

transform [træns'fɔːrm] *v/t* transformar

transformation [trænsfər'meɪʃn] transformação *f*

transformer [træns'fɔːrmər] ELEC transformador *m*

transfusion [træns'fjuːʒn] transfusão *f*

transistor [træn'zɪstər] transistor *m*

transit ['trænzɪt] *n* ***in ~*** em trânsito; ***mass ~*** transporte *m* público

transition [træn'zɪʒn] transição *f*

transitional [træn'zɪʒnl] *adj* de transição

'transit lounge *airport*: área *f* de trânsito

'transit passenger passageiro,-a *m,f* em trânsito

translate [træns'leɪt] *v/t & v/i* traduzir

translation [træns'leɪʃn] tradução *f*

translator [træns'leɪtər] tradutor,a *m,f*

transmission [trænz'mɪʃn] *program, disease*, MOT transmissão *f*

transmit [trænz'mɪt] *v/t* ⟨*pret & pp* ***transmitted***⟩ *news, program, disease* transmitir

transmitter [trænz'mɪtər] *radio, TV*: transmissor *m*

transparency [træns'pærənsɪ] PHOT diapositivo *m*

transparent [træns'pærənt] *adj* transparente; (*obvious*) óbvio

transplant MED **1** [træns'plænt] *v/t* transplantar **2** ['trænsplænt] *n* transplante *m*

transport 1 [træn'spɔːrt] *v/t goods, people* transportar **2** ['trænspɔːrt] *n goods, people*: transporte *m*; ***public ~*** *Brit* transporte *m* público
transportation [trænspɔːr'teɪʃn] *goods, people*: transporte *m*; ***means of ~*** meio *m* de transporte; ***public ~*** transporte *m* público; ***Department of Transportation*** *Am* departamento *m* de transportes
transvestite [træns'vestaɪt] travesti *m*
trap [træp] **1** *n for animal, question, set-up etc* armadilha *f*; ***set a ~ for s.o.*** armar uma armadilha para alguém **2** *v/t* ⟨*pret & pp* ***trapped***⟩ *animal* capturar; *person* pegar; ***be ~ped*** *by enemy, flames, landslide etc* ficar preso
'trapdoor alçapão *m*
trapeze [trə'piːz] trapézio *m*
trappings ['træpɪŋz] *npl power*: insígnias *fpl*
trash [træʃ] (*garbage, poor product*) lixo *m*; (*despicable person*) canalha *m/f*
'trashcan *Am* lata *f* de lixo
trashy ['træʃɪ] *adj goods* sem valor; *novel* ruim
traumatic [trɔː'mætɪk] *adj* traumático
traumatize ['trɔːmətaɪz] *v/t* traumatizar
travel ['trævl] **1** *n* viagem *f*; ***~s*** *pl* viagens *fpl* **2** *v/i* ⟨*pret & pp* ***traveled***, *Brit* ***travelled***⟩ viajar **3** *v/t* ⟨*pret & pp* ***traveled***, *Brit* ***travelled***⟩ *miles* percorrer
'travel agency agência *f* de viagens
'travel agent agente *m* de viagens
'travel bag mala *f* (de viagem)
traveler ['trævələr] *Am* viajante *m*
'traveler's check *Am* cheque *m* de viagem
'travel expenses *npl* despesas *fpl* de viagem
'travel insurance seguro *m* de viagem
traveller *Brit* → ***traveler***
'travel program *on TV etc* programa *m* de viagem **travel programme** *Brit* → ***travel program*** **'travelsick** *adj* nauseado; ***he gets ~*** ele fica enjoado em viagens
trawler ['trɔːlər] *boat* arrastão *m*
tray [treɪ] *food etc*: bandeja *f*; *oven*: fôrma *f*; *printer, copier*: gaveta *f*
treacherous ['tretʃərəs] *adj* traiçoeiro; *roads etc* perigoso
treachery ['tretʃərɪ] traição *f*
tread [tred] **1** *n* passo *m*; *staircase*: degrau *m*; *tire*: banda *f* de rodagem **2** *v/i* ⟨*pret* ***trod***, *pp* ***trodden***⟩ andar
♦**tread on** *v/t s.o.'s foot* pisar
treason ['triːzn] traição *f*
treasure ['treʒər] **1** *n also fig* tesouro *m* **2** *v/t gift etc* apreciar muito
treasurer ['treʒərər] tesoureiro,-a *m,f*
Treasury Department ['treʒərɪ] *Am* Secretaria *f* do Tesouro Nacional
treat [triːt] **1** *n* prazer *m*; ***it was a real ~*** foi um grande prazer; ***I have a ~ for you*** tenho uma surpresa agradável para você; ***it's my ~*** (*I'm paying*) eu vou pagar **2** *v/t materials, illness,* (*behave toward*) tratar; ***~ s.o. to sth*** convidar alguém para algo
treatment ['triːtmənt] tratamento *m*
treaty ['triːtɪ] tratado *m*
treble[1] ['trebl] *n* MUS sopranista *m*
treble[2] ['trebl] **1** *adv* ***~ the price*** o triplo do preço **2** *v/i* triplicar
'treble clef clave *f* de sol
tree [triː] árvore *f*
tremble ['trembl] *v/i* tremer
tremendous [trɪ'mendəs] *adj* (*very good*) tremendo; (*enormous*) enorme
tremendously [trɪ'mendəslɪ] *adv* (*very*) tremendamente; (*a lot*) enormemente
tremor ['tremər] *earth*: tremor *m* de terra
trench [trentʃ] trincheira *f*
trend [trend] tendência *f*; (*fashion*) tendência *f* da moda
trendy ['trendɪ] *adj* em moda; *views, person* moderno
trespass ['trespæs] *v/i* transgredir; ***no ~ing*** entrada proibida
♦**trespass on** *v/t s.o.'s land* entrar sem autorização em; *s.o.'s privacy* transgredir
trespasser ['trespæsər] transgressor,a *m,f*; ***~s will be prosecuted*** os transgressores serão processados
trial ['traɪl] LAW julgamento *m*; *equip-*

ment: teste *m*; ***on ~*** LAW em julgamento; ***have sth on ~*** *equipment* ter algo para testar
trial 'period *employee*: período *m* de experiência; *equipment*: prazo *m* de teste
triangle ['traɪæŋgl] triângulo *m*
triangular [traɪ'æŋgjʊlər] *adj* triangular
tribe [traɪb] tribo *f*
tribunal [traɪ'bjuːnl] tribunal *m*
tributary ['trɪbjəterɪ] *river*: afluente *m*
trick [trɪk] **1** *n to deceive, knack* truque *m*; ***play a ~ on s.o.*** pregar uma peça em alguém **2** *v/t* enganar; ***~ s.o. into doing sth*** enganar alguém para que faça algo
trickery ['trɪkərɪ] trapaças *fpl*
trickle ['trɪkl] **1** *n* escorrimento *m*; *fig money*: pingo *m* **2** *v/i* gotejar
trickster ['trɪkstər] vigarista *m/f*
tricky ['trɪkɪ] *adj* (*difficult*) difícil
tricycle ['traɪsɪkl] triciclo *m*
trifle ['traɪfl] *n* (*triviality*) banalidade *f*
trifling ['traɪflɪŋ] *adj concerns, details* trivial
trigger ['trɪgər] *n gun*: gatilho *m*; *camcorder*: disparador *m*
♦**trigger off** *v/t* desencadear
trim [trɪm] **1** *adj* (*neat*) bem-cuidado; *figure* em forma **2** *v/t* ⟨*pret & pp* ***trimmed***⟩ *hedge* podar; *hair, budget, costs* cortar; (*decorate*) *dress* enfeitar **3** *n* (*light cut*) corte *m* (de cabelo); ***just a ~, please*** *to hairdresser* corte somente as pontas, por favor; ***in good ~*** em boas condições
trimming ['trɪmɪŋ] *clothes*: enfeite *m*; ***with all the ~s*** *dish*: com todas as guarnições; *car*: com todos os acessórios
trinket ['trɪŋkɪt] bugiganga *f*
trio ['triːoʊ] MUS trio *m*
trip [trɪp] **1** *n* (*journey*) viagem *f*; *to stores etc* saída *f*; *touristic* excursão *f* **2** *v/i* ⟨*pret & pp* ***tripped***⟩ (*stumble*) tropeçar **3** *v/t* ⟨*pret & pp* ***tripped***⟩ (*make fall*) fazer tropeçar
♦**trip up 1** *v/t* (*make fall*) dar uma rasteira em; (*cause to go wrong*) confundir **2** *v/i* (*stumble*) tropeçar; (*make a mistake*) cometer um erro
tripe [traɪp] *food* bucho *m*
triple ['trɪpl] → ***treble***^{2}
triplets ['trɪplɪts] *npl* trigêmeos *mpl*
tripod ['traɪpɑːd] PHOT tripé *m*
trite [traɪt] *adj* banal
triumph ['traɪʌmf] *n* triunfo *m*
trivial ['trɪvɪəl] *adj* trivial
triviality [trɪvɪ'ælətɪ] trivialidade *f*
trod [trɑːd] *pret* → ***tread***
trodden ['trɑːdn] *pp* → ***tread***
trolleybus ['trɑːlɪbʌs] trolebus *m*
trombone [trɑːm'boʊn] trombone *m*
troops [truːps] *npl* tropas *fpl*
trophy ['troʊfɪ] troféu *m*
tropic ['trɑːpɪk] trópico *m*
tropical ['trɑːpɪkl] *adj* tropical
tropics ['trɑːpɪks] *npl* trópicos *mpl*
trot [trɑːt] *v/i* ⟨*pret & pp* ***trotted***⟩ trotar
trouble ['trʌbl] **1** *n* (*difficulties*) problemas *mpl*; (*inconvenience*) incômodo *m*; (*disturbance*) confusão *f*; ***go to a lot of ~ to do sth*** ter muitos problemas para conseguir fazer algo; ***no ~!*** não se preocupe; ***get into ~*** *with parents, authorities* arranjar problemas **2** *v/t* (*worry*) preocupar; (*bother, disturb*), *of back, liver etc* incomodar
'trouble-free *adj* sem problemas **'troublemaker** criador,a *m,f* de caso **troubleshooter** ['trʌblʃuːtər] (*mediator*) mediador,a *m,f* de conflitos **'troubleshooting** localização *f* de defeitos
troublesome ['trʌblsəm] *adj* problemático
trousers ['traʊzərz] *esp Brit* calça *f*, *Port* calças *fpl* ***a pair of ~*** uma calça, *Port* umas calças
trout [traʊt] ⟨*pl* ***trout***⟩ truta *f*
truant ['truːənt] gazeteiro *m*; ***play ~*** matar aula, *Port* fazer gazeta
truce [truːs] trégua *f*
truck [trʌk] caminhão *m*, *Port* camião *m*
'truck driver motorista *m* de caminhão, *Port* camionista *m* **'truck farm** *Am* fazenda *f* de horticultura **'truck farmer** *Am* horticultor,a *m,f* **'truck stop** *Am* posto *m* de parada de caminhões, *Port* posto *m* de parada de camiões

trudge [trʌdʒ] **1** *v/i* andar exaustivamente **2** *n* caminhada *f*
true [tru:] *adj* verdadeiro; *friend, American* autêntico; ***come ~** hopes, dream* tornar-se realidade
truly ['tru:lɪ] *adv* sinceramente; ***Yours ~*** sinceramente seu (*or* sua)
trumpet ['trʌmpɪt] trompete *m*
trumpeter ['trʌmpɪtər] trompetista *m/f*
trunk [trʌŋk] *tree, body*: tronco *m*; *elephant*: tromba *f*; (*large case*) baú *m*; *Am car*: porta-malas *m*, *Port* porta--bagagens *f*
trust [trʌst] **1** *n* confiança *f*; FIN fundo *m* de investimentos **2** *v/t* confiar em; ***I ~ you*** eu confio em você
trusted ['trʌstɪd] *adj* confiável
trustee [trʌs'ti:] fiduciário *m*
trustful, **trusting** ['trʌstfl, 'trʌstɪŋ] *adj* confiante
'trustworthy *adj* confiável
truth [tru:θ] verdade *f*
truthful ['tru:θfl] *adj account* verdadeiro; *person* sincero
try [traɪ] **1** *v/t* ⟨*pret & pp* ***tried***⟩ experimentar; LAW julgar; ***~ to do sth*** tentar fazer algo **2** *v/i* ⟨*pret & pp* ***tried***⟩ tentar; ***you must ~ harder*** você tem que se esforçar mais **3** *n* tentativa *f*; ***can I have a ~?*** *food*: posso experimentar?, posso provar?; *at doing sth* posso tentar?
♦**try on** *v/t clothes* experimentar, provar
♦**try out** *v/t new machine, new method* experimentar
trying ['traɪɪŋ] *adj* (*annoying*) incômodo
T-shirt ['ti:ʃɜ:rt] camiseta *f*, *Port* T-shirt *f*
tub [tʌb] (*bath*) banheira *f*; *liquid*: balde *m*; *yoghurt, ice cream*: pote *m*
tubby ['tʌbɪ] *adj* atarracado
tube [tu:b] (*pipe*), *toothpaste, ointment*: tubo *m*; *Brit* metrô *m*, *Port* metro *m*
tubeless ['tu:blɪs] *adj tire* sem câmara de ar
tuberculosis [tu:bɜ:rkjə'loʊsɪs] tuberculose *f*
tuck [tʌk] **1** *n dress*: prega *f* **2** *v/t* (*put*) enfiar
♦**tuck away** *v/t* (*put away*) esconder; (*eat quickly*) devorar
♦**tuck in 1** *v/t children* pôr para dormir **2** *v/i* (*start eating*) começar a comer
♦**tuck up** *v/t sleeves etc* arregaçar; ***tuck s.o. up in bed*** pôr alguém na cama
Tuesday ['tu:zdeɪ] terça-feira *f*
tuft [tʌft] *hair*: mecha *f*, *grass*: moita *f*
tug [tʌg] **1** *n* (*pull*) puxão *m*; NAUT rebocador *m* **2** *v/t* ⟨*pret & pp* ***tugged***⟩ (*pull*) puxar
tuition [tu:'ɪʃn] aulas *fpl*
tulip ['tu:lɪp] tulipa *f*
tumble ['tʌmbl] *v/i* cair
'tumbledown *adj* ruinoso
'tumble-dryer secadora *f* (de roupas)
tumbler ['tʌmblər] *glass* copo *m*; *circus*: acrobata *m/f*
tummy ['tʌmɪ] *fam* barriga *f*
'tummy ache dor *f* de barriga
tumor ['tu:mər] tumor *m*
tumour *Brit* → ***tumor***
tumult ['tu:mʌlt] tumulto *m*
tumultuous [tu:'mʌltʊəs] *adj* tumultuoso
tuna ['tu:nə] atum *m*
tune [tu:n] **1** *n* melodia *f*; ***in ~*** *singer, instrument* afinado; ***out of ~*** desafinado **2** *v/t instrument* afinar
♦**tune in** *v/i radio, TV* sintonizar
♦**tune in to** *v/t radio, TV* pôr no canal
♦**tune up 1** *v/i orchestra, players* afinar **2** *v/t engine* retificar
tuneful ['tu:nfl] *adj* melodioso
tuner ['tu:nər] (*hi-fi*) sintonizador *m*
'tune-up *engine*: retificação *f*
tunic ['tu:nɪk] EDUC túnica *f*
tunnel ['tʌnl] *n* túnel *m*
turbine ['tɜ:rbaɪn] turbina *f*
turbulence ['tɜ:rbjələns] *air travel*: turbulência *f*
turbulent ['tɜ:rbjələnt] *adj weather, life, love affair* turbulento
turf [tɜ:rf] gramado *m*; *piece* grama *f*
Turk [tɜ:rk] turco,-a *m,f*
Turkey ['tɜ:rkɪ] Turquia *f*
turkey ['tɜ:rkɪ] peru *m*
Turkish ['tɜ:rkɪʃ] **1** *adj* turco **2** *n language* turco *m*
turmoil ['tɜ:rmɔɪl] agitação *f*

turn [tɜːrn] **1** *n* (*rotation*) rotação *f*; *road*: curva *f*; *vaudeville*: número *m*; ***take ~s in doing sth*** dar voltas para fazer algo; ***it's my ~*** é a minha vez; ***it's not your ~ yet*** ainda não é a sua vez; ***take a ~ at the wheel*** tomar a vez ao volante; ***do s.o. a good ~*** fazer um favor a alguém **2** *v/t wheel* rodar; *corner* dobrar; ***~ one's back on s.o.*** virar as costas para alguém **3** *v/i driver, car, of wheel* rodar; ***~ right / left here*** vire aqui à direita / à esquerda; ***it has ~ed sour / cold*** azedou / esfriou; ***he has ~ed 40*** ele (já) passou dos quarenta

♦**turn around 1** *v/t object* virar; *company* dar uma virada; COM *order* preparar **2** *v/i person* virar; *driver* dar a volta

♦**turn away 1** *v/t* (*send away*) mandar embora **2** *v/i* (*walk away*) ir embora; (*look away*) desviar o olhar

♦**turn back 1** *v/t edges, sheets* dobrar **2** *v/i walkers etc* voltar; *in course of action* voltar atrás

♦**turn down** *v/t offer, invitation* recusar; *volume, TV* abaixar; *heating* diminuir; *edge, collar* dobrar

♦**turn in 1** *v/i* (*go to bed*) deitar-se **2** *v/t to police* entregar

♦**turn off 1** *v/t radio, TV, heater, engine etc* desligar; *faucet* fechar; *fam sexually* tirar a vontade de **2** *v/i car, driver* virar

♦**turn on** *v/t & v/i radio, TV, heater, engine* ligar; *faucet* abrir; *fam* (*sexually*) excitar

♦**turn out 1** *v/t lights* apagar **2** *v/i* ***as it turned out*** como revelou-se

♦**turn over 1** *v/i in bed* revirar-se; *vehicle* capotar **2** *v/t* (*put upside down*), *page* virar; FIN faturar

♦**turn up 1** *v/t collar* dobrar; *volume, heating* aumentar **2** *v/i* (*arrive*) voltar

turning ['tɜːrnɪŋ] volta *f*

'turning point virada *f*

turnip ['tɜːrnɪp] nabo *m*

'turnout *people*: número *m* de presentes **'turnover** FIN faturamento *m* **turnpike** ['tɜːrnpaɪk] *Am* rodovia *f* com pedágio, *Port* rodovia *f* com pedagem **'turn signal** *Am* MOT pisca-pisca *m* **turnstile** ['tɜːrnstaɪl] porta *f* giratória **'turntable** *record player*: prato *m* **'turn-up** *Brit* bainha *f*

turquoise ['tɜːrkwɔɪz] *adj* turquesa

turret ['tʌrɪt] *castle, tank*: torre *f*

turtle ['tɜːrtl] tartaruga *f* marinha

turtleneck 'sweater suéter *m* de gola rolê, *Port* camisola *f* de gola rolê

tusk [tʌsk] *elephant*: presa *f*

tutor ['tuːtər] *university*: tutor,a *m,f*; (***private***) **~** professor,a *m,f* particular

tutorial [tuː'tɔːrɪəl] *n university*: aula *f* complementar

tuxedo [tʌk'siːdoʊ] *Am* smoking *m*

TV [tiː'viː] TV *f*; ***on ~*** na TV

T'V dinner comida *f* pronta congelada **T'V guide** guia *m* de programas de televisão **T'V program** programa *m* de televisão **TV programme** *Brit* → ***TV program***

twang [twæŋ] **1** *n voice*: som *m* fanhoso **2** *v/t guitar string* dedilhar

tweezers ['twiːzərz] *npl* pinça *f*

twelfth [twelfθ] *n & adj* décimo segundo (*m*)

twelve [twelv] doze

twentieth ['twentɪəθ] *n & adj* vigésimo (*m*)

twenty ['twentɪ] vinte

twenty-four-'seven, 24/7 *adv* 24 horas, 7 dias por semana

twice [twaɪs] *adv* duas vezes; ***~ as much*** o dobro

twiddle ['twɪdl] *v/t* virar; ***~ one's thumbs*** *fig* ficar à toa

twig [twɪg] *n* raminho *m*

twilight ['twaɪlaɪt] crepúsculo *m*

twin [twɪn] gêmeo,-a *m,f*

'twin beds *npl* par *m* de camas de solteiro

twinge [twɪndʒ] *pain*: pontada *f*

twinkle ['twɪŋkl] *v/i stars, eyes* brilhar

twin 'room quarto *m* com duas camas de solteiro

'twin town cidade *f* irmã

twirl [twɜːrl] **1** *v/t* girar **2** *n cream etc*: voluta *f*

twist [twɪst] **1** *v/t* retorcer; ***~ one's ankle*** torcer o tornozelo **2** *v/i road, river* serpear **3** *n rope*: torcido *m*; *road*: curva *f* sinuosa; *plot, story*: virada *f*

twisty ['twɪstɪ] *adj road* sinuoso
twit [twɪt] *fam* bobo,-a *m,f*
twitch [twɪʧ] **1** *n nervous* tique *m* nervoso **2** *v/i* (*jerk*) contrair-se convulsivamente
twitter ['twɪtər] *v/i birds* gorjear
two [tu:] dois, duas; ***the ~ of them*** ambos,-as
two-faced ['tu:feɪst] *adj* falso **'two-piece** *woman's suit* conjunto *m* **'two-stroke** *adj engine* de dois tempos **two-way 'traffic** tráfego de mão dupla
tycoon [taɪ'ku:n] magnata *m*
type [taɪp] **1** *n* (*sort*) tipo *m*; ***what ~ of ...?*** que tipo de ... **2** *v/i* (*use a keyboard*) digitar **3** *v/t with a typewriter* datilografar
'typewriter máquina *f* de escrever
typhoid ['taɪfɔɪd] febre *f* tifóide
typhoon [taɪ'fu:n] tufão *m*
typhus ['taɪfəs] tifo *m*
typical ['tɪpɪkl] *adj* típico; ***that's ~ of you / him!*** isso é típico seu / dele
typically ['tɪpɪklɪ] *adv* tipicamente; ***~ American*** tipicamente americano
typist ['taɪpɪst] datilógrafo,-a *m,f*
tyrannical [tɪ'rænɪkl] *adj* tirânico
tyrannize [tɪ'rənaɪz] *v/t* tiranizar
tyranny ['tɪrənɪ] tirania *f*
tyrant ['taɪrənt] tirano,-a *m,f*
tyre *Brit* → ***tire***[1]

U

ugly ['ʌglɪ] *adj* feio
UK [ju:'keɪ] *abbr* (*of **United Kingdom***) Reino *m* Unido
ulcer ['ʌlsər] úlcera *f*
ultimate ['ʌltɪmət] *adj* (*best, definitive*) definitivo; (*final*) final; (*basic*) essencial
ultimately ['ʌltɪmətlɪ] *adv* (*in the end*) no final das contas
ultimatum [ʌltɪ'meɪtəm] ultimato *m*
ultrasound ['ʌltrəsaʊnd] MED ultra-som *m*
ultraviolet [ʌltrə'vaɪələt] *adj* ultravioleta
um'bilical cord [ʌm'bɪlɪkl] cordão *m* umbilical
umbrella [ʌm'brelə] guarda-chuva *m*
umpire ['ʌmpaɪr] *n* árbitro *m*
umpteen [ʌmp'ti:n] *adj fam* mil e um
UN [ju:'en] *abbr* (*of **United 'Nations***) ONU *f*, Organização *f* das Nações Unidas
unable [ʌn'eɪbl] *adj* ***be ~ to do sth*** (*not know how to*) não saber fazer algo; (*not be in a position to*) não poder fazer algo
unacceptable [ʌnək'septəbl] *adj* inaceitável; ***it is ~ that ...*** é inaceitável que ...
unaccountable [ʌnə'kaʊntəbl] *adj* inexplicável
unaccustomed [ʌnə'kʌstəmd] *adj* ***be ~ to sth*** não estar acostumado a algo
unadulterated [ʌnə'dʌltəreɪtɪd] *adj fig* (*absolute*) puro
un-American [ʌnə'merɪkən] *adj not fitting* pouco americano; *activities* antiamericano
unanimous [ju:'nænɪməs] *adj verdict* unânime; ***be ~ on sth*** estar unânime sobre algo
unanimously [ju:'nænɪməslɪ] *adv vote, decide* unanimemente
unapproachable [ʌnə'proʊʧəbl] *adj person* inacessível
unarmed [ʌn'ɑ:rmd] *adj person* desarmado; ***~ combat*** combate *m* desarmado
unassuming [ʌnə'su:mɪŋ] *adj* despretensioso
unattached [ʌnə'tæʧt] *adj* (*without a partner*) sem compromisso
unattended [ʌnə'tendɪd] *adj vehicle*

abandonado; ***leave sth ~*** deixar algo abandonado
unauthorized [ʌn'ɒːθəraɪzd] *adj* não autorizado
unavoidable [ʌnə'vɔɪdəbl] *adj* inevitável
unavoidably [ʌnə'vɔɪdəblɪ] *adv* inevitavelmente; ***be ~ detained*** ser inevitavelmente detido
unaware [ʌnə'wer] *adj* ***be ~ of*** não estar ciente de
unawares [ʌnə'werz] *adv* de imprevisto; ***catch s.o. ~*** pegar alguém de imprevisto
unbalanced [ʌn'bælənst] *adj also* PSYCH desequilibrado
unbearable [ʌn'berəbl] *adj* insuportável
unbeatable [ʌn'biːtəbl] *adj team* imbatível; *quality* insuperável
unbeaten [ʌn'biːtn] *adj team* invicto
unbeknownst [ʌnbɪ'noʊnst] *adj Am* ***~ to*** sem o conhecimento de
unbelievable [ʌnbɪ'liːvəbl] *adj story, excuse* inacreditável; *fam heat, value* incrível; ***he's ~*** *fam very good / bad* ele é incrível
unbias(s)ed [ʌn'baɪəst] *adj person, opinion* imparcial
unblock [ʌn'blɑːk] *v/t pipe* desentupir
unborn [ʌn'bɔːrn] *adj baby* por nascer
unbreakable [ʌn'breɪkəbl] *adj plates etc* inquebrável; *world record* imbatível
unbutton [ʌn'bʌtn] *v/t* desabotoar
uncalled-for [ʌn'kɒːldfɔːr] *adj* desnecessário
uncanny [ʌn'kænɪ] *adj resemblance* estranho; *skill* inexplicável; (*worrying*) *feeling* inquietante
unceasing [ʌn'siːsɪŋ] *adj* incessante
uncertain [ʌn'sɜːrtn] *adj future, weather, origins* incerto; ***be ~ about sth*** estar inseguro sobre algo
uncertainty [ʌn'sɜːrtntɪ] *of the future* incerteza *f*; ***there is still ~ about ...*** ainda há incertezas sobre ...
unchecked [ʌn'tʃekt] *adj* ***let sth go ~*** deixar algo passar sem controle
uncle ['ʌŋkl] tio *m*
uncomfortable [ʌn'kʌmftəbl] *adj chair, hotel, sitting position* desconfortável; ***feel ~ about sth*** *about decision etc* não sentir-se à vontade com algo; ***I feel ~ with him*** me sinto pouco à vontade com ele
uncommon [ʌn'kɑːmən] *adj* incomum; ***it's not ~*** isso não é estranho
uncompromising [ʌn'kɑːmprəmaɪzɪŋ] *adj* inflexível; intransigente
unconcerned [ʌnkən'sɜːrnd] *adj attitude, parents* indiferente; ***be ~ about s.o. / sth*** ser despreocupado sobre alguém / algo
unconditional [ʌnkən'dɪʃnl] *adj* incondicional
unconscious [ʌn'kɑːnʃəs] *adj* MED, PSYCH inconsciente; ***knock ~*** deixar inconsciente; ***be ~ of sth*** *not aware* estar inconsciente de algo
uncontrollable [ʌnkən'troʊləbl] *adj anger, desire, children* incontrolável
unconventional [ʌnkən'venʃnl] *adj* não convencional
uncooperative [ʌnkoʊ'ɑːpərətɪv] *adj* não cooperativo
uncork [ʌn'kɔːrk] *v/t bottle* desarrolhar
uncover [ʌn'kʌvər] *v/t corpse, plot, remains* descobrir
undamaged [ʌn'dæmɪdʒd] *adj* não danificado
undaunted [ʌn'dɔːntɪd] *adj* ***carry on ~*** seguir destemido
undecided [ʌndɪ'saɪdɪd] *adj question* pendente; ***be ~ about s.o. / sth*** estar indeciso em relação a alguém / algo
undeniable [ʌndɪ'naɪəbl] *adj* inegável
undeniably [ʌndɪ'naɪəblɪ] *adv* inegavelmente
under ['ʌndər] **1** *prep* (*beneath*) debaixo de; (*less than*) menos de; ***it is ~ review / investigation*** está sob revisão / investigação **2** *adv* (*anesthetized*) anestesiado
under'age *adj* ***~ drinking*** o consumo de álcool por menores de idade
'underarm *adv throw* abaixo da altura do ombro
'undercarriage trem *m* de pouso
'undercover *adj agent* secreto
under'cut *v/t* ⟨*pret & pp* **undercut**⟩ COM vender por menos que

'underdog azarão *m*
under'done *adj meat* malpassado
under'estimate *v/t person, skills, task* subestimar
underex'posed *adj* PHOT subexposto
under'fed *adj* subnutrido
under'go *v/t* ⟨*pret* ***underwent***, *pp* ***undergone***⟩ *surgery, treatment* submeter-se a; *experiences, refurbishment* passar por
under'graduate *Brit* estudante *m/f* (de graduação)
'underground 1 *adj passages etc* subterrâneo; POL *resistance, newpaper etc* clandestino **2** *adv work* subterrâneo; ***go ~*** POL passar à clandestinidade; **3** *n Brit* metrô *m*, *Port* metro *m*
'undergrowth vegetação *f*
under'hand *adj (devious)* desonesto
under'lie *v/t* ⟨*pret* ***underlay***, *pp* ***underlain***⟩ *(form basis of)* sustentar
under'line *v/t text* sublinhar
underlying [ʌndər'laɪɪŋ] *adj causes, problems* subjacente
under'mine *v/t s.o.'s position, theory* minar
underneath [ʌndər'ni:θ] **1** *prep* embaixo de **2** *adv* debaixo
'underpants *man*: cueca *f*, *Port* cuecas *fpl*; *woman*: calcinha *f*, *Port* cuecas *fpl*
'underpass *pedestrian*: passagem *f* subterrânea
under'privileged *adj* desprivilegiado
under'rate *v/t* depreciar
'undershirt *Am* camiseta *f*
undersized [ʌndər'saɪzd] *adj* muito pequeno
'underskirt saiote *m*
understaffed [ʌndər'stæft] *adj* sem pessoal suficiente
under'stand *v/t & v/i* ⟨*pret & pp* ***understood***⟩ entender, compreender; ***I ~ that you ...*** eu entendi que você ...; ***they are understood to be in Canada*** se supõe que estejam no Canadá
understandable [ʌndər'stændəbl] *adj* compreensível
understandably [ʌndər'stændəblɪ] *adv* compreensivelmente
under'standing 1 *adj person* compreensivo **2** *n problem, situtation*: entendimento *m*; *(agreement)* acordo *m*; ***on the ~ that ...*** com a condição de que ...
'understatement ***to say he was nervous is an ~*** dizer que ele estava nervoso era dizer pouco
under'take *v/t* ⟨*pret* ***undertook***, *pp* ***undertaken***⟩ *task* empreender; ***~ to do sth*** concordar em fazer algo
undertaker ['ʌndərteɪkər] agente *m* funerário
undertaking [ʌndər'teɪkɪŋ] *(enterprise)* empreendimento *m*; *(promise)* garantia *f*
under'value *v/t* depreciar
'underwear roupas *fpl* íntimas
under'weight *adj person* abaixo do peso normal
'underworld *criminal, in mythology* submundo *m*
under'write *v/t* ⟨*pret* ***underwrote***, *pp* ***underwritten***⟩ FIN subscrever
undeserved [ʌndɪ'zɜ:rvd] *adj* imerecido
undesirable [ʌndɪ'zaɪrəbl] *adj features, changes* não desejável; *person* indesejável; ***~ element*** *person* elemento *m* indesejável
undisputed [ʌndɪ'spju:tɪd] *adj champion, leader* incontestável
undo [ʌn'du:] *v/t* ⟨*pret* ***undid***, *pp* ***undone***⟩ *parcel, wrapping* abrir; *s.o. else's work* desfazer; *buttons, shirt* desabotoar; *shoelaces* desamarrar
undoubtedly [ʌn'daʊtɪdlɪ] *adv* indubitavelmente
undreamt-of [ʌn'dremtəv] *adj riches* inimaginável
undress [ʌn'dres] **1** *v/t patient* despir; *children* tirar a roupa de; ***get ~ed*** despir-se **2** *v/i* despir-se
undue [ʌn'du:] *adj (excessive)* excessivo
unduly [ʌn'du:lɪ] *adv punished, blamed* injustamente; *(excessively)* excessivamente
unearth [ʌn'ɜ:rθ] *v/t remains* desenterrar; *fig (find), secret* descobrir
unearthly [ʌn'ɜ:rθlɪ] *adj* ***at this ~ hour*** a esta hora (inoportuna)
uneasy [ʌn'i:zɪ] *adj relationship, peace*

inquieto; ***feel ~ about*** sentir-se inquieto por causa de
uneatable [ʌn'iːtəbl] *adj* não comestível
uneconomic [ʌniːkə'nɑːmɪk] *adj* não rentável
uneducated [ʌn'edʒəkeɪtɪd] *adj* iletrado
unemployed [ʌnɪm'plɔɪd] *adj* desempregado; ***the ~*** os desempregados
unemployment [ʌnɪm'plɔɪmənt] desemprego *m*
unending [ʌn'endɪŋ] *adj* interminável
unequal [ʌn'iːkwəl] *adj* desigual; ***be ~ to the task*** não estar a altura da tarefa
unerring [ʌn'erɪŋ] *adj judgment, instinct* infalível
uneven [ʌn'iːvn] *adj quality, surface, ground* irregular
unevenly [ʌn'iːvnlɪ] *adv distributed, applied* de forma desigual; ***~ matched*** *contestants* de nível desigual
uneventful [ʌnɪ'ventfl] *adj day, journey* sem incidentes
unexpected [ʌnɪk'spektɪd] *adj* inesperado
unexpectedly [ʌnɪk'spektɪdlɪ] *adv* inesperadamente
unfair [ʌn'fer] *adj decision, treatment* injusto
unfaithful [ʌn'feɪθfl] *adj husband, wife* infiel; ***be ~ to s.o.*** ser infiel a alguém
unfamiliar [ʌnfə'mɪljər] *adj technique, surroundings* desconhecido; ***be ~ with sth*** desconhecer algo
unfasten [ʌn'fæsn] *v/t belt* desatar
unfavorable [ʌn'feɪvərəbl] *adj report, review* negativo; *weather conditions* desfavorável
unfavourable *Brit* → ***unfavorable***
unfeeling [ʌn'fiːlɪŋ] *adj person* insensível
unfinished [ʌn'fɪnɪʃt] *adj* inacabado; ***leave sth ~*** deixar algo inacabado
unfit [ʌn'fɪt] *adj physically* fora de forma; *morally* impróprio; ***be ~ to eat / drink*** não ser comestível / potável
unfix [ʌn'fɪks] *v/t part* soltar, separar
unflappable [ʌn'flæpəbl] *adj fam* calmo
unfold [ʌn'foʊld] **1** *v/t sheets, letter* abrir; *one's arms* descruzar **2** *v/i story etc* desenlaçar; *view* abrir-se
unforeseen [ʌnfɔːr'siːn] *adj* imprevisto
unforgettable [ʌnfər'getəbl] *adj* inesquecível
unforgivable [ʌnfər'gɪvəbl] *adj* imperdoável; ***that was ~ of you*** isso é imperdoável
unfortunate [ʌn'fɔːrʧənət] *adj people* infeliz; *event* lamentável; *choice of words* desacertado; ***that's ~ for you*** é muito azar de sua parte
unfortunately [ʌn'fɔːrʧənətlɪ] *adv* infelizmente
unfounded [ʌn'faʊndɪd] *adj suspicions, complaint* infundado
unfriendly [ʌn'frendlɪ] *adj person* antipático; *hotel* desagradável; *welcome* hostil; *software* complicado
unfurnished [ʌn'fɜːrnɪʃt] *adj* desmobiliado
ungodly [ʌn'gɑːdlɪ] *adj* ***at this ~ hour*** a esta hora inoportuna
ungrateful [ʌn'greɪtfl] *adj* mal-agradecido
unhappiness [ʌn'hæpɪnɪs] infelicidade *f*
unhappy [ʌn'hæpɪ] *adj person, look* triste; (*not content*) *customers etc* descontente; ***be ~ with the service / an explanation*** estar descontente com um serviço / uma explicação
unharmed [ʌn'hɑːrmd] *adj* ileso
unhealthy [ʌn'helθɪ] *adj person* doentio; *conditions, food, atmosphere* insalubre; *economy, balance sheet* pouco saudável
unheard-of [ʌn'hɜːrdəv] *adj* sem precedentes
unhurt [ʌn'hɜːrt] *adj passengers* ileso
unhygienic [ʌnhaɪ'dʒiːnɪk] *adj* anti-higiênico
unification [juːnɪfɪ'keɪʃn] unificação *f*
uniform ['juːnɪfɔːrm] **1** *n* uniforme *m* **2** *adj* uniforme
unify ['juːnɪfaɪ] *v/t* ⟨*pret & pp* ***unified***⟩ unificar
unilateral [juːnɪ'lætərəl] *adj* unilateral
unimaginable [ʌnɪ'mædʒɪnəbl] *adj* inimaginável

unimaginative [ʌnɪ'mædʒɪnətɪv] *adj person, approach* sem imaginação
unimportant [ʌnɪm'pɔːrtənt] *adj* sem importância
uninhabitable [ʌnɪn'hæbɪtəbl] *adj* inabitável
uninhabited [ʌnɪn'hæbɪtɪd] *adj building, region* desabitado
uninjured [ʌn'ɪndʒərd] *adj* não ferido
unintelligible [ʌnɪn'telɪdʒəbl] *adj* ininteligível
unintentional [ʌnɪn'tenʃnl] *adj* sem intenção
unintentionally [ʌnɪn'tenʃnlɪ] *adv* sem querer
uninteresting [ʌn'ɪntrəstɪŋ] *adj* desinteressante
uninterrupted [ʌnɪntə'rʌptɪd] *adj sleep, period* ininterrupto
union ['juːnjən] POL união *f*; (*labor union*) sindicato *m*
unique [juː'niːk] *adj* unico; *fam* (*very good*) extraordinário; ***with his own ~ humor / style*** com seu humor / estilo único
unit ['juːnɪt] *measurement, machine*, MIL unidade *f*; (*part with separate function*) módulo *m*; (*department*) departamento *m*; ***we must work together as a ~*** temos que trabalhar juntos como uma unidade
unit 'cost COM custo *m* unitário
unite [juː'naɪt] **1** *v/t* unir **2** *v/i* unir-se
united [juː'naɪtɪd] *adj* unido
United 'Kingdom Reino *m* Unido
United States (**of A'merica**) Estados *mpl* Unidos (da América)
unity ['juːnətɪ] unidade *f*
universal [juːnɪ'vɜːrsl] *adj* universal
universally [juːnɪ'vɜːrsəlɪ] *adv* universalmente
universe ['juːnɪvɜːrs] universo *m*
university [juːnɪ'vɜːrsətɪ] **1** *n* universidade *f*; ***he is at ~*** ele está na universidade **2** *adj* universitário
unjust [ʌn'dʒʌst] *adj* injusto
unkempt [ʌn'kempt] *adj hair* despenteado; *appearance* descuidado
unkind [ʌn'kaɪnd] *adj* cruel
unknown [ʌn'noʊn] **1** *adj* desconhecido **2** *n* ***a journey into the ~*** uma viagem ao desconhecido
unleaded [ʌn'ledɪd] **1** *adj* sem chumbo **2** *n* gasolina *f* sem chumbo
unless [ʌn'les] *conj* a menos que, a não ser que; ***don't say anything ~ you are sure*** não diga nada a não ser que você tenha certeza; ***~ I am mistaken, that's …*** a menos que eu esteja errado, isso é …
unlike [ʌn'laɪk] *prep* diferente de; ***it's ~ him to drink so much*** ele não costuma beber tanto; ***the photograph was completely ~ her*** na fotografia ela está totalmente diferente
unlikely [ʌn'laɪklɪ] *adj* improvável; ***he is ~ to win*** é improvavél que ganhe
unlimited [ʌn'lɪmɪtɪd] *adj* ilimitado
unlisted [ʌn'lɪstɪd] *adj Am* ***be ~*** não constar na lista telefônica
unload [ʌn'loʊd] *v/t truck, goods* descarregar
unlock [ʌn'lɑːk] *v/t door, gate* abrir
unluckily [ʌn'lʌkɪlɪ] *adv* lamentavelmente
unlucky [ʌn'lʌkɪ] *adj day, choice* fatal; *person* azarado; ***that was so ~ for you!*** que azar o seu!
unmade-up [ʌnmeɪd'ʌp] *adj face* sem maquiagem
unmanned [ʌn'mænd] *adj spacecraft* não tripulado
unmarried [ʌn'mærɪd] *adj* solteiro
unmistakable [ʌnmɪ'steɪkəbl] *adj* inconfundível
unmoved [ʌn'muːvd] *adj emotionally* impassível
unmusical [ʌn'mjuːzɪkl] *adj person* sem musicalidade; *sounds* estridente
unnatural [ʌn'nætʃrəl] *adj behavior, reaction* não natural; ***it's not ~ to be annoyed*** é normal ficar irritado
unnecessary [ʌn'nesəserɪ] *adj* desnecessário
unnerving [ʌn'nɜːrvɪŋ] *adj* enervante
unnoticed [ʌn'noʊtɪst] *adj* desapercebido; ***it went ~*** passou desapercebido
unobtainable [ʌnəb'teɪnəbl] *adj goods* não disponível; TEL inacessível
unobtrusive [ʌnəb'truːsɪv] *adj* discreto
unoccupied [ʌn'ɑːkjʊpaɪd] *adj building, house* desocupado; *post* vacante; *room* vazio; *person* sem ocupação

unofficial [ʌnəˈfɪʃl] *adj* inoficial
unofficially [ʌnəˈfɪʃlɪ] *adv* inoficialmente
unpack [ʌnˈpæk] **1** *v/t* desfazer **2** *v/i* desfazer as malas
unpaid [ʌnˈpeɪd] *adj work* não remunerado
unpleasant [ʌnˈpleznt] *adj* desagradável; ***he was very ~ to her*** ele a tratava muito mal
unplug [ʌnˈplʌg] *v/t* 〈*pret & pp* ***unplugged***〉 *TV, computer* desligar na tomada
unpopular [ʌnˈpɑːpjələr] *adj person* impopular; *decision* malquisto
unprecedented [ʌnˈpresɪdentɪd] *adj* sem precedentes
unpredictable [ʌnprɪˈdɪktəbl] *adj person, weather* imprevisível
unpretentious [ʌnprɪˈtenʃəs] *adj person, style, hotel* despretensioso
unprincipled [ʌnˈprɪnsɪpld] *adj* imoral
unproductive [ʌnprəˈdʌktɪv] *adj meeting, discussion* improdutivo; *soil* infértil
unprofessional [ʌnprəˈfeʃnl] *adj person, behavior* não profissional; *workmanship* amador
unprofitable [ʌnˈprɑːfɪtəbl] *adj* não rentável
unpronounceable [ʌnprəˈnaʊnsəbl] *adj* impronunciável
unprotected [ʌnprəˈtektɪd] *adj borders, machine* sem proteção, desprotegido; ***~ sex*** sexo *m* sem proteção, sexo *m* desprotegido
unprovoked [ʌnprəˈvoʊkt] *adj attack* não provocado
unqualified [ʌnˈkwɑːlɪfaɪd] *adj worker, doctor etc* sem qualificação
unquestionably [ʌnˈkwestʃnəblɪ] *adv* sem dúvida
unquestioning [ʌnˈkwestʃnɪŋ] *adj attitude, loyalty* incondicional
unravel [ʌnˈrævl] *v/t* 〈*pret & pp* ***unraveled***, *Brit* ***unravelled***〉 string desenredar; *knitting* desmanchar; *mystery, complexities* solucionar
unreadable [ʌnˈriːdəbl] *adj book* ilegível
unreal [ʌnˈrɪəl] *adj* irreal; ***this is ~!*** *fam* isto é incrível!
unrealistic [ʌnrɪəˈlɪstɪk] *adj* não realista
unreasonable [ʌnˈriːznəbl] *adj person* irracional; *expectation* exagerado
unrelated [ʌnrɪˈleɪtɪd] *adj issues* sem relação; *people* sem parentesco
unrelenting [ʌnrɪˈlentɪŋ] *adj* implacável
unreliable [ʌnrɪˈlaɪəbl] *adj* não muito confiável
unrest [ʌnˈrest] distúrbios *mpl*
unrestrained [ʌnrɪˈstreɪnd] *adj emotions* sem rédeas
unroadworthy [ʌnˈroʊdwɜːrðɪ] *adj* sem condições de circular
unroll [ʌnˈroʊl] *v/t carpet, scroll* desenrolar
unruly [ʌnˈruːlɪ] *adj behavior* incontrolável; *children* desobediente
unsafe [ʌnˈseɪf] *adj bridge, district, beach* perigoso; ***it's ~ to drink / eat*** é arriscado comer / beber
unsanitary [ʌnˈsænɪterɪ] *adj conditions, drains* insalubre
unsatisfactory [ʌnsætɪsˈfæktərɪ] *adj* insatisfatório
unsavory [ʌnˈseɪvərɪ] *adj* repugnante
unsavoury *Brit* → ***unsavory***
unscathed [ʌnˈskeɪðd] *adj* (*not injured*) incólume; (*not damaged*) intacto
unscrew [ʌnˈskruː] *v/t top* abrir; *something screwed on* desparafusar
unscrupulous [ʌnˈskruːpjələs] *adj* inescrupuloso
unselfish [ʌnˈselfɪʃ] *adj* altruísta
unsettled [ʌnˈsetld] *adj issue* não decidido; *weather, stock market, lifestyle* instável; *bills* não pago
unshaven [ʌnˈʃeɪvn] *adj* não barbeado
unsightly [ʌnˈsaɪtlɪ] *adj* feio
unskilled [ʌnˈskɪld] *adj* não qualificado
unsociable [ʌnˈsoʊʃəbl] *adj* insociável
unsophisticated [ʌnsəˈfɪstɪkeɪtɪd] *adj person, beliefs, equipment* não sofisticado
unstable [ʌnˈsteɪbl] *adj person* lábil; *structure, economy* instável

unsteady [ʌn'stedɪ] *adj on one's feet* cambaleante; *ladder* instável
unstinting [ʌn'stɪntɪŋ] *adj* generoso; ***be ~ in one's efforts / generosity*** não poupar esforços / generosidade
unstuck [ʌn'stʌk] *adj* ***come ~*** *notice etc* escapar; *plan, attempt etc* fracassar
unsuccessful [ʌnsək'sesfl] *adj candidate, attempt etc* malsucedido
unsuccessfully [ʌnsək'sesflɪ] *adv try, apply* sem êxito
unsuitable [ʌn'su:təbl] *adj partner, clothing* inadequado, impróprio; *thing to say* inoportuno
unsuspecting [ʌnsəs'pektɪŋ] *adj* inocente
unswerving [ʌn'swɜ:rvɪŋ] *adj loyalty, devotion* inabalável
unthinkable [ʌn'θɪŋkəbl] *adj* impensável
untidy [ʌn'taɪdɪ] *adj room, desk* desarrumado; *hair* despenteado
untie [ʌn'taɪ] *v/t knot, laces, prisoner* soltar
until [ən'tɪl] **1** *prep* até; ***from Monday ~ Friday*** de segunda a sexta-feira; ***I can wait ~ tomorrow*** posso esperar até amanhã; ***not ~ Friday*** não antes de sexta-feira **2** *conj* até que; ***can you wait ~ I'm ready?*** você pode esperar até que eu esteja pronto?; ***they won't do anything ~ you say so*** eles não vão fazer nada até que você o diga
untimely [ʌn'taɪmlɪ] *adj death* prematuro
untiring [ʌn'taɪrɪŋ] *adj efforts* incansável
untold [ʌn'tould] *adj riches, suffering* indescritível; *story* nunca contado
untranslatable [ʌntræns'leɪtəbl] *adj* intraduzível
untrue [ʌn'tru:] *adj* falso
unused[1] [ʌn'ju:zd] *adj goods* novo
unused[2] [ʌn'ju:st] *adj* ***be ~ to sth*** estar desacostumado a algo
unusual [ʌn'ju:ʒl] *adj person, story* inusitado
unusually [ʌn'ju:ʒəlɪ] *adv* inusitadamente
unveil [ʌn'veɪl] *v/t memorial, statue etc* desvelar
unwell [ʌn'wel] *adj* indisposto
unwilling [ʌn'wɪlɪŋ] *adj* ***be ~ to do sth*** não estar disposto a fazer algo
unwillingly [ʌn'wɪlɪŋlɪ] *adv* contra a vontade
unwind [ʌn'waɪnd] **1** *v/t* ⟨*pret & pp* ***unwound***⟩ *tape* desenrolar **2** *v/i tape* desenrolar-se; *story* desenlaçar; (*relax*) relaxar
unwise [ʌn'waɪz] *adj* imprudente
unwrap [ʌn'ræp] *v/t* ⟨*pret & pp* ***unwrapped***⟩ *gift* abrir
unwritten [ʌn'rɪtn] *adj law, rule* não escrito
unzip [ʌn'zɪp] *v/t* ⟨*pret & pp* ***unzipped***⟩ *dress etc* abrir o zíper de; COMPUT descomprimir
up [ʌp] **1** *adv* em cima; ***~ in the sky / ~ on the roof*** (em cima) no céu / no telhado; ***~ here / there*** aqui / lá em cima; ***be ~*** *out of bed* estar acordado; *sun, prices* estar alto; (*be built*) estar construído; *shelves* estar montada; (*have expired*) estar esgotado; ***what's ~?*** *fam* o que foi?; ***~ to the year 1989*** até o ano de 1989; ***he came ~ to me*** ele veio até mim; ***what are you ~ to these days?*** o que você anda fazendo?; ***what are those kids ~ to?*** o que esses garotos estão tramando?; ***be ~ to something*** (***bad***) estar tramando algo; ***I don't feel ~ to it*** não me sinto em condições para isto; ***it's ~ to you*** a decisão é sua; ***it is ~ to them to solve it*** *their duty* é obrigação deles resolver isto; ***be ~ and about*** *after illness* estar recuperado, estar vencido **2** *prep* em cima; ***further ~ the mountain*** mais em cima da montanha; ***he climbed ~ the tree*** ele subiu na árvore; ***they ran ~ the street*** eles correram pela rua; ***the water goes ~ this pipe*** a água sobe pelo cano; ***we traveled ~ to Recife*** subimos até Recife **3** *npl* ***~s and downs*** altos e baixos *mpl*
upbringing ['ʌpbrɪŋɪŋ] educação *f*
upcoming ['ʌpkʌmɪŋ] *adj* (*forthcoming*) próximo
up'date[1] *v/t file, records* atualizar; ***~ s.o. on sth*** pôr alguém a par de algo
'update[2] *n files, records*: atualização *f*;

U

software: última versão *f*; ***can you give me an ~ on the situation?*** você pode pôr-me a par da situação?
up'grade *v/t computers etc* atualizar; (*replace with new versions*) modernizar; *ticket* fazer um upgrade de; *product* melhorar
upheaval [ʌp'hiːvl] *emotional* comoção *f*; *physical* transtorno *m*; *political, social* agitação *f*
'uphill 1 *adv walk* morro acima **2** *adj* penoso; *struggle* difícil
up'hold *v/t* ⟨*pret & pp* ***upheld***⟩ *traditions, rights* defender, manter; (*vindicate*) confirmar
upholstery [ʌp'hoʊlstərɪ] *padding* estofado *m*; *coverings* tecido *m* para forrar
'upkeep *old buildings, parks etc*: manutenção *f*
'upload *v/t* COMPUT fazer o upload de
up'market *adj Brit restaurant, hotel* de categoria
upon [ə'pɑːn] *prep* → ***on***
upper ['ʌpər] *adj part, atmosphere* superior; *stretches of river* alto; *deck* de cima
'upper class *adj accent, family* de classe alta
upper 'classes *npl* classe *f* alta
'upright[1] 1 *adj citizen* honrado **2** *adv sit* direito
'upright[2], **upright 'piano** *n* piano *m* vertical
'uprising revolta *f*
'uproar (*loud noise*) barulheira *f*; (*protest*) tumulto *m*
'upscale *adj Am restaurant, hotel* de alta categoria
up'set 1 *v/t* ⟨*pret & pp* ***upset***⟩ *drink, glass* derrubar; (*make sad*) perturbar; (*annoy*) chatear **2** *adj emotionally* perturbado; (*annoyed*) chateado; ***get ~ about sth*** ficar perturbado / chateado com algo; ***have an ~ stomach*** estar com dor de barriga
up'setting *adj* (*saddening*) perturbante; (*annoying*) irritante
'upshot (*result, outcome*) resultado *m*
upside 'down *adv* de cabeça para baixo; ***turn sth ~ down*** *box etc* virar algo de cabeça para baixo
upstairs ['ʌpsterz] **1** *adv* no andar de cima **2** *adj room* de andar de cima
'upstart arrivista *m/f*
up'stream *adv* rio acima
'uptake *fam* ***be quick on the ~*** compreender as coisas com facilidade; ***be slow on the ~*** compreender as coisas com dificuldade
up'tight *adj fam* (*nervous*) tenso; (*inhibited*) inibido
up-to-'date *adj information* atualizado; *fashions* atual
'upturn *economy*: melhora *f*
upward ['ʌpwərd] *adv fly, move* para cima; ***~ of 10,000*** acima de 10.000
upwards *Brit* → ***upward***
uranium [jʊ'reɪnɪəm] urânio *m*
urban ['ɜːrbən] *adj* urbano
urbanization [ɜːrbənaɪ'zeɪʃn] urbanização *f*
urchin ['ɜːrʧɪn] moleque *m* de rua, moleca *f* de rua
urge [ɜːrdʒ] **1** *n* impulso *m* **2** *v/t* ***~ s.o. to do sth*** insistir com alguém para fazer algo
◆ **urge on** *v/t* (*encourage*) encorajar
urgency ['ɜːrdʒənsɪ] urgência *f*
urgent ['ɜːrdʒənt] *adj job, letter* urgente; ***be in ~ need of sth*** estar necessitando de algo urgentemente
urinate ['jʊrəneɪt] *v/i* urinar
urine ['jʊrɪn] urina *f*
urn [ɜːrn] urna *f*
Uruguay ['jʊrəgwaɪ] Uruguai *m*
Uruguayan ['jʊrəgwaɪən] **1** *adj* uruguaio **2** *n* uruguaio,-a *m,f*
us [ʌs] *pron* nos; ***that's for ~*** é para nós; ***who's that? – it's ~*** quem é? – somos nós
US [juː'es] *abbr* (*of* ***United States***) **1** *n* Estados *mpl* Unidos da América, EUA **2** *adj* estadunidense
USA [juːes'eɪ] *abbr* (*of* ***United States of America***) Estados *mpl* Unidos da América, EUA
usable ['juːzəbl] *adj* utilizável
usage ['juːzɪdʒ] uso *m*
USB port [juːes'biː] COMPUT porta *f* USB
use 1 [juːz] *v/t tool* utilizar; *skills, knowledge, car, pej person* usar; *word* empregar; *a lot of gas* consumir; ***I***

could ~ a drink *fam* um drinque não seria mal **2** [juːs] *n* uso *m*, utilização *f*; ***be of great ~ to s.o.*** ser de grande utilidade para alguém; ***be of no ~ to s.o.*** não ter nenhuma utilidade para alguém; ***is that of any ~?*** isto serve para algo?; ***it's no ~*** não adianta; ***it's no ~ trying*** não vale a pena tentar, não faz sentido tentar

♦**use up** *v/t* acabar

used[1] [juːzd] *adj car etc* de segunda mão, usado

used[2] [juːst] *adj* ***be ~ to s.o. / sth*** estar acostumado com alguém / algo; ***get ~ to s.o. / sth*** acostumar-se a alguém / algo; ***be ~ to doing sth*** estar acostumado a fazer algo; ***get ~ to doing sth*** acostumar-se a fazer algo

used[3] [juːst] ***I ~ to like / know him*** antes eu gostava dele / conhecia ele; ***I don't work there now, but I ~ to*** eu não trabalho mais lá

useful ['juːsfʊl] *adj* útil

usefulness ['juːsfʊlnɪs] utilidade *f*

useless ['juːslɪs] *adj* inútil; *fam person, machine, computer* imprestável; ***it's ~ trying*** não vale a pena tentar

user ['juːzər] *product*: usuário,-a *m,f*, *Port* utente *m/f*

user'friendly *adj software, device* fácil de utilizar

usher ['ʌʃər] *n wedding*: *responsável por indicar os assentos aos convidados*

♦**usher in** *v/t new era* anunciar

usherette [ʌʃə'ret] *theater etc*: lanterninha *f*, *Port* arrumadora *f*

usual ['juːʒl] *adj* habitual; ***as ~*** como de costume; ***the ~, please*** o de sempre, por favor

usually ['juːʒəlɪ] *adv* normalmente

utensil [juː'tensl] utensílio *m*

uterus ['juːtərəs] útero *m*

utility [juː'tɪlətɪ] (*usefulness*) utilidade *f*; ***public ~*** utilidade *f* pública

u'tility pole *Am* poste *m* telegráfico

utilize ['juːtɪlaɪz] *v/t* utilizar

utmost ['ʌtmoʊst] **1** *adj* extremo, máximo **2** *n* ***do one's ~*** dar o máximo

utter ['ʌtər] **1** *adj* total, completo **2** *v/t sound* emitir

utterly ['ʌtərlɪ] *adv* totalmente, completamente

U-turn ['juːtɜːrn] retorno *m*; *fig policy*: virada *f* de 180 graus

V

V

vacancy ['veɪkənsɪ] *Brit at work* vaga *f*

vacant ['veɪkənt] *adj building* vazio; *position* vacante; *look, expression* vago

vacantly ['veɪkəntlɪ] *adv* vagamente

vacate [veɪ'keɪt] *v/t room* desocupar

vacation [veɪ'keɪʃn] *n Am, Brit university*: férias *fpl*; ***be on ~*** estar em férias; ***go to … on ~*** ir para … de férias

vacationer [veɪ'keɪʃənər] *Am* pessoa *f* que está de férias

vaccinate ['væksɪneɪt] *v/t* vacinar; ***be ~d against …*** estar vacinado contra …

vaccination [væksɪ'neɪʃn] vacinação *f*

vaccine ['væksiːn] vacina *f*

vacuum ['vækjʊəm] **1** *n* PHYS vácuo *m*; *fig* vazio *m* **2** *v/t floors* aspirar

'vacuum cleaner aspirador *m* de pó

'vacuum flask garrafa *f* térmica, *Port* termo *m*

vacuum-'packed *adj* embalado a vácuo

vagabond ['vægəbɑːnd] *n* errante *m*

vagina [və'dʒaɪnə] vagina *f*

vaginal ['vædʒɪnl] *adj* vaginal

vagrant ['veɪgrənt] *n* vagabundo,-a *m,f*

vague [veɪg] *adj answer, wording* não claro; *feeling, resemblance* vago; *taste of sth* leve; ***he was very ~ about it***

ele não foi muito preciso em relação a isso
vaguely ['veɪglɪ] *adv answer,* (*slightly*) vagamente; *possible* bem pouco
vain [veɪn] **1** *adj person* vaidoso; *hope* vão (vã) **2** *n* **in ~** em vão; ***their efforts were in ~*** seus esforços foram em vão
valentine ['væləntaɪn] *card* cartão *m* do dia dos namorados; ***Valentine's Day*** o dia dos namorados
valet **1** ['væleɪ] *n person* camareiro,-a *m,f* **2** ['vælət] *v/t* ***have one's car ~ed*** ter o carro lavado e limpo por dentro
'valet parking serviço *m* de estacionamento
'valet service *clothes*: serviço *m* de lavanderia; *cleaning cars*: lava-carros *m*
valiant ['væljənt] *adj* corajoso
valiantly ['væljəntlɪ] *adv* corajosamente
valid ['vælɪd] *adj* válido
validate ['vælɪdeɪt] *v/t with official stamp* validar; *alibi* confirmar
validity [və'lɪdətɪ] validade *f*
valley ['vælɪ] vale *m*
valuable ['væljʊbl] **1** *adj* valioso **2** *n* **~*s*** objetos *mpl* de valor
valuation [væljʊ'eɪʃn] avaliação *f*; ***at his ~*** segundo a sua estimativa
value ['vælju:] **1** *n* valor *m*; ***be good ~*** ser uma boa compra; ***I didn't get ~ for money*** não valeu pelo preço; ***rise / fall in ~*** aumentar em / perder valor **2** *v/t s.o.'s friendship, one's freedom* valorizar; ***I ~ your advice*** dou (muito) valor a seus conselhos; ***have an object ~d*** mandar avaliar um objeto
'value-added tax *Brit* imposto *m* sobre circulação de mercadorias, *Port* imposto *m* sobre o valor acrescentado
valve [vælv] válvula *f*
van [væn] furgão *m*, *Port* carrinha *f*
vandal ['vændl] vândalo *m*
vandalism ['vændəlɪzm] vandalismo *m*
vandalize ['vændəlaɪz] *v/t* vandalizar
vanguard ['vængɑ:rd] *n* ***be in the ~ of*** *fig* estar na vanguarda de
vanilla [və'nɪlə] **1** *n* baunilha *f* **2** *adj* (de) baunilha
vanish ['vænɪʃ] *v/i* desaparecer
vanity ['vænətɪ] *person*: vaidade *f*; *hopes*: vazio *m*
'vanity case necessaire *m*
vantage point ['væntɪdʒ] *on hill etc* mirante *m*
vapor ['veɪpər] *Am* vapor *m*
vaporize ['veɪpəraɪz] *v/t* vaporizar
'vapor trail *Am airplane*: trilha *f* de condensação
vapour *Brit* → ***vapor***
variable ['verɪəbl] **1** *adj amount* variável; *moods, weather* instável **2** *n* MATH, COMPUT variável *f*
variant ['verɪənt] *n* variante *f*
variation [verɪ'eɪʃn] variação *f*
varicose 'vein ['værɪkoʊs] variz *f*
varied ['verɪd] *adj* variado
variety [və'raɪətɪ] variedade *f*; ***a ~ of things to do*** mil coisas para fazer
various ['verɪəs] *adj* (*several*) vários; (*different*) diversos
varnish ['vɑ:rnɪʃ] **1** *n wood*: verniz *m*; *Brit fingernails*: esmalte *m*, *Port* verniz *m* **2** *v/t wood* envernizar; *Brit fingernails* pintar
vary ['verɪ] ⟨*pret & pp* ***varied***⟩ **1** *v/i* variar; ***it varies*** depende **2** *v/t* variar
vase [veɪz] *n* vaso *m*
vasectomy [və'sektəmɪ] vasectomia *f*
vast [væst] *adj* vasto
vastly ['væstlɪ] *adv* enormemente
VAT [vi:eɪ'ti:, væt] *abbr* (*of* ***value added tax***) *Brit* ICM *m*, *Port* IVA *m*
Vatican ['vætɪkən] Vaticano *m*
vaudeville ['vɔ:dvɪl] *adj Am* teatro *m* de revista
vault[1] [vɒ:lt] *n roof*: abóbada *f*; **~*s*** *pl* (*cellar*) porão *m*
vault[2] [vɒ:lt] **1** *n* SPORT salto *m* **2** *v/t beam etc* saltar
VCR [vi:si:'ɑ:r] *abbr* (*of* ***video cassette recorder***) vídeocassete *m*
veal [vi:l] carne *f* de novilho
veg *Brit* → ***vegetable***
vegan ['vi:gn] **1** *adj* vegano **2** *n* vegano,-a *m,f*
vegetable ['vedʒtəbl] vegetal *m*
vegetarian [vedʒɪ'terɪən] **1** *adj* vegetariano **2** *n* vegetariano,-a *m,f*

vegetarianism [vedʒɪ'terɪənɪzm] vegetarianismo *m*
vegetation [vedʒɪ'teɪʃn] vegetação *f*
vehemence ['viːəməns] veemência *f*
vehement ['viːəmənt] *adj* veemente
vehemently ['viːəməntlɪ] *adv* veementemente
vehicle ['viːɪkl] *also information etc*: veículo *m*
veil [veɪl] **1** *n* véu *m* **2** *v/t* encobrir
vein [veɪn] ANAT veia *f*; ***in this ~*** *fig* nessa linha
Velcro® ['velkroʊ] *n* velcro *m*
velocity [vɪ'lɑːsətɪ] velocidade *f*
velvet ['velvət] *n* veludo *m*
velvety ['velvətɪ] *adj* aveludado
vendetta [ven'detə] rixa *f*
vending machine ['vendɪŋ] máquina *f* de venda automática
vendor ['vendər] LAW vendedor,a *m,f*
veneer [və'nɪr] *wood*: revestimento *m*; *politeness etc*: aparência *f*
venerable ['venərəbl] *adj* venerável
venerate ['venəreɪt] *v/t* venerar
veneration [venə'reɪʃn] veneração *f*
venereal disease [və'nɪrɪəl] doença *f* venérea
venetian 'blind [və'niːʃn] persiana *f*
Venezuela [venə'zweɪlə] Venezuela
Venezuelan [venə'zweɪlən] **1** *adj* venezuelano **2** *n* venezuelano,-a *m,f*
vengeance ['vendʒəns] vingança *f*; ***with a ~*** com mais intensidade
venison ['venɪsn] carne *f* de veado
venom ['venəm] *also fig* veneno *m*
venomous ['venəməs] *snake*, *also fig* venenoso
vent [vent] *n air*: saída *f* de ar; ***give ~ to*** *feelings* expressar
ventilate ['ventɪleɪt] *v/t* ventilar
ventilation [ventɪ'leɪʃn] ventilação *f*
venti'lation shaft poço *m* de ventilação
ventilator ['ventɪleɪtər] ventilador *m*; MED respirador *m*
ventriloquist [ven'trɪləkwɪst] ventríloquo *m*
venture ['ventʃər] **1** *n* (*undertaking*) iniciativa *f*, COM empresa *f* **2** *v/i* aventurar-se
venue ['venjuː] *meeting, concert etc*: sala *f*; *football match etc*: local *m*
veranda [və'rændə] varanda *f*
verb [vɜːrb] verbo *m*
verbal ['vɜːrbl] *adj* verbal
verbally ['vɜːrbəlɪ] *adv* verbalmente
verbatim [vɜːr'beɪtɪm] *adv* literalmente
verdict ['vɜːrdɪkt] LAW veredicto *m*; (*opinion, judgment*) opinião *f*; ***bring in a ~ of guilty / not guilty*** pronunciar o veredicto de culpado / inocente
verge [vɜːrdʒ] *n road*: beira *f*, *Port* berma *f*; ***be on the ~ of …*** *ruin, collapse* estar à beira de …; ***be on the ~ of tears*** estar quase chorando
♦**verge on** *v/t* beirar
verification [verɪfɪ'keɪʃn] verificação *f*; (*confirmation*) confirmação *f*
verify ['verɪfaɪ] *v/t* ⟨*pret & pp* ***verified***⟩ (*check*) verificar; (*confirm*) confirmar
vermicelli [vɜːrmɪ'tʃelɪ] aletria *f*
vermin ['vɜːrmɪn] *npl* pragas *fpl* domésticas
vermouth [vər'muːθ] vermute *m*
vernacular [vər'nækjələr] *n* linguagem *f* coloquial
versatile ['vɜːrsətəl] *adj* versátil
versatility [vɜːrsə'tɪlətɪ] versatilidade *f*
verse [vɜːrs] verso *m*
versed [vɜːrst] *adj* ***be well ~ in a subject*** ser perito em uma matéria
version ['vɜːrʃn] versão *f*
versus ['vɜːrsəs] *prep* SPORT, LAW contra
vertebra ['vɜːrtɪbrə] vértebra *f*
vertebrate ['vɜːrtɪbreɪt] *n* vertebrado *m*
vertical ['vɜːrtɪkl] *adj* vertical
vertigo ['vɜːrtɪgoʊ] vertigem *f*
very ['verɪ] **1** *adv* muito; ***was it cold? – not ~*** estava frio? - não muito; ***the ~ best*** o melhor de todos; ***~ much*** muitíssimo **2** *adj* ***in the ~ act*** em flagrante; ***that's the ~ thing I need*** isso é exatamente o que eu preciso; ***the ~ thought of it*** só de pensar nisso; ***right at the ~ top / bottom*** bem em cima / no fundo
vessel ['vesl] NAUT navio *m*
vest [vest] *Am* colete *m*; *Brit* camiseta *f*, *Port* camisola *f* interior

vestige ['vestɪdʒ] *previous civilization etc*: vestígio *m*; *truth*: indício *m*
vet[1] [vet] *n* (*veterinary surgeon*) veterinário,-a *m,f*
vet[2] [vet] *v/t* ⟨*pret & pp* ***vetted***⟩ *applicants etc* investigar
vet[3] [vet] MIL *Am fam* veterano,-a *m,f*
veteran ['vetərən] **1** *adj* (*old*) antigo; (*old and experienced*) veterano **2** *n* veterano,-a *m,f*
veterinarian [vetərə'nerɪən] *Am* veterinário,-a *m,f*
veterinary surgeon → ***veterinarian***
veto ['vi:toʊ] **1** *n* veto *m* **2** *v/t* vetar
vex [veks] *v/t* (*concern, worry*) preocupar
vexed [vekst] *adj* (*worried*) preocupado; ***the ~ question of …*** a preocupante questão de …
via ['vaɪə] *prep* via
viable ['vaɪəbl] *adj life form, company, plan* viável
vibrate [vaɪ'breɪt] *v/i* vibrar
vibration [vaɪ'breɪʃn] vibração *f*
vicar ['vɪkər] vigário *m*
vicarage ['vɪkərɪdʒ] casa *f* do vigário
vice[1] [vaɪs] vício *m*
vice[2] [vaɪs] *Brit* torninho *m*
'vice president vice-presidente *m/f*
'vice squad divisão *f* de ética e disciplina
vice versa [vaɪs'vɜ:rsə] *adv* vice-versa
vicinity [vɪ'sɪnətɪ] vizinhança *f*; ***in the ~ of*** *the church etc* nas vizinhanças de; *$500 etc* por perto de
vicious ['vɪʃəs] *adj dog* traiçoeiro; *attack, temper* cruel
vicious 'circle círculo *m* vicioso
viciously ['vɪʃəslɪ] *adv* brutalmente
victim ['vɪktɪm] vítima *f*
victimize ['vɪktɪmaɪz] *v/t* vitimar
victor ['vɪktər] vencedor,a *m,f*
victorious [vɪk'tɔ:rɪəs] *adj* vitorioso
victory ['vɪktərɪ] vitória *f*; ***win a ~ over …*** obter uma vitória sobre …
video ['vɪdɪoʊ] **1** *n* vídeo *m*; ***have sth on ~*** ter algo em vídeo **2** *v/t* filmar; (*tape off TV*) gravar da TV
'video camera filmadora *f* **'video cassette** videocassete *m* **'video conference** videoconferência *f* **'video game** videogame *m* **'videophone** videofone *m* **'video recorder** vídeo *m* **'video recording** gravação *f* em vídeo **'videotape** videotape *m*
vie [vaɪ] *v/i* competir
Vietnam [vɪet'næm] Vietnã *m*, *Port* Vietname *m*
Vietnamese [vɪetnə'mi:z] **1** *adj* vietnamita **2** *n* vietnamita *m/f*; *language* vietnamita *m*
view [vju:] **1** *n* vista *f*; *situation*: estimativa *f*; ***in ~ of*** em vista de; ***be on ~*** *paintings* estar exposto ao público; ***with a ~ to doing sth*** visando fazer algo **2** *v/t* ver; *TV program* assistir
viewer ['vju:ər] TV telespectador,a *m,f*
'viewfinder PHOT visor *m*
'viewpoint ponto *m* de vista
vigor ['vɪgər] *Am* (*energy*) vigor *m*
vigorous ['vɪgərəs] *adj person* vigoroso; *shake* forte; *denial* categórico
vigorously ['vɪgərəslɪ] *adv shake* fortemente; *deny* categoricamente
vigour *Brit* → ***vigor***
vile [vaɪl] *adj smell* asqueroso; *thing to do* vil
villa ['vɪlə] mansão *f*
village ['vɪlɪdʒ] aldeia *f*
villager ['vɪlɪdʒər] aldeão *m*, aldeã *f*
villain ['vɪlən] vilão *m*, vilã *f*
vindicate ['vɪndɪkeɪt] *v/t* (*show to be correct*) justificar; (*show to be innocent*) inocentar; ***I feel ~d*** me sinto justificado
vindictive [vɪn'dɪktɪv] *adj* vingativo
vindictively [vɪn'dɪktɪvlɪ] *adv* vingativamente
vine [vaɪn] vinha *f*
vinegar ['vɪnɪgər] vinagre *m*
vineyard ['vɪnjɑ:rd] vinhedo *m*
vintage ['vɪntɪdʒ] **1** *n of wine* vindima *f*; ***it's a good ~*** é uma boa safra **2** *adj* (*classic*) clássico
viola [vɪ'oʊlə] MUS viola *f*
violate ['vaɪəleɪt] *v/t* violar
violation [vaɪə'leɪʃn] *rules, sanctity*: violação *f*, *Am traffic*: infração *f*
violence ['vaɪələns] violência *f*; ***outbreak of ~*** explosão *f* de violência
violent ['vaɪələnt] *adj person, movie,*

gale violento; ***have a ~ temper*** ter um temperamento violento
violently ['vaɪələntlɪ] *adv react* violentamente; *object* veementemente; ***fall ~ in love with s.o.*** apaixonar-se perdidamente por alguém
violet ['vaɪələt] *n color, plant* violeta *f*
violin [vaɪə'lɪn] violino *m*
violinist [vaɪə'lɪnɪst] violinista *m/f*
VIP [viːaɪ'piː] *abbr* (*of* ***very important person***) VIP *m/f*
viper ['vaɪpər] *snake* víbora *f*
viral ['vaɪrəl] *adj infection* virótico
virgin ['vɜːrdʒɪn] virgem *m/f*
virginity [vɜːr'dʒɪnətɪ] virgindade *f*; ***lose one's ~*** perder a virgindade
Virgo ['vɜːrgoʊ] ASTROL Virgem *m*
virile ['vɪrəl] *adj man* viril; *prose* pesado
virility [vɪ'rɪlətɪ] *sexual* virilidade *f*
virtual ['vɜːrtʃʊəl] *adj* virtual
virtually ['vɜːrtʃʊəlɪ] *adv* (*almost*) virtualmente
virtual re'ality realidade *f* virtual
virtue ['vɜːrtʃuː] virtude *f*; ***in ~ of*** em virtude de
virtuoso [vɜːrtʊ'oʊzoʊ] MUS virtuoso,-a *m,f*
virtuous ['vɜːrtʃʊəs] *adj* virtuoso
virulent ['vɪrʊlənt] *adj disease* virulento; *attack, hatred* feroz
virus ['vaɪrəs] MED, COMPUT vírus *m*
visa ['viːzə] visto *m*
vise [vaɪz] *Am* torninho *m*
visibility [vɪzə'bɪlətɪ] visibilidade *f*
visible ['vɪzəbl] *adj object, difference* visível; *anger* evidente; ***not ~ to the naked eye*** invisível a olho nu
visibly ['vɪzəblɪ] *adv different* visivelmente; ***he was ~ moved*** ele estava visivelmente comovido
vision ['vɪʒn] (*eyesight*) vista *f*; REL visão *f*
visit ['vɪzɪt] **1** *n* visita *f*; ***pay a ~ to the doctor / dentist*** visitar o médico / /dentista; ***pay s.o. a ~*** visitar alguém **2** *v/t* visitar; *doctor, dentist* consultar
♦ **visit with** *v/t Am* bater um papo com
visiting card ['vɪzɪtɪŋ] cartão *m* de visita
'visiting hours *hospital*: horário *m* de visitas
visitor ['vɪzɪtər] (*guest, tourist*) visitante *m/f*
visor ['vaɪzər] viseira *f*
visual ['vɪʒʊəl] *adj* visual
visual 'aid recurso *m* visual
visual dis'play unit monitor *m*
visualize ['vɪʒʊəlaɪz] *v/t* visualizar; (*foresee*) prever
visually ['vɪʒʊlɪ] *adv* visualmente
visually im'paired *adj* deficiente visual
vital ['vaɪtl] *adj* (*essential*) vital; ***it is ~ that ...*** é essencial que ...
vitality [vaɪ'tælətɪ] *person*: vitalidade *f*, energia *f*; *city etc*: dinamismo *m*
vitally ['vaɪtəlɪ] *adv* ***~ important*** de importância vital
vital 'organs órgãos *mpl* vitais
vital sta'tistics *woman*: medidas *fpl*
vitamin ['vaɪtəmɪn] vitamina *f*
'vitamin pill pílula *f* de vitamina
vitriolic [vɪtrɪ'ɑːlɪk] *adj humor, criticism* ácido
vivacious [vɪ'veɪʃəs] *adj* vivaz
vivacity [vɪ'væsətɪ] vivacidade *f*
vivid ['vɪvɪd] *adj color* vivo; *memory* vívido; *imagination* fértil
vividly ['vɪvɪdlɪ] *adv* (*brightly*) vivamente; (*clearly*) vividamente
V-neck ['viːnek] decote *m* em V
vocabulary [voʊ'kæbjʊlerɪ] vocabulário *m*
vocal ['voʊkl] *adj* vocal; (*expressing opinions*) expressivo
'vocal cords cordas *fpl* vocais
'vocal group MUS grupo *m* vocal
vocalist ['voʊkəlɪst] MUS vocalista *m/f*
vocals ['voʊklz] ***on ~: Paul McCartney*** vocal: Paul McCartney
vocation [və'keɪʃn] (*calling*) vocação *f*; (*profession*) profissão *f*
vocational [və'keɪʃnl] *adj guidance* vocacional
vodka ['vɑːdkə] vodca *f*
vogue [voʊg] moda *f*; ***be in ~*** estar em moda
voice [vɔɪs] **1** *n* voz *f* **2** *v/t opinions* expressar
voice-activated ['vɔɪsæktɪveɪtɪd] *adj* activado por voz
'voicemail correio *m* de voz
void [vɔɪd] **1** *n* vazio *m* **2** *adj* ***~ of*** ca-

V

rente de
volatile ['vɑːlətəl] *adj personality, situation* volúvel
volcano [vɑːl'keɪnoʊ] vulcão *m*
volley ['vɑːlɪ] *n shots*: salva *f*; *tennis*: voleio *m*
'volleyball voleibol *m*
volt [voʊlt] volt *m*
voltage ['voʊltɪdʒ] voltagem *f*
volume ['vɑːljəm] (*quantity*), *book, radio etc*: volume *m*; *container*: capacidade *f*
'volume control regulador *m* de volume
voluntarily [vɑːlən'terɪlɪ] voluntariamente
voluntary ['vɑːlənterɪ] *adj helper, work* voluntário
volunteer [vɑːlən'tɪr] **1** *n* voluntário,-a *m,f* **2** *v/i* oferecer-se
voluptuous [və'lʌptʃʊəs] *adj woman, figure* voluptuoso
vomit ['vɑːmət] **1** *n* vômito *m* **2** *v/i* vomitar
♦ **vomit up** *v/t* vomitar
voracious [və'reɪʃəs] *adj appetite* voraz
voraciously [və'reɪʃəslɪ] *adv eat, also fig read* vorazmente
vote [voʊt] **1** *n* voto *m*; ***have the ~*** (*be entitled to vote*) ter direito ao voto **2** *v/i* POL votar; ***~ for / against ...*** votar a favor de / contra ... **3** *v/t* ***they ~d him President*** eles o elegeram Presidente; ***they ~d to stay behind*** votaram a favor de ficar atrás
♦ **vote in** *v/t new member* eleger
♦ **vote on** *v/t issue* votar em
♦ **vote out** *v/t of office* destituir em votação
voter ['voʊtər] POL eleitor,a *m,f*
voting ['voʊtɪŋ] POL votação *f*
'voting booth cabine *f* eleitoral
♦ **vouch for** [vaʊtʃ] *v/t truth of sth* dar fé de; *person* responder por
voucher ['vaʊtʃər] cupom *m*
vow [vaʊ] **1** *n* voto *m* **2** *v/t* ***~ to do sth*** prometer fazer algo
vowel [vaʊl] vogal *f*
voyage ['vɔɪɪdz] *n sea, space*: viagem *f*
vulgar ['vʌlgər] *adj person, language* vulgar
vulnerable ['vʌlnərəbl] *adj* vulnerável
vulture ['vʌltʃər] abutre *m*

W

wad [wɑːd] *n cotton etc*: chumaço *m*; *paper etc*: maço *m*; ***a ~ of $100 bills*** um maço de notas de 100 dólares
waddle ['wɑːdl] *v/i* andar como um pato
wade [weɪd] *v/i* ***we ~d out to the island*** fomos até à ilha pela água
♦ **wade through** *v/t book, documents* ler penosamente
wafer ['weɪfər] (*cookie*) bolacha *f* recheada; REL hóstia *f*
'wafer-thin *adj* muito fino
waffle[1] ['wɑːfl] *n to eat* waffle *m*
waffle[2] ['wɑːfl] *v/i* encher lingüiça
wag [wæg] ⟨*pret & pp* ***wagged***⟩ **1** *v/t tail, finger* balançar **2** *v/i tail* abanar
wage[1] [weɪdʒ] *v/t war* travar
wage[2] [weɪdʒ] *n* salário *m*; ***~s*** *pl* salário
'wage earner assalariado,-a *m,f* **'wage freeze** congelamento *m* do salário **'wage negotiations** *npl* negociação *f* salarial **'wage packet** *fig* salário *m*
waggle ['wægl] *v/t ears, loose screw, tooth etc* mexer; *hips* balançar
waggon → ***wagon***
wagon ['wægən] *Am* RAIL vagão *m*; ***be on the ~*** *fam* estar abstinente
wail [weɪl] **1** *n person, baby*: choramingo *m*; *siren*: canto *m* **2** *v/i person, baby* choramingar; *siren* cantar

waist [weɪst] cintura *f*
'waistcoat *Brit* colete *m*
'waistline cintura *f*
wait [weɪt] **1** *n* espera *f* **2** *v/i* esperar; ***we'll ~ until he's ready*** vamos esperar até que ele esteja pronto **3** *v/t meal* esperar para servir; ***~ table*** trabalhar de garçom / garçonete
♦ **wait for** *v/t* esperar por; ***wait for me!*** espere por mim!
♦ **wait on** *v/t* (*serve*) servir
♦ **wait up** *v/i* esperar acordado
waiter ['weɪtər] garçom *m*, *Port* empregado *m*
waiting ['weɪtɪŋ] *n* espera *f*; ***no ~ sign*** placa *f* de parada proibida
'waiting list lista *f* de espera
'waiting room sala *f* de espera
waitress ['weɪtrɪs] garçonete *f*, *Port* empregada *f*
waive [weɪv] *v/t* desconsiderar
wake[1] [weɪk] *v/t & v/i* ⟨*pret* **woke**, *pp* **woken**⟩ ~ (**up**) acordar
wake[2] [weɪk] *ship*: rastro *m*; ***in the ~ of*** *fig* atrás de; ***follow in the ~ of*** seguir
'wake-up call ligação *m* do serviço de despertador
Wales [weɪlz] *n* País *m* de Gales
walk [wɒːk] **1** *n* passeio *m* a pé; (*path*) caminho *m*; ***it's a long / short ~ to the office*** é um longo / curto caminho até o escritório; ***go for a ~*** ir passear; (*hike*) fazer caminhada **2** *v/i* andar; *as opposed to taking the car, bus, etc* caminhar **3** *v/t dog* levar para passear; ***~ the streets*** *walk around* andar pelas ruas
♦ **walk out** *v/i spouse* ir-se; *from theater etc* sair; (*go on strike*) entrar em greve
♦ **walk out on** *v/t spouse, family* abandonar
'walkabout *Brit monarch, politician*: ***go ~*** sair às ruas para encontrar gente
walker ['wɒːkər] (*hiker*) caminhante *m/f*; *baby, old person*: andador *m*; ***be a slow / fast ~*** ser um caminhante lento / rápido
walkie-talkie [wɒːkɪ'tɒːkɪ] walkie-talkie *m*
walk-in 'closet *Am* closet *m* espaçoso
walking ['wɒːkɪŋ] *n as opposed to driving* andar *m*; (*hiking*) caminhadas *fpl*; ***be within ~ distance*** dar para ir a pé
'walking stick bengala *f*
'walking tour caminhada *f*
'Walkman® walkman *m* **'walkout** *n* (*strike*) greve *f* **'walkover** (*easy win*) vitória *f* fácil **'walk-up** *n Am* apartamento *m* sem elevador
wall [wɒːl] *internal* parede *f*, *external* muro *m*; ***go to the ~*** *company* falir; ***drive s.o. up the ~*** *fam* fazer alguém subir pelas paredes
wallet ['wɑːlɪt] carteira *f*
wallop ['wɑːləp] *Brit fam* **1** *n blow* bofetada *f* **2** *v/t* bater; *opponent* dar uma surra em
'wallpaper 1 *n* papel *m* de parede **2** *v/t* revestir com papel de parede
walnut ['wɒːlnʌt] *nut* noz *f*, *tree, wood* nogueira *f*
waltz [wɒːlts] *n* valsa *f*
wan [wɑːn] *adj face* pálido
wander ['wɑːndər] *v/i* (*roam*) perambular; (*stray*) perder-se; *attention* desviar-se
♦ **wander around** *v/i* dar uma volta
wane [weɪn] *v/i interest, enthusiasm* diminuir
wangle ['wæŋgl] *v/t fam* arranjar
want [wɑːnt] **1** *n* ***for ~ of*** por falta de **2** *v/t* querer; (*need*) necessitar; ***~ to do sth*** querer fazer algo; ***I ~ to stay here*** quero ficar aqui; ***do you ~ to come too? – no, I don't ~ to*** você quer vir também? – não, eu não quero; ***you can have whatever you ~*** você pode pegar o que quiser; ***it's not what I ~ed*** não é o que eu queria; ***she ~s you to go back*** ela quer que você volte; ***he ~s a haircut*** ele está precisando de um corte de cabelo **3** *v/i* ***~ for nothing*** não ter o que mais precisar
'want ad anúncio *m* classificado
wanted ['wɑːntɪd] *adj by police* procurado
wanting ['wɑːntɪŋ] *adj* carente; ***be ~ in …*** carecer de …
wanton ['wɑːntən] *adj* maldoso
war [wɔːr] *n* guerra *f*, ***be at ~*** estar em guerra

warble ['wɔːrbl] *v/i bird* gorjear
ward [wɔːrd] *n (child)* tutelado,-a *m,f*; *Brit hospital*: estação *f*
♦ **ward off** *v/t cold* evitar; *attacker, blow* rechaçar
warden ['wɔːrdn] *Am prison*: carcereiro,-a *m,f*; *Brit* diretor,a *m,f* de prisão
warder ['wɔːrdər] *Brit* carcereiro,-a *m,f*
'wardrobe (*clothes*) guarda-roupa *m*; *Brit for clothes* guarda-roupas *m*
warehouse ['werhaʊs] depósito *m*
'warfare guerra *f*
'warhead ogiva *f*
warily ['werɪlɪ] *adv* cautelosamente
warm [wɔːrm] *adj* quente; *welcome, smile* caloroso
♦ **warm up 1** *v/t soup, plates* esquentar; *person, room* aquecer **2** *v/i person, athlete etc* aquecer-se
warmhearted ['wɔːrmhɑːrtɪd] *adj* afetuoso
warmly ['wɔːrmlɪ] *adv dressed* bem agasalhado; *welcome, smile* calorosamente
warmth [wɔːrmθ] calor *m*; *welcome, smile*: cordialidade *f*
'warm-up SPORT aquecimento *m*
warn [wɔːrn] *v/t* prevenir
warning ['wɔːrnɪŋ] advertência *f*; ***without ~*** sem aviso
'warning light luz *f* de advertência
warp [wɔːrp] **1** *v/t wood* deformar; *character* distorcer **2** *v/i wood* deformar-se
warped [wɔːrpt] *adj fig* distorcido
'warplane avião *f* de guerra
warrant ['wɔːrənt] **1** *n* ordem *f* judicial **2** *v/t (deserve, call for)* justificar
warranty ['wɔːrəntɪ] (*guarantee*) garantia *f*, ***be under ~*** estar na garantia
warrior ['wɔːrɪər] guerreiro,-a *m,f*
'warship navio *m* de guerra
wart [wɔːrt] verruga *f*
'wartime período *m* de guerra
wary ['werɪ] *adj* cauteloso; ***be ~ of*** desconfiar de
was [wʌz] *pret sg* → ***be***
wash [wɑːʃ] **1** *n* ***have a ~*** lavar-se; ***that shirt needs a ~*** essa camisa precisa ser lavada **2** *v/t* lavar **3** *v/i* lavar-se
♦ **wash up** *v/i (wash one's hands and face)* dar uma lavada; *Brit* lavar a louça
washable ['wɑːʃəbl] *adj* lavável
'washbasin, 'washbowl pia *f*, *Port* lavatório *m*
'washcloth *Am* toalhinha *f*
washed 'out [wɑːʃt'aʊt] *adj* exausto
washer ['wɑːʃər] *for faucet etc* arruela *f*, → ***washing machine***
washing ['wɑːʃɪŋ] (*clothes washed*) roupa *f* lavada; (*dirty clothes*) roupa *f* suja; ***do the ~*** lavar a roupa
'washing machine máquina *f* de lavar roupa
washing-'up liquid *Brit* líquido *m* para lava-louças
'washroom *Am* banheiro *m*, *Port* casa *f* de banho
wasp [wɑːsp] vespa *f*
waste [weɪst] **1** *n* desperdício *m*; *industrial process*: resíduos *mpl*; ***it's a ~ of time / money*** é perda de tempo / dinheiro **2** *adj* residual **3** *v/t food, money* gastar; *time* perder
♦ **waste away** *v/i* consumir-se
'waste basket cesta *f* de papel
'waste disposal, 'waste disposal unit triturador *m* de lixo
wasteful ['weɪstfʊl] *adj* esbanjador
'wasteland terra *f* desolada **waste 'paper** papel *m* usado **waste 'paper basket** cesta *f* de papel **'waste products** *npl* resíduos *mpl*
watch [wɑːʧ] **1** *n timepiece* relógio *m*; ***keep ~*** ficar de vigia **2** *v/t movie, TV* assistir; (*look after*) olhar; ***the police are ~ing him*** a polícia o está vigiando **3** *v/i* olhar
♦ **watch for** *v/t* esperar
♦ **watch out** *v/i* tomar cuidado; ***watch out!*** cuidado!
♦ **watch out for** *v/t* tomar cuidado com; (*look for*) procurar por
watchful ['wɑːʧfʊl] *adj* atento
'watchmaker relojoeiro,-a *m,f*
water ['wɒːtər] **1** *n* água *f*; NAUT ***~s*** *pl* águas *fpl* **2** *v/t plant* regar **3** *v/i eyes* lacrimejar; ***my mouth is ~ing*** estou com água na boca
♦ **water down** *v/t drink* diluir
'water cannon canhão-d'água *m*

'watercolor *n Am* aquarela *f*
watercolour *Brit* → ***watercolor***
watercress ['wɒːtərkres] agrião--d'água *m*
watered down ['wɒːtərd] *adj fig* leve
'waterfall cachoeira *f*, cascata *f*
watering can ['wɒːtərɪŋ] regador *m*
'watering hole *hum* bar *m*
'water level nível *m* de água **'water lily** ninféia *f* **'waterline** linha *f* de flutuação **waterlogged** ['wɒːtərlɑːgd] *adj earth, field* encharcado; *boat* cheio de água **'water main** cano *m* (de água) principal **'watermark** filigrana *f*, marca-d'água *f* **'water melon** melancia *f* **'water pollution** contaminação *f* da água **'water polo** pólo *m* aquático **'waterproof** *adj* à prova d'água **'watershed** *fig* momento *m* decisivo **'waterside** *n* margem *f*; ***at the ~*** *by lake, sea etc* no litoral **'waterskiing** esqui *m* aquático **'watertight** *adj compartment* estanque *m*; *fig* perfeito **'waterway** hidrovia *f* **'waterwings** *npl* bóia *f* de braço **'waterworks** ***turn on the ~*** *fam* começar a chorar
watery ['wɒːtərɪ] *adj coffee etc* aguado
watt [wɑːt] watt *m*
wave[1] [weɪv] *n sea, hair*: onda *f*
wave[2] [weɪv] **1** *n hand*: aceno *m* **2** *v/i with hand* acenar; ***~ to s.o.*** acenar para alguém **3** *v/t flag etc* agitar
'wavelength RADIO comprimento *m* de onda; ***be on the same ~*** *fig* ter a mesma sintonia
wavy ['weɪvɪ] *adj hair* ondulado; *line* sinuoso
wax [wæks] *n furniture, ear*: cera *f*
way [weɪ] **1** *n* (*method*) método *m*; (*manner*) jeito *m*; (*route*) caminho *m*; ***this ~*** (*like this*) assim; (*in this direction*) nessa direção; ***by the ~*** (*incidentally*) a propósito; ***by ~ of*** (*via*) por; (*in the form of*) como; ***in a ~*** (*in certain respects*) de um certo modo; ***be under ~*** estar em andamento; ***give ~*** (*collapse*) ceder; *Brit* MOT dar prefêrencia de passagem; ***give ~ to*** (*be replaced by*) dar lugar a; ***have one's (own) ~*** impor-se; ***OK, we'll do it your ~*** ok, vamos fazer da sua maneira; ***you lead the ~!*** vai tu à frente!; ***lose one's ~*** perder--se; ***be in the ~*** (*be an obstruction*) estar no caminho; ***it's on the ~ to the station*** fica no caminho da estação; ***I was on my ~ to the station*** eu estava a caminho da estação; ***no ~!*** *fam* de jeito nenhum!; ***there's no ~ he can do it*** é impossivel para ele fazer isto **2** *adv fam* (*much*) muito; ***she paints ~ better*** ela pinta muito melhor; ***it's ~ too soon to decide*** (ainda) é muito cedo para decidir; ***they are ~ behind with their work*** eles estão atrasadíssimos com o trabalho
way 'in *Brit* entrada *f* **way of 'life** modo *m* de vida **way 'out** *n Brit, also Am fig from situation* saída *f*
we [wiː] *pron* nós; ***~ are from Kansas*** somos do Kansas
weak [wiːk] *adj tea, person, currency* fraco
weaken ['wiːkn] **1** *v/t* enfraquecer **2** *v/i* enfraquecer-se
weakling ['wiːklɪŋ] fraco,-a *m,f*
weakness ['wiːknɪs] fraqueza *f*; ***have a ~ for sth*** *liking* ter um fraco por algo
wealth [welθ] riqueza *f*; ***a ~ of*** uma grande quantidade de
wealthy ['welθɪ] *adj* rico
weapon ['wepən] arma *f*
wear [wer] **1** *n* ***~ and tear*** desgaste *m*; ***clothes for everyday / evening ~*** roupas *fpl* do dia-a-dia / de noite **2** *v/t* ⟨*pret* **wore**, *pp* **worn**⟩ (*have on*) usar; (*damage*) desgastar **3** *v/i* ⟨*pret* **wore**, *pp* **worn**⟩ (*wear out*) desgastar-se; (*last*) durar
♦ **wear away 1** *v/i* desgastar-se **2** *v/t* desgastar
♦ **wear down** *v/t* cansar
♦ **wear off** *v/i effect, feeling* passar
♦ **wear out 1** *v/t* (*tire*) cansar; *shoes* gastar **2** *v/i shoes, carpet* desgastar-se
wearily ['wɪrɪlɪ] *adv* cansadamente
wearing ['werɪŋ] *adj* (*tiring*) cansativo
weary ['wɪrɪ] *adj* cansado
weather ['weðər] **1** *n* tempo *m*; ***be feeling under the ~*** não estar se sentindo muito bem **2** *v/t crisis* superar

'weather-beaten *adj face* desgastado (pelo clima) **'weather chart** mapa *m* meteorológico **'weather forecast** previsão *f* do tempo **'weatherman** meteorologista *m/f*, homem *m* do tempo
weave [wiːv] **1** *v/t* ⟨*pret* ***wove***, *pp* ***woven***⟩ tecer **2** *v/i* ⟨*pret & pp* ***weaved***⟩ (*move*) ziguezaguear
web [web] *spider*: teia *f*; ***the Web*** COMPUT a rede
webbed 'feet [webd] pés *mpl* membranosos
'web page página *f* da web
'website site *m* (na internet)
wedding ['wedɪŋ] casamento *m*
'wedding anniversary aniversário *m* de casamento **'wedding cake** bolo *m* de casamento **'wedding day** dia *m* do casamento **'wedding dress** vestido *m* de casamento **'wedding ring** aliança *f* de casamento
wedge [wedʒ] **1** *n to hold sth in place* cunha *f*; *cheese etc*: pedaço *m* **2** *v/t* ***~ a door open*** calçar a porta para que fique aberta
Wednesday ['wenzdeɪ] quarta-feira *f*
wee [wiː] *adj fam* minúsculo; ***a ~ bit*** um pouco; *cake etc*: um pedacinho
weed [wiːd] **1** *n* erva *f* daninha **2** *v/i* arrancar as ervas daninhas
◆ **weed out** *v/t* (*remove*) retirar
'weed-killer herbicida *m*
weedy ['wiːdɪ] *adj fam* franzino
week [wiːk] semana *f*; ***a ~ tomorrow*** uma semana depois de amanhã
'weekday dia *m* da semana
week'end fim *m* de semana; ***on the ~*** no fim de semana
weekly ['wiːklɪ] **1** *adj* semanal **2** *n magazine* semanário *m* **3** *adv* semanalmente
weep [wiːp] *v/i* ⟨*pret & pp* ***wept***⟩ chorar
weepy ['wiːpɪ] *adj* ***be ~*** chorar muito
wee-wee *fam* **1** *n* xixi *m*; ***do a ~*** fazer xixi **2** *v/i* fazer xixi
weigh [weɪ] *v/t & v/i* pesar; ***~ anchor*** levantar âncora
◆ **weigh down** *v/t* ***be weighed down with*** *bags* estar carregado de; *worries* estar cheio de
◆ **weigh on** *v/t* preocupar, engordar
◆ **weigh up** *v/t* (*assess*) estimar
weight [weɪt] peso *m*; ***put on ~*** engordar; ***lose ~*** perder peso
weightlessness ['weɪtlɪsnɪs] falta *f* de gravidade
weightlifter ['weɪtlɪftər] halterofilista *m/f*
weightlifting ['weɪtlɪftɪŋ] halterofilismo *m*
weighty ['weɪtɪ] *adj fig important* de peso
weir [wɪr] barragem *f*
weird [wɪrd] *adj* esquisito
weirdly ['wɪrdlɪ] *adv* estranhamente
weirdo ['wɪrdoʊ] *n fam* esquisitão *m*, esquisitona *f*
welcome ['welkəm] **1** *adj* bem-vindo; ***you're ~!*** de nada!; ***you're ~ to try one*** fique à vontade para provar um **2** *n guests etc*: boas-vindas *fpl*; *fig news, proposal*: recepção *f*; ***they gave us a warm ~*** eles receberam-nos de braços abertos **3** *v/t guests etc* dar as boas-vindas; *fig decision etc* aceitar com prazer
weld [weld] *v/t* soldar
welder ['weldər] soldador *m*
welfare ['welfer] bem-estar *m*; *Am* (*financial assistance*) previdência social *f*; ***be on ~*** *Am* estar recebendo auxílio da previdência social
'welfare check *Am* cheque *m* da previdência social **welfare 'state** estado *m* de bem-estar social **'welfare work** trabalho *m* social **'welfare worker** assistente *m/f* social
well[1] [wel] **1** *adv* bem; ***as ~*** (*too*) também; ***as ~ as*** (*in addition to*) assim como; ***it's just as ~ you told me*** foi bom você ter me contado; ***very ~*** *acknowledging an order* muito bem; *signifying relctant agreement* está bem; ***~, ~!*** *surprise* veja só!; ***~ …*** *uncertainty, thinking* bom … **2** *adj* ***be ~*** estar bem; ***feel ~*** sentir-se bem; ***get ~ soon!*** boas melhoras!
well[2] [wel] *n water, oil*: poço *m*
well-'balanced *adj person, meal* equilibrado **well-behaved** [welbɪ'heɪvd] *adj* bem-comportado **well-'being** bem-estar *m* **well-'built** *adj also*

euph (*fat*) robusto **well-'done** *adj meat* bem passado **well-dressed** [wel'drest] *adj* bem vestido **well-earned** [wel'ɜːrnd] *adj* merecido **well-heeled** [wel'hiːld] *adj fam* rico **well-informed** [welɪn'fɔːrmd] *adj* bem informado **well-'known** *adj* bem-conhecido **well-'made** *adj* bem-feito **well-'mannered** [wel-'mænərd] *adj* educado **well-'meaning** *adj* bem-intencionado **well--'off** *adj* rico **well-'paid** *adj* bem pago **well-read** [wel'red] *adj* lido, versado **well-timed** [wel'taɪmd] *adj* oportuno **well-to-'do** *adj* próspero **'well-wisher** ['welwɪʃər] admirador,a *m,f* **well-'worn** *adj* surrado

Welsh [welʃ] **1** *adj* galês,-esa **2** *n language* galês *m*; ***the ~*** os galeses

went [went] *pret* → **go**

wept [wept] *pret & pp* → ***weep***

were [wer] *pret pl* → **be**

west [west] **1** *n* oeste *m*; ***the West*** (*Western nations*) o Ocidente; (*western part of a country*) o oeste **2** *adj* oeste **3** *adv* para o oeste; ***~ of*** ao oeste de

'West Coast *USA*: costa *f* oeste

westerly ['westərlɪ] *adj direction, wind* oeste

Western ['westərn] *adj* ocidental

western ['westərn] **1** *adj* ocidental **2** *n* (*movie*) (filme *m* de) faroeste *m*

Westerner ['westərnər] ocidental *m/f*

westernized ['westərnaɪzd] *adj* ocidentalizado

westward ['westwərd] *adv* em direção oeste

wet [wet] *adj* úmido; (*rainy*) chuvoso; ***~ paint!*** tinta fresca!; ***be ~ through*** estar encharcado

wet 'blanket *fam* estraga-prazeres *m/f*

'wet suit *diving*: roupa *f* de mergulho

whack [wæk] *fam* **1** *n* (*blow*) bofetada *f* **2** *v/t* bater

whacked [wækt] *adj fam* morto *de cansaço*

whale [weɪl] baleia *f*

whaling ['weɪlɪŋ] caça *f* às baleias

wharf [wɔːrf] *Brit* cais *m*

what [wɑːt] **1** *pron* ◊ *interrogative* que; ***~?*** (*what do you want*) que é?; (*what did you say*) como?; ***~ is that?*** que é isto?; ***~ is it?*** (*what do you want*) que você quer?; ***~ about some dinner?*** que tal um jantar?; ***~ about heading home?*** que tal sairmos?; ***~ for?*** (*why*) para que?; ***so ~?*** e daí? ◊ *relative* ***I don't know ~ he means*** não sei o que ele quer dizer **2** *adj* que; ***~ university are you at?*** em que universidade você está?; ***~ color is your car?*** (de) que cor é seu carro?; ***~ a disaster!*** que desastre!

whatever [wɑːt'evər] **1** *pron* ◊ o que, tudo o que; ***he eats ~ you give him*** come tudo o que lhe derem ◊ (*regardless of*) independentemente de; ***~ happens*** seja lá o que acontecer ◊ ***~ gave you that idea!*** o que é que tenha lhe dado essa idéia ◊ ***is that ok with you? – ~!*** tudo bem por você? – tanto faz! **2** *adj* qualquer; ***you have no reason ~ to worry*** você não tem motivo qualquer para se preocupar

wheat [wiːt] trigo *m*

wheedle ['wiːdl] *v/t fam* bajular; ***~ sth out of s.o.*** conseguir algo de alguém através de bajulação

wheel [wiːl] **1** *n* roda *f*, (***steering***) ***~*** volante *m* **2** *v/t bicycle* empurrar **3** *v/i birds* voar em círculo

♦**wheel around** *v/i* girar

'wheelbarrow carriola *f* **'wheelchair** cadeira *f* de rodas **'wheel clamp** trava *f*

wheeze [wiːz] *v/i* ofegar

when [wen] **1** *adv* quando **2** *conj* quando; ***~ I was a child*** quando eu era criança; ***on the day ~ he arrived*** no dia que ele chegou

whenever [wen'evər] *adv* todas as vezes que

where [wer] **1** *adv* onde; ***~ from?*** de onde?; ***~ to?*** onde? **2** *conj* onde; ***this is ~ I used to live*** aqui é onde eu vivia

whereabouts ['werəbaʊts] **1** *adv* onde **2** *npl* paradeiro *m*

where'as *conj* enquanto

wherever [wer'evər] **1** *conj* onde quer que; ***sit ~ you like*** sente-se onde quer que queira **2** *adv* onde; ~

can he be? onde é que pode estar?

whet [wet] *v/t* ⟨*pret & pp* **whetted**⟩ *appetite* abrir

whether ['weðər] *conj* se

which [wɪʧ] **1** *adj* que, qual; ***~ one is yours?*** qual é o seu? **2** *pron* ◊ *interrogative* qual; ***take one, it doesn't matter ~*** pegue um, não importa qual
◊ *relative* que; ***the mistake ~ you are making*** o erro que está cometendo; ***the way in ~ he said it*** o a maneira em que ele disse isso

whichever [wɪʧ'evər] **1** *adj* qualquer; ***in ~ direction you travel*** em qualquer direção que você viaje **2** *pron* qualquer um/uma; ***take ~ you prefer*** pegue qualquer um/uma que preferir

whiff [wɪf] (*smell*) cheirinho *m*

while [waɪl] **1** *conj* enquanto; (*although*) embora **2** *n* ***a long ~*** um tempão; ***for a ~*** por um tempo; ***I'll wait a ~ longer*** vou esperar um pouco mais

♦**while away** *v/t* passar

whim [wɪm] capricho *m*

whimper ['wɪmpər] **1** *n* lamúria *f* **2** *v/i* choramingar

whine [waɪn] *v/i dog* uivar; *fam* (*complain*) lamentar-se

whip [wɪp] **1** *n* chicote *m* **2** *v/t* ⟨*pret & pp* **whipped**⟩ (*beat*) chicotear; *cream* bater; *fam* (*defeat*) derrotar

♦**whip out** *v/t fam* (*take out*) tirar rapidamente

♦**whip up** *v/t* (*arouse*) impelir; *fam meal* preparar rapidamente

'**whipped cream** [wɪpt] nata *f* batida, chantilly *m*

'**whipround** *fam* vaquinha *f*; ***have a ~*** fazer uma vaquinha

whir, **whirr** [wɜːr] *v/i* zumbir

whirl [wɜːrl] **1** *n* ***my mind is in a ~*** estou com a cabeça girando **2** *v/i* girar

'**whirlpool** *in river* redemoinho *m*; *for relaxation* banheira *f* de hidromassagem

whisk [wɪsk] **1** *n kitchen implement* batedor *m* de claras **2** *v/t eggs* bater

♦**whisk away** *v/t* retirar rapidamente

whiskers ['wɪskərz] *man*: costeleta *f*; *animal*: bigode *m*

whiskey, *Brit* **whisky** ['wɪskɪ] uísque *m*, *Port* whisky *m*

whisper ['wɪspər] **1** *n* sussurro *m*; (*rumor*) boato *m* **2** *v/i & v/t* sussurrar

whistle ['wɪsl] **1** *n sound* assobio *m*; (*device*) apito *m* **2** *v/i & v/t* assobiar

'**whistle-blower** *fam* informante *m/f*

white [waɪt] **1** *n color* branco *m*; *egg*: clara *f*; *person* branco *m* **2** *adj* branco

white 'Christmas Natal *m* branco

white 'coffee *Brit* café *m* com leite

'**white-collar worker** colarinho-branco *m* '**White House** Casa *f* Branca **white 'lie** mentira *f* branca, mentirinha *f* '**white meat** carne *f* branca '**whiteout** *for text* líquido *m* corretor '**whitewash 1** *n* caiação *f*, *fig* encobrimento *m* **2** *v/t* caiar **white 'wine** vinho *m* branco

whittle ['wɪtl] *v/t wood* talhar

♦**whittle down** *v/t* reduzir

whiz, **whizz** [wɪz] *n* ***be a ~ at*** *fam* ser um gênio em

♦**whizz by** *v/i time, car* passar como um raio

♦**whizz past** *v/i time, car* passar como um raio

'**whizzkid** *fam* garoto *m* prodígio

who [huː] *pron* ◊ *interrogative* quem
◊ *relative* que; ***the man ~ lives here*** o homem que mora aqui; ***the man ~ she was speaking to*** o homem com quem ela estava conversando

whodunit, **whodunnit** [huː'dʌnɪt] história *f* de detetive

whoever [huː'evər] *pron* quem quer que seja; ***~ can that be!*** quem quer que possa ser!

whole [hoʊl] **1** *adj* inteiro; ***he drank the ~ lot*** ele bebeu tudo; ***it's a ~ lot easier / better*** é muito mais fácil / muito melhor **2** *n* total *m*; ***the ~ of the United States*** os Estados Unidos todo; ***on the ~*** em geral

whole-hearted [hoʊl'hɑːrtɪd] *adj* incondicional **whole-heartedly** [hoʊl'hɑːrtɪdlɪ] *adv* incondicionalmente '**wholemeal bread** *Brit* pão *m* integral

'**wholesale 1** *adj* por atacado; *fig* indiscriminado **2** *adv* no atacado

wholesaler ['hoʊlseɪlər] atacadista *m/f*
'wholewheat bread *Am* pão *m* integral
wholesome ['hoʊlsəm] *adj* saudável
wholly ['hoʊlɪ] *adv* inteiramente
wholly owned 'subsidiary subsidiária *f* integral
whom [huːm] *pron fml* quem
whooping cough ['huːpɪŋ] coqueluche *f*
whopping ['wɑːpɪŋ] *adj fam* enorme
whore [hɔːr] *n* puta *f*
whose [huːz] **1** *pron* ◇ *interrogative* de quem; **~ *is this?*** de quem é isso? ◇ *relative* cujo,-a; ***a man ~ wife ...*** um homem cuja mulher ...; ***a country ~ economy is booming*** um país cuja economia está crescendo muito **2** *adj* de quem; **~ *bike is that?*** de quem é essa bicicleta?
why [waɪ] *adv interrogative* por que, *Port* porque; *relative* porque; ***that's ~*** isso é porque; **~ *not?*** porque não?
wick [wɪk] pavio *m*
wicked ['wɪkɪd] *adj* malvado
wicker ['wɪkər] *adj* de vime
wicker 'chair cadeira *f* de vime
wicket ['wɪkɪt] *Am station, bank etc*: janelinha *f*
wide [waɪd] *adj street, experience, range* largo; ***be 12 foot ~*** ter 3,6 metros de largura
wide a'wake *adj* totalmente desperto
widely ['waɪdlɪ] *adv used, known* amplamente
widen ['waɪdn] **1** *v/t* ampliar **2** *v/i* alargar-se
wide-'open *adj eyes* arregalado; *window* escancarado
wide-ranging ['waɪdreɪndʒɪŋ] *adj* amplo
'widespread *adj* difundido
widow ['wɪdoʊ] *n* viúva *f*
widower ['wɪdoʊər] viúvo *m*
width [wɪdθ] largura *f*
wield [wiːld] *v/t weapon* empunhar; *power* deter
wife [waɪf] ⟨*pl* ***wives***⟩ esposa *f*, mulher *f*
wig [wɪg] peruca *f*
wiggle ['wɪgl] *v/t hips* balançar; *loose screw etc* abanar
wild [waɪld] **1** *adj animal* selvagem; *flowers* silvestre; *teenager, party* descontrolado; (*crazy*) *scheme* louco; *applause* fervoroso; ***be ~ about ...*** (*keen on*) ser louco por; ***go ~*** (*become very enthusiastic or angry*) ficar louco; ***run ~*** *children* correr à vontade; *plants* crescer selvagem **2** *n* ***the ~s*** as regiões mais remotas
wilderness ['wɪldərnɪs] (*empty place*) região *f* inexplorada; (*garden etc*) matagal *m*
'wildfire *spread like ~* alastrar-se como fogo no palheiro **wild'goose chase** busca *f* inútil **'wildlife** fauna e flora *f*
wildly ['waɪldlɪ] *adv applaud* fervorosamente; *kick* furiosamente; *fam* (*extremely*) loucamente
wilful *Brit* → ***willful***
will[1] [wɪl] *n* LAW testamento *m*
will[2] [wɪl] *n* (*willpower*) vontade *f*
will[3] [wɪl] *v/aux* ***I ~ let you know tomorrow*** você vai ficar sabendo amanhã; **~ *you be there?*** você estará lá?; ***I won't be back until late*** voltarei tarde; ***you ~ call me, won't you?*** você vai me ligar, não vai?; ***I'll pay for this – no you won't*** deixa que eu pago – de jeito nenhum; ***the car won't start*** o carro não quer pegar; **~ *you tell her that ...?*** você pode dizer a ela que ...?; **~ *you have some more tea, sir?*** o senhor aceita mais chá?; **~ *you stop that!*** chega!
willful ['wɪlfl] *adj Am person* teimoso; *action* deliberado
willing ['wɪlɪŋ] *adj* disposto
willingly ['wɪlɪŋlɪ] *adv* de bom grado
willingness ['wɪlɪŋnɪs] disposição *f*
willow ['wɪloʊ] salgueiro *m*
'willpower força *f* de vontade
willy-nilly [wɪlɪ'nɪlɪ] *adv* (*at random*) aleatoriamente
wilt [wɪlt] *v/i plant* murchar
wily ['waɪlɪ] *adj* astuto
wimp [wɪmp] *fam* banana *m/f*
win [wɪn] **1** *n* vitória *f* **2** *v/t* ⟨*pret & pp* ***won***⟩ ganhar **3** *v/i* ⟨*pret & pp* ***won***⟩ vencer
♦ **win back** *v/t* recuperar

wince [wıns] *v/i* estremecer
winch [wıntʃ] manivela *f*
wind[1] [wınd] **1** *n* vento *m*; (*flatulence*) gases *mpl*; ***get ~ of ...*** ficar sabendo de ... **2** *v/t* ***be ~ed*** *by ball etc* ficar sem ar
wind[2] [waınd] ⟨*pret & pp* ***wound***⟩ **1** *v/i road etc* ziguezaguear **2** *v/t* enrolar
♦**wind down 1** *v/i party etc* ficar chato **2** *v/t car window* abrir; *business* encerrar
♦**wind up 1** *v/t clock* dar corda; *car window* fechar; *speech, presentation* finalizar; *business, affairs also company* fechar **2** *v/i* (*finish*) concluir; ***wind up in hospital*** acabar num hospital
'**wind-bag** *fam* tagarela *m/f*
'**windfall** *fig* herança *f* inesperada
'**wind farm** parque *m* eólico
winding ['waındıŋ] *adj* sinuoso
'**wind instrument** instrumento *m* de sopro
'**windmill** moinho *m* de vento
window ['wındoʊ] *also* COMPUT janela *f*; ***in the ~*** *store* na vitrina, *Port* na montra
'**window box** jardineira *f* '**window cleaner** *person* limpador,a *m,f* de janelas '**windowpane** vidraça *f* '**window seat** *plane, train*: assento *m* na janela '**window-shop** *v/i* ⟨*pret & pp* ***shopped***⟩ ***go ~ping*** ir olhar as vitrines das lojas **windowsill** ['wındoʊsıl] peitoril *m*
'**windpipe** traquéia *f* **windscreen** *Brit* → ***windshield*** '**windshield** *Am* pára-brisa *m* '**windshield wiper** *Am* limpador *m* de pára-brisa
'**windsurfer** *person* surfista *m/f*; *board* prancha *f* de windsurf '**windsurfing** windsurf *m* '**wind turbine** turbina *f* eólica
windy ['wındı] *adj weather, day* ventoso; ***it's getting ~*** está ventando, *Port* faz vento
wine [waın] vinho *m*
'**wine bar** bar *m* de bebidas '**wine cellar** adega *f* '**wine glass** taça *f* de vinho '**wine list** carta *f* de vinhos '**wine maker** vinicultor *m* '**wine merchant** comerciante *m* de vinhos
winery ['waınərı] *Am* lagar *m*
wing [wıŋ] *n* asa *f*, SPORT lateral *f*
'**wingspan** envergadura *f*
wink [wıŋk] **1** *n* pestanejo *m*; ***I didn't sleep a ~*** *fam* não preguei os olhos **2** *v/i person* piscar; ***~ at s.o.*** piscar para alguém
winner ['wınər] vencedor,a *m,f*
winning ['wınıŋ] *adj number, team* vencedor; *entry* triunfante
'**winning post** chegada *f*
winnings ['wınıŋz] *npl* prêmio *m*
winter ['wıntər] *n* inverno *m*
winter 'sports *npl* esportes *mpl* de inverno, *Port* desportos *mpl* de inverno
wintry ['wıntrı] *adj* invernal
wipe [waıp] *v/t* enxugar; *tape* apagar
♦**wipe out** *v/t* (*kill, destroy*) destruir; *debt* saldar
wiper ['waıpər] limpador *m* de pára-brisa
wire ['waır] arame *m*; ELEC fio *m*
wireless ['waırlıs] *n* rádio *m*; ***~ network*** rede sem fio; ***~ printer*** impressora *f* sem fio
wire 'netting cerca *f* de arame
wiring ['waırıŋ] *n* ELEC instalação *f* elétrica
wiry ['waırı] *adj person* magro mas musculoso
wisdom ['wızdəm] sabedoria *f*
'**wisdom tooth** dente *m* do siso
wise [waız] *adj* sábio
'**wisecrack** *n fam* brincadeira *f*
'**wise guy** *pej* sabichão *m*, sabichona *f*
wisely ['waızlı] *adv act* sabiamente; *decide, choose* prudentemente
wish [wıʃ] **1** *n* desejo *m*; ***best ~es*** saudações cordiais **2** *v/t* desejar; ***I ~ that ...*** desejo que ...; ***~ s.o. well*** desejar tudo de bom a alguém; ***I ~ed him good luck*** desejei-lhe boa sorte **3** *v/i* ***~ for*** desejar
'**wishbone** *chicken*: osso *m* da sorte
wishful 'thinking ['wıʃfl] desejo *m* ilusório
wishy-washy ['wıʃıwɑːʃı] *adj person* irresoluto; *color* desbotado
wisp [wısp] *hair*: mecha *f*, *smoke*: rastro *m*
wistful ['wıstfl] *adj* nostálgico

wistfully ['wɪstflɪ] *adv* melancolicamente
wit [wɪt] (*humor*) graça *f*; *person* pessoa *f* espirituosa *f*; ***be at one's ~s' end*** estar no fim das forças; ***keep one's ~s about one*** manter a boa calma; ***be scared out of one's ~s*** ficar apavorado
witch [wɪʧ] bruxa *f*
'witchhunt *fig* caça *f* às bruxas
with [wɪð] *prep* com; *cause* de; ***~ a smile / a wave*** com um sorriso / aceno; ***are you ~ me?*** (*do you understand*) você está me entendendo?; ***~ no money*** sem dinheiro; ***shake ~ anger*** tremer de ódio; ***a girl ~ blonde hair*** uma garota com o cabelo loiro
withdraw [wɪð'drɒː] **1** *v/t* ⟨*pret* ***withdrew***, *pp* ***withdrawn***⟩ *complaint, money, troops* retirar **2** *v/i competitor, troops* retirar-se
withdrawal [wɪð'drɒːl] retirada *f*; *drugs*: desintoxicação *f*
with'drawal symptoms *npl* sintomas *mpl* de abstinência
withdrawn [wɪð'drɒːn] *adj person* retraído
wither ['wɪðər] *v/i* murchar
with'hold *v/t* ⟨*pret & pp* ***withheld***⟩ *payment* reter; *permission* recusar
with'in *prep* (*inside*) dentro de; *in expressions of time* em menos de; *in expressions of distance* menos que, dentro de; ***we kept ~ the budget*** ficamos dentro do orçamento; ***~ my capabilities*** dentro das minhas possibilidades; ***~ reach*** ao alcance das mãos
with'out *prep* sem; ***~ a hat*** sem chapéu; ***~ asking*** sem perguntar; ***he left ~ me noticing*** ele saiu sem eu notar
with'stand *v/t* ⟨*pret & pp* ***withstood***⟩ suportar
witness ['wɪtnɪs] **1** *n* testemunha *f* **2** *v/t accident, crime* testemunhar; *signature* autenticar
witness box *Brit* → ***witness stand***
'witness stand *Am* palanque *m* das testemunhas
witticism ['wɪtɪsɪzm] gracejo *m*
witty ['wɪtɪ] *adj* engraçado
wobble ['wɑːbl] *v/i* cambalear
wobbly ['wɑːblɪ] *adj* cambaleante
wok [wɑːk] panela *f* wok
woke [woʊk] *pret* → ***wake***[1]
woken ['woʊkn] *pp* → ***wake***[1]
wolf [wʊlf] **1** *n* ⟨*pl* ***wolves***⟩ lobo *m*; *fig* (*womanizer*) garanhão *m* **2** *v/t* ~ (***down***) engolir
'wolf whistle *n* assobio *m* de paquera
woman ['wʊmən] mulher *f*
woman 'doctor médica *f*
woman 'driver motorista *f*
womanizer ['wʊmənaɪzər] conquistador *m* de mulheres
womanly ['wʊmənlɪ] *adj* feminino
woman 'priest pastora *f*
womb [wuːm] útero *m*
women ['wɪmɪn] *npl* → ***woman***
women's lib [wɪmɪnz'lɪb] emancipação *f* das mulheres
women's libber [wɪmɪnz'lɪbər] feminista *f*
won [wʌn] *pret & pp* → ***win***
wonder ['wʌndər] **1** *n* (*amazement*) assombro *m*; ***no ~!*** não me surpreende!; ***it's a ~ that …*** é suspreendente que … **2** *v/i & v/t* perguntar-se; ***I ~ if you could help*** eu agradeceria se você pudesse me ajudar
wonderful ['wʌndərfʊl] *adj* maravilhoso
wonderfully ['wʌndərflɪ] *adv* (*extremely*) maravilhosamente
wood [wʊd] *n* madeira *f*; *fire, stove*: lenha *f*; (*forest*) floresta *f*
wooded ['wʊdɪd] *adj* arborizado
wooden ['wʊdn] *adj* (*made of wood*) de madeira
woodpecker ['wʊdpekər] pica-pau *m*
'woodwind *npl* MUS instrumentos *mpl* de sopro de madeira **'woodwork** (*parts made of wood*) madeiramento *m*; *activity* carpintaria *f*
wool [wʊl] lã *f*
woolen ['wʊlən] **1** *adj Am* de lã **2** *n* roupa *f* de lã
woollen *Brit* → ***woolen***
word [wɜːrd] **1** *n also* (*promise*) palavra *f*, (*news*) notícia *f*; ***is there any ~ from …?*** há alguma notícia de …?; ***you have my ~*** você tem a minha palavra; ***have ~s*** (*argue*) ter uma discussão; ***have a ~ with s.o.*** ter uma con-

versa com alguém **2** *v/t article, letter* redigir

wording ['wɜːrdɪŋ] redação *f*

'word processing processamento *m* de textos

'word processor (*software*) processador *m* de textos

wore [wɔːr] *pret* → ***wear***

work [wɜːrk] **1** *n* trabalho *m*; ***out of ~*** desempregado; ***be at ~*** estar trabalhando; ***I go to ~ by bus*** eu vou de ônibus para o trabalho **2** *v/i* trabalhar; *machine*, (*succeed*) funcionar; ***how does it ~?*** *device* como isto funciona? **3** *v/t employee* fazer trabalhar; *machine* usar, fazer funcionar

♦ **work off** *v/t bad mood, anger* livrar-se de; *flab* perder

♦ **work out 1** *v/t problem* resolver; *solution* encontrar **2** *v/i at gym* fazer ginástica; *relationship etc* ir bem

♦ **work out to** *v/t* (*add up to*) equivaler a uma soma de

♦ **work up** *v/t enthusiasm* adquirir; *appetite* abrir; ***get worked up*** (*get angry*) ficar fora de si; (*get nervous*) ficar nervoso

workable ['wɜːrkəbl] *adj solution* praticável

workaholic [wɜːrkə'hɑːlɪk] *n fam* workaholic *m/f*, viciado,-a *m,f* em trabalho

'work day (*hours of work*) jornada *f* de trabalho; (*not a holiday*) dia *m* útil

worker ['wɜːrkər] trabalhador,a *m,f*

'workforce força *f* de trabalho

'work hours horário *m* de trabalho

working ['wɜːrkɪŋ] *n* funcionamento *m*

'working class 1 *n* classe *f* trabalhadora **2** *adj* de classe trabalhadora **'working conditions** *npl* condições *fpl* de trabalho **working 'day** *Brit* → ***work day*** **'working hours** *Brit* → ***work hours*** **working 'knowledge** conhecimento *m* básico **working 'mother** mãe *f* que trabalha fora

'workload carga *f* de trabalho **'workman** trabalhador *m* **'workmanlike** *adj* competente **'workmanship** acabamento *m* **work of 'art** obra *f* de arte **'workout** workout *m*, treino *m* **'work permit** permissão *f* de trabalho **'workshop** oficina *f*; (*seminar*) seminário *m* **'work station** estação *f* de trabalho **'worktop** bancada *f*

world [wɜːrld] mundo *m*; ***the ~ of computers / the theater*** o mundo dos computadores / do teatro; ***out of this ~*** *fam* fora de série

'world-class *adj* de classe mundial **World 'Cup** Copa *f* do Mundo **world-'famous** *adj* famoso mundialmente

worldly ['wɜːrldlɪ] *adj* mundano; *person* sofisticado

world 'power potência *f* mundial **world 'record** recorde *m* mundial **world 'war** guerra *f* mundial **'worldwide 1** *adj* mundial **2** *adv* mundialmente

worm [wɜːrm] *n* verme *m*

worn [wɔːrn] *pp* → ***wear***

worn-'out *adj shoes, carpet* gasto; *person* esgotado

worried ['wʌrɪd] *adj* preocupado

worriedly ['wʌrɪdlɪ] *adv* com preocupação

worry ['wʌrɪ] **1** *n* preocupação *f* **2** *v/t* ⟨*pret & pp* ***worried***⟩ preocupar; (*upset*) abalar **3** *v/i* ⟨*pret & pp* ***worried***⟩ preocupar-se; ***don't ~!*** não se preocupe!

worrying ['wʌrɪɪŋ] *adj* preocupante

worse [wɜːrs] *adj & adv* pior

worsen ['wɜːrsn] *v/i* piorar

worship ['wɜːrʃɪp] **1** *n* devoção *f* **2** *v/t* ⟨*pret & pp* ***worshipped***⟩ *also fig* adorar

worst [wɜːrst] **1** *adj & adv* pior **2** *n* ***the ~*** o pior; ***if the ~ comes to the ~*** se o pior acontecer

worst-case scen'ario a pior *f* das hipóteses

worth [wɜːrθ] *adj* ***20 dollars ~ of gas*** 20 dólares de gasolina; ***be ~ …*** *in monetary terms* valer …; ***be ~ reading / seeing*** valer a pena ler / ver; ***be ~ it*** valer a pena

worthless ['wɜːrθlɪs] *adj object* sem valor; *person* imprestável, inútil

worth'while *adj cause* que vale a pena; ***be ~*** valer a pena

worthy ['wɜːrðɪ] *adj* digno; *cause* justo; ***be ~ of*** (*deserve*) merecer
would [wʊd] *v/aux* ***I ~ help if I could*** eu ajudaria se pudesse; ***I said that I ~ go*** eu disse que iria; ***I told him I ~ not leave unless ....*** eu lhe disse que não sairia a não ser que ...; ***~ you like to go to the movies?*** você gostaria de ir ao cinema?; ***~ you mind if I smoked?*** lhe incomoda que eu fume?; ***~ you tell her that ...?*** você poderia dizer a ela que ...?; ***I ~ have told you but ...*** eu teria te contado, mas ...; ***I ~ not have been so angry if ...*** eu não teria ficado tão zangado se ...
wound[1] [wuːnd] **1** *n* ferimento *m* **2** *v/t with weapon, remark* ferir
wound[2] [waʊnd] *pret & pp* → ***wind***[2]
wove [woʊv] *pret* → ***weave***
woven ['woʊvn] *pp* → ***weave***
wow [waʊ] *int* uau
wrap [ræp] *v/t* ⟨*pret & pp* ***wrapped***⟩ *parcel, gift* embrulhar; (*wind*) enrolar; (*cover*) enfaixar
♦ **wrap up** *v/i against the cold* agasalhar-se
wrapper ['ræpər] *candy*: papel *m*; *magazine*: capa *f*
wrapping ['ræpɪŋ], **'wrapping paper** papel *m* de embrulho
wreath [riːθ] coroa *f* de flores
wreck [rek] **1** *n ship, car*: carcaça *f*; ***be a nervous ~*** estar com os nervos à flor da pele **2** *v/t ship* afundar; *car, plans, career, marriage* destruir
wreckage ['rekɪdʒ] *car, plane*: destroços *mpl*; *marriage, career*: ruínas *fpl*
wrecker ['rekər] *Am* guincho *m*
wrecking company ['rekɪŋ] *Am* serviço *m* de reboque
wrench [rentʃ] **1** *n tool* chave *f* inglesa **2** *v/t injure* deslocar; (*pull*) arrancar
wrestle ['resl] *v/i* lutar
♦ **wrestle with** *v/t problems* lutar contra
wrestler ['reslər] lutador *m*
wrestling ['reslɪŋ] wrestling *m*, luta *f* livre
'wrestling match combate *m* de luta livre
wriggle ['rɪgl] *v/i* (*squirm*) balançar; *along the ground* arrastar-se
♦ **wriggle out of** *v/t* livrar-se de
♦ **wring out** *v/t* ⟨*pret & pp* ***wrung***⟩ *cloth* torcer
wrinkle ['rɪŋkl] **1** *n clothes*: prega *f*; *skin*: ruga *f* **2** *v/t & v/i clothes* enrugar
wrist [rɪst] pulso *m*
'wrist watch relógio *m* de pulso
write [raɪt] *v/t & v/i* ⟨*pret* ***wrote***, *pp* ***written***⟩ escrever; *check* preencher
♦ **write down** *v/t* anotar
♦ **write off** *v/t debt* anular; *car* demolir
writer ['raɪtər] escritor,a *m,f*; *song, book*: autor,a *m,f*
'write-up resenha *f*
writhe [raɪð] *v/i* contorcer-se
writing ['raɪtɪŋ] (*handwriting*) letra *f*; (*words, script*) escrita *f*; ***in ~*** por escrito
'writing paper papel *m* para escrever
written ['rɪtn] *pp* → ***write***
wrong [rɒːŋ] **1** *adj* errado; ***be ~*** *person* estar errado; *answer* estar incorreto; *morally* não estar certo; ***what's ~?*** o que há de errado?; ***there's something ~ with the car*** há algo de errado com o carro **2** *adv* incorretamente; ***go ~*** *person* equivocar-se; *marriage, plan etc* não dar certo **3** *n* mal *m*; (*injustice*) injustiça *f*; ***be in the ~*** estar sem razão
wrongful ['rɒːŋfl] *adj* ilícito
wrongly ['rɒːŋlɪ] *adv* erroneamente
wrong 'number número *m* errado
wrote [roʊt] *pret* → ***write***
wrought 'iron [rɔːt] ferro *m* forjado
wrung [rʌŋ] *pret & pp* → ***wring out***
wry [raɪ] *adj* irônico

X

xenophobia [zenoʊ'foʊbɪə] xenofobia *f*
'X-ray ['eksreɪ] **1** *n* raio *m* X **2** *v/t patient, chest* tirar uma radiografia de
xylophone [zaɪlə'foʊn] xilofone *m*

Y

yacht [jɑːt] iate *m*
yachting ['jɑːtɪŋ] iatismo *m*, vela *f*
yachtsman ['jɑːtsmən] velejador *m*
yachtswoman ['jɑːtswʊmən] velejadora *f*
Yank [jæŋk] *n fam* ianque *m/f*
yank [jæŋk] *v/t* puxar
yap [jæp] *v/i* 〈*pret & pp* ***yapped***〉 *small dog* latir; *fam* (*talk a lot*) tagarelar
yard[1] [jɑːrd] *prison, institution etc*: pátio *m*; *Am behind house* quintal *m*; *storage*: depósito *m*
yard[2] [jɑːrd] *measurement* jarda *f*
'yardstick critério *m*
yarn [jɑːrn] *n* (*thread*) fio *m*; *fam* (*story*) história *f* do arco-da-velha
yawn [jɔːn] **1** *n* bocejo *m* **2** *v/i* bocejar
year [jɪr] ano *m*; ***for ~s*** por anos; ***we were in the same ~*** *at school* estávamos na mesma série; ***be six ~s old*** ter 6 anos (de idade)
yearly ['jɪrlɪ] **1** *adj* anual **2** *adv* anualmente
yearn [jɜːrn] *v/i* ***~ to do sth*** ansiar fazer algo
♦ **yearn for** *v/t* desejar ardentemente
yearning ['jɜːrnɪŋ] *n* desejo *m intenso*
yeast [jiːst] fermento *m*
yell [jel] **1** *n* grito *m* **2** *v/i & v/t* gritar
yellow ['jeloʊ] **1** *n* amarelo *m* **2** *adj* amarelo
yellow 'pages *npl* páginas *fpl* amarelas
yelp [jelp] **1** *n* uivo *m* **2** *v/i* uivar
yen [jen] FIN iene *m*
yes [jes] sim
'yesman *pej* pessoa *f* que diz sim para tudo
yesterday ['jestərdeɪ] ontem; ***the day before ~*** anteontem
yet [jet] **1** *adv* ainda; *in questions* já; ***as ~*** ainda; ***have you finished ~?*** você já terminou?; ***he hasn't arrived ~*** ele ainda não chegou; ***is he here ~? – not ~*** ele já chegou? – ainda não; ***~ bigger / longer*** ainda maior / mais comprido **2** *conj* todavia; ***~ I'm not sure*** todavia não estou seguro
yield [jiːld] **1** *n fields etc*: colheita *f*; *investment*: lucro *m* **2** *v/t fruit, good harvest, interest* render **3** *v/i* (*give way*) ceder; *traffic* recuar
yob [jɑːb] *Brit pej* maloqueiro,-a *m,f*
yoga ['joʊgə] yoga *f*
yoghurt ['joʊgərt] iogurte *m*
yolk [joʊk] gema *f* do ovo
you [juː] *pron* **1** *subject* ◊ *singular* você; *plural* vocês; ***are ~ ready, Sue?*** (você) está pronta, Sue?
◊ *familiar* tu; *plural* vocês; ***are ~ ready, Sue?*** (tu) estás pronta, Sue?
◊ *polite singular Port* o senhor, a senhora; *plural* os senhores, as senhoras; ***could ~ possibly tell me …?***

o senhor podia dizer-me …
2 *direct object* o, a, você; *plural* os, as, vocês; ***I saw ~*** eu vi você, eu o/a vi, *Port* eu vi você, eu vi-o/a; *plural* eu vi vocês, eu os/as vi, *Port* eu vi vocês, eu vi-os/as
◇ *familiar* te; *plural* vos; ***I know ~*** eu conheço-te; eu conheço-vos
3 *indirect object* lhe; *plural* lhes; ***I'll send it to ~*** eu envio-lhe isso
◇ *familiar* te; *plural* vos; ***I'll send it to ~*** eu envio-te isso
4 *with prepositions* você; *plural* vocês; ***this is for ~*** isto é para você
◇ *familiar* ti; *plural* vocês; ***these are for ~*** estes são para ti
5 *indefinite* ***~ never know*** nunca se sabe; ***it's good for ~*** faz bem

young [jʌŋ] *adj* jovem
youngster ['jʌŋstər] jovem *m/f*
your [jʊr] *adj* seu, sua; *familiar* teu, tua; ***you should comb ~ hair*** você deveria pentear o cabelo
yours [jʊrz] *pron* seu, sua; *familiar* teu, tua; ***a friend of ~*** seu amigo; ***~ …*** *at end of letter* seu/sua …; ***~ truly*** atenciosamente, seu/sua
your'self *pron* você mesmo,-a; *familiar* tu mesmo,-a; ***did you hurt ~?*** você se machucou?; ***by ~*** sozinho,-a
your'selves *pron* vocês mesmos,-as; ***did you hurt ~?*** vocês se machucaram?; ***by ~*** sozinhos,-as
youth [ju:θ] *n age* juventude *f*; (*young man*) jovem *m*; (*young people*) jovens *mpl*
'youth club clube *m* de jovens
youthful ['ju:θfʊl] *adj* jovem
'youth hostel albergue *m* da juventude
yuppie ['jʌpɪ] *fam* yuppie *m*

Z

zap [zæp] *v/t* ⟨*pret & pp* ***zapped***⟩ *fam* COMPUT (*delete*) deletar; (*kill*) fuzilar; (*hit*) dar um murro; (*send*) enviar
♦**zap along** *v/i fam* (*move fast*) voar
zapped [zæpt] *adj fam* (*exhausted*) acabado
zapper ['zæpər] *TV channels*: controle *m* remoto
zappy ['zæpɪ] *adj fam car, pace* rápido; (*lively, energetic*) vivo
zeal [zi:l] zelo *m*
zebra ['zebrə] zebra *f*
zebra 'crossing *Brit* faixa *f* de pedestres, *Port* passadeira *f*
zero ['zɪroʊ] zero; ***10 below ~*** 10 graus abaixo de zero
♦**zero in on** *v/t* (*identify*) apontar
'zero growth crescimento *m* zero
zest [zest] entusiasmo *m*
zigzag ['zɪgzæg] **1** *n* zigue-zague *m* **2** *v/i* ⟨*pret & pp* ***zigzagged***⟩ ziguezaguear
zilch [zɪltʃ] *fam* nada
zinc [zɪŋk] zinco *m*
zip [zɪp] *Brit* zíper *m*, *Port* fecho *m* (de correr)
♦**zip up** *v/t* ⟨*pret & pp* ***zipped***⟩ *dress, jacket* fechar o zíper de, *Port* correr o fecho de; COMPUT compactar
'zip code *Am* CEP *m*, código *m* de endereçamento postal, *Port* CP, código *m* postal
zipper ['zɪpər] *Am* zíper *m*, *Port* fecho *m* (de correr)
zit [zɪt] *fam on face* espinha *f*
zodiac ['zoʊdɪæk] zodíaco *m*; ***signs of the ~*** signos *mpl* do zodíaco
zombie ['zɑ:mbɪ] *fam* ***feel like a ~*** sentir-se como um zumbi
zone [zoʊn] zona *f*
zonked [zɑ:ŋkt] *adj pej* (*exhausted*) esgotado

zoo [zu:] zôo *m*
zoological [zu:ə'lɑ:dʒɪkl] *adj* zoológico
zoologist [zu:'ɑ:lədʒɪst] zoólogo,-a *m,f*
zoology [zu:'ɑ:lədʒɪ] zoologia *f*
zoom [zu:m] *v/i fam* (*move fast*) passar voando
♦**zoom in on** *v/t* PHOT aproximar o zoom em
'**zoom lens** *nsg* lente *f* zoom
zucchini [zu:'ki:nɪ] *Am* abobrinha *f*

Portuguese verb conjugations

In the following tables verb stems are shown in normal type and verb endings in *italics*. Irregular forms are shown in **bold**.

Grammatical abbreviations

Cond.	*Condicional*, conditional	*Perf.*	*Perfeito*, perfect
Conj.	*Conjuntivo*, subjunctive	*pers.*	person
Fut.	*Futuro*, future	*pl.*	plural
Imperf.	*Imperfeito*, imperfect	*Pres.*	*Presente*, present
Indic.	*Indicativo*, indicative	*Pret.*	*Pretérito*, preterite
Inf.	*Infinitivo*, infinitive	*sg.*	singular
Inf. Pess.	*Infinitivo Pessoal*, personal infinitive	*Mais-que-perf.*	*Mais-que-Perfeito*, pluperfect

Tense formation

The following stems can be used to generate derived forms:

1. The present indicative stem gives
  1.1. the 2nd pers. sg. imperative: **louva, vende, admite** from the 3rd pers. sg. **louva, vende, admite** and
  1.2. the 2nd pers. pl. imperative: **louvai, vendei, admiti** from the 2nd pers. pl. **louvais, vendeis, admitis** by dropping the final **-s**
  1.3. the present subjunctive which is formed from the 1st pers. sg. **louvo, vendo, admito** by changing **o** to **e** or **a**: **louve, venda, admita**

2. The present subjunctive stem, 1st and 3rd pers. sg. and 1st, 2nd and 3rd pers. pl. **louves, louve, louvemos, louveis, louvem; vendas, venda, vendamos, vendais, vendam** or **admitas, admita, admitamos** etc gives the imperative forms of the 1st pers. pl. and 3rd pers. sg. and pl. as well as the *negative* forms of the 2nd pers. sg. and pl.:
não louves, não louve, não louvemos etc; **não vendas, não venda, não vendamos** etc; **não admitas, não admita** etc

3. The 3rd pers. pl. of the *Pretérito Perfeito* **louvaram, venderam, admitiram** gives
  3.1. the future subjunctive by dropping the final syllable **-am: louvar, vender, admitir** [1)]
  3.2. the pluperfect by dropping the final **-m**: **louvara, vendera, admitira**

3.3. the *Pretérito Imperfeito* subjunctive by changing the ending **-ram** to **-sse**:
louvasse, vendesse, admitisse

4. The infinitive **louvar, vender, admitir** gives
   4.1. the *Gerúndio* by replacing the **-r** with **-ndo**:
   louvando, vendendo, admitindo
   4.2. the past participle by changing **-ar** to **-ado, -er** and **-ir** to **-ido**:
   louvado, vendido, admitido
   4.3. the future indicative by adding the present tense endings of **haver**: **louvarei, venderei, admitirei**
   4.4. the conditional by adding the imperfect tense endings of **haver**:
   louvaria, venderia, admitiria

5. All compound tenses are formed using the participle **louvado, vendido, admitido**.

[1] The endings of the future subjunctive are usually identical to those of the personal infinitive. The two forms only differ if the preterite stem of the verb is not the same as the stem of the infinitive, for example: infinitive **fazer**, future subjunctive **fizer**.

1 First Conjugation

⟨**1a**⟩ **louvar** [lo'vaɾ]
No change to the stem in either spelling or pronunciation.

1. Simple tenses

Indicativo

	Presente	Pretérito Imperfeito	Pret. Perfeito Simples
Sg.	louv*o*	louv*ava*	louv*ei*
	louv*as*	louv*avas*	louv*aste*
	louv*a*	louv*ava*	louv*ou*
Pl.	louv*amos*	louv*ávamos*	louv*amos*, *Port* louv*ámos*
	louv*ais*	louv*áveis*	louv*astes*
	louv*am*	louv*avam*	louv*aram*

	Futuro Imperfeito	Condicional Simples	Pret. Mais-que-perfeito Simples
Sg.	louv*arei*	louv*aria*	louv*ara*
	louv*arás*	louv*arias*	louv*aras*
	louv*ará*	louv*aria*	louv*ara*
Pl.	louv*aremos*	louv*aríamos*	louv*áramos*
	louv*areis*	louv*aríeis*	louv*áreis*
	louv*arão*	louv*ariam*	louv*aram*

Conjuntivo

	Presente	Pretérito Imperfeito	Futuro Imperfeito
Sg.	louv*e*	louv*asse*	louv*ar*
	louv*es*	louv*asses*	louv*ares*
	louv*e*	louv*asse*	louvar
Pl.	louv*emos*	louv*ássemos*	louv*armos*
	louv*eis*	louv*ásseis*	louv*ardes*
	louv*em*	louv*assem*	louv*arem*

	Imperativo	Infinitivo Pessoal	
Sg.	—	louv*ar*	
	louv*a* (não louv*es*)	louv*ares*	Particípio
	louv*e*	louv*ar*	louv*ado*
Pl.	louv*emos*	louv*armos*	
	louv*ai* (não louv*eis*)	louv*ardes*	Gerúndio
	louv*em*	louv*arem*	louv*ando*

2. Compound tenses

Active (**ter**, or rarely **haver**, + unchanging participle)

Infinitivo Perfeito: ter louvado (haver louv*ado*)
Gerúndio Perfeito: tendo louv*ado* (havendo louv*ado*)

Indicativo
Pretérito Perfeito Composto: tenho louvado (hei louvado)
Mais-que-perfeito Composto: tinha louvado (havia louvado)
Futuro Perfeito: terei louvado (haverei louvado)
Condicional Composto: teria louvado (haveria louvado)

Conjuntivo
Perfeito Composto: tenha louvado (haja louvado)
Mais-que-perfeito: tivesse louvado (houvesse louvado)
Futuro Perfeito: tiver louvado (houver louvado)

Passive (**ser** + changing participle)

Infinitivo Presente: ser louvado, *Inf. Perfeito*: ter sido louvado
Gerúndio Presente: sendo louvado, *Ger. Perfeito*: tendo sido louvado

Indicativo
Presente: sou louvado, *Imperfeito*: era louvado
Perfeito: fui louvado, *Perf. Composto*: tenho sido louvado
Mais-que-perfeito Simples: fora louvado, *Mais-que-perf. Composto*: tinha sido louvado
Futuro Imperfeito: serei louvado, *Fut. Perfeito*: terei sido louvado
Condicional Simples: seria louvado, *Cond. Composto*: teria sido louvado

Conjuntivo
Presente: seja louvado, *Imperfeito*: fosse louvado
Perfeito Composto: tenha sido louvado
Mais-que-perfeito Composto: tivesse sido louvado
Futuro Imperfeito: for louvado, *Fut. Perfeito*: tiver sido louvado

	Presente do Indicativo	Presente do Conjuntivo	Pret. Perfeito do Indicativo

⟨1b⟩ lavar [la'var]

An unstressed *a* in the infinitive changes to an open *a* [a] when the stress falls on the stem (unless it follows an *m*, *n* or *nh*).

Presente do Indicativo	Presente do Conjuntivo	Pret. Perfeito do Indicativo
lav*o* ['a]	**la**v*e*	lav*ei*
lav*as*	**la**v*es*	etc
lav*a*	**la**v*e*	
lav*amos*	lav*emos*	
lav*ais*	lav*eis*	
lav*am*	**la**v*em*	

⟨1c⟩ levar [le'var]

An unstressed *e* in the infinitive changes to an open *e* [ɛ] when the stress falls on the stem (except for the cases given in ⟨1d⟩).

Presente do Indicativo	Presente do Conjuntivo	Pret. Perfeito do Indicativo
lev*o* ['ɛ]	**le**v*e*	lev*ei*
lev*as*	**le**v*es*	etc
lev*a*	**le**v*e*	
lev*amos*	lev*emos*	
lev*ais*	lev*eis*	
lev*am*	**le**v*em*	

⟨1d⟩ desejar [deze'ʒar] or in Portugal [dəzə'ʒar]

Changes affecting Continental Portuguese. The ə in the infinitive changes, when the stress falls on the stem, to a closed *e* [e] before *m* and *n*, or [ɜ] before *nh*, or [ɜi] before *ch*, *lh* and *j*. The small number of exceptions behave like **levar** ⟨1c⟩.

Presente do Indicativo	Presente do Conjuntivo	Pret. Perfeito do Indicativo
des**e**j*o* ['ɜi]	des**e**j*e*	desej*ei*
des**e**j*as*	des**e**j*es*	etc
des**e**j*a*	des**e**j*e*	
desej*amos*	desej*emos*	
desej*ais*	desej*eis*	
des**e**j*am*	des**e**j*em*	

⟨1e⟩ aprovar [apro'var]

When the stress falls on the stem, unstressed *o* in the infinitive changes to an open *o* [ɔ] with the exception of those cases given at ⟨1f⟩.

Presente do Indicativo	Presente do Conjuntivo	Pret. Perfeito do Indicativo
apr**o**v*o* ['ɔ]	apr**o**v*e*	aprov*ei*
apr**o**v*as*	apr**o**v*es*	etc
apr**o**v*a*	apr**o**v*e*	
aprov*amos*	aprov*emos*	
aprov*ais*	aprov*eis*	
apr**o**v*am*	apr**o**v*em*	

	Presente do Indicativo	Presente do Conjuntivo	Pret. Perfeito do Indicativo

⟨1f⟩ perdoar [peɾ'dwaɾ]
When the stress falls on the stem, unstressed *o* before *n* or *nh* or in final position, or with a few exceptions also before *m*, changes to a closed *o* [o].

Presente do Indicativo	Presente do Conjuntivo	Pret. Perfeito do Indicativo
perd**o***o* ['o]	perd**o***e*	perdo*ei*
perd**o***as*	perd**o***es*	etc
perd**o***a*	perd**o***e*	
perdo*amos*	perdo*emos*	
perdo*ais*	perdo*eis*	
perd**o***am*	perd**o***em*	

⟨1g⟩ adiar [a'dʒiaɾ]
Verbs in *-iar* and *-uar*
When the stress falls on the stem, it falls on the *i* or *u*.

Presente do Indicativo	Presente do Conjuntivo	Pret. Perfeito do Indicativo
ad**i***o* ['i]	ad**i***e*	adi*ei*
ad**i***as*	ad**i***es*	etc
ad**i***a*	ad**i***e*	
adi*amos*	adi*emos*	
adi*ais*	adi*eis*	
ad**i***am*	ad**i***em*	

⟨1h⟩ odiar [o'dʒiaɾ]
Verbs in *-iar*
When the stress falls on the stem, *i* changes to *ei* [ɜj].

Presente do Indicativo	Presente do Conjuntivo	Pret. Perfeito do Indicativo
od**ei***o* ['ɜj]	od**ei***e*	odi*ei*
od**ei***as*	od**ei***es*	etc
od**ei***a*	od**ei***e*	
odi*amos*	odi*emos*	
odi*ais*	odi*eis*	
od**ei***am*	od**ei***em*	

⟨1i⟩ raiar [ha'jaɾ]
Verbs in *-iar*
The *i* forms a diphthong with the preceding vowel and therefore remains unstressed when the stem is stressed.

Presente do Indicativo	Presente do Conjuntivo	Pret. Perfeito do Indicativo
rai*o* ['aj]	**ra**i*e*	rai*ei*
rai*as*	**ra**i*es*	etc
rai*a*	**ra**i*e*	
rai*amos*	rai*emos*	
rai*ais*	rai*eis*	
rai*am*	**ra**i*em*	

	Presente do Indicativo	Presente do Conjuntivo	Pret. Perfeito do Indicativo

⟨1k⟩ boiar [bo'jaɾ]

Verbs in *-oiar*

The *o* takes an accent when the stress falls on the stem and when it is pronounced open. Other forms behave like *raiar* ⟨1i⟩.

Presente do Indicativo	Presente do Conjuntivo	Pret. Perfeito do Indicativo
b**ó**i*o* ['ɔj]	b**ó**i*e*	boi*ei*
b**ó**i*as*	b**ó**i*es*	etc
b**ó**i*a*	b**ó**i*e*	
boi*amos*	boi*emos*	
boi*ais*	boi*eis*	
b**ó**i*am*	b**ó**i*em*	

⟨1l⟩ recear [he'seaɾ]

Verbs in *-ear*

When the stress falls on the stem *e* changes to *ei* [ɜi].

Presente do Indicativo	Presente do Conjuntivo	Pret. Perfeito do Indicativo
rec**ei***o* ['ɜj]	rec**ei***e*	rece*ei*
rec**ei***as*	rec**ei***es*	etc
rec**ei***a*	rec**ei***e*	
rece*amos*	rece*emos*	
rece*ais*	rece*eis*	
rec**ei***am*	rec**ei***em*	

⟨1m⟩ averiguar [averi'gwaɾ]

Verbs in *-guar* and *-quar*

When the stress falls on the stem the u is also stressed and takes an accent in some forms. Brazilian spelling differs as shown from Continental Portuguese in the addition of a dieresis.

Presente do Indicativo	Presente do Conjuntivo	Pret. Perfeito do Indicativo
averig**u***o*	averig**ú***e*	averig**ü***ei* / *Port* averigu*ei*
averig**u***as*	averig**ú***es*	etc
averig**u***a*	averig**ú***e*	
averigu*amos*	averig**ü***emos* / *Port* averigu*emos*	
averigu*ais*	averig**ü***eis* / *Port* averigu*eis*	
averig**u***am*	averig**ú***em*	

	Presente do Indicativo	**Presente do Conjuntivo**	**Pret. Perfeito do Indicativo**

⟨1ma⟩ enxaguar [ẽʃa'gwaɾ]

For verbs in *-guar*, *-quar* compare ⟨1m⟩.
When the stress falls on the stem, Brazilian spelling adds an acute accent to the *a*. Brazilian spelling also adds a dieresis to *u* before *e*.

Presente do Indicativo	Presente do Conjuntivo	Pret. Perfeito do Indicativo
enx**á**gu*o* / *Port* enxag**u***o*	enx**á**g**ü***e* / *Port* enxag**ú***e*	enxag**ü***ei* / *Port* enxag**u***ei*
enx**á**gu*as* / *Port* enxag**u***as*	enx**á**g**ü***es* / *Port* enxag**ú***es*	etc
enx**á**gu*a* / *Port* enxag**u***a*	enx**á**g**ü***e* / *Port* enxag**ú***e*	
enxagu*amos*	enxag**ü***emos* / *Port* enxag**u***emos*	
enxagu*ais*	enxag**ü***eis* / *Port* enxag**u***eis*	
enx**á**gu*am* / *Port* enxag**u***am*	enx**á**g**ü***em* / *Port* enxag**ú***em*	

⟨1n⟩ ficar [fi'kaɾ]

Verbs in *-car*. Final stem consonant *c* changes to *qu* before *e*.

Presente do Indicativo	Presente do Conjuntivo	Pret. Perfeito do Indicativo
fic*o*	fi**qu***e* [k]	fi**qu***ei*
fic*as*	fi**qu***es*	fic*aste*
fic*a*	fi**qu***e*	fic*ou*
fic*amos*	fi**qu***emos*	fic*amos*, *Port* fic*ámos*
fic*ais*	fi**qu***eis*	fic*astes*
fic*am*	fi**qu***em*	fic*aram*

⟨1o⟩ ligar [li'gaɾ]

Verbs in *-gar*. Final stem consonant *g* changes to *gu* before *e*.

Presente do Indicativo	Presente do Conjuntivo	Pret. Perfeito do Indicativo
lig*o*	li**gu***e* [g]	li**gu***ei*
lig*as*	li**gu***es*	lig*aste*
lig*a*	li**gu***e*	lig*ou*
lig*amos*	li**gu***emos*	lig*amos*, *Port* lig*ámos*
lig*ais*	li**gu***eis*	lig*astes*
lig*am*	li**gu***em*	lig*aram*

⟨1p⟩ dançar [dã'saɾ]

Verbs in *-çar*. Final stem consonant *ç* changes to *c* before *e*.

Presente do Indicativo	Presente do Conjuntivo	Pret. Perfeito do Indicativo
danç*o*	dan**c***e*	dan**c***ei*
danç*as*	dan**c***es*	danç*aste*
danç*a*	dan**c***e*	danç*ou*
danç*amos*	dan**c***emos*	danç*amos*, *Port* danç*ámos*
danç*ais*	dan**c***eis*	danç*astes*
danç*am*	dan**c***em*	danç*aram*

	Presente do Indicativo	Presente do Conjuntivo	Pret. Perfeito do Indicativo

⟨1q⟩ saudar [saw'daɾ]

Stem vowels *i* or *u* take an accent when the stress falls on the stem and when preceded by an unstressed vowel.

Presente do Indicativo	Presente do Conjuntivo	Pret. Perfeito do Indicativo
sa**ú**d*o* ['u]	*sa***ú**d*e*	saud*ei*
sa**ú**d*as*	sa**ú**d*es*	etc
sa**ú**d*a*	sa**ú**d*e*	
saud*amos*	saud*emos*	
saud*ais*	saud*eis*	
sa**ú**d*am*	sa**ú**d*em*	

⟨1r⟩ dar [daɾ]

Irregularities in the *Pres. do Indic.* and *Pres. do Conj.*, in particular in the use of the accent; *Pret. Perf.* is regular apart from the 1st pers. sg. which behaves as a regular second conjugation verb.

Presente do Indicativo	Presente do Conjuntivo	Pret. Perfeito do Indicativo
d**ou**	**dê** [e]	d*ei*
dás	**dê***s*	**deste** [ɛ]
dá	**dê**	**deu**
d*amos*	**dê***mos*	**demos** [ɛ]
d*ais*	d*eis*	**destes** [ɛ]
dão	**dê***em*	**deram** [ɛ]

⟨1s⟩ estar [es'taɾ]

Some irregular forms in the *Pres. do Indic.* and in all of the *Pres. do Conj.*; for the *Pret. Perf.*, compare ⟨2v⟩; otherwise regular.

Presente do Indicativo	Presente do Conjuntivo	Pret. Perfeito do Indicativo
est**ou**	este**j***a* [ʒj]	esti**v***e*
est**ás**	este**j***as*	esti**v***este*
est**á**	este**j***a*	este**v***e*
est*amos*	este**j***amos*	esti**v***emos*
est*ais*	este**j***ais*	esti**v***estes*
est**ão**	este**j***am*	esti**v***eram*

2 Second Conjugation

⟨2a⟩ vender [vẽ'deɾ]

No changes to the stem in either spelling or pronunciation.

1. Simple tenses

Indicativo

	Presente	Pretérito Imperfeito	Pret. Perfeito Simples
Sg.	*vendo*	*vendia*	*vendi*
	vend*es*	vend*ias*	vend*este*
	vend*e*	vend*ia*	vend*eu*
Pl.	*vendemos*	*vendíamos*	*vendemos*
	vend*eis*	vend*íeis*	vend*estes*
	vend*em*	vend*iam*	vend*eram*

	Futuro Imperfeito	Condicional Simples	Pret. Mais-que-perfeito Simples
Sg.	*venderei*	*venderia*	*vendera*
	vend*erás*	vend*erias*	vend*eras*
	vend*erá*	vend*eria*	vend*era*
Pl.	*venderemos*	*venderíamos*	*vendêramos*
	vend*ereis*	vend*eríeis*	vend*êreis*
	vend*erão*	vend*eriam*	vend*eram*

Conjuntivo

	Presente	Pretérito Imperfeito	Futuro Imperfeito
Sg.	vend*a*	vend*esse*	vend*er*
	vend*as*	vend*esses*	vend*eres*
	vend*a*	vend*esse*	vend*er*
Pl.	vend*amos*	vend*êssemos*	vend*ermos*
	vend*ais*	vend*êsseis*	vend*erdes*
	vend*am*	vend*essem*	vend*erem*

	Imperativo	Infinitivo Pessoal	
Sg.	—	vend*er*	
	vend*e* (não vend*as*)	vend*eres*	Particípio
	vend*a*	vend*er*	vend*ido*
Pl.	vend*amos*	vend*ermos*	
	vend*ei* (não vend*ais*)	vend*erdes*	Gerúndio
	vend*am*	vend*erem*	vend*endo*

2. Compound tenses

as for the 1st conjugation

	Presente do Indicativo	Presente do Conjuntivo	Pret. Perfeito do Indicativo

⟨2b⟩ abater [aba'ter]

An unstressed *a* in the infinitive changes to an open *a* [a] when the stress falls on the stem.

Presente do Indicativo	Presente do Conjuntivo	Pret. Perfeito do Indicativo
ab**a**t*o* ['a]	ab**a**t*a*	abat*i*
ab**a**t*es*	ab**a**t*as*	etc
ab**a**t*e*	ab**a**t*a*	
abat*emos*	abat*amos*	
abat*eis*	abat*ais*	
ab**a**t*em*	ab**a**t*am*	

⟨2c⟩ beber [be'ber]

An unstressed *e* in the infinitive becomes an open *e* [ɛ] when the stress falls on the stem in the 2nd and 3rd pers. sg. and in the 3rd pers. pl. of the *Pres. do Indic.*, but it is a closed *e* [e] in other forms when the stress falls on the stem.

Presente do Indicativo	Presente do Conjuntivo	Pret. Perfeito do Indicativo
b**e**b*o* ['e]	b**e**b*a* ['e]	beb*i*
b**e**b*es* ['ɛ]	b**e**b*as*	etc
b**e**b*e* ['ɛ]	b**e**b*a*	
beb*emos*	beb*amos*	
beb*eis*	beb*ais*	
b**e**b*em* ['ɛ]	b**e**b*am*	

⟨2d⟩ comer [ko'mer]

An unstressed *o* in the infinitive becomes an open *o* [ɔ] when the stress falls on the stem in the 2nd and 3rd pers. sg. and in the 3rd pers. pl. of the *Pres. do Indic.*, but it is a closed *o* [o] in other forms when the stress falls on the stem.

Presente do Indicativo	Presente do Conjuntivo	Pret. Perfeito do Indicativo
c**o**m*o* ['o]	c**o**m*a* ['o]	com*i*
c**o**m*es* ['ɔ]	c**o**m*as*	etc
c**o**m*e* ['ɔ]	c**o**m*a*	
com*emos*	com*amos*	
com*eis*	com*ais*	
c**o**m*em* ['ɔ]	c**o**m*am*	

⟨2e⟩ resolver [hezow'ver]

A closed *o* [o] changes to an open *o* [ɔ] in the 2nd and 3rd pers. sg. and in the 3rd pers. pl. of the *Pres. do Indic.*

Presente do Indicativo	Presente do Conjuntivo	Pret. Perfeito do Indicativo
resolv*o* ['o]	resolv*a* ['o]	resolv*i*
res**o**lv*es* ['ɔ]	resolv*as*	etc
v**o**lv*e* ['ɔ]	resolv*a*	
resolv*emos*	resolv*amos*	
resolv*eis*	resolv*ais*	
res**o**lv*em* ['ɔ]	resolv*am*	

	Presente do Indicativo	Presente do Conjuntivo	Pret. Perfeito do Indicativo

⟨2f⟩ moer [mwer]

Verbs with unstressed *o* [u] in final stem position have *oi* [ɔj] in the 2nd and 3rd pers. sg. of the *Pres. do Indic.*, and a closed *o* [o] in the other forms when the stress falls on the stem; in some forms they take an accent.

mo*o* ['o]	**mo***a* ['o]	**moí**
mói*s* [ɔj]	**mo***as*	**mo***este*
mó*i* [ɔj]	**mo***a*	**mo***eu*
mo*emos*	**mo***amos*	**mo***emos*
mo*eis*	**mo***ais*	**mo***estes*
mo*em* ['ɔ]	**mo***am*	**mo***eram*

Pret. *Imperf.*: **moí***a*, **moí***as*, **moí***a*, **moí***amos*, **moí***eis*, **moí***am*; *Particípio*: **moí***do*

⟨2g⟩ tecer [te'ser]

Verbs in *-cer*. Final stem consonant *c* changes to *ç* before *o* and *a* (stem as at ⟨2c⟩, unless otherwise indicated).

teç*o*	**teç***a*	**tec***i*
tec*es*	**teç***as*	etc
tec*e*	**teç***a*	
tec*emos*	**teç***amos*	
tec*eis*	**reç***ais*	
tec*em*	**teç***am*	

⟨2h⟩ reger [he'ʒer]

Verbs in *-ger*. Final stem consonant *g* changes to *j* before *a* and *o* (stem as at ⟨2c⟩, unless otherwise indicated).

rej*o* [ɜj]	**rej***a* [ɜj]	**reg***i*
reg*es* [ɛ]	**rej***as*	etc
reg*e*	**rej***a*	
reg*emos*	**rej***amos*	
reg*eis*	**rej***ais*	
reg*em*	**rej***am*	

⟨2i⟩ erguer [er'ger]

Verbs in *-guer*

Final stem consonant *gu* changes to *g* before *a* and *o* (stem as at ⟨2c⟩, unless otherwise indicated).

erg*o*	**erg***a*	**ergu***i*
ergu*es*	**erg***as*	etc
ergu*e*	**erg***a*	
ergu*emos*	**erg***amos*	
ergu*eis*	**erg***ais*	
ergu*em*	**erg***am*	

	Presente do Indicativo	**Presente do Conjuntivo**	**Pret. Perfeito do Indicativo**

⟨2k⟩ crer [krer]
Irregularities with insertion of *i* or use of the circumflex in the present; 2nd pers. pl. of the *Pres. do Indic.* in *-edes*. Otherwise regular.

Presente do Indicativo	Presente do Conjuntivo	Pret. Perfeito do Indicativo
cre**i***o* [ɜj]	cre**i***a* [ɜj]	cr*i*
cr**ê***s* [e]	cre**i***as*	etc
cr**ê**	cre**i***a*	
cre*mos*	cre**i***amos*	
cre**des**	cre**i***ais*	
cr**ê***em*	cre**i***am*	

⟨2l⟩ poder [po'der]
d is replaced by *ss* in the 1st pers. sg. of the *Pres. do Indic.* and in all of the *Pres. do Conj.* Regular in the *Pret. Perfeito.*

Presente do Indicativo	Presente do Conjuntivo	Pret. Perfeito do Indicativo
po**ss***o* ['ɔ]	po**ss***a* ['ɔ]	**pu**d*e*
pod*es*	po**ss***as*	**pu**d*este*
pod*e*	po**ss***a*	**pô**d*e*
pod*emos*	po**ss***amos*	**pu**d*emos*
pod*eis*	po**ss***ais*	**pu**d*estes*
pod*em*	po**ss***am*	**pu**d*eram*

⟨2m⟩ ver [ver]
The same irregularities as at *crer* ⟨2k⟩, except that *j* is inserted instead of *i*. Also the *Pret. Perfeito* follows the 3rd conjugation and the past participle is irregular: **visto**.

Presente do Indicativo	Presente do Conjuntivo	Pret. Perfeito do Indicativo
ve**j***o* [ɜj]	ve**j***a* [ɜj]	**vi**
v**ê***s* [e]	ve**j***as*	**vi***ste*
v**ê**	ve**j***a*	**vi***u*
ve*mos*	ve**j***amos*	**vi***mos*
ve**des**	ve**j***ais*	**vi***stes*
v**ê***em*	ve**j***am*	**vi***ram*

⟨2ma⟩ prover [pro'ver]
As **ver** ⟨2m⟩, but unlike other compounds of **ver** the *Pret. Perfeito* and its derived forms and the past participle are regular: **provido**.

Presente do Indicativo	Presente do Conjuntivo	Pret. Perfeito do Indicativo
provej*o* [ɜj]	provej*a* [ɜj]	prov*i*
prov**ê***s* [e]	provej*as*	etc
prov**ê**	provej*a*	
prov*emos*	provej*amos*	
prove**des**	provej*ais*	
prov**ê***em*	provej*am*	

	Presente do Indicativo	Presente do Conjuntivo	Pret. Perfeito do Indicativo

⟨**2n**⟩ **haver** [a'ver]
Irregularities in the *Presente* and *Pret. Perfeito*.

Presente do Indicativo	Presente do Conjuntivo	Pret. Perfeito do Indicativo
hei	**haj**_a_ [ʒ]	**hou**v_e_
hás	**haj**_as_	**hou**v_este_
há	**haj**_a_	**hou**v_e_
hav_emos_	**haj**_amos_	**hou**v_emos_
hav_eis_	**haj**_ais_	**hou**v_estes_
hão	**haj**_am_	**hou**v_eram_

⟨**2o**⟩ **perder** [per'der]
d changes to *c* in the 1st pers. sg. of the *Pres. do Indic.* and in all the *Pres. do Conj.* Open e [ɛ] in all forms where the stress falls on the stem; otherwise regular.

Presente do Indicativo	Presente do Conjuntivo	Pret. Perfeito do Indicativo
per**c**_o_ [ɛrk]	per**c**_a_ [ɛrk]	perd_i_
perd_es_	per**c**_as_	etc
perd_e_	per**c**_a_	
perd_emos_	per**c**_amos_	
perd_eis_	per**c**_ais_	
perd_em_	per**c**_am_	

⟨**2p**⟩ **valer** [va'ler]
l changes to *lh* [ʎ] in the 1st pers. sg. of the *Pres. do Indic* and in all the *Pres. do Conj.*; otherwise regular.

Presente do Indicativo	Presente do Conjuntivo	Pret. Perfeito do Indicativo
va**lh**_o_ [ʎ]	va**lh**_a_ [ʎ]	val_i_
val_es_	va**lh**_as_	etc
val_e_	va**lh**_a_	
val_emos_	va**lh**_amos_	
val_eis_	va**lh**_ais_	
val_em_	va**lh**_am_	

⟨**2q**⟩ **caber** [ka'ber]
Irregular stem vowel in the 1st pers. sg. of the *Pres. do Indic.*, in all the *Pres. do Conj.* and in the *Pret. Perfeito*.

Presente do Indicativo	Presente do Conjuntivo	Pret. Perfeito do Indicativo
caib_o_	**cai**b_a_	**cou**b_e_
cab_es_	**cai**b_as_	**cou**b_este_
cab_e_	**cai**b_a_	**cou**b_e_
cab_emos_	**cai**b_amos_	**cou**b_emos_
cabeis	**cai**b_ais_	**cou**bestes
cab_em_	**cai**b_am_	**cou**b_eram_

	Presente do Indicativo	Presente do Conjuntivo	Pret. Perfeito do Indicativo

⟨2r⟩ saber [sa'beɾ]
As **caber** ⟨2q⟩ apart from the variation at the 1st pers. sg. of the *Pres. do Indicativo*.

sei [ɜj]	**saib***a*	**sou***be*
sab*es*	**saib***as*	**sou***beste*
sab*e*	**saib***a*	**sou***be*
sab*emos*	**saib***amos*	**sou***bemos*
sab*eis*	**saib***ais*	**sou***bestes*
sab*em*	**saib***am*	**sou***beram*

⟨2s⟩ querer [ke'ɾeɾ]
Omission of *-e* in the 3rd pers. sg. of the *Pres. do Indic.*; subjunctive stem is: **queir-**; irregular *Pret. Perfeito*.

quer*o* ['ɛ]	**queir***a* ['ɜj]	**quis**
quer*es* ['ɛ]	**queir***as*	**quis***este*
quer ['ɛ]	**queir***a*	**quis**
quer*emos*	**queir***amos*	**quis***emos*
quer*eis*	**queir***ais*	**quis***estes*
quer*em* ['ɛ]	**queir***am*	**quis***eram*

⟨2sa⟩ requerer [heke'ɾeɾ]
Stem of the 1st pers. sg. of the *Pres. do Indic.* and the *Pres. do Conj.* **requeir-**, unlike with **querer** ⟨2t⟩ the *Pret. Perfeito*. is regular.

reque**ir***o* ['ɜj]	reque**ir***a* ['ɜj]	requer*i*
requer*es*	reque**ir***as*	etc
reque**r**	reque**ir***a*	
requer*emos*	reque**ir***amos*	
requer*eis*	reque**ir***ais*	
requer*em*	reque**ir***am*	

⟨2t⟩ dizer [dʒi'zeɾ]
z before *a* and *o* is replaced by *g*;
Omission of *-ze-* in the *Fut.* and *Cond.* and omission of *-e* in the 3rd pers. sg. of the *Pres. do Indic.* Irregular *Pret. Perfeito*. *Futuro*: d**ir***ei*, d**ir***ás*, d**ir***á*, d**ir***emos*, d**ir***eis*, d**ir***ão*, *Particípio*: d**it***o*.

dig*o*	dig*a*	diss*e*
diz*es*	dig*as*	diss*este*
diz	dig*a*	diss*e*
diz*emos*	dig*amos*	diss*emos*
diz*eis*	dig*ais*	diss*estes*
diz*em*	dig*am*	diss*eram*

⟨**2u**⟩ **trazer** [tra'zer]
Similar irregularities to **dizer** ⟨2t⟩. Irregular *Pret. Perfeito*. Past participle is regular.
Futuro: tr**a**r*ei*, tr**a**r*ás*, tr**a**r*á*, tr**a**r*emos*, tr**a**r*eis*, tr**a**r*ão*.

Presente do Indicativo	Presente do Conjuntivo	Pret. Perfeito do Indicativo
trag*o*	trag*a*	**troux***e*
traz*es*	trag*as*	**troux***este*
tra**z**	trag*a*	**troux***e*
traz*emos*	trag*amos*	**troux***emos*
traz*eis*	trag*ais*	**troux***estes*
traz*em*	trag*am*	**troux***eram*

⟨**2v**⟩ **fazer** [fa'zer]
z before *a* and *o* is replaced by ç;
Omission of *-ze-* in *Fut*. and *Cond*. and of *-e* in the 3rd pers. sg. of the *Pres. do Indic*. Irregular *Pret. Perfeito*. *Futuro*: f**a**r*ei*, f**a**r*ás*, f**a**r*á*, f**a**r*emos*, f**a**r*eis*, f**a**r*ão*; *Particípio*: f**ei**to.

Presente do Indicativo	Presente do Conjuntivo	Pret. Perfeito do Indicativo
faç*o* [s]	faç*a* [s]	**fiz**
faz*es*	faç*as*	**fiz***este*
fa**z**	faç*a*	**fez** [e]
faz*emos*	faç*amos*	**fiz***emos*
faz*eis*	faç*ais*	**fiz***estes*
faz*em*	faç*am*	**fiz***eram*

⟨**2w**⟩ **ser** [ser]
Most forms are irregular.
Pret. Imperf.: **er***a*, **er***as*, **er***a*, **ér***amos*, **ér***eis*, **er***am*
Imperativo: 2nd pers. sg. **sê**; 2nd pers. pl. **sede**

Presente do Indicativo	Presente do Conjuntivo	Pret. Perfeito do Indicativo
sou	**sej***a* ['ɜj]	**fui**
és	**sej***as*	foste
é	**sej***a*	foi ['oj]
somos ['o]	**sej***amos*	fomos ['o]
sois ['oj]	**sej***ais*	fostes ['o]
são	**sej***am*	foram ['o]

⟨**2x**⟩ **ter** [ter]
Irregularities in the *Presente* and *Pret. Perfeito*. *Pret. Imperf.*: **tinh***a*, **tinh***as*, **tinh***a*, **tính***amos*, **tính***eis*, **tinh***am*

Presente do Indicativo	Presente do Conjuntivo	Pret. Perfeito do Indicativo
tenh*o*	**tenh***a*	**tiv***e*
tens	**tenh***as*	**tiv***este*
tem	**tenh***a*	**tev***e* ['e]
temos	**tenh***amos*	**tiv***emos*
tendes	**tenh***ais*	**tiv***estes*
têm	**tenh***am*	**tiv***eram*

	Presente do Indicativo	Presente do Conjuntivo	Pret. Perfeito do Indicativo

⟨2xa⟩ reter [he'ter]

Compounds of **ter** follow the irregularities of this verb and additionally take an accent in the 2nd and 3rd pers. sg. of the *Pres. do Indic.* and the 2nd pers. sg. of the *Imperativo*. *Pret. Imperf.*: ret**inh***a*, ret**inh***as*, ret**ính***amos* etc.

Presente do Indicativo	Presente do Conjuntivo	Pret. Perfeito do Indicativo
ret**enh***o*	ret**enh***a*	ret**iv***e*
ret**éns**	etc	etc
ret**ém**		
ret*emos*		
ret**endes**		
ret**êm**		

⟨2z⟩ pôr [por]

Irregular in most forms. *Pret. Imperf.*: p**unh***a*, p**unh***as*, p**unh***a*, p**únh***amos*, p**únh***eis*, p**unh***am*; *Particípio*: p**osto**

Presente do Indicativo	Presente do Conjuntivo	Pret. Perfeito do Indicativo
po**nh***o*	po**nh***a*	p**us**
p**ões**	po**nh***as*	p**us***este*
p**õe**	po**nh***a*	p**ôs**
po**mos**	po**nh***amos*	p**us***emos*
po**ndes**	po**nh***ais*	p**us***estes*
p**õem**	po**nh***am*	p**us***eram*

3 Third Conjugation

⟨3a⟩ admitir [adʒimi'tʃir]

No change to the stem in either spelling or pronunciation.

1. Simple tenses

Indicativo

	Presente	Pretérito Imperfeito	Pret. Perfeito Simples
Sg.	admit*o*	admit*ia*	admit*i*
	admit*es*	admit*ias*	admit*iste*
	admit*e*	admit*ia*	admit*iu*
Pl.	admit*imos*	admit*íamos*	admit*imos*
	admit*is*	admit*íeis*	admit*istes*
	admit*em*	admit*iam*	admit*iram*

	Futuro Imperfeito	Condicional Simples	Pret. Mais-que-perfeito Simples
Sg.	admit*irei*	admit*iria*	admit*ira*
	admit*irás*	admit*irias*	admit*iras*
	admit*irá*	admit*iria*	admit*ira*
Pl.	admit*iremos*	admit*iríamos*	admit*íramos*
	admit*ireis*	admit*iríeis*	admit*íreis*
	admit*irão*	admit*iriam*	admit*iram*

Conjuntivo

	Presente	Pretérito Imperfeito	Futuro Imperfeito
Sg.	admit*a*	admit*isse*	admit*ir*
	admit*as*	admit*isses*	admit*ires*
	admit*a*	admit*isse*	admit*ir*
Pl.	admit*amos*	admit*íssemos*	admit*irmos*
	admit*ais*	admit*ísseis*	admit*irdes*
	admit*am*	admit*issem*	admit*irem*

	Imperativo	Infinitivo Pessoal	
Sg.	—	admit*ir*	
	admit*e* (não admit*as*)	admit*ires*	Particípio
	admit*a*	admit*ir*	admit*ido*
Pl.	admit*amos*	admit*irmos*	
	admit*i* (não admit*ais*)	admit*irdes*	Gerúndio
	admit*am*	admit*irem*	admit*indo*

2. Compound tenses

as for the 1st conjugation

	Presente do Indicativo	**Presente do Conjuntivo**	**Pret. Perfeito do Indicativo**

⟨**3b**⟩ **invadir** [ĩva'dʒiɾ]
An unstressed *a* in the infinitive changes to a stressed open *a* [a] when the stress falls on the stem (unless it follows an *m*, *n* or *nh*).

inv**a**d*o* ['a]	inv**a**d*a*	invad*i*
inv**a**d*es*	inv**a**d*as*	etc
inv**a**d*e*	inv**a**d*a*	
invad*imos*	inv**a**d*amos*	
invad*is*	inv**a**d*ais*	
inv**a**d*em*	inv**a**d*am*	

⟨**3c**⟩ **despir** [dez'piɾ]
An unstressed *e* in the infinitive changes to a stressed open *e* [ɛ] in the 2nd and 3rd pers. sg. and in the 3rd pers. pl. of the *Pres. do Indic.*, but the change is to *i* [i] in the 1st pers. sg. and in all of the *Pres. do Conj.*

d**i**sp*o* ['i]	d**i**sp*a*	desp*i*
d**e**sp*es* ['ɛ]	d**i**sp*as*	etc
d**e**sp*e* ['ɛ]	d**i**sp*a*	
desp*imos*	d**i**sp*amos*	
desp*is*	d**i**sp*ais*	
d**e**sp*em* ['ɛ]	d**i**sp*am*	

⟨3d⟩ agredir [agɾe'dʒiɾ]

In some verbs unstressed *e* in the infinitive changes to *i* in all forms of the *Pres. do Indic.* where the stress falls on the stem and in all of the *Pres. do Conj.*

Presente do Indicativo	Presente do Conjuntivo	Pret. Perfeito do Indicativo
agr**i**d*o* ['i]	agr**i**d*a*	agred*i*
agr**i**d*es*	agr**i**d*as*	etc
agr**i**d*e*	agr**i**d*a*	
agred*imos*	agr**i**d*amos*	
agred*is*	agr**i**d*ais*	
agr**i**d*em*	agr**i**d*am*	

⟨3e⟩ sentir [sẽ'tʃiɾ]

Nasalized *e* [ẽ] changes to nasalized *i* [ĩ] in the 1st pers. sg. of the *Pres. do Indic.* and in all the *Pres. do Conj.*

Presente do Indicativo	Presente do Conjuntivo	Pret. Perfeito do Indicativo
s**i**nt*o* ['ĩ]	s**i**nt*a*	sent*i*
sent*es*	s**i**nt*as*	etc
sent*e*	s**i**nt*a*	
sent*imos*	s**i**nt*amos*	
sent*is*	s**i**nt*ais*	
sent*em*	s**i**nt*am*	

⟨3f⟩ dormir [doɾ'miɾ]

Unstressed *o* in the infinitive changes to open *o* [ɔ] in the 2nd and 3rd pers. sg. as well as in the 3rd pers. pl. of the *Pres. do Indic.*, but the change is to *u* [u] in the 1st pers. sg. and in all the *Pres. do Conj.*

Presente do Indicativo	Presente do Conjuntivo	Pret. Perfeito do Indicativo
d**u**rm*o* ['u]	d**u**rm*a* ['u]	dorm*i*
d**o**rm*es* ['ɔ]	d**u**rm*as*	etc
d**o**rm*e* ['ɔ]	d**u**rm*a*	
dorm*imos*	d**u**rm*amos*	
dorm*is*	d**u**rm*ais*	
d**o**rm*em* ['ɔ]	d**u**rm*am*	

⟨3g⟩ polir [po'liɾ]

When the stress falls on the stem, unstressed *o* changes to *u* in the *Pres. do Indic.* and in all the *Pres. do Conj.*

Presente do Indicativo	Presente do Conjuntivo	Pret. Perfeito do Indicativo
p**u**l*o*	p**u**l*a*	pol*i*
p**u**l*es*	p**u**l*as*	etc.
p**u**l*e*	p**u**l*a*	
pol*imos*	p**u**l*amos*	
pol*is*	p**u**l*ais*	
p**u**l*em*	p**u**l*am*	

	Presente do Indicativo	Presente do Conjuntivo	Pret. Perfeito do Indicativo

⟨3h⟩ subir [su'biɾ]
The stem vowel *u* changes to an open *o* [ɔ] in the 2nd and 3rd pers. sg. as well as in the 3. pers. pl. of the *Pres. do Indic.*

Presente do Indicativo	Presente do Conjuntivo	Pret. Perfeito do Indicativo
sub*o*	sub*a*	sub*i*
sob*es* ['ɔ]	etc	etc
sob*e* ['ɔ]		
sub*imos*		
sub*is*		
sob*em* ['ɔ]		

⟨3i⟩ contribuir [kõtribwiɾ]
Verbs with *u* as the final stem vowel take *i* instead of *e* in the 2nd and 3rd pers. sg. of the *Pres. do Indic.* as well as taking an accent in a number of forms, for instance in the *Mais-que-perfeito* and in the *Pret. Imperf.*

Presente do Indicativo	Presente do Conjuntivo	Pret. Perfeito do Indicativo
contribu*o*	contribu*a*	contribu**í**
contrib**ui***s* [ui]	etc	contribu**í***ste*
contrib**ui** [ui]		contribui*u*
contribu**í***mos*		contribu**í***mos*
contribu**í***s*		contribu**í***stes*
contribu*em*		contribu**í***ram*

Pret. Imperf.: contribu**í***a*, contribu**í***as*, contribu**í***a*, contribu**í***amos*, etc.
Futuro do Conj. and *Inf. Pess.*: 2nd pers. sg. contribu**í***res*, 3rd pers. pl. contribu**í***rem*
Imperativo: 2nd pers. pl. contribu**í**; *Participío*: contribu**í**do

⟨3k⟩ destruir [destɾu'iɾ]
Some verbs with *u* as their final stem vowel have, in the *Pres. do Indic.*, both *-uis*, *-ui*, *-uem* and *-óis*, *-ói*, *-oem*; other forms and accents as at **contribuir** ⟨3i⟩.

Presente do Indicativo	Presente do Conjuntivo	Pret. Perfeito do Indicativo
destru*o*	destru*a*	destru**í**
destr**ói***s* (**-ui***s*)	etc	etc
destr**ói** (**-ui**)		
destru**í***mos*		
destru**í***s*		
destr**oe***m* (**-ue***m*)		

⟨3l⟩ cair [ka'iɾ]
Verbs with *a* as final stem vowel conjugate like **contribuir** ⟨3i⟩ with the additional irregularity of the insertion of *i* in the 1st pers. sg. of the *Pres. do Indic.* and in all of the *Pres. do Conj.*

Presente do Indicativo	Presente do Conjuntivo	Pret. Perfeito do Indicativo
ca**i***o* ['kaju]	ca**i***a* ['kaja]	ca**í**
ca**i***s* [kaiʃ]	ca**i***as*	etc
ca**i** [kai]	ca**i***a*	
ca**í***mos*	ca**i***amos*	
ca**í***s*	ca**i***ais*	
ca*em* ['kajẽ]	ca**i***am*	

	Presente do Indicativo	Presente do Conjuntivo	Pret. Perfeito do Indicativo

⟨3m⟩ produzir [pɾodu'ziɾ]

Verbs with stem ending of vowel + *z* do not take *-e* in the 3rd pers. sg. of the *Pres. do Indic.*

Presente do Indicativo	Presente do Conjuntivo	Pret. Perfeito do Indicativo
produz*o*	produz*a*	produz*i*
produz*es*	etc	etc
produz		
produz*imos*		
produz*is*		
produz*em*		

⟨3n⟩ surgir [suɾ'ʒiɾ]

Verbs in *-gir*. Final stem consonant *g* changes to *j* before *a* and *o*.

Presente do Indicativo	Presente do Conjuntivo	Pret. Perfeito do Indicativo
surj*o*	surj*a*	surg*i*
surg*es*	surj*as*	etc
surg*e*	surj*a*	
surg*imos*	surj*amos*	
surg*is*	surj*ais*	
surg*em*	surj*am*	

⟨3o⟩ distinguir [dʒistʃĩ'giɾ]

Verbs in *-guir* and *-quir*. The *u* is silent. Stem ending *gu* or *qu* changes to *g* or *c* [k] before *a* and *o*.

Presente do Indicativo	Presente do Conjuntivo	Pret. Perfeito do Indicativo
disting*o* [g]	disting*a*	distingu*i*
distingu*es*	disting*as*	etc
distingu*e*	disting*a*	
distingu*imos*	disting*amos*	
distingu*is*	disting*ais*	
distingu*em*	disting*am*	

⟨3q⟩ ressarcir [hesaɾ'siɾ]

Verbs in *-cir*. Final c in the stem changes to ç before *a* and *o*.

Presente do Indicativo	Presente do Conjuntivo	Pret. Perfeito do Indicativo
ressarç*o* ['s]	ressarç*a*	ressarc*i*
ressarc*es*	ressarç*as*	etc
ressarc*e*	etc	
etc		

⟨3r⟩ pedir [pe'dʒiɾ]

d changes to ç in the 1st pers. sg. of the *Pres. do Indic.* and in all the *Pres. do Conj.* Where the stress falls on the stem, unstressed *e* in the infinitive changes to open e [ɛ]. Likewise: **medir**.

Presente do Indicativo	Presente do Conjuntivo	Pret. Perfeito do Indicativo
peç*o* ['ɛs]	peç*a* ['ɛs]	ped*i*
ped*es* ['ɛ]	peç*as*	etc
ped*e* ['ɛ]	peç*a*	
ped*imos*	peç*amos*	
ped*is*	peç*ais*	
ped*em* ['ɛ]	peç*am*	

Presente do Indicativo	Presente do Conjuntivo	Pret. Perfeito do Indicativo

⟨3s⟩ proibir [proi'biɾ]
Where stress falls on the stem *i* takes an accent. Likewise: **coibir**.

pro**í**b*o*	pro**í**b*a*	proib*i*
pro**í**b*es*	pro**í**b*as*	etc
pro**í**b*e*	pro**í**b*a*	
proib*imos*	proib*amos*	
proib*is*	proib*ais*	
pro**í**b*em*	pro**í**b*am*	

⟨3t⟩ reunir [heu'niɾ]
When the stress falls on the stem *u* takes an accent.

re**ú**n*o*	re**ú**n*a*	reun*i*
re**ú**n*es*	re**ú**n*as*	etc
re**ú**n*e*	re**ú**n*a*	
reun*imos*	reun*amos*	
reun*is*	reun*ais*	
re**ú**n*em*	re**ú**n*am*	

⟨3u⟩ ouvir [o'viɾ]
The stem *ouv-* changes to *oiç-* ['ois] or *ouç-* ['os] in the 1st pers. sg. of the *Pres. do Indic.* and in all the *Pres. do Conj.*

oiç*o*, **ouç***o*	oiç*a*, **ouç***a*	ouv*i*
ouv*es*	etc	etc
ouv*e*		
ouv*imos*		
ouv*is*		
ouv*em*		

⟨3v⟩ rir [hiɾ]
Some forms are contracted in the *Pres. do Indic.*; otherwise regular.

ri*o*	ri*a*	ri
ris	ri*as*	ri*ste*
ri	ri*a*	ri*u*
ri*mos*	ri*amos*	ri*mos*
rides	ri*ais*	ri*stes*
ri*em*	ri*am*	ri*ram*

	Presente do Indicativo	Presente do Conjuntivo	Pret. Perfeito do Indicativo

⟨3w⟩ vir [viɾ]

Most forms are irregular. *Pret. Imperf.*: **vinh***a*, **vinh***as*, **vinh***a*, **vính***amos*, **vính***eis*, **vinh***am*; *Particípio* and *Gerúndio*: **vind***o*.

Presente do Indicativo	Presente do Conjuntivo	Pret. Perfeito do Indicativo
venh*o* ['ɜ]	**venh***a* ['ɜ]	**vim**
ven*s*	**venh***as*	**vie***ste* ['vjɛ]
vem	**venh***a*	**veio** ['ɜj]
vi*mos*	**venh***amos*	**vie***mos*
vindes	**venh***ais*	**vie***stes*
vêm	**venh***am*	**vie***ram*

⟨3wa⟩ convir [kõ'vir]

Compounds formed with **vir** take an accent in the 2nd and 3rd pers. sg. of the *Pres. do Indic*; otherwise as per **vir**.

Presente do Indicativo	Presente do Conjuntivo	Pret. Perfeito do Indicativo
con**venh***o* ['ɜ]	con**venh***a* ['ɜ]	con**vim**
con**vén***s*	con**venh***as*	con**vie***ste*
con**vém**	con**venh***a*	con**veio** ['ɜj]
convi*mos*	con**venh***amos*	con**vie***mos*
con**vindes**	con**venh***ais*	con**vie***stes*
con**vêm**	con**venh***am*	con**vie***ram*

⟨3x⟩ ir [iɾ]

Almost totally irregular, deriving from more than one stem. *Pret. Imperf.*: **ia, ias** etc, *Futuro*: **ir***ei*, **ir***ás*, **ir***á* etc, *Particípio*: **ido**.

Presente do Indicativo	Presente do Conjuntivo	Pret. Perfeito do Indicativo
vou	**vá**	**fui**
vais	**vás**	**fo***ste* ['o]
vai	**vá**	**foi**
vamos	**vamos**	**fo***mos* ['o]
ides	**vades**	**fo***stes* ['o]
vão	**vão**	**fo***ram* ['o]

⟨3y⟩ parir [pa'rir]

In Portugal as ⟨3b⟩, but 1st and 3rd pers. sg. of the *Pres. do Conj.*: **pára.**

Presente do Indicativo	Presente do Conjuntivo	Pret. Perfeito do Indicativo
par*o*	pára	par*i*
par*es*	par*as*	etc
par*e*	pára	
par*imos*	par*amos*	
par*is*	par*ais*	
par*em*	par*am*	

The Brazilian conjugation differs in some forms.

Presente do Indicativo	Presente do Conjuntivo	Pret. Perfeito do Indicativo
pairo	**paira**	par*i*
par*es*	**pairas**	etc
par*e*	etc	
par*imos*		
par*is*		
par*em*		

Observações sobre o verbo inglês

1 Conjugação indicativa

1.1 **O presente** mantém a mesma forma que o infinitivo em todas as pessoas, menos na terceira pessoa do singular, quando se acrescenta um *-s* à forma infinitiva, por ex. *he brings*. Se o infinitivo termina com um som sibilante (ch, sh, ss, zz), acrescenta-se *-es*, como em *he passes*. Este *s* pode ser pronunciado em duas maneiras diferentes: mudo após uma consoante muda, por ex. *he paints* [peɪnts]; sonoro após uma consoante sonora, por ex. *he sends* [sendz]. Além disso, *-es* se pronuncia de maneira sonora quando o *e* faz parte da terminação da palavra ou quando é a ultima letra do infinitivo, por ex. *he washes* ['wɑːʃɪz], *he urges* ['ɜːrdʒɪz]. No caso de verbos que terminam com *-y*, a terceira pessoa é formada pela substituição do *-ies* pelo *y* (*he worries*, *he tries*). Os verbos que terminam, no infinitivo, com *y* precedido por uma vogal são todos regulares (*he plays*). O verbo *to be* é irregular em todas as pessoas: *I am*, *you are*, *he is*, *we are*, *you are*, *they are*. Três outros verbos tem formas especiais na terceira pessoa do singular: *do* - *he does*, *go* - *he goes*, *have* - *he has*.

Nos outros tempos, os verbos continuam invariáveis em todas as pessoas. **O pretérito** e **o particípio passado** são formados pelo acréscimo do *ed* à forma infinitiva (*I passed*, *passed*), ou simplesmente pelo acréscimo do *-d* ao verbo que termina com *-e* no infinitivo, por ex. *I faced*, *faced*. (Existem vários verbos irregulares; veja a seguir). Esta terminação *-*(*e*)*d* geralmente se pronuncia [t]: *passed* [pæst], *faced* [feɪst]. Porém, no caso de um verbo que termina no infinitvo com uma consoante sonora, com um som consoante ou um *r*, é pronunciada [d]: *warmed* [wɔːrmd], *moved* [muːvd], *feared* [fɪrd]. Quando o infinitivo termina com *-d* ou *-t*, a terminação *-ed* se pronuncia [ɪd]. Quando o infinitivo termina com *-y*, este é substituido por *-ie* e depois se acrescenta *-d*: *try* - *tried* [traɪd], *pity* - *pitied* ['pɪtiːd]. **Os tempos compostos do passado** são formados com o auxiliar *to have* e o particípio passado: **particípio passado** *I have faced*, **mais-que-perfeito** *I had faced*. O **futuro** é formado com o auxiliar *will*, por ex. *I will face*; **o condicional** se forma com o auxiliar *would*, por ex. *I would face*.

Além disso, existe uma forma progressiva para cada tempo, que se forma com o verbo *to be* (= estar) e o particípio presente (veja a seguir): *I am going*, *I was writing*, *I had been staying*, *I will be waiting*, etc.

1.2 Em inglês, **o subjuntivo** é usado muito raramente, e somente em casos muito especiais (*if I were you*, *so be it*, *it is proposed that a vote be taken*, etc.). O subjuntivo presente mantém a forma infinitiva em todas as pessoas: *that I go*, *that he go*, etc.

1.3 Em inglês, **o particípio presente** e **o gerúndio** usam a mesma forma e são construídos com o acréscimo da terminação *-ing* à forma infinitiva: *painting*, *sending*. Porém: 1) quando o infinitivo de um verbo termina com um *e* mudo, este desaparece com o acréscimo da terminação, por ex. *love* - *loving*, *write* - *writing* (as exceções a esta regra: *dye* - *dyeing*, *singe* - *singeing*, retém o último *e* do infinitivo); 2) os particípios presentes dos verbos *die*, *lie*, *vie* etc, são escritos *dying*, *lying*, *vying*, etc.

1.4 Existe uma categoria de verbos que são parcialmente irregulares e que terminam com uma única consoante precedida por uma única vogal acentuada. Para estes verbos, a última consoante é dobrada antes de acrescentar as terminações *-ing* ou *-ed*:

lob	lob*bed*	lob*bing*	compel	compel*led*	compel*ling*
control	control*led*	control*ling*	beg	beg*ged*	beg*ging*
step	step*ped*	step*ping*	stir	stir*red*	stir*ring*

No caso de verbos que terminam com um *-l* precedido por uma vogal não acentuada, a ortografia britânica dobra esta consoante nos particípios passados e presentes, mas a ortografia americana não:

travel travel*led*, *Am* travel*ed* travel*ling*, *Am* travel*ing*

Quando um verbo termina com *-c*, substitui-se *-ck* pelo *c*, depois acrescenta-se a terminação *-ed* ou *-ing*:

traffic traffi*cked* traffi*cking*

1.5 **A voz passiva** é formada da mesma maneira como na língua portuguesa, com o verbo *to be* e o particípio passado: *I am obliged*, *he was fined*, *they will be moved*, etc.

1.6 Quando uma pessoa se dirige em inglês a uma ou várias outras pessoas, somente o pronome *you* é usado, que pode ser traduzido como você ou vocês, tu ou vós.

2 Verbos ingleses irregulares

Você encontrará a seguir as três formas principais de cada verbo: o infinitivo, o pretérito e o particípio passado.

arise - arose - arisen
awake - awoke - awoken, awaked
be (am, is, are) - was (were) - been
bear - bore - borne (1)
beat - beat - beaten
become - became - become
begin - began - begun
behold - beheld - beheld
bend - bent - bent
beseech - besought, beseeched - besought, beseeched
bet - bet, betted - bet, betted
bid - bid - bid
bind - bound - bound
bite - bit - bitten
bleed - bled - bled
blow - blew - blown
break - broke - broken
breed - bred - bred
bring - brought - brought
broadcast - broadcast - broadcast
build - built - built
burn - burnt, burned - burnt, burned
burst - burst - burst
bust - bust(ed) - bust(ed)
buy - bought - bought
cast - cast - cast
catch - caught - caught
choose - chose - chosen
cleave (*cut*) - clove, cleft - cloven, cleft
cleave (*adhere*) - cleaved - cleaved
cling - clung - clung
come - came - come
cost (*v/i*) - cost - cost

creep - crept - crept
crow - crowed, crew - crowed
cut - cut - cut
deal - dealt - dealt
dig - dug - dug
dive - dived, dove [doʊv] (2) - dived
do - did - done
draw - drew - drawn
dream - dreamt, dreamed - dreamt, dreamed
drink - drank - drunk
drive - drove - driven
dwell - dwelt, dwelled - dwelt, dwelled
eat - ate - eaten
fall - fell - fallen
feed - fed - fed
feel - felt - felt
fight - fought - fought
find - found - found
flee - fled - fled
fling - flung - flung
fly - flew - flown
forbear - forbore - forborne
forbid - forbad(e) - forbidden
forecast - forecast(ed) - forecast(ed)
forget - forgot - forgotten
forgive - forgave - forgiven
forsake - forsook - forsaken
freeze - froze - frozen
get - got - got, gotten (3)
give - gave - given
go - went - gone
grind - ground - ground
grow - grew - grown
hang - hung, hanged - hung, hanged (4)
have - had - had
hear - heard - heard
heave - heaved, NAUT hove - heaved, NAUT hove
hew - hewed - hewed, hewn
hide - hid - hidden
hit - hit - hit
hold - held - held
hurt - hurt - hurt
keep - kept - kept
kneel - knelt, kneeled - knelt, kneeled
know - knew - known
lay - laid - laid
lead - led - led
lean - leaned, leant - leaned, leant (5)
leap - leaped, leapt - leaped, leapt (5)
learn - learned, learnt - learned, learnt (5)
leave - left - left
lend - lent - lent
let - let - let
lie - lay - lain
light - lighted, lit - lighted, lit
lose - lost - lost
make - made - made
mean - meant - meant
meet - met - met
mow - mowed - mowed, mown
pay - paid - paid
plead - pleaded, pled - pleaded, pled (6)
prove - proved - proved, proven
put - put - put
quit - quit(ted) - quit(ted)
read - read [red] - read [red]
rend - rent - rent
rid - rid - rid
ride - rode - ridden
ring - rang - rung
rise - rose - risen
run - ran - run
saw - sawed - sawn, sawed
say - said - said
see - saw - seen
seek - sought - sought
sell - sold - sold
send - sent - sent
set - set - set
sew - sewed - sewed, sewn
shake - shook - shaken
shear - sheared - sheared, shorn
shed - shed - shed
shine - shone - shone
shit - shit(ted), shat - shit(ted), shat
shoe - shod - shod
shoot - shot - shot
show - showed - shown

shrink - shrank - shrunk
shut - shut - shut
sing - sang - sung
sink - sank - sunk
sit - sat - sat
slay - slew - slain
sleep - slept - slept
slide - slid - slid
sling - slung - slung
slink - slunk - slunk
slit - slit - slit
smell - smelt, smelled - smelt, smelled
smite - smote - smitten
sneak - sneaked, snuck - sneaked, snuck (7)
sow - sowed - sown, sowed
speak - spoke - spoken
speed - sped, speeded - sped, speeded
spell - spelt, spelled - spelt, spelled (5)
spend - spent - spent
spill - spilt, spilled - spilt, spilled
spin - spun, span - spun
spit - spat - spat
split - split - split
spoil - spoiled, spoilt - spoiled, spoilt
spread - spread - spread
spring - sprang, sprung - sprung
stand - stood - stood
stave - staved, stove - staved, stove
steal - stole - stolen
stick - stuck - stuck
sting - stung - stung
stink - stunk, stank - stunk
strew - strewed - strewed, strewn
stride - strode - stridden
strike - struck - struck
string - strung - strung
strive - strove, strived - striven, strived
swear - swore - sworn
sweep - swept - swept
swell - swelled - swollen
swim - swam - swum
swing - swung - swung
take - took - taken
teach - taught - taught
tear - tore - torn
tell - told - told
think - thought - thought
thrive - throve - thriven, thrived (8)
throw - threw - thrown
thrust - thrust - thrust
tread - trod - trodden
understand - understood - understood
wake - woke, waked - woken, waked
wear - wore - worn
weave - wove - woven (9)
wed - wed(ded) - wed(ded)
weep - wept - wept
wet - wet(ted) - wet(ted)
win - won - won
wind - wound - wound
wring - wrung - wrung
write - wrote - written

(**1**) mas **be born** *nascer*
(**2**) **dove** não é usado em inglês britânico
(**3**) **gotten** não é usado em inglês britânico
(**4**) **hung** para quadro mas **hanged** para assassino
(**5**) O inglês americano geralmente usa somente a forma **-ed**
(**6**) **pled** se usa em inglês americano ou escocês
(**7**) a forma **snuck** se usa somente como forma alternativa familiar em inglês americano
(**8**) a forma **thrived** é mais atual
(**9**) mas **weaved** no senso de se enfiar

Numbers / Números

Cardinal Numbers / Números cardinais

0	zero, *Brit também* nought *zero*	**22**	twenty-two *vinte e dois*
1	one *um, uma*	**30**	thirty *trinta*
2	two *dois, duas*	**31**	thirty-one *trinta e um*
3	three *três*	**40**	forty *quarenta*
4	four *quatro*	**50**	fifty *cinqüenta, Port cinquenta*
5	five *cinco*	**60**	sixty *sessenta*
6	six *seis*	**70**	seventy *setenta*
7	seven *sete*	**71**	seventy-one *setenta e um*
8	eight *oito*	**72**	seventy-two *setenta e dois*
9	nine *nove*	**79**	seventy-nine *setenta e nove*
10	ten *dez*	**80**	eighty *oitenta*
11	eleven *onze*	**81**	eighty-one *oitenta e um*
12	twelve *doze*	**90**	ninety *noventa*
13	thirteen *treze*	**91**	ninety-one *noventa e um*
14	fourteen *catorze*	**100**	a hundred, one hundred *cem*
15	fifteen *quinze*	**101**	a hundred and one *cento e um*
16	sixteen *dezesseis, Port dezasseis*	**200**	two hundred *cento e dois*
17	seventeen *dezessete, Port dezassete*	**300**	three hundred *cento e três*
18	eighteen *dezoito*	**324**	three hundred and twenty-four *trezentos e vinte e quatro*
19	nineteen *dezenove, Port dezanove*	**1000**	a thousand, one thousand *mil*
20	twenty *vinte*	**2000**	two thousand *dois mil*
21	twenty-one *vinte e um*	**1959**	one thousand nine hundred and fifty-nine *mil novecentos e cinqüenta e nove*

1 000 000	a million, one million *um milhão*
2 000 000	two million *dois milhões*
1 000 000 000	a billion, one billion *um bilhão*

Notes / Observações:

i) If **um** or **dois** are used with a following noun, then they must agree (one man **um homem**; one woman **uma mulher**).

ii) 1.25 (one point two five) = 1,25 (um vírgula vinte e cinco)

iii) 1,000,000 (em inglês) = 1.000.000 (in Portuguese)

Ordinal Numbers / Números ordinais

1st	first	1º/1ª	*primeiro / primeira*
2nd	second	2º	*segundo*
3rd	third	3º	*terceiro*
4th	fourth	4º	*quarto*
5th	fifth	5º	*quinto*
6th	sixth	6º	*sexto*
7th	seventh	7º	*sétimo*
8th	eighth	8º	*oitavo*
9th	ninth	9º	*nono*
10th	tenth	10º	*décimo*
11th	eleventh	11º	*décimo primeiro*
12th	twelfth	12º	*décimo segundo*
13th	thirteenth	13º	*décimo terceiro*
14th	fourteenth	14º	*décimo quarto*
15th	fifteenth	15º	*décimo quinto*
16th	sixteenth	16º	*décimo sexto*
17th	seventeenth	17º	*décimo sétimo*
18th	eighteenth	18º	*décimo oitavo*
19th	nineteenth	19º	*décimo nono*
20th	twentieth	20º	*vigésimo*
21st	twenty-first	21º	*vigésimo primeiro*
22nd	twenty-second	22º	*vigésimo segundo*
30th	thirtieth	30º	*trigésimo*
31st	thirty-first	31º	*trigésimo primeiro*
40th	fortieth	40º	*quadragésimo*
50th	fiftieth	50º	*quinquagésimo*
60th	sixtieth	60º	*sexagésimo*
70th	seventieth	70º	*septuagésimo*
71st	seventy-first	71º	*septuagésimo primeiro*
80th	eightieth	80º	*octogésimo*
90th	ninetieth	90º	*nonagésimo*
100th	hundredth	100º	*centésimo*
101st	hundred and first	101º	*centésimo primeiro*
1000th	thousandth	1000º	*milésimo*
1,000,000th	millionth	1 000 000º	*milionésimo*
1,000,000,000th	billionth	1 000 000 000º	*bilionésimo*

Ordinal numbers are adjectives and must agree (the third girl **a terceira menina**). The abbreviated feminine form is 3ª, 4ª etc.

Fractions and other Numbers / Frações e outros números

1/2	one half, a half	*(uma) metade, meio*
1 1/2	one and a half	*um e meio*
1/3	one third, a third	*um terço*
2/3	two thirds	*dois terços*
1/4	one quarter, a quarter	*um quarto*
3/4	three quarters	*três quartos*
1/5	one fifth, a fifth	*um quinto*
3 4/5	three and four fifths	*três e quatro quintos*
1/11	one eleventh, an eleventh	*um onze avos*

The form with *avos* is used in arithmetic for denominators over 10 but not multiples of 10.

seven times as big, seven times bigger	*sete vezes maior*
twelve times more	*doze vezes mais*
first(ly)	*primeiramente*
second(ly)	*em segundo lugar*

Arithmetic / Aritmética

7 + 8 = 15 seven and (*or* plus) eight are (*or* is) fifteen	*sete mais oito é igual a quinze*
10 – 3 = 7 ten minus three is seven, three from ten leaves seven	*dez menos três é igual a sete, três subtraído de dez deixa sete*
2 x 3 = 6 two times three is six	*dois vezes três é igual a seis*
20 ÷ 4 = 5 twenty divided by four is five	*vinte dividido por quatro são cinco*

Dates / Datas

1996 nineteen ninety-six	*mil novecentos e noventa e seis*
2010 two thousand (and) ten	*dois mil e dez*
November 10/11 (ten, eleven), *Brit* the 10th/11th of November	*dia dez/onze de novembro*
March 1 (first), *Brit* the 1st of March	*o primeiro de março*

A B C D E F G H I J K L M N O P Q R S T U V W X Y Z

Headword in **blue**

Entrada em **azul**

blooper ['blu:pər] *Am fam* bobeira *f*

conflict **1** ['kɑ:nflɪkt] *n* (*disagreement, war*) conflito *m* **2** [kən'flɪkt] *v/i* (*clash*) conflitar

International Phonetic Alphabet

Alfabeto Fonético Internacional

clippers ['klɪpərz] *hair*: prendedor *m* de cabelo; *nails*: alicate *m* de unhas; *gardening*: podadeira *f*

Translation in normal characters with gender shown in *italics*

Tradução em caracteres normais com gênero mostrado em *itálico*

assailant [ə'seɪlənt] assaltante *m/f*

Stress shown in headwords

Acentuação mostrada nas entradas

flying 'saucer disco *m* voador

Examples and phrases in ***bold italics***

Exemplos e frases em ***negrito itálico***

discriminate [dɪ'skrɪmɪneɪt] *v/i* **~** ***against*** discriminar; **~** ***between red and green etc*** distinguir entre

Indicating words in *italics*

Indicadores em *itálico*

entry ['entrɪ] entrada *f*; *for competition* participante *m/f*; *in diary, accounts* registro *m*, *Port* registo *m*

Swung dash replaces the entire headword

Til (~) substituindo uma entrada inteira

duress [dʊə'res] coação *f*; ***under ~*** sob coação

earthly ['ɜ:rθlɪ] *adj* terreno; ***it's no ~ use*** *fam* é inútil